LATEST APPROVED METHODS OF TREATMENT FOR THE PRACTICING PHYSICIAN

Edited by

ROBERT E. RAKEL, M.D.

Professor, Department of Family and Community Medicine
Baylor College of Medicine, Houston, Texas

and

EDWARD T. BOPE, M.D.

Family Practice Residency Director, Riverside Family Practice Residency Program
Clinical Professor, Department of Family Medicine
The Ohio State University, Columbus, Ohio

W.B. SAUNDERS COMPANY
An Imprint of Elsevier Science
Philadelphia London New York St. Louis Sydney Toronto

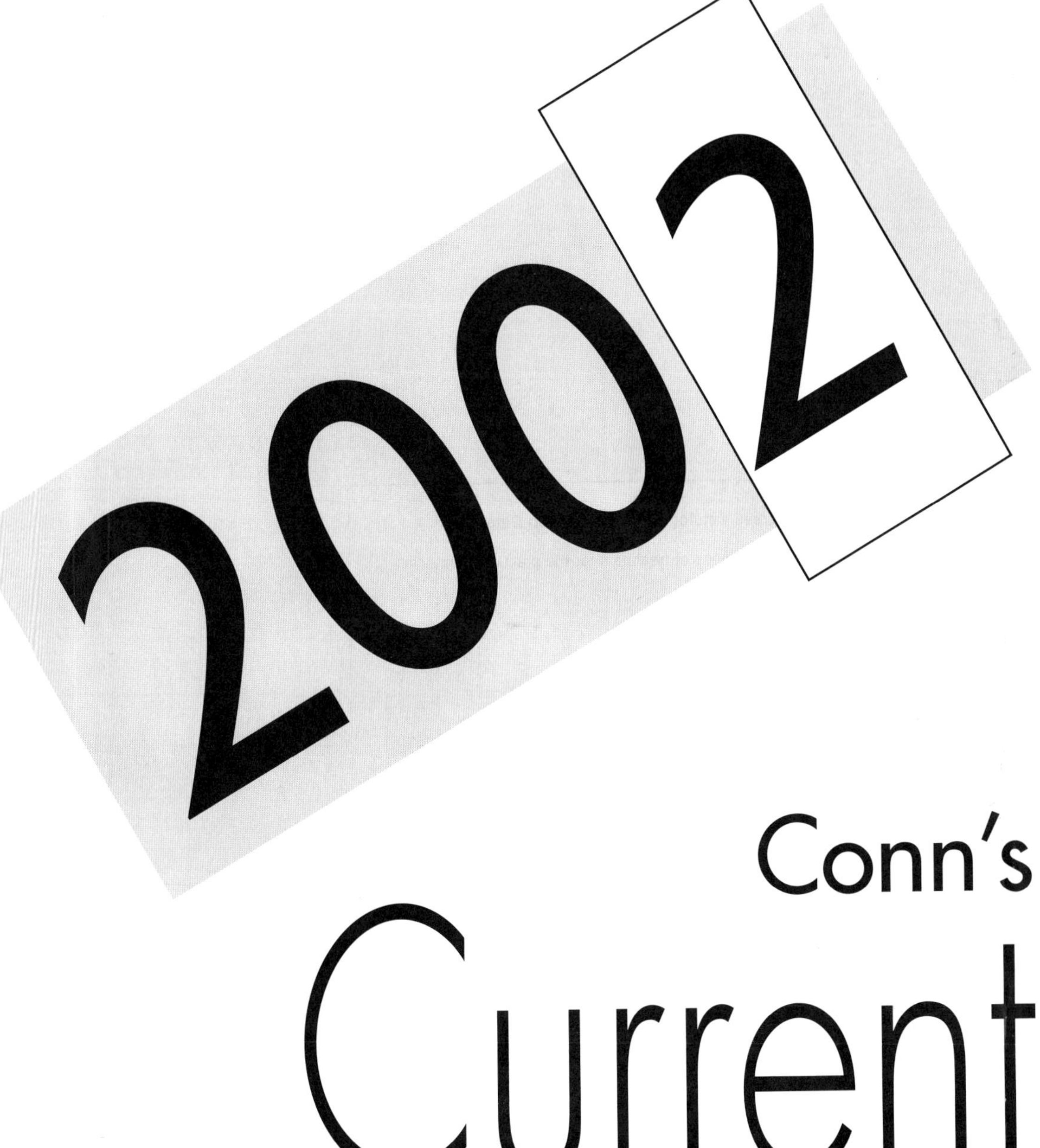

Conn's

Current Therapy

W.B. SAUNDERS COMPANY
An Imprint of Elsevier Science
The Curtis Center
Independence Square West
Philadelphia, Pennsylvania 19106

Library of Congress Cataloging-in-Publication Data

Current therapy; latest approved methods of treatment for the practicing physician.

Editors: H. F. Conn and others

v. 28 cm. annual.

ISBN 0–7216–8744–X

1. Therapeutics. 2. Therapeutics, Surgical. 3. Medicine—Practice.
I. Conn, Howard Franklin, 1908–1982 ed.

RM101.C87 616.058 49–8328 rev*

Acquisitions Editor: Richard Zorab
Developmental Editor: Faith Voit
Production Editor: Amy L. Cannon
Project Manager: Mary Anne Folcher
Senior Illustration Specialist: Peg Shaw
Cover Designer: Ellen Zanolle

CONN'S CURRENT THERAPY 2002 ISBN 0–7216–8744–X

Printed in the United States of America.

Last digit is the print number: 9 8 7 6 5 4 3 2 1

Contributors

WILLIAM T. ABRAHAM, M.D.

Gill Professor of Preventive Cardiology, Chief, Division of Cardiovascular Medicine, and Co-Director, Gill Heart Institute, Division of Cardiovascular Medicine and The Linda and Jack Gill Heart Institute, University of Kentucky; University of Kentucky Chandler Medical Center, Lexington, Kentucky
Congestive Heart Failure

CHARLES W. ACHER, M.D.

Professor of Surgery, University of Wisconsin; Section of Vascular Surgery, University Clinical Science Center, Madison, Wisconsin
Acquired Diseases of the Aorta

PAUL ADAMS, M.D.

Professor of Medicine, University of Western Ontario, London, Ontario, Canada
Hemochromatosis

GABRIEL A. ADELMANN, M.D.

Echocardiography Fellow, The Washington Hospital Center, Washington, D.C.
Mitral Valve Prolapse

DAVID C. AGERTER, M.D.

Chairperson, Department of Family Medicine and Assistant Professor, Mayo Medical School, Mayo Clinic, Rochester, Minnesota
Attention Deficit Hyperactivity Disorder

FARID U. AHMAD, M.D.

Gastroenterologist, Roseburg VA Hospital, Eugene, Oregon
Diverticula of the Gastrointestinal Tract

KENNETH B. AIN, M.D.

Professor of Internal Medicine, Division of Endocrinology and Molecular Medicine, Department of Internal Medicine, University of Kentucky; Director, Thyroid Clinic, Veterans Affairs Medical Center, Lexington, Kentucky
Thyroid Cancer

LOUIS M. ALEDORT, M.D.

The Mary Weinfeld Professor of Clinical Research in Hemophilia, Mount Sinai School of Medicine, New York, New York
Platelet-Mediated Bleeding Disorders

MARILEE C. ALLEN, M.D.

Associate Professor of Pediatrics, The Johns Hopkins University School of Medicine; Associate Director of Neonatology, The Johns Hopkins Hospital; Co-Director of the Neonatal Intensive Care Unit Developmental Clinic, Kennedy-Krieger Institute, Baltimore, Maryland
Care of the High-Risk Newborn

MA'EN A. AL-MRAYAT, M.B.B.S.

Research Fellow in Endocrinology, Imperial College School of Medicine, Specialist Registrar, Endocrinology and Diabetes, St. Mary's Hospital, London, United Kingdom
Hypopituitarism in Adults

COL. ANIL C. ANAND, M.D., D.M.

Associate Professor, Department of Medicine, Armed Forces Medical College, Pune; Senior Adviser, Medicine and Gastroenterology, Base Hospital, Delhi; Cantonment Armed Forces Medical Services, New Delhi, India
Amebiasis

RAMON L. AÑEL, M.D.

Chief Fellow, Rush-Presbyterian-St. Luke's Medical Center and Cook County Hospital, Rush University, Chicago, Illinois
Sepsis and Bacteremia

VERNON ANSDELL, M.D., D.T.M.&H.

Clinical Instructor of Public Health Sciences, University of Hawaii; Internal and Tropical Medicine, Kaiser Permanente, Honolulu, Hawaii
Intestinal Parasites

RODNEY A. APPELL, M.D.

Professor of Urology, Baylor College of Medicine; F. Brantley Scott Chair, St. Luke's Episcopal Hospital, Houston, Texas
Urinary Incontinence

ARAM A. ARABIAN, M.D.

Assistant Professor of Medicine, George Washington University School of Medicine and Health Sciences; Associate Chief Medical Intensive Care Unit, Department of Veterans Affairs Medical Center, Washington, D.C.
Acute Respiratory Failure

JANET N. ARNO, M.D.

Clinical Associate Professor of Medicine, Indiana University School of Medicine; Medical Director, Bell Flower Clinic, Marion County Health Department, Indianapolis, Indiana
Chlamydia Trachomatis

SAM ASIRVATHAM, M.D.

Assistant Professor of Medicine, Mayo Medical School, Senior Associate Consultant, Mayo Clinic, Rochester, Minnesota
Atrial Fibrillation

ROBERT L. ATMAR, M.D.

Associate Professor, Departments of Medicine and Molecular Virology and Microbiology, Baylor College of Medicine; Ben Taub General Hospital, Houston, Texas
Influenza

SUSAN W. AUCOTT, M.D.

Assistant Professor of Pediatrics, The Johns Hopkins University School of Medicine; Medical Director, Neonatal Intensive Care Unit and Fellowship Director, Neonatal-Perinatal Medicine, The Johns Hopkins Hospital, Baltimore, Maryland
Care of the High-Risk Newborn

ROBERT R. BAHNSON, M.D.

Dave Longaberger Chair in Urology, Professor of Surgery, and Director, Division of Urology, The Ohio State University, Columbus, Ohio
Urethral Strictures

RAY BAKER, M.D.

Clinical Assistant Professor, University of British Columbia, Vancouver, British Columbia, Canada
Alcoholism

GEORGE BAKRIS, M.D.

Professor of Preventive Medicine and Internal Medicine, Rush Medical College; Vice-Chairman, Department of Preventive Medicine and Director, Hypertension/Clinical Research Center, Rush-Presbyterian-St. Luke's Medical Center, Chicago, Illinois
Hypertension

HARRISON G. BALL, M.D.

Professor, Department of Obstetrics and Gynecology, University of Massachusetts Medical School; Director, Division of Gynecologic Oncology, UMASS Memorial Medical Center, Worcester, Massachusetts
Management of Endometrial Carcinoma

CHRISTIE M. BALLANTYNE, M.D.

Professor, Section of Atherosclerosis, Department of Medicine, Baylor College of Medicine; Director, Center for Cardiovascular Prevention, Methodist DeBakey Heart Center, Houston, Texas
Hyperlipoproteinemias

LISA BARBA, A.R.N.P.

Dermatology, Mt. Sinai, Miami Beach, Florida
Diseases of the Nails

ROBERT BARBIERI, M.D.

Kate Macy Ladd Professor of Obstetrics, Gynecology and Reproductive Biology, Harvard Medical School; Chairman, Obstetrics and Gynecology, Brigham and Women's Hospital, Boston, Massachusetts
Endometriosis

CLAIRE S. BARLOW, M.B.B.S.

St. Bartholomew's Hospital, West Smithfield, London, United Kingdom
Hodgkin's Disease

PETER F. BARNES, M.D.

Professor of Medicine and Microbiology and Immunology, University of Texas Health Center, Tyler, Texas
Tuberculosis and Nontuberculous Mycobacterial Disease

KURT T. BARNHART, M.D., M.S.C.E.

Assistant Professor, University of Pennsylvania; Attending Physician, Hospital of the University of Pennsylvania, Philadelphia, Pennsylvania
Contraception

RICHARD J. BAROHN, M.D.

Professor and Chair, Department of Neurology, University of Kansas Medical Center, Kansas City, Kansas
Myasthenia Gravis

S. SERGE BAROLD, M.D.

Clinical Professor of Medicine Emeritus, University of Rochester School of Medicine and Dentistry, Rochester, New York; Cardiologist, Broward General Hospital, Ft. Lauderdale, Florida
Heart Block

YOUSRI M. BARRI, M.D.

Assistant Professor, Division of Nephrology, Department of Medicine, University of Arkansas for Medical Sciences; Staff Physician, VA Medical Center, Central Arkansas Veterans Healthcare, Little Rock, Arkansas
Acute Renal Failure

WILLIAM W. BARRINGTON, M.D.

Associate Professor of Medicine and Cardiology, Cardiovascular Institute, University of Pittsburgh Medical Center, Pittsburgh, Pennsylvania
Tachycardias

KENNETH B. BATTS, D.O.

Officer-in-Charge, Clark Health Clinic, Womack Army Medical Center, Fort Bragg, North Carolina
Common Sports Injuries

CRAIG BERGER, M.D.

Assistant Professor, Cornea Service, Department of Ophthalmology, University of South Florida College of Medicine, Tampa, Florida
Conjunctivitis

JEFFREY S. BERNS, M.D.

Associate Professor of Medicine, University of Pennsylvania School of Medicine; Presbyterian Medical Center, Philadelphia, Pennsylvania
Chronic Renal Failure

PELAYO C. BESA, M.D.

Division Head, Radiation-Oncology, Centro de Cancer, and Adjunct Professor, Radiation-Oncology, Facultad de Medicina, Pontificia Universidad Católica de Chile, Santiago, Chile
Hodgkin's Disease: Radiation Therapy

VALÉRIE BIOUSSE, M.D.

Assistant Professor in Neurology, Emory University School of Medicine; Neuro-Ophthalmology Unit, Emory Eye Center, Atlanta, Georgia
Optic Neuritis

ALAIN BITTON, M.D.

Assistant Professor, McGill University; Assistant Physician, Royal Victoria Hospital, McGill University Health Center, Montreal, Quèbec, Canada
Inflammatory Bowel Disease

BRIAN L. BLEAU, M.D.

Director of Endoscopy, St. Joseph's Hospital; Director of Clinical Research, Tacoma Digestive Disease Center, Tacoma, Washington
Bleeding Esophageal Varices

MARGARETA BLOMBÄCK, M.D. PH.D.

Professor Emerita, Karolinska Institutet, Stockholm, Sweden
Disseminated Intravascular Coagulation

RONALD S. BLOOM, M.D.

Professor, Vice-Chairman, Department of Pediatrics, University of Utah, Salt Lake City, Utah
Resuscitation of the Newborn

DAVID E. BLUMENTHAL, M.D.

Staff Physician, Department of Rheumatic and Immunologic Diseases, Cleveland Clinic Foundation, Cleveland, Ohio
Hyperuricemia and Gout

WILLIAM E. BOLGER, M.D.

Associate Professor Otorhinolaryngology, University of Pennsylvania; Chief, Rhinology and Sinus Surgery, Hospital of the University of Pennsylvania, Philadelphia, Pennsylvania
Rhinosinusitis

WILLIAM Z. BORER, M.D.

Director, Clinical Chemistry Laboratory, Thomas Jefferson University Hospital, Philadelphia, Pennsylvania
Reference Intervals for the Interpretation of Laboratory Tests

THOMAS L. BOSSHARDT, M.D.

Cascade Surgical Partners, PLLC, Yakima, Washington
Necrotizing Skin and Soft Tissue Infections

ROBERT H. BOWER, M.D.

Professor and Vice-Chair, Education, Department of Surgery, University of Cincinnati College of Medicine; Chief, Surgical Service, VA Medical Center Cincinnati, Cincinnati, Ohio
Parenteral Nutrition in Adults

JACQUES BRADWEJN, M.D.

Professor and Chairman, Department of Psychiatry, Faculty of Medicine, University of Ottawa; Psychiatrist-in-Chief, Royal Ottawa Hospital and The Ottawa Hospital, Ottawa, Ontario, Canada
Panic Disorder

SIXTEN S. E. BREDBACKA, M.D., PH.D.

Karolinska Institutet; Section Head, Central Operation, St. Goran Hospital, Stockholm, Sweden
Disseminated Intravascular Coagulation

RONALD BRISMAN, M.D.

Associate Professor of Clinical Neurosurgery, College of Physicians and Surgeons of Columbia University; Neurosurgeon, Columbia Presbyterian Medical Center, New York City, New York
Trigeminal Neuralgia

BARBARA J. BROWNE, M.D.

Instructor, Department of Rehabilitation Medicine, Jefferson Medical College; Director of Stroke Rehabilitation and Staff Psychiatrist, Magee Rehabilitation Hospital, Philadelphia, Pennsylvania
Rehabilitation of the Stroke Patient

MARK E. BUBAK, M.D.

Dakota Allergy and Asthma, Sioux Falls, South Dakota
Asthma in Adolescents and Adults

CRAIG A. BUCHMAN, M.D.

Associate Professor, Department of Otolaryngology, University of North Carolina at Chapel Hill, Chapel Hill, North Carolina
Otitis Externa

ROBERT A. BUCKMIRE, M.D.

Assistant Professor of Otolaryngology, University of Pittsburgh School of Medicine, Pittsburgh, Pennsylvania
Hoarseness and Laryngitis

CLAUDE S. BURTON III, M.D.

Assistant Professor, Duke University, Durham, North Carolina
Leg Ulcers

KLAUS J. BUSAM, M.D.

Associate Professor, New York Weill Cornell Center; Associate Attending Pathologist, Department of Pathology, Memorial Sloan-Kettering Cancer Center, New York, New York
Skin Cancer Precursor Lesions

W. RUSSELL BYRNE, M.D.

Associate Professor, Uniformed Services University of Health Sciences, Bethesda, Maryland; Infectious Disease Officer, Medical Division, U.S. Army Research Institute of Infectious Diseases, Fort Detrick, Maryland
Q Fever

CLIFTON W. CALLAWAY, M.D., PH.D.

Assistant Professor of Emergency Medicine, University of Pittsburgh; Attending Physician, UPMC–Presbyterian Hospital, Pittsburgh, Pennsylvania
Cardiac Arrest: Sudden Cardiac Death

CRISTINA R. CAMARA, M.D.

University of Illinois College of Medicine, Chicago, Illinois
Leprosy

SARAH E. CAPES, M.D.

Assistant Professor, Department of Medicine, McMaster University, Hamilton, Ontario, Canada
Thyroiditis

THOMAS CARACCIO, PHARM.D.

Associate Professor of Emergency Medicine, SUNY Stony Brook; Assistant Professor of Pharmacology and Toxicology, New York College of Osteopathic Medicine, Old Westbury; Assistant Professor of Clinical Pharmacy, St. John's University, Jamaica; Director, Long Island Regional Poison and Drug Information Center, Winthrop University Hospital, Mineola, New York
Acute Poisonings

BRUCE R. CARR, M.D.

Paul C. MacDonald Distinguished Chair in Obstetrics and Gynecology, Professor, and Director, Division of Reproductive Endocrinology and Infertility, University of Texas Southwestern Medical Center, Dallas, Texas
Amenorrhea

LAWRENCE S. CHAN, M.D.

Director of Immunodermatology and Assistant Professor of Dermatology, Northwestern University Medical School; Attending Physician, Lakeside Medical Center, VA Chicago Health Care System, Chicago, Illinois
Bullous Diseases

MIRIAM M. CHAN, B.SC., PHARM.D.

Clinical Assistant Professor of Pharmacy, The Ohio State University and Director of Pharmacy Education, Riverside Family Practice Residency Program, Riverside Methodist Hospital, Columbus; Adjunct Assistant Professor of Pharmacy, Ohio Northern University, Ada, Ohio; Affiliate Faculty of Pharmacy Practice, Idaho State University, Pocatello, Idaho
Some Popular Herbal Products

CHRISTINE I. CHEN, M.D.

Lecturer, Department of Medicine, University of Toronto; Hematologist, Princess Margaret Hospital, Toronto, Ontario, Canada
Multiple Myeloma

TONY M. CHOU, M.D.

Associate Professor of Medicine, University of California at San Francisco; Attending Physician, Adult Cardiac Catheter Laboratories, University of California at San Francisco Hospitals and Clinics, San Francisco, California
Acute Myocardial Infarction

CYNTHIA CHRISTY, M.D.

Associate Professor, University of Rochester School of Medicine and Dentistry, Children's Hospital at Strong; Pediatrician and Associate Professor, Rochester General Hospital, Rochester, New York
Viral Respiratory Infections

W. HALLOWELL CHURCHILL, M.D.

Associate Professor of Medicine, Brigham and Women's Hospital, Harvard Medical School, Boston, Massachusetts
Autoimmune Hemolytic Anemia

BARBARA A. CLARK, M.D.

Associate Professor of Medicine, MCP/Hahnemann School of Medicine; Staff Nephrologist, Allegheny General Hospital, Pittsburgh, Pennsylvania
Diabetes Insipidus

KERRY O. CLEVELAND, M.D.

Teaching Staff, Methodist Healthcare of Memphis; Baptist Memorial Healthcare, Memphis, Tennessee
Brucellosis

RICHARD DANIEL CLOVER, M.D.

Professor, School of Medicine, University of Louisville, Louisville, Kentucky
Immunization Practices

ALAN R. COHEN, M.D.

Professor of Pediatrics and Chair, Department of Pediatrics, University of Pennsylvania School of Medicine; Physician-in-Chief, Children's Hospital of Philadelphia, Philadelphia, Pennsylvania
Thalassemia

PHILIP R. COHEN, M.D.

Clinical Associate Professor, Department of Dermatology, University of Texas–Houston Medical School, Houston; Private Practice, Dermatology, The Woodlands, Texas
Nevi

MORTON COLEMAN, M.D.

Clinical Professor of Medicine and Director, Center for Lymphoma and Myeloma, Division of Hematology/Oncology, Weill Medical College of Cornell University; Attending Physician, New York Weill Cornell Medical Center and New York Presbyterian Hospital, New York, New York
Non-Hodgkin's Lymphoma

ROBERT R. CONLEY, M.D.

Associate Professor of Psychiatry and Pharmacy Science, University of Maryland School of Medicine; Director of Treatment Research, Maryland Psychiatric Research Center, Baltimore, Maryland
Schizophrenia

DAVID W. COOKE, M.D.

Assistant Professor of Pediatrics, The Johns Hopkins University School of Medicine, Baltimore, Maryland
Diabetes Mellitus in Children and Adolescents

CAROLYN CRANDALL, M.D.

Assistant Professor of Medicine, University of California at Los Angeles School of Medicine, Department of Medicine, Division of General Internal Medicine, Los Angeles, California
Menopause

JEFFREY CRAWFORD, M.D.

Professor of Medicine, Duke University School of Medicine and Duke University Medical Center, Durham, North Carolina
Primary Lung Cancer

DENNIS CUNNINGHAM, M.D.

Fellow, Pediatric Infectious Diseases, University of Maryland School of Medicine; Medical Staff Member, University of Maryland Medical System, Baltimore, Maryland
Bordetella Pertussis (Whooping Cough)

MARY CURRIER, M.D., M.P.H.

Assistant Professor, University of Mississippi School of Medicine, Jackson, Mississippi; State Epidemiologist, Mississippi State Department of Health
Rabies

JOHN S. CZACHOR, M.D.

Associate Professor of Medicine, Division of Infectious Diseases, Wright State University School of Medicine; Miami Valley Hospital, Dayton, Ohio
Acute Bronchitis and Acute Exacerbation of Chronic Bronchitis

GARY V. DAHL, M.D.

Professor of Pediatrics, Stanford University Medical School, Stanford, California
Acute Leukemia in Childhood

MARK V. DAHL, M.D.

Professor and Chairman, Department of Dermatology, Mayo Clinic Scottsdale, Scottsdale, Arizona
Contact Dermatitis

KENT DAUTERMAN, M.D.

Interventional Cardiology Fellow, Division of Cardiology, University of California at San Francisco, San Francisco, California
Acute Myocardial Infarction

DANIEL DAVIS, M.D.

Assistant Clinical Professor, University of California at San Diego, San Diego, California
Toxic Shock Syndrome

MOLINA DAYAL, M.D., M.P.H.

Fellow, Division of Reproductive Medicine and Surgery, Department of Obstetrics and Gynecology, Hospital of the University of Pennsylvania, Philadelphia, Pennsylvania
Contraception

MARVALYN DECAMBRE, M.D.

University of Connecticut Integrated Program in Urology, Farmington; Resident, Connecticut Children's Medical Center, Hartford, Connecticut
Bacterial Infections of the Urinary Tract in Girls

R. PHILLIP DELLINGER, M.D.

Professor of Medicine, Rush Medical College; Director, Section of Critical Care Medicine, Rush-Presbyterian-St. Luke's Medical Center, Chicago, Illinois
Sepsis and Bacteremia

MARVIN A. DEWAR, M.D., J.D.

Associate Professor, University of Florida College of Medicine; Professor, Community Health and Family Medicine; Vice President, Affiliations, Shands Health Care, Gainesville, Florida
Breast Disorders

CAROL A. DIAMOND, M.D.

Assistant Professor, Pediatric Hematology/Oncology, University of Wisconsin, Madison, Wisconsin
Vitamin K Deficiency

LUIS A. DIAZ, M.D.

Professor and Chairman of Dermatology, University of North Carolina at Chapel Hill, Chapel Hill, North Carolina; Attending, University of North Carolina Hospitals
Pruritus

KARL DOGHRAMJI, M.D.

Associate Professor, Department of Psychiatry and Human Behavior, Jefferson Medical College; Director, Sleep Disorders Center, Thomas Jefferson University Hospital, Philadelphia, Pennsylvania
Insomnia

LT COL MATTHEW J. DOLAN, M.D.

Associate Professor of Medicine, Uniformed Services University of the Health Sciences, Bethesda, Maryland; Chief, Infectious Diseases and Fellowship Program Director, Wilford Hall USAF Medical Center, Lackland AFB, Texas
Cat-Scratch Disease and Bacillary Angiomatosis

STEPHEN DOLAN, M.D.
Assistant Professor of Medicine, Pulmonary/Critical Care Division, Medical College of Wisconsin; Section Chief, Pulmonary/Critical Care Division, Veterans Administration Medical Center, Milwaukee, Wisconsin
Silicosis

DANA WASSON DUNNE, M.D.
Clinical Assistant Professor of Medicine, Yale University School of Medicine; Infectious Diseases Consultant, New Haven Health Department, New Haven, Connecticut
Gonorrhea

ANDREW W. DuPONT, M.D.
Fellow, Division of Gastroenterology, University of Alabama at Birmingham; Birmingham, Alabama
Giardiasis

HERBERT L. DuPONT, M.D.
Clinical Professor, Baylor College of Medicine and The University of Texas–Houston; Chief, Internal Medicine Service, St. Luke's Episcopal Hospital, Houston, Texas
Giardiasis

MARK S. DWORKIN, M.D., M.P.H.T.M.
State Epidemiologist, Illinois Department of Public Health, Chicago, Illinois
Relapsing Fever

LEONARD DZUBOW, M.D.
Professor of Dermatology, University of Pennsylvania, Philadelphia, Pennsylvania
Cancer of the Skin

ASHRAF EL-MITTALLI, M.D.
Fellow, Neurology, University of Texas Medical School, Houston, Texas
Intracerebral Hemorrhage

NATHAN R. EMERY, M.D.
Resident in Ophthalmology, University of South Florida College of Medicine, Tampa, Florida
Conjunctivitis

HARRY P. ERBA, M.D., Ph.D.
Clinical Assistant Professor, University of Michigan, Ann Arbor, Michigan
Acute Leukemia in Adults

KYLE P. ETZKORN, M.D.
Director of Research, Borland-Groover Clinic; Baptist Medical Center, St. Luke's/Mayo Hospital, Jacksonville, Florida
Constipation

JANINE EVANS, M.D.
Yale University School of Medicine; Yale-New Haven Hospital; Hospital of St. Raphael's, New Haven, Connecticut
Lyme Disease

SHEREEN EZZAT, M.D.
Associate Professor of Medicine, University of Toronto; Program Director, Endocrine Oncology, Mount Sinai Hospital, Toronto, Ontario, Canada
Acromegaly

ROBIN L. FAINSINGER, M.D.
Associate Professor, Division of Palliative Care Medicine, Department of Oncology, University of Alberta; Royal Alexandra Hospital; Grey Nuns Hospital, Edmonton, Alberta, Canada
Pain

JOSE N. FAYAD, M.D.
Assistant Professor, Department of Otolaryngology/Head and Neck Surgery, Columbia University College of Physicians and Surgeons; Assistant Professor, New York Presbyterian Hospital; Attending Physician, Manhattan Eye, Ear, and Throat Hospital, New York, New York
Tinnitus

ROBERT D. FECHTNER, M.D.
Associate Professor and Director, Glaucoma Division, Department of Ophthalmology, New Jersey Medical School, University of Medicine and Dentistry of New Jersey, Newark, New Jersey
Glaucoma

RICHARD NEIL FEDORAK, M.D.
Professor of Medicine, University of Alberta; Director, Division of Gastroenterology, University of Alberta Hospital, Edmonton, Alberta, Canada
Malabsorption

PETER J. FENNER, M.D.
Associate Professor, Medical School, James Cook University, Queensland; National Medical Officer, Surf Life Saving Australia, Sydney, New South Wales, Australia
Marine Stings, Bites, and Poisoning

MIGUEL C. FERNÁNDEZ, M.D.
Associate Professor, Division of Emergency Medicine; Medical Director, South Texas Poison Center, The University of Texas Health Science Center at San Antonio, San Antonio, Texas
Snakebite

CRISTINA FERRONE, M.D.
Clinical Fellow in Surgery, Harvard Medical School, Boston, Massachusetts
Chronic Pancreatitis

SYDNEY M. FINEGOLD, M.D.
Emeritus Professor of Medicine and Emeritus Professor of Microbiology, Immunology and Molecular Genetics, UCLA School of Medicine; Staff Physician, Infectious Diseases Section, VA Medical Center, West Los Angeles, Los Angeles, California
Primary Lung Abscess

MARTIN FISHER, M.D.
Professor of Clinical Pediatrics, New York University School of Medicine, New York City; Chief, Division of Adolescent Medicine, Department of Pediatrics, North Shore University Hospital, North Shore–Long Island Jewish Health System, Manhasset, New York
Infectious Mononucleosis

JONATHAN M. FLACKER, M.D.
Assistant Professor of Medicine, Emory University; Director, Grady Geriatrics Center, Grady Health Systems, Atlanta, Georgia
Delirium

FRANKLIN P. FLOWERS, M.D.
Professor, Otolaryngology and Professor, Pathology and Pediatrics, University of Florida College of Medicine, Gainesville, Florida
Viral Diseases of the Skin

HARALD FODSTAD, M.D., Ph.D.
Associate Professor of Neurosurgery, Weill Medical College of Cornell University; Chief of Neurosurgery, New York Methodist Hospital, New York, New York
Hiccup

GREGORY T. FOSSUM, M.D.
Associate Professor of Obstetrics and Gynecology, Jefferson Medical College; Attending Physician, Thomas Jefferson University, Philadelphia, Pennsylvania
Abnormal Uterine Bleeding

NATHAN B. FOUNTAIN, M.D.
Assistant Professor of Neurology and Director, Comprehensive Epilepsy Program, University of Virginia School of Medicine, Charlottesville, Virginia
Seizures and Epilepsy in Adolescents and Adults

MELVIN H. FREEDMAN, M.D.
Professor, Department of Pediatrics, University of Toronto Faculty of Medicine; Senior Staff Physician, Hematology/Oncology and Senior Associate Scientist, Hospital for Sick Children and Research Institute, Toronto, Ontario, Canada
Neutropenia

KENNETH D. FRIEDMAN, M.D.
Associate Medical Director, The Blood Center, Milwaukee, Wisconsin
Therapeutic Use of Blood Components

WILLIAM H. FRISHMAN, M.D.
Barbara and William Rosenthal Professor of Medicine, Professor of Pharmacology, and Chair of Medicine, New York Medical College; Chief of Medicine, Westchester Medical Center, Valhalla, New York
Angina Pectoris

DEBRA L. FROMER, M.D.
Senior Resident, Department of Urology, New York–Presbyterian Hospital, New York, New York
Benign Prostatic Hyperplasia

MICHAEL T. GAMBLA, M.D.
Resident, Division of Urology, The Ohio State University, Columbus, Ohio
Urethral Strictures

BRUCE JAY GANTZ, M.D.
Professor and Head, Department of Otolaryngology–Head and Neck Surgery, University of Iowa College of Medicine; Professor and Head, University of Iowa Hospitals and Clinics, Iowa City, Iowa
Meniere's Disease

GLENN A. GAUNT, M.D.
Resident Physician, Mayo Clinic, Rochester, Minnesota
Antepartum Care

BERNARD GAUTHIER, M.B., B.S.
Professor of Pediatrics, Albert Einstein College of Medicine, Bronx; Attending, Pediatric Nephrology, Schneider Children's Hospital of North Shore–Long Island Jewish Health System, New Hyde Park, New York
Parenteral Fluid and Electrolyte Therapy in Pediatrics

MICHAEL S. GELFAND, M.D.
Clinical Professor of Medicine, University of Tennessee Health Science Center; Chief, Division of Infectious Diseases, Methodist Healthcare, Memphis, Tennessee
Brucellosis; Blastomycosis

HERTZEL C. GERSTEIN, M.D., M.Sc.
Associate Professor, Department of Medicine, McMaster University, Hamilton, Ontario, Canada
Thyroiditis

JAMSHID GHAJAR, M.D., Ph.D.
Associate Professor, Department of Neurosurgery, New York Presbyterian Hospital, Weill Medical College of Cornell University, New York, New York
Acute Head Injuries in Children

GISELLE B. GHURANI, M.D.
Assistant Clinical Faculty, University of Miami School of Medicine; Clinical Fellow in Gynecologic Oncology, Jackson Memorial Medical Center, University of Miami School of Medicine, Miami, Florida
Neoplasms of the Vulva

DEAN GIANAKOS, M.D.
Associate Director, Lynchburg Family Practice Residency, University of Virginia Affiliate Program; Assistant Professor of Clinical Family Medicine, University of Virginia, Lynchburg, Virginia
Chronic Obstructive Pulmonary Disease

BARBARA A. GILCHREST, M.D.
Professor and Chairman, Department of Dermatology, Boston University School of Medicine; Chief of Dermatology, Boston Medical Center, Boston, Massachusetts
Sunburn

RICHARD GLECKMAN, M.D.
Clinical Professor of Medicine, Mount Sinai Medical School, New York, New York; Chairman of Medicine and Chief of Infectious Disease Division, St. Joseph's Regional Medical Center, Paterson, New Jersey
Rocky Mountain Spotted Fever and Ehrlichiosis

CHRISTOPHER G. GOETZ, M.D.
Professor of Neurology, Rush University; Professor, Rush-St. Luke's-Presbyterian Hospital, Chicago, Illinois
Parkinsonism

DAVID B. K. GOLDEN, M.D.
Associate Professor of Medicine, The Johns Hopkins University; Director of Allergy-Immunology, Sinai Hospital, Baltimore, Maryland
Allergic Reactions to Insect Stings

VICTOR R. GORDEUK, M.D.
Professor of Medicine, Center for Sickle Cell Disease, Howard University School of Medicine, Washington, D.C.
Iron Deficiency

DAVID LEE GORDON, M.D.
Associate Professor of Clinical Neurology and Medicine and Director, Emergency Medical Skills and Neurology Training, Center for Research in Medical Education, University of Miami School of Medicine, Miami, Florida
Ischemic Cerebrovascular Disease

JEAN-PAUL GOULET, D.D.S., M.S.D.
Professor and Associate Dean of Research and Graduate Studies, Faculté de Médecine Dentaire, Université Laval, Québec, Québec, Canada
Temporomandibular Disorders

GAIL A. GREENDALE, M.D.
Associate Professor of Medicine, Obstetrics and Gynecology, University of California at Los Angeles School of Medicine, Department of Medicine/Division of Geriatrics, Los Angeles, California
Menopause

JOSEPH GREENSHER, M.D.
Professor of Pediatrics, State University of New York at Stony Brook; Medical Director and Associate Chairman, Department of Pediatrics, Winthrop University Hospital, Mineola; Associate Medical Director, Long Island Regional Poison and Drug Information Center, East Meadow, New York
Acute Poisonings

BRUCE GREENWALD, M.D.
Associate Professor, Department of Pediatrics, New York Presbyterian Hospital, Weill Medical College of Cornell University, New York, New York
Acute Head Injuries in Children

FRANK R. GREER, M.D.
Professor of Pediatrics and Nutritional Sciences, University of Wisconsin; Neonatologist, Meriter Hospital, Madison, Wisconsin
Vitamin K Deficiency

DAVID E. GRIFFITH, M.D.
Professor of Medicine, University of Texas Health Center, Tyler, Texas
Tuberculosis and Nontuberculous Mycobacterial Disease

LEWIS R. GRODEN, M.D.
Associate Professor, Director, Cornea Service, and Director, Residency Program, Department of Ophthalmology, University of South Florida College of Medicine; Medical Director, Lasik Plus Vision Center, Tampa, Florida
Conjunctivitis

JERE D. GUIN, B.M.S., M.D.
Professor Emeritus, University of Arkansas for Medical Sciences; Staff Physician, Baptist Medical Center, St. Vincent's Infirmary, and Arkansas Children's Hospital; Consulting Staff Physician, Arkansas Heart Hospital, Little Rock, Arkansas
Urticaria

KALPANA GUPTA, M.D., M.P.H.
Acting Assistant Professor of Medicine, Division of Allergy and Infectious Diseases, University of Washington, Seattle, Washington
Bacterial Infections of the Urinary Tract in Women

RAYMOND HADDAD, M.D.
Associate Clinical Professor of Medicine, Yale University School of Medicine, New Haven; Chief, Pulmonary Disease, Bridgeport Hospital, Bridgeport, Connecticut
Cough

CAROLINE B. HALL, M.D.
Professor, Children's Hospital at Strong, University of Rochester School of Medicine and Dentistry, Rochester, New York
Viral Respiratory Infections

MURRAY P. HAMLET, D.V.M.
Former Chief, Research Support Division, U.S. Army Research Institute of Environmental Medicine, Natick, Massachusetts
Injuries Due to Cold

ROGER HARTL, M.D.
New York Presbyterian Hospital, Weill Medical College of Cornell University, New York, New York
Acute Head Injuries in Children

DAVID L. HAYES, M.D.
Professor of Medicine, Mayo Medical School; Head, Pacemaker Service and Vice-Chair, Cardiology Division, Mayo Clinic, Rochester, Minnesota
Heart Block

MEGAN RIST HAYMART, B.A.
Medical Student, The Johns Hopkins University Medical School, Baltimore, Maryland
Cirrhosis

PETER W. HEALD, M.D.
Yale University School of Medicine, New Haven, Connecticut
Cutaneous T-Cell Lymphomas

SEÁN HENDERSON, M.D., M.S.
Associate Professor, Department of Emergency Medicine, Keck School of Medicine, University of Southern California, Los Angeles, California
Tetanus

DONALD D. HENSRUD, M.D., M.P.H.
Associate Professor of Preventive Medicine and Nutrition, Mayo Medical School; Consultant, Divisions of Preventive Medicine and Endocrinology, Metabolism, and Nutrition, Mayo Clinic, Rochester, Minnesota
Obesity

H. FRANKLIN HERLONG, M.D.
Associate Dean for Student Affairs and Associate Professor of Medicine, The Johns Hopkins University School of Medicine, Baltimore, Maryland
Cirrhosis

JEROME M. HERSHMAN, M.D.
Professor of Medicine, UCLA School of Medicine; Chief, Endocrinology and Metabolism Division, Veterans Affairs Greater Los Angeles Healthcare System, Los Angeles, California
Hypothyroidism

CARLOTTA H. HILL, M.D.
Clinical Associate Professor and Director, Chicago Regional Hansen's Disease Center, University of Illinois College of Medicine, Chicago, Illinois
Leprosy

BRIAN D. HOIT, M.D.
Professor of Medicine, Case Western Reserve University; University Hospitals of Cleveland, Cleveland, Ohio
Treatment of Pericardial Disease

KATHERINE HOLLAND, M.D., PH.D.
Staff Physician, Section of Pediatric Epilepsy, The Cleveland Clinic Foundation, Cleveland, Ohio
Epilepsy in Infants and Children

MELISA HOLMES, M.D.
Associate Professor, Department of Obstetrics and Gynecology, Medical University of South Carolina, Charleston, South Carolina
Dysmenorrhea

STACY HORN, D.O.
Instructor, Rush University; Instructor, Rush-St. Luke's-Presbyterian Medical Center, Chicago, Illinois
Parkinsonism

ROBERT H. HOWLAND, M.D.
University of Pittsburgh School of Medicine, University of Pittsburgh; Associate Professor of Psychiatry, Western Psychiatric Institute and Clinic, Pittsburgh, Pennsylvania
Mood Disorders

TREVOR A. HOWLETT, M.D.
Honorary Senior Lecturer, University of Leicester Medical School; Consultant Endocrinologist, Leicester Royal Infirmary, Leicester, England
Adrenocortical Insufficiency

RUSSELL HULL, M.B.B.S., M.SC.
Professor of Medicine, University of Calgary; Director, Thrombosis Research Unit, Foothills Hospital, Calgary, Alberta, Canada
Pulmonary Thromboembolism

CHIN HUR, M.D., M.P.H.
Fellow in Medicine, Harvard Medical School, Cambridge; Beth Israel Deaconess Medical Center, Boston, Massachusetts
Gaseousness and Indigestion

HEIDI HWONG, M.D.
Baylor College of Medicine, Houston, Texas
Atopic Dermatitis

ELBA A. IGLESIAS, M.D.
Assistant Professor of Pediatrics, Albert Einstein College of Medicine, Bronx; Attending Physician, North Shore University Hospital, North Shore–Long Island Jewish Health System, Manhasset, New York
Infectious Mononucleosis

MUNAVVAR IZHAR, M.D., D.M.
Attending Physician, Hypertension Section and Clinical Instructor in Medicine, Rush Medical College and Rush-Presbyterian-St. Luke's Medical Center; Chicago, Illinois
Hypertension

ARTHUR D. JACKSON, B.Sc., M.Phil.
Honorary Senior Research Fellow, University of Wales College of Medicine, Cardiff; Associate Specialist in Dermatology, East Cheshire NHS Trust, Macclesfield and Mid Cheshire Hospitals, Crewe, Cheshire, United Kingdom
Warts and Their Management

KOWICHI JIMBOW, M.D., Ph.D.
Professor and Chair, Department of Dermatology, Sapporo Medical University School of Medicine, Dean, Sapporo Medical University School of Medicine, and Dean, Sapporo Medical University Graduate School of Medicine; Chief, Division of Dermatology and Chief, Division of Plastic Surgery, Sapporo Medical University Hospital, Sapporo, Japan
Pigmentary Disorders

DESMOND JOHNSTON, M.B., Ch.B., Ph.D.
Professor of Clinical Endocrinology, Imperial College School of Medicine; Consultant Physician, St. Mary's Hospital, London, United Kingdom
Hypopituitarism in Adults

ERVIN E. JONES, Ph.D., M.D.
Professor and Director of Medical Studies, Department of Obstetrics and Gynecology, Yale University School of Medicine; Professor and Director of Assisted Reproduction, Yale New Haven Hospital, New Haven, Connecticut
Hyperprolactinemia

STEPHEN R. JONES, M.D.
Professor of Medicine, Oregon Health Sciences University; Chief of Medicine, Legacy Health System, Portland, Oregon
Bacterial Infections of the Urinary Tract in Men

PETER J. KAHRILAS, M.D.
Marquardt Professor of Medicine and Chief, Division of Gastroenterology and Hepatology, Northwestern University Medical School; Chief of Gastroenterology and Hepatology, Northwestern Memorial Hospital, Chicago, Illinois
Gastroesophageal Reflux Disease

STEVEN A. KAPLAN, M.D.
Given Foundation Professor of Urology, College of Physicians and Surgeons of Columbia University; Vice Chairman and Administrator, Department of Urology, New York–Presbyterian Hospital, New York, New York
Benign Prostatic Hyperplasia

ILDY M. KATONA, M.D.
Professor of Pediatrics and Medicine, F. Edward Hébert School of Medicine, Uniformed Services University of the Health Sciences, Bethesda, Maryland
Juvenile Rheumatoid Arthritis

TARA KEARNEY, B.Sc., M.B.B.S.
Specialist Registrar/Endocrinology and Diabetes, St. Mary's Hospital, London, United Kingdom
Hypopituitarism in Adults

ROBERT A. KING, M.D.
Professor of Child Psychiatry and Psychiatry, Yale Child Study Center, Yale University School of Medicine; Medical Director, Tourette's Syndrome/OCD Clinic, Yale Child Study Center; Attending, Yale-New Haven Hospital, New Haven, Connecticut
Gilles de la Tourette Syndrome

R. PHILIP KINKEL, M.D.
Medical Director, Mellen Center for Multiple Sclerosis Treatment and Research, Cleveland Clinic Foundation, Cleveland, Ohio
Multiple Sclerosis

JEFFREY T. KIRCHNER, D.O.
Associate Clinical Professor, Family Medicine, Temple University School of Medicine, Philadelphia; Associate Director, Family Practice Residency Program, Lancaster General Hospital, Lancaster, Pennsylvania
Syphilis

MICHAEL B. KIRKPATRICK, M.D.
John L. and Alice Tanner Chair of Pulmonary Medicine, University of South Alabama College of Medicine; Medical Director of Respiratory Therapy, Bronchoscopy, and Pulmonary Function Laboratories, University of South Alabama Medical Center, Mobile, Alabama
Bacterial Pneumonia

CYNTHIA L. KLEINEGGER, D.D.S., M.S.
Assistant Professor, College of Dentistry, University of Iowa, Iowa City, Iowa
Diseases of the Mouth

KENNETH L. KOCH, M.D.
Professor of Medicine, Penn State College of Medicine; Gastroenterology Division, Hershey Medical Center, Penn State University, Hershey, Pennsylvania
Nausea and Vomiting

LARS KOEHLER, M.D.
Senior Registrar and Research Fellow, Department of Rheumatology, Hannover Medical School, Hannover, Germany
Ankylosing Spondylitis and Other Spondylarthritides

KATALIN KORANYI, M.D.
Professor of Clinical Pediatrics, Department of Pediatrics, College of Medicine, Ohio State University; Children's Hospital, Columbus, Ohio
Measles (Rubeola)

DIANA KOSZYCKI, Ph.D.
Associate Professor of Psychiatry, Faculty of Medicine, University of Ottawa; Research Director, Anxiety Disorders Program, Royal Ottawa Hospital, Ottawa, Ontario, Canada
Panic Disorder

DEAN D. KRAHN, M.D., M.S.
Associate Clinical Professor, University of Wisconsin Medical School; Chief, Mental Health Service Line, William S. Middleton Memorial Veterans Hospital, Madison, Wisconsin
Bulimia Nervosa

MARY L. KUMAR, M.D.
Professor of Pediatrics and Pathology, Case Western Reserve School of Medicine; Chief, Pediatric Infectious Diseases, Metrohealth Medical Center, Cleveland, Ohio
Rubella and Congenital Rubella Syndrome

GRACE M. KUO, Pharm.D.
Assistant Professor, Department of Family and Community Medicine, Baylor College of Medicine, Houston, Texas
New Drugs for 2000

ALAN M. LAKE, M.D.
Associate Professor of Pediatrics, The Johns Hopkins University School of Medicine, Baltimore, Maryland
Normal Infant Feeding

KRISTIN E. LAKE, B.S.
Program Project Assistant, Association of Maternal and Child Health Programs, Washington, D.C.
Normal Infant Feeding

PAUL R. LAMBERT, M.D.
Professor and Chair, Department of Otolaryngology–Head and Neck Surgery, Medical University of South Carolina, Charleston, South Carolina
Acute Facial Paralysis

CHARLES N. LANDEN, JR., M.D.
Resident, Department of Obstetrics and Gynecology, Medical University of South Carolina, Charleston, South Carolina
Dysmenorrhea

PHILIP S. LARUSSA, M.D.
Professor of Clinical Pediatrics, Columbia University College of Physicians and Surgeons; Associate Attending Physician, Pediatric Service, New York Presbyterian Hospital, New York, New York
Varicella and Zoster

JAMES F. LECKMAN, M.D.
Neison Harris Professor of Child Psychiatry, Pediatrics and Psychology and Associate Program Director, Children's Clinical Research Center, Yale University School of Medicine; Director of Research, Yale Child Study Center; Attending Physician, Yale New Haven Hospital, New Haven, Connecticut
Gilles de la Tourette Syndrome

JOSEPH I. LEE, M.D., PH.D.
Clinical Instructor, Department of Dermatology, George Washington University Hospital, Washington, D.C.
Condyloma Acuminatum

ANTHONY LEMBO, M.D.
Instructor in Medicine, Harvard Medical School, Cambridge; Beth Israel Deaconess Medical Center, Boston Massachusetts
Gaseousness and Indigestion

JOHN P. LEONARD, M.D.
Assistant Professor of Medicine and Clinical Director, Center for Lymphoma and Myeloma, Division of Hematology/Oncology, Weill Medical College of Cornell University; Medical Director, Oncology Services and Assistant Attending Physician, New York Weill Cornell Medical Center, New York Presbyterian Hospital, New York, New York
Non-Hodgkin's Lymphoma

MITCHELL R. LESTER, M.D.
Fairfield County Allergy, Asthma, and Immunology Associates, Norwalk, Connecticut
Asthma in Children

SEYMOUR R. LEVIN, M.D.
Professor of Medicine, UCLA School of Medicine; Director, Diabetes Program, West Los Angeles VA Medical Center, Greater Los Angeles VA Healthcare System, Los Angeles, California
Diabetes Mellitus in Adults (Type 2 Diabetes)

DONALD P. LEVINE, M.D.
Professor of Medicine and Chief, General Internal Medicine, Wayne State University; Vice-Chief of Medicine, Detroit Receiving Hospital, Detroit, Michigan
Infective Endocarditis

LAURENCE A. LEVINE, M.D.
Professor of Urology, Rush Medical College; Director of Male Sexual Function and Fertility Program, Rush-Presbyterian-St. Luke's Medical Center, Chicago, Illinois
Erectile Dysfunction

EYAL K. LEVIT, M.D.
Clinical Instructor and Fellow in Mohs, Laser, and Dermatologic Surgery, University of Pennsylvania, Philadelphia, Pennsylvania
Cancer of the Skin

MORSE L. LEVY, M.D.
Professor of Dermatology and Pediatrics, Baylor College of Medicine; Chief, Dermatology Service, Texas Children's Hospital, Houston, Texas
Atopic Dermatitis

JAMES T. C. LI, M.D., PH.D.
Professor of Medicine, Mayo Medical School, Rochester, Minnesota
Asthma in Adolescents and Adults

EDWARD N. LIBBY, M.D.
Associate Professor of Internal Medicine, University of New Mexico Health Sciences Center; Staff Physician, University of New Mexico Hospital, Albuquerque, New Mexico
Venous Thrombosis

ROBERT LIBKE, M.D.
Clinical Professor of Medicine and Chief of Infectious Diseases, UCSF-Fresno Medical Education Program, Fresno, California
Coccidioidomycosis

PHIL LIEBERMAN, M.D.
Clinical Professor of Medicine and Pediatrics, University of Tennessee College of Medicine, Memphis, Tennessee
Nonallergic Rhinitis

HENRY W. LIM, M.D.
Professor and Chairman, Henry Ford Hospital, Detroit, Michigan
Sunburn

JEFFREY M. LIPTON, M.D., PH.D.
Professor of Pediatrics, Albert Einstein College of Medicine, New York, Director, Pediatric Hematology/Oncology and Stem Cell Transplantation, Schneider Children's Hospital, New Hyde Park, New York
Aplastic Anemia

T. ANDREW LISTER, M.D.
Director of Cancer Services and Clinical Haematology, St. Bartholomew's Hospital, West Smithfield, London, United Kingdom
Hodgkin's Disease

JINGXUAN LIU, M.D., PH.D.
Chief Resident, Department of Pathology and Hospital Laboratories, University of Massachusetts Memorial Medical Center, Worcester, Massachusetts
Nonimmune Hemolytic Anemias

L. KEITH LLOYD, M.D.
Professor of Surgery (Urology), University of Alabama at Birmingham, Birmingham, Alabama
Epididymitis

KRISTINE M. LOHR, M.D.
Professor of Medicine, University of Tennessee Health Science Center; Associate Chief of Rheumatology, Director, Rheumatology Training Program, and Staff Physician, VA Medical Center, Memphis, Tennessee
Rheumatoid Arthritis

ROGER K. LOW, M.D.

Assistant Professor of Urology and Program Director, Residency Program in Urology, University of California, Davis, Sacramento, California
Urolithiasis

JOSEPH P. LYNCH III, M.D.

Professor of Medicine, Division of Pulmonary and Critical Care Medicine, University of Michigan Medical Center, Ann Arbor, Michigan
Sarcoidosis

JON T. MADER, M.D.

Professor, The University of Texas Medical Branch, Galveston, Texas
Osteomyelitis

KATHRYN MAITLAND, M.D.

Lecturer at Academic Department of Paediatrics, St. Mary's Hospital, Imperial College, London, United Kingdom; Research Fellow, Kemri, Kilifi, Kenya
Malaria

MARC MALKOFF, M.D.

Associate Professor of Neurology and Anesthesiology, University of Texas–Houston, Houston, Texas
Intracerebral Hemorrhage

ASHFAQ MARGHOOB, M.D.

Clinical Assistant Professor, Dermatology Department, State University of New York at Stony Brook, Stony Brook; Assistant Attending Physician, Dermatology Service, Memorial Sloan-Kettering Cancer Center, New York, New York
Skin Cancer Precursor Lesions

THOMAS J. MARRIE, M.D.

Chair, Department of Medicine, University of Alberta; Site Chief, University of Alberta Hospital, Edmonton, Alberta, Canada
Legionellosis (Legionnaires' Disease and Pontiac Fever)

JOAN M. MASTROBATTISTA, M.D.

Associate Professor, University of Texas–Houston Medical School, Houston, Texas
Postpartum Care

CAROL F. McCAMMON, M.D.

Clinical Assistant Professor of Emergency Medicine, Eastern Virginia Medical School, Norfolk, Virginia
Acute Pyelonephritis

KURT A. McCAMMON, M.D.

Assistant Professor of Urology, Eastern Virginia Medical School; Partner, Devine Tidewater Urology, Norfolk, Virginia
Acute Pyelonephritis

MICHAEL T. McCANN, M.D.

Clinical Assistant Professor, Baylor College of Medicine, Houston, Texas
Back Pain

SUSANNA A. McCOLLEY, M.D.

Northwestern University Medical School; Director, Cystic Fibrosis Center, Children's Memorial Hospital, Chicago, Illinois
Cystic Fibrosis

JOSEPH P. McGOWAN, M.D.

Assistant Professor of Medicine, Albert Einstein College of Medicine; Bronx-Lebanon Hospital Center, Bronx, New York
Rat-Bite Fever

MICHAEL A. McGUIGAN, M.D., C.M., M.B.A.

Medical Director, Long Island Regional Poison and Drug Information Center, Winthrop-University Hospital, Mineola, New York
Acute Poisonings

MARILYNNE McKAY, M.D.

Professor Emerita of Dermatology, Emory University School of Medicine, Atlanta, Georgia; Chairman of Dermatology, Lovelace Health System, Albuquerque, New Mexico
Pruritus Ani and Vulvae

PATRICK H. McKENNA, M.D.

Professor of Surgery and Chairman, Division of Urology, Southern Illinois University School of Medicine, Springfield, Illinois
Bacterial Infections of the Urinary Tract in Girls

DAVID S. McKINSEY, M.D.

Clinical Associate Professor of Medicine, University of Kansas, Kansas City, Kansas; Private Practice, Infectious Disease Associates of Kansas City, Kansas City, Missouri
Histoplasmosis

GORDON D. McLAREN, M.D.

Associate Professor of Medicine, Division of Hematology/Oncology, and Chao Family Comprehensive Cancer Center, University of California, Irvine, College of Medicine, Irvine; Staff Physician, Hematology/Oncology Section, VA Long Beach Healthcare System, Long Beach, California
Iron Deficiency

JERRY R. MENDELL, M.D.

Helen C. Kurtz Professor and Chairman of Neurology, The Ohio State University, Columbus, Ohio
Peripheral Neuropathy

ALAN MENDELSOHN, M.D.

Associate Professor of Pediatrics, University of Rochester School of Medicine and Dentistry, Strong Memorial Hospital, Rochester, New York
Congenital Heart Disease

MARIA D. MILENO, M.D.

Assistant Professor of Medicine, Brown University School of Medicine; Director, Travel Medicine Services and Infectious Disease Consulting Staff Physician, The Miriam Hospital, Providence, Rhode Island
Travel Medicine

JAMES S. MILLEDGE, M.D.

Senior Lecturer (Retired), St. Mary's Medical School, Imperial College; Physician Emeritus, Northwick Park Hospital, Harrow, London, United Kingdom
High-Altitude Sickness

JOSEPH I. MILLER, JR., M.D.

Professor of Cardiothoracic Surgery and Chief of General Thoracic Surgery, Emory University School of Medicine; Chief, General Thoracic Surgery, Crawford Long Hospital, Emory University, Atlanta, Georgia
Atelectasis

KARL E. MILLER, M.D.

Associate Professor, Chattanooga Unit, University of Tennessee College of Medicine, Chattanooga, Tennessee
Pelvic Inflammatory Disease

NORMAN S. MILLER, M.D.

Professor of Psychiatry and Medicine, Department of Psychiatry, Michigan State University, East Lansing; Physician in Addiction Unit, St. Laurence Hospital/Sparrow Hospital, Lansing, Michigan
Drug Abuse

PAUL D. MILLER, M.D.
Clinical Professor of Medicine, University of Colorado Medical School, Denver; Medical Director, Colorado Center for Bone Research, Lakewood, Colorado
Osteoporosis; Paget's Disease

JOSEPH L. MILLS, SR., M.D.
Professor of Surgery, University of Arizona Human Sciences Center; Chief, Vascular Surgery and Program Director, Vascular Surgery Fellowship, Tucson, Arizona
Peripheral Arterial Disease

JOHN S. MINASI, M.D.
Chief Scientific Officer, Zassi Medical Evolutions, Inc, Fernandina Beach, Florida
Acute Pancreatitis

ELISABETH I. MINDER, M.D.
Associate Professor, University of Zurich; Head of Department, Central Laboratory, Municipal Hospital Triemli, Zurich, Switzerland
The Porphyrias

DEBRA A. MINJAREZ, M.D.
Colorado Reproductive Endocrinology, Denver, Colorado
Amenorrhea

LAURA J. MURKINSON, M.D.
Assistant Professor, George Washington University School of Medicine; Staff Physician, Children's National Medical Center, Washington, D.C.; Staff Physician, Holy Cross Hospital, Silver Spring, Maryland
Juvenile Rheumatoid Arthritis

HOWARD C. MOFENSON, M.D.
Professor of Pediatrics and Emergency Medicine, State University of New York at Stony Brook, Stony Brook; Professor of Pharmacology/Toxicology, New York College of Osteopathic Medicine, Old Westbury; St. John's University College of Pharmacy, Jamaica; Medical Consultant, Long Island Regional Poison and Drug Information Center, Winthrop University Hospital, Mineola, New York
Acute Poisonings

CULLEN D. MORRIS, M.D.
Senior Resident, General Surgery, Emory University School of Medicine, Atlanta, Georgia
Atelectasis

J. GLENN MORRIS, JR., M.D., M.P.H.T.M.
Professor and Chairman, Department of Epidemiology and Preventive Medicine and Professor of Medicine, University of Maryland School of Medicine, Baltimore, Maryland
Food-Borne Illness

STEEN E. MORTENSEN, M.D.
Assistant Clinical Professor, Kansas University School of Medicine; Chief of Rheumatology, Wichita Clinic, Wichita, Kansas
Bursitis, Tendinitis, Myofascial Pain, and Fibromyalgia

TARIQ MUBIN, M.D.
Fellow in Nephrology, MCP/Hahnemann and Allegheny General Hospital, Pittsburgh, Pennsylvania
Diabetes Insipidus

MAURICE A. MUFSON, M.D.
Professor of Medicine and Chair Emeritus, Joan C. Edwards School of Medicine, Marshall University; Active Staff, St. Mary's Hospital and Cabell-Huntington Hospital, Huntington, West Virginia
Viral and Mycoplasmal Pneumonias

MARK MURPHY, M.D.
Resident, New York Presbyterian Hospital, New York, New York
Tinnitus

VIVEK NARAIN, M.D.
Chief Resident, Wayne State University, Detroit, Michigan
Malignant Tumors of the Urogenital Tract

NANCY J. NEWMAN, M.D.
Professor of Neurology, Ophthalmology, and Neurological Surgery, Emory University School of Medicine; Director, Neuro-Ophthalmology Unit, Emory Eye Center, Atlanta, Georgia
Optic Neuritis

CHARLES R. J. C. NEWTON, M.B., CH.B., M.D.
Senior Lecturer, Institute of Child Health, University of London, London, United Kingdom; Senior Clinical Fellow, Wellcome Trust Research Laboratories, Kilifi, Kenya
Malaria

J. CURTIS NICKEL, M.D.
Professor of Urology, Queen's University; Staff Urologist, Kingston General Hospital, Kingston, Ontario, Canada
Prostatitis

PAUL NYIRJESY, M.D.
Associate Professor, Obstetrics and Gynecology and Medicine (Infectious Diseases), Jefferson Medical College, Philadelphia, Pennsylvania
Vulvovaginitis

JOHN G. OAS, M.D.
Associate Staff and Director, Otoneurology Fellowship Program, Departments of Neurology and Otolaryngology, Cleveland Clinic Foundation; Director, Program of Vestibular and Balance Disorders, Cleveland Clinic Foundation, Cleveland, Ohio
Episodic Vertigo

SUSAN O'BRIEN, M.D.
Professor, University of Texas; Professor, MD Anderson Cancer Center, Houston, Texas
Chronic Leukemias

FRANCIS G. O'CONNOR, M.D.
Assistant Professor, Family Medicine, Uniformed Services University of the Health Sciences; Director, Sports Medicine Fellowship, Uniformed Services University, Bethesda, Maryland
Common Sports Injuries

KEVIN W. OLDEN, M.D.
Assistant Professor of Medicine and Psychiatry, Mayo Medical School, Mayo Clinic, Scottsdale, Arizona
Irritable Bowel Syndrome

ELISE A. OLSEN, M.D.
Professor of Medicine, Division of Dermatology, Duke University Medical Center, Durham, North Carolina
Hair Disorders

CLAUDE H. ORGAN, JR., M.D.
Professor, Department of Surgery, University of California Davis; Alameda County Medical Center, Oakland, California
Necrotizing Skin and Soft Tissue Infections

STEVEN J. ORY, M.D.
Associate Professor of Obstetrics and Gynecology, University of Miami, Miami, Florida
Ectopic Pregnancy

SHAWN S. OSTERHOLT, M.D.
Staff Physician, Blanchfield Army Community Hospital, Ft. Campbell, Kentucky
Hemolytic Disease of the Fetus and Newborn

NINA A. PALEOLOGOS, M.D.

Assistant Professor of Neurology, Northwestern University Medical School, Chicago; Co-Director, Neuro-Oncology, Evanston Hospital, Evanston Northwestern Healthcare, Evanston, Illinois
Brain Tumors

JOHN E. PANDOLFINO, M.D.

Gastroenterology Fellow, Northwestern University; Gastrointestinal Fellow, Northwestern Memorial Hospital, Chicago, Illinois
Gastroesophageal Reflux Disease

JAMES O. PARK, M.D.

Resident, General Surgery, University of Chicago Hospitals, Chicago, Illinois
Tumors of the Stomach

CHARLES J. PARKER, M.D.

Professor of Medicine, University of Utah School of Medicine; Chief, Hematology/Oncology, VA Medical Center, Salt Lake City, Utah
Adverse Reactions to Blood Transfusions

LIBERTO PECHET, M.D.

Professor Emeritus, Medicine and Pathology, University of Massachusetts Medical School; Director, Hematology Laboratory, University of Massachusetts Memorial Medical Center, Worcester, Massachusetts
Nonimmune Hemolytic Anemias

MANUEL A. PENALVER, M.D.

Professor and Chairman, Department of Obstetrics and Gynecology, University of Miami School of Medicine; Chief, Obstetrics/Gynecology Service, University of Miami Jackson Memorial Medical Center, Miami, Florida
Neoplasms of the Vulva

W. JEFFREY PETTY, M.D.

Assistant Chief Resident, Internal Medicine, Duke University Medical Center, Durham, North Carolina
Primary Lung Cancer

MARIAN PETRIDES, M.D.

Assistant Professor of Pathology and Medical Director, Transfusion Service, University of Mississippi Medical Center, Jackson, Mississippi
Thrombotic Thrombocytopenic Purpura

MARCO PICCININNO, M.D.

Assistant, Divisione di Cardiologia, Ente Ospedaliero Ospedali Galliera, Genova, Italy
Hypertrophic Cardiomyopathy

GRAHAM PINEO, M.D.

Professor of Medicine, University of Calgary; Director, Thrombosis Research Unit, Foothills Hospital, Calgary, Alberta, Canada
Pulmonary Thromboembolism

MUNIR PIRMOHAMED, PH.D.

Professor of Clinical Pharmacology, The University of Liverpool; Consultant Physician, The Royal Liverpool University Hospital Trust, Liverpool, Merseyside, United Kingdom
Allergic Reactions to Drugs

LESLIE PLOTNICK, M.D.

Professor, Pediatrics, The Johns Hopkins University School of Medicine, Baltimore, Maryland
Diabetes Mellitus in Children and Adolescents

MITCHELL C. POSNER, M.D.

Associate Professor of Surgery and Chief of Surgical Oncology, University of Chicago Hospitals, Chicago, Illinois
Tumors of the Stomach

JERILYNN C. PRIOR, M.D.

Professor, University of British Columbia, Active Staff, Vancouver Hospital and Health Science Centre, Vancouver, British Columbia, Canada
Premenstrual Symptoms and Signs

JAY B. PRYSTOWSKY, M.D.

Associate Professor of Surgery, Northwestern University Medical School; Attending Staff, Northwestern Memorial Hospital, Chicago, Illinois
Cholelithiasis and Cholecystitis

E. REBECCA PSCHIRRER, M.D., M.P.H.

Assistant Professor, Eastern Virginia Medical School, Norfolk, Virginia
Postpartum Care

RUTH ANNE QUEENAN, M.D.

Assistant Professor of Obstetrics and Gynecology and Residency Program Director, Obstetrics and Gynecology, University of Rochester, Rochester, New York
Vaginal Bleeding in the Third Trimester

THOMAS C. QUINN, M.D.

Professor of Medicine, International Health, and Molecular Microbiology and Immunology, The Johns Hopkins University, Baltimore, Maryland
Psittacosis (Ornithosis)

ERROL J. QUINTAL, SR., M.D.

Xavier University of Louisiana; Medical Staff, Pendleton Memorial Methodist Hospital, New Orleans, Louisiana
Keloids

THOMAS J. RAIFE, M.D.

Associate Medical Director, The Blood Center, Milwaukee, Wisconsin
Therapeutic Use of Blood Components

KIRK D. RAMIN, M.D.

Head, Section of Obstetrics and Associate Professor, Mayo Clinic, Rochester, Minnesota
Antepartum Care

RITA DELIA DIAZ RAMOS, M.D.

Colonia Villa de Cortes, Mexico
Typhoid Fever

DAVID W. RATTNER, M.D.

Associate Professor of Surgery, Harvard Medical School; Chief, Division of General and Gastrointestinal Surgery, Massachusetts General Hospital, Boston, Massachusetts
Chronic Pancreatitis

WILLIAM J. RAVICH, M.D.

Associate Professor, Medicine, Associate Professor, Otolaryngology/Head and Neck Surgery, and Clinical Director, The Johns Hopkins Swallowing Center, The Johns Hopkins University School of Medicine; Active Staff, The Johns Hopkins Hospital, Baltimore, Maryland
Dysphagia

THOMAS E. READ, M.D.

Assistant Professor of Surgery, Section of Colon and Rectal Surgery, Washington University School of Medicine; Attending Surgeon, Barnes-Jewish Hospital, St. Louis, Missouri
Hemorrhoids, Anal Fissure, and Anorectal Abscess and Fistula

TONY REALINI, M.D.

Assistant Professor, Department of Ophthalmology, University of Arkansas for Medical Sciences; Director, Glaucoma Service, Jones Eye Institute, Little Rock, Arkansas
Glaucoma

STEVEN REID, M.B.
Clinical Research Fellow, Guy's King's and St. Thomas School of Medicine and Institute of Psychiatry; Consultant Liaison Psychiatrist, St. Mary's Hospital, London, United Kingdom
Chronic Fatigue Syndrome

MICHAEL F. REIN, M.D.
Professor of Medicine, University of Virginia Health System; Medical Director, Sexually Transmitted Disease Clinic, Thomas Jefferson District Health Department, Charlottesville, Virginia
Nongonococcal Urethritis

MARGARET B. RENNELS, M.D.
Professor of Pediatrics, Clinical Chief, Division of Infectious Diseases, Department of Pediatrics, University of Maryland School of Medicine; Attending Physician, University of Maryland Medical System, Baltimore, Maryland
Bordetella Pertussis (Whooping Cough)

JOHN T. REPKE, M.D.
Chris J. and Marie A. Olson Professor of Obstetrics and Gynecology, University of Nebraska College of Medicine; Chairman, Department of Obstetrics and Gynecology, University of Nebraska Medical Center, Omaha, Nebraska
Hypertensive Disorders of Pregnancy

ADRIAN REUBEN, B.Sc., M.B.B.S.
Professor of Medicine, Medical University of South Carolina, Charleston, South Carolina
Acute and Chronic Viral Hepatitis

ELLEN RICCOBENE, M.D.
Associate Program Director of the Internal Medicine Residency Program, St. Joseph's (ER) Regional Medical Center, Paterson, New Jersey
Rocky Mountain Spotted Fever and Ehrlichiosis

BRUCE W. ROBB, M.D.
Resident, Department of General Surgery, University of Cincinnati College of Medicine; Research Fellow, Shriners Hospital for Burned Children, Cincinnati, Ohio
Parenteral Nutrition in Adults

WILLIAM O. ROBERTS, M.D., M.S.
Associate Clinical Professor, Department of Family Practice and Community Health, University of Minnesota Medical School, Minneapolis; MinnHealth Family Physician, White Bear Lake, Minnesota
Disturbances Due to Heat

LORRAINE RODRIQUEZ, M.D.
Instructor of Obstetrics and Gynecology, Mayo Clinic; St. Luke's, Jacksonville, Florida
Constipation

PRASHANT K. ROHATGI, M.B., B.S.
Professor of Medicine, George Washington University School of Medicine and Health Sciences; Chief, Pulmonary Section, Veterans Affairs Medical Center, Washington, D.C.
Acute Respiratory Failure

KAREN L. ROOS, M.D.
John and Nancy Nelson Professor of Neurology, Indiana University School of Medicine, Indianapolis, Indiana
Bacterial Meningitis

CLARK A. ROSEN, M.D.
Assistant Professor, University of Pittsburgh School of Medicine and Director, University of Pittsburgh Voice Center, Pittsburgh, Pennsylvania
Hoarseness and Laryngitis

TED ROSEN, M.D.
Professor of Dermatology, Baylor College of Medicine; Chief of Dermatology, VA Medical Center, Houston, Texas
Granuloma Inguinale (Donovanosis); Lymphogranuloma Venereum

MARK J. ROSENTHAL, M.D.
Staff Physician, Greater Los Angeles VA (Sepulveda Campus), North Hills, California
Pressure Ulcers

DOUGLAS S. ROSS, M.D.
Associate Professor of Medicine, Harvard Medical School; Associate Physician and Co-Director, Thyroid Associate, Massachusetts General Hospital, Boston, Massachusetts
Hyperthyroidism

RICHARD A. RUDICK, M.D.
Director, Mellen Center for Multiple Sclerosis Treatment and Research, Cleveland Clinic Foundation, Cleveland, Ohio
Multiple Sclerosis

VIOLETA RUS, M.D.
Assistant Professor, Department of Medicine, Division of Rheumatology and Clinical Immunology, University of Maryland Medical School, Baltimore, Maryland
Connective Tissue Disorders

RONALD A. SACHER, M.D.
Professor of Internal Medicine and Pathology, Division of Hematology/Oncology, University of Cincinnati College of Medicine; Director, Hoxworth Blood Center, Cincinnati, Ohio
Pernicious Anemia and Other Megaloblastic Anemias

DANA SACHS, M.D.
Instructor in Dermatology, Weill Medical College of Cornell University; Assistant Member, Dermatology Service, Memorial Sloan-Kettering Cancer Center, New York, New York
Skin Cancer Precursor Lesions

DAVID A. SACK, M.D.
Professor, The Department of International Health, Johns Hopkins University, Baltimore, Maryland; Director, Centre for Health and Population Research, Dhaka, Bangladesh
Acute Infectious Diarrhea

ARTHUR I. SAGALOWSKY, M.D.
Professor of Urology, Chief of Urologic Oncology, and Professor of Surgery, University of Texas Southwestern Medical School; Zale-Lipshy University Hospital and Parkland Memorial Hospital, Dallas, Texas
Genitourinary Trauma

STEVEN A. SAHN, M.D.
Professor of Medicine and Director, Division of Pulmonary and Critical Care Medicine, Allergy and Clinical Immunology, Medical University of South Carolina; Medical Director, Specialty Hospital of South Carolina, Charleston, South Carolina
Pleural Effusion and Empyema Thoracis

YORIKO SAITO, M.D.
Clinical Fellow, Harvard Medical School; Hematology-Oncology Fellow, Dana-Farber/Partners Cancer Care, Boston, Massachusetts
Autoimmune Hemolytic Anemia

RAVI N. SAMY, M.D.
Fellow, Otology, Neurotology, Skull Base Surgery, Department of Otolaryngology/Head and Neck Surgery, University of Iowa, Iowa City, Iowa
Meniere's Disease

DAVID S. SAPERSTEIN, M.D.
Clinical Assistant Professor of Medicine (Neurology), Department of Medicine/Division of Neurology, University of Texas Health Science Center at San Antonio; Chief, Neuromuscular Disease Service, Wilford Hall Medical Center, San Antonio, Texas
Myasthenia Gravis

LAWRENCE SCAHILL, M.S.N., PH.D.
Associate Professor, Yale School of Nursing and Yale Child Study Center, Yale University, New Haven, Connecticut
Gilles de la Tourette Syndrome

ANDREW I. SCHAFER, M.D.
The Bob and Vivian Smith Chair in Medicine, Chairman, Department of Medicine, Baylor College of Medicine; Chief, Internal Medicine Service, The Methodist Hospital, Houston, Texas
Polycythemia Vera

RICK SCHIEBINGER, M.D.
Staff Endocrinologist, Susquehanna Health System, Williamsport, Pennsylvania
Primary Aldosteronism

GEORGE SCHMID, M.D., M.SC.
Department of HIV/AIDS, World Health Organization, Geneva, Switzerland
Chancroid

XIAOYE SCHNEIDER-YIN, PH.D.
Senior Biochemist, Central Laboratory, Municipal Hospital Triemli, Zurich, Switzerland
The Porphyrias

JOHN T. SCHULZ III, M.D., PH.D.
Instructor in Surgery, Harvard Medical School; Assistant Surgeon, Massachusetts General Hospital; Medical and Scientific Staff, Shriners Burns Hospital, Boston, Massachusetts
Burn Injury

RICHARD H. SCHWARTZ, M.D.
Clinical Professor of Pediatrics, George Washington University School of Medicine, Washington, D.C.; Clinical Professor of Pediatrics, University of Virginia School of Medicine, Charlottesville, Virginia; Director of Pediatric Research, Department of Pediatrics, Inova Fairfax Hospital for Children, Falls Church, Virginia
Otitis Media

EILEEN M. SEGRETI, M.D.
Associate Professor, Department of Obstetrics and Gynecology, Virginia Commonwealth University; Medical College of Virginia Hospitals, Richmond, Virginia
Cervical Cancer

SANJIV S. SHAH, M.D.
Assistant Professor of Medicine, Albert Einstein College of Medicine, Beth Israel Medical Center, Bronx, New York
Rat-Bite Fever

SUDHIR V. SHAH, M.D.
Professor of Medicine and Director, Division of Nephrology, University of Arkansas for Medical Sciences; Chief, Renal Medicine Section, Central Arkansas Veterans Healthcare System Hospital, Little Rock, Arkansas
Acute Renal Failure

WIN-KUANG SHEN, M.D.
Professor of Medicine, Mayo Medical School, Mayo Foundation; Professor of Medicine, Staff Consultant in the Division of Cardiovascular Diseases and Internal Medicine, Mayo Clinic, Rochester, Minnesota
Atrial Fibrillation

PHILIP D. SHENEFELT, M.D.
Associate Professor, Division of Dermatology, University of South Florida, Tampa, Florida
Parasitic Diseases of the Skin

MARK E. SHIRTLIFF, PH.D.
Postdoctoral Fellow, Montana State University, Bozeman, Montana
Osteomyelitis

THOMAS C. SHOPE, M.D.
Associate Professor, Department of Pediatrics and Communicable Diseases, University of Michigan; Attending Physician, University of Michigan Health Systems, Ann Arbor, Michigan
Mumps

ABUL K. SIDDIQUE, M.B.B.S., M.P.H.
Senior Scientist, Public Health Sciences Division, International Centre for Diarrhoeal Disease Research, Mohakhali, Dhaka, Bangladesh
Cholera

HELAYNE SILVER, M.D.
Associate Professor, Maternal Fetal Medicine, Brown University; Associate Professor, Maternal Fetal Medicine, Women and Infants Hospital of Rhode Island, Providence, Rhode Island
Hypertensive Disorders of Pregnancy

NALINI SINGH, M.D.
Assistant Clinical Professor of Medicine, UCLA School of Medicine; Physician, Divisions of Ambulatory Care and Endocrinology and Metabolism, Veterans Affairs Greater Los Angeles Healthcare System, Los Angeles, California
Hypothyroidism

STEVEN J. SKOOG, M.D.
Professor of Surgery and Pediatrics, Oregon Health Sciences University, Director, Pediatric Urology, Doernbechers Childrens Hospital, Portland, Oregon
Childhood Enuresis

SHAWN L. SLACK, M.D.
Clinical Assistant Professor of Medicine, Division of Rheumatology, University of Washington, Seattle; Attending Physician, The Everett Clinic, Everett, Washington
Polymyalgia Rheumatica and Giant Cell Arteritis

RAYMOND G. SLAVIN, M.D.
Professor of Internal Medicine, Director, Division of Allergy and Immunology, St. Louis University School of Medicine; Attending Staff, St. Louis University Hospital and John Cochran VA Hospital, St. Louis, Missouri
Hypersensitivity Pneumonitis

DUANE T. SMOOT, M.D.
Associate Professor and Chief, Gastroenterology Division, Department of Medicine, Howard University; Chief, Gastroenterology Division, Department of Medicine, Howard University Hospital, Washington, D.C.
Gastritis and Peptic Ulcer Disease

L. MICHAEL SNYDER, M.D.
Professor in Medicine and Pathology, U Mass Medical School; Chairman, Department of Hospital Laboratories, U Mass/Memorial Health Care, Worcester, Massachusetts
Nonimmune Hemolytic Anemias

JEREMY SOBEL, M.D., M.P.H.
Centers for Disease Control and Prevention, Centers for Disease Control and Prevention, Atlanta, Georgia
Salmonellosis

IRENA SPEKTOR, M.D.
Resident, Department of Dermatology, Emory University, Atlanta, Georgia
Cutaneous Vasculitis

PAOLO SPIRITO, M.D.
Director, Divisione di Cardiologia, Ente Ojpedaziero Ospedali Galliera, Genoa, Italy
Hypertrophic Cardiomyopathy

KEY H. STAGE, M.D.
Associate Professor, University of Texas Southwestern Medical Center at Dallas; Chief of Urology, Parkland Health and Hospital System, Dallas, Texas
Genitourinary Trauma

C. MICHAEL STEIN, M.B., CH.B.
Associate Professor of Medicine and Pharmacology, Vanderbilt University School of Medicine, Nashville, Tennessee
Osteoarthritis

DANIEL T. STEIN, M.D.
Assistant Professor of Medicine, Division of Endocrinology, Diabetes and Metabolism, Albert Einstein College of Medicine, New York, New York
Diabetic Ketoacidosis

MARK S. STEIN, M.B., B.S., PH.D.
Consultant Endocrinologist, Department of Diabetes and Endocrinology, The Royal Melbourne Hospital, Parkville, Victoria, Australia
Hyperparathyroidism and Hypoparathyroidism

LAURENCE D. STERNS, M.D.
Director, Implantable Cardioverter Defibrillator Clinic and Cardiologist/Electrophysiologist, Capital Health Region, Victoria, British Columbia, Canada
Premature Beats

A. KEITH STEWART, M.B., CH.B.
Associate Professor, Department of Medicine, University of Toronto; Director, Toronto General Research Institute and Scott-Whitmore Chair in Hematology and Gene Therapy, Princess Margaret Hospital, Toronto, Ontario, Canada
Multiple Myeloma

CARLOS SUBAUSTE, M.D.
Assistant Professor, Division of Infectious Diseases, Department of Internal Medicine, University of Cincinnati College of Medicine, Cincinnati, Ohio
Toxoplasmosis

JEFFREY R. SUCHARD, M.D.
Assistant Clinical Professor, Division of Emergency Medicine, Department of Medicine, University of California Irvine Medical Center, Orange, California
Spider Bites and Scorpion Stings

SHYAM SUNDAR, M.D.
Professor of Medicine, Institute of Medical Sciences, Banaras Hindu University, Varanasi, India
Leishmaniasis

DAVID L. SWERDLOW, M.D.
Centers for Disease Control and Prevention, Atlanta, Georgia
Salmonellosis

ROBERT A. SWERLICK, M.D.
Associate Professor, Department of Dermatology, Emory University School of Medicine, Atlanta, Georgia
Cutaneous Vasculitis

CYRUS P. TAMBOI, M.D.
Fellow, Gastroenterology, University of Alberta, Edmonton, Alberta, Canada
Malabsorption

NIZAR M. TANNIR, M.D.
Assistant Professor, University of Texas; Assistant Professor, MD Anderson Cancer Center, Houston, Texas
Chronic Leukemias

GUY TAYLOR, M.B., CH.B.
Department of Medicine, Wanganui Hospital, Wanganui, New Zealand
Osteoarthritis

GIRMA TEFERA, M.D.
Assistant Professor, Vascular Surgery, University of Wisconsin; Section of Vascular Surgery, University of Wisconsin Hospital and Clinics, Madison, Wisconsin
Acquired Diseases of the Aorta

MICHAEL E. THASE, M.D.
University of Pittsburgh School of Medicine, Professor of Psychiatry, Western Psychiatric Institute and Clinic, Pittsburgh, Pennsylvania
Mood Disorders

NANCY E. THOMAS, M.D., PH.D.
Associate Professor of Dermatology, University of North Carolina at Chapel Hill; Attending, University of North Carolina Hospitals, Chapel Hill, North Carolina
Pruritus

ALAN G. THORSON, M.D.
Associate Professor of Surgery and Program Director, Section of Colon and Rectal Surgery, Creighton University School of Medicine; Clinical Associate Professor of Surgery, University of Nebraska College of Medicine, Omaha, Nebraska
Tumors of the Colon and Rectum

RICHARD W. TITBALL, B.SC., PH.D.
Defence Evaluation and Research Agency, Salisbury, Wiltshire, United Kingdom
Plague

MARCIA G. TONNESEN, M.D.
Associate Professor of Medicine and Dermatology, School of Medicine, State University of New York at Stony Brook, Stony Brook; Chief, Dermatology, VAMC Northport, Northport, New York
Erythema Multiforme, Stevens-Johnson Syndrome, and Toxic Epidermal Necrolysis

DAVID E. TRACHTENBARG, M.D.
Clinical Professor Family Practice, University of Illinois College of Medicine, Peoria, Illinois
Headache

SCOTT TROXEL, M.D.
Clinical Instructor of Urology, University of California Davis Medical Center; Clinical Instructor, University of California Davis Department of Urology, Sacramento, California
Urolithiasis

ROBIN J. TRUPP, M.S.N., R.N.
Program Manager, Heart Failure Management Program, Division of Cardiovascular Medicine and The Linda and Jack Gill Heart Institute, University of Kentucky; University of Kentucky Chandler Medical Center, Lexington, Kentucky
Congestive Heart Failure

ALEX TSELIS, M.D., PH.D.
Associate Professor, Department of Neurology, Wayne State University School of Medicine; Vice Chief, Neurology, Detroit Receiving Hospital; Staff Neurologist, Harper University Hospital, Detroit, Michigan
Viral Meningitis and Encephalitis

ERNEST A. TURNER, M.D.
Department of Pediatrics, Cook County Children's Hospital, Chicago, Illinois
Sickle Cell Disease and Hemoglobinopathies

ALEX B. VALADKA, M.D.
Associate Professor of Neurosurgery, Baylor College of Medicine; Chief of Neurosurgery, Ben Taub General Hospital, Houston, Texas
Acute Head Injuries in Adults

CARLOS A. VAZ FRAGOSO, M.D.
Medical Director, Gaylord Sleep Services, Gaylord Hospital, Wallingford, Connecticut
Sleep Disordered Breathing

CHARLES S. VIA, M.D.
Professor of Medicine, Rheumatology Division, Department of Medicine, University of Maryland; Baltimore VAMC, Baltimore, Maryland
Connective Tissue Disorders

ADRIANNA VLACHOS, M.D.
Assistant Professor of Pediatrics, Albert Einstein College of Medicine, New York; Associate Head, Stem Cell Transplant Program, Schneider Children's Hospital, New Hyde Park, New York
Aplastic Anemia

NICOLE WAKIM, B.A.
Loyola Stritch School of Medicine, Chicago, Illinois
Tetanus

MCCLELLAN M. WALTHER, M.D.
Staff Physician, National Institutes of Health, Bethesda, Maryland
Pheochromocytoma

BETH A. WAMBACH, M.D.
Otolaryngologist, Private Practice, Holy Cross Hospital, Ft. Lauderdale, Florida
Otitis Externa

JOHN D. WARK, M.B., B.S., PH.D.
Professor of Medicine, Department of Medicine, University of Melbourne; Head, Bone and Mineral Service, Royal Melbourne Hospital, Melbourne, Victoria, Australia
Hyperparathyroidism and Hypoparathyroidism

GREGG WARSHAW, M.D.
Martha Betty Semmons Professor of Geriatric Medicine, Professor of Family Medicine, University of Cincinnati Medical Center, Cincinnati; Medical Director, Maple Knoll Village, Springdale, Ohio
Alzheimer's Disease

GUY WEBSTER, M.D., PH.D.
Professor, Department of Dermatology, Jefferson Medical College, Philadelphia, Pennsylvania
Acne Vulgaris and Rosacea

H. JAMES WEDNER, M.D.
Professor of Medicine, Acting Chief, Division of Allergy/Immunology, Chief, Clinical Allergy/Immunology, Medical Director, The Asthma Center, Washington University School of Medicine; Firm Attending, Barnes-Jewish Hospital, St. Louis, Missouri
Anaphylaxis and Serum Sickness

JEFFREY M. WEINBERG, M.D.
Assistant Clinical Professor of Dermatology, Columbia College of Physicians and Surgeons; Director, Clinical Research Center, St. Luke's-Roosevelt Hospital Center, New York, New York
Fungal Diseases of the Skin

NEIL J. WEISSMAN, M.D.
Associate Professor of Medicine, Georgetown Medical School; Director, Cardiac Ultrasound, Cardiovascular Research Institute, Washington Hospital Center, Washington, D.C.
Mitral Valve Prolapse

MARY JO WELKER, M.D.
Chairperson, Department of Family Medicine, The Ohio State University; The Ohio State University Hospital, Columbus, Ohio
Fever

SIMON WESSELY, M.D.
Professor of Liaison and Epidemiological Psychiatry, Guy's King's and St. Thomas' School of Medicine and Institute of Psychiatry; Honorary Consultant Psychiatrist, Maudsley Hospital, London, United Kingdom
Chronic Fatigue Syndrome

JOSEPH G. WHELAN III, M.D.
Clinical Instructor, Obstetrics and Gynecology, The Johns Hopkins University School of Medicine, Baltimore, Maryland
Uterine Leiomyoma

CHRISTOPHER B. WHITE, M.D.
Professor of Pediatrics, Director, Pediatric Student Education, Medical College of Georgia, Augusta, Georgia
Streptococcal Pharyngitis

MATTHEW P. WICKLUND, M.D.
Wilford Hall Medical Center, San Antonio, Texas
Peripheral Neuropathy

MICHAEL G. WILKERSON, M.D.
Clinical Assistant Professor of Dermatology, University of Oklahoma College of Medicine; Active Staff, Hillcrest Medical Center, Tulsa, Oklahoma
Bacterial Diseases of the Skin

AIMEE WILKIN, M.D., M.P.H.
Instructor of Medicine, The Johns Hopkins School of Medicine, Baltimore, Maryland
Management of the HIV-Infected Patient

TIM WILKIN, M.D.
Post-Doctoral Clinical Fellow, Columbia University, Clinical Fellow, Columbia-Presbyterian Medical Center, New York, New York
Management of the HIV-Infected Patient

PHILLIP M. WILLIFORD, M.D.
Associate Professor of Dermatology, Director of Dermatologic Surgery, Wake Forest University; Staff, North Carolina Baptist Hospital, Winston-Salem, North Carolina
Melanoma

WILLIAM A. WILMER, M.D.
Associate Professor of Medicine, The Ohio State University College of Medicine; Associate Professor of Medicine, The Ohio State University Hospitals, Columbus, Ohio
Primary Glomerular Diseases

HUGH H. WINDOM, M.D.
Associate Clinical Professor of Medicine, University of South Florida, Tampa; Private Practice, Sarasota, Florida
Allergic Rhinitis Caused by Inhalant Factors

WING-YEN WONG, M.D.
Assistant Professor, Pediatrics and Medicine, USC Keck School of Medicine, Los Angeles, California
Hemophilia and Related Disorders

DAVID P. WOOD, M.D.
Professor and Associate Chairman, Department of Urology, Wayne State University, Detroit, Michigan
Malignant Tumors of the Urogenital Tract

LAWRENCE R. WU, M.D.
Assistant Clinical Professor, Duke University School of Medicine; Physician, Duke Hospital, Durham Regional Hospital, Durham, North Carolina
Anxiety Disorders in Primary Care

ELAINE WYLLIE, M.D.
Section Head, Section of Pediatric Epilepsy, The Cleveland Clinic Foundation, Cleveland, Ohio
Epilepsy in Infants and Children

MARTHA M. WYNN, M.D.
Associate Professor, University of Wisconsin; Associate Professor of Anesthesiology, University Hospital and Clinics, Madison, Wisconsin
Acquired Diseases of the Aorta

KIM B. YANCEY, M.D.
Professor and Chairman, Department of Dermatology, Medical College of Wisconsin, Milwaukee, Wisconsin
Skin Diseases of Pregnancy

MICHAEL K. YANCEY, M.D.
Assistant Professor, Uniformed Services University of Health Sciences, Bethesda, Maryland; Director, Perinatal Services and Assistant Chief, Department of Obstetrics and Gynecology, Tripler Army Medical Center, TAMC, Hawaii
Hemolytic Disease of the Fetus and Newborn

WILLIAM F. YOUNG, JR., M.D.
Professor of Medicine, Mayo Medical School; Consultant, Mayo Clinic, Rochester, Minnesota
Cushing's Syndrome

HOWARD A. ZACUR, M.D., PH.D.
Professor, Obstetrics and Gynecology and Division Director, Reproductive Endocrinology and Infertility, The Johns Hopkins University School of Medicine, Baltimore, Maryland
Uterine Leiomyoma

MARTIN ZAIAC, M.D.
Associate Professor, University of Miami, Miami; Program Director, Department of Dermatology, Mt. Sinai, Miami Beach, Florida
Diseases of the Nails

JENNIFER C. ZAMPOGNA, M.D.
Dermatology Resident, University of Florida College of Medicine, Gainesville, Florida
Viral Diseases of the Skin

EDWIN J. ZARLING, M.D.
Associate Professor of Medicine, Loyola University Medical Center, Maywood, Illinois
Diverticula of the Gastrointestinal Tract

HENNING ZEIDLER, M.D.
Director, Department of Rheumatology, Hannover Medical School, Hannover, Germany
Ankylosing Spondylitis and Other Spondylarthritides

JOHN A. ZIC, M.D.
Assistant Professor of Medicine, Dermatology and Director, Vanderbilt University Cutaneous Lymphoma Clinic, Vanderbilt University School of Medicine, Nashville, Tennessee
Papulosquamous Diseases

RICHARD KENT ZIMMERMAN, M.D., M.P.H.
Associate Professor, Family Medicine and Clinical Epidemiology and Health Services Administration, University of Pittsburgh; Staff Physician, East Liberty Family Health Care Center, Pittsburgh, Pennsylvania
Immunization Practices

Preface

This is the 54th annual edition of *Conn's Current Therapy.* Our goal remains the same as when Howard Conn published the first edition in 1949, that is, to provide the busy physician and other health care professionals with a concise, up-to-date, and easy-to-use reference to recent advances in therapy. The focus is on problems frequently encountered in practice and on those less common problems that can be serious if not diagnosed and managed appropriately.

Each year, new authorities provide an entirely new treatment perspective on a myriad of conditions. This ensures that the information in each new edition is fresh and current. The reader is encouraged to compare the favorite method of one authority with that of another in previous editions.

Although our goal is to obtain 100% new material each year, the tight deadlines required for an annual publication are almost impossible to meet. This year we came close, however, with 97.6% of the topics written by new authorities and the remaining 2.4% thoroughly updated.

A new topic added this year is Nonallergic Rhinitis, a common problem in primary care for which specific therapy is available. Important recent changes have also occurred in immunization practices and the management of HIV disease, atrial fibrillation, osteoporosis, and acute leukemia to mention only a few.

Although most of the problems discussed in this book focus on diseases encountered in the United States, a significant number are diseases that may affect U.S. citizens traveling to other countries and immigrants to this country. For this reason, authorities on diseases most common in other countries are invited to present their method of treatment. This year, 38 authors from outside the United States discuss the management of diseases and trauma in articles on Malaria (Kenya), Typhoid Fever (Mexico), Amebiasis (India), Plague (United Kingdom), Cholera (Bangladesh), and Hazardous Marine Animals (Australia). Of the 292 topics in this edition, 38 are written by experts from other countries.

Every manuscript undergoes thorough editorial review by a pharmacist, physician, and multiple editors to ensure accuracy of the material. The treatments recommended are, in the experience of the author, those found to work best. When a recommended drug has not been approved by the FDA for that use, this is indicated by a footnote. This may be because, although the drug has been found to be effective, it has not yet been approved for that use, or perhaps because approval was never requested. It is estimated that half of all prescriptions written are "off-label," meaning they have not received official approval to treat that condition. A recent study of antipsychotics found that 66% were prescribed for off-label indications.[1]

The index has been painstakingly prepared to ensure completeness and to facilitate the rapid recovery of information. Many tables are used to give a maximum amount of information in the most concise manner. Our objective is to make this book an easy-to-use resource of up-to-date information.

REFERENCE

1. Weiss E, Hummer M, Koller D, et al: Off-label use of antipsychotic drugs. J Clin Psychopharmacol 20:695–698, 2000.

Robert E. Rakel, M.D.
Edward T. Bope, M.D.

Contents

SECTION 1. SYMPTOMATIC CARE PENDING DIAGNOSIS

SECTION 2. THE INFECTIOUS DISEASES

SECTION 3. THE RESPIRATORY SYSTEM

SECTION 4. THE CARDIOVASCULAR SYSTEM

SECTION 5. THE BLOOD AND SPLEEN

SECTION 6. THE DIGESTIVE SYSTEM

SECTION 7. METABOLIC DISORDERS

SECTION 8. THE ENDOCRINE SYSTEM

SECTION 9. THE UROGENITAL TRACT

SECTION 10. THE SEXUALLY TRANSMITTED DISEASES

SECTION 11. DISEASES OF ALLERGY

SECTION 12. DISEASES OF THE SKIN

SECTION 13. THE NERVOUS SYSTEM

SECTION 14. THE LOCOMOTOR SYSTEM

SECTION 15. OBSTETRICS AND GYNECOLOGY

SECTION 16. PSYCHIATRIC DISORDERS

SECTION 17. PHYSICAL AND CHEMICAL INJURIES

SECTION 18. APPENDICES AND INDEX

Section 1

Symptomatic Care Pending Diagnosis

PAIN

method of
ROBIN L. FAINSINGER, M.D.
University of Alberta
Edmonton, Alberta, Canada

Pain is a common presenting complaint in a variety of different clinical situations and can be divided into the following categories:

1. Acute pain—common examples would be postoperative pain and pain from an acute injury.
2. Chronic nonmalignant pain—there are countless examples of chronic medical conditions that cause long-standing pain problems, including arthritis, inflammatory bowel disease, headache, and backache.
3. Cancer pain—primary and metastatic disease can cause many pain syndromes.

Although there are specific issues that are unique to these different categories, the overall approach to assessment and management does have significant overlap. A good foundation to a practical understanding of pain management in all its complex presentations is built on a sound fundamental approach to assessment and pharmacologic and nonpharmacologic management.

ASSESSMENT

It can be argued with some justification that, irrespective of a clinician's comprehensive understanding of pharmacologic and nonpharmacologic pain management, this knowledge would be of little value if the assessment is inaccurate in understanding the physiologic and nonphysiologic mechanisms causing the patient to present with a pain syndrome. Failure to adequately assess pain will inevitably lead to inappropriate application of pain management strategies.

In the initial assessment it is essential to include a detailed history, a complete physical examination, a relevant psychosocial assessment, and a subsequent diagnostic workup determined by the circumstances revealed by the initial evaluation. In formulating an approach to management it is helpful to answer the following three questions:

1. What is causing the pain?
2. How bad is the pain?
3. What may complicate pain management (poor prognostic factors)?

What Is Causing the Pain?

In any clinical setting it is necessary to clarify whether the pain is the following:

1. From a major presenting illness (e.g., cancer, arthritis, surgical incision)
2. Indirectly related, such as increasing abdominal pain due to opioid-induced constipation
3. A side effect of treatment, such as chemotherapy-induced neuropathy
4. Unrelated, such as ischemic heart disease or migraine headaches in a patient with known metastatic cancer

Without a disciplined evaluation of all four possibilities, it is very easy to make a mistake early on in the assessment. Although a presenting pain syndrome is likely to be caused by a major known illness such as metastatic cancer, failure to consider the alternative options can easily result in inappropriate management, such as increasing opioid doses for abdominal pain from constipation or assuming the abdominal pain is from a recent surgical incision when a thorough examination might have revealed findings consistent with an acute intra-abdominal complication.

It is also important to characterize the pain as nociceptive or neuropathic. *Nociceptive pain* is a pain syndrome caused by the activation of normal nerve endings. It can be somatic or visceral. Somatic pain is commonly caused by muscle, soft tissue, or bone injury. It is usually well localized, constant or intermittent, and described as gnawing or aching. A common example of visceral pain would be intra-abdominal disease. This is typically poorly localized and can be described by a variety of terms, such as *aching, squeezing,* and *cramping. Neuropathic pain* is caused by injury to the nerve tissue and can be due to peripheral nerve injury, damage to the autonomic nervous system, damage to the central nervous system, or a combination of these three different mechanisms. In peripheral nerve injury there may be a dermatomal distribution. The pain can be described as burning, lancinating, sharp, or shooting radiating pain.

Classification of the many possible pain syndromes has resulted in a task force on taxonomy of the International Association for the Study of Pain. However, from a pharmacologic perspective, the main issue in differentiating neuropathic from nociceptive pain is in determining appropriate management for individual clinical settings. A major controversy has been with regard to the opioid responsiveness of neuropathic pain syndromes. Arguably, there is now sufficient clinical and research experience to conclude that most neuropathic pain syndromes are opioid responsive but may require higher doses than typically reported for nociceptive pain syndromes.

How Bad Is the Pain?

It is often stated that a major barrier to pain management is failure to ask patients whether they are experiencing pain and failure to obtain some measure of pain severity. It is typically recommended that a useful clinical approach is to use either a visual analogue scale or a numerical scale (Figure 1). There are many pain assessment tools described in the literature, but in most clinical settings this simple approach is sufficient. In asking a patient to assess the severity of pain using either a numerical or visual analogue scale, the question can be phrased as to pain at this moment, worst pain in the last 24 hours, best pain control in the last 24 hours, or average pain control over the last 24 hours. It has been suggested that for repeat measurements the best approach is to ask patients to rate their pain at that moment of assessment.

However, it is important to remember that this simple approach is in the end a unidimensional, not a multidimensional, assessment. Some patients are adept at providing an accurate physiologic description of their pain severity, but this is certainly not the case for everyone. This can be demonstrated by the example of a 65-year-old man who states that his pain is 8 on a scale of 1 to 10. What he means is: "My leg hurts like hell where the bone metastases are—give me better pain management." However, another 65-year-old man stating his pain is 8 out of 10 might mean: "My leg hurts a bit, but I feel terrible about my situation. I cannot cope with anything. Are you smart enough to hear my message?"

The complexity of the pain experience was poignantly described by Tolstoy in *The Death of Ivan Ilych* in the following sentence: "It was true, as the doctor said, that Ivan Ilych's physical sufferings were terrible, but worse than the physical sufferings were his mental sufferings, which were his chief torture." It is vital to understand the potential complexity of a patient's pain complaint. It has often been stated that pain is inadequately managed because we do not put sufficient trust in the patient's complaint, as well as the reluctance of physicians to prescribe adequate amounts of effective opioids. However, whereas we should certainly believe that "pain is what the patient says it is," this does not provide a uniform guarantee that every patient's complaint of pain contains only a physiologic mechanism that will always respond if we provide sufficient pharmacologic management.

What May Complicate Pain Management?

Clinicians are often under pressure when managing pain problems to increase the number and strength of pharmacologic options to improve the pain control. However, owing to the complexity of underlying issues, this will not always bring success. In an era in which patients and their families often read in the media that adequate pharmacologic management should provide relief in most settings, it is useful to be aware of the poor prognostic factors that may help to lower expectations of success from pharmacologic management alone and to suggest alternative approaches.

Consider the following scenarios:

A 65-year-old man with prostate cancer and bone metastases presents with pain localized to the right arm and hip. He is able to move comfortably and is oriented and alert. He is responding well to acetaminophen, 325 mg four times a day. He has a stable marriage and home life and no psychiatric history or history of addictive behavior.

A 65-year-old man with prostate cancer and bone metastases complains of a burning, stabbing pain down his right leg. He is reasonably comfortable at rest but cannot move without the pain increasing to the point that movement is severely limited. He shows some evidence of cognitive impairment. His morphine dose has increased from 5 mg every 4 hours to 100 mg every 4 hours over 7 days. He has been divorced three times, lives alone, and has a history of depression and suicide attempts. He has a long history of abuse of alcohol and benzodiazepines.

In the first setting the patient has a nociceptive pain syndrome that is well controlled on low analgesic doses. He also has a history that suggests he has coped well with the stress of life and work to this point. However, in the second scenario the patient has a neuropathic pain, a severe incidental component, difficulty providing an accurate pain history, rapidly escalating opioid doses, and a history suggesting that he does not have the ability to cope well with stress and setbacks.

It has previously been mentioned that neuropathic pain syndromes may require higher opioid doses. It is important to distinguish those patients who have severe incidental pain that significantly impairs function, especially when the background rest pain is adequately managed. Given that the assessment of pain relies heavily on an accurate history, management in a confused patient unable to provide an accurate description of past or present discomfort causes significant problems. In addition, these patients may be at risk from further cognitive deterioration with increasing pharmacologic management. Finally, those patients with a significant history of psychosocial dysfunction may sometimes be at risk of including their suffering in a unidimensional presentation of their pain syndrome. The consequences of attempting to manage this problem with pharmacologic means alone is doomed to failure.

In considering the multidimensional aspects of pain assessment, it is useful to consider the following three steps:

1. Production
2. Perception
3. Expression

The production of pain occurs at the site of injury and cannot be measured directly. The perception of pain occurs at the level of the central nervous system/brain. In clinical settings this cannot be measured. The expression of pain

Visual Analogue Scale (0–10 cm)

No pain ______________________________ Severe pain

Numerical Scale

No pain 0 1 2 3 4 5 6 7 8 9 10 Severe pain

Figure 1. Pain intensity scales.

is the main target of assessment and management. Individual patients with similar injury may still have similar levels of perception but may express different pain intensity levels. Appropriate pain assessment requires consideration of the multiple dimensions of individual expression of pain. Fortunately, in most cases, expression will provide information resulting in good pain control with sound application of pharmacologic principles and options.

PHARMACOLOGIC MANAGEMENT

There have been many advances in both basic and clinical research that have expanded the options for pain management. In some settings, pharmacologic management alone is sufficient; however, there are many pain syndromes in which a variety of approaches using an interdisciplinary team are required. Pharmacologic management has been broken down into three broad categories of pain medications:

1. Nonopioid analgesics such as acetaminophen (Tylenol) and nonsteroidal anti-inflammatory drugs (NSAIDs)
2. Adjuvant analgesics that often have primary indications other than pain
3. A wide variety of opioid analgesics

Nonsteroidal Anti-Inflammatory Drugs

These drugs have analgesic and anti-inflammatory effects caused by inhibiting both peripheral and central cyclooxygenase (COX). Until recently, all of the available NSAIDs inhibited both COX-1 and COX-2. COX-1 produces compounds necessary for normal physiologic function of the stomach, kidneys, and platelets, whereas COX-2 is mainly associated with prostaglandin-mediated inflammation. The long-term benefits of traditional NSAIDs such as ibuprofen (Motrin, Advil) and naproxen (Naprosyn) have been limited by adverse effects such as gastrointestinal hemorrhage and renal impairment. With the arrival of selective COX-2 inhibitors it has been suggested that they may offer analgesia with a decreased incidence of gastrointestinal and renal side effects. While offering clinical potential, the cost benefit of these relatively more expensive drugs, such as celecoxib (Celebrex) and rofecoxib (Vioxx), compared with the relatively inexpensive nonselective NSAIDs is unclear.

NSAIDs are usually indicated for bone and soft tissue pain. Although the maximum dose for analgesic and anti-inflammatory effects for individual NSAIDs has been demonstrated, guidelines regarding selection and dosing remain somewhat empirical. It is important to recognize the problems associated with these drugs in patients at high risk, such as the elderly; those on corticosteroids or anticoagulants; and patients with a previous side effect related to NSAID use. In those patients at increased risk for gastrointestinal side effects in whom an NSAID is deemed necessary, consideration should be given to using gastroprotective treatment such as misoprostol (Cytotec), omeprazole (Prilosec), and H_2 antagonists.

Adjuvant Analgesics

There is a wide variety and sometimes confusing array of pharmacologic options in this category. Typically, they have a primary indication other than for pain but are potentially analgesic for any kind of pain or analgesic in some specific pain syndromes. In individual clinical situations the optimal timing to initiate pain management with an adjuvant analgesic alone or when to add an adjuvant analgesic to an existing pain management regimen is not always clear. However, it is always prudent to minimize polypharmacy to reduce the possibility of side effects. Adjuvant analgesics are often advocated for their opioid-sparing effect. However, if a patient is already on an opioid, optimal titration may achieve adequate pain management without polypharmacy. In other words, if a patient is on morphine, 10 mg every 4 hours, with reasonable pain control, decreasing the opioid dose slightly by using an adjuvant analgesic may provide little clinical benefit other than increasing the risk of side effects by introducing another medication. The variability in response to adjuvant analgesics requires careful individual assessment and occasional sequential therapeutic trials. It is important to remember to discontinue previously instituted medications when no clear benefit to the patient is demonstrated.

The commonly used adjuvant analgesics include corticosteroids, antidepressants, anticonvulsants, oral local anesthetics, muscle relaxants, and bisphosphonates.

*Corticosteroids**

Corticosteroids are commonly indicated for bone, visceral, and neuropathic pain. They have a wide range of effects, including mood elevation, anti-inflammatory activity, antiemetic activity, and temporary appetite stimulation. They may also reduce cerebral and spinal cord edema for the management of intracranial pressure and spinal cord compression. Side effects include oral thrush, increasing hyperglycemia, increased risk of infections, and neuropsychiatric toxicity. The choice of pharmacologic options and dose range is empirical. Short-term use and tapering to the lowest effective clinical dose are generally recommended.

*Tricyclic Antidepressants**

Tricyclic antidepressants are typically used for neuropathic pain. Their analgesic benefit is generally seen at lower doses than when used for the treatment of depression. It is important to clearly inform patients that you are using these agents for their analgesic benefits to avoid misinterpretation by patients and families. The most widely reported experience has been with amitriptyline (Elavil).* The adjuvant analgesic benefits of other antidepressants, in particular the new serotonin selective reuptake inhibitors,* require further research.

*Not FDA approved for this indication.

*Anticonvulsants**

Anticonvulsants have been used for pain management for many years, and there is a wide range of options. Gabapentin (Neurontin)* is a recent introduction that has become increasingly popular. Others include carbamazepine (Tegretol),* phenytoin (Dilantin),* clonazepam (Klonopin),* and lamotrigine (Lamictal).* They are typically used for the treatment of neuropathic pain, and it is recommended that sequential trials for refractory neuropathic pain may be useful.

Oral Local Anesthetics

Local anesthetics can be used orally for neuropathic pain. Side effects are common and include nausea and central nervous system side effects such as ataxia, tremors, or confusion. Patients with a history of heart disease may be at risk for increasing side effects. Mexiletine (Mexitil)* is the most commonly used option, but the use of flecainide (Tambocor)* has also been proposed.

Muscle Relaxant Drugs

These drugs have typically been studied and used in acute pain for musculoskeletal injuries. Their side effects include sedation and anticholinergic problems, but in the acute setting this is probably better tolerated than for chronic pain management. The most popular options include orphenadrine (Norflex), methocarbamol (Robaxin), and cyclobenzaprine (Flexeril).

*Bisphosphonates**

In addition to the usual role for this class of agents in the management of hypercalcemia, they are also indicated for the management of bone pain due to metastatic disease. The commonly used options include clodronate (Bonefos)† and pamidronate (Aredia).* They are generally given in the same doses as used for hypercalcemia and require intravenous administration.

Opioids

The use of opioid analgesics as a major component of the approach to acute and chronic cancer pain has been in general acceptance for decades. However, the role of opioids in chronic nonmalignant pain has been controversial. In recent years there has been an increasing acceptance of the potential benefit to the use of opioids in carefully individualized chronic nonmalignant pain syndromes.

A general approach to opioid management includes an understanding of the three-step World Health Organization ladder approach to pain management. Step One, for mild pain, is to use a mild analgesic such as acetaminophen (Tylenol), with or without the use of other adjuvant analgesics. Step Two, for moderate pain, requires the use of codeine, with or without the use of adjuvant analgesics. Step Three is the use of morphine for severe pain, again with or without the use of adjuvant analgesics. It is helpful to be familiar with a few alternatives.

Guidelines for opioid prescribing include the following:

1. Follow the World Health Organization stepladder approach appropriately. In other words, if a patient has severe pain it is not necessary to start with a weak analgesic.
2. Be aware that opioids are not equivalent and require dose conversion, as does a switch of route from oral to parenteral. It is useful to refer to an opioid equianalgesic table (Table 1). It is important to be aware that opioid conversion tables do not allow for the wide individual differences that exist in clinical practice. Close observation is always required when starting a patient on an opioid for the first time. When switching from one opioid to another, some pain specialists recommend using a conversion table and then decreasing the new opioid by a further 25% to 50%. The commonly used and recommended opioids are codeine, oxycodone, morphine, hydromorphone (Dilaudid), and fentanyl (Duragesic). Methadone (Dolophine) is being increasingly used in the management of both chronic nonmalignant and cancer pain syndromes. In some countries, methadone is being used as a second-line choice after morphine, owing to both availability and cost issues. Methadone has also been reported as extremely useful in difficult pain situations in which patients appear to have increasing analgesic tolerance to high opioid doses or dose-limiting side effects. Caution is advised because methadone appears to be extremely potent in the latter circumstances, with clinicians using dose conversion ratios of 10 to 20 times the potency of morphine (e.g., 1 mg of methadone for every 10–20 mg of morphine equivalent dose). Inexperienced clinicians should seek expert advice before prescribing methadone.

   Other opioids such as meperidine (Demerol) are generally not recommended for chronic use, owing to accumulation of metabolites that cause the potential for increasing side effects. In addition, partial agonists or mixed agonist-antagonist opioids are also not recommended because they have a "ceiling" effect, unlike the usually recommended full opioid agonists.
3. Prescribe and titrate appropriately. This requires regular opioid administration for continuous

TABLE 1. **Approximate Opioid Equianalgesic Dose**

Drug	Oral	SC/IV
Codeine	100 mg	50 mg
Morphine	10 mg	5 mg
Oxycodone	10 mg	5 mg
Hydromorphone	2 mg	1 mg
Meperidine	100 mg	50 mg
Methadone	?	
Fentanyl patch	Use manufacturer's table	

*Not FDA approved for this indication.
†Not available in the United States.

pain, as well as prescription of a dose for breakthrough pain. Breakthrough doses are typically prescribed at approximately 10% of the 24-hour opioid dose. It is important to remember the duration of action of opioids and prescribe appropriate dose intervals. An example would be morphine, 10 mg orally every 4 hours, for a continuous pain syndrome, with morphine, 5 mg orally every hour, as needed for breakthrough pain. Common mistakes would be to use the long-acting formulations available of morphine, hydromorphone, oxycodone, or fentanyl patches when initiating an opioid regimen before having used a short-acting opioid to achieve good pain control. It is difficult to titrate with a long-acting opioid formulation, and these options should be reserved for stable pain syndromes in which the opioid requirements have previously been established using the short-acting option.

4. Common dosing guidelines suggest that the use of three or more doses of breakthrough analgesia in 24 hours requires an appropriate increase in the regular opioid administered. Alternatively, the absence of a need for breakthrough for a period of days may suggest the need to consider a decrease in dose. Regular reassessment based on the guidelines suggested earlier will continue to be helpful in ensuring appropriate opioid management. In situations in which patients are unable to take oral opioids, the use of intramuscular administration should be avoided, owing to the pain associated with repeated use of this route. Suitable alternatives include either intermittent or continuous subcutaneous infusion, the use of rectal opioids, and, less commonly, the use of the intravenous route. For dose-conversion purposes the oral and rectal routes are generally considered similar. As noted in Table 1, when switching from the oral to the parenteral route, it is necessary to use only 30% to 50% of the oral opioid dose.

The common opioid-related side effects are nausea, constipation, somnolence, dry mouth, and pruritus. Nausea is generally temporary and can be adequately managed with appropriate antiemetics such as metoclopramide (Reglan). Constipation tends to persist in most patients remaining on opioids and requires regular laxative regimens, including a stimulant and stool softener. Somnolence tends to be short-lived and does not require management in most patients.

There have been increasing reports of patients receiving opioids developing neuropsychiatric side effects such as myoclonus, hyperalgesia, hallucinations, cognitive impairment, and delirium. These problems appear to occur more frequently in patients receiving high opioid doses for prolonged periods, patients with renal failure, and those with preexisting cognitive impairment or receiving other psychoactive drugs. Whereas opioids continue to be underused for some pain syndromes, there is increasing evidence that inaccurate assessments and overenthusiastic opioid use may be associated with severe neurotoxicity. The use of sequential opioid trials is suggested for patients in whom this problem develops. The inexperienced pain clinician may require advice from a pain expert in these circumstances.

Concerns with regard to physical dependence, addiction (psychological dependence), and tolerance are common to both patients and families and require a clear understanding and explanation. Physical dependence is a normal physiologic response to prolonged pharmacologic opioid administration. Withdrawal symptoms occur if opioids are abruptly stopped or an antagonist is administered. In situations in which patients taking opioids have their pain alleviated by nonpharmacologic approaches, such as surgery or radiation therapy, the opioids should be reduced by 15% to 30% per day, rather than being abruptly discontinued. Addiction is a pathologic/psychologic condition in which patients often take increasing doses to experience psychic effects, such as hallucinations, or cognitive impairment that most individuals would describe as a dysphoria rather than euphoria. Tolerance is understood to be the phenomenon in which increasing opioid doses are required to produce the same analgesic effect. The mechanism is poorly understood, but it is considered to be extremely rare. The most frequent reason for dose escalation is disease progression.

OTHER APPROACHES TO PAIN MANAGEMENT

Intraspinal infusion of analgesics is widely used. There is a remarkable variation in practice patterns surrounding this approach. A recent report by an expert panel, while acknowledging the potential benefit of long-term intraspinal management, concluded that "clinical capabilities have proceeded quickly and far exceed the scientific underpinning of these approaches." They suggested an approach that encourages caution with a critical evaluation of outcomes to ensure favorable results.

A wide variety of anesthetic procedures such as celiac plexus blocks have been recommended and may be useful in well-chosen circumstances. Neurosurgical and orthopedic procedures can also be considered.

Radiotherapy is often useful for the management of bone pain and other syndromes caused by tumor infiltration.

Recommended occupational and physiotherapy modalities include transcutaneous electrical nerve stimulation, acupuncture, massage therapy, relaxation therapy, and supports such as collars and slings for immobilization of fractures.

Considering the potential complexity of pain assessment, as well as the wide variety of pharmacologic and nonpharmacologic approaches, there will inevitably be situations in which the average clinician requires advice and support from pain management specialists and comprehensive multidisciplinary pain programs.

NAUSEA AND VOMITING

method of
KENNETH L. KOCH, M.D.
Pennsylvania State College of Medicine
Hershey, Pennsylvania

Nausea and vomiting are common symptoms that may be acute and severe or chronic and debilitating, or the symptoms range between these extremes. The differential diagnosis of nausea and vomiting is extensive. The pathophysiologic mechanisms of nausea and vomiting remain poorly understood for the specific disorders listed in Table 1. Furthermore, most therapies for the symptoms of nausea and vomiting are supportive, and drug therapies are generally directed toward nonspecific mechanisms of action. Fortunately, nausea and vomiting are usually self-limited, but increasing numbers of patients have chronic, unexplained nausea or nausea induced by a variety of medical and surgical treatments. Moreover, it is now appreciated that nausea is a common symptom in the population, with almost 15% of the individuals surveyed in the United States reporting moderate nausea in the past 3 months.

DEFINITIONS

Several definitions are important to consider. First, *nausea* is a vague, uncomfortable feeling in the stomach associated with an urge to vomit. Nausea is actually quite difficult to describe but may be referred to as a queasiness and "sick to the stomach" sensation. Nausea may be mild or severe, may come in waves, or may be steady and persistent. It is often associated with additional symptoms such as fatigue, lightheadedness, and sweating. Nausea is related to pain in that it is a warning signal of ongoing organ dysfunction. *Vomiting*, the violent expulsion of gastric contents from the stomach, usually relieves the nausea symptoms. *Retching* is the gastrointestinal somatic activities associated with vomiting, but no gastric contents are expelled. *Regurgitation* encompasses the effortless return of liquid and solid gastric contents into the esophagus and the mouth. Regurgitation usually reflects gastroesophageal reflux but may also occur in esophageal obstruction and esophageal motility disorders. *Rumination* is the effortless return of solid foods from the stomach into the mouth in the absence of any abdominal discomfort, heartburn, or nausea.

DIFFERENTIAL DIAGNOSIS OF NAUSEA AND VOMITING: THE 12 CATEGORIES

Causes of nausea and vomiting are listed in Table 1. These diseases and disorders are commonly associated with nausea and vomiting and represent multiple pathophysiologic mechanisms that ultimately involve nausea and vomiting. The exact pathophysiologic mechanisms for triggering nausea and vomiting in most of these entities is unknown. However, a number of general principles should be appreciated. In general, as the nausea intensity increases, the threshold for eliciting the vomiting reflex is exceeded and the vomiting reflex is elicited. Vomiting is completely different from nausea in pathophysiologic terms. The vomiting reflex is organized from the vomiting center, which is located in the medulla and includes the dorsal vagal complex. No specific vomiting center exists, however, inasmuch as several brainstem nuclei are required to integrate the responses of the gastrointestinal tract, respiratory system, pharyngeal muscles, and the somatic musculature to execute an episode of vomiting. That the gastrointestinal portion of the vomiting reflex is abolished by vagotomy indicates the importance of the central efferent limb of this reflex.

TABLE 1. **Differential Diagnosis of Nausea and Vomiting***

Mechanical Obstruction
Stomach, duodenum
Small bowel, colon
Hepatobiliary disease
Pancreatic duct disease
Peptic Disease
Esophagus—GERD
Stomach—gastritis, ulcer, *Helicobacter pylori*
Duodenum—duodenitis, ulcer
Peritoneal Irritation
Peritonitis, cancer, irradiation
Carcinoma
Gastric, ovarian
Hypernephroma
Paraneoplastic syndrome
Metabolic—Hormonal
Diabetes mellitus
Uremia, hypercalcemia
Addison's disease
Hyperthyroidism, hypothyroidism
Pregnancy, progesterone/estrogen
Drugs
Chemotherapy agents, levodopa, digitalis, phenytoin, cardiac antiarrhythmics, NSAIDs, antibiotics, morphine, nicotine, progesterone, estrogen
Ischemic Gastroparesis
Postoperative
Vagotomy with partial/total gastrectomy
Fundoplication, fundic resection
Intestinal Pseudo-Obstruction (visceral neuropathy/myopathy)
Scleroderma, amyloidosis
Idiopathic
CNS Disease
Migraine
Infections
Tumors
Complex partial seizures
Vestibular nerve-brainstem lesions
Parkinson's disease
Psychological/Psychiatric Disorders
Anorexia nervosa
Bulimia nervosa
Rumination, psychogenic nausea (vomiting)
Idiopathic Nausea and Vomiting
With gastroparesis (idiopathic)
Without gastroparesis
Gastric dysrhythmias
Cyclic vomiting syndrome

*May be manifested as acute or chronic symptoms.
Abbreviations: CNS = central nervous system; GERD = gastroesophageal reflux disease; NSAIDs = nonsteroidal anti-inflammatory drugs.

PATHOPHYSIOLOGY OF NAUSEA AND VOMITING

General pathophysiologic mechanisms of nausea include the following: (1) *gastric mucosal irritation*, as produced by peptic ulceration of the esophagus, stomach, or duodenum; (2) *distention or obstruction of the gastrointestinal tract*, as represented by benign or cancerous obstruction of any hollow portion of the gastrointestinal tract from the stomach to the biliary tract to the colon; (3) *duodenal contractility and mucosal serotonin*, which represent mechanisms whereby nausea is produced (the 5-HT_3 antagonists are thought to work in part by blocking the action of serotonin from the duodenal mucosa); (4) *delayed gastric emptying and gastric dysrhythmias*, which are neuromuscular abnormalities of the stomach associated with nausea and vomiting, as typified by diabetic or idiopathic gastroparesis; and (5) *central nervous system mechanisms* of nausea and vomiting, which range from brain tumors and seizures to psychiatric disorders such as bulimia or anorexia nervosa.

CLINICAL EVALUATION OF PATIENTS WITH NAUSEA AND VOMITING

History and Physical Examination

A careful history and physical examination are essential as the physician considers the broad differential diagnosis of nausea and vomiting. The various categories of diseases and disorders listed in Table 1 may be manifested as acute nausea and vomiting, or the nausea and vomiting may appear in a more chronic time frame. Important aspects of the history include careful documentation of any recurrent abdominal pain. *When pain precedes the nausea and vomiting, oftentimes an organic or mechanical reason can be found for the nausea and vomiting.* Therefore, the pain must be understood and a differential diagnosis for that pain considered. Appropriate tests should then be carried out to diagnose the cause of the pain (e.g., acute or chronic appendicitis, acute or chronic cholecystitis).

Morning nausea may suggest the possibility of nocturnal gastroesophageal reflux disease. On the other hand, vomiting in the morning with headache and minimal nausea suggests a central nervous system origin of the symptoms. Neurologic symptoms such as olfactory or staring spells and change in coordination or gait should be sought. Other historical aspects include attention to the content of the vomitus. Hematemesis suggests mucosal diseases of the duodenum, stomach, or esophagus. Bilious vomiting suggests small-bowel obstruction. Vomiting of undigested food suggests a gastric neuromuscular abnormality such as gastroparesis.

Physical examination may reveal clues to a specific diagnosis. Orthostatic hypotension may suggest volume depletion from severe nausea and vomiting, but it may also indicate an autonomic neuropathy. A succussion splash suggests retained gastric fluid. Abdominal distention or local areas of pain may indicate a more acute problem such as bowel perforation or obstruction. An abdominal bruit may indicate an ischemic cause of the abdominal discomfort, nausea, and vomiting. A general neurologic examination should be performed to exclude gross neurologic defects. A pelvic examination should also be performed.

Laboratory and Diagnostic Tests

Laboratory studies should include a complete blood count; determination of electrolyte, amylase, and lipase concentrations; and a liver panel. Pregnancy should be excluded in women of childbearing age. A variety of electrolyte and renal abnormalities may be present if the nausea and vomiting have led to dehydration.

In a patient with acute and severe nausea and vomiting, a computed axial tomographic scan or magnetic resonance image of the head may be indicated if neurologic abnormalities or other central nervous system symptoms are present. If the abdomen is tender or the patient has a pain syndrome, a flat plate and upright view of the abdomen is necessary to exclude obstruction or perforation of the gastrointestinal tract. Computed axial tomography may also be necessary if abdominal symptoms are present. Kidney and pelvic diseases should also be considered.

Other diagnostic tests related to the gastrointestinal tract include upper endoscopy to exclude mucosal abnormalities of the esophagus, stomach, and duodenum that may cause nausea and vomiting. If endoscopy is negative, ultrasound may be needed to determine structural abnormalities in the pancreas or gallbladder.

In patients with chronic symptoms of nausea and occasional vomiting related to meals (dysmotility-like dyspepsia) and negative routine tests, neuromuscular assessment of the stomach may be indicated. These diagnostic studies include electrogastrography, which measures gastric myoelectrical activity (i.e., tachygastrias and bradygastrias), and solid phase gastric emptying studies, which indicate the overall neuromuscular strength of stomach contractions (e.g., gastroparesis).

TREATMENT

General Measures

The initial approach to treatment will reflect the differential diagnosis established for the individual patient. Restoring fluid losses with 0.45% normal saline and a 20-mEq/L potassium chloride supplement is often a necessary first step. Diagnostic tests should be organized according to the differential diagnosis. If gastrointestinal obstruction is present, nasogastric suction may relieve the patient's discomfort and nausea.

Pharmacologic Treatment of Nausea and Vomiting

Progress has been extremely slow in designing drugs with specific mechanisms of actions to stop nausea and vomiting caused by specific diseases or disorders. A list of antinauseant/antiemetic drugs is shown in Table 2. Special success has been achieved in reducing nausea and vomiting induced by cancer chemotherapy agents, the emetogenic potential of which is well known. This type of nausea and vomiting, however, is not a diagnostic dilemma, and successful treatment of drug-induced nausea and vomiting has been achieved by oncologists and other physicians responsible for treating cancers. The 5-HT_3 antagonist drugs listed in Table 2 dramatically reduce the vomiting associated with chemotherapy agents. Of interest, however, these agents have been unsuccessful in controlling chemotherapy-induced nausea or delayed nausea and vomiting. These findings indicate that the 5-HT_3 pathways are more relevant to the acute vomiting reflex induced by chemo-

TABLE 2. **Antinauseant/Antiemetic Drugs**

Agents	Dose/Schedule	Route
Phenothiazines		
Prochlorperazine (Compazine)	5–10 mg q6–8h	PO, IV, IM
	25 mg q6h	PR
Thiethylperazine (Torecan)	10 mg q8h	PO, IV, IM, PR
Substituted Benzamides		
Metoclopramide (Reglan)	5–15 mg q6h	PO, IV, IM
Butyrophenones		
Droperido* (Inapsine)	2.5–5.0 mg q4h	IV, IM
Antihistamines		
Diphenhydramine* (Benadryl)	25–50 mg q4–6h	IV, PO
Promethazine (Phenergan)	25 mg q4–6h	IV, PO
Benzodiazepines		
Diazepam* (Valium)	2–10 mg q6–12h	PO, IV
Lorazepam* (Ativan)	2–6 mg q8–12h	PO
Tricyclic Antidepressants		
Amitriptyline* (Elavil)	25–50 mg hs	PO
Prokinetic		
Cisapride† (Propulsid)‡	10–20 mg ac and hs	PO
Domperidone† (Motilium)	10–20 mg ac and hs	PO
5-HT$_3$ Serotonin Antagonists		
Ondansetron (Zofran)	8–32 mg/24 h§	PO, IV
Granisetron (Kytril)	10 μg/kg/24 h	IV
	2 mg/24 h	PO
Dolasetron (Anzemet)	1.8 mg/kg/24 h	IV
	100 mg/24 h	PO
Corticosteroids		
Dexamethasone	10–20 mg q2–6h	PO, IV
Cannabinoids		
Dronabinol (Marinol)	2.5 mg bid	PO

*Not FDA approved for this indication.
†Not available in the United States.
‡Compassionate clearance use only.
§Dose depends on chemotherapy plans or postoperative nausea treatment plans.
Abbreviations: ac = Before meals (antecibum); bid = twice daily; hs = at bedtime; IM = intramuscular; IV = intravenous; PO = per os; PR = per rectum.

therapy agents than are the pathways that mediate nausea.

For a hospitalized patient with acute nausea and vomiting, several intravenous agents are available that may be effective in the individual patient. Droperidol (Inapsine)* is a potent dopamine antagonist with actions in the central nervous system. Metoclopramide (Reglan) is a dopamine-2 receptor antagonist in the central nervous system and the stomach. Both of these potent antiemetic and antinauseant agents are given early in the hospitalization while intravenous fluids are administered and volume depletion is addressed.

Phenothiazines are the traditional and nonspecific treatments for mild to moderate nausea. Prochlorperazine (Compazine) and the antihistamines diphenhydramine (Benadryl)* and promethazine (Phenergan) may help counteract nausea in some patients. An additional approach is to reduce anxiety with benzodiazepines such as diazepam (Valium)* or lorazepam (Ativan).*

*Not FDA approved for this indication.

For outpatients with chronic nausea and occasional vomiting suggestive of chronic gastric neuromuscular dysfunction, gastroprokinetic agents such as metoclopramide, bethanechol (Urecholine),* and domperidone (Motilium)* should be considered. Unfortunately, cisapride (Propulsid)* has been withdrawn from the market, but it can be obtained through compassionate clearance protocols. Domperidone is not available in the United States but can be procured from Canada and Mexico. The prokinetic drugs are very effective in reducing nausea and vomiting when gastric neuromuscular dysfunction has been documented. Dronabinol (Marinol) is a cannabinoid that has been used for cancer chemotherapy–induced nausea, but little investigation of its use in chronic gastrointestinal neuromuscular disorders has been performed. Finally, in patients with chronic unexplained nausea and vomiting, low-dose amitriptyline (Elavil)* has been shown to decrease nausea in up to 75% of these patients. The mechanism of action of amitriptyline in nausea and vomiting is unknown.

Nondrug Therapies for Nausea and Vomiting

Nondrug treatment of chronic nausea and vomiting includes acupuncture, acupressure, acustimulation, and gastric electrical stimulation or pacing. Acupuncture and acupressure have been used for many years to decrease a variety of symptoms, including nausea and vomiting. A common stimulation point is P6, or Neiguan. Stimulation of this point may be accomplished with pressure or acupuncture needles. In addition, a transecutaneous electrical nerve stimulation–type device is available (ReliefBand) that stimulates the P6 point electrically to reduce the nausea and vomiting associated with pregnancy, motion sickness, and postoperative and chemotherapy-related nausea and vomiting. Finally, gastric pacemakers or electrical stimulation devices with electrodes attached to the gastric corpus and antrum are undergoing investigation. Electrical stimulation appears to reduce the frequency of nausea and vomiting in some patients with refractory and documented gastroparesis.

Dietary Therapy

Patients with acute or chronic nausea and vomiting, especially those with gastric neuromuscular abnormalities, cannot eat regular American diets. Table 3 summarizes a three-step diet for patients with intermittent nausea and vomiting symptoms

*Not FDA approved for this indication.

TABLE 3. **Nausea and Vomiting Diet**

Step 1. Gatorade and Bouillon

Diet

Patients with severe nausea and vomiting should sip small volumes of salty liquids such as Gatorade or bouillon to avoid dehydration. These liquids include salt and sugar in addition to water. Any liquid to be ingested should have some caloric content. A multiple vitamin should be prescribed.

Goal

To ingest 1000 to 1500 mL/d in multiple servings, e.g., 12, 4-oz servings over the course of 12–14 h. 1–2 oz at a time may be sipped to reach approximately 4 oz/h.

Avoid

Citrus drinks of all kinds and highly sweetened drinks. (The acid or hypertonicity may upset the stomach.)

Step 2. Soups

Diet

If Gatorade or bouillon is tolerated, the diet may be advanced to include a variety of soups with noodles or rice and crackers. Peanut butter, cheese, and crackers may be tolerated in small amounts. Caramels or other chewy confections may be tried. These foods should be given in at least 6 divided meals per day. A multiple vitamin should be prescribed.

Goal

To ingest approximately 1500 Cal/d. Patients who can accomplish this goal will avoid dehydration and will ideally ingest enough calories to maintain their weight. In many patients, maintenance of their present weight, not weight gain, is the realistic goal.

Avoid

Creamy, milk-based liquids. (The fat in the meal will delay emptying of the stomach.)

Step 3. Starches, Chicken, and Fish

Diet

Starches such as noodles, pasta, potatoes, and rice are easily mixed and emptied by the stomach. Thus, soups, mashed or baked potatoes, pasta dishes, rice and baked chicken breast, and fish are usually well-tolerated sources of carbohydrate and protein. These solids should also be ingested in 6 small meals per day. A one-a-day vitamin should be prescribed.

Goal

To find a diet of common foods that the patient finds interesting and satisfying and that evoke minimal nausea/vomiting symptoms. As the patient learns what liquids and solids are tolerated, the variety and number of foods that can be enjoyed will increase.

Avoid

Fatty foods, which delay gastric emptying, red meats and fresh vegetables, which require considerable trituration, and pulpy fibrous foods, which promote the formation of bezoars.

from gastric neuromuscular disorders and other diseases in which nausea is a key symptom. After ingestion of food, the stomach must perform "muscular work" to mix, triturate, and empty the nutrients from the stomach into the duodenum. Gastric dysrhythmias and gastric contraction abnormalities interfere with these neuromuscular functions of the stomach. Therefore, the patient's diet must be altered and appropriate foods that are easy to triturate and empty must be selected. In the most severe patients, salty liquids such as bouillon or Gatorade are suggested to avoid dehydration. As symptoms improve, the diet can be advanced to brothy soups with noodles and then finally to solid meals containing starches and white meats which are easier for the stomach to triturate and empty.

For patients with severe and unremitting chronic nausea and vomiting, gastrostomy tubes may be necessary to vent the stomach and prevent multiple vomiting episodes. Jejunostomy tubes may be needed for enteral feeding if nutritional support is required. Some patients with neuromuscular dysfunction of the stomach and small bowel (i.e., intestinal pseudo-obstruction) may require total parenteral nutrition, but efforts should be made to avoid such alimentation because of line sepsis and other complications attendant with this form of nutritional support.

GASEOUSNESS AND INDIGESTION

method of
CHIN HUR, M.D., M.P.H., and
ANTHONY LEMBO, M.D.
Beth Israel Deaconess Medical Center and Harvard Medical School
Boston, Massachusetts

GASEOUSNESS

Excessive "gas" can cause significant discomfort and embarrassment. The symptoms of gaseousness can refer to excessive belching (or eructation), flatus, or even abdominal bloating. In most cases, gaseousness is not due to an increased volume of gas within the gastrointestinal (GI) tract. Unfortunately, we have a limited understanding of the pathogenesis of gaseousness. The lack of useful and clinically available tests to document or refute abnormal gas volume and the patient's strong belief that his or her symptoms are abnormal make successful treatment of gaseousness difficult.

Excessive Belching

Symptoms and Physiology

Occasional belching is a normal physiologic process that allows swallowed air to be removed from the stomach. The normal frequency of belching has not been well documented, but patients who complain of it usually have repetitive and uncontrollable episodes of belching.

The most common cause of excessive belching is excessive air swallowing (*aerophagia*). Swallowing food or even saliva can result in some air entering the upper GI tract. Air can also be swallowed by itself, consciously and unconsciously. Factors that can result in increased aerophagia include stress, gastroesophageal reflux, increased salivary production from excessive sucking on hard candy or chewing gum, and cigarette smoking. Rarely, other upper GI diseases such as peptic ulcer disease, gastroesophageal reflux disease (GERD), and cholecystitis can present as excessive belching.

Treatment

Although belching is usually the result of excessive air swallowing, a complete history and physical examination is important to exclude the rare causes of upper GI disorders that may produce these symptoms (e.g., GERD, peptic ulcer disease, or cholecystitis). If other associated GI symptoms are present, appropriate diagnostic tests should follow. In most patients, no other diagnostic testing is necessary. Rather, the patient should be reassured that the symptom is not associated with an organic disorder.

Dietary modification such as avoiding sucking on hard candies or chewing gum, eating slowly with small swallows, and avoiding carbonated beverages can be suggested, although this has not been sufficiently tested and is usually disappointing in practice. Simethicone and activated charcoal preparations do not seem to be effective. Stress management may be helpful in those patients whose excessive air swallowing seems exacerbated by underlying stress. Other forms of psychotherapy (e.g., cognitive behavioral therapy) should be considered in patients who remain symptomatic.

Excessive Flatus

Symptoms and Physiology

The range of normal volume and frequency of flatus varies widely. Adults pass flatus 10 to 14 times per day for a total volume of 400 to 2500 mL/d.

Rectal gas comes from either swallowed air or from bacterial fermentation. Malabsorption of carbohydrates, which can occur in patients with celiac sprue, pancreatic insufficiency, and short bowel syndrome, can result in increased flatus production. Lactose and fructose are simple sugars found in many foods that are commonly malabsorbed. Likewise, many common starches found in various fruits, vegetables, and flours are not fully absorbed by healthy patients.

Management

The first step is to determine if excessive flatulence is present by having the patient record the frequency of rectal gas passage for 2 weeks. Normal is generally considered to be fewer than 25 episodes of flatus per day.

Patients who pass flatus more than 25 times per day without signs of malabsorption should undergo dietary modification. Specifically, patients should be advised to restrict lactose- and fructose-containing foods. It is virtually impossible to restrict all carbohydrates, but certain carbohydrates that may be malabsorbed include fructose (soft drinks), lactose (dairy), trehalose (mushrooms), raffinose and stachyose (legumes), and resistant starches (fruits, flours, vegetables). A patient diary of foods avoided with concomitant symptoms may be instrumental in determining any salient offending carbohydrates. Patients not responding to dietary modifications should be advised to reduce behaviors associated with excessive air swallowing, including stress, smoking, chewing gum, or sucking on candy.

INDIGESTION (DYSPEPSIA)

Definition and Epidemiology

Indigestion or *dyspepsia* is defined as a persistent or recurrent pain or discomfort centered in the upper abdomen. Other associated characteristics include postprandial fullness, upper abdominal bloating, early satiety, anorexia, nausea, and vomiting. The prevalence in the United States is estimated to be as high as 40%.

Differential Diagnosis

Pelvic ulcer disease accounts for 15% to 25% of patients with dyspepsia. Thirty percent to 60% of these patients will be positive for *Helicobacter pylori* if tested. Nonsteroidal anti-inflammatory drug use accounts for the majority of the remaining patients.

GERD is defined as epigastric burning that radiates substernally. The symptom of substernal radiation is somewhat specific for GERD; however, many patients with GERD may not have the classic radiation but complain solely of epigastric pain or discomfort.

Functional or nonulcer dyspepsia accounts for up to 60% of patients who present with dyspepsia. This syndrome is a diagnosis of exclusion when other organic causes have been excluded. Although up to 40% of patients with irritable bowel syndrome can also have dyspeptic symptoms, isolated functional dyspepsia appears to be a separate syndrome. Various theories or factors that have not been conclusively implicated include *H. pylori* infection, visceral hypersensitivity, and abnormal motility.

Biliary or pancreatic disease can be mistaken for dyspepsia, but a proper history and physical examination should point to these disease processes with further diagnostic tests such as blood work and imaging.

Although gastric and esophageal malignancy is rare (<2%) in patients presenting with dyspepsia, the risk increases with age.

Management

Patients who present with dyspepsia who are older than age 45 should undergo an upper endoscopy to rule out serious processes such as malignancy. Also, any patient who has any alarm features such as unexplained weight loss, anemia, GI bleeding (hematemesis or melena), or a significant examination (tenderness, lymphadenopathy, or jaundice) should also undergo an upper endoscopy.

For patients younger than age 45 without alarm symptoms, empirical testing for *H. pylori* infection either by serology or breath test is a reasonable first step. Alternatively, upper endoscopy with biopsies for

H. pylori may provide the patient added reassurance if the study is negative. If the patient is positive for *H. pylori* infection, he or she should be treated with eradication therapy.

If the tests are negative or the patient's symptoms persist even after an upper endoscopy, various empirical therapies are available. Acid suppression with either an H_2 blocker or proton pump inhibitor should be the first line of therapy. If these do no provide any relief, a promotility agent such as metoclopramide (Reglan) or erythromycin* can be considered. Tricyclic antidepressants such as amitriptyline (Elavil)* have also been used with some anecdotal success. Other behavioral therapies such as biofeedback or hypnosis have not been studied but may be reserved for severely refractory patients.

*Not FDA approved for this indication.

HICCUP

method of
HARALD FODSTAD, M.D., PH.D.
New York Methodist Hospital
Brooklyn, New York

Hiccup (hiccough, *hoquet diabolique,* singultus) is a repeated involuntary, spasmodic, and short-lasting contraction of the diaphragm, accompanied by sudden closure of the glottis. The hiccup spasm may occur from 40 to 100 times per minute. The diaphragm is innervated by the phrenic nerves, which arise in the neck on each side, chiefly from the fourth cervical segment but also from filaments from the third, fifth, and sixth segments.

In its route to its distribution on the undersurface of the diaphragm, each nerve is in close relationship to the deep musculature of the neck, first portion of the subclavian artery, subclavian vein, internal mammary artery, root of the lung, and pericardium and peritoneum. There is also communication with the sympathetic system in the chest, the superior and inferior sympathetic ganglia, and the spinal accessory and hypoglossal nerves. An accessory phrenic nerve may be present in 20% to 75% of cases.

The great majority of hiccup spasms have been reported to be unilateral and confined to the left hemidiaphragm, and men are more often affected than women. The sensation leading to hiccup is mediated by sensory branches of the phrenic and vagus nerves as well as dorsal sympathetic afferents. The principal efferent limb and spasms of the diaphragm are mediated by motor fibers of the phrenic nerve.

ETIOLOGY

Hiccups may be classified as either *transient* (self-limited) or *persistent* (intractable). Conditions associated with transient hiccup are gastric distention, alcohol ingestion, smoking, sudden temperature changes, and emotional stress or excitement.

The etiology of persistent hiccup is obscure. The causes have been localized to the central nervous system, neck, thorax, and abdomen, that is, along the pathways of the phrenic and vagus nerves. In general, hiccups may be triggered by central nervous system lesions or irritation of the phrenic and vagus nerves. Numerous reports have described trauma, infections, inflammations, chemicals, vascular disease, demyelinating disease, arteriovenous malformations, tumors, and hysteria as causative factors. Drugs, blood disease, and cardiac pacemakers may also trigger hiccups. Persistent hiccups have been considered a form of mild myoclonic encephalitis or brainstem encephalitis. They have also presented as a symptom of brainstem tumors. Causes of transient and intractable hiccup are presented in Table 1.

PATHOPHYSIOLOGY

The neuroanatomic locus for hiccup is not known, but the central connection probably consists of an interaction among the brainstem respiratory centers, phrenic nerve nuclei, medullary reticular formation, and the hypothalamus. The existence of a "hiccup center" in the brainstem or in the cervical cord between C3 and C5 has been postulated by several authors. Visceral reflexes such as hiccup, coughing, sneezing, swallowing, and vomiting are invariably connected with the vagus nerve and are considered to follow similar reflex arcs. Hiccup has been classified as a respiratory reflex similar to coughing and as a gastrointestinal phenomenon more similar to the vomiting reflex. Fetal hiccups, which are relatively common, are similar to the gasping reflex. It is well known that hiccups in young infants may affect breathing in clinically significant ways,

TABLE 1. **Causes of Transient and Intractable Hiccup**

Central Nervous System	Peripheral Nerve Involvement
Neoplasms	Postoperative states
Surgery	Gastric distention
Trauma	Myocardial infarction
Infection (e.g., meningitis, encephalitis)	Pericarditis
Cerebrovascular accident	Hiatal hernia
Multiple sclerosis	Esophagitis
Parkinson disease	Hepatitis
Sarcoidosis	Gallbladder disease (e.g., cholecystitis)
Hydrocephalus	Subdiaphragmatic abscess
Syringomyelia	Pancreatitis
Arteriovenous malformation	Tympanic membrane irritation
Metabolic	Infection (e.g., pneumonia, pleurisy)
Toxic (alcohol, medications)	Neoplasms
Uremia	Pulmonary
Diabetes mellitus	Cervical
Electrolyte imbalance	Ear, nose, and throat
Hypocapnia (hyperventilation)	Abdominal
Gout	Mediastinal
Addison disease	Gastritis
Psychological	Ulcer disease
Excitement	Peritonitis
Hysteria	**Pharmacologic**
Stress	Corticosteroids
Malingering	Barbiturates
Idiopathic	Benzodiazepines
Anorexia nervosa	α-Methyldopa (Aldomet)
Enuresis nocturna	Analeptics
	Anesthetics: methohextone*
	Antibiotics: sulfonamides, ceftriaxone (Rocephin), cefotetan (Cefotan), doxycycline (Vibramycin), imipenem/cilastatin (Primaxin)

*Not available in the United States.

but there are no known serious side effects of temporary hiccups.

MANAGEMENT

The different therapeutic approaches to hiccup are equally impressive in their magnitude and variation. Transient hiccups that last only a few minutes rarely require any treatment, but some simple measures may be of help, such as holding the breath, breathing into a paper bag, drinking water, sucking on sugar or candy, compressing the nose while swallowing, pulling on the tongue, putting a finger in the throat, coughing, and sneezing.

Most hiccups will stop when the presumed underlying cause is successfully treated. When the hiccups become persistent or intractable, a variety of pharmacologic agents are available for trial (Table 2). Among these, only chlorpromazine is approved by the Food and Drug Administration for treatment of hiccup at the present time.

TABLE 2. **Pharmacotherapy of Hiccup**

Major Tranquilizers
Chlorpromazine (Thorazine), 25–50 mg IV q6h; if successful, switch to PO at the same dose
Haloperidol (Haldol),* 2–12 mg PO daily
Anticonvulsants
Phenytoin (Dilantin),* 200 mg IV bolus, then 100 mg PO qid
Valproic acid (Depakene),* 15 mg/kg/d PO or rectally
Carbamazepine (Tegretol),* 200 mg PO qid
Magnesium sulfate (magnesium sulfate injection USP),* 2 mL of a 50% solution IM
Central Nervous System Stimulants
Methylphenidate (Ritalin),* 6–20 mg IV bolus
Amphetamine sulfate (Adderall),* 10–20 mg PO bid
Ephedrine sulfate (Marax),* 25 mg PO tid
Anesthetic
Lidocaine (Xylocaine),* 2–4 mg/min continuous IV infusion; Anestacon jelly* used topically in the mouth
Antispastic
Baclofen (Lioresal),* 5–20 mg PO q6–12h
Calcium Channel Blocker
Nifedipine (Adalat),* 10 mg PO bid (escalated to 20 mg tid)
Antidepressant
Amitriptyline (Elavil),* 10 mg PO tid
Serotonin Antagonist
Ondansetron (Zofran),* 4–32 mg IV bolus or 8 mg PO tid
Dopamine Antagonist
Metoclopramide (Reglan),* 10 mg PO q6h or 5–10 mg IM or IV q8h
Dopamine Agonist
Amantadine (Symmetrel),* 100 mg PO daily
Parasympathomimetic
Edrophonium chloride (Tensilon),* 5 mg IV
Parasympatholytics
Atropine sulfate (Atropine sulfate injection USP),* 1 mg IV
Quinidine sulfate,* 200 mg PO q8h

*Not FDA approved for this indication.

Besides a multitude of exotic remedies and pharmaceuticals, the following therapeutic modalities have been tried and recommended with varying results: acupuncture, hypnosis, continuous positive airway pressure, paravertebral block of C3-5 or epidural blockade below C5, pharyngeal stimulation, faradic and galvanic currents, continuous electrophrenic stimulation, blockade, crush and transection of the phrenic nerves, as well as posterior fossa microvascular decompression and electrostimulation of the vagus nerve.

For centuries, trial and error has brought us but a little closer to an effective remedy for persistent hiccups. There is probably no disease that has had more forms of treatment and fewer results from treatment than has intractable hiccups. In 1932, Charles W. Mayo made a statement on persistent hiccups that still seems valid:

> *The amount of knowledge on any subject such as this can be considered as being in inverse proportion to the number of different treatments suggested and tried for it.*

ACUTE INFECTIOUS DIARRHEA

method of
DAVID A. SACK, M.D.
Centre for Health and Population Research
Dhaka, Bangladesh

Acute diarrhea is defined as the passage of an increased number of loose or watery stools in association with other symptoms of intestinal illness, such as abdominal cramps or vomiting. As a general rule, diagnosis can be confirmed by at least three such stools in a day. In industrialized countries, diarrhea is a common inconvenience, affecting people one or two times per year, but it may become a serious condition in certain circumstances, such as when the diarrheal fluid loss is very high, when the symptoms persist and lead to electrolyte imbalance, when the symptoms are accompanied by signs of invasive disease, or when the symptoms represent signs of more serious underlying illness. In developing countries, diarrheal diseases are one of the leading causes of death because the dehydration, if not treated with appropriate rehydration therapy, can quickly lead to death. The number of deaths from diarrhea worldwide is estimated at 2 to 3 million, but this huge number actually represents a sizeable decrease from a decade ago when it was about 5 million. The improvement in the number of deaths is believed to be the result of widespread use of oral rehydration therapy.

Because most cases of diarrhea are self-limiting, the syndrome is divided into acute diarrhea, defined as lasting fewer than 14 days, and persistent diarrhea, in which the symptoms last more than 14 days. This cutoff of 14 days is somewhat arbitrary, but it is a helpful guide in identifying those patients who may require additional investigations. Either acute or persistent diarrhea may have blood (± mucus), and when this occurs the disease is called inflammatory diarrhea or dysentery. Diarrhea without blood in the stool is referred to as secretory or watery diarrhea. Some illnesses, especially those caused by *Shi-*

gella or *Salmonella* species, may start as watery diarrhea and progress to dysentery.

Diarrhea may be caused by a wide variety of infectious agents, but it may also be caused by noninfectious causes, such as laxatives, lactose intolerance, inflammatory bowel disease, pancreatic insufficiency, and irritable bowel syndrome. Among the infectious causes, certain viruses and bacteria are the most common, but parasites may also be considered. Among the viruses, rotavirus is by far the most common cause of diarrhea in infants, but other viruses (e.g., Norwalk-like viruses) are more likely to cause diarrhea in older individuals. Bacteria are much less likely to be the cause of diarrhea in industrialized countries but are common causes in developing countries lacking modern sanitation.

Evaluation of patients with acute diarrhea includes determining several key characteristics. Some of these include age of the patient (because different pathogens tend to infect certain age groups), history of recent travel to developing countries (because bacterial pathogens are much more common in areas of poor sanitation), signs and symptoms of dehydration (because this will determine how aggressive to be with rehydration therapy), history of recent intake of risky foods or water, signs and symptoms of invasive diarrhea (e.g., fever or blood in the stool), history of antibiotic use (because certain agents may infect the gut after use of antibiotics) and duration of symptoms (because chronic symptoms will lead one to consider more chronic conditions). Key physical findings include evaluation for dehydration and evidence of systemic illness. Laboratory tests may be useful in the evaluation of some patients to confirm the presence of blood or pus cells in the stool, to evaluate cases suspected of having infection with *Shigella, Salmonella, Campylobacter, Vibrio, Clostridium difficile*, a parasite, or rotavirus. Although these tests may be useful in selected patients, a pathogen is found only rarely in patients in the United States; and in developing countries, where bacterial pathogens are more common, the facilities and economic resources for such tests are limited. Thus, most mild cases of acute watery diarrhea can be managed without specific laboratory tests. During the search for pathogens, the fundamental management of fluids and electrolytes should not be overlooked.

CLINICAL SYNDROMES

Diarrhea may be classified into different clinical syndromes. These syndromes help to define the pathophysiologic mechanisms, the most likely infectious agents responsible, the treatment needed, and the clinical investigations that may help to further define the illness. These may further be refined depending on specific risk factors, epidemiologic factors, and age groups.

Acute Watery Diarrhea

By far the most common diarrheal syndrome is the sudden occurrence of loose or watery stools. This may be accompanied by nausea, vomiting, loss of appetite, abdominal cramps, and low-grade fever. However, fever greater than 102°F (38.9°C) suggests that the illness is not simply acute watery diarrhea but represents another invasive illness. The stools generally are very watery and of high volume but do not contain blood or mucus. A fecal leukocyte test, if performed, is negative for pus cells.

Within the general category of acute watery diarrhea, a few types in specific groups of patients should be especially noted: infantile diarrhea, elderly diarrhea, traveler's diarrhea, seafood-associated diarrhea, outbreak-associated diarrhea, and cholera-like diarrhea.

INFANTILE DIARRHEA

Infantile diarrhea occurs in nearly all infants during their first 18 months of life, but it usually does not occur during the first 3 months when maternal antibody protects. It continues to cause a large proportion of pediatric hospital admissions in the United States. The illness often starts with vomiting, but then diarrhea becomes the most prominent symptom, along with fussiness and resistance to feeding. The most dangerous complication of infantile diarrhea is the dehydration that may result from the excess loss of diarrhea stool. "Superabsorbent" disposable diapers may mask the large volumes of stool that are being lost and may also obscure the fact that urine output is decreasing. Thus, parents and providers must be alert to the signs of dehydration, including poor skin turgor, dry mucous membranes, increased thirst, and low urine output.

Rotavirus is the most common cause of the infantile diarrhea syndrome in industrialized countries, where it usually occurs during a winter season. In developing countries rotavirus is still the most common agent, but bacterial pathogens, especially enterotoxigenic *E. coli*, are also major causes. Regardless of the specific agent causing the diarrhea, the most important treatment is the restoration of fluids to correct dehydration and maintain hydration until the diarrhea has resolved. Antibiotics and antidiarrheal drugs (e.g., Lomotil or Imodium) should not be used in ordinary infantile diarrhea.

In the United States, few deaths are attributed to infantile diarrhea because it is readily managed with fluid and electrolyte replacement, but it does lead to many hospitalizations and much lost work for the parents and lost days from daycare. Globally, however, infantile diarrhea is estimated to kill about 3 million children each year.

Diarrhea frequently accompanies or follows the use of broad-spectrum antibiotics used to treat other illnesses, such as otitis or pneumonia in young children. These symptoms can usually be managed with oral rehydration solution (Table 1) as needed to prevent dehydration.

DIARRHEA IN THE ELDERLY

Just as dehydration is of great concern in infants, it is also a major problem in the elderly. The agents causing diarrhea in the geriatric age group are more varied. Cali-

TABLE 1. **Preparation of Oral Rehydration Solution**

Constituents to Add (per liter) to Prepare WHO Formula ORS		This Makes a Solution With the Following Composition	
Glucose or	20 g	Carbohydrate	20 g
Rice powder	50 g		40 g
Sodium chloride	3.5 g	Sodium	90 mEq
Potassium chloride	1.5 g	Potassium	20 mEq
Trisodium citrate or	2.9 g	Citrate	20 mEq
Sodium bicarbonate	2.5 g		

Packets of WHO ORS are available in most countries and are to be mixed with clean water using the volumes of water stated on the label. Commercial, ready-to-drink products are more commonly used in the United States and do not require mixing.

Commercial products in industrialized countries (e.g., Pedialyte) will usually contain 25 g of glucose and 45 to 70 mEq of sodium (depending on specific product). CeraLyte contains 40 g of rice carbohydrate and from 50 to 70 mEq of sodium (depending on the specific product).

Abbreviations: ORS = oral rehydration solution; WHO = World Health Organization.

civirus, *Salmonella*, *Clostridium difficile*, and occasionally rotavirus are known to cause diarrhea in both endemic and epidemic forms. Although the diarrhea symptoms are similar to other age groups, the consequences may be much more severe because of the decreased ability of elderly patients to adapt to slightly decreased circulating blood volumes. The diarrheal episode, with some dehydration, may result in cardiovascular complications, such as stroke, heart attack, and mesenteric artery thrombosis. Diarrhea in the elderly is also complicated by more inconvenient nursing care, and the troublesome nursing care and cleaning may take precedence over the recognition that the patient is becoming dehydrated. Urine output and orthostatic blood pressure measurements should be monitored in such patients in addition to observing for other signs of dehydration so that oral or intravenous fluids can be given as needed.

Because nursing homes house many elderly and disabled patients and because enteric pathogens frequently spread in nursing homes, these institutionalized patients are especially at risk from outbreaks of diarrhea. *C. difficile* is of special concern in nursing home patients because these environments typically have exposure to antibiotics that select for *C. difficile* and such patients can easily become infected with this bacterium.

TRAVELER'S DIARRHEA

Persons traveling from industrialized to developing countries are at high risk of developing acute diarrhea. As with other forms of watery diarrhea, it is usually accompanied by abdominal cramps and may also be accompanied by nausea, vomiting, anorexia, and inability to carry out planned activities. Thirty percent to 50% of travelers develop one or more episodes of diarrhea or loose stools during travel to developing countries, although illness sufficiently severe to lead to inability to function is much less common. The most common agent causing this syndrome is enterotoxigenic *Escherichia coli*, but other bacteria and rarely viruses and parasites may also cause these symptoms.

Symptoms of traveler's diarrhea usually last for 3 to 5 days and are self-limited in otherwise healthy people. Treatment includes maintenance of fluids with oral rehydration solution and, in severe cases, use of an antibiotic such as ciprofloxacin (Cipro)* or norfloxacin (Noroxin).* Imodium may be used along with the antibiotic. The antibiotic may be given for 1 to 3 days, but long courses of antibiotic are not needed. Such a course of antibiotic will decrease the duration of diarrhea significantly. Sodium subsalicylate may be used to provide some symptomatic relief for mild cases.

The risk of traveler's diarrhea is less if one follows rules to ensure that food and water are hygienic (e.g., "cook it, peel it, or forget it"); however, even travelers who carefully follow such rules still frequently develop diarrhea. Prophylactic antibiotics can be given to individuals who are at high risk if they are at such risk for a brief time (<3 weeks). Doxycycline* (100 mg/d with food) reduces the risk significantly; however, an increasing proportion of enteric bacteria are resistant to this drug. Frequently, doxycycline is used to prevent malaria and, if given for this purpose, will also prevent most episodes of traveler's diarrhea. Prophylactic norfloxacin (100 mg) or ciprofloxacin (250 mg) daily will prevent nearly all episodes of diarrhea, and either agent is advised for persons who have high risk of complications should they become dehydrated, such as elderly patients or those with cardiovascular disease. Use of such prophylactic antibiotics should be limited to less than 3 weeks; they are given only during days of actual travel, not before or after the travel.

*Not FDA approved for this indication.

SEAFOOD–ASSOCIATED DIARRHEA

Certain diarrhea-causing bacteria are found in seafood, and these should be suspected when the history suggests an association with seafood such as shellfish, raw fish, or other fish that may not be fully cooked. Vibrios, such as *V. parahaemolyticus*, *V. cholerae* including both serogroup O1 and non O1, and other vibrios are especially common in seafood. The risk of *Vibrio* infection is much higher during warmer summer months when seawater temperatures are higher. Persons with immune deficiency who are more susceptible to *Vibrio* infection should avoid raw or undercooked seafood, especially during the summer months. Less commonly associated with seafood are caliciviruses and other enteric bacteria. Other viruses (e.g., hepatitis A) may also be associated with seafood but do not commonly cause diarrhea. Travelers to cholera endemic areas should avoid raw seafood or seafood served cold (e.g., shrimp salad). Even if once cooked, the cold seafood can be again contaminated with utensils or food juices from the kitchen.

OUTBREAK-ASSOCIATED DIARRHEA

Occasionally the history will suggest that the patient may have been infected as part of a common-source outbreak. Such cases should be reported to the local health department immediately so that an outbreak investigation can be carried out. Illness following a "pot luck" meal should especially stimulate questions as to whether others might have also become ill. The Centers for Disease Control and Prevention estimates that each year about 76 million persons experience a foodborne illness in the United States, most of which is diarrheal disease. Many of these occur during common source outbreaks. The most common bacterial agents causing these foodborne infections were *Salmonella*, *Campylobacter*, *Shigella*, and *E. coli*. Identification of such outbreaks can lead to preventative measures to stop the distribution of contaminated food.

CHOLERA SYNDROME

Although rare in industrialized countries, cholera occurs in most developing countries. The occurrence of severe, rapidly progressing, dehydrating diarrhea with "rice-water stools" is the classic presentation for true "cholera gravis" caused by *V. cholerae* serotype O1 or O139, but it may also be caused by enterotoxigenic *E. coli* and by other vibrios. This kind of illness constitutes a life-threatening illness and requires aggressive rehydration.

Dysentery (Inflammatory Diarrhea)

The dysentery syndrome is characterized by loose stools containing blood (sometimes with mucus) and is the result of inflammation of the colon or lower small intestine that leads to frequent loose stools. The patient tends to have the feeling of needing to pass stools frequently, but the volume is very small because the urgency is caused by inflammation of the rectum. Frequently, only small amounts of mucus or pus are passed. Because of the inflammation, patients with dysentery usually have severe cramps; often have fever, body aches, malaise; and may have tenismus (rectal pain that persists even after a stool has been passed). A fecal leukocyte test will reveal many polymorphonuclear leukocytes. In the case of shigellosis or salmonellosis, the illness may start as typical watery diarrhea and then progress to dysentery.

The most common causes for dysentery are *Shigella*, *Campylobacter*, and *Salmonella*. Amebic colitis may cause bloody stools but usually without inflammation, and stool microscopic examination is needed to identify the hematophagous trophozoites of amebiasis.

Antibiotics are indicated for patients with shigellosis, although they are of questionable benefit in infections with *Campylobacter* and *Salmonella*. *Shigella* are now commonly resistant to ampicillin and cotrimoxazole, and the newer quinolones have become the drug of choice for most patients. In developing countries where less expensive antibiotics may have an advantage, knowledge of the antibiotic sensitivities of local or endemic strains should guide immediate therapy. When possible, culture and sensitivity tests should be carried out.

Proctocolitis is a syndrome involving inflammation of only the distal colon leading to passage of small volumes of inflammatory exudates. Agents responsible for the syndrome include *Neisseria gonorrhoeae* and *Chlamydia trachomatis* and are often spread by anorectal intercourse.

Diagnosis of Specific Agents

Recognizing specific pathogens begins with suspecting their presence based on history and physical examination.

ROTAVIRUS

Rotavirus should be suspected in infants and young children, especially during the winter season (although in tropical climates rotavirus occurs year round). The illness often starts with vomiting and then progresses to watery diarrhea. Surveillance shows that nearly every infant is infected with rotavirus before he or she reaches 2 years of age, and 15% to 20% of infants develop diarrhea sufficiently severe to seek care from a provider each year. Pediatricians usually recognize the rotavirus season because many infants may be developing this illness during the same period of the year. There is some variability from year to year and variations in specific locations, but in the United States the "rotavirus season" usually starts in the southwestern states in the late autumn and moves eastward, reaching the eastern states by mid to late winter.

The infection is self-limiting, but children may be ill for several days, and total fluid losses during the illness can be life-threatening unless treated properly. The crucial treatment is the maintenance of fluids and electrolytes using oral rehydration solution, but occasionally children require intravenous fluids. Antibiotics are not needed. Some infants may develop rotavirus infections more than once; however, the first one is usually the most severe and subsequent infections tend to be mild or asymptomatic.

A stool enzyme-linked immunosorbent assay is available to confirm the diagnosis, but the results do not change the treatment of the patient. Patients who must be admitted to a hospital should be under contact precautions to prevent spread of the virus to other patients in the hospital because nosocomial spread is common.

A live, oral vaccine tetravalent vaccine (RotaShield) for rotavirus was introduced to prevent this common infection. The vaccine consisted of a mixture of four reassortant, attenuated, virus vaccine strains. The parent virus for the vaccine originated from a Rhesus monkey. Based on the extensive clinical trials, the vaccine was expected to greatly reduce rates of severe infantile diarrhea and reduce pediatric hospitalizations. Unfortunately, an unanticipated and serious adverse event, intussusception, occurred in a very small proportion of infants who received the vaccine and the vaccine was withdrawn shortly after its introduction. Other vaccines, based on human and bovine strains, are still under development, and it is hoped they will protect without causing intussusception. Epidemiologic evidence suggests that natural infection with human rotavirus does not lead to intussusception, so there is expectation that the other vaccines will be safe.

Rarely, rotavirus causes infection in the elderly, but it may cause mild diarrhea in family members of sick infants who handle their diapers. In immune-suppressed patients, rotavirus infection may cause persistent diarrhea. When persistent, in addition to fluids, a passive antibody via immune milk has proved helpful.

NORWALK-LIKE VIRUS

Norwalk-like virus may cause gastroenteritis in any age group. Generally, the illnesses occur in outbreaks and may affect people in camps and dormitories, who experience acute vomiting and diarrhea. The illness is usually short-lived, lasting a day or two, but outbreaks may involve many people.

VIBRIO CHOLERAE

Cholera is caused by *Vibrio cholerae* serotype O1 or O139. Currently, serotype O1 is found in nearly all developing countries but serotype O139 is only in South Asia, although it may be spreading to other areas. Cholera, sometimes referred to as "epidemic cholera" or "cholera gravis" has major public health importance because of its ability to spread through contaminated food and water and to cause severe watery diarrhea leading to severe dehydration. Deaths from dehydration may occur within a few hours of onset of symptoms even in previously healthy individuals. Contaminated seafood and contaminated water are common vehicles, but many foods have also been implicated. Travelers suspected of having cholera should have a stool culture performed using specific media for this organism, and positive cases should be reported to the authorities. In endemic countries, the numbers of cases are too great to culture all cases and specimens from a sample of cases should be tested to confirm the type of organism and the antibiotic sensitivity patterns. Cases occurring in an area not previously infected should be confirmed and reported to the authorities.

Symptoms include severe watery diarrhea, and often the stool is so watery it loses its fecal character and is like "rice water." Severe cases usually also have severe vomiting, and with increasing dehydration they develop classic signs of acute dehydration proceeding to shock, coma, and death unless treated rapidly. The stools contain large amounts of bicarbonate, and the patients develop severe metabolic acidosis. Muscle cramps may be an especially painful occurrence during the illness.

The symptoms of cholera result from the protein toxin produced by *V. cholerae* that stimulates adenylate cyclase, resulting in increased levels of intracellular cyclic adenosine monophosphate (AMP), chloride secretion, and tremendous outpouring of fluids and electrolytes into the gut lumen. There is essentially no inflammation in the gut and the intestinal mucosal cells remain healthy, but the cholera toxin maximally stimulates their cyclic AMP system. Gm_1 ganglioside is the receptor on the surface of the mucosal cells for the toxin. High titers of antitoxin antibodies can neutralize the toxin by preventing the toxin from reaching its receptor.

Vibrio cholerae that are not serotype O1 or O139, as well as other vibrio species, may also cause diarrhea (as well as systemic infections) in individual patients but do not cause epidemic cholera.

The treatment of cholera includes rapid rehydration, correction of acidosis, replacement of potassium deficit, and antibiotics to shorten the illness and decrease overall purging volumes. Severely dehydrated cholera patients have become dehydrated rapidly, and most of the fluid deficit is from the circulating volume. Thus, intravenous fluids for these severely dehydrated patients need to be given rapidly (in <4 hours) in volumes of about 10% of the body weight to completely restore circulating volumes. Thus, a 50-kg patient will require 5 L in less than 4 hours. Slow or insufficient rehydration may lead to acute renal failure or other complications of shock. The most appropriate intravenous fluid is either lactated Ringer's or another polyelectrolyte solution (e.g., Dhaka solution) that includes a base to correct the acidosis as well as potassium to correct the potassium deficit.

Oral rehydration can be started as soon as the patient is able to drink, even while the intravenous fluids are being given. The best oral rehydration solution for cholera and other severely purging patients is one prepared with rice. Rice ORS is available commercially (CeraLyte), or it can be prepared with homemade ingredients. The electrolytes should be those conforming to the standard oral rehydration solution of the World Health Organization, which contains 90 mEq of sodium, 20 mEq of potassium, and 30 mEq of citrate.

Doxycycline and tetracycline* are the antibiotics of choice for adults, and trimethoprim-sulfamethoxazole (Bactrim) is preferred for children. Other antibiotics can be used for resistant strains.

ENTEROTOXIGENIC ESCHERICHIA COLI

This group of *E. coli* causes illness through the production of a heat-labile enterotoxin (LT) that is similar to cholera toxin, a heat-stable enterotoxin (ST), or both. Either of these toxins leads to secretion of fluid from the small intestine. Frequently, they also express specific colonization factor pili that allow them to colonize the small intestine. In general, the illness is less severe than cholera but individual patients may have an illness that is indistinguishable from cholera. These organisms are among the most common causes of childhood and infant diarrhea in the world and are the leading cause of traveler's diarrhea, but they occur rarely in industrialized countries, usually in the context of a food- or waterborne outbreak.

Treatment is focused on rehydration using the same guidelines as for other watery diarrhea. Antibiotics are not recommended for most cases in endemic settings. However, traveler's diarrhea caused by these organisms is shortened when effective antibiotics are used. The reason for recommending antibiotics for travelers and not for endemic disease in children is the high prevalence of the disease in children, and treatment with antibiotics is simply not practical and would lead to widespread antibiotic overuse.

OTHER FORMS OF E. COLI

Other forms of *E. coli* that may cause diarrheal illness include enteroaggregative *E. coli* (EAEC), enteroinvasive *E. coli* (EIEC), and enterohemorrhagic *E. coli* (EHEC). The EAEC are likely to be common causes of illness in certain areas, but their true importance is still being determined. Other than rehydration, no specific treatment is needed for this illness. The EIEC are very similar to *Shigella* in terms of the virulence properties and clinical illness, and patients with this infection should be managed as if they had shigellosis. The EHEC, which produce a Shiga-like toxin, are fast becoming a major public health problem, with outbreaks of foodborne illness. They can cause severe acute illness, often with severe bloody diarrhea, which may lead to hemolytic-uremic syndrome. The strains appear to be primarily associated with beef and cattle; however, many foods have been vehicles for the transmission of organisms. Risk of EHEC is a major reason to eat beef only if it is well cooked.

SHIGELLA

Shigellae are the organisms that most commonly cause dysentery, or bloody diarrhea, although they may also cause a watery diarrhea syndrome. The genus is divided into four species and multiple serotypes. *S. sonnei* is the most common one in industrialized countries, whereas *S. flexneri* is more common in developing countries. *S. dysenteriae* serotype O1 (Shiga bacillus) may occur in epidemics in developing countries, and these epidemics have become major public health emergencies because the disease is so severe, the strains are often resistant to usual antibiotics, and the disease spreads rapidly. *S. boydii* is generally less common, but the disease is similar to that caused by *S. flexneri*.

Patients with acute dysentery should be assumed to have shigellosis and should be treated accordingly, based on the local patterns of antibiotic sensitivities. Unfortunately, *Shigella* species are becoming increasingly resistant to formerly effective antibiotics. For sensitive strains, ampicillin* or trimethoprim-sulfamethoxazole is effective, but resistant strains will require other antibiotics, such as one of the new quinolones or pivmecillinam.† Nalidixic acid is useful for many strains, but *S. dysenteriae* is now frequently resistant to this drug as well.

CAMPYLOBACTER JEJUNI

Campylobacter jejuni, usually transmitted from poultry, is the most commonly isolated bacterial pathogen isolated in the United States from patients with diarrhea. It can cause either watery diarrhea or dysentery. A benefit from using antibiotics is not clear, especially if the start of treatment is delayed. Erythromycin is generally used if the treatment can begin within the first few days of the onset. Ten percent to 15% of healthy people in developing countries carry *Campylobacter* in their stools, so isolation of such a strain during illness does not necessarily mean that the bacterium is causing the illness in this setting. Occasionally, *Campylobacter* can lead to systemic illness with bacteremia, and these illnesses certainly require appropriate antibiotics according to sensitivity patterns.

Infection with *Campylobacter* has been associated with the subsequent development of Guillain-Barré syndrome. It is believed that certain strains express gangliosides that initiate an autoimmune disease through the process of molecular mimicry. Fortunately, this is a rare complication of *Campylobacter* infection.

SALMONELLA

Salmonella species are frequently associated with foodborne outbreaks and lead to acute diarrhea that is generally watery but may progress to dysentery. Treatment is with appropriate rehydration, but antibiotics are generally not needed except in complicated cases. Rarely, septicemia may occur.

CLOSTRIDIUM DIFFICILE

Clostridium difficile is an anaerobic organism that can produce an enterotoxin leading to colitis. It most commonly occurs after the use of an antibiotic that selects for this organism. This can become a severe infection, especially in the elderly and otherwise compromised hosts. Detection of

*Not FDA approved for this indication.

*Not FDA approved for this indication.
†Not available in the United States.

the toxin from stool specimens is important in detecting this infection. Treatment is with metronidazole (Flagyl), with vancomycin being used for patients who have failed on metronidazole.

REHYDRATION THERAPY

Patients with watery diarrhea lose excessive amounts of fluid. When the fluid loss is mild or moderate, the patient may feel weak and lethargic. When the fluid loss is severe, the condition becomes life threatening. Some illnesses start with mild fluid loss and mild dehydration, but as the illness continues the dehydration worsens. Diarrheal stool is isotonic but contains large amounts of electrolytes. With severe purging, major losses of sodium, bicarbonate, and potassium occur, and these need to be corrected by a rehydration solution that has an electrolyte content similar to the fluid that is lost.

Most patients will improve with oral solutions containing the proper mixture of salts and carbohydrate. Several studies have found complex carbohydrates (e.g., rice starch) to be more effective in severely purging patients and to reduce the purging rate. Although almost any fluid can be used with mild cases, the fluid loss from significant purging should be replaced with oral rehydration solution (e.g., Cera-Lyte, Pedialyte, Infalyte) that contains the proper concentrations of electrolytes and carbohydrates. Soft drinks, sports drinks, and many other commonly used fluids do not have the proper composition of salts, may have excess sugars, or may be hypertonic and are not acceptable for replacing significant loss from diarrhea.

Oral rehydration solution should be given in amounts to correct the fluid loss. A patient who is mildly dehydrated can be assumed to have lost about 5% of body weight, and this volume should be offered to correct the loss. Additional solution should then be given to make up for continuing losses until the illness subsides. If vomiting is a problem, the fluids can still generally be given in small, but frequent, volumes to replace the fluids needed. Additional water and other fluids should be given in addition to the oral rehydration solution to make up for normal physiologic fluid replacement.

With severe dehydration, more aggressive rehydration is needed with intravenous fluids, usually using lactated Ringer's. Saline can be used in an emergency if lactated Ringer's is not available. Patients with severe dehydration can be assumed to have lost about 10% of their body weight, and this loss needs to be corrected. Patients in shock need very rapid administration of fluids, within 1 to 4 hours. Administration of oral rehydration solution can begin as soon as the patient is able to drink to make up for ongoing stool losses. The use of a "cholera cot" can ease assessment of ongoing stool losses and can thus guide the volumes of rehydration fluids that are needed.

SYMPTOMATIC MANAGEMENT

Bismuth subsalicylate (Pepto-Bismol) and loperamide (Imodium) are often used, especially in traveler's diarrhea, to relieve some of the symptoms of diarrhea, but they do not correct the fluid loss nor restore electrolytes. A typical dose of bismuth subsalicylate is two tablets (or 1 tablespoon) every 6 to 8 hours. Patients should be warned that their stools will blacken and that they should avoid overdosing with salicylate. Loperamide is typically given as a 4-mg initial dose, followed by 2 mg every 6 hours until

TABLE 2. **Recommended Antibiotics for Use in Patients With Common Diarrhea Pathogens**

Syndrome	Antimicrobial	Adults	Children
Acute watery diarrhea with no complications		No antibiotic recommended	No antibiotic recommended
Cholera	Doxycycline, single dose	300 mg	Not recommended
	Tetracycline* qid for 3 days	500 mg per dose	12.5 mg/kg per dose
	Ciprofloxacin* bid for 3 days	500 mg per dose	Not recommended
	Trimethoprim-sulfamethoxazole bid for 3 days	TMP 160 mg and SMX 800 mg	TMP 5 mg/kg and SMX 25 mg/kg
Traveler's diarrhea	Ciprofloxacin* bid for up to 3 days	500 mg	Not recommended
	Trimethoprim-sulfamethoxazole bid for 3 days	TMP 160 mg and SMX 800 mg	TMP 5 mg/kg and SMX 25 mg/kg
Shigellosis	Ciprofloxacin* bid for 5 days	500 mg	Not recommended
	Trimethoprim-sulfamethoxazole* bid for 3 days	TMP 160 mg and SMX 800 mg	TMP 5 mg/kg and SMX 25 mg/kg
	Nalidixic acid* qid for 5 days	1 g	15 mg/kg
	Pivmecillinam† qid for 5 days	400 mg	12.5 mg/kg
Giardiasis	Metronidazole* tid for 5 days	250 mg	5 mg/kg
Cyclospora	Trimethoprim-sulfamethoxazole bid for 3 days	TMP 160 mg and SMX 800 mg	TMP 5 mg/kg and SMX 25 mg/kg
Rotavirus		No antibiotic recommended	No antibiotic recommended

*Not FDA approved for this indication.
†Not available in the United States.
Abbreviations: SMX = sulfamethoxazole; TMP = trimethoprim.

symptoms subside. Loperamide should not be given to children or to patients with dysentery.

ANTIMICROBIAL AGENTS

Antimicrobial agents are not needed for most cases of diarrhea but are indicated in a few conditions. These include cholera, shigellosis, severe traveler's diarrhea, *C. difficile* enterocolitis, amebiasis, giardiasis, and *Cyclospora* infection. Immunosuppressed patients may require specific antiviral agents depending on specific infections. A summary of the most common antimicrobial agents is found in Table 2.

CONSTIPATION

method of
KYLE P. ETZKORN, M.D.
Borland-Groover Clinic
Jacksonville, Florida

and

LORRAINE RODRIGUEZ, M.D.
Department of Obstetrics and Gynecology, Mayo Clinic
Jacksonville, Florida

Constipation is a common complaint of patients presenting to their primary care clinician. In the United States it has been estimated that approximately $400 million is spent annually on over-the-counter laxatives. In addition, numerous diagnostic studies and workups are performed every year in the evaluation of constipation, but the exact cost cannot be estimated. In general, most forms of constipation are idiopathic and have little long-term significance, although chronic constipation may have profound impact with respect to a patient's quality of life and can be associated with other disease states.

No true definition exists for constipation. In general, large population studies have suggested that with consumption of an adequate Western diet, at least three bowel movements per week are defined as the norm. *Constipation* thus can be defined as a frequency of defecation fewer than two times a week. In addition to frequency, patients often will complain of difficulty with straining or of change in pattern of bowel frequency and morphology of the stool. In normal subjects, daily stool patterns may vary considerably.

PHYSIOLOGY OF CONSTIPATION

Constipation primarily consists of delayed transit or disordered movement through a segment of the intestine, primarily localized to the colon. In general, constipation can be classified into idiopathic forms, which are noted in the majority of office visits, versus underlying physiologic causes. Several disease states are associated with constipation, including metabolic, endocrine, and neurologic disorders. Table 1 lists several causes of physiologic constipation in patients with systemic illnesses.

The most common endocrine cause of constipation is diabetes. Sixty percent of patients with diabetes may report constipation. In addition, constipation has been associated with hypothyroidism, but usually this is mild and will improve with thyroid replacement. Constipation has been associated with pregnancy and may be related to hormonal changes and the use of iron supplements. Numerous drugs are associated with constipation and should be excluded as a cause (Table 2).

Neurologic disorders have long been established as a cause of constipation. A classic model of this is Hirschsprung disease. In patients with this disease, there is an absence of the rectosphincteric inhibitory reflex. This is secondary to the absence of the intramural ganglion cells of both the submucosal and myenteric plexuses. These patients demonstrate a classic lack of internal anal sphincter relaxation with rectal distention, which can be proved by anorectal motility. Large-rectal biopsies of these patients demonstrate histologic findings with the absence of neurons. Classically, these patients are diagnosed in the first decade of life, but the disease can present in adults too.

Other neurologic causes of constipation may include injury to the lumbosacral spine, meningomyelocele, and spinal anesthesia.

IDIOPATHIC CONSTIPATION

By far, the majority of patients with constipation have the idiopathic type. As such, there is no obvious cause for their symptoms. In these patients, there is an absence of associated disease states or definitive pathophysiology.

Chronic constipation may be manifested in the pediatric population group. In general, when associated disease states have been excluded and chronic idiopathic constipation is diagnosed, the majority of these patients have underlying psychologic factors to be considered. Although behavioral problems may be associated with idiopathic constipation in the pediatric population group, this disorder cannot be confused with psychogenic constipation.

In adults, constipation in its severe form predominantly

TABLE 1. **Diseases Associated With Constipation**

Neurologic Causes
Hirschsprung disease
Chagas disease
Intestinal pseudo-obstruction
Autonomic neuropathy
Neurofibromatosis
Central Neurologic Causes
Multiple sclerosis
Spinal cord lesions
Parkinson disease
Trauma to nervi erigentes
Cerebrovascular disease
Metabolic and Endocrine Disorders
Diabetes mellitus
Hypothyroidism
Hypercalcemia
Hypocalcemia
Pregnancy
Panhypopituitarism
Collagen Vascular Muscle Disorders
Systemic sclerosis
Amyloidosis
Dermatomyositis
Myotonic dystrophy

Table 2. **Drugs That Cause Constipation**

Analgesics	Calcium
Opiates	Barium sulfate
Antihypertensives	Antidepressants
Anticonvulsants	Antipsychotics
Calcium channel blockers	Antiparkinson drugs
Iron supplements	Antispasmodics

occurs in women. Classically, constipation without abdominal pain or bloating differentiates idiopathic constipation from irritable bowel syndrome (IBS). Adults with constipation without features of IBS may complain of infrequent defecation and excessive straining and often will fail minimal therapeutic interventions.

Interestingly, when studied, patients who complain of constipation and who have been unresponsive to conventional therapeutic intervention, such as increasing fiber content, on colonic transit studies are shown to have normal colonic movement. The remaining patients, when studied, demonstrate true slow colonic transit and hence can be described as having colonic inertia. Patients with normal transit times but with complaints of constipation seem to have higher psychologic distress scores as compared with those patients with true colonic inertia, as demonstrated by delayed passage of radiopaque markers.

IRRITABLE BOWEL SYNDROME

As stated earlier, patients with true constipation symptoms must be separated from those with IBS. Patients with IBS classically will have complaints of constipation but with associated features and symptoms of abdominal pain and bloating. Additionally, one must consider other symptoms because patients with IBS may complain of dyspepsia and other generalized symptomatic complaints, which are nonspecific.

CONSTIPATION IN THE ELDERLY

Constipation in the elderly constitutes a real clinical challenge. Often these patients are less mobile and may be bedridden, exacerbating the possibility of constipation. Fecal impaction is often common in this patient population, and inspection for such must be undertaken. In addition, this population tends to abuse laxatives and may be taking numerous medications that can cause or exacerbate constipation.

EVALUATION OF CONSTIPATION

In a patient complaining of constipation, one must first exclude IBS. With such, further questioning must be directed at excluding other associated disease states as causing physiologic constipation. A review of the patient's medical history is a must, as is a thorough review of all prescribed and over-the-counter medication use. Questions should be directed to ascertain whether this is new in onset or present since birth. If present since birth, this may suggest a congenital cause of constipation versus a new physiologic or idiopathic process. Questions about bleeding from the rectum or pain with defection should be asked because this may suggest a structural or mucosal process. In addition, abdominal pain and bloating in association with constipation is important to differentiate true idiopathic constipation from IBS.

Physical Examination

Physical examination should be directed at excluding systemic disease causes of constipation. This includes a detailed neurologic examination, using pinprick of the perianal area to elicit the "anal wink" and digital examination to access rectal tone. A close inspection of the anorectal region should be performed along with digital examination to exclude the presence of pain, which would suggest anal fissure.

Diagnostic Studies

Barium enema may help identify patients with megacolon and Hirschsprung disease. Flexible sigmoidoscopy may help detect lower colonic neoplasms, obstructive lesions, and evidence of chronic laxative abuse. Chronic laxative abuse characteristically can be seen by mucosal changes with a black discoloration known as *melanosis coli.*

Colonic transit studies may be helpful in patients with severe constipation to exclude those with normal colonic transit. Classically, ingested radiopaque markers are used in patients with a high-fiber diet. Then abdominal radiologic studies are performed serially over the next 3 days. The majority of normal patients will pass these markers within 70 hours of oral consumption. Presence of markers beyond 3 days may suggest colonic inertia.

Anorectal manometry is the technique of measuring anal sphincter tone with a manometry catheter placed into the anus. This study may have value in differentiating patients with Hirschsprung disease from those with other neurologic defects. *Defecography* is a technique in which barium is instilled into the rectum and, under fluoroscopy, evacuation is observed by a trained expert. Defecography may have value in patients with complaints of excessive straining during defecation; however, its usefulness is limited by the need for technical and interpretive expertise.

Diagnostic Workup

The majority of patients who present with complaints of constipation need not have a significant diagnostic workup. Once IBS and systemic causes such as diabetes, hypothyroidism, and neurologic causes have been excluded, an attempt at manipulation of the diet may be all that is needed. In addition, a review of all medications and an attempt at eliminating ones that can cause constipation must be considered.

Once other causes of constipation are excluded in patients with severe constipation, in whom simple dietary measures have not resulted in significant improvement, there may be value in further diagnostic workup. In patients who fail conventional pharmacotherapy such as increasing daily fiber intake, a colonic transit study with radiolucent markers may have value, differentiating those patients with true colonic inertia from those with normal colonic movement. In patients with normal studies, this may serve as a reassurance to both the patient and the physician. Unfortunately, in patients with true colonic inertia, as demonstrated by delayed transit of radiolucent markers, dietary manipulations have a poor response. These patients probably should undergo anorectal manometry to exclude sensorimotor causes and imaging of their colon with barium enema and flexible sigmoidoscopy.

TREATMENT

Dietary manipulations are the first step in treating patients with chronic constipation. In general, we first recommend increasing fiber content, to between 20 and 30 g of dietary fiber per day. The use of fiber and the way it alleviates symptoms of constipation have less to do with water retention and more to do with mechanical factors such as the bulking effects of fiber with respect to colonic microbial ecology and the interaction with intraluminal content.

Fiber content in food varies greatly. In patients with severe idiopathic constipation, behavioral approaches may have benefit. This practice is often attempted in children with idiopathic constipation. Behavioral modification is centered on achieving regular evacuations on a scheduled basis in an attempt to eliminate the accumulation and buildup of stool.

Pharmacologic Therapy

Unfortunately, the majority of patients self-medicate with over-the-counter laxatives. Before the initiation of pharmacologic intervention, the clinician must ensure that fecal impaction is not present, and if it is present, it must be cleared. Once impaction is cleared, enemas may have a role. We usually recommend starting with either saline or phosphate (Fleet) enemas, although phosphate enemas should be avoided in patients with renal disease. Mineral oil enemas may be used in more difficult cases, and soapsuds enemas should be avoided.

Laxatives can be considered in patients with more chronic constipation. Laxatives are essentially divided into five major categories: stimulant laxatives, bulk-forming laxatives such as fiber, emollient laxatives, hyperosmolar laxatives, and saline laxatives (Table 3).

Stimulant laxatives are of the most concern for the clinician because their long-term use can render the patient dependent on them, both physiologically and psychologically. Stimulant laxatives include cascara sagrada and bisacodyl-based laxatives and sennosides (e.g., Dulcolax, Ex-Lax). The cascara sagrada laxatives increase fluid electrolyte accumulation in the distal ileum and colon through unknown actions. Phenolphthalein laxatives are stored primarily in the small intestine and undergo an intrahepatic circulation, which may explain their long duration of action.

TABLE 3. **Laxatives for the Treatment of Constipation**

Laxative Class	Recommendation for Adults
Emollient	Docusate (Colace), 50–200 mg/d in divided doses
Fiber	Psyllium (Metamucil), 20–30 g/d
Hyperosmolar agents	70% Sorbitol, 15–45 mL/d
Lavage solutions	Polyethylene glycol–electrolyte solution (GoLYTELY), 250–500 mL/d
Lubricants	Mineral oil, 15–45 mL/d
Saline cathartics	Milk of magnesia, 15–45 mL qhs
Stimulant cathartics	Bisacodyl (Dulcolax), two to four 5-mg tablets qhs

These directly stimulate colonic motor physiology and inhibit the colon's glucose and sodium absorption to increase intraluminal fluid content. In general, we avoid using this class of laxatives.

Bulk-forming laxatives are composed of mostly natural polysaccharides, synthetic polysaccharides, or cellulose derivatives. For their maximum effect, increased water is recommended. Hence, they are somewhat contraindicated in patients on fluid restriction diets. These agents come in a variety of forms as either a powder (Metamucil), biscuit (Metamucil wafer), or tablet (FiberCon). In addition, some tube feeding preparation may have added fiber. These agents are generally safe and well tolerated; minor side effects of bloating and flatulence have been reported, but with continued use, most of these complaints pass. Care should be taken not to use these agents in patients with bowel strictures or obstructions.

Emollient laxatives consist primarily of mineral oil and docusate sodium. Mineral oil may decrease absorption of fat-soluble vitamins A, D, and K. Mineral oil should be administered between meals, and it should be avoided in patients at risk for aspiration because it can cause potentially fatal lipid pneumonia. Docusate sodium (Colace) lowers the surface tension of stool, which subsequently allows the mixing of aqueous and fatty substances, softening stool and permitting easier defecation. In addition, docusate sodium stimulates fluid and electrolyte secretion.

Hyperosmolar agents include polyethylene glycol–electrolyte solution (GoLYTELY) and nonabsorbable sugars such as lactulose and sorbitol. In general, these agents are well tolerated but may have side effects of bloating and flatulence. They can be used on a chronic basis.

Saline laxatives (e.g., milk of magnesia, magnesium citrate) contain nonabsorbable cations and anions that exert an osmotic effect to increase intraluminal water content. These agents should not be used in patients with renal disease or congestive heart failure and should be avoided for chronic use.

Prokinetic agents such as erythromycin,* cisapride (Propulsid),† and metoclopramide (Reglan)* have been used to some extent in helping patients with chronic constipation. None is FDA approved for constipation, and cisapride was recently taken off the United States market.

In general, we start with fiber. If fiber is not successful, we proceed to either a lavage solution or hyperosmolar agent. We avoid stimulant and saline cathartics. In some patients in whom pharmacotherapy and dietary intervention have little success, alternative treatment may include biofeedback training; and in the most severe forms of symptomatic idiopathic constipation, surgery may be contemplated. Surgery can only be contemplated after a thorough workup has excluded other causes of constipation.

*Not FDA approved for this indication.
†Not available in the United States. Taken off the market.

FEVER

method of
MARY JO WELKER, M.D.
Ohio State University
Columbus, Ohio

Fever is common and can be a manifestation of infectious, inflammatory, or malignant disease. It is one of the most common reasons that patients seek medical attention because most patients understand that fever can be the manifestation of significant underlying illness.

DEFINITION

Fever is an elevation in body temperature above normal circadian variation as a result of a change in the thermoregulatory center located in the hypothalamus. Normal body temperature is maintained because the thermoregulatory center balances heat production in the tissues with heat loss. However, when a patient is febrile, the regulatory center has shifted to increase body temperature with increased heat production and decreased peripheral loss. In contrast, hyperthermia is an elevation of body temperature above the hypothalamic setpoint due to insufficient heat dissipation, for example, from exercise or medication.

Although we have been taught that a "normal" temperature is 37°C (98.6°F), the normal temperature for individuals actually spans a range of 36.8° ± 0.4°C (98.2° ± 0.7°F). There is a circadian variation, with the lowest temperatures around 6 AM and the highest around 4 PM. A morning temperature above 37.2°C (98.9°F) and an afternoon temperature above 37.7°C (99.9°F) would be considered a fever.

MEASUREMENT OF FEVER

In recent years, a variety of ways to measure temperature have been explored. Glass mercury thermometers remain the gold standard for evaluation of temperature. However, many patients are unable to read them, and concerns about the dangers of mercury have forced physicians and patients to look for other methods of measurement.

Electronic oral and digital thermometers are now popular. They are generally easy to read and accurate. More recently, TempaDOT strips have also come into use. Infrared ear thermometers have also become popular because they are quick and easy to use. However, their use is controversial because they must be aimed directly at the eardrum and they can also be affected by cerumen. Skin and forehead measurements may be convenient and safe but are not as accurate.

Measurements of temperature with glass thermometers can be done in three sites: sublingual, rectal, and axilla. Sublingual temperatures must be taken with the instrument held under the tongue without biting it and with the lips closed in a kissing fashion. This is difficult for children younger than age 6 years and for elderly individuals. Sublingual temperatures can be unreliable if the patient is mouth breathing or has recently drunk a hot or cold beverage. Rectal temperatures best reflect core temperatures and are preferred to accurately measure temperatures in young children. The axillary site is used in older children and adults as necessary. The thermometer needs to remain in position for 3 to 5 minutes and be allowed to reach a steady state for the reading to be accurate.

CAUSES OF FEVER

Fever is a result of a complex physiologic reaction that results in a cascade of events that produce elevation in body temperature. Pyrogens initiate this reaction. These may be *exogenous pyrogens,* from outside the host, or *endogenous pyrogens,* from inside the host.

Examples of exogenous pyrogens include microorganisms and their products or toxins, drugs in some individuals, and incompatible blood products. Exogenous pyrogens produce fever by activating the endogenous pyrogens. *Endogenous pyrogens* are polypeptides produced by host cells, usually monocytes or macrophages, and examples include interleukin 1 (both α and β), interferon (both α and β), and tumor necrosis factor. The endogenous pyrogens increase the synthesis of prostaglandins in the brain, which then activate the thermoregulatory neurons and increase the setpoint in the hypothalamus. This increase in the setpoint generates reactions in the vasomotor center that increase heat conservation and heat production and cause fever.

CONSEQUENCES OF FEVER

It is known that the growth and virulence of some microorganisms are impaired with fever, and fever has been used in the past to treat certain infections. Some studies have also shown that fever appears to increase the phagocytic effect and bactericidal activity of neutrophils and the cytotoxic effects of lymphocytes. In short, fever probably increases the ability to survive infection.

However, discomfort and other symptoms are a problem for patients. There are increased oxygen consumption, increased caloric requirements, and increased fluid requirements, which can result in weight loss and a negative nitrogen balance. When a pregnant woman has a fever, this increased metabolic demand may cause stress for the fetus during pregnancy and can be teratogenic for the growing fetus during the first trimester. The increased metabolic demand is also stressful for patients with heart disease, lung disease, central nervous system disease, or metabolic disorders.

Fever reduces mental acuity and can produce delirium, stupor, and seizures. It produces tachycardia, increased respiratory rate, and widened pulse pressures. It also causes back pain, generalized myalgia, arthralgia, anorexia, headache, and somnolence. Also distressing are the chills (and sometimes rigor) and sweats that accompany the changes in temperature.

DIFFERENTIAL DIAGNOSIS OF FEVER

Fever can be caused by a variety of illnesses, the most common being infection from organisms that include viruses, bacteria, mycobacteria, fungi, *Rickettsia, Mycoplasma, Chlamydia,* and parasites. Also included in the differential diagnosis are neoplasms, collagen vascular diseases, granulomatous diseases, inherited and metabolic diseases, thermoregulatory disorders, and other miscellaneous diagnoses, including factitious fever.

EVALUATION OF FEVER

The history is an essential part of the evaluation of any patient with fever. The patient's age and the risks related to the fever must be considered. Chronology of symptoms and information about medications taken, including over-the-counter drugs and home remedies, should be detailed. Any pattern to the fever—sustained, intermittent, relapsing—may be important to note. Information about the patient's general health, recent dental or surgical procedures, prosthetic devices, previous illnesses or trauma, transfusions, or immunizations must be elicited. Special attention must be paid to immunocompromised patients. Dietary history about the use of raw or poorly cooked foods or the use of alcohol or other drugs is important. A sexual history is essential, and information about travel, exposure to other people, materials, infectious agents, ticks, and household pets can be helpful. Associated symptoms such as nausea, vomiting, diarrhea, abdominal pain, problems with urination, weight loss, joint pain, or other pain should be part of the review of systems. Finally, family history can also be important for inherited causes of fever.

A complete physical examination is required and may need to be repeated at intervals to determine the cause of the fever. All vital signs are important because patients with fever usually have tachycardia, an increased respiratory rate, and a widened pulse pressure. It is also essential to determine that a fever is present and the extent of the temperature elevation. Skin should be examined to determine any rash, swelling, petechiae, or other lesions. Nail beds should be examined, along with the musculoskeletal system and joints. Eyes, ears, nasal passages and sinuses, and mouth should be examined for any evidence of infection. Lymph nodes in all areas should be palpated. The cardiovascular system, the chest, and the abdomen should be considered carefully as sources of infection. The nervous system should be evaluated for signs of change. A rectal and genital examination should not be overlooked because these areas can be significant sources of infection and fever.

The timing and extent of laboratory data depend on illness severity, diagnostic considerations from the history and physical examination, and immune status. In most cases, the fever is self-limited and little is needed in terms of diagnostic workup. However, if the fever is excessively high or persists for more than a few days, evaluation is necessary. And, if the fever persists for more than 2 weeks, it is considered a fever of unknown origin and will need more extensive testing.

Consider taking a complete blood cell count with a white cell differential in patients with significant or persistent fever. Also consider conducting a urinalysis and an erythrocyte sedimentation rate. Cultures should be done as indicated and may include urine, stool, blood, sputum, and any abnormal fluid or wound. Stool evaluation may also be helpful. Liver function testing may be indicated in some individuals, as well as radiology evaluation as appropriate. More extensive testing is indicated for evaluation of fever of unknown origin and is outside the scope of this article.

TREATMENT

First, differentiate fever from hyperthermia because the treatment of hyperthermia and urgency with which it must be treated is very different from treatment of fever. Then, identify and treat the underlying cause of the fever, if possible.

With hyperpyrexia (fever >41°C [105.8°F]), treatment is indicated and may help to speed the process of resetting the hypothalamic setpoint. Medications are also important in controlling the constitutional symptoms that accompany these fevers and may be helpful because of their analgesic effect as much as their antipyretic effect.

Although elevations in temperature often generate fear and anxiety, with moderate fevers there is little evidence that fever is harmful or that treatment of fever is beneficial. Exceptions might include pregnant women, patients with a history of seizures, and patients with impaired cardiac, pulmonary, or cerebral function. However, treatment of fever does not alter the course of the disease nor does treatment help to make a diagnosis. In fact, treatment can mask the inflammatory features and obscure the important clinical information to be gained by monitoring the upward and downward course of a temperature.

In general, medications control fever in proportion to their ability to inhibit prostaglandin synthesis in the brain. Common medications used for the treatment of fever include aspirin, acetaminophen, and ibuprofen. The first drug to be considered is acetaminophen, which can be given orally or rectally and has an excellent safety record. Ibuprofen is an equally effective alternative, although it appears to have more side effects. Both products come in pills and liquids with varying strength. I recommend using the dosage charts for children. Adult dose is one to two tablets every 4 hours to a maximum of 4000 mg per day of acetaminophen and 3200 mg per day of ibuprofen. Because of the concerns about Reye's syndrome and the greater potential for toxicity, aspirin is not appropriate for use in children and is not usually used as a first-line agent in adults. It may be contraindicated in patients who are allergic to salicylates; who have gastrointestinal upset and/or peptic ulcers, asthma, or bleeding tendencies; or who are on anticoagulant therapy. It is dosed in a manner similar to acetaminophen.

Physical methods may be necessary and justifiable as an adjunct to pharmacologic means of reducing fever, especially in critical situations, and include tepid water sponge baths and cooling ice water packs. Ice water immersion or enemas are not safe and should not be used.

CONCLUSION

Patients with fever and their families should be educated to view fever as a self-limited process that rarely causes harm and appears to be a normal response to infection. They can be encouraged to cope with fever by monitoring its occurrence and using over-the-counter medication for comfort. This can be especially true in children because a child with a normal temperature is more pleasant and will eat and drink more readily than a febrile child. Patients should be given instructions about when to contact their physician about persistent fever and other signs of illness.

COUGH

method of
RAYMOND HADDAD, M.D.
Bridgeport Hospital
Bridgeport, Connecticut

Cough is a normal host defense and protective reflex aimed at clearing the airways and protecting the respiratory tract from excessive secretions or inhaled foreign particles. It is also a common manifestation of respiratory and nonrespiratory disorders that cause significant morbidity, which is one of the most common reasons why patients seek medical attention in the ambulatory setting. Whether cough is a manifestation of a minor illness, such as the common cold, or of a more serious disorder, it can be annoying to the afflicted individual, interfering with work, recreation, sleep, and social interactions.

Cough is initiated by stimulation of receptors located in the epithelium of the upper or lower respiratory tract and in the pericardium, esophagus, diaphragm, pleura, and stomach. These receptors are classified as *mechanical* (stimulated by triggers such as touch or displacement), *chemical* (sensitive to noxious gases or fumes), or *irritant* (responsive to both mechanical and chemical stimuli). Different nerves travel from these receptors to a cough center in the medulla: the *trigeminal nerve* carries impulses from the nose and sinuses; the *glossopharyngeal nerve* from the posterior pharynx; the *phrenic nerves* from the pericardium or diaphragm; and the *vagus nerve* from the larynx, tracheobronchial tree, esophagus, stomach, pleura, and ears.

The cough reflex is completed by efferent nerves carrying outputs from the cough center to the expiratory muscles. These outputs are carried by way of the spinal motor nerves to the diaphragm via the phrenic nerves and finally by the vagus nerve, whose efferents supply the tracheobronchial tree. Inputs from higher cortical centers may be present, which explains why coughs may be involuntarily initiated or transiently suppressed.

Stimulation of the cough reflex results in a deep inspiration with subsequent glottic closure, an increase in pleural and airway pressures, then an opening of the glottis to release that pressure. This process generates high flow rates and shearing forces that help clear the airways of irritants and secretions.

DIAGNOSIS

A rational therapy for cough requires a diagnosis of the underlying cause and a determination of whether the cough is a manifestation of an acute or a chronic process. A targeted history and physical examination (H&P) usually enables one to identify a probable etiology, direct the workup, and ultimately plan the therapy (Table 1). The mode of onset, character, timing, and duration of the cough as well as associated respiratory or systemic symptoms should be noted. Additional data should include a history of cigarette smoking, allergies, workplace exposures, and medication usage, especially angiotensin-converting enzyme (ACE) inhibitors or β-blockers. Table 2 lists some common causes of cough and their associated clinical clues and symptoms.

Although a duration of fewer than 3 weeks is often chosen to define an acute cough, it may persist as long as 8 weeks if it is related to a viral respiratory tract infection. Therefore, it may be advisable to withhold a complete workup unless other causes are also suspected from the H&P. Similarly, testing can be delayed in patients thought to have an ACE inhibitor–related cough until the response to discontinuation of the drug for 4 weeks is assessed.

Cigarette smoking and chronic bronchitis (CB) are common causes of chronic cough; however, it is unusual for affected individuals to complain or to be aware enough of the cough to seek medical attention because they may consider it to be normal. Therefore, when such patients

TABLE 1. **Evaluation of Chronic Cough**

History

Onset, duration, frequency
Factors causing exacerbations or remission
Associated symptoms (see Table 2)
Allergies, seasonal changes
Medication use, especially angiotensin-converting enzyme inhibitors and β-blockers, oral or topical
Environmental causes: tobacco smoke, inhalation of fumes, or inhalation of particles associated with work or hobbies

Physical

Thorough upper respiratory tract and chest examination
Pulsus paradoxus
Changes in neck veins, tracheal shift, adenopathy
Careful cardiac examination (possible occult mitral stenosis)

Other

Chest radiograph
Pulmonary function studies with or without bronchoprovocation if asthma is suspected
Imaging of sinuses if sinusitis is likely
Upper gastrointestinal series/24-hour esophageal pH monitoring if gastroesophageal reflux disease is a possibility
Fiberoptic bronchoscopy, chest computed tomography when a lower respiratory tract cause is suspected

TABLE 2. **Causes Associated With Various Signs and Symptoms**

Clues	Causes
Acute cough*	Upper and lower respiratory tract infections (laryngitis, pneumonia, tracheobronchitis), irritants (environmental, occupational)†
Nocturnal cough	Asthma, gastroesophageal reflux, early congestive heart failure, rhinosinusitis, bronchitis
Sputum	Smoking, chronic bronchitis, respiratory infections
Putrid sputum	Lung abscess, bronchiectasis
Bronchorrhea	Pulmonary edema, alveolar cell cancer
Hemoptysis	Lung cancer, tuberculosis, bronchiectasis, bronchitis
Wheezing	Airway obstruction caused by asthma, chronic obstructive pulmonary disease, foreign body, endobronchial tumor
Crackles	Congestive heart failure, interstitial lung disease, pneumonia
Stridor	Vocal cord dysfunction, laryngeal tumor
Dry cough	Drug-related causes, sarcoidosis, pulmonary fibrosis, tumor, mechanical pressure (aortic aneurysm), interstitial lung disease, psychogenic causes
Fever	Infections (bacterial, mycobacterial, viral, fungal)
Weight loss	Malignancies (lung, mediastinal tumor, metastatic), tuberculosis

*3 weeks.
†Cause chronic cough with prolonged exposure.

are seen for a medical evaluation, they should undergo a thorough workup to exclude other conditions, specifically lung cancer. Several investigators have shown in multiple studies that postnasal drip (PND), asthma, gastroesophageal reflux disease (GERD), and CB, acting individually or in concert, are the most common causes of chronic cough. Hence, unless the H&P directs one to suspect other causes, ancillary testing and empiric therapy should be directed at those conditions, bearing in mind that a positive test does not always predict a favorable response to treatment.

In nonsmokers, PND is the most common cause of an "unexplained" chronic cough, even when throat clearing and nasal or sinus congestion are absent. PND is related to various rhinosinus disorders such as sinusitis, allergic or nonallergic rhinitis, vasomotor rhinitis, or postinfectious rhinitis. An allergy evaluation and four-way view of the sinuses or computed tomography may help identify the underlying cause. However, there is no definite objective test for PND; therefore, cough resolution with a therapeutic trial of an antihistamine (H_1 antagonist) and decongestant is considered diagnostic.

Asthma can present as a nonseasonal, paroxysmal nonproductive cough without wheezing or dyspnea and with a normal spirometry. Bronchoprovocation with methacholine to assess airway hyper-responsiveness is useful in that setting. A positive challenge test is consistent with asthma but does not necessarily mean it is the cause of the cough, unless the cough resolves with specific treatment for asthma.

Cough may be the only manifestation of some patients with GERD, and it is thought to be vagally mediated by an esophagotracheal-bronchial reflex. Barium studies or upper endoscopy may be required when the cough persists after appropriate therapy and when the 24-hour distal esophageal pH monitoring is nondiagnostic. In some studies, cough was the cause of GERD if the patient was a nonsmoker, was not taking ACE inhibitors, had a normal chest radiograph (CXR), and failed therapy for PND or asthma.

A CXR should be obtained early in the workup of all patients with chronic cough in whom the H&P does not provide a plausible cause, especially if a therapeutic trial for a suspected etiology is failing. The CXR can be considered an extension of the physical examination and will help to narrow the differential diagnosis, thereby directing further testing. After the evaluation for chronic cough based on a sequential diagnostic anatomic approach (Figure 1) fails to establish a cause and the patient has not responded to various therapies, one may consider bronchoscopy, computed tomographic scan of the chest, and noninvasive cardiac studies. In general, bronchoscopy has a low diagnostic yield in the assessment of chronic cough unless the CXR is abnormal or an endobronchial lesion is present.

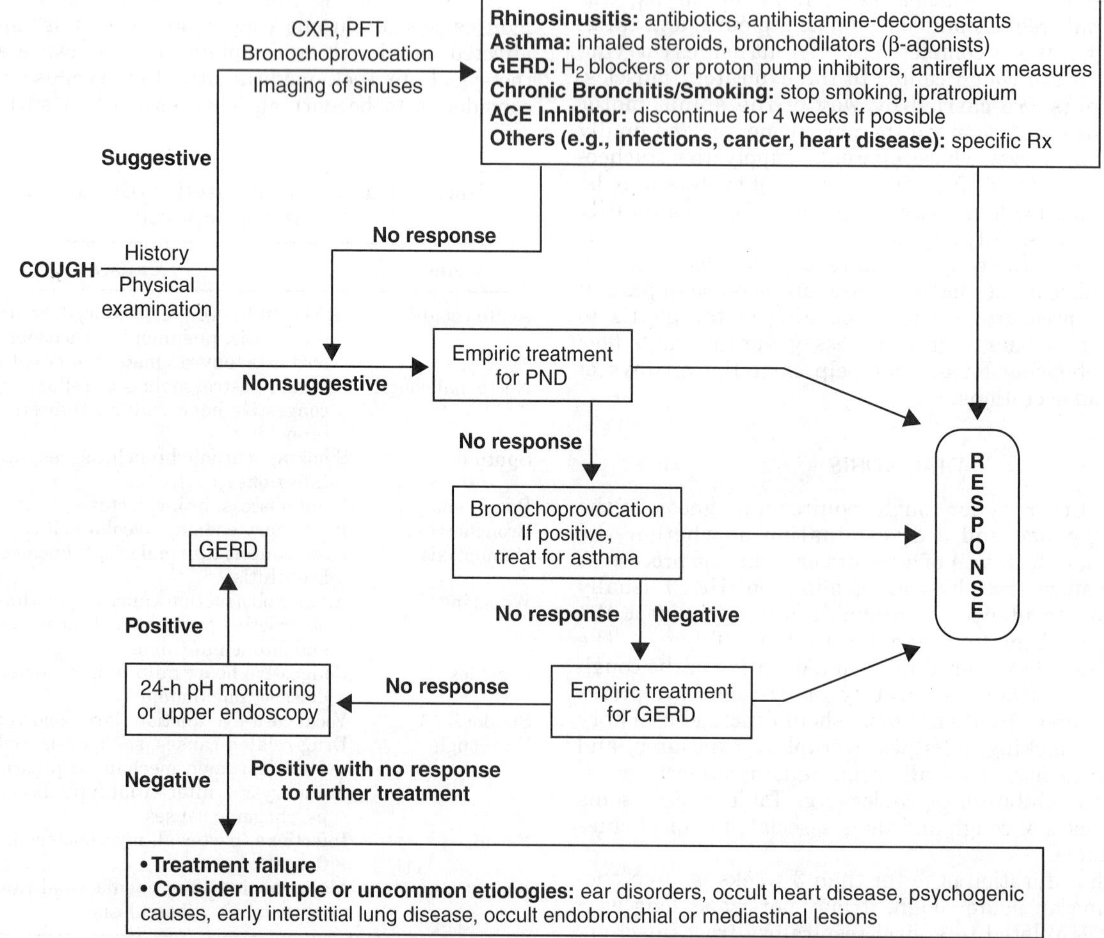

Figure 1. Evaluation of chronic cough in adults. *Abbreviations:* ACE = angiotensin-converting enzyme; CXR = chest radiograph; GERD = gastroesophageal reflux disease; PFT = pulmonary function test; PND = postnasal drip.

TREATMENT OF ACUTE COUGH

The cause of acute cough is most often a viral upper respiratory tract infection (URTI) triggering an inflammation of the airways. In this case, it is a self-limited illness alleviated by simple measures such as demulcents, tea with honey, chicken soup, or menthol-flavored candies, all of which soothe irritated receptors in the oropharynx. When viral rhinosinusitis is accompanied by significant nasal congestion it can lead to PND and cough. Oral decongestants or combination of an older generation H_1 with a decongestant are useful. Examples include pseudoephedrine (Sudafed) 60 mg every 6 hours; dexbrompheniramine maleate (6 mg) with pseudoephedrine (120 mg) (Drixoral Cold & Allergy) every 12 hours; a combination of chlorpheniramine maleate and pseudoephedrine (Chlor-Trimeton 4 or 12 Hour Relief), available in short- and long-acting preparations; and azatadine maleate (1 mg) with pseudoephedrine (120 mg) (Trinalin) every 12 hours.

If a bacterial rhinosinusitis complicates the course of the condition, an appropriate antibiotic is added to provide coverage for *Haemophilus influenzae, Streptococcus pneumoniae,* and *Moraxella.* Agents such as cefuroxime axetil (Ceftin), 250 to 500 mg every 12 hours, or amoxicillin/clavulanate (Augmentin), 875 mg every 12 hours, are effective. In cases of prolonged cough post-URTI, ipratropium bromide (Atrovent) administered by a metered-dose inhaler (MDI) four times a day has been effective.

Caution: The FDA recently issued a recall of products containing phenylpropanolamine, an active ingredient in many over-the-counter decongestant-cough suppressant products.

TREATMENT OF CHRONIC COUGH

Before deciding whether to treat a cough, always consider the risks and benefits of suppressing a cough that may have a beneficial effect in terms of host defenses. However, in most patients with chronic cough, it is such an annoying and disabling symptom that treatment must be initiated, particularly when an underlying cause is found and can be remedied. Figure 1 highlights the major therapeutic strategies for the most common disorders associated with chronic cough.

In PND secondary to nonallergic rhinitis, a combination of sedating antihistamine and decongestant, mentioned earlier, is frequently effective. If the side effects are not well tolerated, use of nonsedating agents with or without intranasal corticosteroid is initiated. Intranasal corticosteroids include beclomethasone 0.084% or 0.042% (Vancenase AQ, Beconase AQ), fluticasone 50 μg/dose (Flonase), and many others. Nonsedating antihistamines with or without pseudoephedrine are especially effective in allergic rhinitis. They include cetirizine (Zyrtec) 5 to 10 mg daily; loratadine (Claritin) 10 mg daily; loratadine with 120 or 240 mg of pseudoephedrine (Claritin-D, Claritin-D 12 Hour, and Claritin-D 24 Hour); fexofenadine (Allegra) 60 mg; and fexofenadine 60 mg with 120 mg of pseudoephedrine (Allegra-D) (Table 3). When chronic suppurative sinusitis is present, antibiotic therapy for as long as 6 weeks may be necessary to prevent relapses.

The mainstay of asthma-related cough consists of inhaled anti-inflammatory agents (corticosteroids), and β-agonists. Multiple preparations are available including beclomethasone (Beclovent), flunisolide (AeroBid), triamcinolone acetonide (Azmacort), flucitasone, and budesonide (Pulmicort). These preparations are supplied in different strengths and usually administered two to four times a day depending on whether it is a short- or long-acting preparation. Albuterol (Proventil, Ventolin) is the most commonly used β-agonist/bronchodilator, given by MDI, four to six times a day as needed. A long-acting preparation such as salmeterol (Serevent) can also be administered by MDI every 12 hours. If this approach fails to lessen the cough, another cause should be considered.

Unlike PND and cough-variant asthma, the response to therapy for cough due to GERD may be delayed as long as 3 to 6 months, particularly if submaximal therapy is used. In addition to taking antacids, H_2 blockers [ranitidine (Zantac), famotidine (Pepcid)], or proton pump inhibitors, [omeprazole (Prilosec), lansoprazole (Prevacid)], patients must adhere to a strict antireflux regimen that includes a high-protein, low-fat diet, elimination of acidic foods and beverages (caffeine), avoidance of meals for 3 hours before bedtime, elevation of the head of the bed, and cessation of smoking. At times, prokinetic therapy with metoclopramide (Reglan) or surgery may be required.

The treatment of cough related to CB due to smoking is tobacco abstinence, which usually results in cough resolution within 4 to 6 weeks. The patient may require a nicotine preparation to suppress the physical symptoms of nicotine withdrawal such as nicotine gum (Nicorette) or patch (Nicoderm CQ). Bupropion (Zyban) and patient education may also be required to achieve abstinence. In patients who remain symptomatic and have airflow limitation, the addition of inhaled ipratropium bromide is useful. Episodes of acute bronchitis or exacerbations of chronic obstructive pulmonary disease will require a short course of oral corticosteroids (40–60 mg of prednisone for 2 weeks) and antibiotics.

NONSPECIFIC THERAPY FOR CHRONIC COUGH

Nonspecific therapy for chronic cough is directed at the symptom rather than the underlying cause. It is considered when cough causes significant morbidity, when the etiology remains elusive, and when specific therapy is noncurative (e.g., unresectable lung cancer, inoperable large aortic aneurysm, and mesothelioma.)

Symptomatic nonspecific cough products can be classified as antitussive or protussive, based on their

TABLE 3. **Nonspecific Therapy for Cough**

Classification	Drug	Dosage	Remarks/Precautions
Protussive			
Expectorant	Guaifenesin (Robitussin)	200–400 mg q 4 h PO	?Effective only at its maximal recommended dosage
Mucolytic	Acetylcysteine (Mucomyst)*	2–3 mL 10% solution NEB	Restricted for in-hospital use
	Dornase alfa (Pulmozyme)*	2.5 mg 12–24 h NEB	Useful in cystic fibrosis
Antitussive			
Afferent limb	Benzonatate (Tessalon)	100 mg q 4–8 h PO	May cause local anesthesia and impair swallowing if chewed
	Lidocaine (Xylocaine)*	3 mL of 4% solution NEB 3–4 times a day	Restricted for procedures (e.g., bronchoscopy) and rarely for intractable cough; systemic toxicity possible
Cough center	NARCOTIC		
	Codeine	10–20 mg q 4–6 h PO	Adverse effects are uncommon with the recommended doses
	Hydrocodone (Hycodan)	5 mg q 4–6 h PO	Higher potency, less constipation, greater addiction potential than codeine
	NON-NARCOTIC		
	Dextromethorphan	10–30 mg q 4–8 h PO	Contraindicated in patients on MAOIs; no narcotic effects
	Diphenhydramine (Benadryl Allergy)	25 mg q 4–6 h PO	The only H_1 antagonist recommended as an antitussive
Efferent limb	Ipratropium (Atrovent)	2–3 puffs q 6 h MDI	Most effective for COPD
Sympathomimetic Decongestant	Pseudoephedrine	60 mg q 4–6 h PO	No hypertensive response at 15–30 mg doses
	Oxymetazoline	2–3 nasal sprays q 12 h	Will cause rebound nasal congestion if used for >4 days
	Phenylephrine	2–3 nasal sprays q 3–4 h	
H_1 Antagonist			
First generation	Chlorpheniramine with pseudoephedrine (Chlor-Trimeton 4 Hour Relief)	4 mg q 4–6 h PO	May produce somnolence
	Dexbrompheniramine with pseudoephedrine (Drixoral Cold and Allergy)	6 mg q 12 h PO	
	Azatidine maleate with pseudoephedrine (Trinalin)	1 mg q 12 h PO	
Second generation	Fexofenadine* (Allegra)†	60 mg q 12 h PO	
	Loratadine (Claritin)*†	10 mg q 24 h PO	No changes in QTc on ECG; drug-drug interaction not yet completely excluded
	Cetirizine (Zyrtec)†	5–10 mg q 24 h PO	

*Not FDA approved for this indication.
†Also available as "D" form with pseudoephedrine.
Abbreviations: COPD = chronic obstructive pulmonary disease; ECG = electrocardiogram; MAOI = monoamine oxidase inhibitor; MDI = metered-dose inhaler; NEB = nebulizer; PO = orally; QTc = corrected QT interval.

mode of action. They are also used as part of the armamentarium of specific therapy, discussed previously. Antitussive agents can act centrally on the cough center and can be either narcotic (codeine, hydrocodone) or non-narcotic (dextromethorphan [Delsym], diphenhydramine [Benadryl]). Some act on the afferent limb of the cough reflex, such as oral benzonatate (Tessalon), inhaled lidocaine (Xylocaine 10% Oral),* or oral naproxen (Anaprox).* Ipratropium bromide–MDI is effective on the efferent limb and effective in chronic obstructive pulmonary disease and post-URTI cough. Agents acting as protussives may enhance cough effectiveness by acting on mucociliary function (dornase alfa [Pulmozyme]*), liquefying mucus (acetylcysteine [Mucomyst]*), or improving expectoration (guaifenesin [Robitussin]). Table 3 shows the doses, indications, and limitations of these agents.

The cause of cough can almost always be identified, but response, even to specific therapy, may be slow. It is always reassuring to the patient when a serious disease is excluded. Efforts at making a specific diagnosis and successfully treating it is rewarding for both patient and physician.

*Not FDA approved for this indication.

HOARSENESS AND LARYNGITIS

method of
ROBERT A. BUCKMIRE, M.D., and
CLARK A. ROSEN, M.D.
University of Pittsburgh Voice Center
Pittsburgh, Pennsylvania

Hoarseness is a common patient complaint that relates to some type of abnormal voice production (dysphonia). Often, hoarseness means something different to patients than it does to the clinician. Thus, further questioning of the patient who is hoarse is required to determine his or her specific voice-related complaints.

Common specific complaints found under the general chief complaint of hoarseness include complete or intermittent voice loss (aphonia), loss of vocal range, and vocal fatigue. Further delineation of the specific problems associated with the voice is required if the patient is a singer. Often, a singer's voice complaints involve loss of singing endurance as well as reduction of vocal range, especially the upper register.

Laryngitis relates to acute voice changes associated with an upper respiratory infection. It involves inflammation of the vocal folds from either infection or trauma (e.g., coughing or screaming). This article primarily focuses on voice changes that last longer than two weeks and, thus, require medical evaluation. Given that hoarseness may represent an early sign of laryngeal cancer, any hoarseness that persists longer than two weeks requires detailed evaluation to ascertain the etiology.

MUSCLE TENSION DYSPHONIA

Muscle tension dysphonia (MTD) is a common voice disorder caused by inappropriate or excessive use of the intralaryngeal and extralaryngeal musculature. Patients with MTD typically present with hoarseness, vocal fatigue, and a globus sensation. The onset of this disorder usually is unknown, but it is often associated with overuse or misuse or is postviral. The condition specifically involves a maladaptive compensatory behavior, often using the extralaryngeal muscles, such as the strap muscles, or muscles within the larynx. This results in hoarseness, neck pain, vocal fatigue, and decreased vocal range and quality. MTD is usually successfully treated with voice therapy. The prognosis for dysphonia from MTD is excellent with voice therapy, which typically requires only 10 to 12 sessions.

NEUROLOGIC VOICE DISORDERS

There are a variety of neurologic disorders that affect voice quality and production. Parkinson's disease, essential tremor, and spasmodic dysphonia are fairly common neurogenic causes of dysphonia. Parkinson's disease causes a classic constellation of communication difficulties consisting of soft voice and rapid, slurred speech. One of the major communication disorder components of Parkinson's disease appears to involve an inability to monitor the patient's own volume, which led to the development of the Lee Silverman Voice Training (LSVT) program. The LSVT program is specialized voice therapy aimed specifically at improving the communication disorder associated with Parkinson's disease and has been shown to be highly efficacious. LSVT is administered by a speech pathologist and requires a specialized form of speech therapy four times a week for 1 month (~16–20 sessions). The improvement gained from using the LSVT program often is best maintained when the patient continues the home exercises on a long-term basis, given that this is a progressive neurologic disease.

Essential Tremor

With essential tremor, hoarseness can result, specifically in the larynx or, more diffusely, throughout the upper airway, digestive tract, and head and neck region. This causes a periodic alteration (tremor) to the voice production that is often mistakenly associated with an aging voice. When this tremor is severe, it can significantly disrupt the normal ability to communicate. The essential tremor is treated first pharmacologically and second with intralaryngeal botulinum toxin injection into the vocal fold musculature.

Spasmodic Dysphonia

Spasmodic dysphonia is a focal dystonia of the laryngeal musculature, usually with unknown etiology. The voice symptoms of this disorder are characterized by severe disruption of the normal fluency of voice production (i.e., voice breaks). Patients typically feel as if they cannot "get their voice out" and often have a "strained/strangled" voice quality and sensation. This disorder is treated successfully with intralaryngeal botulinum toxin injections and sometimes with voice therapy after the injections.

VOICE DISORDERS ASSOCIATED WITH AGING

Voice disorders related to aging are the focus of increasing attention because a growing portion of the aging population remains highly active and the population's life span is increasing. These voice problems are typically related to a loss of muscle bulk or atrophy of the vocal fold musculature, resulting in a weak voice, decreased vocal range, and vocal fatigue. After exclusion of specific or focal neurologic voice pathology, the treatment for this condition is voice therapy; usually 8 to 10 sessions of voice therapy are highly successful (>85%). Some patients who have a voice disorder with severe symptoms due to aging and have significant vocal demands will require vocal fold augmentation, such as lipoinjection of the vocal folds. When needed, this surgery is successful in improving the voices of elderly patients.

VOCAL FOLD LESIONS

Vocal fold nodules, polyps, and cysts are common benign lesions of the true vocal folds causing dysphonia. They can reliably be distinguished from one another only by a thorough laryngoscopic examination, including videostrobolaryngoscopy.

Vocal Nodules

Vocal nodules, often referred to in the singing community as *nodes,* are localized, benign, superficial growths on the medial surface of the true vocal cords that are commonly believed to be the result of a pattern of vocal misuse and abuse. Nodules are bilateral and are usually located at the junction of the anterior one third and the middle one third of the vocal fold. They are most often seen in women aged 20 to 50 years but also are commonly seen in children (boys more than girls) who are prone to excessive loud talking or screaming.

Treatment

Treatment for nodules always involves a course of behavioral voice therapy. Patient compliance is paramount because the therapy is designed to correct the etiologic vocal behaviors. Surgical intervention is inappropriate as a first line therapy. It may be considered, however, in the rare case in which the patient strictly complies with the prescribed course of therapy but is still left with an unacceptable vocal impairment. (If surgery is performed, it must be limited to the most superficial layers of the vocal fold, preserving the uninvolved, surrounding lamina propria.)

Vocal Fold Polyps

Vocal fold polyps are generally unilateral and have a broad spectrum of appearances from pedunculated to sessile. They, too, are thought to result from vocal abuse; however, they can arise from a single episode of abusive behavior or hemorrhage. Polyps typically involve the free (medial) edge of the vocal fold mucosa. Their mass contributes to altered vocal fold vibration, as well as interferes with glottic closure, both of which cause the resultant symptom of dysphonia.

Treatment

Most experts believe that these lesions are most directly related to vocal use and vocal technique and resultant phonotrauma. Treatment is aimed at correcting the underlying causative factors, largely through voice therapy and vocal education. Following voice therapy, if significant dysphonia persists, surgery is indicated, such as a minimally invasive microlaryngoscopic procedure that preserves the uninvolved epithelial cover and surrounding submucosal tissue. When voice therapy and surgery are used appropriately and the patient is compliant, the voice outcome is usually excellent.

Vocal Fold Cysts

Vocal fold cysts are a focal abnormality of the superficial lamina propria and are predominantly unilateral. Intracordal mucous retention cysts are believed to arise after blockage of a glandular duct. Another type of cyst found in the vocal folds, epidermoid cysts, are similar to those found in the skin and tend to be smaller in size. Each variety appears as a well-circumscribed spherical mass beneath intact, normal-appearing epithelial lining.

Treatment

Treatment of vocal fold cysts consists of a surgical microlaryngologic approach. In this approach, a flap of the overlying epithelium is created and will be entirely preserved and returned after removal of the lesion. This approach allows for the return of proper glottic closure and vocal fold vibration previously interrupted by this intracordal mass lesion. Preoperative and postoperative voice therapy is a key component to successful treatment.

Recurrent Respiratory Papilloma

Recurrent respiratory papilloma is a benign neoplastic lesion commonly affecting the glottis and resulting in dysphonia and occasionally airway embarrassment. This papillomatous alteration of the squamous epithelium affects both children and adults and is caused by the human papilloma virus. Lesions may be self-limited or progressive, and, depending on the site of involvement and the size of the patient's airway, symptoms range from mild dysphonia to frank stridor and airway obstruction. Malignant transformation to squamous cell carcinoma is exceedingly rare but has been documented. The course of disease typically involves recurrence and unpredictable remissions. Death from this disease is usually associated with complications of repeated surgical therapy or respiratory failure caused by distal spread of extralaryngeal disease. Aggressive cases in children may require extremely frequent surgical treatments (1–2 per month) or tracheotomy to preserve the airway.

Treatment

Surgical excision of recurrent respiratory papilloma lesions is the mainstay of therapy with either carbon dioxide laser or cold steel excision. Adjuvant medical therapy is also available. The most common of these medications is interferon alfa. Typical doses include 5 million units/m^2 of body surface in a subcutaneous injection on a daily basis to initiate therapy and then 3 million units/m^2 of body surface 3 days a week over 6 months. This treatment regimen has been shown to effectively slow recurrent respiratory papilloma growth, but it is not curative.

Vocal Fold Granuloma

Vocal fold granuloma is characterized by a mass lesion of the glottis located posteriorly near the vocal process of the arytenoids. Granulomas may take on a myriad of appearances from irregular to smooth and pedunculated to broad-based. They are multifactorial in origin, but common correlates include intubation trauma, laryngopharyngeal reflux disease, and vocally abusive behaviors.

Treatment

Treatment of granulomas is similarly multifactorial. Surgical removal of these lesions without further therapy leads to frequent recurrences. Multifaceted treatments, including behavioral modification and gastric acid–lowering medications (proton pump inhibitors) are now the mainstay of therapy. Omeprazole (Prilosec)* starting at 20 mg twice a day is a typical dose. Medical therapy for gastroesophageal reflux disease in conjunction with behavioral voice therapy to eliminate vocally traumatic behaviors has, for the most part, supplanted surgical excision of these lesions and should always be employed before surgical intervention.

Leukoplakia/Erythroplakia

Leukoplakia and *erythroplakia* are terms that refer to discrete areas of abnormal epithelium within the larynx, the normal vocal fold epithelium in a nonkeratinized, stratified squamous cell lining. Alterations in this covering epithelium often appear as discolored (whitish or erythematous) plaques. The altered stiffness and thickness of these areas cause dysphonia that is often the only associated symptom. These changes are often associated with a history of tobacco use.

Treatment

Owing to the risk of premalignant change or frank malignancy, these lesions must be biopsied and submitted for histologic evaluation. Complete excision by delicate phonomicrosurgical techniques is ideal to evaluate surgical margins and to achieve an optimal postoperative voice result. In the case of a circumscribed superficially invasive carcinoma, complete excision may serve as both a diagnostic and therapeutic modality.

Vocal Fold Paralysis (Vocal Fold Immobility)

Normal vocal fold motion involves wide abduction (away from the midline) during inspiration and coordinated glottic closure during phonation and swallowing. When a unilateral vocal fold is found to be immobile, the glottis is generally incompetent in adduction, resulting in some level of dysphonia. Associated vocal fatigue and potential aspiration during swallowing might also be present. In cases of bilateral immobility, the vocal folds are generally found in the paramedian position, allowing for good voice but poor air exchange; thus, patients suffer from airway compromise. When unilateral or bilateral true cord paralysis is diagnosed, a search for the cause should be instituted. The patient's history of systemic disease and past surgical interventions should be elicited. Imaging of the course of neural supply to the larynx, including chest radiograph and computed tomography or magnetic resonance imaging from the skull base through the mediastinum, is necessary to rule out occult neoplastic lesions. Common etiologies of vocal fold immobility include paralysis secondary to vagal or recurrent laryngeal nerve injury from thyroid, carotid, or chest surgery. It must be borne in mind, however, that vocal folds may also be immobile secondary to cricoarytenoid joint dysfunction with an entirely intact nerve supply. Laryngeal electromyelography within 6 months following onset of this problem is helpful in establishing the status of the neural innervation as well as in providing important prognostic information in a timely manner.

Treatment

Treatment for unilateral vocal fold immobility is dependent on the resultant deficits and physiologic impact. Dysphonia in the absence of aspiration may be amenable to both voice therapy and surgical intervention. Therapeutic decision-making is generally based on the patient's desire for an improved voice and on the glottic configuration on laryngoscopic examination. Small glottic chinks associated with an immobile vocal fold in the paramedian position may be well treated with voice therapy alone. Significant dysphonia secondary to a larger glottic gap may be treated with injection laryngoplasty techniques (fat, Gelfoam, or collagen) or medialization laryngoplasty.

Larger levels of glottic incompetence are more

*Not FDA approved for this indication.

likely to require medialization thyroplasty (laryngeal framework surgery) designed to statically position the immobile vocal fold in a phonatory posture. Patients may also benefit from an additional arytenoid adduction procedure to better close the posterior glottic chink. Aspiration is an indication for surgical intervention whether temporary or permanent in scope. This decision must be based on the mechanism of injury and the likelihood of recovery. Procedures to improve closure are employed early in the course of the disease to avoid the potentially devastating complications of aspiration pneumonia.

Laryngopharyngeal Reflux Disease

Reflux laryngitis is caused by the effect of gastric secretions on the mucosal lining of the larynx. The classically described changes include interarytenoid edema and erythema, as well as posterior laryngeal pachyderma (heaped-up thickened tissue). In severe cases, posterior glottic ulceration and granulation tissue are seen. *These changes may be associated with symptoms of heartburn or dyspepsia, but absence of symptoms in no way excludes the clinical diagnosis.* Commonly associated pharyngeal symptoms include excessive thick mucus, throat clearing, globus sensation, and dysphonia. Dysphonia is a result of altered glottic closure and inflammation from the posterior glottic changes. Objective confirmation of pathologic reflux disease is established by means of a multichannel, ambulatory pH probe.

Treatment

Ideal treatment of reflux laryngitis is multifactorial. Lifestyle changes such as elevating the head of the bed, avoiding meals several hours before reclining, and enrolling in weight reduction programs are important in the management of this condition. Dietary controls, including avoidance of acidic foods and those promoting reflux (e.g., tomato-based foods, caffeine, and alcohol), form the core of treatment. Adjuvant medical therapy involves lowering the amount of gastric acid production. Antacids, H_2-blocker agents, and proton pump inhibitors are effective medications, although cases of medication resistance are occasionally seen. With significant glottic changes, aggressive medical therapy might begin with omeprazole (Prilosec)* 20 mg by mouth twice a day in conjunction with the previously mentioned lifestyle and dietary modifications.

Acute Laryngitis

The term *laryngitis* refers to a nonspecific inflammatory condition affecting the larynx and resulting in dysphonia or hoarseness. The causes of this condition are numerous and include all forms of infection or trauma, including viral and bacterial pathogens, intubation trauma, blunt neck trauma, vocal trauma, and laryngopharyngeal reflux disease. In general, an acute voice change persisting for more than 2 weeks is an indication for a laryngeal examination.

Treatment

The therapeutic modality chosen is entirely dependent on the suspected cause of the laryngitis. By far the most common transient cause of this complaint is an inflammation associated with an upper respiratory viral infection. Treatment for this condition should be expectant with attention to good hydration and reduced voice use (not complete voice rest). Bacterial and fungal laryngotracheitis are diagnosed by laryngeal visualization in association with appropriate symptoms. Bacterial infection is suspected with prolonged symptoms of dysphonia, productive cough, and fever and is generally well treated by full-course therapy with a broad-spectrum oral antibiotic that covers oropharyngeal flora. Treatment of fungal laryngitis typically requires a systemic antifungal such as fluconazole (Diflucan) 200 mg by mouth daily for the first day, followed by 100 mg daily for the rest of the prescribed course. These infections are rare unless concurrent steroid use or immunosuppression is present. Topical antifungal preparations (e.g., nystatin [Mycostatin]) may be sufficient for treatment of mild cases. Appropriate treatment for laryngopharyngeal reflux disease is addressed earlier in this article.

*Not FDA approved for this indication.

INSOMNIA

method of
KARL DOGHRAMJI, M.D.
Jefferson Medical College
Philadelphia, Pennsylvania

The simplest and broadest definition of *insomnia* is a difficulty in falling or staying asleep or unrefreshing sleep. Insomnia is a complaint; there are no objective tests to confirm its presence or to quantify its severity. It is present whenever the patient complains of it.

PREVALENCE AND IMPACT OF INSOMNIA

A staggering 50% of adult Americans report having experienced insomnia at some time during their lives. Ten percent experience difficulties with sleep lasting more than 2 weeks at a time, and 5.9 million office visits in 1995 were due to the complaint of insomnia. Insomnia becomes more frequent with age, owing to an increase in medical and psychiatric illnesses in seniors and to a natural deterioration in sleep-generating processes in the brain with aging.

Daytime impairments in individuals complaining of insomnia include drowsiness, diminished memory and concentration, depression, strained relationships, proneness to accidents, and job performance decrement. It appears that these disturbances are caused by not only illnesses that accompany insomnia, such as depression, substance use, and medical illnesses, but also the insomnia process itself because even "pure" insomniacs demonstrate some of these abnormalities in laboratory settings. Conservative estimates suggest that, in the United States, insomnia costs the health care system $30 to $35 billion annually; direct costs account for 40% to 46% of this total.

Despite its frequency and impact, it is quite surprising that only 6% of all insomniacs schedule a visit with their physicians specifically for insomnia. Twenty-four percent address the difficulty with their physicians as a secondary complaint, and most (70%) do not seek medical help for the problem at all. Additionally, most insomnia complaints are not identified or treated in medical settings. Insomniacs remain, therefore, largely an "invisible" population from the standpoint of formal medical practitioners. However, 40% of insomniacs do seek assistance for their malady in the form of over-the-counter sleep aids or alcohol.

INSOMNIA DISORDERS

It is not clear whether insomnia represents a condition in and of itself or whether it is a symptom of underlying conditions. Its occurrence in conjunction with a variety of conditions, and its resolution after the treatment of these conditions, suggests that it is, at least in certain medical settings, a symptom whose cause should be identified by a careful investigation of underlying conditions.

Inadequate Sleep Hygiene

Many individuals unknowingly engage in habitual behaviors that harm sleep. Insomniacs, for example, often compensate for lost sleep by delaying their morning awakening time or by napping, which actually has the effect of further fragmenting nocturnal sleep. Instead, insomniacs should be advised to adhere to a regular awakening time regardless of the amount of sleep and to avoid naps. Although caffeine has a half-life in plasma of 3 to 7 hours, its absorption from the gastrointestinal tract can be erratic and there are wide variations in individual sensitivity to it. Therefore, caffeine consumption should be avoided after noon. Other sleep hygiene measures are outlined in Table 1.

TABLE 1. **Sleep Hygiene Education**

Maintain regular wake time.
Avoid excessive time in bed.
Avoid naps, except if shift worker or elderly.
Expose yourself to bright light while awake.
Use the bed only for sleeping and sex.
Avoid nicotine, caffeine, and alcohol.
Exercise regularly early in the day.
Do something relaxing before bedtime.
Don't watch the clock.
Eat a light snack before bedtime if hungry.

Adjustment Sleep Disorder

Acute emotional stressors, such as a job loss or a hospitalization, often cause insomnia. Typically, however, symptoms remit shortly after the abatement of the stressors. Therefore, this type of insomnia is usually transient and short-term, lasting a few days to a few weeks. Nevertheless, if daytime sleepiness and fatigue develop, and especially if they interfere with daytime functioning, treatment is warranted. Treatment modalities are similar to those outlined for psychophysiologic insomnia (see later). Transient or short-term insomnia also warrants active treatment if a pattern of recurring episodes develops.

Psychophysiologic Insomnia

Once initiated, regardless of cause, insomnia may persist well beyond the resolution of precipitating factors. Thus, a short-term insomnia may develop into a long-term, chronic difficulty with recurring episodes or a constant, daily pattern of insomnia. The insomnia "sets in." Although many factors may be involved, this is usually caused by anticipatory anxiety over the prospect of another night of sleeplessness followed by another day of fatigue (Figure 1). Sufferers often spend hours in bed awake focused on, and brooding over, their sleeplessness, which, in turn, aggravates their insomnia even further. Patients typically have greater difficulty in falling asleep in their own bedrooms and are often amazed to find that they fall asleep more easily when away from home. The optimal treatment for psychophysiologic insomnia is a combination of behavioral strategies and pharmacologic agents, discussed later.

Periodic Limb Movement Disorder and Restless Legs Syndrome

Periodic limb movement disorder (PLMD) is characterized by the repetitive (usually every 20–40 seconds) twitching or kicking of the lower extremities during sleep. Patients usually present with the complaint of interrupted nocturnal sleep or daytime hypersomnolence. They are typ-

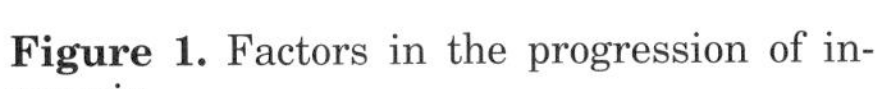

Figure 1. Factors in the progression of insomnia.

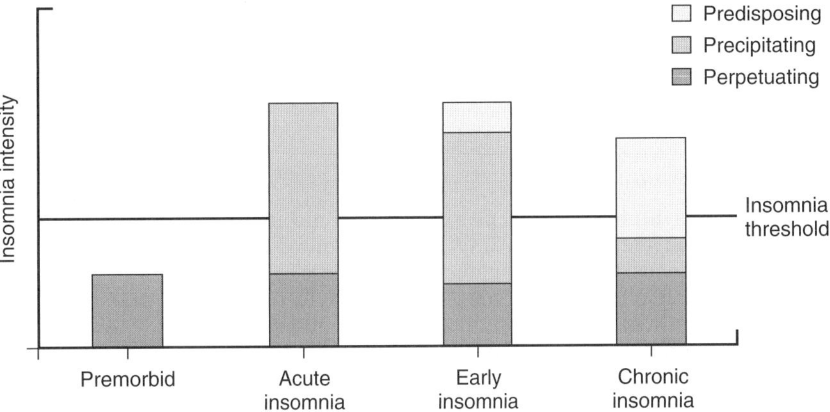

TABLE 2. **Therapy for Periodic Limb Movement Disorder and Restless Legs Syndrome**

Dopaminergic Agents

Carbidopa-levodopa (Sinemet CR),* 25/100–100/400 mg
Bromocriptine (Parlodel),* 5–15 mg
Pergolide (Permax),* 0.05–0.15 mg
Pramipexole (Mirapex),* 0.125–1.0 mg

Benzodiazepines

Clonazepam (Klonopin),* 0.5–2.0 mg
Lorazepam (Ativan),* 1.0 mg
Temazepam (Restoril),* 15–30 mg

Opioids

Propoxyphene (Darvon),* 130–520 mg
Codeine,* 15–240 mg
Tramadol hydrochloride (Ultram)*

Anticonvulsants

Gabapentin (Neurontin),* 100–2700 mg
Carbamazepine (Tegretol),* 200–400 mg

Vitamins and Minerals

Vitamins C,* B_{12}, E
Folate,* magnesium, iron* (serum ferritin <50 μg/L)

*Not FDA approved for this indication.

ically unaware of the movements and the brief arousals that follow and have no lasting sensation in the extremities. The disorder is usually diagnosed during sleep studies conducted to determine the etiology of insomnia. In contrast, patients suffering from the related disorder, restless legs syndrome (RLS), complain of a "creeping" sensation in the lower extremities on reclining. They resort to moving the affected extremity by stretching, kicking, or walking to relieve symptoms. As a result, they complain of intense difficulty in falling asleep or repeated nocturnal awakenings. Most exhibit periodic limb movements during sleep studies. These disorders are more common in middle and older age. They are typically idiopathic yet can be seen during drug withdrawal states, the intake of stimulants and certain antidepressants, chronic renal and hepatic failure, pregnancy, and anemia, among others. To establish a diagnosis in patients who do not have the typical paresthesias, bed partners should be questioned for kicking or jerking movements on the part of the patient. Patients with the disorder should receive a thorough medical evaluation with blood tests for anemia and iron deficiency states.

Treatments are summarized in Table 2. None of these agents has been specifically developed for PLMD/RLS. The dopaminergic agents, although often effective, present the possibility of augmentation (symptoms are felt later in the day), rebound, nausea, and insomnia. The benzodiazepines should be used cautiously to prevent daytime somnolence and tolerance. The opioids are seldom used and present the possibility of tolerance and constipation.

Sleep Apnea Syndrome

The major symptoms of sleep apnea syndrome include interrupted nocturnal sleep, daytime somnolence, and snoring. Predisposing factors include middle age, obesity, male gender, use of central nervous system (CNS) suppressants, and craniofacial abnormalities, among others. The critical pathophysiologic event in the disorder is a collapse of the upper airway at the level of the pharynx, possibly mediated through upper airway muscular laxity. The disorder is associated with cardiovascular abnormalities, such as hypertension, and increased mortality rates. Excessive sleepiness frequently interferes with daytime functioning. Therefore, if suspected, it should be ruled out by polysomnography and managed if diagnosed. Treatments include weight loss, avoidance of CNS depressants, continuous positive airway pressure (CPAP), dental devices, upper airway surgery, and medications.

Drug-Related Sleep Disorders

Drugs that can cause disturbed sleep include certain antidepressants, antihypertensives, antineoplastic agents, bronchodilators, stimulants, corticosteroids, decongestants, diuretics, histamine-2 receptor blockers, and smoking cessation aids. Recreational drugs, such as cocaine, often cause insomnia. Hypnotics and anxiolytics can cause insomnia after long-term use and during the withdrawal phase.

Medical and Psychiatric Sleep Disorders

Many medical and psychiatric disorders interfere with sleep quality. One of the most common psychiatric disturbances responsible for the complaint of insomnia is depression. Eighty percent of depressives suffer from some type of sleep disturbance. Depression can be associated with difficulties in falling asleep, interrupted nocturnal sleep, and early morning awakening, and no one type of insomnia seems to typify sleep in depressives. Insomnia in the depressed patient may be associated with daytime performance decrements and may also lead to noncompliance with antidepressant medications if not addressed rapidly. There are also data suggesting that long-term sleeplessness is associated with an increased risk for the emergence of new psychiatric disorders, most notably major depressive disorder, suggesting the possibility of a bi-directional relationship between insomnia and certain psychiatric disorders, most notably depression.

Antidepressants have variable effects on sleep quality. Although these effects have not been well established in all cases, probable sleep/wakefulness effects of most antidepressants are summarized in Table 3. Many physicians choose the more sedating antidepressants for control of insomnia in depressed patients. This can afford the patient

TABLE 3. **Short-Term Effects of Antidepressants on Sleep/Wakefulness**

Activating Antidepressants

Protriptyline (Vivactil)*
Bupropion (Wellbutrin)*
Most selective serotonin reuptake inhibitors (SSRIs)*
Venlafaxine (Effexor)*
Monoamine oxidase inhibitors*

Sedating Antidepressants

Amitriptyline (Elavil)*
Doxepin (Sinequan)*
Trimipramine (Surmontil)*
Nefazodone (Serzone)*
Trazodone (Desyrel)*
Mirtazapine (Remeron)*

Neural Antidepressants

Citalopram (Celexa)*

*Not FDA approved for this indication.

rapid relief from insomnia, and daytime sedation can be minimized by ensuring evening dosing of the medication. If an antidepressant of the activating class is chosen, insomnia can be dealt with by judicious use of hypnotic agents, discussed earlier. Not much is known about the effects of antidepressants on sleep quality after the first 8 weeks of treatment.

Circadian Rhythm Sleep Disorders

This group of disorders features a disturbance in the coordination between internal and environmental circadian rhythms involving the sleep-wake cycle.

Time zone change (jet lag) syndrome is caused by rapid travel across time zones resulting in a mismatch between the sleep schedules of the body and that of the new environment. Eastward travel results in more severe symptoms than westward travel. The severity of symptoms is also related to the number of time zones crossed; travel across more than two to three times zones surpasses the adaptive capabilities of the body. This often leads to a mismatch between internal body rhythms as well, such as those of temperature, sleep, and hormone secretion. Jet lag countermeasures include the utilization of short-acting hypnotic agents for brief periods of time after arrival in the new locale and maximizing exposure to daylight in the new locale, which has the effect of resetting circadian rhythms with one another and with the environment. Individuals should also be urged to gradually shift their sleep/wake schedules before travel to coincide approximately with those of their destination.

Shift work sleep disorder is especially problematic when sleep times are changed frequently from changing work shifts. This often leads to poor sleep quality immediately after the new shift, which is followed by a period of adaptation. The severity of symptoms is proportional to the frequency with which shifts are changed, the magnitude of each change, as well as the frequency of counterclockwise (phase-advancing) changes. However, even fixed-shift workers who must sleep during the day experience difficulties because daytime noise and light often interfere with the quality of their sleep and because they often change their sleep times on days off of work for social or family events. The elderly are more profoundly affected by rapidly changing shifts. Shift workers should be advised to maximize their exposure to sunlight at times when they should be awake and to ensure that the bedroom is as dark and quiet as possible when they are asleep, which is often during the day. Phototherapy via bright artificial light emanating from especially constructed boxes, or natural sunlight, when administered at critical times can enhance adaptation of internal rhythms to the new shift. If symptoms are not responsive to conventional countermeasures, it may be necessary to devise more rational shift schedules.

In *delayed sleep phase syndrome* individuals fall asleep later than normal evening bedtime hours and awaken later than desired, often extending their bedtimes well into the afternoon. Thus, they typically complain of both insomnia and daytime sleepiness. Sufferers are usually young adults who present for treatment because of diminished school performance resulting from daytime sleepiness or missed morning classes. Prior history reveals a tendency for individuals to be "night owls," preferring to work and play well into the night. They can be distinguished from people who stay up late by choice because of social or occupational needs in that they cannot fall asleep earlier even if they were to try. Phototherapy for 30 minutes to 1 hour early in the morning can advance sleep rhythm on subsequent nights. In *advanced sleep phase syndrome*, which is more common in the elderly, sleep/wake times are advanced in relationship to socially desired schedules. It is responsive to phototherapy in the evening.

MISCELLANEOUS TREATMENTS OF INSOMNIA

Behavioral measures and hypnotic agents are appropriate for a wide variety of insomnia disorders, such as adjustment sleep disorder, psychophysiologic insomnia, shift work and jet lag, and depression, among others. Whereas behavioral measures may take a longer time to implement, they have the advantage of longer-lasting effects than pharmacologic measures. Therefore, pharmacologic agents and behavioral treatments can be instituted from the outset and, once behavioral measures begin to take effect, pharmacologic agents can be withdrawn.

Behavioral Treatments

Relaxation Training. Tension is reduced through electromyographic (EMG) biofeedback, abdominal breathing exercises, or progressive muscle relaxation techniques, among others. Training is usually effective within a few weeks. During EMG biofeedback, the tension of skeletal muscle, typically the temporalis, is monitored electronically and translated into an auditory tone to the patient. The heightened awareness of muscle tension gives the patient direct feedback while engaging in progressive relaxation exercises. These methods are then practiced at home before bedtime.

Cognitive Psychotherapy. This talk therapy strives to identify and dispel thoughts that are tension producing and that have a negative effect on sleep, such as the preoccupation with unpleasant work experiences or examinations at school. During sessions, patients' fears regarding sleeplessness can be overcome by reassurance and by suggestions that they deal with anxiety-producing thoughts during sessions and at times other than bedtime. Other forms of therapy include insight-oriented psychotherapy, which strives to enhance patients' awareness of ongoing psychologic conflicts that stem from prior years and that contribute to sleeplessness through the production of anxiety.

Stimulus Control Therapy. This is well suited for insomniacs who spend a great deal of time in bed brooding over sleeplessness. Patients are asked to use the bed only for sleep (not for reading or watching television) and to not stay in bed trying to sleep for more than 10 to 20 minutes at a time. Rather, they are urged to go into another room and to return to bed only after feeling sleepy. Patients repeat this maneuver as many times as necessary without extending their time in bed beyond the usual arising time. They are also urged to avoid napping. Sleep logs are used to monitor compliance and to assess progress.

Restriction of Time Spent in Bed. This therapy is well suited for insomniacs who wake up repeatedly during the course of the night, such as the elderly. Sleep is monitored through sleep diaries over the course of 2 weeks. On the basis of these diaries, sleep efficiency index is calculated by dividing the average daily time spent asleep over the average daily time spent in bed. As an example, the sleep efficiency of an individual who sleeps, on average, 6 hours per 24-hour day and spends 10 hours in bed during this period of time is 6/10, or 0.6. The physician then asks the patient to lie in bed, on a daily basis, for the time that is equivalent to his or her total sleep time; in this example, that time would be 6 hours. The patient continues to fill out sleep logs and calls the physician every 5 days with log data. If the sleep efficiency during the prior 5 days is less than 85%, no changes are made. However, if the sleep efficiency is greater than 85%, time in bed is increased by 15 minutes by allowing the patient to go bed earlier. No changes are made to the morning awakening time. Patients avoid napping. Over the course of a few weeks, consolidation of sleep is noted along with an increase in quality and the sensation of restorative sleep.

Hypnotic Agents

Sedative-hypnotics are indicated primarily for short-term management of insomnia. The first preparation specifically targeting sleep was chloral hydrate. It is used in daily doses of 500 to 1000 mg, and its sedative effects are mainly due to trichloroethanol, its main metabolite. Its use has been limited, however, by side effects, including daytime hangover, lightheadedness, malaise, ataxia, and nightmares. Its sedative effects are highly magnified when it is administered with alcohol. Chronic use and overdoses have been associated with hepatic damage and fatalities, and sudden discontinuation after chronic use has been associated with delirium, seizures, and death. Barbiturates and related compounds (e.g., glutethimide), although effective hypnotics, have also been limited in usefulness owing to side effects such as daytime somnolence, respiratory suppression when used in high doses, rapid development of tolerance, and high likelihood of interaction with other medications.

More recently introduced agents used exclusively for insomnia are listed in Table 4. These agents have a better side effect profile than do the older agents. The primary pharmacokinetic property that distinguishes them from one another is elimination half-life. Those with a longer half-life include flurazepam (Dalmane) and quazepam (Doral); those with an intermediate half-life include estazolam (ProSom) and temazepam (Restoril). The short half-life hypnotics include triazolam (Halcion), zolpidem (Ambien), and zaleplon (Sonata). Whereas the benzodiazepines bind without selectivity to the types 1 and 2 benzodiazepine receptors, zolpidem and zaleplon (and possibly quazepam) bind selectively to the type 1 receptor. It has been postulated that this selectivity confers the newer agents with some of the side effect advantages that are discussed later, although this connection between mechanism of action at the cellular level and clinical properties has yet to be conclusively established.

Agents with longer elimination half-lives tend to be associated with a greater potential for daytime carryover effects, such as daytime sedation, motor incoordination, amnesia, and slower reflexes. These may lead to performance decrements, automobile accidents, and hip fractures in vulnerable individuals, such as the elderly. Because of its ultra-short half-life, zaleplon is least likely to cause daytime carryover effects when administered at bedtime. At 10-mg doses, its duration of side effects seems to be limited to 4 hours after administration. This property imparts zaleplon with the unique feature of being safely administered in the middle of the night after nocturnal awakenings, as long as the patient is in bed for 4 hours after administration. Some insomniacs feel that this type of usage, whereby they ingest the medication only after they feel the need to do so ("prn"), allows them to use hypnotics more sparingly. Other hypnotics must be used "prophylactically" at the beginning of the night, on a nightly basis until the insomnia problem is thought to have dissipated or until the physician advises the patient to "take a break." On the other hand, the ultra-short half-life of zaleplon makes it less preferred for patients who

TABLE 4. **Hypnotic Agents**

Generic	Trade	Onset	Half-Life (H)	Active Metabolites	Dose (mg)
Benzodiazepines					
Flurazepam	Dalmane	Rapid	40–250	Yes	15, 30
Quazepam	Doral	Rapid	40–250	Yes	7.5, 15
Estazolam	ProSom	Rapid	10–24	Yes	0.5, 1, 2
Temazepam	Restoril	Intermediate	8–22	No	7.5, 15
Triazolam	Halcion	Rapid	<6	No	0.125, 0.25, 0.50
Imidazopyridine					
Zolpidem	Ambien	Rapid	2.5	No	5, 10
Pyrazolopyrimidine					
Zaleplon	Sonata	Rapid	1	No	5, 10, 20

TABLE 5. **Guidelines for the Use of Hypnotic Agents**

1. Define a clear indication and treatment goal.
2. Prescribe the lowest effective dose.
3. Individualize the dose for each patient.
4. Use lower doses with a central nervous system depressant or alcohol.
5. Consider dose adjustment in the elderly and in patients with hepatic or renal disease.
6. Avoid in patients with sleep apnea syndrome, pregnancy, and history of abuse.
7. Limit duration of use.
8. For patients who need longer-term treatment, consider intermittent therapy.
9. Avoid abrupt drug discontinuation (taper).
10. Re-evaluate drug treatment regularly; assess both efficacy and adverse events.

have sleep-interruption insomnia throughout the night and on a nightly basis. A longer elimination half-life agent such as zolpidem may be more predictably efficacious for the entire duration of the night in such cases. Ultimately, the choice of agent should take into consideration the patient's situation, preference, and effects of prior trials with similar agents.

Despite the many advantages of the short elimination half-life hypnotics, they do not offer daytime anxiolysis in patients who are anxious during the daytime. An additional concern, generated primarily regarding triazolam, is the potential for rapid development of tolerance after repeated dosing and for rebound insomnia after abrupt discontinuation. Despite widespread concerns, neither property has been well documented. Nevertheless, both can be minimized by utilizing the medication at the lowest effective dose and for brief periods of time. Additionally, rebound can be controlled by gradually tapering the dosage when discontinuing the drug. Both problems seem to be less prominent with the newest hypnotics, zolpidem and zaleplon, which have been shown not to produce tolerance or rebound after a year of continued use in preliminary trials. Guidelines for the use of hypnotics generally aim toward minimizing abuse, misuse, and addiction by discouraging chronic use (Table 5).

Nonhypnotic "Hypnotics"

Many agents not specifically indicated for insomnia are used for sleep induction. Alcohol may be one of the most widely used agents by insomniacs because it enhances sleepiness and allows for a more rapid onset of sleep. However, it is a poor choice inasmuch as it alters sleep quality, often results in further daytime somnolence, and leads to the rapid development of tolerance. Patients also report unrefreshing and disturbed sleep during use and frequent nocturnal awakenings after discontinuation. Alcohol can also result in further impairment in sleep-related respiration in patients with obstructive sleep apnea syndrome, a disorder commonly seen in insomniacs. Antihistamines and over-the-counter products, whose main active ingredients are antihistamines such as doxylamine and diphenhydramine (Benadryl), suffer from unpredictable efficacy and side effects such as daytime sedation, confusion, and systemic anticholinergic effects. Sedating antidepressants (see Table 3) are effective antidepressants when used at proper clinical doses, yet their use in low doses to control insomnia in nondepressed patients has not been supported by data. Antidepressants are also associated with side effects; in the case of trazodone these include daytime sedation, orthostatic hypotension, and priapism. The tricyclic antidepressants are also, as a class, associated with anticholinergic side effects such as dry mouth, urinary flow difficulties, and cardiac dysrhythmias. Melatonin is a dietary supplement, used in doses of 0.5 to 3000 mg. Anecdotal reports indicate it may be efficacious in certain subtypes of insomnia such as from shift work, jet lag, blindness, and delayed sleep phase syndrome and the elderly. However, melatonin's efficacy has not been conclusively established and is in doubt. Additionally, concerns have been expressed regarding its side effects after the observation of coronary artery tissue stimulation in animals and regarding the purity of available preparations.

EVALUATION OF INSOMNIA

A useful initial step in the evaluation of insomnia is the determination of its etiology. Most short-term insomnias, that is, those lasting a few weeks, are due to situational stressors and respond to sleep hygiene measures. Hypnotic agents may be considered if daytime consequences are apparent, such as sleepiness and occupational impairment, or if the insomnia seems to be escalating. In longer-term insomnias, those lasting more than a few weeks, a more thorough evaluation should be considered, including a general medical and psychiatric history, physical examination, and mental status examination. Additionally, the cardinal symptoms of the disorders described earlier should be asked for, including snoring or anecdotal reports of breathing pauses during sleep (sleep apnea syndrome), restlessness or twitching in the lower extremities (PLMS/RLS), and so on. The bed partner, who may be more aware of such symptoms, should also be questioned. Sleep patterns on weekdays and weekends, bedtime habits, sleep hygiene habits, and drug and medication use should be carefully reviewed. In cases in which the diagnosis is in question, or when treatment of the presumed conditions fails after a reasonable time period, an evaluation at a sleep disorders center may be considered. Once the diagnosis is established, treatment can be conducted with greater confidence.

PRURITUS

method of
NANCY E. THOMAS, M.D., PH.D., and
LUIS A. DIAZ, M.D.
University of North Carolina at Chapel Hill
Chapel Hill, North Carolina

Pruritus (itching) is defined as a sensation that leads one to the desire to scratch. A specific subpopulation of unmyelinated C polymodal neurons carry the sensation of pruritus to specific areas of the brain that then can respond through motor nerves with scratching. Physical or chemical stimuli can act directly on these fibers or release mediators that result in stimulation of the fibers. Histamine mediates many of these stimuli; however, pruritus can be induced independent of histamine. Other potential local mediators include interleukin-2, mast cell–derived proteases, eicosanoids, eosinophil granule proteins, and platelet-activating factor. In addition, it has been shown that the sensation of pruritus can be modified centrally by increases in endogenous opioid agonists and up-regulation of opioid receptors in a histamine-independent manner.

DIAGNOSIS

A thorough history, including the location, duration, severity, and diurnal variation of the pruritus, past medical history, drug history, and history of exposures (to animals, others who are itching, and environmental factors) should be obtained when a patient presents with pruritus. A complete skin examination is also essential, looking for evidence of an eruption and any subtle skin changes, such as xerosis.

When a skin eruption is present, the physician must first determine whether primary lesions are present or whether all the lesions are secondary to scratching, picking, or rubbing. A more specific diagnosis than pruritus can often be rendered by morphologic or histologic examination of the primary lesions (Table 1).

However, some patients present with disorders such as lichen simplex chronicus, localized amyloidosis, postinflammatory hyperpigmentation, and prurigo nodularis that are thought to be secondary to scratching, picking, or rubbing (Table 2). When a patient presents with one of these disorders, the physician must consider whether the disorder is part of another primary pruritic skin condition such as atopic dermatitis secondary to a pruritic systemic disorder or due to a psychologic disorder such as anxiety or depression.

When a pruritic patient has either no skin lesions or only those secondary to pruritus, the cause of the pruritus may be an underlying systemic disorder or a skin condition that, at times, may present without primary lesions (Table 3).

Xerosis is a frequent, often subtle, problem that can lead to pruritus. Elderly patients who previously did not have xerosis often develop it as their skin ages. In addition, patients with atopic diathesis typically have dry "itchy skin" that is reactive to many irritants, such as wool and dust.

Scabies can have few primary or only secondary lesions in patients who scratch vigorously. A scabies prep examination should be considered in any patient with generalized itching or new-onset dermatitis.

HIV-infected patients can present with a number of pruritic skin conditions, such as scabies, bacterial folliculitis, eczematous eruptions, eosinophilic folliculitis, insect bite hypersensitivity, and seborrheic dermatitis. Dry skin is extremely common in this group and is exacerbated by protease inhibitors. In addition, a significant number of patients who have HIV disease suffer pruritus in the absence of discernible skin disease.

In a patient with no primary lesions on skin examination, a complete review of systems and full physical examination to detect any abnormalities such as lymphadenopa-

TABLE 1. **Pruritic Skin Disorders**

Atopic dermatitis	Mastocytosis
Bullous pemphigoid	Miliaria
Candidiasis	Nummular eczema
Contact dermatitis	Parapsoriasis
Cutaneous T cell lymphoma	Pediculosis
Dermatitis herpetiformis	Perforating dermatoses
Dermatographism	Photoeruptions
Dermatophytosis	Pityriasis rubra pilaris
Drug hypersensitivity	Pruritic papules and plaques of pregnancy
Dyshidrotic eczema	Psoriasis
Folliculitis	Scabies and other mites
Impetigo	Seborrheic dermatitis
Insect bites	Transient acantholytic dermatosis
Larva migrans	Urticaria
Lichen planus	Varicella
Lichen sclerosis et atrophicus	Xerosis
Linear IgA dermatosis	

TABLE 2. **Skin Disorders That Can Be Secondary to Pruritus**

Macular and lichen amyloidosis
Lichen simplex chronicus
Postinflammatory hyperpigmentation
Prurigo nodularis

TABLE 3. **Disorders That May Present as Pruritus Without Primary Lesions**

Anorexia nervosa	Hepatobiliary disorders
Aquagenic pruritus	Biliary atresia
Atopy	Cholestasis of pregnancy
Bullous disorders	Drug-induced cholestasis
Bullous pemphigoid	Hepatitis
Dermatitis herpetiformis	Malrotation with cholestasis
Linear IgA dermatosis	Obstructive jaundice
Drug-induced pruritus	Primary biliary cirrhosis
Aspirin	Primary sclerosing cholangitis
Chloroquine	HIV disease
Hydroxyethyl starch infusion	Malignancy
Opioids	Carcinoid
Endocrine disorders	Carcinoma
Diabetes mellitus	Cutaneous T cell lymphoma
Hyperthyroidism/hypothyroidism	Leukemias
Hematologic disorders	Hodgkin lymphoma
Iron deficiency/anemia	Multiple myeloma
Paraproteinemia	Non-Hodgkin lymphoma
Polycythemia vera	Mastocytosis
Infestation and parasites	Notalgia paresthetica
Pediculosis	Pruritus of pregnancy
Onchocerciasis	Renal disorders
Pinworms	Chronic renal failure
Strongyloidiasis	Stroke
Scabies and other mites	

TABLE 4. **Laboratory Workup for Pruritus**

Complete blood cell count with differential
Ferritin
Blood urea nitrogen and creatinine
Fasting blood glucose
Thyroid-stimulating hormone
Liver function tests
Chest radiograph
Stool for parasites
Age-appropriate malignancy workup
Additional tests based on history, review of symptoms, and physical examination

thy and hepatosplenomegaly can provide leads for diagnosis. Laboratory screening for systemic disorders should be considered for pruritus of unknown cause (Table 4). Anemia and thyroid disorders are not uncommon causes of pruritus. Low iron stores even with a normal hematocrit level can be associated with pruritus. Chronic, but not acute, renal failure is associated with pruritus. Conditions that result in cholestasis, including hepatitis with structural damage to the bile ducts, can have associated pruritus. Pruritus is also not uncommon when lymphoma is present.

Based on history and physical examination, additional testing such as serum protein electrophoresis and HIV testing may be indicated. An age-appropriate malignancy workup to rule out carcinoma may also be indicated. At times, skin biopsy, even in the absence of primary lesions, can unmask a disorder such as cutaneous T cell lymphoma, mastocytosis, or scabies. Because the symptom of pruritus can herald the presence of a serious underlying condition, potential causes must be explored rigorously.

TREATMENT

When possible, treatment of the underlying skin or systemic disorder can reduce pruritus. For example, treatment of anemia, thyroid problems, diabetes, and lymphoma often will eliminate pruritus. Anorexia nervosa can have associated pruritus that resolves with sufficient weight gain.

Xerosis, alone or in association with other skin problems such as atopic dermatitis, is often treated with gentle skin care including mild soaps (Dove unscented, Cetaphil) and thick moisturizers (Eucerin, Cetaphil, Aquaphor). These patients then undergo additional workup if their pruritus does not resolve.

TABLE 5. **Topical Treatments for Pruritus**

Calamine lotion
Capsaicin (Zostrix cream)*
Corticosteroids (hydrocortisone, triamcinolone cream)
Doxepin (Zonalon cream)
Emollients (e.g., Eucerin, Aquaphor, Cetaphil)
Lidocaine/menthol (Gold Bond Medicated Itch Cream)
Menthol/camphor (Sarna Anti-Itch lotion)
Oatmeal baths (Aveeno)
Phenol/salicylic acid (Panscol)
Pramoxine (Aveeno Anti-Itch, PrameGel, Itch-X)
Pramoxine/hydrocortisone (Pramosone)
Pramoxine/calamine (Caladryl cream)
Zinc oxide

*Not FDA approved for this indication.

TABLE 6. **Antihistamines Often Used for Pruritus in Adults**

Cetirizine (Zyrtec),*† 10 mg once daily
Cyproheptadine (Periactin),* 4 mg q8h
Diphenhydramine (Benadryl), 25 to 50 mg q6h
Doxepin (Sinequan),* 10 to 25 mg qhs
Fexofenadine (Allegra),*† 60 mg q12h
Hydroxyzine (Atarax), 10 to 25 mg q6h
Loratadine (Claritin),*† 10 mg once daily

*Not FDA approved for this indication.
†FDA indicated for urticaria.

For treatment of symptomatic pruritus, physicians use a variety of topical treatments, many of which are only partially effective (Table 5). Topical pramoxine (Prax lotion) is preferred over topical benzocaine and diphenhydramine (Benadryl) because topical sensitization is believed to be less likely.

Oral antihistamines are often used to treat pruritus even though proof of their efficacy is lacking for many pruritic conditions, such as atopic dermatitis, and their effect is often attributed to sedation (Table 6). Doxepin (Sinequan) is of particular interest because it is both an H_1 and H_2 blocker and believed possibly to be more effective than agents that block only H_1.

Ultraviolet B or A phototherapy and, less frequently, psoralens plus ultraviolet A therapy have been used successfully for symptomatic relief of pruritus due to a number of conditions.

In patients with cholestasis, treatment with bile acid sequestrants cholestyramine (Questran) or colestipol (Colestid) may provide symptomatic relief. Ursodiol (Actigall), which stimulates biliary flow and replaces more hydrophobic bile acids, often decreases pruritus. Rifampin (Rifadin)* is an option for relieving pruritus but must be monitored carefully because it can cause drug-induced hepatitis. Trials of opioid antagonists such as parenteral naloxone (Narcan)* and oral naltrexone (ReVia)* have shown promise for providing symptomatic relief.

Pruritus due to chronic renal failure is not significantly improved by dialysis. Activated charcoal and cholestyramine can be helpful in decreasing pruritus. Some studies have shown that pruritic patients on dialysis with secondary hyperparathyroidism have decreased pruritus after parathyroidectomy. Naltrexone (ReVia)* has been shown to decrease pruritus in dialysis patients.

Trials off certain medication may be necessary to see if pruritus is eliminated because many medications can induce pruritus without a rash, the classic example being opioids. Some medications such as chloroquine may also cause pruritus through stimulation of opioid receptors. Other medications could cause pruritus without rash through a variety of mechanisms, including cholestasis, immunologic hy-

*Not FDA approved for this indication.

persensitivity, photoallergy, and toxicity, or medications could cause pruritus in an idiosyncratic manner.

TINNITUS

method of
JOSE N. FAYAD, M.D.
Columbia University College of Physicians and Surgeons

and

MARK MURPHY, M.D.
New York Presbyterian Hospital
New York, New York

Tinnitus is a common symptom affecting up to 20% of the population older than age 50. An estimated 40 million Americans have experienced head noise, or tinnitus, at some point in their lives. Ten million people are seriously affected by tinnitus, and a million persons are debilitated by this symptom. It may be nothing more than a nuisance to some patients, whereas it may cause others to have suicidal ideas. Tinnitus is most prevalent in patients between the ages of 40 and 70, and it affects men and women equally. A basic understanding of this complex condition is a necessity for all primary care physicians, especially those focusing on the geriatric population. It must be understood that tinnitus itself is not a disease but a symptom, and efforts to ascertain its etiology should be sought.

Tinnitus is loosely defined as noise heard in the absence of acoustic stimuli. It can be subdivided into *subjective* (noise heard only by the patient) or *objective* (noise heard by the patient and observer) tinnitus. Subjective tinnitus is the more common of the two. The patient's presenting complaints and the patient's history guide the physician as to the possible causes and diagnostic tests to be performed.

The character of the tinnitus is the first query made by the physician. Tinnitus may be unilateral, bilateral, "inside the head," pulsatile, ringing, constant, or intermittent. As with any new complaint, the onset, severity, duration, and exacerbating or relieving factors should be determined. A proper otologic history should be taken, with special attention to infections, trauma, hearing loss, noise exposure, stress, and prior otologic procedures. The degree to which the patient is affected should be determined. Does the head noise awaken the patient at night and prevent him or her from sleeping? Does it interfere with the patient's daily activities?

The physician must gain insight into the psychologic status of the patient and evaluate the patient for depression, anxiety, or stress. Stress can play a big role in patients with tinnitus.

Physical examination should include otoscopic examination and tuning fork testing; neurologic examination with special attention to the cranial nerves; and auscultation of the mastoids, carotids, and ears if the tinnitus is pulsatile. In addition, blood pressure recordings should be obtained from both arms.

The importance of audiometry cannot be overemphasized. Any patient presenting with tinnitus should receive a complete audiologic evaluation, including pure tone thresholds for air and bone conduction and speech testing. If the audiogram is normal or shows a symmetric bilateral high-frequency sensorineural hearing loss, usually no further workup is required, and the patient is reassured.

If the patient's presentation is complicated by other medical problems, blood chemistries, thyroid function tests, and other studies deemed valuable by the physician should be obtained. If the patient complains only of unilateral tinnitus, intracranial causes must be ruled out. Magnetic resonance imaging with gadolinium is obtained to rule out an acoustic neuroma. When pulsatile tinnitus is the chief complaint, a vascular cause should be sought.

Temporal bone computed tomography is the study of choice to rule out an erosive process in the area of the jugular foramen. It will also evaluate a retrotympanic mass (glomus tympanicum or jugulare); it will pick up abnormalities of the jugular bulb and/or the carotid artery. It is usually combined with magnetic resonance imaging with gadolinium and sometimes an arteriogram in cases in which a vascular tumor is suspected. When a carotid bruit is auscultated, a carotid artery duplex study is ordered. Table 1 lists some of the more common causes of pulsatile tinnitus, and Table 2 displays common causes of nonpulsatile tinnitus.

TREATMENT

The treatment of tinnitus is based on the underlying pathology. Treatment can be lengthy and frustrating to both the physician and patient. In a review of 69 randomized clinical trials evaluating various treatment modalities ranging from medications to psychotherapy, no treatment has been proven reproducible and effective. Overall, 25% of patients will improve to a great deal, 50% will improve to a moderate degree, and 25% will have no improvement. Few patients will have worsening symptoms.

For metabolic conditions, appropriate correction of the aberrance is the treatment of choice.

Myoclonus of either the soft palate muscle or middle ear muscle (generally described as a "clicking sound," sometimes several times per second) can be treated with muscle relaxants, with botulinum toxin injection of the palate, or by severing the tensor tympani or stapedius muscles.

Benign intracranial hypertension is an often overlooked cause in patients who tend to be obese women; gentle compression of the jugular vein in the neck brings relief of the symptoms. A neuro-ophthalmologic consultation is obtained in these patients.

In cases of paragangliomas of the middle ear or the jugular foramen, total tumor resection is often of benefit. These resections are usually done after tumor embolization.

TABLE 1. **Common Causes of Pulsatile Tinnitus**

Benign intracranial hypertension ("venous hum" tinnitus)
Atherosclerosis of the carotid arteries
Glomus tumor
Vascular malformation: arteriovenous malformation, carotid artery aneurysm
Otosclerosis
Palatal myoclonus
Middle ear muscle (tensor tympani or stapedius) myoclonus
Hypertension

TABLE 2. **Common Causes of Nonpulsatile Tinnitus**

Hearing loss
Noise exposure/acoustic trauma
Acoustic neuroma
Otitis externa and media
Eustachian tube function or dysfunction
Labyrinthitis
Meniere disease
Temporomandibular joint dysfunction
Tension headaches
Stress, depression, anxiety

Medications should also be evaluated as possible etiologic factors and should be changed or terminated if medically feasible. The list of tinnitus-causing medications includes erythromycin, macrolide antibiotics, vancomycin, aminoglycosides, furosemide (Lasix) and other loop diuretics, high-dose aspirin or nonsteroidal anti-inflammatory drugs, chemotherapeutic agents (platinum-containing agents), caffeine, nicotine, and alcohol.

Infections of the outer, middle, and inner ear are often accompanied by tinnitus; treatment of the infection usually relieves the tinnitus.

Meniere disease also poses a unique clinical challenge to the physician. Tinnitus, fluctuating hearing loss, and vertigo compose the classic triad of symptoms. The history and a normal otologic examination are essential in diagnosing this condition. Treatment for Meniere disease is often complex and should be done by an otologist or neuro-otologist.

The vast majority of patients presenting with tinnitus have some degree of sensorineural hearing loss. Many of these patients have become used to the head noise, which they notice at night when it is quiet. Taking the time to explain to these patients that the tinnitus is a manifestation of their hearing loss is usually all that is needed to reassure them.

Victims of acoustic trauma (exposure to brief, high-intensity sounds) and noise-induced trauma (exposure to prolonged, medium to high-intensity sounds) can develop tinnitus. Hearing protection must be discussed at length with these patients.

Stress can be the cause or a major contributing factor to the patient's symptoms. When obtaining a history from the patient, the physician should carefully elicit information about the stresses the patient is experiencing. Difficulties at home, at work, or within the patient's family may cause tinnitus. Counseling these patients may be helpful in eliminating or improving the symptoms. We use the mnemonic CAPPE (chemical, acoustic, pathologic, physical, and emotional) to help identify these stresses (Table 3).

TABLE 3. **CAPPE Mnemonic for Tinnitus Evaluation**

Chemical
Acoustic
Pathologic
Physical
Emotional

Chemical stresses include medications that we mentioned previously. Elimination of some of the medications or changing them could be helpful. We advise our patients to switch to decaffeinated products, quit smoking, and follow healthier diets. Acoustic stresses include chronic noise exposure, acoustic trauma, and hearing loss. We ask our patients who are exposed to occupational noise or loud noises to use hearing protection. Pathologic stresses include infectious, inflammatory, vascular, and neoplastic processes affecting the ear. Diagnosing and specifically treating these conditions as mentioned earlier can be extremely helpful to the patient.

Physical stresses such as vigorous exercise, fever, upper respiratory tract infections, temporomandibular joint dysfunction, tension headaches, and cervical muscle tension may be the cause or an aggravating factor in tinnitus. Treating these conditions will relief the stress associated with these entities. However, emotional stress remains a major contributing factor. Unfortunately for the patient, tinnitus is the result of a vicious cycle. This may induce insomnia, inability to focus, and depression. The cycle must be broken for the patient to feel better. This can be accomplished through various techniques, including stress reduction, biofeedback, psychotherapy, and antidepressant medications, depending on the severity of the symptoms. Amitriptyline (Elavil),* 25 mg orally at bedtime, helps reduce the symptoms of insomnia, stress, and depression.

When no specific cause of tinnitus is ascertained, which is common, several conservative measures can be initiated. The patient should abstain from any caffeine-containing substances (e.g., coffee, tea, and chocolate). Aggravating noises should be avoided, and home masking techniques should be used. The general principle in *masking* is to produce a sound that will overcome the tinnitus. There are several masking techniques available: hearing aids, radios, and masking devices. For example, the radio can be tuned to static at night when the patient is attempting to sleep. The static or "white noise" should be loud enough to mask the tinnitus. Commercial masking devices are also available.

Habituation has also been investigated. The results have been promising. In short, *habituation* is a technique that presents aural stimuli up to 16 hours a day for several months. The premise is that the patient will accommodate to the stimuli.

The use of electrical stimulation via transcutaneous, promontory, and round window stimulation of the cochlea is being investigated. The impetus for these trials was the finding of reduced tinnitus in patients receiving cochlear implants.

CONCLUSION

Tinnitus is an exceptionally common finding throughout the population. Considering the increas-

*Not FDA approved for this indication.

ing prevalence of tinnitus in older individuals, this condition will affect a higher number of patients as the population continues to age. The primary care physician must know the basic presenting complaints of patients suffering from tinnitus. The history, physical examination, and audiometric evaluations are essential in the workup of the patient with tinnitus. Tinnitus is a symptom that is related to many different causes with various contributing factors. Therefore, the primary care physician must know that simple reassurance is adequate for some patients, whereas others need referrals to specialists in dealing with this complex problem.

BACK PAIN

method of
MICHAEL T. McCANN, M.D.
Baylor College of Medicine
Houston, Texas

Although back pain is one of the most common musculoskeletal complaints seen in primary care practices, our understanding of the causes of spine and radicular pain remains poor, leading to empirical treatments, all with limited efficacy. Proper diagnosis from the start is imperative to optimize patient outcomes and minimize the staggering health care and indirect costs associated with these spinal disorders.

A patient who has enough back or neck pain to see a physician is not there because of a muscle strain. Additionally, isolated back pain is usually not a neurologic problem but rather an orthopedic one. Although patients were relatively satisfied with their care for most major illnesses, 20% to 25% of patients surveyed were dissatisfied with their care for back pain. Only headache treatment also received such poor scores. The top reason listed for dissatisfaction with the physician's care was inadequate explanation of the problem. Before we can provide better care, we must change the way we think about spine-related pain.

EPIDEMIOLOGY

Eighty percent of persons will develop back pain that limits the function at some time in their lives. The peak incidence occurs between the ages of 35 and 65 years. This does not correlate with what we would expect anatomically. Based on radiographic evidence of degeneration alone, the incidence should increase linearly with age. In 80% of patients presenting with these complaints, the pain will be self-limited, but 15% to 20% will have pain that has severely restricted function for more than a year. Direct and indirect costs are estimated to be between $80 and $100 billion per year in the United States, and from an insurer's standpoint these costs may exceed all expenditures on pediatric and obstetric care combined. The majority of treatment expenditures are generated by the 20% of patients whose pain does not resolve spontaneously—the sufferers of recurrent or chronic back pain.

PATHOPHYSIOLOGY

Despite their frequent coexistence, radicular extremity symptoms need to be distinguished from referred somatic pain. Radicular pain is caused by evoked ectopic impulses in the dorsal root ganglia, whereas somatic axial and referred pain is caused by noxious stimuli affecting nerve ending receptors in the vertebrae, the joints, the ligaments, and the disks.

The most common cause of lumbar radicular pain is disk herniation (98%); however, nerve compression alone does not offer a satisfactory explanation for the pain produced. In human studies, root compression produces paresthesias and numbness in the extremities but no pain. Isolated lumbar radiculopathy does not cause significant back pain. Additionally, the severity of radicular pain seen with straight leg raising does not correlate with the size of disk herniation or with compression seen on computed tomography (CT). A sensitized root that is compressed does, however, cause extremity pain. Nucleus pulposus placed within the epidural space is inflammatory and produces a 100,000-fold increase in phospholipase A_2 immunoreactivity that can be directly correlated with mechanical hyperalgesia. In the complete absence of root compression, nucleus pulposus stimulates sustained discharges of A delta and A beta fibers in the dorsal root ganglia and causes a conduction delay in the roots. Intravenous methylprednisone prevents this conduction delay. The cause of radicular pain currently appears to be tension in an otherwise chemically mediated sensitized root.

Other vertebral sources of lumbar radicular pain include spinal and lateral recess stenoses caused by facet arthropathies, ligamentous hypertrophy, and spondylolisthesis. Causes that are even more rare include neuromeningeal anomalies, neoplasms, infections, and vascular malformations. Peripheral neuropathies including thoracic outlet, cubital, and carpal tunnel syndromes; piriformis syndrome; and other primary mononeuropathies may also mimic or exist in conjunction with radiculopathies.

Radicular pain is lancinating and shooting, with superficial and deep components that extend in a distinct, but not necessarily dermatomal, band into the extremity. Somatic referred pain is deep, aching, and diffuse. It can overlap with radicular symptoms in the proximal extremities. Pain below the knee that is diffuse may be referred, whereas pain extending distally into the hand or the foot is more likely to be radicular.

Sources of somatic back and neck pain can be from the anterior or the posterior column. Pain generators in the anterior column are primarily the disks and the vertebral bodies. The outer third of a disk's annulus is richly innervated. Tears of these annular fibers produce exquisite sensitivity, even without extrusion of nuclear material into the epidural space. Contained internal annular tears can be extremely painful and result in significant paraspinal spasm and splinting. They are a frequently missed cause of nonspecific back pain because these internal disk disruptions cannot be visualized on routine magnetic resonance imaging (MRI) and CT of the spine. The finding on T2-weighted MRI of a high intensity zone is, however, highly suggestive of a painful annular tear. These disruptions can be definitively diagnosed with manometric provocative CT diskography.

Vertebral compression fractures, whether osteoporotic or pathologic, also contribute to anterior column primary axial pain. Plain radiography will confirm the diagnosis; however, MRI or CT scanning may be necessary to confirm acuteness of a finding and to help rule out metastatic foci. Osteomyelitis or discitis also should be considered in any fracture with associated fever or failure to improve progressively.

The posterior column as a source of back pain includes

the facet joints from the atlanto-occipital articulation caudad to the sacroiliac joints. All are true diarthrodial joints. The surfaces are capped with articular cartilage and are lined with a synovial membrane. These paired innervated structures are subject to degeneration and painful traumatic injuries. In double-blind placebo-controlled studies, the cervical facets appear to be the source of pain in 59% of patients with post whiplash cervicalgia. Estimates in the lumbar spine place the incidence of facet-based low back pain between 15% and 40%. Spondylolisthesis with associated stress fractures of the pars interarticularis may additionally be a source of low back pain. There is often associated fibrosis under the pars defects that involves the traversing nerve roots and may thus produce radicular symptoms without actual compression.

Careful history and examination should help delineate referred cardiac, pulmonary, gastrointestinal, urologic, gynecologic, and vascular sources. Failure to improve, with symptoms out of proportion to objective findings, may be indicative of a pure psychogenic source; however, this is exceedingly rare. More often, psychogenic stressors or underlying personality disorders affect an individual's ability to cope with an otherwise benign condition, treatment response, and functional prognosis.

Finally, central disorders should be considered in a patient with the following "red flag" features:

- Pain at a fixed time every night that prevents sleep
- Significant spontaneous pain at rest aggravated with neck or trunk movement
- Absence of traumatic cause
- Loss of continence
- Positive Babinski sign with clonus and hyperreflexia

Muscle pain and spasm should not be considered the primary sources of the patient's back pain unless all other potential sources have been ruled out and an objective rheumatologic cause has been identified pointing to myositis. In these cases, the muscular pains are often more diffuse, and aggravation occurs with all movements. An antalgic gait from distal degenerative joint disease may cause lumbar muscular aching; however, rarely will the back be the site of greatest pain. This is not to say that muscles cannot be painful but rather that in the majority of cases of primary back pain, they are simply reacting to an underlying derangement in the spine proper.

ASSESSMENT

The goal of the initial assessment is to screen for emergent causes of back or radicular pain, including aneurysms, infections, unstable fractures, tumors, and myelopathy. For all patients presenting with back or radicular pain, the screening history should include weight loss, fevers or infections, and significant change in bowel or bladder function, including incontinence. For patients with neck or upper extremity radicular pain, a history of chest pain or shortness of breath should be added, whereas abdominal symptoms should be included for lumbar pain. The vascular and abdominal screening examinations should be routine in all patients presenting with back or radicular complaints.

Interestingly, physical examination in patients with radicular symptoms is an otherwise poor tool for making a diagnosis. Tumors, cysts, and disk herniations all cause the same clinical signs. Testing, including testing of reflexes, weakness, sensory deficits, and even muscle atrophy, has been shown to lack both sensitivity and specificity in diagnosing disk herniations. Although clinical examination may establish the presence of radiculopathy, the cause of the radiculopathy must be established by other means. Luckily, with the incidence of disk herniation being 98% for the younger patient with radiculopathy, this initial diagnostic impression is fairly accurate. Nonetheless, the same does not hold true in the elderly patient with radiculopathy, nor in the patient with axial pain without radiculopathy. A definitive diagnosis, if required, can be established only by use of specific imaging and interventional procedures for spinal pain.

NATURAL COURSE OF THE DISEASE

For lumbar radicular pain in patients treated conservatively, 50% of patients can expect to experience resolution of radicular symptoms after 4 weeks, and at 12 months, resolution is evident in 49% of males and 33% of females. Unfortunately, 60% to 70% of patients developed back pain at 4 weeks, and this persisted at 12 months regardless of the course of radicular symptoms. For patients treated surgically versus conservatively, at 10 years there appears to be little statistically significant difference in outcome in regard to discogenic radicular pain, with both groups achieving about 60% good results, and poor results occurring in 7% to 8%. This holds true only if surgery is not applied randomly but is applied as a last resort for patients who fail to respond to conservative care.

For cervical radiculopathic symptoms, 70% can be expected to improve with time, and 20% will become asymptomatic. In patients for whom surgery was an option, 90% were improved or only mildly incapacitated at long-term follow-up. Isolated recurrences were seen in 32% of patients, whereas 10% had moderate to severe persistent disability.

Although studies exist detailing overall favorable outcomes for radicular symptoms, the same does not necessarily hold true for mechanical back pain. Whereas 80% of patients appear to experience resolution of initial symptoms no matter what the course of conservative care, 20% develop progressive or unrelenting pain. It appears that approximately 35% of persons will have intermittent recurrences that limit activities.

MANAGEMENT

Radicular Pain Predominating

Taking an algorithmic approach to the patient presenting with radicular symptoms of new onset, if initial history and examination are suggestive of an emergent cause for these symptoms, then appropriate additional diagnostic testing and referral should be done. Indications for urgent surgical interventions are few but include progressive motor deficit and cauda equina syndrome (progressive neurologic deterioration with loss of bowel and bladder function).

Once an emergent source of pain has been ruled out, studies have shown that the primary care physicians who prescribe the least amount of analgesics and who place the fewest restrictions on activities have the best patient outcomes. In many cases, a more aggressive approach may reinforce illness behavior and may foster a fear of future debilitation.

If radicular pain predominates in a minimally distressed patient, simple reassurance and explanation of the natural course of recovery may suffice. Avoiding bed rest and modifying activities to avoid axial loading should be discussed. A 2-week reassessment allows any insidious "red flag" conditions to be picked up, provides reassurance, and allows adjustment of treatment.

For more significantly distressed patients with acute radicular pain, additional analgesics and more frequent follow-up may be required. Although no analgesic regimen has been shown to alter the natural course of recovery, based on the inflammatory pathogenesis of radicular pain, a pulsed dose of prednisone or methylprednisolone (Solu-Medrol) with a taper can be considered over 1 week. In randomized controlled trials, however, the nonsteroidal anti-inflammatory drugs piroxicam (Feldene) and indomethacin (Indocin) did not offer any greater analgesia or enhance recovery more than placebo and are thus not recommended. Limited muscle relaxants and opioid analgesics may be prescribed. The limited course of these prescriptions should be explained to the patient at the outset. No studies exist to support their long-term use; for neuropathic pain, they may actually be contraindicated.

If at follow-up significant progress has not been made and reassessment still lacks red flags, then a 2-week course of active cervical or lumbar stabilization exercises may be considered with continuance as a home program. Again, no scientific studies validate any particular regimen of therapy; however, from a spinal education standpoint and as an impetus to maintaining function, an empirical recommendation can be made. Follow-up should be scheduled, and, if progress is partial, another 2 weeks of therapy could be considered versus simple continuance as a home program.

If failure to improve or deterioration of function occurs, imaging studies would be indicated. An MRI provides the most comprehensive survey of causes for radicular symptoms. It does not, however, guarantee that anatomic changes are definitively the source of a patient's symptoms. In patients younger than the age of 40 years, approximately 30% of asymptomatic volunteers showed disk abnormalities on MRI, whereas 60% to 70% of patients older than 40 had abnormalities. The prevalence of asymptomatic disk protrusions alone ranged from 20% to 40% in patients between the ages of 40 and 60 years.

Evidence-based review of the literature currently does not support the use of electromyography and nerve conduction velocity (EMG/NCV) studies for diagnosis in cases of radiculopathic pain. Pain is mediated through A delta and C fibers, whereas EMG tests activity in A alpha fibers. H and F reflexes similarly lack validity and specificity in clinical trials of radiculopathy, despite proposed theoretical foundations. EMG/NCV testing would be indicated in cases in which peripheral neuropathy or nerve entrapment is suspected and when objective muscle strength testing is suspect.

Recent prospective randomized blinded studies support selective nerve root injection (i.e., fluoroscopically guided transforaminal epidural steroid or epiradicular injection) as the next line of recommended treatment. This highly selective treatment may reduce the need for surgical intervention in up to 59% of the cases. The older regimen of translaminar epidural steroid injections has not been shown to be nearly as efficacious as, and in some studies appears no more effective than, placebo. Partial improvement at 10- to 14-day follow-up would be an indication for repeat injection. Lack of improvement would necessitate additional surgical assessment. An automatic series of three injections is no longer considered a standard of care, and response to a single injection (translaminar or transforaminal) should guide additional treatment.

Long-term management of a patient with radicular pain unrelieved by surgery or a patient for whom surgical options do not exist falls into the realm of neuropathic pain control. Narcotic regimens should be avoided. Medication options are limited; however, gabapentin (Neurontin)* appears to be effective in reducing pain for a large number of patients with both radicular and other sources of neuropathic pain. There are few toxic effects, and it is well tolerated by the majority of patients. With sedation being the most frequent side effect, the dosage should be titrated upward from 100 to 1200 mg three times a day. Other drugs to be considered include mexiletine (Mexitil),* tricyclic antidepressants,* and selective serotonin reuptake inhibitors.* All have been shown to modify neuropathic pain in the presence and the absence of associated depression.

For patients in whom the neuropathic extremity pain far exceeds mechanical back pain despite optimization of all forms of conservative treatment, spinal cord stimulation may be considered. This modality has been shown to be effective in 60% to 70% of patients with neuropathic extremity pain predominating. It is not indicated for mechanical pain. If an outpatient stimulation trial is successful in significantly reducing pain, improving function, and eliminating the need for significant additional analgesic intake, permanent implantation can be performed, usually with an overnight hospital stay. In permanently implanted patients, 70% continue to have approximately 50% improvement in neuropathic pain at 5-year follow-up.

Axial Pain Predominating

For patients with nonurgent axial back or neck pain predominating, again the level of distress helps guide care. Studies regarding early treatment and analgesic regimens for nociceptive back pain lack validity and specificity because early diagnosis is not usually sought, owing to the high incidence of spontaneous improvement. Early treatment thus remains empirical.

In a minimally distressed patient, supportive education and maintenance of activity will support the

*Not FDA approved for this indication.

natural course of recovery. After a 1- to 2-week cooling-off period, if improvement is seen, a course of spinal stabilization exercises would be recommended, followed by a home program to help reduce recurrence.

For the more distressed patient, oral analgesics may be indicated. Because the source of axial pain is nociceptive, nonsteroidal anti-inflammatory drugs should be considered as first-line analgesics, with opioids reserved for very severe pain, again only for limited periods. Failure to improve is not necessarily an indication for continued opioid use. For moderate to severe pain in which a significant inflammatory component is suspected, a bolus or taper dose of corticosteroids over 1 week is often effective, and risks are low with this regimen. Muscle spasms are best managed with gradual stretching and paced activities. In severe cases, however, muscle relaxants may be beneficial, and even a limited course of benzodiazepines should be considered.

If at 2-week reassessment, progress is not seen, physical therapy over 1 month, usually three to four times per week, for range of motion and stabilization exercises should be considered. Partial improvement would be an indication for another month of therapy or, in the motivated patient, another month of a home exercise program.

The goal of therapy is to maintain range of motion, strengthen supportive musculature, and maintain activities of daily living without additional injury. To this end, almost all exercise regimens and modality-based treatments claim efficacy. Validity studies to show that any specific therapy actually alters the natural history remain lacking, however.

Should a patient with primary back or neck pain fail to improve with therapy, screening radiographs may be indicated. Plain radiographs for mechanical back pain should always be obtained, with flexion and extension views to rule out gross instability as well as other mechanical derangements, including spondylolisthesis, spondylolysis, and compression fractures.

Unfortunately, although all radiographic studies of the spine demonstrate anatomic abnormalities, they cannot indicate whether these abnormalities are painful. With physical examination also notoriously unreliable for making a definitive diagnosis, referral for more advanced spinal diagnostic assessment may often be indicated. In many cases, for example, a severely degenerative disk is found to be asymptomatic on provocative diskography, whereas a symptomatic annular disk tear is identified at an adjacent level.

For the 20% of patients in whom function remains limited by back pain despite maximized conservative care, identification of the exact pain source is imperative to improving outcome. These patients are prone to seek numerous opinions, undergo fruitless operations, and pay for unproven modality-based treatments. Physicians tend to make diagnoses based on response to treatment as opposed to the other way around. An early definitive diagnosis allows realistic treatment options and prognosis to be given. Patients can thus adjust their lifestyles to function within the limits imposed by their musculoskeletal condition.

Significant advances have been made in the field of diagnosing back pain. Selected spinal injection techniques have been refined to isolate the exact source of a patient's pain in the majority of cases. Reliability testing can also determine if a patient's complaint has an anatomic basis or if symptom magnification is present.

CT-provocative diskography is the only test available to document internal disk anatomy precisely and to determine if a disk is the source of a patient's back pain. Studies have shown that compared with surgical findings, its anatomic accuracy exceeds MRI and CT myelography. With the use of manometry, intradiskal symptomatic pressures have been shown to correlate with surgical fusion outcome according to approach. Diagnostic facet injections can also precisely identify a symptomatic joint, further helping to determine options for treatment.

New nonsurgical or minimally invasive treatments have been validated, including radiofrequency lesioning (RFTC) for desensitization of painful facet joint arthropathies and intradiskal electrothermal therapy (IDET) for treatment of painful annular disk lesions. Treatment outcomes for both these procedures rely heavily on the information gained through the previously discussed diagnostic tests.

Surgical assessment of isolated axial pain should be reserved for those patients in whom conservative management has failed and who are not candidates for minimally invasive treatment or who have identifiable gross segmental spinal instability. Unlike in radicular pain, decompression alone is unlikely to improve back pain. For mechanical back pain from either a predominant diskogenic or a facetogenic source, the only surgical option is fusion. Poor pain relief is seen most frequently in patients who undergo fusion procedures for back pain based on radiographic findings alone. Additional provocative testing to isolate the actual pain generators and to determine the integrity of surrounding support structures maximizes chances for success. Not all patients are candidates for surgical reconstruction. In many cases, surgical intervention may only serve to worsen a patient's state, and tolerance of symptoms with acceptance of functional limitations is the preferred course.

CONCLUSIONS

Patients presenting with pain of spinal origin should be divided into those with predominantly radicular symptoms and those with primarily mechanical back or neck pain. Back and neck pain in the vast majority of cases originates from derangements of the facets, the disks, or the vertebrae, not the muscles. Failure to respond to outlined conservative management may be expected in up to 20% of patients. For those cases, interventional spinal diagnostic testing should be obtained as soon as possible to avoid unnecessary and unguided treatments.

Identification and isolation of specific spinal pain generators have allowed for the development of minimally invasive treatments. These include epiradicular injections for radiculopathy, RFTC desensitization for facet-based pain, and IDET for diskogenic pain. Decompressive surgery is very effective at relieving severe radicular pain unresponsive to conservative care and injections. Spinal reconstructive surgery for well-diagnosed painful segmental instability remains the definitive treatment for this disorder.

Section 2

The Infectious Diseases

MANAGEMENT OF THE HIV-INFECTED PATIENT

method of
TIM WILKIN, M.D.
Columbia University
New York, New York

and

AIMEE WILKIN, M.D.
Johns Hopkins School of Medicine
Baltimore, Maryland

Twenty years ago, recognition of clusters of *Pneumocystis carinii* pneumonia (PCP) in previously healthy homosexual men led to the first description of the AIDS epidemic. HIV1 causes progressive deterioration of the immune system, primarily through $CD4^+$ lymphocyte depletion. AIDS encompasses a $CD4^+$ count below 200 cells/mm^3 or the presence of opportunistic infections or noninfectious complications that typically occur with a $CD4^+$ count less than 200 cells/mm^3 (Table 1). Remarkable progress has been made in understanding the pathogenesis, immunology, and epidemiology of HIV. The development of pharmaceutical agents targeted at specific sites of the HIV life cycle has revolutionized the care of people infected with HIV, and ongoing exploration of targets for drug and vaccine development holds promise for continued advances in treatment and prevention.

EPIDEMIOLOGY

As of December 2000, 36.1 million people were living with HIV/AIDS worldwide, with 25.3 million in sub-Saharan Africa. The global epidemic is progressing unabated, and many areas of the developing world are suffering from rapidly increasing rates of HIV. Unfortunately, these countries also often lack effective public health infrastructures and the means to afford the therapeutic advances that benefit the developed world. Research into vaccines, microbicides, and behavioral modification offers hope for reducing transmission. Coordinated support from Western governments and major pharmaceutical companies is needed to bring lifesaving treatments to the developing world.

In the United States, an estimated 800,000 to 900,000 people are living with HIV/AIDS, with 470,000 deaths from HIV/AIDS since the beginning of the epidemic. HIV disproportionately affects African and Hispanic Americans, and 70% of the estimated 40,000 new infections in the United States each year occur in these minority groups. Heterosexual transmission is increasingly common, with women now making up approximately 30% of new infections in this country and more than 50% worldwide. Recent reports of increasing unsafe sexual behavior among men who have sex with men are of concern for a resurgence in HIV transmission. The HIV epidemic continues despite the advances in treatment, and it is critical that the medical community properly detect those who are infected and bring them into care. Behavioral risk reduction and early diagnosis of infection must be priorities for all health care providers.

NATURAL HISTORY

In the era before highly active antiretroviral therapy (HAART), the average time from initial infection to the development of AIDS was 10 years, and the mean life expectancy was 12 years. The clinical course of disease is highly variable and depends on host immunologic parameters, viral properties, and genetic factors. Observational studies of men who have sex with men and who acquired HIV infection before the advent of antiretroviral therapy show that progression to AIDS is predicted by both the $CD4^+$ count and plasma HIV viral load (Table 2). The $CD4^+$ count remains the most important marker for determining the risk of opportunistic infections and other complications (see Table 1). The advent of HAART has dramatically altered the clinical course of HIV infection, as manifested by declining morbidity and mortality from AIDS and opportunistic infections. HIV infection may be considered a chronic, manageable illness, but a new spectrum of long-term complications from antiretroviral therapy and liver disease is emerging.

TRANSMISSION OF HIV

Transmission of HIV occurs through sexual contact, from exposure to blood or blood products such as when sharing intravenous needles and drug equipment, and through vertical transmission. Blood, semen, and cervicovaginal fluids are infectious and can transmit HIV infection when in contact with mucous membranes or when the protective barrier of intact skin is breached (as in intravenous injection or needle stick). Vertical transmission from mother to infant can take place in utero, peripartum, or through breast-feeding, with peripartum infection being most likely. One of the great successes of HIV therapy has been a reduction in perinatal transmission to less than 2% of deliveries in women with HIV in the United States. The reduction is due to a combination of factors: prenatal testing, effective antiretroviral therapy, interventions such as cesarean section when the viral load is not fully suppressed, and avoidance of breast-feeding. Factors affecting the risk of sexual transmission include the type of sex act, with receptive anal and vaginal intercourse having the highest risk. The presence of other sexually transmitted diseases (ulcerative and nonulcerative) in either partner also increases transmissibility. A high plasma viral load in the infected partner (independent of gender) is another determinant of risk, and circumcision may have a protective effect. Other behavioral factors include the number of sex partners, anonymous sex partners, trading sex for money or drugs, and illicit drug use. The correct and con-

TABLE 1. **Correlation of CD4+ Count and HIV Complications**

CD4+ Count	Infectious Complications	Noninfectious Complications
>500/mm³	Acute retroviral syndrome Candidal vaginitis	Persistent generalized lymphadenopathy Guillain-Barré syndrome Myopathy Aseptic meningitis
200–500/mm³	Pneumococcal and other bacterial pneumonia Pulmonary tuberculosis Herpes zoster Thrush (oropharyngeal candidiasis) Kaposi's sarcoma Oral hairy leukoplakia	Cervical carcinoma (and CSIL) B-cell lymphoma Anemia Mononeuritis multiplex Idiopathic thrombocytopenic purpura Hodgkin's disease
<200/mm³	*Pneumocystis carinii* pneumonia Disseminated histoplasmosis Coccidioidomycosis Miliary/extrapulmonary TB Progressive multifocal leukoencephalopathy	Wasting Peripheral neuropathy HIV-associated dementia Cardiomyopathy Vacuolar myelopathy Progressive polyradiculopathy Non–Hodgkin's lymphoma
<100/mm³	Disseminated herpes simplex Toxoplasmosis Cryptococcosis Microsporidiosis *Candida* esophagitis	
<50/mm³	Disseminated CMV Disseminated *Mycobacterium avium complex*	CNS lymphoma

Abbreviations: CMV = cytomegalovirus; CNS = central nervous system; CSIL = cervical squamous intraepithelial lesion; TB = tuberculosis.
Adapted from Hanson DL, Chu SY, Farizo KM, Ward JW: Distribution of CD4+ T lymphocytes at diagnosis of acquired immunodeficiency syndrome–defining and other human immunodeficiency virus–related illnesses. The Adult and Adolescent Spectrum of HIV Disease Project Group. Arch Intern Med 155:1537–1542, 1995. Copyright 1995, American Medical Association.

sistent use of condoms or other barrier methods decreases the risk of HIV transmission. Access to methadone clinics and needle exchange programs can reduce risk behavior in intravenous drug users.

KINETICS OF HIV INFECTION

After mucous membrane exposure to HIV, the virus attaches to dendritic cells and is transported to regional lymph nodes. There, it infects T lymphocytes by binding to the CD4 molecule with the use of a coreceptor, CCR5. The virus then disseminates throughout the body and is clinically manifested as acute HIV infection. This initial burst of viremia is controlled by a cytotoxic T-cell response that is followed by the development of HIV antibodies (typically appearing 3 to 12 weeks after exposure). The plasma viral load then settles at a "setpoint." Despite the appearance of a "latent" phase clinically, a tremendous cycle of viral replication, activated CD4+ cell destruction, and repletion ensues. This phase may continue for years even without therapy. Over time, the progressive insult to the immune system overcomes host defenses and the CD4+ count declines. The HIV reverse transcriptase is highly error prone, and mutations in the genome are common. Suboptimal levels of antiretroviral medications lead to incomplete suppression of viral replication and the selection of drug-resistant mutants. Another recent realization is that virus, wildtype and resistant, is archived in long-living quiescent CD4+ cells and other sanctuary sites where currently available therapies are not active.

ACUTE HIV INFECTION

Primary HIV infection is an acute, self-limited, febrile illness that occurs in 50% to 90% of persons infected with HIV (Table 3). Although most patients see a health care provider in primary or emergency care settings during acute HIV infection, the diagnosis is rarely considered and patients are often labeled with "viral syndrome." It is important to consider testing for acute HIV infection in any patient with an unexplained febrile illness or with a suggestive constellation of signs and symptoms because no clear discrimination exists between acute HIV and other viral syndromes. A history of possible exposure to HIV can be helpful, but providers and patients may be uncomfortable discussing behavioral risk factors. Standard testing

TABLE 2. **Percentage of Persons Progressing to AIDS Within 3 Years (and 9 Years) Stratified by CD4+ Count and Viral Load**

	CD4+ <350	CD4+ <500 and >350	CD4+ >500
Viral load 1500–7000	0 (30.6)	4.4 (46.9)	2.3 (33.2)
Viral load 7001–20,000	8.0 (65.6)	5.9 (60.7)	7.2 (50.3)
Viral load 20,001–55,000	40.1 (86.2)	15.1 (78.6)	14.6 (70.6)
Viral load >55,000	72.9 (95.6)	47.9 (94.4)	32.6 (76.3)

Data from the Multicenter AIDS Cohort Study: Mellors JEW, Kingley LA, Rinaldo CR, et al: Quantitation of HIV-1 RNA in plasma predicts outcome after seroconversion. Ann Intern Med 122:573–579, 1995.

TABLE 3. **Signs and Symptoms of Acute HIV**

Symptoms		Signs	
Fever	Myalgias	Pharyngitis	Lymphadenopathy
Sore throat	Arthralgias	Oral/genital ulcers	
Fatigue/ malaise	Night sweats	Oral candidiasis	
		Morbilliform rash	
Headache	Diarrhea	Hepatosplenomegaly	
Neck stiffness			
Laboratory Tests		**Differential Diagnosis**	
Mild transaminase elevations		Infectious mononucleosis	
		Acute toxoplasmosis	
Thrombocytopenia, leukopenia		Hepatitis A	
		"Viral syndrome"	
Decreased CD4+ count		Aseptic meningitis	
CSF lymphocytic pleocytosis			

Abbreviation: CSF = cerebrospinal fluid.

for HIV with enzyme immunoassay and confirmatory Western blot testing will be negative or indeterminate. The two feasible options for diagnosing acute HIV infection are p24 antigen assay and HIV plasma viral load testing. The p24 antigen test has a sensitivity of 88.7% and a specificity of 100%. HIV RNA viral load testing has a sensitivity of 100% and a specificity of 97.4%. True positives by viral load testing in acute infection are typically over 100,000 copies/mL, and false-positive results are usually under 10,000 copies/mL. Making the diagnosis of acute HIV infection can have profound implications. Growing evidence indicates that institution of HAART during acute HIV infection may change the natural history of HIV by preserving HIV-specific immunity and lowering the viral setpoint of chronic infection. Moreover, a patient is extremely infectious during acute HIV infection. An estimated 40% of cases of HIV transmission have a source patient with primary HIV infection. If possible, any patient in whom acute HIV infection is diagnosed should be urgently referred to a research center, where in-depth treatment and immunologic monitoring can improve our understanding of the best treatment approaches for this select group of patients.

TESTING FOR CHRONIC HIV INFECTION

Although HIV infection is often asymptomatic, a number of clinical conditions should prompt HIV testing (Table 4). Assessment of behavioral risk factors should be a standard aspect of routine medical care. Testing for HIV with enzyme immunoassay and confirmatory Western blot analysis is extremely sensitive. New methods of testing, including rapid tests, home test kits, and testing of other fluids such as saliva, will continue to expand opportunities to diagnose HIV infection and provide counseling.

MANAGEMENT OF PATIENTS INFECTED WITH HIV

Baseline Evaluation

A thorough history should cover all past medical and psychiatric illnesses and assessment for symptoms suggestive of current opportunistic infection, neoplasm, or other medical illness. Evaluation for potential psychiatric disorders such as depression is important. A complete evaluation of substance abuse issues and appropriate referral for treatment are also critical to maximize the patient's health and ability to adhere to antiretroviral therapy. Complete ascertainment of all medications and herbal supplements can avoid unfavorable drug interactions with antiretroviral agents. If the patient does not have newly diagnosed HIV infection, a complete history of past antiretroviral therapy, virologic responses to treatment as measured by plasma HIV viral load testing, and immunologic parameters (especially the nadir $CD4^+$ count) is critical to determine the need for antiretroviral therapy and the most appropriate regimen.

Physical examination can show evidence of immunosuppression (see Tables 1 and 2). All women should have a gynecologic examination with cytologic screening if not recently performed, and all patients (particularly those with a $CD4^+$ count below 100

TABLE 4. **Situations in Which HIV Testing Should Be Offered***

Perform HIV testing on all persons who request testing and all pregnant women
Certain Infections
Severe herpetic lesions
Shingles
Community-acquired pneumonia
Recurrent bacterial infection
Infection with unusual organisms
Atypical features of common infections
Other STDs
Oropharyngeal candidiasis
Recurrent vulvovaginal candidiasis
Tuberculosis
Symptoms
Weight loss
Chronic diarrhea
Laboratory Tests
For: ITP, TTP, anemia, leukopenia
Unexplained renal insufficiency
Dermatologic Conditions
Severe psoriasis
Seborrheic dermatitis
Extensive HPV infection
Molluscum contagiosum
Oral leukoplakia
Neurologic Conditions
Neuropathies
Dementia
Gullain-Barré syndrome
Aseptic meningitis
Malignancies
Non–Hodgkin's lymphoma
Hodgkin's disease
Cervical carcinoma
Anal carcinoma

*This list is in addition to persons who report known HIV risk factors and those who have an infection or condition listed in Table 1.

Abbreviations: HPV = human papillomavirus; ITP = idiopathic thrombocytopenic purpura; STDs = sexually transmitted diseases; TTP = thrombotic thrombocytopenic purpura.

cells/mm³) should have dilated funduscopic examination by an experienced ophthalmologist to screen for HIV-related eye diseases.

Laboratory Testing

Baseline laboratory testing should include the following: HIV serology to document HIV status; $CD4^+$ count as a marker of immune status and risk for opportunistic infections; HIV plasma viral load to establish a baseline before therapy; complete blood count to screen for anemia, leukopenia, and thrombocytopenia; serum chemistry panel to screen for hepatitis and to have a baseline before potentially toxic therapies; serum rapid plasma reagin (RPR) test to screen for syphilis; screening for infectious hepatitis with hepatitis C antibody, hepatitis B core antibody, hepatitis B surface antibody, and hepatitis B surface antigen; cytomegalovirus (CMV) antibody to screen for CMV infection (controversial); *Toxoplasma* IgG to screen for the risk of toxoplasmosis; glucose-6-phosphate dehydrogenase level to screen for the risk of hemolytic anemia (especially in high-risk groups); baseline fasting lipid levels before starting antiretroviral medications; tuberculin skin testing; and chest radiograph.

Follow-up laboratory requirements vary depending on the clinical situation. For individuals not receiving antiretroviral therapy, $CD4^+$ counts and HIV viral loads should be measured every 3 to 4 months. For patients receiving therapy, viral load monitoring should be performed after initiation of treatment; the expected decline is a 1.5 to 2 $\log_{10}$ drop by 4 weeks, less than 500 copies/mL by 12 to 16 weeks, and less than 50 copies/mL by 16 to 24 weeks and every 3 months thereafter (target, <50 copies/mL). $CD4^+$ counts are slower to respond to therapy than HIV viral loads, and measurement every 3 months is adequate. In addition, a complete blood count and serum chemistry panel should be performed at least every 3 months to screen for treatment-related toxicities. No consensus has been reached regarding how often to screen for blood lipids, but fasting triglyceride and cholesterol assays every 3 to 6 months may be reasonable. Yearly RPR testing is also recommended.

Substantial fluctuations can be seen in the $CD4^+$ count, so important decisions (for example, starting HAART) should not be made on the basis of a single test result. Likewise, viral load assays can vary by 0.3 to 0.5 $\log_{10}$, and repeat testing should be performed to confirm a rising viral load or a detectable measurement after previous suppression.

Immunizations to consider are pneumococcal vaccine, hepatitis B series, influenza, and tetanus. Generally, HIV patients with $CD4^+$ counts below 200 cells/mm³ are less likely to respond effectively to vaccination, so consideration of withholding vaccines until the $CD4^+$ count is over 200 cells/mm³ or repeating the vaccine after immune reconstitution may be in order. Live-virus vaccines should be avoided. In addition to HIV-specific care and risk assessment, age- and sex-appropriate preventive health screening should be performed.

When to Start Antiretroviral Therapy

One of the critical questions in HIV care is defining the optimal starting point for antiretroviral therapy in asymptomatic individuals with HIV. Antiretroviral therapy in patients with $CD4^+$ counts below 200 cells/mm³ or AIDS-defining illnesses is clearly indicated to restore immune function and slow disease progression. Past enthusiasm for "hit early, hit hard" strategies has been tempered by the complexities of HAART, namely, problems with adherence, drug resistance, the burden of complex medication regimens, and emerging long-term drug toxicities. Current therapies cannot reasonably be expected to eradicate HIV once chronic infection has been established. Recent epidemiologic investigations and extrapolation from the Multicenter AIDS Cohort Study (see Table 2) suggest that therapy can be safely deferred until the $CD4^+$ count falls below 350 cells/mm³. Because waiting for a $CD4^+$ count under 200 cells/mm³ is clearly associated with decreased survival and no firm outcome data support the benefits of initiating therapy with a $CD4^+$ count over 350 cells/mm³, the optimal time to start treatment is probably somewhere in between. The decision to start therapy should be made between the provider and patient after extensive and repeated counseling regarding these issues. The patient's interest in starting therapy and careful evaluation by the provider and patient regarding potential barriers to adherence are critically important. Department of Health and Human Services Guidelines from 2001 reflect the controversy (Table 5).

Adherence

Adherence may be the most important predictor of durable viral suppression with antiretroviral therapy. Rates of success with HAART fall off dramatically with less than 95% adherence. Factors associated with lower adherence include a poor physician-patient relationship, lack of patient education,

TABLE 5. **Guidelines for Starting HAART in Asymptomatic Individuals**

Assess $CD4^+$ and Viral Load	$CD4^+$ <200	$CD4^+$ <350 and >200	$CD4^+$ >350
VL <5000	Recommend Tx	Consider Tx*	Defer Tx
5000 <VL <55,000	Recommend Tx	Recommend Tx	Defer Tx
VL >55,000	Recommend Tx	Recommend Tx	Consider Tx†

*Some experts would consider a delay in therapy given the low rate of progression to AIDS with a viral load less than 5000 even with a $CD4^+$ count between 200 and 350.

†Some experts would recommend starting HAART for all patients with a viral load greater than 55,000 given the greater than 30% progression to AIDS in 3 years, but others would observe patients without an extremely high viral load.

Abbreviations: HAART = highly active antiretroviral therapy; Tx = therapy; VL = viral load.

TABLE 6. **Assessing and Promoting Antiretroviral Therapy Adherence**

Assess the Patient's Understanding of the Disease

Does the patient want to take HAART?
Does the patient readily accept the HIV diagnosis?
Does the patient have an understanding of HIV infection, CD4 count, and viral load?
Does the patient understand the relationship between adherence and drug resistance?

Look for Objective Measures of Adherence

Does the patient keep scheduled clinic appointments?
Is the patient able to adhere to other medications, such as PCP prophylaxis?

Ask About Social Circumstances, Substance Abuse, and Mental Health

Does the patient keep a regular schedule?
Does the patient have other life stressors that make it difficult to adhere to therapy, such as housing issues, a complex work schedule, childcare issues, or physical abuse?
Does the patient have an adequate social support network, friends, family, or coworkers who are aware of the diagnosis and supportive?
Screen for depression and other mental disorders.
Screen for alcohol abuse and illicit drug use.

Measures to Improve Adherence

Education: Can come from the physician, but a multidisciplinary approach including nurses, social workers, support groups, and peer educators can be helpful.
Substance abuse treatment: Alcoholics Anonymous, Narcotics Anonymous, methadone.
Psychiatric care: Establish an alliance with a psychiatrist, therapist, or other mental health professionals so that communication regarding patient care can be improved.
Social work evaluation to address housing, insurance, etc.
Work with the patient to achieve as regular a schedule as possible, and establish exact times for meals and taking medications.
Discuss various drug regimens and weigh patient preference regarding numbers of pills, pill size, food restrictions, and possible side effects.
Warn the patient of potential side effects and outline symptom management principles.
Home nursing or attendants to supervise medications when possible can improve adherence.
Pillboxes and beepers can help remind patients of medications.
Discuss adherence in every follow-up appointment and ask the patient how many doses were missed in the last few days.
Reinforce good adherence by discussing laboratory results.

Abbreviations: HAART = highly active antiretroviral therapy; PCP = *Pneumocystis carinii* pneumonia.

active mental illness or substance abuse, unstable social situations, medication side effects, and high pill burden. Adherence may be assessed by several means—pill counts, memory caps, pharmacy records, patient report (a self-report of poor adherence should be taken seriously)—but none are perfect. Physicians are particularly poor at predicting patient adherence. Even though clinical circumstances sometimes dictate rapid institution of HAART, true antiretroviral emergencies are infrequent, pregnancy and postexposure prophylaxis being notable exceptions. Certainly, in asymptomatic patients, physicians have time to work with patients to establish readiness for therapy. Adherence assessment and counseling should be performed at every visit because compliance can slip over time. Table 6 presents a potential scheme for addressing adherence issues.

STRATEGIES FOR ANTIRETROVIRAL THERAPY

The goal of antiretroviral therapy is durable plasma viral load suppression (currently defined as a plasma viral load below 50 copies/mL on ultrasensitive assay). Such suppression in viral load leads to immunologic improvement (rise in $CD4^+$ count) and prevention of opportunistic infections and death from AIDS. Although numerous drug regimens are successful as initial therapy for HIV, care should be taken to have a rational plan when selecting from the three available classes—nucleoside reverse transcriptase inhibitors (NRTIs), non-nucleoside reverse transcriptase inhibitors (NNRTIs), and protease inhibitors (PIs) (Table 7). Even though the three classes have different resistance patterns, intraclass cross-resistance is common. Using a class-sparing regimen (avoiding either NNRTI or PI use) leaves more potential choices for second-line therapy. Information regarding PI-sparing regimens of two NRTIs plus one NNRTI (such as efavirenz [Sustiva]) or three NRTIs (two NRTIs and abacavir [Ziagen]) is encouraging. These regimens are generally comparable to PI-based regimens in terms of viral suppression, although fewer long-term data are available. The choice of which regimen to start should balance the potential side effect profile, pill burden, compatibility with the patient's schedule, likelihood of pre-existing resistance, predicted drug interactions, and baseline viral load and $CD4^+$ count. Selected potential regimens are presented in Table 8.

Resistance Testing

Antiretroviral therapy without full viral suppression promotes the development of drug resistance by exerting selective pressure on the inherently "mutation-prone" replicative cycle of HIV. The advent of resistance testing through the use of genotypic and phenotypic testing has provided a useful tool to assist in determining the degree of drug resistance in a virologically failing regimen (i.e., detectable, rising viral load). Clinical trials have shown that the use of either test in conjunction with expert interpretation of the test results and previous treatment history provides a better opportunity for a successful salvage regimen than clinical opinion does alone. The genotype reports the mutation pattern in the HIV reverse transcriptase and protease genes, whereas the phenotype measures the ability of the virus to grow in different concentrations of antiretroviral agents. The genotype is less expensive and, in general, has a more rapid turn-around time.

Currently recommended indications for resistance testing are virologic failure during HAART and suboptimal viral suppression after initiation of HAART. Other clinical scenarios in which resistance testing should be considered are acute HIV infection (screen

TABLE 7A. **Nucleoside Reverse Transcriptase Inhibitors**

NRTI*	Dose	Selected Side Effects
Zidovudine (AZT, Retrovir, Combivir, Trizivir)	300 mg q12h Combivir or Trizivir, 1 tablet q12h†	GI upset, headache, anemia,‡ myopathy
Lamivudine (3TC, Epivir, Combivir, Trizivir)	150 mg q12h Combivir or Trizivir, 1 tablet q12h†	Minimal
Stavudine (d4T, Zerit)	40 mg q12h (if >60 kg), 30 mg q12h (if <60 kg)	Neuropathy
Didanosine (ddI, Videx, Videx EC)§	200 mg q12h or 400 mg qd (if >60 kg); 125 mg q12h or 250 mg qd (if <60 kg)	Neuropathy, GI upset,§ pancreatitis
Abacavir (Ziagen, Trizivir)	300 mg q12h, or Trizivir, 1 tablet q12h†	Hypersensitivity reaction‖
Dideoxycytidine (ddC, zalcitabine)¶	0.75 mg tid	Peripheral neuropathy (17% to 30%), pancreatitis

*Renal adjustments are available for all NRTIs except abacavir.
†Combivir is one tablet that contains 300 mg of zidovudine and 150 mg of lamivudine. Trizivir is Combivir with the addition of abacavir, 300 mg.
‡Can treat AZT-associated anemia with erythropoietin; check the hematocrit 2 to 4 weeks after starting treatment and then every 3 months.
§Should be taken on an empty stomach. Doses are for tablets (chewed or dissolved), not powder. Videx EC is preferable because of improved tolerability.
‖The hypersensitivity reaction is characterized by abdominal pain, nausea, vomiting, fever, rash, and malaise. Do not rechallenge; the drug can be fatal if the patient discontinues and then restarts abacavir therapy. Most reactions occur within 6 weeks. Patients must be extensively educated about this side effect.
¶ddC should be avoided because of its side effect profile and decreased efficacy.

for transmission of resistant virus) and pregnancy. Routine testing before starting therapy in chronically infected individuals is not currently recommended. Certain very important limitations to resistance testing should be considered when ordering and interpreting these tests. Both tests require an HIV viral load of at least 1000 copies to reliably assess resistance. Importantly, they only measure resistance to the antiretroviral agents that the patient is currently receiving. In the absence of antiretroviral therapy, drug-resistant mutants become archived in quiescent $CD4^+$ cells and wild-type virus re-emerges. Thus, resistance acquired during past regimens may not be detected. In addition, recognition of mutation patterns is a complex and rapidly evolving process, so expert interpretation of the results in conjunction with the past treatment history is desirable.

Changes in Therapy

Decisions regarding changes in therapy are complex, and a clear rationale for each change along with the risks and benefits of the proposed change should be considered. Many reasons can be found to make a change in therapy. If drug intolerance or the development of long-term complications merits a change in therapy, the offending agent can often be switched without losing viral control (assuming no pre-existing resistance).

TABLE 7B. **Non-Nucleoside Reverse Transcriptase Inhibitors**

NNRTI	Dose	Selected Side Effects
Efavirenz (Sustiva)	600 mg qhs	CNS effects,* rash
Nevirapine (Viramune)	200 mg qd × 14 d, then 200 mg bid	Rash, hepatitis†
Delavirdine (Rescriptor)‡	400 mg q8h	Rash, headache

*CNS effects occur in 25% to 40% and consists of a feeling of dizziness, "disconnected" feeling, and strange dreams, all of which usually decrease within 2 weeks. It is recommended that efavirenz be given at bedtime, and the drug is contraindicated in pregnancy.

†The rash and hepatitis are more common in women. The hepatitis occurs within the first 4 weeks and can be fatal. Stevens-Johnson reaction is reported. Check liver function 2 to 4 weeks after starting therapy.

‡This regimen is used much less commonly because of dosing every 8 hours and rash.

Salvage

In general, construction of a salvage regimen should encompass the following principles: use resistance testing and review of past treatment history to help define drugs to which the virus may be susceptible, consider which medications may have unacceptable side effects, and use at least two or three new drugs to which susceptibility can reasonably be predicted (preferably including a new class, such as an NNRTI after a PI regimen). The addition of one active drug to a failing regimen should be avoided because such a change amounts to monotherapy. Salvage therapy has a much lower rate of success and long-term durability than primary regimens do. The best option is to prevent virologic failure in the first place by close follow-up with ongoing education and support of patients receiving HAART. Despite the availability of three NNRTIs, six NRTIs, and six PIs as of 2001, it is very easy to cycle through all effective regimens without careful planning and attention. Additionally, it is not always feasible to change therapy, and the benefit of a significant rise in $CD4^+$ count without full viral load suppression should not be discounted in patients with a history of opportunistic infection or a low nadir $CD4^+$ count. Novel classes of agents such as fusion inhibitors, integrase inhibitors, and nucleotide analogues and drugs with activity against resistant virus are under development and should expand salvage treatment options.

COMPLICATIONS OF ANTIRETROVIRAL THERAPY

Although an extensive discussion of all possible complications is not feasible, certain drugs have pre-

TABLE 7C. **Protease Inhibitors**

Protease Inhibitors	Dose	Selected Side Effects
Nelfinavir (Viracept)*	1250 mg q12h or 750 mg q8h	Diarrhea, GI upset
Indinavir (Crixivan)†	800 mg q12h (with ritonavir, 100 or 200 mg q12h) or 800 mg q8h	GI upset, increased bilirubin, nephrolithiasis (take with 48 oz of water daily)
Saquinavir SGC (Fortovase)‡	400 mg q12h (with ritonavir, 400 mg q12h) or 1200 mg q8h	GI upset
Amprenavir (Agenerase)§	1200 mg q12h or 600–1200 mg q12h (with ritonavir, 100–200 mg q12h)	Rash, GI intolerance
Lopinavir/ritonavir (Kaletra)‖	400/100 mg q 12h	GI upset, diarrhea
Ritonavir (Norvir)¶	600 mg q12h (not recommended)	GI upset

*Must be taken with food.
†An indinavir/ritonavir combination is preferred because of an improved dosing schedule and pharmacokinetic profile. Indinavir (Crixivan) given alone must be taken on an empty stomach and separated from didanosine (ddI).
‡Saquinavir/ritonavir is preferred because of a smaller pill burden and an improved pharmacokinetic profile.
§Amprenavir alone is eight pills every 12 hours. Co-administration with ritonavir can decrease the pill burden.
‖Increase the dose to 533/133 mg every 12 hours when co-administered with efavirenz and nevirapine.
¶Ritonavir is poorly tolerated at full dose and is primarily used to enhance serum levels of other protease inhibitors through cytochrome P-450 blockade.

dictable side effects that may decrease the attractiveness for a particular patient (see Table 7). Many side effects are more prominent during initiation of therapy, and symptomatic support, including liberal use of antiemetic and antidiarrheal medications, can prevent discontinuation of therapy. Several prominent and developing complications of antiretroviral therapy are reviewed in the following sections.

Neuropathy

Peripheral neuropathy can occur as a complication of HIV infection itself or as a result of drug toxicity. The dideoxynucleosides (dideoxycytidine [ddC], didanosine [ddI], stavudine [d4T]), alone and in combination, have a known risk of precipitating peripheral neuropathy. Patients with pre-existing HIV-related neuropathy are at greater risk. Symptoms can be severe and function limiting. A history of symptoms and a screen for neuropathy should be performed at each routine follow-up. The pathophysiology of NRTI-related neuropathy is uncertain but may be related to mitochondrial toxicity. Sometimes, dose reduction of ddI or d4T stabilizes the symptoms, but often the offending drug has to be replaced with another NRTI. Symptomatic treatment of pain with gabapentin (Neurontin),* lamotrigine (Lamictal),* or low-dose tricyclic antidepressants* can be effective. Narcotics are usually less helpful.

TABLE 8. **Potential Choices for Initial HAART Regimens* (Choose a Dual NRTI Backbone and Either a PI, an NNRTI, or Abacavir)†**

Dual NRTI	NNRTI	PI	Third NRTI
AZT + 3TC (Combivir)	Efavirenz‖	Nelfinavir	Abacavir (use with AZT + 3TC, Trizivir)
d4T + 3TC	Nevirapine¶	Lopinavir/ritonavir	
d4T + ddI‡		Indinavir/ritonavir	
AZT + ddI§		Saquinavir/ritonavir	

*This list does not contain all possible HAART regimens, but rather a list of those more commonly used in clinical practice.
†A triple NRTI regimen, AZT/3TC/abacavir (Trizivir), can be considered in those with a viral load less than 100,000.
‡Higher risk of pancreatitis.
§Not commonly used because of its side effect profile.
‖Contraindicated in pregnancy.
¶Nevirapine is less favorable because of a higher risk of hepatitis and rash.
Abbreviations: AZT = zidovudine; ddI = dideoxyinosine (didanosine); d4T = stavudine; HAART = highly active antiretroviral therapy; NNRTI = non-nucleoside reverse transcriptase inhibitor; NRTI = nucleoside reverse transcriptase inhibitor; PI = protease inhibitor; 3TC = lamivudine.

Lactic Acidosis

Lactic acidosis is a rare complication of NRTIs that has a high mortality rate. The most frequently associated drug is d4T, but lactic acidosis has been reported with all the NRTIs. The mechanism of action may be mitochondrial toxicity, and the syndrome is more likely after 6 months of treatment. Symptoms are nonspecific and include abdominal pain, nausea, and vomiting. Blood lactate levels are elevated and an increased anion gap may be present. Treatment is supportive, and permanent discontinuation of NRTI therapy is in order. Low-level asymptomatic lactic acidemia (below 4 mmol/L) is not uncommon, and appropriate management of this situation is unknown. Lactic acidosis should be considered in any patient taking NRTIs who has unexplained nausea, vomiting, fatigue, and abdominal pain. Currently, monitoring of lactate levels has no role in asymptomatic patients.

Metabolic Complications

Multiple metabolic complications are seen with antiretroviral therapy—peripheral lipoatrophy, central fat accumulation, hyperlipidemia, glucose intolerance—all of which have been pulled together into a syndrome termed *lipodystrophy.* The etiology of this syndrome is unknown, but it is likely that distinctly different processes have been lumped under this term. Lipoatrophy refers to loss of peripheral fat (arms, legs, face, and buttocks) and is most associ-

*Not FDA approved for this indication.

ated with d4T exposure, though not exclusively. No current treatment can effectively restore the fat, but discontinuation of the potentially responsible drug may prevent further destruction. Central fat accumulation is manifested as increased visceral fat, breast enlargement in women, increased waist-hip ratio, or occurrence of a "buffalo hump" and may be related to PI exposure, particularly ritonavir. Testosterone deficiency should be ruled out in men with lipodystrophy. Lipid abnormalities, particularly hypertriglyceridemia, are prominent with HAART and are most strongly linked to PIs. Cardiovascular risk modification is in order, and patients should be treated similar to other people with hyperlipidemia. Substitution of the PI with an NNRTI or NRTI when feasible may help control the lipid abnormalities. If treatment with HMG-CoA reductase inhibitors is needed, pravastatin (Pravachol) should be used because it is not metabolized through the cytochrome P-450 system. Insulin resistance, impaired glucose tolerance, and overt diabetes mellitus have been associated with the use of HAART and again may be related most strongly to PIs.

Drug-Drug Interactions

Polypharmacy is unavoidable in the course of therapy for HIV, and clinicians should recognize that drug-drug interactions frequently occur. Care should be taken to avoid them, modify dosages when needed, or exploit them when appropriate. For example, rifampin (Rifadin), profoundly lowers PI levels, so the two drugs cannot be used concurrently. Rifabutin may be substituted for rifampin, but dose modification of PIs and NNRTIs is needed.

Additionally, herbal supplements such as St. John's wort and garlic can reduce PI levels. Drug interactions are used to advantage when the blood levels of other PIs are boosted by ritonavir (see Table 7C). Drug-drug interactions in HIV care are common and rapidly evolving. Consultation with an experienced pharmacist is recommended and drug interactions can be reviewed at www.hopkins-aids.edu and hivinsite.ucsf.edu.

OPPORTUNISTIC INFECTIONS

Although the dramatic success of HAART is responsible for a decline in the incidence of most AIDS-related complications, PCP, esophageal candidiasis, and *Mycobacterium avium* infection remain the most common opportunistic infections. HIV is not diagnosed in many people until they have significant immunosuppression or an active opportunistic infection has developed. Despite therapy, patients may not experience all the immunologic benefits of treatment or may not adhere to prophylaxis. Evidence continues to accumulate regarding the safety of discontinuing primary and secondary prophylaxis in patients who have achieved sustained and substantial immune reconstitution (typically with $CD4^+$ counts rising above 200 cells/mm^3). Prophylaxis should be resumed promptly if the $CD4^+$ count falls again. The U.S. Public Health Service and the Infectious Diseases Society of America issue joint guidelines regarding risk assessment for opportunistic infection and prophylaxis (*www.hivatis.org*). The best prevention for opportunistic infections is preserving or restoring the immune system with effective HAART. Several of the major opportunistic infections are reviewed in the following sections.

Pneumocystis carinii Pneumonia

P. carinii is an atypical fungus that is a common cause of pneumonia in immunosuppressed HIV patients. Before the advent of prophylaxis, PCP was the initial diagnosis in over 60% of AIDS cases. The risk of PCP increases with a $CD4^+$ count lower than 200 cells/mm^3, and prophylaxis should be initiated when the $CD4^+$ count reaches 200 cells/mm^3. Other indications for prophylaxis are a $CD4^+$ percentage of less than 14, an AIDS-defining illness regardless of the $CD4^+$ count, oral candidiasis, or unexplained fever of over 2 weeks in duration. The agent of choice for prophylaxis is trimethoprim/sulfamethoxazole (Bactrim, Septra), one single-strength or one double-strength tablet per day. Sulfa intolerance is common. (See Table 9 for alternatives.)

PCP is a subacute infection in HIV patients that progresses over a period of several weeks. Symptoms include a nonproductive cough, dyspnea on exertion, and fever. Physical examination may reveal tachypnea, tachycardia, and fever, but pulmonary auscultation is usually normal. Desaturation on exercise pulse oximetry can be helpful. The typical finding on chest radiography is bilateral interstitial infiltrates, although the radiograph is normal in one third of cases. Pneumothorax can be an initial feature or a late complication. Standard expectorated sputum is not helpful for diagnosis. Induced sputum examination performed by experienced personnel may be helpful if positive, but it can be falsely negative as much as 40% of the time. Bronchoalveolar lavage is over 95% sensitive and may also permit the diagnosis of other potential pathogens such as tuberculosis. The mainstay of treatment is also trimethoprim/sulfamethoxazole (Table 9). Therapy usually lasts 21 days and can be given orally if the patient is able to absorb medications. Adjunctive corticosteroids are indicated for moderate to severe PCP to decrease the risk of respiratory failure. Treatment-related toxicities are common, and alternative therapies are available (Table 9).

Toxoplasmic Encephalitis

Toxoplasmic encephalitis can be a devastating consequence of AIDS and typically occurs at $CD4^+$ counts below 100 cells/mm^3. Latent infection can be accurately assessed by testing for IgG to *Toxoplasma gondii* in the blood. Patients seronegative for *Toxoplasma* should be advised to avoid potential sources of infection—poorly cooked meat, outdoor cats, and

TABLE 9. **Treatment of *Pneumocystis carinii* Pneumonia**

Regimens*	Side Effects
Acute Infection	
PRIMARY	
Trimethoprim/sulfamethoxazole (Bactrim, Septra), 15 mg/kg IV or PO trimethoprim and 75 mg/kg/d of sulfamethoxazole divided q6–8h × 21 d†	Neutropenia, rash, GI upset, increased creatinine and potassium
ALTERNATIVES	
Pentamidine (Pentam), 4 mg/kg IV qd × 21 d‡	Pancreatitis, hypoglycemia or hyperglycemia, rash, neutropenia, decreased blood pressure, conduction abnormalities
Clindamycin (Cleocin), 600 mg IV q8h or 300–450 mg PO q6h + primaquine, 30 mg base PO qd × 21 d§	GI upset, neutropenia, diarrhea, *Clostridium difficile*
Trimethoprim (Primsol), 15 mg/kg PO divided q6, + dapsone, 100 mg PO qd × 21 d§	Rash, pruritis, N/V, hemolytic anemia (dapsone)
Trimetrexate (NeuTrexin), 45 mg/m² IV qd, and folinic acid (leucovorin), 20 mg/m² PO/IV q6h, ± dapsone, 100 mg PO qd	Neutropenia, rash, fever
Atovaquone (Mepron), 750 mg PO bid	GI upset, rash
Prophylaxis‖	
PRIMARY	
Trimethoprim/sulfamethoxazole (Bactrim, Septra) 1 DS or 1 SS tablet PO qd¶	Rash, pruritus, hepatitis, neutropenia, hyperkalemia
ALTERNATIVES	
Dapsone, 100 mg PO qd	Rash, neutropenia, hemolytic anemia
Dapsone, 50 mg PO qd, pyrimethamine (Daraprim), 50 mg PO qwk, and + leucovorin, 25 mg PO qwk; or dapsone, 200 mg PO qwk, pyrimethamine, 75 mg PO qwk, and leucovorin, 25 mg PO qwk**	Rash, N/V, hemolytic anemia, megaloblastic anemia, neutropenia
Atovaquone (Mepron), 750 mg PO bid (liquid)	GI upset, rash
Aerosolized pentamidine (NebuPent), 300 mg aerosolized via Respirgard II Nebulizer††	Cough (can give inhaled β-agonist)
Trimethoprim/sulfamethoxazole, 1 DS three times weekly	Neutropenia, rash, GI upset, increased creatinine and potassium

*Check arterial blood gases before starting therapy. When Pa_{O_2} is less than 70 or the alveolar-arterial gradient is greater than 35, use prednisone, 40 mg orally twice daily for 7 days, then 20 mg twice daily for 7 days, and then 10 mg twice daily for 7 days regardless of the regimen (administer 30 minutes before the first dose of antibiotic).

†This regimen has the most experience in the treatment of PCP and should be used if possible.

‡This regimen can be used for patients who are allergic to sulfonamides and have moderate to severe disease.

§Consider using these regimens for patients with mild to moderate PCP who are allergic to sulfonamides. These regimens are equally efficacious.

‖Secondary prophylaxis required after treatment. Primary and secondary PCP prophylaxis can be stopped after the patient has started HAART and is controlling viral replication with a $CD4^+$ count greater than 200 for 3 to 6 months.

¶Most efficacious PCP prophylaxis regimen.

**Only trimethoprim-sulfamethoxazole at a dose of 1 DS daily and dapsone/pyrimethamine/leucovorin protect against toxoplasmosis.

††*Pneumocystis* infection in the apices and in extrapulmonary sites can develop in patients receiving this regimen, and it is less effective when the $CD4^+$ count is less than 50.

Abbreviations: DS = double strength; GI = gastrointestinal; HAART = highly active antiretroviral therapy; N/V = nausea/vomiting; PCP = *Pneumocystis carinii* pneumonia; SS = single strength.

exposure to dirty cat litter without precautions—and should be retested when the $CD4^+$ count falls to 100 cells/mm³. Primary prophylaxis should be initiated in *Toxoplasma* IgG–seropositive patients with a $CD4^+$ count of less than 100 cells/mm³. The prophylactic agent of choice is trimethoprim/sulfamethoxazole, one double-strength tablet per day (Table 10).

The most common initial symptoms of toxoplasmic encephalitis are headaches, seizures, and focal neurologic deficits. The diagnosis is nearly always presumptive and based on brain computed tomographic or magnetic resonance imaging findings of multiple ring-enhancing lesions with surrounding mass effect in an AIDS patient with a positive *Toxoplasma* antibody titer. A trial of anti-*Toxoplasma* therapy is warranted, and failure to respond within 2 weeks should prompt a reconsideration of alternative diagnoses such as central nervous system lymphoma, brain abscess, or progressive multifocal leukoencephalopathy. Treatment consists of sulfadiazine,* pyrimethamine (Daraprim), and folinic acid* (leucovorin). Clindamycin* (Cleocin) is an alternative for sulfa-allergic patients (Table 10). Lifelong suppressive therapy is required. Although reports of stopping secondary treatment after achieving immune reconstitution have appeared, not enough evidence is available to currently recommend this approach.

Mycobacterium Tuberculosis Infection

HIV infection is a major risk factor for tuberculosis reactivation and acquisition. All patients with HIV should have a tuberculin skin test (TST) consisting of the administration of 5 TU of purified protein derivative by the Mantoux method. Anergy testing is not recommended. Induration of 5 mm or larger is

*Not FDA approved for this indication.

TABLE 10. **Treatment of *Toxoplasma gondii* Infection**

Regimens	Side Effects
*Active Treatment**	
PRIMARY	
Pyrimethamine (Daraprim), 200 mg PO × 1, then 75–100 mg PO qd, + folinic acid (leucovorin), 10 mg PO qd, + sulfadiazine, 1–2 g PO q6h × 6 wk	Megaloblastic anemia, neutropenia, rash, pruritus
ALTERNATIVE	
Pyrimethamine + folinic acid (leucovorin) as above + clindamycin (Cleocin), 900–1200 mg IV q6h or 300–450 mg PO q6h × 6 wk†	Megaloblastic anemia, neutropenia, diarrhea, *Clostridium difficile*
Pyrimethamine + folinic acid (leucovorin) as above and 1 of the following: azithromycin (Zithromax), 1200–1500 mg/d, or clarithromycin (Biaxin), 1 g PO bid, or atovaquone, 750 mg PO qid	Megaloblastic anemia, neutropenia, GI upset, rash
Suppression	
PRIMARY	
Pyrimethamine, 25–75 mg qd + folinic acid (10 mg/d), + sulfadiazine, 0.5 mg–1 mg PO q6h	Megaloblastic anemia, neutropenia, rash, pruritus
ALTERNATIVE	
Pyrimethamine + folinic acid (leukovorin) as above + clindamycin (Cleocin), 300–450 mg PO q6h‡	Megaloblastic anemia, neutropenia, diarrhea, *Clostridium difficile*
Prophylaxis§	
PRIMARY	
Trimethoprim/sulfamethoxazole, double-strength tablet PO qd	Rash, pruritus, hepatitis, neutropenia, hyperkalemia
ALTERNATIVE	
Dapsone (Avlosulfon), 50 mg PO qd, + pyrimethamine 50 mg/wk, + folinic acid (leukovorin), 25 mg wk, or dapsone, 200 mg PO qwk, pyrimethamine, 75 mg PO qwk, and folinic acid, 25 mg PO qwk	Rash, nausea/vomiting, hemolytic anemia (check G6PD level)
Trimethoprim/sulfamethoxazole, 1 single-strength tablet PO qd or 1 double-strength tablet PO tiwk	Rash, pruritus, hepatitis, neutropenia, hyperkalemia

*Dexamethasone (Decadron), 4 mg intravenously every 6 hours for significant brain edema/mass effect.
†This is the preferred alternative.
‡Clindamycin/pyrimethamine/leucovorin does not prevent *Pneumocystis carinii* pneumonia.
§Data support stopping primary prophylaxis after a $CD4^+$ count of greater than 100 for 6 months and suppression of the viral load.
Abbreviation: G6PD = glucose-6-phosphate dehydrogenase.

positive and should prompt a chest radiograph and clinical evaluation to rule out active disease. A repeated TST after immune reconstitution may have greater sensitivity. Yearly repeat TST should be considered, particularly in populations at higher risk of infection. Any HIV patient who has close contact with a person with active tuberculosis should receive prophylaxis, regardless of the TST results. Prophylactic regimens include isoniazid (INH, Isotamine) daily or twice a week for 9 months. A 2-month course of prophylaxis with rifampin or rifabutin (Mycobutin) and pyrazinamide (Tebrazid) is effective, but potential drug interactions with PIs and NNRTIs are quite complex and should be carefully assessed in conjunction with expert opinion before treatment. Tuberculosis should be considered in an HIV patient with respiratory symptoms or pneumonia lasting longer than 1 to 2 weeks. Drug interactions with NNRTIs and PIs should be considered during treatment. Treatment of active tuberculosis in the setting of HIV is discussed elsewhere in this book. Extrapulmonary involvement of *M. tuberculosis* infection is common in patients with AIDS and includes lymphadenopathy, abdominal infection, and meningitis.

Disseminated Infection With *Mycobacterium avium* Complex

Disseminated *M. avium* complex (MAC) infection is common in AIDS patients with very low $CD4^+$ counts and causes a wasting febrile illness. Primary prophylaxis should be provided to patients with $CD4^+$ counts of less than 50 cells/mm^3, with the addition of a blood culture for MAC to rule out occult infection at the start of prophylaxis. Azithromycin (Zithromax) or clarithromycin (Biaxin) can be used for prophylaxis, but azithromycin is preferable because of its improved tolerability and fewer drug interactions (Table 11).

Disseminated MAC infection is typically manifested as a chronic disease with fever, night sweats, weight loss, abdominal pain, diarrhea with lymphadenopathy, and hepatosplenomegaly. Laboratory tests may show anemia or pancytopenia secondary to marrow infiltration and increased alkaline phosphatase secondary to infiltration of the liver. The diagnosis can be made by isolator blood culture, bone marrow culture and biopsy, or lymph node biopsy. An emerging syndrome of an inflammatory reaction to MAC can be seen with the initiation of HAART and im-

TABLE 11. **Treatment of *Mycobacterium avium* Complex**

Regimens	Side Effects
Treatment	
PRIMARY	
Clarithromycin (Biaxin), 500 mg PO bid,* + ethambutol (Myambutol), 15 mg/kg/d PO, ± rifabutin (Mycobutin), 300 mg/d PO†	GI upset (Biaxin, Zithromax) Optic neuritis, needs ophthalmologic follow-up (Myambutol)
SECONDARY	
Can substitute azithromycin (Zithromax), 500–600 mg PO qd for clarithromycin	Leukopenia, N/V, uveitis (Mycobutin)
Prophylaxis	
PRIMARY	
Clarithromycin, 500 mg PO bid or azithromycin, 1200 mg PO qwk	GI upset
SECONDARY	
Rifabutin, 300 mg PO qd† Azithromycin, 1200 mg PO qwk, and rifabutin, 300 mg PO qd†	Leukopenia, N/V, uveitis

*Clarithromycin levels are decreased in the presence of rifabutin.
†Rifabutin interacts strongly with protease inhibitors and non-nucleoside reverse transcriptase inhibitors, so dose modification of both drugs is required; check the drug insert before concomitant use.
Abbreviations: GI = gastrointestinal; N/V = nausea/vomiting.

mune reconstitution. A paradoxical worsening of fever and lymphadenopathy may develop, and repeat lymph node biopsy is sometimes required to rule out lymphoma or other causes of lymphadenopathy. Steroids may provide symptomatic relief in the immune reconstitution syndrome. Treatment of disseminated MAC infection usually involves 2 months of three-drug therapy, followed by lifelong two-drug suppressive regimens (Table 11). Discontinuation in asymptomatic patients with good immune restoration and longer than 1 year of anti-MAC treatment may be considered. Resistance to anti-MAC therapy can develop, and expert consultation is advised if patients do not respond to the first-line therapy.

Cytomegalovirus Infection

CMV is a common herpesvirus that rarely causes symptomatic disease in immunocompetent hosts. HIV-positive patients with severely depleted $CD4^+$ counts are at risk for invasive CMV disease, particularly retinitis. Currently, no standard for primary prophylaxis is recognized because of the side effect profile and pill burden of the available agents. Screening eye examinations should be performed when the $CD4^+$ count falls below 50 cells/mm^3. Patients should be advised of warning signs such as increased floaters, decreased visual acuity, or other new visual symptoms and to seek medical attention immediately. The diagnosis is made by the recognition of characteristic retinal lesions. Treatment should be given in conjunction with close ophthalmologic follow-up. Treatment options include induction therapy with ganciclovir (Cytovene) or foscarnet (Foscavir), followed by maintenance therapy. Options for maintenance therapy include ganciclovir ocular implants with oral ganciclovir to protect the contralateral eye and maintenance intravenous dosing of ganciclovir, foscarnet, or cidofovir (Vistide). Ganciclovir has risks of marrow toxicity, particularly neutropenia. Foscarnet and cidofovir can cause renal toxicity and electrolyte disturbances, which may limit their use. The gastrointestinal tract is also a common site for CMV disease and is subject to invasive esophagitis, gastritis, or colitis. Biopsy material should be obtained and examined for the characteristic histopathology.

Discontinuation of secondary prophylaxis for CMV can be considered with a sustained improvement in the $CD4^+$ count above 100 cells/mm^3 and careful ophthalmologic follow-up, but large-scale trials are lacking.

Cryptococcal Meningitis

Cryptococcus neoformans is a ubiquitous fungus that is a common cause of chronic meningitis in HIV patients with $CD4^+$ counts under 200 cells/mm^3. Primary prophylaxis is not routinely recommended. The typical initial symptoms of cryptococcal meningitis are fever and headache. Meningeal signs and focal neurologic deficits may be present. Cerebrospinal fluid (CSF) examination may show lymphocytic pleocytosis, increased opening pressure, and elevated protein and low glucose levels, but it may also demonstrate little evidence of an inflammatory response. The diagnosis can be made by India ink stain, CSF culture, or CSF cryptococcal latex antigen. Serum cryptococcal antigen is 95% sensitive, and a positive serum antigen test should prompt CSF examination and fungal cultures of blood and urine. Headache indicates an elevation in intracranial pressure, and repeated lumbar puncture to relieve symptoms may be needed. Rarely, neurosurgical intervention is necessary to relieve hydrocephalus. The first-line treatment is amphotericin B (Fungizone) at 0.7 to 1.0 mg/kg/d for 4 to 6 weeks if tolerated. Consideration should be given to a follow-up CSF examination.

After 4 to 6 weeks of amphotericin B, oral fluconazole (Diflucan), 400 mg/d, is used to complete 8 to 10 weeks of therapy, followed by 200 mg/d thereafter. Itraconazole* (Sporanox) is associated with a higher rate of relapse. Liposomal preparations of amphotericin B can be substituted if renal toxicity develops. Flucytosine (Ancobon) can be administered during the first few weeks of therapy in addition to amphotericin B, but difficulties in timely measurement of drug levels and the risk of severe mucositis and marrow suppression limit its usefulness. Six to 10 weeks of fluconazole, 400 mg daily, can be used for the treatment of patients with cryptococcosis without meningitis. Lifelong maintenance therapy with fluconazole was required before HAART, but evidence is mounting to support the discontinuation of secondary prophylaxis after immune reconstitution, although such measures cannot be firmly recommended at this point.

Candidiasis

Recurrent mucocutaneous candidiasis is a common illness in patients with AIDS. Oral candidiasis should be treated topically with nystatin (Mycostatin) or clotrimazole (Mycelex) troches whenever possible. Fluconazole should be reserved for second-line therapy to minimize the risk of resistance developing. Esophageal candidiasis is manifested as odynophagia and oral candidiasis and can usually be treated empirically. Failure to respond quickly to treatment should prompt esophagogastroduodenoscopy with biopsy to evaluate for other ulcerative complications (e.g., CMV, aphthous ulcers). Treatment is usually fluconazole, 200 mg daily for 14 to 21 days. Amphotericin B is occasionally required for resistant cases. Recurrent vaginal candidiasis is common in women with HIV at all $CD4^+$ counts. Topical treatments should be used whenever possible and fluconazole reserved for treatment failures. Primary prophylaxis for candidal infections is not recommended. Secondary prophylaxis with fluconazole is reserved for patients with multiple recurrences, but the risk of azole resistance is increased.

Kaposi's Sarcoma

Kaposi's sarcoma is primarily a cutaneous malignancy caused by human herpes virus 8. It is almost exclusively found in male homosexuals with AIDS. Kaposi's sarcoma is usually manifested as a violaceous cutaneous plaque, and biopsy should be performed to distinguish it from bartonellosis. Disseminated disease can occur and produce oropharyngeal lesions, lymph node involvement, and pulmonary or gastrointestinal lesions. Cutaneous disease can be treated with cryotherapy, intralesional vinblastine, irradiation, or topical retinoids. Visceral and extensive cutaneous disease can be treated with systemic chemotherapy or focal irradiation. The institution of HAART and improvement in the $CD4^+$ count can delay disease progression or lead to regression of active lesions.

*Not FDA approved for this indication.

OTHER ASSOCIATED INFECTIONS AND HIV COMPLICATIONS

Hepatitis B

Hepatitis B virus (HBV) has a transmission pattern similar to that of HIV. All patients with HIV should be screened for HBV. Patients with active HBV should be evaluated for treatment. The hepatitis B vaccination series should be offered to HIV patients with no evidence of past exposure.

Hepatitis C

HIV/hepatitis C virus (HCV) co-infection is common, particularly in HIV acquired through blood exposure. Approximately 240,000 people have HIV/HCV co-infection in the United States, or 30% of the HIV population. HIV infection increases the HCV viral load and accelerates the rate of disease progression. Additionally, as HIV survival improves, cirrhosis related to HCV may become more prominent. The effect of HCV on the natural history of HIV is unclear. Although co-infected patients have a higher incidence of hepatotoxicity with HAART, most can safely receive PI-based antiretroviral therapy. Testing for HCV infection should start with enzyme immunoassay for antibody to HCV. Subsequent testing with an HCV RNA test can then confirm infection. A negative HCV RNA test should be repeated 6 to 12 months later. Rarely, HIV/HCV patients with late-stage HIV infection may have a false-negative antibody test. Co-infected patients should be screened for evidence of hepatitis A immunity and vaccinated because of the increased risk of fulminant hepatitis A infection. Alcohol ingestion is contraindicated. Treatment and evaluation should proceed as for HCV patients without HIV, with the caveat that treatment is generally less effective in co-infected patients and clarification of optimal treatment strategies is needed.

Syphilis

All patients with HIV should be screened yearly for syphilis with serum RPR or fluorescent treponemal antibody absorption testing. The clinical course is accelerated with HIV infection. Treatment of primary or secondary syphilis is intramuscular benzathine penicillin (Bicillin L-A), 2.4 million U. If the length of infection is unknown, penicillin should be given intramuscularly weekly for three doses (three doses is recommended by some experts in HIV-positive patients regardless of the stage). Patients with HIV have a higher rate of early neurosyphilis than do HIV-negative patients, and clinicians should maintain a low threshold for spinal fluid examination for VDRL, cell count, and protein level. If an appropriate serologic response to therapy does not occur within 6 to 12 months, CSF examination should be performed. The preferred treatment for neurosyphilis is intravenous aqueous crystalline penicillin, 24 million U/d divided every 4 hours for 14 days, followed by 2.4 million U of intramuscular benzathine penicillin.

Human Papillomavirus–Associated Malignancy

Women with HIV are at higher risk of squamous intraepithelial lesions and invasive cervical cancer. Pelvic examination and a Papanicolaou smear should be performed. If two examinations 6 months apart are normal, yearly examinations can then be performed. Abnormal results should be evaluated and treated as per standard guidelines for all women.

HIV-Associated Neurologic Disease

Progressive multifocal leukoencephalopathy, a devastating subacute neurologic infection with JC virus (polyomavirus family), occurs at a $CD4^+$ count of less than 200/mm^3. It is manifested as weakness, cognitive dysfunction, gait disturbances, and visual impairment and was universally fatal before HAART. Clinicians have treated progressive multifocal leukoencephalopathy with cidofovir (Vistide)*, but firm data are lacking.

HIV-associated dementia occurs in 20% to 30% of untreated patient with AIDS and is initially seen as a chronic subcortical dementia. Lumbar puncture shows increased protein and a mild lymphocytic pleocytosis, and central nervous system imaging shows atrophy. The recommended treatment is with a zidovudine-containing HAART regimen when possible.

*Not FDA approved for this indication.

AMEBIASIS

method of
COL ANIL C. ANAND, M.D., D.M.
Base Hospital, Delhi Cantonment Armed Forces Medical Services
New Delhi, India

Amebiasis refers to illness caused by the protozoan *Entamoeba histolytica*. A disease of worldwide distribution, amebiasis is the third most common cause of parasitic death in the world. Prevalence is high in the developing world (50%–80%), and at least 5% of the "untraveled" population in the United States is infected with *E. histolytica*. It is transmitted primarily by consumption of water contaminated with cysts of *E. histolytica*, although in the urban areas transmission also occurs during sexual contact, through daycare centers caring for children in diapers, and in institutions for the mentally retarded.

AGENT

In the new host, the cyst can survive gastric hydrochloric acid and gives rise to four motile trophozoites, which are potentially pathogenic (Table 1). The incubation period varies from 2 days to 4 months, with an average of 7 days. "Pathogenic" and "nonpathogenic" *Entamoeba* isolates exist as two distinct species, *E. histolytica* and *E. dispar*, which can be differentiated by using monoclonal antibody–based antigen capture enzyme-linked immunosorbent assay.

PATHOLOGY

Trophozoites penetrate epithelial cells and enter the lamina propria of the colon, where radial spread through unresisting submucosal tissue forms a typical flask-shaped ulcer. The invasion leads to lytic necrosis with minimal cellular reaction. The ulcer may spread to muscularis propria and may coalesce with adjacent lesions, thus undermining the mucosa. Later, bacterial invasion is the rule. Occasionally, granulation tissue with eosinophilic, lymphocytic, and fibroblastic accumulations (amebic granulomas or amebomas) may form in the cecum, transverse colon, or sigmoid colon. Less often, secondary infection may lead to gross and histopathologic features similar to those of inflammatory bowel disease.

The amebas penetrate the walls of the mesenteric venules, are swept into the portal stream, and then travel to the sinusoids of the liver. The colonies that form within the liver coalesce to create an amebic hepatic abscess, which contains necrotic liver debris accompanied by variable amounts of blood. Invading amebas are characteristically found at the periphery of such lesions.

A single large abscess is more common (70%) than multiple discrete lesions (30%). An amebic hepatic abscess may rupture into adjacent structures, resulting in empyema, bronchohepatic fistula, pericarditis, or peritonitis. Metastatic amebiasis seeded by hematogenous spread may occur rarely in lungs, brain, spleen, and kidneys or perinephric areas. Cutaneous amebiasis occurs as an ulcerating, granulating lesion that appears in continuity with an area

TABLE 1. **Pathogenesis and Epidemiologic Factors Affecting Invasive Amebiasis**

Pathogenesis

Tissue invasion aided by adhesion and contact-dependent cytolysis of host cells, release of proteases and other degradative enzymes, and amebic phagocytosis. Diarrhea may be partly due to stimulation of secretagogues (such as mucosal prostaglandins).

Gut flora may be a major determinant of invasiveness and pathogenicity.

Predisposing Factors and Persons With Increased Susceptibility

Avitaminosis
Certain dietary components, namely, a diet of wheat or fish
Low socioeconomic status, overcrowding, poor hygiene
Persons living in institutions, the mentally retarded, workers and children in daycare centers
Homosexuals and those with AIDS
Travelers to endemic areas and immigrants from such areas—remain at risk for up to a decade after move from endemic areas

More Fulminant Disease Seen

In children, especially neonates
During pregnancy and postpartum period
In patients with malignancy
With malnutrition
In patients on corticosteroids

of deeper chronic visceral involvement. Most frequently observed is the perineal lesion, which begins as an extension of anorectal ulceration or ameboma.

CLINICAL FEATURES

Intestinal disease may be asymptomatic in about 80% of infected people (Table 2). Chronic nondysenteric colitis, a popular diagnosis in some parts of the world, is a misnomer. These patients are cyst passers who have symptoms due to some other causes, such as irritable bowel syndrome.

Invasive intestinal amebiasis may present with mild diarrhea or fulminant bloody dysentery. In most patients diarrhea is mild, and the stools are mushy to watery, average fewer than 10 a day, and are accompanied by much flatulence. In contrast to the bacillary dysentery, associated systemic manifestations are not marked, although in fulminant cases with secondary infection differentiation may be difficult. Up to 75% of these patients may have peritonitis secondary to leakage through severely diseased colon and have high (>50%) mortality. Less often, such acute fulminant amebiasis may gradually subside spontaneously, with disappearance of blood in the stool and a lessening of diarrhea. Intestinal amebiasis may be complicated by severe bleeding, perforation, stenosis (stricture), or ameboma.

Development of amebic liver abscess does not depend on the severity of enteric symptoms. Local symptoms of pain in the right upper quadrant of the abdomen and varying intensity of liver tenderness draw attention to this complication. Symptoms may be present from 2 weeks to several months before medical attention is sought. The pain is commonly described as a dull or dragging sensation, aggravated by position changes, movement, or deep respiration. On occasion, however, the pain is acute, and tenderness

TABLE 2. **Clinical Characteristics of Amebiasis and Its Treatment of Choice**

Type of Amebiasis	Clinical Presentation	Stool Examination	Serology	Colonoscopy	Interpretation	Remarks and Treatment
Intestinal						
Asymptomatic	Asymptomatic	Cysts +	–	Normal	Infection by nonpathogenic forms or *E. dispar*	No treatment indicated in endemic areas; in high-risk group, use diloxanide furoate.
Chronic nondysenteric	Chronic lower abdominal pain, frequent small loose stools with passage of mucus, alternating constipation and diarrhea, tenesmus or feeling of incomplete evacuation and flatulence	Cysts ±	±	Normal or few nonspecific ulcers	Unlikely to be due to *E. histolytica*	Look for other causes of symptoms, such as irritable bowel syndrome.
Acute amebic dysentery	Mild diarrhea to fulminant bloody dysentery	Cysts ± trophozoites ±	+	Typically flask-shaped ulcers or extensive ulceration similar to bacillary dysentery	Invasive amebic infection; hospitalize in severe cases	Treat with metronidazole and tetracycline.*†
Ameboma	Alteration in bowel habits or frank subacute intestinal obstruction	Cysts ± trophozoites ±	+	Tumorous granuloma with or without typical ulcers in surrounding mucosa	Histology shows granuloma	Treat with metronidazole and tetracycline.*†
Extraintestinal						
Nonsuppurative hepatic	Pain over right hypochondrium, liver enlarged and tender	Cysts ± trophozoites ±	+	Typical ulcers ±	Ultrasound shows no abscess cavity	Treat with metronidazole or chloroquine.*
Amebic liver abscess	Pain over right hypochondrium, fever, past history of diarrhea, liver enlarged and tender, toxic look	Cysts ± trophozoites ±	+ +	Typical ulcers ±	Ultrasound shows one or more abscess cavities	Treat with metronidazole/ dehydroemetine.‡ Add broad-spectrum antibiotics and chloroquine if no response in 48 hours. Drain if required.*
Metastatic abscesses	Abscess anywhere in body often (but not always) in addition to liver abscess	Cysts ± trophozoites ±	+ +	Typical ulcers ±	Imaging confirms abscess	Treat with metronidazole. Drain if required.*

*All cases of tissue amebiasis should also be given a course of luminal amebicide such as diloxanide furoate.
†Not FDA approved for this indication.
‡Investigational drug in the United States.

over the liver or right intercostal spaces is so exquisite that perforation seems incipient.

Systemic symptoms including fever may accompany amebic hepatic abscess. Significant weight loss is common in patients symptomatic for longer than 2 to 3 weeks. The liver is enlarged and tender. Commonly, the right lobe of the liver is involved, and there is a corresponding elevation of the right diaphragm if the superior portion is involved. On the other hand, an abscess of the central or lower portion of the right lobe produces a mass that extends inferiorly, producing pressure effects on adjacent structures. Abscesses of the left lobe are less common (4%–18%) and behave differently. Abscesses have a predisposition to rupture into the pericardium, left pleural space, or abdomen. The patient almost always appears toxic, febrile, and chronically ill.

Poor prognostic markers associated with high risk of death are serum bilirubin greater than 3.5 mg/dL, presence of encephalopathy, hypoalbuminemia (serum albumin <2.0 mg/dL), larger volume, and larger number of abscesses. Complications include secondary bacterial infection (in 10%–30%) by staphylococci, streptococci, and *Escherichia coli;* pleuropulmonary effusions; pericardial penetration; and peritoneal rupture with high (10%) mortality rates.

DIAGNOSIS

The microscopic appearance of stools in amebic colitis is variable. Rarely is there a preponderance of polymorphonuclear leukocytes, as occurs with bacillary dysentery. In the usual patient, blood is not present in the stool in abundance; however, in severe cases of amebic colitis, the stool may be bloody. Charcot-Leyden crystals are commonly seen. Demonstration of *E. histolytica* cysts in stool examination is not a proof of amebiasis because nonpathogenic *E. dispar* may appear exactly similar. Presence of hematophagous trophozoites in dysenteric stools or the material scooped or aspirated from lesions can be considered diagnostic. Culture of amebas with subsequent zymodeme analysis is at best a research tool. In the acute stage, sigmoidoscopy may show punched-out ulcers (pinpoint to 5 mm) separated by intervening normal mucosa.

Serologic tests (Table 3) may be more reliable than stool morphology. Earlier tests, prepared from ameba cultures contaminated with bacteria, gave many false-positive results. However, the specificity of second-generation tests made from bacteria-free antigen has been greatly enhanced and serologic studies have now become a practical aid. Most of the tests are positive in more than 90% of patients with invasive intestinal amebiasis.

A therapeutic trial is a valid diagnostic measure in extraintestinal amebiasis, such as amebic hepatic abscess or visceral lesions (e.g., brain, kidney, lung, or spleen) as well as in cases of colonic ameboma.

Liver abscess is usually associated with moderate leukocytosis and minimal hyperbilirubinemia. Ultrasonography or other imaging methods clinch the anatomic diagnosis. When aspirated, the pus is odorless and bacteriologically sterile. A foul smell should raise suspicion of associated anaerobic infection. From lesions of short duration, the aspirate has a custard-like consistency and the dirty yellow color is streaked with pink or a diffuse red. On exposure to air, the material rapidly darkens to a dark brownish ("anchovy sauce") color. Abscesses of long duration frequently contain thin, yellow, odorless material. The abscess contents should be examined for *E. histolytica* and cultured aerobically and anaerobically to detect secondary infection.

TABLE 3. **Serologic Tests Have Greater Diagnostic Value Than Stool Examination for *Entamoeba histolytica* Morphology**

Test	Remarks
Agar gel diffusion (immunodiffusion)	Test takes about 48 hours; may reflect remote, clinically unimportant disease
Latex agglutination	Test takes 35 to 45 minutes; rheumatoid factor may give false-positive reactions
CIEP	Test takes about 1 hour
Indirect hemagglutination test	1:256 or greater is considered significant, and false-positive results are rare at this titer. Test is laborious and has the disadvantage of requiring fresh sheep red cells
ELISA	Test takes about 1 hour (most popular)
Solid-phase radioimmunoassay for *E. histolytica* antigens	Useful when antigen excess is suspected, but clinical data are presently lacking
Antigen-based tests (CIEP as well as ELISA) in blood, pus, and feces	Antigen titers correlate closely with clinical status of the patient
For differentiating *E. histolytica* versus *E. dispar*	Presence of hematophagous trophozoites; DNA probes (145 bp and 133 bp)

Abbreviations: bp = base pairs; CIEP = countercurrent immunoelectrophoresis; ELISA = enzyme-linked immunosorbent assay.

TREATMENT

The treatment of choice and the drugs used for the treatment of amebiasis are outlined in Tables 2 and 4. Asymptomatic cyst carriers can be treated with diiodohydroxyquinoline, a halogenated hydroxyquinoline, although diloxanide furoate (Furamide [available from CDC]), an anilide derivative, is a safe alternative. Metronidazole, a tissue amebicide, is effective at all sites and is the drug of first choice both in acute intestinal and extraintestinal amebiasis. It is ineffective in the treatment of asymptomatic cyst passers. A luminal amebicide (such as diloxanide) and an antibiotic (tetracycline)* may be used for additional protection in amebic dysentery. For acute amebic colitis, the luminal amebicide can be combined with paromomycin,* tetracycline,* or oxytetracycline.* These drugs alter the bacterial flora, the presence of which is necessary for the normal development of the protozoa. They are also effective against secondary bacterial infection.

For amebic liver abscess, alternatives are oral chloroquine phosphate (Aralen Phosphate), or parenteral dehydroemetine (Dametine).† Chloroquine inhibits DNA synthesis by its action on DNA polymerase. It can also be combined with metronidazole or emetine for enhanced effectiveness. Dehydroemetine (emetine, the original alkaloid from ipecac, is no longer available) exerts an antiparasitic effect by inhibiting

*Not FDA approved for this indication.
†Investigational drug in the United States.

TABLE 4. **Summary of Drugs Commonly Used for Treatment of Amebiasis**

Drug	Comments	Adult Dosage	Pediatric Dosage
Luminal Agents			
Paromomycin (Humatin)	Frequent gastrointestinal disturbances and, rarely, ototoxicity/nephrotoxicity. Useful in pregnancy.	25–35 mg/kg/d PO in 3 divided doses × 7 d	25 mg/kg/d PO in 3 divided doses × 7 d
Iodoquinol (Yodoxin)	Poorly absorbed from the intestinal tract but can cause nausea and cramps. After prolonged usage, optic atrophy/neuritis reported. Because of its iodine content it may interfere with thyroid function tests for more than 1 month.	650 mg PO three times a day × 20 d	30–40 mg/kg/d × 20 d in 3 divided doses (maximum, 2 g/d)
Diloxanide furoate (Furamide)	Safe drug; rarely may cause nausea, vomiting, diarrhea, and urticaria	500 mg PO three times a day × 10 d	20 mg/kg/d in 3 divided doses × 10 d
Agents for Invasive Amebiasis			
ALL TISSUES			
Metronidazole (Flagyl)	Drug of first choice. May cause nausea, vomiting, diarrhea, abdominal cramping, constipation, dry mouth, metallic taste, and headache; convulsive seizures (seizures, ataxia, encephalopathy, and peripheral neuropathy) have been reported occasionally. Potentiates the anticoagulant effects of warfarin (Coumadin). Alcohol consumed during therapy may produce flushing, headache, vomiting, and abdominal cramps. Avoid in pregnancy, particularly in the first trimester. Drug is secreted in maternal milk. Metronidazole, on occasion, can interfere with the determination of serum aspartate aminotransferase activity, resulting in spuriously low values.	750 mg PO three times a day × 10 d 500 mg IV every 8 h × 10 d	30–50 mg/kg/d orally in 3 divided doses × 5–10 d, or 15 mg/kg IV load followed by 7.5 mg/kg (maximum, 2250 mg/d)
Tinidazole	Effects similar to metronidazole	600 to 800 mg two times a day for 5 d	50 to 60 mg/kg (maximum, 2 g) for 3 d
Dehydroemetine†	Effective but more toxic than metronidazole; may cause a fall in blood pressure, elevation of the pulse rate, and the appearance of electrocardiographic abnormalities. It may also produce muscle weakness and cellulitis at the injection site. Less commonly, diarrhea, vomiting, and peripheral neuropathy are noted.	1–1.5 mg/kg/d IM × 5 d (maximum, 90 mg/d)	1–1.5 mg/kg/d IM × 5 d (maximum, 90 mg/d)
BOWEL WALL ONLY			
Tetracycline‡§	For invasive intestinal disease and secondary infection only	500 mg q6h for 10–14 d	Avoid in children
LIVER ONLY			
Chloroquine (Aralen)	May cause nausea, vomiting, abdominal cramps, diarrhea, visual disturbances, blood dyscrasias, and skin eruptions and rarely retinal injury and heart blocks	600 mg base in divided doses × 2 d followed by 150 mg base (one tablet) twice daily for 21 d	10 mg base/kg (maximum, 300 mg base) daily × 2–3 wk

*Other members of the same group include secnidazole|| and ornidazole,|| which can also be used for invasive intestinal amebiasis.
†Investigational drug in the United States.
‡Where tetracycline is contraindicated, doxycycline or erythromycin can be used. In amebic liver abscess, pending culture sensitivity report, broad-spectrum antibiotics with good gram-negative spectrum may be started if secondary infection is suspected.
§Not FDA approved for this indication.
||Not available in the United States.

protein synthesis. It is contraindicated for patients with cardiac, renal, or hepatic (other than amebic) disease. It should also be used with caution in pregnant women, extremely debilitated patients, or the aged. An overdose may produce focal necrosis of the myocardium with subsequent heart failure. Patients undergoing this treatment should be hospitalized and monitored by frequent electrocardiography and blood pressure determinations. The drug should never be given intravenously; even subcutaneous injection is accompanied by marked irritation.

Drainage

Drainage of an abscess (Table 5) can be achieved percutaneously by a No. 14 French, plastic-covered needle with an internal stylet or catheter under ultrasound guidance. The surgical drainage is reserved for left lobe abscesses that cannot be reached percutaneously.

Pregnancy and Amebic Colitis

Despite legitimate concerns about the use of metronidazole in pregnancy, women who develop severe

Table 5. **Features Indicating High Risk of Rupture in Amebic Liver Abscess***

Clinical
Increasing hepatic tenderness
Abscess pointing in the abdominal wall
Pre-rupture syndrome: abdominal distention, ileus, and localized guarding
Poor response to medical therapy
Severe jaundice

Imaging
Very thin rim of liver parenchyma around the abscess cavity
Abscess size >10 cm
Rapidly enlarging abscess
Abscess located in the left lobe or centrally

*Such abscesses should be drained.

amebic colitis should be treated with metronidazole because of their increased risk of developing fulminant colitis. No adverse outcome was noted when this drug was used in pregnancy for trichomoniasis. For milder intestinal disease, a 7-day course of paromomycin is used.

GIARDIASIS

method of
ANDREW W. DuPONT, M.D.
University of Alabama at Birmingham
Birmingham, Alabama

and

HERBERT L. DuPONT, M.D.
St. Luke's Episcopal Hospital
Houston, Texas

Giardiasis is a diarrheal disease caused by *Giardia lamblia*, one of the most prevalent parasites worldwide. *G. lamblia* is a flagellate protozoan responsible for epidemic and sporadic infection in industrialized areas and endemic infection in less developed regions. Transmission occurs through person-to-person contact and ingestion of contaminated food and water. Infection with *G. lamblia* is characteristically asymptomatic, especially in endemic areas; however, when symptomatic giardiasis occurs, it typically manifests as an acute or subacute diarrheal illness. People more prone to symptomatic infection include those experiencing their initial exposure to the protozoan and those with underlying immunodeficiency, hypogammaglobulinemia, and increased gastric pH (e.g., achlorhydria and hypochlorhydria).

EPIDEMIOLOGY

Between 1% and 7% of people living in industrialized regions can be found to be asymptomatically infected with *G. lamblia*. The carriage rate in developing nations is higher, ranging from 5% to 50%. In stools submitted for examination for ova and parasites, the prevalence of *Giardia* is 2% to 5% in industrialized countries and 20% to 30% in developing nations. The important reservoir for transmission of *Giardia* in industrialized areas of the world is water contaminated by infected people and lower mammals. Large community-wide outbreaks occur when central water systems become contaminated with *Giardia* cysts. Infection is also seen in campers and others exposed to lakes and streams, especially in the remote mountainous regions of the United States and Canada where there is suspected contamination from animals (particularly beavers); in infants in daycare centers owing to environmental contamination; and in gay males whose sexual practices facilitate fecal-oral spread.

Travelers to endemic regions are also at high risk for contracting giardiasis. For instance, travelers to St. Petersburg, Russia, have been shown to be at high risk for contracting symptomatic giardiasis. Transmission may also result from ingestion of undercooked foods contaminated with fecal material, as is seen in areas where night soil, or fertilizer made with human excreta, is used.

PATHOPHYSIOLOGY AND CLINICAL MANIFESTATIONS

Giardia lamblia is a low-dose pathogen that can cause symptomatic infection with ingestion of as few as 10 cysts. The infection rate increases to nearly 100% with 10 to 100 cysts. The incubation period in patients who develop symptomatic disease is typically between 1 and 2 weeks but varies between 1 and 45 days. After ingestion, the organism undergoes excystation in the duodenum as a result of exposure to gastric pH and pancreatic enzymes chymotrypsin and trypsin, producing two trophozoites from each cyst. The trophozoites travel down the intestine, attaching to intestinal mucosa by use of a suction cup–like organelle known as the *ventral disk*. Within the crypts of the duodenum and proximal jejunum, the trophozoites replicate asexually by binary fission. The trophozoite stage is responsible for manifestation of disease. The life cycle is completed by encystation in the ileum, possibly as a result of exposure to bile salts or from cholesterol starvation. Cysts are then excreted in the feces.

The majority of people (~60%) infected with *Giardia* will remain asymptomatic and clear the organism spontaneously. In those who develop symptomatic giardiasis, clinical illness can vary widely. Clinical disease can result in acute self-limiting diarrhea, chronic diarrhea, or persistent diarrhea in spite of appropriate therapy; malabsorption; weight loss; and severe life-threatening disease in the immunosuppressed. In children (particularly in the developing world), infection can lead to growth retardation and failure to thrive. The most characteristic symptoms are (1) acute diarrheal illness of brief duration with or without fever, anorexia, nausea, and abdominal cramping; and (2) intermittent or protracted diarrhea with cramps, abdominal pain, bloating, and flatulence. The symptoms of acute disease often mimic other causes of infectious diarrhea; however, in giardiasis, the stool is often pale, greasy, and foul smelling. Mucus is frequently present in stools passed, but gross blood in feces is seen only rarely. Diarrhea with or without overt malabsorption may last for months or even years. Malabsorption may be responsible for substantial weight loss. Even in asymptomatic infection, malabsorption of fats, carbohydrates, sugars, and vitamins may occur. Reduced intestinal disaccharidase activity may persist even after the organism has been eradicated. Lactase deficiency occurs in 20% to 30% of patients.

Giardiasis should be suspected (1) in people who acquire diarrhea during or shortly after trips to Rocky Mountain areas and recreational lakes and ponds; (2) when illness is associated with daycare centers; and (3) in patients with protracted or intermittent symptoms, particularly with a history of malabsorption, flatulence, bloating, foul-smelling stools, or weight loss. Although rare, extraintestinal manifestations of giardiasis including reactive arthropathy, maculopapular rash, urticaria, and aphthous ulcers have been reported.

DIAGNOSIS

The diagnosis of giardiasis is made by identification of cysts or, less frequently, trophozoites in feces, by detection of *Giardia* antigen in stool, or by identification of trophozoites in the small intestine. Examination of a single stool sample has been shown to be 50% to 75% sensitive in establishing the diagnosis of giardiasis. Evaluation of three samples on nonconsecutive days increases sensitivity to 85% to 95%. However, after exposure to *Giardia*, it may take up to 3 weeks before fecal shedding of the organism begins. Also, in many patients, the agent is excreted intermittently, with negative cycles lasting from 20 to 30 days. Immunoassay procedures offer both increased sensitivity and specificity (90%–100%) compared with conventional staining methods and are readily available in commercial kits. These include direct fluorescent antibody assay and enzyme-linked immunosorbent assay.

For patients suspected to have giardiasis clinically but whose stool studies are repeatedly negative, direct examination of small intestinal contents may be necessary to establish the diagnosis. This can be done by esophagogastroduodenoscopy with duodenal aspiration or biopsy. Biopsy, although more invasive, has the potential to diagnose other disease processes that may present with diarrhea and malabsorption, such as Whipple disease, sprue, lymphoma, Crohn disease, and other parasitic infections. The string test or enterotest is another method for diagnosis in which the patient swallows a gelatin capsule attached to a nylon string. The capsule moves to the jejunum where the trophozoites attach. After a period of time, usually between 4 and 12 hours, the string is removed and bile-stained mucus adherent to the string is examined microscopically.

TREATMENT

It is generally accepted that diagnostically proven cases of symptomatic giardiasis should be treated. Multiple effective drug regimens exist, with most patients responding to a single course of treatment (Table 1). Traditionally, the drug of choice has been quinacrine, owing to its efficacy (95%–100% cure rate) and cost. Quinacrine (Atabrine), however, has many established side effects and is difficult to obtain in the United States, although it can be accessed through a few pharmacies (Panorama Pharmacy, Panorama City, California, 800-247-9767, and Priority Pharmacy, San Diego, California, 800-487-7113). Side effects of quinacrine include yellow staining of skin, urine, and sclera; gastrointestinal (GI) upset; dizziness; headache; hemolysis in glucose-6-phosphate dehydrogenase deficiency; exfoliative dermatitis; and reversible psychosis in 0.1% to 1.5% of patients. Quinacrine should be avoided in patients who are pregnant and who have psoriasis, hepatic dysfunction, or a history of psychosis.

Metronidazole (Flagyl)* has largely replaced quinacrine as the drug of choice for most patients with symptomatic giardiasis. Metronidazole may have a cure rate slightly lower (60%–90%) than quinacrine, but it is generally better tolerated. Side effects of metronidazole include metallic taste, frequent upper GI symptoms (e.g., nausea, vomiting), disulfiram-like reaction with alcohol, and, more rarely, drowsiness, ataxia, headache, and peripheral neuropathy, typically with prolonged use. Metronidazole should also be avoided in pregnancy (at least during the first trimester). There has been concern in the past regarding metronidazole mutagenicity in some bacterial species and carcinogenicity in animals, but no increased cancer risk has been established in human beings. An added potential benefit of metronidazole is its effect on enteric anaerobes that may be involved in bacterial overgrowth in some cases of subacute diarrhea and on *Entamoeba histolytica* (although the metronidazole dose for *Giardia* infection is low for this agent), making metronidazole the drug of choice

*Not FDA approved for this indication.

TABLE 1. **Treatment Regimens in Giardiasis***

Drug	Adult Dose	Pediatric Dose	Side Effects	Comments
Metronidazole (Flagyl)†	250 mg tid × 7 d	5–7 mg/kg tid × 7 d	GI (anorexia, nausea), metallic taste, disulfiram-like reaction	Treatment of choice
Quinacrine (Atabrine)	100 mg qid × 5 d	2 mg/kg qid × 5 d	Yellow skin/urine/sclera, GI symptoms (nausea/vomiting), psychosis in 0.1%–1.5%, hemolysis in G6PD deficiency	Difficult to obtain in United States
Tinidazole (Fasigyn)‡	2 g × one dose	50 mg/kg × one dose	Similar to metronidazole	Not yet available in United States
Furazolidone (Furoxone)	100 mg qid × 7–10 d	1.5–2 mg/kg qid × 7–10 d	GI symptoms (nausea/vomiting, diarrhea), hemolysis in G6PD deficiency, disulfiram-like reaction, mild MAOI	Treatment of choice in infants and young children
Paromomycin (Humatin)†	30 mg/kg/d in three to four doses × 10 d	Same	GI symptoms (nausea/vomiting, diarrhea)	Not absorbed, least effective, safe during pregnancy

*See text for indications.
†Not FDA approved for this indication.
‡Not available in the United States.
Abbreviations: G6PD = glucose-6-phosphate dehydrogenase; GI = gastrointestinal; MAOI = monoamine oxidase inhibitor.

for empirical treatment in cases of suspected giardiasis without laboratory confirmation.

Tinidazole (Fasigyn),* another nitroimidazole, has been widely used and has been shown to be effective in a single dose. However, it has not yet been approved for use in the United States. Side effects of tinidazole are similar to those of metronidazole.

Furazolidone (Furoxone) has been shown to be somewhat less effective (<80% cure rate) than metronidazole. It is presently the only drug approved in the United States for treatment of giardiasis. Furazolidone has long been the drug of choice for children, owing to its availability in a suspension form and better taste when compared with other agents. Adverse reactions include GI disturbances, hemolysis in glucose-6-phosphate dehydrogenase deficiency, and disulfiram-like reaction. Furazolidone is also a mild monoamine oxidase inhibitor.

In pregnant women with *Giardia* infection, treatment is not imperative if the patient is gaining weight appropriately. Treatment can be delayed until childbirth because *Giardia* has not been shown to directly affect the developing fetus. When treatment is necessary, paromomycin (Humatin),† a nonabsorbable aminoglycoside, should be used. Because it is almost entirely excreted in the GI tract with negligible absorption, it has little potential for teratogenicity. Paromomycin is the least effective treatment and should not be used in patients with ulcerations of the GI tract owing to possible absorption and nephrotoxicity.

Eradication of giardiasis is often difficult to establish, and treatment failures occur with all standard agents. Treatment failures may result from reinfection, drug resistance, or host immunodeficiency. In patients with persistent or recurrent symptoms, repeat diagnostic evaluation may be of benefit; however, some patients who continue to harbor trophozoites in the small intestine no longer pass cysts in the stool. In patients with recurrent infection, evaluation for possible ongoing or chronic exposure is indicated, including a study of family contacts, sexual practices, and water supply. In cases of treatment failure, patients often respond to increased dose and/or duration, an alternative medication, or a combination of agents.

*Not available in the United States.
†Not FDA approved for this indication.

SEPSIS AND BACTEREMIA

method of
RAMON L. AÑEL, M.D., and
R. PHILLIP DELLINGER, M.D.
Rush-Presbyterian-St. Luke's Medical Center
Chicago, Illinois

Hippocrates used the word *sepsis* in reference to decay or the process of decomposition. It was only in the 20th century with new medical discoveries that the word started to shed its centuries-old association with putrefaction. Sepsis has taken on even more specific meanings in the past 3 decades owing, in large part, to the intense investigative interest in the pathophysiology of this systemic inflammatory response to infection. Recently, it has become increasingly apparent that the clinical manifestations of sepsis result from a fine balance between the proinflammatory response to an infection nidus and the anti-inflammatory response designed to keep the inflammatory process in check. However, despite the advances made in the elucidation and understanding of these responses, the cornerstone of therapy is the identification and treatment of the infection and aggressive supportive care of organ dysfunction. The presence of bacteremia is most useful in definitively establishing the presence of infection and the precise causative organism.

DEFINITION OF TERMS

Sepsis, septicemia, and *septic shock* are some of the terms used loosely, often interchangeably, to describe the progression of a clinically worsening infection. Bacteremia may or may not be present. In order to standardize their use, the American College of Chest Physicians and the Society of Critical Care Medicine, in August 1991, came up with a paper defining these terms:

- *Infection*: A microbial phenomenon characterized by an inflammatory response to the presence of microorganisms or the invasion of normally sterile host tissue by these organisms.
- *Bacteremia*: The presence of viable bacteria in the blood. The presence of other organisms in the blood should be described in like manner—viremia, fungemia, and so forth. Bacteremia can be transient, sustained, or intermittent.
- *Systemic inflammatory response syndrome (SIRS)*: The systemic inflammatory response to a variety of severe clinical insults, including but not limited to infection, pancreatitis, ischemia, multiple trauma and tissue injury, hemorrhagic shock, immune-mediated organ injury, and exogenous administration of inflammatory mediators such as tumor necrosis factor or other cytokines.
- *Sepsis*: The systemic response to infection. This response is similar to SIRS, except that it must result from an infection.
- *Severe sepsis*: Sepsis associated with organ dysfunction, perfusion abnormalities, or hypotension.
- *Septic shock*: Sepsis with hypotension despite adequate fluid resuscitation, in conjunction with perfusion abnormalities.
- *Multiorgan dysfunction syndrome (MODS)*: Presence of altered organ function in an acutely ill patient, such that homeostasis cannot be maintained without intervention. Primary MODS is the direct result of a well-defined insult in which organ dysfunction occurs early and can be directly attributable to the insult itself. Secondary MODS develops as a consequence of a host response and is identified within the context of SIRS.

Recently, the concept of an anti-inflammatory response has also been introduced after demonstrating that traditional anti-inflammatory mediators were also elevated during sepsis; thus, the term *compensatory anti-inflammatory response syndrome (CARS)*.

Although the consensus conference discouraged the use of the term *septicemia* owing to its ambiguity, it is still used by the Centers for Disease Control and Prevention

(CDC) to record vital statistics relating to systemic microbial infections; thus, use of the term persists in various texts.

PATHOPHYSIOLOGY AND CLINICAL MANIFESTATIONS

Sepsis, severe sepsis, and septic shock represent a continuum of clinical manifestations of an infection-induced systemic inflammatory process, with multiorgan dysfunction at the terminal end of the continuum (Figure 1). These manifestations can occur in the absence of bacteremia and positive cultures from the presumed site of infection. The course of sepsis depends on the balance between pro- and anti-inflammatory processes. If the balance is tipped more toward the former, systemic injury and organ dysfunction result from the host's exaggerated inflammatory process. If the latter is favored in excess, it increases the chances for the infection to overwhelm the host or the propensity for a secondary superimposed infectious process to take place. Although the list of pro- and anti-inflammatory mediators is formidable (Table 1), their various interactions are even more overwhelming.

Sepsis begins with a nidus of infection followed by the initiation of an inflammatory response, initially meant to localize the infection. When this process spills over into the bloodstream, a systemic response takes place. The systemic elaboration of various proinflammatory mediators leads to a complex cascade of reactions culminating in a number of classic end-organ responses. In the cardiovascular system, assuming adequate volume resuscitation, the classic description is that of a hyperdynamic state with an increased cardiac index and a low systemic vascular resistance. With overwhelming sepsis, the marked decrease in cardiac contractility and vascular tone renders the patient unresponsive to high levels of vasopressor support. In the lungs, the

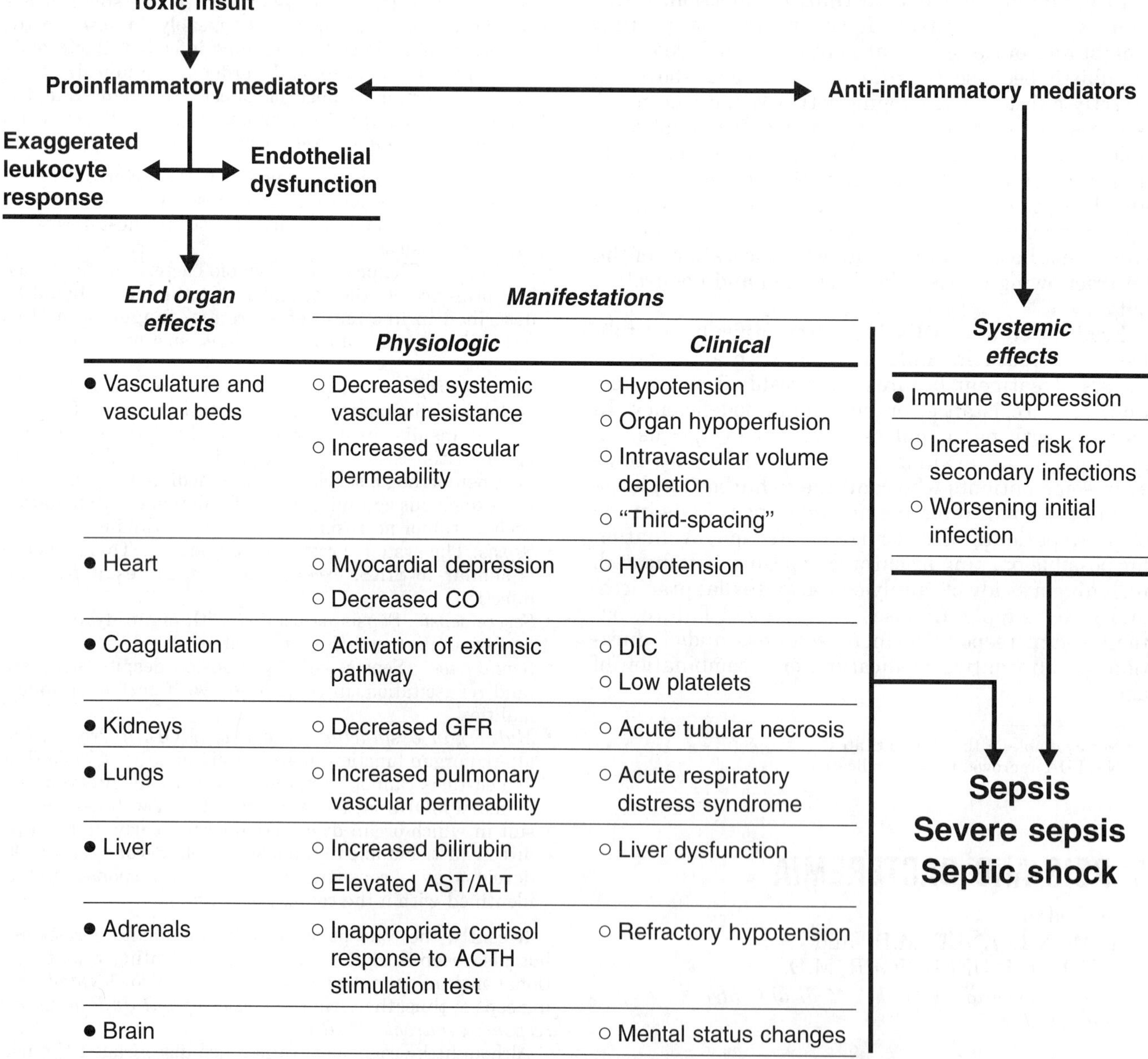

End organ effects	Physiologic	Clinical
• Vasculature and vascular beds	○ Decreased systemic vascular resistance ○ Increased vascular permeability	○ Hypotension ○ Organ hypoperfusion ○ Intravascular volume depletion ○ "Third-spacing"
• Heart	○ Myocardial depression ○ Decreased CO	○ Hypotension
• Coagulation	○ Activation of extrinsic pathway	○ DIC ○ Low platelets
• Kidneys	○ Decreased GFR	○ Acute tubular necrosis
• Lungs	○ Increased pulmonary vascular permeability	○ Acute respiratory distress syndrome
• Liver	○ Increased bilirubin ○ Elevated AST/ALT	○ Liver dysfunction
• Adrenals	○ Inappropriate cortisol response to ACTH stimulation test	○ Refractory hypotension
• Brain		○ Mental status changes

Figure 1. The pathogenesis and clinical manifestations of sepsis. ACTH = adrenocorticotropic hormone; ALT = alanine aminotransferase; AST = aspartate transaminase; DIC = diffuse intravascular coagulopathy; GFR = glomerular filtration rate.

TABLE 1. **Some of the Pro- and Anti-Inflammatory Mediators in Sepsis**

Proinflammatory	Anti-Inflammatory
Endotoxin and other microbial toxins	LPS binding protein
Products of arachidonic acid (thromboxane, prostaglandins, prostacyclin)	Receptors to various cytokines (TNF-R, IL-1R, type II IL-R)
Tumor necrosis factor	Interleukins (4, 10, 13)
Interleukins (1, 6, 8, 15)	Soluble CD-14
G-CSF	Epinephrine and other endogenous catecholamines
Platelet-activating factor	Vasoactive intestinal peptides
Bradykinin and other kinins	TGFβ
Histamine	
Serotonin	
Nitric oxide	
Toxic oxygen metabolites (superoxides, peroxynitrite, hydroxyl species, etc.)	
Protein degradation enzymes (kinases)	
Coagulation factors	
Complement	

Abbreviations: G-CSF = granulocyte colony-stimulating factor; IL = interleukin; LPS = lipopolysaccharide; TNF = tumor necrosis factor.

development of acute lung injury is common owing to the increased vascular permeability induced by proinflammatory cytokines on pulmonary endothelium. This same effect induces third spacing in other vascular beds, leading to subcutaneous edema and ascites, and exacerbates the effect of loss of vascular tone by depleting intravascular volume. Other sepsis-induced end-organ dysfunction includes changes in mentation, renal insufficiency, liver dysfunction, and coagulopathy. Oliguria and lactic acidosis may occur and reflect evidence of organ hypoperfusion.

Bacteremia can be transient or persistent. Transient low-density bacteremia is usually benign. It commonly occurs after brushing the teeth and after a bowel movement and lasts no more than a few minutes. It is also seen after fairly routine minor medical and dental procedures. Persistent bacteremia on the other hand is a pathologic condition. Persistent intermittent bacteremia is seen in conditions in which there is an extravascular collection of infectious material seeding into the bloodstream. However, persistent, sustained bacteremia is usually a hallmark of an endovascular source such as an infected heart valve or vascular fistula.

Metastatic infections to the meninges, large joints, and other serous cavities such as the pericardium can complicate bacteremia. Metastatic abscesses can form practically anywhere and produce signs and symptoms that localize to the organ involved. If the pathogen involved is *Streptococcus* or *Staphylococcus* species, endocarditis can develop as a sequela of bacteremia. In a subgroup of patients, bacteremia can progress to sepsis, depending on the interaction between host factors, the infecting organism, and the environment involved; however, to document bacteremia in a septic patient is not always easy. In patients with sepsis, the presence of bacteremia implies a significantly worse prognosis.

EPIDEMIOLOGY

In the past 20 to 25 years, the number of cases of sepsis has been steadily increasing, and it is expected to continue to do so. The reasons for this are many: increasing use of immunosuppressive therapies, aging of the population, increasing incidence of drug-resistant infections, a growing population of potentially immunocompromised patients such as those with diabetes and cancer, increasing use of invasive devices such as intravascular catheters for monitoring and treatment, and greater availability of life-sustaining devices. Severe sepsis and septic shock are the most common causes of death in intensive care units. The CDC reports sepsis and related syndromes to be the 13th leading cause of death in the United States.

DIAGNOSIS

Differential Diagnosis

Clinically, it is difficult to differentiate sepsis from other causes of SIRS, especially at presentation. The criteria for SIRS (Table 2) outlined by the consensus conference are fairly sensitive but are not specific. The differential diagnosis of noninfectious hyperthermia includes hyperthyroid states, neuroleptic malignant syndrome, hypothalamic insults, drugs, and environmental heat injury. Hypothermia in sepsis is not as frequently recognized as hyperthermia, but it commonly occurs in very young and very old people. Noninfectious causes of hypothermia include endocrine diseases involving the thyroid and pituitary glands, environmental exposure, and drugs. Causes of tachycardia that need to be considered and ruled out promptly are acute myocardial ischemia, acute blood loss, severe dehydration, pulmonary embolism, and anaphylactic reaction. These disorders may also be present with hypotension, mimicking septic shock. A myriad of pulmonary problems can be present with tachypnea as can any hypermetabolic state. Leukocyte count (white blood cell count [WBC]) abnormalities can be found in a variety of clinical situations. Steroids can cause leukocytes to demarginate and reenter the circulating pool, thus increasing the absolute WBC. Stress-induced catecholamine release can also significantly elevate the WBC, which can complicate the diagnosis.

Initial Testing

Patients who are admitted with a clinical impression of sepsis should have a complete laboratory evaluation including complete blood count with differential, complete serum chemistry profile, serum lactate, urinalysis, arterial blood gas, and prothrombin and activated partial thromboplastin times. A chest radiograph is also often warranted together with an electrocardiogram.

TABLE 2. **Criteria* for Systemic Inflammatory Response Syndrome**

Temperature	$<36°C$ *or* $>38°C$
Heart rate	>90 bpm
Respiratory rate *or*	>20 breaths/min
P_{CO_2}	<32 mm Hg
White blood cell count	$>12{,}000$ cells/hpf *or* <4000 cells/hpf *or* $>10\%$ band forms

*Need to satisfy at least two criteria. These represent *acute changes* in the absence of any known cause.
Abbreviation: hpf = high-power field.

Identifying the Source and Etiology of Infection

In patients with suspected sepsis, an exhaustive search for the focus of infection begins with a good history and a thorough physical examination. Any suspicious foci should be subjected to further investigation, and appropriate stains and cultures should be obtained. For blood cultures, there should be a minimum of two sets from two different sites. Each set should have aerobic and anaerobic bottles. Culture media with antibiotic resins may increase the yield if the patient is started on antibiotics before the culture is obtained. In patients with indwelling arterial or venous catheters, samples from each port should be obtained. In severe sepsis and septic shock, blood cultures from patients are positive in 50% to 60% of cases. A Gram stain of sputum is also useful to suggest potential causative organisms. An adequate specimen should contain no more than 25 squamous epithelial cells per low-power (×100) field on the microscope.

Urine cultures should be obtained by a clean-catch method or, if this is not possible, with the use of a clean catheter or via suprapubic aspiration. Urine from a closed collection system with an external or indwelling catheter should not be used for culture.

Stool specimens should also be sent for cultures if a septic-appearing patient has diarrhea. Aspiration from a normally sterile site of fluid that is suspicious for infection should also be performed when appropriate. This includes a spinal tap for a septic patient with altered mental status, a joint aspiration for a suspected septic joint, a peritoneal tap for ascites with possible peritonitis, and a thoracentesis for a possibly infected pleural fluid collection. Areas along the skin surface with evidence of suppuration or necrosis may also be candidates for sampling. In the absence of any localizing signs or symptoms, cultures for blood, sputum, and urine should be sent.

Although information from cultures may not be immediately available, these results are often used to narrow the patient's antibiotic regimen later in the course of therapy. Cultures are preferably obtained before initiation of antibiotics to maximize the diagnostic yield. However, prolonged delays in the initiation of antibiotic therapy are not acceptable.

TREATMENT

Sepsis and Septic Shock

Severe sepsis is a life-threatening illness. Priority should always be given to achieving immediate stabilization. This includes a rapid assessment of airway patency, breathing, and circulation followed by prompt institution of life-sustaining measures to address reversible abnormalities. A more definitive evaluation should follow immediately after stabilization. The primary treatment of patients with sepsis remains antibiotics, source control, and supportive therapy. Although innovative therapy targeted toward modifying the inflammatory response has thus far been unsuccessful, it is hoped that progress will be made in the future.

Antimicrobial Therapy

At the onset of sepsis or septic shock, the etiologic agent is usually presumptive. Initial empirical antibiotic therapy should provide broad coverage for the more common pathogens suspected. Common causative organisms of community-acquired sepsis include *Staphylococcus aureus, Streptococcus pneumoniae*, and *Escherichia coli*. Most nosocomial infections are caused by gram-negative aerobic bacilli, enterococci, coagulase-negative staphylococci, and *S. aureus. Pseudomonas aeruginosa* is frequently associated with neutropenic hosts. Coagulase-negative staphylococci, *S. aureus*, and *Candida* species are the more common organisms seen with indwelling catheters. Bacteremia in immunocompromised and neutropenic patients requires broad-spectrum antibiotics as initial therapy. If opportunistic infections are suspected, the appropriate antimicrobials for the specific opportunistic infections should be added to the regimen. The more unstable a patient becomes, the broader the empirical coverage should be against potential pathogens. Table 3 summarizes general guidelines for the initial selection of antibiotics in cases of sepsis. Empirical coverage for suspected fungal infections should be provided with amphotericin B. Fluconazole may be considered as an alternative if the patient is not severely ill and if *Candida albicans* is deemed the most likely pathogen.

Antimicrobial selection relies heavily on clinical judgment, taking into account the nature of the suspect microorganisms, the possible sources of infection, the patient's co-morbid conditions, the community the patient is coming from, and institutional microbial susceptibility patterns. Gram stain results, which may be obtained within a few minutes after collection of the sample, are helpful in the initial choice of antibiotics.

Supportive Therapy

Patients with severe sepsis and septic shock should be closely monitored in an intensive care setting. An arterial line is recommended in the presence of hemodynamic instability (e.g., need for adrenergic therapy to support blood pressure). In the presence of organ hypoperfusion, an effort to ensure normal oxygen delivery should be made. Use of a pulmonary artery (Swan-Ganz) catheter is controversial but may be useful in the following situations:

1. Verifying that the hemodynamic profile supports sepsis as the cause of hypotension
2. Ensuring adequate left ventricular preload in the hypotensive patient
3. Avoiding excessive volume resuscitation in the patient with acute lung injury
4. Ensuring adequate cardiac output

Rapid infusions of crystalloids or colloids to ensure adequate intravascular volume are the initial therapy of choice in the presence of hypotension or organ hypoperfusion. The addition of vasopressors (e.g., norepinephrine [Levophed], typically starting at 2–4 μg/min, or phenylephrine [Neo-Synephrine], 40–180 μg/min) is necessary for persistent low mean arterial pressure (MAP <60 mm Hg) despite volume replacement. Inotropes (dopamine [Intropin], 5–10 μg/kg/min, or dobutamine [Dobutrex], 2.5–20 μg/kg/min)

TABLE 3. **Empirical Intravenous Antibiotic Selection for Severe Sepsis and Septic Shock**

Source	Recommended Regimen
1. No clinically identifiable source	Antipseudomonal penicillin *or* cephalosporin + aminoglycoside *or* fluoroquinolone (if with renal insufficiency) *or*
but with likely pathogens	Imipenem (Primaxin) as a single agent
(a) Anaerobes	Antipseudomonal penicillin *or* cephalosporin + aminoglycoside *or* fluoroquinolone + clindamycin *or* metronidazole (Flagyl)
(b) *Pseudomonas aeruginosa*	Antipseudomonal penicillin + aminoglycoside *or* fluoroquinolone *or* Imipenem + aminoglycoside *or* fluoroquinolone
2. Community-acquired pneumonia	
(a) Immunocompetent host	Second- and third-generation cephalosporin + macrolide *or* quinolone *or* β-lactam antibiotics with β-lactamase inhibitors
(b) Immunocompromised host	Broad-spectrum coverage as with No.1 Consider empirical coverage for opportunistic infections (mycobacteria, fungi, *Nocardia*, parasites). Also aggressive/invasive diagnostic workup.
(c) Atypicals likely	2(a) *or* 2(b) + erythromycin *or* fluoroquinolone
3. Nosocomial *or* ventilator-associated pneumonia	Broad-spectrum coverage as with No.1
4. Abdominal *or* intra-abdominal	
(a) *P. aeruginosa* unlikely	Imipenem *or* Ampicillin/sulbactam (Unasyn) *or* Ticarcillin/clavulanate (Timentin) *or* Piperacillin/tazobactam (Zosyn)
(b) *P. aeruginosa* likely *or* very severe infections	Ampicillin + metronidazole + aztreonam *or* aminoglycoside *or* Any of the regimens in 4(a) + aminoglycoside *or* Second-generation cephalosporin (cefoxitin, cefotetan) + aminoglycoside
5. Urinary tract	
(a) *P. aeruginosa* unlikely	Third-generation cephalosporin *or* Quinolone
(b) *P. aeruginosa* likely *or* very severe infections	Third-generation cephalosporin + quinolone *or* Either regimen in 5(a) + aztreonam
6. Cellulitis *or* cutaneous abscess	
(a) Methicillin-resistant *Staphylococcus aureus* unlikely	Cefazolin *or* Nafcillin
(b) Methicillin-resistant *S. aureus or* coagulase-negative staphylococcus likely	Vancomycin
7. Necrotizing fasciitis	Any of the regimens in 4(a)
8. Intravascular catheter	Consider removal of catheter *plus*. . .
(a) Outpatient-acquired infection	Third-generation cephalosporin
(b) Methicillin-resistant *S. aureus or* coagulase-negative staphylococcus likely	8(a) + vancomycin
(c) Diabetes	8(b) + quinolone

should be added in the presence of inadequate cardiac output. Hemoglobin should be maintained at a concentration of greater than or equal to 8 g/dL for patients who are not actively bleeding. An initial oxyhemoglobin saturation goal of 95% is reasonable. Although, in theory, packed red blood cell transfusion is an effective means of increasing arterial oxygen content and availability, a randomized study in the intensive care unit showed no difference in outcome between transfusion thresholds of either 7 g/dL or 10 g/dL of hemoglobin in critically ill, nonbleeding patients. There is no evidence that the practice of raising oxygen delivery to supranormal levels has any clinical benefit.

Transfusion of other blood products may be necessary for treatment of patients with coagulopathies and thrombasthenias induced by sepsis. Septic malnourished patients and those who are alcoholic or elderly should be considered for vitamin K supplementation if the prothrombin time is elevated. Thrombocytopenia is common in septic patients. This may or may not be associated with other manifestations of disseminated intravascular coagulopathy (DIC). In the absence of active bleeding or if an invasive or surgical procedure is planned, platelet transfusion is indicated only for patients with counts less than 20,000/mm^3. If the patient is hemorrhaging or if procedures are planned, the platelet count should be kept at or greater than 50,000/mm^3. The treatment for sepsis-induced DIC is the same as for any other cause of DIC. Sepsis-induced coagulopathy is manifested initially and primarily by elevation of the international normalized ratio (INR). In the presence of bleeding and prolongation of the INR, fresh-frozen plasma (FFP) should be administered to reduce the INR below 1.5. When transfused, FFP not only repletes clotting factors but also is an effective colloid for volume resuscitation. FFP should not, however, be used for volume resuscitation in the absence of coagulopathy.

Acute respiratory distress syndrome (ARDS) is a common complication of severe sepsis and requires endotracheal intubation and mechanical ventilation. Sufficient positive end-expiratory pressure (PEEP) should be applied to maximize arterial oxyhemoglobin saturation. It now appears that mechanical ventilation–induced lung injury occurs when either (1) too low a PEEP is used, allowing opening and closing of edematous areas of the lung with each inspiration and expiration; or (2) too high a tidal volume is delivered, causing overinflation of areas of lung with relatively normal compliance. Therefore, the recommendation is to attempt to use minimal PEEP (8–15 cm H_2O) and low tidal volumes (6 mL/kg) in patients with ARDS. PEEP therapy may, however, decrease the cardiac output and predispose the patient to barotrauma.

Dialysis may be required when renal failure accompanies severe sepsis. "Renal-dose" dopamine has been traditionally advocated to "increase renal blood flow" in patients with sepsis. However, the value of this treatment modality is currently questioned because in clinical trials, neither has decrease in the progression of renal dysfunction been shown nor has the need for dialysis been obviated.

Early nutritional support is essential in the management of sepsis. Unless there are specific contraindications (e.g., obstructed gastrointestinal tract, active gastrointestinal bleeding), enteral feeding should be used. If gastric retention becomes a problem, postpyloric feeding should be considered. Patients should also be given prophylaxis for stress-associated gastric ulcers and for deep venous thrombosis.

Source Control

Apparent superficial soft tissue infections may be a harbinger of life-threatening deep tissue infection in need of surgical débridement. Plain radiographs may reveal the presence of subcutaneous gas in these circumstances. Computed tomography (CT) with contrast can also identify necrotic tissue.

Intestinal obstruction can demonstrate characteristic findings on abdominal radiographs. Free air under the diaphragm that may be seen on upright chest or abdominal radiographs is present in patients with perforations of the gastrointestinal tract.

Other special diagnostic scans that can aid in localizing the source of infection include a right upper quadrant ultrasonogram for acalculous cholecystitis or biliary sepsis; echocardiography, particularly via the transesophageal route for localizing cardiac valvular lesions; CT of the sinuses; and CT of the kidneys for detection of perinephric abscesses or emphysematous pyelonephritis.

Innovative Therapy

In the last 3 decades, there has been a flurry of basic research elucidating the complex cascade of inflammatory mediators secreted by immune cells in response to infection. A number of these mediators have been targeted for therapeutic intervention (Table 4). Although some novel anti-inflammatory agents have shown promising results in animal studies, most of them failed to show any clinical benefit in human trials. However, a recently published clinical trial showed a significant reduction in 28-day mortality in patients with severe sepsis treated with drotrecogin alpha, a recombinant form of human activated protein C (rhAPC). Septic patients given rhAPC had a relative risk reduction from dying of 19.4%. This trial represents the first large, multicenter, randomized, double-blind, placebo-controlled study that has demonstrated a statistically significant mortality benefit with the use of a novel agent for sepsis. Drotrecogin alpha is currently awaiting Food and Drug Administration approval.

TABLE 4. **Major Clinical Trials of Anti-Inflammatory Therapy**

Therapy	Sponsor
Human antilipid A MAb*	Centocor
Mouse antilipid A MAb*	Zoma
Antienterobacterial antigen MAb*	Chiron
Interleukin-1 receptor antagonist*	Synergen
Antibradykinin*	Cortech
Anti-PAF*	Ipsen
Anti-TNF MAb*	Bayer/Miles—Noracept I
Anti-TNF MAb*	Bayer/Miles—Intercept
Anti-TNF MAb*	Bayer/Miles—Noracept II
Anti-TNF MAb*	Knoll
Soluble TNF-receptor*	Immunex
Soluble TNF-receptor*	Hoffman-LaRoche
Ibuprofen	NA
NOS Inhibitor*	Glaxo-Wellcome

*Investigational drug in the United States.
Abbreviations: MAb = monoclonal antibody; NA = not available; NOS = nitric oxide synthase; PAF = platelet activating factor; TNF = tumor necrosis factor.

Two other trials have been presented in recent international conferences that showed encouraging results. Although these two studies have not been published and peer-reviewed, study investigators report significant benefit. The first study suggested improved survival with the administration of hydrocortisone (300 mg/d) and fludrocortisone (5 mg/d) for 7 days to septic patients who fail to respond to an adrenocorticotropic (ACTH) stimulation test. The second study utilized a monoclonal antibody to tumor necrosis factor (afelimomab). After a logistic regression analysis for confounders, investigators reported a significant reduction in mortality in septic patients with an interleukin-6 level of greater than or equal to 1000 pg/mL.

Bacteremia

Transient bacteremias resulting from minor medical or surgical procedures or indwelling intravenous or urinary catheters are often undetected. The American Heart Association has published updated guidelines for the prevention of bacterial endocarditis after invasive dental and medical procedures.

Intermittent and sustained bacteremias are of more serious concern. The source should be identified and addressed early. Abscesses should be drained, infected prosthetic devices should be removed, ruptured viscus should be surgically repaired, and gangrenous tissue should be excised. Appropriate antibiotic therapy is usually successful when given promptly for persistent bacteremia caused by infections of the lung and nonobstructive infections of the urinary and biliary tracts. Progression of the disease to sepsis or the presence of a polymicrobial bacteremia often portends a poorer prognosis.

Sepsis, severe sepsis, and septic shock represent the spectrum of inflammatory responses to infection. Although much has been learned about the pathophysiology of these diseases, clinical trials of novel approaches have been disappointing. Management of patients with sepsis remains centered on prompt identification and control of the source of infection, early administration of the appropriate antibiotics, and aggressive supportive care.

Bacteremia, in contrast, is a distinct clinical entity whose treatment is fairly straightforward. Although a small population of bacteremic patients may deteriorate and become septic, the majority do well with appropriate therapy.

BRUCELLOSIS

method of
KERRY O. CLEVELAND, M.D., and
MICHAEL S. GELFAND, M.D.
Methodist Healthcare of Memphis
Memphis, Tennessee

Brucellosis is a zoonotic disease caused by gram-negative coccobacilli from the genus *Brucella*. The disease exists worldwide but is most commonly seen in developing countries. The natural hosts are animals, including cattle, sheep, goats, dogs, camels, and swine. In animals, brucellosis may cause spontaneous abortion.

Human beings may acquire the organism by ingesting unpasteurized dairy products, inhaling infected aerosols, or being in direct contact with secretions and blood of diseased animals.

CLINICAL MANIFESTATIONS

Brucellosis usually manifests as a nonspecific febrile illness with fever, sweats, weight loss, depression, fatigue, and arthralgias, but there may be focal findings, most commonly of the bones and joints, cardiovascular system, central nervous system, or genitourinary system. Commonly, the fever waxes and wanes, leading to the description of the disease as "undulant fever." Mild generalized lymphadenopathy may occur in 10% of patients and 20% to 40% may have mild splenomegaly or hepatomegaly.

Bone and joint manifestations commonly involve the sacroiliac joint. Spondylitis is more frequent in older patients and may be accompanied by a paraspinous abscess. Larger peripheral joints (knees, shoulders, and hips) are involved more frequently than smaller joints. Synovial fluid usually shows elevated proteins and a mononuclear pleocytosis, and the cultures are negative in more than 50% of cases.

Liver functions may be slightly elevated. In hepatic disease due to *Brucella abortus,* biopsy may show noncaseating granulomas similar to those seen with sarcoidosis. Infection with *Brucella melitensis* may resemble viral hepatitis or show granulomas. Liver abscesses are rare but, when seen, are usually due to *Brucella suis*.

Orchitis and epididymitis are the most common genitourinary complications. Unilateral testicular involvement may occur.

Two percent of brucellosis patients also have endocarditis, and this is the most frequent cause of mortality due to this disease. Prolonged antibiotic therapy has been reported to cure this infection, but usually valve replacement is required in addition to antibiotics. Pericarditis may also be seen.

Acute or chronic meningitis may be seen with brucellosis. Signs of meningeal inflammation may be absent. Cerebrospinal fluid usually shows an elevated protein level, normal to low glucose levels, a mononuclear pleocytosis, and negative Gram stain and culture. The presence of specific antibodies in the cerebrospinal fluid is diagnostic. Depression and mental fatigue are common.

Hematologic manifestations are nonspecific. The white blood cell count may be normal or low, mild anemia may exist, and the platelet count is usually normal but may be slightly low. Poorly formed granulomas are found in the bone marrow in 75% of cases.

DIAGNOSIS

To diagnose brucellosis, a high index of suspicion is necessary and a history of animal exposure, unusual food consumption, or travel to an endemic area should be elicited. Definite diagnosis requires isolation of the organism from culture of the blood, bone marrow, or other sources. The organism grows slowly and the laboratory should incubate the cultures for at least 4 weeks. Usually, the diagnosis is made on the basis of rising or high serum antibodies using *B. abortus* antigen, which may not detect antibodies to *Brucella canis*.

TREATMENT

Despite extensive studies, the optimal antibiotic regimen for treatment of brucellosis is disputed. A summary of recommendations is included in Table 1.

The World Health Organization recommends treating acute brucellosis with a 6-week course of doxycycline 200 mg daily and rifampin (Rifadin)* 600 to 900 mg daily. We recommend using doxycycline 100 mg per os (PO) twice daily (bid) for 45 days plus streptomycin 1 g intramuscularly daily for 14 to 21 days. Tetracycline 500 mg PO four times daily may be substituted for doxycycline, but we prefer to use doxycycline owing to a lower incidence of adverse gastrointestinal effects. Gentamicin 3 to 5 mg/kg intravenously or intramuscularly daily may be substituted for streptomycin. Some authorities advocate the use of doxycycline 100 mg PO bid for 45 days. Relapses are common, especially with monotherapy, and should be retreated with combination therapy.

The combination of doxycycline and streptomycin may be more efficacious than doxycycline and rifampin in the treatment of spondylitis and may have a lower rate of relapse. In severe focal infections, such

*Not FDA approved for this indication.

TABLE 1. **Treatment of Brucellosis**

Disease	Recommended	Alternative
Acute brucellosis Adults and children >8 y	Doxycycline 100 mg PO bid × 45 d *plus either* Streptomycin 15 mg/kg IM daily × 14–21 d *or* Gentamicin 3–5 mg/kg IV daily × 14–21 d	Doxycycline 100 mg PO bid *plus* Rifampin*‡ 600–900 mg PO daily × 42 d
Children <8 y	TMP-SMZ 5 mg/kg (of TMP component) PO bid × 45 d *plus* Gentamicin 5–6 mg/kg IV daily × 7 d	Rifampin*‡ 15 mg/kg PO daily × 45 d *plus* Gentamicin 5–6 mg/kg IV daily × 7 d
Focal *Brucella* infections (endocarditis, spondylitis, meningitis, paraspinous abscess)	Doxycycline 100 mg PO bid *and* Rifampin*‡ 600 mg PO daily × 45 d *plus either* Streptomycin 1 g IM daily *or* Gentamicin 3–5 mg/kg IV daily × 14–21 d	Consider surgery Consider ciprofloxacin‡ 750 mg PO bid or ofloxacin‡ 400 mg PO bid as substitute for doxycycline or rifampin*‡
Brucellosis during pregnancy	Rifampin*‡ 600 mg PO daily *plus* TMP-SMZ†‡ 1 DS tablet bid × 2 days	Rifampin*‡ 600–900 mg PO daily × 45 d

Aminoglycoside and quinolone dosage should be adjusted in patients with poor renal function.

*Rifampin should be closely monitored for potential drug interactions.

†TMP/SMZ use in pregnancy should be avoided at term and used with caution earlier during the course of pregnancy.

‡Not FDA approved for this indication.

Abbreviations: DS = double strength; TMP-SMZ = trimethoprim and sulfamethoxazole.

as endocarditis or spondylitis (especially with paraspinous abscess), or in cases of relapse combination therapy with three agents (doxycycline 100 mg PO bid and rifampin* 600 mg PO daily for 45 days with either gentamicin or streptomycin for 14 days) seems reasonable.

Trimethoprim-sulfamethoxazole (TMP-SMZ) (Bactrim)* has been used as a substitute for doxycycline and also as a single agent for prolonged periods (6 months) in the treatment of brucellosis.

In children younger than 8 years of age, TMP-SMZ can be substituted for doxycycline. Another alternative pediatric regimen is the use of rifampin* 15 mg/kg daily in two divided doses for 45 days with gentamicin 5 to 6 mg/kg daily for 7 days.

Treatment of brucellosis in pregnant or nursing mothers should consist of rifampin* 600 mg PO daily for 6 weeks or rifampin 600 mg PO daily plus one double-strength TMP-SMZ tablet PO bid for 4 weeks (if there is little risk of kernicterus).

*Not FDA approved for this indication.

Fluoroquinolones (e.g., ciprofloxacin [Cipro] and ofloxacin* [Floxin]) (as single agents have an unacceptably high rate of failure, but they may prove useful in combination therapy with one or more other agents. Newer macrolides such as azithromycin (Zithromax) appear to have potential for use; however, data from animal studies are less than encouraging and we do not, at present, advocate their use in the treatment of brucellosis.

Rifampin* commonly interacts with other medications. Physicians who prescribe rifampin for treatment of brucellosis should review the patient's other medications for potential interactions.

Surgical treatment is usually needed in cases of endocarditis due to brucellosis. Abscesses of the paravertebral space as well as other large abscesses should probably be drained. In cases of spinal cord impingement, surgical stabilization may be necessary.

*Not FDA approved for this indication.

CONJUNCTIVITIS

method of
LEWIS R. GRODEN, M.D.,
CRAIG BERGER, M.D., and
NATHAN R. EMERY, M.D.
University of South Florida College of Medicine
Tampa, Florida

One of the most common ocular diseases, *conjunctivitis* ("red or pink eye") is usually characterized by an ocular discharge, sometimes with sticking eyelids, a red eye from an injected conjunctiva, and commonly, a foreign body sensation. Vision may be normal or decreased. Causes of conjunctivitis are numerous; they may be bacterial, viral, allergic, or toxic in origin. It is easiest to classify conjunctivitis by speed of onset.

Conjunctivitis may be placed into one of three classifications: *hyperacute* (onset of <12 hours), *acute/subacute* (<4 weeks), or *chronic* (generally lasting >4 weeks). The two most common causes of hyperacute conjunctivitis are *Neisseria gonorrhoeae* and *Neisseria meningitidis*. Noted for its rapid onset with severe purulent discharge, gonococcal conjunctivitis is dramatic in its manifestation. Other signs of the disease include marked chemosis, conjunctival papillae, and palpable preauricular lymphadenopathy. Gonococcal conjunctivitis may occur via direct contact from infected genitalia or in the newborn via infection from the mother's genital tract (ophthalmia neonatorum). Gram stain and culture of conjunctival scrapings should be carried out to search for the characteristic gram-negative intracellular diplococci of *N. gonorrhoeae*. Treatment necessitates both topical and systemic antibiotics because this disease may have systemic complications such as urethritis, arthritis, and even septicemia. This infection is an ophthalmologic emergency because it has the potential to progress to corneal infection and subsequent corneal perforation. Current Centers for Disease Control and Prevention (CDC) treatment guidelines should be followed. Adults require ceftriaxone sodium (Rocephin),* 1 g given intramuscularly daily for 5 days, or penicillin G, 10 million U given intravenously for 5 days. If allergic to penicillin, spectinomycin (Trobicin),* 4 g (10 mL) intramuscularly in two divided doses, or tetracycline hydrochloride, 1.5 g as a loading dose followed by 0.5 g four times a day for 4 days, may be used. Ampicillin, 3.5 g administered orally, with 1.0 g of probenecid given simultaneously, is another alternative. Topical therapy includes penicillin (333,000 U/mL) or bacitracin ointment (500 U/g). Alternatives include tetracycline ophthalmic ointment (1%) or gentamicin sulfate ophthalmic ointment (0.3%) every 2 to 4 hours. Current CDC treatment guidelines should be followed.

Acute forms of conjunctivitis are commonly viral, bacterial, or allergic in origin. Patients with red eyes, a watery mucous discharge, and a history of recent upper respiratory infection or contact with someone with similar symptoms are most likely suffering from viral conjunctivitis. Adenovirus is the likely etiology in these cases. Patients often have red edematous eyelids, pinpoint subconjunctival hemorrhages, and palpable preauricular lymph nodes. More severe cases may have a membrane or pseudomembrane overlying the conjunctiva. Treatment is largely symptomatic. The use of artificial tears every 2 to 4 hours with naphazoline/pheniramine four times per day for itching will bring some relief. If a membrane/pseudomembrane develops or the patient loses vision, the patient should be referred to an ophthalmologist because topical steroid treatment may be required. The use of antibiotics should be avoided in obvious cases of viral conjunctivitis because they will not help and will contribute to the emergence of resistant strains of the normal bacterial flora. Viral conjunctivitis characteristically worsens the first week and may not resolve for 2 to 3 weeks. It is contagious for 10 to 12 days from onset.

Another significant cause of acute conjunctivitis is herpes simplex virus. Primary herpes simplex conjunctivitis, most commonly seen in children 2 months to 6 years of age, is typically manifested as gingivostomatitis, local vesicular lesions on the eyelid, follicular conjunctivitis, palpable preauricular lymphadenopathy, and punctate or dendritic staining of the cornea. Treatment consists of topical ocular antiviral medication, trifluridine 1% (Viroptic) nine times per day or vidarabine 3% ointment (Vira-A) five times per day, cool compresses, and application of an antibiotic ointment such as erythromycin or bacitracin to skin lesions if present.

With symptoms similar to viral conjunctivitis, patients with allergic conjunctivitis often have a history of allergic rhinitis and will characteristically complain of itching and watery discharge. They have red edematous eyelids and conjunctival chemosis without palpable preauricular lymph nodes. In mild cases, signs may be minimal, with symptoms of itchiness predominating. Eliminating the inciting agent is helpful but not always possible. Other treatments include cool compresses, artificial tears (1 drop every 4 to 6 hours), and a vasoconstrictor/antihistamine (naphazoline/pheniramine, 1 drop four times daily [qid]). Other medications, including lodoxamide 0.05% (Alomide), levocabastine (Livostin), ketotifen fumarate ophthalmic solution 0.025% (Zaditor), and cromolyn sodium, may provide relief.

Bacterial conjunctivitis is less common than viral or allergic conjunctivitis. In contrast to viral and allergic conjunctivitis, bacterial conjunctivitis is typically characterized by a purulent discharge. Palpable preauricular lymphadenopathy is uncommon, one of the exceptions being the previously described hyperacute *N. gonorrhoeae* conjunctivitis. Conjunctival chemosis is frequently seen in both forms. The most common causative organisms are *Staphylococcus aureus, Streptococcus pneumoniae*, and in children, *Haemophilus influenzae*. The workup for bacterial conjunctivitis includes obtaining a conjunctival swab for culture and sensitivity testing. One may consider ordering a Gram stain if the symptoms are severe.

Although self-limited in adults, the natural course of the infection will be shortened by the use of topical antibiotic drops. A variety of antibiotics are currently available. The fluoroquinolones ofloxacin (Ocuflox, 1 drop qid) and ciprofloxacin (Ciloxan, 1 drop qid) have a broad spectrum of activity against gram-negative and gram-positive organisms, including *Staphylococcus* and *Pseudomonas* species. Trimethoprim/polymyxin (Polytrim, 1 drop qid), erythromycin (qid), and bacitracin ointments (qid) are also good choices. Of course, antibiotic therapy should be tailored to the culture and sensitivity results.

Patients with conjunctivitis symptoms persisting longer than 4 weeks are classified under the chronic category. Some of the more common etiologies encountered range from chronic immunomodulated mechanisms such as perennial allergic conjunctivitis, contact lens–induced conjunctivitis, vernal conjunctivitis, and atopic conjunctivitis to chronic infectious-based conjunctivitis such as staphylococcal blepharoconjunctivitis.

Perennial allergic conjunctivitis is a type I hypersensitivity reaction usually triggered by an airborne irritant. This condition often has its onset in childhood and patients have bilateral itching, burning, conjunctival hyperemia, and chemosis (conjunctival swelling). In addition, patients will often have an associated rhinitis. Conjunctival scrapings will reveal numerous eosinophils. Treatment is predominantly palliative and involves avoidance of the offending allergen once identified, as well as cool compresses and preservative-free artificial tears (1 drop every 4 to 6 hours). Other measures include topical nonsteroidal anti-inflammatory agents (ketorolac, 1 drop qid), topical mast cell stabilizers (cromolyn sodium, 1 to 2 drops qid), and topical vasoconstrictors.

Vernal conjunctivitis is another hypersensitivity reaction and is characterized by flare-ups often occurring in springtime and showing a greater preponderance in male children. Patients have bilateral itching, burning, mucoid discharge, foreign body sensation, and photophobia. Large papillae may develop on the palpebral conjunctiva, with the upper lid being more commonly affected. Vernal conjunctivitis can extend to involve the cornea (keratoconjunctivitis) and lead to punctate staining (pinpoint areas of epithelial uptake of fluorescein), pannus formation, and ulceration. As with perennial allergic conjunctivitis, treatment involves preservative-free artificial tears, cool compresses, topical mast cell stabilizers, and topical anti-inflammatory drops. More severe cases should be seen by an ophthalmologist because topical steroids or immunomodulating agents may be warranted.

A condition similar to vernal conjunctivitis is atopic keratoconjunctivitis, which can develop in as many as 40% of patients who have atopic dermatitis. Along with the typical redness, burning, and itching, patients will show thickening and scaling of the lids. Other common areas of eczematous involvement (i.e., hands, fingers, scalp) should also be examined. Involvement of the cornea in this disease may potentially be blinding if not treated. Avoidance of the offending irritant and proper lid hygiene are important in treatment. Proper lid hygiene involves warm compresses

*Not FDA approved for this indication.

and gentle scrubbing with a cotton-tipped swab, warm water, and baby shampoo one to two times daily. Topical mast cell stabilizers and systemic antihistamines are also indicated.

Contact lens–induced conjunctivitis is a condition most often seen in patients who wear soft, extended-wear lenses. Symptoms include redness, itching, mucoid discharge, and intolerance to the contact lens. The symptoms can progress to a more severe form of conjunctivitis known as giant papillary conjunctivitis, with large papillae developing on the superior tarsal conjunctiva. Treatment involves discontinuing use of the contact lens, as well as artificial tears, compresses, and mast cell stabilizers. Once the patient's subjective symptoms have resolved, a fitting for new contact lenses is indicated. Changing to daily-wear contact lenses, disposable or gas permeable, as well as better contact lens hygiene, is indicated. These measures often prove effective in resolving symptoms and allow the patient continued use of contact lenses.

Staphylococcal blepharoconjunctivitis is a chronic conjunctivitis, most likely immunologic in etiology. Patients have chronic crusting and scaling lesions of the lids and lashes, which are worse in the morning. Involvement may extend to the cornea and produce punctate staining or even marginal corneal ulcers. Treatment involves warm compresses, lid hygiene, and an antibiotic ointment (bacitracin, erythromycin). Corneal involvement may require topical steroid treatment, and patients should be seen by an ophthalmologist.

VARICELLA AND ZOSTER

method of
PHILIP LaRUSSA, M.D.
Columbia University
New York, New York

Varicella-zoster virus (VZV) is a member of the human herpesvirus family. It causes a primary infection called varicella (chickenpox) that usually occurs in childhood. During this primary infection, the virus establishes latency in the dorsal root ganglia of the spinal cord. The virus may reactivate later in life to cause zoster (shingles).

VARICELLA

Varicella is a highly contagious disease of childhood that is spread by direct contact with lesions or by airborne transmission of large droplets from the oropharynx of infected individuals to susceptible contacts. Secondary attack rates in susceptible siblings after a household exposure to varicella are as high as 90%.

After contact with the mucosa of the upper respiratory tract or the conjunctiva, the virus replicates in the lymphoid tissue of the oropharynx. Four to 6 days later, a small primary viremia allows the virus to spread to reticuloendothelial cells in the liver, the spleen, and other organs, where it is thought to replicate until 10 to 12 days after exposure (1 to 2 days before development of rash). At that time, a larger secondary viremia spreads the virus to the skin. It is during this secondary viremia that the prodromal symptoms of fever, malaise, and irritability are seen and herald the onset of rash. These prodromal symptoms are more pronounced in adolescents and adults than in children.

After an average incubation period of 14 to 16 days after contact (range, 10 to 20 days), lesions develop in three or more successive waves for 3 to 7 days. Development of new lesions for more than 7 days should provoke consideration of an underlying immunodeficiency. Lesions progress through macular, papular, vesicular, and pustular stages. Not all lesions progress to the vesicular stage and beyond. Vesicles dry from the center outward, resulting in an umbilicated appearance. Eventually a scab forms. The scabs will fall off without leaving permanent scars unless a secondary bacterial infection occurs. Vesicles also develop on mucous membranes (oropharynx, conjunctiva, trachea, vagina, and rectum) but rapidly rupture to form shallow ulcers that heal without scab formation. A hallmark of varicella is the presence of lesions in all stages of development at the same time. Rash is often more severe and lesions become confluent in areas of skin where there is local irritation (e.g., diaper rash or under an adhesive bandage).

Lesions appear on the trunk, the face, the scalp, and the extremities, with the greatest concentration on the trunk. Healthy children develop an average of approximately 300 lesions (range, 5 to >500). Secondary cases after a household exposure to a sibling are usually more severe than the primary case. This probably reflects the greater intensity of exposure in this setting compared with more casual contact outside the home. Older adolescents and adults are likely to have more severe cutaneous disease.

Fever usually appears with rash. The height of the fever parallels the severity of rash, and fever may range from undetectable to greater than 105°F (40.6°C). As the appearance of new lesions slows, fever also begins to decline. Other symptoms may include pruritus, headache, malaise, and anorexia.

Clinical manifestations of involvement of other organs are limited, but mild elevations in liver function test results have been reported. Dehydration secondary to poor oral intake and vomiting is occasionally severe enough to warrant hospitalization.

Children are considered to be contagious as long as new lesions continue to appear. Transmission may also occur in the 24- to 48-hour period before the appreciation of rash. This is probably due to spread of virus in large droplets from the oropharynx before development of skin lesions.

Second attacks of varicella are reported but rarely documented. They are usually milder than the primary illness. Although second attacks are more common in immunocompromised children, they have also been seen in healthy children and adults.

Varicella in the immunocompromised host is more likely to be characterized by severe, progressive disease with multiorgan system involvement. Pathologic findings at autopsy after fatal disseminated disease in children with cancer include interstitial pneumonia, hepatitis, splenic involvement, lymphadenitis, enterocolitis, and pancreatitis. An unusual presentation of varicella in immunocompromised children and adults is severe abdominal and back pain that precedes the onset of rash and disseminated disease. The pathogenesis of this pain is not clear.

Initial reports of varicella in highly immunosuppressed HIV-infected children described severe disseminated disease. New lesions appeared for up to 6 weeks after onset of rash and recurred despite antiviral therapy. It is now clear that the relative immunocompetence of HIV-infected children at the time of varicella outbreak correlates with both the severity of varicella and the subsequent risk of developing zoster. In one study, 70% of HIV-infected children with less than 15% $CD4^+$ lymphocytes at the time of varicella infection developed zoster.

Other groups of immunocompromised patients at risk of developing severe varicella include bone marrow, renal, and liver transplant recipients and children receiving high-dose corticosteroid therapy (≥2 mg/kg/d or ≥20 mg/d of prednisone, or the equivalent, in children ≥10 kg, for more than 14 days).

There is conflicting evidence that children with reactive airway disease are at higher risk of developing severe varicella. It is also unclear whether corticosteroids, especially at the doses and duration of treatment used in children with reactive airway disease, increase the risk of severe varicella.

ZOSTER

Zoster (shingles) is caused by the reactivation from the dorsal root ganglia of latent VZV acquired during chickenpox. The distribution of the vesicular rash reflects the dermatome corresponding to the cutaneous distribution of the sensory ganglia from which it reactivated. The incidence and the severity of zoster increase with increasing age. Zoster eventually affects approximately 15% of the population. Younger individuals have rash limited to the involved dermatome with few, if any, sequelae. Older individuals are more likely to develop lesions outside the dermatome and to suffer from postherpetic neuralgia. The risk of developing disseminated zoster and zoster encephalitis is highest in immunocompromised patients and the elderly. Although it is not unusual for older individuals to have a few lesions outside the involved dermatome, the presence of more than 50 extradermatomal lesions indicates that the virus has disseminated. This finding should provoke an investigation of the patient's immunocompetence.

COMPLICATIONS IN HEALTHY CHILDREN AND ADULTS

In the prevaccine era, more than 90% of varicella cases occurred in children 10 years of age or younger. Because most cases of varicella occur in young children, the mean age of children hospitalized with complications of varicella is about 3.8 years, even though complications are more frequent in older children and adults.

Skin and Soft Tissue Complications

The most frequent complications of varicella in healthy children are secondary bacterial infections of skin lesions due to *Staphylococcus* or *Streptococcus*. These can range in severity from impetiginized lesions and bullous impetigo to cellulitis and erysipelas. Scalded skin and toxic shock syndromes secondary to chickenpox have also been described. Septicemia, pneumonia, empyema, osteomyelitis, and suppurative arthritis have also been described. Approximately one third of invasive group A streptococcal infections in children are temporally associated with varicella. The risk of developing invasive disease is highest in the 2-week period after the onset of varicella. The most common presentation is cellulitis, followed by pneumonia, necrotizing fasciitis, and bacteremia without an obvious source. Death may follow severe disease, especially if there is a delay in diagnosis and treatment. Necrotizing fasciitis associated with varicella often requires surgical débridement, fasciotomy, and systemic antibiotic therapy. It is not yet clear whether the risk of invasive group A streptococcal infection in children with chickenpox is increased by the use of ibuprofen (Motrin).

Although complications due to secondary skin infections have been more common in children, pneumonia is more common in adults. Smoking may further increase the risk of pneumonia. Although approximately 15% of adults with varicella have a patchy or diffuse bilateral nodular infiltrate on chest radiography, only one fourth of those with abnormal radiographs have clinical symptoms. The failure to recognize the potential for severe disease has led to delays in instituting therapy and deaths in this group. Mortality in healthy adults with varicella pneumonia has been reported to range from 10% to as high as 40% in pregnant women. Bacterial suprainfection with *Staphylococcus* or *Streptococcus* will increase the risk of a fatal outcome.

Neurologic Complications

Cerebellar ataxia is the most common neurologic complication in children, occurring in 1 of 4000 cases of chickenpox. Symptoms usually develop between 3 and 8 days after the onset of rash, although, rarely, symptoms may develop a few days before the onset of rash. Ataxia may be associated with nystagmus, headache, nausea, vomiting, and nuchal rigidity. The course is self-limited, and recovery is complete.

Encephalitis due to VZV is rare in children. The risk is approximately 1 in 33,000 cases of chickenpox. It may present as depressed levels of consciousness, seizures, headache, and vomiting. Signs of meningeal irritation or cerebral edema and focal signs such as hemiparesis and aphasia may develop. Variation in reported mortality rates from 0% to 35% may reflect inclusion of cases of Reye's syndrome (see later) in this group. Neurologic sequelae, such as paresis, mental retardation, and development of a seizure disorder, may be seen in up to 15% of the survivors.

Other neurologic complications include transverse myelitis, aseptic meningitis, Guillain-Barré syndrome, optic neuritis, and vasculitis and stroke. Febrile seizures, without other neurologic manifestations, have also been reported.

Before the causal association between salicylate use in childhood viral illnesses and Reye's syndrome was appreciated, there were approximately 350 cases of Reye's syndrome reported annually, 20% to 30% of which were associated with varicella. Reye's syndrome is characterized by acute encephalopathy and fatty degeneration of the liver. Mortality was as high as 50%. Reye's syndrome is rare today; in a recent review of complications of varicella, no cases were reported. Unfortunately, some children still receive aspirin during varicella infection, resulting in the rare, but preventable, case of Reye's syndrome.

Neurologic complications in adults are more likely to present as encephalitis, with altered sensorium, seizures, and focal neurologic signs and mortality as high as 35%.

Other Complications

Other rare complications of varicella include nephritis, uveitis, arthritis, carditis, conjunctivitis, orchitis, and the syndrome of inappropriate secretion of antidiuretic hormone. Hemorrhagic varicella with multiorgan system failure is rare in healthy children, but when it does occur, the outcome is usually fatal.

VARICELLA IN PREGNANCY

Two to 3 percent of pregnant women who develop varicella during the first and early second trimester will be delivered of infants who have signs and symptoms of the congenital varicella syndrome. These may include atrophy and scarring of a limb in a zoster-like distribution, microcephaly, microphthalmia, hepatosplenomegaly, and early death. If mothers develop varicella within the 5-day period before birth or up to 2 days afterward, the infant may develop severe or even fatal varicella. This outcome can be prevented by administration of varicella-zoster immune globulin (VZIG) one vial intramuscularly on the first day of life. Infants whose mothers had varicella during pregnancy or who themselves had varicella during the first few months of life are at increased risk of developing zoster during the first year of life. The course is generally uneventful.

MORTALITY

In the prevaccine era, varicella was responsible for 50 to 100 deaths per year in children 15 years of age and younger. Because approximately 4 million cases occurred yearly, the case-fatality rate was low. Although fewer than 5% of varicella cases occur in adults, they are responsible for more than half the deaths due to varicella each year.

TREATMENT

Treatment of chickenpox in healthy children with acyclovir (Zovirax), 20 mg/kg (maximum 800 mg) orally four times a day for 5 days, results in modest improvements in resolution of clinical symptoms. Treatment of adolescents (800 mg orally four times a day for 5 days) and adults (800 mg orally five times a day for 5 days) will significantly improve resolution of symptoms. Therapy should be started within 24 hours of onset of rash. Immunocompromised patients should be started on therapy as soon as possible. The decision to use oral or intravenous therapy will depend on time from onset of rash, severity of symptoms, and degree of immunosuppression. The recommended dose of intravenous acyclovir is 500 mg/m^2 every 8 hours for 5 to 7 days.

Treatment of zoster within 72 hours of onset with acyclovir (800 mg orally five times per day) has resulted in more rapid resolution of symptoms, and in adults 55 years of age and older there has been a reduced risk of postherpetic neuralgia. Immunocompromised patients may be treated with intravenous acyclovir, 10 mg/kg every 8 hours. The duration of therapy will depend on the response to treatment.

Treatment of cerebellar ataxia and encephalitis with antiviral agents is controversial but is recommended by many experts.

Other drugs, such as famciclovir (Famvir) and valacyclovir (Valtrex), have activity against VZV and may be useful in specific situations. Foscarnet (Foscavir) has been useful in the treatment of acyclovir-resistant strains of VZV. Treatment of the immunocompromised patient should be coordinated with an infectious disease specialist.

PREVENTION

Individuals who have had a significant exposure to varicella and who are at high risk of developing severe varicella (i.e., VZV-susceptible immunocompromised patients and susceptible pregnant women; newborns whose mothers experienced onset of varicella within 5 days before and up to 2 days after delivery; premature infants <28 weeks' gestation; premature infants ≥28 weeks' gestation whose mothers are VZV susceptible) should receive VZIG as soon as possible after exposure (1 vial per 10 kg of weight; maximum of 5 vials). It is effective in reducing the likelihood of severe varicella when given up to 72 hours after an exposure (up to 96 hours in immunocompromised patients).

A live attenuated varicella vaccine was approved for use in the United States in 1995. Recommendations for its use include universal immunization of all healthy children at 12 to 18 months of age and of healthy older children and adults who have not yet had varicella. One dose is recommended for children 12 months through 12 years of age and two doses for those 13 years of age or older. The vaccine is contraindicated in children younger than 12 months of age, immunocompromised patients, and pregnant women.

Approximately 5% of vaccinees will develop a vaccine-associated rash, usually 14 to 28 days after immunization, consisting of 6 to 10 papular-vesicular lesions lasting 2 to 3 days. The risk of transmission of vaccine virus from this type of rash to a susceptible contact seems to be extremely small. Unusual vaccine-related complications include severe rash and disseminated visceral disease in inadvertently vaccinated severely immunocompromised patients and rare cases of zoster due to the vaccine virus.

Approximately 85% of vaccinees exposed to varicella in a household setting will be totally protected. The remainder will develop very mild "breakthrough varicella," usually with 30 lesions or less. Data from the Centers for Disease Control and Prevention are showing that the introduction of the vaccine is starting to reduce both the number of cases of varicella and associated hospitalizations. The duration of protection is still under study, but data from Japan and the United States indicate that immunity should be long-lasting.

Varicella vaccine has also proved to be approximately 75% effective when given to healthy individuals within 72 hours after an exposure to varicella. Vaccine has also been safely administered to selected groups of immunocompromised patients (asymptomatic HIV-infected children with CD4$^+$ counts greater than 25%; leukemic children in remission for 9 months or more). Immunization of these children should be considered only in consultation with an infectious disease specialist.

FUTURE CONSIDERATIONS

A combined measles-mumps-rubella/varicella (MMRV) vaccine is likely to become available within the next few years. This vaccine will help reduce the number of injections in an already crowded immunization schedule and will likely improve the immune response to varicella because children will probably receive two doses of MMRV. Studies are in progress to determine whether a high-potency "zoster vaccine" can reduce the incidence or the severity of zoster in individuals who had varicella as children and are now in age groups at higher risk of developing zoster (i.e., ≥60 years of age). It is hoped that the VZV-specific booster effect of vaccination will reduce the likelihood of reactivation.

CHOLERA

method of

ABUL K. SIDDIQUE, M.B.B.S., M.P.H.
International Centre for Diarrhoeal Disease Research, Bangladesh
Mohakhali, Dhaka, Bangladesh

Cholera is recognized as the most severe of all diarrheal diseases. The disease has been known since earliest recorded history in the region of the Ganges river delta that is now primarily Bangladesh and a small part of India. The modern history of cholera began in 1817 when a violent epidemic broke out in the lower Ganges river delta and spread out of its Asiatic "home" to involve the entire world in the form of seven pandemics. More than 1½ centuries have elapsed since the first pandemic of cholera invaded the world. Even today, the distribution of cholera has remained nearly worldwide.

EPIDEMIOLOGY

Understanding the epidemiology of cholera has always been a challenge. The bacterium responsible for the human disease was first recognized in 1884 and was named *Vibrio cholerae*, which was further grouped as O1 on the basis of its serologic characteristics. *V. cholerae* O1 was further differentiated into classic and El Tor biotypes because of certain biologic identification tests. Each biotype can be further classified into the serotypes Ogawa and Inaba.

The causative organism of cholera was not identified until the fifth pandemic. Therefore, the serotypes and the biotypes causing the first four pandemics are not known for certain. Evidence, however, suggests that the fifth and the sixth pandemics were caused by classic biotypes of *V. cholerae* O1. For nearly 80 years, the classic biotype of *V. cholerae* O1 dominated the spectrum of cholera on a global scale. However, in 1906, a new type of *V. cholerae* was detected at the El Tor Quarantine Station in the Sinai desert. It was named the El Tor biotype. The organism caused small epidemic outbreaks in Indonesia for nearly 30 years. In 1961, the El Tor cholera began to move out of Indonesia in the form of the seventh pandemic and covered nearly the entire world; it reached Latin America in 1991.

V. cholerae biotype El Tor shares most of the known virulence properties of classic *V. cholerae*. Thus, people living in an area endemic for classic cholera are at least partially immune to El Tor cholera. Despite this, El Tor caused large epidemics in these partially immune populations and completely displaced all classic strains during the current (seventh) pandemic.

At a time when considerable ground was thought to have been gained in understanding the epidemiology of *V. cholerae* O1, an epidemic of cholera broke out on the Indian subcontinent in 1992. It was caused by an unknown strain of *V. cholerae* non-O1, designated as O139 Bengal. *V. cholerae* O139 has cell wall antigens that are different from the O1 serogroup. People living in areas endemic for O1 did not have significant immunity against infection with the O139 vibrios. Therefore, the entire world is essentially nonimmune to this new vibrio. The epidemiologic characteristics and recent changes in molecular characteristics of *V. cholerae* O139 suggest that this strain has pandemic potential. Despite many years of study, it is still not known how *V. cholerae* spreads around the world in pandemic form, what determines its seasonality, and what determines evolution of the epidemic cholera strains.

PATHOPHYSIOLOGY

In human beings, cholera infection occurs after ingestion of food or water contaminated with the organism *V. cholerae*. The infective dose is high (10^6). The organisms are highly acid labile and most are killed in the acidic environment in the stomach.

The small intestine is the primary site of infection. *V. cholerae* colonizes the intestinal epithelium but does not invade epithelial cells or cause any structural alteration to the epithelium.

After successful adhesion and colonization, the organism produces a potent enterotoxin. The massive diarrhea caused by *V. cholerae* is produced by this enterotoxin. The toxin increases chloride and bicarbonate secretion into the intestinal lumen by crypt cells and decreases villous absorption of sodium chloride. The increased chloride and bicarbonate are associated with an increased and passive transfer of water across the mucosal surface into the gut lumen, resulting in accumulation of a large amount of water and electrolytes (Table 1). The amount of fluid reaching the colon from the small intestine exceeds the reabsorptive capacity of the colon. The result is the profuse watery diarrhea that characterizes cholera.

CLINICAL FEATURES

The incubation period ranges from several hours to 5 days. The clinical manifestations of infection with *V. cholerae* vary from asymptomatic infection to severe diarrhea. Many infected patients have mild diarrhea that cannot be distinguished from other milder forms of diarrhea.

A small proportion of cholera-infected people develop severe manifestations of the disease (Table 2). Patients may have rapid onset of illness; their duration of diarrhea before hospitalization could be up to 12 hours. Voluminous quantities of largely painless and effortless electrolyte-rich white and opalescent ("rice water") stools are passed. In severe cholera, the rate of diarrhea may quickly reach 500 to 1000 mL/h, leading to tachycardia, hypotension, and hypovolemic shock. There may be absence of peripheral pulses and undetectable blood pressure. Skin turgor is poor, giving the skin a doughy consistency. The eyes are sunken, and the hands and feet become wrinkled, as after long immersion ("washer woman's hands"). Patients become restless and extremely thirsty. Oliguria may be present until dehydration and electrolyte deficiencies are corrected. Mental status remains unchanged in most adult patients; therefore, they remain well oriented but apathetic, even in the face of severe hypovolemic shock.

Vomiting is almost universal at the onset of illness. Early symptoms include anorexia, abdominal discomfort, and simple diarrhea. Stools of cholera patients may initially contain fecal matter or bile, although patients with high

TABLE 1. **Electrolyte and Glucose Composition of Cholera Stool and of Fluids Used for Hydration of Patients With Cholera**

Fluid	Na^+ (mmol/L)	Cl^- (mmol/L)	K^+ (mmol/L)	HCO_3 (mmol/L)	Glucose or Dextrose (mmol/L)	Osmolality (mOsm/L)
Cholera Stool						
Adult	130	100	20	44	0	300
Children	100	90	33	30	0	300
Oral Rehydration						
Glucose ORS	90	80	20	30	111	331
Rice ORS	90	80	20	10*	50 g rice powder	288
Intravenous Fluids						
Lactated Ringer's	130	109	4	28	0	271
Dhaka solution	133	98	13	48	0	292
Normal Saline	154	154	0	0	0	308

*Citrate.
Abbreviation: ORS = oral rehydration solution.

purging rates quickly develop rice water stool, which can have a fishy odor. Some patients complain of intestinal cramping, which is presumably due to bowel distention. Patients with mild forms of the disease usually only develop diarrhea and vomiting. Patients with more severe forms of the disease may develop some degree of dehydration. The features of dehydration dominate the appearance of patients with cholera (see Table 2). Painful muscle cramps may occur, probably resulting from hypokalemia.

LABORATORY DIAGNOSIS

Using vibrio culture, biochemical methods, and serologic methods, laboratory diagnosis of cholera infection is confirmed. Stool samples from stool specimens or rectal swabs, preferably collected before the patient starts antibiotic therapy, are inoculated onto thiosulfate citrate bile salts sucrose agar or tellurite, taurocholate, and gelatin agar media and incubated overnight at 37°C for culture. Identification of *V. cholerae* is done by biochemical tests. For serologic diagnosis, specific antisera of *V. cholerae* O1 and O139 are commonly used.

Treatment

Because there were no adequate treatments of any kind until the early 1900s, mortality rates of 50% to 70% were recorded during the early cholera pandemics. Severe dehydration is responsible for deaths due to cholera infection, and prevention of such deaths can only be achieved by rehydration using appropriate fluid therapy. Advances made in the treatment of cholera in the last 3 decades have greatly improved the chances of averting death from the disease. The main objective of cholera treatment, therefore, is to replace the lost water and electrolytes and to maintain their normal level until diarrhea stops. This can be achieved through oral rehydration therapy or intravenous rehydration therapy. The methods of rehydration are determined through clinical assessment of the degree of dehydration (see Table 2).

Oral rehydration therapy is preferred for patients who are mildly dehydrated or who are moderately dehydrated but do not have excessive purging and

TABLE 2. **Method of Clinical Assessment of Dehydration of Cholera Patients**

Objective Measure	Physical Attribute	Dehydration: *None*	Dehydration: *Some*	Dehydration: *Severe*
Look at	General condition	Well, alert	**Restless, irritable**	**Lethargic or unconscious, floppy**
	Eyes*	Normal	Sunken	Very sunken and dry
	Tears	Present	Absent	Absent
	Mouth and tongue†	Moist	Dry	Very dry
	Thirst	Drinks normally, not thirsty	**Thirsty, drinks eagerly**	**Drinks poorly or not able to drink**
Feel	Skin pinch‡	Skin goes back to normal quickly	**Skin goes back to normal slowly**	**Skin goes back to normal very slowly**
Decide		The patient has no sign of dehydration.	If the patient has two or more signs, including at least one sign shown in boldface, there is some dehydration.	If the patient has two or more signs, including at least one sign shown in boldface, there is severe dehydration.

*In some infants and children, the eyes normally appear somewhat sunken. It is helpful to ask the mother if the child's eyes are normal or more sunken than usual.
†Dryness of the mouth and tongue can also be palpated with a finger. The mouth may always be dry in a child who habitually breathes through the mouth. The mouth may be wet in a patient with dehydration owing to recent vomiting or drinking.
‡Skin pinch is less useful in infants or children with *Marasmus* (severe wasting) or *kwashiorkor* (severe undernutrition with edema) or in obese children.

vomiting. Correction of severe dehydration by intravenous therapy should be followed by oral rehydration therapy for maintenance of hydration.

Glucose-based oral rehydration salt packets, which can replace the electrolytes lost by cholera patients (see Table 1), have been made available by the World Health Organization and by commercial firms in countries where watery diarrhea is endemic. The solution made out of the oral rehydration salt packets should be administered in a volume sufficient to match ongoing stool losses and insensible losses. For mild dehydration, oral rehydration solution (ORS) is given in a volume of 50 mL/kg within 4 hours. In patients with moderate dehydration, twice this volume (100 mL/kg) should be given in the same amount of time. In children younger than 2 years of age, 50 to 100 mL of oral fluid should be given after each loose stool as fluid maintenance therapy. The volume should be 100 to 200 mL for older children. Adults should drink as much as they want over the suggested amount.

The effectiveness and safety of the currently formulated glucose ORS are universally recognized. However, recently, cereal-based formulations, such as rice-based ORS, have been gaining ground as an effective method of oral rehydration in the treatment of cholera. Rice-based hypo-osmolar ORS with reduced sodium concentration has been shown to be markedly effective in reducing total stool output, shortening duration of diarrhea, and promoting consumption of ORS, particularly in children with cholera.

Cholera, however, continues to be a medical emergency. A patient with cholera-produced severe dehydration may die within a few hours unless treatment is provided quickly. All severely dehydrated patients should be rehydrated with appropriate intravenous fluids (see Table 1). At the time of initial treatment, when rapid fluid replacement is necessary to correct hypovolemia and acidosis, intravenous fluids with the correct composition of electrolytes given in the required volume can efficiently avert death. For adults, intravenous rehydration should be accomplished as rapidly as possible, initially at a rate of 30 mL/kg infused within a half hour, then 70 mL/kg over the next 2.5 hour. Children should receive intravenous rehydration at a rate of 30 mL/kg in the first hour, then 70 mL/kg in the next 5 hours. Once patients are fully hydrated, intravenous therapy may be discontinued and oral rehydration should be initiated and continued until diarrhea stops. For patients with high purging rates (>10 mL/kg/h) and for those with persistent vomiting, intravenous fluid therapy may need to be continued even during the maintenance phase.

Antibiotics are often prescribed to treat cholera. The aim of antibiotic therapy is to shorten the fecal excretion of vibrios, reduce the transmissibility of the disease, and diminish the duration of diarrhea. The choice of antibiotic should be determined by susceptibility of the drug to *V. cholerae* infection and based on other factors such as very young age and pregnancy. In case of adults, a single 300-mg dose of doxycycline is as effective as a multiple-dose course of tetracycline* (500 mg every 6 hours for 3 days). Pregnant women with cholera should be treated with erythromycin* (500 mg every 6 hours for 3 days). Children are treated with erythromycin, 50 mg/kg, every 6 hours for 3 days.

THE FUTURE OF CHOLERA

The advances made in microbiology, improvement of treatment methods, and implementation of appropriate cholera-prevention measures have not led to the effective control of cholera worldwide. Experience has shown that introduction of cholera into a country cannot be prevented. Mankind and the environment have always been and will always be the ultimate test for survival of the disease. High population density is one of the factors thought to be associated with both the origin of the pandemics and existence of high levels of endemic cholera in the Ganges delta. The disease survives where the human environment is degraded by poverty and overcrowding, spreads as people travel, and thrives when human conflicts and disasters displace populations. The global resurgence and persistence of cholera underscore the importance of effective cholera control.

Despite efforts to create vaccines to control cholera, up to the present time, no highly effective vaccine exists. The current cholera vaccine gives only limited protection and does not prevent asymptomatic infections. Because even natural infection does not provide complete and long-lasting immunity against reinfection with the El Tor strain, an effective vaccine will have to be more immunogenic than natural infection. The appearance of the new strain O139 in the Indian subcontinent, where high levels of natural immunity to cholera exist, suggests that evolutionary changes in the bacteria may permit the organism to evade natural and vaccine-induced immunities. This further increases the challenges for developing a successful vaccine against the disease. Eradication of cholera will be difficult to achieve because it has environmental reservoirs. A better understanding of the ecologic determinants for persistence of *V. cholera* in the environment will improve prevention strategies.

*Not FDA approved for this indication.

FOOD-BORNE ILLNESS

method of
J. GLENN MORRIS, Jr., M.D., M.P.H.T.M.
*University of Maryland School of Medicine
Baltimore, Maryland*

Food-borne disease is a continuing public health problem in the United States. Although numbers from different sources vary widely, it has been estimated that food-borne pathogens cause up to 76 million illnesses each year, with over 300,000 hospitalizations and 5000 deaths. There are concerns that the magnitude of the problem is growing because of the increasing globalization of the U.S. food supply (with the corresponding dependence on fresh fruits and vegetables grown in countries where the level of sanitation may not match that of the United States), the concentration of production into a smaller number of large companies (increasing the opportunity for cross-contamination), the increasing reliance on "fast foods" and restaurants, and the decreasing emphasis on food safety education and adherence to traditional food safety practices in home kitchens.

Table 1 provides a list of the most common etiologies of food-borne illness. A more exhaustive listing is available in the Centers for Disease Control and Prevention (CDC) publication "Diagnosis and Management of Foodborne Illness: A Primer for Physicians," which can be downloaded at *www.cdc.gov/mmwr/preview/mmwrhtml/rr5002al.htm.* As noted in Table 1, etiologies include viral, bacterial, and parasitic agents and "natural toxins." Specific data on mushroom-associated syndromes are provided in Table 2.

TABLE 1. **Food-Borne Illnesses**

Etiologic Agent	Estimated U.S. Food-Borne Cases/Year*	Incubation	Signs and Symptoms	Associated Foods	Treatment
Viral Agents					
Calicivirus (Norwalk-like agents)	~9,200,000	24–48 h	Nausea, vomiting, watery diarrhea; may be fever	Fecally contaminated foods, ready-to-eat foods touched by infected food workers, shellfish	Fluids, antimotility agents
Rotavirus, astrovirus	~39,000 each	1–3 d	Vomiting, watery diarrhea, low-grade fever	Same	Same
Hepatitis A	~4200	30 d (range, 15–50 d)	Dark urine, jaundice, flulike symptoms, diarrhea	Same	Same
Bacterial Agents					
Campylobacter jejuni	~2,000,000	2–5 d	Diarrhea, cramps, fever, vomiting; may be bloody diarrhea Sequela: Guillain-Barré syndrome	Raw and undercooked poultry, unpasteurized milk, contaminated water	Fluids; antibiotics (ciprofloxacin [Cipro], 500 mg PO bid × 3 d, or azithromycin [Zithromax], 500 mg PO qd) may be of benefit early in course
Salmonella (nontyphoidal)	~1,300,000	1–3 d	Diarrhea, fever, abdominal cramps, vomiting; occasional bloody diarrhea Sequela: septicemia	Raw or undercooked poultry, contaminated eggs *(Salmonella enteritidis),* unpasteurized milk or juice, contaminated raw fruits or vegetables	Fluids; antibiotics *not* indicated unless extraintestinal spread (or immunocompromised host at risk for extraintestinal spread); for invasive/extraintestinal disease, ciprofloxacin, 500 mg PO bid × 5–7 d
Clostridium perfringens	~250,000	8–16 h	Watery diarrhea, nausea, abdominal cramps; fever rare	Meats, poultry, gravy; often precooked	Fluids, supportive care
Staphylococcal food poisoning	~190,000	1–6 h	Sudden onset of severe nausea and vomiting; may be diarrhea	Unrefrigerated or improperly refrigerated meat, potato and egg salad, cream pastries	Fluids, supportive care
Escherichia coli O157:H7 and STEC	~94,000	1–8 d	Diarrhea, often bloody; abdominal pain and vomiting; little or no fever Sequela: hemolytic-uremic syndrome	Undercooked beef (esp. hamburger), unpasteurized milk and juice, raw fruits and vegetables (sprouts)	Fluids, supportive care; *antibiotics contraindicated*
Shigella	~90,000	24–48 h	Abdominal cramps, fever, diarrhea; stool may contain blood and mucus	Fecally contaminated food or water, ready-to-eat foods touched by infected food workers	Fluids, supportive care. Treat with ciprofloxacin, 500 mg PO bid × 3 d, or TMP/SMZ (Bactrim), DS PO bid × 3 d
Yersinia enterocolitica	~87,000	24–48 h	Diarrhea and vomiting, fever, abdominal pain; may cause pseudoappendicitis syndrome	Undercooked pork, unpasteurized milk	Fluids, supportive care; antibiotics if suggestion of invasive disease (ciprofloxacin, 500 mg PO bid × 3 d, TMP/SMZ, DS PO bid × 3 d, or ceftriaxone [Rocephin], 2.0 g IV qd)
Food-borne streptococcus	~51,000	24–48 h	Pharyngitis	Contamination of foods by infected food workers	Pen V PO × 10 d, or azithromycin, 500 mg PO qd × 5 d
Bacillus cereus	~27,000	Emetic toxin: 1–6 h Diarrheal toxin: 10–16 h	Sudden onset of nausea and vomiting; diarrhea may be present Abdominal cramps, watery diarrhea, nausea	Improperly refrigerated/rewarmed cooked and fried rice Meats, stews, gravies; often precooked	Fluids, supportive care

TABLE 1. **Food-Borne Illnesses** *Continued*

Etiologic Agent	Estimated U.S. Food-Borne Cases/Year*	Incubation	Signs and Symptoms	Associated Foods	Treatment
E. coli, enterotoxigenic	~24,000	1–3 d	Watery diarrhea, abdominal cramps, some vomiting	Water or food contaminated with human feces	Fluids; antibiotics in severe cases (ciprofloxacin, 500 mg PO bid × 3 d; TMP/SMZ)
Vibrio cholerae (nonepidemic/ non-O1/O139), *Vibrio parahaemolyticus*	~5200	6–72 h	Watery diarrhea; occasionally bloody diarrhea	Raw or undercooked shellfish, seafood	Fluids; doxycycline, 100 mg PO bid × 3 d in severe cases
Vibrio vulnificus		1–4 d	Sepsis in patients with liver disease or those who are immuno-compromised; possible diarrhea	Same	Minocycline (Minocin), 100 mg PO q12h, and cefotaxime (Claforan), 2.0 g IV q8h
Listeria	~2500	GI: 9–48 h; invasive disease: 2–6 wk	Fever, muscle aches, and nausea or diarrhea. Pregnant women may have mild flulike illness, with infection leading to premature delivery or still birth. Elderly or immunocompromised patients may have bacteremia or meningitis	Fresh soft cheese, unpasteurized milk, ready-to-eat deli meats, hot dogs	Fluids for gastroenteritis; for invasive disease, ampicillin, 2 g IV q4–6h, or TMP/SMZ
Botulism	~60	12–72 h	Blurred vision, dysphagia, descending muscle weakness; may be vomiting, diarrhea	Home-canned foods with low acid content; foods where anaerobic growth possible	Supportive care. Botulinum antitoxin helpful if given early in course of illness. Call (404) 639-2206 or (404) 639-3753 workdays or (404) 639-2888 nights and weekends
Parasitic Agents					
Giardia lamblia	~200,000	1–4 wk	Acute or chronic diarrhea, flatulence, bloating	Untreated surface water, contamination of foods by water or infected food worker	Metronidazole (Flagyl), 250 mg PO tid × 5 d
Toxoplasma gondii	~110,000	6–10 d	Generally asymptomatic; cervical lymphadenopathy and/ or flulike illness may develop in 20% Immunocompromised patients: CNS disease Pregnant women: fetal CNS infection	Undercooked meats, including pork, lamb, venison; contact with cat fecal material	Asymptomatic infections: no treatment Pregnant women (first 18 weeks' gestation): spiramycin,† 3 g qd, obtained from FDA, (301) 827-2335 Immunocompromised hosts: pyrimethamine (Daraprim) plus sulfadiazine, folinic acid
Cryptosporidium parvum	~30,000	2–28 d	Cramping, abdominal pain, watery diarrhea; fever and vomiting may be present and may be relapsing	Contaminated water, vegetables, fruits, unpasteurized milk	Supportive care
Cyclospora cayetanensis	~15,000	1–11 d	Fatigue, protracted diarrhea; often relapsing	Imported berries, contaminated water, lettuce	TMP/SMZ, DS PO bid × 7 d
Natural Toxins					
Ciguatera fish poisoning		GI: 2–12 h	Abdominal pain, nausea, vomiting, diarrhea; in severe cases, may be hypotension and bradycardia	Large predacious tropical reef fish: barracuda, grouper, red snapper, amberjack	Supportive care, atropine and blood pressure support; IV mannitol (20% solution, 1 g/kg piggybacked over 30 min) reported to be lifesaving in severe cases
		Neurologic: 12 h–5 d	Paresthesias, pain and weakness in legs, temperature reversal		In chronic cases, amitriptyline‡ (Elavil) may be beneficial
Scombroid (histamine toxicity)		1 min–3 h	Flushing, rash; burning sensation of skin, mouth	Improperly refrigerated "scombroid" fish, including tuna, mahi-mahi	Supportive care, antihistamine
Paralytic shellfish poisoning		30 min–3 h	Paresthesias, ataxia, dysphagia, mental status changes, hypotension; respiratory paralysis in severe cases	Scallops, mussels, clams, cockles harvested from beds exposed to blooms of the dinoflagellate *Alexandrium;* occurs primarily in Alaska, Pacific Northwest, California, and Maine	Supportive care

*Estimates of disease incidence (rounded to two significant figures) from Mead PS, Slutsker L, Dietz V, et al: Food-related illness and death in the United States. Emerg Infect Dis 5:607–625, 1999.

†Investigational drug in the United States.

‡Not FDA approved for this indication.

Abbreviations: CNS = central nervous system; DS = double-strength tablet; FDA = Food and Drug Administration; STEC = Shiga toxin–producing *E. coli*; TMP/SMZ = trimethoprim/sulfamethoxazole.

Adapted from Diagnosis and management of foodborne illnesses: A primer for physicians. MMWR Morb Mortal Wkly Rep 50 (RR02):1–69, 2001.

TABLE 2. **Mushroom Syndromes**

Syndrome (Toxin)	Incubation	Symptoms	Mushrooms
Anticholinergic syndrome (muscarine)	30 min–2 h	Sweating, salivation, lacrimation, bradycardia, hypotension	*Inocybe* species
Delirium (ibotenic acid, muscimol isoxazole)	20–90 min	Dizziness, ataxia, incoordination, hyperactivity	*Clitocybe* species *Amanita* species
Hallucination (psilocin, psilocybin)	30–60 min	Mood elevation, hallucination	*Psilocybe* species *Panaeolus* species
Disulfiram-like (coprine)	30 min after alcohol	Headache, nausea, vomiting	*Coprinus* species
Hepatic failure (gyromitrin)	2–12 h	Nausea, vomiting, hemolysis, hepatic failure, seizures	*Gyromitra* species
Hepatorenal (amatoxins and phallotoxins)	6–24 h	Abdominal pain, vomiting, diarrhea, renal and hepatic failure	*Amanita phalloides*
Nephritis (orellanine)	3–5 d	Thirst, nausea, headache, abdominal pain, renal failure	*Corinarius* species

It is now thought that viruses are the most common cause of food-borne disease (accounting for approximately 80% of cases), with calicivirus (including Norwalk and Norwalk-like agents) being the most common viral etiologic agent. Bacterial pathogens account for approximately 13% of food-borne cases, and parasitic agents, about 7%. *Campylobacter* is the most common bacterial cause of food-borne illness; it has been estimated that 2.0 million food-borne *Campylobacter* infections occur each year in the United States.

The risk of hospitalization or death associated with food-borne illness varies by pathogen. Reflecting the high frequency with which it occurs, food-borne calicivirus may cause up to 20,000 hospitalizations per year—but relatively few deaths. Among bacterial food-borne pathogens, *Salmonella* is the most common cause of hospitalization (estimated 15,000/y) and deaths (estimated 550/y). Food-borne *Campylobacter* may be responsible for some 10,000 hospitalizations per year (including an estimated 1500 hospitalizations for Guillain-Barré syndrome, which has been linked with previous *Campylobacter* infections). However, the estimated fatality rate associated with *Campylobacter* infection is low (probably fewer than 100 deaths per year). In contrast, *Listeria* causes some 500 deaths per year in this country. The *Listeria* data are based largely on culture data from sites other than stool because laboratories do not routinely culture stool samples for the presence of the organism; however, recent data suggest that *Listeria* may also be a significant cause of food-borne gastroenteritis. It has been estimated that *Toxoplasma* is responsible for 375 food-borne deaths per year based on the estimate that 50% of all *Toxoplasma* infections are food-borne.

Rates of reported cases for most food-borne pathogens are highest in children younger than 1 year, a finding that may reflect increased susceptibility to infection in infants. It may also reflect the increased likelihood that infants will be taken to a physician when they are having diarrhea and, when taken to a physician, that a stool culture or other stool examination will be performed. For both *Campylobacter* and *Salmonella*, cases are most commonly reported in infants; however, the rate of infection with *Salmonella* in infants is higher than that of *Campylobacter*, and *Campylobacter* infection rates in persons aged 20 years and older are two to three times those for *Salmonella* (i.e., among bacterial food-borne pathogens, an infant is more likely to have *Salmonella*, whereas an adult is two to three times more likely to be infected with *Campylobacter*). Hospitalizations and deaths tend to be concentrated in the very young and very old because of increased susceptibility to both dehydrating diarrheal illness and invasive disease. For pregnant women, *Listeria* and *Toxoplasma* pose particular risks related to their direct risk to the fetus.

Occurrence of a food-borne illness is suggested when multiple people with a common food history become ill simultaneously. However, failure to identify multiple cases does not exclude the diagnosis of food-borne disease: symptomatic food-borne illness may occur in only one person in a group—or only one person may eat the contaminated food. With the advent and increasing use of molecular typing techniques, it is being increasingly recognized that many isolated cases of illness are indeed part of larger outbreaks, with pathogens moving in "clonal waves" through populations. Because of increasing globalization of the food supply and reliance on "big agriculture" rather than smaller farmers and producers, illness with a common source may occur among persons in multiple states (and countries).

Points in the history that may be important in suggesting the etiologic agent causing a food-borne illness include symptoms (vomiting, diarrhea, bloody diarrhea, neurologic manifestations, sepsis syndromes), the incubation period, the implicated food (and its preparation), and recent travel. Care should be taken to exclude syndromes such as inflammatory bowel disease. Diarrheal illness in persons with a history of travel to less developed parts of the world (i.e., "traveler's diarrhea") is often caused by enterotoxigenic strains of *Escherichia coli*. Persons with a history of recent shellfish ingestion should enkindle a high degree of suspicion of *Vibrio* infection. *Salmonella* and *Campylobacter* infections are often linked with undercooked chicken (or cross-contamination in a kitchen where raw chicken has been handled); *Yersinia* is more common in pigs. *Listeria* cases have been linked with fresh soft cheeses, ready-to-eat deli meats, and hot dogs (all of which should be avoided by pregnant women). Local variations in the incidence of specific pathogens may also be noted. For example, incidence rates for *Campylobacter* are substantively higher in California than in Maryland, whereas the incidence of *Salmonella* in Maryland is higher than that of *Campylobacter*. Similarly, it has been suggested that the incidence of infection with *E. coli* O157:H7 is higher in the midwest than on the east coast of the United States.

Identification of an etiologic agent almost always requires isolation of the organism from the patient or food or its identification in appropriate clinical or food samples. Suspected outbreaks of food-borne illness should be reported immediately to the local health department. The health department may have access to resources not available to individual practitioners to allow the etiologic agent to be identified, and prompt involvement of the health department may permit interventions to be undertaken to prevent other persons from becoming ill. Persons with known food-borne illness should not be involved in food preparation (and, for infants and young children, should not return to daycare settings) until symptoms have resolved and/or cultures (for bacterial pathogens) have become negative; specific criteria for return to work or school/daycare may vary from locale to locale and should be obtained from the local health department.

APPROACHES TO THERAPY

Illnesses associated with foodborne pathogens can in general be divided into those that cause (1) a short-incubation vomiting syndrome, (2) gastroenteritis with diarrhea as a primary manifestation, (3) neurologic symptoms, and (4) systemic manifestations.

Short-Incubation Vomiting Syndrome

Short-incubation vomiting syndromes are generally caused by ingestion of a preformed emetic toxin. Most cases are due to staphylococci or (less commonly) *Bacillus cereus*. Management is supportive and includes fluids as needed. Symptoms generally resolve within 12 to 24 hours with no sequelae.

Gastroenteritis With Diarrhea as a Primary Manifestation

The single most important element in management of gastroenteritis is the prevention of dehydration, regardless of the etiologic agent. World Health Organization guidelines call for the use of oral rehydration solution containing 3.5 g NaCl, 1.5 KCl, 2.5 g $NaHCO_3$ and 20 g glucose in 1 L of boiled water. In the United States, Pedialyte (which has a slightly lower sodium concentration) is a reasonable alternative. The key factor, from a physiologic standpoint, is the use of a solution containing both sugar and salt. Parenteral rehydration may be necessary for persons with vomiting or severe dehydration, although oral rehydration is still possible.

Most food-borne cases are caused by viruses, with symptoms that are mild and self-limited. In addition to maintaining adequate hydration, use of an over-the-counter antidiarrheal agent such as loperamide (Imodium) may be helpful (the over-the-counter dosage is two 2-mg capsules, followed by one 2-mg capsule after each subsequent loose bowel movement, not to exceed four 2-mg capsules per day). Loperamide is contraindicated in patients with blood or mucus in their stool or if antibiotic-associated colitis is a possibility. Bismuth subsalicylate (Pepto-Bismol),* 2 tablespoons or 2 tablets every 30 to 60 minutes, not to exceed eight doses, may also be useful in controlling the symptoms of gastroenteritis. For patients with severe vomiting, the use of promethazine (Phenergan) or prochlorperazine (Compazine) administered by rectal suppository may be beneficial. Antibiotics should not be used, except as outlined in the following text.

Cases in which diarrhea is combined with blood and/or mucus are more likely to be caused by bacterial agents. As noted earlier, *Campylobacter* is the most common bacterial cause of food-borne disease, particularly in adults. Limited studies suggest that erythromycin given early in the course of illness is beneficial in reducing the severity of symptoms associated with *Campylobacter* gastroenteritis. However, at a practical level, identification of the organism by stool culture takes several days. Under these circumstances, ciprofloxacin is the preferred initial empirical therapy because it has activity against other bacterial causes of food-borne diarrhea.

Although ciprofloxacin (Cipro) is the drug of choice for invasive *Salmonella* infections, antibiotics are *not* recommended for normal, healthy adults with *Salmonella* gastroenteritis because antibiotics (including ciprofloxacin) have been shown to prolong asymptomatic carriage of the organism after resolution of the symptoms (i.e., prolonged convalescent carriage). Current data suggest that antibiotics may actually be harmful in infections with *E. coli* O157:H7 and other Shiga toxin–producing *E. coli*. Based on these observations, *antibiotics should be used only in severe cases of suspected bacterial diarrhea or in suspected bacterial cases involving immunocompromised hosts*. If it is thought that illness is being caused by *E. coli* O157:H7 or other shiga toxin–producing *E. coli*, antibiotics should *not* be administered. Antibiotic resistance is an increasing problem with many of these pathogens: the most recent data indicate that 17% of *Campylobacter* organisms are now resistant to ciprofloxacin. Stool cultures should always be obtained *before* starting antibiotic therapy to identify the pathogen and assess its susceptibility to the antibiotic being used.

Neurologic Syndromes

Neurologic syndromes associated with food-borne disease are generally caused by preformed toxins present in food. Botulism, caused by botulinal toxin produced by *Clostridium botulinum*, produces a characteristic syndrome of descending paralysis starting with diplopia and dysphagia and progressing (in severe cases) to respiratory paralysis. Cases in the United States have been associated primarily with improper home canning of low-acid foods, although toxin production may occur in any setting that promotes the germination of botulinal spores and then provides an appropriate anaerobic environment for growth of the organism. Botulinal spores are present in raw honey and, in an immature human intestinal tract, may germinate and produce toxin (infant botulism); for this reason, honey should not be fed to infants. In cases of botulism, administration of botulinal antitoxin early in the course of illness may be

*Not FDA approved for this indication.

beneficial. Antitoxin is available from the CDC. If botulism is suspected for any reason, the CDC should be called immediately for consultation and, if necessary, for shipment of antitoxin at (404) 639–2206 or (404) 639–3753 workdays or (404) 639–2888 nights and weekends.

Ciguatera fish poisoning results from the ingestion of fish containing ciguatoxin; the toxin is produced by a dinoflagellate on tropical coral reefs, is passed up the food chain and becomes concentrated in large, predacious fish (such as barracuda, 70% of which, in some locales, may be toxic). Clinically, in persons who ingest toxic fish, a syndrome may develop that is characterized initially by gastrointestinal complaints (diarrhea, vomiting) lasting 1 to 3 days, followed by the onset of paresthesias, fatigue, and other neurologic manifestations, which may last for 1 to 2 weeks (or longer). In the South Pacific, deaths have been associated with ciguatera fish poisoning; in this setting, data suggest that acute intravenous administration of mannitol* (Osmitrol) (20% solution given as 1 g/kg over a 30-minute period by piggyback) can reduce the severity of symptoms and may be lifesaving. Management is otherwise based on symptoms. Persons with long-term, chronic manifestations may be helped by amitriptyline (Elavil).*

Several other natural toxin–associated syndromes have been described, including paralytic shellfish poisoning (associated with harvesting of clams, mussels, and other shellfish in areas where blooms of the toxin-producing dinoflagellate *Alexandrium* have occurred, most commonly seen in Alaska, Maine, and the Pacific Northwest), neurotoxic shellfish poisoning (associated with the production of brevetoxin by red tides along the Florida, Gulf, and mid-Atlantic coasts), diarrhetic shellfish poisoning (described primarily from Europe), and amnesic shellfish poisoning (associated with the presence of domoic acid in shellfish; the only documented human cases have been along the St. Lawrence River in Canada). Certain fish (tuna, mahi-mahi), mostly in the scombroid group, may undergo bacterial decomposition of muscle with the release of histamine if not properly refrigerated after being caught. If subsequently eaten, the fish causes a tingling, "peppery" sensation in the mouth, with a typical histamine-like reaction including paresthesias and flushing. Symptoms resolve within a matter of hours, with no sequelae; antihistamines may speed recovery.

Toxins present in mushrooms have been associated with several different syndromes (Table 2). Most of these syndromes produce nausea, vomiting, and abdominal pain accompanied by neurologic symptoms. In all mushroom poisoning, gastric emptying and activated charcoal may be administered to aid in removal of the toxin; cathartics such as magnesium citrate or sodium sulfate speed transit through the gut. Atropine is the treatment for muscarine-containing mushrooms, which produce an anticholinergic syndrome of sweating, salivation, lacrimation, and bradycardia. *Amanita* species cause confusion, restlessness, and dizziness. Ataxia, stupor, and convulsions are seen in severe cases. Physostigmine (Antilirium),* 0.5 to 1.0 mg intramuscularly or intravenously, can be used in serious cases. The mood elevation, hallucinations, and hyperkinetic activity seen with *Psilocybe* and *Panaeolus* species can be treated with benzodiazepines. *Gyromitra* species cause nausea and vomiting followed by hemolysis with methemoglubinemia and hepatic failure. Amatoxins and phallotoxins produce vomiting and diarrhea, followed by renal and hepatic failure several days later. Thioctic acid is a partial antidote, and hemoperfusion may be useful. Consultation with local poison control centers is recommended in all such cases.

*Not FDA approved for this indication.

Systemic Syndromes

Certain food-borne pathogens are associated with sepsis syndromes in persons with specific underlying medical conditions and/or immunosuppression. *Vibrio vulnificus*, a common organism in shellfish harvested from warmer (>20°C) water, can cause "primary septicemia" (sepsis without an obvious source of infection) in persons who are immunosuppressed or who have underlying liver disease. Clinically, patients with hypotension, a history of recent consumption of raw oysters, and characteristic bullous skin lesions should be assumed to be infected with *V. vulnificus* pending culture results; therapy with the combination of minocycline and ceftriaxone is currently recommended. For the elderly, *Listeria* is a well-recognized cause of sepsis and central nervous system infections. Both *Listeria* and *Toxoplasma* can cause infection in a fetus and, consequently, represent major risks for pregnant women. Food may also serve as the vehicle of transmission for streptococci (from infected food handlers) that cause typical streptococcal pharyngitis.

*Not FDA approved for this indication.

NECROTIZING SKIN AND SOFT TISSUE INFECTIONS

method of
THOMAS L. BOSSHARDT, M.D.
Cascade Surgical Partners PLLC
Yakima, Washington

and

CLAUDE H. ORGAN, Jr., M.D.
University of California, Davis
Oakland, California

Necrotizing soft tissue infections (NSTIs) encompass a diverse disease process charact[illegible]zed by extensive, rapidly progressive soft tissue inflammation and necrosis. NSTIs have been recognized for many years but seem to be increasing as evidenced by recent published reports. Despite advances in diagnosis and treatment, they often continue to be associated with a fulminant course and high morbidity and mortality rates. These infections comprise a spectrum of diseases ranging from skin necrosis to life-threatening infections involving the fascia and muscle with systemic toxicity. They vary in predisposing and causative factors, anatomic location, type of offending bacteria, and level of tissue involvement.

Many terms are used to describe problem presentations. The original description of "hospital gangrene" was made by Joseph Jones in 1871 following his experience during the U.S. Civil War. Additional terms used in the past included *Fournier gangrene, acute hemolytic* Streptococcus *gangrene,* and *gas gangrene* (clostridial myonecrosis). The term *necrotizing fasciitis* was popularized by Wilson in 1952. The terminology of NSTIs is of secondary concern when one is challenged by a patient with the aggressive form of this illness. Primary emphasis must be given to rapid recognition and appropriate treatment. A high index of suspicion leads to early diagnosis, aggressive surgical intervention, and appropriate antimicrobial therapy; these are essential steps in reducing the mortality of NSTIs.

PRESENTATION AND DIAGNOSIS

The presentation of NSTIs is highly variable and can range from sepsis with obvious skin involvement to minimal cutaneous manifestations with disproportionate underlying necrotizing fasciitis. The usual clinical presentation begins with localized pain and a deceptively benign appearance. Clinical clues that may assist in establishing an early diagnosis are edema beyond the area of erythema, small skin vesicles, crepitus, absence of lymphangitis, and pain out of proportion to skin changes. Additional local signs suggesting deep infection include cyanosis or bronzing of the skin, induration, dermal thrombosis, and epidermolysis or dermal gangrene. Classic signs of fever, diffuse crepitus, and shock are late signs. Once large blisters and gangrene develop, the infectious process is already at an advanced stage.

It is essential to recognize risk factors early. Multiple risk factors increase the probability of a life-threatening infection. These co-morbid conditions include diabetes mellitus, peripheral vascular disease, malnutrition, malignancy, an immunocompromised state (AIDS, steroid therapy), obesity, and chronic alcohol or intravenous drug abuse. In the urban setting, intravenous and subcutaneous injection of illicit substances has become a more prevalent risk factor and should raise suspicion.

The etiologies for NSTIs are not always obvious, and often the initiating event is surprisingly minor. The most common etiologies include postoperative wound complications, penetrating and blunt trauma, cutaneous infections, intravenous or subcutaneous illicit substance injection, perirectal abscesses, and strangulated hernias. Primary infections, also called *idiopathic,* are uncommon and occur in the absence of an identifiable etiology.

Establishing an early diagnosis depends on a high index of suspicion and a willingness to proceed with appropriate treatment. Laboratory studies commonly encountered include significant leukocytosis, hyponatremia, and hypocalcemia. Plain radiographs of the area may demonstrate subcutaneous air and confirm the diagnosis but are usually not necessary. There has been recent interest in the use of computed tomography and magnetic resonance imaging (MRI) to aid in diagnosis. MRI is more sensitive in detecting soft tissue inflammation and necrosis. However, rapidly obtaining an MRI scan may not always be feasible. Additional useful tools in selected cases include fine needle aspiration with immediate Gram stain and frozen section analysis to identify necrosis. We contend that early and aggressive surgical intervention should not be delayed by these ancillary studies in most cases. At exploration, the diagnosis can be confirmed by the finding of necrotic fascia with the absence of gross pus, and by easy finger dissection along the fascial planes.

BACTERIOLOGY

The bacteriology of NSTIs is well recognized, and the infectious process is independent of specific bacteria. Recently reported series reveal that most NSTIs are polymicrobial, involving organisms behaving synergistically. Anaerobes, skin flora, and gram-negative rods are commonly encountered. Necrosis occurs secondary to bacterial toxins, tissue ischemia, and vascular thrombosis.

Monomicrobial NSTIs are usually caused by hemolytic group A streptococcus, *Staphylococcus aureus,* or clostridial species. Group A streptococcal NSTIs not uncommonly involve younger patients, involve the extremities, and are associated with a streptococcal toxic shock–like syndrome. There has been a recent rise in cases of necrotizing fasciitis caused by group B streptococcus. Marine vibrio species have also been associated with NSTIs.

TREATMENT

NSTIs must be treated aggressively and rapidly and as potentially life-threatening emergencies. Previous studies have documented the efficacy of a unified approach to successful treatment. The essential elements of treatment are resuscitation, antimicrobial therapy, surgical débridement, and supportive care. Patients must undergo resuscitative measures with invasive monitoring to achieve fluid, electrolyte, and hemodynamic stability. Massive volumes of fluid are often required secondary to third-spacing and sepsis.

Antimicrobial therapy consists of broad-spectrum antibiotics. Empiric coverage with high-dose penicillin G, an aminoglycoside, and clindamycin (Cleocin) or metronidazole (Flagyl) is recommended. Single agent coverage with imipenem/cilastatin (Primaxin) or an extended-spectrum penicillin with a β-lactamase inhibitor is an alternative choice. Antibiotics are adjusted once cultures are reported. Tetanus status must be addressed.

Surgical débridement is paramount and must be performed early and aggressively. It should not be delayed if the patient is in septic shock. Débridement is best performed using general anesthesia, and all necrotic tissue must be excised. Débridement is considered adequate when finger dissection no longer easily separates the subcutaneous tissue from the fascia. The deep muscle should be inspected. Parallel counter incisions may be made if indicated to exclude additional spread of infection. Amputation may be necessary for massive involvement of an extremity. The wound is packed open and kept moist with saline or 0.25% sodium hypochlorite (Dakin solution). Patients should undergo re-exploration and débridement every 24 hours or earlier if indicated until progression of the necrosis has been halted.

Postoperatively, patients are monitored in the intensive care unit until stable. Intravenous antibiotics are continued and early nutritional support is initiated. Physical therapy can be started once sepsis has resolved. Wound coverage should be delayed until the infection has clinically resolved and healthy granulation tissue is present. Split-thickness skin grafts usually provide coverage, although more extensive wounds may require a flap procedure.

Controversy surrounds the routine use of hyperbaric oxygen (HBO) in treating NSTIs. Supporters claim a decrease in mortality when infections involve anaerobic bacteria, specifically clostridial species. However, no survival benefit has been well demonstrated by a prospective, randomized trial for HBO in treating nonclostridial NSTIs. Its use may delay appropriate and adequate surgical débridement. For these reasons, HBO should be considered an adjunctive therapy and in no way should replace or diminish the importance of proper surgical management.

Despite advances in intensive medical care, mortality rates for NSTIs remain substantial. Recent large series continue to demonstrate rates in excess of 20%. The number of risk factors present, extent of infection, delay in initial débridement, and degree of organ system dysfunction at admission have been shown to be predictors of outcome. Retrospective reviews clearly demonstrate that a delayed presentation and débridement both contribute to the high mortality rates. Time is a critical element in successful management of NSTIs, and delays must be avoided.

TOXIC SHOCK SYNDROME

method of
DANIEL DAVIS, M.D.
University of California, San Diego

Toxic shock syndrome (TSS) is a model for toxin-mediated syndromes and affords a unique opportunity to witness the unadulterated effects of immune system stimulation. Indeed, the clinical manifestations of TSS result from various inflammatory mediators that are released in response to a relatively minor infection. Although TSS is historically associated with menstruation and tampon use, a nonmenstrual toxic shock syndrome (NMTSS) is described after surgery, postpartum, and in association with skin and bone infections, burns and open dermatologic lesions, and respiratory tract infections including sinusitis. Since the early 1980s, the ratio of menstrual toxic shock syndrome (MTSS) to NMTSS has steadily decreased. As the pathophysiology of TSS and other toxin mediated diseases is better elucidated, new diagnostic and therapeutic avenues of research are revealed and the basic workings of the immune system are more fully understood.

HISTORIC PERSPECTIVE

In 1978, Todd and associates described a series of children with relatively minor skin and wound infections but with an unusual cluster of symptoms characterized by fever, hemodynamic instability, and a sunburn-like rash followed by desquamation of the palms and soles. Although this represented the first formal description of TSS, sepsis syndromes have been recognized for centuries, with one author speculating that TSS may have been responsible for the plague in Athens that ended the Golden Age. Following the initial description of TSS, most reports have involved menstruating females. These early papers documented a 98% incidence of *Staphylococcus* from endovaginal culture specimens of patients with TSS, and in 1981 two groups independently identified the causative toxin—pyogenic exotoxin C and enterotoxin F—in 91% and 94% of isolates, respectively. These were later demonstrated to be the same toxin, which was renamed toxic shock syndrome toxin-1 (TSST-1).

Over 90% of initial TSS cases were associated with tampon use, and certain compositions were found to dramatically increase the risk of TSS. The removal from the market of tampons made of cross-linked carboxymethylcellulose and polyester foam in 1980 along with increased awareness among physicians and patients led to a decrease in MTSS. A similar syndrome of streptococcal TSS has been described following superinfection of varicella lesions but with higher morbidity and mortality than that reported for staphylococcal TSS; interestingly, the causative exotoxin is structurally very similar to TSST-1. Staphylococcal TSS has also been implicated in the pathophysiology of Kawasaki disease and scarlet fever.

PATHOPHYSIOLOGY

Development of TSS involves three distinct stages: local proliferation of toxin-producing bacteria at the site of infection, production of toxin, and exposure of this toxin to the immune system with a resultant immune response. The inciting infection may be relatively insignificant, especially with endovaginal foci, where only a minimal amount of discharge or the presence of a tampon may be all that precedes the development of TSS.

Staphylococcus aureus can be isolated from 5% to 10% of endovaginal cultures in normal females, 10% to 15% of which can produce TSST-1; thus, the prevalence of TSST-1–producing *S. aureus* colonization within the general population is approximately 1%. In contrast, *S. aureus* has been isolated from over 90% of endovaginal culture specimens in females with MTSS, and over 90% of these specimens produce TSST-1. The use of tampons, intrauterine devices, and contraceptive sponges can affect all three stages of TSS development, with a ratio of 33:1 for tampon use versus nonuse. Vaginal conditions during menstruation and tampon use contribute to the proliferation of toxin-producing *S. aureus* through elevations in vaginal temperature and pH, retention of endometrial blood in the vaginal canal, and alterations in vaginal flora. Furthermore, menstruation and tampon use raise the partial pressures of both oxygen and carbon dioxide, enhance the proliferation of *Escherichia coli*, and facilitate binding of cations such as magnesium, all of which stimulate TSST-1 production.

Tampons, intrauterine devices, and contraceptive sponges facilitate toxin exposure to the immune system through microscopic tissue injury, local inflammation, and retrograde flow of endometrial blood into the uterus. Vaginal delivery results in tissue injury that can stimulate the development of postpartum NMTSS. Once TSST-1 has been exposed to local and circulating immune cells, an inflammatory cascade is initiated, with fever, hypotension, and multi-organ dysfunction resulting from the effects of inflammatory mediators, such as tumor necrosis factor (TNF) and interleukin 1 (IL-1). In addition, TSST-1 appears to act as a superantigen, activating and stimulating mitosis in T cells, suppressing neutrophil migration and immunoglobulin secretion, inducing interferon production, increasing susceptibility to endotoxins, and enhancing oxygen radical formation. More recent research indicates that TSST-1 interferes with the normal mechanisms by which lymphocytes differentiate in response to antigenic stimulation.

CLINICAL PRESENTATION

Despite the availability of assays for TSST-1, TSS remains a clinical diagnosis, with specific criteria outlined in Table 1. The key features of TSS include high fever, a diffuse sunburn-like rash, and end-organ dysfunction. Desquamation of the palms and soles typically occurs several weeks later. The onset of MTSS is typically in the middle or at the end of a menstrual period, with over 90% of cases associated with tampon use. Skin and respiratory infections are usually clinically apparent before the development of NMTSS.

Postpartum NMTSS most often occurs within a week of delivery and is usually preceded by vaginal discharge suggestive of endometritis; postpartum NMTSS may also occur in association with mastitis. Tables 2 and 3 list many of the clinical and laboratory findings with TSS. In addition, pancreatitis, adult respiratory distress syndrome (ARDS), myocardial suppression, heart block, and high-output failure may occur as a result of inflammatory mediators or from the direct effect of TSST-1.

Culture specimens from the initial focus of infection may be positive for *S. aureus*; however, this is not required for the diagnosis of TSS. Increased availability of assays for TSST-1 may help confirm clinical suspicions. Their clinical utility has been limited due to prolonged turnaround times; however, recent evidence suggests that rapid polymerase chain reaction assays may soon become available and have demonstrated excellent sensitivity and specificity. Blood, urine, and CSF culture specimens should be obtained, and alternative diagnoses should be considered, including Rocky Mountain spotted fever, legionnaires' disease, toxic epidermal necrolysis, rheumatic fever, leptospirosis, rubeola, Lyme disease, Epstein-Barr virus, or disseminated fungal infections.

TABLE 1. **Toxic Shock Syndrome: Defining Criteria**

1. Fever with temperature greater than or equal to 38.9°C (102.0°F)
2. Diffuse macular erythematous rash
3. Desquamation after 1–2 weeks in survivors
4. Hypotension with systolic blood pressure less than or equal to 90 mm Hg or orthostatic syncope
5. Involvement of three or more of the following organ systems:
   - Gastrointestinal—vomiting or diarrhea
   - Muscular—myalgias or elevated creatine phosphokinase (twice normal)
   - Mucous membranes—vaginitis, pharyngitis, conjunctivitis
   - Renal—elevated BUN or creatinine level (twice normal) or 5 or more WBC per HPF in urine without urinary tract infection
   - Hepatic—elevated total bilirubin, SGOT, or SGPT (twice normal)
   - Hematologic—platelets less than or equal to 100,000/mm^3
   - Central nervous system—disorientation or altered level of consciousness without focal neurologic findings (when fever and hypotension are absent)
   - Cardiopulmonary—ARDS, pulmonary edema, new 2d- or 3d-degree heart block, or myocarditis
6. Negative throat or cerebrospinal fluid culture results (positive *Staphylococcus aureus* blood cultures do not exclude TSS)
7. Negative serologic studies for Rocky Mountain spotted fever, leptospirosis, and rubeola

Abbreviations: ARDS = adult respiratory distress syndrome; BUN = blood urea nitrogen; HPF = high-power field; SGOT = serum glutamic oxaloacetic transaminase; SGPT = serum glutamic pyruvic transaminase; TSS = toxic shock syndrome; WBC = white blood cell.

TABLE 2. **Signs and Symptoms in Toxic Shock Syndrome**

Signs/Symptoms	Prevalence in TSS (%)
Constitutional	
Fever	100
Rash (with desquamation)	100
Myalgias	97
Chills/rigors	55
Arthralgia	28
Gastrointestinal	
Vomiting	89
Diarrhea	88
Abdominal tenderness	75
Head and Neck	
Pharyngitis	73
Throat pain	71
Conjunctivitis	60
Strawberry tongue	50
Neurologic	
Headache	77
Photophobia	60
Altered level of consciousness	59
Genitourinary	
Vaginitis	40
Adnexal tenderness	26

Abbreviation: TSS = toxic shock syndrome.
From Sweet RL, Gibbs RS: Toxic shock syndrome. In Sweet RL, Gibbs RS (eds): Infectious Diseases of the Female Genital Tract. Baltimore, Williams and Wilkins, 1995, pp 321–340.

TREATMENT

As with any ill patient, the first priorities are stabilization of airway, breathing, and circulation. Although most patients with TSS have no pulmonary manifestations, early or prolonged ARDS is a strong predictor of mortality, and early intubation and mechanical ventilation should be instituted with the onset of respiratory distress or pulmonary edema. Oxygen should be administered to any patient with TSS. Aggressive fluid resuscitation is required in virtually all patients with TSS, beginning with normal saline or lactated Ringer's solution. Pressors and invasive monitoring are indicated for resistant hypotension, tachycardia, or evidence of end-organ hypoperfusion. Coagulopathy may require the use of fresh frozen plasma, cryoprecipitate, or platelet transfusion. Electrolyte abnormalities are common, and acute renal insufficiency may require temporary or permanent hemodialysis.

TABLE 3. **Laboratory Abnormalities in Toxic Shock Syndrome**

Laboratory Abnormality	Prevalence in TSS (%)
Electrolytes	
Metabolic acidosis	83
Hypokalemia	78
Hypocalcemia	70
Increased serum creatinine	65
Decreased phosphorus	58
Azotemia	53
Hyponatremia	47
Hematologic	
Anemia	61
Leukocytosis	59
Prolonged prothrombin time	55
Thrombocytopenia	53
Prolonged partial thromboplastin time	46
Urinary	
Pyuria	82
Proteinuria	59
Microhematuria	59
Liver Function Tests	
Decreased total protein	82
Increased SGOT	77
Increased LDH	57
Increased SGPT	48

Abbreviations: LDH = lactate dehydrogenase; SGOT = serum glutamic oxaloacetic transaminase; SGPT = serum glutamic pyruvic transaminase; TSS = toxic shock syndrome.

From Sweet RL, Gibbs RS: Toxic shock syndrome. In Sweet RL, Gibbs RS (eds): Infectious Diseases of the Female Genital Tract. Baltimore, Williams and Wilkins, 1995, pp 321–340.

A 10% mortality rate has been reported with TSS, usually from ARDS, intractable hypotension, or renal failure; however, in most patients, the symptoms resolve within 48 to 72 hours. Poor prognosticators include ARDS and refractory hypotension, both associated with mortality rates of up to 50%. Streptococcal TSS is associated with mortality rates of 30% to 60%. Mild residual cognitive deficits with electroencephalogram abnormalities have been reported in up to 50% of patients.

The rate of TSS recurrence is approximately 30% to 50%, typically occurring within 2 months of the primary illness but with a milder course. Anti-staphylococcal antibiotics have not been demonstrated to alter the clinical course of TSS but can decrease recurrence rates to 25% to 33%. Broad antibiotic coverage is indicated for the first 48 to 72 hours until other serious bacterial infections can be ruled out with negative culture results or serologic studies. In addition, the suppression of TSST-1 synthesis has been targeted using the combination of an antistaphylococcal agent and either clindamycin (Cleocin) or gentamicin, both of which can inhibit bacterial protein synthesis. Patients with MTSS should be counseled to avoid tampons and intrauterine devices in the future.

Acetaminophen has been used both for patient comfort and to control hyperthermia. Cyclooxygenase inhibitors, such as ibuprofen, have been used in patients with TSS to attempt to modulate the deleterious effects of prostaglandins and other arachidonic acid metabolites; however, recent literature has suggested that nonsteroidal anti-inflammatory drugs may actually increase the progression to TSS by enhancing production of TNF. Glucocorticoids have been used to attenuate the inflammatory response, but results have not supported their empirical use unless adrenal insufficiency is suspected. Intravenous immunoglobulin has shown some promise in both animal and human trials and is currently being used in some centers for severe cases. Specific monoclonal antibodies are also being developed against TSST-1. In addition, interleukin therapy (IL-4, IL-6, IL-10, and IL-11) has demonstrated efficacy in decreasing TSST-1–induced cytokine production.

TSS is the best understood of the toxin-mediated syndromes, with clinical manifestations resulting from the immune response to a relatively mild infection. Although newer assays exist to detect the presence of specific exotoxins, the diagnosis of TSS remains clinical. Suspicion of TSS should be raised in a septic patient without an obvious source of infection to explain the clinical presentation, especially in the presence of a sunburn-like rash. Supportive therapy remains the standard of care, with antibiotics used to prevent recurrence, although newer immune-based therapies are being developed that may help in the treatment of TSS and other inflammatory syndromes in the future.

INFLUENZA

method of
ROBERT L. ATMAR, M.D.
Baylor College of Medicine
Houston, Texas

Influenza occurs in annual epidemics in temperate climates and causes excessive morbidity and mortality. Epidemics usually occur during late fall or winter, but recently, small outbreaks also have been noted in travelers during summer. Infection is transmitted person to person by aerosol or close contact, and the incubation period typically is 1 to 3 days. Illness attack rates are highest in school-aged children, whereas mortality rates are highest in people older than 65 years of age.

Influenza is caused by an RNA virus with a segmented genome. There are two types (A and B) that are responsible for epidemic disease, and among the influenza A viruses there are multiple subtypes (e.g., H1N1, H3N2). Two surface glycoproteins, hemagglutinin (HA) and neuraminidase (NA), are targets for antibodies that can prevent infection, and it is change in these proteins that is responsible for the epidemiologic patterns of influenza infection. Minor antigenic changes in HA and NA are caused by point mutations in the genes encoding these proteins. This "antigenic drift" occurs in both influenza A and B viruses and leads to a portion of the population not having sufficient levels of antibody to prevent infection with the new variant, resulting in the occurrence of annual epidemics. Recent excess mortality in the United States associated with epidemic influenza has ranged from 10,000 to more than 40,000 deaths annually.

A second epidemiologic pattern is seen with influenza A viruses when major antigenic changes occur to the HA, leading to a worldwide epidemic (*pandemic*). Exchange (reassortment) of genes between human and avian influenza A viruses during a dual infection produces a new strain that can replicate efficiently in human beings and to which most, if not all, people are susceptible.

Four such antigenic shifts occurred during the 1900s: in 1918 (H1N1), 1957 (H2N2), 1968 (H3N2), and 1977 (H1N1). The emergence of the shift variant was associated with the disappearance of the preceding variant, with the exception of the H1N1 reappearing in 1977. Excess mortality is generally much higher during periods of pandemic influenza, having been as high as 500,000 deaths in 1918–1919. The reemergence of H1N1 viruses in 1977 was not associated with mortality rates in excess of that seen with interpandemic influenza, probably because of residual immunity in the population resulting from past infection with H1N1 strains (in people born before 1957).

The occurrence of epidemic influenza within a community is heralded by an increase in school absenteeism and visits to health care facilities for febrile respiratory illness. Increases in industrial absenteeism, hospitalization rates for pneumonia and influenza, and mortality rates follow. Regional and national surveillance networks also monitor the circulation of influenza viruses, and these surveillance data are useful in guiding the empirical treatment of febrile acute respiratory disease.

CLINICAL MANIFESTATIONS AND COMPLICATIONS

Influenza-associated illness is classically associated with the presence of both respiratory and systemic symptoms. In adolescents and adults, there is an abrupt onset of systemic symptoms such as fever, chills, headache, myalgia, malaise, and anorexia. Respiratory symptoms, including cough, nasal congestion or rhinorrhea, and sore throat, are seen simultaneously or develop a short time later. Hoarseness, tracheal and chest pain, and conjunctival injection also may occur. The acute febrile illness generally lasts for 3 to 5 days, but cough and general lassitude may persist for up to several weeks. Among children, other clinical syndromes, including bronchiolitis, croup, pneumonia, otitis media, and febrile seizures, are also seen in addition to the febrile respiratory illness just described. Gastrointestinal symptoms, including nausea, vomiting, and abdominal pain, occur more commonly in children than in adults. In geriatric patients, lethargy, confusion, lassitude, and fever may be the only features present.

The most common complications of influenza include otitis media, sinusitis, bronchitis, and pneumonia. Each of these complications may be associated with the primary virus infection or may be the result of a secondary bacterial infection. Secondary bacterial infection should be suspected when fever recurs in association with increasing local symptoms and signs after a period in which the patient appears to be improving. Although pneumococcal pneumonia is the most common secondary bacterial pneumonia, the relative frequency of *Staphylococcus aureus* pneumonia is increased compared with periods when influenza is not in the community. Other complications include exacerbations of asthma and chronic obstructive pulmonary disease, myositis, myocarditis, and central nervous system manifestations. Reye syndrome, an illness associated with fatty degeneration of the liver and cerebral edema, occurs rarely and is associated with the use of salicylate-containing medications.

DIAGNOSIS

There are a number of other respiratory viruses and infectious agents that can cause a clinical syndrome (influenza-like illness) similar to that of influenza virus. Influenza virus infection is likely in people with an influenza-like illness when influenza virus is known to be circulating in the community. In such a setting, 70% to 80% of influenza-like viruses have been associated with influenza virus infection. A definitive diagnosis requires the use of virus-specific assays.

A number of rapid diagnostic assays are currently available for the detection of influenza viruses in respiratory secretions. The most rapid assays use enzyme immunoassay techniques to detect the presence of specific viral proteins or detect virus-specific NA activity in clinical specimens. Results are available as early as 30 minutes after collection of the respiratory specimen. These assays can be performed in the physician's office.

Some assays distinguish between type A and B viruses whereas others do not. Direct and indirect immunofluorescent tests require more equipment and expertise, and they are usually performed in hospital-based or reference clinical virology laboratories. In general, immunofluorescent assays take longer to perform than enzyme immunoassays, with results not being available for at least several hours after specimen collection. The specificity of the rapid diagnostic assays is generally high (>90%). The sensitivity of the assays ranges from 60% to 90%, being somewhat higher in children than adults.

The gold standard for detection of influenza virus infections is virus isolation using embryonated eggs or cell culture monolayers. The most commonly assayed specimens are nasal washes or aspirates, pharyngeal swabs, or nasopharyngeal swabs, with a combination of nasal and pharyngeal specimens being optimal. Other specimens that can yield virus include throat gargles, sputum, and bronchoalveolar lavage. The respiratory sample should be placed in a viral transport medium and transported to the laboratory on wet ice. Storage of the specimen (in viral transport medium) at 4°C for up to several days does not significantly alter the likelihood of isolating influenza viruses, although the detection of other respiratory viruses may be adversely affected. Most influenza viruses are isolated within 3 to 7 days of inoculation.

Serologic assays are a third method for identifying influenza virus infection. These assays are the least valuable clinically because paired sera must be collected 2 to 4 weeks apart before the assay can be performed, but serologic assays are an important tool for epidemiologic studies. Nucleic acid detection methods (such as reverse transcription/polymerase chain reaction assays) are not generally available.

PREVENTION AND TREATMENT

Vaccine

Trivalent inactivated influenza virus vaccine is the principal means for the prevention of influenza and its complications. The vaccine is composed of virus antigens from three influenza virus strains: A/H1N1, A/H3N2, and B. The virus strains included in the vaccine are selected to be those most likely to be circulating in the current season based on the results of worldwide surveillance. Each of the vaccine strains is grown in embryonated chicken eggs, rendered noninfectious (*inactivated*) with a chemical agent, and partially purified. The vaccine virus can then be used in a whole-virus vaccine (WVV) (Fluzone) or processed further to disrupt virus particles (subvirion; Fluogen, FluShield, Fluzone) or to purify the HA and NA from the virions (purified surface antigen; Fluvirin). Subvirion- and purified surface antigen–containing vaccines are referred to collectively as split-virus vaccines (SVVs). Each vaccine is standardized to contain 15 μg of HA antigen from each of the vaccine strains in a 0.50-mL dose. WVVs and SVVs have similar efficacy rates, but WVVs are associated with an increased frequency of fever compared with SVVs in children 12 years of age and younger. Thus, only SVVs should be used in this age group. The vaccine is administered intramuscularly. Table 1 contains the recommended doses and vaccines to be used in different age groups. Children younger than 9 years receiving trivalent inactivated influenza virus vaccine for the first time should receive a second vaccine dose approximately 1 month after the initial dose.

Influenza virus vaccine is indicated for people older than 6 months of age who are at the greatest risk for complications related to influenza virus infection. People at greatest risk include those older than age 50 years, residents of nursing homes or chronic care facilities, people with chronic disorders of the pulmonary or cardiovascular system (including asthma), people with chronic medical conditions (e.g., diabetes mellitus, kidney disease, hemoglobinopathy, immunosuppression), people receiving chronic aspirin therapy (thus having an increased risk of developing Reye syndrome), and women in the second or third trimester of pregnancy. Health care workers and other people (e.g., household members) who come into close contact with high-risk individuals also should be vaccinated. In addition, vaccine can be provided to any person who wishes to decrease his or her likelihood of becoming infected with influenza. Vaccine should not be administered to anyone with a known history of anaphylactic hypersensitivity to eggs or to other components in the vaccine or to people who have developed Guillain-Barré syndrome within 6 weeks of a previous vaccination (see later). Vaccination should be delayed in people with acute febrile illnesses until their symptoms have abated.

Timing of influenza vaccination is targeted toward achieving the highest levels of antibody at a time when influenza virus is likely to be in the community. Influenza vaccine induces peak serum antibody levels 1 to 2 months after vaccination, with levels declining thereafter. Because influenza epidemics are most likely to occur in December and January, vaccination should be given in October and early November. Vaccine efficacy is 70% to 90% in preventing disease in healthy adults younger than 65 years of age. In older adults, the vaccine is less effective in preventing illness but is as much as 70% to 80% effective in preventing the need for hospitalization and in preventing death as a complication.

TABLE 1. **Dose and Inactivated Trivalent Influenza Vaccine Products for Different Age Groups**

Age Group	Product	Dose
6–35 mo	SVV	0.25 mL*
3–12 y	SVV	0.50 mL*
≥13 y	WVV or SVV	0.50 mL

SVV, split-virus vaccine; WVV, whole-virus vaccine.
*A second dose of vaccine is recommended 1 month after the first in children younger than 9 years of age receiving the vaccine for the first time.

The most frequent side effect of influenza vaccine is soreness at the injection site, developing in 10% to 64% of people and lasting 1 or 2 days. Systemic features, such as fever, malaise, and myalgia, occur in less than 10% of people. Such symptoms usually begin 6 to 12 hours after vaccination, last 1 to 2 days, and can be relieved with acetaminophen. Hypersensitivity reactions, including anaphylaxis, occur rarely after influenza vaccination. Although these immediate allergic reactions may be associated with any component of the vaccine, traces of residual egg protein are thought to be the most frequent cause, leading to the recommendation that people with severe egg allergy should not receive the vaccine. The risk of Guillain-Barré syndrome may be increased slightly in the 6 weeks after vaccination (≈1 additional case per million people vaccinated). However, the potential benefits from the prevention of influenza-related complications, hospitalization, and death are much greater than the risk of developing Guillain-Barré syndrome.

New approaches to improving the efficacy of influenza vaccination are being evaluated in clinical studies. One promising approach is the use of live attenuated influenza virus vaccine (LAIV),* given intranasally. LAIV has the advantage of not requiring an intramuscular injection, increasing its acceptability among certain groups, and inducing local mucosal immunity. LAIV may soon be available for clinical use.

Antivirals

There are currently four antivirals licensed for treatment of influenza. The antivirals belong to two different classes of drugs based on their mechanism of action. The M2 inhibitors amantadine (Symmetrel) and rimantadine (Flumadine) are active only against influenza A viruses. M2 inhibitors block proton ion channels (the M2 protein) in the virus membrane, preventing virus uncoating and initiation of infection. NA inhibitors, such as zanamivir (Relenza) and oseltamivir (Tamiflu), are active against both influenza A and B viruses. NA inhibitors block the activity of the viral NA or sialidase. This enzyme removes sialic acid residues from the surface of the infected cell, allowing the virus to bud from the cell without forming large viral aggregates. The enzyme also has a role in helping the virus pass through the overlying

*Investigational drug in the United States.

mucus layer so that it can infect the respiratory epithelium.

All four drugs are approved for the treatment of acute influenza A virus infection. The NA inhibitors may also be used to treat acute influenza B virus infection. Infection with influenza A and B viruses cannot be distinguished clinically, so the selection of an antiviral agent should be influenced by knowledge of which viruses are circulating in the community and/or by the results of rapid diagnostic assays. Treatment should be started within 2 days from onset of illness. The magnitude of therapeutic benefit increases as the interval from symptom onset to initiation of treatment decreases. The average reduction in clinical illness is 1 to 3 days for each of the drugs. Use of the NA inhibitors also has been associated with decreased complication rates and decreased use of antibiotics associated with influenza virus infection.

All four drugs also are effective when given prophylactically, although influenza vaccine remains the primary means for prevention of influenza. An antiviral agent might be used prophylactically in a variety of circumstances, including in people at high risk who are vaccinated after influenza virus is circulating in the community, in people with immune deficiencies who are expected to have an inadequate immune response to vaccination, as postexposure prophylaxis (e.g., after introduction of influenza into a family), to control influenza outbreaks in institutional settings, and in people for whom influenza vaccine is contraindicated. Prophylactic efficacy is similar for each of the drugs, ranging from 70% to 90%. Table 2 lists the Food and Drug Administration–approved indications for each drug and recommended drug doses by age group.

TABLE 2. **Recommended Prophylaxis and Treatment Regimens for Influenza Antiviral Medications***

Antiviral [Route of Administration]	Prophylaxis Regimen	Treatment Regimen
M2 inhibitors (influenza A virus only)		
Amantadine (e.g., Symmetrel) [oral]	Age 1–9 years: 5 mg/kg/d up to 150 mg in two divided doses Age 10–64 years: 100 mg bid Age ≥65 years: ≤100 mg qd	Age 1–9 years: 5 mg/kg/d up to 150 mg in two divided doses Age 10–64 years: 100 mg bid Age ≥65 years: ≤100 qd
Rimantadine (Flumadine) [oral]	Age 1–9 years: 5 mg/kg/d up to 150 mg in two divided doses Age 10–64 years: 100 mg bid Age ≥65 years 100 mg qd	Age ≤13 years: NR Age 14–64 years: 100 mg bid Age ≥65 years: 100 mg qd
Neuraminidase inhibitors (influenza A and B viruses)		
Zanamivir (Relenza) [inhalation]	NR	Age ≥7 years: 10 mg bid
Oseltamivir (Tamiflu) [oral]	Age >13 year: 75 mg qd	Age >1 year: ≤15 kg, 30 mg bid >15–23 kg, 45 mg bid >23–40 kg, 60 mg bid >40 kg and adults, 75 mg bid

*FDA approved indications as of 4/1/2001.
Abbreviation: NR = no recommendation by FDA for this indication/age group.

The four drugs have different side effect profiles. Both amantadine and rimantadine are associated with central nervous system complaints (e.g., nervousness, lightheadedness, difficulty concentrating). These effects are more common with amantadine, occurring in 10% to 15% of people. Gastrointestinal complaints (anorexia, nausea) occur in 1% to 3% of people. More serious side effects (e.g., delirium, hallucinations, seizures) have been observed in association with high serum amantadine levels. Increased serum levels are more likely to occur in geriatric patients and in people with impaired renal function because amantadine is cleared by renal mechanisms. Thus, dosage adjustment is recommended with renal insufficiency; rimantadine is cleared by both renal and hepatic mechanisms, and dosage reduction (by half) is recommended only in advanced renal failure.

Zanamivir is infrequently associated with side effects. However, clinically significant bronchospasm has been observed after its use in people with pulmonary disease (asthma, chronic obstructive pulmonary disease). If zanamivir is used in patients with obstructive lung disease, the patient should be told to have a fast-acting inhaled bronchodilator readily available and to discontinue the drug and inform his or her physician if breathing problems develop.

Oseltamivir is associated with an increased frequency of nausea and vomiting. These side effects are more prominent when the drug is taken on an empty stomach and with the first dose of drug. Few people being treated for influenza discontinue the drug because of these side effects.

Drug resistance to the four drugs occurs. With the M2 inhibitors, resistance is more likely to develop in pediatric patients and in immunocompromised patients. Transmission of virus resistant to the M2 inhibitors leads to illness indistinguishable from that caused by susceptible virus (i.e., virus is not attenuated). In contrast, although resistance to the NA inhibitors has been recognized, drug-resistant viruses are significantly attenuated, and it is not clear whether they can be transmitted to or cause illness in human beings.

Other Measures

Additional treatment can be given for symptom management: oral hydration; acetaminophen to treat fever, myalgia, and headache; nasal decongestants; and an antitussive for cough. Aspirin should be avoided because of the risk of Reye syndrome. Antibiotic therapy should not be given prophylactically and should be used only to treat secondary bacterial infections.

LEISHMANIASIS

method of
SHYAM SUNDAR, M.D.
Banaras Hindu University
Varanasi, India

Leishmaniasis comprises several diverse clinical syndromes caused by obligate intracellular protozoa belonging to the genus *Leishmania*. It causes three broad groups of disorders: visceral leishmaniasis (VL, kala-azar), cutaneous leishmaniasis (CL), and mucocutaneous leishmaniasis (MCL). Although most clinical syndromes are zoonotic and are transmitted from animal reservoirs through *Phlebotomus* sandfly vectors, major VL foci in India and Sudan are anthroponotic. There are 21 *Leishmania* species responsible for these disorders. About 350 million people are at risk in 88 countries around the world, and an estimated 2 million new cases occur every year. Of these, 1.5 million people suffer from CL, and 500,000 suffer from VL.

VISCERAL LEISHMANIASIS

Visceral leishmaniasis is also known as kala-azar (Hindi meaning "black fever") and if untreated is almost always fatal. Most (90%) of the disease occurs in India, Nepal, and Sudan; however, it also occurs in Brazil, Africa, and the Mediterranean region. This syndrome is typically characterized by fever (often with rigor and chills), splenomegaly, and pancytopenia. Once clinical VL sets in, patients become emaciated and are prone to develop secondary infections such as pneumonia, tuberculosis, and amebic or bacillary dysentery. In India and Sudan, VL may be followed by development of post–kala–azar dermal leishmaniasis (PKDL), which is characterized by development of nodules and hypopigmented macules. This occurs in up to half the patients in Sudan, although the number is much less (3%–5%) in India. Contrary to Sudanese PKDL, in which ulceration and secondary infections are common, in Indian PKDL ulceration does not occur.

*HIV-*Leishmania *Co-Infection*

In areas around the Mediterranean basin such as Spain, Italy, Greece, southern France, and sub-Saharan Africa (Ethiopia, Kenya, Sudan), HIV-*Leishmania* co-infection is common. Atypical presentation of VL (e.g., absence of hepatosplenomegaly, fever, or lymphadenopathy and gastrointestinal manifestations) may be seen in these patients, and the presence of other opportunistic infections may complicate the picture.

CUTANEOUS LEISHMANIASIS

Old World anthroponotic CL is caused by *L. tropica*, and zoonotic CL is caused by *L. major, L. aethiopica*, and dermotropic *L. infantum*; New World CL is caused by *L. mexicana* complex, comprising *L. mexicana, L. amazonensis*, and *L. venezuelensis*, and *Viannia* subgenus *L. Viannia braziliensis* complex, constituted by *L. Viannia guyanensis*, *L. Viannia panamensis*, *L. Viannia braziliensis*, and *L. Viannia peruviana*. In all types of CL, the common feature is development of a papule followed by ulceration of the skin with raised borders, usually at the site of the bite by the vector. These ulcers develop a few weeks to months after the bite. There can be satellite lesions, especially in *L. major* and occasionally in *L. tropica* infections; regional lymphadenopathy, pain, pruritus, and secondary bacterial infections might occur occasionally. If the immunity is good, usually there is spontaneous healing in *L. tropica, L. major*, and *L. mexicana* lesions. In some patients with anergy to *Leishmania*, the skin lesions of *L. aethiopica, L. mexicana*, and *L. amazonensis* infections progress to diffuse cutaneous leishmaniasis, characterized by spread of the infection from the initial ulcer, usually on the face, to involvement of the whole body with nonulcerative nodules.

MUCOSAL LEISHMANIASIS

In *L. Viannia braziliensis* complex infections, cutaneous lesions may be followed by mucosal spread of the disease simultaneously or even years later. It is characterized by thickening, and erythema of the nasal mucosa, typically starting at the junction of the nose and the upper lip. Later, ulceration develops with destruction of the nasopharynx, exposing the larynx to full view through the nose. There is no spontaneous healing, and death might result from severe respiratory tract infections from massive destruction of the pharynx.

IMMUNOLOGY

After inoculation by the vector, the parasite is taken up by the dendritic cells or the macrophages; these cells, as in any intracellular infection, process the antigen for presentation to the Th cells. These macrophages or dendritic cells probably determine the future course of infection and disease. If activated by a predominantly Th1 type of response driven by interleukin-12 and mediated by interleukin-2 and interferon γ, the parasites are killed and healing results; on the other hand, a predominantly Th2 type of response, mediated by interleukin-10 and interleukin-4, leads to progressive VL. In cutaneous leishmaniasis as well, a Th1 response leads to healing of lesions, a positive leishmanin skin test (LST), and high in vitro proliferative response of peripheral blood mononuclear cells (PBMC) to the challenge of leishmanial antigen. On the contrary, a Th2 response leads to progressive disease, negative LST, and absence of a proliferative response of PBMCs to leishmanial antigen challenge.

DIAGNOSIS

Diagnosis of leishmaniasis requires the recovery of the organisms from the lesions, either in smears or in cultures. In VL, most often the diagnosis is made by demonstration of amastigotes in tissue smears from spleen, bone marrow, liver, or lymph node. Splenic smear examination remains the most (>98%) sensitive method, although splenic tear and hemorrhage are potentially fatal risks. Similarly, in cutaneous leishmaniasis, amastigotes can be demonstrated in the skin scrapings, aspirates from skin lesions or lymph nodes, or touch preparations of histology specimens. In both VL and CL, in vitro culture can improve the sensitivity. In recent years, DNA diagnosis using polymerase chain reaction has been increasingly employed; however, reproducibility and field applicability have to be proved before widespread application. Of the various serologic tests employed in the diagnosis of VL, two are potentially useful: (1) the direct agglutination test (DAT), in which stained promastigotes are used, and (2) a rapid strip test based on recombinant k39 antigen (39 amino acids, conserved in the kinesin region of the amastigotes of *L. donovani chagasi*). Their simplicity (no equipment needed), easy field applicability, and inexpensive cost are the major advantages. Batch-to-batch antigen variation with the DAT needs to be ironed out before its widespread use. An inherent disadvantage of these antibody-based tests, is their inability to predict cure or relapses. In CL and MCL, serologic examination is often negative; however, LST is positive in most of the cases.

TREATMENT

In general, treatment of leishmaniasis is far from satisfactory. Most antileishmanial drugs are toxic and have to be given parenterally for prolonged periods. Controlled clinical trials have been few and far between. The multiplicity of organisms and the varying response to the drug treatment in different geographical regions make the situation worse, because extrapolation of results of one trial to another region is not possible.

In VL, once successful therapy is instituted, there is a prompt return of temperature to normal (except in infusion-related pyrexia with amphotericin B), decrease in the splenic size, and recovery of blood cell counts (hemoglobin, white blood cell counts, and platelets) toward normal. A short-term cure can be declared if no parasites are seen at the end of treatment (or 2 weeks later). Because relapses are common with this illness, patients should be followed for at least 6 months before a long-term definite cure is pronounced.

In CL, effective treatment results in the flattening of the raised margins of the ulcer followed by re-epithelization and healing with scarring. As in its VL counterpart, however, relapses occur in the beginning, mostly at margins of the healed lesions.

Pentavalent Antimonials (Sb^v)

Since the early 1940s, pentavalent antimonials have been the anchor of treatment for leishmaniasis, and in most parts of the world these compounds are used to treat all forms of leishmaniasis. There are two pentavalent antimony compounds: sodium antimony gluconate (Pentostam),* available as multidose vials in the concentration of 100 mg/mL, and meglumine antimoniate (Glucantime),* available in a concentration of 85 mg/mL. These drugs are administered either intravenously or intramuscularly. Side effects are quite common and include arthralgias, myalgias, increased levels of hepatic transaminases, pancreatitis, and electrocardiographic changes (decrease in the height of the T wave and inversion). Occasionally, however, severe cardiotoxicity, manifested by a concave ST segment and prolongation of the QTc to more than 0.5 msec, ventricular ectopic beats, runs of ventricular tachycardia, torsades de pointes, ventricular fibrillation, and death, can occur.

For VL, Sb^v should be used in doses of 20 mg/kg for 28 to 30 days without any upper limit. For CL both Old World (*L. major* or *L. tropica*) and New World (*L. mexicana* or *L. braziliensis* complexes) types should be treated with Sb^v, 20 mg/kg for 20 days. In an effort to decrease the adverse reactions to Sb^v, several workers have employed a lower dose, 5 mg/kg for 30 days, with good results in New World CL; instead of the systemic route, intralesional Sb^v injections (0.2–0.8 mL/lesion) up to 2 g have been used to good effect. Addition of allopurinol (Zyloprim)* or granulocyte-macrophage colony-stimulating factor to Sb^v therapy has been shown to offer additional benefit, but these alternatives remain to be proven in well-designed controlled clinical trials.

*Not available in the United States.

Pentamidine Isethionate

This drug is a polyamine compound, and during the 1980s it was used successfully to treat Sb^v-refractory patients with VL in India in a dose of 4 mg/kg intramuscularly or by slow intravenous infusion. Usually, 15 to 20 injections were needed. With the passage of time, however, the efficacy of pentamidine (Pentan)* has declined, and now only 69% to 78% of patients can be cured, even after using up to 33 doses. It is also an expensive and toxic drug and may cause transient hyperglycemia, irreversible insulin-dependent diabetes mellitus, hypoglycemia, shock, sterile injection abscess, and so on. Cardiac toxicity leading to fatal arrhythmias and deaths is also seen with this drug. Declining response, high cost, and serious toxicity have led to its decreased use in India. Elsewhere in the world, pentamidine is seldom used to treat VL.

Many workers have recently demonstrated the efficacy of pentamidine in both Old and New World CL and MCL, albeit mostly in uncontrolled clinical trials in small numbers of patients. In Old World CL, three injections of pentamidine (4 mg/kg on alternate days) cured 73% of patients, whereas in Colombian CL, four to seven injections of 2 to 3 mg/kg of pentamidine cured 84% to 96% of patients. In MCL caused by *L. braziliensis*, using a dose of 4 mg/kg on alternate days, eight injections produced a cure rate of 87% of patients in one study, whereas in another study, the mean total doses of 2140 mg† and 2872 mg† cured 90% and 94% of patients, respectively.

Amphotericin B

Amphotericin B is a polyene antibiotic that has been used extensively in the treatment of Sb^v-refractory patients in India with good results. This agent inhibits biosynthesis of ergosterol-like sterols, which are membrane sterols for both fungi and *Leishmania*, leading to increased membrane permeability and ultimate killing of *Leishmania* organisms.

Amphotericin B deoxycholate is used in doses of 0.75 to 1.0 mg/kg in 5% dextrose infusions at a rate

*Not FDA approved for this indication.
†Exceeds dosage recommended by the manufacturer.

of 15 to 20 infusions daily or on alternate days. Infusion-related hyperpyrexia, rigor, and thrombophlebitis occur often. Other uncommon toxicities include hypokalemia, renal dysfunction, hepatic toxicity, bone marrow suppression, myocarditis, and sudden death. Response to the treatment is excellent; the long-term cure rate is almost 100%. Successful treatment of MCL with amphotericin B has also been noted in patients form Bolivia and Peru.

Lipid-Associated Amphotericin B

To improve the tolerability of amphotericin B, lipid formulations have been developed in which deoxycholate has been replaced by other lipids. Basically, these formulations work on the principle that after infusion, lipid-associated amphotericin B is taken by the cells of the reticuloendothelial system, thus reducing toxicity as well as targeting drug delivery to the very cells that harbor the organism. Renal uptake of these drugs is poor, and thus nephrotoxicity is minimal. With these formulations, it has been possible to deliver a large quantity of amphotericin B over a short time. Three such lipid-associated formulations of amphotericin B are commercially available: (1) liposomal amphotericin B (AmBisome; Gilead Sciences, Foster City, Calif), (2) amphotericin B lipid complex (Abelcet [ABLC]; Liposome Company, Princeton, NJ), and (3) amphotericin B colloidal dispersion (Amphocil [ABCD; Amphotec]; Sequus Pharmaceuticals, Menlo Park, Calif). All three preparations have been tested successfully in visceral leishmaniasis.

Abelcet and AmBisome have been investigated for treatment of visceral leishmaniasis in sufficient patients to derive meaningful conclusions. In our four clinical trials with Abelcet, this drug was found to be very safe, and infusion reactions and other toxicities were minimal. It was possible to infuse a cumulative dose of 10 mg/kg within 24 hours. A total dose of 10 to 15 mg/kg could cure 90% to 100% of patients, and duration of therapy could be compressed to 2 to 5 days.

AmBisome is approved in several European countries for primary treatment of VL. The U.S. Food and Drug Administration approved it recently and recommended a total dose of 21 mg/kg, whereas in Europe, Africa, and South America, 18 mg/kg or more is considered adequate. AmBisome, 0.75 mg/kg for 5 days, cured 89% of Indian VL patients in long-term follow-up. Mild infusion-related fever and rigor were seen in one third of patients, and no other systemic toxicity occurred.

Amphotec is the third lipid formulation used in VL; however, the experience is limited because it caused severe side effects in children younger than 6 years. Although five and seven doses of 2 mg/kg cured 90% and 100% of patients, respectively, the high incidence of side effects is a major drawback. The high cost of these lipid amphotericin B formulations prohibits their use in developing countries, where most of VL exists. In CL, there are stray reports that AmBisome, 2 to 3 mg/kg for 20 days (total dose 2 to 5 g), was able to cure five of six (83%) patients with mucosal leishmaniasis unresponsive to Sb^v.

Aminosidine (Paromomycin)

Aminosidine,* an aminoglycoside, has been combined with antimony to reduce the duration of therapy, and a dose ranging from 12 to 20 mg/kg/day has been used with successful reduction in the duration of therapy to 17 to 21 days. In India, aminosidine alone at 16 mg/kg/day for 21 days cured 93% of patients. In CL, it has been used in *L. braziliensis* infection: 20 mg/kg/day for 20 days cured 93% of patients. In ML, 16 mg/kg/day for 20 days resulted in long-term cure of only 33% of patients. In Colombia, 22.5 mg/kg/day for 14 days cured only half of the patients; similarly, in CL in Belize, 14 mg/kg/day for 20 days cured only 59%.

Because it is an aminoglycoside, potential adverse reactions of aminosidine include nephrotoxicity and eighth cranial nerve toxicity; however, these side effects have been very uncommon. Unfortunately, this drug is not available commercially.

Oral Drugs

Oral treatment has obvious advantages, and for several decades oral drugs have been tried without success. A new oral antileishmanial compound, miltefosine, is likely to be the first oral drug to be used extensively in the treatment of leishmaniasis.

Miltefosine

Miltefosine (Miltex)* is an alkyl phospholipid and was developed as an antitumor agent, but when administered orally it was poorly tolerated, with significant gastrointestinal adverse events in phase I and II antitumor studies. In its first clinical trial for kala-azar, a phase I dose-ranging study, we tested oral miltefosine (50-mg capsules, [Asta Medica, Germany]) in 30 patients, including 14 with Sb^v failure. The total dose ranged from 700 to 7000 mg. It was administered over 28 days, and doses of 100 to 150 mg were found to be safe and well tolerated, resulting in cure in 14/15 (93%) of patients. Lower doses were ineffective, and higher doses were not tolerated. Gastrointestinal side effects such as vomiting and diarrhea were dominant adverse reactions. Subsequently, three phase II studies, including a World Health Organization (WHO)–sponsored multicenter trial, led to the following conclusions: (1) mild to moderate gastrointestinal side effects such as vomiting were seen in about one half to two thirds of the patients; (2) mild drug-induced diarrhea occurred in a small number of patients; (3) a daily dose of 100 to 150 mg for 4 weeks cured more than 95% of patients; and (4) treatment for either 3 or 4 weeks at 100 mg/day cured almost all patients. Transient elevation of he-

*Not available in the United States.

patic enzymes and nephrotoxicity (in high doses) may occur. A WHO-sponsored phase III trial with 100 mg of miltefosine for 4 weeks is now nearing completion, and results are encouraging, with a likely cure rate of greater than 95%. Miltefosine is also being evaluated for cutaneous leishmaniasis in Colombia and Guatemala and has shown promise in a pilot study.

WR6026

WR6026 (Sitamaquine),* a primaquine analogue with high antileishmanial activity, was developed in the United States at the Walter Reed Army Institute of Research for malaria several decades ago. The first clinical trial in Kenya showed that a dose of 1 mg/kg/day for 4 weeks resulted in 4 of 8 (50%) patients being cured. More trials are under way.

Ketoconazole

Ketoconazole (Nizoral),† the first imidazole compound (a class of drugs that inhibits ergosterol biosynthesis in *Leishmania* and fungi), has been used for treatment (600 mg daily for 4 weeks) of CL due to *L. mexicana mexicana* in Guatemala and resulted in 89% cure; however, it was ineffective in CL due to *L. braziliensis* (30% cure rate) and *L. tropica* infections. Itraconazole (Sporanox),† 200 mg/d for 4 to 8 weeks, cured 79% of those with Old World CL. The role of allopurinol† in either VL or CL remains unproven for lack of controlled clinical trials. In Colombia, in a double-blind placebo-controlled trial, allopurinol was no better than placebo in *L. panamensis* CL.

HIV-Visceral Leishmaniasis Co-Infection

Treatment of VL in a setting of HIV co-infection remains essentially the same as in an immunocompetent patient, with some differences in the outcome. Conventional amphotericin B (0.7 mg/kg/day for 28 days) may be more effective in achieving initial cure as compared with Sb^v (20 mg/kg/day for 28 days), although in some studies similar results have been reported. By using high-dose AmBisome (4 mg/kg/day on days 1–5, 10, 17, 24, 31, and 38), a high cure rate is possible. These co-infected patients have a tendency to experience relapse within a year, however. For prevention of relapse the role of maintenance chemotherapy needs further study.

Local Treatment of Cutaneous Leishmaniasis

Local treatment of CL is with intralesional Sb^v injecting each lesion (0.2–0.8 mL intermittently for several weeks), and cure rate has been reported to be more than 70% in both Old and New World CL. Paramomycin† (15%) ointment in combination with methylbenzethonium chloride (MBC; 5%–12%) twice daily for 10 to 20 days cures most patients in Israel and Equador. Burning sensations, pruritus, and vesicle formation are quite common with this combination. In another formulation MBC has been replaced by urea (10%). Local imidazole creams (miconazole [Monistat],* clotrimazole [Lotrimin]†) have also been tested in CL without much benefit. Cryotherapy, heat therapy, and direct current electrotherapy are the other methods used for treating CL. Lack of well-controlled clinical trials, self-healing of lesions, and parasitic variations limit the applicability of various local treatments.

*Investigational drug in the United States
†Not FDA approved for this indication.

*Not available in the United States.

LEPROSY
(Hansen's Disease)

method of
CARLOTTA H. HILL, M.D., and
CRISTINA R. CAMARA, M.D.
University of Illinois College of Medicine
Chicago, Illinois

Leprosy or *Hansen's disease* is a chronic infectious disease of the skin and peripheral nerves caused by *Mycobacterium leprae*. It currently affects more than 640,000 people worldwide, and an estimated 2 million people are permanently disabled as a result of it. About 150 new cases are seen annually in the United States. Most new cases in the United States have occurred among immigrants from leprosy endemic areas, such as Southeast Asia, Central Africa, and South and Central America.

The causative organism, *M. leprae*, is a slow-growing, gram-positive, acid-fast obligate intracellular bacillus with a doubling time of 11 to 13 days. Although it cannot be cultivated in vitro, it can multiply in mouse footpads, armadillos, and monkeys. The infected patient is thought to be the most important reservoir of the organism, which has a predilection for peripheral nerves and skin of the cooler parts of the body. Hansen's disease has a long incubation period ranging from 3 months to several decades; the average incubation is 3 to 5 years. Although not proven, the most commonly accepted theory is that it is spread by the respiratory route because nasal discharge from patients with untreated multibacillary leprosy often contains large numbers of bacilli.

Patients infected with *M. leprae* present with a spectrum of clinical manifestations that are determined by the individual's cellular immune response to the bacilli. The communicability of leprosy is thought to be very low, with about 95% of people not susceptible to it. Indeterminate leprosy may develop initially in people who are susceptible to infection. Clinically, the indeterminate lesion is a hypopigmented macule that may or may not have a sensory deficit. If diagnosed, it is always treated even though it may be self-healing. If the host is unable to mount a definite immunologic response to cure, the disease progresses.

On one end of the spectrum, tuberculoid leprosy patients (TT in the Ridley-Jopling classification) express extensive cell-mediated immunity. Therefore, hypoesthetic macules or plaques, often with raised borders and central clearing, are solitary or few (not more than three). Lesions are characterized histologically by well-developed epithelioid granulomas surrounded by a cuff of T lymphocytes that express T helper 1 (TH1) cytokine profiles.

TABLE 1. **World Health Organization Treatment**

Single Dose/Single Lesion
Rifampin* 600 mg
Ofloxacin* 400 mg
Minocycline* 100 mg
Paucibacillary: 6-Month Treatment
Rifampin* 600 mg q month, supervised
Dapsone 100 mg q day
Multibacillary: 12-Month Treatment
Rifampin* 600 mg q month, supervised
Clofazimine 300 mg q month, supervised; 50 mg q day
Daspone 100 mg q day

*Not FDA approved for this indication.

On the other end of the spectrum, patients with lepromatous leprosy have markedly reduced or absent cell-mediated immunity against *M. leprae* and manifest with multiple skin-colored or erythematous nodules or widespread patches and plaques. The lesions histologically show replacement of the dermis with foamy macrophages. The T cells' inability to respond to *M. leprae* antigen is expressed by lack of migration and proliferation at the site of antigen deposition and lack of cytokine production. As a result, the macrophages are not activated, with growth and replication of the bacilli in an uncontrolled manner within them.

Between the two extremes is the borderline spectrum, which can range from borderline tuberculoid, midborderline, or borderline lepromatous.

A simpler clinical classification by the World Health Organization (WHO) is now gaining popularity (Table 1). It has three major categories:

1. Single lesion with sensory loss, which is referred to as *single lesion paucibacillary*
2. *Paucibacillary leprosy,* with two to five lesions
3. *Multibacillary leprosy,* with more than five lesions

The bacteriologic index is useful in quantifying the number of bacteria in the biopsy specimens and skin smears and in assessing the progress of the patient under treatment. Results are expressed in a semi-logarithmic scale: 0 has no bacilli in 100 oil immersion fields and 6+ has at least 1000 bacilli per oil immersion field. Patients with paucibacillary leprosy tend to have negative results on skin smear studies. Currently, all patients with positive skin smear results are considered to have multibacillary disease and are treated appropriately.

TREATMENT

Antileprosy Drugs

Treatment is directed at the infection and, if present, at the reactional state. Requirements for antimycobacterial agents should include ability to penetrate the lipid-rich cell wall, activity against slow-growing or dormant intracellular bacteria, compatibility with other agents, and low toxicity for long-term administration. The three main drugs used to treat leprosy include rifampin (Rifadin),* which is highly bactericidal; and dapsone and clofazimine (Lamprene), which are weakly bactericidal alone but more active when taken together. Also effective although not as bactericidal as rifampin are ofloxacin (Floxin),* clarithromycin (Biaxin),* and minocycline (Minocin).* Multidrug treatment (MDT) regimens were developed to minimize drug resistance to single agents and to potentiate the bactericidal effects of the drugs when taken together. Patients should be made aware of the pigmentary changes induced by clofazimine before initiation of therapy.

*Not FDA approved for this indication.

The WHO MDT regimens arose in response to increasing resistance to dapsone monotherapy in the early 1980s. These regimens have proved to be highly successful and are now the standard antileprosy therapy throughout most of the world. The seventh WHO Expert Committee on Leprosy recommended the use of a solitary dose of rifampin* (600 mg), ofloxacin* (400 mg), and minocycline* (100 mg) (ROM) for single-lesion paucibacillary leprosy. The rationale was that most paucibacillary leprosy cases presenting with only one skin lesion have a high tendency to heal without any specific treatment. Because it is not possible to identify those who will develop progressive disease, all such cases need to be treated. This single-dose regimen was recommended for use by programs detecting 1000 or more single-lesion cases annually.

The WHO-recommended standard regimen for paucibacillary leprosy is rifampin,* 600 mg once a month supervised and dapsone 100 mg daily for 6 months (completed within 9 months). The WHO standard regimen for multibacillary leprosy is rifampin* 600 mg once a month supervised, dapsone 100 mg daily, and clofazimine 300 mg once a month supervised and 50 mg daily for 12 months (completed within 18 months). These regimens have proven to be highly successful with relapse rates of only about 1%. Multibacillary patients starting with a high bacillary index (BI) are more likely to experience slow clearance of bacilli and to have a significant BI at the end of 12 months compared with those starting with a low BI. These multibacillary patients may need additional treatment. Relapsed patients, almost without exception, respond to re-treatment with the same drug combination, indicating that the exacerbation in their condition was due to insufficient treatment or compliance. Thus, if relapse occurs, the patient should be re-treated with the same regimen.

At the National Hansen's Disease Center (NHDC) in Baton Rouge, Louisiana, recommended standard treatment regimens are longer than those recommended by WHO, and rifampin is given daily instead of monthly (Table 2). The NHDC standard regimen for paucibacillary disease in adults is rifampin* 600 mg and dapsone 100 mg both taken daily for 1 year. The NHDC standard multibacillary regimen consists of rifampin* 600 mg, dapsone 100 mg, and clofazimine 50 mg all taken daily for 2 years. The total duration may need to be extended if BI is greater than 4 at the onset of treatment or positive at the end of treatment, since these patients have a higher

*Not FDA approved for this indication.

TABLE 2. **National Hansen's Disease Center Regime**

Treatment	Post-Treatment Follow-Up
Paucibacillary: 1-Year Treatment	
Dapsone 100 mg q day Rifampin* 600 mg q day	Every 6 mo for 2 y, then annually for 3 y
Multibacillary: 2-Year Treatment	
Dapsone 100 mg q day Rifampin* 600 mg q day Clofazimine 50 mg q day	Every 6 mo for 2 y, then annually for 8 y

*Not FDA approved for this indication.

risk for relapse. Finally, if a patient refuses to take clofazimine to avoid the temporary pigmentation caused by it, 100 mg of minocycline* or 400 mg of ofloxacin* daily may be substituted. However, the patient should be strongly encouraged to take clofazimine owing to its potent antibacterial activity when given with dapsone and owing to its antireactional activity, which decreases the chance that erythema nodosum leprosum will develop.

FOLLOW-UP

Patients who are receiving standard therapy and who have no reactions or complications may be seen monthly. Routine laboratory follow-up studies include a complete blood cell count, blood urea nitrogen (BUN), creatinine level, liver function tests, and urinalysis. After the first year of treatment, drug toxicity is uncommon. Reactive episodes of varying severity are more likely to occur during the first 2 years of therapy and may require weekly or more frequent follow-up visits. After therapy is completed and the danger of reaction is significantly decreased, the patients are observed less frequently. After completion of therapy, follow-up visits should occur every 6 months for the first 2 years, then annually for a total of 5 years of observation for paucibacillary patients, 10 years for multibacillary patients. Patients should be advised to return immediately if there are new skin lesions, progressive motor or sensory loss, neuritis, iritis, or evidence of reaction.

Clinically, the skin lesions gradually clear within the first year. The BI on skin scrapings or biopsy specimens falls very gradually (½ to 1 BI per year). If possible, skin scrapings should be done from three or four of the most active sites including any new lesions, if present, yearly. Routine biopsies are not recommended unless the patient develops new lesions.

REACTIONS

As much as 50% of patients with Hansen's disease have their disease course punctuated by acute exacerbations of tissue destructive inflammatory processes termed *reactions,* which can be a major cause of nerve damage. Reactions are caused by the immune response to bacterial antigens released with the destruction of bacilli and may occur before, during, or after completion of therapy. They may be triggered by infection, pregnancy, or other stress. Although they are most common in the first 2 years of treatment, reactions tend to be less frequent in regimens including clofazimine. MDT should be continued during reactive episodes, although it may be necessary to decrease the dosage of rifampin to once a month (if the patient was receiving it daily) to lessen its effects on corticosteroids, which are the mainstay in the treatment of reactions.

*Not FDA approved for this indication.

Reversal Reactions

Reversal reactions (also called *type 1 reactions*) are a type of delayed hypersensitivity response. They occur most commonly in borderline lepromatous, midborderline, or borderline tuberculoid patients and are clinically characterized by abrupt onset of edema and erythema of pre-existing lesions that may lead to ulceration. Occasionally, new tumid lesions arise in clinically normal skin. Edema of the hands and feet and systemic symptoms may be seen as well. Neuritis manifesting as exquisitely tender and thickened regional nerve areas may occur. High doses of corticosteroids (60 mg/d prednisone) can usually control the reaction within a few days. However, if neuritis is present, at least 3 months of therapy is necessary. During this time, prednisone may be tapered until the lowest possible maintenance level is reached or until it can be discontinued altogether, although it is possible that prednisone may need to be continued for years.

Erythema Nodosum Leprosum

Type 2 reaction (erythema nodosum leprosum) occurs almost exclusively in borderline lepromatous and lepromatous leprosy patients. It manifests with fever and the sudden appearance of tender erythematous nodules, usually over extensor surfaces of the body. Systemic manifestations include neuritis, iritis, orchitis, lymphadenitis, and arthralgias. Treatment consists of corticosteroids, which may help prevent permanent nerve damage. Prednisone is usually given at a rate of 60 mg per day, with gradual tapering to an alternate-day regimen.

Thalidomide (Thalomid) is also effective. Because of its extreme teratogenicity, it cannot be given to women of child-bearing age except under the most stringent guidelines. It is usually given at a dosage of 300 to 400 mg daily for an acute episode and the reaction is usually controlled within 2 to 3 days. The dosage is then tapered to a maintenance level of about 100 mg daily. Some patients may need to take it for months to years before it can be discontinued without recurrence of the reaction. Clofazimine, with its longer onset of action, is usually given in conjunction with prednisone and may be of value in chronic cases of erythema nodosum leprosum. A typical starting dose is 100 mg two to three times daily with tapering after a response to 100 mg or less within 12 months. Gastrointestinal symptoms usually limit the use of higher dosages.

Lucio Reaction

The Lucio phenomenon is a rare type of reaction seen almost exclusively in patients from Mexico and Central America. It occurs in the setting of diffuse non-nodular lepromatous leprosy and often develops before treatment is initiated. It consists of hemorrhagic infarcts, clinically seen as crops of necrotic lesions with serrated margins. Ulceration is common below the knees. New lesions may cease within 1 week of beginning rifampin. Corticosteroids are helpful.

MULTIDISCIPLINARY APPROACH NEEDED FOR OPTIMAL TREATMENT

The primary goal of Hansen's disease treatment should be the prevention of nerve damage, deformity, and disability by early diagnosis and treatment and effective treatment of reactions. Achieving this goal may require medical specialists working in conjunction with the primary care physician. The myriad of other complications associated with leprosy require vigilance on the part of both the primary health care provider and the patient. A significant proportion of disability in leprosy can be attributed to loss of protective sensation, which predisposes the patient to injury and infection. Likewise, loss of motor innervation leading to muscle weakness may manifest as claw hand or foot drop. Management and prevention of the problems arising from nerve injury require the skills of physical and occupational therapists, podiatrists, and surgeons. Patient education regarding frequent inspection of involved skin and the use of protective apparatus such as splints and gloves is of utmost importance.

Silent neuritis, progressive loss of nerve function developing without pain or tenderness and outside of the context of reactions, may occur both during and after treatment and should be monitored by periodic screening of nerve function of the hands and feet. In patients with recent loss of function, treatment with corticosteroids in dosages appropriate for reactions should be instituted to avoid permanent nerve damage. Iridocyclitis is a medical emergency, and patients with any evidence of eye problems are treated best by an ophthalmologist. Orchitis may develop in males, especially during reactions, and fertility may be compromised.

CONTROL

WHO recommends examining all people in the household at the time the patient is diagnosed. WHO recommends advising them of the signs and symptoms of leprosy and to return to the doctor's offices should these occur. Many programs, however, repeat contact examination every year for a few years. Chemoprophylaxis is generally not recommended. Keeping in touch with patients until the recommended follow-up period after treatment as well as rapid retrieval of people who leave treatment is also vital. Health education of both patients and the general public may help not only to detect cases but also to diminish the stigma of the disease. The WHO's goal of reducing Hansen's disease to below 1 per 10,000 population at the national level is within reach this century.

MALARIA

method of
KATHRYN MAITLAND, M.D., and
CHARLES R. J. C. NEWTON, MBChB., M.D.
Wellcome Trust Research Laboratories
Kilifi, Kenya

Malaria is one of the most common and important parasitic diseases worldwide. In 1996, the World Health Organization (WHO) estimated that malaria was responsible for 500 million episodes of clinical infection and 2.7 million deaths. Although there are four species known to naturally infect humans, only *Plasmodium falciparum* is potentially lethal. The greatest burden of *P. falciparum* malaria falls on sub-Saharan Africa, where more than 90% of the world's malaria deaths occur, almost entirely in children younger than 5 years old. Measures to eradicate malaria have been ineffective. During the late 1950s and 1960s, coordinated mass action, particularly with the use of DDT, showed great achievements in malaria control in many areas of the world, but only limited successes were achieved in Africa. A more rational approach to malaria control has focused on the provision of insecticide-impregnated bed nets and access to early treatment. Throughout the world, many countries are reporting an increasing number of cases of imported malaria, largely owing to increased long-distance travel coupled with increased malaria transmission secondary to failing malaria control programs, drug resistance, and global warming.

GEOGRAPHIC DISTRIBUTION

Although indigenous malaria has been recorded as far north as Russia and as far south as Argentina, the current limits of malaria transmission fall far short of these extremes. Within the malaria-endemic areas, there are large areas free of malaria because transmission depends on local environmental and other conditions. *P. falciparum* is the most common species throughout the tropics and the subtropics, but *P. vivax* has the widest geographic range; it is prevalent in many temperate zones but also in the subtropics and the tropics. *P. malariae* is patchily present over the same range as *P. falciparum* but is much less common, and *P. ovale* is found chiefly in tropical Africa (Table 1).

TRANSMISSION

Natural transmission of malaria infection occurs through exposure to the bites of infective female *Anopheles* mosqui-

TABLE 1. **Brief Summary of Malaria Endemic Areas of the World**

Areas	Malaria Risk	Countries	*P. falciparum*	Chloroquine-resistant *P. falciparum*	Benign Malarias
Europe	No risk				
Former Soviet Union	Limited	Azerbaijan, Georgia, Tajikistan	No		Exclusively *P. vivax*
USA/Canada	No risk				
Central America		All countries: Belize,* Costa Rica, El Salvador, Guatemela,* Honduras,* Mexico, Nicaragua,* Panama*	Limited risk*	Reported in Panama only	Mostly *P. vivax*
Caribbean	Limited	Haiti, Dominican Republic	*P. falciparum* rural areas only	Reported in Haiti	
Tropical South America		Bolivia, Brazil, Colombia, Ecuador, French Guyana, Guyana, Paraguay, Peru, Surinam, Venezuela	All areas except Paraguay	All areas except Surinam and Venezuela	*P. vivax* all areas; exclusive in Paraguay
Temperate South America	No risk except Argentina				*P. vivax* only
Pacific Islands/ Oceania		Papua New Guinea, Solomon Islands, Vanuatu. No malaria in countries beyond 20°S and 170°E	Significant risk	Reported in all areas	All areas *P. vivax; P. malariae* plus *P. ovale* in Papua, New Guinea
Australia and New Zealand	No risk				
North Africa/ Middle East (incl. Turkey)		All areas: Afghanistan,* Algeria,† Egypt,* Morocco,† Oman, Syria,† Turkey,† Yemen*	Limited risk*	Reported	Mostly *P. vivax*†
Sub-Saharan Africa		All areas except southern tip and Reunion, St. Helena, Seychelles, Lesotho Isles	Predominant species in most areas	In many areas highly chloroquine-resistant strains	*P. vivax*: Sudan and Mauritius; *P. malariae*, *P. ovale* elsewhere
Indian continent	All countries but absent in Maldives	Bangladesh, Bhutan, India, Nepal, Pakistan, Sri Lanka	Significant risk	Reported in all areas	*P. vivax* all areas; exclusive in Nepal
Southeast Asia and Far East	Wide variation within region and countries: Cambodia,‡, China,† Indonesia, Laos, Myanmar‡, Sabah (Malaysia), Thailand‡, Vietnam‡		Significant risk but only in very rural areas and not in tourist areas	Multidrug resistance‡	Mostly *P. vivax*†

*Indicates countries where *P. falciparum* occurs.
†Indicates countries where *P. vivax* occurs.
‡Multidrug-resistant *P. falciparum* present.

toes. Anophelines bite between dusk and dawn (whereas *Aedes* and some *Culex* mosquitoes will bite during the day and do not transmit malaria). Congenital infection is uncommon and can occur in nonimmune individuals. Infection, however, may also be transmitted accidentally, such as from a blood transfusion when the donor harbors malaria parasites or between drug addicts sharing the same hypodermic needle. Cases of malaria have also been described in inhabitants living near airports ("airport malaria") who have been inoculated by infective mosquitoes from malarious areas.

NATURAL INFECTION AND IMMUNITY

In general, when an infected mosquito bites, motile sporozoites are injected into the blood that invade the liver within 30 minutes. The parasite multiplies within the liver and releases thousands of merozoites, which invade red blood cells. In *P. vivax* and *P. ovale* malaria, a proportion of sporozoites differentiate into hypnozoites, which may remain dormant within the hepatocyte for months or years before giving rise to late relapses. Within the red blood cell, merozoites of all species mature and multiply by asexual replication to produce erythrocytic schizonts. With schizont rupture, neo-merozoites are released into the circulation to invade fresh erythrocytes, leading to amplification of the parasite biomass by repeated episodes of intraerythrocytic multiplication. In the human, asexual stages (trophozoites and schizonts) are responsible for clinical infection. Gametocytes *do not* cause clinical disease. The incubation period (time between inoculation and first clinical symptom) varies between species and with immunity and antimalarial medication. The incubation period for *P. falciparum* is generally 9 to 14 days; that for *P. vivax* is 12 to 17 days (although primary attack may occur up to 6 to 12 months after inoculation); that for *P. ovale* is 16 to 18 days; and that for *P. malariae* is 18 to 40 days. The development of immunity is slow, and it takes years of repeated exposure for immunity to malaria to become established. Currently, there are no effective vaccines available against malaria.

IMPORTED MALARIA AND THE TRAVELER

In the past 20 years, air travel has increased by almost 7% per year and is predicted to increase by more than 5% a year during the next 20 years. In 1995, in the United States the Centers for Disease Control and Prevention (CDC) received reports of 1167 cases of malaria, an increase of 15% from 1994. Of these, 48% were due to *P. vivax* and 39% were due to *P. falciparum;* most of the latter came from Africa. A retrospective study of patients presenting to the Hospital for Tropical Diseases in London showed that in those travelers who had returned from Africa in the previous 6 months, 61% of fevers were due to malaria. A recent meta-analysis of available data showed that 90% of travelers who are infected with malaria do not become unwell until they return home. Most cases of malaria, especially if diagnosed and treated early in the course of the illness, remain uncomplicated; however, in 12% the clinical course is severe and life-threatening, with a case-fatality rate in adult travelers of 2% to 6%. Most of these deaths were due to delays in diagnosis.

CLINICAL MALARIA

Malaria should be considered in any patient presenting with a fever who has traveled to or come from an endemic area. Although most patients present within a few months of their return, presentation can be delayed, particularly in the semi-immune, those who have taken prophylaxis, and *P. vivax, P. ovale,* and *P. malariae* infections. The usual presentation is with fever, but sometimes there can be nonspecific symptoms, particularly in children, such as cough, headache, malaise, vomiting, and diarrhea. Common supportive findings in malaria include splenomegaly, mild thrombocytopenia, anemia, and mild jaundice.

PARASITOLOGIC DIAGNOSIS

In general, any fever starting within 8 days of arrival to a malarial endemic area is probably *not* malaria. Three thick films taken 12 hours apart exclude most malarial infections in any patient exposed to malaria. If clinical suspicion is high, further films are warranted. Thick films are necessary to diagnose malaria, and a thin film is required to define species and stages. Failure to prepare and rigorously examine a thick film may lead to a false-negative malaria film, especially in nonimmune patients, who often present with scant parasitemias. The microscopist should examine 100 thick-film high-magnification fields. Despite this, some scanty infections may escape detection. There are a number of other tests that are used to detect parasitemia. The tests detect parasite-derived histidine-rich protein 2 (HRP-2) (e.g., *Para*Sight F, ICT malaria Pf, parasite lactate dehydrogenase [OptiMal]), or parasite nuclear material (quantitative buffy coat [QBC]) (Table 2). Polymerase chain reaction is useful, especially for low-level parasitemia, but it is time-consuming, is expensive, and requires considerable experience.

MILD OR SEVERE FALCIPARUM MALARIA

Of the four types of malaria in humans, only *P. falciparum* has the potential to transmit severe life-threatening disease. Initial workup should include parasite density, blood cell count, platelet count, electrolyte studies (including calcium), blood gas analysis, lactate and glucose determinations, liver function tests, clotting time, blood cultures, and C-reactive protein and glucose-6-phosphate dehydrogenase (G6PD) tests. The presence of any of the features in Table 3 indicates severe malaria. These patients ideally should be transferred to a high-dependency unit or an intensive care ward, and their cases warrant immediate discussion with an infectious disease specialist.

DIFFERENTIAL DIAGNOSIS

Although malaria should be suspected in any illnesses presenting in a traveler to an endemic area, 25% to 40% of fevers are caused by less exotic causes, such as sickle cell crisis, streptococcal pharyngitis, glandular fever (Epstein-Barr virus), influenza, sinusitis, urinary tract infection, pneumonia, meningitis, and other viral illnesses. Other imported causes of fever should be considered (Table 4). In any patient presenting with pyrexia of unknown origin, it is worth considering HIV, amebic liver abscess, leishmaniasis (bone marrow aspirate), tuberculosis (plus chest radiograph and Mantoux test), brucellosis, fungal infection, or malignancy.

TREATMENT

If the infective species of malaria is not known or the infection is mixed (e.g., *P. falciparum* and *P.*

TABLE 2. **Some Tests Used for the Diagnosis of Malaria**

Test	Manufacturer	Sensitivity (Range) %	Specificity (Range) %	Comments
ParaSight F	Becton Dickinson	94 (86–97)	94 (88–99)	*P. falciparum* only
ICT Malaria pf	ICT Diagnostics	90 (89–93)	98 (97–100)	*P. falciparum* only
OptiMAL	Flow, Inc.	93 (83–97)	99 (92–100)	Differentiates between *P. falciparum* and *P. vivax*
QBC	Becton Dickinson	90 (83–98)	96 (84–98)	Species differentiation difficult

Abbreviation: QBC = quantitative buffy coat.

TABLE 3. **Clinical and Laboratory Features of Severe Malaria**

Clinical Complications	Laboratory Complications
Depressed conscious state (of any degree)	Parasite density ≥2%
Repeated or prolonged convulsions	Schizonts in the peripheral blood film
Respiratory distress	Acidosis (pH <7.3) or lactate >2 mmol
Adult respiratory distress syndrome	Hypoxemia ± hypercapnia
Shock	Hypoglycemia
Signs of spontaneous bleeding	Prolonged clotting time ± thrombocytopenia
Bacterial infections	Anemia (hemoglobin <7.5 g/dL)
Jaundice	Bilirubin >40 μmol/L
Acute renal failure	Hemoglobinuria
Hematuria	

ovale), initial treatment should be for falciparum malaria. Doses are calculated per milligram of base for chloroquine (Aralen) and per milligram of salt for quinine.

Mild and Uncomplicated Malaria

Benign Malarias (P. vivax, P. ovale, P. malariae)

Chloroquine is the drug of choice, although some strains of *P. vivax* have now been described that display limited resistance to chloroquine. For *P. vivax* and *P. ovale,* treatment of latent forms requires primaquine. Higher doses are required for the Oceanic strains. Check for G6PD deficiency before starting primaquine treatment, because severe hemolysis is likely in those with reduced G6PD activity. In G6PD-deficient individuals, primaquine can be given in reduced dose (Table 5). Mefloquine (Lariam) has been shown to treat benign malarias, and halofantrine (Halfan) is active against *P. vivax;* However, radical cure (killing the hepatic stages) is still required with primaquine.

Uncomplicated P. falciparum *Malaria*

In most parts of the world, chloroquine resistance is widespread, and the use of chloroquine for the treatment of falciparum malaria is no longer recommended. All patients with *P. falciparum* malaria should be admitted for assessment and initiation of treatment. The patient should be regularly assessed to establish that features of severe malaria do not develop (see Table 3). Parasite density should be checked twice daily to ensure parasitologic cure. In general, the first-line treatment of uncomplicated malaria is quinine sulfate, mefloquine, or atovaquone/proguanil (Malarone). Quinine treatment should be followed by pyrimethamine/sulfadoxine (Fansidar), doxycycline (Vibramycin), or clindamycin (Cleocin).* Halofantrine may be given as an alternative, but it has been associated with severe cardiotoxicity. A specialist's opinion should be sought regarding the second-line therapy for treatment failures or in cases presenting from Southeast Asia (where quinine resistance is common). In the case of clinical or parasitologic deterioration, consider treatment with artemesinin derivatives in conjunction with mefloquine.

Severe *P. falciparum* Malaria

The *Cinchona* alkaloids (quinine dihydrochloride or quinidine gluconate) remain the first-line treat-

*Not FDA approved for this indication.

TABLE 4. **Common Imported Causes of Fever**

Diagnosis	Features	Differentiating Features
Dengue	Short incubation period (2–10 days) Headache, retro-orbital pain, myalgia	Rash, intense myalgia, neutropenia, thrombocytopenia
Typhoid	Fever (often low grade), cough, headache, gastrointestinal disturbance. Incubation period: 3 weeks to 2 months	Chest signs, tender abdomen, low white blood cell count, rose spots, and relative bradycardia (often not useful)
Hepatitis A, B, or E	Fever and jaundice, lethargy	Incubation period, serology, transaminases associated with malaria often of much lower intensity
Leptospirosis	Fever, sore throat, conjunctivitis Jaundice and liver failure less common	Exposure to water (e.g., rafting in Thailand)
Schistosomiasis	Katayama fever (9 days–5 weeks post exposure)	Eosinophilia, water exposure, or walking barefoot
Tick-bite fever (typhus)	Fever, macular rash (including soles and wrist), headache, myalgia	History of bite with eschar and positive serology for rickettsia
Amebic liver abscess	Subacute, fever, weight loss, history of diarrhea often absent	Neutrophilia; Chest radiograph shows right basal changes; liver ultrasound diagnostic
Leishmaniasis	Fever, hepatosplenomegaly, pancytopenia 6 weeks to 6 months (or longer)	Trephine bone marrow
Meningococcal disease	Fever, rash	Travel to endemic area or pilgrims to Mecca (hajj) festival

Table 5. **The Drug Treatment of *P. vivax, P. ovale,* and *P. malariae* Malaria in Children**

Drug	Adults	Children
Chloroquine*	600 mg (four 150-mg tablets) stat	10 mg base/kg stat then 5 mg/kg at 8, 24, and 36 hours
	300 mg after 12, 24, and 36 hours	
Primaquine		
Normal G6PD activity	15 mg daily for 14–21 days Use 20 mg for 14 days in patients returning from Oceania	0.25 mg base/kg daily for 14–21 days 0.33 mg/kg for 14 days in patients returning from Oceania
G6PD deficiency	30 mg once weekly for 8 weeks	500–750 μg/kg/wk for 8 weeks

*Either chloroquine phosphate (250 mg salt = 156 mg base) or chloroquine sulfate (200 mg salt = 147 mg base) may be used.
Abbreviation: G6PD = glucose-6-phosphate dehydrogenase.

ment of severe falciparum malaria, although alternative drugs, particularly the artemisinin derivatives, should be considered in patients returning from areas with documented quinine resistance. Supportive and adjunctive therapies are covered at the end of this section.

Antimalaria Treatment

Quinidine Gluconate

In America, a CDC review concluded, in 1991, that parenteral quinidine gluconate (Quinadex)* was the drug of choice for treatment of complicated *P. falciparum* infections. Since that time, intravenous quinine has been unavailable for treatment. Quinidine gluconate is given as a loading dose and by continuous infusion (Table 6) until quinine sulfate can be taken by mouth. Its properties are similar to those of quinine dihydrochloride. It should be given in conjunction with doxycycline, pyrimethamine/sulfadoxine, or clindamycin.* See Table 7 for malaria prophylaxis regimens.

Quinine Dihydrochloride

Parenteral quinine is prescribed as quinine dihydrochloride (122 mg of salt contains 100 mg of quinine base) made up in 5% or 10% dextrose. Intramuscular quinine can be given if intravenous access is not possible. The pharmacokinetics of intravenous and intramuscular quinine is similar, so the same doses apply. Local toxicity of the intramuscular route is avoided if the loading dose is diluted 1:1 with normal saline solution or sterile water and the dose is divided and administered into both thighs (not buttocks). Subsequent doses can be alternated between thighs.

Interactions and Main Complications

Mefloquine is a synthetic analogue of quinine, and the *quinine loading dose should be omitted if the patient has taken mefloquine prophylaxis* in the previous 24 hours or has received a treatment dose within the previous 3 days. The main complications of quinine and quinidine are hypoglycemia, cardiotoxicity, hypotension, heart block and ventricular arrhythmias, and cinchonism (tinnitus, deafness, headache, nausea, and visual disturbances). Patients should be monitored for hypoglycemia and QT interval prolongation. Quinine infusion should be reduced or stopped if the corrected QT interval becomes prolonged by more than 25% of the baseline value and should be reduced to every 12 hours in severe cinchonism or renal impairment.

*Not FDA approved for this indication.

Artemisinin Derivatives

In severe malaria, parenteral artesunate can be given intravenously on an alternative basis. Artemether* is formulated in peanut oil base and is given intramuscularly; it must never be given parenterally or to anyone with a history of peanut allergy. Artemisinin derivatives are given in conjunction with mefloquine or doxycycline. The usual length of treatment is 1 to 7 days. Shorter courses may be possible if mefloquine treatment is introduced when the patient is still tolerating oral medication, but if combined with doxycycline, then the treatment should be given for 7 days.

Complications and Management

Hyperpyrexia increases the risk of convulsions, particularly in children, and should be treated with antipyretics, although this may delay parasitic clearance.

Hypoglycemia is a common complication of severe malaria, particularly in children and pregnant women, and is exacerbated by quinine infusion. Quinine or quinidine† should therefore be reconstituted in 5% to 10% dextrose.

Secondary bacterial infection (meningitis/pneumonia/septicemia) occurs, and empirical antibiotics are warranted. Lumbar puncture may be delayed in the acute phase of cerebral malaria, especially in the presence of focal (in particular, brainstem) neurologic signs and until increased intracranial pressure has been excluded.

Convulsions should be treated in the conventional manner (i.e., a stepwise approach from benzodiazepines to intravenous loading doses of phenytoin [Dilantin]). Exclude hypoglycemia as a cause of convulsions.

*Not available in the United States.
†Not FDA approved for this indication.

TABLE 6. **Drug Treatment of *P. falciparum* Malaria**

Drug	Oral Treatment of Uncomplicated Malaria	Parenteral Treatment of Complicated Malaria
Quinine	Quinine sulfate 10 mg salt/kg q8h for 7 days Adults: 600 mg q8h *Plus one of the following*: Doxycycline 200-mg loading dose, then 100 mg daily for 6 d (drug of choice for Southeast Asian and Fansidar-resistant strains). In children >8 y give 3 mg/kg for 7 d Pyrimethamine/sulfadoxine (Fansidar) P = 1.5 mg/kg; S = 30 mg/kg single dose (adults: 3 tabs; children ≤4 y: ½ tab; 5–6 y: 1 tab; 7–9 y: 1½ tabs; 10–14 y: 2 tabs) Clindamycin* 10 mg/kg bid for 3–7 d	Quinine hydrochloride: loading dose 20 mg salt/kg IV over 4 h, then 10 mg/kg IV q8h with electrocardiographic monitoring and switch to oral quinine when able to tolerate *Plus one of the following*: Doxycycline, Fansidar, clindamycin (dose as for uncomplicated malaria)
Quinidine gluconate (Quinaglute)*		Loading dose: 10 mg/kg over 1 h followed by a 0.02-mg/kg/min continuous infusion until parasites are cleared *Plus one of the following:* Doxycycline, Fansidar, clindamycin
Malarone (atovaquone and proguanil)†	Total daily dose (A = 15–20 mg/kg; P = 6–8 mg/kg) Adults: 4 tabs daily for 3 d Children daily dose for 3 d: 11–20 kg: 1 tab; 21–30 kg: 2 tabs; 31–40 kg: 3 tabs; >40 kg: adult dose	
Mefloquine (Lariam)†	15 mg base/kg followed by a second dose of 10 mg/kg 8–24 h later	
Halofantrine (Halfan)†	8 mg/kg given 6 hours apart for three doses Adults: 500 mg q6h for three doses. Repeat treatment 1 wk later in nonimmune individuals	
Multidrug-resistant P. falciparum or *Second-Line (Treatment Failure)*		
Artemether‡ mefloquine	4 mg/kg/d for 3 days taken in combination with mefloquine single dose 15–25 mg/kg on day 3	3.2 mg/kg IM stat then 1.6 mg/kg IM once daily for 7 d Given in combination with mefloquine or doxycycline
Artemether‡ doxycycline	Artemether (4 mg/kg/d) for 7 d when combined with doxycycline (see dose earlier)	
Artesunate‡ mefloquine or doxycycline	4 mg/kg/d for 3 d taken in combination with mefloquine single dose 15–25 mg/kg on day 3 or doxycycline (see dose earlier)	2.4 mg/kg IV followed by 1.2 mg/kg at 12 and 24 h, then 1.2 mg/kg/d for 7 d Given in combination with mefloquine or doxycyline

*Not FDA approved for this indication.
†Not necessary to give doxycycline, Fansidar, or clindamycin after mefloquine, Malarone, or halofantrine.
‡Not available in the United States.

Increased intracranial pressure may occur and should be treated with mannitol (Osmitrol) (loading dose followed by continuous infusion) in the absence of shock or impaired renal function, although its efficacy is not proven. The effect of corticosteroids on increased intracranial pressure remains unproven.

Severe malaria anemia may occur. All patients with malaria will have some reduction of hemoglobin levels. Most patients remain stable and do not require transfusion. The decision to transfuse may be influenced by the parasitemia level and the clinical condition of the patient. In general, transfusion should be considered if the hemoglobin level falls below 7.5 g/dL.

Shock or severe acidosis may be a complicating factor. In adults, shock can be defined by hypotension (<2 SD mean blood pressure), but in children hypotension is a late feature of shock. Early signs include tachycardia and evidence of impaired perfusion (prolonged capillary refill, decreased urine output, or decreased consciousness). Treatment is with conventional bolus doses of resuscitation fluids, and consideration is given to artificial ventilation and inotropic support.

Respiratory distress in severe malaria is multifactorial (lactic acidosis is a common cause in children, but pulmonary edema and adult respiratory distress syndrome are more common in adults).

TABLE 7. **Malaria Prophylaxis Regimens**

Drug	Usage	Adult	Child Dosage	Comments
Mefloquine (Lariam)	Recommended for most areas	250 mg (one tablet) every week	Weekly dose: 5–19 kg: ¼ tab 20–30 kg: ½ tab 31–45 kg: ¾ tab >45 kg: 1 tab	Not recommended for persons with epilepsy, seizure disorders, severe psychiatric disorders, cardiac conduction abnormalities, early pregnancy (safe beyond first trimester)
Malaron (atovaquone and proguanil)	Alternative to mefloquine	Children >40 kg and adults: one adult tablet daily	Pediatric tablets 11–20 kg: 1 tab 21–30 kg: 2 tabs 31–40 kg: 3 tabs	Few side effects. Only need to take for 7 d after return from malaria endemic area
Doxycycline	Alternative to mefloquine (SE Asia, Oceania)	100 mg/d	Children > 8y 2 mg/kg/d (max: 100 mg/d)	Contraindicated in children <8 y of age, pregnant women, and lactating women
Chloroquine + proguanil	Alternative (Africa), if mefloquine or doxycycline cannot be used	Chloroquine, 300 mg once/week Proguanil, 200 mg/d	Fraction of adult dose (chloroquine weekly, proguanil daily) <2 mo: ⅛; 2–12 mo: ¼; 1–5 y: ½; 6–11 y: ¾	Proguanil is not sold in the United States but is available in Canada, Europe, and Africa. Less effective than mefloquine or doxycycline. Safe throughout pregnancy

Impaired clotting or disseminated intravascular coagulopathy is treated with fresh frozen plasma and platelet transfusions.

Impaired renal function is indicated by falling urine output and elevated levels of blood urea nitrogen and serum creatinine and can be treated conservatively. Hypovolemia should be treated until the central venous pressure is more than 5 mm Hg. Established renal failure should be treated with dialysis.

Other Adjunctive Therapies

Corticosteroids and heparin are contraindicated. The role of other ancillary therapies such as prostacycline,* dextran,* pentoxifylline (Trental),* and anti–tumor necrosis factor antibodies* remains unknown.

Exchange Transfusion

Although numerous accounts have been published reporting successful use of exchange transfusion in the treatment of severe malaria, these should be treated with some caution, owing to the positive reporting bias. Despite these concerns, exchange transfusion should be considered in the following circumstances:

- Parasitemia greater than 10% in the absence of any signs of severe disease
- Parasitemia of 2% to 10% in the presence of other signs of severe disease
- Any parasite density, if mature forms (schizonts) are seen in the peripheral film

It is recommended that a 1 or 2 volume exchange should be performed either manually or using an automated cell cycler. The aim is to reduce the parasitemia to less than 2%.

*Not FDA approved for this indication.

Notes on Antimalarial Agents for Nonsevere Falciparum Malaria

Chloroquine

Resistance to chloroquine (Aralen) is now extensive, and this drug cannot be relied on alone to produce a radical cure. In endemic areas, chloroquine is still used, especially where resistance is low grade, because the degree of immunity in patients contributes to the eradication of parasites. Chloroquine is still used to treat benign nonfalciparum malaria. Common complications include pruritus, nausea, diarrhea, and exacerbation of psoriasis.

Amodiaquine

Amodiaquine* belongs to the 4-aminoquinolone group of antimalarials, which also includes chloroquine. Its activity is similar to that of chloroquine, but it retains some activity against chloroquine-resistant strains of *P. falciparum*. Its side effects are more common, and it should never be used for malaria prophylaxis. Side effects include toxic hepatitis and agranulocytosis (occurring in 1:2000 people taking amodiaquine prophylactically).

Pyrimethamine/Sulfadoxine

Pyrimethamine is formulated in fixed combination with sulfadoxine (Fansidar). Resistance is well established in Southeast Asia and is rapidly emerging in Africa. The drug is well tolerated and is safe in pregnancy but should not be given to anyone with a history of sulfonamide sensitivity. The therapeutic and parasitologic response to treatment is usually slower than that of chloroquine. Other combinations of more rapidly eliminated antifolates and sulfones are being developed.

*Not available in the United States.

Cinchona Alkaloids: Quinine and Quinidine

Quinine and quinidine* are schizonticidal and result in longer parasite clearance times. Oral quinine is prescribed as quinine sulfate (121 mg of the salt, quinine sulfate, contains 100 mg of base) and is given for 7 days, unless vomiting is problematic; then it should be given as an intravenous infusion. Almost all patients will develop mild cinchonism, which makes it a difficult drug to use on outpatients owing to poor compliance. In severe cinchonism, the dose can be reduced to every 12 hours. Treatment should continue until parasite clearance has been achieved for 24 hours, and complete eradication can be ensured if given with one of the following antimalarials: doxycycline, pyrimethamine/sulfadoxine, or clindamycin.* One major side effect of quinine, hypoglycemia, is unusual when given orally in uncomplicated falciparum infection, except when treating pregnant women, in whom glucose levels should be monitored.

Mefloquine

Mefloquine (Lariam) is an excellent drug for treating uncomplicated chloroquine-resistant malaria. (It has no parenteral form.) Common side effects are nausea, vomiting, dysphoria, dizziness, sleep disturbance, and weakness. The gastrointestinal side effects are more common in children, and adults are more prone to neuropsychiatric side effects. Serious neuropsychiatric effects (seizures, encephalopathy, and psychosis) occur in 1:200 whites and blacks and 1:1000 Asians; these effects are self-limiting.

Atovaquone/Proguanil

In July 2000, the U.S. Food and Drug Administration approved atovaquone/proguanil (Malarone) for the prevention and treatment of malaria in adults and children. Atovaquone is a broad-spectrum antiprotozoal drug and acts by inhibition of parasite mitochondrial electron transport. It is highly effective against *P. falciparum* but has a high recrudescence rate when used alone. In combination with proguanil, it is highly effective and well tolerated. It is available in many countries for malaria prevention and treatment of acute, uncomplicated malaria caused by chloroquine-resistant *P. falciparum*. It is a safe drug with few side effects (usually abdominal pain, anorexia, nausea, vomiting, diarrhea, and coughing). Malarone is available in a fixed-dose combination in adult-strength (250 mg of atovaquone and 100 mg of proguanil hydrochloride per tablet) and pediatric-strength (62.5 mg of atovaquone and 25 mg of proguanil hydrochloride per tablet) forms. Limited data are available to date on the efficacy of Malarone for the treatment of benign malaria species, although treatment efficacy was high in small numbers of patients with *P. vivax* malaria treated with Malarone. It should be followed by primaquine for treatment of the persistent liver stage.

*Not FDA approved for this indication.

Halofantrine

Halofantrine is an excellent drug in the treatment of multidrug-resistant infections, but cardiotoxicity has limited its use. Cross-resistance of mefloquine has been reported. The absorption is erratic but can be increased by taking it with fatty foods. Halofantrine causes prolonged ventricular repolarization, manifesting as prolonged QT interval, and can cause ventricular fibrillation in patients with latent prolonged QT interval. A 12-lead electrocardiogram should be obtained before treatment to ensure that the patient has a normal QT interval. Halofantrine is available only as an oral preparation.

Artemisinin Derivatives

Artemisinin derivatives drugs are rapidly effective and well tolerated. They are all available in oral formulations. Artemether* and artesunate* are artemisinin derivatives and are five times more potent than the parent compound; however, they should always be given in conjunction with slower-acting antimalarials to prevent the development of resistance. Neither artemether nor artesunate is licensed in the United Kingdom or the United States; however, both have been used extensively in malarious areas, where they appear to be safe and highly effective.

HOW CAN MALARIA AND OTHER TRAVEL-RELATED ILLNESSES BE PREVENTED?

Before traveling to a foreign country for any reason, a traveler should visit his or her medical practitioner or travel center to inquire about necessary vaccinations and a prescription for antimalarial drugs. Up-to-date advice should be obtained, and the following sources are useful:

Centers for Disease Control and Prevention (United States): http://www.cdc.gov/travel/

Department of Health (United Kingdom): http://www.calaib.co.uk/launch-it/travax.htm

World Health Organization: http://www.who.int/ith/english/index.htm

The following advice should be given to anyone traveling to malaria-endemic areas:

1. Prevent mosquito and other insect bites.
   a. Wear suitable clothing that covers arms and legs (including feet) from dusk to dawn.
   b. Use diethyltoluamide (DEET) or dimethyl phthalate insect repellent on exposed skin, and use insect repellents in the room.
   c. Sleep under an insecticide (permethrin or deltamethrin)-impregnated bed net if living accommodation is not adequately screened.
   d. Sleep in air-conditioned rooms if possible.
2. Take the prophylactic antimalarial drug as prescribed, without missing doses, for 2 to 3 weeks before travel and 4 weeks after leaving a malari-

*Not available in the United States.

ous area (except for Malarone, which needs to be taken for only 1 week after). Chemoprophylaxis is not 100% effective, however.
3. If fever or flulike symptoms develop while traveling or for up to 1 year after return, malaria needs to be excluded; inform the doctor that exposure to malaria may have occurred.
4. Carry antimalarial agents for presumptive treatment if traveling in areas where immediate medical attention is not available.

CONCLUSION

Physicians should be familiar with diagnosis, management, and potential complications of malaria because it is likely that the number of cases of imported malaria seen annually will rise. Currently, there is no effective vaccine, and travelers should be advised on prevention of mosquito bites and compliance with the up-to-date recommendations for prophylaxis, as well as the symptoms of malaria.

BACTERIAL MENINGITIS

method of
KAREN L. ROOS, M.D.
Indiana University School of Medicine
Indianapolis, Indiana

Bacterial meningitis is an acute purulent infection within the subarachnoid space. More than the subarachnoid space is involved, however, and bacterial meningitis is frequently complicated by an altered level of consciousness, seizure activity, cranial nerve palsies, and stroke.

Before the availability of the *Haemophilus influenzae* type b (Hib) conjugate vaccines in 1987, Hib was the most common cause of bacterial meningitis in the United States. The incidence of *H. influenzae* meningitis has declined dramatically since 1987. At present, the most common causative organisms of community-acquired bacterial meningitis in children and adults are *Streptococcus pneumoniae* and *Neisseria meningitidis*. An increase in the incidence of meningococcal infection has been noted on college campuses. There has been a major change in the epidemiology of pneumococcal disease, with the global emergence and increasing prevalence of penicillin-resistant and cephalosporin-resistant strains of *S. pneumoniae*. In 1998, approximately 44% of clinical isolates of *S. pneumoniae* in the United States had intermediate or high levels of resistance to penicillin. Meningitis caused by strains of *N. meningitidis* with moderate or relative resistance to penicillin and decreased susceptibility to ampicillin has been reported worldwide. Group B streptococcus (or *Streptococcus agalactiae*) was previously primarily a meningeal pathogen in the neonatal age group. Meningitis resulting from this organism is increasingly reported in individuals older than 50 years of age, particularly individuals with chronic illness. In the mid-1980s, a combination of a third-generation cephalosporin and ampicillin was recommended for the empirical therapy of bacterial meningitis. Ampicillin was used in the empirical regimen to cover *Listeria monocytogenes*, which had emerged as a predominant causative organism of bacterial meningitis in individuals with impaired cell-mediated immunity from AIDS, organ transplantation, malignancy, or immunosuppressive therapy. The present use of trimethoprim-sulfamethoxazole (Bactrim) as prophylaxis for *Pneumocystis carinii* pneumonia has decreased the incidence of meningitis resulting from *L. monocytogenes*. This change and the emergence of penicillin-resistant and cephalosporin-resistant strains of *S. pneumoniae* have changed the recommendations for the empirical therapy of bacterial meningitis.

CLINICAL PRESENTATION

The classic triad of symptoms and signs of meningitis is fever, headache, and stiff neck. Nausea, vomiting, photophobia, and lethargy are also common complaints. A stiff neck, or nuchal rigidity, is present when the neck resists passive flexion. An elderly patient may have a stiff neck from arthritis or from a central nervous system degenerative disease such as Parkinson's disease. In these patients, the neck resists lateral rotation as well as passive flexion. The presence or absence of the Brudzinski sign may also be helpful in elderly patients to distinguish between a stiff neck from meningitis and that from another cause. The Brudzinski sign is elicited with the patient in the supine position and is positive when passive flexion of the neck results in spontaneous flexion of the hips and knees.

Meningitis in children either presents as a subacute infection that gets progressively worse over several days and was preceded by an upper respiratory infection or otitis media or can appear as an acute fulminant illness that develops rapidly in a few hours. Pneumonia may precede the development of symptoms of meningitis in an adult. Seizure activity occurs in approximately 40% of patients. Focal or generalized seizure activity may occur as part of the initial presentation of bacterial meningitis or any time during the course of the illness.

The rash of meningococcemia begins as a diffuse, erythematous, maculopapular rash resembling a viral exanthem, but the skin lesions of meningococcemia rapidly become petechial. Petechiae are found on the trunk and lower extremities, in the mucous membranes and conjunctivae, and, occasionally, on the palms and soles. Other infectious diseases that may manifest with a petechial, purpuric, or erythematous maculopapular rash similar to that of meningococcemia include enteroviral meningitis, Rocky Mountain spotted fever, bacterial endocarditis, echovirus type 9 viremia, West Nile fever encephalitis, and pneumococcal or *H. influenzae* meningitis. The location of the rash predominantly on the trunk and lower extremities is typical of meningococcemia.

Increased intracranial pressure is an expected complication of bacterial meningitis and is the major cause of obtundation and coma in this disease. The most common signs of increased intracranial pressure in bacterial meningitis are an altered (especially deteriorating) level of consciousness and papilledema. The symptoms and signs of bacterial meningitis in the neonate are often subtle and nonspecific and include fever, lethargy, poor feeding, respiratory distress, irritability, vomiting and diarrhea, seizures, and a bulging fontanelle.

DIAGNOSIS

When the clinical presentation is suggestive of bacterial meningitis, blood cultures should be obtained and empirical antimicrobial therapy initiated immediately. A cranial magnetic resonance imaging (MRI) or computed tomography (CT) scan can be obtained followed by lumbar puncture. The necessity of neuroimaging before lumbar puncture has been debated for years. If the neurologic examination shows no focal deficits, the level of consciousness is normal, and there is no evidence of papilledema, it is safe to perform lumbar puncture without imaging the brain first. The clinical presentation rapidly may become complicated by a deteriorating level of consciousness and seizure activity, however, and the appearance and management of these complications are better tolerated by the physician if neuroimaging has been obtained before lumbar puncture. If the patient is being treated with antibiotics, there is no risk in delaying lumbar puncture until after neuroimaging is performed. Antibiotic therapy for several hours before lumbar puncture does not alter the cerebrospinal fluid (CSF), white blood cell count, or glucose concentration so significantly that the possibility of bacterial meningitis is not suspected, and it is not likely to sterilize the CSF so that the organism cannot be identified on Gram stain or grown in culture. MRI is preferred over CT because of its superiority in showing areas of cerebral edema and ischemia. The meninges enhance diffusely after the administration of gadolinium. This is a nonspecific abnormality, however, and occurs in any process in which there is an increase in permeability of the blood-brain barrier.

The diagnosis of bacterial meningitis is made by examination of the CSF. The classic CSF abnormalities in bacterial meningitis are as follows: (1) increased opening pressure, (2) pleocytosis of polymorphonuclear leukocytes, (3) decreased glucose concentration, and (4) increased protein concentration.

Opening pressure should be measured in the lateral recumbent position because the sitting position does not allow accurate measurement of CSF pressure. The normal range of opening pressure for infants and children up to 6 years old is 10 to 120 mm H_2O; for children and adults, 10 to 180 mm H_2O; and for obese adults, 10 to 250 mm H_2O. The number of white blood cells in CSF varies normally with age. The upper limit of normal for neonates for CSF total white blood cell count is 22 per mm^3 in full-term neonates, 30 per mm^3 in infants 0 to 8 weeks old, and 5 per mm^3 in infants older than 8 weeks of age. In newborns, about 60% of the cells in normal uninfected CSF are polymorphonuclear leukocytes, and 40% are mononucleated cells. In children and adults, the normal white blood cell count in uninfected CSF ranges from 0 to 5 mononuclear cells (lymphocytes and monocytes) per mm^3. In normal uninfected CSF, there should be no polymorphonuclear leukocytes; however, with the use of the cytocentrifuge, an occasional polymorphonuclear leukocyte may be seen. If the total white blood cell count is less than 5, the presence of a single polymorphonuclear leukocyte may be considered normal. In patients with bacterial meningitis, there are 10 to 10,000 white blood cells per mm^3 in CSF, with a predominance of polymorphonuclear leukocytes. A normal CSF glucose concentration is 45 to 80 mg/dL in patients with a blood glucose concentration of 70 to 120 mg/dL. Values less than 45 mg/dL are abnormal, and a CSF glucose concentration of 0 mg/dL is not unusual in patients with bacterial meningitis. Use of the CSF/serum glucose ratio corrects for hyperglycemia, which may mask a decreased CSF glucose concentration. The CSF glucose concentration is low when the CSF/serum glucose ratio is less than 0.6. A CSF/serum glucose ratio less than or equal to 0.31 is highly predictive of bacterial meningitis. It takes approximately 4 hours for the CSF glucose concentration to reach equilibrium with the blood glucose concentration after the administration of glucose; an ampule of 50% dextrose in water (50 mL of 50% glucose) before lumbar puncture, as commonly occurs en route to, or in, the emergency department, is unlikely to alter the CSF glucose concentration significantly, unless more than a few hours have passed between glucose administration and lumbar puncture. Normal CSF protein values are less than 45 mg/dL. The CSF protein concentration is increased in bacterial meningitis, but this is a nonspecific abnormality. The CSF protein concentration is increased in any process that increases the blood-brain permeability.

Gram stain is positive in 70% to 90% of untreated cases of bacterial meningitis. CSF polymerase chain reaction (PCR) tests are not as useful in the diagnosis of bacterial meningitis as they are in the diagnosis of viral central nervous system infections. A PCR assay is available for all of the common meningeal pathogens, but their sensitivity and specificity have not been defined.

The latex particle agglutination test for the detection of bacterial antigens of *S. pneumoniae, N. meningitidis*, Hib, group B streptococcus, and *Escherichia coli* K1 strains in the CSF is useful for making a rapid diagnosis of bacterial meningitis and in detecting the disease in patients who have been pretreated with oral or parenteral antibiotics, in whom Gram stain and CSF culture are negative. The latex particle agglutination test has a specificity of 96% for *S. pneumoniae* and 100% for *N. meningitidis*. It has a sensitivity of 69% to 100% for the detection of *S. pneumoniae* in CSF and a sensitivity of 33% to 70% for the detection of bacterial antigens of *N. meningitidis* in CSF. A negative latex particle agglutination test for bacterial antigens does not rule out bacterial meningitis. The Limulus amebocyte lysate assay is a rapid diagnostic test for the detection of gram-negative endotoxin in CSF and for making a diagnosis of gram-negative bacterial meningitis. This test is reported to have a sensitivity of 99.5% and a specificity of 86% to 99.8%. CSF bacterial culture is positive in 80% of untreated cases.

Lumbar puncture should be performed with a 22- or 25-gauge needle, and a minimum amount of CSF should be removed for analysis. Approximately 6 mL of CSF is sufficient to obtain cell count and glucose and protein concentrations, Gram stain and culture, and latex agglutination. An additional 1 mL of CSF can be sent to the PCR laboratory for viral DNA analysis, because viral encephalitis is the leading disease in the differential diagnosis of bacterial meningitis.

If there are skin lesions, biopsy specimens of these should be obtained. The rash of meningococcemia results from the dermal seeding of organisms with vascular endothelial damage, and biopsy may reveal the organism on Gram stain.

DIFFERENTIAL DIAGNOSIS

The leading disease in the differential diagnosis of bacterial meningitis is viral meningoencephalitis, including herpes simplex virus (HSV) encephalitis and the arthropod-borne viral encephalitides. The clinical presentation of HSV encephalitis includes hemicranial headache and fever with one or a combination of the following: behavioral abnormalities, focal or generalized seizure activity, and focal neurologic deficits (disturbance of language, hemiparesis with greater involvement of face and arm, or superior quadrantic visual field defects). The symptoms of HSV encephalitis typically evolve over several days. Patients with HSV encephalitis usually have MRI abnormalities. On T_2-weighted and fluid-attenuated inversion recovery (FLAIR) images, high–signal-intensity lesions may be seen in the medial and inferior temporal lobe extending up into the insula. There is a distinctive electroencephalographic pattern in HSV encephalitis consisting of periodic stereotyped sharp and slow wave complexes from one or both temporal areas that occur at regular intervals of 2 to 3 seconds. Examination of the CSF reveals an increased opening pressure, a lymphocytic pleocytosis of 5 to 500 cells per mm^3, a mild to moderate elevation in the protein concentration, and a normal or mildly decreased glucose concentration. CSF viral cultures for HSV-1 are almost always negative. The PCR technique for HSV DNA in CSF is typically positive early in infection, with a decline after the first week. PCR obtained from bloody CSF may result in a false-negative result. Antibodies to HSV appear in CSF approximately 8 to 12 days after the onset of symptoms and can be detected for at least 30 days.

During the summer and early fall months when mosquitoes are biting, arthropod-borne (arbovirus) viral encephalitis is in the differential diagnosis. In the United States, the La Crosse virus and St. Louis encephalitis virus are the most common causes of arbovirus encephalitis. Eastern equine encephalitis virus causes the most severe arbovirus encephalitis, and the fatality rate is high. Japanese encephalitis virus is the most common cause of arthropod-borne human encephalitis worldwide.

Patients with arthropod-borne viral encephalitis may have an influenza-like prodrome of malaise, nausea and vomiting, myalgias, and fever before symptoms of encephalitis, which include headache, confusion, disorientation, irritability, stupor, and convulsions. Neuroimaging is normal, or there may be nonspecific abnormalities in arboviral encephalitis. Examination of the CSF shows a polymorphonuclear leukocytic pleocytosis early in infection with a shift to a lymphocytic or mononuclear pleocytosis later in the illness. The CSF glucose concentration is normal. The diagnosis is made by showing a fourfold or greater rise in antibody titer between acute and convalescent sera or the isolation of the virus from tissue, blood, or CSF.

Viral meningitis is in the differential diagnosis only if the clinical presentation is limited to fever, headache, and stiff neck. Patients with viral meningitis do not have focal neurologic deficits, an altered level of consciousness, or seizure activity. Polymorphonuclear leukocytes may predominate in CSF early in viral meningitis, but thereafter, lymphocytes predominate, and the glucose concentration is normal. The tests on CSF that best identify the causative organism of viral meningitis are viral cultures, reverse-transcriptase PCR (RT-PCR) for enteroviral RNA, and PCR for HIV RNA and HSV-2 DNA.

Focal infectious intracranial mass lesions, including brain abscess, subdural empyema, and epidural abscess, should be included in the differential diagnosis. If a focal infectious mass lesion is suspected by the clinical presentation or examination, a lumbar puncture should not be performed until a mass lesion has been ruled out by either MRI or CT scan. A bacterial brain abscess typically appears as an expanding mass lesion rather than an infectious process. The most common symptom is headache, which is characterized as a constant, dull, aching sensation that is hemicranial or generalized and becomes progressively worse. Fever is present in only 50% of patients at the time of diagnosis. New-onset focal or generalized seizure activity is the presenting sign in 25% to 30% of patients. A focal neurologic deficit, such as a hemiparesis, is part of the initial presentation in more than 60% of patients. A subdural empyema appears with fever and a progressively worsening headache that is initially localized to the side of the subdural infection. As the empyema evolves, focal neurologic deficits, seizures, and signs of increased intracranial pressure develop. Contralateral hemiplegia is the most common focal neurologic deficit. If untreated, the increasing mass effect from a subdural empyema and increase in intracranial pressure cause progressive deterioration in consciousness, leading to stupor and then coma. A cranial epidural abscess manifests with severe hemicranial headache and fever. The presence of a focal infectious mass lesion is ruled out by neuroimaging.

The classic presentation of a subarachnoid hemorrhage is the explosive onset of a severe headache or a sudden transient loss of consciousness followed by a severe headache. Nuchal rigidity and vomiting are frequently present; therefore, subarachnoid hemorrhage is included in the differential diagnosis of bacterial meningitis. A dilated nonreactive pupil is suggestive of a subarachnoid hemorrhage from an aneurysm of the posterior communicating artery. When a subarachnoid hemorrhage has occurred, CT scan may show blood in the basal cisterns. If the CT scan is normal, examination of the CSF is indicated. Red blood cells are present in the CSF within minutes of the rupture of an intracranial aneurysm. A sample of the bloody CSF should be centrifuged. In a subarachnoid hemorrhage, the supernatant is a yellow, or xanthochromic, color within 2 to 4 hours of the subarachnoid hemorrhage.

TREATMENT

Empirical Antimicrobial Therapy

Antimicrobial therapy is initiated when bacterial meningitis is suspected, before the results of CSF Gram stain and culture and antimicrobial susceptibility tests are known. The most common causative organisms of community-acquired bacterial meningitis in children and adults are *S. pneumoniae* and *N. meningitidis*. Empirical therapy should be based on the possibility that penicillin-resistant and cephalosporin-resistant pneumococci are the causative organisms of the meningitis and should include a third-generation cephalosporin, either ceftriaxone (Rocephin) (pediatric dose, 100 mg/kg/d in a 12-hour dosing interval; adult dose, 2 g every 12 hours) or cefotaxime (Claforan) (pediatric dose, 200 mg/kg/d in a 4- to 6-hour dosing interval; adult dose, 2 g every 4 hours), plus vancomycin (Vancocin) (pediatric dose, 40 to 60 mg/kg/d in a 6- or 12-hour dosing interval; adult dose, 500 mg every 6 hours or 1 g every 12 hours). Ampicillin should be added to the empirical regimen for coverage of *L. monocytogenes* in individuals with impaired cell-mediated immunity because of chronic illness, organ transplantation, pregnancy, AIDS, malignancies, or immunosuppressive therapy, if they have not been on trimethoprim-sulfamethoxazole prophylactic therapy. Enteric gram-negative bacilli are the causative organisms of meningitis that is associated with chronic and debilitating diseases, such as diabetes, cirrhosis, or alcoholism. Enteric gram-negative bacillary meningitis is treated with a third-generation cephalosporin. In hospital-acquired meningitis and in neurosurgical patients, in whom staphylococci and gram-negative organisms are possible causative organisms, empirical therapy should include a combination of vancomycin and ceftazidime (Fortaz). Ceftazidime should be substituted for ceftriaxone or cefotaxime in neurosurgical patients and in

TABLE 1. **Antimicrobial Therapy for Bacterial Meningitis**

		Total Daily Dose	
Organism	**Antibiotic**	*Pediatric (Dosing Interval)*	*Adult (Dosing Interval)*
Streptococcus pneumoniae			
Sensitive to penicillin	Penicillin G	0.2 million U/kg (q4h)	20–24 million U/d (q4h)
	or		
	Ampicillin	200–300 mg/kg/d (q4h)	12 g/d (q4h)
Relatively resistant to penicillin	Ceftriaxone	100 mg/kg/d (q12h)	4 g/d (q12h)
	or		
	Cefotaxime	200 mg/kg/d (q4h)	12 g/d (q4h)
Resistant to pencillin	Vancomycin	40–60 mg/kg/d (q6–12h)	2 g/d (q6–12h)
	plus		
	Cefotaxime *or* ceftriaxone		
	with or without		
	Intraventricular vancomycin	10 mg/d	20 mg/d
Neisseria meningitidis	Penicillin G		
	or		
	Ampicillin		
Gram-negative bacilli (*Escherichia coli*, *Klebsiella* species, *Haemophilus* species, but not *Pseudomonas aeruginosa*)	Cefotaxime *or* Ceftriaxone		
P. aeruginosa	Ceftazidime	150–200 mg/kg/d (q8h)	8 g/d (q8h)
Staphylococci			
Methicillin-sensitive	Nafcillin	150–200 mg/kg/d (q4h)	12 g/d (q4h)
Methicillin-resistant	Vancomycin		
	with or without		
	Intraventricular vancomycin		
Streptococcus agalactiae	Penicillin G		
Listeria monocytogenes	Ampicillin		
	with or without		
	Gentamicin	7.5 mg/kg/d (q8h)	5 mg/kg/d (q8h)

neutropenic patients because *Pseudomonas aeruginosa* may be the meningeal pathogen, and ceftazidime is the only third-generation cephalosporin with sufficient activity against *P. aeruginosa* in the central nervous system. The empirical therapy of neonatal bacterial meningitis should include a combination of ampicillin plus cefotaxime or ampicillin plus gentamicin to cover *S. agalactiae, E. coli, L. monocytogenes*, and *Klebsiella pneumoniae*.

Specific Antimicrobial Therapy

Table 1 lists the specific antimicrobial agents that are recommended when the results of bacterial culture and antimicrobial susceptibility tests are known. The pediatric and adult doses of each antibiotic are provided. Table 2 lists the recommended antimicrobial therapy of neonatal bacterial meningitis.

Meningococcal Meningitis

Penicillin G or ampicillin can be used for meningococcal meningitis. All CSF isolates of *N. meningitidis* should be tested for penicillin and ampicillin susceptibility. If antimicrobial susceptibility testing shows that the isolate is a relatively penicillin-resistant strain of meningococci and in areas with a high prevalence of meningococci with decreased susceptibility to penicillin, cefotaxime or ceftriaxone should be used. A 7-day course of intravenous antibiotic therapy is adequate for most uncomplicated cases of meningococcal meningitis. The index case and all close contacts should receive chemoprophylaxis with a 2-day regimen of rifampin (Rimactane) (adult dose, 600 mg every 12 hours for 2 days; pediatric dose [children >1 year old], 10 mg/kg every 12 hours for 2 days). Rifampin should not be used in pregnant women. Adults can alternatively be treated with 1 dose of ciprofloxacin (Cipro), 750 mg, or azithromycin (Zithromax), 500 mg. Close contacts are defined as individuals who have had contact with oropharyngeal secretions through kissing or through sharing toys, beverages, or cigarettes.

TABLE 2. **Antimicrobial Therapy for Neonatal Bacterial Meningitis**

Organism	**Antimicrobial Agent**
Group B streptococcus	Ampicillin + aminoglycoside
	or
	Penicillin + aminoglycoside
Escherichia coli	Cefotaxime + aminoglycoside
Listeria monocytogenes	Ampicillin + aminoglycoside
Staphylococcus aureus	Methicillin or vancomycin
Staphylococcus epidermidis	Vancomycin
Citrobacter diversus	Ampicillin

Pneumococcal Meningitis

Antimicrobial therapy of pneumococcal meningitis is initiated with a third-generation cephalosporin and vancomycin. All CSF isolates of *S. pneumoniae* should be tested for sensitivity to penicillin and the third-generation cephalosporins. Once the results of antimicrobial susceptibility tests are known, therapy can be modified accordingly (see Table 1). For *S. pneumoniae* meningitis, an isolate is defined as penicillin-susceptible when the minimal inhibitory concentration (MIC) is less than or equal to 0.06 μg/mL, to be relatively resistant to penicillin when the MIC is 0.1 to 1.0 μg/mL, and to be resistant to penicillin when the MIC is greater than 1.0 μg/mL. An isolate of *S. pneumoniae* with MICs for cefotaxime or ceftriaxone greater than or equal to 0.5 to 1.0 μg/mL is considered to have intermediate resistance to the cephalosporins, and an isolate with a MIC greater than or equal to 2 μg/mL is considered to be highly resistant. Vancomycin is initially given by parenteral administration, but consideration should be given to using intraventricular vancomycin in patients not responding to parenteral vancomycin. Cefepime (Maxipime) is a broad-spectrum fourth-generation cephalosporin with in vitro activity similar to that of cefotaxime or ceftriaxone against *S. pneumoniae* and *N. meningitidis*. In clinical trials, cefepime has been shown to be equivalent to cefotaxime in the treatment of pneumococcal and meningococcal meningitis. Meropenem (Merrem) is a carbapenem antibiotic structurally related to imipenem but reportedly with less seizure proclivity than imipenem. Meropenem shows good activity against penicillin-resistant pneumococci in vitro, but the number of patients enrolled in clinical trials of meropenem in bacterial meningitis has not been sufficient to date to assess its efficacy against penicillin-resistant pneumococci or its epileptogenic potential. For pneumococcal meningitis, a repeat lumbar puncture should be performed 24 to 36 hours after the initiation of antimicrobial therapy to document eradication of the pathogen. A 2-week course of intravenous antimicrobial therapy is recommended for pneumococcal meningitis.

Gram-Negative Bacillary Meningitis

The third-generation cephalosporins, cefotaxime, ceftriaxone, and ceftazidime, are equally efficacious for the treatment of gram-negative bacillary meningitis, with the exception of *P. aeruginosa*. Ceftazidime is the drug of choice for *P. aeruginosa* meningitis. A 3-week course of intravenous antibiotic therapy is recommended for meningitis caused by gram-negative bacilli.

Staphylococcal Meningitis

Meningitis caused by *Staphylococcus aureus* or coagulase-negative staphylococci is treated with nafcillin (Nafcil) or oxacillin (Bactocill). Vancomycin is the drug of choice for methicillin-resistant staphylococci and for patients allergic to penicillin. The CSF should be monitored during therapy, and if the CSF continues to yield viable organisms after 48 hours of parenteral therapy, intrathecal or intraventricular vancomycin can be added (see Table 1).

Adjunctive Therapy

A meta-analysis of randomized, concurrently controlled trials of dexamethasone (Decadron) therapy in patients with childhood bacterial meningitis published from 1988 to 1996 confirmed benefit for Hib meningitis if begun with or before antibiotics and suggested benefit for children with pneumococcal meningitis. The American Academy of Pediatrics recommends the consideration of dexamethasone for bacterial meningitis in infants and children 2 months of age and older. The recommended dose is 0.6 mg/kg/d in four divided doses (0.15 mg/kg per dose) given intravenously for the first 4 days of antibiotic therapy. Clinical trials of dexamethasone therapy in adults with bacterial meningitis are ongoing. Scientists working in the area of the molecular basis of neurologic injury in bacterial meningitis are in favor of the use of dexamethasone because of its beneficial effect in inhibiting the synthesis of the inflammatory cytokines. There has been concern that dexamethasone may decrease the penetration of vancomycin into the CSF, but this has not been supported by clinical experience.

PREVENTION

The Advisory Committee on Immunization Practices recommends that college freshmen be vaccinated against meningococcal meningitis with the tetravalent (MenA,C,W135,Y) meningococcal polysaccharide vaccine. MenC polysaccharide vaccine would also be effective. There has been an increasing incidence of meningococcal infection outbreaks on college campuses. Most of these have been caused by serogroup C *N. meningitidis*, which is potentially preventable by vaccine. During an outbreak of meningococcal disease, individuals who have not been previously vaccinated should be treated with chemoprophylaxis (see earlier). Of secondary cases of meningococcal disease, 33% develop within 2 to 5 days of appearance of the index case. Vaccination is not a substitute for chemoprophylaxis to prevent secondary disease because there is an insufficient amount of time for optimal effect of vaccination, which requires approximately 1 to 2 weeks for good antibody production.

Vaccination against the pneumococcus is recommended for three at-risk populations: adults older than age 65, adults with chronic underlying diseases (cardiopulmonary diseases, renal diseases, diabetes mellitus, splenectomy, or CSF fistula), and immunocompromised patients older than 10 years of age. Individuals infected with HIV should also be vaccinated against the pneumococcus.

INFECTIOUS MONONUCLEOSIS

method of
ELBA A. IGLESIAS, M.D., and
MARTIN FISHER, M.D.
North Shore–Long Island Jewish Health System
Manhasset, New York

Infectious mononucleosis (IM) was first described as a clinical entity in the early 1900s. Pharyngitis, fever, fatigue, and lymphadenopathy are just some of the clinical findings associated with this very complex disease. Since that time, there has been an expanding fund of knowledge pertaining to IM. Research continues to be conducted to study the clinical spectrum of disease to aid in making the diagnosis and in hopes of reducing morbidity associated with the complications of IM.

ETIOLOGY

Epstein-Barr virus (EBV) was first discovered as a cause of IM in the 1960s. EBV is known to infect B lymphocytes, leading to their uncontrolled proliferation. EBV has been linked to diseases such as Burkitt lymphoma and other lymphoproliferative disorders. Infection is spread from person to person through respiratory droplets. The virus may remain dormant in salivary glands and may periodically reactivate. This may lead to shedding of the virus in the saliva of infected individuals.

Although IM has mostly been associated with EBV, other infectious agents, including cytomegalovirus, adenovirus, human immunodeficiency virus, human herpesvirus 6, and *Toxoplasma gondii*, may lead to a very similar clinical syndrome. Approximately 90% of patients who have the classic clinical symptoms of IM have acute EBV infection. Much of the following discussion pertains to EBV-related IM, because this has been the most widely studied and is seen most often clinically.

EPIDEMIOLOGY

More than 90% of adults worldwide test positive for past EBV infection. The peak incidence of IM occurs in the adolescent age group. EBV is transmitted through oropharyngeal secretions and more rarely through blood products. IM has been known in the past as the "kissing disease," secondary to one of its modes of transmission. The incubation period is between 30 and 50 days. Shedding of the virus is known to occur from the oropharynx for months and then decreases gradually. EBV has not been found to be transmitted easily in the home but is easily transmitted to sexual partners. Individuals with acquired immunodeficiency syndrome (AIDS), as well as other immunodeficiency states, are known to have higher rates of viral shedding. They are also at risk of developing lymphomas related to defective regulation of EBV infection. An example of this, as mentioned earlier, is Burkitt lymphoma. Primary EBV infection leads to a protective immunologic response. Therefore, individuals who are re-exposed are not susceptible to reinfection.

CLINICAL MANIFESTATIONS

EBV infection has a wide range of clinical presentations. Infection can range from asymptomatic seroconversion to more severe clinical syndromes. Symptoms of IM may include fever, malaise, lymphadenopathy, fatigue, and exudative pharyngitis. Lymphadenopathy may be diffuse, usually occurring in the anterior and posterior cervical chains and in the occipital nodes. Fever may be as high as 104°F (40°C). Malaise and fatigue usually persist throughout the entire course of the acute illness. Fatigue may be the only presenting symptom in IM and can be disabling, with a prolonged course.

Splenomegaly occurs in most patients (up to 100% of those who have been studied by ultrasonography) but is detectable on palpation in only 20% to 40% of patients. Hepatitis, occasionally with clinical manifestations, may also be a presenting symptom of acute IM, and up to 90% of patients have elevated transaminase levels. Symptoms of IM usually peak 7 days after the onset of illness and last an average of 2 to 3 weeks. Lymphadenopathy and splenomegaly may persist for weeks after the acute illness. A rash may develop in patients with IM receiving the antibiotic ampicillin. In children, the usual manifestation of IM may be only that of an upper respiratory tract infection.

DIAGNOSIS

Along with the above mentioned clinical manifestations, laboratory tests may help in making the diagnosis of EBV-induced IM. Heterophile antibodies, which are IgM antibodies that bind to red blood cells from non human species (such as sheep), are very useful in making the initial diagnosis. The longer the time from the onset of symptoms, the higher the percentage of people who have a positive heterophile antibody test. Most people older than 4 years of age will have a positive heterophile test by the end of the first week of symptoms. The accuracy of the test also varies according to which test kit is used, with sensitivity and specificity varying among the various commercially available tests. Heterophile antibodies may be positive for up to 1 year from the onset of symptoms.

Other virus-specific antibody tests are useful in confirming the diagnosis of acute EBV-IM, especially in cases that are not clinically obvious. IgG and IgM antibodies to the viral capsid antigen aid in the diagnosis of acute versus past EBV infection. IgM antibodies develop quickly at the onset of infection, generally by 1 to 2 weeks, and may persist for weeks to months. They are usually not detectable by 6 months after infection. Therefore, testing positive for IgM antibodies is indicative of a recent infection. IgG antibodies are usually detectable several weeks after the onset of infection and have a lifetime persistence. Therefore, the presence of IgG antibodies, along with negative findings for IgM antibodies, is indicative of past infection. Anti-EBNA antibodies (to the EBV nuclear antigen) usually develop 6 to 12 weeks after acute infection and have a lifetime persistence.

Other laboratory findings consistent with IM include atypical lymphocytosis, mild thrombocytopenia, and, occasionally, mild hemolytic anemia. Leukocytosis may be seen during the first 1 to 2 weeks, with subsequent leukopenia for the remainder of the acute illness. Abnormalities may be found in the urine, such as proteinuria, pyuria, and hematuria. Reports have indicated that up to one third of patients with IM are found to be concomitantly infected with group A β-hemolytic streptococci in the throat, although many of these patients may be only carriers.

THERAPY/MANAGEMENT

Management of IM is mostly supportive. Bed rest may be recommended for those with a more severe acute illness or a prolonged course. Fever reduction with acetaminophen or ibuprofen is recommended. Splenic rupture is a known complication of IM, and patients are therefore advised to avoid exercise or contact sports for a period of at least 4 weeks. Evaluation of the spleen with ultrasonography has been recommended by some authorities after 1 month of acute illness in athletes who wish to resume sports activities. Health care providers may recommend resumption of daily activities on improvement or resolution of symptoms.

Corticosteroids are used in the treatment of IM, but usually only in cases of more severe illness. Although they have been shown to shorten the duration of symptoms, such as fever and malaise, corticosteroids are not recommended in uncomplicated IM. Corticosteroids are extremely beneficial in severe cases with upper airway obstruction (see later). The effectiveness of corticosteroids for other complications, such as hemolytic anemia or neurologic disease, is controversial. Acyclovir* (Zovirax) has also been studied as a treatment modality for IM. Studies have shown, however, that although oropharyngeal viral shedding is decreased during treatment, complications of IM are not found to be less in patients treated with acyclovir, and patients do not have a significant decrease in symptoms.

COMPLICATIONS

Splenomegaly, although detectable by palpation in few patients, is detectable ultrasonographically in nearly all patients with IM and usually resolves in 1 month. Splenic rupture, a potentially fatal complication of IM, has been reported in the literature. Thankfully, this occurs rarely. Nearly all cases of splenic rupture occur 4 to 21 days after the onset of symptoms. This complication may be easily diagnosed with the aid of ultrasonography in a patient who is hemodynamically unstable and needs emergency intervention. The presence of intraperitoneal fluid is indicative of a ruptured spleen. Splenectomy is required in most cases, although conservative management (using a catheter to drain a hematoma) has been shown to be successful in some situations.

Upper airway obstruction is another potentially life-threatening complication of IM. Patients usually present with severe lymphadenopathy, pharyngitis, and difficulty speaking or swallowing. These patients usually require inpatient monitoring with corticosteroid treatment, intravenous fluids, and close observation. On occasion, establishment of an airway may be necessary.

Other rare complications of IM have been reported in organ systems other than the spleen and the respiratory tract. These include nervous system complications such as cranial nerve palsies and encephalitis. Myocarditis and pleuritis have each been reported in rare cases of EBV-associated IM. Clinically significant renal and hepatic complications have also been seen in acute cases of EBV-associated IM but are extremely rare.

*Not FDA approved for this indication.

OUTCOME

Most patients with acute IM return to full functioning within several weeks or months after the onset of illness. Some patients report feeling a persistent low level of fatigue for 6 to 12 months. Several studies have suggested that psychological status at the onset of illness may affect the severity and the duration of symptoms. Chronic fatigue syndrome, which at one time was thought to be due to an ongoing EBV infection, is now believed to be an independent entity, although viral illnesses may serve as the precipitant for the onset of symptoms in many patients with chronic fatigue and EBV is undoubtedly one of the viruses that may play that role. A separate entity, referred to as chronic active EBV infection, is reported in rare patients; it has a high level of mortality, and its susceptibility may have a familial basis. This entity is marked by a severe and persistent illness, organ system diseases (including pneumonitis, hepatitis, bone marrow hypoplasia, and uveitis), and evidence of EBV antigens in body tissues. This last condition should not be confused with either routine mononucleosis, which is almost always associated with a full recovery, or the chronic fatigue syndrome, which has a multifactorial etiology and is not due to EBV per se.

CHRONIC FATIGUE SYNDROME

method of
STEVEN REID, M.B., and
SIMON WESSELY, M.D.
Guy's, King's and St. Thomas' School of Medicine and Institute of Psychiatry
London, United Kingdom

Chronic fatigue syndrome (CFS) denotes an illness of uncertain etiology characterized by severe, disabling fatigue. In recent years, it has attracted a resurgence of interest, at the same time becoming the subject of controversy regarding its cause and management. In addition to fatigue, CFS may be associated with musculoskeletal pain, sleep disturbance, impaired concentration, and headaches. Together, these symptoms form the basis of the widely used case definition developed by the Centers for Disease Control and Prevention (Table 1). The severity and duration of CFS vary considerably from patient to patient, but many experience a substantial decline in physical and cognitive functioning.

EPIDEMIOLOGY

Fatigue is a medical complaint in one in five primary care visits. A smaller number of patients suffer from idiopathic chronic fatigue, and community-based and primary care–based studies have reported the prevalence of CFS to be 0.2% to 2.6%, depending on the definition and exclusion criteria used. In contrast to those patients attending spe-

TABLE 1. **International Consensus Definition of Chronic Fatigue Syndrome**

A. Clinically evaluated, unexplained, persistent or relapsing chronic fatigue (>6 months' duration) that is of new or definite onset (has not been lifelong); is not the result of ongoing exertion; is not substantially alleviated by rest; and results in substantial reduction in previous levels of occupational, educational, social, or personal activities

B. Four or more of the following symptoms are concurrently present for >6 months:
   1. Impaired memory or concentration
   2. Sore throat
   3. Tender cervical or axillary lymph nodes
   4. Muscle pain
   5. Multijoint pain
   6. New headaches
   7. Unrefreshing sleep
   8. Postexertion malaise

Exclusionary Clinical Diagnoses
- Any active medical condition that could explain the chronic fatigue
- Any previously diagnosed medical condition whose resolution has not been documented beyond reasonable clinical doubt and whose continued activity may explain the chronic fatiguing illness
- Psychotic major depression; bipolar affective disorder; schizophrenia; delusional disorders; dementias; anorexia nervosa; bulimia nervosa
- Alcohol or other substance abuse within 2 years prior to the onset of the chronic fatigue and at any time afterward

From Fukuda K, Straus SE, Hickie I, et al: The chronic fatigue syndrome: A comprehensive approach to its definition and study. Ann Intern Med 121:953–959, 1994.

cialist clinics, community samples show no association of CFS with socioeconomic status or particular ethnic group. Women, however, are at increased risk of developing CFS, with a relative risk of 1.3 to 1.7, depending on diagnostic criteria used.

ETIOLOGY

Despite considerable research effort and several hypotheses, the cause of CFS remains poorly understood. Endocrine abnormalities—low levels of cortisol and a blunted adrenal response to stress—in many patients have led to a disturbance of the hypothalamic-pituitary-adrenal axis being posited as a cause of the symptoms experienced in CFS. Whether these abnormalities are causal or epiphenomena is yet to be established. Also, these findings are not universal in CFS patients. Alterations in immune function have been found in some patients, but the findings have been inconsistent and nonspecific, so again, any causal role remains speculative.

CFS is frequently attributed to viral infection, but epidemiologic studies have not demonstrated any association with common, everyday infective agents. Specific infections such as Epstein-Barr virus, toxoplasmosis, cytomegalovirus, and Q fever can, however, precipitate prolonged periods of fatigue. What is unclear is whether these infections are specific causative agents or are acting as triggers in predisposed individuals.

The relationship between depression and CFS is complex. Many depressed patients complain of prolonged fatigue, and depression is common in CFS populations. As well as similarities, there are significant differences between the two illnesses. Patients with CFS often do not show the cognitions typically associated with depression—low self-esteem, hopelessness, suicidal ideation—and studies of neurotransmitter and neuroendocrine function in the two conditions emphasize a distinction. Depression is an indicator of poorer outcome in CFS.

CFS shares many similarities with other medically unexplained syndromes such as fibromyalgia, irritable bowel syndrome, and multiple chemical sensitivity. Of particular importance in all of these illnesses are patients' health beliefs and attributions. Evidence suggests that these factors may influence the development of symptoms as well as their outcome.

ASSESSMENT

The management of CFS is by necessity collaborative, and key to this is the establishment of a positive relationship with the patient, beginning at the assessment.

Unfortunately, when patients with chronic fatigue consult medical practitioners, often these patients are confronted with disbelief or are reassured that there is nothing physically wrong and that their symptoms are "all in the mind." Understandably, this leads to resentment and a distrust of the medical profession, with the patient seeking alternatives either within the general medical sphere or in more unorthodox circles. Therefore, an important first step in management is to validate the patient's experience of symptoms and allow him or her to air difficulties that may have been experienced in previous medical encounters. It is also important to take note of any abnormal or unusual beliefs the patient may describe while avoiding collusion with them. Negotiating illness beliefs is a key aspect of treatment in CFS.

Fatigue is a common feature of a wide range of medical disorders, but most disorders can be excluded on clinical grounds and by using simple screening tests. The need to rule out an organic disorder must also be balanced with the potential adverse consequences of continued investigation. The importance of an adequate history cannot be overemphasized. In addition to detailing the nature and development of the presenting complaint, the history should include a comprehensive account of the patient's background, including family history, past medical and psychiatric history, employment, and financial situation. The mental state and physical examinations are both of central importance to making a diagnosis. The aim of the mental state examination is not only to exclude clearly distinguishable diagnoses such as psychotic illness but also to identify disorders such as anxiety and depression, which have significant implications for treatment.

It is also important to identify potential obstacles to recovery. This requires exploration of the patient's illness beliefs, coping strategies, and prior experience of medical care, as well as attitudes of caregivers or family members. A thorough physical examination is always appropriate, and abnormal findings such as pyrexia or lymphadenopathy merit further investigation and should not be ascribed to CFS. There may be evidence of prolonged physical inactivity on examination, such as muscle wasting and postural hypotension, which indicate the severity of the illness.

A careful history and examination should preclude the need for all but a minimum of investigations in patients presenting with chronic fatigue, and it should be remembered that there is no diagnostic test for CFS (Table 2). Special investigations should be conducted only if specifically indicated because they may paradoxically lead to an increase in concern about the possibility of abnormal results and have the potential to result in iatrogenic harm themselves. They should also be considered in the presence

TABLE 2. **Recommended Investigations for the Fatigued Patient**

Routine Investigations
Complete blood cell count
Erythrocyte sedimentation rate or C-reactive protein
Urea and electrolytes
Thyroid function tests
Urine protein and glucose
Special Investigations
Epstein-Barr virus serology
Toxoplasmosis serology
Cytomegalovirus serology
HIV serology
Chest radiograph
Creatine phosphokinase
Rheumatoid factor
Cerebral magnetic resonance imaging (for demyelination)

of the following circumstances: extremes of age; significant weight loss; recent foreign travel; absence of mental fatigue/fatigability.

A diagnosis of CFS should be made on a pragmatic basis; that is, the patient complains of chronic physical and mental fatigue and manifests substantial disability in the absence of identifiable organic disease. A diagnosis provides the patient with a coherent (although simply descriptive) label for his or her illness and should be given in the context of understanding that the cause of the illness is poorly understood but that treatment is available and recovery possible. The acronyms ME and CFIDS are to be avoided because *myalgic encephalomyelitis* is a misleading term that implies a known disease process and there is no consistent evidence to justify the addition of "immune dysfunction" to the diagnosis. There will also be fatigued patients who do not quite meet the case definition for CFS but who may still benefit from this approach to treatment.

TREATMENT

The principal aim of treatment is to reduce functional disability, and emphasis should be on rehabilitation rather than cure. Management follows a few basic principles, but the CFS population includes many people with differing needs. Therefore, treatments, which can be broadly divided into general and specific (Table 3), should be tailored to the individual patient.

General education about CFS is necessary for most patients and for some may be all that is required. The reality of the illness and its associated symptoms should be acknowledged while emphasizing that there is no specific underlying, ongoing disease process (i.e., this is not like HIV). The next step is to agree on a model for thinking about the illness that encompasses the many factors, both physical and psychologic, involved in its development and persistence. The purpose of this is to demonstrate to patients how, by modifying these factors, they can influence the outcome of their illness. A helpful analogy is that of being involved in a hit-and-run accident, emphasizing the futility of searching for a cause but the importance of rehabilitation. Patients may also be reassured that CFS is not associated with mortality and that people can improve and recover but that they have a significant role to play in this. For most, this will include a gradual increase in activity levels, overcoming previous and present avoidance behavior. Advice also needs to be given on the importance of reducing stressors from employment or lifestyle that may be contributing to symptoms and hindering recovery.

Pharmacologic Treatments

Patients who have a co-morbid depressive illness should be offered treatment with antidepressants, whether it is considered a primary or secondary problem. For patients who are not depressed, the evidence for the use of antidepressants is unclear. Tricyclic antidepressants* do, however, have analgesic properties* and may also be beneficial in patients complaining of insomnia.* To minimize side effects (commonly dry mouth, constipation, postural hypotension), the patient should be started at the lowest possible dose, such as 10 mg of amitriptyline (Elavil)* or imipramine (Tofranil),* which may be increased incrementally. For depressed patients, the dosage aimed for will be 150 to 300 mg daily (divided if necessary). In nondepressed patients complaining of myalgia or insomnia, lower dosages are often effective. Selective serotonin reuptake inhibitors* and other more recently developed antidepressants have the advantage of being more easily tolerated and may also have an alerting effect, but their analgesic properties are less clear.

Although many other drug treatments have been evaluated in the management of CFS, there is as yet insufficient evidence to recommend their use routinely.

Nonpharmacologic Treatments

These treatments consist of a combination of educational and behavioral interventions, which can be used without recourse to a specialist clinic.

*Not FDA approved for this indication.

TABLE 3. **Treatment of Chronic Fatigue Syndrome**

General
Accept illness
Educate about the illness
Encourage self-help and normal activity
Treat co-morbid psychiatric illness
Pharmacologic
Consider antidepressant medication
Avoid untested treatments
Nonpharmacologic
Goal setting
Sleep hygiene
Graded activity schedule
Cognitive-behavioral therapy
Other psychotherapies if indicated

Graded activity is central to the treatment of CFS. As part of the assessment, levels of activity should be monitored by using a diary. Many patients with CFS initially overdo attempts to exercise, become severely fatigued, and develop a pattern of overactivity and underactivity. Other patients avoid all levels of exercise and may develop features of deconditioning. Therefore, before any exercise plan is advised, it is necessary to stabilize current activity levels, which may even mean an overall reduction. A plan of gradually increasing exercise can then be tailored accordingly. Activities should be set at an attainable level, and the patient should be made aware that initially symptoms may worsen but will subsequently lessen. The first steps may involve simple tasks, such as getting out of bed or going to the toilet unaided, and at this stage involvement of a partner or caregiver in supervising management can be helpful. Periods of adequate rest should also be included in the activity schedule.

Sleep disturbance occurs commonly in CFS and may have a considerable impact on the patient's ability to participate in daily activities. A number of measures can be taken to correct abnormal sleep patterns. Daytime naps should be avoided, as should stimulants such as caffeine or nicotine in the evening. The bedroom should be used only for sleep and intimacy and not for other activities such as eating or watching television. Time spent in bed should be curtailed to the actual time spent sleeping, the aim being to build up a mild sleep debt that increases the patient's ability to stay asleep. Should these measures not prove sufficient, it may be necessary to consider a sedative antidepressant.

For some patients, interpersonal problems and psychosocial difficulties may make progress with treatment difficult. For such patients, supportive therapy and graded activity may be insufficient and referral for specialist treatment may be required. There is now considerable research backing the effectiveness of cognitive-behavioral therapy, which, in addition to including the principles of treatment already discussed, places an emphasis on the reappraisal of illness beliefs. Other psychotherapies, such as family therapy and psychodynamic therapy, may have a role in the management of some patients, if specifically indicated.

In patients who have a long history of severely impaired functioning or who have proved consistently resistant to treatment, management is essentially supportive with infrequent but regular contact. The aim with this approach is to at least reduce further deterioration and limit unnecessary or repeated investigations and treatments.

PROGNOSIS

Most studies of prognosis in CFS have focused on people attending specialist clinics, who are likely to have a poorer prognosis. Outcome appears to be influenced by the presence of psychiatric disorders and beliefs about causation and treatment (Table 4).

TABLE 4. **Perpetuating Factors in Chronic Fatigue Syndrome**

Depression and anxiety
Lack of physical fitness
Sleep disorder
Chronic life stresses and difficulties
Inaccurate or unhelpful illness beliefs
Avoidance of activities

Twenty percent to 50% of adults with the disorder will show some improvement after 1 to 2 years, but few will return to their previous level of functioning. Children generally have a better outlook, with the majority showing definite improvement when followed up in the longer term.

MUMPS

method of
THOMAS C. SHOPE, M.D.
University of Michigan Health Systems
Ann Arbor, Michigan

Mumps is an acute, contagious viral infection of childhood, characterized by abrupt, painful swelling of one or both parotid glands and fever. The incubation period is 18 days with a range of 12 to 25 days. Before widespread use of mumps vaccine (circa 1970), the illness occurred in annual epidemics, generally in focal clusters, and usually in midwinter to early spring. Now the illness occurs only sporadically. The name may derive from the English verb *mump*, "to be sulky or to grimace," or the noun meaning "lump."

Mumps was described in the writings of Hippocrates and subsequently was viewed primarily as a cause of epidemic illness among the military during times of mobilization (in fact, in older literature the illness is referred to as epidemic parotitis). The viral etiology of mumps was established in landmark studies of Johnson and Goodpasture in 1934. They reported successful transmission of mumps from filtrates of patient's saliva to rhesus monkeys. In 1946, Enders propagated mumps virus in tissue culture and speculated that virus attenuation could lead to development of a live-virus vaccine. By 1966, Hilleman, working with virus obtained from saliva of his daughter Jeryl Lynn, reported successful development of the attenuated, live-virus vaccine in use today (licensed in 1967).

The clinical manifestations of mumps are variable. Typically, mumps begins after a prodrome (1–7 days) that may include fever, anorexia, myalgia, and malaise. Swelling involves single or multiple salivary glands, often progressing asynchronously among the glands. Swollen glands may be tender (presenting as an earache without otitis) and generally continue to enlarge for 2 to 3 days before swelling subsides over the next few days. Look for swelling of the parotid gland to obliterate the angle of the mandible and push the lower portion of the ear pinna up and away from the head. Inflammation of the Stensen or Wharton ducts supports the diagnosis. Fever peaks (sometimes at 40°C [104°F]) with the peak of salivary gland swelling. Nausea and vomiting, a manifestation of pancreatitis, can be pernicious. In addition to salivary gland involvement, meningitis, associated with photophobia and headache, is common. Meningitis is not generally followed by lasting pathology. Be aware that mumps meningitis occurs in up to 30% of patients without parotitis. Among postpubertal females, mastitis is common and oophoritis is rare. Among postpubertal males, orchitis occurs in as many as 25% to 30% of cases. Orchitis may be followed by unilateral or, rarely, bilateral testicular atrophy but, in contrast to popular lore, is not commonly associated with sterility. Hearing loss, especially unilateral, has been rarely noted after mumps. Finally, as many as a third of people with mumps antibody never had clinical signs of mumps.

Parotid swelling can be caused by other viruses (parainfluenza, enteroviruses, cytomegalovirus, and Epstein-Barr virus), bacteria (*Staphylococcus*, pneumococci, and gram-negative bacilli), drugs (iodides and phenothiazines), obstruction from stones or tumors, and a wide variety of other diseases. Bacterial etiology should be strongly suspected in a patient who is toxic or who has a purulent discharge from the Stensen duct. Cervical lymphadenitis can be differentiated from parotitis with careful examination to determine the location of the facial swelling. In difficult cases, ultrasonography or computed tomography will differentiate lymph nodes from salivary glands. Mumps is a clinical diagnosis, and laboratory diagnosis is often not helpful. The virus can be readily isolated in tissue culture from saliva, urine, and cerebrospinal fluid, but this will take several days to accomplish. Serology can be used to confirm cases and to sort out questions of susceptibility. The serum amylase value is elevated but may represent production from salivary glands or pancreas.

TREATMENT

The optimal treatment of mumps is prevention. Live, attenuated mumps vaccine is recommended for children after 1 year of age and is generally included with measles and rubella vaccines as MMR. Given as recommended, the vaccine is safe, is unassociated with reactions, and induces protective immunity in greater than 95% of recipients. Because not every child will respond, a second dose of vaccine (as MMR) is routinely given to children between 4 and 6 years of age, before school entry when exposure risk increases. Treatment of clinical mumps is supportive; there are no antiviral drugs approved for use against mumps virus. Pain associated with parotitis can be managed with analgesics such as acetaminophen or ibuprofen. Pain associated with orchitis may require codeine or meperidine (Demerol) in addition to testicular support and possibly ice packs. Treatment with corticosteroids for salivary gland inflammation, orchitis, mastitis, or meningitis shows no beneficial effect. The vomiting that sometimes accompanies mumps may require careful fluid monitoring. Keep in mind that fluids chosen for replacement, such as citrus juice, may cause additional parotid pain and not be well tolerated. Bed rest to prevent complications is of no proven value.

OTITIS EXTERNA

method of
CRAIG A. BUCHMAN, M.D.
University of North Carolina at Chapel Hill
Chapel Hill, North Carolina

and

BETH A. WAMBACH, M.D.
Holy Cross Hospital
Ft. Lauderdale, Florida

Otitis externa (OE) is an inflammatory process of the external auditory canal (EAC) that encompasses a wide spectrum of diseases, ranging from mild dermatitis to necrotizing skull base osteomyelitis. It is important to be familiar with the various forms of OE so that appropriate treatment can be instituted.

The EAC is lined with skin throughout the entire length, with adnexal structures (apocrine and exocrine glands) being limited to the lateral portion of the canal. Cerumen is formed from secretions from these glands combined with exfoliated skin. The ear canal is normally self-cleaning in that the exfoliated skin migrates laterally along with cerumen from the tympanic membrane to the external auditory meatus. The skin and the cerumen provide a protective barrier against infection. Disruption of the normal protective layer by instrumentation such as a cotton-tipped applicator, especially in the presence of a moist environment, can lead to infection and inflammation.

ACUTE OTITIS EXTERNA

Acute OE is usually caused by a bacterial infection of the EAC. This condition has commonly been referred to as "swimmer's ear" because of the common association with water exposure. *Pseudomonas* species and *Staphylococcus aureus* are the two most frequently isolated pathogens in routine cases of acute OE. Clinically, acute OE presents as rapid onset of otalgia, accompanied by pruritus, hearing loss, and discharge. There is often a recent exposure to water or mechanical trauma to the EAC. On physical examination, the hallmark findings include marked tenderness to manipulation of the auricle and the tragus. The EAC skin may also be edematous and erythematous, often with a purulent discharge. It may be impossible to visualize the tympanic membrane because of the edema of the EAC.

Treatment of acute OE involves gentle cleaning of the debris from the EAC under direct visualization and application of a topical antimicrobial agent. Numerous ototopical preparations are available for the treatment of patients with acute OE (Table 1). Important considerations in choosing an ototopical preparation for acute OE include antimicrobial sensitivity of the offending organism(s), adverse reactions, status of the tympanic membrane, delivery, and cost. Most of the commercially available formulations include either acetic acid (2%) (VōSol), antibiotics (aminoglycoside,* polymyxin B, quinolone), hydrocor-

*Not FDA approved for this indication.

TABLE 1. **Ototopical Agents**

Product Name	Acid	Antiseptic	Antibiotic	Antifungal	Anti-Inflammatory	Carrier
Ciloxan* solution (ophthalmic)	Hydrochloric		Ciprofloxacin			
Cipro HC Otic	Acetic	Alcohol	Ciprofloxacin	Polysorbate	Hydrocortisone	
Coly-Mycin S Otic	Acetic		Polymyxin E Neomycin	Polysorbate 80	Hydrocortisone	
Cortisporin Otic solution	Hydrochloric	Alcohol	Polymyxin B Neomycin		Hydrocortisone	
Cortisporin Otic suspension		Alcohol	Polymyxin B Neomycin	Polysorbate 80	Hydrocortisone	
Cresylate		M-cresyl acetate				Propylene glycol
Debrox	Citric					Carbamide peroxide
Floxin Otic solution	Hydrochloric	Benzalkonium chloride	Ofloxacin			
Lotrimin solution*				Clotrimazole		Propylene glycol
Otic Domeboro	Acetic and boric					
Pediotic		Cetyl alcohol	Polymyxin B Neomycin		Hydrocortisone	Propylene glycol Mineral oil
TobraDex suspension* (ophthalmic)	Sulfuric		Tobramycin		Dexamethasone	
VōSol HC Otic	Acetic Citric	Alcohol			Hydrocortisone	Propylene glycol
VōSol Otic	Acetic	Alcohol				Propylene glycol

*Not FDA approved for this indication.
From American Academy of Otolaryngology–Head and Neck Surgery Foundation Inc, Alexandria, Virginia.

tisone, or some combination thereof. Nearly all the preparations demonstrate significant activity against *Pseudomonas* species as well as *S. aureus*. Table 1 shows each of the available preparations with the constituent elements. Acetic acid and aminoglycoside-containing preparations are potentially ototoxic and should be used with caution when the tympanic membrane is not intact or its status is unknown. Furthermore, neomycin application may result in skin erythema and swelling in as many as 5% to 10% of patients. Currently, ofloxacin otic drops (Floxin Otic) are the only drops with U.S. Food and Drug Administration approval for use in the middle ear. To date, there have been no demonstrated ototoxic effects of either ofloxacin or ciprofloxacin drop preparations in either human or animal studies.

I prefer acetic acid preparations for routine cases of acute OE when the tympanic membrane is intact. Acetic acid is bactericidal by way of its ability to change the pH of the EAC. This substance is highly effective, is well tolerated, has few side effects, and avoids the issue of developing antimicrobial resistance. The other agents are reserved for more complicated cases, such as when the ear canal is completely obstructed, the tympanic membrane is perforated or its status is unknown, a resistant organism is present, necrotizing OE is suspected, the disease involves the patient's only hearing ear, or the patient is immunocompromised.

If edema of the canal interferes with the delivery of drops, an expandable sponge wick should be inserted so that the drops will be able to coat the length of the canal. This wick is removed after 3 to 5 days. The use of the drops should be continued for at least 3 days after resolution of symptoms. Systemic antibiotics to cover *Pseudomonas* (e.g., ciprofloxacin) or *S. aureus* (e.g., cephalexin) should be considered if there is severe cellulitis extending outside the EAC. During the treatment period, patients should keep the ear dry except for the application of drops. Culture is indicated if there has been no response to adequate therapy or the patient is immunocompromised. Biopsy of the EAC should also be considered when therapy has failed or when necrotizing otitis externa or malignancy is suspected.

Prevention

To prevent acute OE, it is important to teach patients to avoid using cotton-tipped applicators or hairpins to clean their ear canals. Not only does this traumatize the canal skin, but it also removes the cerumen, which provides a protective function. Patients with intact tympanic membranes who have persistent EAC pruritus should be taught to use a combination of half rubbing alcohol (70% isopropyl) and half vinegar (acetic acid) to irrigate their ears one to two times per week. Should this exacerbate the symptoms, the EAC can be moisturized with baby oil, skin lotion, or hydrocortisone cream when inflammation is present. Swimmers and patients who wear hearing aids may be at increased risk of developing acute OE because their EACs may have a tendency to be moist. These patients can also use the vinegar and alcohol preparation after swimming or weekly.

FUNGAL OTITIS EXTERNA

Fungal infections of the EAC (otomycosis) are also a common cause of both acute and chronic otitis externa. *Aspergillus* and *Candida* are the two most frequently isolated species. Clinically, otomycosis usually manifests as pruritus of the EAC with or without otalgia and hearing loss. Physical examination reveals the characteristic hyphae of *Aspergillus* species (black, yellow, or gray) and *Candida* (white) in an erythematous EAC. Treatment involves meticulous cleaning and topical medications. When the tympanic membrane is intact, acetic acid (vinegar) and alcohol irrigations twice a day are highly effective. The acetic acid is bactericidal, the alcohol acts as a drying agent, and the irrigation provides manual débridement of the fungal elements. Clotrimazole drops (Lotrimin) and nystatin (Mycostatin) powder may also be useful for cases when *Candida* appears to be the offending agent. For recalcitrant cases, a mixture of chloramphenicol,* sulfanilamide, and amphotericin B (Fungizone) can be used. This preparation is highly effective in nearly all cases of otomycosis. Management of fungal otitis also involves avoidance measures to keep the EAC intact and dry.

HERPES ZOSTER

Herpes zoster is the most common viral infection to involve the EAC. The patient will complain initially of severe burning pain and will subsequently develop vesicles 3 to 7 days later. When the infection involves not only the skin of the EAC but also the facial nerve, causing paresis, then Ramsay Hunt syndrome is present. Treatment involves topical débridement and drops to avoid bacterial superinfection and systemic acyclovir (Zovirax). Corticosteroids are added when facial paralysis is present.

DERMATITIS

Often, dermatologic diseases can cause otitis externa. They usually take the form of chronic EAC inflammation and symptoms. The goals of treatment are to clear up any acute bacterial superinfection with antibiotic drops and then to treat the underlying disease. Seborrheic dermatitis has been treated by many authors as follows: (1) Apply tar shampoo to the meatus and the EAC; (2) blow the EAC dry to remove moisture; (3) apply three drops of 2% acetic acid; and (4) apply topical corticosteroid cream. This regimen should be repeated for 7 days.

NECROTIZING OTITIS EXTERNA

Necrotizing otitis externa, also known as malignant otitis externa, is a virulent infection that starts in the EAC and can extend through the temporal bone to cause skull-base osteomyelitis. This disorder is most common among immunocompromised patients and diabetics and can be a life-threatening problem. The patient usually presents with progressive, severe deep-seated otalgia, purulent discharge, and granulation tissue at the posteroinferior EAC. The disease may progress to involve the cranial nerves (most commonly VII, X, and XI). Diagnosis is suspected in any immunocompromised patient or diabetic with otitis externa that is refractory to standard therapy or when the just listed signs are present. The diagnosis is strengthened by the demonstration of osseous erosion on computed tomography of the temporal bone. In addition, gallium and technetium-99 scintigraphy will help determine the extent of inflammation and bony involvement, respectively. Treatment consists of cleaning the EAC, performing a biopsy of any granulation tissue to rule out cancer, and obtaining culture and sensitivity information on the offending organism. *Pseudomonas aeruginosa* is the most commonly isolated organism. Ototopical drops with antipseudomonal coverage (e.g., ofloxacin) are applied, and a wick is placed when necessary. Broad-spectrum, double intravenous antibiotic coverage for *Pseudomonas* (e.g., ceftazidime [Fortaz] and gentamicin) is started and usually lasts up to 6 weeks. The underlying process (i.e., diabetes or immunodeficiency) is managed. The ear is cleaned frequently under microscopic guidance. Selected patients with limited disease may be managed with oral ciprofloxacin (Cipro), 750 mg twice daily, along with topical anti-*Pseudomonas* drops and close follow-up. To avoid relapse, antibiotic therapy should be continued until the patient is asymptomatic, the EAC appears normal, and gallium scanning indicates resolution of temporal bone inflammation. Technetium-99 scintigraphy may stay positive for years and thus is not useful in disease monitoring. Surgical débridement is rarely indicated and is reserved for those patients with a deteriorating clinical course despite medical intervention, abscess formation, or sequestrectomy of devitalized bone.

OTHER LESIONS

Bullous external otitis is a painful disease in which bullae form along the medial bony EAC. These bullae are typically hemorrhagic. Cultures have yielded *Pseudomonas* as well as *Mycoplasma pneumoniae*. Management involves adequate pain control, sometimes decompression of the tense bullae, and oral and topical antibiotics.

Furunculosis is a localized infection of a hair follicle at the lateral EAC along the superior meatus caused by *S. aureus*. Treatment often involves incision and drainage, as well as systemic (e.g., cephalexin) and topical antibiotic drops.

Perichondritis and chondritis are infections of the perichondrium and the cartilage of the auricle. These infections may result from trauma to the auricle or from direct extension of an otitis externa infection. Necrosis of the cartilage may occur if this is not treated appropriately. Treatment involves débridement and topical and oral antibiotics covering *Pseu-*

*Not FDA approved for this indication.

domonas species. If the infection spreads to involve the soft tissue around the ear, the patient should be admitted for therapy with intravenous anti-*Pseudomonas* antibiotics, combined with anti-*Pseudomonas* drops.

PLAGUE

method of
RICHARD W. TITBALL, B.Sc., Ph.D.
Defence Evaluation and Research Agency
Salisbury, United Kingdom

Plague is a disease of human beings caused by the gram-negative bacterium *Yersinia pestis*. It is generally accepted that there have been three pandemics of plague. The first, the Justinian plague, occurred in 540 AD. The second pandemic, often referred to as the *Black Death,* lasted for 2 centuries, killing more than one third of the population of Europe. The third pandemic emerged in Southeast Asia during the latter part of the 19th century.

There are at least 2000 reported cases of plague throughout the world today, and these cases are considered to be the vestigial remnants of the third pandemic. These cases occur predominantly in Southeast Asia, in the southwestern United States, and in Madagascar and other areas in Africa. The bacterium persists in the environment in these areas in rodent reservoirs such as the ground squirrel in California and the marmot in Southeast Asia. These infected rodents appear to suffer from a chronic and protracted disease. In other animal hosts and in human beings, plague is an acute and often fatal disease.

Outbreaks of bubonic plague are often a consequence of contact between human beings and fleas that have fed on infected animals. A variety of events might predispose to this. Natural disasters such as floods and earthquakes often result in infected rodents being driven out of their normal environment and colonizing human habitation. The continuing encroachment of human beings into areas where plague foci exist might also allow human beings to be in contact with infected rodents. Hikers, hunters, and campers in some parts of the world are considered to be at special risk of contacting infected rodents. Finally, because domesticated animals are also at risk of contracting plague, veterinarians in some parts of the world are considered to be at risk of catching the disease directly from infected animals.

Pneumonic plague, in which the disease can be transmitted from infected host to susceptible host by the airborne route, is rarely seen today. It is the likely form of disease that would be seen after the illegitimate use of *Y. pestis* as a bioterrorist weapon. Pneumonic plague was certainly common at the height of the plague pandemics and is the most infectious form of the disease. During the Surat outbreak of plague (India, 1994), there was great concern that pneumonic plague could be transmitted from person to person during air travel from India. This route of transmission remains a cause for concern and could allow the rapid spread of disease.

CLINICAL FEATURES

Bubonic plague usually occurs after a bite from an infected flea. Exceptionally, infection occurs via open wounds, for example, if a trapper skins an infected animal carcass. The incubation period is typically 2 to 6 days, and the patient develops a fever, headache, and chills. The classic feature of bubonic plague is the appearance of a swollen and exquisitely tender bubo. The bubo can reach the size of a hen's egg and occurs within the lymph node draining the original site of infection (often the inguinal or femoral lymph node). There may be lesions at the original site of infection and gastrointestinal involvement with nausea, vomiting, pain, and diarrhea. Occasionally, the bacteria disseminate from the initial focus of infection, resulting in a septicemic plague without the appearance of buboes. Patients with this form of the disease present with a high fever and hypotension. A septicemia might also occur in the later stages of bubonic plague, and meningeal involvement is possible. In cases of sepsis, bacteria in blood might reach high levels (up to 10^8/mL). The hematogenous dissemination of bacteria can result in colonization of the lungs, with a resultant pneumonia resulting in pneumonic plague.

Of these three forms of disease, bubonic plague is the easiest to manage. In contrast, septicemic and pneumonic plagues are often fatal. Of great concern is the potential for person-to-person transmission of pneumonic plague by coughing and sneezing. Pneumonic plague transmitted in this way is characterized by the remarkable speed with which the disease develops. Typically, the time from infection to death is 1 to 3 days.

DIAGNOSIS

Y. pestis should be considered as the etiologic agent in individuals who have been in areas of the world where plague is endemic and who present with sudden onset of fever associated with lymphadenitis, sepsis, or pneumonia. Blood samples reveal an elevated white blood cell count (10,000–20,000 cells/mm^3), with neutrophils predominating. Bacteriologic diagnosis can be made from aspirates taken from a bubo or from blood or sputum samples. Care should be taken when taking these samples, especially if pneumonic plague is suspected. Samples should be handled in a microbiologic laboratory equipped to work with containment level 3 pathogens. The most straightforward analysis involves Gram or Wayson staining of air-dried smears on microscope slides. After staining, *Y. pestis* cells appear as small gram-negative rods with a characteristic bipolar staining (safety pin appearance). However, this appearance is not in itself diagnostic for *Y. pestis,* and other pathogens such as *Burkholderia pseudomallei* have a similar appearance. An additional rapid test for *Y. pestis* involves the negative staining of films with India ink, which reveals heavily encapsulated bacteria.

A variety of confirmatory tests for *Y. pestis* have been proposed, including the use of fluorescent antibody to the capsular antigen, passive hemagglutination tests, polymerase chain reaction, and enzyme-linked immunoassay. However, many of these tests are not available outside of a specialist laboratory. Culture on Congo red agar, ideally at 26°C to 28°C, results in the appearance of colonies with a pigmented central region and paler margins. However, culture methods are generally considered to be too slow (typically taking 48 hours) in the context of the rapid progression of the disease, and a presumptive diagnosis should be made before such tests are carried out.

Patients with plague should be placed in strict respiratory isolation, at least until pneumonic disease is discounted. As a class 1 notifiable disease, cases must be reported both to the national health authorities and to the World Health Organization in Geneva, Switzerland.

PROPHYLAXIS AND PREVENTION

Because most plague is contracted from fleas that have fed on infected wild rodents, it is important to minimize contact between wild rodents and human beings in areas of the world where plague is endemic. Rodent control measures might be considered as an important element of any plague control program.

Family members and other people who have been in close contact with individuals suffering from plague should be kept under surveillance for at least 8 days. It may be appropriate to use tetracycline or doxycycline prophylactically in these individuals, especially if the primary case is pneumonic plague. In children and pregnant women, trimethoprim-sulfamethoxazole (Bactrim, Septra) can be used.

A killed whole cell vaccine is produced by Commonwealth Serum Laboratories of Australia for use in human beings. This vaccine does not provide good protection against pneumonic plague, and three doses are required over a period of 6 months for the primary course of immunization. This vaccine might be of use to protect individuals who are traveling to areas of the world where the disease is endemic or in areas of the world where there is recurrent or intense plague activity. However, vaccination is not a requirement for travel to any part of the world. The vaccine is not suitable for postexposure use.

TREATMENT

Successful treatment of plague depends on the commencement of therapy during the early stages of the disease. In cases of bubonic plague treated with antibiotics, the fatality rate is generally less than 5%. In contrast, septicemic and pneumonic plague are notoriously difficult to treat effectively, partly because of the rapidity with which the disease develops and the difficulties of making an early diagnosis. For all antibiotics, a 10-day course is recommended and is important to prevent relapse.

Streptomycin (30 mg/kg/d) is the antibiotic of choice, given daily intramuscularly as two doses. In the absence of streptomycin, gentamicin should be considered. Tetracycline (40 mg/kg/d) can be given orally as four daily doses. Ciprofloxacin (Cipro)* (20–40 mg/kg twice daily) is effective for preventing and treating experimental bubonic or pneumonic plague in mice. However, successful therapy of pneumonic disease is dependent on the start of treatment within 24 hours of infection. The utility of ciprofloxacin for treating disease in human beings has not been evaluated. For the treatment of plague meningitis, intravenously administered chloramphenicol (Chloromycetin) is the antibiotic of choice at a loading dose of 25 mg/kg/d, followed by 60 mg/kg/d in four doses.

Improvement in the condition of patients is seen within 2 to 3 days, but buboes may remain for several weeks after successful treatment. A strain of *Y. pestis* resistant to tetracycline, streptomycin, chloramphenicol, and sulfonamides has recently been isolated from a case of bubonic plague in Madagascar. Therefore, the failure of a patient to respond to antibiotic treatment should alert the clinician to the possibility of an antibiotic-resistant strain of *Y. pestis*.

*Not FDA approved for this indication.

PSITTACOSIS
(Ornithosis)

method of
THOMAS C. QUINN, M.D.
Johns Hopkins University School of Medicine
Baltimore, Maryland

Psittacosis is primarily a disease of birds caused by *Chlamydia psittaci*, and human beings become infected through direct exposure to infected birds. The disease is therefore solely a zoonosis and is seen primarily in people with direct contact with birds, such as pet shop owners and employees, poultry workers, pigeon fanciers, falconers, taxidermists, veterinarians, and abattoir workers. Anyone in contact with an infected bird or animal is at risk. Human cases occur both sporadically and as outbreaks. Psittacosis attracted considerable attention as a result of a pandemic in 1929 to 1930. In the preantibiotic era, the case-fatality rate approached 20%. Psittacosis is now recognized as an occupational hazard to those exposed to infected turkeys in poultry processing plants. *C. psittaci* is also an important pathogen in domestic mammals, causing a number of conditions, such as abortion and arthritis, that have considerable economic impact.

Chlamydia organisms are obligate intracellular bacteria that consist of four species: *C. trachomatis*, *C. pneumoniae*, *C. psittaci*, and *C. pecorum*. They are differentiated from other bacteria by their unique developmental cycle, which involves two morphologic forms: the elementary body, a metabolically inert form that is adapted to extracellular survival, and the reticulate body, a metabolically active form that replicates intracellularly by binary fission. *C. psittaci* infects primarily the upper respiratory tract and eventually disseminates to the reticuloendothelial cells of the spleen and liver. Invasion of the lung probably takes place by way of the bloodstream rather than through direct extension from the upper air passages. Histologically, the infected areas of the alveolar spaces are filled with fluid, erythrocytes, and lymphocytes. The respiratory epithelium of the bronchi usually remains intact, whereas more infiltration is present within the alveoli and in the reticuloendothelial system of the liver and spleen.

Infected birds may be asymptomatic or severely ill. They may exhibit anorexia, emaciation, dyspnea, and diarrhea, frequently with closed eyes and ruffled feathers. The infection in the birds may spontaneously relapse or remit, although it is during periods of illness that the birds excrete large numbers of organisms. Discharge from their beaks and eyes, as well as from feces and urine, is infective, and the feathers and the dust around their cages become contaminated. Humans become infected by the respiratory route, by direct contact, or by aerosolization of infected discharges or dust. Although most human exposure comes from birds, mammals also become infected. Disease has occurred in ranchers after exposure to infected cows, goats, and sheep. Abortion in sheep has been followed by abortion in women who assist in lambing, and endocarditis has occurred with both avian and nonavian strains. Human-to-human transmission is rare, and isolation of infected patients is not required.

CLINICAL MANIFESTATIONS

The clinical manifestations of psittacosis are extremely variable. The incubation period is 5 to 15 days after exposure. The onset may be either insidious or abrupt, and the clinical manifestations may be nonspecific. Fever is present in nearly all cases and may be as high as 40°C (104°F). Headache is almost always present and is associated with a nonproductive cough, but the cough frequently appears 3 to 5 days after onset of fever. The patient may complain of myalgia, arthralgias, lethargy, mental depression, agitation, insomnia, and disorientation. Gastrointestinal complaints include abdominal pain, nausea, vomiting, and diarrhea.

Clinical signs most frequently reported are fever, pharyngeal erythema, rales, and hepatosplenomegaly. The pulse rate is slow in relation to the fever. Hepatosplenomegaly in patients with acute pneumonitis should suggest the possibility of psittacosis. Jaundice is a rare but ominous finding reflecting severe hepatic involvement. A faint macular rash referred to as Horder spots simulates the rose spots of typhoid fever. Other dermatologic lesions are erythema multiforme, erythema marginatum, erythema nodosum, and urticaria.

Cardiac complications may include pericarditis, occasionally with effusion and tamponade; myocarditis; and culture-negative endocarditis. In cases of endocarditis, *Chlamydia* organisms have been demonstrated histologically in both aortic and mitral valves and have been grown from the blood. Thrombophlebitis is not unusual, and pulmonary infarction has been reported in rare instances. Neurologic consequences include cranial nerve palsy, cerebellar involvement, transverse myelitis, confusion, meningitis, encephalitis, transient focal neurologic signs, and seizures. Cerebrospinal fluid is usually normal, but a small number of white blood cells, predominantly lymphocytes, may be seen, and the protein level may be elevated.

The white blood cell count is usually normal or slightly elevated with an increase in lymphocytes. Hepatic enzymes may be elevated in 50% of cases. Chest radiographs often show an infiltrate, usually confined to a single lower lobe, that is usually patchy in appearance but can be hazy, diffuse, homogeneous, lobar, atelectatic, wedge shaped, nodular, or miliary.

DIAGNOSIS

Diagnosis of psittacosis should be considered in anyone with pneumonia or a severe systemic illness who has had a history of contact with birds. The differential diagnosis is extensive and depends on the manifestation. The typhoidal picture is suggestive of one of the causes of the mononucleosis syndrome, typhoid fever, brucellosis, tularemia, influenza, and subacute bacterial endocarditis. Respiratory signs and symptoms plus headache and myalgias are suggestive of causes of atypical pneumonia such as viral pneumonia; Q fever; *Legionella*, *Mycoplasma*, or *Chlamydia pneumoniae* pneumonia; or miliary tuberculosis. Helpful clues to psittacosis when present are relative bradycardia, rash, and hepatosplenomegaly. The diagnosis is confirmed by isolation of the causative microorganism or by serologic studies. *C. psittaci* is difficult to isolate and requires tissue culture in an experienced laboratory. Serologic diagnosis is confirmed by a fourfold increase in titer to at least 1:32 on a complement fixation assay. An acute specimen and a convalescent specimen should always be tested. *C. trachomatis*, *C. psittaci*, and *C. pneumoniae* share a common genus-specific group antigen that can cross-react serologically, which is a problem because *C. pneumoniae* is a more common cause of pneumonia. A microimmunofluorescent test can help differentiate antibody to each of the three species, and polymerase chain reaction of sputum can help detect and rapidly differentiate all three species, but both assays are available only in research laboratories at this time.

TREATMENT

The preferred treatment for adults with psittacosis is doxycycline (Vibramycin), 100 mg twice daily, or tetracycline, 500 mg four times a day for 10 to 21 days. Azithromycin (Zithromax),* 500 mg the first day followed by 250 mg daily thereafter for 10 days, or clarithromycin (Biaxin),* 250 to 500 mg twice daily for 2 weeks, may be efficacious, although there is little experience with these agents. Erythromycin,* 500 mg four times daily, is an alternative treatment, but it is less effective than the tetracyclines. Penicillins, cephalosporins, and sulfonamides are ineffective. With appropriate treatment, patients generally improve within 24 to 48 hours, and the rate of mortality among untreated patients has dropped to less than 1%.

Preventive measures should include quarantine and long-term antibiotic prophylaxis for all imported birds. Many birds, however, are imported without adequate antibiotics. All cases of psittacosis should be reported and fully investigated, and all ill birds should be treated with antibiotics.

*Not FDA approved for this indication.

Q FEVER

method of
W. RUSSELL BYRNE, M.D.
U.S. Army Research Institute of Infectious Diseases
Fort Detrick, Maryland

BACKGROUND AND EPIDEMIOLOGY

Q fever is a febrile, usually self-limited illness that most commonly results from direct or indirect exposure to infected livestock, particularly sheep, cattle, and goats. This can occur on farms or ranches or in slaughterhouses or research laboratories. In the United States and Canada, a few cases have been attributed to exposure to domestic cats.

Q fever is caused by *Coxiella burnetii*, a highly infectious rickettsia-like organism with a worldwide distribution. Infection in humans is usually caused by inhalation of infected aerosols. Large numbers of organisms are produced in the placenta of infected animals, and human cases frequently occur as a result of exposure to animals giving birth.

The high infectivity of *C. burnetii* is caused either by a

spore form that can survive in the environment and initiate infection for weeks or months after an infected animal is no longer present or by transport of the organism on an inanimate surface, such as clothing. Airborne carriage of the *C. burnetii* spore form may cause outbreaks of Q fever in individuals who live or work in the general vicinity of infected animals or at sites miles distant from a source.

Individuals at risk for acquisition of Q fever include people who live or work on or in the vicinity of ranches or farms that harbor infected animals. Workers in slaughterhouses or research laboratories are also at risk if infected animals are present.

CLINICAL FEATURES

The incubation period of Q fever is usually about 2 weeks, although it may vary from 10 days to 6 weeks. Fever, chills, headache, and myalgias are the most common symptoms. Cough may also be present. Neurologic signs and symptoms have been observed in up to one quarter of patients with acute Q fever. Untreated acute Q fever usually lasts 2 weeks or less. Malaise and easy fatigue lasting months after acute infection have been reported in up to one fifth of patients.

Physical findings are generally nonspecific. Laboratory abnormalities are usually characterized by elevated liver function test results, and patients may present with a clinical and laboratory picture consistent with acute hepatitis.

Chronic Q fever, usually manifested by endocarditis or granulomatous hepatitis, probably develops in less than 1% of acute infections. Q fever endocarditis usually develops in the setting of a pre-existing cardiac valvular abnormality.

DIAGNOSIS

The diagnosis of Q fever is usually accomplished by serologic testing for antibodies to *C. burnetii*. Significant antibody titers are not consistently identifiable until 2 to 3 weeks into the illness. Convalescent antibody titers, measured 2 to 3 months after onset of illness, typically demonstrate a fourfold increase or greater. Chronic infection almost always induces significant antibody titers; the diagnosis of chronic Q fever should be considered doubtful in the absence of this finding.

The identification of even a single case of Q fever should prompt an epidemiologic investigation to determine the cause of infection. There are almost always numerous undiagnosed cases of Q fever associated with an index case, and control measures may well prevent additional cases.

TREATMENT

Acute Q Fever

Tetracyclines are recommended as the first choice for the treatment of acute Q fever. Doxycycline (Vibramycin), 100 mg orally twice a day for 10 to 14 days, is preferred because of ease of administration and patient tolerance. Tetracycline, 500 mg orally four times daily, may also be used.

Fluoroquinolones, such as ofloxacin (Floxin),* 200 mg orally three times daily, may also be useful, but a treatment course of 14 to 21 days is recommended.

*Not FDA approved for this indication.

Among the macrolides, erythromycin* is recommended, at a dose of 500 mg orally four times daily for 10 to 14 days. Azithromycin (Zithromax)* and clarithromycin (Biaxin)* have also been used successfully, but experience with these antibiotics for the treatment of Q fever is very limited.

Rifampin (Rifadin)* has also been used effectively for the treatment of acute Q fever, both individually and in combination with erythromycin* (for severe disease). The dose of rifampin used has been 300 mg orally one to two times per day for 10 to 14 days.

Chronic Q Fever

Chronic Q fever is usually treated for at least 2 years with a combination of antibiotics, such as doxycycline plus one of the fluoroquinolones* or rifampin,* or a fluoroquinolone* plus rifampin.* Recently, a combination of doxycycline, 100 mg orally twice a day plus hydroxychloroquine (Plaquenil),* 200 mg orally three times a day, has been shown to be effective and may be more effective than a combination of doxycycline plus ofloxacin.* Q fever endocarditis usually requires the surgical replacement of the affected valve.

Prevention and Control

Although reporting of Q fever cases to public health departments is not a legal requirement in all states, notification should be done so that a source of infection can be identified and appropriate control measures initiated.

An effective vaccine (Q-Vax)† is available in Australia but not in the United States.

Animals (e.g., sheep, cattle, or goats) that are associated with a high risk of infection with *C. burnetii* and are intended for use in research laboratories should be screened by serologic testing before shipment so that appropriate control measures can be taken.

*Not FDA approved for this indication.
†Not available in the United States.

RABIES

method of
MARY CURRIER, M.D., M.P.H.
Mississippi State Department of Health
Jackson, Mississippi

Rabies is a viral zoonotic disease for which the natural reservoirs are carnivorous animals and bats. The rabies virus causes an encephalitis that has been described in literature since antiquity in both humans and animals. Proposed causes and preventive measures have been diverse and plentiful throughout the ages. Causes have ranged from a pestilence in the air to "dog tongue worm." Prevention measures and treatment included cauterization of bite wounds, cutting and removal of part of the attachment of a dog's tongue (where the "worm" that causes rabies was supposed to reside), eating of a cock's brain, and bathing in hot oil. Ancient Greeks called rabies *lyssa,* meaning "madness," from whence came the name of the genus *Lyssavirus,* which contains the rabies virus.

Rabies is estimated to cause more than 50,000 deaths per year worldwide. The majority of these cases occur in tropical and subtropical regions. In countries that can afford domestic animal vaccination and control programs, the incidence of human rabies is very low. It is estimated that more than $300 million is spent each year on rabies detection, prevention, and control in the United States. This includes the cost of postexposure prophylaxis for about 40,000 Americans annually. Human rabies is rare in the United States. It has been suspected that cases have gone undiagnosed, because in many encephalitis cases the cause is never identified. In the California Encephalitis Project, however, in which extensive testing of encephalitis cases occurred, none of the 112 cases of presumptively infectious origin were found to include rabies.

EPIDEMIOLOGY

Until the 1960s, the majority of reported cases of animal rabies in the United States were diagnosed in domestic animals. The incidence in domestic animals has decreased, and now more than 90% of cases occur among wild animals. The domestic animals most commonly found to be rabid are cats, cattle, and dogs. Rodents, rabbits, and opossum are rarely found to be rabid and have not been documented in association with human disease. The principal rabies hosts today in the United States are wild carnivores and bats. Raccoons, skunks, and foxes are the terrestrial animals most often found to be rabid in the United States today, with Hawaii being the only state remaining consistently rabies free. Rabies is epizootic among raccoons in the eastern United States extending south to Alabama. Raccoons accounted for 41% of reported rabid wildlife species in 1999. It is regionally enzootic in foxes and skunks and throughout the United States among bats. Wild animals are the most important potential source of infection in humans and domestic animals in the United States.

In most countries in Asia, Africa, and South America, dogs are the major species with rabies and pose the greatest risk of rabies transmission to humans. Among the 42 human cases of rabies that have occurred in the United States from 1980 through 2000, 13 (31%) were associated with rabies virus variants found in domestic dogs abroad.

Recently, individuals with human rabies in the United State have acquired the virus most commonly from bat exposure. Of the 42 cases in the past 21 years, 26 (62%) were associated with the rabies virus variant found in insectivorous bats. Five human rabies cases occurred in 2000, four of which were associated with the bat variant of the rabies virus. In all four, there was a history of bat exposure reported by the patient or the family, but in only one was there a history of an actual bat bite. In the 26 bat virus–associated cases, 14 patients had a history of bat exposure and an additional 2 had a definite bite. This suggests either a lack of understanding of the risks associated with bat exposure or that a bat bite may be imperceptible but adequate to transmit the rabies virus.

Although eight cases of human-to-human transmission have occurred through corneal transplants, no other documented human-to-human transmission from bite or nonbite exposure has been laboratory-confirmed.

VIROLOGY

Rabies virus is one of the "bullet-shaped" viruses, flat on one end and rounded on the other, that make up the Rhabdoviridae family. The genus *Lyssavirus* includes the rabies virus, Lagos bat virus, Mokola virus, Duvenhage virus, European bat virus 1 and 2, and Australian bat virus, which are all associated with acute encephalitis. All but rabies virus are restricted to the Old World. The major components of the rabies virus are nonsegmented, negative-stranded RNA and a surrounding envelope (membrane). The membrane is covered with glycoprotein spikes that are involved in attachment and fusion to nerve cells. The virus is highly neurotropic, and infection is nearly completely restricted to the nervous system, without a viremic phase throughout the course of infection in animals and humans.

PATHOGENESIS

Transmission of rabies virus occurs when infected saliva of a host enters an uninfected animal, usually through a bite. Other methods of transmission have been documented but are rare and include mucous membrane exposure, corneal transplantation from an infected person, or aerosolization of the virus in unusual circumstances in which a large amount of virus is present in a confined space such as a laboratory or a bat-colonized cave. When the virus enters the body, it enters an eclipse phase, in which it remains undetectable by fluorescent antibody staining, virus isolation, or electron microscopy for days to months. During this time, the virus is susceptible to host immune defenses. The virus may then enter the peripheral nerves directly or may multiply in the muscle tissue before entry. It is taken up into the peripheral nerves and transported to the central nervous system via retrograde axoplasmic flow. Once it reaches the central nervous system, it disseminates rapidly. The virus then travels passively back out to peripheral nerves. This is the time during which the salivary glands become infected. The period of cerebral infection is when classic rabies symptoms develop.

CLINICAL HUMAN RABIES

The incubation period for rabies varies from days to years. Most cases occur within 30 to 90 days of the original exposure. Duration of the incubation period varies depending on the site of the bite (proximity to the central nervous system and enervation of the bite site), the quantity of virus inoculated, the rabies virus strain, and host factors such as age and immune status. Early symptoms may include paresthesias, pain, and pruritus at the site of the bite, although the wound is usually healed by that time. These symptoms may be due to arrival of the virus at the spinal cord. Local symptoms are followed by nonspecific flulike symptoms, including malaise, fever, or headache, that may last for days. Progression from these prodromal symptoms to encephalopathy and death occurs over the 10 to 30 days from symptom onset.

In 80% of patients, the classic or encephalitic ("furious") form of rabies develops. Patients exhibit anxiety, confusion, and agitation, progressing to delirium, hallucinations, and insomnia. They display autonomic dysfunction (hypersalivation, piloerection, cardiac arrhythmias, and priapism in males) and "hydrophobia." With hydrophobia, on swallowing, the diaphragm and other respiratory muscles contract painfully for 5 to 15 seconds, conditioning the patient to fear water. Initially, the hydrophobia is triggered by attempting to drink water, but as the disease progresses even the mention of water will cause an episode. The patient may remain intermittently lucid but within days will progress to paralysis, coma, and death.

In 20% of patients, the paralytic ("dumb") form of the disease develops. In these patients, the spinal cord is more involved than the brain. The patient develops numbness, pain, weakness, and then flaccid paralysis, which often progresses from the bitten extremity to the rest of the body.

LABORATORY DIAGNOSIS

The standard laboratory test for determining whether animals have rabies is the direct fluorescent antibody (DFA) test performed on fresh brain tissue. It is rapid and reliable and has been standardized over 40 years of use. Fluorescence-labeled rabies antibody is added to brain tissue and binds to the rabies antigen. Unbound antibody is washed away, and the areas where antigen and antibody are bound fluoresce bright green when viewed through a fluorescence microscope.

DFA or reverse transcriptase-polymerase-chain reaction (RT-PCR) may be used to confirm rabies in a human patient by examining a skin biopsy from the nape of the neck. Virus can be found at the base of the hair follicle in the cutaneous nerves. Saliva may be tested using viral isolation or RT-PCR methods. Serum and cerebrospinal fluid may be tested for the presence of antibodies (keeping in mind that rabies immune globulin [RIG] or previous rabies vaccination may cause the serum antibody test to be positive), but these tests may be positive later than tests that look for the virus directly. Autopsy or biopsy specimens of neural tissue will show histologic changes, including mononuclear infiltration, perivascular cuffing of lymphocytes or polymorphonuclear cells, lymphocytic foci, Babès nodules, and Negri bodies. A more sensitive and specific method of detecting rabies in formalin-fixed tissues is immunohistochemistry, which uses specific antibodies to detect rabies virus inclusions.

MANAGEMENT

Once clinical signs of rabies appear, the disease is almost universally fatal and the only treatment is supportive. Eight patients with clinical rabies have been documented to survive, and all had received some sort of pre-exposure prophylaxis before the onset of symptoms. At least six had permanent neurologic sequelae. Pre-exposure prophylaxis, including wound treatment and passive and active immunization, when applied correctly and in a timely manner, is uniformly effective.

Pre-exposure vaccination should be offered to persons in groups at high risk of exposure to rabies, such as veterinarians, animal handlers, animal control and wildlife workers, and laboratory workers who perform rabies research, rabies biologicals production, or rabies diagnostic testing. Additionally, any person who is likely to come in contact with potentially infected animals, such as spelunkers who visit caves with many bats or travelers to countries with endemic rabies where modern rabies biologicals for pre-exposure prophylaxis are not immediately available should consider pre-exposure vaccination. As a rule, travelers visiting rabies-endemic countries for a month or more should consider pre-exposure prophylaxis.

Pre-exposure prophylaxis in the United States consists of 1.0 mL of human diploid cell vaccine (HDCV, Imovax), rabies vaccine adsorbed (RVA), or purified chick embryo cell vaccine (PCEC, RabAvert) given intramuscularly in the deltoid (or in the thigh if the patient is an infant). HDCV also has an intradermal formulation that may be used for pre-exposure prophylaxis, for which the dose is 0.1 mL. Three doses of vaccine should be given, one each on days 0, 7, and 21 to 28. Persons with continuous exposure, such as rabies research laboratory workers and rabies biologicals production workers, should have rabies antibody testing every 6 months. Persons with frequent possible exposures, such as spelunkers, veterinarians, and animal control and wildlife workers in rabies-endemic areas, should have testing performed at 2-year intervals. Booster vaccine doses should be given, if necessary, to maintain an acceptable titer of virus-neutralizing antibody.

There are several questions that should be asked when considering pre-exposure prophylaxis of a patient. First, what kind of exposure occurred? Bites are by far the most likely method of transmitting the virus, but transmission can also occur through saliva or other infectious material, such as neural tissue, contaminating open skin lesions, or mucous membranes. Contact with animal feces, urine, or blood or petting or otherwise touching the infected animal without exposure to the saliva does not constitute an exposure.

Second, what were the circumstances of the bite? Animals that attack without provocation are more likely to be rabid than those that inflict a bite after a provoked attack. Generally, feeding or attempting to handle an animal is considered provocation.

Third, what kind of animal exposed the patient? Dogs, cats, and ferrets that have bitten or otherwise exposed a person can be observed for 10 days. If they remain free of signs of rabies and are eating and drinking, no prophylaxis is needed for the patient because the animal could not have been shedding virus in the saliva at the time of the exposure and still remain healthy at the end of the 10-day period. If the animal develops illness during the period of observation, it should be evaluated by a veterinarian and reported to the health department. If the illness is suggestive of rabies, the animal should be euthanized and the head removed and promptly sent under refrigeration (do not freeze) to a qualified laboratory. If laboratory testing and results are delayed, pre-exposure prophylaxis should be initiated but may be discontinued if DFA testing is negative. The risk of rabies from an animal appropriately vaccinated is very small. If the animal is not available for observation, the local or state health department should be consulted to determine the risk of rabies in the geographic area.

Bites from wild terrestrial carnivores, especially raccoons, skunks, and foxes (the terrestrial animals most often infected with rabies), should be considered possible exposures to rabies virus. The animal should be euthanized and the brain tested for rabies at a qualified laboratory. Pre-exposure prophylaxis should be initiated if laboratory testing and results are delayed. If the immunofluorescence testing is negative, pre-exposure prophylaxis may be discontinued. If the animal is not available for testing, the series of prophylactic vaccinations should be completed. Holding wild carnivores for 10 days to observe for signs of rabies is not reliable and is unsatisfactory management.

Bat exposure has been the most common cause of rabies in humans in the United States recently. Pre-exposure prophylaxis should be initiated with any suspected bite, scratch, or mucous membrane exposure from a bat. If a bat is found in proximity to humans and exposure cannot be ruled out—such as when a bat is found in the room with an unattended child or a sleeping, intoxicated, or mentally impaired person—pre-exposure prophylaxis should be considered. All bats thought to have exposed humans should be submitted for laboratory testing.

Small rodents (e.g., squirrels, hamsters, guinea pigs, gerbils, chipmunks, rats, and mice) and lagomorphs (rabbits and hares), as well as opossum, are rarely found to be infected with rabies virus and have never been associated with a human case. In areas with epizootic raccoon rabies, woodchucks have accounted for a large proportion of the rodent rabies reported to the Centers for Disease Control and Prevention. The state or local health department should be consulted before initiation of pre-exposure prophylaxis due to rodent exposure.

Livestock are a special problem for which there are few data on the timing of viral shedding. Depending on the circumstances of the bite (or other exposure), it may be appropriate to observe the offending animal for 10 to 14 days, as is done with domestic animals. Although livestock can be infected and can transmit the virus, the disease is not endemic among them, and a documented human case from livestock has not occurred since the mid-1900s. The local or state health department should be consulted regarding the risk of rabies among livestock in a given area.

The first step in postexposure rabies prevention is to clean the wound immediately with soap and water and irrigate it with an antiviral agent such as povidone-iodine. The full dose of rabies immune globulin (RIG; Imogam, BayRab), 20 IU/kg, should be infiltrated around the wound site. If not all the RIG can be given around the site of the wound, the rest should be administered intramuscularly at a site distant from the vaccine site. Vaccine (HDVC, RVA, or PCEC), 1.0 mL, should be administered intramuscularly in the deltoid area (or outer thigh in infants) on days 0, 3, 7, 14, and 28. The vaccine should not be administered in the gluteal area.

For patients who have received pre-exposure vaccine, the wound should be cleansed with soap and water and irrigated with an antiviral agent. Vaccine (HDVC, RVA, or PCEC), 1.0 mL, should be administered intramuscularly in the deltoid area (or outer thigh in infants) on days 0 and 3. The vaccine should not be administered in the gluteal area. RIG is not indicated and, in fact, is contraindicated.

Outside the United States, other rabies vaccines may be available, such as purified duck embryo vaccine* and purified Vero cell rabies vaccine.* Also, purified equine rabies immune globulin (ERIG)* may be available where RIG is not. Nerve tissue vaccine* should be used only when there is no alternative, because it is reported to induce neuroparalytic reaction in 1 in 200 to 2000 persons. Unpurified antirabies serum of equine origin,* which may be found in some areas where RIG and ERIG are not available, is associated with higher rates of adverse events, including anaphylaxis.

The best method of prevention of human rabies is through domestic animal control and vaccination, which provide a buffer between the endemic rabies in wild animals and in humans. Wild animals should not be maintained as pets, and bats should be excluded from human dwellings.

---

*Not available in the United States.

RAT-BITE FEVER

method of
JOSEPH P. McGOWAN, M.D.
Bronx-Lebanon Hospital Center
Bronx, New York

and

SANJIV S. SHAH, M.D.
Beth Israel Medical Center
New York, New York

The term *rat-bite fever* is used to describe two distinct diseases with different causative agents: a bacillary form caused by *Streptobacillus moniliformis* and a spirillary form (also known as *Sodoku*) caused by *Spirillum minor*. Rat-bite fever usually occurs sporadically with a worldwide distribution. It is more common in resource-poor areas, where unsanitary conditions persist. *S. moniliformis* accounts for most cases in the United States. It is usually transmitted to human beings after a bite or scratch from rats, other rodents (e.g., mice, squirrels, gerbils), or animals that feed on them such as weasels, dogs, and cats. Rodent bites account for less than 1% of animal bites and occur most often in children younger than age 12. Adults with mental or physical impairment are also at risk. The bites usually occur at night during sleep and in squalid conditions. Infection of laboratory personnel who handle rodents has been described and accounts for half of all recently reported cases of rat-bite fever in the United States. Handling dead rodents can also be a means of transmission. The possibility of mucosal transmission was raised by a recent case report of a 12-year-old boy who developed culture-confirmed *S. moniliformis* septic arthritis of the hip, most likely from close contact with his pet rat, which he was fond of kissing on the lips.

Ten percent to 100% of laboratory rats and 50% to 100% of wild rats may asymptomatically carry one of the causative organisms as part of their nasopharyngeal flora. The risk of developing rat-bite fever has been estimated to be 10% after being bitten by a rat. However, the true incidence of the disease is unknown because it is not a reportable condition to the Centers for Disease Control and Prevention. Many rat bites go unreported, and episodes of the syndrome may not be recognized. In addition, widespread use of antibiotics after bites may abort the infection.

S. moniliformis has also been associated with an epidemic form, called *Haverhill fever*, that is spread by the consumption of raw milk or water that has been contaminated by rat urine or other secretions, rather then by direct contact or bite.

ORGANISMS/MICROBIOLOGY

S. moniliformis is a facultative anaerobic, pleomorphic, gram-negative curved rod. It is not acid fast and nonencapsulated. It tends to form chains with interspaced beadlike gram-variable swellings from which the name *moniliformis* is derived. *S. moniliformis* requires the supplementation of media with 10% to 20% serum, ascitic fluid, or blood to grow. Growth in serum-supplemented thioglycolate broth produces typical "cottonball" colonies. The organism will grow on blood or chocolate agar in 3 to 5 days, is catalase-, oxidase-, indole-, and urease-negative, and has a distinctive fatty acid composition profile on gas chromatography. Growth is inhibited by sodium polyanethol sulfonate (SPS), which is an anticoagulant in most aerobic blood culture bottles. Therefore, bacteremia with this organism may be missed unless blood is cultured in SPS-free or resin-containing bottles. The organism can adopt a cell-wall deficient L-phase that renders it resistant to penicillin; this may account for some reports of therapeutic failure if the transformation occurs in vivo.

S. minor is a short, thick, flagellated, gram-negative rod that cannot be cultured on artificial media. Diagnosis often requires inoculation of blood, obtained at the height of a febrile episode, into mice and guinea pigs. Peritoneal fluid from the animals is examined daily under darkfield microscopy for typical organisms.

CLINICAL SYNDROMES

Rat-bite fever is an acute or chronically relapsing illness. *S. moniliformis* usually has an incubation period of 1 to 4 days, which can rarely extend as long as 3 weeks after exposure. The wound tends to heal uneventfully, and there may be some mild regional lymphadenitis. The disease is heralded by sudden onset of fever that can relapse at irregular intervals, headache, and an erythematous maculopapular rash of the distal extremities (often involving the palms and soles) that begins when the initial fever lessens after about 48 hours. The rash lasts an average of 6 days (ranging from 1–21 days) and will desquamate in about 20% of cases. Pustules and petechiae have been described in some cases. Asymmetric migratory polyarthritis, which is usually sterile, occurs in more than half of the cases and is diagnostically helpful. Examination of the joint fluid reveals leukocytosis with a polymorphonuclear cell predominance. Cough, sore throat, chills, myalgia, nausea, and vomiting may also be present. Up to 25% of patients will have a false-positive nontreponemal test for syphilis. Focal septic complications have been described and include septic arthritis (of the hip, wrists, ankles, and knees), infective endocarditis, meningitis, brain and other abscesses, splenic and renal infarcts, pneumonia, pericarditis, prostatitis, and chorioamnionitis.

The spirillary form (*S. minor*) of the disease is somewhat distinct, with a longer incubation period, more localized symptoms, and lack of the polyarthritis commonly seen in the bacillary form. The incubation period of rat-bite fever caused by *S. minor* ranges from 1 to 6 weeks. Localized inflammation including ulceration of the bite is common, followed by paroxysmal fever, localized lymphadenitis and pain on the affected limb, and dark red maculopapular eruption of the palms and soles. Splenomegaly may be noted. Up to six or eight febrile episodes may occur of 2 to 4 days' duration interspersed with asymptomatic periods of similar length before spontaneous resolution. Arthritis is rarely seen. Chronic cases of spirillary fever, with recurring symptoms over years, have been described.

Haverhill fever, named after the site of the initial report from Haverhill, Massachusetts, in 1926, is caused by *S. moniliformis* and has been reported in outbreaks in the United States and England during which no direct contact by patients with rats could be ascertained. The latter epidemic, which occurred at a girls' boarding school, involved 304 patients and was believed to be associated with contaminated drinking water. Consumption of unpasteurized milk, ice cream, and other milk products has also been implicated as a possible source of transmission. The syndrome, also known as erythema arthriticum epidemicum, includes abrupt onset of fever, headache, centrifugal rash, and arthralgia.

DIAGNOSIS

The diagnosis must begin with clinical suspicion in a patient with fever, arthritis, and rash involving the palms and soles. If history of rat bite is absent, the diagnosis is usually made after the unanticipated growth of the organism from blood or joint tissue. The bacillary form of the disease may be diagnosed with culture of infected material, including blood, abscess, and biopsy material. Culture can be difficult because the organism may adopt a nutritionally fastidious L-form. The microbiology laboratory should be notified that rat bite fever is suspected. Blood, inoculated into blood culture media, may suffice as the organism's requirement for body fluids for growth. Prior antibiotic therapy and the presence of SPS in blood culture media may reduce the yield of culture. Specific streptobacillus serology is neither reliable nor readily available.

Laboratory diagnosis of *S. minor* is difficult because it cannot be easily cultured. The organism has been demonstrated in biopsy samples of the skin lesion and regional lymph nodes, exudate, and blood (by Giemsa or Wright stain or darkfield microscopy); however, the yield is low.

The differential diagnosis of rat-bite fever includes febrile illnesses associated with rash and/or arthralgias such as Rocky Mountain spotted fever and other rickettsial illnesses, coxsackievirus B and Epstein-Barr virus infection, leptospirosis, syphilis, Lyme disease, rheumatoid arthritis, and systemic lupus erythematosus.

TREATMENT

Death from untreated rat-bite fever has been reported to occur in up to 10% of cases, usually associated with endocarditis due to *S. moniliformis*. In vitro, penicillin demonstrates the most activity against *S. moniliformis*. Ampicillin* and cephalosporins* are also very active. For patients with penicillin allergy, tetracycline, streptomycin,* chloramphenicol,* and erythromycin* are alternatives. Ciprofloxacin (Cipro)* has modest activity. Organisms transformed to the L-phase will be penicillin resistant but

*Not FDA approved for this indication.

will remain susceptible to tetracycline and streptomycin.

Penicillin is the drug of choice for both the bacillary and the spirillary forms of the disease. Intravenous penicillin, at a dose of 1.2 to 2.4 million units per day for a minimum of 7 days, followed by a week of oral penicillin V or amoxicillin* is recommended for treatment of uncomplicated cases. Complicated cases, such as those with endocarditis, require up to 20 million units of aqueous penicillin G intravenously for 4 to 6 weeks. In patients with penicillin allergy, tetracycline (500 mg every 6 hours), doxycycline (intravenously or orally), or the cephalosporins* (in the absence of a type 1 hypersensitivity reaction to penicillin) may be used. Chloramphenicol* is a therapeutic alternative in children younger than the age of 8 who are allergic to penicillin. Streptomycin* (7.5 mg/kg intramuscularly every 12 hours) can also be given, but patients should be carefully monitored for signs of ototoxicity. If penicillin-resistant *S. moniliformis* has been clinically isolated, streptomycin or tetracycline (both of which are active against the L-forms) may be added to regimens. A Jarisch-Herxheimer reaction may occur during treatment of *S. minor.*

Prophylactic use of penicillin V, 500 mg orally every 6 hours for 3 days, after rat bite has been advocated. However, the efficacy of this strategy is unknown. Wounds should be thoroughly cleansed with soap and water, and administration of tetanus prophylaxis should be considered as indicated.

*Not FDA approved for this indication.

RELAPSING FEVER

method of
MARK S. DWORKIN, M.D., M.P.H.T.M.
Illinois Department of Public Health
Chicago, Illinois

Relapsing fever is characterized by recurring episodes of fever and nonspecific symptoms (e.g., headache, myalgia, arthralgia, and abdominal complaints). Usually, episodes last several days and are then interrupted by cessation of symptoms. Untreated patients have experienced up to 13 febrile episodes. The illness is caused by infection with *Borrelia* species (spirochetes) that extensively vary their surface antigens. Relapsing fever spirochetes are transmitted to humans by exposure to infected lice (*Pediculus humanus*) or the bite of an infected tick (*Ornithodoros* species). The mean incubation period is 7 days (range, 4–18 days or more). *Borrelia recurrentis* causes louse-borne relapsing fever (LBRF, or epidemic relapsing fever). Spirochetes are introduced by crushing the louse (e.g., when scratching), which releases the insect's infected hemolymph and contaminates abraded or normal skin and mucous membranes.

EPIDEMIOLOGY

LBRF is associated with poor hygiene and catastrophic events; an estimated 15 million cases and more than 5 million deaths occurred in Africa, Eastern Europe, and Russia during the 20th century. Tick-borne relapsing fever (TBRF, or endemic relapsing fever) is found throughout most of the world. It is endemic in the western United States, southern British Columbia, the plateau regions of Mexico, Central and South America, the Mediterranean, Central Asia, and most of Africa. The tick vectors, *Ornithodoros* species, are argasid (soft) ticks that have nocturnal feeding habits and painless bites. The primary reservoirs of *Borrelia* are rodents (e.g., deer mice, chipmunks, squirrels, and rats). Unlike the body louse, which lives only several weeks, *Ornithodoros* ticks may live many years between blood meals and may harbor spirochetes for prolonged periods.

In Texas, cases have been associated with entering caves where the tick *O. turicata* harbors *B. turicatae*. In most other western states and southern British Columbia, *B. hermsii* is transmitted by *O. hermsii* at varying elevations; patients often report exposure in rustic cabins where rodent's nests may harbor these ticks. *B. parkeri* may also cause TBRF in the United States, and other species are responsible elsewhere in the world. Borreliae have also been transmitted by blood transfusion, intravenous drug use, and blood contamination of skin.

TBRF differs from Lyme disease, caused by a *Borrelia* species (*B. burgdorferi*), in important ways. For example, the reported Lyme disease vectors in the United States (*Ixodes scapularis* and *I. pacificus*), their geographic distribution, and the methods of preventing Lyme disease differ considerably from TBRF.

CLINICAL MANIFESTATIONS

The clinical manifestations of TBRF and LBRF are similar, although not identical. The frequency of occurrence of the clinical manifestations of TBRF is presented in Table 1. Alteration of sensorium is common. Persons with LBRF are more likely to have jaundice; central nervous system involvement; petechiae on the trunk, the extremities, and the mucous membranes; epistaxis; and blood-tinged spu-

TABLE 1. **Manifestations of Tick-Borne Relapsing Fever in the United States**

Sign or Symptom	Frequency, %
Headache	94
Myalgia	92
Chills	88
Nausea	76
Arthralgia	73
Vomiting	71
Abdominal pain	44
Confusion	38
Dry cough	27
Eye pain	26
Diarrhea	25
Dizziness	25
Photophobia	25
Neck pain	24
Rash	18
Dysuria	13
Jaundice	10
Hepatomegaly	10
Splenomegaly	6
Conjunctival injection	5
Eschar	2
Meningitis	2
Nuchal rigidity	2

tum. In addition to the manifestations presented in the table, iridocyclitis, cranial nerve palsy, myocarditis, and rupture of the spleen may rarely occur. The average length of the first episode is 3 days for TBRF and 5.5 days for LBRF. The average period from the first episode to the first relapse is 7 days for TBRF and 9 days for LBRF. The patient may have symptoms such as malaise during afebrile intervals. Relapsing fever in a pregnant woman may lead to spontaneous abortion, premature birth, or neonatal death.

There may be great individual variability among relapsing fever cases. Although the relapsing nature of the disease is consistent, one person may present with apparent meningitis whereas another may appear to have influenza, a febrile gastrointestinal illness, or perhaps no physical findings. A careful history of the present illness, physical examination, and consideration of relapsing fever in the differential diagnosis are keys to avoiding misdiagnosis.

The differential diagnosis of infectious diseases causing fevers that may relapse or have biphasic patterns includes Colorado tick fever, yellow fever, dengue fever, African hemorrhagic fevers (e.g., Lassa), lymphocytic choriomeningitis, brucellosis, malaria, leptospirosis, chronic meningococcemia, rat-bite fever, ascending (intermittent) cholangitis, and infection with echovirus 9 and *Rochalimaea* species. A history of travel, place of residence, and animal exposures is useful in patients who have these fever patterns.

Jarisch-Herxheimer Reaction

The Jarisch-Herxheimer reaction, an acute exacerbation of the patient's symptoms, may occur on initial treatment of relapsing fever with an effective antibiotic. During this reaction, the spirochetes rapidly disappear from the circulation. Symptoms often include hypotension, tachycardia, chills, rigors, diaphoresis, and marked elevation of the temperature. The reaction typically begins within 1 to 4 hours of the first dose of antibiotic, and the symptoms may be very severe. Patients with this reaction have been known to say that they felt as if they were going to die. When possible, patients with LBRF who develop the Jarisch-Herxheimer reaction should be transferred to an intensive care unit for close monitoring of fluid balance, measurements of arterial and central venous pressure, and monitoring of myocardial function. Patients with TBRF should also be closely monitored. Corticosteroids and nonsteroidal anti-inflammatory agents have not been shown to prevent or modify this reaction significantly. Tetracyclines nearly always produce a Jarisch-Herxheimer reaction in LBRF. Death has been reported as a complication of the reaction, most often secondary to cardiovascular collapse.

Generally, death occurs more frequently in untreated LBRF than in TBRF; however, a patient's nutritional status may play a significant role in the outcome. LBRF often occurs in the setting of famine or overcrowding where nutrition may be poor and additional diseases may complicate the diagnosis or the disease course. The fatality rate for LBRF is 5% in treated persons and is much lower for TBRF.

DIAGNOSIS

Cases of relapsing fever are confirmed when spirochetes are visualized in a peripheral blood thin smear or dehemoglobinized thick smear or buffy coat preparations stained with Wright, Giemsa, or acridine orange stain. Also, the motility of the organism can be best witnessed with a fresh specimen visualized with darkfield microscopy. Peripheral smears are more often positive for spirochetes in LBRF than in TBRF. Therefore, repeating phlebotomy, especially during periods of fever preceding or during a relapsing "crisis," may be necessary to confirm the diagnosis. Three main factors may contribute to poor detection on a peripheral smear: (1) the microscopists inexperience, (2) increased use of automated differentials, and (3) examination of blood in the asymptomatic interval when spirochetes are absent from the circulation or their level is below the level of detection. Manual examination of a peripheral smear should be performed in the setting of an appropriate exposure history when a patient has flulike symptoms (especially high fever and severe headache) and when laboratory results demonstrate a normal or mildly elevated white blood cell count, increased segmented neutrophils, and thrombocytopenia.

Spirochetes may also be visualized in bone marrow, cerebrospinal fluid, or spleen. Other methods of diagnosis include the finding of a typical clinical history combined with positive serology results (indirect fluorescent antibody test or enzyme-linked immunosorbent assay confirmed by Western blot). Serologic false-positive results for Lyme disease (*B. burgdorferi*) and syphilis (*Treponema pallidum*) may occur. The spirochetes may be cultured from blood using specialized medium.

Other laboratory findings are not diagnostic. These include thrombocytopenia; a normal or modestly elevated leukocyte count, sometimes with increased immature cells ("left shift"); elevated serum bilirubin levels; proteinuria; microhematuria; and prolonged prothrombin time and partial thromboplastin time.

TREATMENT

Relapsing fever spirochetes are very sensitive to antibiotics, and antimicrobial resistance is uncommon. Treatment options for adults are summarized in Table 2. The likelihood of producing the Jarisch-Herxheimer reaction with one drug versus another is not well understood. Antibiotics other than those

TABLE 2. **Treatment Options for Relapsing Fever in Adults**

Medication	Tick-Borne Relapsing Fever (7-Day Adult Dosage Schedule)	Louse-Borne Relapsing Fever (Single Adult Dose)
Oral		
Chloramphenicol†	500 mg q6h‡	500 mg‡
Doxycycline	100 mg q12h	100 mg
Erythromycin†	500 mg q6h	500 mg
Tetracycline†	500 mg q6h	500 mg
Parenteral*		
Chloramphenicol†	500 mg q6h‡	500 mg‡
Doxycycline	100 mg q12h	100 mg
Erythromycin†	500 mg q6h	500 mg
Penicillin G (procaine)†	600,000 IU daily	600,000 IU
Tetracycline†	250 mg q6h	250 mg

*Parenteral medication should be continued until oral medication is tolerated. If oral medication is tolerated at the time of diagnosis, parenteral medication may not be necessary.
†Not FDA approved for this indication.
‡Rarely used in the United States.

listed in the table have not been investigated and should be avoided. For LBRF, single-dose therapy is generally recommended. A 7-day (or 10-day) course of therapy is generally used for TBRF. There is insufficient information available on the possible efficacy of single-dose therapy for TBRF. Intravenous medication should be administered when oral medication is not tolerated.

Children younger than 8 years of age and pregnant women should be treated with penicillin or erythromycin. The Jarisch-Herxheimer reaction in children has been reported to be milder than in adults. Monitoring of patients who have taken the first dose of antibiotic has generally been recommended for the first 12 hours.

PREVENTION

Prevention of TBRF includes avoiding rodent- and tick-infested dwellings and infested natural sites such as animal burrows or caves. Rodent-proofing of homes and vacation cabins and assessing and limiting rodent-friendly environments around homes may be performed with the consultation of local health department environmental health specialists and pest removal services. Chemical treatment of rodent-infested areas is available and should be administered by pest control specialists. Contact with ticks and potential animal vectors should occur only while wearing gloves. Wearing clothing that protects skin from tick access (e.g., long pants and long-sleeved shirts) and applying insect repellents (e.g., permethrin) to exposed skin and clothing may help prevent this disease. Protection during sleeping in a potentially infested dwelling may best be provided by use of topical repellents. Prevention of LBRF occurs through control of lice by promoting personal hygiene and systematic delousing with DDT or lindane powder. Control of epidemics also involves widespread antibiotic use and possibly antibiotic prophylaxis with doxycycline, 100 mg twice weekly.

LYME DISEASE

method of
JANINE EVANS, M.D.
Yale University School of Medicine
New Haven, Connecticut

EPIDEMIOLOGY

Lyme disease, a systemic illness caused by the spirochete *Borrelia burgdorferi*, is the most common tickborne disease in the United States. More than 128,000 cases have been reported to health authorities in the United States since 1982, when a systematic national surveillance was initiated. It is likely that the true number of cases of Lyme disease is significantly greater because many do not fulfill the Centers for Disease Control and Prevention (CDC) case definition, and Lyme disease is often underreported. Although cases have been reported from 48 states, the disease occurs mostly in distinct and geographically limited areas. Over 90% of reported cases come from eight states located in the Northeast, the upper Midwest, and the Pacific Coast.

Lyme disease occurs worldwide. However, most cases occur in temperate regions and coincide with the distribution of the principal vector, ticks of the *Ixodes ricinus* complex: *Ixodes scapularis* in the eastern and upper midwestern United States; *Ixodes pacificus* in California; *I. ricinus* in Europe; and *Ixodes persulcatus* in Eastern Europe and Asia.

The *I. scapularis* tick has a three-stage, 2-year life cycle. Transovarial passage of *Borrelia burgdorferi* occurs at a low rate. Ticks become infected with spirochetes by feeding on a spirochetemic animal, typically small mammals, during larval and nymphal stages. In highly endemic areas, from 20% to more than 60% of *I. scapularis* carry *B. burgdorferi*. Human beings are only incidental hosts of the tick; contact is typically made in areas of underbrush or high grasses but may occur in well-mown lawns in endemic areas. Lyme disease occurs predominantly during May through July when nymphal *I. scapularis* ticks feed. Animal models show that transmission is unlikely to occur before a minimum of 36 hours of tick attachment and feeding.

B. burgdorferi displays phenotypic and genotypic diversity and has been classified into three separate genospecies: *species I*, which includes all strains studied thus far from the United States and some European and Asian strains, are termed *Borrelia burdorferi sensu stricto*; *species II*, which are termed *Borrelia garinii*; and *species III*, *Borrelia afzelii*, which are found in Europe and Asia. *B. afzelii* seems primarily associated with a chronic skin lesion, acrodermatitis chronica atropicans, which is rare in the United States.

CLINICAL MANIFESTATIONS

Lyme disease primarily affects the skin, heart, joints, and nervous system. Clinical features of Lyme disease are typically divided into three general stages: early localized, early disseminated, and late persistent infection. These stages may overlap, most patients do not exhibit all of them, and seroconversion can occur in asymptomatic individuals but is rare with strict surveillance. The illness usually begins with a skin lesion, erythema migrans (EM), and associated symptoms (early localized), sometimes followed weeks to months later by neurologic or cardiac abnormalities (early disseminated) and weeks to years later by arthritis. Chronic neurologic and skin involvement also may occur years after onset (late persistent).

Early Localized Disease

Erythema migrans, the hallmark of early localized disease, appears as an expanding erythematous papule or macule, sometimes with central clearing, at the site of a deer tick bite. EM lesions have been reported in 60% to 90% of individuals with well-documented Lyme disease. Typically, the lesion is flat, warm, and not painful. Sometimes it may become indurated, warm, and pruritic. The outer borders are red, generally well demarcated, and without scaling. Variations may occur (e.g., multiple rings). Central clearing is associated with lesions that have been present for longer duration. With time, the lesion expands centrifugally, presumably related to the outward migration of the organisms. With time, EM lesions may become quite large (>5 cm). Lesions are often located in intriginous areas such as the groin, buttocks, axilla, and popliteal fossa, as well as the waist and thigh, areas where clothing ends. EM lesions occur 1 to 36 days (median, 7–10 days) after a deer tick bite. Only 14% to 32% of patients with EM recall a tick bite. If left untreated, the rash disappears without scarring several days to weeks after onset; in treated patients, resolution typically occurs faster. Most patients (up to 80%) have associated systemic complaints, including fatigue, myalgias, arthralgias, headache, fever and/or chills, and stiff neck. In early localized disease, these symptoms tend to be mild. The most common objective physical findings associated with this stage are fever and lymphadenopathy. Occasionally, Lyme disease can produce a febrile, flulike syndrome (e.g., myalgias, arthralgias, headache, stiff neck, and/or fatigue) without an associated EM rash.

EM-like rashes have been reported from many southern U.S. states. Whether such rashes represent cases of Lyme disease is controversial. The Lone Star tick (*Amblyomma americanum*) appears to be an important vector in the transmission of the Lyme disease–like infections because it accounts for 95% of the human tick bites in some regions with reported cases. It is uncertain if *B. burgdorferi* infection is the responsible agent because it has rarely been isolated from local reservoir animals, patients typically do not have serologic evidence of exposure, and cultures of biopsy specimens failed to grow the organism. It is possible that these rashes are secondary to a different but related spirochetal infection.

Early Disseminated Disease

In some patients the spirochetes disseminate hematogenously to multiple sites, causing characteristic clinical features. Secondary annular lesions, sites of metastatic foci of *Borrelia* in the skin, develop within days of onset of EM in about half of U.S. patients. They are similar in appearance to EM but are generally smaller, migrate less, and lack indurated centers.

Cardiac involvement occurs in up to 10% of untreated patients. Transient and varying degrees of atrioventricular block several weeks to months after a tick bite are the most common manifestations. Other features are pericarditis, myocarditis, ventricular tachycardia, and, on rare occasions, a dilated cardiomyopathy; valvular disease is not seen. Carditis is typically mild and self-limited, although patients may present quite dramatically in complete heart block and some may require the insertion of a temporary pacemaker. In most cases, carditis resolves completely, even without treatment with antibiotics. Treatment of carditis is indicated to prevent the development of late manifestations of the disease.

In addition to musculoskeletal "flulike" symptoms, mild hepatitis, splenomegaly, sore throat, nonproductive cough, testicular swelling, conjunctivitis, and regional and generalized lymphadenopathy may sometimes occur during early stages.

Early neurologic involvement occurs in 15% to 20% of untreated patients and appears within 2 to 8 weeks after the onset of disease. Manifestations include cranial nerve palsies, meningitis or meningoencephalitis, chorea, and peripheral neuritis or radiculoneuritis, in various combinations. Unilateral or bilateral seventh nerve palsies are the most common neurologic abnormalities. Presenting symptoms depend on the area of the nervous system involved: patients with meningitis present with fever, headache, and a stiff neck; those with Bannwarth syndrome (primarily in Europe) develop severe and migrating radicular pain lasting weeks to several months; and those with encephalitis have concentration deficits, emotional lability, and fatigue. Analysis of cerebrospinal fluid (CSF) from patients with early central nervous system (CNS) involvement typically reveals a lymphocytic pleocytosis. Specific antibodies against *B. burgdorferi* may also be present and concentrated in the CSF relative to the serum concentration; they are useful to confirm disease. In general, neurologic abnormalities last for months but usually resolve completely.

In Europe, patients occasionally develop a solitary cutaneous lesion called *Borrelia* lymphocytoma with follicles resembling those seen in lymph nodes. It has been reported to occur in less than 10% of individuals in most series. Lymphocytomas appear most often as a red or violaceous solitary lesion on the ear or nipple; sometimes, more widespread lesions may be seen. Patients usually have associated regional lymphadenopathy; generalized symptoms are typically absent. Lesions promptly resolve with antibiotic therapy; if untreated, they may last months and even years.

Late Disease

Late manifestations of Lyme disease typically occur months to years after the initial infection (mean, 6 months). In the United States, arthritis is the dominant feature of late Lyme disease, reported in approximately 60% of untreated individuals. The initial pattern of involvement may be migratory arthralgias (early), followed later by intermittent attacks of arthritis. Large joints, particularly the knee, are most commonly involved. Swelling is often prominent, with large effusions and Baker cysts. However, small joints may be affected and a few patients have had symmetric polyarthritis. Attacks of arthritis, which generally last from weeks to months, typically recur for several years and decrease in frequency over time. Systemic symptoms such as fever do not accompany bouts of arthritis, in most cases.

Synovial fluid specimens usually demonstrate white blood cell counts that vary from 500 to 110,000 cells/mm^3, with an average of 25,000 cells/mm^3, predominantly polymorphonuclear leukocytes. Joint fluid protein ranges from 3 to 8 g/dL.

A small subgroup of patients with Lyme arthritis develop a prolonged, potentially erosive arthritis unresponsive to antibiotics. These patients often have major histocompatibility class II gene products (HLA-DR4) accompanied by strong serum IgG responses to *Borrelia* outer surface proteins A or B (OspA or OspB). Repeated courses of treatment with antibiotics have not been demonstrated to improve clinical outcome.

A chronic neurologic syndrome may occur months to years after disease onset and involve the central or peripheral nervous system. Typically, the neurologic features consist of a radiculoneuropathy, encephalopathy, or, rarely, encephalomyelitis. Peripheral nervous system involvement is characterized by paresthesias and electrophysiologic evidence of axonal polyneuropathy. Lyme encephalopathy, a rare neuropsychiatric disorder, predominantly affects memory and concentration. Cognitive dysfunction, headache, affective changes, seizures, ataxia, and chronic fatigue have all been reported. Because these complaints are often nonspecific and may be associated with post-Lyme syndromes, it is important to look for and document evidence of ongoing *B. burgdorferi* infection. Lymphocytic pleocytosis is uncommon in late neurologic disease, but increased intrathecal *B. burgdorferi*–specific antibodies and/or elevated CSF protein may well be present. Polymerase chain reaction assays have been applied to CSF specimens but are not very sensitive. Single-photon emission computed tomography (SPECT) may detect reduced cerebral perfusion, especially in frontal subcortical and cortical region, but are nonspecific and abnormalities should not be used as the sole criterion for diagnosis. Careful evaluation with neuropsychological testing can help to distinguish cognitive abnormalities in Lyme disease from those associated with chronic fatigue states and depression.

Other late findings (years) associated with this infection include a chronic skin lesion—acrodermatitis chronica atrophicans, well known in Europe but rare in the United States. These lesions appear as violaceous infiltrated plaques or nodules, especially on extensor surfaces, that eventually become atrophic. One third of patients experience an associated polyneuropathy, usually sensory. *B. burgdorferi* have been isolated from skin biopsy specimens of acrodermatitis chronica atrophicans.

Ocular lesions in Lyme disease are rare but have involved every portion of the eye and vary depending on the stage of disease. The most common ophthalmic presentations in early disease include conjunctivitis, photophobia, and neuro-opthalmologic manifestions due to cranial nerve palsies. The most severe ocular manifestations occur in late stages: they include episcleritis, symblepharon, keratitis, iritis, choroiditis, panuveitis, and retinal vasculitis.

INFECTION IN CHILDREN

Children have the highest incidence of Lyme disease, likely owing to a greater risk of exposure. The clinical spectrum is similar to that of adults. Most children present for medical attention with EM lesions. Younger children typically have EM lesions on either the head or neck, whereas in older children the extremities are the most common site. Children appear to recover more completely from active infection with *B. burgdorferi*. Most studies have indicated that long-term outcomes in children are excellent.

INFECTION DURING PREGNANCY

Intrauterine transmission of *B. burgdorferi* is uncommon, usually occurring in cases of obvious disseminated infection during pregnancy. No uniform pattern of congenital anomaly has been reported. Prenatal exposure to Lyme disease has not been found to be associated with an increased risk of adverse pregnancy outcome.

DIAGNOSIS

The diagnosis of Lyme disease relies on the presence of characteristic clinical features and supporting serologic test results. Although spirochetes have been isolated from a variety of patient specimens, culture or direct visualization of *B. burgdorferi* is difficult and frequently yields negative results. In response to the need for a uniform definition, the CDC, in association with state health departments, developed a national surveillance case definition for Lyme disease. The criteria were intended to be used for epidemiologic surveillance and for comparing the results of treatment in different trials. Because the criteria are biased toward certainty in the diagnosis of Lyme disease, strict application in clinical practice may result in underdiagnosis and unnecessary delay in treatment. Serologic confirmation is the most practical and widely used laboratory aid currently available. Laboratory testing is best used to confirm a diagnosis of Lyme disease. Valid interpretation of test results depends on sound clinical evidence that Lyme disease is present. Disease predictive value calculations demonstrate that when tests are ordered without regard for clinical features (i.e., used as a screening test) the positive predictive value is only 7%, even under ideal testing conditions. The positive predictive value rises to more than 96% when patients with a good clinical history for Lyme disease are tested.

IgM antibodies generally develop within 2 to 4 weeks after the onset of infection, peak after 6 to 8 weeks of illness, and decline to the normal range after 4 to 6 months of illness in most patients. Antibodies of the IgG class are usually measured within 6 to 8 weeks after the onset of disease and peak after 4 to 6 months. In some patients, IgG levels remain elevated indefinitely.

An immunologic response can be detected within weeks of onset of the disease using either an indirect immunofluorescence assay (IFA) or an enzyme-linked immunosorbent assay (ELISA). ELISA tests are preferred because they are more sensitive and reproducible. Most ELISA assays use extracts of sonicated whole *B. burgdorferi* as antigen. Purified *B. burgdorferi* proteins have also been used as substrates. Currently available commercial tests vary in sensitivity and specificity; hence, identical serum samples sent simultaneously to different laboratories may yield different results. In the best of circumstances, false-positive and false-negative results occur.

Immunoblotting has been advocated as a method of distinguishing true-positive ELISA results. Antibodies directed against specific *Borrelia* proteins are identified. Because many proteins on *B. burgdorferi* are shared with other organisms, false-positive results may also occur with immunoblots. Criteria for interpretation of immunoblot results have been established.

When serologic testing is indicated, authorities recommend testing initially with a sensitive first test, either an ELISA or an IFA test, followed by testing with the more specific Western immunoblot test to corroborate equivocal or positive results obtained with the first test. Although antibiotic treatment in early localized disease may blunt or abrogate the antibody response, patients with early disseminated or late-stage disease usually have strong serologic reactivity.

B. burgdorferi can be cultured from 80% or more of biopsy specimens taken from early EM lesions. However, the diagnostic usefulness of this procedure is limited because of the need for a special bacteriologic medium (modified Barbour-Stoenner-Kelly medium) and protracted observation of cultures.

Polymerase chain reaction (PCR) has been used to amplify genomic DNA of *B. burgdorferi*. Sensitive and specific PCR assays have been developed. Recent application of a PCR method on skin biopsy specimens resulted in an 80% positive rate from patients with EM lesions and a 92% positive rate from patients with acrodermatitis chronica atrophicans. PCR assays of synovial fluid specimens have proved valuable in studying patients with Lyme arthritis. PCR techniques have also been applied to blood, urine, and CSF specimens but, to date, the results have been disappointing. The major problem in using the PCR technique is the issue of false-positive results. Proper handling of specimens is required to avoid contamination. Interpretation of PCR results is reliable only when the tests are performed in laboratories where appropriate precautions are taken.

TREATMENT

The goal of antibiotic therapy in Lyme disease is to eradicate the causative organism and reduce the risk of developing serious late manifestations of infection. Lyme disease is most responsive to treatment with antibiotics early in the course of infection. Current treatment recommendations are based on the results of published scientific studies and on clinical experience. The appropriate endpoint in antibiotic treatment is not always clear, owing to the persistence of certain symptoms and difficulty in proving when the organism has been fully eradicated. Better understanding of the etiology of persistent symptoms after treatment will likely result in improved therapies. The treatment regimens outlined here represent guidelines (Table 1).

Treatment of early stages of Lyme disease with oral antibiotics is adequate in the majority of patients. In patients with acute disseminated Lyme

TABLE 1. **Treatment Guidelines**

Disorder	Antibiotic Regimen	Comments
Erythema migrans	Amoxicillin,* 500 mg three times daily for 14–21 days	Pediatric dose is 50 mg/kg/d three times daily.
	Doxycycline (Vibramycin), 100 mg twice daily for 14–21 days	Effective against human granulocytic ehrlichiosis; not recommended for children younger than 9 years of age or for pregnant or lactating women
	Cefuroxime axetil (Ceftin), 500 mg twice daily for 21 days	
	Tetracycline,* 500 mg four times daily for 14–21 days	Not recommended for children younger than 9 years of age or for pregnant or lactating women
	Azithromycin (Zithromax),* 500 mg daily for 7–10 days	Less effective than other regimens
Early disseminated disease (without neurologic, cardiac, or joint involvement)	Initial treatment is the same as for erythema migrans except duration of treatment is 21–28 days.	
Two types of neuroborreliosis		
Isolated seventh nerve palsy	Initial treatment is the same as for erythema migrans except duration of treatment is 21–28 days.	
All other neurologic manifestations (including meningitis, radiculoneuritis, peripheral neuropathy, encephalomyelitis, chronic encephalopathy)	Ceftriaxone (Rocephin),* 2 g/d for 14–30 days	30-Day regimen associated with fewer relapses in patients with chronic encephalopathy
	Penicillin G,* 20 million units daily for 14–28 days	Pediatric dose: 200,000–400,000 units/kg/d q4h
	Cefotaxime sodium (Claforan), 2 g q8h for 14–28 days	Pediatric dose: 90–180 mg/kg/d
	Doxycycline, 100 mg twice daily (oral or intravenous) for 14–28 days	No published experience in the United States
Carditis	Doxycycline, 100 mg orally twice daily for 21 days	For first-degree heart block, PR interval <0.3 s.
	Amoxicillin,* 500 mg three times daily	For first-degree heart block, PR interval <0.3 s.
	Ceftriaxone,* 2 g/d for 14–30 days	Optimal duration of therapy is unknown.
	Penicillin G,* 20 million units daily for 14–30 days	Optimal duration of therapy is unknown; drug is given in divided doses every 4 hours.
Arthritis	Amoxicillin* and probenecid,* 500 mg four times daily for 30–60 days	Oral regimens should be limited to patients without evidence of neurologic involvement; oral treatment may be extended for 60 days if no response to 30-day course.
	Doxycycline, 100 mg two times daily for 30–60 days	
	Cefuroxime axetil, 500 mg twice daily for 30–60 days	For patients with doxycycline and penicillin allergy
	Ceftriaxone,* 2 g daily for 14–30 days	
Lyme disease in pregnancy	Amoxicillin,* 500 mg three times daily for 21 days	For early localized disease only
	Penicillin G,* 20 million units daily for 14–28 days	Given in divided doses every 4 hours
	Ceftriaxone,* 2 g/d for 14–28 days	
Asymptomatic tick bite	No treatment recommended	For pregnant women, a 10-day course of amoxicillin may be considered.

*Not FDA approved for this indication.

disease but without meningitis, oral doxycycline appears to be equally as effective as parenteral ceftriaxone (Rocephin)* in preventing the late manifestations of disease. Initial studies of treatment for early Lyme disease reported that therapy with phenoxymethyl penicillin,* erthromycin,* and tetracycline,* in doses four times a day for 1 to 20 days shortened the duration of symptoms of early Lyme disease. Phenoxymethyl penicillin and tetracycline were superior to erythromycin in preventing serious late manifestations of disease. Subsequent clinical trials have proven amoxicillin* and doxycycline to be equally efficacious. Concomitant use of probenecid has not been definitively shown to improve clinical outcome and is associated with a higher incidence of side effects. Doxycyline is effective in treating the agent of human granulocytic ehrlichiosis, an organism also transmitted by *I. scapularis* ticks; amoxicillin is not. Cefuroxime axetil (Ceftin), an oral second-generation cephalosporin, has been shown to be effective in treating early Lyme disease; azithromycin (Zithromax),* an azilide analogue of erthromycin, is somewhat less so. The prognosis for patients treated during early stages of Lyme disease is excellent. Jarisch-Herxheimer–like reactions, an increased discomfort in skin lesions, and temperature elevation occurring within hours after the start of antibiotic treatment have been encountered in 14% of patients treated during early Lyme disease. They typically occur within 2 to 4 hours of starting therapy, are more common in disseminated disease, and are presumably due to rapid killing of a large number of spirochetes.

Minor symptoms including arthralgia, fatigue, headaches, and transient facial palsy are common after treatment and generally resolve over a 6-month period. The etiology of these symptoms is unclear: it may be the result of retained antigen rather than persistence of live spirochetes. Persistent symptoms are more common in adults, patients treated when in disseminated or late stages of disease, and individuals who have had long delays before receiving antibiotic therapy.

The optimal treatment of Lyme carditis is unknown, and, to date, no studies have been performed focusing specifically on treatment of carditis. Several oral and intravenous antibiotic regimens have been successful. Thirty-day courses of oral antibiotics such as amoxicillin,* 500 mg orally three to four times a day, or doxycycline, 100 mg two times per day, are likely sufficient to treat milder forms of cardiac involvement such as first-degree heart block with PR intervals less than 0.3 second. Hospitalization with cardiac monitoring is indicated for patients with first-degree heart block with longer PR intervals, higher-degree heart block, or evidence of global ventricular impairment. Intravenous antibiotics such as penicillin G,* or ceftriaxone* are recommended for such patients. Insertion of a temporary pacemaker should be considered in patients with severe and

*Not FDA approved for this indication.

symptomatic heart block, although permanent pacing is rarely indicated. The use of adjuvant corticosteroids or salicylates should be reserved for patients with prolonged dense heart block to speed recovery and reduce the risk of permanent conduction system defects.

Intravenous antibiotics are recommended for all cases of neuroborreliosis except isolated seventh nerve palsy. Patients presenting with a Bell-like palsy who have features that suggest possible CNS involvement, such as high fever, headache, or stiff neck, should undergo a lumbar puncture looking for evidence of more extensive disease. The most experience in the treatment of CNS Lyme disease has been with aqueous penicillin and third-generation cephalosporins. Although optimal duration of therapy is unknown, it is recommended that patients be treated for 2 to 4 weeks. The risk of relapse of Lyme encephalopathy is reduced when intravenous therapy with antibiotics is extended to 4 weeks.

Lyme arthritis has been successfully treated with both oral and parenteral antibiotics, but failures have occurred with both regimens. Unless CNS involvement is present, first-line treatment with 1 or 2 months of doxycycline, 100 mg twice a day, or amoxicillin,* 500 mg three times a day, is recommended. Complete resolution of arthritis may be delayed as long as 3 months or more after completion of treatment with antibiotics. In patients who do not respond to one or more courses of antibiotics, immunomodulatory therapy or arthroscopic synovectomy is recommended. Persistent Lyme arthritis eventually resolves over several years regardless of the regimen chosen.

PREVENTION

Recommended personal protective measures against tick bites include avoiding areas highly infested with deer ticks; wearing light-colored clothing, long-sleeved shirts, and long pants; tucking pant legs into socks; using a tick repellent on clothing and exposed skin; and performing regular body checks for ticks. All of these strategies require significant self-motivation.

The risk of infection from a deertick bite in a Lyme disease endemic area is low. In mice, infected ticks have been attached for over a 36-hour period before significant risk of developing Lyme disease occurred. In a controlled double-blind study of patients with tick bites, no patient asymptomatically seroconverted, no treated patient developed EM, and the 2 of 182 untreated patients who did develop EM were successfully treated with oral antibiotics. These results support marking and watching a tick bite and, should EM develop, treating it early, when antibiotics are most effective.

The results of two large clinical trials reported that vaccination using recombinant OspA preparations was safe and efficacious. LYMErix, a recombinant

*Not FDA approved for this indication.

OspA vaccine, has been approved by the Food and Drug Administration for the prevention of Lyme disease in individuals older than age 16. Recommendations for the use of the Lyme disease vaccine have been made by the CDC and the Committee on Infectious Disease.

CONCLUSION

Lyme disease is the most common tick-borne disease in the United States. The overall trend has been an average annual increase in cases since surveillance was initiated by the CDC in 1982. Most individuals with Lyme disease are diagnosed early with erythema migrans and respond well to short courses of oral antibiotics. In patients who present with later stages of illness, the diagnosis is based on sound clinical evidence of disease and supported by serologic testing. The stage and organ system involved guide the selection of an antibiotic regimen. Successful eradication of the infecting organism, *B. burgdorferi*, appears to occur in the majority of patients with Lyme disease using these treatment guidelines.

Patients with persistent symptoms after antibiotic therapy, particularly those with previous evidence of disseminated disease, pose a difficult management problem. Most persistent symptoms are likely due to retained antigens and are not the result of persistent infection; in some patients symptoms are due to noninfectious sequelae such as fibromyalgia. In the former patients, resolution of symptoms occurs over the course of weeks to months and does not require prolonged courses of antibiotics; in the latter, treatment is that of the associated syndrome. Rarely, persistent or recurrent symptoms are due to continued or recurrent infection and require additional courses of antibiotics. Such patients require careful diagnostic evaluation to determine the need for additional treatment.

RUBELLA AND CONGENITAL RUBELLA SYNDROME

method of
MARY L. KUMAR, M.D.
Case Western Reserve School of Medicine
Cleveland, Ohio

BACKGROUND AND EPIDEMIOLOGY

Rubella is a self-limited viral infection characterized by fever and rash. Its major morbidity occurs when infection in pregnancy results in transplacental transmission of virus to the developing fetus. First described in 1941, congenital rubella was initially characterized by congenital cataracts, deafness, and heart disease following first-trimester maternal rubella. The spectrum of congenital rubella syndrome (CRS) was further expanded during the rubella pandemic in 1963 and 1964 to include growth retardation, hepatitis, thrombocytopenia and purpura, chronic encephalitis, endocrinopathies, and other sequelae.

Since the introduction of rubella vaccine in 1969, the incidence of rubella and CRS in the United States has decreased by more than 99%. Despite the dramatic success of rubella immunization programs in the United States and other developed countries, endemic and epidemic rubella continues to occur throughout the world. In countries without rubella immunization programs, rubella epidemics occur in 4- to 7-year cycles, an epidemiologic phenomenon noted in developed countries in the prevaccine era. In 1995, a World Health Organization (WHO) survey found that only 78 of 214 countries (36%) had a national rubella policy; WHO estimates that more than 200,000 cases of CRS occur every year. A recent WHO study revealed rates of CRS in developing countries from 0.6 to 2.2 per 1000 births, similar to rates in developed countries before universal rubella immunization. Considering the high cost of caring for a child with CRS, the cost-benefit ratio for rubella vaccine is enormous, particularly when it is administered in combination with measles vaccine.

Recently, WHO has reiterated the feasibility of worldwide rubella eradication. Most important, rubella is a human virus that does not infect other species. Additionally, the current rubella vaccine is highly effective in preventing rubella and CRS, and it can be administered in combination with measles vaccine. Clearly, new global vaccine initiatives are required to expand worldwide vaccine coverage to prevent the tragedy of devastating intrauterine infection, which can occur when rubella infects women who are pregnant.

CLINICAL FEATURES

Postnatally Acquired Rubella

After exposure to rubella virus in a susceptible host, viral replication begins during the 14- to 21-day incubation period. Infectivity peaks just before onset of clinical symptoms. Approximately 25% to 50% of infections may be asymptomatic. In children, the first sign of illness is rash. In adolescents and adults, rash is usually preceded by a 1- to 5-day prodrome with low-grade fever, headache, malaise, mild respiratory symptoms, and lymphadenopathy. Nodes most frequently involved are suboccipital, postauricular, and cervical.

The rash of rubella has no pathognomonic features. It usually appears first on the face and then spreads rapidly to the neck, the trunk, and the extremities. Rash erupts and disappears more quickly than in measles, typically with a duration of 3 days ("3-day measles"). Unless the rash is unusually severe, there is no desquamation as it fades.

Joint symptoms are more common in adolescents and adults than in children. Typically, joint symptoms appear as rash is fading. Joint inflammation may be mono- or polyarticular and may consist of arthralgia or frank arthritis. Typically, joint symptoms resolve completely in 5 to 10 days.

Complications of postnatally acquired rubella, other than congenital infection, are rare. Encephalitis is estimated to occur in 1 in 6000 cases, in contrast to 1 in 1000 with measles. Hematologic complications, including thrombocytopenia or purpura, rarely occur.

Congenital Rubella

Congenital rubella represents a disseminated multisystem infection in the immunocompromised fetus. Fetal infection occurs following maternal viremia, placental infection, and subsequent fetal viremia. The timing of maternal infection affects the frequency and the severity of fetal involvement. Women infected in the first 2 months of gestation have an 80% to 100% chance of giving birth to infants who are either severely affected or spontaneously aborted. Maternal infection in the third month of gestation leads to congenital rubella in 50% to 80% of cases, whereas fetuses infected in the fourth month are affected in 35% to 66% of cases. Infection between the 16th and 20th weeks may result in isolated hearing abnormalities. Infection after the 20th week of gestation rarely causes defects. Previous rubella immunity confers protection to pregnant women and is the cornerstone of the current rubella immunization strategy.

The classic congenital rubella syndrome first described by Gregg in 1941 was characterized by cataracts, deafness, and congenital heart disease. During the epidemic in the 1960s, the availability of rubella-specific laboratory tests led to a more detailed understanding of the adverse outcomes following rubella in pregnant women, including an increased risk of spontaneous abortions and stillbirths. The spectrum of rubella embryopathy includes abnormalities in virtually every organ system. Rubella-infected infants are frequently growth retarded at birth and remain growth stunted. Eye defects in addition to cataracts include glaucoma, retinopathy, and microphthalmia. Hearing loss may be present in combination with other abnormalities or may occur as an isolated defect, particularly when maternal infection occurs after the 16th week of gestation. Other abnormalities of the nervous system include microcephaly and panencephalitis. Mental retardation may be mild to profound. Severe progressive neurologic deterioration during the second decade of life may occur, reflecting the chronicity and the persistence of intrauterine rubella infection. Infants with CRS may appear normal at birth but subsequently develop late sequelae involving any of the potentially infected organ systems.

DIAGNOSIS

Clinical overlap with other viral illnesses, including parvovirus B19, necessitates specific laboratory tests for confirmation of clinically suspect cases. Particularly when infection is a concern in pregnant women, accurate laboratory diagnosis is of paramount importance. Properly performed and interpreted, serologic tests for rubella-specific IgG and IgM antibodies will usually be able to confirm or rule out recent infection. For IgG antibody tests, a fourfold or greater increase in titer between acute and convalescent sera denotes recent infection. With rubella-specific IgM tests, detection of antibody in a single serum sample usually indicates recent infection.

Determination of whether intrauterine rubella infection is present in a rubella-infected pregnant woman presents the greatest diagnostic challenge. Possible methods of diagnosis include detection of rubella-specific IgM antibody in fetal blood obtained by ultrasound-guided percutaneous umbilical blood sampling; however, rubella-specific IgM antibody may not be detectable, particularly before 22 weeks of gestation. Additional laboratory tests involve chorionic villus or amniotic fluid sampling, tested by either culture or polymerase chain reaction amplification. Consultation with a perinatologist familiar with the complexities of diagnosis of possible intrauterine infection can be helpful.

If congenital rubella is suspected at birth, additional laboratory tests are recommended. Pharyngeal secretions, urine, and cerebrospinal fluid remain culture positive for weeks to months, reflecting the persistent nature of intrauterine infection. Rubella virus can be readily isolated when samples are cultured appropriately. The laboratory should always be informed that rubella is suspected, because additional testing following inoculum into tissue culture is required to identify rubella specifically. In addition to culture, polymerase chain reaction techniques and serologic tests may be helpful. The presence of rubella-specific IgM in a newborn is highly suggestive of congenital infection; however, one must remember that both false-negative and false-positive results occur. An increase in the titer of rubella-IgG antibody or persistence for 6 months of life or longer is also suggestive of congenital infection.

TREATMENT AND MANAGEMENT

There is no specific treatment for rubella. Prevention of infection in pregnant women is best accomplished by active immunization. If rubella exposure occurs in pregnant women, careful follow-up, including appropriately timed serologic tests, is critical to determine if infection has occurred. Administration of immunoglobulin to exposed pregnant women is not recommended because passive immunoprophylaxis may modify maternal infection but not prevent fetal infection.

If serologic tests indicate maternal rubella infection in the first half of pregnancy, many perinatologists recommend additional fetal tests in an effort to determine whether fetal infection has occurred. Other experts advise pregnancy termination if serologic tests indicate rubella has occurred in early pregnancy.

VACCINE

In the United States, rubella vaccine has been available since 1969. Since 1979, RA27/3 vaccine has been the strain used extensively throughout most of the world and exclusively in the United States. Originally isolated from a rubella-infected fetus, RA27/3 was attenuated by passage in diploid human fibroblasts. The vaccine is highly immunogenic, with protective levels of neutralizing antibody in more than 95% of vaccine recipients. Adverse events are infrequent, particularly in young children. Transient arthritis has been described and may occur in approximately 15% of adults. A recent study from the Center for Disease Control and Prevention's Vaccine Safety Datalink Project determined that there was no evidence of chronic arthropathies in women immunized with RA27/3 vaccine. Transient thrombocytopenia has been described after RA27/3 vaccination. A decrease in blood platelet levels occurs in approximately 1 in 3000 after wild-type infection, whereas the rate reported in vaccine recipients is 10-fold lower.

Since 1989, rubella vaccine in the United States has been administered as a component of the two-dose measles, mumps, and rubella (MMR) schedule, with the first dose at 12 to 15 months of age and the second dose at 4 to 6 or 11 to 13 years. Rubella immunization continues to be recommended for women of childbearing age and may be administered immediately postpartum in women who test negative for rubella IgG during pregnancy. Rubella vaccine may be given after delivery to women who received blood products or $Rh_o(D)$ immune globulin (RhoGAM). Vaccine immunogenicity may be decreased in women who have received blood products or D immunoglobulin, and a serologic test 6 to 8 weeks after vaccination to assess seroconversion is recommended. Breast-feeding is not a contraindication to postpartum immunization. Contraception methods should be provided to avoid pregnancy, which rarely occurs in the immediate postpartum period.

Additional strategies to achieve universal rubella immunization include administration of vaccine to college students, military recruits, and all persons who work in health care, educational facilities, and child care centers. In these populations, routine serologic testing before vaccination to determine rubella immune status is not necessary.

Because rubella vaccine is a live attenuated virus, pregnancy remains a contraindication to immunization; however, the risk of fetal complications from rubella vaccine is extremely low. A follow-up study of women inadvertently given rubella vaccine in early pregnancy revealed that 2% of infants had inapparent infection; none had evidence of disease. Other contraindications to rubella immunization include recent administration of immunoglobulin or immunocompromising disorders associated with the cell-mediated immune dysfunction of viral infections. Rubella vaccine may be given to most HIV-infected patients, however, unless they are severely immunocompromised.

MEASLES
(Rubeola)

method of
KATALIN KORANYI, M.D.
Ohio State University
Columbus, Ohio

Measles (rubeola) is a highly contagious viral disease manifested by fever, cough, coryza, conjunctivitis, Koplik spots, and a rash. It is now only rarely seen in the United States and other industrialized countries, but in areas of the world where measles vaccine is not always available, the disease continues to cause significant morbidity and mortality. Malnutrition and underlying immunodeficiencies increase the severity of the disease. Before immunization programs, the entire cohort of birth, close to 4 million persons, contracted measles every year in the United States. In developing countries, measles still causes 1 million deaths every year.

PATHOGENESIS AND CLINICAL COURSE

Measles virus is a single-stranded RNA virus from the paramyxovirus family, the same family to which respiratory syncytial and mumps viruses belong. Lipid solvents such as ether or chloroform, heat, cold, and extremes of ultraviolet light inactivate the measles virus. Although only one antigenic type is known, minor antigenic shifts occur in the various strains of the measles virus. These shifts, however, do not seem to compromise lifelong immunity, and second cases are very rare. Measles virus infects only humans and primates. Transmission occurs by direct contact with respiratory droplets and, less commonly, by airborne spread. Infectious droplets can persist for over 1 hour in the environment. The disease peaks in the late winter and spring, and in the prevaccine era, biennial peaks were observed. The incubation period is generally 8 to 10 days from exposure, and the greatest period of communicability is during the prodromal stage (7–10 days after exposure) to 4 days after appearance of the rash. The virus enters the nasopharynx, attaches to the respiratory mucosa, and spreads to the regional lymphatics. Low-grade viremia from the lymph nodes occurs on the second or third day after exposure. The virus continues to replicate in local and distant lymph nodes, from which a secondary viremia occurs about 10 days after infection, and active replication of the measles virus takes place throughout the body, including the respiratory tract, skin, and other organs. This period of active replication coincides with symptoms of the prodromal stage, including fever, a harsh brassy cough, nonpurulent conjunctivitis, and coryza. Photophobia is common, hence the custom to confine the infected individual to a dark room. One to 2 days into the prodromal stage, Koplik spots appear as tiny, bluish dots in the buccal mucosa and herald the appearance of rash by 1 to 2 days. This period is marked by extensive viral damage to the respiratory mucosa, and the individual is very contagious. The rash begins 4 to 5 days after onset of the prodromal stage as a maculopapular eruption with a burgundy color that spreads in a cephalocaudal distribution. The rash becomes confluent over the face and trunk and may occasionally be hemorrhagic. It lasts for about 4 to 5 days and is followed by a fine, branny desquamation. At the height of the rash, the other symptoms (hacking cough, fever, and malaise) intensify. Cervical lymphadenopathy and pharyngitis may be present. Diarrhea is especially severe in children from developing countries. "Black measles" is more common in children from developing countries and is manifest by pneumonia and diffuse intravascular coagulopathy. Within 4 to 5 days after onset of the rash, viral shedding ceases and the individual is no longer contagious.

COMPLICATIONS

Because of extensive damage to the respiratory mucosa, complications such as otitis, sinusitis, croup, and viral "giant cell" or bacterial pneumonia occur often, most commonly in young children. The risk of contracting encephalitis is 1 in 1000 cases of measles; about 20% of those affected are left with permanent brain damage. Clinical manifestations of encephalitis include fever, headache, vomiting, and changes in mental status. The etiology of measles encephalitis is unclear but is most likely an autoimmune reaction; however, measles virus has occasionally been found in the cerebrospinal fluid. A much less common, but fatal complication of measles is subacute sclerosing panencephalitis, which is due to a persistent central nervous system infection. The overall risk of death from measles is 1 in 3000 cases. Children younger than 5 years and those with immunodeficiency disorders such as leukemia and HIV infection have an increased risk of fatality. Malnutrition, especially vitamin A deficiency, contributes to the complications of measles.

DIAGNOSIS

Measles virus infection can be diagnosed by demonstrating the presence of measles IgM antibody in the patient's serum or by a fourfold rise in measles IgG antibody in paired sera collected 2 to 4 weeks apart. Measles virus can be isolated from nasopharyngeal secretions, urine, or blood.

MANAGEMENT OF MEASLES

Measles virus is susceptible in vitro to ribavirin* (Virazole), but no controlled clinical studies have been conducted. Ribavirin has on occasion been administered by the intravenous and aerosol routes to immunocompromised children with severe measles. Generally, treatment is symptomatic and consists of oral fluids, humidification of the environment, and occasional use of antitussives for the cough. Acetaminophen can be recommended to manage the fever and for the child's comfort. Antimicrobials are indicated for the treatment of specific bacterial complications. The World Health Organization recommends the administration of vitamin A to all children from communities where vitamin A deficiency is a recognized problem. Vitamin A treatment of children with measles in developing countries has decreased morbidity and mortality. In the United States, however, vitamin A deficiency is not a severe problem, but low serum concentrations of vitamin A have been found in children with severe measles. The American Academy of Pediatrics Committee on Infectious Diseases recommends that vitamin A supplementation be considered in the following circumstances:

- Children 6 months to 2 years of age who are hospitalized with measles and have complications such as pneumonia, croup, or diarrhea. Limited data are available regarding the safety of vitamin A in children younger than 6 months.
- Children older than 6 months with measles and risk factors such as immunodeficiency, ophthalmic evidence of vitamin A deficiency, malabsorption, malnutrition, or recent immigration from areas where measles causes high mortality.

Vitamin A is available in oral capsules and for parenteral administration. For children older than 1 year, the dose of vitamin A is 200,000 IU orally. For children between 6 months and 12 months of age 100,000 IU of vitamin A is given. Administration of vitamin A may be associated with headache and vomiting for a few hours. Two additional doses of 200,000 IU of vitamin A are recommended for children with ophthalmologic evidence of vitamin A deficiency at 24 hours, and then 4 weeks later.

Airborne isolation is recommended for 4 days after onset of the rash in otherwise healthy children and for the duration of the illness in immunocompromised patients. Isolation alone is not effective in preventing transmission to household contacts because virus is excreted before the onset of clinical symptoms.

*Not FDA approved for this indication.

ACTIVE IMMUNIZATION

The measles vaccine licensed in the United States is a live attenuated strain of the virus prepared in chick embryo cell culture. It is generally given as a combination vaccine consisting of MMR (measles, mumps, and rubella) (M-M-R II) or MR (measles and rubella) (M-M-Vax II). A monovalent formulation (measles only) (Attenuvax) is also available. MMR is recommended for routine childhood immunization at 12 to 15 months of age. Serum antibodies against measles develop in 95% of children when the vaccine is given at 12 months of age and in 98% when it is given at 15 months of age. A small percentage of individuals lose their immunity after several years. A second dose of MMR before school entry at 4 to 5 years of age provides long-term immunity against measles in more than 99% of persons who receive two doses separated by at least 4 weeks. In special circumstances, such as travel to an area where measles is endemic, children between the ages of 6 and 11 months should be immunized with MMR. Children who have received one dose of MMR before their first birthday should receive two additional doses of the vaccine. Older children and adults not immunized against measles should receive two doses of the vaccine at least 4 weeks apart. High schools, colleges, and other institutions for education beyond high school should require that all students have documentation of physician-diagnosed measles, birth before 1957, receipt of two doses of measles vaccine, or serologic evidence of immunity.

Measles vaccine can be effective if given within 72 hours of exposure. Vaccine is the intervention of choice during outbreaks in schools and daycare centers. Immunoglobulin can be effective when administered within 6 days of exposure. Immunoglobulin is particularly indicated for susceptible household contacts, such as children younger than 1 year of age, pregnant women, and persons with immunodeficiency disorders. It can prevent or modify measles in a susceptible, exposed individual. Adverse events after measles immunization include fever in 5% to 15% of susceptible vaccinees between 6 and 12 days after MMR immunization. Mild and transient rash is seen in 5% of recipients. Thrombocytopenia is a very rare complication of MMR vaccine. Overall, it is estimated that severe adverse reactions occur in 3 of every 100,000 doses of the vaccine. MMR immunization does not cause sudden infant death syndrome or childhood autism. Contraindications to MMR immunization include pregnancy, anaphylactic reaction to neomycin, and immunodeficiency states. Persons with HIV infection who are not severely immunosuppressed or symptomatic should receive the vaccine because measles infection can often be fatal in HIV-infected individuals. Tuberculosis skin testing is not necessary before measles immunization is administered because the vaccine does not reactivate tuberculosis. The vaccine and tuberculosis skin test can be administered the same day. Immunoglobulin preparations may interfere with the antibody response to measles vaccine. For suggested intervals between immunoglobulin or blood product administration and measles immunization, the *Red Book Report* of the Committee on Infectious Diseases should be consulted. A history of egg allergy is not a contraindication to measles immunization. Skin testing for egg allergy is not predictive of a reaction to MMR vaccine. Children who experienced an anaphylactic reaction to measles vaccine should not be reimmunized but, instead, require serologic testing to determine whether they are susceptible. Pregnant women should not receive measles vaccination, and those vaccinated should avoid becoming pregnant for 3 months. Minor febrile illnesses, breast-feeding, or pregnancy in mothers of children requiring vaccination does not constitute a contraindication. To control an outbreak, every suspected case of measles should be reported to local health departments and efforts made to confirm the diagnosis.

TETANUS

method of
SEÁN O. HENDERSON, M.D.
LAC+USC Medical Center, University of Southern California
Los Angeles, California

and

NICOLE WAKIM, B.A.
Loyola Stritch School of Medicine
Chicago, Illinois

ETIOLOGY AND EPIDEMIOLOGY

Clostridium tetani is a gram-positive, rod-shaped, anaerobic bacillus that causes tetanus, a disorder of the nervous system that, if left untreated, is highly fatal. Ubiquitous in nature, this saprophytic organism is commonly found in dirt, dust, rust, and feces of animals and human beings. Historically, in the United States, tetanus has been known to affect African American men of the rural south, men older than 50, women without formal schooling or in institutionalized careers, and individuals without military experience. More recently, women have been removed from this group, although recent immigrants and intravenous drug users (particularly Latino intravenous drug users in California) have been added. Despite the availability of tetanus toxoid, worldwide endemic areas still report approximately 5 cases of neonatal tetanus per 1000 live births.

Tetanus is a disease that is almost entirely preventable with appropriate vaccination and wound management. The incidence of tetanus in underdeveloped countries far outweighs that of the United States owing to better living conditions and routine immunizations shortly after birth (6–8 weeks) in the United States. From 1995 to 1997, only 124 cases were reported in the United States.

However, regardless of immunization status, anyone can be susceptible if the appropriate conditions, such as a grossly infected wound, exist. Tetanus tends to be found in patients with acute injuries to the skin such as abrasions, lacerations, puncture wounds, intravenous drug entry sites, and surgery. Tetanus has been associated with abortion, childbirth (owing to an infected umbilical stump from unsanitary procedures), animal bites, insect stings, burns, frostbite, ear infections, corneal foreign bodies, splinters, self-tattooing, and body piercing.

Even though some wounds may contain evidence of *C. tetani*, not all patients are afflicted with tetanus. Generally, the bacteria favors an environment with a low oxidation-reduction potential to convert the spore into the toxin-producing (vegetative) form. The *incubation period of tetanus,* the time from inoculation to presentation of symptoms, ranges from days to months. The severity of the symptoms depends in large part on the amount of organism inoculated as well as the amount of toxin produced by that organism load. The median incubation period is 7 days; typically, the shorter the incubation period the more severe the disease, the more aggressive the treatment must be, and the poorer the prognosis.

PATHOPHYSIOLOGY

Once the bacteria find a suitable environment, they grow, sporulate, and lyse to release toxins including tetanospasmin and tetanolysin. Tetanospasmin is accountable for the clinical manifestations of tetanus. The neurotoxin, encoded on a plasmid, is believed to enter the nervous system either through bloodborne delivery or retrograde intraneuronal transport. Eventually, tetanospasmin enters the central nervous system via peripheral nerves and prevents the release of the neurotransmitters γ-aminobutyric acid (GABA) and glycine from inhibitory fibers. Thus, inhibitory signals are blocked and muscular rigidity and muscle spasms ensue. Tetanolysin's role remains unclear, but some speculate it may somehow support the activity of tetanospasmin.

The shorter the peripheral nerve, the faster the neurotoxin may enter the central nervous system. Therefore, the earliest symptoms are manifested in the face, causing classic lockjaw (*trismus*) and occasionally a sneering grin due to prolonged spasms (*risus sardonicus*). Tetanospasmin also inhibits the release of acetylcholine, norepinephrine, and enkephalins at the motor end plates, causing autonomic dysfunction and sympathetic overactivity. Unfortunately, once the neurotoxin has attached to the neurons, treatment with antitoxin is ineffective; thus, new nerve junctions must be formed to regain normal function.

Four forms of tetanus have been described clinically. The most common form is *generalized tetanus.* The distinguishing symptom on presentation is trismus or lockjaw followed by generalized rigidity and spasms of the muscles in the face, neck, back (*opisthotonos*), and abdominal region. *Localized tetanus* is a second form of the disease in which spasms occur only in the region of the wound. In most cases, patients with such localized symptoms fare better than those with systemic symptoms. *Cephalic tetanus* results from an injury to the head, or alternatively from an ear infection, and leads to cranial nerve deficiencies and trismus. This form of the disease has been known to progress into generalized tetanus.

Neonatal tetanus is a final form of tetanus that affects newborns in the first weeks of life. This form is very uncommon in the United States because most mothers are immunized and pass some degree of passive immunity to the fetus. For those mothers who are not immunized, as is the case in many underdeveloped countries, there is a higher risk for their children to develop neonatal tetanus. In fact, neonatal tetanus is the most common form of tetanus worldwide and caused more than 390,000 deaths in

1994. This form of tetanus has a high mortality rate (90%) due to generalized spasms and rigidity affecting the child's ability to nurse. The source of the infection is attributed to the umbilical stump, which has been contaminated during the usually unsterile birthing process. Some suggest that at least two doses of tetanus toxoid be administered to any woman of childbearing age to eliminate neonatal tetanus completely.

PROPHYLAXIS

Childhood Immunization

Tetanus immunization typically consists of a series of childhood immunizations with diphtheria and tetanus toxoids and acellular pertussis vaccine (DTaP) or diphtheria and tetanus toxoids and pertussis vaccine (DTP) at 2, 4, and 6 months. This is followed by a fourth injection between the 15th and 18th months and a booster at age 5 years. Further boosters are given every 10 years or as needed. Tetanus and diphtheria toxoids adsorbed, for adult use (Td), is preferred for boosters in patients older than age 11 if it has been at least 5 years since the last dose of DTP or DTaP.

Immunization in People Older Than 7 Years of Age

Primary tetanus immunization for patients older than 7 years consists of two doses of Td intramuscularly at least 4 weeks apart followed by a third dose 6 to 12 months later. Boosters should follow every 10 years or as needed. The elderly deserve special consideration in that they may have a decreased immunologic memory, which requires more frequent immunization.

Postexposure Antitetanus Prophylaxis

Wounds are typically considered tetanus prone if they meet one of the following criteria:

- More than 6 hours old
- Stellate
- Deeper than 1 cm
- Secondary to a missile injury, crush injury, or burn
- Devitalized tissue
- Contaminated with foreign material, such as dirt or saliva

If the patient has such a wound and has a reliable history of complete tetanus immunization (>3 doses), a follow-up dose of Td may be given if more than 5 years have elapsed since the previous booster.

If the patient has an incomplete immunization history (<3 doses) or is unreliable, Td is given (DT for patients <7 years of age) as well as tetanus immunoglobulin (TIG) 250 U intramuscularly. In this patient, tetanus toxoid stimulates antibody production in the body to remove the circulating toxin released by *C. tetani*, a phenomenon that takes several weeks. Human TIG provides passive immunity in the interim.

DIAGNOSIS

The initial diagnosis of tetanus is clinical, is obtained by a thorough history (including all past immunizations), and is based on physical presentation. The increased muscle tone associated with the disease may first manifest as difficulty in chewing. Trismus, the most common symptom, occurs in approximately 75% of the patients and is often accompanied by other presenting complaints such as neck stiffness or rigidity, dysphagia, restlessness, and reflex spasms. Uncontrolled spasms of the respiratory muscles may lead to a need for mechanical ventilation. As the disease progresses, autonomic dysfunction characterized by cardiac dysrhythmias, tachycardia, bradycardia, hypertension, hypotension, peripheral vasoconstriction, fever, and diaphoresis occur.

Routine laboratory testing generally does not help establish the diagnosis. Culture results are unreliable: the wound of a tetanus-inflicted patient may provide no trace of *C. tetani*, whereas the wound of another patient with no symptoms of tetanus may have positive culture results. Acute tetanus titers are only accurate if obtained before any therapy with human tetanus immune globulin (HTIG) begins. However, waiting for tetanus titer results in a patient who is critically ill is inappropriate and may compromise patient care. Other diagnostic tests, such as white blood cell counts, creatine kinase levels, electroencephalography, and cerebrospinal fluid examination are nonspecific.

One test, with a sensitivity of 94% and a specificity of 100%, involves trying to evoke the gag reflex from patients. In tetanus, the masseter muscles spasm before eliciting a gag, causing the patient to bite on the tongue blade. Several colleagues have recognized the need for a rapid bedside test for the diagnosis of tetanus, but to date, no such test exists.

Differential Diagnosis

The main use of laboratory testing is to rule out other disease processes in the differential diagnosis. Strychnine poisoning closely mimics tetanus but lacks abdominal rigidity and trismus. Generalized muscle spasms can also be attributed to meningitis, status epilepticus, psychiatric disorders, hypocalcemia, and an acute abdomen. Trismus can commonly be confused with tooth abscess or orofacial infection, mandibular dislocation, and abscess of the retropharyngeal or peritonsillar origin. Drugs such as phenothiazines and metoclopramide may cause dystonic reactions similar to those seen in tetanus.

TREATMENT

Once tetanus is suspected, aggressive therapy is warranted regardless of the severity of the initial presentation. Due to the prolonged and meticulous treatment necessary in tetanus, the patient should remain under close observation in the intensive care unit. To avoid irritation of the patient and subsequent spasms or cardiovascular sequelae, the patient should be kept in a dark, quiet room. Initial therapy should be directed toward airway maintenance; because laryngeal spasms are a known complication, the airway should be protected early in the course of the disease. Pretreatment of the patient with paralytic agents and benzodiazepines will facilitate airway maintenance. To avoid spasms from the prolonged periods of tracheal suction and intubation (>7–10 days), a tracheostomy is often the best choice.

Options for the treatment of these characteristic muscle spasms includes benzodiazepines, baclofen (Lioresal), and, in severe cases, paralytics. The most commonly used medications are the benzodiazepines, which are used to relax the spastic muscles and sedate the patient. Benzodiazepines target GABA-A receptors and suppress the disinhibition of excitatory neural pathways in the central nervous system. Although lorazepam (Ativan) has the longest duration of action of benzodiazepines, a midazolam (Versed) infusion is preferred for prolonged therapy because it is not suspended in propylene glycol, a cardiotoxic solution. Although intrathecal benzodiazepines have been suggested as alternative therapy, they have also been criticized for having a sedating effect that is too heavy and for having associated toxicity.

Baclofen, a GABA-B agonist, may be an alternative to benzodiazepines. This drug does not cross the blood-brain barrier well and therefore must be given as an intrathecal infusion. Baclofen is less sedating than benzodiazepines and is nontoxic with a short half-life, allowing titration of its effects. The patient's response to baclofen varies based on the position of the catheter, severity of the disease, number of GABA-B receptors, and time from onset of symptoms to baclofen therapy. In addition to reducing generalized spasms, baclofen normalizes heart rate and blood pressure. Patients benefit most from 500 to 2000 μg of intrathecal baclofen per day when no previous benzodiazepines have been given. Doses of 2000 μg or more may cause problems with blood pressure, heart rate, and respiratory drive.

As far as other neuromuscular blocking agents for patients with artificial ventilation are concerned, there is disagreement as to whether vecuronium (Norcuron) or pancuronium (Pavulon) is best. The latter is more cardiovascularly active with an accompanying tachycardia that may be poorly tolerated by an already unstable patient with tetanus.

One of the other medications that may be used in the acute treatment of a tetanus patient's spasticity is dantrolene (Dantrium), which causes muscle relaxation by interfering with the release of calcium from the smooth endoplasmic reticulum. Dantrolene should not be given for more than 60 days owing to the toxic effects it has on the liver.

The autonomic instability associated with tetanus may be treated with any number of suggested therapies. High-dose continuous magnesium sulfate may be effective because it inhibits the release of norepinephrine and epinephrine from the adrenal glands, thus eliminating catecholamine stimuli on the nervous system. Epidural blockade with bupivacaine (Marcaine) decreases urinary catecholamine levels, leading to less frequent and less severe blood pressure fluctuations. Morphine (Duramorph) reduces α-adrenergic sympathetic tone and lowers sympathetic efferent discharge allowing for stabilization of the cardiovascular and nervous system.

Although propranolol* previously was used to counter the sympathetic overactivity associated with tetanus, it has been associated with pulmonary edema and cardiac arrest in various case reports. Metoprolol (Lopressor)* is an effective alternative to propranolol, both for oral and intravenous use, to control hypertension and tachycardia. Clonidine (Catapres)* has been suggested for treatment of the autonomic nervous system dysfunction, whereas atropine* has been used for cardiac stabilization.

*Not FDA approved for this indication.

Finally, corticosteroid use is not yet recommended, although some studies have noted a lower mortality rate for patients with tetanus who were administered prednisolone over those who were not.

Once respiratory and autonomic stability have been attained, the goal is to neutralize the tetanospasmin circulating in the system. The earlier the treatment with human tetanus immune globulin is instituted, the better the chances for full recovery because HTIG neutralizes the circulating toxin. For patients with high-risk wounds, 250 IU HTIG is administered before surgical débridement and as soon as the airway and spasms are controlled. For patients with severe tetanus, 500 IU HTIG is sufficient and as effective as larger doses. Because HTIG does not cross the blood-brain barrier to reach the toxin affecting the anterior horn cells, intrathecal injection has been proposed; however, the efficacy of this route is unknown. Tetanus toxoid should also be administered to stimulate antibody production as either a booster or a primary immunization series. The HTIG and the toxoid should be administered on opposite deltoid muscles.

Débridement and irrigation of the wound follow neutralization of the toxin and immunization. For débridement of the wound, 2.0 cm around the wound margins should be excised. Additionally, abscesses should be drained and excised. Antibiotic therapy is used to destroy the vegetative form of *C. tetani*. Cephalosporins, macrolides, tetracyclines, imipenem (Primaxin), penicillin, and metronidazole (Flagyl) all target the bacteria.

Penicillin has been shown to antagonize GABA receptors and should not be considered a first-choice therapy. Alternatively, metronidazole 500 mg is effective and may be given every 8 hours either intravenously or by mouth. During the prolonged treatment and recovery periods associated with this disease, preventive measures against gastrointestinal and decubitus ulcers, as well as deep venous thrombi, must be implemented.

*Not FDA approved for this indication.

BORDETELLA PERTUSSIS
(Whooping Cough)

method of
DENNIS CUNNINGHAM, M.D., and
MARGARET B. RENNELS, M.D.
University of Maryland School of Medicine
Baltimore, Maryland

BACKGROUND

Whooping cough refers to the classic presentation of pertussis. Symptoms begin with rhinorrhea, lacrimation, and cough suggestive of a viral upper respiratory infection (catarrhal stage). The frequency and the severity of coughing episodes increase, eventually developing into repetitive series of coughs following a single expiration (paroxysmal stage). Post-tussive emesis is common, especially in infants. After paroxysmal coughing attacks, older children and adults may have an inspiratory whoop, caused by deep inhalation against a partially closed glottis. During coughing attacks, patients may appear in distress and exhausted. Typically, patients appear well between attacks. Coughing attacks gradually decrease in frequency and intensity (convalescent phase). Patients remain afebrile throughout the illness unless secondary infection ensues.

Detailed accounts of epidemics in Europe during the 16th century describe classic pertussis. Bordet and Gengou identified *Bordetella pertussis* as the etiologic agent of pertussis in 1906. Eldering and Kendrick isolated *B. parapertussis* in 1936 and showed that it caused a similar illness. Approximately 95% of whooping cough cases are due to *B. pertussis,* and the remaining 5% are caused primarily by *B. parapertussis. B. bronchiseptica* also has been reported occasionally to cause a whooping cough–type illness.

Pathogenesis

Members of the *Bordetella* genus are aerobic gram-negative organisms with a pleomorphic appearance on Gram stain. *Bordetella* species have a high degree of genetic homology, and classification of species is based on proteins expressed by the organisms. *B. pertussis* and *B. parapertussis* have greater than 98% genetic homology. The primary difference is that *B. pertussis* produces pertussis toxin. *B. pertussis* is strictly a human pathogen; *B. parapertussis* has been isolated from domesticated animals with respiratory symptoms, and *B. bronchiseptica* primarily infects animals. Illness from infection with *B. pertussis* is more severe and prolonged than that due to *B. parapertussis* or *bronchiseptica.*

Bordetella virulence factors include fimbriae, filamentous hemagglutinin, pertussis toxin (PT), lipo-oligosaccharide, pertactin, adenylate cyclase toxin, and tracheal cytotoxin. PT is a protein expressed on the outer surface that serves as an adhesive between bacteria and respiratory ciliated epithelial cells. PT also induces lymphocytosis, inhibits leukocyte function, and sensitizes tissue to histamine. As a response to PT, white blood cell counts can range from 12,000 to 80,000 cells per microliter of blood. Additional attachment factors include the two surface proteins, pertactin and filamentous hemagglutinin, as well as fimbriae. Tracheal cytotoxin produces local damage to the tracheal lining. Adenylate cyclase toxin is an extracellular protein that inactivates leukocytes and produces local damage similar to that caused by tracheal cytotoxin. The inflammatory process induced by PT, lipo-oligosaccharide, and tracheal cytotoxin results in the accumulation of cellular debris. Ciliary movement ceases when *Bordetella* binds to respiratory cells. The resultant inability to clear secretions combined with local destruction of the respiratory mucosa contributes to the development of secondary bacterial pneumonia. Patients with fever or abnormal respiratory status between coughing attacks require a chest radiograph. Seizures or encephalopathy may occur. The most likely mechanism is severe hypoxia during paroxysmal coughing. Additional complications include pneumothorax, epistaxis, subdural hematomas, hernias, and rectal prolapse, all of which result from increased intrathoracic pressure generated by coughing. Young patients may require critical care, including tracheal intubation with mechanical ventilation, because of respiratory distress.

Incidence

There are approximately 50,000,000 cases per year worldwide resulting in 350,000 deaths annually. The true incidence and case-fatality rate are probably underestimated. The majority of infections (90%) occur in developing countries. Children younger than 6 months of age have the highest mortality and morbidity. Young maternal age and prematurity increase the risk of dying from pertussis. For this reason, most infants in the U.S. younger than 6 months of age are admitted for treatment. The age distribution of U.S. cases in 1997 was 18% in patients younger than 3 months, 24% in those less than 6 months, and 43% recorded in children younger than 5 years of age. Despite effective pertussis vaccines, the disease remains endemic with regional epidemics occurring in cycles of 3 to 5 years. Small respiratory airborne droplets effectively transmit organisms. The attack rate for susceptible household contacts is estimated to range from 80% to 100%.

Natural History

The incubation period ranges from 7 to 21 days, followed by a 1- to 2-week catarrhal stage. The duration of the paroxysmal stage ranges from 1 to 6 weeks, and the convalescent period typically lasts 2 to 3 weeks. Duration of classic illness is between 6 and 10 weeks. Although coughing usually ceases at the end of the convalescent stage, other respiratory infections may trigger paroxysmal coughs for a several-month period. The majority of pertussis cases are atypical and never diagnosed. In infants younger than 6 months of age, weak inspirations rarely cause a whoop. Infants usually present with episodes of apnea and bradycardia, occasionally accompanied by a seizure. Feeding may precipitate a coughing attack, making infants and toddlers refuse food and potentially require parenteral nutrition.

Studies in healthy adults showed that one quarter of those with cough lasting more than 7 days have laboratory-confirmed pertussis. Adolescents and adults are often susceptible to pertussis because protection following immunization wanes over a 5- to 10-year period. Adolescents and adults may serve as a source of infections in young children. For this reason, booster immunizations of adolescents and young adults are being considered.

DIAGNOSIS

The differential diagnosis of pertussis includes infections caused by *Mycoplasma pneumoniae, Chlamydia trachomatis,* and *Chlamydia pneumoniae.* Noninfectious diagnoses include cystic fibrosis or pulmonary disease resulting in lymphadenopathy that compresses large airways. Only infections from *B. pertussis* have marked lymphocytosis. *Mycoplasma* and *Chlamydia* usually cause a staccato-like repetitive cough, with tachypnea noted between episodes of coughing. Adenovirus was thought to cause a pertussis-like syndrome, but more recent evidence suggests that it co-infects patients with pertussis. It is not clear whether adenovirus increases the severity of disease.

The gold standard for diagnosis of pertussis is culture of the organism or identification by specific fluorescent antibody staining. Fluorescent staining is positive for both *B. pertussis* and *B. parapertussis.* Cross-reacting antibodies prevent speciation by this method. Agglutination antibodies to fimbriae can distinguish between species and strains. Cultures obtained during the catarrhal stage have the greatest chance of detecting pertussis. Bacteria counts gradually decline after the first cough. Twenty-one days after the first cough, bacteria are nondetectable. Usually, pertussis is diagnosed clinically from the presence of cough, post-tussive emesis, whooping, and lymphocytosis. For patients not cultured or patients with negative cultures, comparing antibody titers in samples of acute and convalescent serum may help make a diagnosis. At this time, only research laboratories provide this test, and it is not approved for clinical diagnosis. Polymerase chain reaction assays have a high sensitivity in research laboratories, but there is no pertussis technique currently approved for clinical diagnosis.

Technique is critical when obtaining a culture for *Bordetella.* A specimen of posterior nasopharyngeal mucous membranes is required. Acceptable techniques include using a swab or aspiration after irrigation with sterile fluid. Aspiration is useful in infants and small children. Use only Dacron or calcium alginate swabs. Fatty acids in cotton will inhibit growth of *Bordetella* and result in false-negative cultures. Insert a swab into the posterior nasopharynx and keep it there for 15 to 30 seconds, slowly rotating the swab. On removal, the tip of the swab should be placed in Regan-Lowe transport medium and immediately delivered to the laboratory. Extended time in the transport medium decreases the chance for a positive culture. Cultures require incubation for 10 to 14 days. Health care providers should wear a mask and an eye shield when culturing because the procedure frequently triggers a coughing attack.

TREATMENT

Treating a patient early in the course of the catarrhal stage may decrease the duration of disease and symptoms. More important, treatment eradicates the organism and potentially decreases infectivity. The drug of choice is oral erythromycin (40 to 50 mg/kg/d in four divided doses; maximum 2 g/d for 14 days). There is no evidence to suggest that either the estolate or the base formulation of erythromycin is superior for treating pertussis. Historically, erythromycin has been the drug of choice to treat pertussis, despite a lack of data supporting its efficacy. In light of case reports suggesting an association between pyloric stenosis and erythromycin use in infants, physicians should explain the small risk of this complication to parents and describe symptoms of pyloric stenosis. The recommended second-line agent is trimethoprim-sulfamethoxazole (Bactrim) for 14 days (10 to 12 mg/kg/d divided into two doses, maximum 320 mg/d) although there are little data to prove efficacy. Azithromycin* at 10 mg/kg on day one (maximum 500 mg) and 5 mg/kg on days 2 through 5 (maximum 250 mg) is equally efficacious for sterilizing nasopharyngeal cultures; however, this does not prove that azithromycin is as effective as erythromycin for treating pertussis.

Evidence for and against treating pertussis with glucocorticoids* exists. Without additional information, corticosteroids should be considered only in severely ill patients requiring critical care. β-agonists* have decreased the frequency of cough in a few patients, but there is no clear evidence to recommend them. Preliminary studies on the use of pertussis hyperimmunoglobulin suggest good efficacy in decreasing symptoms, but there is no licensed pertussis hyperimmunoglobulin.

Because contacts of patients with pertussis are at high risk of becoming infected, erythromycin treatment is recommended to prevent secondary cases (40 to 50 mg/kg/d divided into 4 doses; maximum dose 2 g/d). Prophylaxis with antimicrobials is recommended for household members and close contacts such as child care providers. There is no evidence that treating an entire school class is of any benefit. Children younger than 7 years of age who are not immunized or who have had fewer than four doses of the vaccine should receive diphtheria, tetanus, and acellular pertussis (DTaP) vaccine. Unimmunized children should follow the recommended vaccination schedule. Of those children who develop pertussis, more than 50% have delayed or absent immunizations.

VACCINATION

Development of vaccines to protect infants from pertussis started in the mid-20th century. Initially, a whole-cell vaccine (inactivated bacteria) combined with diphtheria and tetanus toxoids (DTwP) was used, and it dramatically decreased the number of cases in developed countries. Because of the whole-cell vaccine's reactogenicity, research focused on acellular vaccines. Acellular vaccines consisting of various *Bordetella* antigens had fewer instances of systemic reactions, fever, fussiness, decreased activity, and hypotonic hyporesponsive episodes.

Acellular vaccines were also combined with diphtheria and tetanus toxoids (DTaP). Efficacy for whole-cell and acellular pertussis vaccines is in the range of 70% to 90%. Limited evidence suggests that the acellular vaccine provides longer immunity because of T cell–mediated immunity. Acellular vaccines are licensed for children younger than 7 years of age. Each dose of DTaP consists of 0.5 mL administered intramuscularly. The current immunization schedule for the United States recommends administration of DTaP at 2, 4, 6, and 15 to 18 months and between 4 and 6 years of age. If feasible, the same product should be used throughout the series. If the initial formulation is unknown or unavailable, use of a formulation by another manufacturer is acceptable.

Contraindications to pertussis vaccination include anaphylactic reaction to a previous dose or new-onset encephalopathy within a week of vaccination. Precautions–reactions to the vaccine without permanent sequelae—include seizures within 72 hours, severe and inconsolable crying lasting at least 3 hours and occurring within the first 48 hours after vaccination, hypotonic-hyporesponsive episodes, and fever greater

*Not FDA approved for this indication.

*Not FDA approved for this indication.

than 40.5°C (104.8°F). If a child has any history of these conditions, the physician should discuss with the parents the risk of immunization against the risk of contracting pertussis. There is no contraindication to vaccinating children with a mild febrile illness, patients with a known stable seizure disorder, or children with a relative who had an adverse effect to the vaccine.

Pertussis remains a significant cause of mortality and morbidity in both the developed and the undeveloped world. Vaccination with DTaP or DTwP is necessary to prevent increased incidence and deaths; countries that suspended immunization had large increases in incidence. For more detailed information regarding therapy, consult the local health department or *The Red Book 2000* (Report of the Committee on Infectious Diseases) published by the American Academy of Pediatrics, Elk Grove Village, Illinois.

IMMUNIZATION PRACTICES

method of
RICHARD DANIEL CLOVER, M.D.
University of Louisville
Louisville, Kentucky

and

RICHARD KENT ZIMMERMAN, M.D., M.P.H.
University of Pittsburgh
Pittsburgh, Pennsylvania

Vaccination has been tremendously successful in decreasing the incidence of vaccine-preventable diseases in the United States. For example, the total number of measles cases among U.S. children dropped from 458,083 in 1964, the year before widespread use of measles vaccine, to 100 in 1999 (provisional total). Cases of *Haemophilus influenzae* type B (Hib) disease among children in the U.S. have also dropped dramatically, from an estimated 20,000 annually before introduction of Hib vaccine to fewer than 33 in 1999.

HEPATITIS B VACCINE

It is estimated that 128,000 to 320,000 persons in the United States are infected annually with hepatitis B virus (HBV), according to the Centers for Disease Control and Prevention (CDC) (unpublished data). The number of persons chronically infected with HBV in the United States, each of whom is potentially infectious, is estimated to be 1.25 million. HBV infection is much more likely to become chronic when acquired early in life than when acquired during adulthood: chronic HBV infection develops in 90% of those infected as infants, 30% to 60% of those infected before the age of 4 years, and only 5% to 10% of those infected as adults.

The hepatitis B vaccines (e.g., Recombivax HB) currently produced in the United States are manufactured by recombinant DNA technology using baker's yeast and do not contain human plasma. The vaccination schedule is given in Figure 1.

For infants born to mothers with positive or unknown hepatitis B surface antigen (HBsAG) status, postexposure prophylaxis, including both hepatitis B immune globulin and hepatitis B vaccine, should be initiated within 12 hours of birth, regardless of gestational age. These infants should receive their second and third doses of vaccine at 1 to 2 months and 6 months of age. If the mother is chronically infected with HBV, the infant should be tested for HBsAG and antihemoglobin S at 9 to 15 months of age.

For infants who weigh less than 2 kg at birth whose mother is known to be HBsAG negative, the first dose of hepatitis B vaccine should be delayed until the infant weighs 2 kg, because seroconversion rates are lower in infants born prematurely with birth weights less than 2 kg and are lower still in those with birth weights of less than 1 kg.

DIPHTHERIA, TETANUS, AND PERTUSSIS (DTP) VACCINE

Diphtheria is an acute toxin-mediated disease caused by *Corynebacterium diphtheriae*. Transmission is often person-to-person from the respiratory tract. Rarely transmission may occur from skin lesions. The disease can involve almost any mucus membrane. In general, it is classified based on the site of infection (i.e., anterior nasal, tonsillar pharyngeal, laryngeal, cutaneous, ocular, or genital). Complications include myocarditis, neuritis, airway obstruction, and death.

Tetanus is an acute, often fatal disease caused by an exotoxin produced by *Clostridium tetani*. It is characterized by generalized rigidity and convulsive spasms of the skeletal muscles. The organisms normally enter the body through a wound. In the presence of low-oxygen conditions, the spores germinate. Complications of tetanus include laryngospasm, fractures of the spine or the long bones, hyperactivity of the autonomic nervous system, and death.

Pertussis is transmitted primarily by respiratory droplets and is highly contagious: From 70% to 100% of susceptible household contacts and 50% to 80% of susceptible school contacts will become infected following exposure. Pertussis complications include seizures, encephalopathy, and pneumonia, which occurs in about 15% of cases and is the leading cause of death from pertussis. Encephalopathy is fatal in approximately one third of cases and causes permanent brain damage in another one third.

In U.S. studies, DTP vaccination was found to be 70% to 90% effective in preventing pertussis, 97% effective in preventing diphtheria, and 100% effective in preventing tetanus. In studies conducted in Europe, DTaP vaccines (with an acellular pertussis component) demonstrated efficacies for preventing pertussis between 59% and 89%, and DTP vaccines had efficacies from 36% to 98%.

DTaP vaccines have approximately one quarter to one half the common adverse events associated with

Recommended Childhood Immunization Schedule United States, January - December 2001

Vaccines[1] are listed under routinely recommended ages. Bars indicate range of recommended ages for immunization. Any dose not given at the recommended age should be given as a "catch-up" immunization at any subsequent visit when indicated and feasible. Ovals indicate vaccines to be given if previously recommended doses were missed or given earlier than the recommended minimum age.

Age ▶ / Vaccine ▼	Birth	1 mo	2 mos	4 mos	6 mos	12 mos	15 mos	18 mos	24 mos	4-6 yrs	11-12 yrs	14-18 yrs
Hepatitis B[2]	Hep B #1											
		Hep B #2				Hep B #3					(Hep B[2])	
Diphtheria, Tetanus, Pertussis[3]			DTaP	DTaP	DTaP		DTaP[3]			DTaP	Td	
H. influenzae type b[4]			Hib	Hib	Hib	Hib						
Inactivated Polio[5]			IPV	IPV		IPV[5]				IPV[5]		
Pneumococcal Conjugate[6]			PCV	PCV	PCV	PCV						
Measles, Mumps, Rubella[7]						MMR				MMR[7]	(MMR[7])	
Varicella[8]							Var				(Var[8])	
Hepatitis A[9]									Hep A — in selected areas[9]			

Approved by the Advisory Committee on Immunization Practices (ACIP), the American Academy of Pediatrics (AAP), and the American Academy of Family Physicians (AAFP).

Figure 1.

1. This schedule indicates the recommended ages for routine administration of currently licensed childhood vaccines, as of November 1, 2000, for children through 18 years of age. Additional vaccines may be licensed and recommended during the year. Licensed combination vaccines may be used whenever any components of the combination are indicated and its other components are not contraindicated. Providers should consult the manufacturers' package inserts for detailed recommendations.
2. *Infants born to HBsAg-negative mothers* should receive the 1st dose of hepatitis B (Hep B) vaccine by age 2 months. The second dose should be at least 1 month after the first dose. The third dose should be administered at least 4 months after the first dose and at least 2 months after the second dose but not before 6 months of age for infants.
   Infants born to HBsAg-positive mothers should receive hepatitis B vaccine and 0.5 mL hepatitis B immune globulin (HBIG) within 12 hours of birth at separate sites. The second dose is recommended at 1–2 months of age and the third dose at 6 months of age.
   Infants born to HBsAg-positive mothers should receive hepatitis B vaccine and 12 hours of birth. Maternal blood should be drawn at the time of delivery to determine the mother's HBsAg status; if the HBsAg test is positive, the infant should receive HBIG as soon as possible (no later than 1 week of age).
   Infants born to mothers whose HBsAg status is unknown should receive hepatitis B vaccine within 12 hours of birth. Maternal blood should be drawn at the time of delivery to determine the mother's HBsAg status; if the HBsAg test is positive, the infant should receive HBIG as soon as possible (no later than 1 week of age).
   All children and adolescents who have not been immunized against hepatitis B should begin the series during any visit. Special efforts should be made to immunize children who were born in or whose parents were born in areas of the world with moderate or high endemicity of hepatitis B virus infection.
3. The fourth dose of DTaP (diphtheria and tetanus toxoids and acellular pertussis vaccine) may be administered as early as 12 months of age, provided 6 months have elapsed since the third dose and the child is unlikely to return at age 15–18 months. Td (tetanus and diphtheria toxoids) is recommended at 11–12 years of age if at least 5 years have elapsed since the last dose of DTP, DTaP, or DT. Subsequent routine Td boosters are recommended every 10 years.
4. Three *Haemophilus influenzae* type b (Hib) conjugate vaccines are licensed for infant use. If PRP-OMP (PedvaxHIB or ComVax) is administered at 2 and 4 months of age, a dose at 6 months is not required. Because clinical studies in infants have demonstrated that using some combination products may induce a lower immune response to the Hib vaccine component, DTaP/Hib combination products should not be used for primary immunization in infants at 2, 4, or 6 months of age, unless FDA-approved for these ages.
5. An all-IPV schedule is recommended for routine childhood polio vaccination in the United States. All children should receive four doses of IPV at 2 months, 4 months, 6–18 months, and 4–6 years of age. Oral polio vaccine (OPV) should be used only in selected circumstances. (See *MMWR* May 19, 2000/49 (RR-5), 1–22.)
6. The heptavalent conjugate pneumococcal vaccine (PCV) is recommended for all children 2–23 months of age. It also is recommended for certain children 24–59 months of age. (See *MMWR* October 6, 2000/49(RR-9); 1–35).
7. The second dose of measles, mumps, and rubella (MMR) vaccine is recommended routinely at 4–6 years of age but may be administered during any visit, provided that at least 4 weeks have elapsed since receipt of the first dose and that both doses are administered beginning at or after 12 months of age. Those who have not previously received the second dose should complete the schedule by the 11–12 year visit.
8. Varicella (Var) vaccine is recommended at any visit on or after the first birthday for susceptible children, that is, those who lack a reliable history of chickenpox (as judged by a health care provider) and who have not been immunized. Susceptible persons 13 years of age or older should receive second doses, given at least 4 weeks apart.
9. Hepatitis A (Hep A) is shaded to indicate its recommended use in selected states and/or regions, and for certain high risk groups; consult your local public health authority. (See *MMWR* October 1, 1999/48(RR-12): 1–37.)

For additional information about the vaccines listed above, please visit the National Immunization Program Home Page at http://www.cdc.gov/nip/ *or call the National Immunization Hotline at 800–232–2522 (English) or 800–232–0233 (Spanish).*

DTP vaccines; furthermore, the rates of adverse events are similar for DTaP and DT vaccines. Minor adverse events associated with DTP vaccination include localized edema at the injection site, fever, drowsiness, and fretfulness. Uncommon adverse events are persistent crying for 3 or more hours following DTP vaccination, an unusual high-pitched cry, seizures, and hypotonic-hyporesponsive episodes. It is generally accepted that on rare occasions a child may have an anaphylactic reaction to DTP, and in these cases further doses of DTP or DTaP are contraindicated.

DTaP is recommended for all children because of the reduced incidence of reactions when compared with DTP. DTaP is strongly recommended over DTP for children with a family history of seizures. Although DTaP has fewer reactions following the first three doses, recent data suggest that frequency of reactions is similar with the fourth and fifth doses. Premature infants should be vaccinated with full doses at the appropriate chronologic age.

Completing the recommended series is important for optimal efficacy. For instance, one study found that the efficacy of whole-cell vaccine, based on a case definition of a cough of at least 14 days with paroxysms, whoop, or vomiting, is 36% after one dose, 49% after two doses, and 83% after three doses.

HAEMOPHILUS INFLUENZAE TYPE B VACCINES

Haemophilus influenzae type B (Hib) bacteria are spread by respiratory droplets and secretions. In unvaccinated populations, Hib is the most common cause of bacterial meningitis in preschool children. Since the introduction of Hib vaccines, there has been a dramatic decrease (95%) in the rate of invasive Hib disease in children in the United States.

Three conjugate Hib vaccines—PRP-OMP (PedvaxHIB), HbOC (HibTITER), and PRP-T (OmniHIB/ActHIB)—approved for use in infants in the U.S. have estimated efficacies of 93% to 100% for a completed series. Adverse reactions to conjugate Hib vaccines are generally mild and include erythema, tenderness, or induration at the injection site.

All children younger than 60 months (after which the risk of invasive Hib disease is significantly lower) should be vaccinated against Hib according to the recommended schedule shown in Table 1 for the particular Hib vaccine chosen. Hib vaccines should not be given before 6 weeks of age because they may induce immune tolerance, preventing adequate antibody response to further doses of Hib vaccine. Administration of Hib conjugate vaccines from different manufacturers results in antibody titers as good as or better than are seen with the same vaccine used throughout the series. Interchanging conjugate Hib vaccines is now considered fully acceptable.

TABLE 1. **Detailed Vaccination Schedule for *Haemophilus influenzae* Type B Conjugate Vaccines**

Vaccine	Age at First Dose (mos)	Primary Series	Booster
HbOC or PRP-T	2–6	3 doses, 2 mo apart	12–15 mo
	7–11	2 doses, 2 mo apart	12–18 mo
	12–14	1 dose	2 mo later
	15–59	1 dose	—
PRP-OMP	2–6	2 doses, 2 mo apart	12–15 mo
	7–11	2 doses, 2 mo apart	12–18 mo
	12–14	1 dose	2 mo later
	15–59	1 dose	—
PRP-D (Connaught)	15–59	1 dose	—

Abbreviations: HbOC = Hib vaccine conjugated with a pediatric dose of diphtheria toxoid; PRP-D = Hib vaccine conjugated with a pediatric dose of diphtheria toxoid; PRP-OMP = Hib vaccine conjugated with *Neisseria meningitidis* group B; PRP-T = Hib vaccine conjugated with tetanus toxoid.

Adapted from Epidemiology and Prevention of Vaccine-Preventable Diseases, 4th ed. Atlanta, Ga, Centers for Disease Control and Prevention, September 1997; p 110.

POLIOVIRUS VACCINE

Poliovirus is quite infectious, and transmission to susceptible household contacts occurs in 73% to 96% of infections, depending on the contact's age. Poliovirus vaccination programs have resulted in dramatic decreases in disease incidence: Circulation of indigenous wild polioviruses ceased in the United States in the 1960, and the last case of wild poliomyelitis contracted in the United States was reported in 1979. In 1994, the Americas were declared free of indigenous poliomyelitis.

Two vaccines are currently available to prevent poliomyelitis: inactivated poliovirus vaccine (IPV) and oral poliovirus vaccine (OPV). IPV cannot cause poliomyelitis but is administered by injection and offers less intestinal immunity. OPV has the advantage of easier administration, induces early intestinal immunity, and confers probably lifelong protection from poliomyelitis in almost all recipients. The main disadvantage of OPV is that the oral polioviruses can revert to a more virulent form and cause vaccine-associated paralytic poliomyelitis (VAPP). The overall risk of VAPP is quite small: 1 case per 2.4 million doses of OPV distributed. When VAPP occurs in healthy vaccine recipients, it is usually after the first dose of vaccine (1 case per 750,000 first doses). VAPP also occurs in contacts and among immunodeficient persons, especially those with B-cell disorders.

The Advisory Committee on Immunization Practices (ACIP), American Academy of Pediatrics, and American Academy of Family Physicians now recommend that all doses of poliovirus vaccine should be IPV. OPV is recommended by the World Health Organization for global eradication efforts and provides the earliest mucosal immunity. IPV should be used for the primary vaccination of adults 18 years of age or older.

MEASLES, MUMPS, AND RUBELLA (MMR) VACCINE

Measles is transmitted person-to-person by respiratory droplets and also by smaller aerosolized droplets that can spread through ventilation systems within a building and are infective for at least 1 hour. Infected persons may transmit the disease 4 days before and 4 days after the appearance of the rash. Following the introduction of measles vaccine in 1963, the incidence of measles dropped by more than 98%, although a major epidemic from 1989 to 1991 caused 55,467 reported cases and 136 deaths.

The measles vaccine contains live, highly attenuated virus. Following measles vaccination, seroconversion rates are 95% for children vaccinated at 12 months of age and 98% for children vaccinated at 15 months of age.

When measles outbreaks occurred among school-aged children in the U.S. in the 1980s despite high vaccination levels, measles vaccination guidelines were reassessed. Studies have found that failure of seroconversion after the initial dose of measles vaccine occurs at a rate of 2% to 5%. In 1989, the ACIP recommended a second dose of measles-containing vaccine at age 4 to 6 years (entry to kindergarten or first grade) to provide protection for most of those who did not respond to the initial measles vaccination.

VARICELLA VACCINE

Varicella in children is typically a self-limited benign illness. Complications can occur, however, and the disease is highly contagious, as indicated by secondary household attack rates as high as 90% in unvaccinated household contacts. Communicability (by the respiratory route) begins 1 to 2 days before the rash develops and lasts until all lesions have formed crusts. Most children who need hospitalization due to varicella are immunologically normal. Varicella is more severe in infants and adults than in children, as seen by age-specific hospitalization rates of 103 per 10,000 cases in infants, 23 per 10,000 cases in 1- to 4-year-olds, and 65 per 10,000 cases in to 29-year-olds. Because the incidence of varicella is so high in young children, they suffer the highest hospitalization rate: The largest number of annual hospitalizations for varicella (2814) is in 1- to 4-year-olds. Routine vaccination of children 12 to 18 months of age was determined to be a cost savings to society.

The varicella vaccine currently available (Varivax) contains live attenuated virus and is highly immunogenic: Almost all (97%) children 1 to 12 years of age seroconvert after one dose. The ACIP concluded that varicella vaccination provides 70% to 90% protection against infection and 95% protection against severe disease for 7 to 10 years after vaccination. Furthermore, if children who have been vaccinated contract varicella, the clinical course is milder.

Adverse events following varicella vaccination consist principally of pain and erythema at the injection site. After vaccination, 4% to 6% of recipients report a generalized varicella-like rash consisting of a few (median five) lesions. Children with leukemia who were immunized have transmitted the virus to others; however, the virus does not become more virulent. The risk of herpes zoster is lower following vaccination than following naturally acquired varicella.

Catch-up varicella vaccination is recommended for children between 18 months and 12 years of age who do *not* have a history of varicella. Varicella vaccine is approved in adolescents (≥13 years of age) and adults without a history of chickenpox on a 2-dose schedule; the doses should be spaced 4 to 8 weeks apart. The vaccine is heat sensitive and must be stored at −15°C (+5°F) or colder. Vaccine not used within 30 minutes after being reconstituted should be discarded.

Vaccinees who develop a varicelliform rash following vaccination might be contagious; hence they should avoid contact with individuals at high risk for complications of varicella, such as immunocompromised persons. If contact does occur, however, it is not necessary to give the immunocompromised contact varicella-zoster immune globulin (VZIG) because the virus in the vaccine is attenuated.

PNEUMOCOCCAL CONJUGATE VACCINE

Streptococcus pneumoniae causes approximately 17,000 cases of invasive disease per year among children younger than 5 years, including 700 cases of meningitis and 200 deaths. The highest rates of invasive pneumococcal disease occur among young children, especially those 2 years of age or younger. In the United States, the most common manifestation of invasive pneumococcal disease among young children is bacteremia without a known site of infection, which accounts for approximately 70% of cases of invasive pneumococcal infections among children 2 years of age or younger. *Streptococcus pneumoniae* has become the leading cause of bacterial meningitis in the United States. Children younger than 1 year have the highest incidence of pneumococcal meningitis, which is approximately 10 per 100,000.

There are subsets of children who are at increased risk of pneumococcal infections. High rates of invasive pneumococcal disease are reported among African Americans, Alaskan natives, and specific American Indian populations compared with whites. Children with functional or anatomic asplenia and children who are infected with HIV have significantly higher rates of invasive pneumococcal disease than do otherwise healthy children. Furthermore, out-of-home daycare increases the risk of invasive pneumococcal disease and acute otitis media among children.

The ACIP previously recommended 23-valent pneumococcal polysaccharide vaccines for use among children 2 years of age or older who have high rates of disease. In February 2000, a seven-valent pneumococcal polysaccharide-protein conjugate vaccine (PCV7) was licensed for use among infants and young children. Conjugation of polysaccharides to proteins changes the nature of the antipolysaccharide response from T independent to T dependent. This antigen complex stimulates a T helper cell response, leading to a substantial primary response among infants and a strong booster response at re-exposure. The conjugate pneumococcal vaccine is highly efficacious. PCV7 was 97.4% (95% Confidence Interval [CI], 82.7%–93.9%) and 93.9% (95% CI, 79.6%–98.5%) efficacious against vaccine serotypes among children who were fully or partially vaccinated, respectively. The study further demonstrated a decrease in the incidence of pneumonia, acute otitis media, and use of antibiotics. The duration of protection after vaccination with PCV7 is unknown. Booster responses have been clearly demonstrated 18 to 20 months after primary vaccination. Additional studies of PCV7 with longer follow-up periods are needed.

Adverse effects of PCV7 include local reactions and low-grade fever. PCV7 vaccination resulted in less-frequent local reactions than DTwP (containing whole-cell pertussis) vaccine but more frequent local reactions than DTaP vaccine and the control vaccine. Except for erythema, no pattern of increasing local reactogenicity with subsequent doses of PCV7 has been reported. Fever of 38.0°C (100.4°F) or higher 48 hours or less after vaccination was more common among children who received PCV7 concomitantly with DTaP vaccine and other recommended vaccines than among those who received the control vaccine. Febrile seizures after vaccination were slightly more common in the PCV7 group; however, the majority of events occurred when whole-cell pertussis vaccine was administered concurrently with PCV7.

In October 2000, the recommendations of the ACIP regarding the use of PCV7 were published. Currently, the ACIP recommends that the vaccine be used for all children aged 2 to 23 months and for children aged 24 to 59 months who are at increased risk of pneumococcal disease (i.e., children with sickle cell disease, HIV infection, or other immunocompromising illnesses or chronic diseases). The ACIP also recommends that the vaccine be considered for all children aged 24 to 59 months, with priority given to (1) children aged 24 to 35 months, (2) children who are Alaskan natives or of American Indian or African American decent, and (3) children who attend group daycare centers. In addition, among children aged 24 to 59 months for whom polysaccharide vaccine is already recommended, ACIP recommends vaccination with pneumoconjugate vaccine followed 2 months or more later by the 23-polysaccharide vaccine. PCV7 has not been studied sufficiently among older children or adults to make recommendations for its use among persons older than 5 years.

HEPATITIS A

Hepatitis A continues to be one of the most frequently reported vaccine-preventable diseases in the United States, despite the licensure of hepatitis A vaccine (Havrix) in 1995. The reported incidence of hepatitis A is highest among children 5 to 14 years of age, with approximately one third of reported cases involving children younger than 15 years of age. Many more children have unrecognized asymptomatic infection and can be the source of infection for others. Hepatitis A incidence varies by race and ethnicity, with highest rates among American Indians and Alaskan natives and lowest rates among Asians; rates among Hispanics are higher than among non-Hispanics. These differences in rates most likely reflect differences in the risk of infection related to factors such as differences in socioeconomic levels and living conditions and more frequent contact with persons from countries where hepatitis A is endemic. An estimated 100 persons die as a result of acute liver failure due to hepatitis A yearly. Although the case-fatality rate for fulminant hepatitis A among persons of all ages with acute hepatitis A reported to the CDC is approximately 0.3%, the rate is 1.8% among adults older than 50 years of age. Persons with chronic liver disease are at increased risk of developing fulminant hepatitis A.

Hepatitis A virus infection is acquired primarily by the fecal-oral route through either close person-to-person contact with an infected person or ingestion of contaminated food or water. Depending on conditions, the virus can be stable in the environment for months. On rare occasions, the virus has been transmitted by transfusion of blood or blood products. Both licensed vaccines are highly immunogenic in children aged 2 to 18 years and in adults. Protective antibody levels developed in 94% to 100% of individuals 1 month after the first dose and in essentially 100% after the second dose. Available data indicate that hepatitis A vaccine is immunogenic in children younger than 2 years of age who do not have passively acquired maternal antibodies. The efficacy of the hepatitis A vaccine is between 94% and 100%. The ACIP's 1996 recommendations on the prevention of hepatitis A focused primarily on vaccinating persons in groups shown to be at high risk of infection (e.g., travelers to countries with high or intermediate disease endemism, men who have sex with men, injectable drug users, and persons with clotting factor disorders), persons with chronic liver disease, and children living in communities with high rates of disease. In October 1999, the ACIP added the recommendation for routine vaccination of children in states, counties, or communities with rates that are equal to or greater than 20 cases per 100,000 population. In states, counties, or communities with rates exceeding 10 but less than 20 cases per 100,000 population, routine vaccination of children may be considered.

The most frequently reported side effects include soreness at the injection site, warmth at the injection site, and headache. Review of the data from multiple sources for more than 5 years regarding adverse events from an estimated 65 million doses of hepatitis A vaccine administered worldwide did not find any serious adverse events among children or adults that could be definitely attributed to hepatitis A vaccine.

INFLUENZA VACCINE

In each of 10 recent influenza epidemics in the United States, estimated deaths totaled more than

20,000. Furthermore, during some epidemics of influenza type A, there have been approximately 172,000 hospitalizations attributable to influenza and pneumonia. The cost of a severe influenza epidemic is estimated to be $12 billion.

Partly because they have a higher incidence of chronic medical conditions, the elderly have the highest age-specific case-fatality rate from influenza: More than 90% of deaths due to influenza occur in persons 65 years of age or older. In one study of the elderly, influenza vaccination resulted in a 27% to 39% reduction in the number of hospitalizations (depending on the year studied) due to acute or chronic respiratory conditions and, in 1 year, a 37% reduction in the number of hospitalizations due to congestive heart failure.

Beginning each September, when vaccine for the upcoming influenza season becomes available, all persons 50 years of age or older who are seen by health care providers should be offered influenza vaccine so that vaccination opportunities are not missed. Persons 6 months of age or older may receive influenza vaccine.

PNEUMOCOCCAL VACCINE (POLYSACCHARIDE VACCINE)

Pneumococcal disease causes an estimated 3000 cases of meningitis, 50,000 cases of bacteremia, and 500,000 cases of pneumonia annually in the United States. Most (60%–87%) cases of pneumococcal bacteremia in adults are associated with pneumonia, and the rate of bacteremia is highest in persons 65 years of age and older. Despite appropriate therapy, the overall case-fatality rate for pneumococcal bacteremia is 15% to 20% among adults; this climbs to approximately 30% to 40% for elderly patients.

All persons 65 years of age and older should receive one dose of pneumococcal vaccine unless they are known to have received vaccination within the past 5 years. A prime opportunity for vaccination in this age group is at hospital discharge: In one study, 61% to 62% of persons aged 65 years or older who were hospitalized with pneumonla had been discharged from a hospital within the previous 4 years.

LATE VACCINATIONS

If the vaccination schedule is interrupted, it does not need to be restarted. Instead, the schedule should be resumed using minimal intervals between doses (Table 2).

VACCINATION PROCEDURES

Contraindications

There are two permanent contraindications to administering a dose of vaccine: (1) severe allergy to a vaccine component or anaphylactic reaction to a previous dose of the vaccine and (2) for pertussis vaccine, encephalopathy without a known cause within 7 days of a dose. Contact dermatitis from neomycin, however, is a delayed-type (cell-mediated) immune response and is not a contraindication to vaccination. If the pertussis component is withheld

TABLE 2. **Age for Initial Childhood Vaccinations and Minimum Interval Between Vaccine Doses, by Type of Vaccine***

Vaccine	Minimal Age for Dose 1	Minimal Interval From Dose 1 to 2	Minimal Interval From Dose 2 to 3	Minimal Interval From Dose 3 to 4
DTaP (DT)†	6 wk	4 wk	4 wk	6 mo
Combined DTP-Hib‡	6 wk	1 mo	1 mo	6 mo
Hib (primary series)				
HbOC	6 wk	1 mo	1 mo	‡
PRP-T	6 wk	1 mo	1 mo	‡
PRP-OMP	6 wk	1 mo	‡	
Pneumococcal conjugate	6 wk	1 mo	1 mo	‡
Poliovirus	6 wk	4 wk	4 wk	‖
MMR	12 mo	1 mo		
Hepatitis B	Birth	1 mo	2 mo**	
Varicella	12 mo	4 wk		

*The minimal acceptable ages and intervals may not correspond with the *optimal* recommended ages and intervals for vaccination. For current recommended routine schedules, see the annual Recommended Childhood Immunization Schedule of the United States.

†The total number of doses of diphtheria and tetanus toxoids should not exceed six each before the seventh birthday.

‡The booster doses of Hib and pneumococcal conjugate vaccines that are recommended following the primary vaccination series should be administered no earlier than 12 months of age *and* at least 2 months after the previous dose.

§For unvaccinated adults at increased risk of exposure to poliovirus with <3 months but >2 months available before protection is needed, three doses of inactivated poliomyelitis vaccine should be administered at least 1 month apart.

‖If the third dose is given after the third birthday, the fourth (booster) dose is not needed.

¶Although the age for measles vaccination may be as young as 6 months in outbreak areas where cases are occurring in children <1 year of age, children initially vaccinated before the first birthday should be revaccinated at 12 to 15 months of age, and an additional dose of vaccine should be administered at the time of school entry or according to local policy. Doses of MMR or other measles-containing vaccines should be separated by at least 1 month.

**This final dose is recommended at least 4 months after the first dose, no earlier than at 6 months of age.

Abbreviations: DT = diphtheria and pertussis; DTaP = diphtheria, tetanus, and acellular pertussis; DTP = diphtheria, tetanus, and pertussis; HbOC = Hib vaccine conjugated with a pediatric dose of diphtheria toxoid; Hib = *Haemophilus influenzae* type B; MMR = measles, mumps, and rubella; PRP-OMP = Hib vaccine conjugated with *Neisseria meningitidis* group B; PRP-T = Hib vaccine conjugated with tetanus toxoid.

Adapted from Epidemiology and Prevention of Vaccine-Preventable Diseases, 6th ed. Atlanta, Ga, Centers for Disease Control and Prevention, 2000.

because of a contraindication or precaution, then pediatric DT is administered instead, except in the case of true anaphylaxis, in which case the diphtheria and the pertussis components are permanently contraindicated.

Four conditions are temporary contraindications to vaccination: severe acute illness, immunosuppression, pregnancy, and recent receipt of blood products. Severe acute illness usually warrants postponement of vaccination until the patient has recovered from the acute phase.

Immunosuppression due to an immune deficiency disease or malignancy or therapy with high-dose corticosteroid drugs, alkylating agents, antimetabolites, or radiation is a contraindication to administration of a live vaccine (although HIV-infected persons who are not severely immunosuppressed should receive MMR vaccine when indicated). Inactivated vaccines may be given to immunosuppressed persons because they do not contain live organisms that can replicate; however, immunosuppression may decrease the response to vaccination.

Pregnancy is a contraindication to administration of live-virus vaccines because of the theoretical risk of damage to the fetus. Women should avoid becoming pregnant within 3 months of receiving MMR or rubella vaccine and within 1 month of mumps or varicella vaccination. Inadvertent administration of a live-virus vaccine during pregnancy is not an indication for pregnancy termination because there are no data to link live-virus vaccination with increased risk of fetal malformations. Vaccines may be given to breast-feeding mothers.

Recent administration of blood products can interfere with development of an immune response to a live-virus (but not inactivated-virus) vaccine. CDC information has been published that describes when various vaccines may be administered in such cases.

Precautions

Precautions for vaccination are conditions that *may* increase the risk of a serious or life-threatening adverse event or may compromise the ability of the vaccine to produce immunity. Generally, the vaccine is withheld or postponed in such situations; however, the decision whether to vaccinate in such cases is made by weighing the individual patient's risk of acquiring the disease against the risk of the adverse event (or inability to produce immunity). Certain infrequent adverse events occurring after pertussis vaccination are contraindications to further doses: (1) temperature of 40.5°C (105°F) or higher within 48 hours of a previous dose (not due to another identifiable cause); (2) collapse or shocklike state (hypotonic-hyporesponsive episode) with 48 hours of a previous dose; (3) persistent, inconsolable crying lasting 3 hours or more occurring within 48 hours of a previous dose; or (4) convulsions within 3 days of a previous dose.

DTaP vaccination should be postponed for infants with an evolving neurologic disorder, unevaluated seizures, or a neurologic event between doses of pertussis vaccine. Vaccination should be resumed after evaluation and treatment of the condition.

Vaccine Information Statements for Patients

Under the Public Health Service Act, health care providers who administer any vaccine containing diphtheria, tetanus, pertussis, measles, mumps, rubella, poliovirus, varicella, hepatitis B, or *Haemophilus influenzae* type B antigens are required to provide a copy of the relevant Vaccine Information Statements (VISs) to the patient before vaccination. These VISs may be downloaded from the CDC website: www.cdc.gov/nip/publications/vis.

Interchangeability of Vaccines From Different Manufacturers

Vaccines from different manufacturers can be given interchangeably if there is a serologic test for the disease that shows if a person is protected, as is the case for hepatitis B and Hib. No data are yet available on the safety or the efficacy of acellular pertussis vaccination when different brands are administered for the first three doses. Thus, when possible, use of the same brand of acellular pertussis vaccine for sequential doses is preferred. When a child who started the series with one brand is due for another dose and the office stocks a different brand, however, it may be used.

Simultaneous Vaccination and Combination Vaccines

Most vaccines will be efficacious and safe when administered simultaneously with another vaccine, except for (1) yellow fever and cholera vaccine, which should be administered at least 3 weeks apart and (2) cholera and plaque vaccines, which should be given on separate occasions to avoid augmentation of adverse events.

TRAVEL MEDICINE

method of
MARIA D. MILENO, M.D.
The Miriam Hospital
Providence, Rhode Island

There are about 520 million international travelers each year; 40 million travel to underdeveloped parts of the world. Of the approximately 15 million Americans who travel abroad each year, about half go to the developing world. Short-term consultants and tourists and, to a greater extent, longer-term travelers and resident expatriates are exposed to diseases and environmental factors that are not present, or are at least rare, in the United States. In response to these hazards, travel medicine has emerged as a distinct medical specialty that is now increasingly based on scientific data. Advising travelers has become a specialist's task because preventive measures have become more complex owing to the changing epidemiology of diseases, the problem of antimicrobial resistance, and the increase in travel to remote and exotic destinations. It is estimated that for every 100,000 travelers who go to the developing world for 1 month, 50,000 will develop a health problem, 8000 will be sick enough to see a physician, 5000 will be confined to bed, 1100 will be incapacitated, 300 will have to be hospitalized during the trip or upon return, 50 will have to be evacuated or repatriated, and 1 will die. Several well-written texts are devoted to the topics summarized in this article.

Travel medicine deals with both the prevention of travel-related disorders and the diagnosis and treatment of exotic, primarily tropical diseases. Travel medicine specialists provide specific resources for travelers and present a broad variety of ways to effectively minimize risks of both common and potentially life-threatening illnesses.

Specialized strategies are available for high-risk travelers, including those traveling off the usual tourist routes, backpackers, and foreign-born persons who are returning to visit friends and family. The process of delivering formalized travel health advice includes gathering pertinent information from the patient, evaluating potential risks, making an individualized plan, and providing careful teaching, counseling, and prophylaxis.

A professional group for travel and tropical medicine specialists is the American Committee on Clinical Tropical Medicine and Travelers' Health. Although there are no specialty boards for travel or tropical medicine, the American Society of Tropical Medicine and Hygiene (ASTMH) and this society's American Committee on Clinical Tropical Medicine prepare an annual certification examination to assess and recognize individual excellence in training and knowledge. Meeting educational criteria in the field, including experience abroad, and passing the examination lead to a certificate of knowledge in Clinical Tropical Medicine and Travelers' Health.* Another organization dealing with all aspects of travel medicine is the International Society of Travel Medicine (ISTM).†

Internists may be the initial contacts for travelers. Healthy individuals with a straightforward itinerary may be cared for at this level, given a certain amount of travel medicine knowledge on the part of their personal physician. Individuals with complicated medical problems may benefit from an evaluation of their medications to optimally regulate any existing health problems. Persons with complicated itineraries, travel that includes malaria-endemic regions, and travelers with underlying medical problems should be referred to the nearest formal travel clinic. Travel clinics have been established at many medical centers nationwide. The enormous increase in travel, particularly to developing countries, has resulted in a need for specific medical information regarding disease risks. Travel medicine information can be obtained from health departments at various government levels, which are in turn supported with information from the Centers for Disease Control and Prevention (CDC). Most health departments refer travelers to designated travel medicine clinics, which can properly facilitate specific education and preparation for travel to the developing world.

*Information on ASTMH activities and the certification examination may be obtained from the American Society of Tropical Medicine and Hygiene, 60 Revere Drive, Suite 500, Northbrook, Illinois 60062; phone: 847-480-9592; fax: 847-480-9282.

†Information on ISTM activities may be obtained from ISTM Secretariat, PO Box 871089, Stone Mountain, Georgia 30087; phone: 770-736-7060; fax: 770-726-6732.

PRE-TRAVEL ADVICE

Ideally, travelers should undergo a pre-travel physical examination if they have serious medical problems, are planning a long or physically demanding trip, or are planning to reside abroad. This examination is best accomplished by the personal physician, who is familiar with the traveler and his or her health history. A medical summary and a copy of recent pertinent laboratory tests, electrocardiograms, or chest radiographs should be taken along by the traveler. Engraved bracelets or health cards with a brief summary of any serious medical conditions can be obtained from a number of sources. Travel medicine clinics can often provide the names of well-recognized English-speaking physicians overseas in case of illness while abroad. The traveler's health insurance should be reviewed to determine whether coverage applies to conditions acquired while traveling, to hospitalization abroad, or to medical evacuation from foreign countries.

In some countries, over-the-counter drugs often lack label warnings. Travelers must be cautioned that potentially dangerous drugs and chemicals may be included in such preparations, including chloramphenicol (Chloromycetin), sulfa drugs, butazolidin,* and aminopyrine,* among others. Travelers with chronic illnesses should carry a sufficient supply of required drugs.

PREPARATION OF AN INDIVIDUALIZED MEDICAL KIT

Components of a traveler's medical kit vary according to pre-existing and other potential needs. Useful general items include a thermometer, bandages, gauze, tape, a bactericidal soap solution, aspirin, antacids, anti–motion sickness drug, and a mild laxative or suppository for constipation. A nasal decongestant and saline nose drops and eyedrops may be useful during flight. An antihistamine may be taken for allergies. Cough medicine and other liquids should be carried in tightly stoppered plastic bottles.

*Not available in the United States.

Antibiotic, antifungal, and anti-inflammatory ointments may be included. Salt tablets may be helpful in hot, humid climates; a sunscreen should be included. In general, antibiotics, other than those for self-treatment of diarrhea, should not be given to the average traveler. If sufficiently ill, the traveler would be better served by consulting a local physician, except in remote areas where medical assistance is not readily available.

MALARIA PREVENTION

With the emergence and continued spread of malaria that is resistant to chloroquine and other drugs and the complexities of malarial prophylactic drugs (e.g., contraindications and toxic side effects), physicians may find it very difficult to offer appropriate advice to travelers. Travel medicine centers have access to information updated weekly and sometimes daily regarding resistant malaria to facilitate decisions on the best drug and antimosquito measures for particular travelers. Malaria is probably the greatest hazard to travelers in many parts of the developing world, and expert opinion is required to give optimal protection. (See also the article on malaria.)

Personal Protection Measures Against Mosquito Bite

No current antimalarial drug regimen guarantees protection against malaria. Prevention of malarial infection requires great attention to personal protection measures against mosquito bites. These measures are as important as an antimalarial drug prescription, if not more so!

Malaria transmission by mosquitoes occurs primarily between dusk and dawn. During these hours, measures to reduce contact with mosquitoes are an essential adjunct to drug prophylaxis in the prevention of malaria. These measures include (1) remaining in well-screened areas; (2) using mosquito nets impregnated with permethrin; (3) wearing clothes that cover most of the body; (4) applying insect repellents containing diethyltoluamide (DEET)—optimally a 20% to 35% concentration of lotion on all exposed body parts; (5) using permethrin spray (Nix)* in clothing as an insecticide; and (6) using a flying-insect spray containing pyrethrum in living areas. Travel medicine centers spend a great deal of time describing the use of the best products currently available to prevent insect exposures.

Drug Prophylaxis

Plasmodium falciparum is the malaria species that causes the most serious disease. This parasite is almost universally resistant to chloroquine (Aralen) and, to a lesser extent, other available antimalarial drugs. *P. falciparum* remains sensitive to chloroquine only in Central America, Haiti, the Dominican Republic, and parts of the Middle East. In these areas, a weekly 500-mg dose of chloroquine phosphate (equal to a 300-mg base) can be used for prophylaxis. In the United States, generic chloroquine phosphate is unavailable, and only oral Aralen in a 500-mg tablet can be obtained. Other tablet and liquid preparations are available abroad. Chloroquine is considered safe for use in pregnancy.

Recently, chloroquine-resistant *P. vivax* malaria has been reported from Indonesia, Papua New Guinea, parts of Southeast Asia, and Latin America. For protection against chloroquine-resistant *P. falciparum* malaria, there are four available regimens currently recommended by American experts.

Mefloquine (Lariam). This drug is the most widely used and effective regimen of the four; however, high-level mefloquine resistance is carried by *P. falciparum* parasites along the Thai-Cambodian and Thai-Myanmar borders. Rarely confirmed cases of resistance in tropical Africa and other malarious areas have been reported. The adult dosage is a 250-mg tablet taken weekly; dosages for children and infants are reduced. Mefloquine is considered safe for use during the second and third trimesters of pregnancy and is apparently also safe in the first trimester when this drug is indicated to reduce malaria infection. There has been considerable controversy over the safety of mefloquine, particularly in relation to the incidence of neuropsychiatric side effects, such as convulsions and hallucinations; however, comparative studies have shown that the adverse effects of mefloquine are similar in frequency and quality to those of chloroquine. Reported side effects of mefloquine include insomnia, bad dreams, dizziness, headache, anxiety, and gastrointestinal symptoms. The more serious toxic psychosis occurs in approximately 1 in 10,000 users. Long-term use of mefloquine by Peace Corps volunteers in Africa showed it to be well tolerated. Contraindications to mefloquine include a history of epilepsy, serious psychiatric disorder, or cardiac conduction system abnormalities, particularly prolonged QT_C intervals.

Mefloquine is not recommended for emergency self-treatment of malaria because of the frequency of potentially serious side effects (hallucinations and convulsions) associated with higher dosages used for malaria (1250 mg).

Doxycyline. For persons unable to tolerate mefloquine or who have a contraindication to its use, and in areas where malaria has considerable resistance to mefloquine, doxycycline* (100-mg daily dose) can be used by adults and children older than 8 years of age. This drug cannot be used by pregnant women or by children younger than 8 years of age. Potential adverse effects include photosensitivity in about 2% of users, vaginal candidiasis, and gastrointestinal effects, such as esophageal ulceration when taken without food.

Atovaquone/Proguanil (Malarone). The newest choice for prevention of malaria is the oral, once-

*Not FDA approved for this indication.

*Not FDA approved for this indication.

daily combination agent atovaquone/proguanil that was approved by the U.S. Food and Drug Administration in August 2000. In three placebo-controlled clinical trials in endemic areas, atovaquone/proguanil was highly effective in preventing *P. falciparum* malaria. Studies done in nonimmune travelers are now complete and show the same protective efficacy as in other studies and improved tolerability over mefloquine or chloroquine with proguanil. Atovaquone/proguanil is indicated for the prevention of *P. falciparum* malaria, including areas where chloroquine resistance has been reported, and it represents an alternative to mefloquine or doxycycline. Protective efficacy against *P. vivax* in nonimmune individuals is only 81%, and terminal prophylaxis is indicated if Malarone is used for prolonged travel to regions where *P. vivax* or *P. ovale* is prevalent.

Malarone is a category C drug not yet indicated for use in pregnancy, although more studies are under way. The adult dosage includes 250 mg of atovaquone and 100 mg of proguanil. This adult-strength tablet is taken daily with food from 1 day before travel to 7 days after travel. The most commonly reported adverse events attributed to atovaquone/proguanil were headache and abdominal pain, which occurred at rates comparable to those of placebo. In clinical trials for prevention of malaria, only 3 of 381 adults abandoned the trial owing to treatment-related adverse events. A pediatric formulation exists as tablets that are one quarter the strength of the adult tablets. Atovaquone/proguanil is contraindicated in individuals with known hypersensitivity to atovaquone or proguanil. Administration of rifampin, tetracycline, and metoclopramide is associated with reduced plasma concentrations of atovaquone, and co-administration is not recommended.

Chloroquine Used With Proguanil (Paludrine).*† A weekly dose of chloroquine phosphate (as described earlier) plus a 200-mg daily dose of proguanil has been recommended as malaria prophylaxis for many years. Both these drugs are considered safe during pregnancy and for all age groups. Proguanil is not available in the United States, but it is available by prescription in Canada and Europe and usually over the counter in Africa. This combination is the least effective of the available regimens. Travelers using this combination may need an emergency self-treatment regimen, such as a treatment dose of atovaquone/proguanil (four tablets once a day for 3 days). Atovaquone/proguanil should replace the use of the chloroquine/proguanil combination for prophylaxis.

Almost all these regimens must be taken regularly while the traveler is in a malarious area and for 4 weeks after departure from the area. Atovaquone/proguanil must be taken only 7 days after exposure, however. Doxycycline and atovaquone/proguanil may be started 1 day before entering malarious areas, whereas chloroquine and mefloquine should be started 1 to 3 weeks before travel to a malarious area to ensure adequate blood levels of the drugs on arrival and tolerance of them. Because more than 75% of adverse reactions to mefloquine are apparent by the third dose, first-time users of mefloquine might ideally begin taking the drug 3 weeks before departure. Long-term travelers benefit from the convenience that the weekly dosing regimen of mefloquine offers.

*Combination not FDA approved for this indication.
†Not available in the United States as a single agent.

Primaquine. Some new drug regimens for multidrug-resistant *P. falciparum*–related malaria are being evaluated but are not yet approved for use in the United States. These include a daily 30-mg base dose of primaquine and a related 8-aminoquinoline agent, tafenoquine.*

Primaquine prophylaxis eliminates *P. vivax* and *P. ovale* hypnozoite forms from the liver so that a future attack will not occur when administration of the previously mentioned drugs is completed. Primaquine in a base dose of 15 mg daily for 14 days is given after completion of routine drug prophylaxis. Primaquine for terminal prophylaxis is not indicated for all travelers, and the decision to administer it must be made on an individual basis. The intensity and the duration of the traveler's exposure to *P. vivax* or *P. ovale* must be considered. Primaquine is not generally recommended for travelers with relatively short-term (less than 1 month) exposure, because late relapses rarely occur in such persons owing to minimal exposure. Before any use of primaquine, glucose-6-phosphate dehydrogenase deficiency must be ruled out. Primaquine is contraindicated during pregnancy. Terminal prophylaxis with primaquine is not universally effective; relative resistance of strains of *P. vivax* to the drug has been documented in Oceania, Southeast Asia, and parts of Latin America.

Even with all these measures, particularly if they are not used carefully, it is still possible to contract malaria. Travelers who develop fever during travel or within 3 years after return from a malarious area should be promptly evaluated for possible malaria infection. Research is continuing on malaria vaccines, but one is not expected for some years.

REQUIRED AND RECOMMENDED IMMUNIZATIONS

Vaccine requirements listed by country are published by the CDC in *Health Information for International Travel.* A number of commercial computer programs are also available. Daily updates regarding outbreaks and new information for travel medicine specialists are incorporated into the day-to-day advice offered to travelers.

Yellow fever vaccine is given only in travel clinics and other state-licensed official vaccination centers. Because this vaccine is live and requires cold storage, it is viable and used for only 60 minutes after reconstitution. Certain other vaccines are difficult to obtain or come only in multiple-dose vials and are thus

*Not available in the United States.

more cost-effective at busy travel clinics and government facilities; these include meningococcal meningitis, plague, Japanese encephalitis, and rabies vaccines.

Required Immunizations

Yellow Fever. Yellow fever occurs in parts of tropical Africa and South America, and the vaccine may be required for entry into countries in these regions or for travelers wishing to enter other countries after visiting regions where the disease is endemic. The vaccination must be validated in the correct section of the yellow International Certificate of Vaccination. Yellow fever vaccine is contraindicated in anyone with altered immune status or a known hypersensitivity to eggs, in children younger than 9 months of age, and in pregnant women. These persons should be given a letter of contraindication on an official letterhead and must be warned not to enter any area with active yellow fever infection. A single dose is effective for at least 10 years, and side effects are minimal.

Cholera. In 1988, the World Health Organization (WHO) dropped the requirement for cholera vaccine, and the International Certificate of Vaccination no longer has a special section for cholera. Cholera vaccine is not recommended for most travelers, even those going to cholera epidemic areas, because the currently available injectable inactivated vaccine is not very effective in preventing cholera. Unfortunately, cholera epidemics continue to occur, but the risk of travelers acquiring cholera is low.

Occasionally, certain officials whom travelers may meet on entering particular countries will ask to see evidence that the travelers have received cholera vaccine. A waiver can be written on the International Certificate, which should bear an official stamp. Travelers should practice appropriate hygiene in handling food and water to prevent cholera as well as numerous other enteric diseases. Two new oral cholera vaccines* have been developed; both are effective and better tolerated and provide high-level protection, at least for several months. Neither of these vaccines appears to offer protection against the 0139 serogroup of *Vibrio cholerae,* which is the strain responsible for much of the world's endemic cholera. These vaccines are not yet available in the United States, and recommendations for their use in travelers have not yet been formulated.

Smallpox. In 1983, the WHO deleted smallpox from the list of diseases subject to the International Health Regulations. Smallpox vaccine* is not available routinely any longer, and vaccination is not indicated for any international traveler.

Recommended Immunizations

Certain vaccines are recommended for protection against diseases prevalent in many parts of the world (Table 1). For children, routine childhood immunizations should be up to date before travel is undertaken. (See the article on immunization practices.)

Hepatitis A Vaccine. Hepatitis A is the most common vaccine-preventable disease encountered by unprotected travelers to developing countries. Two hepatitis A vaccines are now available in the United States. Havrix (GlaxoSmithKline, Research Triangle Park, NC) and Vaqta (Merck & Co., Whitehouse Station, NJ), each given in a two-dose series 6 to 12 months apart, are expected to provide long-term, possibly lifetime protection against infection. These vaccines are available in both adult and pediatric formulations. Children older than 2 years of age can receive the vaccine. After administration of an initial single dose of either vaccine, protective immunity can be assumed by 4 weeks, if not sooner. Ideally, the vaccine should be given 2 weeks before entering an endemic region; however, concurrent administration of immune serum globulin is unnecessary, even if travelers are leaving sooner than 2 weeks from the day of immunization.

Hepatitis B Vaccine. Hepatitis B is more prevalent in some parts of the developing world and is a particular hazard for travelers who have contact with blood or have sexual contact with local residents. Recent data suggest that increasing numbers of travelers may engage in other activities while abroad that pose a theoretical risk for acquisition of hepatitis B, such as dental work, tattooing, acupuncture, and riding in unsafe vehicles. A recombinant hepatitis B vaccine series is highly recommended for long-stay travelers and for frequent short-term travelers to the developing world. Both available U.S.-licensed vaccines can be given in a standard three-dose series over a 6-month period; however, Engerix-B (GlaxoSmithKline) is approved for an accelerated course of three monthly doses, with a fourth booster given 12 months after the first dose. Discussion of hepatitis B risks provides the optimal time to address safety while driving as well as safe-sex practices, including use of condoms in all sexual encounters to avoid acquisition of sexually transmitted diseases, including hepatitis B and HIV infection.

A more accelerated dosing schedule (0, 7, and 21 days), with a booster dose administered after 1 year, is offered to individuals who present just weeks before they must leave for an extended trip with high-risk situations. Data showing protection at 30 days have already been published. Hepatitis B vaccine is safe and effective, but its relatively high cost and extended dosing schedules pose difficulties. Studies are in progress to evaluate combined hepatitis A and B vaccines.

Immune Globulin. This is an alternative to hepatitis A vaccine when single short-term protection is needed against hepatitis A. Persons traveling for less than 3 months are protected by a single intramuscular dose of 0.02 mL/kg. Hepatitis A vaccine, although more expensive, is much more cost-effective and longer lasting for the longer-term or frequent traveler.

*Not available in the United States.

TABLE 1. **Dosing Schedules for Commonly Used Vaccines for Travel**

Vaccine	Primary Series	Booster Interval
Hepatitis A (Havrix, Vaqta)	One dose for adults and children older than 2 y	1 dose 6 to 12 mo after first, predicted to protect for 10 y or more
Hepatitis B (Engerix-B) (accelerated schedule) *or* Hepatitis B (Recombivax) (standard schedule)	Three doses at 0, 30, and 60 d	A fourth dose is recommended at 12 mo
Immune globulin (IG) (hepatitis A protection)	One dose IM in the gluteus muscle (2-mL dose for 3-mo protection; 5-mL dose for 5 mo); pediatric dose, 0.02 mL/kg for 3-mo trip; 0.06 mL/kg for 5-mo trip	At 3- to 5-mo intervals
Japanese encephalitis (JEV) (Japanese manufacturer, Biken)	Three doses on days 0, 7, and 30 (1 mL SC for children older than 3 y; 0.5 mL SC for children younger than 3 y)	After 3 y
Measles/mumps/rubella (MMR)*	One dose† SC at 15 mo of age	Booster measles vaccine at 4–6 y old; boost measles vaccine once in adult life before international travel for people born in or after 1957
Meningococcus† (A/C/Y/W-135)	One dose†	After 3 years
Plague†	First and second doses given 1–3 mo apart; third dose given 5–6 mo after second dose	Booster if the risk of exposure persists
Poliomyelitis, enhanced-potency inactivated (eIPV) (killed vaccine; safe for all ages)	Single dose at ages 2, 4, and 6–18 mo and 4–6 y	Once before travel in areas of risk
Poliomyelitis, oral (OPV) (attenuated live virus)*	Single dose at ages 2, 4, and 6–18 mo and 4–6 y	Once before travel in areas of risk
Rabies, human diploid cell vaccine (HDCV) *or* Rabies, purified chick embryo cell vaccine (PCEC) *or* Rabies vaccine adsorbed (rhesus diploid cell with aluminum) (RVA)	Three doses (1-mL doses IM in deltoid areas) on days 0, 7, and 21 or 28	With frequent exposure risk, booster after 2 y or test serum for antibody level
Tetanus and diphtheria toxoids adsorbed (Td) (for children older than 7 y of age and for adults)	Three doses (0.5 mL SC or IM); first and second dose given 4–8 wk apart; third dose at 6–12 mo after second dose	Routinely every 10 y
Typhoid, oral (Vivotif)	One capsule PO every other day (>6 y)	5 y
Typhoid, Vi capsular polysaccharide vaccine (Typhim Vi)	Single dose (>2 y)	2 y
Varicella (Varivax)	One dose for children younger than 13 y; two doses for susceptible persons older than 13 y	None currently recommended
Yellow fever (YF-Vax)*	One dose (0.5 mL SC) for those over 9 mo of age	10 y
Cholera, parenteral	Two doses 1 wk or more apart (0.5 mL SC or IM); pediatric dose 0.3 mL for 5–10 y of age, 0.2 mL for 6 mo–4 y of age	6 mo
Cholera, live oral CVD 103-HgR	One dose PO on an empty stomach for child older than 2 y	6 mo (optimal booster schedule not yet determined)

*Caution: May be contraindicated in patients with any of the following conditions: pregnancy; leukemia; lymphoma; generalized malignancy; immunosuppression due to HIV infection; or treatment with corticosteroids, alkylating drugs, antimetabolites, or radiation therapy.

†See manufacturers' package insert and text for detailed recommendations on dosage and schedule.

Abbreviations: IM = intramuscular; PO = orally; SC = subcutaneous.

Adapted from Jong EC, McMullen R: The Travel and Tropical Medicine Manual, 2nd ed. Philadelphia, WB Saunders, 1995.

Influenza Vaccine. Persons considered at high risk of serious influenza infection who are traveling to areas of the world where epidemic influenza is present should receive the influenza vaccine.

Japanese Encephalitis Vaccine. Rare cases of Japanese encephalitis have occurred in resident expatriates and travelers to certain parts of the Far East and Southeast Asia where this disease is endemic or, at times, epidemic. The risk of infection is much greater in rural agricultural regions than in urban areas; in some areas, the risk is seasonal. A three-dose vaccine series is recommended for persons spending more than 1 month in endemic areas during the transmission season, especially if travel includes rural areas, and for certain shorter-term travelers to areas where epidemics occur and risk is high.

The vaccine for Japanese encephalitis is associated with moderately frequent local and mild systemic side effects and uncommonly with more serious allergic reactions. The rate of serious reactions in American citizens is 2 to 6 per 1000 vaccine recipients, and reactions are more common in persons with a history of asthma. These reactions may be delayed in onset for up to 10 to 14 days.

Measles Vaccine. The risk of contracting measles is much greater in the developing world than in the United States, and for younger children traveling to measles-endemic areas the age at immunization should be lowered from the usual 15 months to 6 months. A second dose of measles vaccine should then be given at the age of 12 to 15 months. Adults born in the United States or before 1957 are considered immune to measles, but persons born after 1957 who travel abroad should have assured protection against measles. Travelers who have not previously received two doses of measles vaccine and who do not have a history of measles infection should receive one dose of measles vaccine, unless there is a contraindication. Some individuals born between 1963 and 1967 may have received killed measles vaccine and may not have mounted a sufficient immune response. This has placed approximately 900,000 persons in the United States at risk of atypical measles infection, a severe disease that may simulate Rocky Mountain spotted fever or meningococcemia.

Meningococcal Meningitis Vaccine. Meningococcal meningitis is endemic worldwide, but, in particular areas, seasonal epidemics caused by *Neisseria meningitidis* serogroup A and C occur. In the sub-Saharan Sahel region of Africa, epidemics occur almost yearly during colder dryer months. Meningitis is very uncommon in travelers, but immunization with the quadrivalent A,C,Y,W135 vaccine is recommended for all travelers to countries in the "meningitis belt" during epidemic seasons. Pilgrims to Saudi Arabia for the haj are required to have proof of having received this vaccine. Outbreaks of meningococcal meningitis serogroup B also occur, but there is currently no vaccine available against this serogroup.

Plague Vaccine. The usual traveler to plague-endemic countries is at very low risk of infection. Most outbreaks have occurred in more remote areas. Certain travelers at high risk for this disease should consider plague immunization. These include mammalogists, ecologists, and other field workers who have regular contact with wild rodents or fleas in plague-enzootic or plague-epizootic areas. There is limited availability of plague vaccine, and it does not protect against pneumonic plague.

Polio Vaccine. Poliovirus transmission has been interrupted in the Americas, but wild poliovirus continues to circulate in other parts of the world. Polio remains a definite hazard to travelers to polio-affected areas of the world, such as Asia, Africa, and India. Most adult travelers have had a basic polio vaccine series during childhood, and a single dose of enhanced-potency injectable vaccine is recommended once as an adult, preferably before travel. This is expected to give lifelong protection, and no need for further supplementary doses has been established.

Rabies Vaccine. Relatively few countries can be considered rabies free. For travelers to rabies-endemic countries such as India who may be at high risk of infection, primarily from dog bites, a three-dose intramuscular pre-exposure rabies vaccine series may be recommended. These might include young children, joggers, bikers, people working with animals, field workers, and persons in remote areas who are distant from facilities where adequate post-exposure treatment can be obtained. Avoidance of direct contact with animals should be emphasized, including instructions not to pet or feed small animals. Pre-exposure immunization offers valuable added protection when rabies exposure occurs, and the need for human rabies immune globulin, often difficult to obtain, is eliminated. Administration of two postexposure vaccine doses is still required, however.

Tetanus-Diphtheria (Td) Vaccine. It is essential for everyone, traveling or not, to maintain immunity against tetanus and diphtheria by receiving a booster dose at 10-year intervals. Most travelers already received primary diphtheria-pertussis-tetanus (DPT) vaccine during childhood. For travelers to underdeveloped parts of the world, documentation of a booster dose within 5 to 10 years is suggested. For boosters, persons older than the age of 7 years receive Td vaccine, which has a smaller amount of diphtheria toxoid. A travel-associated risk of diphtheria infection has been present in Russia and the new independent states, where epidemics occurred in the past.

Tick-Borne Encephalitis Vaccine.* This viral infection of the central nervous system is transmitted by ticks in forested areas of central and eastern Europe and the former Soviet Union. This vaccine is not available in the United States, but an effective vaccine may be obtained in Europe and can be considered for travelers or residents who are at risk of exposure in forested areas of countries where the disease is endemic, such as southern Germany.

Tuberculosis/Bacille Calmette-Guérin (BCG) Vaccine. BCG vaccine is rarely recommended except for some long-term travelers, but the worldwide increase in multidrug-resistant tuberculosis may reawaken interest in this vaccine. It is a live vaccine that has the potential for dissemination in recipients with compromised immunity.

Typhoid Vaccine. Typhoid fever is endemic in the developing world, and typhoid vaccine is recommended for travelers to those areas with substandard hygienic practices involving water and food. Two vaccines are recommended in the United States, and both provide about 70% protection. An oral, live-attenuated vaccine is administered in capsules, with one capsule taken every other day for four doses; a booster series is required every 5 years for those still

*Not available in the United States.

at risk. A parenteral capsular polysaccharide vaccine given in a single dose provides protection for 2 years.

Typhus Vaccine. Typhus vaccine* is no longer recommended and is not available in the United States.

Varicella Vaccine. International travelers who do not have a history of chickenpox or evidence of immunity to varicella-zoster virus should consider receiving this vaccine, especially if close personal contact with local populations is expected.

Immunizations During Pregnancy and Breast-Feeding

Pregnancy is not a contraindication to the administration of toxoid vaccines, killed or inactivated vaccines, or serum immune globulin when clear risk of infection is present. Live measles-mumps-rubella, varicella, and oral typhoid vaccines are contraindicated during pregnancy. Yellow fever vaccine administration is contraindicated during pregnancy unless exposure to yellow fever virus during travel is unavoidable. Breast-feeding does not adversely affect immunizations and is not a contraindication to administering any vaccine. Neither killed nor live vaccines affect the safety of breast-feeding for mothers or infants.

Vaccination in Altered Immunocompetence

Immunocompromised travelers require a closely individualized approach to vaccine protection during travel. Advice varies based on the type and the severity of each underlying cause of immunosuppression.† Some individuals may simply not mount a protective immune response to certain vaccines, whereas others could potentially acquire disseminated disease from such vaccine administration. In general, killed or inactivated vaccines and immune serum globulin are not contraindicated for immunocompromised travelers. Measles vaccine is recommended for some immunosuppressed travelers; however, some persons infected with HIV who had very suppressed immune systems developed measles pneumonitis after administration of measles vaccine. Oral polio vaccine has been phased out of use and certainly should not be given to either any immunocompromised persons or household or other close contacts. Except in extremely unusual situations of high infection risk, yellow fever vaccine is contraindicated in immunosuppressed travelers.

TRAVELER'S DIARRHEA

Traveler's diarrhea affects up to half the travelers from industrialized countries who visit the developing world. Fever, abdominal cramping, or vomiting may also occur along with diarrhea. Traveler's diarrhea is usually contracted by eating food containing bacterial pathogens, drinking contaminated water, or coming into contact with infected persons. The syndrome can be caused by bacteria, viruses, or parasites. The most common cause is infection with enterotoxigenic *Escherichia coli,* which is usually self-limited with resolution of symptoms after several days. Other relatively common causes are *Campylobacter, Shigella,* and *Salmonella* species. Viruses and parasites are less common causes.

Recommended preventive measures include (1) eating only well-cooked hot foods; (2) avoiding vegetable salads, unpeeled fruit, and ice cubes; (3) boiling drinking water for 3 minutes; (4) disinfecting water with iodine tablets or filters that incorporate iodine resin; (5) avoiding dairy products such as soft cheese whose safety is questionable; and (6) avoiding custards, cream pastries, mayonnaise products, and raw or poorly steamed shellfish.

Prophylaxis

Most authorities agree that prophylactic antibiotics should not be routinely recommended because the potential risks of allergic reactions and antibiotic-associated colitis may outweigh the benefit. Bismuth subsalicylate (Pepto-Bismol) in a dosage of two tablets four times a day for periods of less than 3 weeks is a safe and effective way of reducing the occurrence of traveler's diarrhea by approximately 65% in persons at risk. Travelers already using salicylates should not use bismuth subsalicylate prophylaxis.

Treatment

The most important intervention for traveler's diarrhea is the correction of fluid and electrolyte losses. This can be only partially accomplished by drinking tea, broth, or carbonated beverages. Better yet are oral rehydration electrolyte mixtures that are mixed with potable water to prepare a more favorable replacement fluid (e.g., one containing sodium, potassium, bicarbonate, and glucose). For most patients, this is the only treatment necessary because of the usual short duration and self-limitation of diarrhea caused by enterotoxigenic *E. coli.* When bowel movements are frequent and abdominal cramps are troublesome, antisecretory or antimotility agents may be used. Bismuth subsalicylate liquid, taken in a dose of 1 ounce every 30 minutes for a total of eight doses, is effective because of its antisecretory effect. Loperamide (Imodium) is an over-the-counter synthetic opioid with an antimotility effect. It is taken by adults as a 4-mg loading dose, followed by 2 mg orally after each loose bowel movement, to a maximal daily dose of 16 mg. Adding a single dose of a fluoroquinolone (i.e., 500–750 mg of ciprofloxacin [Cipro]) to loperamide may shorten the duration of symptoms to 24 hours. If significant diarrhea persists after these measures are begun or it is accompanied by

*Not available in the United States.

†Detailed discussions of the approach to compromised travelers can be found in Mileno MD, Bia FJ: The compromised traveler. Infect Dis Clin North Am 12:369–412, 1998.

blood and mucus in the stool or high fever, antibiotic treatment is indicated. If medical care is not available and the possibility of this situation has been discussed with a physician before travel, emergency self-treatment is appropriate. The most effective antibiotics that are active drugs against the common bacterial pathogens are the fluoroquinolones. A 3-day course accompanied by adequate hydration may be instituted.

Diarrhea that develops after a traveler's return home is more likely to be caused by a pathogenic intestinal protozoan and should be evaluated for that possibility.

OTHER CONSIDERATIONS AND MEDICAL IMPLICATIONS OF TRAVEL

Pre-travel education can help address the environmental risks of travel. The form of counseling is tailored to the topics that are pertinent to each traveler as well as to his or her level of understanding. Sometimes simple measures can prevent or treat many conditions associated with travel.

Flying. Jet lag, barotrauma, and motion sickness can be problems for international travelers. About 1 day is necessary to readjust the body clock for each time zone change. Sleeping pills such as benzodiazepines or melatonin* may help improve sleep during travel and after arrival. Chewing or swallowing during ascent and descent or feeding young children at these times can help prevent barotrauma.

Motion sickness can be prevented with diphenhydramine (Benadryl), meclizine (Antivert), or a scopolamine transdermal disk (Transderm Scōpe). Keeping eyes fixed on still, distant objects and increasing air flow around the face while seated in the center of the vehicle can help. Prolonged sitting in airliners can lead to venous stasis and the potential for pulmonary emboli. It is best to move around the cabin during flight, avoid dehydration, and minimize alcohol consumption to prevent stasis.

Respiration. Individuals with cardiopulmonary conditions or a baseline PaO_2 of less than 70 mm Hg may benefit from supplemental oxygen during high-altitude commercial flights, because atmospheric pressure in the cabin results in a PaO_2 of approximately 65 mm Hg in healthy individuals. Also, aside from heavy air pollution as a risk of travel to many places, there may be a tuberculosis risk, which may necessitate tuberculosis skin testing before and after travel for some individuals going abroad.

Acclimatization. Gradual ascent is the cornerstone for prevention of altitude sickness. Current recommendations are to avoid abrupt ascents to altitudes higher than 3000 m (10,000 ft) and to spend two or three nights at 2500 to 3000 m before further ascent. Initially, moderate activity and avoidance of alcoholic beverages, tobacco, and excessive food are helpful in acclimatizing to high altitude. Increased water intake is necessary at high altitudes because of respiratory losses. Acetazolamide (Diamox), at a dose of 125 mg twice a day taken 24 hours before ascent and continued for the first few days at the higher altitude, can prevent altitude illness.

Sun and Heat Disorders. Protection against strong ultraviolet light can be accomplished by applying a broad-spectrum sunscreen to exposed skin to protect against both ultraviolet A and ultraviolet B sunlight. Sunscreens with a sun protection factor (SPF) of 30 offer an optimal period of protection. Parsol-containing products work best against ultraviolet A light. Heatstroke and sunstroke can be avoided by limiting prolonged exposure to the sun, avoiding overly strenuous exercise, drinking extra fluids, and adding salt to food. Rapid cooling is the mainstay of treatment.

Fresh Water and Seawater-Related Illness. Swimming precautions should be defined, such as avoidance of swimming or wading in fresh, nonchlorinated water to prevent schistosomiasis in endemic regions, especially if the water is stagnant or slow flowing. Eating predatory shellfish may cause ciguatera poisoning regardless of adequate cooking. Scuba divers should be certified and should follow established guidelines for flying after diving.

POST-TRAVEL CARE

Physicians at a travel clinic should have the capability to recognize, diagnose, and treat unusual infections contracted during travel. Evaluation by a physician is usually unnecessary for persons who remain healthy during and after short-term travel. Travelers who have undertaken long-term travel, as well as expatriate residents from the developing world, should receive medical evaluation even if they are asymptomatic. This testing should include a physical examination, complete blood cell count, blood chemistry profile, tuberculin skin test, and stool examinations for ova and parasites. If exposure has occurred, serologic testing can be performed for such infections as HIV and schistosomiasis. Both travelers and physicians must always consider previous travel in the evaluation of symptoms that appear months or, rarely, years after return home. Significant symptoms include fever, chills, sweats, fatigue, or persistent diarrhea. Other diagnoses, diagnostic methods, and treatment for symptomatic returnees are fully described in textbooks on travel and tropical medicine.

TOXOPLASMOSIS

method of
CARLOS SUBAUSTE, M.D.
University of Cincinnati College of Medicine
Cincinnati, Ohio

Toxoplasma gondii is a protozoan of worldwide distribution that commonly infects mammals and birds. Infection

*Not FDA approved for this indication.

is characterized by two stages: *acute* (recently acquired) and *chronic* (latent). Depending on the geographic locale, it is estimated that between 3% and 67% of the adult population in the United States is chronically infected with the parasite. *T. gondii* infection in human beings is usually asymptomatic. However, disease (toxoplasmosis) occurs in some cases, especially in the immunodeficient patient and fetus.

T. gondii exists in three forms: tachyzoite, tissue cyst (containing bradyzoites), and oocyst (containing sporozoites). The oocyst form of the parasite is produced during the sexual cycle, which only occurs in the intestine of felines (the definitive host). Oocysts are shed in the feces of infected felines. In contrast, tachyzoites and tissue cysts occur in all intermediate hosts (including people) and felines. People become infected with *T. gondii* mainly by ingesting poorly cooked or raw meat (pork, lamb) containing tissue cysts or consuming vegetables or other food products contaminated with oocysts. After ingesting tissue cysts or oocysts, bradyzoites or sporozoites, respectively, are released into the intestinal lumen and infect surrounding cells where they become tachyzoites. Cells containing intracellular tachyzoites circulate in the blood and lymphatic system, causing dissemination of the infection. Development of cell-mediated immunity is associated with disappearance of tachyzoites and formation of tissue cysts. Any organ can contain tissue cysts, but this form of the parasite is more readily detected in the central nervous system (CNS) and myocardial, skeletal, and smooth muscle. Chronically infected individuals appear to carry tissue cysts for life.

Cell-mediated immunity is necessary for keeping infection quiescent. Thus, chronically infected patients who become immunocompromised (e.g., through AIDS, Hodgkin's disease, or administration of immunosuppressive agents) are at risk for reactivation of their infection. Toxoplasmosis in this setting usually manifests as toxoplasmic encephalitis. However, these patients may also present with extracerebral toxoplasmosis (usually ocular and/or pulmonary disease) with or without encephalitis.

Fetuses can acquire *T. gondii* infection through the transplacental route. Congenital toxoplasmosis can occur when pregnant women become acutely infected with *T. gondii* or when chronic infection is reactivated due to underlying disorders that cause immunosuppression. The incidence of congenital toxoplasmosis in the United States ranges from 1 in 1000 to 1 in 8000 live births.

DIAGNOSIS

The diagnosis of *T. gondii* infection is made with serologic studies. The most commonly used serologic tests are those that detect anti–*T. gondii* IgG and IgM antibodies. IgG antibodies can be detected with the Sabin-Feldman dye test (considered the gold standard), indirect fluorescent antibody (IFA), agglutination, or enzyme-linked immunosorbent assay (ELISA) tests. Although IgG titers peak within 1 to 2 months after infection, measurable levels of these antibodies persist for life. Tests that detect anti–*T. gondii* IgM antibodies (double-sandwich ELISA, IFA, immunosorbent assay) are frequently used for the diagnosis of acute infection. The usefulness of these tests comes from the fact that absence of anti–*T. gondii* IgM virtually excludes a recent infection in immunocompetent patients. Although IgM antibodies usually disappear a few weeks or months after infection, they can remain elevated for more than 1 year. Thus, the presence of anti–*T. gondii* IgM antibodies does not necessarily indicate that the infection was acquired recently. This issue is of utmost importance in the evaluation of pregnant women because congenital toxoplasmosis in immunocompetent women occurs almost exclusively when infection is acquired during gestation (recently acquired).

The pitfalls in the interpretation of serologic tests indicate that an accurate diagnosis of acute *T. gondii* infection often requires performing a panel of additional tests in a reference laboratory. Recent *T. gondii* infection is likely when serial specimens obtained at least 3 weeks apart and tested in parallel show an increase in IgG titers (at least fourfold), and/or by the presence of elevated IgM, IgA, or IgE titers in conjunction with an acute profile in the differential agglutination test.

The presence of anti–*T. gondii* IgG antibodies in an HIV-infected patient indicates that this individual is at risk for developing toxoplasmosis. Therefore, all HIV-positive patients should undergo serologic testing for *T. gondii* infection. Between 97% and 100% of AIDS patients with toxoplasmic encephalitis have anti–*T. gondii* IgG antibodies in their serum. Hence, the absence of antibodies against the parasite strongly argues against a diagnosis of toxoplasmic encephalitis.

In the United States, the vast majority of patients with AIDS-associated toxoplasmosis lack detectable anti–*T. gondii* IgM antibodies because this illness represents reactivation of a chronic infection. Results of *T. gondii* serologic studies should be interpreted with caution in transplant recipients who are chronically infected with *T. gondii*. Rising titers of IgG and IgM antibodies may be observed in these patients in the absence of clinical evidence of toxoplasmosis.

Definitive diagnosis of toxoplasmosis in immunodeficient patients ultimately relies on histologic studies. A brain biopsy that reveals the presence of tachyzoites and tissue cysts in areas of inflammation is diagnostic of toxoplasmic encephalitis. In addition, tachyzoites may be identified in cytocentrifuge preparations of cerebrospinal fluid (CSF) and bronchoalveolar lavage. Isolation of the parasite from tissue biopsy specimens or body fluids (CSF, blood, bronchoalveolar lavage fluid) is also diagnostic of toxoplasmosis. Isolation studies may not be helpful for a rapid diagnosis of toxoplasmosis because it may take up to 6 weeks to obtain results. Polymerase chain reaction (PCR)-based detection of *T. gondii* DNA from appropriate sites has been used to diagnosis toxoplasmosis in HIV-infected patients. However, a positive PCR result can occur in blood samples from patients unlikely to have toxoplasmic encephalitis.

TREATMENT

The need for and duration of therapy depend on the clinical manifestations of toxoplasmosis, immune status of the patient, and pregnancy status of the patient. With few exceptions, therapy for toxoplasmosis requires a combination of chemotherapeutic agents. Currently available anti–*T. gondii* regimens are not active against the tissue cyst form. Pyrimethamine (Daraprim) is considered the cornerstone in the treatment of toxoplasmosis. The combination of pyrimethamine (a dihydrofolate reductase inhibitor) plus sulfadiazine (a dihydrofolate synthase inhibitor) has been the regimen of choice. This regimen produces sequential blocks in the pathway of folic acid synthesis, resulting in synergistic activity against tachyzoites. Sulfonamides other than sulfadiazine and trisulfapyrimidines* are less effective against *T. gondii*.

Because pyrimethamine is a folate antagonist, the most common side effect is dose-related bone marrow suppression. Mammalian cells can be preferentially rescued by administration of folinic acid (also called *leucovorin*). Thus, patients receiving pyrimethamine should be placed on a daily oral dose of 10 to 20 mg of folinic acid and have complete blood cell and platelet counts measured twice weekly. Higher doses may be necessary in patients with persistent bone marrow suppression. Folic acid should not be used because it may impair the anti–*T. gondii* activity of pyrimethamine.

The intolerance to sulfonamides seen especially in AIDS patients has underscored the need for alternative regimens against toxoplasmosis. The combination of pyrimethamine plus clindamycin (Cleocin)† has proven effective in AIDS patients with toxoplasmic encephalitis. Other drugs with activity against *T. gondii* are discussed later.

Acute Infection in Immunocompetent Patients

Symptoms develop in only 10% to 20% of immunocompetent individuals who become infected with *T. gondii*. Toxoplasmosis in these patients usually manifests as lymphadenopathy with or without constitutional symptoms. The diagnosis is confirmed by serologic evidence of recent *T. gondii* infection. Toxoplasmic lymphadenopathy is a self-limited disease. Therefore, patients with this form of toxoplasmosis require antimicrobial therapy only if symptoms are severe and persistent. Pyrimethamine plus sulfadiazine is considered the regimen of choice. A loading dose of 200 mg of pyrimethamine is administered orally in two divided doses on the first day. This is followed by 25 to 50 mg per day orally. Sulfadiazine is administered as a loading dose of 75 mg/kg (up to 4 g) orally followed by a daily dose of 100 mg/kg (up to 6 g) divided in two to four doses. Treatment is usually continued for 2 to 4 weeks followed by reassessment of the patient's condition. Infections acquired from transfused blood or through a laboratory accident may be severe and therefore should be treated.

Ocular Toxoplasmosis in Immunocompetent Patients

Approximately 35% of cases of chorioretinitis in the United States are caused by *T. gondii* infection. Most cases of toxoplasmic chorioretinitis represent reactivation of congenital infection rather than acute infection. Ocular toxoplasmosis usually becomes clinically evident during the second and third decades of life. The presence of characteristic retinal lesions in a patient with serologic evidence of *T. gondii* infection (usually chronic) is considered diagnostic. Identification of *T. gondii* DNA in vitreous fluid with PCR is a useful diagnostic tool in atypical cases. Patients with toxoplasmic chorioretinitis may be treated with pyrimethamine plus sulfadiazine for 4 weeks. Clindamycin* (300 mg every 6 hours), either alone or in combination with pyrimethamine or sulfadiazine, has also been effective. It appears that atovaquone (Mepron) (750 mg four times a day for 3 months) is an effective alternative for treatment of ocular toxoplasmosis. Systemic corticosteroids are added to the regimen when chorioretinitis involves the macula, optic nerve head, or papillomacular bundle. Despite treatment, relapse occurs in 13% to 30% of patients. Relapse requires reinstitution of therapy.

*Not available in the United States.
†Not FDA approved for this indication.

Acute Infection in Pregnant Women

Acute *T. gondii* infection in pregnant women is usually asymptomatic. The importance of *T. gondii* infection in this population is that it can lead to congenital toxoplasmosis. In immunocompetent pregnant women, transplacental transmission to the fetus occurs almost exclusively when infection is acquired during gestation. Maternal infection acquired 6 to 8 weeks before conception can very rarely lead to fetal infection. If the acute infection in the mother goes untreated, congenital infection occurs in approximately 15% of fetuses when the maternal infection is acquired during the first trimester, 30% when acquired in the second trimester, and 60% when acquired in the third trimester. The earlier in pregnancy that transmission to the fetus occurs, the more severe the outcome.

A positive anti–*T. gondii* IgM does not necessarily indicate a recently acquired infection. Therefore, the first step to take when a pregnant woman's IgM results in a commercial laboratory are positive is to request confirmatory testing in a reference laboratory (see earlier). If additional serologic tests indicate that *T. gondii* infection was acquired recently, the patient should be started on spiramycin.† Spiramycin (available through the Food and Drug Administration) at a dose of 1 g orally three times a day appears to reduce the incidence of fetal infection by about 60%.

The next step is to determine whether fetal infection has occurred (prenatal diagnosis). Currently, PCR-based assays for the detection of *T. gondii* DNA in amniotic fluid are considered by many authorities to be the gold standard. Another method of prenatal diagnosis is based on detection of parasite-specific IgM, IgA, and IgE antibodies in fetal serum obtained by percutaneous umbilical cord sampling. However, serologic studies must be interpreted with caution because of the possibility of contamination with maternal blood. Fetal ultrasonography should be performed periodically to determine if intracranial calcifications or hydrocephalus have developed.

If prenatal diagnosis reveals that the fetus is in-

*Not FDA approved for this indication.
†Investigational drug in the United States.

fected, a regimen effective for the treatment of congenital toxoplasmosis should be started. Spiramycin does not cross the placenta. Thus, this drug is unlikely to optimally control infection in the fetus. Treatment of the infected fetus is achieved by administering pyrimethamine-sulfadiazine-folinic acid to the pregnant woman during the second and third trimester. Because of potential teratogenicity, pyrimethamine should not be administered in the first 16 weeks of pregnancy. If there is no evidence of fetal infection, spiramycin should be continued until delivery.

Congenital Toxoplasmosis

The clinical consequences of congenital *T. gondii* infection are varied. Spontaneous abortion may occur. The baby may be born with no apparent sequelae, or he or she may have problems such as clinically overt neurologic or generalized disease (chorioretinitis, hydrocephalus, intracranial calcifications, hepatosplenomegaly, jaundice, anemia). Although most congenitally infected babies appear normal at birth, this subclinical infection is associated with subsequent chorioretinitis, seizure disorder, and psychomotor and mental retardation. Early treatment reduces the development of these sequelae.

Babies born with serologic evidence of congenital *T. gondii* infection should be treated regardless of whether or not they have symptoms at birth. These patients should receive pyrimethamine (2 mg/kg for 2 days, then 1 mg/kg per day for 2–6 months, followed by 1 mg/kg three times a week) plus sulfadiazine (50 mg/kg twice a day) plus folinic acid (10 mg three times a week) for a total of 12 months. Patients with high protein concentrations in the CSF (1 g/dL or higher), and/or sight-threatening chorioretinitis should receive prednisone (0.5 mg/kg twice a day) until resolution of these abnormalities. Response to therapy should be monitored with repeated serologic, neuroradiologic, and ophthalmologic evaluations and CSF analysis if indicated.

Toxoplasmosis in Immunocompromised Patients

T. gondii is a major opportunistic pathogen in HIV-infected patients. The most common presentation of toxoplasmosis in these patients is necrotizing encephalitis. In the United States, between 8% and 16% of HIV-infected individuals have antibodies against *T. gondii*. If primary prophylaxis against toxoplasmosis is not administered, toxoplasmic encephalitis will develop in 20% to 47% of dually infected patients. The vast majority of AIDS patients with toxoplasmic encephalitis have $CD4^+$ T cell counts less than 100/mm^3. Patients with toxoplasmic encephalitis usually present with focal neurologic abnormalities of subacute onset, frequently accompanied by nonfocal signs and symptoms (e.g., headache, altered mental status, or fever). Motor weakness is the most common focal neurologic sign. Patients may also present with cranial nerve palsies, speech disturbances, visual field defects, sensory disturbances, cerebellar signs, focal seizures, and movement disorders.

Lymphoma of the CNS is the most common differential diagnosis of toxoplasmic encephalitis in AIDS patients. Neuroradiologic studies represent the cornerstone in the diagnosis of toxoplasmic encephalitis and are usually helpful to distinguish this illness from CNS lymphoma. Magnetic resonance imaging (MRI) and computed tomography (CT) scans of patients with toxoplasmic encephalitis typically reveal multiple enhancing cerebral lesions. Basal ganglia and the hemispheric corticomedullary junction are the areas most commonly involved. Whether brain lesions are multiple or single has important implications in the diagnosis. The presence of a single lesion raises the possibility of a diagnosis other than toxoplasmic encephalitis (CNS lymphoma). MRI is more sensitive than CT for the detection of brain lesions, especially in patients who lack focal neurologic symptoms. Therefore, if at all possible, MRI should be performed in patients suspected to have toxoplasmic encephalitis. If a CT scan reveals a single brain lesion, MRI should be performed to determine if other lesions are present. Although patients with toxoplasmic encephalitis can have a single brain lesion on an MRI, this presentation is highly suggestive of CNS lymphoma.

Newer neuroradiologic tests appear to be useful in the differential diagnosis between tumor (CNS lymphoma) and infection in AIDS patients. Positron-emission tomography (PET) reveals areas of decreased glucose metabolism in brains of patients with toxoplasmic encephalitis, whereas areas of increased glucose metabolism are observed in patients with CNS lymphoma. Thallium 201 (^{201}Tl) brain single photon emission computed tomography (SPECT) is another radiologic study that is highly sensitive and specific for the diagnosis of tumors and thus helpful in differentiating CNS lymphoma from toxoplasmic encephalitis. Foci of increased ^{201}Tl uptake are seen in patients with CNS lymphoma but not in those with toxoplasmic encephalitis. PET and brain SPECT should be considered in the evaluation of patients with single brain lesions on MRI.

A definitive diagnosis of toxoplasmic encephalitis is based on identification of the parasite in the brain with histopathologic studies. However, in an effort to avoid brain biopsies, it has become standard practice to initiate empiric anti–*T. gondii* therapy on patients with probable toxoplasmic encephalitis. Although MRI and CT scan findings are not pathognomonic of toxoplasmic encephalitis, the presence of multiple brain lesions in AIDS patients who are seropositive for anti–*T. gondii* antibodies allows for a presumptive diagnosis of toxoplasmic encephalitis. Brain biopsy should be considered in the following situations: patients who are seronegative for anti–*T. gondii* antibodies; an MRI reveals a single brain lesion (especially if PET or ^{201}Tl brain SPECT are compatible with a tumor); or despite adequate anti–*T. gondii* therapy, there is no clinical improvement by 10 to 14 days or there is deterioration by day 3.

Toxoplasmosis in AIDS patients can also present as chorioretinitis and pneumonitis. These forms of toxoplasmosis may or may not be associated with toxoplasmic encephalitis. Pulmonary toxoplasmosis usually manifests as a prolonged fever, cough, dyspnea, and radiologic findings that mimic *Pneumocystis carinii* pneumonia.

Treatment of toxoplasmosis in AIDS patients has two phases: acute stage therapy and maintenance treatment. Acute therapy should be administered for at least 3 weeks; 6 weeks is recommended in patients with severe illness or when significant clinical and/or neuroradiologic response has not been achieved. Maintenance therapy should be continued for life to avoid relapse.

Pyrimethamine plus sulfadiazine has been the standard regimen for treatment of toxoplasmic encephalitis (Table 1). Between 65% and 90% of patients will exhibit an initial response to this regimen. Unfortunately, approximately 40% of patients discontinue these drugs because of side effects. The need for alternative therapy for toxoplasmic encephalitis prompted the evaluation of pyrimethamine plus clindamycin.* This antibiotic combination is as effective as pyrimethamine plus sulfadiazine during the acute phase of therapy of toxoplasmic encephalitis.

Neurologic improvement usually occurs within the first week of therapy. Most patients will also experience radiologic improvement by the third week of treatment. Therefore, neuroradiologic study should be repeated 2 to 4 weeks after initiation of therapy. These studies should be repeated earlier in patients who fail to show clinical evidence of improvement.

*Not FDA approved for this indication.

TABLE 1. **Guidelines for Acute or Primary Treatment of AIDS Patients With Toxoplasmic Encephalitis**

Drug	Dosage
Recommended Regimens	
Pyrimethamine (Daraprim)	200 mg loading followed by 50–75 mg q24h PO
Folinic acid	10–20 mg q24h PO, IV, or IM
plus	
Sulfadiazine	1–1.5 g q6h PO
or	
Clindamycin (Cleocin)*	600–1200 mg q6h IV or PO
Alternative Regimens	
Trimethoprim-sulfamethoxazole (Bactrim, Septra)	5 mg (trimethoprim component)/kg q6h PO or IV
Pyrimethamine and folinic acid *plus one of the following:*	As in recommended regimen
Clarithromycin (Biaxin)*	1 g q12h PO
Atovaquone (Mepron)*	750 mg q6h PO
Azithromcyin (Zithromax)*	1200–1500 mg q24h PO
Dapsone	100 mg q24h PO

*Not FDA approved for this indication.

Modified from Subauste CS, Remington JS: AIDS-associated toxoplasmosis. In Sande MA, Volberding P (eds): The Medical Management of AIDS, 6th ed. Philadelphia, WB Saunders, 1999, pp 379–398.

The mortality rate among patients with toxoplasmic encephalitis treated with an appropriate antimicrobial regimen ranges between 1% and 25%.

Few studies suggest that trimethoprim* and sulfamethoxazole (TMP-SMZ) (Bactrim, Septra) may be effective for acute therapy of toxoplasmic encephalitis. However, this antibiotic combination exhibits less in vitro and in vivo anti–*T. gondii* activity than pyrimethamine plus sulfadiazine. Therefore, TMP*-SMZ is currently not recommended as first-line drug for acute therapy of toxoplasmic encephalitis.

Poor tolerance of anti–*T. gondii* regimens is a significant problem in AIDS patients. Rash is a common adverse reaction to pyrimethamine plus sulfadiazine. It appears that patients with non–life-threatening dermatologic reactions may be treated with continuation of sulfadiazine and administration of antihistamines. Rash and diarrhea are frequent side effects to pyrimethamine plus clindamycin,* whereas bone marrow suppression can occur with any combination that contains pyrimethamine. Some investigators propose sulfonamide desensitization in patients who cannot tolerate both sulfadiazine and clindamycin.*

Effective antimicrobial regimens are needed for patients intolerant to pyrimethamine plus sulfadiazine and pyrimethamine plus clindamycin.* A number of agents have been shown to exhibit anti–*T. gondii* activity in vitro and in animal models of toxoplasmosis, as well as to be effective in few case reports. However, additional studies are required before these investigational agents can be recommended routinely as therapy for toxoplasmosis. If these agents are to be used for treatment of toxoplasmic encephalitis, they should be administered in combination with pyrimethamine (see Table 1).

Azithromycin (Zithromax)* and clarithromycin (Biaxin)* are effective either in vitro or in a murine model of toxoplasmosis. A small study of AIDS patients with toxoplasmic encephalitis reported that clarithromycin* plus pyrimethamine resulted in clinical and radiologic response rates of 80% and 50%, respectively. Another pilot study of pyrimethamine plus azithromycin* reported an overall response rate of 65%.

Atovaquone exhibits in vitro and in vivo activity against both the tachyzoite and the tissue cyst forms of *T. gondii*. A small study indicated that 66% of patients with toxoplasmic encephalitis treated with atovaquone alone had a favorable clinical response during the acute phase of therapy. In addition, atovaquone may be effective in patients intolerant to pyrimethamine plus either sulfadiazine or clindamycin.* Unfortunately 50% of patients treated with atovaquone alone relapse during the maintenance phase of therapy.

Corticosteroids can be administered to patients with toxoplasmic encephalitis with cerebral edema and intracranial hypertension. However, the duration of corticosteroid administration should be as short as possible (preferably no more than 2 weeks).

*Not FDA approved for this indication.

Steroid therapy may make it difficult to ascertain if improvement in the patient's condition is secondary to control of the infection by antimicrobial agents. Anticonvulsants should not be administered prophylactically; rather they should be used only if seizures occur.

Although the data are limited, it appears that AIDS patients with extracerebral toxoplasmosis respond to therapy with pyrimethamine plus sulfadiazine or pyrimethamine plus clindamycin.* The mortality rate in patients with pulmonary or disseminated toxoplasmosis may be higher than in patients with toxoplasmic encephalitis alone.

Neither pyrimethamine plus sulfadiazine nor pyrimethamine plus clindamycin* eradicate tissue cysts of *T. gondii*. Persistence of the cyst form of the parasite may explain the high relapse rate seen in AIDS patients who discontinue therapy. In the era before HAART (highly active anti-retrovial therapy) the relapse rate of toxoplasmic encephalitis in patients who did not receive maintenance therapy was 50% to 80% at 12 months. Thus, AIDS patients with toxoplasmic encephalitis who complete a primary course of therapy and who have had a favorable response to therapy should receive anti–*T. gondii* agents for life. Usually, the same drugs used for acute therapy are continued but at lower doses. Additional study is needed to see if it is safe to discontinue maintenance therapy in patients who responded to HAART.

The combination of pyrimethamine plus sulfadiazine appears to be the most effective regimen for prevention of relapse of toxoplasmic encephalitis. It is not clear how pyrimethamine plus clindamycin* compares to pyrimethamine plus sulfadiazine during maintenance therapy. Although one study reported a higher rate of relapse in patients treated with pyrimethamine plus clindamycin,* these patients received a low dose of clindamycin (1.2 g/day). Pyrimethamine plus sulfadiazine but not pyrimethamine plus clindamycin* prevent *P. carinii* pneumonia.

Pyrimethamine-sulfadoxine* (Fansidar) has been reported to be effective as maintenance therapy. Alternatives for patients who do not tolerate conventional regimens include pyrimethamine alone, or pyrimethamine plus either dapsone, atovaquone, clarithromycin* or azithromycin* (Table 2). Approximately 33% of patients on maintenance therapy will experience a relapse of toxoplasmic encephalitis, which is usually due to poor compliance.

Toxoplasmosis can also occur in immunocompromised individuals who are not infected with HIV. Toxoplasmosis has been associated with cancer (usually Hodgkin's disease and other hematologic malignancies), organ transplantation, and administration of immunosuppressive agents. Toxoplasmosis in this setting may be secondary to reactivation of a chronic infection (patients with cancer, recipients of a bone marrow transplant, patients treated with immunosuppressive agents), or represent a newly acquired infection (seronegative patients who receive a solid organ from a seropositive donor). Although encephalitis is the most common presentation of toxoplasmosis in these patients, myocarditis, pneumonia, and chorioretinitis may also occur. Toxoplasmosis in non-AIDS immunodeficient patients is treated with pyrimethamine plus sulfadiazine until 4 to 6 weeks after clinical evidence of toxoplasmosis resolves (usually for at least 6 months). Immunodeficient patients with serologic evidence of an acute *T. gondii* infection should be treated with pyrimethamine plus sulfadiazine for 6 weeks. Chronic asymptomatic infection does not require treatment.

*Not FDA approved for this indication.

TABLE 2. **Guidelines for Maintenance Treatment of AIDS Patients With Toxoplasmic Encephalitis**

Drug	Dosage (PO)
Recommended Regimens	
Pyrimethamine* *and*	25–50 mg q24h
sulfadiazine	500–1000 mg q6h
Pyrimethamine *and*	25–50 mg q24h
clindamycin†	600 mg q6h
Pyrimethamine/sulfadoxine† (Fansidar)	25 mg/500 mg (1 tablet) tiw
Alternative Regimens	
Pyrimethamine alone	50 mg q24h
Pyrimethamine *plus one of the following:*	25–50 mg q24h
Dapsone	100 mg biw
Atovaquone	750 mg q6h
Clarithromycin†	1000 mg q12h
Azithromycin†	1200–1500 mg q24h

*Folinic acid 10–20 mg q24h is recommended for all patients receiving pyrimethamine to help ameliorate the hematologic side effects associated with pyrimethamine.

†Not FDA approved for this indication.

Modified from Subauste CS, Remington JS: AIDS-associated toxoplasmosis. In Sande MA, Volberding P (eds): The Medical Management of AIDS, 6th ed. Philadelphia, WB Saunders, 1999, pp 379–398.

PREVENTION (PRIMARY PROPHYLAXIS)

All patients who are seronegative for *T. gondii* antibodies and who have evidence of deficient cellular immunity or are pregnant should be educated about appropriate precautions to take to prevent acquisition of *T. gondii* infection. These patients should be instructed to eat meat only if it is well cooked, and to wash their hands after touching undercooked meat. Fruits and vegetables should be washed prior to consumption. In addition, patients should avoid contact with materials that may be contaminated with cat feces (avoid the litterbox, wear gloves during gardening). If possible, seronegative recipients should receive transplanted organs from seronegative donors. If this is not feasible, patients who receive organs from seropositive donors should be treated with pyrimethamine 25 mg daily for 6 weeks.

Despite the availability of effective antimicrobial regimens, AIDS patients in whom toxoplasmic encephalitis develops have a mortality rate of 70% at 12 months. This poor prognosis provides an argu-

TABLE 3. **Regimens Used for Primary Prophylaxis Against Toxoplasmosis**

Drug	Dosage (PO)
Trimethoprim/sulfamethoxazole	1 DS* tab qd 2 DS tab tiw
Pyrimethamine-dapsone†	Pyrimethamine 50 mg qw; dapsone 50 mg qd Pyrimethamine 50 mg biw; dapsone 100 mg biw Pyrimethamine 75 mg qw; dapsone 200 mg qw
Pyrimethamine/sulfadoxine†‡§ (Fansidar)	3 tab every 2 weeks 1 tab biw

*DS, double strength.

†Folinic acid 25 mg qw is recommended for all patients receiving pyrimethamine to help ameliorate the hematologic side effects associated with pyrimethamine.

‡Each tablet contains pyrimethamine 25 mg, sulfadoxine 500 mg.

§Not FDA approved for this indication.

Modified from Subauste CS, Remington JS: AIDS-associated toxoplasmosis. In Sande MA, Volberding P (eds): The Medical Management of AIDS, 6th ed. Philadelphia,WB Saunders, 1999, pp 379–398.

ment for primary prophylaxis against toxoplasmic encephalitis. Primary prophylaxis is recommended in *T. gondii* seropositive patients with CD4$^+$ T cell counts less than 100/mm^3 regardless of clinical status, and in patients with CD4$^+$ T cell counts less than 200/mm^3 if an AIDS-defining opportunistic infection or malignancy develops.

Numerous studies have reported the efficacy of TMP-SMZ, pyrimethamine-dapsone, and pyrimethamine-sulfadoxine* in the prevention of toxoplasmic encephalitis in AIDS patients (Table 3). TMP (160 mg)-SMZ (800 mg) once a day is the regimen most commonly used because of its efficacy for the prevention of *P. carinii* pneumonia. Discontinuation of primary prophylaxis is associated with a low risk of toxoplasmic encephalitis in patients on HAART whose CD4$^+$ T cell count increased to greater than or equal to 200/mm^3 for at least 3 months.

At present, it is not known if administration of antimicrobial agents to HIV-infected pregnant women who are chronically infected with *T. gondii* would prevent parasite transmission to the fetus. The current recommendation is that these women receive spiramycin† (1 g three times a day) during the first trimester if their CD4$^+$ T cell counts are less than 200/mm^3. Pyrimethamine plus sulfadiazine or TMP-SMZ may be considered after the 17th week of gestation.

Routine serologic screening of pregnant women has been recommended in an effort to prevent congenital toxoplasmosis. Serologic studies for *T. gondii* should be evaluated no later than the 10th or 12th week of gestation. Patients who have seronegative results should undergo retesting at the 20th to 22nd week and then again near term.

*Not FDA approved for this indication.

†Investigational drug in the United States.

CAT-SCRATCH DISEASE AND BACILLARY ANGIOMATOSIS*

method of
LT. COL. MATTHEW J. DOLAN, M.D.
Wilford Hall USAF Medical Center
Lackland AFB, Texas

Cat-scratch disease is most commonly identified with a lymphadenitis associated with close contact or a scratch from a cat. Debré first described this syndrome in 1950, but the search for the etiology did not reach a conclusion until the 1990s, when *Bartonella henselae* was shown to be the causative microbe. Work during the 1990s further demonstrated that *B. henselae* and *Bartonella quintana* could cause bacillary angiomatosis. Contemporary research is showing an expanding spectrum of disease due to these and other *Bartonella* species and is revealing an elaborate zoonotic epidemiology involving human beings, domestic and wild animals, and ectoparasites.

EPIDEMIOLOGY

Although early epidemiologic work in pediatric practices emphasized cat-scratch disease as primarily a disease of children, later work by the Centers for Disease Control and Prevention showed that roughly half of the cases occur in adults and that there is an increased rate of cases in the fall and winter months. The rate of infection in domestic cats (in some cases reaching 30%–50%) has been shown to correspond to cat flea density in the United States. Cats younger than 1 year tend to have higher rates of bacteremia and have been identified epidemiologically as risk factors for human infection. Although cat fleas are competent vectors for transmission of *B. henselae* infections among cats, their role in transmission from cats to human beings is not clear. The proportion of cases that are transmitted directly from cats to people by minor trauma or secretions versus the proportion vectored by cat fleas is unknown. The question remains an important one for prevention because flea control will obviously not prevent direct transmission from cats to human beings.

Contact with cats and cat fleas likewise is a risk factor for bacillary angiomatosis caused by *B. henselae.* When *B. quintana* is the cause of bacillary angiomatosis, however, head or body lice, homelessness, and low socioeconomic status were more likely risk factors than contact with cats and cat fleas.

CLINICAL MANIFESTATIONS

Patients with cat-scratch disease typically present with tender lymphadenitis, often following a flulike illness. The nodes progressively enlarge over days to weeks, in some cases becoming quite bulky, even up to several centimeters in diameter. They are typically very tender, and the overlying skin may become warm and erythematous. A minority of nodes progress to frank fluctuance. When a surgical biopsy is performed, such as in the case of massive adenopathy to rule out lymphoma, the involved node or node cluster is intensely inflamed, matted, and adherent. The pattern of involved nodes is usually a single site or region

*The views expressed herein are those of the authors and do not reflect the official policy of the Department of Defense or other departments of the U.S. government. All material in this chapter is in the public domain, with the exception of any borrowed figures or tables.

(i.e., ipsilateral epitrochlear and axillary sites). An inoculation papule or eschar can be found with a careful physical examination on the involved extremity in about half of the cases. Patients rarely mention the inoculation papule to the examining physician.

An increasing number of reports describe ocular involvement with *B. henselae.* Unilateral conjunctivitis, often with a conjunctival granuloma and tender ipsilateral preauricular lymph node, constitute Parinaud oculoglandular syndrome, a long-appreciated manifestation of cat-scratch disease. Confusion can occur with adenovirus infection, which can also cause conjunctivitis and preauricular adenopathy. Neuroretinitis often presents as a unilateral severe decrease in visual acuity sometimes occurring after a flulike illness. Patients are usually afebrile at presentation. Examination early on shows optic disk edema, followed in a few days by the appearance of a macular star. Chorioretinitis and uveitis have also been described. Significant vision loss has occurred from branch retinal artery and vein occlusion.

Neurologic syndromes due to *B. henselae* infection include aseptic meningitis, encephalitis, and postpartum coma. Convulsions occurred in 46% of children with encephalitis in one study. Complete recovery from untreated encephalitis is the rule, although rare cases with residual sequelae have been noted. Cranial and peripheral nerve involvement have also been described.

Bartonella species are recognized as responsible for an increasing share of fever of unknown origin and culture-negative endocarditis cases. Conversely, patients can have persistent or relapsing bacteremia or endocarditis without fever. Persistent bacteremia should prompt an echocardiographic evaluation for endocarditis. Even in the absence of endocarditis, however, bacteremia may be difficult to eradicate, having a propensity to relapse asymptomatically after therapy in both human beings and felines.

Bacillary angiomatosis typically presents as angiomatous nodular or papular lesions that somewhat resemble the skin lesions of verruga peruana, caused by *Bartonella bacilliformis.* Bacillary angiomatosis is overwhelmingly found in immunocompromised patients, particularly those with HIV infections. The cutaneous lesion can be mistaken for Kaposi sarcoma on physical examination. Clumps of bacteria may be seen in Warthin-Starry silver stained tissue, in contrast to cat-scratch biopsy specimens, in which bacteria are rare to absent.

The liver can be involved in bacillary angiomatosis or in peliosis hepatis, particularly in patients with HIV infection. The illness presents as fever, malaise, and weight loss, with an elevation of serum alkaline phosphatase level. *Mycobacterium avium-intracellulare* infection presents similarly in late-stage HIV infection. Although bacillary angiomatosis of the skin is equally attributable to *B. henselae* and *B. quintana,* disease of the liver and lymph node is usually caused by *B. henselae.* Bone disease is usually a result of *B. quintana* infection. *Bartonella* species can also cause pulmonary nodules.

DIAGNOSIS

Diagnosis of cat-scratch disease is normally made on the basis of typical findings on physical examination and a history of cat or cat flea exposure and is confirmed by serology. The cat-scratch disease skin test is of historical interest only and has no role in contemporary diagnosis. In a patient with cat-scratch disease, the indirect immunofluorescence assay (IFA) had a sensitivity of 88% and a specificity of 94%. Even in culture-proven cases, occasional patients never produce antibody detectable by IFA or enzyme immunoassay. Although the IFA test does not distinguish between *B. henselae* and *B. quintana* infections, that distinction is not necessary for making therapeutic decisions. Enzyme immunoassay tests for the diagnosis of *B. henselae* infection have been marketed but appear to correlate poorly with the clinically validated IFA test. Polymerase chain reaction has been used for diagnosis in research laboratories and will likely be commercially available in the future.

Histopathology for cat-scratch disease shows stellate granulomas, perivascular mixed cellular infiltrates, and multinucleated giant cells. Biopsy is not usually performed to establish a diagnosis of cat-scratch disease but rather to exclude a diagnosis of lymphoma.

Culture of *B. henselae* from lymph nodes is usually not possible with needle aspiration, and it is only occasionally achievable with an excisional biopsy. To culture biopsy material, a heavy inoculum should be applied to a hematin-enriched blood agar plate, which should be incubated at 35°C to 37°C in 5% to 10% CO_2 for 4 to 6 weeks. *Bartonella* may be isolated from ethylenediaminetetraacetic acid (EDTA)-anticoagulated blood using a single freeze-thaw or with a lysis-centrifugation technique. Automated blood culture systems routinely fail to detect growth of *B. henselae,* so weekly acridine orange staining or subculturing of blood is necessary to detect the organism.

TREATMENT AND PREVENTION

Treatment of the previously described diseases is directed by the syndrome, not by the determination of whether the etiologic organism was *B. henselae* or *B. quintana* (Table 1). The impact of therapy ranges from excellent in bacillary angiomatosis and neuroretinitis to minimal in lymphadenitis. In the latter, the inflamed, enlarged nodes typically return to normal in 2 to 6 months. One study showed a significantly more rapid reduction in node size using azithromycin (Zithromax). In contrast, patients with neuroretinitis who are only able to count fingers often have full return of normal visual acuity within days of starting therapy, although there are no controlled studies to address this.

Although the optimal duration of therapy has not been defined, relapses of disease after short course therapy of 1 to 2 weeks are common. The organism resides in erythrocytes and endothelial cells in vivo, and antimicrobial agents with good intracellular penetration are likely needed for successful therapy. Significant infections should be treated for 4 to 6 weeks, similar to therapy for the genetically related organism *Brucella.* Unfortunately, in vitro susceptibility testing in axenic media appears to have little correlation with in vivo therapy results. Intracellular susceptibility testing systems appear to confirm the utility of tetracycline, macrolides, quinolones, and possibly gentamicin. The toxicity of aminoglycosides limits their usefulness for lymphadenitis.

Immunosuppressed people might reduce the risk of infection with *B. henselae* by using good flea control, avoiding rough play with cats, and selecting cats older than 1 year old as pets. Cat-associated wounds should be washed promptly and cats should not be

TABLE 1. **Antimicrobial Therapy for *Bartonella henselae* Infection**

Antibiotic	Dose/Route	Notes
Cat-Scratch Disease		
Clarithromycin (Biaxin)	*Adults:* 500 mg bid for 4–6 wk *Children:* 7.5 mg/kg bid or 4–6 wk	
Doxycycline (Vibramycin, Doryx)	*Adults and children >8 y:* 100 mg bid for 4–6 wk	Do not use tetracyclines in children aged <8 y.
Levofloxacin (Levaquin)*	*Adults and children >8 y:* 500 mg bid for 4–6 wk	
Ciprofloxacin (Cipro)*	*Adults and children >8 y:* 500–750 mg PO bid for 4–6 wk	
Rifampin (Rifadin, Rimactane)	*Adults:* 300 mg PO bid or tid for 4–6 wk *Children:* 10–20 mg/kg PO divided into two to three doses daily for 4–6 wk	Consider in combination with another antibiotic.
Retinitis		
Doxycycline (Vibramycin, Doryx)	*Adults and children >8 y:* 100 mg bid for 4–6 wk	Do not use tetracyclines in children aged <8 y.
or		
Ciprofloxacin (Cipro)*	*Adults and children >8 y:* 500–750 mg PO bid for 4–6 wk	
or		
Levofloxacin (Levaquin)*	*Adults and children >8 y:* 500 mg bid for 4–6 wk	
plus		
Rifampin (Rifadin, Rimactane)	*Adults:* 300 mg PO bid or tid for 4–6 wk *Children:* 10–20 mg/kg PO divided into two to three doses daily for 4–6 wk	
Bacillary Angiomatosis		
Erythromycin (E-Mycin, Erythrocin)	500 mg qid for 2–4 mo	Duration of therapy depends on response.
Doxycycline (Vibramycin, Doryx)	100 mg bid for 2–4 mo	Consider suppressive therapy for patients with HIV infection.
Clarithromycin (Biaxin)	500 mg bid for 2–4 mo	

*Not FDA approved for this indication.

allowed to lick cuts or wounds of HIV-infected people. There is no recommendation to test cats for infection, treat asymptomatic cats, or declaw animals.

There has been excellent clinical experience with macrolides and tetracyclines for bacillary angiomatosis. Long-term suppressive therapy should be considered in patients with HIV infection.

SALMONELLOSIS*

method of
JEREMY SOBEL, M.D. M.P.H., and
DAVID L. SWERDLOW, M.D.
Centers for Disease Control and Prevention
Atlanta, Georgia

Nontyphoidal salmonellosis is the second most common enteric bacterial infection in the United States. About 35,000 culture-confirmed cases are reported each year, and it is estimated that 1.4 million cases occur annually, including 16,400 hospitalizations and 580 deaths. In most cases, nontyphoidal *Salmonella* causes a self-limited febrile gastroenteritis, but in susceptible individuals, life-threatening extraintestinal syndromes may occur. The incidence of culture-confirmed *Salmonella* infections is highest in infancy and peaks at 159.5/100,000 per year in the second month of life. Rates decrease abruptly after infancy and remain relatively constant throughout adult life at about 12/100,000 per year, with a slight increase after age 70.

It is estimated that 95% percent of *Salmonella* infections are food-borne. The natural reservoirs of nontyphoidal *Salmonella* are the intestines of warm-blooded animals and reptiles, and human infection is caused by consuming contaminated foods of animal origin or other foods that have been contaminated by animal fecal material, such as fruits and vegetables, or by direct contact with animals. Direct person-to-person transmission is rare.

Serotyping is an extremely useful tool for understanding the epidemiology of *Salmonella*. About 2500 serotypes of *Salmonella* are known as defined by the presence of surface O and H antigens. Different serotypes may occupy different natural reservoirs, and therefore changes in trends of serotype incidence in humans reflect either changes in the natural reservoir or changes in exposure experienced by humans. For example, *Salmonella* serotype *enteritidis* can colonize the egg-laying hen ovary, whence it can be transmitted vertically to the chicken egg and thence to the human consumer. From the 1970s to the mid-1990s, the proportion of human *S. enteritidis* infections in the United States increased from less than 5% to almost 30%, largely because of the consumption of contaminated eggs. The large increase in the number of eggs infected with *S. enteritidis* may have occurred as a result of consolidation of the egg industry, industrial-scale farming, and vaccination of chickens against competing pathogens, which set the stage for the spread of *S. enteritidis* among flocks. Recently, implementation of control measures along the continuum from egg farm to consumer has dramatically reduced the incidence of this serotype. Recent increases in human infection with *Salmonella marina* and other serotypes associated with reptiles reflect the growing popularity of pet reptiles such as iguanas.

The most common sources of *Salmonella* infection are eggs, poultry, and meat. However, infections from other sources are increasing, including fruits such as melons and cantaloupes, unpasteurized orange juice, and vegetables such as alfalfa sprouts. Outbreaks from milk contaminated after pasteurization and processed breakfast cereal have also occurred recently. These outbreaks can reveal the ways in which animal fecal matter can contaminate assorted classes of foods not of animal origin and underscore the importance of ongoing surveillance and outbreak investigation in the identification of vulnerabilities of the food supply and the development of appropriate control measures.

Multiply resistant strains of *Salmonella typhimurium* and *Salmonella newport* are an increasing proportion of all cases of salmonellosis; approximately 10% of *Salmonella* infections in 1999 were caused by multiply resistant strains. The increasing antimicrobial resistance in *Salmonella* is a consequence of the widespread use of antibiotics in farm animals. Addressing this problem requires promoting the prudent veterinary use of antimicrobial agents and restricting the types of antibiotics used for nontherapeutic purposes to antibiotics not important in human medicine.

CLINICAL FEATURES (SYNDROMES)

Typically, nontyphoidal *Salmonella* produces a self-limiting febrile gastrointestinal illness in which dehydration is the principal clinical concern. In susceptible individuals, however, severe, life-threatening syndromes may arise. Susceptible individuals include infants (in which the overall incidence of *Salmonella* infections is highest), the elderly, and persons with immunosuppressive conditions such as HIV/AIDS, diabetes, chronic liver disease, or sickle cell disease; immunosuppressive chemotherapy or radiotherapy related to cancer or organ transplantation; achlorhydria related to gastric surgical procedures or anti-acid medications; and endovascular abnormalities (Table 1). Several *Salmonella* serotypes appear to be more likely to cause extraintestinal and invasive disease: *Salmonella choleraesuis, Salmonella dublin, Salmonella virchow* and *S. typhimurium*. Some, such as *S. enteritidis*, are particularly likely to cause invasive illness in a compromised host. However, most cases of extraintestinal syndromes of salmonellosis are attributable to host-related susceptibilities, as well as increased pathogenicity of a particular *Salmonella* serotype.

TABLE 1. **Susceptibility and Risk Factors for Severe Gastroenteritis and Extraintestinal Syndromes**

Host Factors
Age
Neonatal
>50 y
Immunosuppressive Conditions
HIV/AIDS
Sickle cell disease
Malignancy
Diabetes mellitus
Lymphoproliferative disease
Organ transplantation
Immunosuppressive Therapy
Steroids
Chemotherapy
Radiotherapy
Transplant-related immunosuppressive medications
Recent antimicrobial treatment
Endovascular Abnormalities
Atheroma
Aneurysm
Prosthesis
Valvular abnormalities
Disruption of Host Intestinal Flora
Recent antimicrobial treatment
Bowel surgery
Decreased Gastric Acidity
Primary achlorhydria
Gastric surgery
Anti-acid medications
Pathogen Factors
Serotypes Associated With Bacteremia and Invasive Disease
Salmonella virchow
Salmonella choleraesuis
Salmonella dublin
Salmonella enteritidis (in immunocompromised patients)

Gastroenteritis

Most nontyphoidal *Salmonella* infections result in a self-limited febrile diarrheal illness that is indistinguishable from that caused by other bacterial enteric pathogens. The incubation period between ingestion of the bacteria and the onset of illness varies from 6 to 72 hours. Symptoms include diarrhea, abdominal cramps, fever, nausea, or vomiting. The diarrhea may be nonbloody, occur several times per day, and not be very voluminous, although in severe cases it may be frequent, bloody and/or mucoid, and of high volume. Clinicians should be aware that patients seeking medical care probably represent those with more severe symptoms than average. Polymorphonuclear leukocytes are typically seen in the stool. Fever generally occurs in the 38°C to 39°C range. Vomiting is less common than diarrhea. Headaches, myalgias, and arthralgias are often reported as well. Whereas the diarrhea typically lasts 24 to 72 hours, patients often report fatigue and other nonspecific symptoms lasting 7 days or longer.

Blood cultures are rarely (5%) positive in immunocompetent individuals with diagnosed *Salmonella* gastroenteritis; the percentage is higher in immunocompromised individuals, in whom the risk is also greater for metastatic spread to sterile sites and consequent life-threatening complications. Rarely, *Salmonella* can produce a pseudoappendicitis syndrome resembling that caused by *Yersinia enterocolitica* and manifesting as an acute abdomen.

Excretion of *Salmonella* in feces decreases precipitously with resolution of the diarrhea, but it may continue for several weeks to months. Excretion is more prolonged in neonates; however, chronic carriage, a rare event, is described only in adults.

Bacteremia and Extraintestinal Syndromes

As noted, bacteremia occurs in 5% of immunocompetent adults with *Salmonella* gastroenteritis and more frequently in the immunocompromised. *Salmonella* endocarditis is a rare event that occurs in 5% of patients with bacteremia and should therefore be suspected in patients with persistent bacteremia and a high proportion (>50%) of positive blood cultures. *Salmonella* appears to have an affinity for endothelial tissue, particularly atherosclerotic plaque and aneurysms, which places older patients at higher risk. The most common source of arterial *Salmonella* infection is the abdominal aorta. Prolonged or recurrent fever after gastroenteritis, especially in patients with a known abdominal aneurysm or with abdominal, chest, or back pain or a history of aortic grafting, should raise suspicion of this high-mortality condition.

Salmonella may cause localized infections in most anatomic regions. The most common intra-abdominal site is the spleen, particularly in patients with sickle cell disease. Soft tissue infections may be associated with hematomas from preceding trauma. *Salmonella* pneumonia is rare and usually caused by hematogenous spread or extension from a splenic abscess. *Salmonella* meningitis occurs in neonates and children, as well as adults, and neonates are at particular risk for severe complications, recurrent infections, and permanent disability. Focal central nervous system infections have been encountered principally in HIV/AIDS patients.

Salmonella osteomyelitis arises from hematogenous spread after gastroenteritis. Sickle cell disease is the most common predisposing co-morbidity, but other immunosuppressive conditions, as well as trauma, are also associated with the condition. Infectious arthritis usually occurs in patients with immunosuppressive conditions and most frequently affects the knee. Reactive arthritis is an autoimmune sequela of enteric bacterial infection that involves inflammation of multiple joints, possibly in combination with uveitis and urethritis. Reactive arthritis is strongly associated with the HLA-B27 antigen and occurs typically about 2 to 3 weeks after gastroenteritis in 1% to 7% of patients. Symptoms generally resolve after several weeks but, in a minority of cases, may persist for months or years and be debilitating.

TREATMENT

The primary objective in treating *Salmonella* gastroenteritis is to prevent dehydration and electrolyte imbalance by replenishing fluids and electrolytes. In mild to moderate cases, this goal is best accomplished with oral rehydration solutions and, in severe cases, by initial intravenous rehydration followed by oral rehydration. Pepto-Bismol is effective in reducing abdominal cramping and the frequency of diarrheal stools. Dairy products, caffeinated or carbonated drinks, and fatty foods tend to worsen abdominal cramps and should be avoided. Antimotility drugs may be used in treating mild diarrhea, but it should be kept in mind that diarrhea is a normal response to invasive colonic bacterial infection. Antimotility drugs should be avoided in the presence of fever and bloody or mucoid stool and not given to elderly patients who are at risk for ileus, toxic megacolon, and perforation.

Stool culture may add relatively little to the clinical management of uncomplicated *Salmonella* gastroenteritis, but clinicians should keep in mind that detection and control of *Salmonella* by the public health system depends on diagnosis by culture. Collection of stool samples from persons with febrile diarrhea serves a vital public health function and should be performed whenever no burden is placed on the patient.

Treatment of uncomplicated *Salmonella* gastroenteritis in otherwise healthy children and adults does not require antimicrobial therapy. Meta-analysis of 12 clinical trials has clearly shown no reduction in the duration of illness, diarrhea, or fever in otherwise healthy adults and children treated with antimicrobials. In fact, antimicrobial therapy appears to increase the rate of relapse and long-term carriage and is also associated with drug-related adverse effects.

Antimicrobial therapy is indicated for adult patients who are severely ill, require hospitalization, are septic or immunocompromised, have anatomic vascular abnormalities, or are at risk for atherosclerosis because of age older than 50 years (Table 2). For severe gastroenteritis, fluoroquinolones are the first-line choice of treatment in adults (e.g., ciprofloxacin [Cipro], 500 mg every 12 hours for 3 to 5 days), with excellent response and documented reduction of the duration of illness. Alternative regimens include aminopenicillins, ceftriaxone (Rocephin), or cefotaxime (Claforan).

TABLE 2. **Considerations Regarding Therapy for Salmonellosis**

No Antimicrobial Therapy
Gastroenteritis with nonbloody, nonmucoid diarrheal stools; mild to moderate dehydration
Consider Antimicrobial Therapy
Gastroenteritis with bloody or mucoid stools
and risk factors for severe illness (see Table 1)
or severe dehydration
or requires hospitalization for another reason

Antimicrobial therapy is also indicated for newborns, particularly if the mother had diarrheal illness preceding or during birth, and for children who are severely ill, are septic or require hospitalization, are immunocompromised, or have anatomic vascular abnormalities. Approved treatments include trimethoprim-sulfamethoxazole (Bactrim), ampicillin, cefotaxime, and ceftriaxone. Fluoroquinolones are not approved for pediatric use because in animal trials this class of compounds damaged the cartilaginous end plates of long bones. However, accumulating evidence from treatment of children with quinolones for multidrug-resistant *Salmonella typhi* and other infections suggests that this adverse affect may not occur in humans. Some authorities recommend using fluoroquinolones for children with severe salmonellosis.

Antimicrobial resistance is a growing problem in *Salmonella* because of extensive injudicious use of antimicrobial agents to treat farm animals. In both the United States and the United Kingdom, *S. typhimurium* DT-104, commonly resistant to ampicillin, chloramphenicol, streptomycin, sulfonamides, and tetracycline, has become the most common subtype of *S. typhimurium*. In the United Kingdom, fluoroquinolone resistance appeared in *S. typhimurium* DT-104 isolates in the early 1990s after licensing of this class of drugs to treat farm animals. In the United States, ceftriaxone-resistant *S. typhimurium* and *S. newport* have recently emerged. When antimicrobial treatment is contemplated, stool cultures and antimicrobial susceptibility testing for *Salmonella* should be performed and treatment regimens adjusted accordingly.

CONTROL AND PREVENTION

Individuals can protect themselves to a certain extent from salmonellosis by avoiding risky exposure and maintaining good hygiene. Such measures are particularly important for persons at increased risk for infection and severe complications of infection (see Table 1). Avoiding raw animals foods such as undercooked or raw meat, unpasteurized milk, poultry, eggs, and fish and careful hand washing after handling these items are key practices. Eating pasteurized eggs and irradiated ground beef will reduce the risk. Households with children younger than 5 years should not own reptile pets. Careful hand washing after contact with farm animals and reptiles is important as well. More rigorous recommendations have been made by the U.S. Public Health Service (*Morbidity and Mortality Weekly Report*, August 20, 1999, 48(RR10):1–59) for persons with HIV/AIDS and are applicable to persons with other immunocompromising conditions.

Public health officials are charged with the prevention and control of salmonellosis by conducting surveillance for illness and antimicrobial resistance, which is possible only if *Salmonella* infections are detected through positive stool cultures. Obtaining such samples from persons with febrile gastroenteritis serves a critical public health function, as well as benefiting patients who ultimately need antimicrobial therapy.

TYPHOID FEVER

method of
RITA DELIA DIAZ RAMOS, M.D.
Colonia Ville de Cortes
Mexico

DEFINITION

Typhoid fever is an acute systemic illness caused by *Salmonella typhi* that is confined to humans. Complications and relapses are common. Clinical presentation has a broad spectrum depending on age. Illness may be severe, with prominent systemic symptoms such as high fever, abdominal discomfort, malaise, and headache. Children frequently present with constipation or diarrhea and nonproductive cough. Intestinal ischemia can cause bleeding ileitis, ulcers, and perforation. The gallbladder is an important reservoir for *S. typhi*. Key bacterial factors in typhoid fever pathogenesis include dose, acid tolerance, intestinal epithelial invasion, monocyte-macrophage interaction, and survival. The bacteria are highly invasive in the small intestine, penetrating through the mucosal epithelium to the lamina propria and eventually reaching the reticuloendothelial system. After an 8- to 14-day incubation period, they precipitate a systemic illness. The mortality rate in untreated patients is about 10%. Most of the patients developed an effective immune response involving a mix of cell-mediated, humoral, and mucosal elements. Monocyte-macrophage interaction with bacteria is an essential property that allows dissemination of the bacteria to the bloodstream through the thoracic duct.

S. typhi is a facultative, aerobic, motile, gram-negative bacillus. It is acquired through contaminated food or water. Typhoid fever is included in enteric fever produced by other *Salmonella* species (*S. enteritidis, S. paratyphi A, B,* and *C*).

EPIDEMIOLOGY

Typhoid fever is a common infection in developing countries, where water contaminated by sewage is implicated in transmission. Persons from developed countries usually acquire infection during travel to endemic areas. The peak incidence is observed among school-aged children and young adults. Transmission in endemic areas has had an annual frequency up to 1200 per 100,000 individuals. These areas include India, Indonesia, sub-Saharan Africa, and some countries of South and Central America. In the past few years, typhoid fever in the United States has become uncommon (35,994 cases per year in 1920 and 300 to 400 cases since 1968) as compared with nontyphoidal salmonellosis. Control is related to improved food hygiene and water treatment The estimated attack rate during Mexican travel is considered low (0.002%) compared with the highest attack rates in areas such as Peru (0.017%), India (0.011%), Pakistan (0.01%), Chile (0.006%), and Haiti (0.004%). The case-fatality rate in the preantibiotic era was 10% to 20%. Chloramphenicol therapy caused this rate to drop below 1%. Since 1972, *S. typhi* strains with plasmid-encoded resistance to chloramphenicol, trimethoprim-sulfamethoxazole, and amoxicillin appeared and, in the 1990s, began to disseminate throughout Asia and northeast Africa. Fluoroquinolone-resistant strains have also emerged.

COMPLICATIONS

Typhoid fever is a systemic illness with a wide clinical spectrum. Approximately 10% of patients not receiving antimicrobial therapy will experience a relapse. Perforation is the most frequent complication (3%–5%) in the third week. Intestinal bleeding may present as occult blood in the stools at the end of second week (in 10% to 20% of cases). Circulatory collapse in severely ill patients is another important complication. The long-term carrier state is related to inadequate antimicrobial treatment. Hepatitis, cholecystitis, myocarditis, pericarditis, endocarditis, pneumonitis, bronchitis, neuropsychiatric complications, anemia, disseminated intravascular coagulation, and hemolytic-uremic syndrome could all be part of the clinical spectrum of disease.

DIAGNOSIS

Typhoid fever diagnosis requires isolation of *S. typhi* from blood or bone marrow aspirates. It is also useful to culture stool, rose spots, urine, and gastric and intestinal secretions. Children produce higher isolation (60%) in stool culture than do adults (20%–30%) at the end of the first week of acute illness. Ideally, blood, bone marrow, stool, and duodenal string cultures increase the isolation rate to more than 90%. After convalescence, 10% of the patients are still eliminating *S. typhi* in feces, and 1% do so for more than 12 months (long-term carrier state). The female gender and biliary abnormalities predispose one to the long-term carrier state. High titer of Vi antigen is associated with this state, which also is a predisposing factor in gallbladder carcinoma.

Less definite, but more rapid, evidence of infection can be obtained by demonstrating the presence of *S. typhi* antigens or antibodies in blood and body fluids. The tube-agglutination test developed by Widal and Sicard (1896) involves the search for agglutinins in the patient's serum. It may be performed with a careful choice of antigen; both O and H antibodies can be selectively measured. This method should be used in addition to other more reliable tests. A fourfold increase in antibodies to *S. typhi* O, H, or Vi antigens provides support for a typhoid fever diagnosis. After vaccination in endemic areas, high levels of antibodies are found in healthy people. Immunoassays detect O or Vi antigens of *S. typhi* in blood or urine by means of enzyme-linked immunosorbent assay, conglutination, immunoelectrophoresis, or genetic identification via DNA probes or polymerase chain reaction amplification of *S. typhi* genes. Unfortunately, these tests have demonstrated low sensitivity and specificity.

Common hematologic findings are leukopenia, anemia, and thrombocytopenia. Other findings include hyponatremia, hypokalemia, and elevated liver function test results and muscle enzyme levels.

THERAPY

Prompt antimicrobial treatment is very important to avoid complications and reduce the duration of disease. There are a large number of useful antibiotics, and optimal therapy depends on the patient's condition. Supportive measures in severe cases (including hepatitis, myocarditis, and sepsis) are as important as antimicrobial therapy.

Chloramphenicol (Chloromycetin) has been effective for typhoid fever since 1948 and is considered the treatment of choice. Later studies showed similar efficacy with other first-line antibiotics (amoxicillin [Amoxil],* furazolidone [Furoxone],* trimethoprim/sulfamethoxazole [Bactrim]*) and second-line antibiotics such as cefotaxime, ceftriaxone (Rocephin),* cefoperazone (Cefobid),* ceftizoxime (Cefizox),* cefpirome,† cefixime (Suprax)* azithromycin (Zithromax),* and fluoroquinolones.* Chloramphenicol is effective by means of the oral route, is inexpensive, and reduces fever in 48 to 72 hours and mortality from 20% to 1%. The emergence of resistance, the bacteriostatic efficacy, and the increased relapse rate (10%–15%), in addition to bone marrow toxicity (agranulocytosis incidence of 1 per 10,000), however, make other effective therapy preferable. Before 1970, a few sporadic isolated instances of chloramphenicol-resistant *S. typhi* were reported. The first epidemic caused by a chloramphenicol-resistant plasmid-mediated strain occurred in Mexico in 1972. Since 1989, multidrug-resistant outbreaks have been reported.

Third-generation cephalosporins are effective with 7 to 14 days of therapy. Although aztreonam has shown efficacy against *S. typhi*, this drug is not commonly used. Azithromycin has shown efficacy in high doses (1 g/d), but duration of illness is prolonged.

Fluorinated quinolones are highly effective in typhoid fever treatment, increasing cure rate and causing rapid defervescence. Ciprofloxacin (Cipro), ofloxacin (Floxin), norfloxacin (Noroxin), and fleroxacin† have been effective in clinical trials. Unfortunately, resistance to quinolones has been reported. Ciprofloxacin remains the drug of choice for multidrug-resistant *S. typhi*, however. Fluoroquinolones* show the same efficacy, although optimal duration of treatment is not established. Table 1 summarizes the most common agents used in typhoid fever therapy. Bactericidal antibiotics such as third-generation cephalosporins or fluoroquinolones must be included for immunocompromised patients. Unnecessary use of quinolones could induce positive selection for resistant strains and decrease their efficacy.

*Not FDA approved for this indication.
†Not available in the United States.

For those in the long-term carrier state, treatment includes surgery for anatomic abnormalities (with biliary or kidney stones) after antibiotic therapy.

Amoxicillin* (100 mg/kg/d) and trimethoprim-sulfamethoxazole* (160/800 mg every 12 hours) are effective in elimination of the long-term carrier state after 6 weeks (80%). Quinolones have also been successful in eliminating the long-term carrier state. In a urinary carrier of schistosomes, praziquantel (Biltricide) is recommended in addition to adequate antibiotic therapy.

In severe cases, mostly those associated with shock, stupor, and coma, high doses of dexamethasone (Decadron) (3 mg/kg) infused intravenously over 30 minutes, followed by eight additional doses of 1 mg/kg every 6 hours, reduce the case-fatality rate (10%).

PREVENTION

Useful strategies to interrupt the transmission of *S. typhi* are (1) identify and eliminate the bacteria from patients with acute illness or from carriers; (2) prevent transmission by means of adequate antibiotic therapy, sanitation, water and food hygiene control, safe disposal of infected urine and feces, and health education programs for infected people and food handlers; and (3) install transmission control measures in people at risk of infection. These measures include supplying adequate information to travelers so that they avoid drinks and foods with low-

*Not FDA approved for this indication.

TABLE 1. **Antibiotic Therapy for Typhoid Fever**

Drug	Route	Pediatric Dosage	Adult Dosage
Chloramphenicol	O, IV, IM	50–100 mg/kg qid	500–750 mg qid
Amoxicillin†	O, IV, IM	50–100 mg/kg qid	500–1000 mg qid
TMP/SMX†	O, IV	8/40 mg/kg bid	160/800 mg bid
Ceftriaxone†	IV, IM	75–100 mg/kg bid	1–2 g bid
Cefotaxime	IV, IM	100 mg/kg q6–8h	1–2 g q6–8h
Cefoperazone†	IV, IM	50–100 mg/kg bid	1–2 g bid
Cefpirome*	IV	N/A	1–2 g bid
Cefixime†	O	8–10 mg/kg bid	200–400 mg bid
Ciprofloxacin	O	20–30 mg/kg bid	500 mg bid
Ciprofloxacin	IV	15–20 mg/kg bid	200–400 mg bid
Ofloxacin†	O	15 mg/kg bid	400 mg bid
Pefloxacin*	O, IV	N/A	400 mg bid
Norfloxacin†	O	N/A	400 mg bid
Fleroxacin*	O, IV	N/A	400 mg qid
Aztreonam†	IM	90–120 mg/kg qid	1 g bid/qid
Azithromycin†	O	5–10 mg/kg qd	1 g qd

*Not available in the United States.
†Not FDA approved for this indication.
Abbreviations: IM, intramuscular; IV, intravenous; O, oral; TMP/SMX, trimethoprim/sulfamethoxazole.

quality purification (improperly cooked foods, fresh salads, and drinks in endemic areas).

VACCINES

Typhoid vaccination is not universally indicated, not even in endemic countries. It is specifically recommended for people in high-risk jobs, such as microbiology laboratory workers who work with *S. typhi*, those with household contacts, food handlers, and, in some cases, travelers.

The first available typhoid vaccine was created more than 100 years ago. There have been many attempts to produce an ideal vaccine for typhoid fever, with poor results. Three typhoid vaccine formulations are licensed in the United States.

An oral (enteric-coated) live attenuated vaccine (Vivotif Berna; Berna Products, Coral Gables, Fla.) is manufactured from the Ty21a strain of *S. typhi*. This vaccine stimulates local intestinal immunity by blocking infection at its earliest state, but disease is reacquired with high doses; adults and children older than 6 years require four capsules, one per day 1 week before exposure, with revaccination every 5 years. Side effects include mild diarrhea and abdominal pain. Ty21a vaccine in a liquid formulation for children 3 years of age or older (Vivotif Berna Liquid; Swiss Serum and Vaccine Institute, Berne, Switzerland) had better results than the enteric-coated presentation, and only three doses are required.

Capsular polysaccharide vaccine is given by intramuscular administration (Typhim VI; produced by Pasteur Merieux Serums and Vaccines for Connaught Laboratories, Swiftwater, Pa). It is prepared with purified Vi antigen and contains the cell surface Vi polysaccharide from *S. typhi* Ty2 strain. A single intramuscular injection (0.5 mL) at least 2 weeks before exposure is required. It is not recommended in children younger than 2 years old.

A heat-phenol-inactivated vaccine for subcutaneous use (manufactured by Wyeth-Ayerst Laboratories, Philadelphia, Pa) is the oldest typhoid vaccine and is highly reactogenic, causing fever, headache, severe local pain, or swelling. More severe reactions have been reported, such as hypotension and shock.

An acetone-inactivated vaccine* for parenteral use is available only to the British Army.

All these vaccines show the same efficacy, 50% to 80%. The protection rate is very low even with a large dose, with a short protection period (2–5 years). An ideal future typhoid vaccine would be an oral, single-dose, inexpensive formulation with minimal adverse reactions and high efficacy.

---

*Not available in the United States.

ROCKY MOUNTAIN SPOTTED FEVER AND EHRLICHIOSIS

method of
RICHARD GLECKMAN, M.D., and
ELLEN RICCOBENE, M.D.
St. Joseph's Regional Medical Center
Paterson, New Jersey

ROCKY MOUNTAIN SPOTTED FEVER

Rocky Mountain spotted fever (RMSF), the most serious of the tick-borne rickettsial diseases, is caused by the gram-negative, pleomorphic, coccobacillary intracellular bacterium, *Rickettsia rickettsii*. The term *RMSF* is deceiving, however, because the greatest incidence of the disease occurs in the Carolinas and Oklahoma, usually but not exclusively between April and September. Considered a disease of rural or suburban environments, the infection has also been detected in urban areas, such as New York City and Philadelphia.

In the United States, this disease is transmitted by *Dermacentor* variables (dog tick) in the East and parts of the West Coast and by *Dermacentor andersoni* (wood tick) in the Rocky Mountain states. After the bite of the adult tick (which is painless and often unnoticed) or while crushing an infected tick during removal from persons or domestic animals, the rickettsiae spread through the lymphatics and the blood vessels, invade and multiply within the endothelial and smooth muscle cells of blood vessels, and cause vascular permeability and vasculitis. The organism has the potential to attack every organ.

The incubation period is 2 to 14 days after the tick bite, with a mean of 7 days. Patients initially experience fever, headache, myalgia, and, less commonly, nausea, vomiting, or diarrhea. Additional manifestations that can develop include cardiovascular (hypovolemic hypotension, arrhythmia), pulmonary (dyspnea, cough, adult respiratory distress syndrome), hepatobiliary (hepatomegaly), hematologic (lymphadenopathy, splenomegaly), renal (prerenal azotemia, acute tubular necrosis), ocular (conjunctivitis), neurologic (stupor, meningismus, ataxia, photophobia, transient deafness, cranial nerve palsies, paresthesias, seizures) and soft tissue (gangrene) abnormalities.

The hallmark of the disease is rash (initially, erythematous 1 to 4 mm macular lesions), which starts most often on the ankles and the wrists and then appears on the palms, the soles, and the trunk. As the rash evolves, it becomes more defined and maculopapular or petechial. Skin necrosis and gangrene can occur. Fewer than 50% of patients experience rash during the first 3 days of illness, and some patients, approximately 10% (particularly blacks and older individuals), never experience a rash.

Abnormalities of the complete blood count (e.g., anemia, thrombocytopenia), traditional blood chemistry tests (hyponatremia; elevated levels of aspartate transaminase, lactic dehydrogenase, and creatine phosphokinase), and the cerebrospinal fluid are noted in some patients and indicate the multisystemic nature of RMSF, but these altered studies have no specific diagnostic value.

The nonspecific nature of the early manifestations, the failure to recognize or remember the tick bite, the frequent absence of or delay in the characteristic rash, the relative infrequency of RMSF, and the protean manifestations that can develop all contribute to the diagnostic challenge and a delay in diagnosis.

The differential diagnosis is extensive and consists of

those disorders unassociated with petechial rash (including meningitis or encephalitis, enterocolitis, infectious mononucleosis, bronchitis or pneumonia, ehrlichiosis, leptospirosis, hepatitis, and typhoid as well as diseases associated with a petechial rash (including meningococcemia, atypical measles, coxsackievirus or echovirus infections, Hantavirus pulmonary syndrome, idiopathic or thrombotic thrombocytopenic purpura, drug eruptions, endocarditis, and acute leukemia).

It is of interest that considerable resources have been dedicated to the diagnosis of Lyme disease, a virtually nonfatal and often overdiagnosed condition. In contrast, RMSF, a potentially fatal tick-borne rickettsial disease affecting 600 to 1200 individuals per year in the United States, has not engendered the investment of talent and funding necessary to produce an early, clinically useful diagnostic test. Cultivation of the organism from blood, serologic and immunologic tests to detect antibody, and immunohistochemical tests performed on skin lesions are research tests, performed exclusively at reference laboratories and incapable of confirming the diagnosis within the first days of clinical expression. In essence, because the case-fatality ratio is 20%, unless the disorder is treated early and with correct antibiotic therapy (even when the patient is young and previously well), the disease must be considered in any patient experiencing a febrile disorder accompanied by headache or myalgia (with or without a rash) who may have had a recent tick exposure (although approximately 12% of patients report no known exposure to ticks or their habitats). Risk factors for a fatal outcome include the following: age of more than 40 years, delay in diagnosis, delay in initiating therapy, shock, seizures, coma, jaundice, hepatomegaly, and acute renal failure. Fulminant disease is experienced disproportionately in African Americans with glucose-6-phosphate dehydrogenase deficiency.

TREATMENT

Treatment consists of doxycycline (Vibramycin), in an adult dose of 100 mg every 12 hours supplemented by adjunctive measures dictated by the patient's clinical condition (e.g., oxygen therapy and mechanical ventilation for adult respiratory distress syndrome or hemodialysis for acute tubular necrosis; Swan-Ganz catheter insertion to manage fluid administration and assess hemodynamic status; intracranial pressure monitoring for individuals with encephalitis-related coma). Patients with diminished state of consciousness require measures to attempt to prevent aspiration and pressure ulcers. Doxycycline is administered for at least 1 week. Adult pregnant women should receive chloramphenicol (Chloromycetin), 500 mg intravenously every 6 hours, rather than intravenous doxycycline. Patients can develop permanent neurologic sequelae consisting of hemiplegia, deafness, and cranial neuropathies.

Preventive measures include avoiding walks through bushy vegetation, keeping pets tick free, using tick repellant, checking for ticks (particularly the scalp and the pubic and axillary hair), and removing ticks properly.

EHRLICHIOSIS

Ehrlichia belong to the family Rickettsiaceae and, although similar, have a separate genus, named for the German bacteriologist Paul Ehrlich. *Ehrlichia* are obligate intracellular gram-negative bacteria that divide to form clusters of bacteria within cytoplasmic vacuoles called morulae, from the Latin word for mulberry. *Ehrlichia* are tick-borne zoonoses that infect phagocytic bone marrow–derived cells in mammalian hosts.

In 1987, *Ehrlichia chaffeensis* the species responsible for human monocytic ehrlichiosis (HME), was identified. More than 1500 cases of this disease have been reported in more than 30 states, primarily in the south central and southeastern United States. *E. chaffeensis* infection is acquired from the bite of the Lone Star tick, *Amblyomma americanum*, with a peak incidence in May to July. White-tailed deer and possibly dogs are important reservoirs.

In 1994, human granulocytic ehrlichiosis (HGE) was identified. The species has yet to be described but is similar to *E. equi* and *E. phagocytophila*. More than 600 cases have been reported in 13 states. The peak incidence occurs between May and August, when nymphal stage ticks are questing. Adult ticks quest in the autumn months but, owing to their larger size, are easier to detect and remove. As the name implies, the HGE agent infects granulocytes, but nonhematologic cell lines may also become infected in severe disease. *Ixodes scapularis*, the deer tick, is the primary tick vector in the northeastern and upper midwestern United States. *I. scapularis* may also transmit *Borrelia burgdorferi* and *Babesia microti*, and 6% to 21% of patients with HGE have also been found to have serologic evidence of these organisms. The white-footed mouse and the white-tailed deer are the important host mammal reservoirs in the eastern and midwestern United States. The vector in the Pacific western states is *Ixodes pacificus*, the black-legged tick. The vector in western Europe is *Ixodes ricinus*, the sheep tick.

Other ehrilicheal species that have been identified in humans include *E. canis*, *E. ewingii*, and *E. sennetsu* (found exclusively in Asia). It is probable that additional ehrlichial disease affecting humans will be identified.

The clinical presentation of ehrlichiosis ranges from asymptomatic (found in some studies to be as high as two thirds of patients) to a mild, self-limiting illness or a potentially fatal multisystemic illness. Approximately 40% of patients may require hospitalization, most notably patients of advanced age, patients with concomitant chronic illnesses, or those in whom the diagnosis is delayed.

After transmission from a tick bite, *Ehrlichiae* invade their target cells, the hematopoietic and lymphoreticular systems. Seven to ten days after transmission, patients typically present to a physician after the development of a nonspecific febrile (39°C/102°F) illness with chills, headache, myalgias, and malaise. The majority of patients give a history of tick exposure. Given a history of a tick bite, the differential diagnosis should also include Rocky Mountain spotted fever, relapsing fever, tularemia, lyme disease, Colorado tick fever, and babesiosis.

Routine laboratory testing is helpful diagnostically. In the first 7 days of illness, most patients will manifest leukopenia (1300 to 4000 cells/μL) and thrombocytopenia (usually 50,000 to 140,000 platelets); both cell lines reach a nadir at about day 7. Thereafter, counts return toward baseline, even while clinical symptoms persist. In the first 7 days, serum chemistry results will reveal a two- to fourfold elevation in hepatic transaminase levels. Light microscopic examination of peripheral smears treated with Wright stain may reveal morulae and thus provide immediate evidence of the diagnosis. Morulae are detected most frequently within the first week of illness and may be seen in 20% to 80% of patients with HGE and in as few as 7% of patients with HME. A presumptive diagnosis based on epidemiologic and clinical factors offers an opportunity to initiate empirical treatment.

If not recognized, the disease may develop into a multisystemic illness with a wide differential diagnosis. A minority of patients may develop a nonspecific erythematous rash, which may be maculopapular or petechial and is more commonly seen in patients with HME and in children. Patients may also develop nausea, vomiting, arthralgias, a nonproductive cough, and confusion. In severe illness, cough, diarrhea, and lymphadenopathy may occur. Severe complications include respiratory failure, renal insufficiency, central nervous system changes (confusion), gastrointestinal hemorrhage, and death. Further diagnostic studies may reveal an infiltrate on chest radiography, cerebrospinal fluid pleocytosis (mostly lymphocytes), and an increase in protein. Pulmonary edema and adult respiratory distress syndrome may occur late in infection. A decreased intravascular volume may result in acute tubular necrosis. Advanced disease may also mimic thrombotic thrombocytopenic purpura.

A presumptive diagnosis based on history and clinical findings may be confirmed with further laboratory tests. Indirect immunofluorescent assay is diagnostic if a fourfold or greater increase in antibody titer is found, but this may take weeks to occur. Successful isolation of the agent in blood culture is possible but is laborious and available only at a few research centers. Amplification of specific DNA by polymerase chain reaction analysis and demonstration of the presence of morulae in peripheral blood are more timely and also diagnostic. None of these tests is 100% sensitive. Rapid tests (dot-blot or enzyme immunoassay) may be available in the future.

Doxycycline and tetracycline have both been proven to have in vivo and in vitro efficacy in the treatment of this disease. Doxycycline has a better pharmacokinetic profile (lipid solubility and long half-life) and patient tolerability. It is given to patients 8 years of age or older at 100 mg twice daily orally or intravenously for 14 days. Response is usually seen in 1 to 2 days, and another diagnosis should be considered in patients who do not respond. Children younger than 8 years of age may receive a shorter course. Clinical experience with rifampin is limited, but rifampin may be used in pregnant women for 7 to 10 days.

If exposure to ticks is possible, use of insecticide sprays and protective clothing may be preventative. Removal of ticks within 24 hours aids in the prevention of transmission.

Section 3

The Respiratory System

ACUTE RESPIRATORY FAILURE

method of
ARAM A. ARABIAN, M.D., and
PRASHANT K. ROHATGI, M.D.
*Veterans Affairs Medical Center
Washington, D.C.*

Acute respiratory failure is an inability to adequately oxygenate the blood and/or remove carbon dioxide in the setting of acute respiratory acidosis (pH <7.30). Many disorders can lead to acute respiratory failure, such as infection of the lung parenchyma, ventilation/perfusion ($\dot{V}/\dot{Q}$) mismatch of any etiology, airway obstruction, pneumothorax, shunting, and neuromuscular diseases. The two common broad categories, however, are acute lung injury (ALI) caused by diffuse alveolar epithelial-capillary membrane damage and acute respiratory failure in patients with chronic bronchitis, emphysema, and other airway obstructive diseases.

Criteria for ALI are a $Pa{O_2}/F{I}{O_2}$ ratio of 300 or less, bilateral infiltrates on chest radiography in a pattern consistent with pulmonary edema, and a pulmonary artery occlusion pressure of 18 mm Hg or less. When the ALI is of greater degree, the term *acute* (or adult) *respiratory distress syndrome* (ARDS) is used and defined as ALI is, but with a $Pa{O_2}/F{I}{O_2}$ equal to or less than 200

Acute respiratory failure in patients with underlying chronic airway obstruction is deemed to be present when the patient has an acute drop in $Pa{O_2}$ greater than 10 to 15 mm Hg and/or hypercapnia in association with an arterial pH below 7.30.

GENERAL PRINCIPLES FOR TREATING ACUTE RESPIRATORY FAILURE

Initial evaluation should consider the ABCs of cardiopulmonary resuscitation. Are the airways sufficiently patent? Is breathing adequate? Is the circulation adequate? Mechanical obstruction of the upper airway is usually obvious, but stridor has been misinterpreted as wheezing and bronchodilators given inappropriately. When upper airway obstruction is present, rapid measures must be taken to reverse this condition and may include, depending on the cause, removal of a foreign body, institution of therapy to reduce airway edema, endotracheal intubation if feasible, and even tracheostomy if necessary. Lower airway mechanical obstruction usually requires rigid bronchoscopy for removal of aspirated foreign bodies. Patency can be ensured and the airway protected by intubation of the trachea.

Initial therapy in acute respiratory failure is directed at ensuring adequate gas exchange and oxygen delivery to tissues by administering controlled supplemental oxygen to provide sufficient oxygenation, which must be confirmed by arterial blood gas evaluation or pulse oximetry if pH and $Pa{CO_2}$ are not in question. Adequate $Pa{O_2}$ and $Pa{CO_2}$ only ensure adequate gas exchange; they do not ensure adequate oxygen delivery to tissues. Adequate tissue oxygenation requires that the hematocrit and cardiac output be sufficient.

When spontaneous ventilation is inadequate, mechanical ventilation is necessary. It is important to set the ventilator to minimize the work of breathing until the underlying cause of the respiratory failure is identified and treatment begun. It is not always necessary that the patient be intubated; instead, noninvasive positive-pressure ventilation may be used via a tight-fitting mask if the patient is awake, is not in danger of vomiting, does not have copious secretions, and can tolerate a face mask. Such ventilation is most appropriate when the respiratory failure is expected to be rapidly reversed.

Adequate circulation and oxygen-carrying capacity must be ensured. It is not usually necessary to use a pulmonary artery catheter to distinguish cardiogenic from noncardiogenic pulmonary edema or to measure cardiac output. Satisfactory cardiac output can generally be determined clinically by assessing not only the heart rate and blood pressure but also urine output, mentation, and temperature and perfusion of the extremities. The hemoglobin level should be checked and packed red blood cells transfused if necessary to ensure that the oxygen content is acceptable.

ACUTE RESPIRATORY DISTRESS SYNDROME

Diagnosis

The clinical diagnosis of ARDS is complex and depends on a combination of clinical, radiologic, and physiologic findings, which together present a unique description of the disorder (Table 1).

The etiology of ALI/ARDS is diverse and can be divided into conditions that cause direct or those that cause indirect damage to the alveolar epithelial-capillary membrane (Table 2). The most common direct cause initiating ARDS is pneumonia, and the most common indirect cause producing ARDS is sepsis from any source. Indirect injury to the alveolar epithelial-capillary membrane is a consequence of unregulated overexpression of a systemic inflammatory response, with proinflammatory mediators overwhelming the anti-inflammatory mediators. The pathophysiologic consequences of alveolar capillary and alveolar epithelial injury are shown in Figure 1.

Clinically, dyspnea is always present and patients are hypoxemic. The inciting event may precede the onset of ARDS by hours or by a day or two. Physical examination shows the patient to be tachypneic and tachycardic, with evidence of increased work of breathing with the use of accessory muscles of respiration. Auscultation of the lungs usually reveals crackles in dependent portions of the lung, but a normal examination is not uncommon. Other clinical findings are related to the underlying disorder responsible for the development of ARDS.

The typical standard *radiographic* representation of established ARDS is small lung volumes with diffuse, bilat-

TABLE 1. **Criteria for Diagnosing Acute Respiratory Distress Syndrome**

Proper Clinical Setting
Catastrophic event
Direct pulmonary injury
Indirect pulmonary injury
Respiratory distress
Tachypnea
Exclusions
Left ventricular failure
Pulmonary capillary wedge pressure ≥18 mm Hg
Chest Radiograph
Diffuse alveolar infiltrates
Physiologic Change
PaO_2/FIO_2 ≤300 for ALI
PaO_2/FIO_2 ≤200 for ARDS
Compliance of 50–97 mL/cm H_2O for ALI
Compliance ≤50 mL/cm H_2O for ARDS

Abbreviations: ALI = acute lung injury; ARDS = acute respiratory distress syndrome.

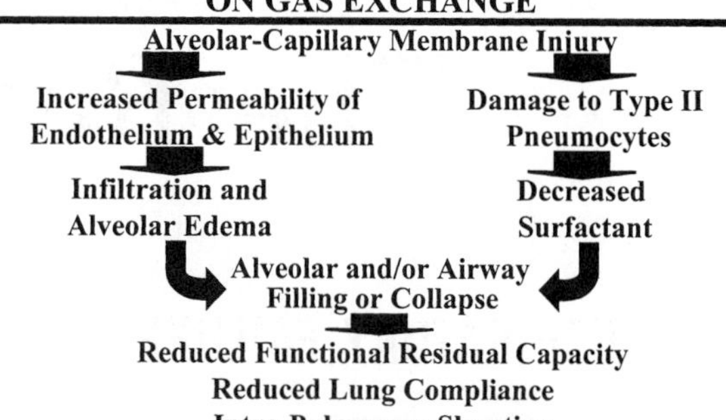

Figure 1. Pathophysiologic consequences of injury to alveolar capillary and alveolar epithelium.

eral alveolar infiltrates with or without air bronchograms (Figure 2). Although not applicable in all situations, some patterns can help distinguish the radiographic representation of ARDS from cardiogenic pulmonary edema. Normal heart size, the presence of air bronchograms, the absence of septal lines (Kerley B lines), and the absence of pleural effusions are useful differentiating features that indicate ARDS.

The pattern on chest computed tomography is more variable than that seen on a projection radiograph. In the early phase of the disease, the edema fluid accumulates evenly and produces homogeneous lung density; however, with time and as patients are mechanically ventilated in the supine position, the pattern on computed tomography is usually nonuniform, with ground-glass opacities or consolidation in the most dependent areas, especially the peripheral portions of the lung, and more normal aeration in the nondependent areas. Partial resolution of passive collapse of the dependent lungs takes place rapidly on prone positioning.

The *physiology* of ARDS shows reduced compliance as a consequence of alveolar flooding and alveolar atelectasis. Unfortunately, respiratory system compliance can be measured only when the patient is intubated and receiving mechanical ventilation and is therefore not useful in the clinical diagnosis of ARDS. Severe hypoxemia is primarily due to intrapulmonary shunting.

TABLE 2. **Clinical Disorders Associated With the Development of Acute Respiratory Distress Syndrome**

Direct Lung Injury
Common causes
Pneumonia
Aspiration
Less common causes
Toxic inhalation, including high-concentration oxygen
Pulmonary contusion
Radiation
Emboli—amniotic fluid, air, fat
Near drowning
Indirect Lung Injury
Common causes
Sepsis
Severe massive trauma
Less common causes
Acute pancreatitis
Drugs, both therapeutic and illicit
Eclampsia
Multiple blood transfusions
Post–cardiopulmonary bypass
Leukoagglutinin reaction

Not included are other causes of noncardiogenic pulmonary edema, such as neurogenic conditions, high altitude, and near-drowning, because they usually resolve more rapidly than typical ARDS.

Therapy

Unfortunately, no specific therapeutic interventions can correct or hasten recovery of the alveolar epithelial-capillary membrane damage. As a consequence, the general principles of management in ARDS are to (1) treat the underlying disorder responsible for producing ARDS, (2) prevent further damage to the alveolar epithelial-capillary membrane (avoid hypotension, hyperoxia, ventilator-associated lung damage, pneumonia, line sepsis, etc.), (3) permit the lung to heal spontaneously (adequate nutrition, avoidance of pulmonary barotrauma, etc.), and (4) prevent complications (venous thromboembolism, gastrointestinal bleeding, pulmonary barotrauma, etc.) while supporting the patient during this catastrophic illness, which carries a mortality of approximately 40%. The major components of supportive care are correction of tissue hypoxia and maintenance of fluid balance.

Correction of Tissue Hypoxia. The aim of therapy is to prevent tissue hypoxia by improving tissue oxygen transport. Tissue oxygen transport is a function of cardiac output and arterial oxygen content, which in turn is dependent on the hemoglobin level and arterial oxygen saturation. The aim is to optimize both these factors without producing adverse effects, such as oxygen toxicity, ventilator-associated lung damage, and fluid overload. Because the hypoxemia in ARDS is primarily due to intrapulmonary shunting, it is not usually corrected by supplemental

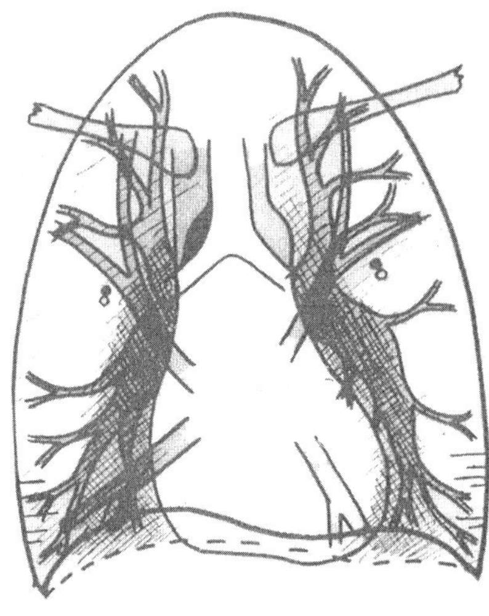

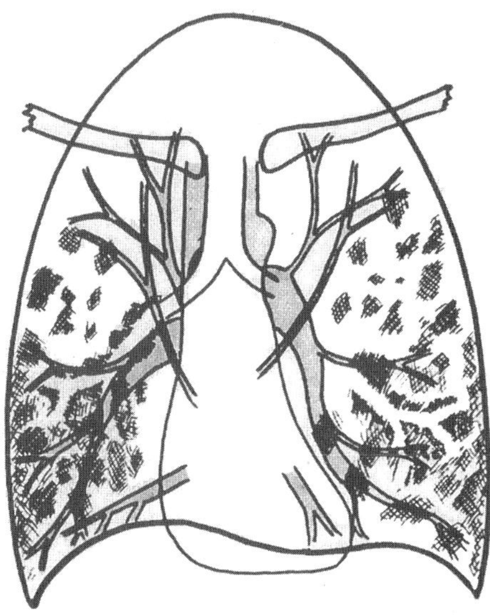

Figure 2. Typical radiographic representation of hydrostatic pulmonary edema and established acute respiratory distress syndrome.

oxygen. *Presently, mechanical ventilation is the most important modality available to treat ARDS.* Most patients require not only mechanical ventilation but also the addition of positive end-expiratory pressure (PEEP); these interventions assume much of the work of breathing resulting from the high ventilatory requirements and poor lung compliance and they support and improve oxygenation. The use of sedation and, infrequently, neuromuscular blocking agents may be necessary to obtain optimal patient-ventilator interaction.

Treatment should begin with the patient receiving 100% oxygen from a volume-cycled mechanical ventilator in the assist/control mode and tidal volume set to 6 to 10 mL/kg of predicted weight at a rate that allows an inspiratory-to-expiratory ratio of 1:1 to 1:3. If the plateau pressure exceeds 35 cm H_2O, tidal volume can be reduced in stepwise fashion up to 5 to 6 mL/kg . Plateau pressures exceeding 35 cm H_2O have been associated with volutrauma, biotrauma, and perhaps barotrauma. PEEP is used in a range of 5 to 15 cm H_2O when the FIO_2 is greater than 0.5 for more than a few hours. Theoretically, any FIO_2 greater than ambient air is toxic; however, clinical experience suggests that an FIO_2 up to 0.4 can be tolerated for prolonged periods without obvious harm and that an FIO_2 of 0.6 appears to avoid progression of alveolar epithelial-capillary membrane damage. PEEP should be instituted immediately if the FIO_2 must be above 0.6 to maintain a PaO_2 greater than 60 mm Hg. Higher levels of PEEP usually require invasive monitoring of cardiac output and, possibly, prophylactic placement of bilateral chest tubes. If hemodynamic parameters remain stable, PEEP should not be reduced until the FIO_2 is less than 0.5. In the event that mechanical ventilation with a high tidal volume, respiratory rate, and PEEP does not result in a PaO_2 greater than 60 mm Hg, the patient should be turned to a prone position.

Pharmacologic interventions in ARDS have been ineffective except in very specific instances. The use of corticosteroids may benefit patients with long-bone fractures if given before the onset of ARDS. They may also benefit patients with *Pneumocystis carinii* pneumonia and hypoxemia. Corticosteroids have been found to produce profound resolution of ARDS when it is due to acute eosinophilic pneumonia, the diagnosis of which is suggested by high numbers of eosinophils in blood and/or bronchoalveolar lavage fluid. Corticosteroid use (2–4 mg prednisone/kg/d) may also be considered a week after the onset of ARDS when no clinical improvement has been seen and the patient is considered to be in the fibroproliferative phase of ARDS. Although the literature is replete with pharmacologic therapies, none have clearly shown reduced mortality.

If standard therapies fail and the underlying, inciting cause of ARDS cannot be reversed, thought can be given to the use of extracorporeal life support, also known as extracorporeal membrane oxygenation. The indications for instituting this procedure are an alveolar-arterial oxygen gradient greater than 600 mm Hg, a PaO_2/FIO_2 ratio less than 70 on 100% O_2, and a pulmonary shunt greater than 30% despite optimal therapy. This treatment should be carried out in a center with experience in this technique.

Fluid Management. Conflicting therapeutic goals have to be balanced when considering the administration of fluids. The need to restrict fluid to decrease pulmonary edema has to be balanced against maintaining adequate cardiac output and oxygen delivery while increasing PEEP. Earlier use of vasopressors should be considered if the patient is having problems maintaining adequate tissue perfusion despite restoration of intravascular volume.

Prevention of Pneumonia. Prevention of nosocomial pneumonia is a major priority, and any manipulation of the ventilator tubing and suctioning of the endotracheal tube should be done using sterile technique. The major determinant of the prognosis of ARDS is the ability to diagnose and treat the underlying cause.

Pneumonia as the initiating or complicating factor in ARDS is difficult to distinguish from ARDS without pneumonia. ARDS without pneumonia can cause radiographic infiltrates, fever, and purulent sputum with colonization by pathogenic organisms. Absolute criteria for the diagnosis of pneumonia would be histologic evidence of infection from the lung; however, obtaining such evidence is not practical, and therefore a positive blood culture, cavitation seen on the chest radiograph, or infection in the pleural space is considered diagnostic of bacterial pneumonia. Obtaining quantitative culture from protected brush specimens or bronchoalveolar lavage fluid is invasive and helpful only if the patient had not previously been receiving antibiotics. It is usually just as beneficial to know the bacterial flora of your institution and begin administering empirical broad-spectrum antibiotics to which these organisms are sensitive. Specimens should be sent for culture before starting antibiotic therapy if bacterial infection is suspected. Growth of a predominant organism may allow the initiation of specific therapy and thus avoid the prolonged use of broad-spectrum antibiotics.

Survival of patients with ARDS depends on several factors. The ability to interrupt the underlying cause is paramount. The presence of nosocomial pneumonia with ARDS increases mortality substantially, up to 90%. If other organs show signs of failure, mortality is markedly increased. When insufficiency in any organ is detected, prompt therapy should be instituted. Mortality approaches 100% when signs of failure or insufficiency are detected in four organs. After recovery of a patient with severe respiratory insufficiency, the lung may return to fairly normal function and radiographic appearance, but the process may take 6 months or more.

MANAGEMENT OF ACUTE RESPIRATORY FAILURE IN CHRONIC OBSTRUCTIVE AIRWAY DISEASE

Assessment

Factors that increase symptoms and worsen preexisting emphysema, chronic bronchitis, or a combination of both, grouped together as chronic obstructive airway disease (COAD), thereby precipitating acute respiratory failure, are listed in Table 3. In a large proportion of cases, a precipitating factor is never established. Most exacerbations, however, are due to upper respiratory tract viral infection and environmental factors such as pollution. The assumption that the increased morbidity and purulence is due to bacterial infection is probably not true; however, we still give these patients a course of antibiotics that are effective against common bacterial pathogens—*Streptococcus pneumoniae, Haemophilus influenzae*, and *Moraxella catarrhalis*—when no evidence of pulmonary infiltrates can be seen on chest radiographs.

TABLE 3. **Precipitating Factors in Acute Respiratory Failure Secondary to Chronic Obstructive Pulmonary Disease**

Common	Uncommon
Bronchopulmonary infections	Sedatives
Environmental pollutants	β-Adrenergic blockers
Pulmonary embolism	Dehydration
Left ventricular failure	Metabolic alkalosis
Pneumothorax	Improper oxygen use

While initiating therapeutic measures, it is important to determine the patient's baseline arterial blood gases and, in particular, the presence and severity of hypercapnia. If this information is not available, an approximation of $PaCO_2$ can be back-calculated from the first pH and $PaCO_2$ determined during the acute episode. This calculation is performed by using the reciprocal relationship in which a 0.08 change in pH is caused by a 10–mm Hg change in $PaCO_2$ in an acute situation, the assumption being that the pH was normal before deterioration. Serum bicarbonate can also be used to extrapolate the $PaCO_2$ inasmuch as bicarbonate increases by about 4 mEq/L for every 10–mm Hg chronic elevation in $PaCO_2$.

Therapy

The aim is to treat the precipitating factor, if known, relieve hypoxemia while avoiding CO_2 elevation, decrease airway obstruction, and prevent muscle fatigue and the need for mechanical ventilation.

Controlled Oxygen Therapy. The intent of controlled O_2 therapy is to maintain PaO_2 around 60 mm Hg, which would produce over 90% hemoglobin saturation. Because hypoxemia in these patients is mostly due to ventilation perfusion inequality, it responds readily to small amounts of supplemental oxygen. Most hypercapnic patients will have a small rise in $PaCO_2$ with supplemental oxygen, but it is very important (1) that uncontrolled oxygen not be given to patients with hypercapnia because of the danger of inducing CO_2 narcosis and (2) that intermittent oxygen be avoided in hypercapnic patients because of the danger of producing life-threatening hypoxemia. Controlled oxygen can be given by nasal prongs at a flow of 1 to 2 L/min or, better still, by using a face mask with a Venturi device.

Relieve Airway Obstruction. Besides providing encouragement to cough and clear secretions, hydration, mucolytics, and treatment of infection may also help. Bronchodilators are the mainstay of therapy for relieving airway obstruction, and the medication used must be individualized. Many patients with COAD will respond to anticholinergics, but others will have a better response to β-adrenergics. To avoid intubation and mechanical ventilation the use of both is justified, and when the patient is having a severe episode, these medications should be given continuously until ventilation is satisfactory or the patient has symptoms from the inhaled bronchodilators, usually noted as tachyarrhythmias. Theophylline derivatives do not usually provide any additional benefit in acute respiratory failure.

The use of systemic glucocorticoids is indicated in patients with acute respiratory failure in COAD. They are indicated for those who have responded to them in the past, those with seasonal variation in respiratory symptoms, those in whom the exacerbation has followed a period of rapid weaning from steroids, and those who have eosinophils in their sputum. In patients without known steroid responsiveness, their use is indicated for a short duration. They should be started promptly, and when the acute episode has resolved, their dose should be rapidly tapered with attention to the return of dyspnea, in which case steroid administration should be restarted or increased and tapered more slowly. Inhaled steroids presently have no role in acute respiratory failure in COAD.

Relieve Muscle Fatigue. In a cooperative and alert patient, noninvasive mechanical ventilation can be used to provide rest to respiratory muscles and improve alveolar ventilation, with the aim of reducing hypercapnia and improving hypoxemia. This goal requires a tight-fitting face or nasal mask, the latter being safer if the patient can control the tendency to mouth-breathe. The mechanical device can be a bilevel positive airway pressure (Bi-PAP) unit or a standard mechanical ventilator. The ventilator mode should be one that is comfortable for the patient, and supplemental O_2 is added as necessary to ensure a $Pa{O_2}$ of at least 55 mm Hg.

Mechanical Ventilation. When mechanical ventilation is needed, care must be taken to prevent lowering the $Pa{CO_2}$ to normal in a patient who retains CO_2. The goals should be a satisfactory $Pa{O_2}$ (>55 mm Hg) and a $Pa{CO_2}$ that matches the patient's baseline $Pa{CO_2}$. Care must be taken to not overventilate the patient so that the elevated bicarbonate is reduced to normal. The use of PEEP at low levels to keep the airways open is justified to overcome auto-PEEP, but PEEP above a few centimeters of water pressure is not justified because it will increase an already markedly elevated functional residual capacity and put respiratory muscle mechanics at a disadvantage. Attention must be given to the amount of inspiratory pressure required to ventilate lungs that are already overdistended and have increased compliance, the danger being barotrauma and development of pneumothorax and pneumomediastinum. Finally, the rate should be set to ensure that the patient maintains a spontaneous rate above that set by the ventilator to prevent muscle wasting.

Most patients can be removed from mechanical ventilation when the episode that brought on the dyspnea has resolved Only a minority of patients require slow weaning and coaxing from the ventilator. Studies have shown that the most effective means of weaning is the use of T-piece trials. The patient is removed from the ventilator for varying periods, with removal terminated by the presence of stress such as agitation, hypertension, tachycardia, tachypnea, and deteriorating gas exchange. When such complications occur, the patient is again ventilated mechanically until rested and another trial is instituted. This procedure is continued until the patient is successfully removed from mechanical ventilation without signs or symptoms of stress. If these trials are not tolerated, pressure support trials may be instituted with the amount of pressure support reduced periodically to gradually remove the patient from mechanical ventilation.

ATELECTASIS

method of
JOSEPH I. MILLER, Jr., M.D., and
CULLEN D. MORRIS, M.D.
Emory University School of Medicine
Atlanta, Georgia

Atelectasis is diminished gas within the lung associated with a decrease in lung volume and, often, collapse of alveoli. It is a common cause of hypoxemia in hospitalized patients and results from right-to-left shunting and ventilation/perfusion ($\dot{V}/\dot{Q}$) mismatching. Predisposing conditions include an inability to achieve an adequate inspiratory effort, obesity, pre-existing airway disease, and intrabronchial obstruction. The clinical significance of atelectasis is directly related to its duration, the extent of collapse, and the pre-existing pulmonary reserve of the patient. Four mechanisms of atelectasis are recognized: resorption (most common), adhesion, relaxation or compression, and cicatrization (Table 1). Likewise, four patterns of atelectasis occur: total lung, lobar, or segmental; platelike (discoid); round; and generalized or diffuse.

Whether an individual becomes hypoxemic depends heavily on the vigor of the pulmonary hypoxic vasoconstrictor response. Atelectasis most frequently accompanies conditions that limit respiratory excursion, and therefore the patient may experience no specific symptoms or may complain of varying degrees of dyspnea. Occasionally, the patient will have a cough mediated by vagal stretch receptors in the lung. Atelectasis in postsurgical patients develops in the first 48 hours after surgery, and the condition is often worse on the third or fourth postoperative day as the effects accumulate.

Objectively, the patient often has a low-grade fever, and this finding is almost always present in postsurgical patients. In atelectasis of acute onset, tachypnea and tachycardia may be prominent. On physical examination, the physician may find dullness to percussion, egophony, decreased breath sounds, and elevation of the diaphragm. Diffuse microatelectasis may produce dependent end-inspiratory crackles that improve after coughing. The extent of alveolar collapse and right-to-left shunting is apparent in arterial blood gas determinations, which will reveal a low $Pa{O_2}$ and initial hypocapnia.

The chest radiograph is a valuable tool in the diagnosis of atelectasis, and findings vary with the severity of the

TABLE 1. **Causes of Atelectasis**

Resorption/Airway Obstruction
- Mucous plugs
- Blood clots
- Intrabronchial tumor or lesion
- Foreign body aspiration
- External bronchial compression (tumor or lymphadenopathy)
- Endotracheal tube malposition

Microatelectasis
- Adult respiratory distress syndrome
- Respiratory distress syndrome of the newborn
- Acute radiation pneumonitis
- Smoke inhalation
- Prolonged shallow breathing (neuromuscular weakness, obesity, pain)
- Pulmonary embolism

Relaxation/Compression
- Pneumothorax/hydrothorax
- Pulmonary mass or bulla
- Round atelectasis
- Pleural effusion
- Dependent (gravity) atelectasis

Cicatrization
- Pulmonary fibrosis (interstitial disease, old age)
- Chronic infection

abnormality. In addition to its ability to rule out other causes of respiratory dysfunction, radiography may disclose certain dependable radiologic signs of atelectasis. Displacement of the interlobar fissures that form the boundary of an atelectatic lobe and crowding of vessels and bronchi are two "direct signs" of atelectasis on chest radiographs. A local increase in opacity, elevation of the hemidiaphragm, mediastinal displacement, compensatory overinflation of the ipsilateral lung, and displaced hila are five reliable "indirect radiologic signs" of atelectasis.

Computed tomography is rarely necessary in the diagnosis of atelectasis, except in the case of round atelectasis. Round atelectasis is localized peripheral lung collapse near a thickened pleura, with "comet tail" extensions of curvilinear-appearing vessels and bronchi extending toward the hilum. This benign lesion may be confused with a neoplasm.

Proper prevention of atelectasis in all patients is aimed at achieving appropriate inspiratory depth and secretion clearance. Important risk factors include postsurgical recovery, obesity, chronic airway disease, secretion retention, neuromuscular weakness, and pain. Patients who have sustained chest trauma are another high-risk group. Postoperatively, patients should be provided with enough pain medication and persuasion to breath deeply, cough, use an incentive spirometer, and avoid immobility. Patients should use an incentive spirometer every 2 to 4 hours, beginning in the immediate postoperative period as circumstances allow. Occasional judicious use of bronchodilators such as albuterol* (Proventil), 1.25 to 2.5 mg nebulized every 4 to 8 hours, may help prevent atelectasis in susceptible patients.

Treatment of atelectasis begins with identification and management of the cause. Mobilization, periodic deep breathing, and incentive spirometry will help expand collapsed airways. Chest physiotherapy will stimulate vigorous coughing and drainage of secretions. Some physicians propose using intermittent positive-pressure breathing as treatment of atelectasis, but this technique may cause gastric distention, and incentive spirometry is just as effective and less expensive. In recalcitrant cases, nasotracheal aspiration with a sterile catheter may be attempted in awake patients. However, this treatment may contaminate the lower airway with nasopharyngeal flora, and it is not recommended for routine care.

If conservative measures fail or when secretions become copious and tenacious and hypoxemia persists, fiberoptic bronchoscopy should be attempted. Fiberoptic bronchoscopy may be used earlier in critically ill patients who cannot clear secretions by other methods or in patients with total lung atelectasis. Total lung atelectasis in a patient with a history of chest trauma (recent or delayed) may herald a missed tracheobronchial injury and mandates urgent diagnosis with fiberoptic bronchoscopy.

Atelectasis is a common cause of hypoxemia from right-to-left shunting. Its presence warrants a search for the cause. Prevention starts with identifying risk factors, and treatment is initially conservative. After re-expansion of the involved tissue, a prophylactic respiratory program should be instituted to prevent recurrence.

*Not FDA approved for this indication.

CHRONIC OBSTRUCTIVE PULMONARY DISEASE

method of
DEAN GIANAKOS, M.D.
Lynchburg Family Practice Residency
Lynchburg, Virginia

Chronic obstructive pulmonary disease (COPD) is a term that refers to patients who have either chronic bronchitis or emphysema, and progressive airflow obstruction on spirometric examination. *Chronic bronchitis* is usually defined in clinical terms: patients have cough, usually with sputum production, for 3 months in 2 consecutive years. *Emphysema,* on the other hand, is anatomically defined: patients have abnormal enlargement of airways distal to terminal bronchioles as well as destruction of alveolar walls. Clinically, emphysema patients usually have dyspnea on exertion, hyperinflation on physical examination and chest radiographs, and reduced diffusion capacity on pulmonary function testing.

In reality, most COPD patients are smokers who have elements of both emphysema and chronic bronchitis, and present with varying degrees of dyspnea, cough, expectoration, and progressive airflow obstruction on spirometry. Some COPD patients also have an asthmatic component characterized by airway inflammation and partial reversibility of airflow obstruction. Some asthma patients have partial irreversibility of expiratory flow. However, most clinicians do not include asthma in the definition of COPD unless there is progressive decline of airflow over time.

COPD is the fourth leading cause of death in the United States and the 12th most prevalent disease worldwide. The most common cause, cigarette smoking, accounts for over 80% of cases. Air pollution, passive smoking, α_1-antitrypsin deficiency, and other unknown causes account for the rest. For unclear reasons, COPD develops in only 15% of regular smokers. This group experiences accelerated loss of lung function.

Historical clues to the diagnosis of COPD include smok-

TABLE 1. **American Thoracic Society Staging of Disease Severity in Chronic Obstructive Pulmonary Disease**

Stage	FEV_1 (%)
Mild	>49
Moderate	35–49
Severe	<35

ing history, cough, dyspnea (particularly with exertion), expectoration, wheezing, and frequent upper respiratory infections. Physical examination may reveal pursed lip breathing, accessory muscle use, wheezes, decreased breath sounds, and prolonged expiratory times. As previously noted, diagnosis hinges on evidence of airflow obstruction on spirometry (forced expiratory volume in 1 second [FEV_1]/forced vital capacity [FVC] <70%); severity of disease is based on FEV_1 values (Table 1). Although chest radiographs, additional pulmonary function tests (lung volumes and diffusing capacity of lung for carbon monoxide [DLCO]), and chest computed tomography scans are not necessary for diagnosis, they may help exclude other conditions or confirm the diagnosis of COPD.

OUTPATIENT MANAGEMENT OF CHRONIC OBSTRUCTIVE PULMONARY DISEASE

The primary goals of outpatient care for patients with COPD are listed:

- Enhance quality of life
- Minimize further decline of lung function
- Prevent acute exacerbations

The patient-physician relationship should be a collaborative one, with patients making informed decisions under the guidance of their physicians. Ideal outpatient treatment is reviewed in the following sections.

Supportive, Collaborative Relationship

This obvious point needs to be reiterated. There is no cure for COPD. An empathic, caring physician can help patients cope with not only the acute exacerbations but also the many psychosocial issues that arise from living with a chronic illness.

Smoking Cessation

Unless COPD patients quit smoking, they not only risk accelerated decline of lung function but also have increased risk of lung cancer and other medical problems. Physicians have a significant role to play in offering encouragement and education regarding the risks of smoking. Nicotine patches, gum, or nasal sprays can alleviate nicotine withdrawal effects.

The oral antidepressant bupropion (Zyban) can be taken in 150-mg doses once daily for 3 days, then 150 mg can be taken twice daily for 7 to 12 weeks. It is contraindicated in patients with seizures or eating disorders but may be the most effective treatment today, although long-term abstinence data are not available. Patients should be encouraged to talk frequently to their physicians during the cessation process, and to join support groups to help them cope with withdrawal from cigarettes.

Immunizations

Patients with COPD should receive an influenza vaccine every year. They should also receive a one-time vaccination against pneumococcus (Pneumovax). Patients aged 65 and older should be revaccinated if they received their first vaccination more than 5 years previously and were younger than 65 years old at the time of original vaccination.

Bronchodilators

Bronchodilators are the mainstay of pharmacologic therapy for COPD. They can be divided into three groups: β agonists, anticholinergics, and theophylline. For patients with few symptoms and mild disease, short-acting β-agonist drugs such as an albuterol metered-dose inhaler (MDI) (with a spacer), two puffs every 4 to 6 hours as needed, may suffice. Nebulized forms of albuterol are no more effective than metered-dose forms, although some patients prefer the former.

For patients with more significant disease, albuterol MDI in combination with the anticholinergic drug ipratropium (Atrovent), has been shown to be more effective than either drug used alone. A combination inhaler, Combivent, contains both of these drugs and can be used two puffs every 6 hours. Alternatively, ipratropium, two to four puffs every 6 hours, in combination with albuterol, two puffs every 4 to 6 hours as needed, can be used. Longer acting β-agonist inhalers (salmeterol [Serevent], two puffs every 12 hours) have also proved useful, particularly in patients with nocturnal symptoms. In fact, one recent study suggested that it may be better than ipratropium and should be considered a first-line treatment for COPD.

For patients unresponsive to these bronchodilators or unable to use inhalers or nebulizers, oral preparations of theophylline (Slo-bid) may be helpful. The usual starting dose for theophylline is 200 mg every 12 hours, with the goal of maintaining a theophylline level of 8 to 12 mg/mL. Like the β agonists, theophylline can cause nervousness and palpitations. In addition, at higher serum levels, nausea, vomiting, and seizures can occur. It is important to review potential drug interactions because theophylline interacts with many other drugs.

Other Considerations in Outpatient Management

Inhaled Steroids

The use of inhaled steroids for COPD is controversial. However, a recent study suggested that inhaled fluticasone (Flovent) 500 μg twice daily decreases acute exacerbations and slows decline in respiratory health status (no effect on rate of FEV_1 decline). As more studies emerge, inhaled steroids may become a more important arm of therapy. In the meantime, a trial of inhaled steroids, particularly in those patients who have a reversible component of airflow obstruction, may be reasonable.

Oral Steroids

Short bursts of steroids (10–14 days) have been shown to be beneficial to control COPD exacerbations. See Table 2 for indications for hospitalization. However, long-term steroid therapy for patients with COPD is not recommended unless patients experience improvement in FEV_1 after a 2-week trial of therapy (e.g., prednisone 40 mg/d for 2 weeks). Only 20% of patients with COPD will be candidates for steroids. When used, the drug should be tapered to the lowest effective dose to avoid side effects such as cataracts, osteoporosis, hyperglycemia, and weight gain.

Antibiotics

Clinical evidence of infection—change in sputum character, fever, leukocytosis, or infiltrate on chest radiograph—suggests the need for antibiotics. Older antibiotics such as tetracycline, amoxicillin, or trimethoprim-sulfamethoxazole may be as effective as some of the newer agents. However, in patients with more significant underlying COPD and severe symptoms, the newer fluoroquinolones, macrolides, amoxicillin clavulanate (Augmentin), or second-generation cephalosporins are probably more appropriate.

Oxygen Therapy

Patients with Pa_{O_2} less than or equal to 55 mm Hg, as well as patients with a Pa_{O_2} of 56 to 59 mm Hg and evidence of cor pulmonale, should receive long-term oxygen therapy. In these patients, oxygen therapy has been shown to reduce mortality.

TABLE 2. **American Thoracic Society Indications for Hospitalization of Patients With Chronic Obstructive Pulmonary Disease**

1. Patient has acute exacerbation characterized by increased dyspnea, cough, or sputum production, plus one or more of the following:
   - Inadequate response of symptoms to outpatient management
   - Inability to walk between rooms (patient previously mobile)
   - Inability to eat or sleep due to dyspnea
   - Conclusion by family and/or physician that patient cannot manage at home, with supplemental home care resources not immediately available
   - High risk co-morbid condition, pulmonary (e.g., pneumonia) or non-pulmonary
   - Prolonged, progressive symptoms before emergency visit
   - Altered mentation
   - Worsening hypoxemia
   - New or worsening hypercarbia
2. Patient has new or worsening cor pulmonale unresponsive to outpatient management
3. Planned invasive surgical or diagnostic procedure requires analgesics or sedatives that may worsen pulmonary function
4. Co-morbid condition, e.g., severe steroid myopathy or acute vertebral compression fractures, has worsened pulmonary function

Pulmonary Rehabilitation

Pulmonary rehabilitation programs, including exercise training and patient education, have been shown to improve the quality of life for patients with COPD.

Anxiety and Depression

Many patients with COPD experience anxiety and depression as they cope with dyspnea, functional limitations, and the difficulties of living with a chronic illness. Physicians should offer psychosocial support, counseling referral, pulmonary rehabilitation, and appropriate medications as needed.

Air Travel

Many patients with COPD can safely travel by air. For most patients, 1 to 2 L of oxygen per nasal cannula above baseline use will suffice. However, patients with co-morbid conditions and severe disease need to be carefully evaluated before recommending air travel. Consultation with a specialist may be necessary.

Surgical Options

Some patients with COPD have benefited from lung volume reduction surgery, a procedure in which emphysematous lung is removed. This surgery is thought to increase the elastic recoil of the lung and improve the mechanical advantage of the diaphragm. However, it is not considered standard therapy for COPD. An ongoing National Institutes of Health study may better clarify which patients are the best candidates for this operation. Patients with severe COPD (especially α_1-antitrypsin deficiency patients) who also have limited life expectancy (<3 years), minimal co-morbid disease, and are younger than 65 years may be candidates for lung transplantation. This operation can improve quality of life for certain patients. Before transplantation evaluation, referral to a pulmonary specialist is recommended to ensure that medical management has been maximized.

Ethical Issues

Ideal outpatient treatment includes discussions with the patient about prognosis, advance directives, and wishes regarding mechanical ventilation and other means of life support. Acute respiratory failure by itself does not necessarily portend a poor outcome. Prognosis depends on, among other things, severity of illness, co-morbid conditions, and functional status. The patient's preferences for or against life support should be respected, unless the decision compromises the physician's integrity.

Nutrition

Patients with COPD are often malnourished. Physicians should encourage them to achieve ideal body weight by eating well-balanced meals and taking nutritional supplements as needed.

Sleep

Routine sleep studies are not indicated for patients with COPD. Awake Pa_{O_2} levels usually predict the need for nocturnal oxygen therapy. However, sleep studies should be considered in patients with COPD suspected of having obstructive sleep apnea or unexplained cor pulmonale.

INPATIENT MANAGEMENT OF CHRONIC OBSTRUCTIVE PULMONARY DISEASE

The primary goals of inpatient care of COPD patients are to reverse or eliminate the precipitating factors of an exacerbation (i.e., congestive heart failure, pneumonia, upper respiratory viral infections, or pneumothorax), to restore patients to prehospital functional status, and to reinforce outpatient goals as the patient recovers. Table 2 refers to American Thoracic Society guidelines for hospitalization of patients with COPD. In cases of persistent hypoxemia and worsening respiratory acidosis, admission to an intensive care unit (with frequent clinical assessment and arterial blood-gas [ABG] analysis and preparation for possible ventilatory support) must be considered.

Like outpatient management, bronchodilators and steroids remain the cornerstones of inpatient management of COPD.

Bronchodilator Therapy

As in outpatient management, combination therapy with albuterol and ipratropium is indicated. More frequent administration of an albuterol MDI or nebulization treatments (every 1–2 hours as needed) may be required for patients on the verge of respiratory failure.

Steroids

Recent data show that systemic glucocorticoid treatment improves clinical outcomes (shorter hospital stays and reduced airflow obstruction) among patients hospitalized for COPD exacerbations. Methylprednisolone (Solu-Medrol) 60 to 125 mg intravenously every 6 hours usually suffices. When the patient's condition stabilizes, the steroid can be converted to oral form and the dose tapered over 10 to 14 days.

Antibiotics

For a more complete review, see the section on outpatient management. For sicker patients with evidence of infection, consider intravenous antibiotics. Also consider sputum cultures to guide antibiotic choice in patients with severe exacerbations or patients unresponsive to empiric therapy.

Oxygen

Use ABG levels to monitor oxygen therapy and the possible development of respiratory acidosis. Titrate oxygen to keep Pa_{O_2} above 55 and oxygen saturations greater than 88%. This level of oxygen saturation should be maintained even in the presence of carbon dioxide retention. However, when titrating oxygen levels, the physician must carefully watch for the development of respiratory failure and frequently assess the need for ventilatory support.

Noninvasive Mechanical Ventilation

Physicians should consider this mode of respiratory support for patients with significant respiratory acidosis and clinical signs of fatigue. Initial inspiratory mask pressures of 15 cm and expiratory pressures of 5 cm can later be adjusted per ABG analysis. If the patient does not tolerate the mask or respiratory failure worsens, endotracheal intubation with mechanical ventilation is indicated, assuming that the patient desires invasive, respiratory support.

Most patients with COPD are smokers who have evidence of both chronic bronchitis and emphysema and who present with varying degrees of dyspnea, cough, expectoration, and progressive airflow obstruction on spirometry. A collaborative, patient-centered approach goes a long way toward helping these patients live fulfilling lives. Bronchodilators, steroids, antibiotics, and supplemental oxygen remain the cornerstones of medical therapy, and along with continuous patient education and pulmonary rehabilitation, help to improve the patient's quality of life. Certain patients may be candidates for lung transplantation or lung volume reduction surgery.

CYSTIC FIBROSIS

method of
SUSANNA A. McCOLLEY, M.D.
Cystic Fibrosis Center, Children's Memorial Hospital
Chicago, Illinois

Cystic fibrosis (CF) is the most common life-shortening genetic disease in whites, with a frequency of approximately 1:3300 live births in the United States. It occurs in all ethnic groups; unique gene mutations occur in different populations. CF is an autosomal recessive disorder caused by mutations in the cystic fibrosis transmembrane regulator (*CFTR*) gene, discovered in 1989. *CFTR* codes for a membrane-bound protein that conducts chloride through the apical membrane of epithelial cells and serves as a regulator of other apical membrane ion channels. Defective *CFTR* causes abnormalities in sodium and chloride transport in multiple organs. The major clinical manifestations of CF are seen in the sinopulmonary tract, the digestive system, the reproductive tract, and the sweat glands.

CF may be diagnosed from a variety of clinical findings. Approximately 15% of newborns with CF exhibit meconium ileus, a disorder of impacted meconium in the intestine, which causes bowel obstruction and, sometimes, intestinal volvulus or atresia. Others are diagnosed from failure to gain weight, steatorrhea, acute or chronic respiratory symptoms (e.g., cough, wheezing, or pneumonia), or a combination of these findings. Important, although rarer, presentations include obstructive jaundice, hyponatremia and metabolic alkalosis, nasal polyposis, chronic sinusitis, recurrent acute pancreatitis, and male infertility due to congenital absence of the vas deferens. An increasing number of patients are being diagnosed by newborn screening methods, which are currently employed in a number of states, or by prenatal diagnostic techniques. Although the majority of affected individuals are diagnosed in the first year of life, 20% are diagnosed after the fifth birthday and a growing number of cases are being diagnosed in adults.

The diagnosis of CF requires documentation of clinical features or a family history of CF and at least one of the following:

1. Sweat chloride greater than 60 mmol/L by quantitative pilocarpine iontophoresis on two occasions
2. Demonstration of two CF-causing *CFTR* mutations by blood or buccal mucosal cell analysis
3. Demonstration of abnormal potential difference across the nasal mucosa.

Appropriate measurement of sweat chloride by pilocarpine iontophoresis requires complex methodology and is best performed at centers that frequently perform such testing. It is impractical for most community hospitals and freestanding laboratories. A sweat conductivity test (Wescor Sweat-Chek) is a highly sensitive screening test; positive tests must be confirmed by a pilocarpine iontophoresis sweat test or another method described previously. *CFTR* mutation screening is specific but relatively insensitive as a first-line test because although more than 900 *CFTR* gene mutations cause CF, only 90 to 120 can be efficiently screened by current techniques. The accuracy of genetic testing depends on the ethnic origin of the patient; cases in 90% of Northern European whites and 97% of Ashkenazic Jews will be ascertained, whereas accuracy is much lower in Hispanic, African American, and Asian populations. Nasal potential difference measurements are primarily used as a research tool at large CF centers; this technique is used primarily in atypical cases with negative or borderline sweat chloride measurements and lack of a confirmatory CF genotype.

MAINTENANCE THERAPY

The major goals of maintenance or preventive therapy for CF are to maintain normal nutritional status, to decrease the frequency of symptomatic respiratory infections (pulmonary exacerbations), and to slow the decline in pulmonary function over time. During the past several decades, these maintenance strategies have resulted in a significant increase in life expectancy for individuals with CF. General maintenance therapy should include age-appropriate health maintenance visits, including routine immunizations and annual influenza vaccination. CF-specific maintenance therapy, discussed later, should be overseen during regularly scheduled visits in a specialized care center staffed by a multidisciplinary care team. In the United States, the Cystic Fibrosis Foundation provides oversight of and accreditation for CF centers.

PULMONARY THERAPY

Cystic fibrosis causes chronic pulmonary infection and inflammation that result in bronchiectasis and declining pulmonary function over time. Chronic cough; production of thick, tenacious sputum; and physical examination findings of chest hyperexpansion, crackles, and digital clubbing occur as a result. Lung disease causes premature death in more than 90% of affected individuals. The onset and the clinical course of pulmonary symptoms in individuals with CF is highly variable; however, recent studies demonstrate that even asymptomatic infants with CF have profound neutrophilic inflammation in the lungs. Strategies to aid mucociliary clearance, decrease sputum viscosity, decrease inflammation, and decrease burden of infection in the lung are mainstays of therapy. Commonly used drugs are listed in Table 1.

For the majority of patients with CF, airway clearance techniques are prescribed, which aid in loosening secretions from airway walls, and coughing or postural techniques are used to increase sputum clearance and improve pulmonary function. Manual percussion and postural drainage have historically been most widely used; these techniques require a trained caregiver but are effort independent for the patient, making them useful during infancy and early childhood. Older children and adults benefit from techniques that can be performed independently. An active cycle of breathing and autogenic drainage requires training from an expert respiratory therapist and a motivated patient but requires no special devices. Positive expiratory pressure devices, the Flutter device, intrapulmonary percussive ventilation, and high-frequency chest wall oscillation (the ThAIRapy Bronchial Drainage System) are other independently administered options. Patients should be assessed by an experienced respiratory therapist before prescription of such devices and periodically thereafter.

In CF, sputum viscosity is greatly increased by the presence of DNA in sputum, which results from degradation of neutrophils in the airways. Dornase alfa (Pulmozyme) (recombinant human DNAse 1), given by inhalation once daily, improves sputum viscosity, improves FEV_1 modestly, and decreases the frequency of pulmonary exacerbations requiring intravenous antibiotic therapy.

Because profound airway inflammation contributes significantly to the decline in pulmonary function over time in CF, anti-inflammatory agents have been studied. Prednisone, at a dose of 1 mg/kg every other day, improves lung function modestly but has side effects, including a long-term decrease in height. High-dose ibuprofen has been demonstrated to decrease FEV_1 decline in CF; dosing must be based on pharmacokinetic studies. Renal insufficiency or failure has been reported during ibuprofen administration; renal function must be monitored and the drug held when patients are receiving concomitant aminoglycoside therapy. Inhaled corticosteroids and

TABLE 1. **Pulmonary Maintenance Therapy**

Drug or Drug Class	Dose	Comments
β Agonists Short acting (e.g., albuterol [Proventil]) Long acting (e.g., salmeterol [Serevent])	Short acting: 2–4 puffs via MDI or 2.5 mg albuterol or equivalent via nebulizer before airway clearance and as needed Long acting: 2 puffs via MDI or 1 puff via diskhaler bid	
Dornase alfa (rhDNase, Pulmozyme)	2.5 mg via nebulizer qd	Use manufacturer's recommended nebulizer and compressor.
Ibuprofen (Motrin)	20–30 mg/kg/dose q12h	Pharmacokinetic studies must be performed before initiation and every 24 months and/or when body weight increases by 25%. Monitor renal function and gastrointestinal symptoms. Stop medication during intravenous aminoglycoside administration. Do not substitute generic products.
Tobramycin for inhalation (TOBI)	300 mg bid, 28 days on therapy followed by 28 days off	Use manufacturer's recommended nebulizer and compressor.
Prednisone	1 mg/kg qod	Use for a maximum of 24 months. Monitor for glucose intolerance, cataracts, and decreased linear growth velocity.

Abbreviation: MDI = metered-dose inhaler.

cromolyn sodium are widely prescribed but have not undergone evaluation in large clinical trials.

Chronic pulmonary infection with *Pseudomonas aeruginosa* occurs in the majority of affected individuals. Strategies to eradicate *P. aeruginosa* infection temporarily and to suppress the organism have been employed with increasing frequency during the past decade. Tobramycin for inhalation (TOBI) is a proprietary formulation of preservative-free tobramycin; chronic intermittent administration improves FEV_1 and decreases the risk of symptomatic pulmonary exacerbation in *P. aeruginosa*–infected patients older than 5 years of age with a baseline FEV_1 of 25% to 75% predicted.

Specific manufacturers' recommendations for nebulizer and compressor use with inhalational drugs should be followed. Patients and their caregivers should be taught appropriate care and replacement of nebulizers to avoid contamination and poor nebulizer output.

NUTRITIONAL THERAPY

Individuals affected with CE should eat a high-calorie diet with unrestricted fat and liberal salt. Caloric requirements are at least 120%, and may exceed 150%, of the recommended daily allowance for age. Malnourished patients and those with advanced lung disease require additional calories and often benefit from supplements delivered orally or by nasogastric or gastrostomy tube. Growth and weight maintenance should be monitored, and dietary advice should be overseen by an experienced dietitian.

Most individuals with CF have pancreatic insufficiency and require pancreatic enzyme supplementation for adequate digestive function. Enzymes should be titrated to optimal clinical effect within the guidelines delineated in Table 2. Excessive doses of pancreatic enzymes are associated with the development of fibrosing colonopathy, which causes colonic stricture and usually requires surgical therapy. Because pancreatic enzymes lose efficacy in an acid environment, addition of an H_2 antagonist or a proton pump inhibitor may be helpful in enhancing enzyme effectiveness without increasing dose.

Supplementation of fat-soluble vitamins is necessary to avoid vitamin deficiency in CF. All patients should receive multivitamins, preferably formulations with water-miscible A, D, E, and K. Additional A, D, E, or K supplements are needed when deficiency states or certain complications, such as cirrhosis, exist. Annual monitoring of vitamin A and E levels is recommended.

COMPLICATIONS

Pulmonary Complications

The most common complication of CF is pulmonary exacerbation; approximately one in three affected individuals will require hospitalization for this complication in any given year. Pulmonary exacerbation is defined as an increase in cough and sputum production, usually accompanied by other clinical findings, such as new or increased crackles on physical examination, weight loss, and decline in FEV_1. Fever and radiographic findings of lobar pulmonary infiltrates only occasionally occur. Treatment includes antibiotics and increased administration of airway clearance techniques; nutritional rehabilitation is also important because pulmonary exacerbation is accompanied by both increased metabolic demands and anorexia.

Antibiotic therapy should be selected based on results of a sputum or pharyngeal culture that is processed appropriately for the detection of CF-related organisms. This processing must include special media for isolation of *Burkholderia cepacia* and for avoiding overgrowth of *P. aeruginosa* in the detection

TABLE 2. **Nutritional Maintenance Therapy**

Drug	Dosage	Comments
Multivitamins with water-miscible vitamins A, D, E, and K (ADEK, Vitamax)	Infants: 1 mL liquid/d (ADEK only) Children <10 years: 1 tablet/d or 2 mL/d Adults and children ≥10 years: 2 tablets/d	Most patients receiving these preparations will not require additional vitamin A, D, E, or K. Monitor vitamin levels annually.
Vitamin A	1,500–10,000 IU/d	Treatment of vitamin A deficiency requires higher doses for short-term repletion.
Vitamin E	5–10 IU/kg/d (maximum 400 IU)	
Vitamin K	2.5–5 mg twice weekly	Needed for patients with liver disease. Many experts recommend vitamin K supplementation during the first 12 months of life and during prolonged antibiotic therapy.
Pancreatic enzymes (Pancrease, Ultrase, Creon, Pancrecarb)	500–2,500 lipase units/kg/meal; ½ usual dose with snacks	Do not exceed 10,000 lipase units/kg/d. Do not substitute generic products.
Cimetidine (Tagamet)*	10–40 mg/kg/d divided q6h	Not FDA approved for this indication.
Ranitidine (Zantac)*	3–5 mg/kg/d divided q12h	Not FDA approved for this indication.
Omeprazole (Prilosec)*	2.5–20 mg qd to bid	Not FDA approved for infants and young children. Doses <10 mg may be prepared by opening capsules or by preparation of an extemporaneous suspension.

*Not FDA approved for this indication.

of *Staphylococcus aureus*. Mucoid phenotypes of *P. aeruginosa* should be reported. Initial antibiotic choice is usually based on a culture obtained during a routine medical encounter; guidelines recommend that all patients have a culture at least annually and as indicated based on clinical course. Antibiotics may be given orally, by inhalation, or intravenously; the route of administration depends on the severity of exacerbation and underlying lung disease, the specific organisms targeted, and other individual considerations, such as previous response to therapy. Intravenous therapy for *P. aeruginosa* should include two antibiotic agents, usually a β-lactam and an aminoglycoside; generally, a course of 14 to 21 days is needed. Intravenous antibiotic therapy can be administered at home to an adequately stable patient who has good adherence and the ability to perform enhanced airway clearance in the home setting. Commonly prescribed antibiotics are listed in Table 3.

Infection with antibiotic-resistant organisms is a significant problem in CF. *B. cepacia* is an inherently resistant gram-negative plant pathogen that may cause a sepsis syndrome or rapidly declining lung function. Other inherently resistant organisms include *Stenotrophomonas maltophilia* and *Alcaligenes xylososidans*. Methicillin-resistant *S. aureus* and multiply resistant strains of *P. aeruginosa* also challenge clinicians.

Other pulmonary complications include hemoptysis, pneumothorax, and respiratory failure. Minor hemoptysis is usually a symptom of pulmonary exacerbation and requires antibiotic therapy; many clinicians withhold airway clearance techniques until frank bleeding has stopped. Major hemoptysis is treated with bronchial artery embolization. Pneumothorax, unless very small, rarely responds to conservative therapy. Thoracostomy tube placement and pleurodesis are often required. Lung transplantation is frequently performed in patients with chronic respiratory failure; waiting times for organs may be greater than 2 years, so recognition of patients who are likely to die within several years is critical in making timely referrals. Noninvasive ventilation through bilevel positive airway pressure may help alleviate dyspnea and may help stabilize blood gases in patients awaiting transplantation. Expert palliative care is essential for patients in the terminal phases of illness.

Upper Airway Disease

Although chronic inflammatory changes of the paranasal sinuses are almost always detectable in individuals with CF through radiographic techniques, symptoms are variable. Medical or surgical therapy should therefore be reserved for patients who have both significant symptoms and radiographic findings. Nasal polyposis occurs in approximately 3% of patients; it tends to recur after surgical therapy, which is reserved for patients with significant obstructive symptoms or refractory sinusitis.

Diabetes Mellitus

Approximately 15% of affected individuals develop diabetes; rare in individuals younger than 10 years of age, the risk increases with age. Insulin deficiency is present, but ketoacidosis is rare. Thus, CF-related diabetes is distinct from either type 1 or type 2 diabetes. Many teenagers and young adults with CF have glucose intolerance manifested as intermittent hyperglycemia, which may become clinically significant during pulmonary exacerbation, corticosteroid therapy, or other forms of stress. Screening of random blood glucose levels is recommended annually in stable patients and during pulmonary exacerbation. An increasing number of CF centers perform routine oral glucose tolerance testing. Insulin is the treat-

TABLE 3. **Antibiotics for Treatment of Pulmonary Exacerbation***

Drug	Dose	Comments
Aminoglycosides		Monitor for renal and ototoxicity
Tobramycin (Nebcin)	7.5–15 mg/kg/d IV divided q8h or q24h	Monitor drug levels: Trough ≤2 μg/mL Peak 8–12 μg/mL (q8h regimen)
Gentamicin (Garamycin)	7.5–15 mg/kg/d IV divided q8–q12h	Monitor drug levels: Trough ≤2 μg/mL Peak 8–12 μg/mL
Amikacin (Amikin)	30 mg/kg/d IV divided q8–12h	Monitor drug levels: Trough ≤10 μg/mL Peak 25–40 μg/mL
β Lactams		
PENICILLINS		
Dicloxacillin (Diclox)	25–45 mg/kg/d PO divided q12h (maximum dose: 875 mg q12h)	
Nafcillin (Nafcil)	50–100 mg/kg/d IV q4–6h (maximum dose: 12 g/d)	
Piperacillin (Pipracil)	400–600 mg/kg/d IV divided q4–6h (maximum dose: 24 g/d)	
Piperacillin/tazobactam (Zosyn)	400–600 mg/kg/d IV divided q4–6h (maximum dose: 24 g/d)	
Ticarcillin (Ticar)	400–600 mg/kg/d IV divided q4–6h (maximum dose: 24 g/d)	
Ticarcillin/clavulanic acid (Timentin)	400–600 mg/kg/d IV divided q4–6h (maximum dose: 24 g/d)	
OTHER β LACTAMS		
Cephalexin (Keflex)	50–100 mg/kg/d PO divided q6h (maximum dose: 2 g/d)	
Ceftazidime (Fortaz)	150–300 mg/kg/d IV divided q8h (maximum dose: 6 g/d)	
Aztreonam (Azactam)	150–200 mg/kg/d IV divided q8h (maximum dose: 8 g/d)	
Imipenem (Primaxin)	60–100 mg/kg/d IV divided q6h (maximum dose: 4 g/d)	
Meropenem (Merrem)	120 mg/kg/d IV divided q8h (maximum dose: 4 g/d)	
Fluoroquinolones		
Ciprofloxacin (Cipro)	20–50 mg/kg/d PO divided bid–tid 10–15 mg/kg/d IV divided q12h	
Levofloxacin (Levaquin)	500 mg PO qd (adults)	Dosage not established for children
Other Antibiotics		
Trimethorrim-sulfamethoxazole (Bactrim, Septra)	8–10 mg/kg/d PO of trimethoprim divided q8–12h 10–20 mg/kg/d IV of trimethoprim component divided q6h	
Azithromycin (Zithromax)	10 mg/kg/d PO first day (maximum dose: 500 mg) 5 mg/kg/d PO days 2–5 (maximum dose 250 mg)	
Doxycycline (Vibramycin, Doxy-tab, Dynacin)	4–6 mg/kg/d PO divided bid	Do not use in children <8 years of age
Clindamycin (Cleocin)	20–40 mg/kg/d PO divided q8h	
Vancomycin (Vancocin)	30–60 mg/kg/d IV divided q12h (maximum dose: 2 g/d)	Reserve for use with resistant organisms (e.g., methicillin-resistant *Staphylococcus aureus*)
Colistin (Colymycin)	5–7 mg/kg/d IV divided q8h (maximum dose: 100 mg q8h)	Neurotoxicity and nephrotoxicity may occur; usually reserved for highly resistant *Pseudomonas aeruginosa* infections

*Assumes normal renal function.

ment of choice for CF-related diabetes; calorie and fat intake should not be restricted.

Gastrointestinal Complications

Distal intestinal obstruction syndrome is a common complication. It is believed to occur because of dehydration of distal ileal and colonic secretions, usually in conjunction with malabsorption, leading to increased fecal mass. Presenting symptoms include abdominal pain, sometimes with constipation or frank obstipation. A palpable mass of fecal material may be present on physical examination. Radiographic images reveal abundant fecal material throughout the colon. Although mild cases may be treated with stool softeners, oral hydration, and adjustment of enzyme dosage, more significant disease requires hospitalization, intravenous hydration, and bowel cleansing using a balanced intestinal lavage solution (such as GoLYTELY), generally through a nasogastric tube. Enemas with *N*-acetylcysteine (Mucomyst) may be helpful if severe distal impaction is present.

Gastroesophageal reflux disease occurs in many affected individuals and is particularly problematic in infants and patients with severe lung disease. H_2

blocking agents, proton pump inhibitors, and prokinetic agents are helpful in managing this disorder; occasional patients require surgical therapy.

The liver is affected in CF; virtually all patients have elevation of serum alkaline phosphatase levels; many have elevated hepatic enzyme levels; and 2% to 5% develop severe cirrhosis. Liver transplantation is an accepted therapy for patients with adequate pulmonary function. Ursodeoxycholic acid (Actigall) at a dose of 20 mg/kg/day improves transaminase level elevation, but its long-term impact on development of cirrhosis is unknown.

Pancreatitis may occur in CF; it is more common in patients with pancreatic insufficiency. Treatment includes pain management and bowel rest; rarely, surgical resection is required. Rarer but important gastrointestinal complications of CF include appendicitis, intussusception, and fibrosing colonopathy. Recently, an increased risk of gastrointestinal tract malignancy in adults with CF was reported in a large epidemiologic study.

Osteoporosis

Osteopenia, osteoporosis, pathologic fractures, kyphosis, and scoliosis occur in CF. Patients with severe lung disease or malnutrition and those on long-term corticosteroid therapy are at increased risk. Maintenance of normal body weight and adequate calcium, vitamin D, and vitamin K intake are important preventive measures. Bisphosphonate therapy appears promising but remains under evaluation.

SLEEP DISORDERED BREATHING

method of
CARLOS A. VAZ FRAGOSO, M.D.
Gaylord Hospital
Wallingford, Connecticut

Sleep disordered breathing (SDB) describes a heterogeneous group that includes nonapneic snoring, obstructive sleep apnea-hypopnea syndrome (OSAHS), central sleep apnea (CSA), and various forms of central and peripheral alveolar hypoventilation. This discussion is limited to obstructive SDB, which represents a continuum ranging from snoring to OSAHS. In the setting of a laboratory measured apnea-hypopnea index (AHI) greater than or equal to 5 is termed *OSAHS,* commonly referred to as *sleep apnea.* If the AHI is less than 5, it is termed *nonapneic snoring.*

PUBLIC HEALTH

It is imperative to evaluate driving risk in SDB (Table 1). OSAHS has an odds ratio of 6.3 for a sleep-related accident. In one study, continuous positive airway pressure (CPAP) in OSAHS reduced the number of motor vehicle accident hospital days from 885 to 84 during a 12-month period before and after CPAP therapy. In other studies, 3% of sleep-related motor vehicle accidents involved large trucks with drivers who had a twofold to threefold risk for OSAHS. Truck drivers are prone to SDB because they tend to be middle-aged men who are overweight, have broad necks, and work varying shifts. Truck driving is considered the most dangerous occupation in the United States with 857 deaths in 1997.

SDB can lead to cognitive dysfunction and contribute to poor work performance. A study of 201 medical students taking examinations in internal medicine identified snoring as a risk factor for failing. In a study of 50 patients with severe OSAHS, most showed cognitive impairment with deficits in thinking, perception, memory, communication, or ability to learn new information. In another study, an AHI of 15 (moderate OSAHS) was equivalent to a reduction in psychometric efficiency of 5 additional years of age or to 50% of that typically seen with sedative-hypnotic use. Depression and delirium have also been reported in OSAHS with subsequent reversal after treatment with CPAP.

SDB may result in a poor medical outcome and higher health care utilization. Snoring, for example, has an increased prevalence in patients with hypertension and cardiovascular and cerebrovascular disease. Snoring is also common in pregnancy (23%) and may lead to fetal growth retardation. It can be a sign of pregnancy-induced hypertension, and, in preeclampsia, CPAP attenuates sleep-induced increments in blood pressure. OSAHS can be especially devastating. It has many systemic manifestations (Table 2) and, at an apnea index greater than or equal to 20, the 8-year survival rate is only 63%.

PATHOPHYSIOLOGY

Obstructive SDB is characterized by upper airway instability due to anatomic narrowing and sleep-induced reductions in neuromuscular control. Common anatomic findings in SDB include excessive parapharyngeal wall adipose tissue and increases in the size of the tongue, soft palate, and uvula. These are typically related to obesity and reduce the lateral diameter of the upper airway. Other relevant abnormalities include a high, arched hard palate with maxillary constriction; tonsillar hypertrophy; micrognathia; retrognathia; or acromegaly. Chronic rhinosinusitis may

TABLE 1. **Driving Risk in Obstructive Sleep Apnea-Hypopnea Syndrome**

Assessment of driving risk requires an awareness of licensing criteria in one's own state.
The following may assist in decision-making:
Patients with a sleep disorder as defined by the American Academy of Sleep Medicine International Classification need to be reported to a licensing authority if they are . . .

1. Sleepy as reflected . . .
   by an Epworth Sleepiness Scale Score >8, *or*
   by an average sleep latency of <10 min on a Multiple Sleep Latency Test, *or*
   as judged by the clinical history
2. *and* have a history of a motor vehicle accident or close call as judged by the clinical history
3. *and* whose treatment as judged by the clinical history cannot be expeditiously implemented (within 2 months of diagnosis) *or*
   is unsuccessful *or*
   is refused by the patient *or*
   the patient is unwilling to restrict driving until effective treatment is instituted

Data from Am J Respir Crit Care Med 1994, 150:1463–1473; JAMA 1998, 279:1908–1913.

Table 2. **Complications of Obstructive Sleep Apnea-Hypopnea Syndrome**

Excessive daytime sleepiness
Neuropsychiatric impairment
Reduced cognition or mood, delirium
Erectile dysfunction
Secondary sleep enuresis
Sleep-related gastroesophageal reflux
Awakening headaches
Peripheral neuropathy
Cardiovascular morbidity
Systemic or pulmonary hypertension, right ventricular dysfunction, myocardial infarction, congestive heart failure, cardiac arrhythmias
Cerebrovascular accidents

also exacerbate SDB by increasing upper airway resistance and predisposes to mouth breathing during sleep, which can lead to abnormal airway dynamics favoring pharyngeal collapse and posterior migration of the tongue.

There are often multiple sites of anatomic narrowing in SDB. In a study of 64 patients with OSAHS, the most common site was at the level of the soft palate (81%), but there were also multiple (60%) and secondary (66%) sites of narrowing. This, in part, explains the limited response of SDB to site-specific interventions in contrast to CPAP, which stabilizes the entire upper airway.

Neuromuscular control of the upper airway in SDB is complex but can be summarized as follows: *the principle upper airway dilator muscle is the genioglossus.* In the awake individual with reduced upper airway patency, there is a compensatory increase in genioglossus activity. When asleep, the compensation is reduced, resulting in a collapsible upper airway and obstructive SDB. The etiology of this sleep-induced loss of compensation is unknown. Habitual snoring, due to repetitive vibratory injury, further perpetuates neuromuscular instability by inducing progressive local neurogenic lesions.

Laboratory manifestations of upper airway instability include snoring and hypoventilation. Snoring, however, is neither necessary for, nor diagnostic of, clinically significant SDB. On polysomnography (PSG), there may be sleep fragmentation characterized by electroencephalographic-defined arousals subsequent to an increase in respiratory effort, snoring, or obstructive hypoventilation (Table 3). Obstructive hypoventilation can be further complicated by cardiac arrhythmias and hypoxemia, the severity of which depends on the duration and frequency of respiratory events, baseline oxygen stores in the lung, and co-morbidity.

The clinical manifestations of upper airway instability are derived from chronic sleep deprivation and vascular injury. The responsible mechanisms include chronic sleep fragmentation, recurrent sleep-induced hypoxemia, and repetitive activation of the sympathetic nervous system. At a molecular level, there is involvement of various cytokines, atrial natriuretic factor, and hyperleptinemia.

Nonapneic Snoring

Thirty-four percent of adults report snoring, and 19% are so loud they can be heard through a closed door. Most do not have OSAHS and are, thus, categorized as having nonapneic snoring (AHI <5). Nonapneic snoring is not a benign diagnosis given its association with adverse medical outcomes, cognitive impairment, and difficult bedroom arrangements. In one study, elimination of snoring translated to an additional 62 minutes of sleep per night for the spouses of snorers. Nonapneic snoring has also been identified as an independent risk factor for excessive daytime sleepiness (EDS). This specifically refers to the upper airway resistance syndrome (UARS) (see Table 3), which is a known cause of EDS and may contribute to the development of hypertension. UARS is a possibility in the setting of nonapneic snoring with complaints of fatigue or EDS, and laboratory-defined respiratory effort-related arousals (RERAs). The diagnosis can be a problem because UARS may not always be associated with snoring or RERAs, but only with fatigue or drowsiness.

Treatment of nonapneic snoring emphasizes preventive measures, which are identical to those outlined in the section, Treatment of Obstructive Sleep Apnea-Hypopnea Syndrome. CPAP therapy is also a consideration but is reserved for symptomatic snoring, that is, UARS. Unfortu-

Table 3. **Laboratory Definitions of Obstructive Sleep-Disordered Breathing**

Respiratory Event	Definition	Physiologic Consequence
RERA (adult)	EEG-based arousals associated with increased respiratory effort or snoring. The respiratory effort is best determined by esophageal balloon manometry but may also be assessed by qualitatively analyzing inspiratory airflow morphology, magnitude of respiratory effort, or the presence of snoring in the 1–3 breaths before an EEG arousal.	Sleep fragmentation Nonrestorative sleep
Obstructive Apnea (adult)	a ≥10-s cessation in flow despite continued respiratory effort.	Sleep-induced hypoventilation
Hypopnea (adult)	>30%–50% reduction in flow (≥10 s) associated with a ≥3% O_2 desat or with an EEG arousal. It is obstructive if associated with paradoxical breathing, snoring or arousals.	Sleep-induced hypoventilation
AHI (adult)	The number of apneas and hypopneas per hour of sleep. AHI ≥5 confirms OSAHS.	Sleep-induced hypoventilation Sleep fragmentation Nonrestorative sleep
RERA Index (adult)	The number of RERAs per hour of sleep. RERA Index ≥10–15 with an AHI <5 suggests UARS.	Sleep fragmentation Nonrestorative sleep

Abbreviations: AHI = apena-hyponea Index; EEG = electroencephalogram; Index = average per hour of sleep; OSAHS = obstructive sleep apnea-hypopnea syndrome; RERA = respiratory effort related arousals; UARS = upper airway resistance syndrome.

nately, the CPAP acceptance rate in nonapneic snoring averages less than 20%. In the absence of drowsiness or fatigue, there is no role for CPAP in nonapneic snoring.

Treatment of snoring as a socially disruptive behavior may also include external nasal dilation (e.g., Breathe Right strips), adjustable mandibular advancement devices (e.g., Herbst or Klearway), and site-specific ear, nose, and throat interventions. Site-specific interventions include adenotonsillectomy, uvulopalatopharyngoplasty, laser-assisted uvulopalatoplasty, and radiation frequency volumetric reduction of the soft palate (somnoplasty). These procedures can reduce the intensity of snoring and its antisocial complications. However, before surgery, OSAHS should be excluded because the patient may develop silent SDB given the subsequent elimination of snoring as a marker of disease activity. These treatments remain to be validated in UARS.

DIAGNOSIS OF OBSTRUCTIVE SLEEP APNEA-HYPOPNEA SYNDROME

In the United States, 2% of women and 4% of men have symptomatic OSAHS, defined as an AHI of ≥5 associated with EDS. Of these, less than 10% have ever sought medical attention. Another 10% of adult females and 25% of adult males have asymptomatic OSAHS.

History and Physical Examination

Historic factors identify those at risk for OSAHS. These include snoring, obesity, observed SDB, hypertension, and EDS. The latter is reflected in an Epworth Sleepiness Scale score of greater than 8, a self-administered questionnaire measuring perceived drowsiness. Clinical judgment is necessary because these risk factors lack 100% sensitivity or specificity. For example, the combination of snoring, obesity, observed SDB, and hypertension has a sensitivity of 50% to 85% and a specificity of 30% to 70% for predicting OSAHS. Obesity with a large neck establishes the greatest risk, with a threefold increase for OSAHS. Clinical tools such as the Berlin Questionnaire, which address snoring behavior, obesity, hypertension, and wake-time drowsiness or fatigue, may be used to identify those at risk. Although relevant to medical care, the physical examination is limited. In a study of 200 patients with OSAHS, only 3 had a correctable anatomic abnormality.

Polysomnography

PSG records multiple physiologic parameters at the patient's usual major sleep schedule (Level I study) (Table 4). The PSG determines the presence and severity of SDB. An AHI greater than or equal to 5 is confirmatory of OSAHS. The AHI is also assessed specific to rapid eye movement (REM) sleep. For example, a REM-specific AHI greater than or equal to 15 over at least 30 minutes of REM sleep is a validated cause of EDS even if the overall AHI is normal at less than 5.0. This defines REM-specific OSAHS. A cautionary note regarding PSG is advised. In a study of 37 patients with OSAHS undergoing two consecutive PSGs, 22% were only correctly diagnosed on the second night, and 32% demonstrated an AHI that varied by 10 or more. Such data reflect variability in sampling during supine and REM sleep and confounding variables such as the previous week's sleep-wake schedule and recent use of sedative-hypnotics or alcohol. This emphasizes the importance of pursuing a second PSG in patients at high risk for SDB if results of the first PSG are negative.

Laboratory testing for SDB is expensive. Traditionally, the diagnostic and therapeutic (CPAP) components are performed on two separate nights of testing. To limit cost, split-night PSGs have been advocated as a means to reduce the number of laboratory-based PSGs. It combines into one night both diagnostic and therapeutic evaluations while using a diagnostic AHI threshold of 20 to 40. However, up to 25% of planned split-night PSGs will not meet criteria for initiating CPAP on that same night, despite CPAP's subsequent demonstrated need. This is a consequence of the diagnostic and therapeutic requirement to sample during supine and REM sleep. In general, when CPAP titrations are for fewer than 3 hours of sleep, CPAP prescription can lead to subtherapeutic or excessive pressure levels. Additionally, compliance with CPAP is lower for split-night studies, averaging a nightly use of 3.8 versus 5.2 hours for full-night titrations. As a result, split-night PSGs should be considered successful only if the diagnostic AHI is greater than or equal to 20, CPAP titrations include at least 3 hours of sleep, and there is adequate sleep sampling during REM and in the supine position.

Unattended ambulatory sleep studies have also been proposed as a cost-effective strategy. The American Academy of Sleep Medicine advocates home-based sleep apnea screening with either Level II or III testing (see Table 4). Recordings that only use oxygen saturation as measured by pulse oximetry (Spo_2) are not reliable as a screening tool. Indications for ambulatory studies are limited to a diagnostic assessment in the following situations:

1. When the patient has severe symptoms consistent with OSAHS, treatment is urgent, and standard PSG is not readily available

TABLE 4. **Laboratory Diagnosis of Obstructive Sleep-Disordered Breathing**

Data	Level of Laboratory Evaluation			
	I	*II*	*III*	*IV*
Sleep laboratory, technologist attended	X			
Home-based, unattended		X	X	
Sleep staging (EEG, EOG, chin EMG)	X	X		
Respiratory indices (airflow, respiratory effort, Spo_2, snoring)	X	X	X	
Spo_2				X
Cardiac rhythm (ECG)	X	X	X	
Pulse rate				X
Leg EMG	X	X		
Body position (sensor or observed)	X	X	X	

Abbreviations: ECG = electrocardiogram; EEG = electroencephalography (typically, central, occipital); EMG = electromyography (chin, right and left legs, ± arms); EOG = electro-oculography (right and left eye movements); Level I = traditional sleep laboratory evaluation; Levels II, III, IV = various forms of unattended home-based studies; Spo_2 = O_2 saturation by pulse oximetry.

2. When the patient is unable to be studied in the laboratory (e.g., nonambulatory)

3. When the clinician needs to evaluate the patient's response to therapy (e.g., diagnosis and treatment had been established by previous standard PSG)

Secondary Diagnostic Needs

Although the vast majority of patients with OSAHS have an idiopathic form, there are various medical conditions that may secondarily cause obstructive SDB. This would necessitate further diagnostic testing specific to that disorder, including evaluations for hypothyroidism, acromegaly, extrathoracic upper airway obstruction (e.g., vocal cord paralysis, goiter), and neurologic disorders (e.g., Shy-Drager syndrome, poliomyelitis, myotonic dystrophy).

PREVENTION OF OBSTRUCTIVE SLEEP APNEA-HYPOPNEA SYNDROME

Prevention includes controlling weight, establishing good sleep hygiene, undergoing positional therapy, avoiding alcohol and sedative-hypnotics, treating nasal congestion, and ensuring a euthyroid state (Table 5). With regard to obesity, a 10% reduction in weight can lead to a 30% improvement in SDB. In fact, up to 11% of obese patients with OSAHS may achieve a normal AHI in response to weight loss. Caution is advised because 46% have recurrence of their OSAHS despite maintaining weight loss. Weight reduction may also lead to lower and better-tolerated CPAP levels.

Chronic rhinosinusitis can have important implications in SDB. In children, it can result in mandibular deficiency, leading to anatomic narrowing of the upper airway and increased nasopharyngeal resistance. Measures targeting rhinosinusitis may thus improve upper airway stability. These can include allergy evaluation, nonsedating antihistamines, topical nasal steroid inhalers, immunotherapy, and/or antibiotics, as clinically indicated.

Sleep deprivation and sedatives reduce neuromuscular control of the upper airway. As a result, sleep hygiene promoting sufficient sleep time can ameliorate sleep quality and upper airway stability. Similarly, alcohol should be avoided within 6 hours of bedtime and at doses in excess of 1.5 to 2.0 mL/kg. Sedative-hypnotics are also to be avoided whenever clinically feasible.

Hypothyroidism is an infrequent but potentially relevant cause of OSAHS. It reduces respiratory drive and neuromuscular control and patency of the upper airway. In a study of 336 patients with suspected OSAHS, routine screening of thyroid-stimulating hormone and free T4 concentrations identified four new patients (1.41%) with subclinical hypothyroidism. In another study, it was concluded that screening was cost-effective despite only 2.4% of OSAHS patients having undiagnosed hypothyroidism.

Sleep disordered breathing can have a predilection for the supine position. It is characterized by a supine AHI that is greater than or equal to twice the nonsupine AHI or by observations of supine-specific snoring or RERAs. Such SDB lends itself to positional therapy. This may include a fanny pack filled with tennis balls oriented toward the back, a wedged pillow, a knapsack stuffed with towels, a tennis ball within a sock sewn to the back of a pajama top, or posture alarms. In an 8-week study using posture alarms, more than half of the patients with supine-dependent OSAHS normalized their AHI. However, without the alarms, only half were able to maintain nonsupine sleep, and how long this response is sustainable remains unknown.

TREATMENT OF OBSTRUCTIVE SLEEP APNEA-HYPOPNEA SYNDROME

Options include pressurization of the upper airway (CPAP), orthodontics, or surgery (see Table 5). Of these, only CPAP and tracheostomy have been shown to reduce mortality related to OSAHS.

TABLE 5. **Treatment of Obstructive Sleep-Disordered Breathing**

Diagnosis	AHI	Preventive	Oral Appliance	CPAP	Surgery
Nonapneic snoring Without fatigue or drowsiness	<5	Yes	Yes (if antisocial)	No	Yes—site specific (if antisocial)
		.... First assess response to prevention prior to prescribing another intervention			
UARS Snoring with fatigue or drowsiness	<5 (RERAs >10/hr)	Yes	Not validated	Yes (Preferred)	Not validated
		.... First assess response to prevention prior to prescribing another intervention			
Mild OSAHS Without fatigue, drowsiness, or cardiovascular risk ... with antisocial snoring	5–15 nadir SpO_2 >85%	Yes	Yes (If supine–dependent or after failed UP3)	Yes (Preferred)	Yes—site specific (If CPAP intolerant)
		.... First assess response to prevention prior to prescribing another intervention			
Mild OSAHS With fatigue, drowsiness, nadir SpO_2<85%, or cardiovascular risk	5–15	Yes (Together with another intervention)	Yes (If supine dependent or after failed UP3)	Yes (Preferred)	Yes—site specific (If CPAP intolerant)
Moderate-Severe OSAHS	≥15	Yes (Together with another intervention)	Yes (If CPAP intolerant)	Yes (Preferred)	Yes—site specific (If CPAP intolerant)

Abbreviations: AHI = apnea-hypopnea index; CPAP = continuous positive airway pressure; OSAHS = obstructive sleep apnea-hypopnea syndrome; RERAs = respiratory effort-aroused arousals; UARS = upper airway resistance syndrome.

Pressurization of the Upper Airway

The most frequently prescribed treatment is CPAP given its level of validation, simplicity, and cost advantage. It administers airflow typically at room air oxygen concentrations and in a continuous mode. The airflow is generated by a small portable air compressor and is delivered through a hose connected to a small nasal or oronasal mask. CPAP pressurizes the nasopharynx, oropharynx, and hypopharynx, simulating a pneumatic splint and increasing the lateral diameter of the upper airway. Flow is titrated to an optimal pressure with the goal of eliminating upper airway collapsibility and restoring sleep architecture. Acceptance rates for CPAP average 70% to 80%. In those accepting such therapy, compliance rates, in the largest series to date, average 90% after 3 years and 85% after 7 years. Other studies report lower compliance but these still compare favorably to other medical disorders requiring indefinite treatment. Follow-up for CPAP, including telephone calls, written information, and support groups, can maximize compliance. In those having difficulties, it is critical that the mask be fitted appropriately. With a properly fitted mask, there is less skin breakdown, there are fewer air leaks, and there are fewer claustrophobic responses of lower magnitude. If there is refractory nasal congestion, epistaxis, or dryness, heated-in-line humidification should be instituted. This has also been shown to improve compliance, whereas cold-passover humidifiers do not.

Up to 20% to 30% of patients become intolerant to CPAP. This may be a result of perceived expiratory resistance, CPAP-induced hypoventilation, refractory air leaks, aerophagia, or chest discomfort. In such settings, bilevel positive airway pressure (BiPAP) is considered because it may result in a lower mean nasal pressure. It achieves this by reducing expiratory pressures while optimizing inspiratory pressures. In fact, it is when the inspiratory pressure exceeds expiratory levels by more than 6 cm H_2O that one sees an improvement in compliance relative to CPAP. Future alternatives may also involve an autoPAP system, which works by varying the applied pressure in response to snoring or flow limitation. Putative advantages include a lower mean nasal pressure and improvements in sleep quality and compliance. There is a need, however, for autoPAP systems to undergo larger validation studies, especially in patients with cardiopulmonary disease, hypoventilation syndromes, air leaks, minimal snoring, or mild OSAHS.

Orthodontics

Oral appliances have a role in mild OSAHS and supine-dependent OSAHS (see Table 5). One such appliance is an adjustable mandibular advancement device. In a study of 44 patients, it reduced the AHI to less than 10 in 81% of patients with mild OSAHS. However, only 60% of those with moderate and 25% of those with severe OSAHS achieved an AHI less than 10. Efficacy has also been demonstrated in supine-dependent OSAHS or after a failed uvulopalatopharyngoplasty (UP3). Relative contraindications to the device include an elongated soft palate, elongated and engorged uvula, significant tonsillar hypertrophy, periodontal disease, and temporomandibular syndrome. In supine-dependent OSAHS, a tongue-retaining device (TRD) may also be effective. In a study of 15 patients with an overall AHI of 30.7 (supine-specific AHI, 63.9) treated with both positional therapy and a TRD, 12 patients reduced their AHI to less than 10. Although not as effective as CPAP, oral appliances are usually preferred by patients because of greater comfort. Complications related to oral appliances are infrequent but may include excessive salivation, mouth dryness, malocclusion, or temporomandibular joint syndrome.

Surgery

Surgery in OSAHS is site-selective and, in general, is considered after failed CPAP therapy. If a type 1 (retropalatal) collapse is noted, a UP3 may be effective. If there is a type 3 (retroglossal) collapse, a mandibular osteotomy with genioglossus advancement, hyoid myotomy, and resuspension of the hyoid bone onto the superior edge of the larynx (MOHM) is advised. In a type 2 collapse (retropalatal and retroglossal collapse), a combined UP3 and MOHM is suggested. This approach has a reported success rate of 60% defined as a postoperative AHI less than 20 or a 50% reduction in the preoperative AHI. In 6 months, if the patient does not achieve efficacy, a maxillary and mandibular osteotomy with maxillary and mandibular advancement is considered. With this phased protocol, greater than 90% success has been reported (preoperative AHI, 68.3; final postoperative AHI, 8.4). Complications related to this phased protocol are infrequent and transient but may include pain, bleeding, infection, palatal stenosis, paresthesia, nasal speech, mild loss of taste, and nasal reflux.

Other available surgical options include the following: In patients with OSAHS associated with a high arched hard palate and maxillary constriction, a study of 10 patients using rapid maxillary expansion (RME) demonstrated a reduction in the AHI from 19 to 7. The RME may be achieved with a fixed orthodontic appliance or be surgically assisted (maxillary osteotomies). With regard to adenotonsillectomy, its role in adults is very limited as primary treatment for OSAHS. It is more effective in prepubertal children, but there is significant recurrence of OSAHS in adult life. Currently, there is no role for a laser-assisted uvulopalatoplasty in OSAHS while the role of somnoplasty needs further validation. Nasal reconstructive surgery, for example, septoplasty, although necessary as an adjunct to CPAP, is of limited value in treating SDB. The most effective surgical treatment remains a tracheostomy. It bypasses the upper airway obstruction but is reserved for refractory

TABLE 6. **Referral Guidelines for Obstructive Sleep-Disordered Breathing**

1. **Incorporate Sleep-Based Clinical Tools as Part of Primary Care**
   - Berlin Questionnaire (Ann Intern Med 1999; 131:485–491)
   - Epworth Sleepiness Scale (Sleep 1991; 14:540–545)
   - A 2-wk sleep log: Catalogs daily bedtime, arise time, and the estimated sleep onset latency, sleep time, and number of awakenings; frequency and duration of napping; time of evening meal; latest time of caffeine, alcohol, or nicotine consumption.
2. **When Referring to the Sleep Laboratory, Provide the Appropriate Clinical Information**
   - Indications for testing
   - A medical history and physical examination
   - The above-outlined clinical tools
3. **Referrals to a Sleep Specialist May Be Required If Any of the Following Occurs**
   - The PSG fails to be definitive
   - The clinical response to CPAP is incomplete
   - There is intolerance to CPAP

Abbreviations: CPAP = continuous positive airway pressure; PSG = polysomnograph.

cases given its morbidity, wound care, and low patient preference.

OTHER TREATMENT CONSIDERATIONS

A word of caution is warranted regarding hypoxemia in OSAHS because there may be a high prevalence for a patent foramen ovale (PFO). In one study, 33 of 48 patients with OSAHS had a detectable PFO. Although it is inappropriate to advocate routine screening for a PFO in OSAHS, one should be alert to this possibility in patients with sleep-induced hypoxemia refractory to CPAP or unexplainably disproportionate to the AHI. The treatment of hypertension in OSAHS also merits consideration. Recent work has demonstrated β blockers (atenolol) to be effective relative to amlodipine, enalapril, hydrochlorothiazide, and losartan.

There are other available treatments but these are more appropriate for obesity-hypoventilation syndrome (medroxyprogesterone [Provera]*, CSA (acetazolamide [Diamox]*), peripheral alveolar hypoventilation (O_2), and Cheyne-Stokes variant of CSA in CHF (O_2, theophylline*). There has been an interest in serotoninergic mechanisms as a treatment, but this approach remains clinically insignificant. In a study of 20 patients with OSAHS, paroxitene only reduced the AHI from 36.3 to 30.2 ($P = 0.021$).

CONCLUSION

The evaluation of SDB should be part of general preventive care. This ensures the appropriate management of SDB, thereby improving public health and a patient's well-being. Table 6 outlines referral guidelines using clinical tools that may be applied by ancillary office staff.

*Not FDA approved for this indication.

PRIMARY LUNG CANCER

method of
W. JEFFREY PETTY, M.D., and
JEFFREY CRAWFORD, M.D.
Duke University School of Medicine and the Duke University Medical Center
Durham, North Carolina

Despite improvements in prevention, detection, and therapy, lung cancer causes more deaths than any other cancer. Worldwide, lung cancer is responsible for 17.8% of cancer deaths. In recent years, there have been numerous developments in lung cancer research, and it is hoped that these will lead to more effective treatment. Although improvements in therapy remain an active area of research, two fundamental issues in reducing the mortality of lung cancer are the elimination of tobacco use and the detection of cancers at an early stage.

ETIOLOGY

Tobacco smoke induces the majority of lung cancers. People who smoke cigarettes increase their risk of developing lung cancer almost 20-fold. The type of tobacco, the amount of daily use, the depth of inhalation, and the age at onset have all been correlated with the magnitude of risk of developing lung cancer. Second-hand smoke also increases the risk of lung cancer, although the magnitude of increase is not as great, on the order of two- to threefold for people who live with a smoker. Similarly, cigar use, which has become popular in recent years, also increases the risk of lung cancer, although the magnitude of risk is not as great as that for cigarette use.

The carcinogenic compounds in tobacco smoke appear to be polycyclic aromatic hydrocarbons, nitrosamines, and other gas-phase components that have not been identified. The exact mechanism by which the carcinogens in tobacco smoke induce lung cancer is not known, but they appear to increase DNA methylation, which may, in turn, alter gene expression and contribute to tumorigenesis. Both tumor specimens and samples of lung tissue from smokers have an increased level of DNA methylation, which is not seen in lung biopsy specimens from nonsmokers. Chromosomal abnormalities have been found in lung cancers as well. The most common of these is a deletion of the short arm of chromosome 3. Excessive DNA methylation and this deletion often coexist, but a cause-and-effect relationship has not been established.

PATHOLOGY

Lung cancer can be divided into two major groups, small cell and non–small cell. Non–small cell lung cancer accounts for 80% of all lung cancer, and small cell lung cancer accounts for the remaining 20%. The pathologic differentiation between these two groups is based on cell size as well as nuclear characteristics and mitotic rate. Occasionally, the morphologic characteristics alone are indeterminate, and cell surface markers can be helpful in differentiating whether a tumor is truly small cell or non–small cell. Small cell cancer often overexpresses the neural cell adhesion molecule (NCAM) but not the epidermal growth factor receptor (EGFR), whereas non–small cell lung cancer often overexpresses EGFR but not NCAM.

Non–small cell lung cancer is further divided into histologic subtypes that may present differently but currently do not guide therapy: squamous cell carcinoma, adenocarcinoma, bronchoalveolar carcinoma, large cell carcinoma, and spindle cell carcinoma. Squamous cell carcinomas are centrally located tumors that are more likely to cause hemoptysis and obstruction than the other subtypes. Adenocarcinomas are increasing in prevalence for unknown reasons and are more common in women than in men. Bronchoalveolar carcinoma is a subtype of adenocarcinoma that spreads rapidly within the lung and usually presents as an infiltrative lesion. Large cell carcinomas are usually located peripherally and are believed to be part of the continuum of neuroendocrine tumors that includes carcinoid and small cell lung cancer, but large cell carcinoma is treated clinically as non–small cell lung cancer. In 1997, the World Health Organization (WHO) guidelines defined a new subdivision of non–small cell lung cancer, spindle cell carcinoma, which has morphologic characteristics similar to sarcoma.

EPIDEMIOLOGY

The epidemiology of lung cancer has been tightly linked to cigarette use, which is responsible for approximately 90% of lung cancers. Since the U.S. Surgeon General's report in 1964, the prevalence of cigarette use in the United States has been steadily declining. Unfortunately, despite previous reports to the contrary, the increased risk of lung cancer from smoking does not appear to be reversible. This means that the large and growing number of former smokers constitute a population who will remain at increased risk of the development of lung cancer and would be appropriate patients for screening and chemopreventive trials.

Despite the overall progress in smoking cessation, some disturbing trends in cigarette use have developed in recent years. Perhaps the most disturbing trend is increasing use in young people, especially young African Americans. From 1991 to 1999, the prevalence of smoking among high-school students has increased from 27.5% to 34.8%. Because the increased risk of lung cancer appears to be durable, the impact of this high prevalence of smoking among young people will likely be seen for years to come.

SCREENING FOR LUNG CANCER

Screening is an area of research that has had renewed vigor. Initial screening studies for lung cancer used chest radiography with or without sputum cytologic analysis and failed to find a benefit for screening. The largest of these was the Mayo Lung Project, which found no mortality advantage for screening but has been criticized because of numerous shortcomings, including poor compliance with screening and the lack of a control arm that was not screened. Despite these shortcomings, because no mortality benefit was seen in this or in other smaller studies, screening for lung cancer with either chest radiography or sputum cytologic examination has not been recommended for more than a decade.

Using the modern technology of low-dose spiral computed tomography (CT) of the chest, the Early Lung Cancer Action Project has published the baseline characteristics of a screening study for patients at high risk of lung cancer. At the baseline screening, the superiority of spiral CT over regular chest radiography for the detection of early lung cancer was evident. In total, 2.5% of patients enrolled were found to have resectable lung cancer, and the majority of these tumors were not detectable by chest radiography. Even though these results are encouraging, the study design is limited by the lack of a control group and a study group that is highly selected. The results of this baseline screening, however, have been sufficiently encouraging to spur larger controlled trials to evaluate the potential mortality benefit of screening larger populations with low-dose spiral CT of the chest.

TREATMENT

Non–Small Cell Lung Cancer

Staging and Prognosis

The clinical and pathologic staging of non–small cell lung cancer carries great significance for both prognosis and therapy. All patients who are diagnosed with non–small cell lung cancer should undergo staging with CT evaluation of the chest and upper abdomen, including the adrenal glands, which are common sites of metastasis. A contrast medium–enhanced CT of the brain and radionucleotide bone scan should also be performed in all patients, other than possibly those with stage IA disease. The presence of either brain metastases or significant bone metastases may preclude surgery and may direct initial therapy to irradiation rather than chemotherapy. If indeterminate lesions are found on these staging scans, either biopsy or positron emission tomography may be necessary to determine whether a radiographic abnormality represents metastatic disease.

If no metastatic disease is found on staging scans and the tumor is believed to be resectable, mediastinoscopy is often helpful to determine the pathologic extent of mediastinal lymph node involvement. For purposes of pathologic staging, the mediastinal lymph nodes are categorized by station. The mediastinum is divided into nine stations that are characterized by anatomic landmarks visible during mediastinoscopy. Pathologic involvement of multiple mediastinal nodal stations or contralateral mediastinal nodes often precludes resection, although definitions of resectability are variable.

Staging for non–small cell lung cancer uses the TNM system that is described in Tables 1 and 2. In stage I and II non–small cell lung cancer, prognosis for 5-year survival gradually worsens with the extent of disease. Currently, surgery is the only therapy recommended for early-stage lung cancer.

Stage III non–small cell lung cancer is divided into IIIA and IIIB based on the extent of lymph node involvement and the characteristics of the primary tumor. The significance for therapy is that stage IIIA disease is often resectable, whereas stage IIIB disease is largely unresectable. The definition of mediastinal lymph node stations helps define resectability based on the number of nodal stations involved. Even microscopic involvement of more than one station is believed to correlate with a poor prognosis from surgery alone. The role of surgery with neoadjuvant therapy is currently being evaluated in a number of clinical trials for patients with stage IIIA disease who have mediastinal lymph node involvement.

TABLE 1. **TNM Classification of Lung Cancer**

Tumor

T1 The tumor is 3 cm or smaller and is located distal to a lobar bronchial orifice. If the tumor is contained within the bronchial wall, it can be located within 2 cm of the carina and still be considered a T1 tumor. It cannot involve any of the structures listed for T2, T3, or T4 tumors.

T2 The tumor is larger than 3 cm, abuts the visceral pleura, or is associated with obstructive atelectasis or pneumonitis that involves the hila but not the entire lung. The tumor must be located more than 2 cm from the carina and cannot involve the structures listed for T3 and T4 tumors.

T3 The tumor either invades parietal pleura, mediastinal pleura, pericardium, chest wall, or diaphragm or is located within 2 cm of the carina and extends through the bronchial wall. The tumor may cause obstruction of the entire lung but cannot involve the carina itself.

T4 The tumor either invades myocardium, great vessels, trachea, esophagus, vertebral body, mediastinum, or carina or is associated with a malignant pericardial effusion, pleural effusion, or satellite nodules confined to the primary tumor–containing lobe of the lung.

Lymph Nodes

N0 No lymph nodes are involved.

N1 Ipsilateral hilar, peribronchial, or intrapulmonary lymph nodes are involved.

N2 Ipsilateral mediastinal or subcarinal nodes are involved.

N3 Any scalene or supraclavicular lymph nodes are involved, or contralateral mediastinal or hilar lymph nodes are involved

Distant Metastasis

M0 No distant metastases are present.

M1 A distant metastasis is present. This includes metastases to the contralateral lung or lobes of the ipsilateral lung other than the primary tumor–containing lobe.

Modified from Mountain CF: Revisions in the international system for staging lung cancer. Chest 111:1710–1717, 1997.

Stage IIIB disease constitutes a heterogeneous group of patients: those with malignant effusion and those without. Documentation of malignant effusion does not require cytologic evaluation; rather, any bloody or exudative effusion is classified as malignant in the setting of newly diagnosed lung cancer unless proven otherwise. Patients without malignant effusions often have disease that can be localized within a radiation port and have a better prognosis, which may in part be due to the delivery of combined modality therapy.

Patients with stage IIIB disease with malignant effusion and those with stage IV disease have a similar prognosis. Five-year survival is poor for both, about 1%. In general, there are also no significant differences in therapy between these groups other than the use of local measures such as drainage and sclerotherapy for the treatment of the effusion itself.

TABLE 2. **Staging of Non–Small Cell Lung Cancer**

Stage	TNM Subset	5-Year Survival (%)
IA	T1, N0, M0	67
IB	T2, N0, M0	57
IIA	T1, N1, M0	55
IIB	T2, N1, M0	39
	T3, N0, M0	38
IIIA	T1–3, N2, M0	23
	T3, N1, M0	25
IIIB	T4, any N, M0	7
	Any T, N3, M0	3
IV	Any T, any N, M1	1

Modified from Mountain CF: Revisions in the international system for staging lung cancer. Chest 111:1710–1717, 1997.

Stage I and II Disease

Surgery is the backbone of therapy for early-stage lung cancer. Lobectomy with lymph node dissection is usually the best resection. In the past, thoracotomy was required for the majority of these procedures, but mediastinoscopy and thoracoscopic lobectomy are much better tolerated and appear to have similar efficacy. Wedge resections have been performed in the past but have higher failure rates, so, whenever possible, lobectomy should be performed as long as the patient has adequate pulmonary reserve to tolerate the procedure.

The addition of chemotherapy or radiation therapy is not recommended for this group of patients. Delivery of either postoperative chemotherapy or radiation therapy is difficult and carries significant morbidity. When evaluated in a meta-analysis called the PORT (postoperative radiation therapy) meta-analysis, postoperative radiation therapy demonstrated a lack of efficacy and even a worsening of survival for patients with stage I and II disease. As for adjuvant chemotherapy, Le Chevalier's meta-analysis found mixed results, and certain chemotherapeutic agents significantly worsened survival. Delivery of neoadjuvant chemotherapy, however, causes less morbidity, and several small trials have suggested that platinum-based regimens may improve survival in this setting. Overall, the neoadjuvant chemotherapy is more promising than adjuvant chemotherapy for early-stage lung cancer, but neither is recommended as standard therapy outside a research protocol.

Stage IIIA Disease

Stage IIIA disease is a heterogeneous group and the subject of significant research efforts. Currently, there is no set protocol by which all patients with stage IIIA disease should be treated, and the criteria used to determine whether a patient has resectable or unresectable disease are variable. In the past, one frequently used scheme for separating resectable from nonresectable disease was based on the size of mediastinal lymph nodes on CT. Those patients with multiple bulky nodes (bulky IIIA) were believed to have unresectable disease, and those without enlarged nodes or only a few mildly enlarged lymph nodes (nonbulky IIIA) were believed to have resectable disease. Unfortunately, the size of lymph nodes on CT may not correlate with pathologic involvement. Large nodes can be reactive, and normal-sized nodes can harbor disease.

Another guideline for identifying resectable stage

IIIA lung cancer accounts for the inaccuracy of diagnosis based on lymph node size and is based on the pathologic extent of mediastinal lymph node involvement. Patients are divided into those without positive mediastinal (N2) lymph nodes, those with positive N2 nodes at a single station, and those with positive N2 nodes at multiple stations. To discriminate among these, mediastinoscopy is usually necessary. There are some data that suggest positron emission tomography is also accurate for evaluation of mediastinal lymph nodes, but mediastinoscopy is considered the gold standard and is recommended for the majority of patients before surgical resection. For patients who undergo this procedure, the mediastinal node sampling should be performed systematically, or a complete mediastinal node dissection should be performed. Random sampling of enlarged nodes does not appear to be as sensitive as these two techniques.

Patients with N2 nodes positive at a single station and those with no positive N2 nodes (similar to nonbulky IIIA) may be candidates for surgery. This decision is dependent on multiple factors, including the patient's age and ability to tolerate surgery in addition to the resectability of the tumor itself. Many institutions are currently investigating the role of neoadjuvant chemotherapy with or without radiation therapy for patients with resectable stage IIIA lung cancer, and this appears to be beneficial. Even though a mortality benefit has not been proven, patients with IIIA disease who did not receive preoperative radiation, particularly those with mediastinal lymph node involvement, are frequently given postoperative radiation therapy to reduce the risk of local and regional recurrence. This subgroup of patients did not have worsened survival in the PORT meta-analysis, and radiation therapy techniques have substantially improved since the trials used for the meta-analysis were performed.

Patients with N2 nodes positive at multiple stations (similar to bulky IIIA) or those with contralateral mediastinal nodes are generally not considered to be candidates for surgery. Treatment with combined modality therapy using cisplatin-, carboplatin-, or platinum-based chemotherapy and radiation therapy is recommended for these patients, as it is for patients with unresectable IIIB non–small cell lung cancer. A more meaningful term for the composite group of unresectable IIIA and unresectable IIIB is locally advanced unresectable non–small cell lung cancer.

Stage IIIB Disease

Almost all patients with this stage of disease are not candidates for surgical resection unless they have a resectable T4 tumor without significant mediastinal adenopathy. Combination therapy with concurrent irradiation and chemotherapy has demonstrated the greatest efficacy in treating this group of patients. Radiation therapy has been accepted as a standard for patients with unresectable disease for many years. Although there are no randomized controlled data to prove a survival benefit from radiation therapy, the rate of local progression without radiation therapy is high and often necessitates administration of radiation therapy when it is not given initially.

The addition of chemotherapy to radiation therapy had been demonstrated to improve median survival in multiple meta-analyses. A recent large randomized study from Japan compared concurrent chemotherapy and radiation therapy with sequential therapy and found that concurrent therapy improved response rate, median survival, and 5-year relapse-free survival. Many more studies of concurrent and sequential therapy are still ongoing.

Overall, combined therapy with radiation and a platinum-containing chemotherapy regimen is recommended for the majority of patients with locally advanced, unresectable non–small cell lung cancer. Although the data supporting benefit from concurrent rather than sequential administration are not definitive, it is reasonable to offer concurrent therapy to patients with adequate performance status. After initial courses of chemotherapy and radiation therapy are completed, additional administration of docetaxel (Taxotere) has been reported to improve further 1-year survival and is being evaluated in randomized trials.

Stage IV Disease

Patients with stage IV non–small cell lung cancer are not candidates for surgery with curative intent unless they have resectable thoracic disease and a solitary resectable brain metastasis. Most patients with this stage of disease are candidates for only chemotherapy, with palliative radiation as necessary. The prognosis is poor, with a 5-year survival rate of approximately 1%. With modern chemotherapy, the median survival and 1-year survival rates have improved, but the 5-year survival remains poor.

The role of chemotherapy in this setting has undergone careful scrutiny with numerous meta-analyses that demonstrate a small but significant improvement in median survival and 1-year survival. Platinum-based chemotherapy improves median survival to 6 to 8 weeks and improves 1-year survival from 15% to 25%. Newer regimens containing one platinum-based agent and one newer agent have demonstrated 1-year survival rates as high as 40% to 50%. These newer agents include gemcitabine (Gemzar), paclitaxel (Taxol), docetaxel (Taxotere), vinorelbine (Navelbine), and irinotecan (Camptosar).* The newer agents were recently compared with a large four-arm trial in which each was given with a platinum-based agent. There were no statistically significant differences in median survival or 1-year survival among them. The most common dose-limiting toxicity for these regimens is myelosuppression, although occasionally neurotoxicity can become dose limiting. Choosing an initial regimen is based largely on patient and physician preferences. The combination of

*Not FDA approved for this indication.

carboplatin (Paraplatin)* and paclitaxel is the most widely used initial therapy in the United States, whereas the combination of cisplatin (Platinol)* and gemcitabine is the most widely used in Europe.

When progression of disease after initial therapy occurs, the options for further therapy are guided largely by the location of recurrence and patient symptoms. For patients who progress with either brain metastases or symptomatic disease in bone or lung, radiation therapy is the most appropriate second step. If patients have measurable progression of disease that does not necessitate radiation therapy, a second course of chemotherapy may improve symptoms and modestly prolong survival. Docetaxel is currently approved for this indication. Further therapy beyond first- and second-line chemotherapy can be offered if the tumor has been repeatedly responsive to previous chemotherapy. In this setting, enrollment in a phase I clinical trial would also be appropriate for patients with adequate functional status.

Small Cell Lung Cancer

Pathophysiology

Small cell lung cancer has distinctly different biologic behavior than non–small cell lung cancer. Small cell lung cancer spreads much more rapidly and is treated as a systemic disease even when it appears to be surgically resectable. Fortunately, it is much more chemoresponsive than non–small cell lung cancer. Before the use of chemotherapy for the treatment of this disease, 5-year survival rates were extremely poor. Now, with the combination of chemotherapy and radiation therapy, survival rates have improved, with recent reports of up to 26% 5-year survival for limited-stage disease. Although 5-year survival for extensive disease remains poor, median survival has improved greatly with the use of chemotherapy.

Surgery has a limited role in the treatment of small cell lung cancer. There are occasional patients who present with a single pulmonary nodule and have no evidence of mediastinal lymph node involvement who may be candidates for surgical resection followed by chemotherapy and radiation therapy. Because small cell lung cancer spreads so rapidly, these patients are uncommon and have not been well studied.

Staging

The goal of staging of small cell lung cancer is to determine whether the involved lung and lymph nodes can be encompassed within a single radiation port. If it can, it is termed *limited stage;* if it cannot, it is termed *extensive stage.* If distant metastases are found, it is considered extensive stage, whether or not the thoracic disease could be encompassed within a single radiation port.

Because small cell lung cancer metastasizes rapidly, all patients should undergo staging scans that include the common locations of metastasis even if the thoracic disease appears to be limited. These will serve as a reference to document response to therapy and may be important to direct initial radiation therapy. The usual evaluation includes CT of the chest and upper abdomen including the adrenals, contrast medium–enhanced CT or magnetic resonance imaging of the brain, and a radionucleotide bone scan.

Limited-Stage

Treatment of limited-stage small cell lung cancer has improved significantly with the progress of chemotherapy and radiation therapy. Initially, chemotherapy was based on alkylating agents, but etoposide was found to produce significantly higher response rates. The combination of cisplatin and etoposide has been used for more than 20 years and continues to be one of the options for front-line treatment. This regimen has been compared with carboplatin and etoposide in a randomized trial, which revealed similar response rates. The advantage of carboplatin and etoposide found in this trial was that the side effect profile was significantly better with much less nausea, so many oncologists are now using carboplatin and etoposide as standard front-line treatment. Several of the new chemotherapeutic agents, including gemcitabine,* paclitaxel,* topotecan, vinorelbine, docetaxel, and irinotecan,* have also demonstrated significant activity against small cell lung cancer, but their role in therapy is still reserved for patients who experience relapse after an initial response to therapy.

Radiation therapy offers significant benefit in limited-stage small cell lung cancer and has demonstrated a 5-year survival benefit in controlled clinical trials. Whether chemotherapy and radiation therapy should be administered concurrently or sequentially has been debated. Concurrent administration may necessitate a reduction in the dose intensity of chemotherapy, but response rates and median survival appear to be improved. In general, chemotherapy and radiation therapy should be administered concurrently with radiation therapy started early in the course of treatment.

Extensive-Stage Cancer

Unlike limited-stage small cell lung cancer, extensive-stage small cell cancer almost always recurs after an initial response to therapy, with 5-year survival of 1%. Although there has been some suggestion that 5-year survival was seen more commonly in patients with brain metastases as the only site of extrathoracic disease, this has not been borne out in more recent studies.

Treatment of extensive-stage small cell lung cancer revolves around chemotherapy with radiation therapy given mainly for palliation of symptoms. Chemotherapy greatly improves median survival for patients with extensive-stage small cell cancer even though it is usually not curative. Median survival

*Not FDA approved for this indication.

*Not FDA approved for this indication.

without therapy is 4 to 6 weeks, whereas median survival with therapy is 7 to 9 months. As with limited-stage small cell cancer, etoposide appears to be the most active agent and is frequently given with either carboplatin or cisplatin.

As discussed in the preceding section, a number of newer chemotherapeutic agents have demonstrated activity against small cell lung cancer. Their role in extensive-stage disease is also largely reserved for treatment of relapse. Clinical trials have attempted additional courses of non–cross-resistant chemotherapy after initial response to front-line therapy. These have produced more toxicity without a significant impact on median survival or 5-year survival. There are numerous ongoing trials studying new combinations of concurrent and sequential therapy in this setting, but none has proven superior to treatment with a platinum and etoposide followed by observation and treatment of relapse. Other investigational treatments for patients with small cell lung cancer include vaccine trials and immunotherapy trials for those who achieve complete response to initial therapy.

Prophylactic Cranial Irradiation

Prophylactic cranial irradiation (PCI) has been demonstrated to improve median survival and 3-year survival by 5.4% in patients with limited-stage small cell cancer who achieve a complete response to therapy. For young patients with adequate functional status and a complete response to therapy, PCI should probably be offered to afford the greatest chance of cure. Unfortunately, some patients tolerate cranial irradiation poorly, particularly elderly patients and patients with poor performance status. The decision regarding PCI needs to be individualized based on the patient's preferences and ability to tolerate the therapy.

TARGETED CANCER THERAPY

For many years, scientists have been trying to identify a single biochemical pathway in cancer that is a sine qua non. Unfortunately, human malignancies have not afforded such a single pathway that bears this significance. Rather, a large number of oncogenes, tumor suppressor genes, and replicative signal pathways have been identified in human malignancies during an explosion of molecular and cell biology research. This astounding diversity of mechanisms is fascinating from the perspective of basic science and will likely have an impact on clinical science in the near future. Compounds that target specific extracellular growth factors, cell surface proteins, intracellular signaling proteins, angiogenesis, and the cellular genome have been developed by numerous pharmaceutical companies and are now being tested in clinical trials.

In phase I trials, several of these agents have already demonstrated activity against lung cancer, but all are associated with some degree of toxicity. The advantage they may offer in the future is that most do not cause myelosuppression, which is the current dose-limiting toxicity of lung cancer chemotherapy. To use these targeted therapies most effectively, we will need to develop our knowledge of molecular epidemiology in lung cancer and develop better tests for these molecular targets in individual cancer specimens.

COCCIDIOIDOMYCOSIS

method of
ROBERT LIBKE, M.D.
University of California–San Francisco—Fresno Medical Education Program
Fresno, California

Coccidioidomycosis is an illness caused by the fungus *Coccidioides immitis*. This fungus grows well in soil in conditions found in the arid and semiarid regions of the southwestern United States and in a few places in Central and South America. Under proper conditions, the fungus produces an abundance of arthroconidia, which are very light and are easily carried in the air.

Infection occurs when arthroconidia are inhaled and, in the host, are converted to spherules, which reproduce by endosporulation. The primary infection is almost always in the lung. In the great majority of cases, the infection is quickly contained and remains confined to a limited area of the lung. In a few cases the organism is more aggressive and rapidly produces a diffuse pneumonia with an acute respiratory distress syndrome (ARDS)–like picture that may be fatal. In other cases, the pulmonary lesions heal but the organism is spread to other organs in the body through the blood or lymphatic channels. When this happens, the disease is considered to be disseminated and takes on a different character.

The pathology of infection with *C. immitis* is dimorphic, like the fungus. The body initially reacts to the arthroconidia and the endospores with an acute inflammatory reaction similar to that seen in acute bacterial infections. Reaction to the mature coccidioidal spherules is a granulomatous one similar to that seen in tuberculosis. Clinically, coccidioidomycosis reflects both of those processes; that is, it can have features of both acute and chronic infection.

CLINICAL MANIFESTATIONS

The primary infection in the lung is asymptomatic in the majority of instances. When symptomatic, it resembles many other acute lower respiratory tract infections. In some cases, however, clues are present that raise the suspicion of coccidioidomycosis:

- Radiologic finding of hilar adenopathy on the side of the airspace consolidation
- Significant eosinophilia in the differential leukocyte count
- Certain dermatoses (erythema nodosum, erythema multiforme, or a morbilliform maculopapular eruption)
- Failure to show a clinical response to conventional antibiotic therapy

Recovery from the primary pulmonary infection may be complete or may leave chronic residuals of either a cavity or a granuloma. Some cavities heal spontaneously within 2 years of the primary infection. Others are complicated by secondary infection, recurrent hemoptysis, or, rarely, rupture into the pleural space. Occasionally, these complications are severe enough to warrant lobectomy, but this is the exception rather than the rule (except in cavity rupture). Unlike tuberculosis, the chronic cavitary residuals of primary pulmonary coccidioidomycosis rarely progress. When they do, the progressive fibrocavitary disease may be indistinguishable from tuberculosis in radiographs.

The residual granuloma is only significant because of the difficulty of distinguishing it from a carcinoma of the lung when it is first discovered on a routine chest radiograph. If the patient is younger than 40 years of age or the lesion is calcified (coccidioidal granuloma calcify in <20% of cases), the lesion can be considered benign and possibly followed with serial chest radiographs. Occasionally, organisms recovered from the lesion on computed tomography–guided fine-needle aspiration allow the pathologist to make the diagnosis without tissue biopsy. Otherwise, enough tissue must be obtained by transbronchial, thoracoscopic, or open biopsy to allow the pathologist to make a diagnosis.

Dissemination is considered to occur when clinically apparent lesions are found outside the thoracic cavity. The most common sites of dissemination are the skin, lymph nodes, skeleton, synovia, and central nervous system. Almost any organ, however, can be involved. Dissemination may be focal, multifocal, or diffuse.

The two most serious forms are diffuse dissemination and focal dissemination to the central nervous system. Before the advent of effective therapy, those two forms were almost always fatal. Even now, with effective antifungal agents, these two conditions carry a significant mortality rate. Dissemination usually occurs with the primary infection and only rarely as a late complication of a chronic pulmonary lesion. Cumulative clinical experience during the 10 decades since the first description of coccidioidomycosis now allows the clinician to predict with some accuracy the likelihood of dissemination.

Coccidioidomycosis is unique among infectious illnesses in that human beings have a genetically determined resistance to dissemination of the organism. This resistance is found most commonly in whites and least frequently in Filipinos. In between, in descending order of frequency of inherited resistance, are Asians, Native Americans, Hispanics, and African Americans. Infection in infancy and infection in the second or third trimester of pregnancy carry a high risk of dissemination, as does infection in persons with immunocompromised status. Clinical clues to the development of dissemination are a rapid rise in complement-fixing antibodies to a titer of 1:32 or greater, a prolonged febrile primary illness (>4 weeks), or the development of mediastinal adenopathy on chest radiography. The risk of dissemination is so high in patients with prolonged fever and mediastinal adenopathy that treatment is advisable before actual evidence of dissemination occurs. The same can be said for infection in infants and in immunocompromised patients. Otherwise, the risk of dissemination is a matter of clinical judgment in weighing the number of unfavorable factors such as race, pregnancy, and complement-fixation titers.

DIAGNOSIS

The diagnosis of coccidioidomycosis is established by finding the distinctive organism microscopically, in culture specimens of tissue or body fluids, or with serologic studies. Occasionally, one is fortunate enough to establish the diagnosis when a previously negative skin test result converts to a positive result or by finding a positive skin test result in a person who has only recently lived or traveled in an endemic area. Otherwise, the skin test is of no diagnostic value. In particular, a negative skin test result should never be interpreted as excluding the possibility of a coccidioidal illness.

Serologic reactions are the tests most frequently used for the diagnosis of coccidioidal infection—the best are both specific and sensitive. Some of the serologic tests are designed to detect IgM antibodies (the earliest and most evanescent); others detect IgG antibodies (which persist much longer and are quantitatively related to the severity of the infection), and others detect both.

The most reliable techniques for detecting IgM antibodies are the tube precipitin test, the immunodiffusion technique, and an enzyme immunoassay. The most reliable tests for IgG antibodies are the complement fixation test and an immunodiffusion test. The magnitude of the complement fixation titer or IgG quantitative immunodiffusion has the great advantage of being related to the severity of infection and therefore is useful in observing the progression or resolution of the disease.

In patients with extrapulmonary spread, biopsy of lesions or aspiration of fluid from abscesses or joints may not only establish the diagnosis of coccidioidomycosis but also confirm the presence of dissemination. Cerebrospinal fluid (CSF) examinations are needed to evaluate for coccidioidal meningitis. Differential and total blood cell counts, glucose and protein level measurements, and CSF complement fixation titers should be done. Fungal culture results of CSF specimens are rarely positive in patients with proven meningitis and should not be relied on for diagnosis.

TREATMENT

Treatment is not considered necessary for patients with uncomplicated primary infection. When the infection appears to be unusually severe and is progressing to an ARDS-like picture, however, it is prudent to undertake immediate diagnostic tests and initiate treatment with intravenous amphotericin B (Fungizone). For patients with diabetes mellitus, in the third trimester of pregnancy, of Filipino ancestry, and who are immunocompromised, treatment of primary coccidioidomycosis with an azole is prudent.

There is general agreement that disseminated disease is always an indication for treatment. For a time, amphotericin B was the only effective medication. Now there are at least three other agents that have demonstrated effectiveness in both in vitro and clinical trials, namely, ketoconazole, fluconazole, and itraconazole. All three have the big advantage of being sufficiently absorbed from the gastrointestinal tract to achieve serum concentrations that are effective. Fluconazole (Diflucan)* and itraconazole (Sporanox)* appear to have an advantage over ketoconazole (Nizoral) in having considerably less toxicity and as good or better therapeutic effectiveness in initial clinical trials. Fluconazole is less dependent on gastric

*Exceeds dosage recommended by the manufacturer.

acidity for absorption and has the additional theoretical advantage of readily passing the blood-brain barrier to achieve good concentration in the CSF. So far no direct comparative study has been done between itraconazole and fluconazole to determine any superiority in therapeutic effectiveness between the two drugs.

Treatment with fluconazole or itraconazole should start with 200 mg per day and should be increased to tolerance to a maximum of 800 mg* per day. Because the half-life of both of those drugs is very long, they can be administered in one dose or divided into a twice-daily dosage schedule. The length of treatment is entirely dependent on the clinical course and probably should be continued for several months following complete clinical resolution. Relapse following cessation of therapy is common, and some patients may require lifelong treatment. When given for threatened rather than clinically evident dissemination, the course of treatment can often be shortened.

From reports in the medical literature, toxicity appears to be greater with itraconazole than with fluconazole. The major unwanted side effects of the former are nausea and vomiting, edema, and hypertension. Fluconazole is also effective in the treatment of coccidioidal meningitis. It has been used as sole therapy in doses of 400 to 1000 mg* per day. Control of disease with improvement in CSF parameters has occurred in the majority of patients, but relapse has been frequent when therapy has been stopped. It is now our policy when treating patients with coccidioidal meningitis with fluconazole to continue it indefinitely and possibly lifelong. When used in conjunction with intrathecal amphotericin, fluconazole may shorten the duration of intrathecal therapy.

When dissemination is diffuse and rapid or an ARDS-like pulmonary picture develops, the mortality rate is high regardless of the type of therapy used. Initial control of severe dissemination with intravenous amphotericin B is recommended because it may have more rapid onset of action than other agents. Amphotericin B is given intravenously in a concentration of 0.1 mg/mL over 1 to 2 hours daily. It is customary to start with a small dose of 10 mg and increase it by 20-mg increments up to a daily dose of 50 mg. The dosage can be escalated more rapidly when the patient is desperately ill or when the clinical course is deteriorating rapidly.

Toxic side effects are almost universal and should be anticipated by giving acetaminophen 650 mg and diphenhydramine (Benadryl) 50 mg to lessen the rigors that frequently accompany the intravenous infusion. When this combination fails to control rigors, 25 mg of meperidine (Demerol) given as a slow intravenous bolus is often successful. Nausea and vomiting can frequently be ameliorated with antiemetic agents, such as prochlorperazine (Compazine) or trimethobenzamide (Tigan). Renal tubular acidosis with hypokalemia, hypomagnesemia, mild metabolic acidosis, and azotemia is also a predictable result of continued amphotericin treatment. The metabolic acidosis is rarely significant enough to require attention, but the serum potassium, magnesium, and creatinine levels must be monitored frequently until the response to treatment appears to be stable. Potassium can be replaced orally but sometimes requires very large doses. Magnesium replacement may also be required and usually can be done orally. Daily amphotericin should be discontinued when the serum creatinine level exceeds 3.0 and can be restarted and given less frequently when the creatinine level drops below 2.5. After 0.5 g of amphotericin has been given, administration can often be reduced to three times a week instead of daily. This makes outpatient administration quite practical for most patients. The clinical course and response to treatment should determine the total dosage of amphotericin. When given for threatened dissemination rather than clinically evident dissemination, 0.5 g is often enough. For clinically apparent dissemination, anywhere from 1 to 4 g or more may be required.

Newer liposomal forms of amphotericin (Abelcet, AmBisome) have reduced side effects compared with the older colloidal dispersion form of amphotericin B (Fungizone). Liposomal amphotericin may be considered if patients have severe immediate reactions such as hypotension, bronchospasm, and persistent uncontrollable rigors to the standard form of amphotericin. In addition, patients with preexisting renal dysfunction may be candidates for treatment with these newer agents because they seem to be less nephrotoxic. Doses of 3 to 5 mg/kg of the liposomal formulations are given intravenously (IV) over 1 to 2 hours daily. The possibility of reduced side effects must be balanced with the dramatic increase in cost of the liposomal forms.

When amphotericin B is used for primary treatment in patients with coccidioidal meningitis, it is customary to give a total dose of 0.5 to 1.0 g IV amphotericin over several weeks. Since IV amphotericin B will not give a sustained response in patients with meningitis, it is also necessary to give intrathecal*† (cisternal or intraventricular) amphotericin‡ for an indefinite period as determined by the lumbar fluid parameters as well as the clinical response. It is desirable to continue intrathecal therapy until the lumbar fluid returns to normal and then for an additional 3 to 6 months. Cisternal injection is the preferred route of administration whenever possible. The starting dose is 0.05 mg, which is increased daily to the largest dose tolerated or a maximum of 0.5 mg. After achieving a stable dose, the frequency of administration can be reduced to three times a week and, after lumbar fluid parameters have returned to normal, to once or twice a week.

*Exceeds dosage recommended by the manufacturer.

*Not yet approved for use in the United States.
†Exceeds dosage recommended by the manufacturer.
‡Not FDA approved for this indication.

HISTOPLASMOSIS

method of
DAVID S. McKINSEY, M.D.
*University of Kansas
Kansas City, Missouri*

Histoplasmosis is caused by *Histoplasma capsulatum*, a thermal dimorphic fungus that exists as a mold in the environment but converts to a yeast at body temperature. Although cases of histoplasmosis have occurred in all five continents, the major endemic area is in the Ohio and Mississippi River valleys in the United States. *H. capsulatum* has an extensive natural reservoir in decaying vegetation and soil, particularly in areas contaminated by starling, chicken, or bat guano. Infection occurs after airborne microconidia are inhaled into the alveoli, convert to yeast, and spread to contiguous alveoli and then to hilar and mediastinal lymph nodes and the bloodstream. Cases occur either sporadically or in epidemics, which have been reported after activities such as spelunking or cleaning chicken coops, bird roosts, or parks.

CLINICAL MANIFESTATIONS

Most infections with *H. capsulatum* are asymptomatic and go unrecognized, but there are a variety of forms of symptomatic infection. Acute pulmonary histoplasmosis presents as a flulike illness associated with fever, chills, malaise, headache, myalgias, nonproductive cough, vague substernal discomfort, and patchy pulmonary infiltrates, often with ipsilateral hilar lymphadenopathy. Milder cases generally resolve spontaneously, but more severe cases can lead to respiratory failure. Chronic pulmonary histoplasmosis occurs in patients who have underlying chronic obstructive pulmonary disease and causes weight loss, fatigue, dyspnea, productive cough, hemoptysis, and unilateral or bilateral upper lobe pulmonary infiltrates that sometimes cavitate; the clinical presentation mimics that of chronic pulmonary tuberculosis.

Disseminated histoplasmosis is a rare disorder that is seen either in people at the extremes of age or in individuals with impaired cellular immunity due to HIV infection or immunosuppressive therapy. Symptoms include fever, weight loss, malaise, nonproductive cough, and diarrhea; physical examination reveals hepatosplenomegaly and, in some cases, painless oral ulcers or nodular skin lesions. Disseminated histoplasmosis in the HIV infected patient is a subacute febrile wasting illness. About half of patients have cough, dyspnea, and bilateral pulmonary infiltrates; in these patients, the clinical presentation mimics that of *Pneumocystis carinii* pneumonia. Physical examination findings include generalized lymphadenopathy, hepatosplenomegaly, skin lesions, or oral ulcers. In approximately 5% of patients, the clinical presentation is fulminant and is associated with multiple organ system failure, resembling gram-negative bacterial sepsis.

Several other manifestations of histoplasmosis can occur due to inflammatory responses to *H. capsulatum*. During acute histoplasmosis, such inflammatory processes include pericarditis, polyarthritis, and erythema nodosum. A mediastinal granuloma is a cystic mediastinal structure that occurs rarely during acute histoplasmosis due to an intense inflammatory reaction within mediastinal lymph nodes and can obstruct the trachea, bronchi, esophagus, or great vessels.

A *histoplasmoma* is an asymptomatic pulmonary nodule caused by a healed focus of *H. capsulatum* infection. Its principle significance is that the radiographic appearance is virtually identical to that of a malignant neoplasm, with the exception that histoplasmomas often contain calcifications. Occasionally, calcified material from a histoplasmoma erodes into a bronchus, resulting in expectoration of a stone (broncholithiasis). Mediastinal fibrosis is a rare life-threatening complication that is characterized by an exuberant fibrotic reaction within the mediastinum. Potential complications include esophageal compression, superior vena cava syndrome, constrictive pericarditis, or trapping of a lung.

DIAGNOSIS

Useful diagnostic tests include complement fixation and immunodiffusion serology, *H. capsulatum* polysaccharide antigen (HPA), culture, and histopathologic studies of biopsy or necropsy specimens. Histoplasmin skin testing is useful only for epidemiologic purposes because a positive test result cannot differentiate between remote and active infections.

Acute pulmonary histoplasmosis is diagnosed by complement fixation serology testing, which is positive in approximately 85% of cases. However, titers may not become positive until up to 6 weeks after symptoms begin, and the specificity of this test is low in endemic areas where many of the population have had prior asymptomatic infection. Results of urine and serum HPA testing and sputum culture often are negative in patients with acute pulmonary histoplasmosis.

In chronic pulmonary histoplasmosis, serologic results are positive in more than 90% of cases and sputum cultures grow *H. capsulatum* 30% to 60% of the time. HPA generally cannot be detected in serum or urine.

Disseminated histoplasmosis is diagnosed by positive serum or urine HPA results; visualization of organisms in bone marrow, liver, lymph nodes, or other tissues; positive results of blood culture (using the lysis-centrifugation technique) or cultures of tissue specimens; or by serologic studies, results of which are positive in 70% of cases.

TREATMENT AND PREVENTION

General Considerations

After the diagnosis of histoplasmosis is established, the clinician must address several questions:

Is the process likely to be self-limited or is antifungal therapy warranted?

If treatment is indicated, can an oral azole antifungal drug be used, or is intravenous (IV) amphotericin B therapy necessary?

If an azole drug is to be prescribed, which of the three available drugs is preferred?

If amphotericin B therapy is necessary, should I use conventional amphotericin B or a lipid preparation?

Some forms of histoplasmosis are self-limited and do not require antifungal therapy. Most cases of acute pulmonary histoplasmosis are asymptomatic or minimally symptomatic and resolve spontaneously within a few weeks. Pulmonary histoplasmomas represent healed self-contained foci of infection for which treatment is unnecessary. Pericarditis, polyarthritis, and erythema nodosum respond to anti-inflammatory therapy but not to antifungal treatment. For other forms of histoplasmosis (e.g., progressive acute pneumonia, chronic pneumonia, and disseminated infection), antifungal therapy is warranted.

Azole antifungal drugs with activity against *H. capsulatum* include itraconazole (Sporanox, oral and IV), ketoconazole (Nizoral, oral), and fluconazole (Diflucan, oral and IV). Itraconazole has the best in vitro activity against *H. capsulatum*, has been shown to be more effective than fluconazole for treatment of both chronic pulmonary histoplasmosis and disseminated histoplasmosis, and is considered the preferred azole drug. Ketoconazole has an unfavorable toxicity profile at the doses necessary to treat histoplasmosis and is no longer recommended. Fluconazole could be considered as a treatment option if a patient is unable to take itraconazole because of intolerance, poor absorption, or drug interactions.

Amphotericin preparations include conventional amphotericin B deoxycholate (Fungizone, IV) liposomal amphotericin B (AmBisome, IV), amphotericin B lipid complex (Abelcet, IV), and amphotericin B colloidal dispersion (Amphotec, IV). Conventional amphotericin B is highly effective but has a number of undesirable properties. It can cause phlebitis of peripheral veins, chills, fever, headache, nausea, renal insufficiency, hypokalemia, and hypomagnesemia. Liposomal amphotericin B is less toxic than conventional amphotericin B, and in a clinical trial, it was shown to be significantly more effective for treatment of severe disseminated histoplasmosis in patients with AIDS; however, it is far more expensive. Amphotericin B lipid complex and amphotericin B colloidal dispersion have not been studied for treatment of histoplasmosis. Because of cost considerations, conventional amphotericin B is the preferred agent except for patients with renal insufficiency or for HIV-infected patients who have severe disseminated histoplasmosis; in these cases, liposomal amphotericin B therapy is warranted.

For treatment recommendations, see Table 1.

TABLE 1. **Treatment of Histoplasmosis**

Form	Treatment*
Acute Pulmonary	
Mild, duration <4 wk	None
Moderate or duration >4 wk	Itraconazole 200 mg/d for 6–12 wk
Severe (respiratory failure)	Amphotericin B 0.7 mg/kg/d for 10–14 d, then itraconazole 200 mg/d for 10 wk Consider prednisone 60 mg burst and taper for 2 wk
Mediastinal Granuloma	None, or Itraconazole 200 mg/d or bid for 6–12 mo
Chronic Pulmonary	Itraconazole 200 mg/d or bid for 12–24 mo, or Amphotericin B 0.7 mg/kg/d (total dose ≤35 mg/kg/d), or Fluconazole 200–400 mg/d for 12–24 mo
Disseminated, HIV Seronegative	
Mild-moderate	Itraconazole, 200 mg/d or bid for 6–18 mo, or Fluconazole, 400–800* mg/d for 6–18 mo
Severe	Amphotericin B 0.7 mg/kg/d (total dose ≤35 mg/kg), or Liposomal amphotericin 3–5 mg/kg/d until stable, then itraconazole 200 mg/d or bid
Disseminated, HIV Seropositive	
Mild-moderate	Itraconazole 200 mg tid† for 3 d, then 200 mg bid for 12 wk, then 200 mg/d indefinitely, or Fluconazole 800 mg/d for 12 wk, then 400–800 mg/d indefinitely, or Amphotericin B 0.7 mg/kg/d for 2 wk, then 50 mg weekly or every other week indefinitely
Severe	Liposomal amphotericin B 3–5 mg/kg/d for 7–14 d, then itraconazole 200 mg bid for 10 wk, then itraconazole 200 mg/d indefinitely

*In order of preference.
†Exceeds dosage recommended by the manufacturer.

Acute Pulmonary Histoplasmosis

Many cases resolve without treatment. For patients who have not improved after a few weeks of observation, oral itraconazole therapy (200 mg daily) should be administered for 6 to 12 weeks. In those patients for whom hospitalization is necessary for management of respiratory failure due to diffuse pulmonary infiltrates, the treatment of choice is conventional amphotericin B, 0.7 mg/kg/day (or, if the patient has renal insufficiency, liposomal amphotericin 3–5 mg/kg/day). Amphotericin therapy should be continued for 10 to 14 days and then oral itraconazole should be administered to complete a 12-week treatment course. In such cases, a concomitant 2-week 60 mg burst and taper course of prednisone therapy may decrease the inflammatory response to the infection, and thus hasten resolution of respiratory failure.

Chronic Pulmonary Histoplasmosis

Because most untreated cases progress and cause permanent lung damage, treatment is recommended. Although amphotericin B therapy is effective, azole therapy is much more convenient and thus is preferred. The standard treatment regimen is itraconazole, 200 mg daily or twice daily for 12 to 24 months. A serum itraconazole concentration should be measured 2 to 4 hours after a dose to ensure adequate absorption; a concentration above 1 μg/mL is considered to be in the therapeutic range, and if the concentration is lower either the dose should be increased or the formulation should be changed from capsules to oral suspension (which is absorbed better).

Disseminated Histoplasmosis in HIV-Seronegative Patients

Patients with mild to moderately severe infection should be treated with oral itraconazole 200 mg once or twice daily for 6 to 18 months, and a serum itraconazole concentration should be documented to be within the therapeutic range as described previously. If the patient is unable to take itraconazole, fluconazole can be used; the dose is 400 mg or 800 mg* once daily. For patients who are severely ill, amphotericin B therapy (0.7–1.0 mg/kg/day) is recommended. After clinical stabilization, the patient can be treated with oral itraconazole to complete the 6- to 18-month course of therapy. Urine HPA concentrations should be measured every 3 months; declining values indicate response to treatment.

Disseminated Histoplasmosis in Patients With AIDS

Treatment is divided into two phases: an initial 12-week induction phase followed by lifelong maintenance therapy. For mild-to-moderate cases, oral itraconazole is the preferred induction therapy (200 mg thrice daily for 3 days as a loading dose, then 200 mg twice daily for 12 weeks). Fluconazole is less effective but can be used in patients who are unable to take itraconazole; the dose is 800 mg* daily. Patients with severe cases should be treated with liposomal amphotericin B, 3 to 5 mg/kg daily for 2 weeks and then itraconazole 200 mg twice daily for 10 weeks. For long-term maintenance therapy, treatment options (in order of preference) include itraconazole 200 mg daily or twice daily, amphotericin B 50 mg IV weekly or every other week, or fluconazole 400 or 800 mg daily. Urine HPA levels should be measured every 3 months or if a relapse is suspected. It is unclear if maintenance therapy can be discontinued if a patient responds well to highly active antiretroviral therapy; that is, if there is a substantial increase in CD4 count. An ongoing clinical trial is assessing this issue.

Mediastinal Granuloma and Fibrosing Mediastinitis

Although mediastinal inflammation can be self-limited, in patients with obstruction of the airways, esophagus, or great vessels it is reasonable to administer antifungal therapy. Treatment options include oral itraconazole 200 mg once or twice daily for 6 to 12 months or IV amphotericin B 0.7 mg/kg daily for 2 to 4 weeks. In cases of major airway obstruction, concomitant prednisone therapy (40–80 mg daily for 2 weeks) may be useful. For severe, refractory cases surgical resection of the mediastinal mass could be done, although this is rarely necessary. Mediastinal fibrosis generally has a much more indolent onset than granulomatous mediastinitis. Although antifungal therapy is unlikely to be beneficial for this chronic fibrotic process, in view of the progressive and life-threatening nature of the illness some authorities recommend a 12-week course of itraconazole therapy, 200 mg daily or twice daily.

Prophylaxis

In HIV-infected patients with CD4 counts below 100/μL who reside in areas where rates of histoplasmosis are high, itraconazole primary prophylaxis (200 mg daily) is effective.

*Exceeds dosage recommended by the manufacturer.

BLASTOMYCOSIS

method of
MICHAEL S. GELFAND, M.D.
Methodist Hospitals
Memphis, Tennessee

Blastomycosis (Gilchrist's disease) is an uncommon, noncontagious subacute or chronic systemic fungal infection caused by the dimorphic fungus *Blastomyces dermatitidis*.

Blastomycosis is endemic in areas of North America adjacent to the Mississippi and Ohio Rivers, the Midwestern states, and the Canadian provinces bordering the Great Lakes. Most cases are reported from Mississippi, Arkansas, Kentucky, Tennessee, and Wisconsin. This disease is also reported from Africa, Mexico, and Central and South America. Hyperendemic areas and point-source outbreaks have been reported.

Clinical illness is more common in men, but self-limited infection during the outbreaks is independent of age, gender, and race. Dogs are highly susceptible to blastomycosis and may develop the disease before or at the same time as their owners. Occupational and recreational activities along streams and rivers may bring susceptible individuals into contact with areas with warm moist soil enriched with decaying organic matter, where the fungus is likely to grow. Inhaled spores from the mycelial form of the fungus establish a pulmonary focus of infection. The pulmonary form of blastomycosis is the most common and clinically dominant form of the disease. Lymphohematogenous dissemination from the lungs may occur, and other commonly involved sites include the skin, bones, and male genitourinary tract. Dissemination and multisystem involvement occur more often in immunocompromised individuals.

Histologically, blastomycosis is manifested by suppuration and granulomas that present simultaneously and to a variable degree. Skin and mucous membrane lesions show pseudoepitheliomatous hyperplasia and may mimic a malignancy.

The clinical picture of blastomycosis ranges from an asymptomatic state to an acute, subacute, or chronic pneumonia to a disseminated infection. Acute pulmonary blastomycosis develops after an incubation period of 30 to 45 days and resembles a nonspecific community-acquired pneumonia with pleuritic chest pain, fever, and cough with purulent sputum production. Chest radiography shows a lobar, interstitial, or alveolar infiltrate.

Spontaneous recovery from acute pulmonary blastomycosis is documented in the literature, but the rate is uncertain.

Subacute or chronic pneumonia is the most common manifestation of blastomycosis. Patients often receive several courses of oral antibiotics without success. Clinically and radiographically it resembles tuberculosis, other fungal infections, or bronchogenic carcinoma. Low-grade fever and cough, sometimes with hemoptysis and weight loss, are the usual clinical features. Radiographically, air-space and masslike infiltrates are usually present, with predominant involvement of the upper lobes. Cavitation can occur. Perihilar mass lesions have led to confusion with malignancy and subsequent lobectomy or even pneumonectomy in some patients. A fulminant form of pneumonia with miliary or diffuse pulmonary infiltrates and acute respiratory distress syndrome has been described in both immunocompetent and immunocompromised patients, with a high mortality rate of up to 50%.

Laryngeal blastomycosis is not uncommon and has a clinical and histopathologic appearance resembling squamous cell carcinoma. Extrapulmonary blastomycosis can occur with or without pulmonary disease. Skin lesions are the most common form of extrapulmonary blastomycosis. Verrucous lesions suggestive of squamous cell skin carcinoma and, less commonly, skin ulcers can be present. Osteomyelitis can mimic tuberculosis, especially when occurring in the vertebral bodies. Bone disease is more difficult to treat and more likely to relapse.

The prostate and epididymis are the most common sites of genitourinary blastomycosis in men. Sexual transmission of blastomycosis to a female partner has been reported.

Cerebral abscesses and chronic meningitis are the central nervous system (CNS) manifestations of blastomycosis.

Blastomycosis in immunocompromised patients (e.g., with AIDS, transplants, or leukemia) is a more severe and fulminant disease with a higher mortality rate (up to 40%) and slower response to therapy. Relapses are frequent and long-term suppressive therapy with itraconazole (Sporanox) or intermittent amphotericin B (Fungizone) is usually recommended. In AIDS patients, restoration of immune function with highly active antiretroviral therapy may allow discontinuation of suppressive therapy, provided that the CD4 count is above 200/μL.

A definitive diagnosis of blastomycosis requires isolation of the organism from a clinical specimen. Blastomycosis is never a colonizer, and isolation from any clinical specimen indicates infection. Sputum, a bronchoscopy specimen, exudate from a skin lesion, or a biopsy sample can be cultured on enriched agar at 30°C.

Identification of mycelial cultures with exoantigen tests or DNA probes and conversion of culture to the yeast phase at 37°C are both used in clinical microbiology laboratories.

A presumptive diagnosis can be made by visualization of the typical yeast forms (broad-based budding yeasts) in a clinical specimen (e.g., sputum or exudate). In an appropriate clinical setting, this is sufficient to initiate therapy while awaiting the culture results. A wet slide preparation of sputum or exudate can be examined directly after digestion with 10% potassium hydroxide solution or with calcofluor white stain. Cytologic examination of the bronchoscopy specimen is very helpful. Biopsy specimens are usually stained with Gomori methenamine silver stain (GMS) and/or periodic acid–Schiff stain (PAS). If the radiographic pulmonary infiltrate is highly atypical for blastomycosis, I recommend bronchoscopy to exclude tuberculosis and, particularly in smokers, an investigation for bronchogenic carcinoma, even in patients with sputum smear results positive for blastomycosis-like yeast. Clinically available serologic tests are not very sensitive or specific and are not clinically helpful in most cases. Skin testing materials for blastomycosis are not commercially available.

TREATMENT

Although spontaneous resolution of acute pulmonary blastomycosis has been reported, it is unpredictable; therefore, I treat all patients with blastomycosis with antifungal agents. Immediate initiation of treatment is especially important in patients with progressive pulmonary, extrapulmonary, and disseminated disease and in immunocompromised patients with blastomycosis (Table 1). Treatment options include amphotericin B (Fungizone and lipid forms, e.g. Abelcet or AmBisome) and azoles, such as ketoconazole (Nizoral), itraconazole (Sporanox), and fluconazole (Diflucan).*

Amphotericin B is the standard treatment for severe, life-threatening forms of blastomycosis. Itraconazole is an effective alternative for patients with mild-to-moderate pulmonary and extrapulmonary disease. Azoles should not be used for patients with severe, life-threatening, or CNS disease. Azoles are contraindicated in pregnant women (embryotoxic and teratogenic potential), and amphotericin B should be used in pregnant women with blastomycosis. Amphotericin B should be the initial treatment in immunocompromised patients. Patients with severe, life-threatening blastomycosis, CNS disease, or disease progression despite azole therapy and those who are unable to tolerate azole therapy should be treated with amphotericin B.

Ketoconazole was the first azole proven to be effective in patients with mild-to-moderate blastomycosis. Cure rates of up to 80% were documented with doses of 400 to 800 mg* per day. Higher doses are more likely to produce side effects, and the usual initial dose is 400 mg per day. The dose can be increased in 200-mg increments up to maximum of 800 mg† per day if the response is not satisfactory. Treatment should be given for at least 6 months.

Itraconazole is highly effective for the treatment of blastomycosis. Clinical studies have documented cure rates of 90% or greater with a daily dose of 200 mg to 400 mg of itraconazole. Treatment is usually started with 400 mg per day for the first few days and then continued with a daily dose of 200 mg. The dose can be increased by 100 mg to a maximum daily dose of 400 mg if the response is not satisfactory. The treatment should be continued for at least 6 months. Itraconazole is more expensive than ketoconazole but appears to be more efficacious and better tolerated, and itraconazole has replaced ketoconazole for the treatment of non–life-threatening blastomycosis.

Both ketoconazole and itraconazole require gastric acid for absorption, and inadequate absorption and

*Not FDA approved for this indication.
†Exceeds dosage recommended by the manufacturer.

TABLE 1. **The Treatment of Blastomycosis**

Type of Disease	First Choice	Alternative Therapy
Pulmonary		
Severe	Amphotericin B. Start with 0.7–1.0 mg/kg/d for a total dose of 2 g*	Change to itraconazole 200–400 mg/d after the patient is stable and has received at least 500 mg of amphotericin B.
Mild to moderate	Itraconazole, 200–400 mg/d†	Ketoconazole, 400–800 mg/d‡ or fluconazole, 400–800 mg/d.†
Disseminated		
CNS	Amphotericin B, 0.7–1.0 mg/kg/d for a total dose of 2.0–2.5 g	If unable to tolerate full course of amphotericin B, consider fluconazole‡ 800§ mg/d.†
Non-CNS		
Severe	Amphotericin B. Start with 0.7–1.0 mg/kg/d for a total dose of 2 g*	Change to itraconazole 200–400 mg/d after the patient is stable and has received at least 500 mg of amphotericin B.
Mild to moderate	Itraconazole, 200–400 mg/d†	Ketoconazole, 400–800 mg/d‡ or fluconazole‡, 400–800§ mg/d.†
Immunocompromised Host	Amphotericin B. Start with 0.7–1.0 mg/kg/d for a total dose of 2 g*	Indefinite suppressive therapy (after amphotericin B) with itraconazole, 200–400 mg/d or fluconazole,§ 800 mg/d (if CNS involvement)

*After the patient is clinically stable, decrease amphotericin B dosage to 0.5–0.7 mg/kg/d.
†Treatment with an azole should be for a minimum of 6 months (12 months if bone disease).
‡Exceeds dosage recommended by the manufacturer.
§Not FDA approved for this indication.
Abbreviation: CNS = central nervous system.

therapeutic failures can occur in patients taking antacids, H_2-receptor antagonists, and proton-pump inhibitors. If the patient is known to be achlorhydric, checking the serum level of the azole, administering it with an acidic cola beverage, or using a solution form of itraconazole is advisable. The oral solution form of itraconazole is more expensive and less palatable, but it is better absorbed and can be taken in a fasting state. The use of hepatic enzyme inducers (rifampin, phenytoin [Dilantin], carbamazepine [Tegretol]) has been shown to markedly increase the hepatic metabolism of both itraconazole and ketoconazole and may result in therapeutic failure. If azole is to be continued, either checking azole serum levels or switching to another non–enzyme-inducing cotherapy is essential. Alternatively, amphotericin B can be substituted for the azole.

Other significant drug interactions have been observed with cyclosporine (Sandimmune), tacrolimus (Prograf), digoxin (Lanoxin), warfarin (Coumadin), midazolam (Versed), triazolam (Halcion), and phenobarbital.

Life-threatening ventricular arrhythmias can occur when ketoconazole and itraconazole are combined with cisapride (Propulsid)* and the nonsedating antihistamines (e.g., terfenadine [Seldane],* astemizole [Hismanal]*), and concurrent administration of these agents is contraindicated.

Nausea and vomiting can be side effects with ketoconazole and itraconazole and are dose dependent. Taking these drugs with meals or dividing the daily dose may help. Hormonal abnormalities are more common with ketoconazole and may include gynecomastia, oligospermia, impotence, and abnormal uterine bleeding. Edema and hypokalemia can occur with ketoconazole. Severe hepatic toxicity is unusual with both agents, but I routinely check monthly liver function tests, at least for the first few months of therapy. An intravenous form of itraconazole is now available and may be useful for short-term therapy in patients unable to take oral azoles (e.g., perioperatively), but severely ill patients should be treated with amphotericin B.

*Not available in the United States.

Relapses after azole therapy are more common than after amphotericin B and are reported in the range of 10% to 14%. I usually continue to observe patients for at least 1 year after the completion of therapy. Breakthroughs and relapses with CNS blastomycosis have been reported with azole therapy in patients who initially did not have clinical CNS disease. Attention to CNS complaints and a high index of suspicion therefore is essential when using azoles for blastomycosis.

Fluconazole* is less efficacious than itraconazole and is comparable to ketoconazole in blastomycosis therapy when used in a dose of 400 mg to 800 mg† daily. Fluconazole is well absorbed in the absence of gastric acid, drug interactions are less frequent, and the side effects are less common and milder than those with ketoconazole and itraconazole. Unlike other azoles, fluconazole penetrates well into the CNS and may be an alternative therapy for blastomycosis patients with CNS disease who are intolerant of amphotericin B.*

Amphotericin B is the treatment of choice for patients who are immunocompromised; have severe, life-threatening, or CNS disease; are pregnant; or

*Not FDA approved for this indication.
†Exceeds dosage recommended by the manufacturer.

have disease progression with or are unable to tolerate azole therapy.

A total of at least 1.5 g of amphotericin B results in lowest rates of relapse (<4%); I usually give a course of at least 2 g of amphotericin B. In patients with severe, life-threatening (such as acute respiratory distress syndrome), or CNS disease, I start treatment with an amphotericin B dose of 0.7 to 1 mg/kg/d. Less seriously ill patients or those who fail to improve with azole or are unable to tolerate azole drugs are usually given 0.5 to 0.7 mg/kg/d. In these less seriously ill patients without CNS disease, I administer 500 to 1000 mg of amphotericin B, and if the patient is clinically stable, I switch to itraconazole to complete the course of treatment.

Because of the high rates of relapse, even after amphotericin B therapy, of blastomycosis in AIDS patients and patients continuing on immunosuppressive therapy, I continue itraconazole indefinitely in these patients. Fluconazole* (except with CNS involvement or itraconazole intolerance) and ketoconazole are not recommended in this setting. Amphotericin B, especially in high doses and for prolonged therapy, is often associated with significant side effects. Phlebitis is prevented by using a peripherally inserted central catheter or a central venous line. Infusion toxicity (e.g., fever, chills) often abates after the first few doses and can be controlled with premedication (acetaminophen, diphenhydramine) and intravenous meperidine (Demerol). Renal impairment is the most significant problem and may result in interruption of therapy. Infusion of 1000 mL of saline before amphotericin B and avoidance of other nephrotoxins (e.g., aminoglycosides, intravenous contrast) are recommended. Patients experiencing severe renal toxicity may benefit from lipid forms of amphotericin B, but the clinical experience in severe forms of blastomycosis is limited.

*Not FDA approved for this indication.

PLEURAL EFFUSION AND EMPYEMA THORACIS

method of
STEVEN A. SAHN, M.D.
Medical University of South Carolina
Charleston, South Carolina

PLEURAL EFFUSIONS

Pleural effusions are common in the practice of medicine because they result not only from primary diseases in the chest but also from organ dysfunction below the diaphragm (cirrhosis) and systemic diseases (systemic lupus erythematosus). When a patient presents with a pleural effusion, suspected from the physical examination and confirmed by chest radiography, it affords an opportunity for the clinician to diagnose, definitively or presumptively, the cause of the disease by means of a simple bedside or office procedure—thoracentesis.

Analysis of 20 to 30 mL of fluid aspirated from the chest cavity can provide important clinical information when used in conjunction with history, physical examination, and other laboratory findings. Only about 25% of patients can be diagnosed definitively by pleural fluid analysis, however, and an additional 55% to 60% can be diagnosed presumptively, leaving 15% to 20% of patients undiagnosed following the initial analysis of pleural fluid. Only by finding malignant cells, purulent fluid, a specific organism, high levels of triglycerides (chylothorax), lupus erythematosus cells, an elevated amylase level (pancreatic disease, malignancy or esophageal rupture), or a pleural fluid/serum creatinine of greater than 1.0 (urinothorax) can a definitive diagnosis be established. With undiagnosed effusions, observation may be appropriate, but in some, a diagnosis needs to be pursued more vigorously through thoracoscopy or thoracotomy.

TREATMENT

Not all patients presenting with a pleural effusion require immediate thoracentesis. For example, a patient with classic congestive heart failure who presents with orthopnea, paroxysmal nocturnal dyspnea, jugular venous distention, a left ventricular S3 gallop, bilateral basilar crackles, and a chest radiograph that shows cardiomegaly and bilateral effusions (left greater than right) should be treated for congestive heart failure. Only if treatment does not lead to appropriate resolution should thoracentesis be performed. If on admission the patient with presumed congestive heart failure has fever, pleuritic chest pain, hemoptysis, a unilateral pleural effusion, bilateral effusions of disparate size, or hypoxemia inappropriate for the clinical condition, however, immediate thoracentesis should be done. The patient who presents with a secure clinical diagnosis (i.e., viral pleurisy) and a minimal pleural effusion can have thoracentesis delayed pending the clinical outcome. If it is deemed necessary to obtain pleural fluid with a small volume of fluid or loculation, thoracentesis should be performed under ultrasound guidance.

Diagnostic Factors

An important deductive step in diagnosis is to determine whether the effusion is a transudate or an exudate. Transudates result from imbalances in hydrostatic and oncotic pressure and are seen in congestive heart failure, hepatic hydrothorax, nephrotic syndrome, other causes of hypoalbuminemia, atelectasis, peritoneal dialysis, constrictive pericarditis, and trapped lung. Exudative effusions, which encompass a larger differential diagnosis, are due to inflammatory processes that result in increased capillary permeability (e.g., pneumonia) and disease of the lymphatic system (malignancy), which blocks removal of fluid from the pleural space. The major categories of exudative pleural effusions include infection, malignancy, connective tissue disease, endocrine dysfunction, lymphatic abnormalities, movement of fluid from the peritoneal to the pleural space, and iatrogenic causes (see Table 1).

TABLE 1. **Causes of Exudative Pleural Effusions**

Column 1	Column 2	Column 3
Infections	**Malignancy**	**Connective Tissue Disease**
Bacterial pneumonia	Carcinoma	Lupus pleuritis
Tuberculous pleurisy	Lymphoma	Rheumatoid pleurisy
Parasitic infection	Mesothelioma	Mixed connective tissue disease
Fungal disease	Leukemia	Churg-Strauss syndrome
Atypical pneumonias	Chylothorax	Wegener granulomatosis
Nocardia, Actinomyces infections	**Other Inflammatory Causes**	Familial Meditterranean fever
Subphrenic abscess	Pancreatitis	**Endocrine Dysfunction**
Hepatic abscess	Benign asbestos pleural effusions	Hypothyroidism
Splenic abscess	Pulmonary embolism	Ovarian hyperstimulation syndrome
Hepatitis	Radiation therapy	**Lymphatic Abnormalities**
Spontaneous esophageal rupture	Uremic pleurisy	Malignancy
Iatrogenic Causes	Sarcoidosis	Yellow nail syndrome
Drugs	Post–cardiac injury syndrome	Lymphangiomyomatosis (chylothorax)
Esophageal perforation	Hemothorax	**Movement of Fluid from Abdomen to Pleural Space**
Esophageal sclerotherapy	Adult respiratory distress syndrome	Pancreatitis
Central venous catheter misplacement/migration	**Increased Negative Intrapleural Pressure**	Pancreatic pseudocyst
Enteral feeding tube in pleural space	Atelectasis	Meigs' syndrome
	Trapped lung	Carcinoma
	Cholesterol effusion	Chylous ascites
		Urinothorax

From Sahn SA: Diagnostic value of pleural fluid analysis. Semin Respir Crit Care Med 16:272, 1995.

A fluid is usually exudative if the pleural fluid protein concentration is greater than 3.0 g/dL, the pleural fluid/protein ratio is greater than 0.5, the pleural fluid lactate dehydrogenase level is greater than two thirds of the upper limits of normal for serum lactate dehydrogenase, or the pleural fluid cholesterol is greater than 60 mg/dL. If none of these criteria is present, the fluid is usually transudative. None of these tests is 100% sensitive and specific; therefore, the clinician must interpret the pleural fluid findings in the context of the clinical presentation.

The total nucleated cell count is virtually never diagnostic; however, counts of more than 50,000/μL are usually found only in parapneumonic effusions. Exudative pleural effusions from bacterial pneumonia, acute pancreatitis, and lupus pleuritis usually have total nucleated cell counts of greater than 10,000/μL, whereas chronic exudates, as seen in tuberculous pleurisy and malignancy, usually have nucleated cell counts of less than 5000/μL. When the nucleated cell differential of the exudate effusion shows more than 80% lymphocytes, the differential diagnosis includes tuberculous pleurisy, chylothorax, lymphoma, yellow nail syndrome, chronic rheumatoid pleurisy, sarcoidosis, and trapped lung. When greater than 10% of nucleated cells are eosinophils, the usual causes are pneumothorax, hemothorax, benign asbestos pleural effusion, pulmonary embolism with infarction, parasitic disease, fungal disease, drug-induced disease, and malignancy, both carcinoma and Hodgkin disease.

A low pleural fluid pH (<7.30), measured with a radiometer (like arterial blood pH), narrows the differential diagnosis to empyema, esophageal rupture, rheumatoid pleurisy, malignancy, tuberculous pleurisy, and lupus pleuritis. These same diagnoses are found when the pleural fluid glucose is low (<60 mg/dL or pleural fluid/serum ratio <0.5). A pleural fluid amylase greater than the upper limits of normal for serum amylase or a pleural fluid/serum amylase ratio of greater than 1.0 is found only with acute pancreatitis, pancreatic pseudocyst, esophageal rupture, or carcinoma.

EMPYEMA THORACIS

Empyema is defined as pus in a body cavity; therefore, empyema thoracis is pus in the pleural space. Pus assumes its character because it is composed of coagulable pleural fluid, cellular debris, fibrin, and collagen and appears as a thick, yellow-white, opaque fluid. Empyema is the end stage of a parapneumonic effusion (associated with pneumonia) and generally develops 2 to 3 weeks following the clinical presentation of pneumonia. Empyema forms only in untreated or inadequately treated patients. If pneumonia is treated shortly after symptoms begin with the appropriate antibiotic, it is unlikely that a parapneumonic effusion will develop and even less likely that empyema will occur.

The management of a parapneumonic effusion is relatively straightforward in the early (exudative) and late (organizational/empyema) stages but is problematic in the intermediate (fibrinopurulent) stage. All patients with empyema require drainage of the pleural space to resolve pleural sepsis and to prevent severe pleural fibrosis. This can be accomplished with chest tube or small-bore catheter drainage, usually aided by image guidance, with or without fibrinolytic therapy. Patients with multiloculated empyema will need drainage via thoracoscopy or standard thoracotomy.

In the exudative stage, the pleural fluid is free-flowing and occupies less than one third of the hemithorax. The pleural fluid is a slightly turbid, sterile, neutrophil-predominant exudate with a pH of greater than 7.30 and glucose of greater than 60 mg/dL. Administration of antibiotics will result in resolution of the effusion in 1 to 2 weeks without pleural space sequelae.

In the fibrinopurulent stage, which occurs about 5 to 10 days after clinical symptoms of pneumonia, several factors need to be considered before making a judgment regarding the need for drainage. Clinical features that increase the likelihood that drainage should be done include prolonged symptoms, anaerobic infection, failure to respond to antibiotic therapy, virulence of the pathogen, and an effusion of more than 40% of the hemithorax. Pleural fluid findings suggesting the need for drainage of the nonpurulent exudate include pH of less than 7.30, glucose of less than 40 mg/dL, lactate dehydrogenase of more than 1000 IU/L, or a positive Gram stain or culture.

The primary care physician should seek immediate pulmonary or thoracic surgery consultation when the patient presents in or progresses to the fibrinopurulent stage. Delay in treatment results in increased morbidity, mortality, and cost.

PRIMARY LUNG ABSCESS

method of
SYDNEY M. FINEGOLD, M.D.
VA Medical Center West Los Angeles
Los Angeles, California

A lung abscess is a cavity, 2 cm or more in diameter, containing pus and necrotic debris. It reflects infection with a large microbial load (e.g., acute aspiration), a failure in microbial clearance (e.g., bronchial obstruction), or both.

ETIOLOGY

The principal predisposing conditions and background factors are noted in Table 1. Anaerobic bacteria of the indigenous oropharyngeal flora are involved in 90%, half with nonanaerobes also. The principal anaerobes are pigmented and nonpigmented *Prevotella, Fusobacterium,* and *Peptostreptococcus. Bacteroides fragilis* group strains occur in 7% of cases. Among the nonanaerobes, streptococci, *Staphylococcus aureus,* and gram-negative bacilli (especially *Klebsiella pneumoniae*) are prominent; the latter two are often hospital acquired. *Nocardia* and *Rhodococcus* occur in immunocompromised hosts, and *Paragonimus westermani* and melioidosis are usually acquired in the Far East or Indonesia.

CLINICAL MANIFESTATIONS

There is an insidious onset in many patients; additional clues are involvement of dependent lung segments, predisposition to aspiration, and periodontal disease. Putrid sputum is noted in half of patients, and hemoptysis may be seen. Weeks to months of malaise and low-grade fever may occur, as well as cough, weight loss, and anemia. On occasion, the picture is acute. Patients with lung abscess due to *S. aureus* or gram-negative bacilli may have a fulminant course and often manifest chills. In edentulous people, lung abscess is uncommon and suggests carcinoma.

DIAGNOSIS

The classic radiographic appearance of lung abscess is a cavity with an air-fluid level. Microbiologic studies are desirable in sicker patients because so many different organisms may cause lung abscess and antimicrobial resistance is a problem. Expectorated sputum cannot be used for culture because large numbers of anaerobes are present in the indigenous flora and even *S. aureus* and gram-negative bacilli frequently colonize the oropharynx in institutionalized patients. Empyema fluid constitutes an excellent source for anaerobic (and aerobic) culture. Two approaches suitable for respiratory tract secretion culture are performing bronchoalveolar lavage and using a protected specimen brush with quantitation of results.

TREATMENT

Antimicrobial therapy and drainage are the keystones of treatment; identification and treatment of underlying processes are also important. Prolonged therapy (1–3 months or more) is important to prevent relapse. The initial antimicrobial choice is empirical but should be guided by the Gram stain and the likely bacteriology of the infection and then adjusted as culture and susceptibility data become available.

Some 40% of certain anaerobic gram-negative rods (*Prevotella, Bacteroides* species, and some fusobacteria) produce β-lactamases and are resistant to penicillin G. Clindamycin (Cleocin) has given better clinical results than penicillin. Although some anaerobic cocci, clostridia, and *B. fragilis* group strains are resistant to clindamycin, it generally gives good results in lung abscess patients who are not seriously ill. The dosage is 600 mg every 6 hours given intravenously initially; when the patient is improved, 300 mg is given orally every 6 hours. Cefoxitin (Mefoxin),

TABLE 1. **Primary Lung Abscess**

Predisposing Conditions
Reduced level of consciousness
Dysphagia
Nasogastric tube interference with cardiac sphincter
Endotracheal intubation
Major Background Factors
Alcoholism
Seizure disorders
General anesthesia
Cerebrovascular accidents
Esophageal disease
Nasogastric tube feeding
Drug addiction
Periodontal disease, gingivitis

despite the resistance of some clostridia and *B. fragilis* group strains, may also give good results in patients with only moderately severe disease. Dosage is 1 to 2 g intramuscularly or intravenously every 4 to 6 hours. When penicillin is used, it should be used in high dosage (12 million units per day intravenously in average-sized adults with normal renal function) and in combination with metronidazole (Flagyl), 2 g intravenously per day in four divided doses, or clindamycin. Metronidazole alone may be ineffective because of resistance of aerobic bacteria, *Actinomyces*, and some anaerobic streptococci. After improvement, one can use ampicillin (Omnipen, Totacillin) or amoxicillin (Amoxil, Trimox, Wymox) plus metronidazole orally, each in a dose of 500 mg every 6 to 8 hours. Imipenem (Primaxin) or meropenem (Merrem) and β-lactam/β-lactamase inhibitor combinations such as ticarcillin and clavulanic acid (Timentin), piperacillin/tazobactam (Zosyn), ampicillin/sulbactam (Unasyn), and amoxicillin/clavulanate (Augmentin) are active against essentially all anaerobes and many of the nonanaerobes important in lung abscess. Newer quinolones with good activity versus most anaerobes and other potential pathogens have not yet been adequately studied.

Postural drainage is important. Bronchoscopy may help in effecting good drainage, removal of foreign bodies, and diagnosis of tumor.

Persistence of high fever after 72 hours, or lack of change in sputum production or character or in the radiograph over 7 to 10 days, suggests unappreciated obstruction, empyema, or resistant organisms. Surgical resection of necrotic lung may occasionally be needed if the response to antimicrobial agents is poor or if airway obstruction limits drainage. In poor surgical risks, percutaneous drainage of lung abscess may be useful.

PROGNOSIS

The mortality rate is 5% to 10%. Patients with large abscesses (>6 cm), progressive pulmonary necrosis, obstructing lesions, aerobic bacterial infection, immune compromise, old age, and debility, and with treatment delays, have higher mortality and more complications.

OTITIS MEDIA

method of
RICHARD H. SCHWARTZ, M.D.
Inova Fairfax Hospital for Children
Falls Church, Virginia

Otitis media is among the three most common outpatient diagnoses in infants and young children between 6 and 36 months of age. It is particularly common in the very young. One child out of five may experience at least three recurrent attacks of acute otitis media (AOM) during infancy. Antibiotics have greatly reduced the number of serious complications of AOM, and today 20% of all antibiotic prescriptions written for children of this age are for the treatment of middle ear disease. At the same time, the emergence of antibiotic resistance has led to other problems, including recurrent and chronic infection.

DIAGNOSIS

Many children with AOM do not complain of pain; fever is likewise not necessarily present. The following behavioral criteria do generally correlate with AOM, as demonstrated by the recovery of bacterial pathogens during tympanocentesis.

- Irritability or crankiness, whining, or crying
- Anorexia or sleep disturbance
- Rubbing or tugging at the auricle or digging the index finger into the auditory meatus
- Complaints of a feeling of fullness of the middle ear
- Diminished hearing capacity

Prerequisites for accurate diagnosis include (1) a well-maintained halogen light source; (2) properly designed otoscopic specula (3-mm, 4-mm, and 5-mm) that can be inserted 5 to 6 mm into the ear canal; (3) skilled use of stainless steel, blunt aural curets, disposable plastic curets, or aural lavage to remove ear wax and skin; (4) firm restraint of the patient's arms and legs; and (5) application of alternate negative and positive pressure with a pneumatic otoscope. The principal pneumo-otoscopic signs of AOM are fullness, bulging, or opacification of the tympanic membrane as well as reduced mobility. Another important sign may be spontaneous acute otorrhea from a ruptured eardrum or through a tympanostomy tube. The color of the membrane is of minor importance; likewise, diffusion or absence of the light reflex is no longer believed to be a reliable criterion for the diagnosis of AOM.

When the diagnosis is in doubt, an impedance instrument (tympanometry) or an acoustic reflectometer may be useful in detecting middle ear effusion. Wax impactions and narrow ear canals in infants may reduce the reliability of these techniques; in this case, they should be coupled with pneumatic otoscopy.

The clinical practice guidelines issued in 1997 by the Centers for Disease Control and Prevention and the American Academy of Pediatrics should be used to ensure the appropriate diagnosis and avoid unnecessary use of antibiotics.

PATHOGENESIS

Respiratory syncytial, parainfluenza, and influenza viruses have major roles in the pathogenesis of AOM. The five most common pathogens, in descending order, are *Streptococcus pneumoniae, Haemophilus influenzae, Moraxella catarrhalis, Streptococcus pyogenes,* and *Staphylococcus aureus.* Other factors that have a role in the pathogenesis of AOM include exposure to cigarette smoke, face-to-face or hand-to-mouth contact with other children and with adults, and allergies. Anatomic features associated with AOM include the length and the angulation of the eustachian tube and, possibly, the presence of chronically infected lymphoid tissue in the nasopharynx.

TREATMENT

In general, the more virulent the bacteria and the greater the child's pain and fever, the greater the importance of treatment with antibiotic and antipyretic/analgesic agents.

Antibiotics. Amoxicillin remains the antibiotic of choice for treatment of AOM in most areas of the United States. The initial dosage generally ranges between 55 and 90 mg/kg/d in two or three divided doses. For children 3 years of age or older who are not otitis prone, a recently recommended truncated (5-day) course of amoxicillin may be appropriate. Amoxicillin is not a good choice if the patient is allergic to penicillins, has taken it or another β-lactam antibiotic within the past month, or is very otitis prone. For these children, an expanded-spectrum macrolide antibiotic is a reasonable alternative. One such agent is azithromycin (Zithromax), 10 mg/kg/d as a single dose on day 1, followed by 5 mg/kg/d on days 2 through 5.

Antibiotic resistance is a growing problem; for example, at present, 20% to 40% of *S. pneumoniae* clinical isolates are drug-resistant strains. The most appropriate alternative agents for the treatment of drug-resistant *S. pneumoniae* are (1) amoxicillin/clavulanate (Augmentin), 50 to 75 mg/kg/d of the 200- or 400-mg/5 mL suspension in two divided doses; (2) cefdinir (Omnicef) 14 mg/kg/d in two divided doses or cefuroxime axetil (Ceftin) suspension, 30 mg/kg/d in two divided doses; or (3) ceftriaxone (Rocephin) injection, 50 mg/kg/d with a maximum volume of 1 mL per site. Several studies have shown excessive numbers of early recurrences of AOM after a single injection of ceftriaxone; for this reason, the agent should be injected for 2 or 3 days, for a total dose of 100 to 150 mg/kg.

Tympanocentesis should be considered after tandem failure of antibiotics (e.g., amoxicillin followed by amoxicillin/clavulanate or cefuroxime) or after failure of several doses of intramuscular ceftriaxone.

Antipyretics/Analgesics. Patients in significant pain, especially those whose pain interferes with sleeping, should receive an analgesic. These include acetaminophen syrup (15 mg/kg every 4 hours), ibuprofen suspension (10 mg/kg every 6–8 hours), acetaminophen with codeine syrup (1.0 mg/kg per dose of the codeine component), or, for infants, paregoric syrup (one drop per pound of body weight). Pain can also be reduced by applying a heating pad to the ear or instilling warmed vegetable oil into the ear canal. Topical anesthetic drops containing benzocaine in glycerin can relieve pain if the eardrum is intact. Decongestant-antihistamine drug combinations are not effective in treating AOM.

RE-EVALUATION

After 48 to 72 hours of appropriate antibiotic therapy, the child should exhibit a decrease in otalgia or fussiness and a significant reduction in fever. Should severe symptoms continue, prompt re-evaluation is essential. Otherwise, routine re-evaluation is not needed for children older than 2 or 3 years of age and those with unilateral AOM. Re-evaluation is likewise not needed in asymptomatic infants who are scheduled to return for routine check-ups within 3 months. A clinically improving child with a past history of otitis media with effusion (OME) or a young child with bilateral AOM should have a follow-up visit in 2 or 3 months.

OTHER MANAGEMENT CONSIDERATIONS

Acute Otorrhea

Acute otorrhea may be caused by a perforated tympanic membrane or liquefaction of cerumen. It may be spontaneous or may exude from a tympanostomy tube. Bacterial pathogens associated with acute otorrhea respond well to customary oral antibiotics. Recent studies show that instillation of fluoroquinolone otic drops alone may relieve otorrhea associated with a patent tympanostomy tube.

The Otitis-Prone Child

The descriptor *otitis-prone* may be used to refer to a child who has had more than two episodes of AOM in a 6-month period or more than three episodes in 12 months. (An antibiotic failure or a case of secretory otitis media does not count.) Children most likely to be otitis prone include those in child care settings or who live in households with adults who smoke tobacco; those who had their first episode of AOM before the fourth month of life; infants not breast-fed for at least 3 months and those who bottle feed in a prone position; children who are highly allergic to certain foods; and those who have chronic mucopurulent rhinorrhea. Certain orofacial anomalies, such as cleft palate, may make a child more susceptible to a middle ear infection.

In addition to removal of manageable risk factors, management includes a trial of pneumococcal vaccine (for children older than 2 years), annual influenza vaccinations for older children, and a therapeutic trial of antireflux medications.

Some children may benefit from a daily dose of prophylactic antibiotic during the otitis season. Traditional prophylactic regimens include sulfisoxazole, 30 mg/kg administered at bedtime, or amoxicillin, 13 mg/kg per dose.

Otitis Media with Effusion

Following a course of antibiotic therapy, between 50% and 70% of children will develop OME. The mean duration of this condition is 12 weeks. OME is seasonal, peaking in December through May in the mid-Atlantic states. Risk factors for OME are the same as those associated with being otitis prone. Associated conductive hearing loss is usually mild, but if the condition is bilateral and lasts more than 4 months, it may interfere with the child's hearing and learning. Impedance testing may be used to complement pneumatic otoscopy in these patients. Tympanometry and acoustic reflectometry are valuable adjuncts.

Children with OME should be followed over time; there is usually no need for antibiotics or other medication. Environmental management solutions such as those recommended for the otitis-prone child should be followed. By 90 days, the cutoff point for the onset of chronic OME, all but 10% of these cases will resolve.

Deserving special attention are children with bothersome symptoms that interfere with sleep, balance, and hearing. They should be referred for an audiogram or an emittance test approximately 60 days after the OME developed or earlier if hearing impairment seems significant. If hearing acuity has substantially declined, the child is not speaking clearly, or language milestones have been delayed, placement of tympanostomy tubes or a therapeutic trial of corticosteroids may be warranted.

Children with no underlying problems (e.g., craniofacial abnormalities, pre-existing hearing loss) should be referred to an otolaryngologist if the condition has not resolved in 60 days. Patients with minimally symptomatic bilateral effusions should be followed for about 120 days; those with minimally symptomatic unilateral effusions may be followed for 180 days before being referred to an otolaryngologist.

ACUTE BRONCHITIS AND ACUTE EXACERBATION OF CHRONIC BRONCHITIS

method of
JOHN S. CZACHOR, M.D.
Wright State University School of Medicine
Dayton, Ohio

Bronchitis can be defined as an inflammatory process involving the lower respiratory tract. It ranks as one of the most common diagnoses encountered in outpatient primary care medicine, accounting for nearly 30% of all antibiotic prescriptions written for infectious diseases. Bronchitis has been clinically divided into acute and chronic forms.

ACUTE BRONCHITIS

Acute bronchitis has classically been defined as a brief respiratory illness lasting fewer than 15 days in patients without underlying chronic lung disease. Clinical manifestations include cough with or without sputum production, as well as substernal chest discomfort but lacking the physical or radiologic findings of pneumonia. Acute bronchitis more commonly occurs during the winter months, and the vast majority of cases are viral in origin. Bacterial causes occur infrequently, responsible for only approximately 10% of cases (Table 1). Inhalation of toxic or irritating substances, such as air pollution or occupational exposures, may initiate an acute bronchitis syndrome.

Pathophysiology

During acute bronchitis the mucous membranes of the bronchial tree become hyperemic and edematous, resulting in airway narrowing. Excessive mucus production is common. Although extensive destruction of respiratory epithelium occurs only with influenza, some degree of impaired mucociliary clearance is found in all patients. Increased airway reactivity and airway resistance are part of the syndrome and may persist for 6 to 8 weeks. This hyperreactivity is time limited and mimics the spirometric changes seen with asthma. It is possible that repetitive acute bronchitis infections may be a contributing factor in the genesis of chronic obstructive pulmonary disease.

Diagnosis

The diagnosis of acute bronchitis is usually one of exclusion. The differential diagnosis includes such infectious causes as pneumonia, sinusitis, and nasopharyngeal infections and such noninfectious considerations as allergic rhinitis, an aspirated foreign body, and asthma. Cough, which is a universal symptom, lasts longer than other symptoms, and almost 20% of patients will have cough persisting beyond 2 weeks. Other findings of upper airway infection are routinely noted, and wheezing may be present as well. Body temperature is seldom elevated dramatically.

The nature of sputum production, whether it is based on the color, consistency, or through the types of inflammatory cells identified, may provide clues to infecting organisms, but it is not an accurate predictor of whether bacteria are responsible for the condition. Hemoptysis may occur; however, it is usually limited to minor blood streaks within the sputum representing the inflammatory changes throughout the bronchial mucosa. Large amounts of bloody sputum should prompt the investigator to evaluate for an alternative diagnosis.

To distinguish between acute bronchitis and pneumonia, chest radiographs are necessary in those patients who have high fever or signs of pneumonia on physical examination. This diagnostic separation of acute bronchitis from pneumonia is critical because antibiotic therapy for acute bronchitis is seldom warranted. Other routine laboratory tests are not helpful in establishing the diagnosis or in guiding therapeutic decisions.

TREATMENT

Because the overwhelming portion of acute bronchitis is viral in etiology, therapy should initially be directed toward symptom relief: antipyretics, anti-

TABLE 1. **Etiology of Acute Bronchitis**

Common
Rhinovirus
Coronavirus
Influenza virus
Adenovirus
Uncommon
Respiratory syncytial virus
Parainfluenza virus
Herpes simplex virus
Mycoplasma pneumoniae
Chlamydia pneumoniae
Bordetella pertussis
Unclear
Haemophilus influenzae
Streptococcus pneumoniae

tussives, hydration, and rest. Cessation of cigarette smoking and avoidance of other inhaled noxious stimuli is imperative. If bronchospastic symptoms predominate, then there may be a role for inhaled β_2-adrenergic bronchodilators.

The value of antibacterial agents for the treatment of acute bronchitis has not been confirmed, and their use is not recommended for immunocompetent patients without underlying medical illnesses. Unfortunately, almost 70% of patients with acute bronchitis receive antibiotics despite this recommendation. Antibiotic therapy for acute bronchitis should be reserved for those patients with severe or persistent disease, usually greater than 14 days' duration, with an emphasis on treating *Mycoplasma* and *Chlamydia* infections, as well as pertussis. Factors in addition to prolonged duration of illness that may result in antibiotic administration include elderly age, significant co-morbid conditions, or especially severe symptoms. An essential component to reduce antibiotic abuse and misuse is effective communication with the patient about the lack of benefit, potential side effects, and burgeoning antimicrobial resistance associated with improper antibiotic use. Treatment of acute bronchitis caused by influenza virus is warranted during influenza outbreaks. Amantadine (Symmetrel), rimantadine (Flumadine), zanamivir (Relenza), and oseltamivir (Tamiflu) all are effective therapeutic options if administered within 48 hours.

ACUTE EXACERBATION OF CHRONIC BRONCHITIS

Chronic bronchitis is defined as a productive cough on a daily basis for at least 3 months during a minimum of 2 consecutive years. Chronic bronchitis is a significant factor in the production of chronic airway obstruction leading to chronic obstructive pulmonary disease. Patients with preexisting chronic bronchitis may suffer an acute exacerbation of their illness without an objectively documented cause for the decompensation. The major risk factor for chronic bronchitis is cigarette smoking, with other issues such as occupational environmental exposures and childhood respiratory tract infections playing a role.

PATHOPHYSIOLOGY

As mucociliary clearance effectiveness is reduced by smoking, mucus volume, and viral infections, various bacteria become colonizers of the lower respiratory tract. This stimulates an inflammatory response from the host, producing progressive airway damage mediated by irreversible bronchial wall thickening and hypertrophy of mucus glands. This damage predisposes to more frequent infections, with more colonization, resulting in continued host defense impairment and further airway damage.

The role of bacterial infection in acute exacerbation of chronic bronchitis is controversial. Meta-analysis has shown a small but statistically significant clinical and physiologic improvement for patients treated with antibiotics. Patients with reduced lung function, advanced age, co-morbid conditions, and frequent recurrences of chronic bronchitis demonstrate an increased risk for mortality and should be treated accordingly.

DIAGNOSIS

An acute change in the respiratory status, often accompanied by cough with increased volume and viscosity of sputum, signals the onset of acute exacerbation of chronic bronchitis. A chest radiograph is essential to rule out pneumonia. Sputum Gram stain and culture may not be helpful because viruses are usually the instigators of infection. Bacteria are isolated in approximately 50% of cases, but they may reflect colonization. Organisms frequently encountered in patients with chronic bronchitis may be linked to lung function: at an FEV_1 above 50% predicted values, *Streptococcus pneumoniae* is the most commonly isolated bacteria, but a shift toward *Haemophilus influenzae* and *Moraxella catarrhalis* occurs once forced expiratory volume in 1 second (FEV_1) is less than 50%, and eventually Enterobacteriaceae predominate once the FEV_1 dips below 35%.

TREATMENT

Because the role of bacterial infection in acute exacerbation of chronic bronchitis remains unclear, and because many of these episodes resolve spontaneously, it has been suggested that only certain groups of patients receive antimicrobial therapy. Therefore, it is imperative to identify those patients who are at particular risk. Patients who have demonstrated improvement with antibiotics generally were older, had reduced lung function, had multiple recurrences of chronic bronchitis, and possessed significant nonrespiratory co-morbid conditions. Similarly, a role for antibiotic treatment in patients with acute exacerbation of chronic bronchitis has been established if at least two of the three following symptoms are present: increased dyspnea, increased sputum volume, and increased sputum purulence. Patients with type 1 produce all three manifestations, patients with type 2 demonstrate any two of the three complaints, whereas patients with type 3 have only one of these symptoms. In patients with type 1 and type 2 with more than three exacerbations of chronic bronchitis per year the use of antibiotics is warranted.

Which antibiotic to prescribe remains problematic. Many options abound, and the issue of increasing bacterial resistance is a serious consideration. Although earlier studies suggested that tetracycline/doxycycline, amoxicillin, and trimethoprim-sulfamethoxazole (TMP-SMZ) are effective, newer broad-spectrum agents that possess activity directed against drug-resistant pneumococci and β-lactamase–producing strains of *H. influenzae* and *M. catarrhalis* appear useful as well. Even though these newer antibiotics are more expensive, cost-effective analysis demonstrated a reduction in the therapeutic failure rate, a decreased need for hospitalization, and a greater duration between exacerbations. The overall result was a net cost savings.

Ancillary measures should not be ignored when treating chronic bronchitis. Smoking cessation (both short-term and long-term), reviewing vaccination status for pneumococcal and influenza vaccine and their subsequent appropriate administration if needed, and the symptomatic use of inhaled β_2-adrenergic agonists and anticholinergics are indicated for successful therapy. Short courses of systemic glucocorticosteroids are clinically relevant as well. Occasionally, intubation and mechanical ventilation is required for severe acute respiratory failure.

BACTERIAL PNEUMONIA

method of
MICHAEL B. KIRKPATRICK, M.D.
University of South Alabama College of Medicine
Mobile, Alabama

Bacterial pneumonia, defined as a bacterial infection of the lung parenchyma, can be classified into community-acquired pneumonia, nosocomial pneumonia, and nursing home–acquired pneumonia. In the United States, the annual incidence of pneumonia in the population is approximately 1.5%, resulting in about 4 million cases of pneumonia annually. Each year about 15%, or 600,000, of these patients with community-acquired pneumonia will be hospitalized. The mortality of hospitalized community-acquired pneumonia is 13% to 14%. The mortality of community-acquired pneumonia treated on an outpatient basis is assumed to be exceedingly low (<1%). Ninety percent of the mortality of community-acquired pneumonia occurs in patients 65 years of age or older. Overall, pneumonia is the sixth leading cause of death in the United States.

Nosocomial pneumonia, defined as pneumonia occurring in a hospitalized patient more than 48 hours after admission, is the second most common nosocomial infection and carries a mortality of 20% to 50%. More than 80% of nosocomial pneumonia occurs in intubated mechanically ventilated patients and is commonly referred to as *ventilator-associated pneumonia*.

Nursing home–acquired pneumonia is increasing in incidence because of the increasing elderly population residing in nursing homes and assisted living facilities. In this population, pneumonia is second only to urinary tract infection as the cause of bacterial infections and may carry a mortality of 20% to 40%.

DIAGNOSIS

The diagnosis of pneumonia is based on typical symptoms and findings on physical examination along with abnormal laboratory results. The symptoms of pneumonia typically include cough, sputum production, fever, dyspnea, and pleuritic chest pain. Although cough is a feature of pneumonia in greater than 90% of episodes, sputum production may be present in only about 60% of these patients. Pleuritic chest pain is reported by 50% to 60% of adults aged 18 to 44 years but is reported by fewer than one third of elderly patients. Pneumonia may be accompanied by hemoptysis in 15% to 20% of patients, but unless the infection is accompanied by lung necrosis (e.g., necrotizing pneumonia or lung abscess), is usually minor. Physical examination reveals fever in 90% of young adults; however, up to 50% of elderly, debilitated patients may be afebrile on presentation. Lung examination reveals crackles in up to 80% of patients, but signs of consolidation occur in only about 25% of patients. Tachypnea is uncommon in younger patients but occurs in 65% to 70% of elderly, debilitated patients and may be the only clinical clue to the presence of pneumonia as the cause of the elderly patient's illness. Extrapulmonary signs and symptoms include headache, myalgias, pharyngitis, nausea, vomiting, and diarrhea. Elderly nursing home patients may present predominantly with altered mental status, decreased oral intake, and volume contraction.

Laboratory abnormalities include a new pulmonary infiltrate on chest radiography and leukocytosis or leukopenia. With rare exceptions (such as the occasional AIDS patient with *Pneumocystis carinii* pneumonia), a new or progressive pulmonary infiltrate by chest radiography is essential to the diagnosis of pneumonia. Diagnostic criteria for entry of patients into pneumonia studies usually require a pulmonary infiltrate by radiography plus one or two of the following features: (1) fever or hypothermia, (2) productive cough, or (3) leukocytosis or leukopenia.

Severe pneumonia occurs in about 15% of patients hospitalized for community-acquired pneumonia and is usually defined as illness severe enough to require admission to an intensive care unit. Clinical features of severe community-acquired pneumonia include altered mental status, hypotension, tachypnea (respiratory rate >30 breaths per minute), tachycardia (heart rate >125 beats per minute), oliguric renal failure, severe hypoxemia (Pa_{O_2} <60 mm Hg while breathing room air), and multilobar involvement on chest radiography. The mortality of severe community-acquired pneumonia is 35% to 40%. The most common complication of severe community-acquired pneumonia is hypoxemic respiratory failure requiring intubation and mechanical ventilation.

The diagnosis of nosocomial pneumonia requires onset of pneumonia more than 48 hours after hospital admission. Clinical criteria for the diagnosis of nosocomial pneumonia in the incubated mechanically ventilated patient (ventilator-associated pneumonia) are a new or progressive pulmonary infiltrate accompanied by fever, purulent tracheobronchial secretions, and leukocytosis. Because other disorders in these patients can cause these abnormalities (e.g., pulmonary embolism, atelectasis, pulmonary hemorrhage), some authorities recommend invasive diagnostic techniques such as bronchoscopy with quantitative cultures of pulmonary specimens to better identify both the presence and etiology of ventilator-associated pneumonia. Some studies have indicated that up to 50% of people suspected of having ventilator-associated pneumonia based on the just described clinical criteria may actually have other noninfectious disorders identified when invasive testing is pursued. Nevertheless, there is no current consensus among authorities whether noninvasive or invasive testing is most appropriate in these patients.

The signs and symptoms of nursing home–acquired pneumonia are similar to those of community-acquired pneumonia except that elderly, debilitated patients are more likely to present with an altered mental status, decreased oral intake, and volume contraction and as many as 50% of these patients may be afebrile on presentation.

Essential diagnostic studies in patients with pneumonia,

in addition to examination, routine laboratory studies, and chest radiography, include blood cultures from two different sites and collection of sputum for Gram stain, culture, and sensitivity before administration of antibiotics. In individual patients, further diagnostic studies such as urine assay for *Legionella* antigen and/or pneumococcal antigen, serum for acute phase serology of atypical organisms (e.g., *Chlamydia*, *Legionella*, *Mycoplasma*, and viruses), testing of respiratory secretions for the presence of viral antigens such as influenza and respiratory syncytial virus, or culture of respiratory secretions for *Legionella* and respiratory viruses may be indicated. Invasive diagnostic procedures such as flexible bronchoscopy, transthoracic needle aspiration, transtracheal aspiration, and surgical lung biopsy are usually reserved for specific situations.

ETIOLOGY

Identifying the microbiologic etiology of pneumonia allows for narrow targeted antimicrobial therapy and assists in epidemiologic studies. Unfortunately, most prospective pneumonia studies fail to identify the etiology in 30% to 50% of patients. Definitive diagnostic criteria for identifying the etiology of pneumonia include (1) culture of a pathogen from a normally sterile body site such as blood or pleural fluid, (2) culture or identification by other means of organisms that are thought not to colonize and consequently are assumed to always be pathogenic if found (*Mycobacterium tuberculosis*, *P. carinii*, *Legionella* species, influenza viruses A and B, respiratory syncytial virus, and certain fungi such as *Histoplasma*, *Coccidioides*, and *Blastomyces*), and (3) identification of pathogenic organisms by either specific antigen detection techniques such as for influenza and respiratory syncytial virus or documented by an increase in specific immune response such as a fourfold IgG antibody titer increase between acute and convalescent serum specimens.

The identification of bacteria from sputum specimens (by Gram stain or culture) may indicate a probable diagnosis but cannot be considered definitive because bacterial pathogens can colonize the oropharynx and, consequently, recovery of these organisms from sputum may not represent the pathogen causing the pulmonary infection.

Based on diagnostic criteria similar to those noted earlier, studies in North America and Europe have consistently identified *Streptococcus pneumoniae* to be the most common pathogen in community-acquired pneumonia. Other important bacterial causes include *Haemophilus influenzae*, gram-negative bacilli, and the atypical pathogens including *Chlamydia*, *Mycoplasma*, and *Legionella* (Table 1). The etiology remains unknown in 30% to 50% of patients.

TABLE 1. **Microbial Etiology of Community-Acquired Pneumonia**

Streptococcus pneumoniae	20%–50%
Haemophilus influenzae	5%–15%
Staphylococcus aureus	5%
Gram-negative bacilli	5%–10%
Mycoplasma species	2%–10%
Chlamydia species	2%–10%
Legionella species	1%–5%
Aspiration	2%–10%
Viruses	5%
Unknown	30%–50%

Severe community-acquired pneumonia is most commonly caused by *S. pneumoniae*, gram-negative bacilli, *Legionella* species, or *Staphylococcus aureus*. Approximately 50% of patients with severe community-acquired pneumonia will have no specific etiology identified.

Aspiration pneumonia, defined as bacterial pulmonary infection caused by aspiration of oropharyngeal contents, is almost always a mixed flora infection composed of anaerobic and microaerophilic bacteria. The diagnosis of aspiration pneumonia is usually a clinical diagnosis based on (1) a patient's predisposition to aspiration of oropharyngeal contents (substance abuse, alcoholism, seizure disorder, recent general anesthesia) and (2) typical radiographic location (posterior segments of the upper lobes and superior segments of the lower lobes). Because the organisms involved are part of the normal oropharyngeal flora, a definitive microbiologic diagnosis requires invasive procedures such as bronchoscopy, transthoracic needle aspiration, or transtracheal aspiration, and, consequently, this diagnosis is usually made clinically.

The most common etiology of nosocomial pneumonia occurring during the first 4 to 5 days of hospitalization includes the pneumococcus and *H. influenzae*. Thereafter, gram-negative bacilli *Escherichia coli*, *Klebsiella*, *Proteus* species), *S. aureus* (including methicillin-resistant *Staphylococcus*), and *Legionella* become of more concern. Patients with prolonged hospitalization are at increased risk of colonization and infection with more drug-resistant organisms such as *Acinetobacter*, *Serratia*, and vancomycin-resistant *Staphylococcus* as well as yeasts and fungi.

Nursing home–acquired pneumonia may be caused by the usual community-acquired pathogens such as pneumococcus and *H. influenzae*, but these patients have an increased incidence of pneumonia caused by gram-negative organisms such as *E. coli* and *Klebsiella*, as well as aspiration pneumonia. Outbreaks of pneumonia occasionally occur in nursing home facilities (as well as other closed populations) and may be caused by *S. pneumoniae*, influenza virus, *Legionella*, or *Mycobacterium tuberculosis*.

MANAGEMENT

The initial decision regarding community-acquired pneumonia is treatment location, that is, hospitalization or outpatient treatment. In the past, almost all patients with pneumonia were hospitalized for treatment, but, in recent years, outpatient treatment has been preferred when possible. Although much of the initial impetus for outpatient therapy was financial (inpatient treatment of pneumonia costs 15 to 20 times more than outpatient treatment), other reasons to prefer outpatient treatment when possible include the following:

1. Studies indicate that most patients prefer outpatient therapy.
2. New antibiotics (especially the quinolones) achieve equivalent blood levels whether taken orally or given intravenously.
3. Outpatient treatment allows the patient to avoid any risk of nosocomial complications such as infections or medication errors.
4. Studies show that even when severity of illness is equivalent, patients treated as outpatients have a shorter recovery period and return to usual activities sooner.

Although a physician's subjective assessment of pneumonia severity (e.g., a patient does or does not "look sick") is valuable, recent studies have attempted to identify objectively quantifiable criteria that would assess risk of death. Although these studies were designed to identify risk of mortality from pneumonia, these criteria may be useful in determining the most appropriate location of therapy (i.e., outpatient versus hospital treatment). Criteria that indicate an increased risk for mortality from pneumonia include the following:

1. Age and co-morbid diseases such as cancer, congestive heart failure, liver and kidney disease, or cerebrovascular disease
2. Abnormal physical examination findings such as altered mental status, respiratory rate greater than 30 breaths per minute, heart rate greater than 125 beats per minute, systemic hypotension
3. Laboratory abnormalities, including multilobe involvement on chest radiography, parapneumonic effusion, $Pa{O_2}$ less than 60 mm Hg on room air, white blood cell count greater than 30,000/mL or less than 4,000/mL, blood urea nitrogen greater than 30 mg/dL, and bacteremia, especially with *S. pneumoniae*.

A patient with none of the listed co-morbidities, physical examination abnormalities, or laboratory abnormalities would likely be a good candidate for outpatient therapy. Whatever location of treatment is determined, obtaining laboratory studies and administering appropriate antibiotics in a timely manner are essential. Indeed, the Health Care Financing Administration Pneumonia Quality Indicators include the acquisition of blood cultures before antibiotic therapy and the administration of appropriate antibiotics within 8 hours of the patient's initial presentation. Although objective criteria for predicting mortality assist in the determination of treatment location, the physician's ultimate decision must also include the patient's psychological, social, and economic status such as ability to buy medicines, social support system, and probability of compliance with therapy.

Initial antibiotic therapy for pneumonia is almost always empirical based on the pathogens most likely to be responsible for an individual's pneumonia. Consequently, initial empirical therapy for pneumonia will vary considerably based on the classification of pneumonia as community-acquired, nosocomial, or nursing home–acquired. Recommendations for empirical antibiotic therapy of community-acquired pneumonia continue to evolve largely because of the concern over the increasing incidence of penicillin-resistant *S. pneumoniae*. Based on the current standard definition of penicillin susceptibility (minimal inhibitory concentration for 90% of organisms <0.1 μg/mL), approximately 30% of invasive pneumococcal disease is caused by penicillin-resistant *S. pneumoniae*. Thus far, published studies have not clearly indicated an increased mortality in patients with penicillin-resistant pneumococcal pneumonia even when treated with antibiotics to which the pneumococcus was not fully susceptible. Nevertheless, it seems intuitive to prefer the use of antibiotics with good in vitro activity against penicillin-resistant pneumococci.

Antibiotic Treatment

Initial antibiotic regimens will depend on the likelihood of the microbiologic etiology, which in turn is influenced by location (community-acquired pneumonia, nosocomial pneumonia, nursing home–acquired pneumonia), severity of illness, and whether aspiration pneumonia is a possibility.

For outpatient community-acquired pneumonia in a patient younger than 50 years of age, treat with either clarithromycin (Biaxin), 500 mg orally twice daily, azithromycin (Zithromax), 500 mg for 1 day followed by 250 mg a day for 5 days orally, or doxycycline (Vibra-Tabs), 100 mg twice daily orally. For outpatient treatment in patients older than age 50 or with co-morbid disease (e.g., congestive heart failure, liver or kidney disease, neoplastic disease, diabetes mellitus), give cefuroxime (Ceftin), 500 mg twice daily orally, or cefpodoxime (Vantin), 200 mg twice daily orally, or a newer quinolone antibiotic (levofloxacin [Levaquin], 500 mg/d, or gatifloxacin [Tequin], 400 mg/d, or moxifloxacin [Avelox], 400 mg/d) (Table 2).

The hospitalized patient with community-acquired pneumonia who does not require admission to an intensive care unit can be treated with either cefu-

TABLE 2. **Antibiotics for Community-Acquired Pneumonia***

Outpatients
Age < 50
Macrolide or doxycycline (orally)
Age > 50 or co-morbid diseases
Cefuroxime or cefpodoxime or a quinolone (orally)
Hospitalized Patient (not severely ill)
Cefuroxime or ceftriaxone or cefotaxime *plus* a macrolide (if allergic to β-lactams may use a quinolone as a single drug)
Severe (Intensive Care Unit) Pneumonia
Ceftriaxone or cefotaxime *plus* a macrolide or quinolone
Aspiration Pneumonia
Clindamycin† with or without a quinolone

*Specific drugs below; see text for dosages:
Macrolides = clarithromycin (Biaxin), azithromycin (Zithromax)
Cefuroxime (PO = Ceftin, IV = Zinacef), doxycycline (Vibra-Tabs)
Cefpodoxime (Vantin), ceftriaxone (Rocephin)
Cefotaxime (Claforan)
Quinolones = levofloxacin (Levaquin), gatifloxacin (Tequin), moxifloxacin (Avelox)
Clindamycin (Cleocin)

†Not FDA approved for this indication.

roxime (Zinacef), 500 mg every 8 hours intravenously, or ceftriaxone (Rocephin), 1 g intravenously every 24 hours, or cefotaxime (Claforan), 1 or 2 g every 8 hours intravenously, plus either a macrolide (clarithromycin or azithromycin) or a newer quinolone (levofloxacin, gatifloxacin, or moxifloxacin).

For severe community-acquired pneumonia requiring admission to an intensive care unit use ceftriaxone or cefotaxime plus either quinolone or a macrolide.

If aspiration pneumonia is suspected, use clindamycin (Cleocin),* 900 mg every 8 hours intravenously, with or without a quinolone.

Empirical antibiotic treatment of nosocomial pneumonia will depend on the patient's location (medical or surgical ward versus intensive care unit), duration of hospitalization, and local resistance patterns of nosocomial organisms. Generally, treatment will include coverage for gram-positive organisms, including *S. aureus*, enteric gram-negative organisms, and *Legionella* species. Prolonged hospitalization may increase the risk of drug-resistant organisms such as methicillin-resistant *S. aureus* and resistant gram-negative bacilli such as *Pseudomonas aeruginosa* and *Acinetobacter baumannii.*

Initial antibiotic treatment of patients with nursing home–acquired pneumonia can follow the same guidelines as treatment of community-acquired pneumonia, but one must maintain a higher index of suspicion that these patients may have an increased risk of gram-negative pneumonia and anaerobic pneumonia (from aspiration).

Many hospitalized patients with community-acquired and nursing home–acquired pneumonia can be switched from parenteral to oral antibiotics within 2 to 3 days of admission. Criteria for switch to oral therapy include adequate patient oral intake and a functioning gastrointestinal tract, decrease of temperature toward normal, decreasing white blood cell count, and decrease in dyspnea with a respiratory rate less than 25 breaths per minute. When possible, the oral antibiotic should be the same as the parenteral drug or an oral antibiotic with equivalent spectrum of activity. It is not necessary to continue hospitalization of the patient for 24 hours on oral antibiotics; recent studies have not found any benefit of this practice. The conventional duration of antibiotic treatment of community-acquired pneumonia and nursing home–acquired pneumonia is 10 to 14 days. Pneumonia caused by atypical organisms such as *Chlamydia*, *Mycoplasma*, and *Legionella* should be treated for 14 to 21 days. The conventional duration of treatment for nosocomial pneumonia is 14 to 15 days except for pneumonia from *Legionella*, which is treated for 14 to 21 days.

COMPLICATIONS AND RESOLUTION

Potential significant complications of pneumonia include complicated parapneumonic effusion or empyema, respiratory failure requiring intubation and mechanical ventilation, sepsis syndrome with shock and multiple organ dysfunction, metastatic infections or contiguous spread, hemoptysis, and lung necrosis and/or cavitation (necrotizing pneumonia). Although sterile parapneumonic effusions may occur in 40% to 50% of patients with pneumonia, only about 5% will have an empyema or complicated parapneumonic effusion requiring a drainage procedure. If the thickness of the parapneumonic effusion is less than 1 cm on a lateral decubitus chest radiograph the risk of empyema is minimal. If pleural fluid thickness is greater than 1 cm on a lateral decubitus film, then a diagnostic thoracentesis should be performed. The presence of gross pus, organisms identified by Gram stain or culture, or a pH less than 7.1 indicate the need for drainage. Hypoxemic respiratory failure that may progress to acute respiratory distress syndrome is the most common cause for admission to the intensive care unit for the patient with community-acquired pneumonia. Sepsis syndrome with shock and multiple organ dysfunction is the second most common cause for admission of these patients to an intensive care unit and is particularly associated with bacteremic pneumococcal pneumonia. Metastatic infections such as meningitis, endocarditis, or septic arthritis, as well as contiguous spread to the mediastinum or pericardium, are dreaded potential complications of bacterial pneumonia. Although hemoptysis is usually minor, patients with necrotizing pneumonia (e.g., lung abscess) can have major bleeding or even life-threatening hemoptysis.

The radiographic resolution of pneumonia depends on both the host and the etiology of the pneumonia. Patients younger than age 50 without co-morbid diseases will usually have radiographic resolution within 2 to 4 weeks. Older patients and patients with either underlying lung disease or the co-morbid diseases mentioned earlier may have delayed radiographic resolution up to 6 to 8 weeks. Additionally, radiographic resolution of *Legionella* may be very prolonged with up to 20% of these patients having residual radiographic abnormalities even after 4 to 5 months. Slowly resolving or nonresolving pneumonia may be caused by host abnormalities, resistant or unusual pathogens, or noninfectious disorders that mimic pneumonia. Delayed resolution of pneumonia commonly occurs in elderly, debilitated patients as well as in patients with underlying cardiopulmonary diseases, malnutrition, diabetes mellitus, and liver and kidney diseases. On occasion, delayed resolution may be the result of endobronchial obstruction such as from a tumor or foreign body. Resistant pathogens or unexpected pathogens, such as a fungal pneumonia or tuberculosis, should be considered in patients with delayed resolution of their pneumonia. Also, a number of noninfectious pulmonary disorders may mimic pneumonia. These include pulmonary embolism, alveolar hemorrhage syndromes, hypersensitivity pneumonitis, drug-induced lung disease, and neoplasia and must be considered in the differential diagnosis of nonresolving pneumonia.

*Not FDA approved for this indication.

PREVENTION

Every effort should be made to administer pneumococcal vaccine to individuals at risk, as recommended by the Advisory Committee on Immunization Practices. Likewise, annual influenza vaccination should be administered to all patients at risk for complications from influenza, as well as health care workers, household members of patients who are at high risk, and all persons age 50 years or older.

VIRAL RESPIRATORY INFECTIONS

method of
CYNTHIA CHRISTY, M.D., and
CAROLINE B. HALL, M.D.
University of Rochester School of Medicine and Children's Hospital at Strong
Rochester, New York

Viral respiratory infections are among the most common infections of humans. The average preschool child has 6 to 10 colds per year, and older adolescents and adults average 2 to 4 colds per year. These illnesses are an important cause of discomfort and costs associated with absenteeism from work and school. Most illnesses are self-limited, but some are accompanied or followed by complications such as reactive airway disease, otitis media, and sinusitis.

The viruses involved in upper respiratory infections (URIs) belong to several groups, most notably orthomyxovirus (influenza), paramyxovirus (parainfluenza and respiratory syncytial viruses), picornaviruses (rhinoviruses and enteroviruses), coronaviruses, and adenoviruses. Rhinoviruses are the most important cause of URIs, accounting for as many as 40% of episodes. Rhinoviruses are prevalent throughout the year, whereas influenza, coronavirus, and respiratory syncytial viruses peak in the winter. URIs more often occur during the colder months than the warmer months in temperate climates. These infections are more common in children than adults, in part because children have less experience with exposure to many of the major causative agents and thus less immunity. Symptoms usually last 7 days in 50% of children, but 5% to 10% have symptoms for 10 days without other complications being recognized. These agents are spread from person to person, most commonly by large-particle aerosols from close contact with an infected person, or by contact with contaminated fomites. Infection acquired by small particle aerosols from individuals at greater distances appear to be less common for many of the major respiratory agents, such as rhinoviruses.

The most common manifestations of URIs include rhinorrhea, nasal congestion, sore throat, and cough. Other problems such as myalgia, pharyngitis, laryngitis, croup, bronchitis, bronchiolitis, and pneumonia may occur. Up to 70% of individuals infected with rhinovirus develop eustachian tube dysfunction soon after viral inoculation. Viral infections commonly cause acute inflammatory phase changes in the sinuses. Eighty-seven percent of young adults in one study demonstrated abnormalities of paranasal sinuses on computed tomography during the acute phase of illness. Infections with any of these viruses may also increase airway reactivity to cold or pollutants and exacerbate pre-existing reactive airway disease.

Illnesses due to respiratory viruses are usually self-limited, but complications such as croup, bronchiolitis, and pneumonia can be life threatening. Several antiviral medications are available for treatment of acute influenza and for severe bronchiolitis and pneumonia in children. Secondary bacterial infections involving the paranasal sinuses and middle ear, and less commonly the bronchi and lungs, may develop a few days into the illness, often as the viral infection is improving, and respond to antibiotic therapy.

TREATMENT

Many over-the-counter cough and cold preparations are marketed for relief of the common symptoms of nasal congestion, rhinorrhea, and cough. Little evidence, however, supports the efficacy of these over-the-counter products in ameliorating the symptoms of URIs in children.

Children and adults often use acetaminophen and ibuprofen to control the fever and malaise accompanying colds. Studies have shown variable effects on duration and viral shedding, but in one study no significant difference in viral shedding occurred among those treated with aspirin, acetaminophen, ibuprofen, or placebo.

Systemic decongestants, including pseudoephedrine and phenylephrine, are often used to treat the congestion associated with URIs. In the year 2000, the use of phenylpropanolamine was associated with an increased risk of hemorrhagic strokes. The pharmaceutical companies producing these products thus have voluntarily withdrawn products containing phenylpropanolamine from the market. In adults, decongestants have proved effective in reducing nasal congestion and sneezing, but no studies have documented their effect in children. Side effects of decongestants include irritability, sleeplessness, hypertension, tachycardia, nausea, vomiting, and seizures. Topical decongestants, such as oxymetazoline, are beneficial in reducing nasal congestion in adults initially, but use beyond a few days is associated with rebound congestion. Topical phenylephrine does not decrease nasal congestion in children.

Antihistamines are commonly used to treat cold symptoms, even though histamine levels in nasal secretions have been shown to not increase during URIs. Some studies in adults suggest that the first-generation antihistamines (e.g., triprolidine, diphenhydramine, hydroxyzine, and chlorpheniramine) benefit the symptoms and duration of rhinoviral URIs. Side effects can include dry mouth, blurred vision, tachycardia, arrhythmias, and urinary retention. The beneficial effects of chlorpheniramine may be explained by the anticholinergic effects of first-generation antihistamines, which specifically decrease nasal secretions. A randomized double-blind trial of an antihistamine-decongestant combination versus placebo in children 6 months to 5 years of age with URIs showed no improvement in cough, rhinorrhea, or nasal congestion in the treated group but found that many of the treated children, 47% versus 27%, were asleep 2 hours after treatment. More than half the children were better 2 days later regardless of whether they received drug treatment or placebo.

An anticholinergic nasal spray, ipratropium bromide, effectively decreases nasal discharge associated with the common cold for children 5 years or older. However, side effects, which include excessive dryness of the nose, throat, nosebleeds, and headache, limit its usefulness.

Although the cough reflex is helpful in clearing secretions in the airways, to the infected individual, cough is often a major discomfort and concern. This may be controlled by narcotic cough syrups containing codeine or hydrocodone, which act centrally to suppress cough. Side effects, however, are common, including nausea, vomiting, constipation, dizziness, and palpitations. These agents may also cause respiratory depression. Dextromethorphan, a narcotic analogue, as well as codeine, suppresses cough in adults without central nervous system effects when used in appropriate doses. Excessive doses can depress respirations. In one study in children 18 months to 12 years of age, no difference in the frequency of cough was observed among three groups receiving either placebo, dextromethorphan, or codeine. By 3 days, the cough was improved in all patient groups. No well-controlled studies exist documenting the efficacy of narcotics or dextromethorphan in treating cough in children. The American Academy of Pediatrics recommends education of parents about the lack of efficacy and possible side effects of these drugs.

Expectorants are common ingredients in cough and cold preparations. Guaifenesin (glycerol guaiacolate) is used to help thin secretions, although controlled studies have shown no change in sputum amount or consistency with the use of guaifenesin.

Some studies in adults have suggested that early treatment with zinc gluconate lozenges can shorten the duration of a cold. Treatment may be effective if begun early, within 24 hours of the onset of symptoms, and requires taking lozenges five to six times per day. Many patients find this regimen difficult, and common side effects include a bad taste, nausea, irritation of the oropharynx, and diarrhea. Zinc lozenges were not effective in treating cold symptoms in children and adolescents in grades 1 through 12 enrolled in two suburban school districts in one study.

OTHER THERAPIES

Vitamin C has been suggested as ameliorating and preventing symptoms associated with the common cold, but very large doses need to be taken early in the course to prevent symptoms.

Physicians often recommend humidified air for symptomatic relief, although controlled studies have shown no benefit from air inhalation therapies.

Bulb suction of nasal secretions remains a key therapy for infants with cold symptoms. Effectiveness of suctioning is improved by using saline nose drops to loosen the mucus. Saline nose drops are available over-the-counter or can be made by dissolving a teaspoon of salt in 2 cups of water.

Antibiotics have no effect on the clinical course of viral infections. They may, however, be needed to treat complications such as otitis media and sinusitis.

PREVENTION

In view of the limited effectiveness of therapeutic measures, can the common cold be prevented? Frequent hand washing reduces transmission of colds. Recent data of the use of a waterless alcohol gel hand sanitizer in the classroom significantly reduced the illness-related rate of absenteeism for elementary school students. Immunization is available currently only for the prevention of influenza. Because more than 100 rhinovirus serotypes exist, the development of a vaccine to prevent the most common causative agents would be a challenge.

Modest clinical benefit with the use of some over-the-counter cold and cough medications has been observed in adults, but similar studies in children have not shown benefit. The best treatment of colds is patience by the patient and physician and explanation by the physician of the cause and pathogenesis of a "cold."

VIRAL AND MYCOPLASMAL PNEUMONIAS

method of
MAURICE A. MUFSON, M.D.
Marshall University
Huntington, West Virginia

Viruses and mycoplasmas give rise to interstitial pneumonias that are historically grouped as "atypical pneumonias" because their clinical and epidemiologic characteristics differ from "typical" bacterial pneumonias. *Mycoplasma pneumoniae*, the dominant human mycoplasmal pathogen of the respiratory tract, is the most common atypical pneumonia treatable with antibiotics. It accounts for one fourth to one third of community-acquired pneumonias in adults managed on an ambulatory basis but few pneumonias in persons admitted to the hospital.

Influenza virus infection is the dominant viral respiratory tract infection and the only one associated with high case-fatality rates. It accounts for more morbidity and deaths than all other respiratory viruses as a group. A small proportion of persons infected with influenza virus, mainly those with underlying heart and lung disease, develop a primary community-acquired pneumonia. Community-acquired pneumonias due to respiratory syncytial virus, parainfluenza viruses, and other viruses occur less frequently in adults, and, unlike influenza virus, they rarely cause death. Among infants and children, viral pneumonias occur very often, more so than bacterial pneumonias, owing mainly to respiratory syncytial virus, parainfluenza viruses, influenza virus, coronavirus, and adenovirus.

TABLE 1. **Target Population, Diagnostic Tests, and Recommended Drug Therapy for Viral and Mycoplasmal Pneumonias**

Pathogens	Target Population* Children	Target Population* Adults	Rapid Diagnostic Test Antigen Test	Rapid Diagnostic Test Antibody Test	Distinctive Clinical Findings	Recommended Drugs†
Primary Respiratory Tract						
MYCOPLASMAL						
Mycoplasma pneumoniae	+ +	+ + + +		IgM Cold agglutinins		Doxycycline or a macrolide or a fluoroquinolone
VIRAL						
Influenza viruses A and B	+ +	+ + + +				Zanamivir or oseltamivir; rimantadine or amantadine
Respiratory syncytial virus	+ + + +	+ +	EIA, IFA			Ribavirin
Parainfluenza viruses	+ + + +	+	EIA, IFA			
Coronaviruses	+ + +	+	IFA			
Adenoviruses	+ + + +	+ +	IFA			
Other Respiratory Tract						
VIRAL						
Varicella-zoster virus	+	+	DFA		Yes	Acyclovir
Herpes simplex virus	R	R	DFA		Yes	Acyclovir
Cytomegalovirus		R	Shell vial, IFA			Ganciclovir
Measles (rubeola) virus	R	R	DFA		Yes	

*Frequency of occurrence: R = rare; + infrequent to + + + + very common.
†See text for dosages and routes of administration.
Abbreviations: DFA = direct immunofluorescent antibody; EIA = enzyme immunoassay; IFA = indirect immunofluorescent antibody; shell vial = specimen centrifuged onto tissue culture cells in small glass vial, incubated, and stained 24 to 48 hours later by IFA. The tests listed can be done routinely in a hospital laboratory.

MYCOPLASMAL PNEUMONIA

Mycoplasma pneumoniae (historically referred to as Eaton agent until it was identified as *Mycoplasma*) is the only mycoplasmal pathogen of pneumonia (Table 1). It occurs among all age groups but most often in young adults and begins insidiously with fever, dry cough, fatigue, headache, and anorexia. The chest radiograph shows an interstitial pneumonia that is usually unilateral but sometimes bilateral and accompanied by few auscultatory findings. About one fifth of cases are complicated by pleural effusion. The clinical findings are insufficient to distinguish it from other atypical pneumonias or, in some instances, ambulatory bacterial pneumonias. A rapid diagnostic test can identify specific *M. pneumoniae* IgM antibody (ImmunoCard Mycoplasma) in less than 1 hour. Detection of cold agglutinin levels greater than about 1:80 in an acute-phase serum is presumptive evidence of this infection. The isolation of *M. pneumoniae* on agar from respiratory secretions or the demonstration of a diagnostic antibody increase in paired sera requires too much time to be useful for treatment decisions.

TREATMENT

The treatment of infection with *M. pneumoniae* involves two aspects, supportive care and effective antibiotic therapy. Supportive care in this type of pneumonia (and the viral pneumonias) aims to alleviate fever, reduce headache, and relieve cough. Adequate hydration and bed rest for fatigue are advised. Mycoplasmas are susceptible in vitro to broad-spectrum antibiotics, including doxycycline, macrolides, and fluoroquinolones. In any individual case, antibiotic susceptibility tests are unlikely to be done because isolation of the organism takes too long; in addition, they are not necessary because antibiotic resistance is rare. *M. pneumoniae* pneumonia can be treated with (1) doxycycline (Vibramycin), 100 mg orally twice daily for 14 days; (2) a macrolide, for example, erythromycin (Ilosone), 500 mg orally every 6 hours for 14 days; azithromycin (Zithromax), 500 mg orally on day 1 and 250 mg orally each day for 5 to 7 more days, or clarithromycin (Biaxin), 500 mg* orally twice daily for 14 days; or (3) a fluoroquinolone, for example, levofloxacin (Levaquin) 500 mg orally daily for 14 days, moxifloxacin (Avelox), 400 mg orally daily for 14 days, or gatifloxacin (Tequin), 400 mg orally daily for 14 days.

When the clinical picture is consistent with *M. pneumoniae* or another ambulatory atypical pneumonia and the diagnosis cannot be confirmed by laboratory tests, start treatment on an empirical basis with doxycyline, a macrolide, or a fluoroquinolone. These antibiotics will also cover the other atypical pneumonias due to *Chlamydia pneumoniae, Chlamydia psittaci*, and *Legionella* pathogens.

VIRAL PNEUMONIAS

Influenza virus infection causes a primary pneumonia, although complicating bacterial infection can develop in the course of influenza pneumonia. Influenza pneumonia begins abruptly with high fever, headache, myalgias, tracheobronchitis, and cough, all signaling the severity associated with "the flu."

*Exceeds dosage recommended by the manufacturer.

Rales and rhonchi also occur. The chest radiograph shows interstitial pneumonia. The case-fatality rate in influenza virus pneumonia is high. Elderly persons and persons with underlying heart and lung disorders, diabetes, or immune disorders are at highest risk of dying of influenza pneumonia. During epidemics of influenza, the diagnosis of influenza pneumonia can usually be suspected from clinical findings, but it can (and should) be confirmed by diagnostic tests because of the availability of several drugs for the treatment of this infection. A rapid enzyme immunoassay (Directigen Flu A + B) detects influenza viral antigen in respiratory tract secretions in about 1 hour (see Table 1).

Influenza virus pneumonia should be treated supportively to alleviate fever, reduce headache, relieve cough, and hydrate adequately. Bed rest is recommended for fatigue, and oxygen is given as needed. It is a serious disease, especially in older persons who should be hospitalized for treatment.

Two classes of drugs effective for the treatment of uncomplicated influenza virus infection include competitive inhibitors of neuraminidase of types A and B—zanamivir (Relenza), 10 mg every 12 hours by inhalation for 5 days, and oseltamivir (Tamiflu), 75 mg orally twice daily for 5 days; and blockers of M2 potein of type A only—rimantadine (Flumadine), 100 mg orally twice daily for 7 days (100 mg once a day in elderly persons), and amantadine (Symmetrel), 200 mg orally once a day until 1 to 2 days after illness subsides. However, no data exist to support their use in influenza virus pneumonia. They do not prevent the development of pneumonia when administered for uncomplicated influenza illness. These drugs must be given within 48 hours of the onset of illness and preferentially only when influenza virus infection is confirmed by laboratory tests.

Respiratory syncytial virus pneumonia in infants and children usually requires treatment in the hospital (see Table 1). Deaths rarely occur among healthy children. In children with underlying lung disease, however, it can be a serious and fatal disease, and these children should be treated with ribavirin (Virazole) delivered by aerosol generator in an oxygen tent. The dose is 20 mg/mL of ribavirin in sterile water, sufficient to fill the generator, administered over an 18-hour period for 3 to 7 days depending on the severity of illness.

No specific drugs are available for pneumonias due to parainfluenza viruses, coronaviruses, and adenoviruses (see Table 1). Immunocompromised and HIV–infected persons are at high risk of developing pneumonia with varicellae-zoster, measles, and cytomegalovirus infections, although some immunocompetent persons do develop varicella pneumonia. Pneumonia accompanying varicellae-zoster and herpes simplex virus infections in adolescents and adults can be treated with acyclovir (Zovirax), 10 mg/kg intravenously every 8 hours (20 mg/mL for children 3 months to 12 years of age) for 10 days. Cytomegalovirus pneumonia, can be treated with ganciclovir (Cytovene), 5 mg/kg intravenously every 12 hours for 14 to 21 days, administered over 1 hour; use reduced doses in renal-impaired persons. No specific antiviral drugs are available for treatment of measles pneumonia.

LEGIONELLOSIS

(Legionnaires' Disease and Pontiac Fever)

method of
THOMAS J. MARRIE, M.D.
Walter C. Mackenzie Health Sciences Centre
Edmonton, Alberta, Canada

There are now more than 42 recognized species of *Legionella,* about half of which have been shown to cause disease in humans. *Legionella pneumophila,* of which there are 15 serogroups, accounts for most of these infections. Other important species include *Legionella micdadei, Legionella bozemanii, Legionella dumoffi,* and *Legionella longbeachae.* Legionellaceae are fastidious gram-negative rod-like microorganisms that require special media for cultivation in the laboratory.

EPIDEMIOLOGY

Legionella species (aquatic microorganisms) are found in low concentrations in many water sources. Under certain circumstances (water temperatures of 32°C to 45°C (89.6°–113°F), stagnant water, presence of biofilms in pipes, various amebae in natural water systems), the concentration of these organisms may be amplified.

Infection in humans occurs when water containing the organism is aerosolized, inhaled, or aspirated by a susceptible host. Exposure to contaminated aerosols from cooling towers, respiratory therapy equipment, showers and faucets, whirlpool spas, decorative fountains, ultrasonic mist machines in the supermarket, saunas, and hot tubs has resulted in isolated cases and outbreaks of legionnaires' disease. Recently in the United States, cases of legionnaires' disease due to *L. longbeachae* have been associated with exposure to contaminated potting soil. Risk factors for sporadic cases of legionnaires' disease include recent travel with an overnight stay outside the home, recent domestic plumbing repairs, and host factors such as renal or liver failure, tobacco smoking, diabetes, systemic malignancy, and other immunosuppressive states.

CLINICAL MANIFESTATIONS

Legionellosis may present as two clinically distinct syndromes: legionnaires' disease and Pontiac fever. Legionnaires' disease manifests as pneumonia, which can range from mild to life-threatening. Many of the clinical features of legionnaires' disease are indistinguishable from other pneumonias. Rapidly progressive pneumonia in a young, otherwise healthy adult should always raise the suspicion of legionnaires' disease. The following clinical features are seen in legionnaires' disease more commonly than they are in other forms of pneumonia: higher temperature (often up to 41°C [105.8°F]), diarrhea, and central nervous system manifestations, including headache, confusion, and cerebellar signs.

Pontiac fever is a self limited, influenza-like illness that often occurs in outbreaks among individuals who share exposure from a common water source. Pontiac fever results from the effects of the lipopolysaccharide of the microorganism and is not an infection.

DIAGNOSIS

The key to the diagnosis of legionnaires' disease is a high index of clinical suspicion. Isolation of the microorganism, the gold standard for diagnosis, can be performed from sputum, pleural fluid, lung tissue, or bronchial washings. Cultivation requires a special medium (buffered charcoal yeast extract agar) and a degree of technical expertise. Three to 5 days are required to detect growth of the organism. Unfortunately, 25% to 75% of patients with *Legionella* pneumonia do not expectorate sputum. Using serologic testing as a gold standard, the sensitivity of sputum culture is less than 10%; however, the yield is higher in specialized laboratories and when endotracheal aspirates are used. Direct fluorescent antibody testing can be used to detect *Legionella* in specimens of respiratory secretions. The sensitivity is higher than that for sputum culture.

About 80% of patients with *L. pneumophila* serogroup 1 infection excrete *Legionella* antigen in the urine. This antigen can be detected using an enzyme immunoassay or a radioimmunoassay. In culture-proven *L. pneumophila* serogroup 1 infection, the sensitivity is high (86% to 93%), and the specificity is close to 100%. Antigen is detectable in the urine early in the disease and may persist for weeks and rarely for up to 1 year.

Polymerase chain reaction testing for detection of legionella DNA is available at some centers, but currently it is expensive and lacks standardization. A major advantage is that it can detect DNA of all species of *Legionella*.

Serologic tests (acute and 6- to 8-week convalescent serum samples) are useful for epidemiologic purposes. They are not of much value for management of acute disease. This test is only about 40% sensitive. Although IgM antibodies appear earlier in the course of infection, fewer than 50% of patients have diagnostic titers at 1 week.

THERAPY

Pontiac fever is a self-limited illness for which specific therapy is rarely required. Prompt treatment of legionnaires' disease is essential for best results, because delay in therapy is associated with increased mortality. In one study, patients who died from legionnaires' disease had erythromycin started a median of 5 days after onset of symptoms (range, 1 to 10), versus a median of 1 day for those who survived (range, 1 to 5). Many regimens for initial treatment of community-acquired pneumonia include antibiotics that are effective against legionnaires' disease. Furthermore, at hospitals where nosocomial legionnaires' disease is known to occur, one should consider empirical treatment of patients with nosocomial pneumonia for *Legionella*.

Fluoroquinolones such as ciprofloxacin (Cipro), levofloxacin (Levaquin), moxifloxacin (Avelox), gatifloxacin (Tequin), and newer macrolides such as azithromycin (Zithromax) and clarithromycin (Biaxin) show superior activity against *Legionella* when compared with erythromycin. Azithromycin can be given intravenously and is associated with a lower rate of phlebitis than is erythromycin. In addition, it does not interact with immunosuppressive agents such as cyclosporine (Sandimmune) or tacrolimus (Prograf). In the past, anecdotal clinical data suggested that the addition of rifampin (Rifadin) to erythromycin for patients seriously ill with legionnaires' disease improved outcomes. Other antibiotics with activity against *Legionella* include doxycycline, quinupristin/dalfopristin (Synercid)*, and the new ketolides HMR 3647† and HMR 3004†, which are currently under investigation. Our current preferred therapy for serious *Legionella* infections is given in Table 1.

TABLE 1. **Preferred Therapy for Serious Legionella Infections**

First Choice
Levofloxacin (Levaquin), 500 mg IV qd
Azithromycin (Azithromax), 500 mg IV qd
Second Choice
Erythromycin, 1 g IV q6h, plus rifampin (Rifadin), 600 mg po qd

As patients improve, therapy can be switched from intravenous to oral. If intravenous erythromycin is used, step-down to oral therapy should be with azithromycin or clarithromycin. Rifampin alone is not recommended because of the rapid emergence of *Legionella* resistant to this agent.

I recommend 10 days of treatment with azithromycin rather than a 3- or 5-day course, which is recommended in other settings. Immunosuppressed patients should receive 21 days of treatment with any of the agents listed.

A suspected outbreak of legionnaires' disease should always be reported to health authorities for investigation of a common source. Cases of nosocomial legionnaires' disease should be reported to infection control authorities in the hospital, and an investigation should be carried out to determine the source of the *Legionella* (e.g., contaminated potable water or aerosols from a contaminated potable water tower).

*Not FDA approved for this indication.
†Investigational drug in the United States.

PULMONARY THROMBOEMBOLISM

method of
GRAHAM PINEO, M.D., and
RUSSELL HULL, M.B.B.S., M.Sc.
University of Calgary
Calgary, Alberta, Canada

Death from pulmonary embolism occurs in approximately 100,000 patients per year in the United States, and pulmonary embolism contributes to the death of another 100,000 patients. Pulmonary embolism represents the third most common cause of cardiovascular death after acute myocardial infarction and stroke and is the most common preventable cause of death in hospitalized patients. Although pulmonary embolism frequently develops in hospitalized patients with one or more co-morbid disorders, this condition may develop in otherwise healthy individuals after orthopedic surgery or trauma or in pregnancy. Effective prophylaxis is available for most of these situations, but venous thromboembolism can occur unexpectedly in ambulatory patients, particularly if they have been exposed to risk factors in the preceding months. When venous thromboembolism occurs, it is important that an accurate diagnosis be established by the use of the appropriate objective tests, so that treatment can be instituted immediately. The first indication that venous thromboembolism has occurred may be a massive pulmonary embolus that, unfortunately, can be fatal within a short time in up to a third of patients. This discussion is devoted to the diagnosis and management of patients presenting with pulmonary embolism. The diagnosis, prevention, and management of patients presenting with deep-vein thrombosis is presented elsewhere.

ETIOLOGY AND PATHOGENESIS

Pulmonary embolism originates from thrombi in the deep veins of the leg in 90% or more of patients. Other less common sources of pulmonary embolism include the deep pelvic veins, renal veins, inferior vena cava, right side of the heart, and the axillary veins. Most clinically important pulmonary emboli arise from proximal deep venous thrombosis (DVT) of the leg. Recent data indicate that upper extremity DVT may also lead to clinically important pulmonary embolism. DVT and/or pulmonary embolism are referred to collectively as venous thromboembolism.

Multiple epidemiologic studies, particularly in hospitalized patients, have identified a number of clinical factors that predispose to venous thromboembolism. Common risk factors for venous thromboembolism are shown in Table 1. Activated protein C resistance is the most common hereditary abnormality predisposing to venous thrombosis. The defect is due to substitution of glutamine for arginine at residue 506 in the factor V molecule, making factor V resistant to proteolysis by activated protein C. The gene mutation is known as factor V Leiden and follows autosomal dominant inheritance. Factor V Leiden is present in approximately 5% of the normal population, in 16% of patients with a first episode of DVT, and in up to 35% of patients with idiopathic DVT. Prothrombin 20210 A is a more recently identified gene mutation predisposing to venous thromboembolism. It is present in approximately 2% of apparently healthy individuals and in 7% of those with DVT. Homocysteinemia (sometimes referred to as hyperhomocysteinemia) predisposes to both venous and arterial thrombosis through mechanisms that are poorly understood. The same applies to patients with the antiphospholipid syndrome and heparin-induced thrombocytopenia. In approximately 50% of patients with idiopathic DVT, an inherited abnormality cannot be detected, indicating that other gene mutations are present and may have an etiologic role. Indeed, several new defects predisposing to thrombosis have been described in the past few years.

TABLE 1. **Clinical Risk Factors Predisposing to the Development of Venous Thromboembolism**

Surgical and nonsurgical trauma	Inherited or acquired abnormalities
Previous venous thromboembolism	Activated protein C resistance
Immobilization	Protein C deficiency
Malignant disease	Protein S deficiency
Heart disease	Antithrombin deficiency
Leg paralysis	Prothrombin mutant
Age (>40 y)	Elevated factor VIII levels
Obesity	Homocysteinemia
Estrogens	Anticardiolipin syndrome
Parturition	Heparin-induced thrombocytopenia
Varicose veins	

CLINICAL FEATURES

Pulmonary embolism occurs in 50% of patients with objectively documented proximal venous thrombosis. Many of these emboli are asymptomatic. The clinical importance of pulmonary embolism depends on the size of the embolus and the patient's cardiorespiratory status. Usually only part of the thrombus embolizes, and 70% of patients with pulmonary embolism detected by angiography have detectable DVT of the legs at presentation. DVT and pulmonary embolism are not separate disorders but a continuous syndrome of venous thromboembolism, in which the initial clinical presentation may be symptoms of either DVT or pulmonary embolism. Strategies for the detection of venous thromboembolism can include tests for the detection of pulmonary embolism (lung scanning, pulmonary angiography or spiral computed tomography) or tests for DVT of the legs (ultrasound, impedance plethysmography, or venography).

The clinical features of acute pulmonary embolism include the following syndromes, which may overlap:

1. Transient dyspnea and tachypnea in the absence of other clinical features
2. Syndrome of pulmonary infarction or congestive atelectasis (also known as ischemic pneumonitis or incomplete infarction), including pleuritic chest pain, cough, hemoptysis, pleural effusion, and pulmonary infiltrates on chest radiograph
3. Right-sided heart failure associated with severe dyspnea and tachypnea
4. cardiovascular collapse with hypotension, syncope, and coma (usually associated with massive pulmonary embolism)
5. Several less common and nonspecific clinical presentations, including unexplained arrhythmia, resistant cardiac failure, wheezing, cough, pyrexia, anxiety/apprehension, and confusion.

All of the above clinical features are nonspecific and may be caused by a variety of cardiorespiratory disorders. Objective testing is mandatory to confirm or exclude the presence of pulmonary embolism. Attempts have been made to categorize patients using pretest probabilities of low, intermediate, and high, with or without measurement of the D-dimer and combining them with ventilation-perfusion lung scan patterns to streamline the diagnostic approach to patients with suspected pulmonary embolism. At this time, the use of pretest clinical probabilities for the diagnosis of pulmonary embolism has not been as successful as those for the diagnosis for DVT and is useful in only the minority of patients presenting with suspected pulmonary embolism.

LABORATORY FEATURES

Venous thromboembolism is associated with nonspecific laboratory changes that make up the acute-phase response to tissue injury. This response includes elevated levels of fibrinogen and factor VIII, increases in the leukocyte and platelet counts, and systemic activation of blood coagulation, fibrin formation, and fibrin breakdown, with increases in the plasma concentrations of prothrombin fragment 1.2, fibrinopeptide A, complexes of thrombin-antithrombin III, and D-dimer. All of these changes are nonspecific and may occur as the result of surgery, trauma, infection, inflammation, or infarction. None of the reported laboratory changes can be used to predict the development of venous thromboembolism.

The fibrin breakdown fragment D-dimer can be measured by an enzyme-linked immunosorbent assay (ELISA) or by a latex agglutination assay. Some of these assays have a rapid turnaround time, and some are quantitative. The D-dimer may be useful as an exclusionary test for patients with suspected venous thromboembolism. A positive result is highly nonspecific.

DIAGNOSIS

Differential Diagnosis in Pulmonary Embolism

The differential diagnosis in patients with suspected pulmonary embolism includes multiple cardiopulmonary disorders for each of the clinical syndromes. For the presentation of dyspnea and tachypnea, this includes atelectasis, pneumonia, pneumothorax, acute pulmonary edema, bronchitis, bronchiolitis, and acute bronchial obstruction. For the syndrome of pulmonary infarction (e.g., pleuritic chest pain, hemoptysis), this includes pneumonia, pneumothorax, pericarditis, pulmonary or bronchial neoplasm, bronchiectasis, acute bronchitis, tuberculosis, diaphragmatic inflammation, myositis, muscle strain, and rib fracture. For the clinical presentation of right-sided heart failure, this includes myocardial infarction, myocarditis, and cardiac tamponade. For cardiovascular collapse, this includes myocardial infarction, acute massive hemorrhage, gram-negative septicemia, cardiac tamponade, and spontaneous pneumothorax.

Objective Testing For Pulmonary Embolism

The key tests include lung scanning, pulmonary angiography, and objective testing for proximal DVT. The diagnostic approach is summarized in Figure 1.

Perfusion lung scanning is the key diagnostic test for patients with suspected pulmonary embolism. A normal perfusion scan excludes important pulmonary embolism. An abnormal perfusion scan, however, is nonspecific and can occur in conditions that produce either increased radiographic density (e.g., pneumonia, atelectasis, pleural effusion) or a regional reduction in ventilation (e.g., chronic obstructive lung disease, acute asthma, bronchial mucous plugs, bronchitis—conditions frequently associated with normal radiography).

Ventilation imaging improves the specificity of an abnormal perfusion scan by differentiating between embolic occlusion of the pulmonary vasculature and perfusion defects occurring secondary to a primary disorder of ventilation. Recent prospective clinical trials show the basic premise—that is, perfusion defects that ventilate normally (ventilation-perfusion mismatch) are caused by pulmonary embolism, but matching ventilation-perfusion abnormalities are caused by other conditions—to be incorrect.

Ventilation lung scanning is helpful only if the perfusion defect is segmental or greater and is associated with ventilation mismatch. Pulmonary angiography shows that such patients have a high probability (≥86%) of pulmonary embolism. Other abnormal findings on lung scans, such as matching ventilation-perfusion defects (either segmental or subsegmental), subsegmental defects with ventilation mismatch, or perfusion defects that correspond to an area of increased density on the chest radiograph (nondiagnostic perfusion scan), are associated with a 20% to 40% frequency of pulmonary embolism. Therefore, further investigations, including pulmonary angiography and objective tests for venous thrombosis, must be carried out in patients with nondiagnostic ventilation-perfusion scan findings.

Using the Prospective Investigation of Pulmonary Embolism Diagnosis (PIOPED) criteria, if the lung scan shows a high probability pattern, the patient is treated with anticoagulants. If the pattern is normal, the patient requires no further testing or treatment. Unfortunately, the majority of patients have nondiagnostic patterns (formerly termed indeterminate, intermediate, and low probability lung scan patterns). In these patients, further investigation will depend on whether the patients have adequate

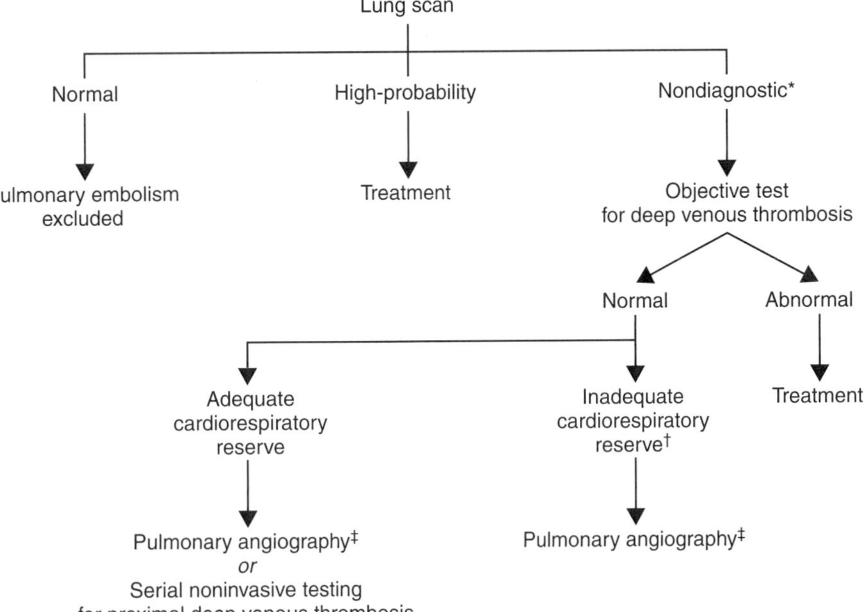

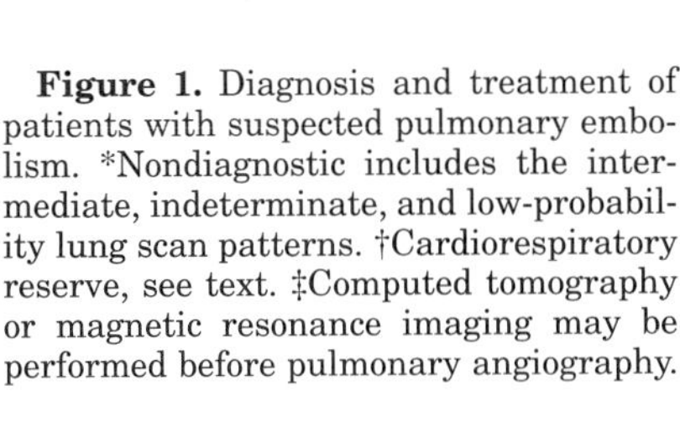
Figure 1. Diagnosis and treatment of patients with suspected pulmonary embolism. *Nondiagnostic includes the intermediate, indeterminate, and low-probability lung scan patterns. †Cardiorespiratory reserve, see text. ‡Computed tomography or magnetic resonance imaging may be performed before pulmonary angiography.

cardiorespiratory reserve. Objective testing for DVT is useful in patients with suspected pulmonary embolism, particularly those with nondiagnostic lung scan results (indeterminate, intermediate, or low-probability categories). The detection of proximal venous thrombosis by objective testing provides an indication for anticoagulant treatment, regardless of the presence or absence of pulmonary embolism, and avoids the need for further testing. A negative result by objective testing for DVT does not exclude the presence of pulmonary embolism. If the patient has adequate cardiorespiratory reserve, then serial noninvasive testing for proximal venous thrombosis may be used as an alternative to pulmonary angiography. Inadequate respiratory reserve is defined as the presence of syncope, hypotension (blood pressure less than 90 mm Hg), pulmonary edema, clinical finding of right-sided heart failure or echocardiographic finding of right ventricular hypokinesis, acute tachyarrhythmia, severe hypoxemia (Po_2 <50 mm Hg) or severe respiratory insufficiency (Pco_2 >45 mm Hg; FEV_1 <1.0, vital capacity <1.5 L).

Pulmonary angiography is the accepted diagnostic reference standard for pulmonary embolism. The diagnosis is established if an intraluminal filling defect is a constant finding on multiple films or if abrupt termination (cutoff) of a vessel greater than 2 to 5 mm in diameter is a constant finding on multiple films. Other abnormalities, such as oligemia, vessel pruning, and loss of filling of small vessels, are nonspecific and occur in a variety of conditions, including pneumonia, atelectasis, bronchiectasis, emphysema, and pulmonary carcinoma.

In recent years the diagnostic resolution of pulmonary angiography has been markedly improved and the risk to the patient decreased by the use of selective catheterization with repeated injections of small volumes of dye. This is a safe technique in the absence of severe chronic pulmonary hypertension or severe cardiac or respiratory decompensation. Clinically significant complications, including tachyarrhythmias, endocardial or myocardial injury, cardiac perforation, cardiac arrest, and hypersensitivity reactions to contrast medium, occur in fewer than 3% to 4% of patients.

The rationale is that the clinical objective in such patients is to prevent recurrent pulmonary embolism, which is unlikely in the absence of proximal venous thrombosis. For patients with inadequate cardiorespiratory reserve, the clinical objective is to prevent death and morbidity from an existing embolus, and further testing for the presence or absence of pulmonary embolism is needed.

Both spiral computed tomography (CT) and magnetic resonance imaging (MRI) are promising approaches for the diagnosis of pulmonary embolism. Spiral CT is highly sensitive for large emboli (segmental or greater arteries) but is less sensitive for emboli in subsegmental pulmonary arteries. Such emboli may be clinically important in patients with inadequate cardiorespiratory reserve. MRI appears to be highly sensitive for pulmonary embolism. However, two recent studies documented significant interobserver variation in the sensitivity, ranging from 70% to 100%. The safety of withholding anticoagulant treatment in patients with negative results by spiral CT or MRI has not been established by prospective clinical trials incorporating long-term follow-up. Therefore, spiral CT and MRI are useful tests for ruling in the diagnosis of pulmonary embolism if positive results are obtained, but the validity of negative results remains uncertain. The role of spiral CT in the diagnosis of pulmonary embolism is being assessed by a multicenter clinical trial funded by the National Institutes of Health (PIOPED II).

The assay for plasma D-dimer is potentially useful to exclude pulmonary embolism, based on a high negative predictive value reported in studies using a validated assay such as the Vidas DD assay. However, further studies are required to establish the place of D-dimer testing and, in particular, to evaluate the safety of withholding anticoagulant treatment in patients with suspected pulmonary embolism who have a negative D-dimer result.

TREATMENT

The objectives of treatment in patients with venous thromboembolism are (1) to prevent death from pulmonary embolism, (2) to prevent recurrent venous thromboembolism, and (3) to prevent the postphlebitic syndrome. The anticoagulant drugs heparin, low-molecular-weight heparin (LMWH), and warfarin constitute the mainstay of treatment for venous thrombosis. The use of graduated compression stockings for 24 months significantly decreases the incidence of the post-thrombotic syndrome. Furthermore, the incidence of the post-thrombotic syndrome is decreasing in recent years, suggesting that the more efficient treatment of venous thromboembolism and the prevention of recurrent DVT are having a positive impact on this complication.

Treatment With Unfractionated Heparin

Until recently, the accepted anticoagulant therapy for venous thromboembolism was a combination of continuous intravenous unfractionated heparin and oral warfarin. More recently, subcutaneous LMWH has been used in place of unfractionated heparin for the initial treatment of venous thromboembolism. Either of these agents must be used for a minimum of 5 days and until the international normalized ratio (INR) is therapeutic on 2 consecutive days. A few exceptions include patients who require immediate medical or surgical interventions such as thrombolysis or surgical procedures or patients with a very high risk of bleeding, in which case the heparin may be continued for a longer period of time before warfarin treatment is initiated.

It has been established from experimental studies and clinical trials that the efficacy of heparin therapy depends on achieving a critical therapeutic level of heparin within the first 24 hours of treatment. Patients who fail to achieve a therapeutic activated partial thromboplastin time (APTT) threshold within 24 hours have a significantly higher incidence of recurrent venous thromboembolism over the subsequent 3 months. The critical therapeutic level of heparin as measured by the APTT is 1.5 times the mean of the control value or the upper limit of the normal APTT range. This corresponds to a heparin blood level of 0.35 to 0.70 by the antifactor Xa assay.

Unless a prescriptive heparin nomogram is used, many patients will fail to achieve therapeutic APTT levels within the first 24 to 48 hours. Two such heparin nomograms have been evaluated prospectively in clinical trials. These heparin nomograms are shown in Tables 2 and 3.

TABLE 2. **Intravenous Heparin Dose Titration Nomogram According to the APTT**

APTT (sec)	Rate Change (mL/h)	Dose Change (IU/24 h)*	Additional Action
≤45	+6	+5760	Repeated APPT† in 4–6 h
46–54	+3	+2880	Repeated APTT in 4–6 h
55–85	0	0	None‡
86–110	−3	−2880	Stop heparin sodium treatment for 1 h; repeated APTT 4–6 h after restarting heparin treatment
>110	−6	−5760	Stop heparin treatment for 1 h; repeated APTT 4–6 h after restarting heparin treatment

*Heparin sodium concentration 20,000 IU in 500 mL = 40 IU/mL.
†With the use of Actin-FS thromboplastin reagent (Dade, Mississauga, Ontario, Canada).
‡During the first 24 h, repeated APTT in 4–6 h. Thereafter, the APTT will be determined once daily, unless subtherapeutic.
Abbreviation: APTT = activated partial thromboplastin time.
Adapted from Hull RD, Raskob GE, Rosenbloom D, et al: Optimal therapeutic level of heparin therapy in patients with venous thrombosis. Arch Intern Med 152:1589–1595, 1992. Copyright 1992, American Medical Association.

Complications of Heparin Therapy

The main adverse effects of heparin therapy include bleeding, thrombocytopenia, and osteoporosis. Patients at particular risk of bleeding are those who have had recent surgery or trauma or who have other clinical factors that predispose to bleeding on heparin, such as peptic ulcer, occult malignancy, liver disease, hemostatic defects, obesity, age older than 65 years, and female gender.

The management of bleeding on heparin therapy will depend on the location and severity of bleeding, the risk of recurrent venous thromboembolism, and the APTT. Heparin should be discontinued temporarily or permanently. Patients with recent venous thromboembolism may be candidates for insertion of an inferior vena cava filter. If urgent reversal of heparin effect is required, protamine sulfate can be administered.

Heparin-induced thrombocytopenia is a well-recognized complication of heparin therapy, usually occurring within 5 to 10 days after heparin treatment has started. One percent to 2% of patients receiving unfractionated heparin will experience a fall in platelet count to less than the normal range or a 50% fall in the platelet count within the normal range. In the majority of cases, this mild to moderate thrombocytopenia appears to be a direct effect of heparin on platelets and is of no consequence. However, 0.1% to 0.2% of patients receiving heparin develop an immune thrombocytopenia mediated by IgG antibody directed against a complex of platelet factor 4 and heparin.

TABLE 3. **Weight-Based Nomogram for Initial Intravenous Heparin Therapy***

	Dose (IU/kg)
Initial dose	80 bolus, then 18/h
APTT <35 sec (<1.2×)	80 bolus, then 4/h
APTT 35–45 sec (1.2–1.5×)	40 bolus, then 2/h
APTT 46–70 sec (1.5–2.3×)	No change
APTT 71–90 sec (2.3–3.0×)	Decrease infusion rate by 2/h
APTT >90 sec (>3.0×)	Hold infusion 1 h, then decrease infusion rate by 3/h

*Figures in parentheses show comparison with control.
Abbreviation: APTT = activated partial thromboplastin time.
Adapted from Raschke RA, Reilly BM, Guidry JR, et al: The weight-based heparin dosing nomogram compared with a "standard care" nomogram: A randomized controlled trial. Ann Intern Med 119:874–881, 1993.

The development of thrombocytopenia may be accompanied by arterial or venous thrombosis, which may lead to serious consequences such as death or limb amputation. The diagnosis of heparin-induced thrombocytopenia, with or without thrombosis, must be made on clinical grounds, because the assays with the highest sensitivity and specificity are not readily available and have a slow turnaround time.

When the diagnosis of heparin-induced thrombocytopenia is made, heparin in all forms must be stopped immediately. In those patients requiring ongoing anticoagulation, several alternatives exist; the agents most extensively used recently are the heparinoid danaparoid (Orgaran)* or hirudin.

Osteoporosis has been reported in patients receiving unfractionated heparin in dosages of 20,000 U/d (or more) for more than 6 months. Demineralization can progress to the fracture of vertebral bodies or long bones, and the defect may not be entirely reversible.

Low-Molecular-Weight Heparin

Heparin currently in use clinically is polydispersed unmodified heparin, with a mean molecular weight ranging from 10 to 16 kd. In recent years, low-molecular-weight derivatives of commercial heparin have been prepared that have a mean molecular weight of 4 to 5 kd.

The LMWHs commercially available are made by different processes (such as nitrous acid, alkaline, or enzymatic depolymerization), and they differ chemically and pharmacokinetically. The clinical significance of these differences, however, is unclear, and there have been very few studies comparing different LMWHs with respect to clinical outcomes. The doses of the different LMWHs have been established empirically and are not necessarily interchangeable. Therefore, at this time, the effectiveness and safety of each of the LMWHs must be tested separately.

The LMWHs differ from unfractionated heparin in numerous ways. Of particular importance are the following: increased bioavailability (>90% after subcutaneous injection), prolonged half-life and predictable clearance enabling once-or twice-daily injection, and predictable antithrombotic response based on body weight permitting treatment without laboratory monitoring. Other possible advantages are their abil-

*Not FDA approved for this indication.

ity to inactivate platelet-bound factor X_a, resistance to inhibition by platelet factor IV, and decreased effect on platelet function and vascular permeability (possibly accounting for less hemorrhagic effects at comparable antithrombotic doses).

There has been hope that the LMWHs will have fewer serious complications, such as bleeding, osteoporosis, and heparin-induced thrombocytopenia, when compared with unfractionated heparin. Evidence is accumulating that these complications are indeed less serious and less frequent with the use of LMWHs. The LMWHs all cross-react with unfractionated heparin; therefore, they cannot be used as alternative therapy in patients who develop heparin-induced thrombocytopenia. The heparinoid danaparoid* possesses a 10% to 20% cross-reactivity with heparin, and it can be used safely in patients who have no cross-reactivity.

In a number of early clinical trials (some of which were dose finding), LMWHs given by subcutaneous or intravenous injection were compared with continuous intravenous unfractionated heparin, with repeat venography at day 7 to 10 being the primary endpoint. These studies demonstrated that LMWHs were at least as effective as unfractionated heparin in preventing extension or increasing resolution of thrombi on repeat venography.

Subcutaneous unmonitored LMWHs have been compared with continuous intravenous heparin in a number of clinical trials for the treatment of proximal venous thrombosis using long-term follow-up as an outcome measure. These studies have shown that LMWHs are at least as effective and safe as unfractionated heparin in the treatment of proximal venous thrombosis. Pooling of the most methodologically sound studies indicates a significant advantage for LMWHs in the reduction of major bleeding and mortality. More recent studies have indicated that LMWHs used predominantly out of hospital were as effective and safe as intravenous unfractionated heparin given in hospital. Also, LMWHs are as effective as intravenous heparin in the treatment of patients presenting with pulmonary embolism. Economic analysis of treatment with LMWHs versus intravenous heparin demonstrated that LMWHs were cost-effective for treatment in hospital as well as out of hospital.

At present, two LMWHs are approved for venous thromboembolism in the United States and four are available in Canada. As these agents become more widely available for treatment, they will undoubtedly replace intravenous unfractionated heparin in the initial management of patients with venous thromboembolism.

Oral Anticoagulant Therapy

Oral anticoagulant therapy is begun together with initial heparin or LMWH therapy and overlapped for 4 to 5 days. Oral anticoagulant treatment is continued for 3 to 6 months in patients with a first episode of proximal venous thrombosis or pulmonary embolism. Stopping oral anticoagulant treatment at 4 to 6 weeks results in a high incidence (12%–20%) of recurrent venous thromboembolism during the following 12 to 24 months. Oral anticoagulant treatment should be continued for 1 year to indefinitely in patients with a second episode of objectively documented venous thromboembolism. Stopping treatment at 3 months in these patients results in a 20% incidence of recurrent venous thromboembolism during the following year and a 5% incidence of fatal pulmonary embolism.

The optimal duration of oral anticoagulant treatment for different patient subgroups is the subject of ongoing investigation. Long-term follow-up studies indicate that patients with a first episode of proximal venous thrombosis who receive treatment for 3 months have a 25% incidence of recurrent venous thromboembolism during the subsequent 5 years. The patients at high risk of recurrent thromboembolism are those with idiopathic thrombosis, an inhibitor deficiency state such as protein C or S deficiency, antithrombin deficiency, the anticardiolipin antibody syndrome, and cancer. Patients with advanced cancer remain at continued risk, and treatment should be continued indefinitely in these patients. Patients with idiopathic DVT should be treated for at least 6 months. Treatment beyond 6 months for patients with a first episode of idiopathic thrombosis or for those who have continuing risk factors has the potential to reduce recurrent venous thromboembolism, but it also has the risk of major bleeding, including fatal bleeding. The relative risk-benefit of extending treatment beyond 6 months for patients with a first episode of idiopathic venous thromboembolism with full-dose warfarin (INR 2.0–3.0) or low-dose warfarin (INR 1.5–2.0) awaits the results of ongoing clinical trials.

MASSIVE PULMONARY EMBOLISM

Patients with acute massive pulmonary embolism usually have a dramatic presentation with the sudden onset of severe shortness of breath, hypoxemia, and right ventricular failure. Symptoms include central chest pain, often identical to angina, severe dyspnea, and, frequently, syncope, confusion, or coma. Examination reveals a patient in severe distress with tachypnea, cyanosis, and hypotension. The marked increase in pulmonary vascular resistance leads to acute right ventricular failure with the presence of large A waves in the jugular veins and a right ventricular diastolic gallop. With pulmonary hypertension there is marked right ventricular dilatation with a shift of the intraventricular septum, decreasing cardiac output, and further decrease in coronary perfusion, and this frequently results in cardiorespiratory arrest. If patients with a massive pulmonary embolus survive, they are acutely threatened by any further pulmonary thromboembolism.

The emergency management of massive pulmo-

*Not FDA approved for this indication.

nary embolism includes the use of intravenous heparin; the use of oxygen, with or without mechanical ventilation, which may include positive end-expiratory pressure, volume resuscitation; and the use of inotropic agents and vasodilators. In addition to these supportive measures, specific treatment options for massive pulmonary embolism include thrombolysis; pulmonary thrombectomy, with or without cardiopulmonary bypass support; transvenous catheter embolectomy or clot dissolution; and insertion of an inferior vena caval filter.

Thrombolytic Treatment

Thrombolytic therapy is indicated for patients with pulmonary embolism who present with hypotension and/or syncope and for patients with pulmonary embolism who have clinical findings of right ventricular failure or echocardiographic evidence of right ventricular hypokinesis. Thrombolytic therapy provides more rapid lysis of pulmonary emboli and more rapid restoration of right ventricular function and pulmonary perfusion than anticoagulant treatment. An effective regimen is 100 mg of recombinant tPA by intravenous infusion over 1 to 2 hours. An alternative is the use of streptokinase, 250,000 units over 30 minutes followed by 100,000 units/h for up to 24 hours.

The role of thrombolytic agents in the management of acute massive pulmonary embolism remains controversial. Although there is a more rapid dissolution of venous thromboemboli, the risk of serious bleeding remains a concern. Until there is a clearly demonstrated benefit in both morbidity and mortality from well-controlled prospective randomized clinical trials, the question of risk-benefit will remain. In the meantime, the use of thrombolytic agents has become simpler with the use of echocardiography or spiral CT to confirm the diagnosis, the use of short-term or bolus infusion of thrombolytic agents into peripheral veins rather into the pulmonary artery, the elimination of monitoring by laboratory tests, and treatment on the medical ward rather than in the intensive care unit. The fact that a high percentage of acute massive pulmonary emboli are occurring after surgery despite the fact that effective prophylactic regimens are available against venous thromboembolism indicates that greater efforts must be taken to ensure that these prophylactic measures are being applied in a more uniform fashion.

Pulmonary Embolectomy

Pulmonary embolectomy is occasionally indicated in the management of massive pulmonary embolism. This is defined as the sudden occurrence of a massive embolus producing severe cardiovascular decompensation with severe hypotension, oliguria, and hypoxia refractory to aggressive treatment. A somewhat more generous indication would be an obstruction of more than 50% of the pulmonary vasculature, arterial oxygen saturation less than 60 mm Hg, systolic blood pressure less than 90 mm Hg, and urine output of less than 20 mL/h.

The role of pulmonary embolectomy remains unclear and will depend in part on the ready availability of a surgical team. Patients who are not candidates for thrombolysis (e.g., recent surgery) or who have not responded to maximal medical therapy may be candidates for pulmonary embolectomy. However, the recent report of successful thrombolysis with intrapulmonary urokinase in patients treated within 10 days of surgery casts further doubt on the need for this somewhat radical procedure. Alternatives to pulmonary thrombectomies such as catheter tip embolectomy or catheter tip fragmentation are available in specialized centers.

Inferior Vena Caval Interruption

Insertion of an inferior vena caval filter is indicated for the folling patients:

1. The patient with acute venous thromboembolism and an absolute contraindication to anticoagulant therapy
2. The rare patient with massive pulmonary embolism who survives but in whom recurrent embolism may be fatal
3. The rare patient who has objectively documented recurrent venous thromboembolism during adequate anticoagulant therapy
4. The patient with recent (<6 weeks) proximal venous thrombosis who requires emergency surgery.

The insertion of a vena caval filter is effective for preventing important pulmonary embolism. However, the use of a filter results in an increased incidence of recurrent DVT 1 to 2 years after insertion (increase in cumulative incidence at 2 years from 12% to 21%). If it is not contraindicated, long-term anticoagulant treatment should be administered after placement of a vena caval filter to prevent morbidity from recurrent DVT.

SARCOIDOSIS

method of
JOSEPH P. LYNCH III, M.D.*
University of Michigan Medical Center
Ann Arbor, Michigan

Sarcoidosis, a multisystem granulomatous disease of unknown etiology, has an extremely variable clinical expression and course. Pulmonary manifestations are most common, but virtually any organ can be affected. The histologic hallmark of sarcoidosis is non-necrotizing granulomas; varying degrees of fibrosis may be present. Interactions between T helper/inducer ($CD4^+$) cells and mononuclear phagocytes drive the granulomatous process, but the precise signals influencing evolution of the disease have not

*Supported in part by National Institutes of Health Grant 1P50HL46487

been elucidated. The natural history and prognosis of sarcoidosis are highly variable. Spontaneous remissions occur in nearly two thirds of patients. In 10% to 30% of patients, the course is chronic, with progressive damage or dysfunction of affected organs. A waxing and waning course over months or years may be seen. Fatalities occur in 1% to 4% of patients, typically as a result of respiratory failure or central nervous system (CNS) or myocardial involvement. Although only a minority of patients with sarcoidosis require treatment, treatment is essential for patients with severe, chronic, or progressive disease to avert serious late sequelae. However, given the high rate of *spontaneous* remissions, indications for therapy are controversial.

INDICATIONS FOR TREATMENT

Indications for treatment should be circumscribed. The decision to treat is based on the severity, acuity, and duration of symptoms, site of involvement, chest radiographic stage, and evolution of the disease (in the absence of therapy). Patients with debilitating symptoms, critical organ involvement (e.g., cardiac, CNS, eye), severe impairment in pulmonary function tests, or an accelerated course should be treated immediately (typically with corticosteroids). When symptoms are not severe and critical organs are not involved, the decision to treat may be deferred for up to 6 to 12 months because spontaneous remissions may occur within that time frame. Chronic, persistent disease warrants therapy if symptoms or significant organ dysfunction is present. For patients with pulmonary sarcoidosis, assessment of chest radiographic stage has prognostic value. The chest radiographic staging system is defined as follows: 0, normal; I, bilateral hilar lymphadenopathy (BHL) *without* parenchymal infiltrates; II, BHL *plus* parenchymal infiltrates; and III, parenchymal infiltrates *without* BHL. Treatment is rarely required for radiographic stage I disease because spontaneous remissions occur in 60% to 85% of patients in this context. Further, most patients with persistent BHL remain asymptomatic and do not require treatment. In contrast, stage II or III disease may persist or worsen over time and necessitate treatment. Spontaneous remission occurs in only 30% to 70% of patients with stage II and in less than 20% of patients with stage III sarcoidosis. Patients with *persistent* stage II or III disease lasting more than 6 to 12 months and chronic symptoms or pulmonary dysfunction should be treated because spontaneous remissions are unlikely to occur beyond this point. Earlier treatment is warranted for patients with severe or debilitating symptoms. Therapy is rarely beneficial when advanced parenchymal distortion, honeycombing, or fibrosis is present. Immediate treatment with corticosteroids is warranted for life-threatening or sight-threatening organ involvement (e.g., cardiac, CNS, eye). A trial of corticosteroids should be offered for disfiguring cutaneous sarcoid (lupus pernio), hypersplenism, persistent hypercalcemia, or progressive or symptomatic sarcoidosis involving the lungs or extrapulmonary sites (Table 1).

TABLE 1. **Sarcoidosis: Indications for Treatment According to Site of Involvement**

Central nervous system (brain, spinal cord)
Heart (arrhythmias, heart block, cardiomyopathy)
Eye (posterior uveitis, recurrent anterior uveitis)
Persistent pulmonary infiltrates on chest radiograph (stage II or III) plus symptoms
Disfiguring cutaneous sarcoid (lupus pernio)
Splenic involvement (hypersplenism, abdominal pain, massive splenomegaly)
Hepatic involvement (cholestatic jaundice, severe abdominal pain)
Chronic hypercalcemia
Chronic hypercalciuria with end-organ complications (e.g., nephrocalcinosis, nephrolithiasis)
Chronic, symptomatic extrapulmonary sarcoidosis (any organ)

CORTICOSTEROIDS

Corticosteroids are the cornerstone of therapy for sarcoidosis. Short-term responses are often dramatic, but long-term efficacy is controversial. Toxicities of corticosteroids may be appreciable, particularly with long-term use. Despite extensive published data, interpretation of the efficacy of therapy is difficult because of the high rate of spontaneous remissions, lack of standardization of criteria for response, differing dosages and duration of therapy, and heterogeneous populations of patients.

In several large nonrandomized series, favorable responses to corticosteroids were noted in 40% to 85% of patients. However, relapses occurred in 15% to 73% of patients after discontinuation of therapy. Thus, despite initial responses, the *long-term* impact of corticosteroids on altering the natural history of the disease is unproven.

Several prospective, randomized placebo-controlled trials in the United States, Europe, and Japan in the 1970s and 1980s failed to show benefit from early corticosteroid treatment in pulmonary sarcoidosis. These "negative" studies reflect study designs because patients included in these randomized trials were usually asymptomatic, had normal or minimally impaired pulmonary function, and had stage I or II chest radiographs, features that predict high rates of spontaneous remission. Despite their limitations, these studies affirmed that *routine* use of corticosteroids for patients with *asymptomatic* or *minimal* disease is not appropriate. However, these studies do not address the role of corticosteroids for *symptomatic* patients with severe or progressive disease. In fact, patients with more severe disease or symptoms were excluded from these studies and were often empirically treated with corticosteroids, with purported benefit.

Although the long-term benefit of corticosteroids is unproven, the anti-inflammatory effects of corticosteroids may prevent loss of pulmonary function and avert late sequelae in patients with persistent granulomatous inflammation. One multicenter randomized trial in England published in 1996 evaluated 149 patients with stage II or III sarcoidosis. Patients were initially observed *without* treatment for 6 months, at which time patients with *persistent* radiographic infiltrates were randomized to receive long-term corticosteroids (for 18 months) or no treatment (unless symptoms mandated corticosteroid therapy). Of the original cohort, 91 patients were excluded because of spontaneous improvement in chest radiographs (58 patients) or treatment with corticosteroids for persistent or progressive symptoms (33 patients). The remaining 58 patients with *persistent* radiographic infiltrates at 6 months were randomized to the respective treatment arms. At long-term follow-up, pulmonary function was improved in the long-term corticosteroid cohort when compared with controls receiving placebo (some also received corticosteroids for clinical indications). These data support treating patients with persistent stage II or III sarcoidosis but only *after* an appropriate observation period (e.g., 6–12 months).

The optimal dose or duration of corticosteroid therapy has not been studied in randomized trials. However, high doses of corticosteroids for prolonged periods are associated with untoward adverse effects and are rarely appropriate. The dose and duration of therapy should be individualized according to the severity of the illness and the site of involvement. I initiate therapy with 40 mg of prednisone daily (or equivalent) for 1 month and taper to 40 mg every other day within 2 to 4 months if the disease is controlled. Higher doses (1 mg/kg/d) are warranted for cardiac or CNS sarcoidosis. Objective parameters are essential to monitor response to therapy. Responses are usually evident within 4 to 12 weeks of initiation of therapy. Patients who fail to respond within 3 months are unlikely to respond to a more protracted course of therapy. Therapeutic failures may reflect an inadequate dose of therapy, irreversible disease, noncompliance, or intrinsic corticosteroid resistance. Among nonresponders, the corticosteroid dosage is rapidly tapered and discontinued. These patients may be candidates for alternative immunosuppressive or cytotoxic agents (discussed later). Patients responding to corticosteroid therapy are maintained on prednisone, in a tapering dose, for a total course of 12 to 18 months. The rate of taper is individualized according to clinical response and the presence or absence of side effects. For non–life-threatening sarcoidosis, I try to taper prednisone therapy to 30 mg on alternate days within 3 to 6 months and to 20 mg on alternate days within 9 months. Low-dose prednisone (5–15 mg on alternate days) is continued for an additional 6 to 9 months to minimize the chance of relapse. Relapses require reinstitution of daily high-dose corticosteroids. Some patients relapse each time that the steroid dose is tapered below a critical threshold. Such patients should be treated long-term (sometimes indefinitely) with low-dose alternate-day prednisone. Immunomodulatory agents may be used in patients experiencing adverse effects from corticosteroids.

Inhaled Corticosteroids

Inhaled coprticosteroids may have a limited role in patients with suspected endobronchial sarcoidosis, but data confirming efficacy are lacking. One placebo-controlled, double-blind randomized trial showed no benefit of high-dose inhaled corticosteroids for pulmonary sarcoidosis. Another placebo-controlled study suggested a possible steroid-sparing effect. Inhaled corticosteroids are expensive but relatively nontoxic. An empirical trial of inhaled corticosteroids (for 2–4 months) is reasonable for patients with cough, wheezing, or bronchial hyperreactivity. Inhaled corticosteroids are not adequate for severe pulmonary sarcoidosis.

TABLE 2. **Therapy for Sarcoidosis**

Corticosteroids (first line)
Topical for superficial involvement (e.g., conjunctivitis, episcleritis, skin, endobronchial)
Systemic (oral prednisone) for parenchymal involvement
IV pulse methylprednisolone for fulminant CNS disease
Immunosuppressive or Immunomodulatory Agents (second line, steroid sparing)
(e.g., methotrexate, azathioprine, hydrochloroquine) Reserve for:
Failing corticosteroids
Steroid adverse effects
High risk for steroid side effects
Cyclophosphamide (oral or pulse intravenous)
Reserve for CNS sarcoidosis refractory to corticosteroids and immunosuppressive agents
Organ Transplantation (renal, liver, heart, lung)
Only if aggressive medical therapy fails
Radiation Therapy
Reserve for localized, CNS mass lesions unresponsive to aggressive medical therapy

Abbreviation: CNS = central nervous system.

OTHER IMMUNOSUPPRESSIVE AND CYTOTOXIC AGENTS

Immunosuppressive, cytotoxic, and antimalarial agents with immunomodulatory properties may be used to treat patients failing or experiencing adverse effects from corticosteroid therapy. Randomized, controlled trials are lacking and the best agent has not been elucidated (Tables 2 and 3).

Methotrexate (Rheumatrex)*

Methotrexate (MTX), a folic acid antagonist with immunosuppressive and anti-inflammatory effects, may be efficacious for sarcoid patients failing therapy or experiencing unacceptable side effects from corticosteroids. MTX can be given orally or intramuscularly (7.5–20 mg once weekly); both routes are comparable in efficacy. Favorable responses have been cited with MTX for sarcoidosis involving the lungs, skin, muscles or joints, CNS, and diverse extrapulmonary sites. An empirical trial for 4 to 6 months is reasonable. I continue therapy *beyond* 6 months only for patients manifesting *objective* and unequivocal improvement. The effects of MTX are not sustained;

*Not FDA approved for this indication.

TABLE 3. **Therapeutic Options for Sarcoidosis**

Corticosteroids

Prednisone, 40 mg/d PO (or equivalent) for 4 wk, gradual taper
Dose: prednisone, 1 mg/kg/d PO for CNS or cardiac involvement
IV pulse methylprednisolone (up to 1 g daily for 2–3 d) for severe CNS disease

Methotrexate*

Dose: 7.5–20 mg once weekly (PO or IM)
Concomitant folic acid, 1 mg/d PO (to reduce toxicity)

Azathioprine*

Dose: 1–3 mg/kg/d PO (maximal dose, 200 mg)

Cyclophosphamide*†

Dose: 1–2 mg/kg/d PO (maximal dose, 150 mg)
IV pulse (0.75–1.5 g once monthly)

Hydroxychloroquine*

Dose: 200 mg once or twice daily PO

Cyclosporine‡

Dose: 3–6 mg/kg/d PO

*Not FDA approved for this indication.
†Reserve for severe disease refractory to corticosteroids and other immunosuppressive agents (e.g., methotrexate or azathioprine).
‡Reserve as part of combination therapy for severe disease refractory to combination therapy with corticosteroids and immunosuppressive agents.
Abbreviation: CNS, central nervous system.

relapses are frequent after cessation of therapy, but re-treatment is usually efficacious.

Enthusiasm for the use of MTX should be tempered by its toxicities. Side effects require discontinuation of therapy in 3% to 15% of patients. Symptoms may be attenuated or ablated by reducing the dose or by concomitant administration of folic acid (1 mg/d). The most common adverse effects include: nausea, vomiting, diarrhea, dyspepsia (10% to 40%); stomatitis (2% to 8%); rash or alopecia (1% to 4%); megaloblastic anemia, leukopenia, or thrombocytopenia (1% to 4%); and hypersensitivity pneumonia (2% to 7%). MTX is teratogenic and induces abortions. As with all immunosuppressive agents, the risk of opportunistic infections is heightened with MTX, particularly when steroids are administered concomitantly. MTX is not carcinogenic. A worrisome complication of chronic use of MTX is hepatic injury (including cirrhosis). Risk factors for hepatotoxicity include: cumulative dose greater than 3 g, pre-existing hepatic disease, diabetes mellitus, excessive alcohol use, obesity, renal failure, and advanced age. Alternative agents are advised for patients with these risk factors. Serial transaminases (aspartate aminotransferase [AST] and alanine aminotransferase [ALT]) should be measured every 6 to 8 weeks in patients receiving MTX. Sustained or progressive rises in AST or ALT (to twice the normal range) warrant dose reduction or cessation of therapy. Unfortunately, liver enzymes do not reliably predict hepatoxicity, and cirrhosis may develop even when liver enzyme levels are normal. Surveillance liver biopsies may detect subclinical toxicity, but the value of surveillance biopsies is debatable. Given the potential risk for cirrhosis as a late complication of MTX use, I limit the course to a *total cumulative* dose of 3 g.

Azathioprine* (Imuran)

Azathioprine, a purine analogue with pleiotropic immunosuppressive effects, may be used in corticosteroid-refractory sarcoidosis or as a corticosteroid-sparing agent in patients experiencing or at high risk for corticosteroid adverse effects. Azathioprine is administered orally (1 to 3 mg/kg/d; maximum, 200 mg/d). Randomized studies have not been conducted, but favorable responses have been cited, even in patients failing corticosteroid treatment. In many studies, interpretation of the efficacy of azathioprine has been clouded by the concomitant use of corticosteroids. As with MTX, a 4- to 6-month trial of azathioprine is advised before abandoning this agent. Long-term therapy (months to years) may be necessary for responding patients who show a propensity for relapse after cessation of therapy.

Azathioprine is usually well tolerated, but adverse effects require discontinuation of therapy in 2% to 3% of patients. Principal toxicities include: bone marrow suppression, gastrointestinal symptoms, rash, mucosal ulcerations, heightened susceptibility to infections, and idiosyncratic reactions (fever, rash, arthralgias). Serious hepatotoxicity or pancreatitis is a rare complication (<0.5%). Bone marrow toxicity is dose dependent. Complete blood counts, differential, and platelet counts should be obtained within 2 weeks of initiation of azathioprine and every 4 to 8 weeks with chronic therapy. Leukopenia (<3000/mm^3) or thrombocytopenia (<100,000/mm^3) mandates dose reduction. I measure liver function tests (AST, ALT) within 4 weeks of initiation of therapy and at 3- to 4-month intervals thereafter. Azathioprine is less oncogenic than the alkylating agents but is associated with an increased risk of cutaneous and cervical carcinoma and lymphoproliferative disorders. This risk probably reflects the intensity of immunosuppression rather than a direct oncogenic effect.

Cyclophosphamide (Cytoxan)*

Cyclophosphamide, an antineoplastic alkylating agent with potent immunosuppressive properties, is rarely used to treat sarcoidosis, but anecdotal success has been cited, even in patients failing corticosteroid or other immunosuppressive therapy. Cyclophosphamide can be administered orally (1–2 mg/kg/d) or as an intravenous "pulse" (0.75–1.5 g) once monthly. Toxicities of cyclophosphamide are substantial and include: infertility; gastrointestinal, mucosal, pulmonary, and bone marrow toxicities; hemorrhagic cystitis; heightened susceptibility to infection; alopecia; and induction of neoplasia. Cyclophosphamide suppresses all cell lines in the bone marrow and is more toxic in this regard than MTX or azathioprine. Progressive pancytopenias and myelodysplasia may occur with long-term use. Transitional cell carcinoma of the bladder develops in 2% to 15% of patients

*Not FDA approved for this indication.

receiving long-term oral cyclophosphamide. The risk of bladder cancer increases when the cumulative dose exceeds 80 g and may persist for years, even after discontinuing therapy with cyclophosphamide. Cyclophosphamide is also associated with an increased risk of hematologic malignancies (e.g., lymphomas, leukemias) and other neoplasms. Because of its myriad potential toxicities (including oncogenesis), I rarely use cyclophosphamide for sarcoidosis. However, intravenous pulse cyclophosphamide has a role in patients with CNS sarcoidosis refractory to corticosteroids and other agents (e.g., MTX, azathioprine, antimalarials).

Chlorambucil (Leukeran)*

Chlorambucil, an alkylating agent related to cyclophosphamide, was used in the 1970s and 1980s to treat corticosteroid-refractory sarcoidosis, with anecdotal success. Chlorambucil is teratogenic and oncogenic and has myriad toxicities (e.g., bone marrow suppression, gastrointestinal toxicity, oral ulcers, rash, opportunistic infections, interstitial pneumonia). Because of its oncogenicity, chlorambucil should not be used to treat sarcoidosis.

Cyclosporine*

Cyclosporine, an immunosuppressive agent that inhibits T helper cell activation and proliferation, has been used in corticosteroid-recalcitrant sarcoidosis, but results were disappointing. In one randomized trial, the combination of cyclosporine (5 to 7 mg/kg/d) plus prednisone was no more effective than prednisone alone. Cyclosporine is exceedingly expensive (>$500 per month) and is nearly invariably toxic. Principal toxicities include: nephrotoxicity (5%–30%), hypertension (11%–50%), hirsutism (50%–70%), and CNS toxicities (10%–20%). Cyclosporine has no role as primary therapy for sarcoidosis. Oral cyclosporine *combined* with corticosteroids or other immunomodulatory drugs (e.g., MTX, azathioprine, antimalarials) may be considered for use as salvage therapy in severe sarcoidosis refractory to multiple agents.

Antimalarials

Antimalarial drugs (e.g., chloroquine [Aralen],* hydroxychloroquine [Plaquenil]*) inhibit several facets of the immune response (e.g., antigen presentation and cytokine production), concentrate in cells of the reticuloendothelial system and melanin-containing tissue (e.g., skin, spleen, kidney, leukocytes), and have been used, with anecdotal success, to treat sarcoid-induced hypercalcemia or sarcoidosis involving the skin, bone, lungs, CNS, and other extrapulmonary sites. Chloroquine is more potent than hydroxychloroquine but is rarely used because of potential serious ocular toxicity. Hydroxychloroquine is less toxic and may used to treat patients with sarcoidosis who are failing treatment or experiencing adverse effects from corticosteroids, as an adjunctive (steroid-sparing) agent, or as primary therapy for cutaneous sarcoidosis (particularly lupus pernio). The initial dose is 200 mg twice daily for the first 6 months. If remissions are achieved, 200 mg once daily may be adequate for maintenance therapy. Hydroxychloroquine has an exceptionally long half-life; responses are often delayed for 2 or more months. A 6-month trial is advised before abandoning this agent. Hydroxychloroquine is well tolerated; adverse effects require discontinuation of therapy in less than 5% of patients. Ocular toxicity, the major complication of antimalarials, is rare with hydroxychloroquine. Corneal deposits or blurred vision may occur with long-term use but reverse with cessation of therapy. Serial examinations by an ophthalmologist are advised every 6 to 9 months while taking hydrochloroquine. Other principal side effects include: nausea, vomiting, bloating; cutaneous changes (pruritus, urticaria, rash, skin hyperpigmentation); and headache, insomnia, or nervousness. Antimalarials should not be used in pregnancy or in children. Combining an antimalarial with corticosteroids or immunosuppressive agents may enhance the immunomodulatory effects in comparison with any of these agents used alone.

Nonsteroidal Anti-inflammatory Agents

Nonsteroidal anti-inflammatory agents may palliate myalgias or arthritis in patients with acute inflammatory forms of sarcoidosis (e.g., in the context of erythema nodosum, fever, Löfgren's syndrome). These drugs have no role in treating serious manifestations of sarcoidosis.

Novel Agents

Pentoxifylline (Trental),* an immunodulatory agent that inhibits the synthesis of cytokines important in the pathogenesis of sarcoidosis (e.g., tumor necrosis factor and TH_1 cytokines), has been tried in untreated or corticosteroid-refractory sarcoidosis, with anecdotal success. Thalidomide, a sedative withdrawn from the market in 1962 because of teratogenic effects, has immunomodulatory properties, and favorable responses have been cited in a few patients with sarcoidosis. Data are sparse and the role (if any) of pentoxifylline or thalidomide as therapy for sarcoidosis needs to be studied.

Organ Transplantation

Organ transplantation (e.g., renal, liver, heart, or lung) is an accepted therapeutic option for patients with end-stage organ failure secondary to sarcoidosis. Lung transplantation may be lifesaving for sarcoid patients with severe respiratory insufficiency

*Not FDA approved for this indication.

*Not FDA approved for this indication.

refractory to medical therapy. One- and 2-year survival rates are similar to those after lung transplantation in nonsarcoid recipients, with a 2-year survivorship rate of 60% to 75%. Recurrent sarcoid granulomas within lung allografts are common after transplantation but do not usually cause symptoms. Because transplant recipients receive immunosuppressive therapy for life, the intensity of the granulomatous response may be attenuated.

TREATMENT OF SPECIFIC SITES OF INVOLVEMENT

Lung and Bronchi

Although the clinical spectrum of sarcoidosis is protean, pulmonary manifestations typically dominate. Abnormalities on chest radiographs are present in more than 90% of patients. Cough or dyspnea may be prominent with endobronchial or lung involvement. Chronic pulmonary sarcoidosis evolving over years may cause inexorable destruction of the alveolar architecture and irreversible loss of lung function. Fatal respiratory insufficiency develops in 1% to 3% of patients with sarcoidosis. Treatment is indicated for patients exhibiting severe or progressive pulmonary involvement, particularly when lung function deteriorates. However, spontaneous remissions occur in 50% to 60% of patients, so treatment should be circumscribed. Certain features (e.g., lupus pernio, osseous involvement, nephrocalcinosis, chronic uveitis) predict a low rate of spontaneous remission (<20%), whereas erythema nodosum, acute polyarthritis, fever, and stage I disease (i.e., Löfgren's syndrome) are associated with a high rate of spontaneous remission (>85%). The chest radiographic stage is a good but not entirely reliable predictor of prognosis. For example, spontaneous remission occurs in 60% to 85% of patients with radiographic stage I sarcoidosis, whereas spontaneous remission rates are lower with stage II (30%–70%) or stage III (10% to 20%) disease. The course of sarcoidosis is usually evident within 1 to 2 years after diagnosis. The vast majority (>85%) of spontaneous remissions occur within this time frame. Treatment is rarely necessary for stage I but is often necessary to prevent devastating sequelae in patients with stage II or III disease.

Whom and when to treat are difficult decisions. Asymptomatic patients with normal pulmonary function do not require treatment, even with abnormal chest radiographs. A trial of therapy is warranted for symptomatic patients, but the decision can often be delayed for 6 to 12 months to see whether spontaneous remission will occur. For patients with persistent symptoms and pulmonary infiltrates, delaying therapy beyond this point may result in irreversible fibrocystic changes. Pulmonary function tests and chest radiographs are performed at 3- to 4-month intervals to gauge evolution of the disease and determine the need for therapy. Spirometry and flow-volume loops to measure forced vital capacity and forced expiratory volume in 1 second are cost-effective tests to judge the course of the disease (and in treated patients, to assess response to therapy). More complex measurements (e.g., lung volumes, diffusing capacity, exercise studies) are reserved for *selected* patients. Treatment should be considered for patients with severe or progressive symptoms (e.g., cough, dyspnea), declining or significant impairment in lung function, or persistent stage II or III sarcoidosis after an initial observation period (e.g., 6–12 months). Although computed tomographic (CT) scans are not necessary in the *routine* evaluation or management of sarcoidosis, high-resolution thin-section CT scans may be helpful in *selected* patients with stage II or III disease to discriminate active alveolitis (i.e., granulomatous inflammation) from irreversible fibrosis. Ground-glass opacities, nodules, or alveolar opacities suggest granulomatous inflammation, which may reverse with therapy. In contrast, honeycombing, cysts, coarse broad bands, distortion, or traction bronchiectasis indicate fibrosis and a low likelihood of response to therapy.

Corticosteroids are the cornerstone of therapy for pulmonary sarcoidosis. I initiate treatment with prednisone at 40 mg/d for 4 weeks, with subsequent taper guided by clinical response and toxicities. For patients failing corticosteroid therapy, I consider azathioprine, MTX, or hydroxychloroquine (for a 6-month trial). Inhaled steroids have little or no role in severe pulmonary sarcoidosis, but they may be used in patients with cough, bronchial hyperreactivity, and suspected endobronchial involvement.

Extrapulmonary Involvement (Selected Sites)

Cardiac Involvement

Cardiac involvement may give rise to sudden death, arrhythmias, cardiomyopathy, or pericardial effusions. Clinically evident cardiac disease is recognized antemortem in 2% to 5% of patients with sarcoidosis; much higher rates are cited in necropsy studies. Because of the potentially lethal nature of cardiac sarcoidosis, aggressive therapy is essential. Initial treatment is high-dose corticosteroids (prednisone, 1 mg/kg/d or equivalent, with gradual taper. For severe or fulminant cases, high-dose intravenous pulse methylprednisolone (Solu-Medrol) is advised. After a response is achieved, I often add azathioprine or hydroxychloroquine for their steroid-sparing effects. Long-term (possibly indefinite) treatment is required to prevent recrudescent disease. Patients with complete heart block or serious arrhythmias should receive a permanent implantable pacemaker-debrillator in addition to medical therapy.

Central Nervous System Involvement

CNS involvement is noted in 2% to 8% of patients with sarcoidosis and can be devastating. Sarcoidosis has a predilection for the cranial nerves (particularly the seventh facial nerve), hypothalamus, pituitary gland, and optic chiasm, but any portion of the brain or spinal cord can be involved. Strokes, quadriparesis, or devastating sequelae may ensue. A definitive diagnosis of CNS sarcoidosis is difficult because CNS lesions are not often amenable to biopsy. A presumptive diagnosis of CNS sarcoidosis can be made provided that the clinical context is appropriate, noncaseating granulomas are documented at non-CNS sites, and magnetic resonance images reveal enhancing lesions after gadolinium administration. Management of CNS sarcoidosis is similar to the management of cardiac sarcoidosis. Patients with CNS sarcoidosis who are failing corticosteroid or other immunosuppressive drug therapy should be treated with intravenous pulse cyclophosphamide. Radiation therapy is reserved for localized, space-occupying lesions refractory to medical therapy.

Ocular Sarcoidosis

Ocular involvement occurs in 10% to 30% of patients with sarcoidosis during the course of the disease. Superficial manifestations (e.g., conjunctivitis, episcleritis) may be treated with topical corticosteroids. Posterior uveitis or recurrent anterior uveitis can cause visual loss and necessitates systemic corticosteroids.

Skin Involvement

Skin lesions occur in 10% to 30% of patients with sarcoidosis during the course of the disease. Lupus pernio, characterized by violaceous lesions of the face (principally the nose and perioral regions) can be disfiguring. Treatment with corticosteroids (systemic, topic, or intralesional), hydroxychloroquine, or immunosuppressive agents may be tried, but dermatologic lesions are often refractory to therapy.

Hepatic and Splenic Sarcoidosis

Asymptomatic involvement of the liver occurs in 40% to 80% of patients, but symptoms from hepatic sarcoidosis are uncommon (2%–6%). Rare manifestations include: cholestatic jaundice, portal hypertension, hepatic failure, and cirrhosis. Asymptomatic involvement of the spleen is common (38%–77%), but symptoms from splenic involvement (e.g., abdominal pain, portal hypertension, splenic rupture, and pancytopenias) are noted in only 2% to 5% of sarcoid patients. Corticosteroids are first-line therapy for symptomatic hepatic or splenic sarcoidosis (initial dose, 40 mg prednisone daily for 4 weeks, with gradual taper). Serial measurements of alkaline phosphatase or transaminases are useful to gauge the response to therapy for hepatic sarcoidosis. Abdominal CT scans are helpful for determining the extent of splenic (or hepatic) disease and response to therapy. Hydroxychloroquine achieves high concentrations in the spleen and may be useful as adjunctive therapy. Splenectomy may be warranted for massive, symptomatic splenomegaly refractory to medical therapy.

Osseous Sarcoidosis

Symptomatic bone involvement occurs in 1% to 4% of patients with sarcoidosis. Lytic, punched-out lesions involving the small bones of the hands or feet are characteristic; sclerotic lesions are rarely observed. Treatment with corticosteroids, hydroxychloroquine, or immunosuppressive agents may be tried but is usually ineffective.

Disorders of Calcium Metabolism

Hypercalcemia occurs in 2% to 4% of patients with sarcoidosis, and hypercalciuria, in 15% to 40%. Nephrolithiasis and nephrocalcinosis are complications of chronic hypercalcemia and hypercalciuria. Corticosteroids (20–40 mg daily with taper) are highly efficacious. Hydrochloroquine may also be effective. Oral ketoconazole has been tried, with anecdotal success.

Treatment of sarcoidosis requires paying careful attention to the course of the disease over months or even years and balancing the risk-benefit profile of therapeutic agents. Failure to treat patients with chronic, progressive disease may result in inexorable loss of function and even death. However, overaggressive use of corticosteroids may lead to debilitating adverse effects. The use of immunosuppressive or immunomodulatory agents may allow a reduction in the corticosteroid dose while maintaining remission. Patients with chronic, relapsing disease requiring unacceptably high doses of steroids may benefit from creative strategies using combinations of agents.

SILICOSIS

method of
STEPHEN DOLAN, M.D.
Medical College of Wisconsin
Milwaukee, Wisconsin

Silicosis is a pneumoconiosis that arises from long-standing silica exposure. The pneumoconioses are non-neoplastic lung diseases that result from the chronic inhalation of mineral dust, usually in a workplace environment. Silicosis refers to a slowly progressive fibrosing nodular lung disease that results from the inhalation of crystalline silica. Silica or silicon dioxide (SiO_2) composes 25% of the Earth's crust and exists in nature in both amorphous and crystalline forms. Amorphous silica includes the natural glasses and is much less toxic than crystalline silica. Free silica is a pure crystalline form of silicon dioxide that contains the silicon-oxygen tetrahedron and exists in a number of polymorphs. Alpha quartz is the most important polymorph in, and accounts for the majority of, human disease. Other forms include cristobalite and tridymite, which are less common but more fibrogenic. The silicates are complexes of silicon dioxide and the cations of sodium, potassium, calcium, aluminum, and magnesium. They are less fibrogenic than silica and evoke a distinctly different pulmonary response when inhaled. During high-temperature processing, however, noncrystalline silica can be converted to the crystalline silica, cristobalite, as occurs in the processing of diatomaceous earth and in certain applications of ceramic fibers. Despite its known toxicity, an estimated 2 million U.S. workers annually are exposed to hazardous concentrations of crystalline silica, including more than

100,000 in high-risk settings. Workers at risk include sandblasters, miners, tunnelers, silica millers, abrasives and flour workers, ceramics workers, glassmakers, quarry and foundry workers, stonecutters, polishers, and carvers. Sandblasting historically has been the most at-risk occupation. In Europe, sandblasting with silica has been banned for the past 40 years. This has given rise to the development of multiple nonsilica abrasives that are available as alternatives to silica for sandblasting and are advocated by industrial hygienists.

The development of any pneumoconiosis is a function of the size of the particle inhaled, the magnitude and duration of exposure, and the physiochemical properties of the particle. Particles greater than 10 μm are usually filtered and removed by the upper respiratory tract with its mucociliary transport system. Those particles less than 5 μm reach the distal airway and the lung parenchyma, where they are phagocytized by alveolar macrophages and incorporated into phagosomes. In contrast to other mineral dusts, silica particles are toxic to the phagocytes' lysosomal membranes, resulting in rupture, cell injury, and cell death. On phagocytosis, alveolar macrophages become activated, resulting in recruitment of lymphocytes, release of proinflammatory cytokines, and an influx of neutrophils. These recruited neutrophils degranulate, releasing toxic oxygen radical species that result in lipid membrane injury and result in cell death. Disruption of type I alveolar epithelial cells ensues, leading to type II pneumocyte hyperplasia, fibroblast recruitment, and hyalinization.

The characteristic pathologic feature on lung biopsy is the silicotic nodule. A peribronchiolar, whorled collection of collagen is surrounded by macrophages, fibroblasts, and lymphocytes. Refractile particles can be seen at the center of the lesion. Perinodular emphysematous regions develop and may coalesce to form macroscopic blebs. If these blebs are subpleural, they may rupture into the pleural space, leading to spontaneous pneumothoraces, which occur with increased frequency in patients with silicosis.

CLINICAL MANIFESTATIONS

The diagnosis of silicosis can be established when there is historical evidence of occupational silica dust exposure, a typical chest radiographic pattern, and the absence of an alternative diagnosis. Lung biopsy is reserved for those cases in which the exposure history is not straightforward or is forgotten and the radiographic pattern is not typical. The clinical forms of silicosis are divided into four subgroups, according to exposure history, rate of progression of symptoms, and chest radiographic findings. These include simple silicosis, accelerated silicosis, chronic silicosis or progressive massive fibrosis, and acute silicosis or silicoproteinosis. In simple silicosis, which is the most common form of silica-induced lung disease, there is a 10- to 20-year exposure history. Typical symptoms include the insidious onset of breathlessness with exertion. A chronic productive cough may precede or accompany breathlessness and may be attributed to the disease itself or associated tobacco use. The typical radiographic pattern is that of a bilateral upper lobe nodular infiltrate, with nodular opacities ranging from 1 to 3 mm in diameter. Calcification of hilar lymph nodes may occur in up to 10% to 15% of exposed individuals, revealing a characteristic eggshell calcification pattern that is suggestive of but not pathognomonic for silicosis. In accelerated silicosis, there is a more intense exposure history and a shorter latency period of 5 to 7 years. The chest radiograph reveals a diffuse reticulonodular infiltrate without upper lobe predominance. Progressive massive fibrosis is an advanced chronic form of simple silicosis in which the rounded opacities have coalesced to large irregular masslike lesions. The middle and lower lobes become involved, and there is an associated reticular infiltrate, heralding the development of pulmonary fibrosis. Interestingly, fibrosis has been found to progress long after exposure has ceased. Very intense exposure with poor respiratory protection can cause acute silicosis or silicoproteinosis, which can develop within months to a few years after exposure and can lead to respiratory insufficiency. The radiographic pattern is that of diffuse perihilar alveolar infiltrates with ground-glass opacities. Histopathologic findings also differ from classic silicosis, with dense material that stains with periodic acid–Schiff filling the air spaces (resembling pulmonary alveolar proteinosis). A variant of simple silicosis is Caplan syndrome, which is the presence of pneumoconiosis in a patient with underlying rheumatoid arthritis. Characteristically, the chest radiograph reveals multiple large lung nodules that may cavitate; these are termed *necrobiotic nodules*. They are seen against a background of typical silicotic nodules and usually occur in patients with rheumatoid nodules on the extensor surfaces of their extremities.

In simple silicosis, pulmonary function studies may be normal. With more advanced disease, a mixed obstructive and restrictive ventilatory defect is seen. In progressive massive fibrosis, a severe restrictive ventilatory defect occurs, along with diffusion abnormalities and resting hypoxemia, both of which may lead to pulmonary hypertension and cor pulmonale. The degree of pulmonary function impairment is generally believed to be related to the severity of radiographic abnormalities.

TREATMENT

Currently, there is no recognized specific treatment for silicosis once the disease is established. Prevention at the workplace, vaccination, and symptom control are the mainstays of therapy. Some have advocated the use of corticosteroids for acute silicosis. For chronic well-established silicosis or progressive massive fibrosis, corticosteroids have not been found to be of benefit. All patients should receive annual influenza vaccination and skin testing for tuberculosis if they are nonreactors, as well as a one-time pneumococcal vaccination. Smoking cessation should be actively pursued. For those with an obstructive component on their pulmonary function studies, inhaled bronchodilators may help with breathlessness. Supplemental oxygen should be offered to those with resting or exertional hypoxemia.

For centuries, the association between tuberculosis and silicosis has been well recognized. The mechanism by which silicotics predispose to the development of tuberculosis remains unclear. Leading theories include impaired T-cell immunity or altered macrophage phagocytic function resulting from the ingestion of silica crystals. It is often difficult to distinguish infection with *Mycobacterium tuberculosis* from progression of the underlying disease. For those with constitutional symptoms and evidence of radiographic progression, a thorough search for tuberculosis is warranted. This should include skin testing, induced sputum analysis, and, if necessary, fiberoptic bronchoscopy with bronchoalveolar lavage and possibly transbronchial biopsy. For those found to have latent tuberculosis infection (positive skin test <10 mm of induration and no culture evidence of *M. tuberculosis*), chemotherapy to include isoniazid plus rifampin for 4 months is currently recommended. For those with active tuberculous disease (positive culture), four-drug chemotherapy to include isoniazid, rifampin pyrazinamide, and ethambutol (Myambutol) is recommended for initial therapy until results of sensitivity tests are known.

Silicosis is a reportable disease. Underreporting by physicians is unfortunately commonplace and impairs the ability to track demographic trends. There are strict industry standards for occupational mineral dust exposure. The National Institute for Occupational Safety and Health advocates regular industrial hygiene inspections for high-risk workplace environments, with a maximum permissible exposure limit of 100 μg/mm^3 for respirable silica dust. Regular screening of workers at risk is also advocated and should include both a baseline chest radiograph and spirometry. This should be repeated at regular intervals during the worker's entire career. Those found to have silicosis should be removed from the workplace.

Despite being recognized since antiquity, silicosis remains an important occupational lung disease worldwide. With no effective treatment, physicians should work alongside industrial hygienists and engineers to recognize high-risk occupations and encourage improved efforts at prevention.

HYPERSENSITIVITY PNEUMONITIS

method of
RAYMOND G. SLAVIN, M.D.
Saint Louis University School of Medicine
Saint Louis, Missouri

Hypersensitivity pneumonitis is a disease process caused by sensitivity to an inhaled organic dust. In the acute form, associated with intermittent intense exposure to the organic dust, the individual responds 4 to 6 hours later with low-grade fever, chills, chest pain, cough, and dyspnea. In the chronic form, associated with prolonged, low-grade exposure, the clinical presentation is more insidious, with progressively increasing cough, dyspnea, malaise, weakness, and weight loss.

The antigens responsible for hypersensitivity pneumonitis include thermophilic actinomycetes, fungi, amebae, animal proteins, and chemicals. One should also keep in mind medications such as amiodarone (Cordarone) and chlorambucil (Leukeran). Although the majority of cases are occupational in nature, such as farming, mushroom picking, and grain loading, offending antigens may contaminate home heating or cooling units or be associated with hobbies such as pigeon breeding.

The diagnosis of hypersensitivity pneumonitis should be suspected in any patient presenting with interstitial pneumonitis or pulmonary fibrosis. Pulmonary function testing reveals a largely restrictive component, including decreases in pulmonary compliance and in carbon monoxide diffusing capacity. A careful history eliciting the onset of symptoms after exposure with remission on avoidance together with positive serum precipitins to the appropriate antigen is presumptive evidence of hypersensitivity pneumonitis.

THERAPEUTIC APPROACH

Avoidance

Clearly the most important aspect in the management of hypersensitivity pneumonitis is recognition and avoidance of the causative antigen. Hypersensitivity pneumonitis ultimately may be a fatal disease because of progressive respiratory insufficiency. It is estimated that five acute episodes will be followed by pulmonary damage and progressive disease. Therefore, it is vital to make the diagnosis early and institute environmental precautions to prevent the inexorable progression to pulmonary fibrosis. A number of interventions will decrease the formation of antigens in conducive environments. For example, the growth of thermophilic *Actinomyces* spores in compost can be suppressed by treatment with a 1% solution of propionic acid. Water that remains for long periods of time in older air conditioners or humidification units may become a fertile source for the growth of thermophilic organisms. Therefore, the water needs to be changed and the units cleaned on a regular basis.

In occupational situations in which organic dust generation is inevitable, efforts should be made to reduce the workers' exposure through mechanical handling of dusty material, improved ventilation, and electrostatic air purifiers. The use of personal dust respirators or masks is limited because of inconvenience. The best device available has a maximal filtering capacity of 99% for fine particles. The remaining 1% can produce new attacks in highly sensitive individuals. If the disease is not yet manifest, a filter with 95% filtering capacity such as a 3M disposable mask model 8710 or reusable model 7200 is adequate.

When these environmental control measures cannot be carried out or are inadequate, the patient should be removed from that work area. This may entail a change in the workplace or type of work or, in extreme cases, a change in occupation. If the diffusing capacity has not returned to normal in 3 months, the individual should be advised to leave that particular workplace permanently.

Therapy

In most cases of hypersensitivity pneumonitis, no treatment is necessary other than avoidance of the causative antigen (Table 1). Corticosteroid therapy, however, can greatly accelerate clinical improvement and should be instituted in very ill patients with gross radiographic or physiologic abnormalities such as hypoxemia. Oral therapy with prednisone in an initial daily dose of 40 to 60 mg is usually adequate and should be continued until there is significant

TABLE 1. **Treatment of Hypersensitivity Pneumonitis**

Acute Form
Remove patient from exposure; may entail hospitalization
Oxygen
Prednisone, 40–60 mg/d with slow tapering
Supportive measures—rest, antitussives, antipyretics
Repeated Acute or Subacute Form
Decrease exposure as much as possible
Long-term corticosteroid therapy emphasizing alternate-day therapy
Chronic Form
Trial with corticosteroids but continue only if radiographic findings and physiologic testing indicate a response.

clinical, radiographic, and pulmonary function test evidence of improvement. The prednisone dosage then may be tapered slowly over a period of 4 to 6 weeks until resolution of clinical and radiologic signs is complete. In cases of severe hypoxemia, oxygen should be administered in amounts sufficient to keep the partial pressure of oxygen level between 60 and 100 mm Hg. Other supportive measures include rest, antitussives, and antipyretics.

The dramatic response of hypersensitivity pneumonitis to corticosteroids may be a two-edged sword. The rapid relief afforded by corticosteroids may result in a false sense of security, so much so that the patient may return to the same work environment. Re-exposure will result in progression of the disease. It therefore must be emphasized and re-emphasized to the patient that corticosteroids are not a substitute for antigen identification and avoidance.

The chronic form of hypersensitivity pneumonitis occurring because of repeated acute episodes or long-term, low-grade exposure can be treated with corticosteroids, but this should be continued only if radiographic findings and physiologic testing indicate a beneficial response.

RHINOSINUSITIS

method of
WILLIAM E. BOLGER, M.D.
University of Pennsylvania
Philadelphia, Pennsylvania

Sinusitis is one of the most common medical conditions physicians encounter. Each year about 20 million cases of acute bacterial sinusitis occur in the United States, accounting for about 7% to 12% of all antibiotic prescriptions. Health care costs are significant when over-the-counter medication costs, time lost from employment, and cost of surgery are considered. This common and significant problem is managed largely by primary care physicians; it is estimated that family practitioners, pediatricians, and internists manage more than 85% of cases. It is therefore imperative that primary care physicians have a solid understanding of this important condition.

Sinusitis presents in many ways and has different underlying causes. Traditionally, sinusitis is classified as acute if the symptoms have been present for less than 3 weeks and chronic if present for greater than 8 weeks. There are inherent shortcomings in this classification scheme, because it is an oversimplification to classify sinusitis solely on the basis of symptom duration; however, this basic designation is clinically useful and well engrained in medical practice.

Acute sinusitis is widely considered a bacterial infection of a paranasal sinus cavity associated with obstruction of mucus drainage from the sinus. Acute bacterial sinusitis is usually preceded by a viral upper respiratory tract infection. Viral-induced inflammation causes nasal and sinus mucosal edema, which can lead to obstruction of the sinus ostia and secondary bacterial infection. Although the term *sinusitis* is used most frequently, the term *rhinosinusitis* may more correctly describe the associated nasal disorders (Table 1). Typical presenting symptoms include nasal congestion, nasal obstruction, facial pain or pressure, headache, rhinorrhea, postnasal drip, and, less commonly, fever.

The diagnosis is made largely based on clinical history because physical findings available in the primary care setting are limited. The patient's general appearance is important, and palpation of the sinus can be helpful. Unfortunately, examination of the nose with an otoscope yields little information because only the most anterior surface of the inferior turbinate and septal mucosa can be seen. A diagnosis of sinusitis cannot be made reliably with this instrument. Transillumination is not helpful because it is notoriously inaccurate; however, sinus radiographs can be valuable in cases of acute sinusitis. They can demonstrate an air-fluid level within the maxillary or frontal sinuses, but plain sinus radiographs work less well for the sphenoid and ethmoid sinuses. Diagnostic cultures are difficult to obtain in a primary care setting because nasal swabs are not representative of sinus disease. Therefore, the diagnosis is made largely on clinical grounds, and treatment is based empirically.

TREATMENT

Empirical therapy for acute sinusitis is based on microbiologic studies of maxillary sinus aspirates during infection. Many series have demonstrated that the most common pathologic organisms in acute sinusitis are *Streptococcus pneumoniae, Haemophilus influenzae,* and *Moraxella catarrhalis.* Typical first-line agents for sinusitis include amoxicillin for mild cases. If the sinusitis is moderate in severity, amoxicillin/clavulanate (Augmentin), at 500 mg three times daily of the amoxicillin component, is an excellent agent. Cefuroxime (Ceftin), at 500 mg twice daily, is also an acceptable agent for patients with mild to moderate sinusitis. If the patient is allergic to penicillin, trimethoprim-sulfamethoxazole (TMP/

TABLE 1. **Symptoms and Signs of Sinusitis**

Major	Minor
Nasal congestion/obstruction	Halitosis
Postnasal drainage	Fever
Facial pressure, congestion, or pain	
Headache	
Anosmia, olfactory loss	

SMX), one double-strength tablet twice daily, azithromycin (Zithromax), 250 mg once daily, or clarithromycin (Biaxin), 500 mg twice daily, can be used. Because the cost of therapy is increasingly being considered, amoxicillin and TMP/SMX are attractive. If a patient does not respond in 72 hours, then reevaluation is indicated, and a change in antibiotic is considered. If symptoms fail to resolve and sinusitis becomes chronic, further evaluation is warranted.

If sinusitis progresses, it can extend from the paranasal sinus cavities into the orbit or the central nervous system. This may be signaled by proptosis, chemosis, gaze restriction, visual change, severe headache, change in mental status, nausea and vomiting, forehead redness, and swelling. Should this occur, detailed imaging and consultation with an otolaryngologist are strongly recommended. Intravenous antibiotics are appropriate for such cases. Surgery for acute sinusitis is usually reserved for infections that threaten to spread outside the sinus cavities.

A challenge primary care physicians face is distinguishing acute bacterial sinusitis from self-limited uncomplicated viral upper respiratory tract infection (URI). Patient presentation and symptoms are similar. The distinction is largely based on severity and duration of symptoms. Viral URI symptoms usually begin to abate during the first week. If symptoms persist for 10 to 14 days, then acute bacterial sinusitis should be considered. A change in the color of nasal mucus from clear to yellow is not a specific sign of acute bacterial rhinosinusitis. In viral URI, an inflammatory response occurs within the nasal mucosa, which includes an influx of white blood cells. This produces an inflammatory exudate that is responsible for the yellow mucus color and is not necessarily bacterial in origin. Primary care physicians face pressure from patients to prescribe antibiotics to treat this nasal exudate; however, they are also under increasing pressure from the microbiology community not to prescribe antibiotics in light of the mounting problem of antimicrobial resistance. Fortunately, most cases of viral URI resolve spontaneously, and it is estimated that 46% of cases of acute bacterial sinusitis also resolve spontaneously.

Primary care physicians are further challenged to distinguish acute sinusitis from other entities that may present similarly. Acute exacerbations of chronic sinusitis are relatively common and can usually be distinguished by history. More concerning are sinonasal tumors that obstruct the sinus ostia and present initially as acute sinusitis. To diagnose these tumors early, a high index of suspicion needs to be maintained. If sinusitis symptoms do not clear fully or recur repeatedly, imaging with computed tomography may be helpful. Also of concern are invasive fungal sinus conditions. In the past, these have been relatively uncommon; however, now more than ever, primary care physicians are caring for increasing numbers of patients in various immunocompromised states. Patients with diabetes mellitus, patients undergoing chemotherapy, patients receiving posttransplant immunosuppressive therapy, and patients taking systemic corticosteroids need to be followed more closely. Early imaging and referral to an otolaryngologist are important considerations for these patients.

Chronic Sinusitis

When sinus symptoms persist for longer than 8 weeks, the condition is considered chronic. The major symptoms of chronic sinusitis are nasal congestion, nasal obstruction, headache, facial pain and pressure, and olfactory disturbance. Halitosis is a less common symptom, and fever occurs rarely. The pathophysiology of chronic sinusitis is not fully elucidated but is evolving. The ostiomeatal complex has been identified as a key location for sinus obstruction. Nasal endoscopy and endoscopic sinus surgery within the ostiomeatal complex have increased diagnostic accuracy, reduced surgical morbidity, and increased surgical success. The role of inflammation is increasingly being recognized and is an area of active research. The next major advances in understanding sinusitis will come from elucidating the inflammatory mechanisms involved in this disease.

The diagnosis of chronic sinusitis is often made based on clinical history alone in the primary care setting (Figure 1). Sinus radiographs are rarely helpful and are not recommended. A coronal computed tomography scan of the paranasal sinuses is extremely useful. It can demonstrate the presence, the extent, and the location of disease within the eight sinuses. Transillumination is highly insensitive, and ultrasonography provides variable results and is not recommended.

Empirical therapy with oral antibiotics, initiated in the primary care setting, is recommended. Therapy is based on the most common causative organisms, *Staphylococcus* species and anaerobes. Appropriate antibiotic agents include amoxicillin/clavulanate, 500 mg orally three times daily, cefuroxime, 500 mg orally twice daily, and, if the patient is allergic to penicillin, clindamycin (Cleocin), 300 mg orally three times daily, or clarithromycin, 500 mg orally twice daily. A longer course of antibiotic therapy is typically recommended in chronic sinusitis. A 14- to 21-day course is appropriate; a longer course can be considered if the patient has not been on any therapy, whereas shorter courses can be used for patients who show a rapid clinical response or who have received multiple recent antimicrobial treatments.

The response to therapy is an important diagnostic and prognostic indicator. Should the patient not respond, referral to an otolaryngologist is helpful. In the otolaryngologist's office, diagnostic sinonasal endoscopy can be performed, which can identify nasal polyps, tumors, and pathologic nasal secretions. Cultures of pathologic secretions can be obtained, and culture-directed antibiotic therapy can be given. Endoscopic cultures have shown a high correlation (85.7%) with the bacteria present within the maxil-

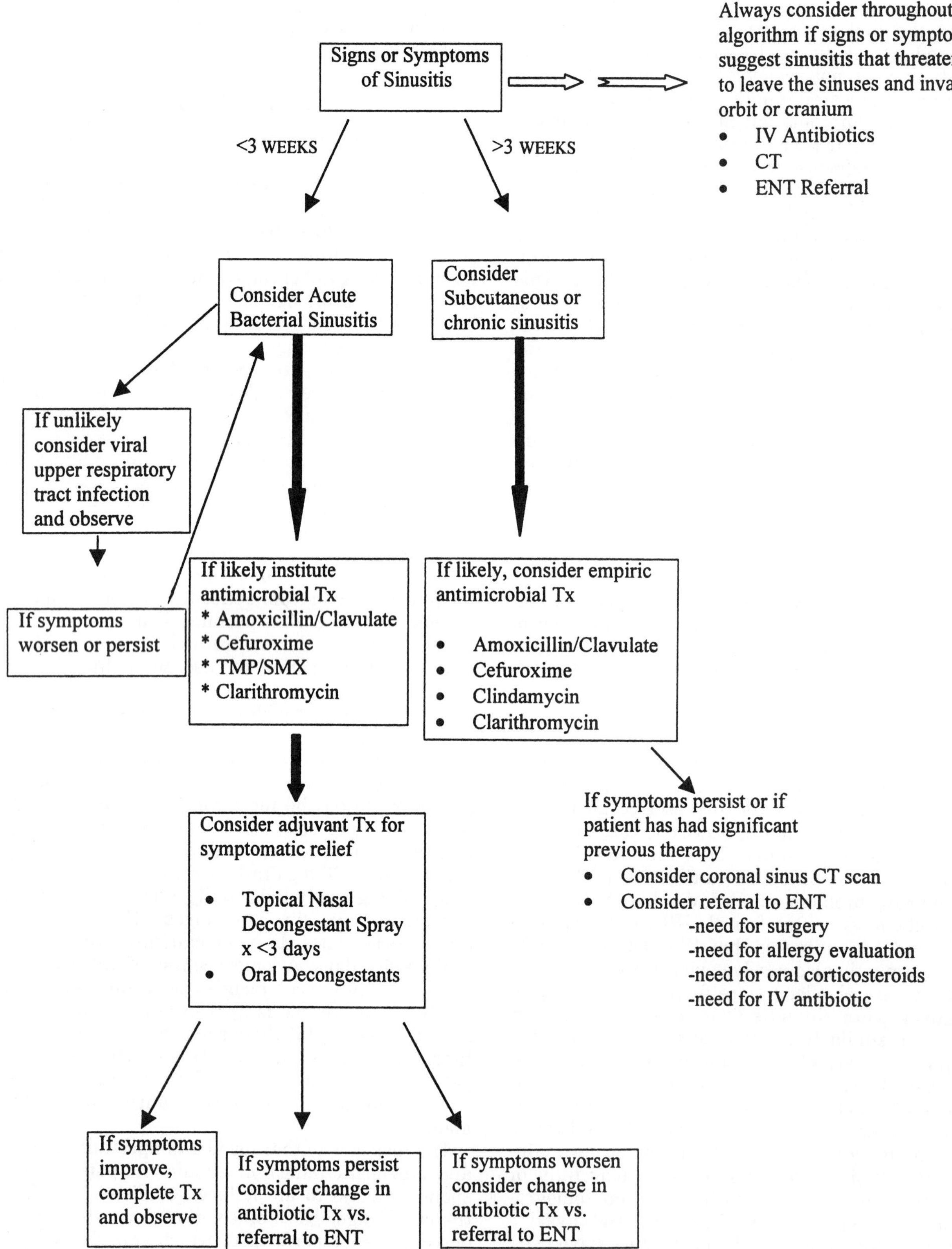

Figure 1. Algorithm for treatment of a patient with the signs or symptoms of sinusitis. *Abbreviations:* CT = computed tomography; ENT = ear, nose, and throat physician; IV = intravenous; TMP/SMX = trimethoprim-sulfamethoxazole; Tx = treatment.

lary antrum. In practical terms, endoscopic cultures give the practitioner a fairly accurate representation of ostiomeatal region bacteriology. Oral antibiotic selection is relatively simple once one can direct therapy based on culture data. Endoscopic cultures are especially important in patients who have had previous sinus surgery because gram-negative organisms (particularly *Pseudomonas*), *Staphylococcus aureus*, coagulase-negative *Staphylococcus* species, and β-lactamase–producing organisms predominate.

As previously mentioned, sinusitis is largely discussed as an infectious disease or as an obstruction of the ostiometal complex; however, other pathologic mechanisms are evident. Patients with aspirin sensitivity and asthma can have an associated inflammatory condition of the nose and the sinuses manifested by sinonasal polyposis that is difficult to treat. Environmental allergies may contribute to a heightened state of nasal reactivity, which can predispose to sinusitis. Another form of chronic sinusitis is allergic fungal sinusitis. In this condition, patients suffer from extensive sinonasal polyposis and produce an eosinophilic mucus. Fungus can be recovered from the sinuses at surgery. Total serum IgE can be elevated as well as serum-specific IgE to the recovered fungus. Inflammation is increasingly being recognized as an important factor in allergic fungal sinusitis and other forms of chronic sinusitis. In these forms of sinusitis, antibiotics are not the sole treatment, and a multidisciplinary approach is recommended.

Several interesting investigations may lead to new hope for patients with chronic sinusitis and for physicians caring for these patients. Recent reports indicated that one class of antibiotics, the macrolides, may have interesting immunomodulating properties in addition to their antibacterial effect. Erythromycin may act as a biologic modulator that inhibits interleukin 8 (IL-8), an important inflammatory mediator (cytokine) secreted by nasal inflammatory cells in patients with chronic rhinosinusitis. Topical treatment for chronic rhinosinusitis is increasingly being considered in selected refractory cases of sinusitis. Several other investigators are currently investigating a variety of topical antibiotics and different delivery mechanisms for topical therapy in the sinuses, such as aerosolization, nebulization, and sustained release of polymers. Formal published reports of these experiences are anxiously awaited.

In patients who do not respond to antibiotic therapy or endoscopic surgery, new treatments are being tried. Oral corticosteroids are effective for polypoid variants of chronic sinusitis because they provide temporary resolution of disease and relief of symptoms. Desensitization immunotherapy to specific fungal species is being tried in patients with allergic fungal sinusitis and continues to show promise. Recent reports indicate a possible link between chronic rhinosinusitis and gastroesophageal-associated reflux. A significant improvement in sinus disease has been noted when reflux is treated appropriately. Further studies in this regard should be revealing.

In conclusion, sinusitis is a common condition caused by a variety of infectious, anatomic, and inflammatory factors. Successful treatment is achieved through accurate diagnosis and effective medical therapy in the primary care setting in the vast majority of cases. Complementary otolaryngologic specialty care is useful for chronic and recalcitrant cases and those acute cases that threaten to spread from the confines of the paranasal sinuses.

NONALLERGIC RHINITIS

method of
PHIL LIEBERMAN, M.D.
University of Tennessee College of Medicine
Memphis, Tennessee

EPIDEMIOLOGY

Rhinitis is defined as inflammation of the membranes lining the nose. The symptoms include sneezing, nasal congestion, postnasal drainage, and anterior rhinorrhea. Chronic rhinitis may be allergic or nonallergic in origin. Nonallergic rhinitis is distinguished from its allergic counterpart by the absence of a clinically relevant IgE antibody response to aeroallergens. Thus, the diagnosis of chronic nonallergic rhinitis is one of exclusion. Nonallergic rhinitis is not a single disorder but consists of a variety of syndromes that manifest the abovementioned symptoms and share a single characteristic, the absence of allergy.

The frequency of nonallergic rhinitis and of the various syndromes that make up this broad class of disease is estimated to be 17% to 57% of all rhinitis patients worldwide (Table 1).

Based on the findings of one of the studies listed in Table 1, conducted by the National Rhinitis Classification Task Force, a nationwide epidemiologic survey of patients in the outpatient setting is currently under way. This survey, which uses a patient screening tool for rhinitis, is being conducted in 25,000 office-based nonallergy practices nationwide. This study is aimed at developing better epidemiologic data on the incidence of allergic, nonallergic, and mixed (allergic and nonallergic) disease and at assessing the usefulness of the rhinitis screening tool in diagnosing rhinitis. Interim data in 3500 patients show that 32% of patients have allergic rhinitis, 22% have nonallergic rhinitis, and 46% have mixed rhinitis.

Nonallergic rhinitis is more prevalent in adults older than the age of 20 (approximately 70%), whereas allergic disease is more common in patients younger than the age of 20. Female gender may also be a risk factor for nonallergic rhinitis.

PATHOPHYSIOLOGY AND CLASSIFICATION

Vasomotor Rhinitis

Nonallergic rhinitis is classified into distinct syndromes based on etiologic and cytologic features (Table 2). Vasomotor rhinitis (VMR), or idiopathic perennial nonallergic rhinitis, is the most common of these syndromes (61%). The term *vasomotor* implies a vascular or neurologic dysfunction but is perhaps a misnomer, because no mechanism of production has been established. The syndrome is unrelated to allergy, infection, structural lesions, systemic dis-

TABLE 1. **Frequency of Occurrence of Rhinitis**

Investigator (year)	N	Rhinitis Type		
		Allergic, %	*Mixed, %*	*Nonallergic, %*
Mullarkey (1980)*	142	48	Not studied	52
Enberg (1989)†	152 (128)‡	54	16§	30
Togias (1990)‖	362	83	Not studied	17
ECRHS (1999)¶	1412	75	Not studied	25
NRCTF (1999)**	975	43	34	23

*Mullarkey MF, Hill JS, Webb DR: Allergic and nonallergic rhinitis: Their characterization with attention to the meaning of nasal eosinophilia. J Allergy Clin Immunol 65:122–126, 1980.
†Enberg RN: Perennial allergic rhinitis: A retrospective review. Ann Allergy 63:513–516, 1989.
‡Diagnosis determined in only 128.
§16% had positive skin test but no allergic component.
‖Togias A: Age relationships and clinical features of nonallergic rhinitis. J Allergy Clin Immunol 85:182, 1990.
¶European Community Respiratory Health Survey.
**National Rhinitis Classification Task Force.

ease, or drug use. VMR probably results from multiple causes. The symptoms are similar to those of allergic rhinitis without the pruritus. VMR is characterized by nonspecific nasal hyperreactivity on exposure to nonimmunologic stimuli. Mucosal biopsy can reveal increases in mast cells similar to those seen in allergic rhinitis but with no increase in goblet cells. Stimuli include changes in temperature or relative humidity, ingestion of alcohol, strong odors, and airborne irritants. Hyperreactivity of the nasal mucosa to capsaicin, histamine, and methacholine in vivo has been demonstrated.

Nonallergic Rhinitis Eosinophilia Syndrome

Nonallergic rhinitis eosinophilia syndrome (NARES), first described in 1981, is characterized by increased nasal eosinophilia and makes up 15% to 20% of cases of nonallergic rhinitis. The pathophysiology is not understood. Patients present with profuse watery rhinorrhea and nasal pruritus. Eosinophilia, the hallmark of this syndrome, may contribute to nasal mucosal dysfunction owing to the release of major basic protein and eosinophil cationic protein. These toxins damage nasal ciliated epithelium and prolong mucociliary clearance, increasing the propensity for infection. Recurrent infection appears to be a predisposing factor for the development of nasal polyps, although the pathogenesis of polyp development is unknown. Nasal polyps are often associated with nasal eosinophils; consequently, concerns have been raised that nasal eosinophilia may be a precursor to the aspirin-induced tetrad syndrome (NARES, asthma, sinusitis, and nasal polyps). BENARS

TABLE 2. **Classification of Nonallergic Rhinitis Based on Etiologic and Cytologic Features**

Perennial Nonallergic Rhinitis (Inflammatory)	Noninflammatory, Nonallergic Rhinitis	Structurally Related Rhinitis
Eosinophilic nasal disease (NARES, BENARS)	Rhinitis medicamentosa Topical decongestants Systemic medications	Septal deviation, turbinate deformation, nasal valve dysfunction, obstructive adenoid hyperplasia
Basophilic/metachromatic nasal disease	Reflex-induced rhinitis (bright light or other physical modalities)	Neoplastic and non-neoplastic tumors
Infectious disease	Vasomotor rhinitis Irritant rhinitis Cold air rhinitis Gustatory rhinitis	Miscellaneous (choanal atresia/stenosis, trauma, foreign body, malformation, cleft palate, adenoid hypertrophy)
Nasal polyps Aspirin intolerance Chronic sinusitis Churg-Strauss syndrome Young syndrome (sinopulmonary disease, azoospermia) Cystic fibrosis Kartagener syndrome (bronchiectasis, chronic sinusitis, nasal polyps) Atopic rhinitis	Rhinitis sicca	
Immunologic nasal disease (non-IgE–mediated or secondary to systemic immunologic disorders) Sjögren syndrome Systemic lupus erythematosus Relapsing polychondritis Churg-Strauss syndrome Sarcoidosis Wegener granulomatosis	Metabolic (estrogen-related, hyperthyroid, acromegaly)	

Abbreviations: BENARS = blood eosinophilia nonallergic rhinitis syndrome; NARES = nonallergic rhinitis with eosinophilia syndrome.

(blood eosinophilia nonallergic rhinitis syndrome), a related disorder that accounts for approximately 4% of all nonallergic rhinitis cases, is associated with an increase in blood eosinophils.

Basophilic/Metachromatic Nasal Disease

A subcategory of nonallergic rhinitis is basophilic/metachromatic cell nasal disease, or nasal mastocytosis. Mast cell infiltration (>2000/mm^3) requires, like NARES, a histologic diagnosis. Likely symptoms include profuse rhinorrhea and congestion without significant sneezing or pruritus. The cause of this syndrome is unknown.

Drug-Induced Rhinitis

Nonallergic rhinitis can be induced by multiple drugs. The term *rhinitis medicamentosa* is commonly used to describe the rebound nasal congestion that occurs with overuse of decongestant nasal sprays as well as cocaine abuse. Underlying rhinitis can lead to this type of overuse. The rebound swelling of this disorder is the result of interstitial edema, not vasodilation.

A number of oral agents, such as antihypertensives, hormones, and other drugs, can also cause rhinitis. In addition, eyedrops, via transit through the nasal-lacrimal duct, can also produce this syndrome.

Endocrine-Induced or Hormonally Induced Rhinitis

Oral contraceptives, estrogen replacement therapy, pregnancy, hypothyroidism, and acromegaly can cause rhinitis. Pregnancy can produce rhinitis characterized mainly by congestion due to increased blood volume in combination with hormonally induced vasodilation. Hypothyroidism and acromegaly both can cause turbinate hypertrophy.

Gustatory Rhinitis

Rhinitis can be due to an overly sensitive cholinergic reflex, which can be triggered by eating (gustatory rhinitis) or cold air (skier's/jogger's nose). This form of rhinitis is characterized by profuse watery rhinorrhea that begins within minutes of eating or exposure to cold air.

DIAGNOSIS

The differential diagnosis of rhinitis can be difficult given the often-indistinguishable symptoms of nonallergic and allergic rhinitis, the number of patients presenting with mixed rhinitis, and the multiple syndromes that make up nonallergic rhinitis.

Physical examination is not helpful in distinguishing between allergic and nonallergic disease but is essential in the evaluation of structural problems such as septal deviations, septal perforations, polyps, and tumors.

The features that distinguish nonallergic from allergic disease in terms of the history are seen in Table 3. The definitive diagnosis rests on the presence or the absence of clinically important IgE-mediated reactions to aeroallergens. The test of choice in this regard is the allergy skin test; however, a positive test does not rule out the presence of nonallergic disease and must be evaluated for significance in light of the history. On the other hand, negative tests establish the presence of nonallergic rhinitis by exclusion.

MANAGEMENT

Management of chronic nonallergic rhinitis (Table 4) can be difficult because some cases are relatively resistant to therapy. The mainstay of treatment is pharmacologic, but, of course, avoidance of triggers is helpful.

Two pharamacologic approaches can be taken to the treatment of vasomotor rhinitis—nonspecific broad-based therapy aimed at multiple symptoms or therapy tailored to specific symptoms. Owing to the variability of vasomotor symptoms, nonspecific treatment may be preferable.

Nonspecific, Broad-Based Treatment. Broad-based treatment includes the topical antihistamine

TABLE 3. **Differential Diagnosis of Rhinitis**

Manifestation	Allergic Rhinitis	Chronic Nonallergic Rhinitis
Age of onset	<20 y of age	>20 y of age
Seasonality	Seasonal variations: spring and fall	Usually perennial but not infrequently worse during weather changes, such as during fall and early spring
Exacerbating factors	Allergen exposure	Irritant exposure, weather conditions
Nature of symptoms		
Pruritus	Common	Rare
Congestion	Common	Common
Sneezing	Prominent	Usually not prominent but can be dominant in some cases
Postnasal drainage	Not prominent	Prominent
Other related manifestations (e.g., allergy, conjunctivitis, atopic dermatitis)	Often present	Absent
Family history	Usually present	Usually absent
Physical appearance	Variable, classically described as pale, boggy, swollen mucosa but may appear normal	Variable, erythematous
Allergy testing	Allergy skin tests always positive	Allergy skin tests negative or not clinically significant
Nasal eosinophilia	Usually present	Present 15%–20% of the time (NARES)

Abbreviations: NARES = nonallergic rhinitis with eosinophilia syndrome.

TABLE 4. **Management of Nonallergic Rhinitis**

Broad-Based Pharmacologic Control	Comments
Second-generation antihistamines	Azelastine nasal spray is the only second-generation antihistamine with FDA approval for nonallergic rhinitis
Azelastine hydrochloride (Astelin nasal spray)	
Intranasal corticosteroids	The three intranasal corticosteroids are the only corticosteroids with FDA approval for nonallergic rhinitis
Beclomethasone dipropionate (Beconase, Beconase AQ, Vancenase, Vancenase AQ)	
Fluticasone propionate (Flonase nasal spray)	
Budesonide (Rhinocort, Rhinocort Aqua)	
Oral decongestants	Useful only for nasal stuffiness
Ipratropium bromide (Atravent)	Useful only for rhinorrhea
Intranasal saline solution	
Surgery	Reserved for recalcitrant cases
Turbinectomy	For nasal congestion
Parasympathectomy	For increased secretions

Abbreviation: FDA = Food and Drug Administration.

azelastine (Astelin) or topical corticosteroids, the only two forms of therapy demonstrated to be of use for the management of nonallergic rhinitis. Azelastine is the only antihistamine approved for use in both allergic and nonallergic rhinitis. The antihistaminic and anti-inflammatory activities of azelastine have been shown to produce a high response rate (82% to 85%) in vasomotor rhinitis, to improve all associated rhinitis symptoms (congestion, rhinorrhea, postnasal drainage, and sneezing) and to have a rapid onset of action. In addition, three topical corticosteroids are approved for use in the treatment of nonallergic rhinitis: budesonide, fluticasone, and beclomethasone. There are no comparative studies that assess the relative efficacy of any of these drugs, and the choice of therapy remains speculative.

Symptom-Specific Therapy. For treatment tailored to specific symptoms, decongestants are first-line therapy for patients whose symptoms are obstructive. Decongestants, however, have no effect on other manifestations such as rhinorrhea or sneezing.

The topical anticholinergic agent ipratropium bromide (Atrovent) is first-line treatment for vasomotor rhinitis with a predominant symptom of rhinorrhea. Anticholinergics primarily affect rhinorrhea, with only modest effects on congestion. The only intranasal anticholinergic agent available in the U.S. is ipratropium bromide in a 0.03% solution for use in chronic nonallergic rhinitis. Ipratropium bromide can be used alone or in combination with topical nasal corticosteroids. The benefits of this particular therapeutic combination appear to be additive compared with the use of either drug alone. Ipratropium has minimal side effects (infrequent episodes of nasal dryness and minor epistaxis).

Topical saline solution alone or in combination with other therapies may provide additional relief from the symptoms of postnasal drainage, sneezing, and congestion in vasomotor rhinitis. In patients with vasomotor rhinitis who do not respond to pharmacotherapy, several surgical approaches have been successful.

Other Therapeutic Approaches

Surgical approaches that divide the parasympathetic supply to the nasal mucosa, thereby reducing nasal secretion, are endoscopic vidian nerve section and electrocoagulation of the anterior ethmoidal nerve. In cases in which the predominant symptom is congestion, turbinectomy is a treatment option.

Rhinitis of pregnancy is a particularly challenging therapeutic problem. The major principle that guides therapy for this disorder is caution in medication use. First-line treatment should include the safest therapies, such as steam inhalation, saline solution nasal sprays, and avoidance of irritants. Unfortunately, rhinitis of pregnancy can often be recalcitrant, responding only to topical corticosteroids.

Treatment of rhinitis medicamentosa requires withdrawal from the topical decongestant, the oral agent, or the eyedrops as well as treatment of the underlying rhinitis. This is often best accomplished with a 1-week tapering course of an oral glucocorticoid, with gradual discontinuation of the decongestant spray beginning on the second or third day of treatment. Administration of a topical corticosteroid spray can also begin on the third day of treatment and should be maintained subsequently. Oral decongestants can be used as needed.

The presence of nasal eosinophilia in patients with chronic nonallergic rhinitis is generally regarded as a good prognostic indicator for response to treatment with topical corticosteroids. Patients with NARES with massive eosinophilic infiltration also may require intermittent use of oral glucocorticoids to control symptoms.

Treating Mixed Rhinitis

Once a differential diagnosis of mixed rhinitis has been confirmed, empirical treatment with a topical broad-based agent effective in both allergic and nonallergic rhinitis (e.g., azelastine or an intranasal corticosteroid) is a reasonable choice for first-line therapy. Other agents such as oral decongestants or ipratropium can be used adjunctively as indicated.

STREPTOCOCCAL PHARYNGITIS

method of
CHRISTOPHER B. WHITE, M.D.
Medical College of Georgia
Augusta, Georgia

Streptococcal pharyngitis is a frequent problem encountered by the primary care physician. Despite its frequency, differences of opinion still exist about the optimal methods of diagnosis and management of "strep throat." This article discusses the microbiology, epidemiology, clinical presentation, diagnosis, and management of streptococcal pharyngitis, emphasizing practical information that is useful to the practicing physician.

MICROBIOLOGY

Streptococcus pyogenes are facultative anaerobic gram-positive cocci that produce a characteristic β-hemolysis when grown on blood agar. In 1932, Rebecca Lancefield classified β-hemolytic streptococci into groups based on antigenic differences in cell wall carbohydrates. Although some serogroups of β-hemolytic streptococci have multiple species, *S. pyogenes* is the only species of group A streptococci (GAS). To date, groups A to H and K to V have been designated, although groups A, B, C, D, and G are the species most frequently found in people. The structure of *S. pyogenes* includes a complex cell wall containing M-protein, a major virulence factor. Group A streptococci can be further classified into more than 100 serotypes based on the M-protein. The organism can also elaborate streptolysins, streptokinase, hyaluronidase, and a variety of other toxins including streptococcal pyrogenic exotoxins A and C, which are responsible for scarlet fever and streptococcal toxic shock syndrome. Although GAS can cause a variety of clinical infections, the remainder of this article deals with streptococcal pharyngitis.

EPIDEMIOLOGY

Streptococcal pharyngitis occurs in people of all ages and is caused by the transmission of infectious respiratory tract secretions. Probably because of the close personal contact that occurs in school, the majority of infections occur in school-age children in late autumn, winter, and spring. Similarly, the crowded living conditions found in military barracks and boarding schools can also facilitate transmission of this infection. Foodborne outbreaks of streptococcal pharyngitis have occurred, associated with ingestion of contaminated foods prepared by infected food handlers. Fomites and household pets are not vectors of infection.

Acute rheumatic fever (ARF) may develop 2 to 4 weeks after an untreated streptococcal pharyngeal infection. Before the 1950s, ARF was estimated to occur in 3% of patients with GAS pharyngitis, although it now occurs in less than 1 case per 100,000 children in the United States. Acute poststreptococcal glomerulonephritis can occur after streptococcal pharyngitis or skin infections, even in patients promptly treated with antibiotics. The epidemiology of both of these nonsuppurative poststreptococcal diseases mirrors the epidemiology of streptococcal infections in children regarding seasonality and associated age.

There are several situations in which GAS may be detected in the throat but the patient is not at risk of developing ARF. The first example is that of school-age children who are colonized but not infected with GAS. In some surveys, throat culture specimens of asymptomatic school children during the winter have shown GAS prevalence rates of 15% to 25%. These children, referred to as streptococcal carriers, are not at risk for acquiring ARF, and they do not transmit infection to others. A second example is GAS-infected children younger than 3 years. Children in this age group with a streptococcal upper respiratory infection present with a protracted febrile illness known as streptococcosis, which is characterized by coryza and a serous rhinitis but not pharyngitis.

CLINICAL PRESENTATION

The symptoms of streptococcal pharyngitis typically begin abruptly with fever, headache, sore throat, abdominal pain, nausea, and/or vomiting. Patients with coryza, cough, hoarseness, or conjunctivitis frequently complain of sore throat but rarely have streptococcal infection. The physical examination findings that are most consistent with GAS pharyngitis include tonsillopharyngeal erythema, tonsillar exudate, soft palate petechiae, a beefy red swollen uvula, and tender anterior cervical lymphadenopathy.

Some patients with GAS pharyngitis develop a fine, red, sandpaper-like papular eruption accentuated in the groin and axilla, accompanied by a "strawberry tongue" and circumoral pallor. This scarlatiniform rash, when present, strongly suggests GAS pharyngitis, although *Arcanobacterium haemolyticum* infection is possible in adolescents and young adults as well. Patients with conjunctivitis, stomatitis, or discrete ulcers on the buccal mucosa or soft palate are unlikely to have streptococcal disease.

The most common causes of pharyngitis are listed in Table 1. In the majority of instances, differentiation of viral causes from GAS pharyngitis is straightforward, based on the signs and symptoms previously noted. However, even world-renowned experts in GAS disease will only correctly

TABLE 1. **Infectious Causes of Pharyngitis**

Etiologic Agent	Common Clinical Presentation	Relative Frequency
Viruses		
Adenovirus	Pharyngoconjunctival fever	+ + + +
Coronavirus	Common cold	+ +
Epstein-Barr virus	Infectious mononucleosis	+ +
Influenza virus	Influenza	+ +
Parainfluenza virus	Croup, common cold	+ +
Rhinovirus	Common cold	+ +
Cytomegalovirus	Infectious mononucleosis	+
Herpes simplex virus	Gingivitis, stomatitis, pharyngitis	+
Respiratory syncytial virus	Common cold, bronchiolitis	+
Bacteria		
Group A streptococci	Pharyngitis, scarlet fever	+ + + +
Group C, G streptococci	Pharyngitis	+ +
Arcanobacterium haemolyticum	Pharyngitis, scarlatinaform rash	+
Neisseria gonorrhoeae	Pharyngitis	+
Corynebacterium diphtheriae	Diphtheria	±
Francisella tularensis	Oropharyngeal tularemia	±
Treponema pallidum	Secondary syphilis	±
Other		
Chlamydia pneumoniae	Pharyngitis, bronchitis, pneumonia	+
Mycoplasma pneumoniae	Pharyngitis, bronchitis, pneumonia	+
Toxoplasma gondii	Flulike illness, infectious mononucleosis	+

predict patients with and without streptococcal pharyngitis approximately 75% of the time. Thus, if there is any question about a patient's diagnosis, a throat swab should be obtained and tested for the presence of GAS organisms.

DIAGNOSIS

Confirmation of the clinical presentation of streptococcal pharyngitis requires finding GAS organisms in the tonsillopharyngeal tissues. However, the presence of GAS in the throat does not prove that the patient has streptococcal pharyngitis. Many school-age children will be asymptomatic GAS carriers during the school year. If a GAS carrier develops a sore throat from a viral upper respiratory tract infection and the physician performs a throat culture just to be sure that the child does not have streptococcal pharyngitis, the patient may be mislabeled as having a GAS infection. Many patients referred to infectious disease specialists for evaluation of recurrent streptococcal infections are actually GAS carriers with recurrent upper respiratory tract infections. Thus, the diagnosis of streptococcal pharyngitis requires the presence of GAS in the throat and the clinical symptoms consistent with this infection.

The throat culture is the traditional method of detecting GAS in the tonsillopharyngeal tissues. Secretions from the throat swab are plated on sheep blood agar plates and incubated overnight at 35°C to 37°C. β-hemolytic, catalase-negative organisms that are inhibited by a disk containing 0.04 U of bacitracin can be presumptively identified as GAS. A more accurate method, commonly performed in microbiology laboratories, is to confirm these organisms as GAS using a group-specific cell wall carbohydrate antigen detection kit. The yield of positive culture results can be increased by any of the following: incubating negative plates an additional 24 hours, incubating plates in 5% carbon dioxide or a candle jar, incubating plates anaerobically (impractical), or using selective culture media.

Rapid antigen detection tests (RADTs) have made it possible to detect the group A carbohydrate antigen directly from a throat swab in as few as 15 minutes. The tests are easier to perform and interpret than a throat culture. Early RADTs using latex agglutination were relatively insensitive, but newer tests using enzyme immunoassay, optical immunoassay, and chemiluminescent DNA probes have been developed that are much more sensitive and specific.

A patient with a positive RADT result likely has GAS in the tonsillopharyngeal tissues, and no confirmatory testing is needed. However, even though the throat culture only has a sensitivity of 85% to 90%, the majority of experts continue to recommend that all patients with a negative RADT have a back-up throat culture performed for confirmation. If future peer reviewed studies can confirm that a particular RADT is as sensitive as the throat culture, back-up throat culture confirmation of a negative result should be unnecessary. Physicians must understand, however, that each RADT is different, and the performance results of one RADT are not applicable to another one, even though both may use a similar technology.

Regardless of the test used, no GAS will be detected unless an accurate specimen is obtained. The swab must be gently rubbed against both tonsils and the posterior pharyngeal wall, sites with the highest concentration of organisms. Properly done, this procedure should stimulate a gag reflex, causing the tongue to elevate and a strong desire to move away from the swab. To avoid obtaining an inadequate specimen, especially in children, a tongue blade should be used in all patients. If a self-contained culturing device is used, such as the Culturette, care should be taken not to break the liquid ampule because this will decrease the sensitivity of the culture or the RADT.

TREATMENT

Antibiotic treatment of streptococcal pharyngitis will usually produce rapid clinical improvement in most patients within 24 hours. However, even without treatment, most patients will be clinically better in 3 to 5 days. Therefore, to ensure good compliance, it is critical that the patient or patient's guardian understands the major reason for the antibiotic treatment of streptococcal pharyngitis is the prevention of ARF, which requires that antibiotics be taken for the full course of therapy.

Table 2 lists the major available options for the treatment of GAS pharyngitis. Several points deserve emphasis:

1. Penicillin V potassium remains the treatment of choice, although some physicians prefer amoxicillin suspension for younger patients because it tastes better and the improved taste presumably would improve compliance.
2. A macrolide is recommended for penicillin-allergic patients. Erythromycin is preferred, but azithromycin (Zithromax), although more expensive, has the advantage of having fewer gastrointestinal adverse reactions, and it also requires only five doses for treatment.
3. Even with excellent compliance, 10% to 15% of patients may relapse after completing their treatment course. The reasons for relapse are controversial and beyond the scope of this discussion. However, oral cephalosporins probably have a slightly higher treatment success rate than penicillins, even though there has never been a reported case of penicillin-resistant GAS. Many physicians prefer to treat patients who relapse after a course of penicillin with a first-generation cephalosporin, whereas others simply retreat with another course of penicillin or amoxicillin.

Compliance with oral antibiotics can be improved by decreasing either the number of daily doses or the duration of therapy. A large single-daily dose of amoxicillin for 10 days has been shown to be as effective as standard therapy. A 6-day course of amoxicillin has reportedly been effective but cannot be recommended until confirmed by additional studies. Twice-daily cefpodoxime (Vantin) and cefdinir (Omnicef) have both been approved by the Food and Drug Administration for short-course (5-day) treatment of GAS pharyngitis. However, like all the extended spectrum cephalosporins, these drugs are much more expensive and offer no significant benefit over conventional therapies.

FOLLOW-UP EXAMINATION

Physicians who obtain culture specimens from clinically asymptomatic patients after treatment will commonly discover GAS still present in the pharyn-

TABLE 2. **Antibiotic Treatment of Streptococcal Pharyngitis**

Antibiotic	Pediatric Dose	Adolescent/ Adult Dose	Mode	Duration	Cost*	Comments
Recommended Choices						
Penicillin V potassium (Penicillin VK)	250 mg bid or tid	500 mg bid or tid	oral	10 d	$	
Benzathine Penicillin G (Bicillin L-A)	600,000 U (<60 lb) 1.2 million U (>60 lb)	1.2 million U	IM	1 d	$$	Painful. Useful in patients where compliance may be a problem.
Amoxicillin (Amoxil)	250 mg bid	500 mg bid	oral	10 d	$	Suspension tastes better than Penicillin VK.
	50 mg/kg/d or 750 mg qd	750 mg qd	oral	10 d	$	
Erythromycin ethyl succinate (E.E.S.)	40 mg/kg/d bid to qid	400 mg bid	oral	10 d	$$	GI side effects are common.
Erythromycin estolate (Ilosone)	20–40 mg/kg/d bid to qid		oral	10 d	$$	Less GI side effects. Not recommended for adults due to possible hepatotoxicity.
Alternate Choices						
Amoxicillin-clavulanate (Augmentin)	40 mg/kg/d tid		oral	10 d	$$$$	
Azithromycin (Zithromax)	12 mg/kg/d qd	250 mg qd	oral	5 d	$$$	
Cephalexin (Keflex)	250 mg bid or tid	500 mg bid or tid	oral	10 d	$	
Cefadroxil (Duricef)	30 mg/kg/d qd	1000 mg qd	oral	10 d	$$$	
	30 mg/kg/d bid		oral	4 d	$$$	Not FDA approved for short course treatment.
Cefdinir (Omnicef)	14 mg/kg/d qd	600 mg qd	oral	10 d	$$$$	
	7 mg/kg/d bid		oral	5 d	$$$$	
Cefixime (Suprax)	8 mg/kg/d qd	400 mg qd	oral	10 d	$$$$	
Cefpodoxime (Vantin)	10 mg/kg/d bid	100 mg bid	oral	5 d	$$$$	
Cefuroximeaxetil (Ceftin)	20 mg/kg/d bid		oral	5 d	$$$	Not FDA approved for short course treatment.
Clarithromycin (Biaxin)	15 mg/kg/d bid		oral	10 d	$$$$	
Clindamycin (Cleocin)	20 mg/kg/d tid	300 mg tid	oral	10 d	$$$$	

*Cost (based on treating a 25-kg child).
Abbreviations: $ = <$10; $$ = $11–25; $$$ = $26–50; $$$$ = >$50; GI = gastrointestinal.

geal tissues. These patients are likely GAS carriers and are not at risk to develop ARF or transmit the infection to others. Therefore, patients who respond clinically to antibiotic therapy should not undergo follow-up throat cultures. Identification and treatment of GAS pharyngeal carriers are indicated in the following few circumstances:

1. During outbreaks of ARF or poststreptococcal glomerulonephritis
2. When a case of GAS toxic shock syndrome or necrotizing fasciitis has occurred in a household contact
3. When multiple episodes of GAS pharyngitis continue to occur within a family despite appropriate therapy
4. When tonsillectomy is being considered because of chronic GAS carriage
5. When a family has excessive anxiety about recurrently positive GAS throat culture results

Eradication of GAS carriage has been accomplished with a 10-day course of any of the following regimens: oral clindamycin (Cleocin), amoxicillin-clavulanate (Augmentin), or the combination of penicillin (or a cephalosporin) and rifampin. Once a negative throat culture result has been obtained, physicians should not perform another culture unless clinically indicated.

SUMMARY

Streptococcal pharyngitis is a common infection in school-age children. Confirmation of GAS in the tonsillopharyngeal tissues is readily accomplished by performing a RADT or throat culture on a properly obtained throat swab. Judicious use of the throat culture or RADT will minimize the problems caused by identifying streptococcal carriers. Infected patients will respond rapidly to a variety of inexpensive antibiotics; therefore, compliance must be emphasized to minimize the risk of developing ARF.

TUBERCULOSIS AND NONTUBERCULOUS MYCOBACTERIAL DISEASE

method of
PETER F. BARNES, M.D., and
DAVID E. GRIFFITH, M.D.
University of Texas Health Center at Tyler
Tyler, Texas

TUBERCULOSIS

Tuberculosis is one of the most common infectious diseases in the world, causing an estimated 1.9 million deaths annually. Although the incidence of tuberculosis is declining in the United States, drug-resistant tuberculosis that responds poorly to therapy is increasingly common, and substantial transmission of tuberculosis continues to occur. Therefore, it is essential that physicians promptly diagnose tuberculosis and institute appropriate therapy.

Clinical Manifestations

PULMONARY TUBERCULOSIS

Pulmonary tuberculosis in adults generally causes subacute or chronic fever, weight loss, night sweats, and cough, sometimes with hemoptysis. The physical examination usually does not show evidence of consolidation, and the chest radiograph typically shows upper lobe infiltrates, with or without cavitation. This presentation can mimic that of a lung neoplasm. Therefore, tuberculosis should be considered in all patients with suspected lung cancer, particularly if fever is present. The diagnosis of tuberculosis is often missed in the following situations:

1. The patient has acute tuberculous pneumonia, manifested by acute onset of symptoms, a toxic appearance, and a chest radiograph showing unilobar or multilobar alveolar infiltrate. Tuberculosis should be considered whenever bacterial pneumonia does not respond to antibiotics.
2. The chest radiograph shows predominantly middle or lower lobe disease.
3. The patient has extensive tuberculosis, often with respiratory failure, and the chest radiograph shows diffuse alveolar infiltrates.

EXTRAPULMONARY TUBERCULOSIS

The most common sites of extrapulmonary tuberculosis are the pleura, lymph nodes, and genitourinary system. Pleuritis is usually an acute or subacute illness characterized by fever, pleuritic chest pain, and cough. The pleural effusion is usually unilateral, sometimes blood-tinged, but rarely grossly bloody. It is typically an exudate with a mononuclear cell predominance, but it may be a transudate in patients with underlying diseases that cause transudates, such as chronic liver disease. Pleural fluid eosinophilia (>10%) is rare and suggests an alternative diagnosis.

Tuberculous lymphadenitis typically presents as subacute to chronic swelling of the cervical nodes, often with fever and weight loss. In genitourinary tuberculosis, dysuria, hematuria, and flank pain are noted in only 40% to 70% of patients, and fever and weight loss are uncommon. Sterile pyuria or hematuria suggest the diagnosis. Many women have coexistent tuberculosis and bacterial infections, and tuberculosis should be considered when pyuria or hematuria persist despite elimination of bacterial infection.

Tuberculous meningitis is a rare but life-threatening manifestation of disease. Patients usually present with several days to weeks of fever, headache, and altered mental status. The cerebrospinal fluid generally shows a low glucose level, a high protein level, and 100 to 1000 cells/mm^3. These cells are predominantly mononuclear, although polymorphonuclear cells may predominate early in the course of disease.

Miliary tuberculosis is the hematogenous dissemination of *Mycobacterium tuberculosis* to multiple organs, and the diagnosis is often based on chest radiographic findings of tiny nodules throughout both lung fields. In 10% to 40% of cases, the chest radiograph reveals nonspecific abnormalities. The lungs, bone marrow, and liver are frequently involved sites. Miliary disease should be considered in patients with fever, weight loss, and unexplained pancytopenia or liver test abnormalities.

Special Populations

HIV INFECTION

Most HIV-infected tuberculosis patients are unaware of their HIV status, and many do not acknowledge HIV risk factors. Therefore, HIV testing is recommended for all patients with tuberculosis. In HIV-infected people with tuberculosis, typical chest radiographic findings are mediastinal adenopathy, pleural effusions, and a miliary pattern, whereas apical disease and cavities are uncommon. Extrapulmonary tuberculosis, particularly lymphadenitis and miliary disease, is more frequent in HIV-infected patients than in immunocompetent ones.

CHILDREN

Tuberculosis in children usually causes no respiratory symptoms. Characteristic chest radiographic changes are mediastinal adenopathy, sometimes with parenchymal changes secondary to bronchial obstruction by enlarged lymph nodes.

Diagnosis of Tuberculosis

PULMONARY TUBERCULOSIS

A presumptive diagnosis of tuberculosis usually depends on finding acid-fast bacilli (AFB) in a clinical specimen. The sputum AFB smear is not sensitive or specific because positive results are obtained in only 50% of patients with pulmonary tuberculosis and in some patients with nontuberculous mycobacterial disease. The sensitivity of the AFB smear varies with chest radiographic findings. If there is extensive alveolar infiltrate or cavitation, 98% of cases are AFB+. If there is only interstitial or lower lobe infiltrate, nodules or scarring, only 50% of cases are AFB+. Negative smear results in this latter situation do not exclude tuberculosis. Because AFB smears are not specific, confirmation of the diagnosis generally requires culture, which should be performed in all patients to identify those with drug-resistant tuberculosis. In a minority of cases, culture results are negative and the diagnosis is based on clinical and radiographic findings, combined with a response to antituberculosis therapy.

If sputum AFB smear results are negative but tuberculosis is suspected, bronchoscopy should be performed to obtain bronchoalveolar lavage fluid, as well as tissue by transbronchial biopsy. AFB or granulomata are present in 50% to 70% of patients, providing a rapid diagnosis. Children are often unable to produce sputum, in which case gastric washings for AFB and mycobacterial culture should be done.

EXTRAPULMONARY TUBERCULOSIS

In patients with extrapulmonary tuberculosis, the chest radiograph shows evidence of active or prior tuberculosis in only 50% of cases. Depending on the site of suspected tuberculosis, large volumes of relevant body fluids should be obtained for AFB smear and mycobacterial culture. At least 100 mL of pleural or peritoneal fluid, three early morning voided urine samples of 100 mL each, or 10 mL of cerebrospinal fluid should be evaluated whenever possible. Even with large volumes, the yield of the AFB smear in body fluids is low. If pleural or peritoneal fluid study results are negative, tissue biopsy should be performed because AFB smear results are more often positive in tissue than in body fluids, and granulomatous inflammation can provide presumptive evidence of tuberculosis.

Fine-needle aspiration or excisional biopsy of lymph nodes is indicated in suspected tuberculous lymphadenitis. An intravenous pyelogram is recommended to help diagnose genitourinary tuberculosis because characteristic abnormalities, such as ureteral strictures and calyceal narrowing, are seen in 60% to 90% of patients. For suspected miliary disease, bronchoscopic studies or liver or bone marrow biopsies are used most frequently. Diagnostic tests should be directed toward the organs involved, based on clinical and laboratory findings.

NUCLEIC ACID AMPLIFICATION TESTS

The *M. tuberculosis* Direct test (Gen-Probe, San Diego, Calif.) and the Amplicor test (Roche Molecular Systems, Branchburg, NJ) permit rapid diagnosis of tuberculosis by detecting ribosomal RNA and DNA of *M. tuberculosis*, respectively. These tests are more sensitive and specific than the AFB smear. However, they are expensive and do not replace the AFB smear or mycobacterial culture.

A positive sputum AFB smear result is an important indicator of infectivity, and culture is essential to determine drug susceptibility. Both nucleic acid amplification tests are approved for AFB+ sputum samples because the sensitivity and specificity are greater than 95%. The *M. tuberculosis* direct test is approved for AFB-negative sputum samples, but sensitivity is lower than that in AFB+ samples and negative test results do not exclude tuberculosis. These tests are not approved for extrapulmonary samples. Nucleic acid amplification tests are most useful in the following situations:

- Patients with AFB+ sputum in whom the clinical suspicion of tuberculosis is low. If the nucleic acid amplification test result is negative, therapy can be administered for nontuberculous mycobacterial disease, and not for tuberculosis.
- Patients with AFB-negative sputum in whom the clinical suspicion of tuberculosis is moderate or high and in whom results of the nucleic acid amplification test will affect the decision to give antituberculosis therapy or to perform invasive diagnostic procedures. For example, in a patient with suspected miliary tuberculosis, a positive nucleic acid amplification test will prompt initiation of antituberculosis therapy and avoid bronchoscopy.

NOTIFICATION OF PUBLIC HEALTH OFFICIALS

Physicians are legally bound to notify public health officials of cases of suspected or confirmed tuberculosis. Laboratories report cases with positive results on AFB smears or mycobacterial cultures. However, when the diagnosis of tuberculosis is based only on clinical, radiographic, and/or histologic findings, the treating physician must report the case to the appropriate authorities.

Tuberculin Skin Test

The tuberculin skin test measures the delayed-type hypersensitivity response to *M. tuberculosis* antigens, which is positive in people with an intact immune response and prior exposure to *M. tuberculosis* or to environmental mycobacteria. The skin test should be placed by the intradermal Mantoux method, and not by multiple puncture tests, which are unreliable. The test should be read after 48 to 72 hours by a health care professional, not by the patient.

When tuberculin skin testing is performed to evaluate the diagnosis of tuberculosis disease, 5 mm of induration is considered a positive result. A positive test result is not diagnostic of tuberculosis but provides supportive evidence, together with clinical and chest radiographic findings. A negative tuberculin skin test alone does not exclude the diagnosis and is common in extensive tuberculosis and in immunosuppressed patients. However, a negative tuberculin skin test with positive control skin tests argues strongly against the diagnosis of tuberculosis.

When tuberculin skin testing is used to identify people with latent tuberculosis infection (LTBI), testing should be targeted to those who would benefit from therapy to prevent progression to disease. This includes people at high risk for recent infection and those at high risk for progression of LTBI to disease (Table 1). Tuberculin skin testing of low-risk groups is discouraged. The threshold for a positive test varies from 5 to 15 mm, as detailed later. Interpretation of the skin test is unaffected by prior vaccination with bacille Calmette-Guérin.

TREATMENT OF LATENT TUBERCULOSIS INFECTION

Selection of Patients for Treatment

Treatment reduces the likelihood of progression of LTBI to disease but can cause adverse effects, includ-

TABLE 1. **People in Whom Targeted Tuberculin Skin Testing Should Be Performed**

High Risk of Recent Infection	High Risk for Progression of Latent Tuberculosis Infection to Disease
Contacts of tuberculosis patients	HIV infection
Residents and employees of high-risk congregate settings*	Organ transplants
Persons who immigrated from high-prevalence countries in previous 5 y	Immunosuppressive therapy (≥ equivalent of ≥15 mg/d of prednisone)
Mycobacteriology laboratory personnel	Fibrotic chest radiograph lesions of prior tuberculosis
Children and adolescents exposed to high-risk adults	Intravenous drug use
Age <5 y	Specific high-risk medical conditions†

*Prisons and jails, long-term facilities for the elderly, health care facilities, residential facilities for patients with AIDS, homeless shelters.

†Diabetes mellitus; chronic renal failure; silicosis; leukemia; lymphoma; cancer of the head, neck or lung; weight loss ≥10% of ideal body weight; gastrectomy; jejunoileal bypass.

ing fatal hepatotoxicity. People with severe acute or chronic liver disease and those with prior adequate treatment for tuberculosis or for LTBI should generally not be treated. However, some experts treat HIV-infected patients with significant recent exposure to tuberculosis despite prior therapy for LTBI.

Before treating LTBI, it is imperative to exclude active tuberculosis because treatment with isoniazid (INH) may cause drug resistance. Patients should be questioned about symptoms of tuberculosis, and a chest radiograph should be obtained. In asymptomatic people with normal or stable chest radiographs, LTBI can be treated. If symptoms are present or the stability of the radiographic findings is uncertain, sputum cultures should be obtained. Never start such a patient on INH alone. If there is enough clinical suspicion of tuberculosis to send samples for mycobacterial culture, do not treat for LTBI until culture results are available. The patient should either receive no therapy if the likelihood of tuberculosis is low or four antituberculosis drugs if the likelihood of tuberculosis is high.

Treatment of LTBI is recommended at a lower threshold of tuberculin sensitivity in people at high risk for progression of LTBI to disease:

1. Highest risk group. HIV-infected people with recent close contact with a tuberculosis patient or a history of a positive tuberculin skin test result should be treated for presumed LTBI, regardless of tuberculin skin test results, that is, even with no induration.
2. High-risk group. These patients should be treated if the tuberculin skin test result is equal to or greater than 5 mm.
   - Severely immunocompromised patients, including HIV-infected people, organ transplant recipients, and people receiving the equivalent of greater than 15 mg/d of prednisone for more than 1 month.
   - Close contacts of infectious tuberculosis patients.
   - People with fibrotic chest radiographic changes of prior tuberculosis, excluding minimal apical scarring or small calcified granulomas.
3. Moderate-risk group. These people should be treated if the tuberculin skin test result is equal to or greater than 10 mm.
   - Intravenous drug users.
   - People with certain medical conditions (e.g., diabetes mellitus, chronic renal failure, silicosis, weight loss greater than 10% of ideal body weight, malnutrition, gastrectomy, jejunoileal bypass, leukemia, lymphoma, head and neck cancer, lung cancer).
   - People who immigrated from high-prevalence countries in the previous 5 years.
   - Residents and employees of high-risk congregate settings (e.g., prisons, jails, health care facilities, homeless shelters).
   - Mycobacteriology laboratory personnel.
   - All children younger than 5 years, and people older than 18 years exposed to high-risk adults.
   - People with documented skin test conversion (≥10 mm increase in size) in the previous 2 years.
4. Low-risk group. Although tuberculin testing should be minimized in low-risk people, some testing is performed, for example, in newly employed health care workers. In people with none of the above risk factors, a skin test result greater than 15 mm is considered positive, but no national recommendations are provided on treatment. We believe that the following guidelines are reasonable.
   - The patient should be informed of the benefits and risks of treatment.
   - Treatment is recommended for people younger than 35 years but not for people older than 50 years.
   - For people 36 to 50 years old, the decision is individualized, based in part on the patient's wishes.
   - Treatment is favored for people in whom development of tuberculosis may cause extensive spread of disease, for example, an employee in an AIDS hospice.

Treatment Regimens

Table 2 shows the recommended regimens for treatment of LTBI, in order of preference for most cases. INH for 9 months is preferred because it is more effective than INH for 6 months. There is more experience with INH than with the other regimens, and INH costs far less than the other agents. Directly observed preventive therapy with twice-weekly INH is preferred in high-risk groups. If INH cannot be given for 9 months, 6 months is acceptable, except in HIV-infected people, children younger than 18 years, and people with fibrotic chest radiographic lesions. Because rifampin (RIF) interacts with many antiretroviral agents, rifabutin may be substituted for RIF in some HIV-infected patients.

Baseline liver tests should be measured in those with risk factors for drug-induced hepatotoxicity (prior or current liver disease, HIV infection, alcoholism, pregnancy, or postpartum state) and perhaps in patients receiving chronic medications. To evaluate for adverse drug reactions, patients taking INH or RIF alone should be seen monthly, and those taking RIF and pyrazinamide (PZA) should be seen every 2 weeks. In patients with baseline liver test abnormalities or with risk factors for drug-induced hepatotoxicity, liver tests should be measured monthly if they are receiving INH or RIF, and every 2 weeks if they are receiving RIF and PZA. Treatment should be discontinued if jaundice or other symptoms and signs of hepatotoxicity develop, or if the transaminase lev-

TABLE 2. **Regimens for Treatment of Latent Tuberculosis Infection**

Regimen	Daily Dose	Twice-Weekly Dose	Duration
INH*	Adult: 5 mg/kg Child: 10–20 mg/kg Maximum: 300 mg	Adult: 15 mg/kg Child: 20–40 mg/kg Maximum: 900 mg	9 mo
INH*	Adults only 5 mg/kg Maximum: 300 mg	Adults only 15 mg/kg Maximum: 900 mg	6 mo
RIF and PZA†	Adults only RIF 10 mg/kg Maximum: 600 mg PZA 15–20 mg/kg Maximum: 2 g	Not recommended	2 mo
RIF‡	Adult: 10 mg/kg Child: 10–20 mg/kg Maximum: 600 mg	Not recommended	Adult: 4 mo Child: 6 mo

*To reduce the likelihood of peripheral neuropathy, pyridoxine is given with INH to pregnant and nursing women, to patients with a poor diet, and to patients with seizures or illnesses that predispose to neuropathy, such as diabetes mellitus, alcoholism, malnutrition, and HIV infection.

†Used in the following situations: exposure to an INH-resistant source case, INH intolerance, persons are available for treatment for >2 but <6 months, for example, persons incarcerated or hospitalized for this duration.

‡Little experience with this regimen; used only in adults who cannot take INH because of intolerance or an INH-resistant source case, and who cannot tolerate PZA; children who cannot take INH because of intolerance or an INH-resistant source case.

Abbreviations: INH = isoniazid; PZA = pyrazinamide; RIF = rifampin.

els are more than five times the upper limit of normal.

For pregnant women at high risk for progression of LTBI to tuberculosis, especially those with HIV infection or recent tuberculosis infection, LTBI should be treated with INH, even during the first trimester. For women with a lower risk of disease, some experts treat LTBI after delivery. For pregnant patients who cannot tolerate INH or who are exposed to an INH-resistant source case, RIF for 4 months can be given. RIF and PZA for 2 months may be considered in HIV-infected patients after the first trimester. PZA should be avoided in HIV-negative pregnant women.

TREATMENT OF TUBERCULOSIS DISEASE

Initial Therapy

Because the AFB smear is relatively insensitive and therapy should not be delayed until culture results are available, empiric antituberculosis therapy is advised in AFB smear-negative patients in whom there is moderate or high suspicion of tuberculosis, particularly if disease is extrapulmonary. Risk factors for drug-resistant tuberculosis are previous antituberculosis therapy and immigration from high-prevalence countries. In the United States, most tuberculosis patients should be treated initially with INH, RIF, PZA, and ethambutol (EMB; Myambutol). EMB is withheld only in regions where the prevalence of INH resistance is less than 4% and the patient has no risk factors for drug-resistant tuberculosis. Drug susceptibility testing should be done on all initial *M. tuberculosis* isolates, and EMB can be discontinued if the isolate is susceptible to INH and RIF.

Treatment of Drug-Susceptible Tuberculosis

INH, RIF, and PZA is given for 2 months, followed by INH and RIF for 4 months, using the dosages shown in Table 3. This regimen cures more than 95% of patients. If PZA is not given for the first 2 months, INH and RIF are given for 9 months. Although streptomycin (SM) is considered a first-line drug, it is generally used only when one or more of the other agents cannot be used because of drug resistance, intolerance, or toxicity. If patients respond well to therapy, treatment is given daily for 2 weeks, then twice weekly thereafter. If patients respond slowly, daily therapy should be prolonged. All therapy, particularly twice-weekly doses, should be directly observed by public health personnel, if resources permit. If the clinical or microbiologic response to therapy is poor (positive culture results after 2 months of therapy), treatment is given for more than 6 months. For patients with a good bacteriologic response and who have completed a 6-month INH and RIF-containing regimen, routine follow-up is not needed.

To reduce development of drug resistance, adults on self-administered therapy should receive the drug combinations rifampin-isoniazid (Rifamate) (150 mg INH/300 mg RIF) or rifampin-isoniazid-pyrazinamide (Rifater) (50 mg INH/120 mg RIF/300 mg PZA). The daily rifampin-isoniazid-pyrazinamide dosage is 4 tablets in patients weighing less than 45 kg, 5 tablets in patients 45 to 54 kg, and 6 tablets in those over 54 kg.

Special Situations

Extrapulmonary Tuberculosis

Extrapulmonary tuberculosis in adults is treated in the same way as pulmonary tuberculosis. In children with meningitis, skeletal disease, or miliary disease, INH and RIF are continued for a total of 12 months because of insufficient data with shorter regimens.

Drug-Resistant Tuberculosis

Drug-resistant tuberculosis should be treated only in consultation with physicians with expertise in this area. Treatment is usually prolonged and second-line

TABLE 3. **Dosages and Adverse Effects of First-Line Antituberculosis Drugs**

Drug	Daily Dose	Twice-Weekly Dose	Adverse Reactions
INH*	Adult: 5 mg/kg Child: 10–20 mg/kg Maximum: 300 mg	Adult: 15 mg/kg Child: 20–40 mg/kg Maximum: 900 mg	Hepatotoxicity, peripheral neuropathy, rash, anorexia, nausea, vomiting, insomnia, somnolence
RIF	Adult: 10 mg/kg Child: 10–20 mg/kg Maximum: 600 mg	Adult: 10 mg/kg Child: 10–20 mg/kg Maximum: 600 mg	Hepatotoxicity, thrombocytopenia, flulike syndrome, rash, orange secretions; increases metabolism of many drugs, such as methadone and coumadin; oral contraceptives not effective with rifampin
PZA	15–30 mg/kg Maximum: 2 g	50–70 mg/kg Maximum: 4 g	Nausea, vomiting, hepatotoxicity, arthralgias, gout, rash
EMB†	15–25 mg/kg	50 mg/kg	Decreased red-green color discrimination, visual acuity
SM	Adult: 15 mg/kg Child: 20–40 mg/kg Maximum: 1 g	Adult: 25–30 mg/kg Child: 25–30 mg/kg Maximum: 1.5 g	Auditory, vestibular and renal toxicity, hypokalemia, hypomagnesemia

*To reduce the likelihood of peripheral neuropathy, pyridoxine is given with INH to pregnant and nursing women, to patients with a poor diet, and to patients with seizures or illnesses that predispose to neuropathy, such as diabetes mellitus, alcoholism, malnutrition, and HIV infection.
†Dosage of EMB should be based on lean body mass.
Abbreviations: EMB = ethambutol; SM = streptomycin.

agents are less effective and more toxic than first-line drugs.

HIV-Infected Patients

Patients with HIV infection and drug-susceptible tuberculosis respond well to standard therapy. However, because cure rates are reduced with suboptimal therapy, directly observed therapy is recommended in all cases. Because of the potential for drug interactions, health care providers treating tuberculosis and those treating HIV infection must communicate closely. Factors such as HIV viral load and patient commitment to therapy should be evaluated to determine if antiretroviral therapy is indicated. If patients are not candidates for antiretroviral therapy, standard antituberculosis therapy is used. If patients are currently receiving antiretroviral therapy or if future antiretroviral therapy is planned, interactions between rifamycin and antiretroviral agents must be considered. Because recommendations are complex and evolving, a physician knowledgeable about these interactions should guide therapy. In some patients, rifabutin is substituted for RIF.

Patients with tuberculosis who are receiving antiretroviral therapy have enhanced cell-mediated immunity and can develop paradoxical reactions during antituberculosis therapy, manifest by fever, lymphadenopathy, and tissue inflammation. These reactions can be managed with brief courses of nonsteroidal anti-inflammatory agents or corticosteroids.

Pregnancy

INH, RIF, and EMB are used initially, avoiding PZA because of inadequate teratogenicity data. EMB is discontinued if organisms are susceptible to INH and RIF. Because PZA is not used, INH and RIF are given for 9 months. SM is avoided because it can cause congenital deafness. Breast-feeding is safe because the concentrations of antituberculosis drugs in breast milk are low.

Monitoring During Therapy

Baseline liver tests, a complete blood cell count, and serum creatinine and uric acid levels are recommended in all patients. The response to therapy, adherence to therapy, and potential for drug toxicity should be monitored, as outlined in Table 4. Patients should be questioned monthly for symptoms of hepatotoxicity and other adverse reactions (see Table 3). Nonadherence is the most common cause of treatment failure and relapse, and adherence must be monitored in all patients (see Table 4).

Hospitalization and Isolation

Most patients with tuberculosis who are clinically stable, are likely to adhere to therapy, and live in stable family settings can be treated as outpatients without increasing the risk of transmission of tuberculosis to household contacts, probably because they were infected before diagnosis. Hospitalization is advised if nonadherence is suspected, if any household contacts are highly susceptible such as infants or immunocompromised people, or if the patient's living situation will expose new contacts to infection, for example, homeless people.

Hospitalized patients with suspected or confirmed pulmonary or laryngeal tuberculosis should be placed in respiratory isolation. Ideally, isolation is continued until sputum AFB smear results are negative for 3 consecutive days if drug-susceptible tuberculosis is suspected, or until three negative culture results are obtained if drug-resistant tuberculosis is suspected. When the number of respiratory isolation rooms is not adequate, patients should be prioritized:

1. Patients with AFB+ sputum smears have highest priority.
2. If patients have the same AFB smear status, those with drug-resistant tuberculosis have priority.
3. Patients who have received the shortest duration of therapy have priority.

TABLE 4. **Monitoring During Antituberculosis Therapy**

Tests	Frequency and Interpretation
AFB smear and culture	Every 2 wk until culture result is negative, and one after completion of therapy; culture results are negative in 90% of cases after 2 mo of therapy; if culture results are positive, nonadherence, drug resistance, or malabsorption should be considered, and an expert should be consulted
Drug susceptibility	If clinical or microbiologic response is poor
Chest radiograph	1. After 2–3 mo, if culture results are negative; resolving abnormalities confirm the diagnosis of tuberculosis 2. If the response to therapy is poor, the chest radiograph may suggest other diagnoses
Clinical evaluation	Every 1–2 wk until the patient improves clinically; then monthly to assess for adverse reactions
Liver tests	Monthly in patients at increased risk for hepatotoxicity (alcohol users, HIV infection, underlying liver disease or liver test abnormalities, age >35); discontinue antituberculosis drugs if patients develop signs of hepatotoxicity or if transaminase levels are >5 times the upper limit of normal
Visual acuity, red-green discrimination	Monthly in patients receiving ethambutol
Auditory testing	Monthly in patients receiving streptomycin
Serum creatinine	Every 1–2 wk for first 4 wk, then monthly in patients receiving streptomycin
Serum uric acid	1. At least monthly to evaluate adherence in patients receiving PZA who are not on DOT; levels should be above baseline levels in adherent patients 2. Monthly in patients receiving PZA who have a history of gout
Pill counts	At each clinic visit in patients not receiving DOT
Urine sample for color	At each clinic visit in patients not receiving DOT; urine should be orange-red in patients who are taking RIF

NONTUBERCULOUS MYCOBACTERIAL DISEASE

Clinical Manifestations and Diagnosis of Pulmonary Disease

The lung is the most common site of infection due to nontuberculous mycobacteria (NTM) in immunocompetent people. NTM are acquired from the soil and water, and patients with lung disease due to NTM are not contagious. Cavitary lung disease due to NTM causes apical fibronodular infiltrates that mimic tuberculosis, occurring primarily in men with underlying obstructive lung disease. Noncavitary lung infection due to NTM causes mid and lower lung field fibronodular infiltrates, typically in elderly, nonsmoking females with no underlying lung disease. The diagnosis of noncavitary disease due to NTM, particularly *Mycobacterium avium* complex (MAC), is suggested by high-resolution computed tomography scan findings of clusters of small nodules in the lung periphery, associated with ectatic changes of the draining bronchi.

To diagnose NTM lung disease, at least three sputum and/or bronchial wash specimens must be obtained for AFB smear and mycobacterial culture, fulfilling one of the following criteria:

- One culture-positive sample is either heavily AFB+ or heavily culture-positive.
- At least three culture results are positive over 1 year, regardless of AFB result.
- If the radiographic presentation is unusual or sputum analysis is nondiagnostic, a lung biopsy demonstrates granulomatous inflammation or a positive culture result.

These guidelines emphasize long-term follow-up, with collection of multiple respiratory specimens for AFB and mycobacterial culture, so that the diagnosis can be made in patients with subtle or slowly progressive noncavitary disease. Potentially pathogenic isolates of NTM should not be prematurely dismissed as "colonizers." For questionable cases, expert consultation should be obtained. Because disease due to NTM may be rapidly progressive in immunosuppressed hosts, these guidelines are best applied to evaluation of infections with NTM, especially MAC, in immunocompetent hosts.

TREATMENT OF PULMONARY DISEASE DUE TO NONTUBERCULOUS MYCOBACTERIA IN PATIENTS WITHOUT HIV INFECTION

Mycobacterium avium Complex

The most common cause of lung disease due to NTM in the United States is MAC, which is treated with regimens based on clarithromycin (Biaxin) or azithromycin (Zithromax). Dosages and adverse drug reactions are shown in Table 5. Susceptibility of MAC to clarithromycin in vitro correlates with the response to treatment, whereas susceptibility to other agents does not. Initial therapy should include at least three drugs: clarithromycin or azithromycin; rifabutin or RIF; and EMB. SM two to three times weekly during the first 2 to 3 months of therapy should be considered in addition for extensive or life-threatening disease. Because thrice-weekly regimens are as effective as daily therapy and are not associated with emergence of macrolide resistance, we favor intermittent regimens for most patients. The optimal duration of therapy for MAC lung disease is not well defined, but we believe that treatment should be

TABLE 5. **Dosages and Adverse Effects of Drugs Used Frequently for Treatment of *Mycobacterium avium* Complex**

Drug	Daily Dose	Thrice-Weekly Dose	Adverse Reactions
Clarithromycin (Biaxin)	500 mg bid	1000 mg	Nausea, vomiting, diarrhea, hepatitis, decreased hearing
Azithromycin (Zithromax)	250 mg	500 mg	Nausea, vomiting, diarrhea, hepatitis, decreased hearing
Rifabutin (Mycobutin)	150–300 mg	300 mg	Nausea, vomiting, hypersensitivity, hepatitis, polymyalgia, polyarthralgia, leukopenia, uveitis
Rifampin	600 mg	600 mg	See Table 3
Ethambutol*	25 mg/kg × 2 mo; then 15 mg/kg	25 mg/kg	See Table 3
Streptomycin	750–1000 mg	750–1000 mg	See Table 3

*Dosage of ethambutol should be based on lean body mass.

continued until sputum culture results are negative for at least 10 months, emphasizing the importance of collecting multiple sputum samples during therapy.

Significant toxicity can result from the drugs used to treat MAC disease, especially rifabutin (see Table 5), and clinical monitoring is essential. For patients receiving clarithromycin or azithromycin, transaminase and gamma glutamyl transferase levels should be measured monthly for the first 3 months, and then if symptoms of possible hepatotoxicity develop. For patients receiving rifabutin, the leukocyte count and transaminase levels should be measured every few months. Monitoring for RIF, EMB, and SM is performed as for treatment of tuberculosis. RIF is better tolerated than rifabutin but induces hepatic enzyme levels that metabolize clarithromycin and lower its blood levels. This may favor development of clarithromycin resistance, although this has not yet been observed. We believe that RIF should be substituted for rifabutin in most cases. Patients tolerate better regimens that include neither rifabutin nor RIF, such as clarithromycin and EMB. However, it is uncertain if this constitutes adequate therapy and prevents emergence of clarithromycin resistance.

Some patients, especially elderly people with other illnesses, do not tolerate therapy of MAC disease, and it is reasonable to withhold treatment in patients with indolent disease. For patients who are macrolide-intolerant or who have macrolide-resistant organisms, a salvage regimen might include INH 300 mg/d, rifabutin or RIF, and EMB, with SM for the initial 3 to 6 months of therapy. Although clofazimine* and the quinolones have been advocated for use in MAC disease, there is little or no evidence of their clinical efficacy.

Mycobacterium kansasii

The second most common cause of lung disease due to NTM in the United States is *Mycobacterium kansasii*, which causes disease that closely mimics tuberculosis. Susceptibility in vitro to RIF is the best predictor of successful therapy. Essentially all untreated strains are susceptible to RIF, but isolates from previously treated patients can show RIF resistance. Interpretation of susceptibility testing of *M. kansasii* in vitro to drugs other than RIF is difficult because the drug concentrations tested are those used for *M. tuberculosis*, and these may not be appropriate for *M. kansasii*. For previously untreated patients, resistance to drugs such as INH and SM in vitro does not predict a poor clinical response to these agents. For previously treated patients, resistance in vitro may be clinically significant, and consultation from a specialist should be obtained to guide therapy.

The recommended treatment regimen for *M. kansasii* lung disease is RIF, INH, and EMB for 18 months, with at least 12 months of negative sputum culture results. PZA is not active against *M. kansasii*. Clarithromycin has activity against *M. kansasii* in vitro and in vivo, and may facilitate shorter and/or intermittent treatment regimens. For patients with RIF-resistant *M. kansasii*, treatment may include clarithromycin, EMB at 25 mg/kg/d throughout therapy, sulfamethoxazole (Gantanol) 1 g three times daily, and high-dose INH (900 mg/d) with pyridoxine (vitamin B_6). SM two to three times weekly can also be added for severe or life-threatening disease.

Mycobacterium abscessus and Other Mycobacteria

The third most common cause of lung disease due to NTM in the United States is *Mycobacterium abscessus*. The clinical presentation closely resembles that of noncavitary MAC disease. Unfortunately, treatment of *M. abscessus* disease is often ineffective. The only oral agents that are active against this organism are clarithromycin and azithromycin. Parenteral agents with activity include amikacin (Amikin), imipenem (Primaxin), and cefoxitin (Mefoxin). A reasonable approach is to attempt monotherapy with clarithromycin or azithromycin, which may arrest the disease but seldom yields long-term sputum conversion. For patients who do not respond, a specialist should be consulted. Unfortunately, addition of parenteral agents has not significantly enhanced the response to therapy.

Other NTM that rarely cause disease include *My-*

*Not available in the United States.

cobacterium fortuitum, *Mycobacterium simiae*, and *Mycobacterium xenopi*, all of which can be treated with clarithromycin and other agents, preferably in consultation with a specialist.

Role of Surgery

Surgery is an important adjunct to therapy for a few carefully selected patients with cavitary disease due to NTM, usually MAC, and patients with limited disease due to *M. abscessus*. The indications for surgery are varied, but include patients who fail therapy because macrolide resistance has developed. Intraoperative and postoperative complications are common, and close follow-up and aggressive drug therapy are required after surgery.

DISSEMINATED NONTUBERCULOUS MYCOBACTERIAL DISEASE IN IMMUNOCOMPROMISED PATIENTS

Prophylaxis to prevent disseminated MAC disease is indicated for HIV-infected adults and adolescents with CD4 cell counts less than 50 cells/μL. It is essential to exclude disseminated MAC disease before starting prophylaxis with a single drug, which can result in development of macrolide resistance. Azithromycin 1200 mg weekly is the drug of choice because of the convenient dosage schedule, minimal side effects, absence of significant interactions with other drugs, and low cost. Clarithromycin 500 mg twice daily is an alternative. Rifabutin is effective but is used less often because of side effects and drug interactions with antiretroviral agents. For patients in whom the CD4 cell count increases to more than 100 cells/μL and HIV viral burden is suppressed for more than 3 to 6 months, prophylaxis can be discontinued.

We favor treatment of disseminated MAC disease with a macrolide (clarithromycin or azithromycin), EMB, and rifabutin, administered daily. Elimination of rifabutin from this regimen is acceptable because it does not affect treatment outcome and minimizes adverse drug effects and drug interactions with antiretroviral agents. However, without rifabutin, clarithromycin resistance is more likely to emerge. Although lifelong therapy is currently recommended, guidelines are evolving and discontinuation of therapy may be reasonable in patients with sustained increases in CD4 cell counts and suppressed HIV viral burden, as in the case of prophylaxis.

The treatment of pulmonary or disseminated *M. kansasii* disease in HIV-infected patients is the same as that for patients without HIV infection. Rifabutin can be substituted for RIF to minimize interactions with antiretroviral agents. Disseminated *M. chelonae* infection in patients receiving corticosteroids or other immunosuppressive drugs is treated with clarithromycin alone.

TREATMENT OF LYMPHADENITIS AND SOFT-TISSUE INFECTIONS

Localized lymphadenitis due to NTM, usually MAC, can be cured by surgical excision alone. The regimens used to treat pulmonary MAC disease are effective for patients with lymphadenitis that is too extensive for surgical excision or that had an inadequate response to surgery. Soft-tissue infections with *M. abscessus* usually result from penetrating injury and can be treated with surgical débridement and clarithromycin monotherapy. *M. marinum* infections can be successfully treated with single agents, such as clarithromycin, doxycycline (Vibramycin), trimethoprim/sulfamethoxazole (Bactrim, Septra), or with the combination of RIF and EMB.

Section 4

The Cardiovascular System

ACQUIRED DISEASES OF THE AORTA

method of
CHARLES W. ACHER, M.D.,
GIRMA TEFERA, M.D., and
MARTHA M. WYNN, M.D.
University of Wisconsin
Madison, Wisconsin

Aneurysm formation, dissection, plaque hemorrhage, and occlusion comprise the acquired conditions of the aorta. The diseases resulting in these conditions include genetic abnormalities of connective tissue such as Marfan and Ehlers-Danlos syndromes, vasculitides such as Takayasu disease, systemic lupus erythematosus, giant cell arteritis, degenerative aortic disease (i.e., atherosclerosis), bacterial aortitis, and trauma. The expression of these disease processes in the human life cycle is modified by a complex interaction of environmental and genetic factors that determine severity and age of onset in a very intricate interaction, leading to a broad and unpredictable spectrum of clinical presentations. Marfan syndrome is an example of a heritable genetic fibrillin defect located on the 15th chromosome that leads to abnormal connective tissue formation in the aorta, making it weaker than normal. Familial aggregations of aortic occlusive disease and aneurysm formation are clearly identified and may be related to known heritable factors such as lipid abnormalities, diabetes, or abnormalities of the immune system or matrix protein production.

Environmental factors such as smoking, stress, and diet can accelerate this predisposition to aortic wall degeneration so that it develops decades sooner than would normally occur. The ultimate expression of this degeneration as aneurysm, occlusion, plaque hemorrhage, or dissection is poorly understood within a particular individual, however.

Diagnosis of aortic disease has been greatly enhanced with rapid computed tomography and magnetic resonance image scanning with three-dimensional reconstructive angiography to identify vascular anatomy. These diagnostic modalities plus transesophageal echocardiography have significantly reduced the necessity of using higher-risk invasive angiography for evaluating patients with aortic diseases.

Minimally invasive endovascular treatment options for aortic disease have become increasingly available (e.g., the recently approved aortic endografts for aneurysmal disease). Percutaneous balloon angioplasty with or without stent placement has been used successfully for a number of years in selected clinical presentations. It is clear that the more complex the aortic disease, the less satisfactory these minimally invasive procedures are, with frequent complications and long-term failures. As useful as these newer techniques appear to be, there is no evidence that they pose less treatment risk, and modular devices have a disturbing rate of rupture and mechanical failure both early and late in follow-up. This is a rapidly evolving field of research and development, however, and better devices with lower profiles for easier placement and better durability will undoubtedly enhance clinical effectiveness and safety.

Effective elective treatment of aortic disease can be compromised because of cardiac, pulmonary, and renal disease, which are the primary causes of operative morbidity and mortality. Complete evaluation of these systems is mandatory before treatment to determine if treatment risk can be reduced by correction or improvement of cardiac, pulmonary, or renal function preoperatively. Patients presenting acutely have little opportunity for risk modification.

AORTIC OCCLUSIVE DISEASE

Lower extremity claudication is the most common presentation of infrarenal aortic occlusive disease. The indication for revascularization is limiting or disabling claudication, limb-threatening ischemia with or without tissue loss, or complete aortic occlusion to the renal arteries with renal artery stenosis. If the patient does not have limb-threatening ischemia and is satisfied with limitations imposed by claudication, there is no absolute indication for revascularization. Atherosclerosis is by far the most frequently associated condition, and most patients are heavy smokers. In younger patients (<50 years), just the distal aorta and the proximal iliac arteries may be involved (Leriche syndrome), whereas older patients commonly have more extensive involvement of the iliac and the femoral arteries. Renal and visceral arteries are commonly involved in the elderly patient, leading to significant ischemic nephropathy, hypertension, and, occasionally, visceral ischemic symptoms. Women in their 20s and 30s may have Takayasu aortitis as the underlying disorder, but it is not uncommon to see male and female smokers with hyperlipidemia in their 30s and early 40s with advanced atherosclerotic occlusive disease of the aorta. More recently, homocystinemia has been implicated in patients with occlusive atherosclerosis. Homocystinemia can be treated with folic acid and B vitamins. Rarely, aortic occlusive disease involves the suprarenal or the descending thoracic aorta and may be caused by large calcified aortic plaques or Takayasu aortitis.

After confirming occlusive disease by means of physical examination for pulses and bruits, noninvasive testing with ankle/brachial index (ABI) and pulse volume recordings is used to assess the severity of ischemia and the level of occlusive disease. An ABI of less than 0.30 is considered limb threatening. In diabetic patients, who commonly have calcified noncompressible arteries, the ABI is artificially elevated and less helpful. This noninvasive testing, supplemented with magnetic resonance angiography, can avoid the necessity for standard arteriography in most patients. Intra-arterial angiography gives the most precise anatomic detail but may be associated with a significant risk of complications in patients with ischemic nephropathy or "shaggy aortas."

TREATMENT

The standard treatment for occlusive aortic disease is aortoiliac or femoral bypass from the infrarenal aorta with a bifurcated Dacron or Teflon graft through a midline abdominal incision. If the aorta is completely occluded to the renal arteries, suprarenal aortic cross-clamping combined with aortic endarterectomy is necessary. If significant renal artery stenosis is present, endarterectomy of the renal arteries is also done. This type of bypass is the most durable method of revascularization, with 5-year patency of more than 90% and 10-year patency of 80%. The severity of iliac and femoral artery occlusive disease can adversely affect long-term graft function. The operative mortality risk for this procedure if patients are properly evaluated for surgery should be less than 3%. The presence of significant pulmonary or cardiac disease may preclude a direct surgical approach, necessitating an extra-anatomic axillobifemoral bypass. In the clinical circumstance of a hostile abdomen or a previously infected infrarenal graft, a bypass from the distal thoracic aorta to the femoral arteries can be done, with excellent long-term patency.

Extensive aortic endarterectomy is an option in selected patients with atherosclerotic occlusive disease and may be the treatment of choice in patients with visceral and renal artery stenosis or suprarenal atherosclerotic occlusion. In patients younger than 50 years of age, aortic endarterectomy has a high failure rate and should not be done.

Percutaneous transluminal angioplasty with or without stenting has limited applicability in aortic occlusive disease but may be effective for treatment of localized stenotic lesions of the aorta. Percutaneous transluminal angioplasty and stenting are not advisable for complete aortic occlusion, shaggy aortic disease, or heavily calcified aortas because of the high complication rate.

Occlusive disease of the suprarenal aorta due to aortitis is treated with a bypass from the descending thoracic aorta proximal to the stenosis to a suitable location in the abdominal aorta. If the stenotic portion extends to the aortic arch, an extra-anatomic graft from the ascending to the abdominal aorta may be required. In some patients with extensive vasculitis, revascularization of the renal or the visceral vessels is necessary.

ANEURYSMS

Infrarenal aneurysms are the most common and usually occur in individuals older than 55 years of age with advanced degenerative aortic disease. Thoracic aneurysms most commonly occur in a similar age group but also are seen in younger patients with heritable disorders such as Marfan syndrome, nonheritable marfanoid-like aortopathy (cystic medial disease), or vasculitis. Ninety percent of patients with aneurysms are smokers, which is believed to accelerate aneurysm development greatly through a variety of mechanisms, from direct aortic wall damage with abnormal collagen remodeling to increased activity of metalloproteases from inflammatory cellular infiltrates. Inflammatory aneurysms have an extremely prolific inflammatory cell infiltrate in the aortic wall; the inflammatory response spreads to the periaortic tissues and can cause ureteral and visceral obstruction. This inflammatory variant of degenerative aneurysms always occurs in heavy smokers and presents technical problems in repair because of the dense inflammatory tissue. Chronic aortic dissections also become aneurysmal in about 40% of patients. From 5% to 15% of aneurysms are familial, which has been linked to abnormal collagen and elastin production, similar to Ehlers-Danlos syndrome. Trauma and infection lead to aneurysm formation by rapid direct aortic wall destruction. In the case of aortic infection (mycotic aneurysms), the bacterial source may be external, such as salmonella food poisoning, or something overlooked, such as severe periodontal disease resulting in frequent bacteremia. Without some pre-existing abnormality, however, bacteria rarely colonize the aortic wall.

The incidence of infrarenal aneurysms is about 6% after the age of 60 years, with a gender ratio of 5:1 (male to female); however, only one third of these are greater than 4 cm in diameter. With increasing age, the incidence advances to approximately 10% of individuals older than 80 years of age. Aortic aneurysms occur in all anatomic regions of the aorta: infrarenal, ascending thoracic, descending thoracic, thoracoabdominal, and aortic arch, in order of frequency. The incidence of thoracoabdominal aneurysms is estimated to be 0.02% of the population, occurring equally by gender with a bimodal age distribution.

The primary risk of aortic aneurysms is death from rupture. The risk of rupture can be determined when wall tension (T) exceeds the tensile strength of the aortic wall according to Laplace's law:

$$T = \text{Diameter} \times \text{Pressure/Wall Thickness}$$

Twenty percent of the aneurysms treated are ruptured, but it is estimated that only 15% of patients with ruptured aneurysm survive long enough to be considered for treatment. The average diameter of a ruptured aneurysm is 8 cm whether in the thoracic or the abdominal aorta, with very few ruptures occurring with an aneurysm diameter of less than 5 cm but many more occurring with diameters of greater than 6 cm. Thoracic and abdominal aortic aneurysms have similar natural histories and expansion rates (about 4 mm per year after reaching 4 cm in diameter). It is considered prudent to treat an abdominal aortic aneurysm greater than 5.5 cm in diameter unless cardiac or pulmonary disease precludes safe treatment. Fusiform thoracic aneurysms are usually treated at diameters of 6 cm or greater because of the greater operative risk. These rules do not apply to mycotic aneurysms, which can rupture at any size, and saccular aneurysms, which are unpredictable at smaller diameters. In recent randomized trials from Great Britain and the United States, there was no survival advantage to treating asymptomatic infrarenal aneurysms smaller than 5.5 cm in diameter.

Treatment

Aortic aneurysms are repaired by replacing the aneurysmal portion of the aorta with a synthetic Dacron or Teflon graft. The technique and the risks of placing this graft depend on which anatomic region of the aorta needs replacement and the cause and acuity of the aneurysm.

Abdominal Aneurysms of the Infrarenal, Juxtarenal, and Suprarenal Aorta

Most abdominal aneurysms are infrarenal and are usually repaired through a transabdominal incision with the patient under general anesthesia with or without supplementary epidural anesthesia. A Dacron or a Teflon tube or a bifurcated graft is sewn to the aorta with nonabsorbable monofilament sutures below the renal arteries. The iliac arteries are involved with aneurysmal or occlusive disease in less than 30% of patients; this allows a tube graft 70% of the time, which simplifies and shortens the surgery. The inferior mesenteric artery is reimplanted in 5% of patients to avoid colonic ischemia. In 5% to 10% of patients, renal bypass or endarterectomy is done for ischemic nephropathy and hypertension from significant renal artery stenosis. The risk of death from elective repair should be 1% to 5%, but the risk of other nonlethal complications is 20% to 30%. Most are pulmonary complications due to chronic obstructive pulmonary disease. Other complications include bleeding, myocardial infarction, renal failure, colonic ischemia, urinary sepsis, and lower extremity arterial thrombosis. The mortality associated with treating ruptured aneurysms averages 50%. In juxtarenal and suprarenal aneurysms and aneurysms requiring renal endarterectomy, suprarenal aortic cross-clamping is necessary; in most reports, this increased the risk of surgical mortality.

Repair of infrarenal aneurysms is in the midst of a minirevolution of minimally invasive techniques, which include endovascular aortic stent grafts inserted with catheter guidewire techniques from the femoral arteries and minilaparotomy with or without laparoscopy. With the recent U.S. Food and Drug Administration approval of endovascular stent grafts, their use in repair has increased dramatically. It is clear, however, that without proper patient selection, the risk of complications and mortality exceeds that of standard repair. Additionally, there has been a disturbing mechanical failure of modular endografts, with aneurysm ruptures occurring despite successful placement. The incidence of failure from endoleaks increases with time, which requires lifelong surveillance for device malfunction. Therefore, it seems prudent to use endografts in older patients with limited life spans or in those patients with excessive surgical risk due to comorbid conditions who meet the anatomic criteria for device placement. This is a rapidly evolving field, which is in the middle of defining its usefulness in the treatment of aortic aneurysms. There are no significant data on minilaparotomy as an alternative to endografting or standard techniques. There are reliable reports that by (1) shortening the postoperative recovery pathway with metoclopramide (Reglan), for gastric emptying and bowel motility; (2) early removal or no use of nasogastric tubes; (3) proper pain control with epidural or patient-controlled analgesia; and (4) early ambulation, the size of the abdominal incision is irrelevant to the length of stay and recovery.

Another approach to the infrarenal aorta is the lateral extraperitoneal approach, which is especially useful in patients with a hostile abdomen and in those with juxtarenal and suprarenal aneurysms.

Thoracic Aneurysms

Thoracic aneurysms consist of aneurysms of the ascending aorta, the aortic arch, the descending thoracic aorta, and occasionally all three areas. Aortic dissection accounts for a significant number of patients requiring repair of the ascending aorta, whereas most arch and descending thoracic aneurysms are degenerative. Aortic plaque hemorrhage most commonly occurs in a nonaneurysmal descending thoracic aorta and is unstable in most patients, leading to rupture or dissection. Aneurysm location and extent determine the technical options for repair. Femorofemoral cardiopulmonary bypass is needed for aneurysms that involve the ascending aorta or the aortic arch. Hypothermic circulatory arrest with retrograde cerebral perfusion through the superior vena cava is used for arch replacement. Ascending and arch aneurysms require a median sternotomy approach, whereas descending thoracic aneurysms are repaired through a left thoracotomy. Occasionally, with involvement of the arch and the descending thoracic aorta, the repair is staged, with an elephant trunk or reverse elephant trunk technique employed as the first procedure. Replacement of the descending thoracic aorta can be done with or without bypass with similar results. In patients with aortic valve stenosis or insufficiency, a composite valve graft is used, with the coronary arteries attached directly to the valve conduit (Bentall technique) or with bypass off the valve conduit (Cabrol technique). The mortality of elective thoracic aneurysm repair is 10% to 15% owing to the increased complexity of the repair and the presence of co-morbid conditions (valve disease, coronary artery disease). Pulmonary complications from chronic obstructive pulmonary disease are common, and stroke occurs in up to 10% of patients when the aortic arch is replaced. There is a 1% to 4% risk of paraplegia with elective descending thoracic aneurysm repair, which can double in patients with rupture. As in those with abdominal aneurysms, most patients with rupture die before treatment can be given.

There are a few promising self-expanding endografts on the verge of Food and Drug Administration approval for treatment of descending thoracic aortic aneurysm, dissection, and trauma. These devices may have significant impact on treatment of acute type B dissections and descending thoracic aneurysms, but few data are available to confirm the usefulness of this approach in treatment. Hopes are high, however.

Thoracoabdominal Aortic Aneurysms

Thoracoabdominal aortic aneurysms (TAAAs) involve the thoracic and the abdominal aortas. They stand apart from other aneurysms because of the complexity and the risk of repair. Mortality of elective repair is 10% to 20%, and the risk of paraplegia historically has been 5% to 40% (average 15%), depending on the extent of aortic replacement and the acuity of clinical presentation (rupture or dissection). Advanced age (>80 years), acuity, and severe ischemic nephropathy significantly increase the risk of death from aneurysm repair. The factors associated with aneurysm formation are similar to those for other aortic aneurysms, and smoking with chronic obstructive pulmonary disease is a common association. The Crawford classification is used to group TAAAs by paralysis risk. Crawford type I involves the descending thoracic aorta and the upper abdominal aorta to the renal arteries. Type II involves the descending thoracic aorta and the abdominal aorta below the renal arteries. Type III aneurysms involve the distal descending thoracic aorta and the abdominal aorta, and type IV involves all of the abdominal aorta. In Crawford's experience, the risk of paralysis with aortic repair, with or without assisted circulation and with selective intercostal reimplantation, was as follows: type I, 10%; type II, 20%; type III, 5%; and type IV, 2%. With acute rupture or dissection, the risk of paraplegia doubled for any Crawford type of lesion.

Repair is done through a thoracoabdominal incision with graft inclusion and reattachment of the visceral and the renal vessels to the aortic graft with Carrel patches. Atriofemoral bypass to perfuse the visceral and the renal vessels is advocated by many surgeons and does reduce systemic acidosis but has not been associated with a decrease in mortality, paraplegia risk, or renal failure. The renal or the visceral arteries require endarterectomy or bypass for occlusive disease in 30% of patients. There is strong evidence that aggressive renal revascularization and renal cooling during aneurysm repair significantly reduce the risk of renal failure, which historically exceeds 10%. Spinal cord protective strategies, which have significantly reduced the risk of paralysis, include cerebrospinal fluid drainage and systemic or regional hypothermia. Hypothermia may be moderate, with ambient surface cooling, or profound, with circulatory arrest. Circulatory arrest with complete anticoagulation with heparin, however, increases the risk of bleeding and mortality in most clinical reports. Steroids and inhibitors of endogenous endorphins and excitatory neurotransmitters reduce paralysis risk synergistically when used with cerebrospinal fluid drainage and hypothermia, and these adjuvants in combination result in the most reductions in paraplegia risk. Atriofemoral bypass and selective intercostal reimplantation have not demonstrated effectiveness in reducing paralysis risk in TAAA repair. With the recent advances in operative and perioperative management, elective mortality has decreased to 5% and paralysis risk to 5% in selected centers. The best results are obtained in those centers with a dedicated and designated anesthesia and surgical team with specialized training and experience in treating aneurysms of this complexity and risk.

Aortic Dissection

Aortic dissection is caused by a disruption of the intima and the media of the aortic wall (a tear), which results in a splitting of the media generated by blood under pressure. Commonly, two flow channels develop, with reentry of the dissecting channel (false lumen) back into the true lumen. The false lumen usually has a spiral course down the aorta, making the actual flow channel orientation difficult to determine. The immediate cause of the aortic tear is predominantly uncontrolled hypertension, but an underlying aortopathy is present in most patients. Dissection also occurs under normal physiologic conditions in patients with Marfan syndrome. Dissection is lethal in 90% of patients if untreated. It is the most common aortic emergency, but the diagnosis is also the most often missed. Presenting symptoms are usually very severe (10/10) chest pain or interscapular back pain of sudden onset, which can simulate myocardial ischemia. Involvement of the brachiocephalic vessels can cause stroke, and dissection into the abdomen can cause visceral, renal, and lower extremity ischemia. Occasionally, dissections present with paraplegia from interruption of intercostal arteries. The most common lethal event is rupture of the aorta into the pericardium or the thorax or interruption of myocardial blood flow with myocardial infarction due to occlusion of the coronary arteries.

Dissections are classified by their point of origin and their distal extent. Both the older DeBakey and the newer Stanford classification systems are used. A Stanford type A dissection starts in the ascending aorta or the aortic arch and may or may not extend distally to the descending thoracic or abdominal aorta. Type A dissections are considered surgical emergencies because there is no effective nonsurgical management. Stanford type B dissections begin at or distal to the left subclavian artery and may remain confined to the thoracic aorta or extend into the iliac arteries. Type B dissections have the option of medical management with intravenous antihypertensives and β-blockers. DeBakey type I and II dissections are equivalent to Stanford type A lesions and DeBakey type III to Stanford type B dissections.

Accurate identification of the starting point of a dissection is essential to proper treatment. The most sensitive tests for determining this are the computed tomography scan with contrast and three-dimensional reconstruction and the magnetic resonance angiogram with three-dimensional reconstruction. Transesophageal echocardiography has also become popular as the initial diagnostic study, but its precision is operator dependent. Standard arteriography is important for identifying branch vessel obstruction but may not show the dissection's origin if the false lumen is thrombosed. Once the diagnosis is confirmed, immediate control of the blood pressure is the highest priority. Stanford type A aneurysms should then be immediately repaired. This requires femorofemoral bypass and, if the arch needs replacement, hypothermic circulatory arrest. Because the aortic wall is disrupted, the Dacron or the Teflon graft has to be sutured to the aortic wall with a felt strip or pledgets to secure the disrupted wall at both ends of the interposition graft. The goal of repair is to redirect blood flow down the true lumen, which usually re-establishes flow to arteries that have been compromised by the dissected septum.

Stanford type B aneurysms can be managed medically in an intensive care unit, where the patient can be closely monitored for any change in clinical condition that might prompt surgical intervention. The indications for surgical intervention include rupture; branch vessel occlusion leading to visceral, renal, or lower extremity ischemia; continued pain; and aneurysmal dilation threatening rupture. The standard surgical repair is to replace a short segment of the proximal descending thoracic aorta, securing the split aortic layers so that blood flow is redirected down the true lumen. This requires felt strips or pledgets to secure the layers together, to which the graft is sutured. Most intercostals remain open in acute dissections; unless the aorta is sequentially cross-clamped during repair, exsanquination may occur from backbleeding intercostal arteries. Reattachment of intercostals in acute repair is problematic because of the disruption of the aortic wall. If the dissected aorta is too dilated, a longer segment of the aorta requires replacement and, occasionally, the entire thoracoabdominal aorta. Many surgeons lower the risk of paralysis and renal failure during surgical repair by employing retrograde perfusion of visceral and intercostal vessels during aortic replacement using atriofemoral or femorofemoral bypass. Like TAAAs, the more aorta replaced, the less effective this strategy.

The operative mortality rate for repair of acute aortic dissections is 15% to 25%. Only Stanford type B (DeBakey type III) dissection repair carries the risk of paraplegia, which is low (4%) for short-segment replacements but may be as high as 80% for total thoracoabdominal reconstruction in the acute setting. Because of this increased morbidity, total replacement of acute type B dissections is avoided if at all possible by most surgeons. Nonsurgical management of acute type B dissections with β-blockers and antihypertensives (esmolol [Brevibloc] and sodium nitroprusside or nitroglycerin) carries a mortality risk of 5% to 10%. The goal of treatment is to keep the systolic blood pressure lower than 110 mm Hg and the heart rate lower than 80 beats per minute. Such drastic lowering of blood pressure can lead to encephalopathy with confusion and disorientation, decreased renal function, ileus, and increased pulmonary shunt with hypoxia. Fifty percent of medically managed patients require intubation with mechanical ventilation and intensive care unit stays of 5 to 7 days. Nonsurgical management fails 15% of the time, necessitating surgical intervention.

Lesser revascularization procedures, such as femorofemoral, visceral and renal, or axillofemoral bypasses, can be quite effective in the acute setting if the patient is too debilitated for primary aortic surgery. Angiographic fenestration and branch artery stenting to re-establish blood flow have been reported anecdotally.

Mycotic Aneurysms

Mycotic aneurysms are caused by a variety of bacteria that colonize aortic plaque through blood-borne bacteremia. *Staphylococcus aureus*, *Streptococcus viridans*, and *Salmonella* account for most infections, with other gram-negative bacteria involved in less than 10% of patients. Every patient with a mycotic aneurysm should be investigated for bacterial endocarditis, although *Salmonella* is not usually associated with endocarditis. The diagnosis is usually delayed, sometimes for weeks, because of the indolent nature of the endovascular infection, with lassitude, fever, and weight loss. Diagnosis is made most often with computed tomography scan or arteriography, which may show multiple saccular aneurysms or a large nonspecific aneurysm. The infected aorta may be well beyond the confines of the aneurysm. Once the diagnosis is established or suspected, broad-spectrum antibiotic coverage should be initiated after blood cultures have been obtained and surgical repair has been attempted. Treatment involves débridement of all the infected tissue with or without replacement of the aorta, depending on the anatomic location of the infection. Many mycotic aortic aneurysms involve the distal thoracic and abdominal aorta and require in situ aortic replacement with revascularization of renal and mesenteric vessels. Cure of the infection can be expected with *Streptococcus* and *Salmonella*, but treatment of *Staphylococcus* has a high failure rate owing to recurrent infection. The eventual mortality rate is greater than 50% even when the initial surgery is successful. In patients with the option of complete aortic excision and extra-anatomic bypass, the recurrent infection risk is lower.

Traumatic Aortic Aneurysms

Deceleration injury with aortic transection, whether from a motor vehicle accident or a fall, is a lethal event in most instances. Of the few patients who survive transport to a trauma center, many have multiple coincident injuries of the brain, long bones, spine, and abdominal organs that also require urgent attention. The initial diagnostic suspicion usually results from the chest radiograph, which shows a wide mediastinum and loss of prominence of the aortic knob. Computed tomography scan or arteriography is used to define the area of injury. The timing of repair is determined by the severity of the aortic tear and other injuries. Once the injury is diagnosed, repair should be carried out as soon as feasible. Aortic repair is best done through a fourth or fifth interspace left thoracotomy. A short interposition graft is usually necessary, although in children and younger adults, a primary repair can sometimes be accomplished. This is one instance in which assisted circulation with femorofemoral bypass can reduce the risk of paralysis (16% to 4% in a multicenter trial) from aortic occlusion if the aortic occlusion time is prolonged (>30 minutes). Aortic occlusion time in these patients is a function of surgical experience and ability, however, and with expedient repair, paraplegia risk is significantly reduced with or without assisted circulation. Eighty-five percent of patients are younger than 50 years of age, and death in these patients is usually caused by rupture from delayed diagnosis and repair or associated injuries. Elderly patients die more often from cardiopulmonary failure secondary to the stress of aortic repair.

ANGINA PECTORIS

method of
WILLIAM H. FRISHMAN, M.D.
New York Medical College
Valhalla, New York

Angina pectoris is defined as an uncomfortable feeling in the chest, the jaw, the shoulder, the back, or the arm that is typically aggravated by exertion or emotional stress and is relieved by nitroglycerin. Angina usually occurs in patients with coronary artery narrowing; however, it can also occur in patients with valvular heart disease, hypertrophic cardiomyopathy, and uncontrolled hypertension. It can be present in patients with normal coronary arteries (syndrome X) who have endothelial cell dysfunction and spasm (Prinzmetal's angina). Angina of cardiac origin needs to be differentiated from chest pain caused by disorders of the esophagus, the lungs, or the chest wall.

The important features of anginal chest discomfort are its location, its relationship to exercise, its character, and its duration. The discomfort is typically described as originating in the retrosternal area, but it frequently radiates across the precardium, up the neck, and down the ulnar surface of the left arm or down both arms. The chest discomfort may be associated with or even overshadowed by dyspnea, fatigue, lightheadedness, and mild epigastric discomfort. Terms used to describe angina include heaviness, pressure, squeezing, crushing, or a strangling sensation. Pain may vary in intensity from mild localized discomfort to severe pain. Typical angina begins gradually during exercise and is usually relieved within 3 minutes of rest. The discomfort may last up to 10 minutes or even longer after very strenuous exercise or emotional duress. Chest pain lasting for more than 30 minutes may suggest an acute myocardial infarction (MI). Angina pectoris is typically induced by cardiac exertion related to increased myocardial oxygen demands that result from exercise or other stressors; it is relieved by rest. Emotional stress may be another provocative stimulus for angina.

Angina pectoris is further classified as stable or unstable. Unstable angina is important in that its presence predicts a much higher short-term risk of an acute MI. Unstable angina is defined as angina that presents in three different ways: rest angina, severe new-onset angina, or increasing angina. Patients with unstable angina can also be subdivided according to their short-term risk. Patients at high or moderate risk often have coronary plaques that have recently ruptured, and these individuals are susceptible to developing an MI. These patients will require intensive therapy in an inpatient setting. In contrast, low-risk patients with unstable angina have a short-term risk not different from that of patients with stable angina.

In the evaluation of patients with angina pectoris, a detailed history of chest pain is taken. The presence of risk factors for coronary artery disease (CAD) should be determined. Cigarette smoking, hyperlipidemia, diabetes, hypertension, and a family history of premature CAD are all important. In addition, a past history of cerebrovascular or peripheral vascular disease will increase the likelihood of CAD.

The cardiac examination is often normal in patients with stable angina; however, an examination made during an episode of pain can reveal an S_4 or S_3 sound, a mitral regurgitant murmur, a paradoxically split S_2 sound or bibasilar rales, or a chest wall heave that disappears when the pain subsides. The general examination may also identify evidence of atherosclerosis in noncoronary vascular beds, xanthelasma, tendon xanthomas, and elevated blood pressure. Physical signs of anemia, thyrotoxicosis, fever, infection, arrhythmias, and substance abuse may be present.

A wide variety of noninvasive tests are available to establish CAD as the most likely cause of angina pectoris. These evaluations also help to quantitate the severity of ischemic heart disease and other causes of angina pectoris, such as aortic stenosis and hypertrophic cardiomyopathy.

The first part of any noninvasive evaluation is the resting electrocardiogram (ECG). Findings can be normal or can show an infarct pattern or an ischemic repolarization pattern suggestive of underlying CAD. Exercise testing is useful to confirm the diagnosis of CAD in patients with angina and to establish the risk of a subsequent coronary event. Exercise thallium scintigraphy and technetium-99m sestamibi imaging are useful tests when conventional exercise ECG stress testing results in diagnostic uncertainty. Myocardial perfusion scintigraphy following pharmacologic stress caused by adenosine or dipyridamole is particularly useful for patients who cannot exercise adequately. Exercise echocardiography and pharmacologic stress echocardiography with dobutamine have a sensitivity similar to that of nuclear testing. Compared with the exercise ECG, imaging stress tests are particularly useful in patients with bundle branch block, intraventricular conduction defects, left ventricular hypertrophy, or preexcitation syndromes in which ST and T wave abnormalities are present on the baseline ECG. In patients with angina who have evidence of a previous MI, measurement of the left ventricular ejection fraction is necessary to determine prognosis and to select appropriate therapy. In such patients, an exercise ECG stress test in combination with resting echocardiography or gated blood pool scanning can be performed. Stress echocardiography and recently gated myocardial perfusion imaging can accomplish two goals—assessing the ischemic burden and assessing the left ventricular ejection fraction. For predicting the presence or the absence of CAD in patients with angina pectoris, the specificity and the sensitivity of ST segment abnormalities obtained with 24- to 48-hour ambulatory ECG monitoring are lower than are seen with stress ECG. Similarly, the role of electron beam computed tomography in evaluating coronary artery calcification in patients with angina pectoris remains controversial. Coronary angiography is often recommended in patients with unstable angina if there is a moderate to severe risk of MI. Coronary angiography in patients with stable angina that is severe and refractory to medical therapy will provide information on the extent of coronary artery narrowing and will guide correction of the disease by means of angioplasty, stents, and bypass surgery.

Other diagnostic tests that will aid in the management of patients with angina pectoris include fasting blood sugar analysis, determination of total cholesterol, low-density lipoprotein (LDL) and high-density lipoprotein (HDL) cholesterol analysis, triglyceride level determination, and routine hematologic and thyroid function tests to exclude anemia or abnormal thyroid function, which can be associated with worsening angina. Homocysteine concentrations should be measured in patients with a strong family history of CAD, and C-reactive protein level should be measured as a prognostic indicator in patients with unstable angina.

PATHOPHYSIOLOGY

Stable angina is usually associated with a chronic atherosclerotic narrowing of at least one coronary artery, where the plaque disease is stable. The plaques in patients with unstable angina have recently ruptured, and there is a strong thrombotic predisposition with advanced vessel narrowing and myocardial ischemia.

Angina occurs when there is inadequate myocardial perfusion to meet the oxygen needs of the myocardium. Myocardial oxygen demand is enhanced by increases in heart rate, systemic blood pressure, myocardial contractility, and left ventricular size. Myocardial oxygen supply is dependent on coronary blood flow, intraluminal coronary patency, coronary perfusion pressure, the hemoglobin oxygen content of the blood, and the duration of systole.

Coronary stenoses of more than 75% of the cross-sectional area of a coronary artery can result in myocardial ischemia and angina when the myocardial energy requirements are high, as in physical exercise. The threshold for ischemia is reduced as the severity of the obstruction increases if there is inadequate collateral circulation, or because of thrombosis formation or associated vasospasm of a coronary artery. Myocardial oxygen demands can be increased by fever, sepsis, anemia, and hyperthyroidism, which can also lower the ischemic threshold. Under normal physiologic situations, the coronary circulation is autoregulated to maintain constant myocardial perfusion in the face of changing perfusion pressures. Abnormalities in the vascular endothelium, as seen in coronary atherosclerosis, will inhibit any of the compensatory coronary vasodilatory processes associated with nitric oxide and adenosine production, whereas vasoconstrictor mediators, such as endothelin, will become more prominent in their action.

TREATMENT OF STABLE ANGINA

The treatment of stable angina has two major purposes. The first is to prevent MI and death, thereby increasing the length (quantity) of life. The second is to reduce symptoms of angina and the occurrence of ischemia, which should improve the quality of life.

Therapy aimed at the prevention of death has the highest priority. When there are two therapeutic approaches available, the therapy that best prevents death should be recommended. For instance, in patients with left main CAD, bypass surgery would be recommended because it prolongs life. In patients with mild angina and single-vessel disease, medical therapy is a reasonable option when compared to coronary angioplasty and stenting or coronary bypass surgery.

Pharmacotherapy to Prevent Myocardial Infarction and Death

Antiplatelet therapy is recommended in all patients with angina pectoris and CAD. The risk of MI and death is reduced by 25% in patients with stable angina, and aspirin use will also reduce the short- and long-term risk of fatal and nonfatal MI in patients with unstable angina. The recommended daily dose is 75 to 160 mg in patients older than 65 years of age and 325 mg in patients younger than 65. Aspirin exerts an antithrombotic effect by inhibiting cyclooxygenase and thromboxane synthesis.

In the presence of contraindications to aspirin, the thienopyridine derivatives, clopidogrel (Plavix) and ticlopidine (Ticlid),* are recommended. These drugs act as antiplatelet agents by preventing the adenosine diphosphate–mediated activation of platelets by selectively and irreversibly inhibiting the binding of adenosine diphosphate to its platelet receptors. In a randomized trial that compared clopidogrel, 25 mg daily, to aspirin, 325 mg daily, in patients at risk of ischemic events, clopidogrel appeared to be slightly more effective in decreasing the combined risk of MI, vascular disease, and death. Patients with stable angina pectoris were not specifically evaluated, however. Because of a more favorable side effect profile, clopidogrel may be preferred over ticlopidine, which has also been shown to be useful in the secondary prevention of vascular events.

Dipyridamole (Persantine)* is a pyridopyridimine derivative that exerts vasodilatory effects on coronary resistance vessels and also has antiplatelet effects. The drug can enhance exercise-induced myocardial ischemia in patients with stable angina and should not be used by itself as antiplatelet therapy.

Long-term antithrombotic therapy with warfarin can be considered because abnormalities in fibrino-

*Not FDA approved for this indication.

lytic function and increased thrombogenicity have also been documented in patients with angina pectoris. There is limited experience with chronic use of low-molecular-weight heparin in daily subcutaneous injections in patients with angina. Low-intensity oral anticoagulation with warfarin (Coumadin) combined with aspirin has been shown to reduce the risk of ischemic events in patients with risk factors for atherosclerosis, but no angina. The combination of aspirin and low-dose warfarin for the prevention of recurrent MI was not shown to be more beneficial than aspirin alone. The addition of warfarin to aspirin should certainly be considered in patients with atrial fibrillation or when significant left ventricular dysfunction is present.

The use of lipid-lowering agents, specifically the 3-hydroxy-3-methylglutaryl coenzyme A (HMG-CoA) reductase inhibitors (statins), has been shown to reduce mortality and cardiovascular morbidity in patients with established CAD, including patients with angina pectoris. Therapy should be used to reduce the LDL cholesterol level to less than 100 mg/dL and to raise HDL cholesterol level. The specific reduction of high triglyceride levels with drugs has not been shown to have an impact on survival. The benefits of the statins extend beyond cholesterol reduction and may also include improved endothelial cell functioning and an anti-inflammatory action. Clinical studies are ongoing to see whether statins can raise the threshold for myocardial ischemia while relieving angina symptoms.

β-Blockers and angiotensin-converting enzyme (ACE) inhibitors should be given to both diabetic and nondiabetic patients with angina pectoris, with or without hypertension or heart failure, to reduce the risk of subsequent cardiovascular events and strokes. ACE inhibitors are themselves not antianginal agents, but a study using ramipril (Altace), 10 mg daily in patients at risk of cardiovascular events, showed a reduction in strokes, MI, and deaths. As yet, there is no evidence to show that the angiotensin II receptor blockers would have the same benefit as the ACE inhibitors.

There is also no evidence that the use of antioxidant vitamins such as vitamins C and E can improve survival. Estrogen administration with and without progesterone should not be given to postmenopausal women with angina pectoris until more definite data from ongoing clinical trials are available. Chelation therapy is probably of no clinical value in patients with angina pectoris.

ANTIANGINAL AND ANTI-ISCHEMIC THERAPY

Coexisting conditions that aggravate myocardial ischemia and angina symptoms should be identified and managed (e.g., anemia, thyrotoxicosis, hypertension). Patients with angina should avoid stressful situations, and behavioral psychotherapeutic and psychopharmacologic interventions should be considered for patients with severe anxiety and depression. Sexual intercourse does not need to be restricted if patients are symptom free. Sildenafil (Viagra) can be used for male impotence as long as patients have not taken nitrates in the past 24 hours. Inclement weather, especially excessive cold, wind, or heat, should be avoided. Meals and the postabsorption state should not coincide with other physical stresses. Vigorous or strenuous exercise that can be expected to cause angina should be avoided, and instead, patients should be encouraged to engage in regular moderate isotonic exercise.

β-Adrenergic Blocking Drugs

β-Adrenergic blocking drugs are the first-line treatment for the long-term management of the symptoms of angina pectoris. Activation of the β-adrenergic receptors by catecholamines is associated with an increase in heart rate, contractility, blood pressure, and atrioventricular conduction. β-Blockers cause a decrease in heart rate, contractility, and arterial pressure, both at rest and during exercise, thereby reducing myocardial oxygen demands. A longer diastolic filling time is associated with a slower heart rate, which can allow for greater cardiac perfusion. With these effects, the drugs will relieve angina symptoms and the need for sublingual nitroglycerin while augmenting the exercise time until myocardial ischemia. In addition, β-adrenergic blocking drugs improve survival, particularly in patients who have survived an MI.

When the dose is titrated to achieve clinical benefit, virtually all β-blockers—whether they have partial agonist activity, β_1-selective actions, membrane stabilizing activity, and general or selective β-blocking properties—will improve exercise tolerance and relieve anginal symptoms. β-Adrenergic blocking drugs are frequently combined with nitrates or slow-release dihydropyridine calcium antagonists to achieve greater symptom relief while minimizing the adverse hemodynamic effects of both drugs. For instance, nitrates tend to increase heart rate, which is attenuated by the concurrent use of β-blockers.

The absolute contraindications to the use of β-blockers are severe bradycardia, high-degree atrioventricular block, and unstable left ventricular failure. Relative contraindications include bronchial asthma, severe mental depression, peripheral vascular diseases, and vasospastic angina. Most diabetic patients tolerate β-blockers, although the drugs should be used with caution in patients who require insulin and are prone to hypoglycemia. Fatigue, lethargy, insomnia, nightmares, worsening claudication, and impotence are frequently experienced side effects. The mechanism of fatigue is not known.

Calcium Antagonists

Calcium antagonists reduce the transmembrane flux of calcium via the calcium channels. They include the newer second-generation vasoselective dihydropyridine agents and nondihydropyridine drugs, such as verapamil (Calan), diltiazem (Cardizem), and bepridil (Vascor). All calcium antagonists have negative inotropic actions, and they can reduce smooth muscle tension in the peripheral blood vessels to cause vasodilation. Dilation of the epicardial coronary arteries is the principal mechanism for the beneficial effect of calcium antagonists in the treatment of vasospastic angina. Calcium antagonists also reduce myocardial oxygen requirements by reducing the systemic vascular resistance and the arterial pressure. The negative inotropic and chronotropic effects of calcium antagonists vary in intensity with the drug being used (e.g., diltiazem and verapamil usually lower the resting heart rate; the dihydropyridines do not). Calcium antagonists are therefore useful for the treatment of both myocardial supply and myocardial demand ischemia. Randomized trials have shown that calcium antagonists are equipotent to β-blockers in the treatment of vasospastic angina. It is recommended that calcium antagonists (e.g., dihydropyridines) be used in combination with β-blockers when initial treatment with β-blockers is not successful or as a substitute for β-blockers when initial treatment leads to unacceptable side effects. The calcium antagonist bepridil (a combined sodium-calcium channel blocker) is approved for use in drug-refractory angina pectoris.

Overt decompensated heart failure is a relative contraindication to the use of calcium antagonists. Bradycardia, sinus node dysfunction, and atrioventricular nodal block are contraindications to the use of heart rate–lowering calcium antagonists. Side effects of calcium antagonists include constipation, peripheral edema, hypotension, and headache. Bradycardia and heart block can occur with rate-lowering calcium antagonists.

Nitrates

Nitrates are the oldest drugs available for the short- and long-term management of angina. They are endothelium-independent vasodilators that produce beneficial actions in patients with angina by reducing the myocardial oxygen requirements while augmenting coronary perfusion. The drugs reduce left ventricular volume and arterial pressure while dilating both large epicardial coronary arteries and collateral vessels. They are useful in patients with vasospastic angina. Sublingual nitroglycerin tablets or nitroglycerin spray are used for the immediate relief of effort and rest angina and also can be used prophylactically to avoid ischemic episodes with exercise. The use of long-acting oral agents or transcutaneous drug delivery can provide long-term antianginal control, but a nitrate-free interval of about 8 hours is required to prevent pharmacologic tolerance.

The most common side effects with nitrates are headache, hypotension, and syncope. The use of the phosphodiesterase V inhibitor, sildenafil citrate (Viagra), is contraindicated in patients receiving nitrates. Nitrates can be used in combination with β-blockers and calcium antagonists to provide greater antianginal efficacy. As monotherapy, long-acting calcium antagonists are preferable to long-acting nitrates because of their sustained 24-hour action.

Combination Therapy

Combination therapy with β-blockers, nitrates, and calcium blockers is indicated when monotherapy does not provide maximal relief of anginal symptoms. Special care needs to be taken when β-blockers are combined with diltiazem and verapamil, especially in patients with myocardial conduction abnormalities or left ventricular dysfunction. The additional benefit of combining different antianginal drugs is not always evident, and a recent study suggests that an observed improvement in anginal symptoms may be related to the clinical response of the new drug and not the additive action. There is little evidence to suggest that triple therapy provides any benefit over one or two drugs. In severe disabling angina, the sodium-calcium channel antagonist bepridil may be combined with β-blockers and nitrates to achieve additional antianginal effects.

Other Therapies

Chelation therapy, garlic, and acupuncture are not recommended for the treatment of angina. Although some studies have found benefit with exertional counterpulsation, it is not recommended as a proven treatment. Although some studies have suggested an inflammatory cause of coronary atherosclerosis, the standard use of antibiotics is not recommended. Studies are in progress to evaluate statins and estrogen (because of their effects on endothelial function) as treatments for symptomatic myocardial ischemia.

Myocardial Revascularization

Coronary angiography is indicated in patients with stable angina with poorly controlled symptoms despite medical therapy and in those patients with high-risk stress tests, particularly when there is evidence of left ventricular dysfunction. Depending on the anatomic findings on angiography (extent of coronary disease, left ventricular dysfunction), patients can undergo percutaneous transluminal coronary angioplasty with stenting or coronary artery bypass surgery. Patients with minimal CAD or inoperable disease should remain on medical therapy. The revascularization procedures will result in an immediate relief of coronary obstructions, and 90% or more of patients will achieve relief of anginal symptoms. Coronary restenosis remains a frequent complication of angioplasty with or without stenting. For patients having triple-vessel or left main CAD, bypass surgery will have an advantage over angioplasty regarding survival and long-term angina relief. For non–left main single-vessel coronary disease, there is no apparent survival advantage when comparing medical therapy with revascularization procedures.

Recent studies have suggested that transmyocardial laser revascularization can provide relief of anginal symptoms in patients unable to undergo the usual revascularization procedures. This procedure is associated with a high mortality rate, and its actual clinical benefits remain in question.

MANAGEMENT OF VASOSPASTIC AND UNSTABLE ANGINA

Patients with vasospastic or rest angina should be treated with coronary dilators such as nitrates and calcium antagonists to relieve vasospasm. β-Blockers can be used as part of a combination regimen with coronary vasodilators, but never as monotherapy.

Unstable angina, which is often associated with unstable plaque disease and coronary thrombosis, has a worse prognosis than stable angina. Based on a patient's clinical presentation, patients can be assigned into high-, intermediate-, and low-risk categories for death or MI. The short-term treatment of unstable angina includes interventions to control pain, reduce myocardial oxygen demand, and improve coronary perfusion.

Intravenous or sublingual nitroglycerin is used initially, switching patients to oral or topical nitrates when they become asymptomatic. β-Blockers are indicated in patients at high risk of adverse events and should be administered first intravenously and then maintained orally to a target heart rate of 50 to 60 beats per minute. Calcium channel blockers are useful as adjunctive treatments when pain relief is not achieved. Short-acting dihydropyridines (e.g., nifedipine [Adalat]) should never be given without concomitant β-blocker therapy.

Aspirin should be started immediately at an initial dose of 160 to 325 mg, and a 300-mg loading dose of clopidogrel (Plavix) should be given to those patients who cannot take aspirin. A recent study showed that clopidogrel plus aspirin may be more effective than aspirin alone. Intravenous heparin should be started immediately in all patients at high or intermediate risk. Recent studies have shown that low-molecular-weight heparin can be used as a substitute treatment for standard heparin, and it can be administered subcutaneously to produce a sustained and reproducible anticoagulation response. The risk of bleeding with low-molecular-weight heparin is not any lower than that seen with standard heparin. In addition, intravenous glycoprotein IIb/IIIa platelet antagonists should be given as adjuncts to heparin and aspirin. The IIb/IIIa inhibitors can be continued during coronary angiography and percutaneous coronary interventions. Thrombolytic agents have not been shown to be useful in patients with unstable angina.

Patients with unstable angina with an intermediate or a high risk of death or MI (unstable ECG, high C-reactive protein levels) should undergo coronary angiography within 24 hours, and, depending on the anatomic findings, a revascularization procedure should be performed. This approach appears to reduce mortality and morbidity compared with continuous medical therapy. Patients presenting with a low risk of MI can be treated medically, and angiography may not be necessary unless symptoms cannot be relieved. In patients with refractory angina symptoms, intra-aortic balloon augmentation may be necessary to support them through angiography and revascularization procedures.

CONTROL OF RISK FACTORS FOR ATHEROSCLEROSIS

All patients presenting with stable or unstable angina and those who have undergone revascularization procedures for angina require aggressive management of risk factors for atherosclerosis on an ongoing basis. These interventions include treatment of hypertension according to the Sixth Report of the Joint National Committee for the Prevention, Detection, Evaluation, and Treatment of High Blood Pressure (JNC-VI) guidelines, attempting to reduce systolic blood pressure to less than 140 mm Hg in nondiabetics and less than 130 mm Hg in diabetics. Other interventions include smoking cessation therapy, management of diabetes, and exercise training programs. Lipid-lowering therapy, using statins as a first-line treatment, should be dosed to reduce the level of LDL cholesterol to less than 100 mg/dL, while attempting to raise HDL cholesterol levels. The benefit of plasma triglyceride lowering has not been demonstrated. Weight reduction should be encouraged, especially when there is associated hypertension, hyperlipidemia, or diabetes mellitus. Patients should be prescribed a type II American Heart Association diet, which allows less than 30% of total calories to be fats, one third or less of which can be saturated fats. Increased homocysteine levels are associated with risk of CAD. Patients with CAD and elevated homocysteine levels should receive folic acid to reduce homocysteine level, even though clinical trials have not yet proven definitive benefits for the clinical outcome.

There is no evidence of benefit from taking antioxidant vitamins such as vitamins C and E. Alcohol consumption in moderation (approximately one or two drinks daily) may be beneficial in reducing CAD risk; however, the medical problems of excessive alcohol intake will outweigh any benefit and should be discouraged.

Finally, the psychological problems of patients with CAD need to be addressed, including recognition and treatment of clinical depression and use of interventions directed at psychosocial stress reduction.

Patients with angina need close follow-up from a supportive caregiver, with careful monitoring of symptoms, functional capacity, and CAD risk factor profiles. Patients also need to be educated about the significance of a change in clinical symptoms, the importance of taking their prescribed medications, and the value of maintaining a healthy lifestyle in the years to come.

CARDIAC ARREST: SUDDEN CARDIAC DEATH

method of
CLIFTON W. CALLAWAY, M.D., Ph.D.
University of Pittsburgh
Pittsburgh, Pennsylvania

Cardiovascular disease is the leading cause of death in North America. Sudden and unexpected cardiovascular collapse, also known as *cardiac arrest,* is a major contributor to this mortality. *Sudden cardiac death* (SCD) is defined as death occurring less than 24 hours after the onset of cardiac symptoms. Using this broad definition, the annual mortality from SCD in the United States approaches 400,000. As many as 250,000 individuals die suddenly outside of the hospital. These deaths are referred to as out-of-hospital cardiac arrests (OOHCAs). For many patients, sudden collapse is the first symptom of a cardiac event. Furthermore, many people with cardiac arrest are not suffering from acute coronary artery ischemia at the moment of collapse, even though coronary artery disease may be present. Paradoxically, victims of SCD and OOHCA in particular are often completely well minutes before their collapse, yet these individuals are among the most critically ill patients cared for by physicians.

SCD is a two-organ disease, involving primarily the heart and the brain. Although the entire body is ischemic during cardiac arrest, most other organs can recover from periods of ischemia that are devastating to the highly oxygen-dependent heart and brain. The heart can be plagued both by dysrhythmias and by failure of myocardial contractility resulting from intracellular energy depletion. Impaired contractility can persist for extended periods after resuscitation. The brain undergoes almost immediate loss of energy when blood flow stops, and both active and necrotic forms of cellular death can be triggered by periods without blood flow lasting more than 4 or 5 minutes. Brain cell death can continue to occur for hours or days after restoration of blood flow.

Most cases of SCD result from dysrhythmias. Tachyarrhythmias and ventricular fibrillation (VF) are the most common disturbances in survivors of SCD. Cases of SCD resulting from bradyarrhythmias tend to have poorer prognoses. If treated soon after onset, VF is reversible by electrical shock (defibrillation). Because this definitive therapy exists for VF, the highest survival rates are noted in patients in whom the initial dysrhythmia was VF.

MODERN THERAPY AND SURVIVAL AFTER SCD

Before 1960, OOHCA was a uniformly fatal event. At that time, many clinicians combined their cumulative experience about resuscitation and intensive care in the operating room with already extensive animal data and synthesized recommendations for a set of procedures for cardiopulmonary resuscitation (CPR). Perhaps the most important version of these recommendations follows:

*A*irway management
Artificial *b*reathing
Artificial *c*irculation

These ABCs of resuscitation were promulgated by Jude, Kouwenhoven, and Safar. In particular, these recommendations incorporated artificial breathing without endotracheal intubation and closed-chest compressions without thoracotomy. Thus, CPR could be performed by clinicians outside of the operating room and even by lay people. This approach to resuscitation was easily taught and has formed the core of education about emergency response for 4 decades.

After the introduction of CPR and advanced life support in the 1960s, survival from OOHCA increased. Detailed statistics were first collated in the 1970s, at which time it appeared that between 5% and 10% of patients with OOHCA survived to hospital discharge, with significant variations among communities. Survival rates of less than 1% are reported in some large cities, whereas unique communities such as Seattle report survival rates as high as 18%. Conversely, when one considers only arrests in which VF is the primary arrhythmia, survival rates of 30% or greater are reported.

It is important to consider what endpoint is considered "survival" when interpreting outcome data about SCD. For example, data from many different systems indicate that as many as 30% of subjects who experience SCD have pulse restored at some point during resuscitation attempts and thus have a short-term survival. A smaller proportion survives to hospital admission. Furthermore, the same data indicate an overall survival to hospital discharge of only about 7%. In most hospital systems, 80% to 90% of individuals who survive to hospital discharge enjoy an acceptable quality of life. The excellent neurologic status among patients discharged from the hospital reflects the fact that poor neurologic recovery often leads to death in the hospital. Supporting this idea, many subjects (60%) who are initially resuscitated from cardiac arrest die within 48 to 72 hours of hospitalization. Few data about long-term survival (12 months or more) are available, but survivors do have a higher death rate during the months after their initial event.

The specific procedures for CPR and intensive care after SCD have not changed significantly since their introduction in 1960. The procedures for advanced cardiac life support have been codified in the form of guidelines by the Emergency Cardiac Care Committees of the American Heart Association. These guidelines have been revised with increasing scientific rigor and are now a good example of an evidence-based approach to a clinical problem. Nevertheless, there have been no subsequent breakthrough insights into improving survival such as occurred in 1960. Reflecting this fact, survival to hospital discharge after SCD has not increased since 1975 in communities such as Seattle that have maintained detailed statistics and have even declined in large cities such as Los Angeles.

Principles of Resuscitation

Resuscitation after SCD is based on two physiologic principles: electrical therapy of dysrhythmias and increasing myocardial perfusion. During cardiac arrest, the electrical activity of the heart may be disorganized or absent. Defibrillation or pacing may restore an organized rhythm. However, the ischemic myocardium will not be able to contract because of the loss of high-energy phosphates and disruption of ionic gradients. Perfusion of the myocardium with oxygenated blood may restore the metabolic well-being of the myocardium to a point sufficient for maintaining organized electrical and mechanical activity. After restoration of cardiac contractility, subsequent therapy may be directed at improving neurologic recovery.

Defibrillation

Shocks are administered for external defibrillation by pads or paddles placed across the chest. A direct current shock delivering 2 to 4 J/kg (200–400 J in an adult) is administered during VF. This shock depolarizes the myocardium for a few seconds. The goal of this procedure is that the depolarized myocardium will resume organized electrical activity through its innate conduction system. Most external defibrillators deliver *monophasic* (single direction of current flow) electrical shocks, yet internal devices employ circuitry that delivers *biphasic* (rapidly alternating direction of current) shocks. The biphasic shocks provide more effective depolarization of the heart with less energy, allowing for smaller batteries. Under carefully controlled conditions, the lower-energy biphasic shocks appear to cause less post-shock myocardial dysfunction. However, whether this technical advantage of biphasic shocks over monophasic shocks translates into actual improvement in clinical outcome is debatable.

The success rate of defibrillation attempts declines with duration of VF. In the electrophysiology laboratory in which defibrillation is attempted within seconds after the onset of VF, induced VF can be terminated by a single shock more than 90% of the time and is rarely refractory to repeated shocks. This responsiveness declines with each minute that the heart is ischemic after the onset of VF. One rule of thumb is that the efficacy of defibrillation attempts declines 10% per minute delay. In the case of OOHCA, where delay in arrival of equipment for defibrillation is an inherent obstacle, defibrillation attempts rarely begin in fewer than 4 minutes after a patient collapses. Consequently, only 25% of shocks delivered to patients with OOHCA successfully convert VF to an organized rhythm (Figure 1). Moreover, in many cases of SCD, a shock will convert VF into asystole. This post-shock asystole may be less amenable to resuscitation than asystole encountered in primary bradyasystolic arrests.

The high efficacy of early compared with late shocks delivered has driven much of the design of modern emergency cardiac care. Even before the advent of invasive cardiac procedures, coronary care units increased survival of patients recovering from acute coronary syndromes by placing these patients close to defibrillators. Likewise, the introduction of paramedics throughout the United States was justified by their ability to bring defibrillation directly to the patient with SCD outside the hospital. Both the number and geographic placement of paramedics have been directed by the goal of reaching patients with OOHCA in as short a time as possible.

Automated Defibrillation

One strategy to improve the success of defibrillation in SCD is to expedite the arrival of a defibrillator to the patient. Increasing automation available in defibrillators has decreased the training required of their operators. Several studies have demonstrated the feasibility and utility of enabling minimally trained providers to operate automatic external defibrillators (AEDs). In these studies, AEDs were provided to emergency medical technicians and first responders, including police officers, fire fighters, and security personnel. Recently, interest has developed in the placement of public access defibrillators. These AEDs are positioned in high traffic public places such as airports, shopping malls, and office buildings. Some training is then offered to the individuals who are regularly in those places but who are not traditionally considered first responders, such as flight attendants, retail clerks, and office managers. Nevertheless, the hardware for these devices remains expensive ($3000 per unit), and the actual benefit of widespread deployment, especially of public access defibrillators, is the subject of ongoing clinical trials.

As in most diseases, prevention of sudden death would be much more effective and less costly than advanced treatment. There are identifiable populations at risk in whom it is possible to implant automatic internal cardiac defibrillators (AICDs). Individuals with ventricular dysrhythmias identified in the electrophysiology laboratory and individuals with cardiomyopathy have a decreased incidence of sudden death as a result of AICD placement. In general, survivors of ventricular arrhythmias, individuals with low ejection fractions, and individuals recognized to have repolarization abnormalities may benefit from electrophysiologic evaluation. In most studies, implantation of an AICD affords greater improvement in survival than long-term treatment with an antiarrhythmic drug.

Delayed Defibrillation

Another strategy to increase the success of defibrillation attempts in VF that lasts more than a few minutes is the provision of CPR. Although CPR performed without airway adjuncts or drug administra-

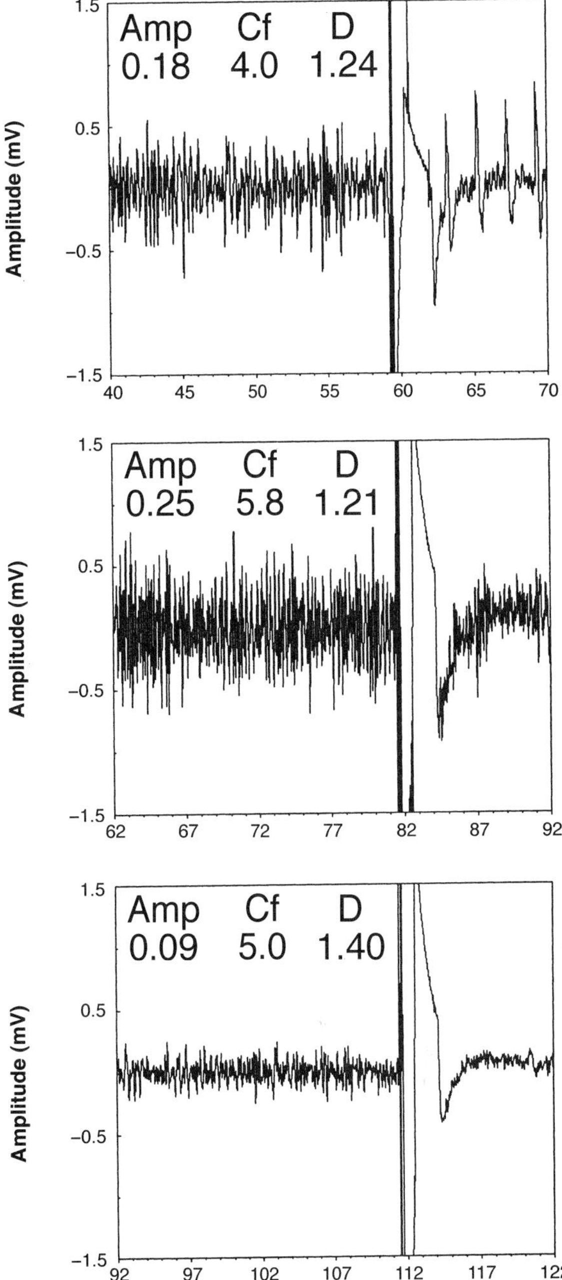

Figure 1. Electrical shocks have varying efficacy for returning ventricular fibrillation (VF) to an organized rhythm. Tracings recorded by automatic external defibrillators placed on patients with sudden cardiac death are depicted. The mean amplitude (Amp) in millivolts, centroid frequency (Cf) in hertz, and fractal dimension (D) of each tracing are indicated. Early, "coarse" VF (*top*) has a high amplitude with a low Cf and D and is frequently converted to an organized rhythm by a shock. In cases in which early VF is not defibrillated (*middle*), the amplitude of VF declines after the shock, perhaps indicating myocardial injury. Late, "fine" VF (*bottom*) has a low amplitude and higher Cf and D. The shock applied to late VF results in asystole.

tion produces only a fraction of normal myocardial perfusion, this small amount of blood flow can slow the metabolic decay of the heart. Thus, CPR can increase the success rate of shocks and the likelihood that the myocardium will contract once it is defibrillated. A recent clinical trial suggested that 90 seconds of CPR preceding the first shock in OOHCA increased the likelihood of successful defibrillation and survival. This benefit was most pronounced in the subgroup of patients in whom first treatment was delayed more than 4 minutes after receipt of the emergency call. These data suggest that all victims of SCD should receive a brief period of artificial reperfusion before defibrillation.

It would be desirable to provide artificial reperfusion before defibrillation in subjects with prolonged VF, while avoiding delays for subjects for whom immediate defibrillation would succeed. Clinical experience indicates that VF decays from early, "coarse" VF that is responsive to shocks to a late, "fine" VF that is refractory to shocks (see Figure 1). However, the large variation in interpretation between providers precludes altering therapy based on this distinction. Quantitative analysis of the electrocardiographic waveform can substitute for this clinical impression. Amplitude and frequency measures of the VF waveform have been used in laboratory investigations but have limited clinical use. Nonlinear tools for signal analysis also can distinguish early and late VF as well as predict likelihood of defibrillation success. It is conceivable that these quantitative tools could help guide the timing of defibrillation in SCD.

Antiarrhythmic Drugs

Few data support the use of antiarrhythmic drugs during resuscitation of the heart in VF. Drugs that have been used intravenously over the past few decades include lidocaine, 1 mg/kg boluses up to 3 mg/kg, bretylium (Bretylol), 5 mg/kg boluses up to 10 mg/kg, and procainamide, 30 mg/min up to 17 mg/kg. Lidocaine also can be administered intratracheally. Each of these agents has benefit for preventing the development of VF in a beating heart. However, no drug will correct VF by itself, and there is no evidence indicating that these drugs improve the success of electrical defibrillation attempts. Amiodarone (Cordarone), 150 to 300 mg intravenously as a bolus, does produce a modest increase in survival to hospital admission when administered during VF. However, amiodarone has not been shown to increase survival to discharge.

Organized bradyarrhythmias and tachyarrhythmias may be more amenable to pharmacologic treatment. In the setting of SCD, tachyarrhythmias are by definition unstable and should be treated with synchronized electrical cardioversion (200 J or more). Ventricular tachycardia may respond to intravenous lidocaine, procainamide, or, if it has features of torsades de pointes, even magnesium, 2 to 4 g intravenous bolus. Although the ventricular response to supraventricular tachycardia can be slowed by treatment of the atrioventricular node with calcium channel blockers, β-blockers, or digoxin, none of these drugs is appropriate for administration during cardiovascular collapse. Heart block or sinus bradycardia may respond to the chronotropic effects of epinephrine, 0.01 to 0.03 mg/kg, or atropine, 1 to 3 mg. In other instances, bradyarrhythmias are secondary to the poor metabolic state of the heart during hypoxia and ischemia. Thus, artificial perfusion for a few minutes will increase the rate and effectiveness of cardiac activity. When conduction system injury has occurred, transthoracic pacing or transvenous pacing is appropriate.

Artificial Coronary Perfusion

CPR consists of airway management, artificial ventilation, and chest compressions. The airway is optimally protected by an endotracheal tube, although the head-tilt–jaw-thrust maneuver can also open the airway. Surrogate devices such as Combitubes or laryngeal masks provide partial airway protection and facilitate ventilation. Regurgitation is common during chest compressions, and a definitive airway is preferred. Positive-pressure ventilation is provided at volumes sufficient to expand the chest (8–10 mL/kg) at rates of 10 to 15 breaths per minute via rescue breathing, self-inflating bag, demand valve, or ventilator. Chest compressions are accomplished by compressing the sternum toward the spine 80 to 100 times per minute. Compression expels blood into the aorta, and the relaxation of the chest permits venous return.

Resuscitation success is determined by the quality of myocardial perfusion during CPR. Coronary perfusion pressures during CPR of less than 15 mm Hg usually preclude any restoration of myocardial contraction. Myocardial blood flow occurs only during relaxation of the ventricle during CPR (Figure 2). Thus, CPR should be optimized to increase the *diastolic* or "relaxation" pressure rather than the *systolic* or "compression" pressure. Relaxation pressures are affected by arterial tone, which determines the rate of runoff of blood from the aorta into the periphery. Carbon dioxide excretion by the lungs is related to pulmonary blood flow during CPR and thus indirectly related to myocardial perfusion. Thus, capnography performed during CPR can assess the adequacy of artificial perfusion. Persistently low end-tidal carbon dioxide measurements during CPR usually predict failure of resuscitation.

Pressor agents are administered during CPR to increase systemic resistance, thereby promoting coronary perfusion (Figure 3). At the same time, increased systemic vascular resistance can also shunt blood more effectively to the brain. Epinephrine, 0.01 to 0.1 mg/kg, is typically administered every 3 to 5 minutes intravenously. Escalating doses of epinephrine are theoretically superior for increasing coronary perfusion, but they increase post-reperfusion complications. The result is that no net benefit was afforded by high doses of epinephrine in clinical tri-

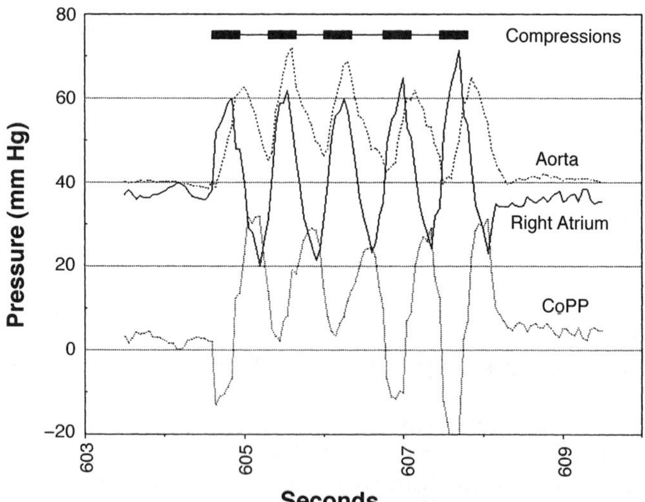

Figure 2. Coronary perfusion occurs during the relaxation phase of cardiopulmonary resuscitation. Pressure tracings from catheters in the aorta and in the right atrium are depicted. Coronary perfusion pressure (CoPP) is calculated as aortic–right atrial pressure. Chest compressions cause increased pressure in both the atrium and the aorta, resulting in no pressure gradient and no myocardial perfusion. During relaxation between compressions when the chest reexpands, atrial pressure falls more quickly than aortic pressure, resulting in a positive pressure gradient (25–30 mm Hg at peak) that perfuses the heart.

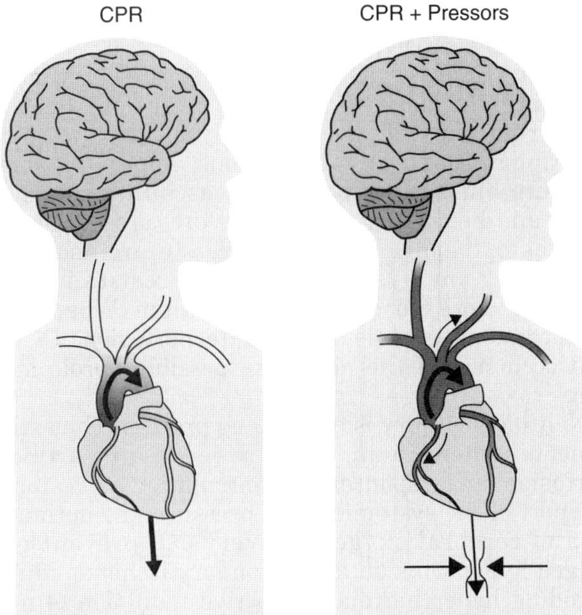

Figure 3. Pressors promote arterial tone and reduce the rate of fall of aortic pressure during the relaxation phase of cardiopulmonary resuscitation (CPR). The decreased runoff of blood from the central aorta during the relaxation phase results in an increased coronary perfusion pressure and better myocardial perfusion. Cross-clamping or occluding the descending aorta would produce the same effect. When peripheral arterial tone is completely collapsed, adequate coronary perfusion pressure will not be generated by CPR.

als. Another pressor with less toxicity is vasopressin. Recent experience suggests vasopressin may surpass epinephrine as the pressor of choice. Small clinical trials demonstrate a large increase in survival when 8-L-arginine vasopressin, 20 IU intravenously, is administered early during CPR. Other pressors such as phenylephrine and norepinephrine remain to be investigated clinically.

Closed-chest cardiac massage is less effective at circulating blood than is open-chest cardiac massage (OCCM). Given that the adequacy of perfusion determines the success of resuscitation, it is appropriate to consider OCCM for SCD if capnography or other measures suggest perfusion is inadequate. "Semi-open" techniques employing plungers or cups inserted through small incisions have been proposed to mimic the efficacy of OCCM. There are limited clinical data about these devices, and left lateral thoracotomy probably remains the quickest technique most familiar to surgeons and emergency physicians. This approach for OCCM can also permit more efficient internal defibrillation. However, the procedural risk of these heroic measures must be balanced against the expectation of neurologic recovery. Thus, OCCM should be considered early after collapse, if at all.

Occlusion of the descending aorta is an alternative strategy that can promote myocardial and cerebral blood flow. This approach is widely used in the form of an intra-aortic balloon pump to bolster poor cardiac output after invasive cardiac procedures. Introduction of balloon catheters into the aorta through the femoral artery can markedly improve CPR efficacy. Likewise, cross-clamping of the aorta during OCCM substitutes for pressors during CPR.

Promoting Neurologic Recovery

CPR can open the window of survival for the brain much longer than 5 minutes. However, no amount of prolongation is sufficient unless spontaneous circulation is restored. Therefore, the foremost priority is resuscitation of cardiac contractility. Histologic signs of neuronal death appear hours to days after reperfusion. This delay between the injury and the appearance of cell death suggests a window of opportunity in which to intervene.

Determination of neurologic status after SCD should not be attempted during the first day after resuscitation. Coma is expected to follow brain ischemia lasting more than a few moments. Some subjects who are initially unconscious may awaken over the next 2 to 3 days. The prognostic value of neurologic examinations after resuscitation increases for at least 72 hours after the initial injury. Because it is not possible to prospectively ascertain which patients will awaken after resuscitation, it is reasonable to provide maximal support and effort to all subjects for at least 48 to 72 hours after resuscitation. At that point, failure to emerge from coma or improve neurologically has greater predictive value for adverse outcome. One exception might be the situation in which a subject who is resuscitated is known to have had poor premorbid function. The additional insult of SCD and resuscitation would essentially preclude any possibility that this individual will recover to a level of functioning better than pre-coma status, and limitation or withdrawal of support might be considered.

The period of no flow during cardiac arrest triggers neuronal death by transient energy failure, free radical generation, and excitatory amino acid release. All of these stressors return to near-normal levels within minutes after restoration of circulation. These stressors subsequently trigger a cascade of new gene expression and signal transduction over the first 24 to 72 hours of reperfusion. Although many antioxidant drugs and excitatory amino acid antagonists have been touted for improving neurologic outcome after cardiac arrest, they would be expected to be beneficial only if delivered before collapse or within moments of restoring circulation. Moreover, it may be unreasonable to expect that blockade of one stressor will prevent other stressors from producing damage on their own. Interventions targeted at the subacute phase of gene expression and signal transduction remain to be explored.

After restoration of circulation, some areas of the brain exhibit persistent hypoperfusion. This ongoing "secondary ischemia" can worsen brain injury. A brief episode of controlled hypertension, along with optimization of blood rheology, can overcome this delayed hypoperfusion. Therefore, a 10- to 15-minute period of controlled hypertension (mean arterial pressure of

130–150 mm Hg) shortly after restoration of circulation should be induced with titrated infusions of pressors (dopamine [Intropin], 5–20 μg/kg/min, or norepinephrine [Levophed], 2–10 μg/min). Frequently, the residual effects of catecholamines administered and released during resuscitation will accomplish this effect. Avoiding hypotension or hemoconcentration during the acute recovery period will also prevent secondary injury.

The injured or ischemic brain is sensitive to temperature. Even mild fever can exacerbate injury and must be scrupulously avoided during the recovery period after resuscitation. Conversely, mild brain cooling produces a greater benefit than any single drug. In fact, replication of some early studies suggesting neuroprotective roles for particular drugs found that these drugs actually reduced body temperature. These drugs had no additional benefit for the brain when temperature was meticulously controlled. Hypothermia is safest and most efficacious when induced to a mild level (32°C–34°C) for at least 24 hours. This intervention can reduce brain metabolic requirements and free radical and excitatory amino acid damage as well as alter subsequent signal transduction and gene expression. The more quickly a patient is cooled after collapse, the greater the potential for benefit.

Inducing hypothermia in the survivor of cardiac arrest is not difficult because of the stunning of brain thermoregulatory centers. Most survivors are already mildly hypothermic and simply must not be rewarmed. Technically difficult attempts to quickly cool the brain may be unnecessary given recent laboratory studies indicating that prolonged, mild hypothermia can improve neurologic recovery even if initiated hours after reperfusion. Clinical trials of induced hypothermia for patients resuscitated from SCD employ cooling blankets, fans, and other conventional techniques.

CONCLUSION

SCD is potentially reversible if aggressive treatment is initiated within minutes of collapse. Because many SCD patients were without debilitating disease before collapse and because many survivors of SCD enjoy acceptable quality of life, aggressive therapy is warranted. Initial treatment is organized around two simultaneous activities: restoration of appropriate organized electrical activity and artificial perfusion of the heart. Subsequent care is focused on hemodynamic stabilization and prevention of ongoing neurologic injury.

Restoration of organized electrical activity for the heart in VF can be accomplished by rapid defibrillation within the first few minutes of arrest and by artificial perfusion followed by defibrillation for more prolonged cardiac arrest. Organized electrical activity that is too slow may respond to artificial perfusion, chronotropic drugs such as epinephrine and atropine, or electrical pacing. Organized electrical activity that is too fast and without perfusion may respond to electrical cardioversion.

Chest compressions and positive-pressure ventilations are the basis of artificial perfusion. Because myocardial blood flow occurs only during the relaxation phase of chest compressions, improving aortic pressure during this phase increases the amount of brain and heart perfusion. Therefore, pressor agents such as epinephrine and vasopressin are useful for increasing the systemic vascular resistance and shunting more blood to the myocardium. When chest compressions provide inadequate perfusion, OCCM and occlusion of the aorta are possible heroic measures to consider.

Neurologic injury is an ongoing process. The extent of acute ischemic injury may be reduced by artificial perfusion until spontaneous circulation is restored. Support of the systemic blood pressure and optimization of cerebral oxygen delivery can prevent prolonged hypoperfusion and secondary ischemic injury. Avoiding hyperthermia and active induction of mild (32°C–34°C) hypothermia can improve brain recovery.

To increase survival after SCD, each step leading from collapse to hospital discharge must be optimized. Thus, it is reasonable to examine the effects of interventions on intermediate outcome variables. For example, increasing the success of defibrillation can increase the proportion of subjects with return of circulation. Similarly, increasing successful resuscitation of the heart can increase the proportion of subjects who survive to hospital admission. Finally, any interventions that promote neurologic recovery can significantly increase the percentage of admitted patients that are discharged from the hospital. Failure at any step in this process may completely mask the beneficial effects of intervention at another step. Thus, an aggressive, longitudinally integrated approach to the victim of SCD holds the greatest promise for reducing this type of mortality.

ATRIAL FIBRILLATION

method of
SAM ASIRVATHAM, M.D., and
WIN-KUANG SHEN, M.D.
Mayo Clinic
Rochester, Minnesota

Atrial fibrillation currently affects about 2.2 million patients in the United States. The prevalence of this disorder increases with age from 0.5% in the fifth decade to about 9% in octogenarians. Although atrial fibrillation is generally considered to be a benign arrhythmia, particularly when compared with rhythm disorders of ventricular origin, it is not without untoward sequelae, thus requiring therapy.

Atrial fibrillation is an independent risk factor for stroke and is associated with a fourfold to fivefold higher risk than that in the unaffected population. This rhythm disorder is incriminated in approximately 75,000 strokes per year and is the major cause of embolic stroke. Whether atrial fibrillation is an independent marker for mortality other than through the propensity (from other associated cardiovascular diseases) for stroke is debated. Some studies suggest a 1.5-fold to twofold increased risk of mortality even after adjusting for other cardiovascular disorders. Perhaps the most compelling reason for treating patients for atrial fibrillation is the associated symptoms of fatigue, decreased exercise tolerance, uncomfortable palpitation, dizziness, presyncope, and precipitation of angina. Symptoms vary greatly in severity, ranging from minimal or absent (particularly in patients who are otherwise healthy) to severe and disabling (particularly in patients with coexisting structural heart disease).

Because atrial fibrillation is primarily a disease of the elderly, with the aging of the population, its prevalence would be expected to increase. There appears, however, to be an increased incidence and prevalence of atrial fibrillation in recent years not accounted for by the aging of the population alone. Furthermore, there is also now an increased awareness of the syndrome of paroxysmal atrial fibrillation and its attendant symptoms.

Therapy, therefore, is largely directed at the elimination of symptoms and the prevention of serious complications, such as heart failure (tachycardia-induced cardiomyopathy) and thromboembolism.

APPROACH TO TREATMENT

In contemplating therapy for a patient with atrial fibrillation, after excluding treatable or reversible causes of atrial fibrillation (Table 1), three important questions must be considered:

1. *What is the reason for the patient's symptoms?* Patients may be symptomatic from rapid ventricular rates, from slow ventricular rates, from the uncomfortable feeling of irregular heart rates, or because of the loss of atrioventricular synchrony. Ascertaining this can be aided by correlating with monitoring techniques and is essential for rational therapy (Table 2).
2. *What type of atrial fibrillation does the patient have?* Atrial fibrillation may be chronic, persistent, or paroxysmal. Paroxysmal forms of atrial fibrillation in younger subjects without significant heart disease are most amenable to potential curative focal radiofrequency ablation in the pulmonary veins (Table 3).
3. *What, if any, untoward sequelae need to be prevented?* Thromboembolism or tachycardia-induced cardiomyopathy may occur.

TABLE 1. **Associated and Potentially Reversible Causes of Atrial Fibrillation**

Cardiac
Valvular heart disease
Cardiomyopathy
Hypertension
Wolff-Parkinson-White syndrome*
Atrial tachycardia/flutter degenerating into atrial fibrillation*
Noncardiac
Thyrotoxicosis
Alcohol
Stimulant drugs
Pulmonary disease

*Ablation may eradicate atrial fibrillation.

TABLE 2. **Approach to Therapy for Atrial Fibrillation**

Question / Cause	Therapy
1. What is the reason for the patient's symptoms?	
Rapid ventricular rates →	Rx—AV node–blocking drugs —AV node ablation
Slow ventricular rates →	Rx—Pacemaker
Irregularity of heart beats →	Rx—AV node ablation —Maintain sinus rhythm
Loss of AV synchrony →	Rx—Obtain and maintain sinus rhythm
2. Is there a definitive therapy based on the type of atrial fibrillation? →	see Table 3
3. What complications need to be prevented?	
Stroke →	Rx—Anticoagulation —? Maintain sinus rhythm
Tachycardia-induced cardiomyopathy →	Rx—AV node ablation —AV node–blocking drugs

Abbreviation: AV = atrioventricular.

PHARMACOLOGIC RATE CONTROL

Although urgent cardioversion is required for hemodynamic instability, persistent angina, and patients with critical aortic stenosis, most symptoms can be controlled with prompt decrease in ventricular response rate.

Initial control is usually effected with an intravenous agent (Table 4). In our practice we choose β-blockers preferentially in patients with existing anxiety and other high-catecholamine states. In the presence of bronchospasm or other contraindications to β-blockers, calcium channel blockers such as intravenous verapamil (Calan) or diltiazem (Cardizem) are effective. Intravenous digoxin is often combined with these agents so as to decrease their dose and avoid hypotension. Digoxin is particularly useful when there is coexisting heart failure and borderline hypotension. Intravenous calcium can be used to offset the hypotension caused by calcium channel blockers if needed.

For long-term rate control, it is important to remember that digoxin is not as effective during the awake and active hours, when catecholamines primarily drive the ventricular response rates during atrial fibrillation. Thus, for active patients, digoxin alone is usually not effective; the judicious use of β-blockers and/or calcium channel blockers so as to achieve heart rates low enough to avoid symptoms and yet not blunt appropriate increases in heart rates with exercise is preferred.

Achieving adequate rate control with drugs may be difficult when underlying heart disease and ventricular dysfunction result in hypotension and thus the inability to tolerate pharmacologic efforts. Certain clinical situations such as chronic obstructive lung disease, patients on β-agonists, thyrotoxicosis, and decompensated heart failure may make adequate rate control impossible to achieve. Further-

TABLE 3. **Types of Atrial Fibrillation**

Type	Features	Therapeutic Impact
Acute	Initial presentation usually highly symptomatic	
Chronic	Patient remains in atrial fibrillation	Usually restoration of sinus rhythm not feasible
Vagal	Often nocturnal associated with slow ventricular response rates	Consider disopyramide Avoid digoxin
Paroxysmal	Younger patients without structural heart disease, short repetitive self-limited episodes lasting from minutes up to 1 week	Consider focal radiofrequency ablation in the pulmonary veins
Secondary to other arrhythmias	Younger patients; starts as a regular tachycardia but degenerates into a regular palpitation	Effective treatment of Wolff-Parkinson-White syndrome or atrial flutter eliminates atrial fibrillation

more, in certain patients, rate control is not adequate to alleviate symptoms, particularly in patients with diastolic dysfunction such as with hypertrophic cardiomyopathy, in which restoration of sinus rhythm may be paramount.

CARDIOVERSION AND MAINTAINENCE OF SINUS RHYTHM

The optimal therapeutic goal in treating atrial fibrillation is to restore and maintain sinus rhythm.

Acute Cardioversion

In general, for a patient with a first episode of atrial fibrillation, acute cardioversion is undertaken without the use of chronic antiarrhythmic therapy. Acute conversion may be effective with synchronous direct-current shock or the use of antiarrhythmic drugs (Table 5). The likelihood of successful conversion is 50% to 60% for ibutilide (Corvert) and procainamide and 80% to 90% at 1 hour for propafenone. When using ibutilide, it is critical to not use this drug in the presence of a prolonged QT interval or simultaneously with other drugs that can prolong the QT interval.

In our practice, we use direct cardioversion as a first-line approach after appropriate precautions to avoid thromboembolic sequelae (see later). For refractory cases, ibutilide (presumably to decrease defibrillation threshold and to prevent reinitiation of atrial fibrillation), alternative skin patch positions, biphasic waveform shock, and, occasionally, internal cardioversion are used.

TABLE 4. **Initial Rate Control for Atrial Fibrillation**

Agent	Dosage
Calcium channel blockers	
Diltiazem (Cardizem)	0.25 mg/kg IV over 2 minutes; repeat 0.35 mg/kg in 15 minutes if desired heart rate response not achieved and begin continuous infusion between dose of 5–15 mg/h.
Verapamil (Calan, Isoptin)	5–10 mg IV over 2 minutes; repeat with 10 mg after 30 minutes if needed.
β-Blockers	
Esmolol (Brevibloc)	0.5 mg/kg/min IV over 1 minute followed by a 4-minute maintenance infusion of 0.05 mg/kg/min. A maintenance drip at this dose can be used if increasing the dose is desired. A re-bolus needs to be done.
Metoprolol (Lopressor)*	5 mg IV over 2 minutes; repeat every 5 minutes to a total dose of 15 mg.
Digoxin (Lanoxin)	0.25–0.50 mg IV followed by 0.25 mg IV every 4–8 hours not to exceed 1 mg in 24 hours.

*Not FDA approved for this indication.

CHRONIC ANTIARRHYTHMIC THERAPY

In patients with more than one episode of atrial fibrillation who proved to be intolerant to rate control and anticoagulation, consideration is given to chronic antiarrhythmic therapy. The drug efficacy for class IA agents to maintain sinus rhythm is approximately

TABLE 5. **Acute Chemical Conversion to Sinus Rhythm**

Agent	Dosage and Use
Procainamide (Pronestyl)*	10–12 mg/kg typically 1 g IV over 30 minutes
Propafenone (Rythmol)*	800 mg PO as a single dose or 2 mg/kg IV over 10 minutes (IV form not available in United States)
Ibutilide (Corvert)	1 mg IV over 10 minutes; repeat in 10 minutes if sinus rhythm not achieved and QT interval not prolonged.
Amiodarone (Cordarone)*	5 mg/kg IV over 30 minutes followed by 1200 mg over 24 hours

*Not FDA approved for this indication.

50% at 1 to 2 years and is similar for class IC agents. Amiodarone (Cordarone),* a class III drug, has a slightly better chance of maintaining sinus rhythm at 60% at 2 years.

Quinidine

Although quinidine (Quinaglute, Quinidex) (class IA) is effective for both chemical cardioversion of atrial fibrillation and sinus rhythm maintenance, in a meta-analysis of six randomized control trials of quinidine, the total mortality in the quinidine group was significantly higher (2.9% versus 0.8%); this finding has raised serious concerns about the proarrhythmic potential of the drug. Furthermore, quinidine can cause hypotension, diarrhea, and serious proarrhythmia from QT internal prolongation. Quinidine also has potential to increase the ventricular rate by its anticholinergic action on the atrioventricular (AV) node and/or by converting atrial fibrillation to slow atrial flutter with one-to-one conduction. Because of these unfavorable side effects, quinidine is used less frequently in today's practice in treating atrial fibrillation.

Procainamide

Procainamide (Pronestyl)* (class IA) is similar to quinidine in its efficacy as well as the propensity for hypotension, significant proarrhythmic potential, and paradoxical increase in ventricular response rates. Gastrointestinal side effects are less common than with quinidine, but procainamide can cause agranulocytosis and central nervous system side effects and induce a lupus-like syndrome. The utility of procainamide is usually limited in selected situations, such as postoperative atrial fibrillation, when intravenous drug administration is desirable. The intravenous formulation of procainamide has been available in the United States for more than 20 years.

Disopyramide

Disopyramide (Norpace)* differs from other class IA drugs in its profound anticholinergic and negatively inotropic effects. These effects can be used with benefit in patients with vagally mediated atrial fibrillation (athletic patients with heightened vagal tone) as well as in patients with significant diastolic dysfunction (patients with hypertrophic cardiomyopathy).

Propafenone

The efficacy of propafenone (Rythmol)* (class IC) has been studied extensively; this agent is one of the most frequently used drugs for sinus rhythm maintenance. Acute administration is relatively safe, and no deaths or life-threatening tachyarrhythmias have been reported in several studies. This has led to suggestions that selected patients without structural heart disease could use propafenone for acute cardioversion and subsequent rhythm maintenance at home. Severe bradyarrhythmias including sinus arrest and high-grade AV block have been reported with propafenone use, and noncardiac adverse effects such as gastrointestinal symptoms and a metallic taste can occur. Propafenone has weak β-blocking properties.

*Not FDA approved for this indication.

Flecainide

Flecainide (Tambocor) (class IC) is similar to propafenone in its efficacy and safety but lacks its β-blocking properties. Because of the increased mortality observed in patients with coronary artery disease and compromised ejection fraction when flecainide was used for the suppression of asymptomatic premature ventricular contractions and nonsustained ventricular tachycardia, and because of its moderate negative inotropic effect, flecainide has been primarily reserved for treating atrial fibrillation in patients with a structurally normal heart.

Sotalol

Sotalol (Betapace) (class III) is effective for long-term maintenance of sinus rhythm in 50% to 60% of patients. Its reverse use dependence makes it less effective at rapid rates, but its overall efficacy is similar to that of quinidine and propafenone. Sotalol's propensity to cause QT interval prolongation is worsened at higher doses, and with coexisting hypokalemia and bradycardia. Furthermore, dose reduction is required in patients with renal dysfunction.

Dofetilide

Dofetilide (Tikosyn) is a class III agent that has recently become available for clinical use in the United States. It has an efficacy for acute cardioversion of atrial fibrillation of about 31% at 6 hours. Importantly, dofetilide has not been associated with increased mortality in patients with left ventricular dysfunction or after myocardial infarction. Hemodynamic changes are minimal during acute administration of this drug.

Amiodarone

Amiodarone (Cordarone)* is an antiarrhythmic drug with multiple actions on several facets of cardiac depolarization and repolarization. Amiodarone is quite effective in sinus rhythm maintenance and is superior to other antiarrhythmic drugs at 2 years (60%). The major advantage of amiodarone is that it has little or no negative inotropic effect and is well tolerated in patients with congestive heart failure. The major disadvantage, however, is serious and po-

*Not FDA approved for this indication.

tentially life-threatening noncardiac toxicity, including lung and liver toxicity, whereas corneal deposits and thyroid toxicity occur more frequently but are not life threatening. The dose of amiodarone to maintain sinus rhythm is lower than that used to treat ventricular dysrhythmias. At the lower dose, usually 200 mg/d, incidence of amiodarone-mediated toxicity is significantly reduced.

In our practice, propafenone, flecainide, and sotalol are typically used to maintain sinus rhythm in patients without structural heart disease, whereas amiodarone and, more recently, dofetilide are used in patients with decreased ventricular function. The outright poor efficacy of antiarrhythmic drugs coupled with their serious cardiac and noncardiac toxicity makes maintenance of sinus rhythm a formidable task.

ANTICOAGULATION

The issue of anticoagulation needs to be addressed in all patients with atrial fibrillation. The annual incidence of stroke in elderly patients with nonvalvular atrial fibrillation is approximately 5%; by comparison, the rate is 1% for similar populations in sinus rhythm. Nearly all randomized trials have shown that anticoagulation in patients with nonrheumatic atrial fibrillation reduces the risk of stroke to levels comparable to those in the general population. Thus, all patients with atrial fibrillation in the absence of a definite contraindication should be either on aspirin, 325 mg/d, or on warfarin (Coumadin). After a decision to proceed with anticoagulation, a choice between aspirin and warfarin must be made. Based on the data from four large multicenter trials, it is clear that warfarin is superior to aspirin in preventing stroke in high-risk populations. Higher risk is associated with age older than 65 years and the presence of one or more of the following conditions: hypertension, prior myocardial infarction, prior stroke, mitral valve stenosis, congestive heart failure, thyrotoxicosis, dilated or hypertrophic cardiomyopathy, prior surgical repair of an atrial septal defect, and diabetes mellitus. Table 6 outlines the decision-making process regarding anticoagulation based on these factors. When warfarin is used, the International Normalized Ratio (INR) should be maintained between 2 and 3. An INR of less than 2 does not effectively decrease the risk of stroke, whereas an INR of more than 3 significantly increases the risk, particularly in the elderly.

TABLE 6. **Choosing the Mode of Anticoagulation for Patients With Atrial Fibrillation**

Age (y)	Risk Factors*	Therapy
<65	Present	Warfarin (INR 2–3)
<65	Absent	None or aspirin
≥65	Present	Warfarin (INR 2–3)
≥65	Absent	Warfarin (INR 2–3)

*See text.
Abbreviation: INR = International Normalized Ratio.

Anticoagulation for Cardioversion

The risk of thromboembolism with acute cardioversion in patients with atrial fibrillation that has been present for fewer than 48 hours is comparable to that of the general population and is quite low (0.8%). For patients with atrial fibrillation longer than this or of unknown duration, anticoagulation for 3 to 4 weeks before attempts at cardioversion (either electrical or chemical) is necessary. Present evidence suggests that transesophageal echocardiography is effective in excluding atrial thrombi and allows earlier cardioversion in patients with atrial fibrillation of unknown duration. Thrombi are detected in around 15% of patients in this setting. Although definitive data from large studies are pending, this approach is being increasingly used. It is critical that anticoagulation be continued for at least 4 to 6 weeks after cardioversion because the risk of thromboembolism continues after cardioversion both because of mechanical atrial stunning and the risk of recurrent atrial fibrillation.

NONPHARMACOLOGIC APPROACHES TO MANAGING ATRIAL FIBRILLATION

Atrioventricular Node Ablation

For patients who are symptomatic from rapid or highly variable ventricular rates during atrial fibrillation, AV node ablation with pacemaker implantation is effective in relieving these symptoms and improving the quality of life. Furthermore, exercise tolerance and, in patients with tachycardia-induced cardiomyopathy, left ventricular function have been shown to improve after ablation. A major concern with this approach has been the creation of permanent pacemaker dependence and its potential negative effect on survival, but in one large study, it was demonstrated that long-term survival is comparable to that of control populations.

Maze Procedure

The surgical Maze procedure is effective in 80% to 90% of patients in maintaining sinus rhythm in the long term. The major drawback of this procedure is the requirement for open heart surgery, which may be accompanied by a 2% to 3% mortality risk, prolonged hospital stay, and other associated morbidities. There is an increased need for chronic pacing in 2% to 5% of patients after the surgical Maze procedure.

The Catheter Maze Procedure

Initial reported success with mimicking the surgical Maze procedure with an endocardial catheter-based process has not been reproducible, and this procedure has been largely abandoned because of lack of efficacy and prohibitive risks of cardiac perforation and stroke. Feasibility of this approach with investigational catheters will continue to evolve.

Pacemaker Techniques

Pacing techniques under evaluation to help prevent atrial fibrillation, particularly in patients with paroxysmal atrial fibrillation, including dual-site right atrial pacing, Bachmann bundle pacing, and coronary sinus pacing, have looked promising in initial studies. Such alternative methods of pacing should be considered in patients with atrial fibrillation who are receiving a pacemaker for an established condition.

Implantable Atrial Defibrillators

Implanted defibrillators that can be used to internally convert atrial fibrillation to sinus rhythm are being investigated. Although effective, the widespread use of such devices is limited by the pain associated with defibrillation. Furthermore, these are not effective in patients with frequently recurring paroxysms of atrial fibrillation but may be combined with other modalities of therapy.

Focal Ablation in the Pulmonary Veins

Perhaps the most increasingly widespread and intriguing nonpharmacologic therapy for atrial fibrillation is the targeted ablation of triggering foci in the pulmonary veins. In patients with spontaneous recurrences of atrial fibrillation after cardioversion or with repeated occurrences of atrial fibrillation, the earliest activating site (triggering focus) is mapped using multiple electrode-tipped catheters in both atria and the pulmonary veins. In up to 85% of patients with paroxysmal atrial fibrillation, a triggering focus can be identified in the pulmonary veins (usually the superior pulmonary veins). Either ablation of the triggering site or circumferential ablation at the ostium of the pulmonary veins so as to electrically dissociate the vein from the left atrium has been reported to effectively "cure" patients of this dysrhythmia in up to 50% of cases. Although several unanswered questions exist, including those regarding the optimal site for ablation in patients without spontaneous atrial fibrillation, the long-term effectiveness, the long-term risk for stroke, the ideal energy source, and the ideal methods for preablation selection of patients, this therapy is presently considered a major breakthrough in the nonpharmacologic therapy for atrial fibrillation.

CONCLUSION

Atrial fibrillation is the most common dysrhythmia associated with significant morbidity and mortality, with a major socioeconomic burden on the health care system. Mechanisms of atrial fibrillation are complex in a heterogeneous patient population. Great strides have been made in treating patients with atrial fibrillation in the areas of rate control, maintenance of sinus rhythm, and stroke prevention. A "cure," however, may be possible in only a few selected patients. Basic (e.g., arrhythmogenic mechanisms, atrial remodeling, genetic predisposition) and clinical (e.g., new antiarrhythmic agents, oral antithrombin agents, mapping and ablation devices) investigations are vigorously moving forward. Treating atrial fibrillation is more challenging than ever before because new therapeutic modalities are developed at a rampant pace. The ultimate goal of treating patients, however, should remain the same—the most effective therapy at the lowest risk with evidence-based strategy.

PREMATURE BEATS

method of
LAURENCE D. STERNS, M.D.
Implantable Cardioverter Defibrillator Clinic
Victoria, British Columbia, Canada

Atrial and ventricular premature beats (APBs and VPBs, respectively) are normal physiologic events in every human being. However, occasionally, these beats may arise from unknown cardiac pathology and together with this pathology could adversely affect the patient's prognosis. This chapter will address the presentation of a patient with premature beats as well as the differentiation between atrial and ventricular ectopy. A stepwise approach to the investigations and therapy is also presented. The underlying goals throughout are to maximize patient prognosis while minimizing patient symptoms.

PRESENTATION

Patients with premature beats may present with asymptomatic or symptomatic ectopy. Asymptomatic premature beats may be picked up as an incidental finding on routine investigations such as a physical examination, electrocardiography, or another test requiring monitoring. At times the patient will find them on a community testing machine such as a blood pressure monitor or heart monitor on exercise equipment. Sometimes they will detect "skipped beats" on taking their own pulse.

Patients may complain of many symptoms that are attributed to ectopic beats, even if those symptoms may not be related to the ectopy. These symptoms may include the following:

- Palpitations
- Shortness of breath
- Cough
- Chest pain
- Light-headedness
- Syncope
- Exercise intolerance

Many of these symptoms occur most often at rest because that is when patients are most likely to notice cardiac irregularities. Often the symptoms are worse when the patient is lying on the left side because this is the position that brings the heart closest to the chest wall and makes the person more aware of the beat. The symptoms are also affected by many noncardiac factors, such as anxiety, meals, fever, menstrual cycles, and medications.

Cough is more frequently a symptom of VPBs because it causes a reverse pressure wave in the pulmonary veins when the normal atrial contraction occurs against the mitral valve that has been closed from the VPB. This pressure wave stimulates stretch receptors in the lungs that trigger the cough reflex. Most other symptoms can occur from premature beats of either atrial or ventricular origin.

ELECTROCARDIOGRAPHIC DIAGNOSIS AND DIFFERENTIATION

An electrocardiogram (ECG) is the best way to differentiate APBs and VPBs. A 12-lead ECG capturing the ectopic beats is most accurate; however, a rhythm strip from a monitor or Holter recorder can often provide enough information. APBs are most often identified as a P wave complex occurring before the next expected sinus beat, frequently with a P wave morphology different than that of the intrinsic sinus beat. In general, most APBs will be followed by a narrow QRS complex, or, in the case of an underlying bundle-branch block, a QRS complex the same as the usual sinus QRSs. However, if the APB follows closely after the preceding QRS complex, it is possible that the QRS complex after the APB will have a different bundle-branch block morphology. This occurs because one or the other of the infra-Hisian bundles may be refractory at the time of conduction of the APB, leading to conduction down only one of the bundles and a subsequent bundle-branch block pattern. It is also possible that either the atrioventricular (AV) node itself or both of the main infra-Hisian bundles could be refractory at the time of the APB, leading to no QRS complex. This could be read inappropriately as AV nodal block. Alternately, if the APB is hidden in the preceding T wave, the delay until the next sinus beat could be inappropriately interpreted as a sinus pause.

VPBs are usually identified as wide-complex beats falling before the next expected sinus beat. In contrast to APBs, there is no early atrial contraction preceding the QRS. Occasionally, VPBs will occur just after a sinus beat but before the normal QRS complex. In these cases, the initial part of the QRS complex will be from the ectopic focus and the latter part from the usual conduction pathway, leading to a "fusion" complex. The concept of premature beats does not really apply during atrial fibrillation because the irregularity of the rhythm precludes predicting when the next beat would be due. However, wide-complex beats with their suspected origin in the ventricle during atrial fibrillation are still frequently referred to as VPBs.

One way to differentiate between an APB with aberrant conduction and a VPB is by the timing of the next sinus beat. An APB by definition excites the atrium and will usually penetrate into the sinus node, "resetting" the node early and advancing the timing of the next expected sinus beat. As a result, the time from the sinus beat before the APB to the sinus beat after the APB is less than the expected time for two cardiac cycles. This is termed a *noncompensatory pause*. In contrast, a VPB may not occur early enough to enter into the His-Purkinje system, conduct up the AV node, and then conduct through the atrium to the sinus node before it fires for the next expected sinus beat. The sinus node will therefore depolarize on time, but usually it does not conduct to the ventricle because of the recent activation of the AV node from the VPB. As such, there is no resetting of the sinus node and the following sinus beat is delivered at the time expected. The timing of the sinus beat before the VPB to the sinus beat after the VPB is therefore exactly twice the normal sinus interval. This is termed a *compensatory pause*.

ATRIAL PREMATURE BEATS

Clinical Significance

APBs alone are benign, although in some cases they may cause symptoms, including palpitations, shortness of breath, exercise intolerance, and, rarely, dizziness. However, they can become more clinically significant if they induce atrial fibrillation or supraventricular tachyarrhythmia. These arrhythmias may be much more symptomatic and could cause more significant problems, such as the risk of stroke or syncope. These arrhythmias are covered in separate chapters.

Pathophysiology

APBs can be caused by anything that irritates or stretches the atrium. This could include pericarditis, congestive heart failure, pulmonary hypertension, chronic obstructive pulmonary disease, mitral valve disease, or cardiomyopathy. Exogenous stimulants such as caffeine, alcohol, and nicotine, or other drugs such as bronchodilators, can also trigger APBs. They can also be stimulated by high endogenous catecholamines such as with stress or other systemic illness.

Investigations

Patients with frequent APBs should be investigated to rule out any potential initiating factors such as thyrotoxicosis, significant lung disease, or pericarditis. A thyroid-stimulating hormone determination, electrolyte panel, magnesium and calcium determinations, hemoglobin, and chest radiograph should be done in all patients. A Holter monitor may be of value to determine the frequency of the APBs and to see if there are other associated arrhythmias such as atrial fibrillation. Other tests, such as an echocardiogram, should be considered if the history is suggestive of structural heart disease or if the APBs are found to degenerate into atrial fibrillation.

Treatment

The best treatment of uncomplicated APBs is reassurance to the patient that the irregularities that he or she feels are not dangerous and that the risk of serious problems is exceedingly low. Often, with such reassurance patients will gradually become less aware of the irregular pulse over time and the symptoms will clear. It is worth recommending a decrease in stimulants such as caffeine and smoking, and the patients should avoid drinking large quantities of alcohol. Use of other stimulating medications such as bronchodilators and theophylline should be minimized if possible.

If the patient still has symptoms after these conservative measures, then suppression of the ectopy can be attempted with β-blockers such as metoprolol (Lopressor),* 25 to 50 mg bid, or atenolol (Tenormin),* 25 to 50 mg/d. This will usually decrease catecholamine-dependent APBs, but it may not affect the number of ectopic events that occur at rest. The other possible benefit of treatment with β-blockers is a decrease in the intensity of the beat after the APB, because there is a longer diastolic interval before this beat from the noncompensatory pause and therefore more filling of the heart. This postectopic beat would therefore have a greater preload and, through increased Starling forces, a greater force and volume of contraction that is often felt by the patient. The β-blocker will decrease this force of contraction and often minimize the symptoms. If a patient cannot tolerate β-blockers, then calcium channel blockers such as verapamil, 240 mg/d, or diltiazem, 240 mg/d, could provide a similar benefit (Table 1).

Rarely, patients will continue to be symptomatic and more aggressive antiarrhythmic therapy is necessary. It is important to stress to the patient that antiarrhythmic drug or ablation therapy does carry risk, whereas the APBs alone are usually benign. The treatment in this case may be worse than the disease. However, if the patient's symptoms warrant, then antiarrhythmic drugs such as flecainide (Tambocor), 50 to 100 mg bid or propafenone (Rythmol), 150 to 300 mg bid could be tried. These drugs have a significant potential for proarrhythmia in patients with structural heart disease and therefore should only be used in patients with structurally normal hearts. In patients with ischemic or structural heart disease, sotalol (Betapace), 40 to 80 mg bid to tid could be tried. However, sotalol should be used with caution because it carries a small risk of a potentially life-threatening polymorphic ventricular tachycardia called torsades de pointes. This is especially worrisome in those who are elderly, female, and of smaller stature and in patients who have congestive heart failure, have renal failure, or are on diuretics that could decrease potassium levels. Amiodarone (Cordarone),* 100 to 200 mg/d (after an appropriate loading regimen of 400 mg bid for 2 weeks), is a very effective antiarrhythmic with a very low risk of causing dangerous proarrhythmia. However, it can produce side effects, including bradycardia, increased heart block, corneal deposits, skin photosensitivity, and the possibility of long-term effects on the thyroid and liver; thus, amiodarone should be used only when the clinical situation is significant enough to warrant its use.

*Not FDA approved for this indication.

In certain cases of very frequent APBs that have a single morphology, the origin of the APBs can be mapped in an electrophysiology laboratory and ablated to eliminate the arrhythmia. This has been done most often when the APBs also occur in runs of symptomatic ectopic atrial tachycardia and when they lead to atrial fibrillation, but it can be used for very symptomatic atrial ectopy as well.

VENTRICULAR PREMATURE BEATS

Clinical Significance

Asymptomatic VPBs are frequently found on routine clinical evaluation of healthy, asymptomatic people. The incidence increases with age and with the presence of structural heart disease. In some cases,

*Not FDA approved for this indication.

TABLE 1. **Initial and Secondary Therapy for Symptomatic Premature Beats of Atrial or Ventricular Origin***

Premature Beat Origin	Structural Heart Disease	Initial Therapy	Secondary Therapy
Atrial	No	β-Blockers Calcium blockers	Class IC drugs Class III drugs Ablation
Atrial	Yes	β-Blockers Calcium blockers	Class III drugs
Ventricular	No	β-Blockers Calcium blockers	Class IC drugs Class III drugs Ablation
Ventricular	IHD − EF >35%	β-Blockers	Class III drugs
Ventricular	IHD − EF <35%	Amiodarone	β-Blockers
Ventricular	DCM	β-Blockers	Amiodarone
Ventricular	HCM, ARVC	Consult a specialist	

*The calcium blockers referred to in this table include verapamil and diltiazem only. Class IC drugs include propafenone and flecainide. Class III drugs include sotalol and amiodarone.

Abbreviations: ARVC = arrhythmogenic right ventricular cardiomyopathy; DCM = dilated cardiomyopathy; EF = ejection fraction; HCM = hypertrophic cardiomyopathy; IHD = ischemic heart disease.

VPBs will be the first marker of ischemic or other types of heart disease; however, the vast majority of people with VPBs will have a structurally normal heart.

Pathophysiology

The majority of VPBs are benign, possibly owing to stimulation or activation of automatic cells that reside within the ventricles or His-Purkinje system. VPBs may be stimulated by the same factors that cause APBs, including caffeine, alcohol, and some sympathomimetic medications. However, other more disconcerting causes of VPBs include coronary artery disease with ischemia and various cardiomyopathies. These possible causes include idiopathic dilated cardiomyopathy as well as other more unusual forms, such as hypertrophic cardiomyopathy (HCM) and arrhythmogenic right ventricular cardiomyopathy (ARVC, sometimes called ARVD—*arrhythmogenic right ventricular dysplasia*). The reason why these other causes may be of more concern is the potential negative prognosis from the conditions, from both the conditions themselves and the possible initiation of lethal ventricular arrhythmias from the VPBs. It is therefore very important to rule out these conditions before addressing the VPBs.

Approach to the Patient

A complete history must be done to search for any symptoms of coronary artery disease, and an evaluation of the risk factors for the development of atherosclerosis should be performed. A family history is important to consider other types of inheritable conditions such as HCM, ARVC, or the long QT syndrome. If a patient has a family history of these conditions or of unexplained sudden cardiac death, VPBs must be much more vigorously investigated. Symptoms of possible associated conditions such as thyrotoxicosis must be considered and ruled out on history and laboratory evaluation.

The physical examination must be thorough to examine for signs of any atherosclerosis or indicators of structural heart disease, including the provocable murmurs of hypertrophic obstructive cardiomyopathy (HOCM) or mitral valve prolapse. If there is any suggestion or suspicion of heart disease, then further investigations must be carried out, including a treadmill test to look for ischemia or exercise potentiation of arrhythmias and an echocardiogram to rule out structural abnormalities. Further investigations such as perfusion scanning with thallium or sestamibi or cardiac catheterization would be reserved for those with abnormalities on the initial tests. Baseline laboratory investigations should also include determination of thyroid-stimulating hormone, hemoglobin, electrolytes, magnesium, calcium, blood urea nitrogen, and creatinine.

ECG documentation of the VPBs is mandatory to make the diagnosis and may help to delineate the cause of the ectopic beats. The morphology of the VPBs may be of value to a specialist in determining their origin. If all of the VPBs are of a single morphology on the ECG, there is usually a focal site that is causing the beats that may possibly be explained or ablated by an electrophysiologist if necessary. If the VPBs are of several different morphologies, they may be due to a more diffuse process that could have an impact on the prognosis. A Holter monitor is a valuable tool in evaluating patients with VPBs. It allows a determination of the frequency and morphology of the beats as well as their relationship to activity and rest. The Holter monitor will often help in ruling in or out a correlation between symptoms and the ectopic beats themselves. A patient who is found to have palpitations and VPBs may not actually have symptoms from the VPBs but rather palpitations from awareness of his or her regular heart beat and asymptomatic ectopic beats.

Therapy

Normal Heart

If no structural heart disease is found in the workup of the patient, the most likely diagnosis is benign ventricular ectopy. As the name suggests, this is ventricular ectopy from usually a single focus that can be extremely bothersome but is not known to lead to more dangerous arrhythmias. In these patients, reassurance is the best therapy, along with an explanation of the fact that their symptoms are real but common and not dangerous. Patients should also be counseled to decrease intake of caffeine and alcohol and to quit smoking. By following such advice, patients frequently find that their symptoms subside significantly even if the VPBs do not go away. Moreover, removing stress and anxiety surrounding the VPB symptoms will frequently decrease patients' endogenous catecholamine levels, which will also decrease the frequency and intensity of the ectopic beats.

In some patients no amount of reassurance and education will alleviate the symptoms and other therapy is necessary. In these patients it is again important to recognize the benign nature of the condition and to make sure that the treatment is not worse than the disease. The initial medical therapy should be a β-blocker such as metoprolol,* 25 to 50 mg PO bid or atenolol,* 25 to 50 mg/d PO OD (see Table 1). This will frequently decrease the frequency of the VPBs. Even if it does not decrease their frequency, the drug will decrease the intensity of the accentuated beats after the compensatory pause, which decreases patient awareness of the arrhythmia. If the patient cannot tolerate β-blockers, an alternate would be long-acting verapamil (Calan, Isoptin)* or diltiazem (Cardizem),* 120 to 240 mg/d.

In patients with ongoing symptoms despite all of the previously mentioned measures, referral to a specialist may be in order. An electrophysiologist may

*Not FDA approved for this indication.

be able to offer alternate therapies, including radiofrequency catheter ablation of some ectopic ventricular foci, or in some instances may recommend more powerful antiarrhythmic drugs. The routine use of antiarrhythmic drugs in a patient with a structurally normal heart may harbor a risk of proarrhythmia, giving the patient an unnecessary risk of significant morbidity or mortality.

Structural Heart Disease

Patients with structural heart disease must be considered differently because of their potentially worse prognosis and different responses to medications. If premature beats lead to investigations revealing HCM or right ventricular dysplasia, the patient should be referred to a specialist for evaluation of the risk of sudden death and any possible treatment. If investigations reveal a diagnosis of ischemic heart disease or dilated cardiomyopathy, the prognosis usually depends on the severity of the underlying disease.

If the patient has relatively well preserved left ventricular function (ejection fraction >40%), the risk of the VPBs is usually quite low, regardless of the number of VPBs seen on evaluation. In these cases, the best treatment is usually a β-blocker, which will often decrease the frequency of the VPBs and protect the patient from adverse events from the underlying disease. In some cases the patient will have significant symptoms from the VPBs that are not resolved by the β-blocker. In this case, switching to sotalol,* 40 to 80 mg bid to tid could be used for β-blocker protection and symptom relief. Sotalol should be used with caution in patients who are elderly, are female, are of small stature, or have renal dysfunction because of the risk of proarrhythmia. In these patients, amiodarone* may be more effective and safer, with a loading dose of 400 mg bid for 2 weeks, then a maintenance dose of 300 to 400 mg/d. Other antiarrhythmic drugs such as the class IC drugs should not be used in this patient population because of the risk of increased mortality. The Cardiac Arrhythmia Suppression Trial (CAST) examined the use of these agents to decrease VPBs and hopefully decrease mortality in patients with ischemic heart disease. Unfortunately, the treatment group in this trial had greater than three times the mortality of the placebo group, indicating an increased risk of sudden death with the use of these agents in patients with ischemic heart disease. This study seemed to indicate that the VPBs are a marker for sudden death in some patients but are not actually the trigger that causes it, because suppression of the VPBs does not improve the prognosis.

In patients with low ejection fractions and frequent VPBs, there seems to be a significant increase in the risk of sudden cardiac death. In these patients there is good evidence that treatment not only decreases symptoms but also improves prognosis. In the landmark Canadian Amiodarone Myocardial Infarction Trial (CAMIAT) and European Myocardial Infarction Amiodarone Trial (EMIAT), patients with ischemic heart disease and either low ejection fractions or frequent VPBs were randomized to amiodarone or placebo. These studies showed a significant decrease in arrhythmic death in those patients on treatment versus placebo and a decrease in total mortality in the group with the lowest ejection fractions. Therefore, patients with low ejection fractions and frequent VPBs should be considered for treatment with amiodarone, regardless of their symptomatic status, to improve their prognosis. There also seemed to be a synergistic effect between amiodarone and β-blockers noted in these studies, indicating that patients should be treated with both agents if possible.

In patients with poor ejection fractions (<35%) and frequent or more advanced ventricular ectopy including runs of nonsustained ventricular tachycardia, there is good evidence that there is an extremely high risk of sudden arrhythmic death. In the Multicenter Automatic Defibrillator Implantation Trial (MADIT) and Multicenter Unsustained Tachycardia Trial (MUSTT), these patients were evaluated with electrophysiologic testing to see if sustained ventricular tachycardia could be induced. If sustained ventricular tachycardia could be induced and was not easily suppressed with medications, then the patients were treated with either an implantable cardioverter defibrillator (ICD) or more conventional therapy, including antiarrhythmic drugs. In both of these studies, the patients treated with prophylactic implantation of an ICD had a significantly lower mortality than patients treated with drugs. It is routine practice now to evaluate patients with ischemic heart disease, low ejection fractions, and nonsustained ventricular tachycardia with an electrophysiologic study; and if inducible ventricular tachycardia is found, a prophylactic ICD should be inserted. Further studies are being carried out looking at all patients with low ejection fractions to see if ICD or amiodarone can improve their prognosis regardless of ventricular ectopy.

*Not FDA approved for this indication.

HEART BLOCK

method of
S. SERGE BAROLD, M.D.
Broward General Hospital
Ft. Lauderdale, Florida

and

DAVID L. HAYES, M.D.
The Mayo Clinic
Rochester, Minnesota

There are many causes of heart block, but progressive idiopathic fibrosis of the conduction system is the most common cause of chronic acquired atrioventricular (AV) block, related to an aging process of the cardiac skeleton. Barring congenital AV block, Lyme disease is the most common cause of reversible third-degree AV block in young individuals and it is usually AV nodal. Before implantation of a permanent pacemaker, reversible causes of AV block such as Lyme disease, athletic heart, hypervagotonia, sleep apnea, ischemia, and drug, metabolic, or electrolyte imbalance must be excluded. Table 1 outlines the classification used in the 1998 American College of Cardiology/American Heart Association (ACC/AHA) guidelines for pacemaker implantation. The indications for permanent pacing in *symptomatic* patients with second- or third-degree AV block are often straightforward. The decision to implant a pacemaker in *asymptomatic* patients is more difficult and requires knowledge of the pathophysiology and natural history of AV block (Tables 2 and 3).

ANATOMIC AND ELECTROPHYSIOLOGIC CONSIDERATIONS

The specialized conduction system below the AV node consists of the bundle of His proximally and the three intraventricular fascicles distally: the right bundle branch, the anterior (superior) division of the left bundle branch, and the posterior (inferior) division of the left bundle branch (Figure 1). Although the left bundle branch does not exist as two discrete anatomic divisions, this functional separation is a useful concept clinically and electrocardiographically. Left anterior hemiblock (LAH) causes left axis deviation and left posterior hemiblock (LPH) causes right axis deviation in the frontal plane. Disease in any one of the three fascicles is of little clinical significance. When the electrocardiogram (ECG) shows evidence of block in two fascicles (bifascicular block), only one pathway remains for AV conduction. Bifascicular block may be identified on the ECG when there is right bundle branch block (RBBB) with LAH, RBBB with LPH, or left bundle branch block (LBBB). In bifascicular block without documented second- or third-degree AV block, the functional status of the third fascicle cannot be evaluated from the ECG.

TABLE 1. **Standard ACC/AHA Format for Device Indications**

Class I	Conditions for which there is evidence and/or general agreement that a given procedure or treatment is beneficial, useful, and effective
Class II	Conditions for which there is conflicting evidence and/or a divergence of opinion about the usefulness/efficacy of a procedure or treatment
Class IIa	Weight of evidence/opinion in favor of usefulness/efficacy
Class IIb	Usefulness/efficacy less well established by evidence/opinion
Class III	Conditions for which there is evidence and/or general agreement that a procedure/treatment is not useful/effective and in some cases may be harmful

Adapted from ACC/AHA Guidelines for Implantation of Cardiac Pacemakers and Antiarrhythmia Devices: A Report of the American College of Cardiology/American Heart Association Task Force on Practice Guidelines (Committee on Pacemaker Implantation). *J Am Coll Cardiol* 1998;31:1175–1209. Copyright 1998 by the American College of Cardiology and American Heart Association, Inc. Permission granted for one time use. Further reproduction is not permitted without permission of the ACC/AHA.

TABLE 2. **Indications for Pacing in Acquired AV Block in Adults**

Class I

A. Permanent or intermittent complete AV block at any anatomic level in the absence of reversible causes, regardless of symptoms
B. Permanent or intermittent asymptomatic type II second-degree AV block
C. Permanent or intermittent second-degree AV block regardless of the type or the site of block, with symptomatic bradycardia
D. Asymptomatic type I or advanced second-degree AV block at intra-His or infra-His levels
E. Exercise-induced second or complete AV block regardless of symptoms but in the absence of reversible ischemia
F. Complete AV block or documented progression of AV block or His-Purkinje disease of any degree in patients with neuromuscular diseases (e.g., myotonic muscular dystrophy, Kearns-Sayre syndrome, limb-girdle dystrophy of Erb, and peroneal muscular atrophy. (Progression could be any number of electrocardiographic changes, such as first-degree AV block to second-degree AV block, bifascicular block to intermittent or chronic trifascicular block and so on.)
G. Atrial fibrillation, atrial flutter, or rare cases of supraventricular tachycardia with AV block and bradycardia associated with congestive heart failure or periods of asystole >3.0 seconds or escape rates <40 beats per minute or alternating tachycardia and bradycardia difficult to control pharmacologically. The bradycardia must be unrelated to drugs known to impair AV conduction.

Class II

A. Symptomatic first-degree AV block (i.e., when hemodynamic and symptomatic states are attributable to marked prolongation of the PR interval at rest and with exercise)

Class III

A. Asymptomatic first-degree AV block
B. Asymptomatic type I second-degree AV block at the supra-His (AV nodal) level

Adapted from ACC/AHA Guidelines for Implantation of Cardiac Pacemakers and Antiarrhythmia Devices: A Report of the American College of Cardiology/American Heart Association Task Force on Practice Guidelines (Committee on Pacemaker Implantation). *J Am Coll Cardiol* 1998;31:1175–1209. Copyright 1998 by the American College of Cardiology and American Heart Association, Inc. Permission granted for one time use. Further reproduction is not permitted without permission of the ACC/AHA; and Hayes DL, Barold SS, Camm AJ, Goldschlager NF: Evolving indications for permanent cardiac pacing: An appraisal of the 1998 American College of Cardiology/American Heart Association Guidelines. Am J Cardiol 82:1082–1086, 1998.

During 1:1 AV conduction the diagnosis of trifascicular block can only be made in rare situations involving alternating RBBB and LBBB or RBBB with alternating LAH and LPH.

INTRACARDIAC RECORDINGS

The His bundle potential is easily recorded with an electrode catheter passed from the femoral vein to the level of the tricuspid valve. The A wave reflects depolarization of the low right atrium, the V deflection is produced by ventricular depolarization near the recording catheter, and the H deflection is generated by rapid transmission of depolarization through the bundle of His and appears between the A and V waves (see Figure 1). The AH interval (normal is 60–140 ms) basically reflects AV nodal conduction (rarely intra-atrial delay), and the HV interval (normal is 35–55 ms) reflects the conduction time from the His bundle to the beginning of ventricular activa-

TABLE 3. **Indications for Permanent Pacing Intraventricular Conduction Blocks**

Class I

A. Bundle branch block* or bifascicular block with intermittent or stable second or complete AV block associated with symptomatic bradycardia (see Table 2)
B. Bundle branch block* or bifascicular block with intermittent or stable type II second-degree AV block without symptoms (see Table 2)
C. Bundle branch block* or bifascicular block with intermittent or stable infranodal block without symptoms: type I second-degree, advanced second-degree, or complete AV block† (see Table 2)
D. Trifascicular block during 1:1 AV conduction regardless of symptoms such as alternating left bundle branch block and right bundle branch block or fixed right bundle branch block with alternating left anterior hemiblock and left posterior hemiblock
E. Exercise-induced second or complete AV block regardless of symptoms, but without demonstrable ischemia as a cause of AV block (see Table 2)
F. Bradycardia (or phase 4) dependent second- or third-degree infranodal AV block either spontaneous or induced by carotid sinus massage or electrically induced atrial or ventricular extrasystoles during an electrophysiologic study

Class II

A. Bundle branch block* or bifascicular block with syncope that is not proved to be due to complete AV block, but other possible causes of syncope are not identified especially when HV ≥70 ms
B. Markedly prolonged HV interval (≥100 ms) regardless of symptoms
C. Infra-His block induced by atrial pacing
D. Infra-His block induced by ventricular pacing (fatigue phenomenon)

Class III

A. Hemiblock, bundle branch block, or bifascicular block without second-degree or complete AV block or symptoms
B. Hemiblock, bundle branch block, or bifascicular block with (or without) first-degree AV block without symptoms

*There is no need to state whether this is left bundle branch block or right bundle branch block because left bundle branch block is bifascicular block. Right bundle branch block is described as bundle branch block rather than unifascicular block to avoid confusion with left anterior (fascicular) hemiblock or left posterior (fascicular) hemiblock.

†The term *trifascicular block* used in the ACC/AHA guidelines to describe this entity is redundant.

Adapted from ACC/AHA Guidelines for Implantation of Cardiac Pacemakers and Antiarrhythmia Devices: A Report of the American College of Cardiology/American Heart Association Task Force on Practice Guidelines (Committee on Pacemaker Implantation). *J Am Coll Cardiol* 1998;31:1175–1209. Copyright 1998 by the American College of Cardiology and American Heart Association, Inc. Permission granted for one time use. Further reproduction is not permitted without permission of the ACC/AHA.

tion, that is, the His-Purkinje system. Bifascicular block is associated with a normal HV interval if conduction in the third fascicle remains intact. Consequently, a prolonged HV interval strongly suggests delayed conduction in all three fascicles. However, HV delay may occasionally be within the His bundle itself or due to a combination of delay in the His bundle and the three fascicles. Prolongation of the PR interval in the ECG is an unreliable indicator of bifascicular or trifascicular disease because it may be due to prolongation of the AH and/or HV intervals. Consequently, RBBB + LAH + first-degree AV block should not be designated as trifascicular block unless invasive recordings demonstrate prolongation of the HV interval. Finally, asymptomatic patients with bundle branch block do not require determination of the HV interval because the risk of developing complete AV block is very low, at 1% to 2% per year.

The development of second- or third-degree His-Purkinje block in an electrophysiologic "stress test" performed by gradually increasing the atrial rate by pacing is an insensitive sign of conduction system disease but constitutes an indication for pacing because it correlates with a high incidence of third-degree AV block or sudden death. Almost all cases of exercise-induced AV block are due to disease of the His-Purkinje system, with a poor prognosis. In most of these patients incremental atrial pacing demonstrates tachycardia-dependent His-Purkinje block. Rarely, exercise-induced AV block is caused by myocardial ischemia that does not require pacing unless ischemia cannot be alleviated. Finally, a drug challenge with procainamide that depresses His-Purkinje conduction may be used to provoke HV interval prolongation or actual His-Purkinje block in susceptible patients and define the need for a pacemaker.

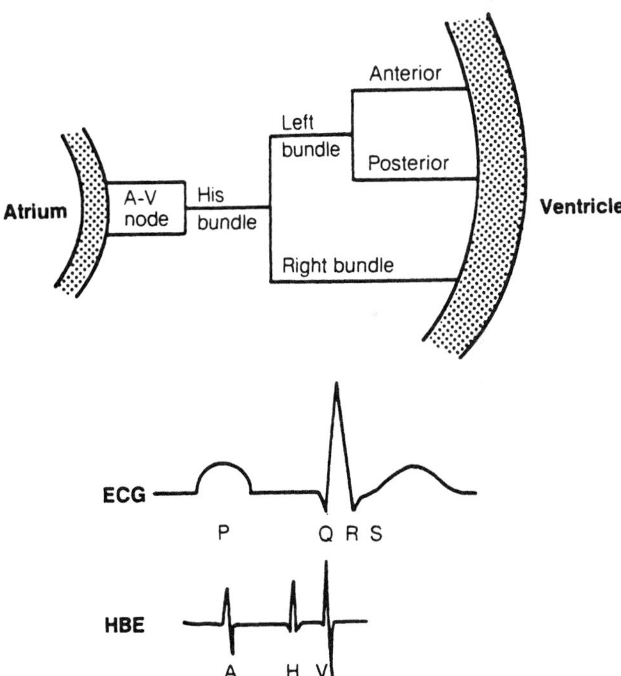

Figure 1. Diagrammatic representation of the atrioventricular conduction system. The bundle branch system consists of a three-pronged system (two on the left side and one on the right side). At the bottom, the surface ECG is depicted simultaneously with a His bundle electrogram (HBE). The HBE is recorded near the septal leaflet of the tricuspid valve. A = depolarization of the low atrium; H = depolarization of the His bundle; V = depolarization of the upper ventricular septum. The AH interval reflects AV nodal conduction, and the HV interval reflects conduction within the His-Purkinje system. The normal HV interval is 35 to 55 ms. A prolonged HV interval indicates delayed conduction in all three prongs of the conduction system and/or the His bundle. With His-Purkinje disease the HV interval (but not the surface QRS complex) remains normal as long as one of the three prongs conducts normally. (From Barold SS: Pacemaker treatment of bradycardias and selection of optimal pacing modes. Contemp Treat Cardiovasc Dis 1:123, 1997. Lippincott Williams & Wilkins©.)

COMPLETE AV BLOCK

In complete AV block there is total failure of conduction from atrium to ventricle and the atrial rate exceeds the ventricular rate. In acquired chronic AV block, the site of block is usually in the His-Purkinje system, with an escape wide QRS ventricular rhythm at 20 to 40 beats per minute in contrast to an escape rate of 40 to 60 beats per minute seen in AV nodal block. Table 2 outlines the indications for pacing in acquired AV block in adults that best reflect current practice. Complete AV block with a rate greater than 40 beats per minute in asymptomatic patients designated as a Class II indication in the 1998 ACC/AHA guidelines is really a Class I indication in practice (see Table 2). In this context, one may ask whether the patient is truly asymptomatic and whether the patient and/or clinician is certain of this. There is no definitive evidence regarding the long-term stability of the escape rate. For example, is an escape rate of 41 to 45 beats per minute prognostically different than a rate of 36 to 40 beats per minute? It is not the escape rate that is critical to stability but rather the site of origin of the escape rhythm (i.e., junctional or ventricular); rate instability may not be predictable or obvious. Irreversible acquired complete heart block should be a Class I indication.

SECOND-DEGREE AV BLOCK

The electrocardiographic patterns of type I and type II describe the behavior of the PR intervals (in sinus rhythm) in sequences (with at least two consecutive conducted PR intervals) where a *single* P wave fails to conduct to the ventricles.

Type I Block (Wenckebach or Mobitz Type I)

Type I second-degree AV block is defined as the occurrence of a single nonconducted P wave associated with inconstant PR intervals before and after the blocked impulse provided there are at least two consecutive conducted P waves (i.e., 3:2 AV block) to determine behavior of the PR interval. The PR interval after the blocked impulse always shortens provided the P wave is conducted to the ventricle. The term *inconstant* PR or AV intervals is important because the majority of type I sequences are atypical and do not conform to the traditional teaching about the mathematical behavior of the PR intervals. The description of "progressive" prolongation of the PR interval is misleading because PR intervals may shorten or stabilize and show no discernible or measurable change anywhere in a type I sequence. Atypical type I structures can therefore exhibit a number of consecutive PR intervals showing no discernible change in the terminal portion before the single blocked impulse (Figure 2). In such an arrangement the first conducted PR interval after the blocked impulse is always shorter. Slowing of the sinus rate does not interfere with the diagnosis of type I block, whereas it does with type II block, as discussed later. In contrast, an increase in the sinus rate does not interfere with the diagnosis of both type I and type II blocks.

Site of Block. In *narrow QRS type I block*, the block is in the AV node in almost all the cases. Intra-Hisian narrow QRS type I block is rare. Type I block can be physiologic, especially during sleep in normal individuals with high vagal tone, and these people do not need to be considered for treatment. Outside of

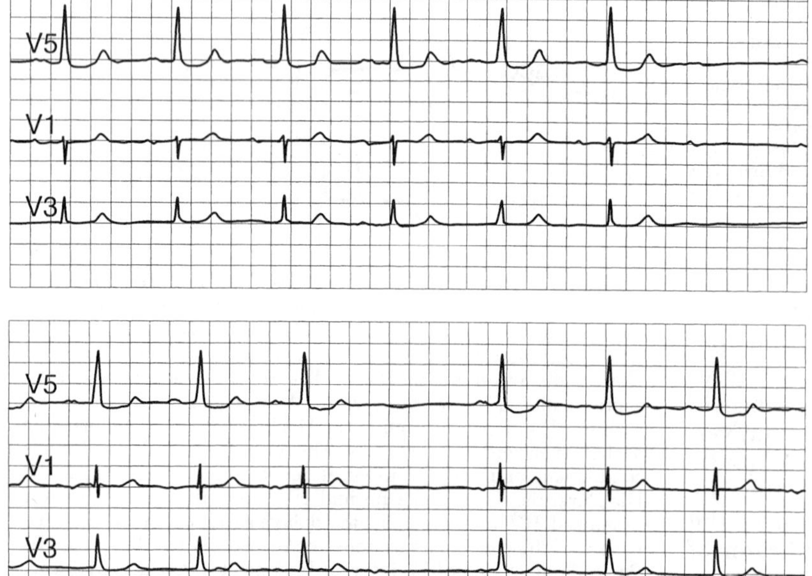

Figure 2. Two examples of narrow QRS complex atypical type I second-degree AV block registered in three-lead Holter recordings. *Top*, There is sinus arrhythmia. The last three PR intervals before the nonconducted P wave are constant. The diagnosis of type II block is untenable because the first PR interval on the left is shorter than the ones immediately before the block. Actually, the first postblock P wave was conducted (not shown) with a shorter PR interval compared with the one before the block. The pattern is consistent with type I second-degree AV block. *Bottom*, The three PR intervals before the blocked P wave are constant. The postblock PR interval is slightly shorter. The second postblock PR interval is longer than the first postblock PR interval and the last PR interval is very slightly longer than the second postblock PR interval. The pause is slightly shorter than two (PP) intervals. This makes the diagnosis of type I block. Applying the strict definition of type II block to these two situations avoids the diagnosis of type II second-degree AV block. © Mayo Clinic.

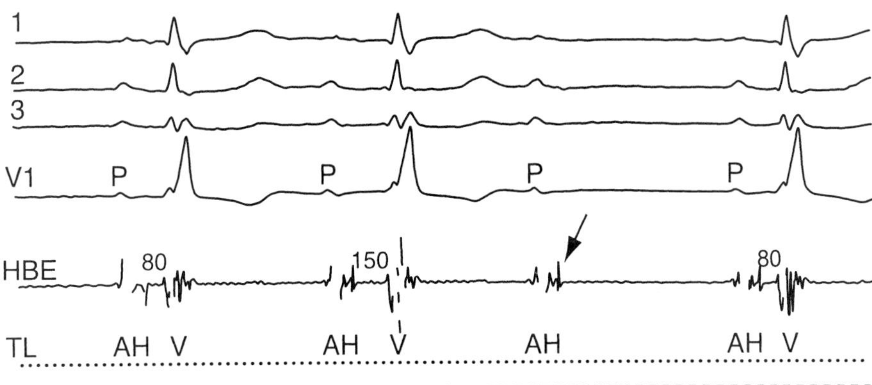

Figure 3. Sinus rhythm with second-degree Type I 3:2 infranodal AV block and right bundle branch block. Note that the AH interval remains constant. The HV interval increases from 80 ms (after first P wave) to 150 ms (after second P wave). The third P wave is followed by an H deflection but no QRS complex. AV block occurs in the His-Purkinje system below the site of recording of the His bundle potential (*arrow*). Note the shorter PR interval after the nonconducted P wave, a feature typical of Type I second-degree AV block. *Abbreviations:* A = atrial deflection; H = His bundle deflection; HBE = His bundle electrogram; P = P wave; TL = time lines 50 ms; V = ventricular deflection. (From Barold SS: Pacemaker treatment of bradycardias and selection of optimal pacing modes. Contemp Treat Cardiovasc Dis 1:123, 1997. Lippincott Williams & Wilkins ©.)

acute myocardial infarction, type I block and bundle branch block (QRS ≥ 0.12 s) occur in the His-Purkinje system in 60% to 70% of the cases (Figure 3). Yet many still believe that type I blocks are all AV nodal and therefore basically benign. It is widely believed that the prognosis of infranodal type I block is as serious as that of type II block and a permanent pacemaker is generally recommended in both types regardless of symptoms (see Table 2). On this basis patients with type I block and bundle branch block should undergo an invasive study to determine the level of second-degree block.

Type II Block (Mobitz Type II)

Type II second-degree AV block is defined as the occurrence of a single nonconducted P wave associated with constant PR intervals before and after the blocked impulse, provided the sinus rate or the PP interval is constant and there are at least two consecutive conducted P waves (i.e., 3:2 AV block) to determine behavior of the PR interval. The pause encompassing the blocked P wave should equal two (PP) cycles. The PR interval is either normal or prolonged but remains constant (Figure 4). Type II block cannot be diagnosed whenever a single blocked impulse is followed by a shortened postblock PR interval or no P wave at all. In this situation it is either a type I pattern or an unclassifiable sequence. Stability of the sinus rate is a very important criterion because a vagal surge can cause simultaneous sinus slowing and AV nodal block, generally a benign condition, that can superficially resemble type II second-degree AV block. In the presence of sinus arrhythmia, the diagnosis of type II block may not be possible if there is sinus slowing, especially if the block occurs in one of the longer cycles.

Site of Block. Type II block according to the strict definition always occurs in the His-Purkinje system and is a Class I indication for pacing (see Table 2). The QRS complex is wide (≥ 0.12 s) in 70% to 80% of cases. Type II block has not yet been convincingly demonstrated in the AV node.

Fixed-Ratio Block

A 2:1 AV block can be AV nodal or in the His-Purkinje system. It cannot be classified as type I or type II block because there is only one PR interval to examine before the blocked P wave. The 2:1 AV block is best considered as "advanced block" for the purpose of classification, as are AV blocks that are 3:1, 4:1, and so on. The site of the lesion in 2:1 block can often be determined by seeking the company 2:1 AV block keeps. An association with either type I or type II helps localization of the block according to the correlations already discussed. Outside acute myocardial infarction, sustained 2:1 and 3:1 AV blocks with a wide QRS complex occur in the His-Purkinje system in 80% of cases and 20% in the AV node (see Table 2). It is inappropriate to label nodal 2:1 or 3:1 AV block as type I block and infranodal 2:1 or 3:1 AV block as type II block because the diagnosis of type I and type II blocks is based on ECG patterns and not on the anatomic site of block. When stable sinus rhythm and 1:1 AV conduction is followed by sudden AV block of several impulses (>1) and all the PR intervals before and after the block remain constant, infranodal block is strongly suggested with the need for a pacemaker.

SYMPTOMATIC BUNDLE BRANCH BLOCK

Patients presenting with syncope and bundle branch block require an electrophysiologic study (EPS) because sustained monomorphic ventricular tachycardia is the cause of symptoms in 20% to 30% of cases, especially in association with structural heart disease. A markedly prolonged HV interval

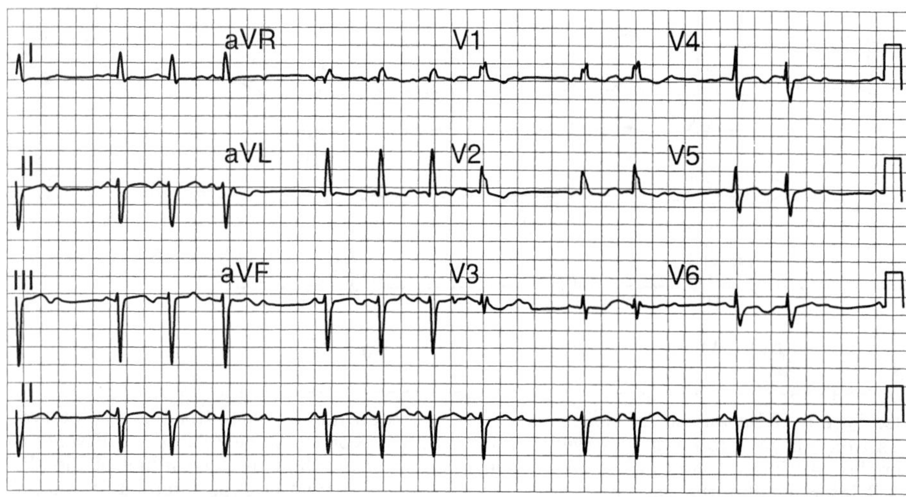

Figure 4. Sinus rhythm with second-degree type II AV block in the presence of right bundle branch block and left anterior hemiblock. There are tiny q waves in V_2 and V_3 probably related to left anterior hemiblock rather than old anterior myocardial infarction. Note that the sinus rate is constant and the PR interval after the blocked beat remains unchanged. (From Barold SS: Pacemaker treatment of bradycardias and selection of optimal pacing modes. Contemp Treat Cardiovasc Dis 1:123, 1997. Lippincott Williams & Wilkins ©.)

(≥100 ms) identifies patients with a higher risk of developing complete AV block and the need for a pacemaker. An EPS can be defined by a process of exclusion by which patients might benefit from pacing in the presence of HV prolongation (≥70 ms) and no other electrophysiologic abnormality (see Table 3).

FIRST-DEGREE AV BLOCK

During markedly prolonged anterograde AV conduction, the close proximity of atrial systole to the preceding ventricular systole produces the same unfavorable hemodynamic consequences as continual retrograde ventriculoatrial conduction during ventricular pacing. Patients with a markedly prolonged PR interval may or may not be symptomatic at rest. They are, of course, more likely to become symptomatic with mild to moderate levels of exercise when the PR interval does not shorten appropriately and atrial systole occurs progressively closer to the previous ventricular systole. The 1998 ACC/AHA guidelines include symptomatic first-degree AV block as a Class IIA indication for dual-chamber pacing to restore optimal AV synchrony (see Table 2). This recommendation does not apply to patients with dilated cardiomyopathy, a long PR interval, and congestive heart failure.

ACUTE INFERIOR MYOCARDIAL INFARCTION

AV block in inferior myocardial infarction (MI) is relatively benign because it occurs in the AV node and occasionally in the His bundle. Type I second-degree AV block often precedes complete AV block. In complete AV block, the AV junctional rhythm exhibits a narrow QRS complex in over 70% of cases with an adequate rate (50 to 60/min), often without associated hemodynamic compromise. The AV block is transient and often resolves within a week. Temporary pacing is indicated in second- or third-degree AV block only in the presence of an excessively slow ventricular rate (<40), ventricular arrhythmia requiring antiarrhythmic agents, hypotension, signs of hypoperfusion, or congestive heart failure. Patients with AV block and right ventricular MI require dual-chamber pacing

Permanent Pacing. Permanent pacing is almost never needed in inferior MI and narrow QRS AV block. Pacemaker implantation should be considered only if second- or third-degree AV block persists for 14 to 16 days (Table 4). The use of permanent pacing is required in only 1% to 2% of all the patients who develop acute second- or third-degree AV block regardless of thrombolytic therapy.

ACUTE ANTERIOR MYOCARDIAL INFARCTION

Second- or third-degree AV block is almost invariably preceded by an intraventricular conduction disorder. AV block in anterior MI involves the His-Purkinje system and occasionally occurs in the form of second-degree AV block (Mobitz type II, 2:1, or higher-degree AV block) before the appearance of complete heart block. Type I second-degree AV block may occur in the His-Purkinje system and almost invariably progresses to 2:1 and complete AV block. All patients with second- or third-degree heart block need temporary pacing, although the mortality is quite high; improvement of eventual survival is controversial because the conduction disturbances generally occur in patients with very large infarcts. Nevertheless, pacing protects against hypotension that may minimize infarct extension and malignant ventricular arrhythmias, particularly when dual-chamber pacing is employed.

Prophylactic temporary pacing is generally recommended in the presence of new RBBB with LAH, RBBB with LPH, LBBB with first-degree AV block, and alternating RBBB and LBBB because of the higher risk of progression to complete AV block. The role of pacing for RBBB with normal axis or LBBB with normal PR interval is more controversial. Preexisting RBBB or LBBB is usually not an indication for temporary pacing. The advent of reliable external

TABLE 4. **Indications for Permanent Pacing After Acute Myocardial Infarction**

Class I

A. Persistent or transient second-degree or complete AV block in the His-Purkinje system
B. Alternating left bundle branch block and right bundle branch block with 1:1 AV conduction

Class II

Persistent advanced or complete AV block at the AV node (longer than 16 days)

Class III

A. Transient AV conduction disturbances without intraventricular conduction defects
B. Transient AV block in the presence of isolated left anterior hemiblock
C. Acquired left anterior hemiblock, bundle branch block, or bifascicular block with or without first-degree AV block, but in the absence of second-degree or complete AV block
D. Transient second-degree or complete AV block and associated bundle branch block in acute inferior myocardial infarction*

*Transient AV block in inferior myocardial infarction is virtually always in the AV node or His bundle and almost never requires permanent pacing even if associated with permanent bundle branch block. Therefore, transient advanced AV block and associated bundle branch block should not be classified as a Class I indication, unless there is firm evidence of transient second- or third-degree AV block in the His-Purkinje system.

Adapted from ACC/AHA Guidelines for Implantation of Cardiac Pacemakers and Antiarrhythmia Devices: A Report of the American College of Cardiology/American Heart Association Task Force on Practice Guidelines (Committee on Pacemaker Implantation). *J Am Coll Cardiol* 1998;31:1175–1209. Copyright 1998 by the American College of Cardiology and American Heart Association, Inc. Permission granted for one time use. Further reproduction is not permitted without permission of the ACC/AHA.

transcutaneous pacing has diminished the need in many patients for prophylactic temporary right ventricular pacing in acute MI, an important consideration in patients treated with thrombolytic therapy and anticoagulants.

Permanent Pacing. Patients who develop bundle branch block and transient second- and third-degree AV block during anterior MI have a high in-hospital mortality rate and are at a high risk of sudden death after hospital discharge. Sudden death usually is due to malignant ventricular tachyarrhythmias and less commonly related to the development of complete AV block with prolonged ventricular asystole. The use of permanent pacing in patients with transient trifascicular AV block or bilateral (alternating) bundle branch block is still controversial, but most workers recommend it with the aim of preventing sudden death from asystole despite the return of 1:1 AV conduction (see Table 4). Permanent pacing is not indicated in patients with acute anterior MI and residual bundle branch or bifascicular block without documented transient second- or third-degree AV block because there is no appreciable risk of late development of complete AV block. Measurement of the HV interval does not predict which patients will develop progressive conduction system disease. The very high 1-year mortality of patients with new and persistent RBBB (worse with associated LAH) in the thrombolytic era suggests that the benefit of prophylactic defibrillators (with pacemakers) should be investigated.

VAGALLY MEDIATED AV BLOCK

Vagally mediated AV block occurs in the AV node and differs from neurally mediated (malignant vasovagal) syncope, where head-up tilt testing causes sinus arrest and rarely predominant AV block. Vagally induced AV block can occur in otherwise normal individuals and also in patients with cough, swallowing, hiccups, micturition, and so on when vagal discharge is enhanced. EPS in vagally mediated AV block is basically normal. Vagally mediated AV block is characteristically paroxysmal and often associated with sinus slowing. As a rule, AV nodal block is associated with obvious irregular and longer PP intervals and is bradycardia *associated* (not bradycardia dependent); that is, both AV block and sinus slowing result from vagal effects. An acute increase in vagal tone may occasionally produce AV block without preceding prolongation of the AH interval (constant PR), giving the superficial appearance of a type II AV block mechanism (i.e., no PR prolongation before the blocked beat). In this situation, AH prolongation may occur during the initial several beats when AV conduction resumes. Vagally induced block is occasionally expressed in terms of constant PR intervals before and after the blocked impulse, an arrangement that may lead to an erroneous diagnosis of the more serious type II block if sinus slowing is ignored. Sinus slowing can sometimes be subtle because the PP interval may increase by as little as 0.04 second.

AV BLOCK IN ATHLETES

Severe sinus bradycardia and second-degree (including type I) and third-degree AV block can occur at rest or after exercise in athletes and lead to symptoms such as lightheadedness, syncope, or even Stokes-Adams attacks. These changes are considered secondary to increased parasympathetic (hypervagotonia) and decreased sympathetic tone on the sinus and AV nodes related to physical training. Most patients become asymptomatic after physical deconditioning. Mobitz type II second-degree AV block (always infranodal) does not occur in otherwise healthy athletes.

TACHYCARDIAS

method of
WILLIAM W. BARRINGTON, M.D.
Cardiovascular Institute of the University of Pittsburgh Medical Center
Pittsburgh, Pennsylvania

The human heart can beat rapidly for a multitude of reasons. Sometimes, the beating is in response to the excitement of an athletic competition, whereas at other times, it may signal the onset of a life-threatening cardiac event. This wide range of causes of tachycardia and the differences between those with a benign prognosis and those with a malignant prognosis make tachycardia a topic worthy of further discussion.

This article provides one approach to the diagnosis and treatment of tachycardia using tools available to the average clinical practitioner. This approach begins with the identification of the type of tachycardia.

IDENTIFICATION OF TACHYCARDIA TYPE

In the strictest sense, any heart rate greater than 100 beats per minute (bpm) is a *tachycardia,* but most clinically significant tachycardias have a ventricular rate greater than 120 bpm. Examination of electrocardiographic (ECG) tracings during tachycardia provides measurements of the ventricular rate, P wave, and QRS complex morphology and allows analysis of the relationship between atrial and ventricular activity. These findings are the starting points for determining whether the tachycardia is supraventricular or ventricular in origin.

In a *supraventricular tachycardia (SVT),* the supraventricular activity drives the ventricular response. This means that some structure at or above the level of the atrioventricular (AV) valves is required for maintenance of the rhythm. These rhythms cannot proceed without involving the sinus node, atria, AV node, or AV junction. This fact is reflected in the names used to identify the types of SVT noted in Figure 1.

These rhythms typically have a "narrow" QRS complex (<100 ms in duration) but can show a widened QRS if the patient has an underlying fixed bundle branch block or some type of functional bundle branch block (aberrant conduction). Frequently, an association is noted between the atrial and ventricular activity, but this finding is not sufficient to establish the diagnosis of SVT. For example, atrial fibrillation is one type of SVT that fails to show evidence of AV association due to the absence of discernible P waves on ECG recordings. This rhythm is covered elsewhere in this book.

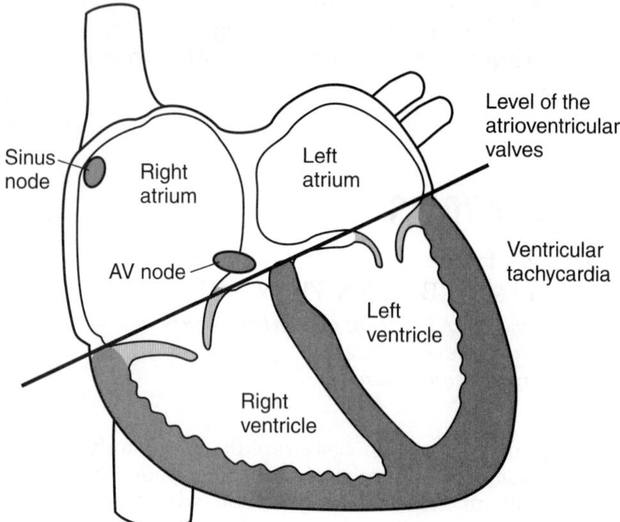

Figure 1. Anatomic localization of supraventricular and ventricular tachycardia.

In contrast, the ventricular response in *ventricular tachycardia (VT)* is driven by signals generated from structures below the anatomic level of the AV valves such as the His-Purkinje system or, more commonly, the ventricular muscle. Supraventricular structures are not required to maintain this rhythm, and AV nodal blockade has no effect on the ventricular rate.

Typically, the QRS complex during VT is wide (120 ms or more in duration). VT may exhibit ventricular-atrial association. This type of 1:1 QRS complex to P wave ratio occurs when ventricular activation passes "backward" in the AV node to generate a P wave in response to the QRS. The presence of dissociation between the atrial and ventricular activity, however, is sufficient to classify a wide complex rhythm as ventricular tachycardia.

In general, SVT has a more favorable prognosis than VT, thus placing the tachycardia into one of these two groups has clinical significance. This process begins by examining the width of the QRS complex on the tachycardia ECG tracings.

Narrow Complex Tachycardia

If the QRS complex during tachycardia is "narrow," the rhythm is supraventricular in origin and can be more specifically classified by examining the P wave morphology, PR interval duration, and ventricular response from ECG recordings obtained during both tachycardia and normal rhythm. This approach is diagrammed in Figure 2 for the most common SVTs.

If a P wave is discernible during tachycardia, the analysis proceeds along the lefthand limb of the diagram. Initially, the P wave morphology and PR interval recorded during tachycardia are compared with those recorded during normal rhythm. If the P wave and PR interval are similar, the SVT is a variety of sinus tachycardia (appropriate, inappropriate, or sinus node reentry). If the tachycardia exhibits three or more distinct P-wave morphologies, then it is classified as a multifocal atrial tachycardia. If the tachycardia has not been specifically classified by this point in the algorithm, additional analysis is required.

If a P wave is not discernible during tachycardia, the analysis proceeds down the righthand limb of the diagram. If the ventricular response is not regular, the rhythm can be classified as atrial fibrillation. If the ventricular response is regular, the P waves may not be visible because they are buried in the QRS complex during tachycardia. The algorithm still leaves atrial flutter, an ectopic atrial-junctional tachycardia, AV nodal reentry tachycardia (AVNRT), and AV reentry tachycardia (AVRT) as diagnostic possibilities.

Information from the patient's history may narrow the choices at this point. For instance, if the tachycardia is paroxysmal in nature and starts or stops suddenly, it most likely has a reentrant mechanism. This observation is consistent with sinus node reentry tachycardia, AVNRT, AVRT, and some ectopic atrial or junctional tachycardias. In comparison, a tachycardia that is more persistent in nature and appears to gradually speed up and slow down is most likely caused by an automatic mechanism (related to the slope of phase 4 of the action potential). Normal sinus tachycardia is the most common example of an automatic tachycardia, but this behavior can also be seen with some ectopic atrial or junctional tachycardias.

Finally, if the type of tachycardia is still uncertain, it may be helpful to examine the response of the tachycardia

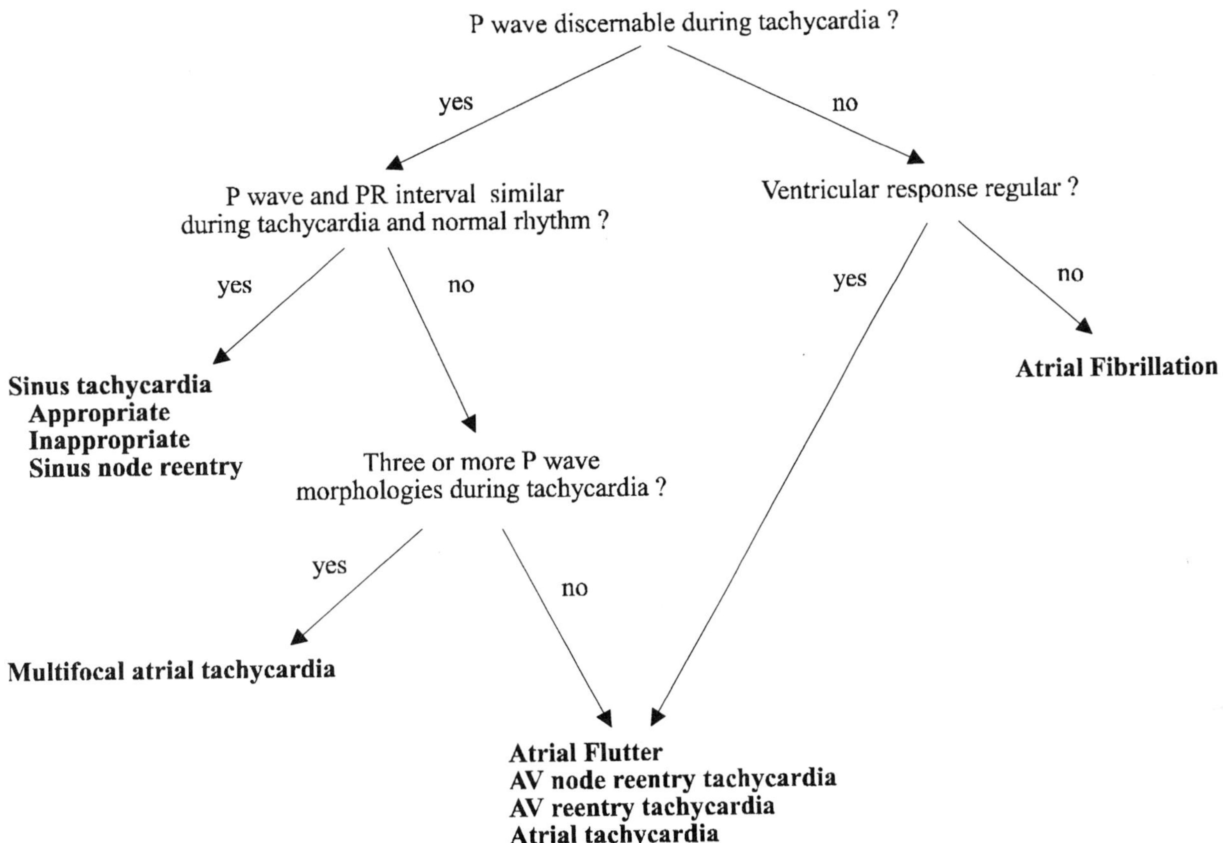

Figure 2. Evaluation of narrow complex tachycardia.

to physiologic or pharmacologic interventions. For years, vagal stimulation via carotid sinus massage or the Valsalva maneuver has been used to terminate SVTs, and the response to these interventions may determine if the AV node is involved in the rhythm. In many cases, these maneuvers have been replaced by intravenous adenosine (Adenocard). The response of various tachycardias to adenosine is shown in Table 1.

In brief, if the tachycardia terminates (both the P wave and QRS complex stop), the tachycardia is sinus node reentry, AVRT, AVNRT, or, in some cases, an ectopic atrial tachycardia. If administration of adenosine transiently suppresses the rhythm (temporarily stopping or slowing the rhythm), the tachycardia is most likely sinus tachycardia, although some ectopic atrial rhythms behave in this manner. Finally, if adenosine results in transient AV nodal block that reveals the underlying atrial activity, it may be easier to establish a diagnosis of atrial flutter or another atrial tachycardia.

In some cases, the adenosine appears to have no effect on the narrow complex tachycardia. This may be due to the fact that the adenosine has not reached the myocardium before being metabolized. In this situation, either the site of intravenous access should be moved to a more central location or a larger dose of adenosine should be administered.

If these steps have not provided sufficient information to diagnose the patient's SVT and either a more specific diagnosis is required or the patient wishes to pursue possible curative procedures such as radiofrequency catheter ablation, refer the patient to a cardiac electrophysiologist for further evaluation.

TABLE 1. **Response of Narrow Complex Tachycardia to Adenosine**

Tachycardia Terminates	Transient Suppression of Tachycardia	Transient AV Block Revealing Atrial Activity
Sinus node reentry AV reentry (associated with WPW) AV node reentry Some ectopic atrial tachycardias	Sinus tachycardia Some ectopic atrial tachycardias	Atrial flutter Some ectopic atrial tachycardias

Abbreviations: AV = atrioventricular; WPW = Wolff-Parkinson-White syndrome.

Wide Complex Tachycardia

If the QRS complex during tachycardia is not less than 100 msec in duration, it is classified as a wide complex tachycardia (WCT), and the differentiation between SVT and VT is more problematic. A WCT is one of three types of rhythm: (1) VT, (2) SVT with aberrancy (a fixed or functional bundle branch block), or (3) a "pre-excited" tachycardia.

The first step is to assess the patient's clinical situation. If the patient has a history of coronary artery disease with a prior myocardial infarction and some depression of left ventricular function, the WCT is considered VT until proven otherwise. This type of patient should be referred to an electrophysiologist for evaluation and treatment. Other factors in the patient's history that favor the diagnosis of

VT are dilated or hypertrophic cardiomyopathy, repaired valvular or congenital heart disease, and either a familial or acquired long QT syndrome. In contrast, if the ECG during normal rhythm shows evidence of a delta wave, the diagnosis of SVT with aberrancy or preexcited tachycardia becomes more likely.

Patient history aside, the ECG recording is still important in establishing the diagnosis of VT. Algorithms have been developed and guidelines have been proposed to help the clinician differentiate ventricular tachycardia from other WCTs. Unfortunately, these approaches frequently use a 12-lead ECG obtained during the WCT (which is not often available) or rely on statistical probabilities of one finding being more or less common in SVT than VT. Physiologically, VT does not require any involvement of the structures above the level of the AV valves; therefore, finding evidence of AV dissociation is the strongest proof that a WCT is ventricular in origin.

Establishing the presence of AV dissociation can be difficult and frequently requires examination of long ECG recordings obtained during the WCT (Figure 3). Sometimes the evidence of dissociated P waves is obvious on the tracing, but at other times, the tracings only show indirect evidence of AV dissociation in the form of fusion or capture beats.

If the diagnosis of VT has been eliminated, the rhythm is either an SVT with aberration or a preexcited tachycardia, and the algorithm outlined in Figure 2 can be used to further classify the rhythm. The response to adenosine, however, is slightly more complex in the case of a wide complex tachycardia (Table 2). The differences between the adenosine responses summarized in Tables 1 and 2 occur when an accessory bypass tract is used in the antegrade direction to conduct the signal from the atrial to the ventricular side of the AV valves (Figure 4). This antegrade conduction through the accessory bypass tract has the effect of generating a delta wave in each of the QRS complexes and is responsible for the increased width of the

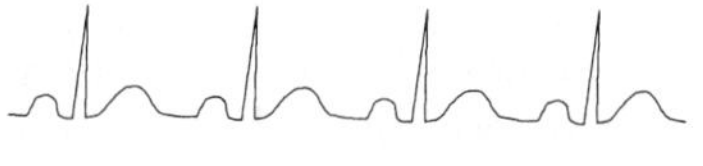

Normal sinus rhythm

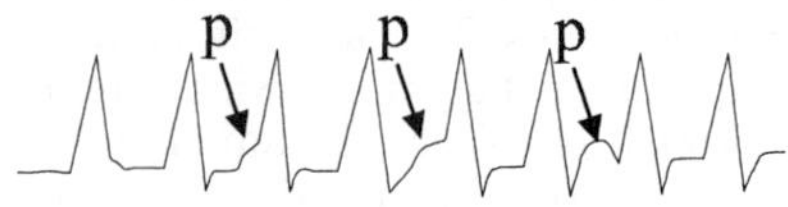

VT with AV dissociation

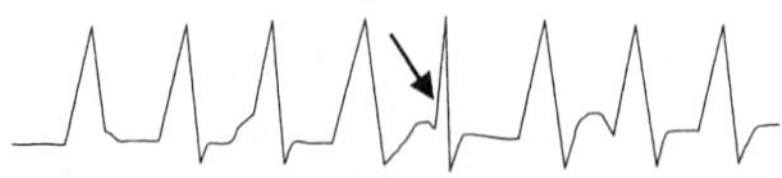

VT with fusion beat

VT with capture beat

Figure 3. Recordings made during wide complex tachycardia showing AV dissociation, fusion beats, and capture beats.

TABLE 2. **Response of Wide Complex Tachycardia to Adenosine**

Tachycardia Terminates	No Effect on Tachycardia	Transient AV Block Revealing Atrial Activity
Sinus node reentry with aberration	VT	Atrial fibrillation or flutter with aberration
AV reentry with aberration	Atrial tachycardia with accessory bypass tract (WPW)	Some ectopic atrial tachycardias with aberration
Antidromic tachycardia using retrograde AV node	Atrial flutter with accessory bypass tract (WPW)	**Transient Suppression of Tachycardia**
AV node reentry with aberration	Antidromic tachycardia using two accessory bypass tracts	Sinus tachycardia with aberration
Some ectopic atrial tachycardias with aberration		Some atrial tachycardias with aberration
Adenosine sensitive VT		

Abbreviations: AV = atrioventricular; VT = ventricular tachycardia; WPW = Wolff-Parkinson-White syndrome.

QRS complex during tachycardia. Because the accessory bypass tract is usually insensitive to adenosine, several new responses can be seen.

An AVRT that uses an accessory bypass tract in the antegrade direction is termed *antidromic tachycardia.* If an accessory bypass tract is used only in the antegrade direction and the retrograde limb of the circuit uses the AV node (see Figure 4*B*), administration of adenosine will block the AV node and terminate the tachycardia. If, however, the patient has more than one accessory pathway, the tachycardia can use different bypass tracts for antegrade and retrograde conduction. This situation leaves the AV node out of the reentry circuit; thus, adenosine will not terminate the tachycardia. In a similar vein, if the patient has some other type of tachycardia that does not terminate with adenosine and happens to have an accessory bypass tract that is not part of the tachycardia circuit (the "innocent bystander" accessory pathway), adenosine will not stop the tachycardia. In these types of cases, the patient is likely to benefit from further electrophysiologic evaluation.

GENERAL APPROACHES TO TREATMENT

Until the late 1980s, the treatment of tachycardias relied on medications. Initially, little more than digoxin was available but as medicinal chemistry improved, potent antiarrhythmic drugs were developed and shown to be useful in preventing many types of tachycardia. Several classification schemes have been proposed for these drugs, but the Vaughn Williams classification scheme remains the one most familiar to clinical practitioners, despite its shortcomings. This classification is summarized in Table 3 as a reference for the specific recommendations made next.

In the case of SVTs, alternative and in many cases curative treatments have emerged. This alternative is referred to as RF catheter ablation. The procedure involves an invasive electrophysiology study in which a steerable, large-tipped ablation catheter is introduced into the cardiac chambers. Mapping is performed on the endocardial surface, and a critical re-

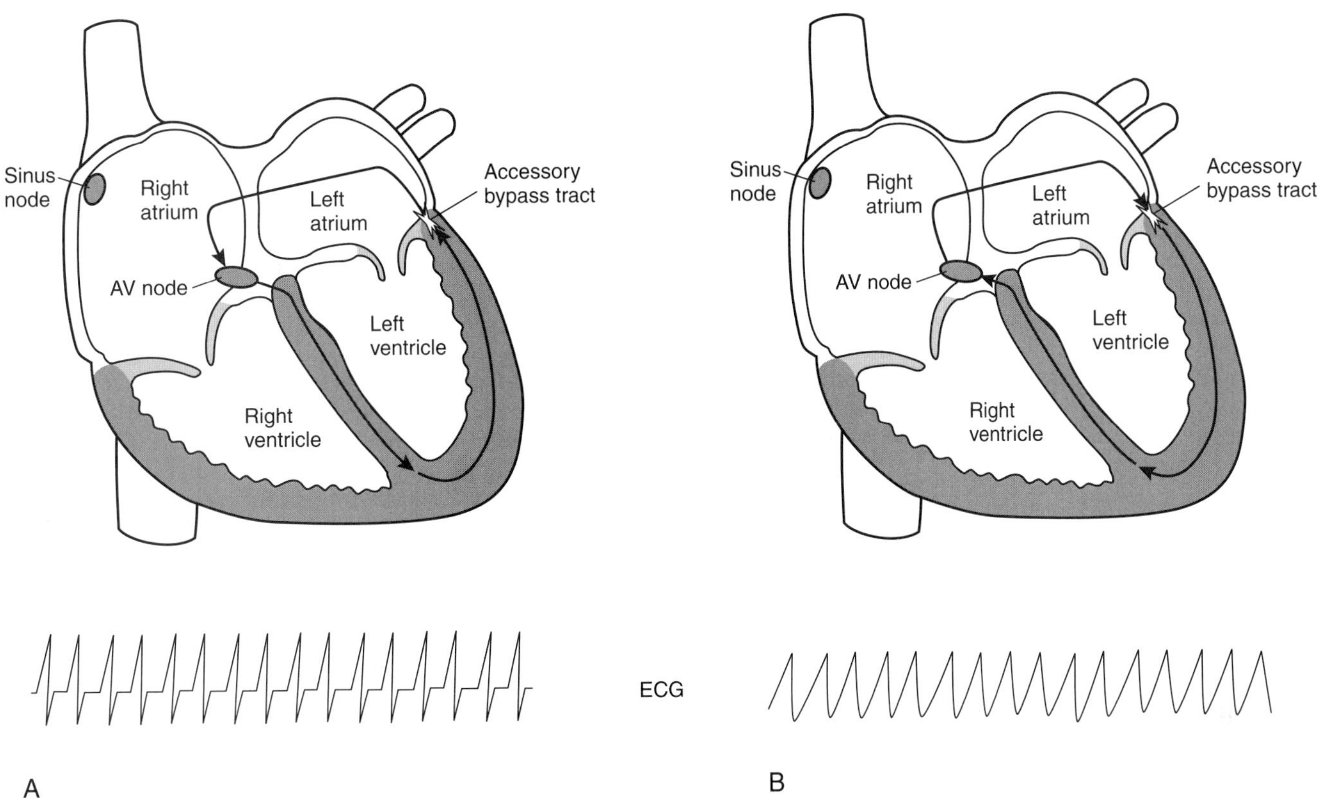

Figure 4. Reentry circuit of AV reentry tachycardia. *A,* Orthodromic tachycardia; *B,* antidromic tachycardia.

gion or portion of the tachycardia circuit is localized. The catheter tip is then placed adjacent to this location, and RF energy is delivered through the catheter for 30 to 60 seconds. The heating that accompanies the delivery of RF energy eliminates the electrical activity of the underlying tissue, making it impossible for the tachycardia to occur. Several studies have shown a greater than 95% cure rate for cases of

TABLE 3. **Vaughn Williams Antiarrhythmic Drug Classification**

Class	Actions	Examples
I	*Sodium Channel Blockers*	
A	Prolongation of action potential duration Modest sodium channel effects	Procainamide (Pronestyl) Quinidine (Quinaglute) Disopyramide (Norpace)
B	Shortens or no change in action potential duration Less potent sodium channel effect	Lidocaine (Xylocaine) Mexiletine (Mexitil) Tocainide (Tonocard) Phenytoin (Dilantin)*
C	Mild prolongation or no change in action potential duration Potent sodium channel effect	Propafenone (Rythmol) Flecainide (Tambocor)
II	*β-Adrenergic blockers*	Propranolol (Inderal) Atenolol (Tenormin) Metoprolol (Lopressor)
III	*Potassium Channel Effects* Prolong action potential duration	Amiodarone (Cordarone) Bretylium Sotalol (Betapace) Ibutilide (Corvert) Dofetilide (Tikosyn)
IV	*Calcium Channel Blockers*	Diltiazem (Cardizem) Verapamil (Calan, Isoptin)

*Not FDA approved for this indication.

AVNRT (Figure 5*A*) and AVRT (Figure 5*B*) associated with the Wolff-Parkinson-White syndrome. Although the current rates of success are lower for some other types of SVT and most varieties of VT, RF ablation remains an attractive option for people who would otherwise be committed to a lifetime of antiarrhythmic drug therapy.

The treatment of ventricular tachycardia has also evolved over the last decade, with implantable cardioverter-defibrillators (ICDs) rapidly becoming the treatment of choice. This is based on several randomized clinical trials that documented increased survival in patients treated with an ICD compared with those treated with any of the current antiarrhythmic drugs.

APPROACHES TO TREATMENT OF SPECIFIC TACHYCARDIAS

Sinus Tachycardia

Sinus tachycardia is characterized by a P wave morphology and PR interval similar to those observed in normal sinus rhythm and consists of three distinct entities. *Appropriate sinus tachycardia* is the most common variety and occurs in response to physiologic stressors such as anemia, dehydration, fever, or hyperthyroidism. In this case, treatment is correction of the underlying stress.

In other instances, the sinus rate is persistently elevated and shows an exaggerated response to even minimal physiological stress. This nonparoxysmal sinus tachycardia is classified as *inappropriate sinus tachycardia.* The mechanism of this tachycardia remains unclear but is likely either a primary abnormality of the sinus node or a manifestation of autonomic dysfunction. Initial therapy consists of high-dose β-blocker therapy, typically 160 to 320 mg/d of propranolol (Inderal),* or 100 to 200† mg/d of atenolol (Tenormin).* If this therapy fails, it may be possible to obtain some symptomatic relief by ablating the region of the sinus node with RF energy.

The final variety of sinus tachycardia is paroxysmal in nature and is termed *sinus node reentry tachycardia.* This rhythm is caused by a reentrant circuit located near or in the sinus node and may be acutely terminated by intravenous adenosine or calcium channel blockers. The most useful drugs for the prevention of recurrences are digoxin* and calcium channel blockers such as diltiazem (Cardizem), and verapamil (Calan). Intravenous amiodarone (Cordarone)* has shown some efficacy in preventing reinduction of this rhythm in the electrophysiology laboratory, but it is unclear if this finding shows a role for other class III antiarrhythmic drugs in the management of this disorder. Sinus node reentry has been successfully ablated at some centers and remains an option if drugs are ineffective or poorly tolerated.

Multifocal Atrial Tachycardia

Multifocal atrial tachycardia (MAT) is characterized as a supraventricular rhythm that demonstrates at least three distinct P wave morphologies with variable PP, RR, and PR intervals. The rhythm is most commonly seen in very ill patients who often have chronic obstructive pulmonary disease or coronary artery disease. Hypokalemia, hypomagnesemia, theophylline, and β-agonists have been associated with exacerbations of this tachycardia, and some cases respond to acute treatment with verapamil, metoprolol, or esmolol.

*Not FDA approved for this indication.
†Exceeds dosage recommended by the manufacturer.

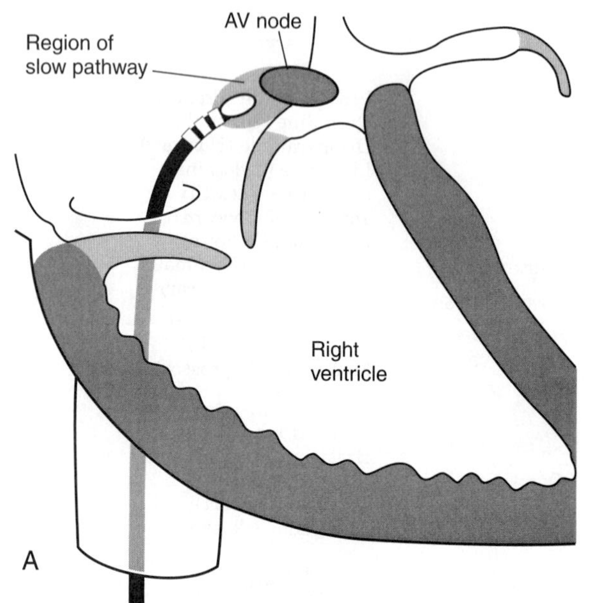

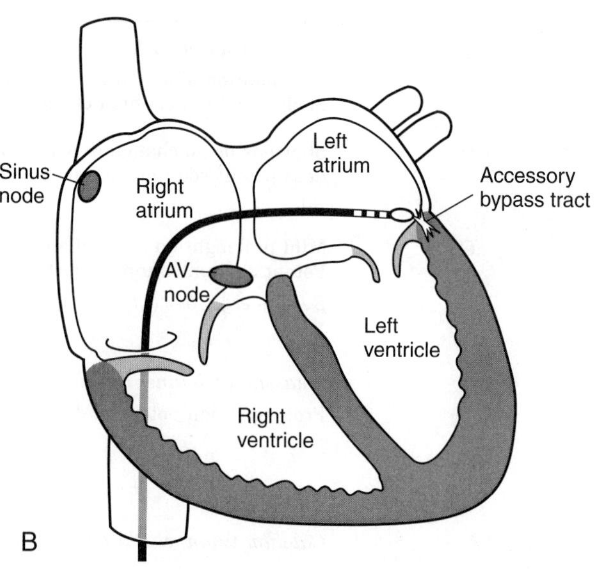

Figure 5. Radiofrequency catheter ablation techniques. *A,* Slow pathway ablation for AV node reentry via the inferior vena cava approach. *B,* Left-sided accessory bypass tract ablation via the transseptal approach.

The mechanism is thought to be increased automaticity due to a hyperadrenergic state; therefore, chronic therapy consists of treating the underlying illness that leads to the hyperadrenergic state.

Atrial Fibrillation and Flutter

These conditions are covered elsewhere in this book and will not be reviewed here.

Atrioventricular Nodal Reentry Tachycardia

AVNRT is the most common cause of a regular, narrow complex tachycardia, accounting for as much as 80% of the cases of paroxysmal atrial tachycardia (PAT). This tachycardia is more common in women than men and typically presents in the fourth or fifth decade of life. If a 12-lead ECG is obtained during tachycardia, the presence of a new r′ in lead V1, a new S in leads II and III, or aVF is highly suggestive of AVNRT.

Interventions that increase vagal tone such as carotid massage and the Valsalva maneuver are useful for termination of acute episodes. AV nodal blocking agents such as adenosine, verapamil, diltiazem, or quick-acting β-adrenergic blockers are all effective as well. Adenosine has emerged as the agent of choice and can be administered peripherally in bolus doses of 6 or 12 mg. If central venous access is available, adenosine has been effective in doses as small as 3 mg. Intravenous diltiazem in a dose of 0.15 to 0.45 mg/kg is another option for acute termination.

Chronic drug therapy involves the use of classes I and III antiarrhythmic drugs in addition to calcium channel or β-adrenergic blockers. The class IC agents flecainide (Tambocor), up to 200 mg twice a day, and propafenone (Rythmol), 150 to 300 mg three times a day, are safe and effective choices in patients without structural heart disease. Sotalol (Betapace), 160 to 480 mg/d in divided doses, and the class IA drugs are also effective, but side effects or inconvenient dosing schedules lead many patients to discontinue these regimens.

Many patients now are opting to avoid drug therapy entirely by proceeding with RF catheter ablation. The electrophysiologic basis of AVNRT is well understood, and the procedure to cure the rhythm (see Figure 5*A*) is over 90% successful. Clearly, ablation should be pursued if medical therapy fails to prevent symptomatic episodes of AVNRT, but the low risk and high success rate of the procedure has lead many patients to opt for this as first line therapy.

Atrioventricular Reentry Tachycardia

AVRT is a macro-reentrant tachycardia associated with the Wolf-Parkinson-White syndrome. In this case, an additional AV connection that bypasses the AV node (hence the term *accessory bypass tract*) makes up one or more limbs of the reentry circuit. If the tachycardia has a "narrow" QRS complex, the reentry circuit uses the AV node to conduct the signal from the atrium to the ventricle and is termed *orthodromic tachycardia* (see Figure 4*A*). On the other hand, if the signal passes from the atrium to the ventricle via the accessory bypass tract, the tachycardia will be "wide" and is termed *antidromic tachycardia* (see Figure 4*B*).

Acute termination is best accomplished with adenosine administered via a peripheral intravenous line in a rapid bolus dose of 6 to 12 mg. If this is ineffective or the patient is unstable, direct current cardioversion should be employed.

Drug therapy for the AVRTs consists of the class IA, IC, and III antiarrhythmic drugs because these agents all slow conduction over the accessory pathway as well as the AV node. Class IC agents such as flecainide (50–200 mg twice a day) or propafenone (150–300 mg three times a day) are particularly effective at eliminating ECG evidence of the delta wave in some cases. The next most commonly employed antiarrhythmic drug is sotalol, which appears to be effective in divided doses of 160 to 320 mg per day.

Increasingly, RF catheter ablation is employed early in the treatment of AVRT. The electrophysiologic basis of AVRT (and the Wolff-Parkinson-White syndrome) is well understood, and the procedure to cure the rhythm (depicted as the ablation of a left-sided accessory bypass tract; see Figure 5*B*) is over 90% successful. Although most experts agree that asymptomatic Wolff-Parkinson-White syndrome does not require therapy, ablation should be considered if medical therapy fails to prevent symptomatic episodes of AVRT.

Ectopic Atrial Tachycardias

Ectopic atrial tachycardias are a diverse group that is distinct from AVNRT and AVRT and are the least common type of supraventricular tachycardia. They may be paroxysmal or incessant in nature; have a reentrant, automatic, or "triggered" mechanism; and become better or disappear over time. If the tachycardia is due to an automatic mechanism, it may be very difficult to control with medical therapy. Although flecainide, sotalol, and amiodarone have shown some success, the class IA drugs and digoxin have been uniformly ineffective in treating the automatic atrial tachycardias. If the rapid ventricular response is the main problem with this tachycardia, β-adrenergic blockers and calcium channel blockers may decrease the ventricular response to a manageable rate but are unlikely to eliminate the rhythm.

RF catheter ablation is an alternative therapy regardless of the mechanism of the atrial tachycardia, but the success rate is variable depending on the location of the tachycardia.

Ventricular Tachycardia

VT is the type of tachycardia that is driven by impulses below the level of the AV valves and is most commonly associated with coronary artery disease. Currently, any patient who is a survivor of sudden cardiac death, has sustained VT, or has nonsustained VT and a depressed ejection fraction should be referred to a cardiac electrophysiologist for further evaluation and possible placement of an ICD.

In the setting of normal LV function, the mortality from ventricular arrhythmias is quite low and simple PVCs are frequently treated only with reassurance and β-adrenergic blockers. If these measures are incapable of adequately suppressing the ventricular ectopy, antiarrhythmic drug therapy can be tried, but the risk of antiarrhythmic drug therapy to the patient must be weighed against the risk of the continued ventricular ectopy.

Ablation is also being employed in the treatment of VT and will become more successful as our knowledge of the underlying mechanisms improves.

CONGENITAL HEART DISEASE

method of
ALAN MENDELSOHN, M.D.
Centocor
Malvern, Pennsylvania

Defects of the cardiovascular system are among the most commonly identified congenital lesions, particularly in the premature and stillborn infant, with an incidence of 8 to 12 per 1000 live births. Many patients with significant congenital heart lesions are asymptomatic for the first 6 to 8 weeks of life because of elevated pulmonary vascular resistance. The causes of congenital heart defects are many and include multifactorial genetic and environmental interactions (up to 90%), significant chromosomal abnormalities (5%, e.g., trisomy 21, trisomy 18), or single mutant gene syndromes with incomplete penetrance. Other factors that influence the occurrence of congenital heart lesions are maternal conditions such as infections, diabetes mellitus, systemic lupus erythematosus, or maternal medications.

PHYSIOLOGY OF CONGENITAL HEART DEFECTS

Left-to-Right Shunts

Intracardiac and extracardiac flow from the systemic circulation to the pulmonary circulation is described as a left-to-right shunt. From a physiologic standpoint, this allows oxygenated blood to recirculate through the pulmonary circulation without first entering the peripheral arterial circulation. Four important and interrelated physiologic factors influence the volume of blood shunting from left to right in the postnatal period and hence symptomatology:

1. Absolute diameter of the defect (e.g., patients with small ventricular septal defects [VSDs] are usually symptom-free)
2. Location of the defect within the cardiovascular system (atrial versus ventricular level shunts)
3. Differences in pressures between the two connected chambers or vessels (e.g., large patent ductus arteriosus [PDA] with an initially large pressure gradient between the aorta and pulmonary artery [PA])
4. Portion of the cardiac cycle in which the majority of shunting occurs (e.g., diastolic flow through atrial septal defects usually produces fewer symptoms than shunts in patients with abnormal systolic flow patterns of similar volumes)

Ventricular Septal Defect

Errors in formation of any of the four elements of the ventricular septum (muscular, outflow, inlet, perimembranous) occur in 30% to 40% of patients who have congenital heart lesions, making them the most common congenital cardiac defect. The most common type of VSD (75%–80%) occurs in the perimembranous region (in the outflow tract of the left ventricle immediately beneath the aortic valve). Muscular VSDs are the second most common type (≈20%). Inlet VSDs (5%) lie beneath the septal cusp of the tricuspid valve and are referred to more commonly as VSDs of the atrioventricular canal. Outlet VSDs (infundibular or supracristal VSDs) occur in all population groups but have a higher incidence in patients originally from the Pacific rim. Early identification of these defects is important because of associated aortic valve prolapse and aortic insufficiency.

CLINICAL PRESENTATION

In patients who have small VSDs, regardless of location, few symptoms are identified. Patients tend to have normal growth and development except for the onset of a new murmur. Patients who have moderate to large VSDs may present both with a new murmur and symptoms of congestive heart failure (CHF). In some neonates or infants with significant VSDs, poor weight gain or development may be the sole manifestation.

PHYSICAL EXAMINATION

In the majority of patients, heart sounds are normal. In most children with small defects, soft systolic regurgitant murmurs are heard on auscultation. These murmurs are well localized to the region of the defect. Such murmurs tend to be of mid to high frequency, reflecting significant differences in pressures between left and right ventricles. Paradoxically, children with small septal defects may have loud harsh regurgitant murmurs. Such loud systolic murmurs in a child with a small VSD can be differentiated from similar murmurs in the child with a large defect by the following:

1. Lack of symptomatology in the child with a small defect
2. Absence of a diastolic component in the child with a small defect
3. Absence of pulmonary hypertensive changes on physical examination
4. Absence of a gallop rhythm or rumble
5. Differences in murmur frequency (i.e., higher frequency, smaller defect)

Patients with more symptomatic defects may demonstrate a hyperdynamic precordium and increases in their heart sounds. Diastolic rumbles may occur secondary to increased filling of the left atrium.

TESTING

In patients with small hemodynamically insignificant VSD, the electrocardiogram (ECG) tends to remain normal. In some children who have inlet VSDs, a leftward and superior QRS axis (0 to −90 degrees) may be identified. Patients who have large defects and normal pulmonary vascular resistance may demonstrate increases in ventricular and atrial voltages. Chest radiography (CXR) defines cardiac size and pulmonary vascular changes. Two-dimensional (2-D) echocardiographic images and Doppler flow studies can be helpful in localizing the defect for future planning. Cardiac catheterization may be performed to determine the size of the physiologic shunt and any concomitant PA hypertension and to define contiguous structures or multiple defects.

Therapy

Seventy-five percent to 90% of small perimembranous VSDs and 90% to 95% of small muscular VSDs undergo spontaneous closure or diminution in size within the first 2 years of a child's life. Spontaneous closure of inlet or outlet defects is rare. Follow-up is indicated routinely to detect continuing spontaneous closure and to reinforce the importance of prophylactic antibiotics to prevent endocarditis.

Treatment of patients with symptomatic VSDs includes diuretic agents (i.e., furosemide and/or thiazide agents) or afterload reduction with angiotensin-converting enzyme inhibitors. Surgical intervention is indicated in patients unresponsive to medical therapy. Pulmonary vascular obstructive disease does not usually occur in patients who have moderate to large defects operated on when younger than 2 years of age. The location of the defects, symptoms, and presence of associated cardiovascular conditions influence the timing of corrective surgery. Surgical closure is indicated in patients with perimembranous VSD who become symptomatic or have a defect that fails to regress spontaneously. Standard surgical intervention for single lesions yields success rates of 99%; significant mortality of less than 5%; and morbidity including arrhythmias (right bundle branch block or atrioventricular block), small residual VSDs or patch leaks, and progressive pulmonary hypertension. The management of patients who have multiple VSDs remains controversial. Primary closure, interventional catheter techniques, and palliative surgery all may have a role in treatment. Despite advances in diagnosis and surgical treatment, morbidity and mortality remain high in this subgroup of patients.

ATRIAL SEPTAL DEFECTS

Atrial septal defects constitute 7% to 10% of all congenital heart lesions. Ostium primum (atrioventricular canal defects) and ostium secundum (central) atrial septal defects are the most common, constituting 75% to 80% of atrial lesions. Defects in formation of the embryologic sinus venosus or coronary sinus may lead to atrial septal defects in 5% of cases. Sinus venosus defects often are associated with partial anomalous pulmonary venous return, particularly of the right upper pulmonary veins.

Clinical Presentation

The majority of patients who have atrial septal defects present with a heart murmur with or without a history of pulmonary disease. Symptoms tend to be nondescript but involve some changes in pulmonary function such as recurrent asthma mildly responsive to standard medical therapy or multiple respiratory infections. In adolescents and adults, the initial manifesting symptoms may be palpitations, sensed extra beats, or chest pain.

Physical Examination

The telltale signs on physical examination are widening and fixed splitting of the second heart sound (also heard in patients with complete right bundle branch block). Most patients will have a soft systolic flow murmur heard best along the left upper sternal border. However, in many patients, no significant abnormalities may be noted.

Testing

Classically, patients demonstrate a volume overload pattern (regular sinus rhythm pattern in leads V_1, V_2, and V_3R) with mild-to-moderate right-axis deviation and mild first-degree heart block. CXR may demonstrate variable cardiomegaly and increase in pulmonary vascular markings. Echocardiography is valuable in determining the location and size of the defect and associated anomalies of the pulmonary veins. There is little role for diagnostic cardiac catheterization or angiography.

Therapy

For the asymptomatic patient with a large defect, elective surgery is usually performed after the age of 4 or 5 years, although if the child is symptomatic, surgical repair can be performed sooner. Complications of surgery include atrial dysrhythmias, residual septal leaks, and postpericardiotomy syndrome. Over the past 30 years, interventional cardiologists have shown that small central ostium secundum defects can be closed by means of the transcatheter route. Typically, patients who have smaller nonrepaired atrial septal defects remain active and asymptomatic and may only have symptoms of pulmonary hypertension or dysrhythmias in late adulthood. Pulmonary hypertension occurs in only a small proportion of adult patients.

ATRIOVENTRICULAR SEPTAL DEFECTS

Abnormalities of the endocardial cushion can cause defects of the atrial septum or ventricular septum or combined atrial and ventricular lesions with concomitant abnormalities of the atrioventricular valves (i.e., tricuspid, mitral valves). This type of lesion often is seen in children who have Down syndrome.

Clinical Presentation and Physical Examination

Patients with isolated ostium primum defects present similarly to patients with ostium secundum defects. In the patient with normal chromosomes and complete defects, clinical histories are similar to those of patients with other large left-to-right shunts. CHF is uncommon in the neonate and young infant with ostium primum defects. Abnormalities of the second heart sound and physical examination may be similar to those of an ostium secundum defect. In many patients with an ostium primum defect, significant mitral insufficiency may produce an apical regurgitant murmur. Early in the clinical course, the physical examination in the patient with a complete defect is similar to that of the patient who has an isolated large VSD. Development of increasing frequency and amplitude of the second heart sound, lack of splitting of the second heart sound, and/or disappearance of the murmurs may signify early onset of pulmonary hypertension.

Testing

The ECG in these patients is dominated by a leftward and superior QRS axis (0 to −90 degrees), with the remainder similar to that seen with ostium secundum atrial septal defects. CXR may appear similar to that of patients with other atrial septal defects. Echocardiography usually confirms the diagnosis and reveals any other associated valvular defects, particularly clefts of the mitral valve. Cardiac catheterization may be indicated to supplement insufficient echocardiographic images or to evaluate pulmonary hemodynamics.

Therapy

Standard diuretic therapy and/or afterload reduction using angiotensin-converting enzyme inhibitors usually is the treatment of choice for children with complete defects early in the patient's course, even before symptoms of CHF develop. In the presence of poor ventricular function, positive inotropes such as digoxin may be added. The surgical repair of such complete and partial lesions is similar to that already described except for the use of pericardial patch material rather than artificial materials. Surgical repair for complete defects usually is mandated within the first 2 to 6 months of life. The mitral valve cleft can also be repaired at the same time, usually by suture closure. Ostium primum defects currently are not amenable to transcatheter device closure.

PATENT DUCTUS ARTERIOSUS

The incidence of PDA (a fetal vessel between main PA and aorta) beyond 48 hours of life is 1 in 5000 live births and is more common (up to 80%) in premature infants. PDA may be associated with first-trimester rubella infection.

Clinical Presentation

The majority of patients with a small PDA are asymptomatic and come to medical attention because of a continuous murmur along the upper sternal border. In the rare patient, the initial presentation may be that of acute bacterial endocarditis or stridor secondary to tracheal compression. A small number of patients who have murmurs thought to be benign are found to have small-caliber PDA on echocardiography.

Physical Examination

Patients with a small PDA present with mildly increased pulses and a widened pulse pressure on sphygmomanometry. A continuous murmur of variable intensity is usually heard just below the left clavicle. Neonates with a PDA may present with a short systolic ejection murmur along the left upper sternal border rather than a continuous murmur. Patients with a large PDA may present with CHF.

Testing

The ECG in these patients varies from normal to a pattern of left atrial and ventricular volume overload. Similarly, patients with a small ductus tend to have normal cardiac silhouettes and trivial to mild increases in pulmonary vascular markings on CXR. 2-D echocardiography documents the PDA and rules out any ductal dependent lesions (e.g., tetralogy of Fallot, significant valvar obstruction) not fully manifested at the time of the examination.

Therapy

Medical therapy for the patient who has a hemodynamically significant PDA is similar to that for other left-to-right shunt lesions. In the neonatal population, diuretic therapy may be indicated, but other treatments include vascular volume restriction and the use of prostaglandin inhibitors, such as indomethacin. Beyond the neonatal period, the treatment of choice is complete occlusion of the PDA by simple ligation and division of the PDA. Portsmann described techniques for transcatheter occlusion of the PDA in the late 1960s. In many centers, coil embolization of the PDA has become the treatment of choice because of its low cost compared with open thoracic surgery, the low incidence of residual shunts, and the ability to reposition coils. Treatment of the small hemodynamically insignificant PDA is controversial. The issue of the "silent" echocardiographically documented PDA raises an even more interesting issue. Most cardiologists will not advocate either surgical or transcatheter closure of such lesions.

OBSTRUCTIVE LESIONS

As a group, obstructive lesions of either the right or left ventricular tract constitute 30% of congenital heart lesions. Generally, severe stenoses in the neonatal period are associated with significant CHF symptoms and/or cyanosis, depending on the location of the lesion within the cardiopulmonary circulation.

Right Ventricular Outflow Tract Obstruction

Right ventricular obstruction occurs anatomically below (e.g., muscular obstruction), at (e.g., fused leaflets), or above (e.g., hypoplasia) the pulmonary valve in 10% of patients with congenital heart disease (CHD). The association between myxomatous, dysplastic valvar pulmonary stenosis, and Noonan syndrome is high.

Clinical Presentation and Physical Examination

In the neonatal period, patients may present with symptomatology of right-sided heart failure or cyanosis. In the majority of older patients, pulmonary stenosis is diagnosed on routine physical evaluation of an ejection murmur and is well tolerated. Commonly, a variable systolic ejection click (decreasing during inspiration and increasing during expiration) is heard that helps to differentiate valvar pulmonary stenosis from either subvalvar (infundibular) or supravalvar pulmonary stenosis, conditions in which a click is absent. The loudness of the murmur may not necessarily correlate with the severity of the stenosis, particularly in the presence of poor cardiac output.

Testing

The ECG is normal in 40% to 50% of patients with mild valvar obstruction. With increasing disease severity, a more rightward QRS axis and associated increased right ventricular voltages are identified. On CXR, there may be enlargement of the main PA segment or "post-stenotic dilation" that varies inversely with the degree of obstruction. Echocardiography is the primary tool in defining the presence and severity of stenosis, intrinsic valvar abnormalities, and the degree of compensatory right ventricular pathology. Doppler-derived transvalvar gradients have been shown to correlate well with those directly measured during cardiac catheterization.

Therapy

Cardiac catheterization and concomitant balloon valvuloplasty between 2 and 4 years of age is considered the treatment of choice for most cases of valvar pulmonary stenosis. Most recent studies have demonstrated that successful balloon valvuloplasty results in significant reduction of the systolic gradient (residual gradient <25 mm Hg) in 70% to 85% of patients with no recurrent stenosis for up to 10 years of follow-up. Interventional therapy in the symptomatic neonate usually follows stabilization with prostaglandin E_1 and is technically more challenging with less favorable results. Surgical valvulotomy with patch angioplasty of the supravalvar stenosis or infundibular muscle resection may be indicated. Most cardiologists believe that mild valvar pulmonary stenosis has a benign course and does not require treatment except for antibiotic prophylaxis for bacterial endocarditis. This view has been borne out by long-term studies in more than 400 patients.

Subvalvar Pulmonic Stenosis

Mechanical obstruction in this condition may be attributable to a discrete fibrous or fibromuscular ring. Clinical features and ECG and CXR findings are similar to those in patients who have valvar pulmonary stenosis. The physical examination differs from valvar disease by the absence of the systolic ejection click. Therapy for this lesion tends to be surgical because balloon valvuloplasty has not proven to be effective in resolving gradients.

Supravalvar Pulmonic Stenosis

Stenosis of the main PA is rarely an isolated lesion, more often occurring in conjunction with hypoplasia of the branch PAs in conditions such as Alagille syndrome, Williams syndrome, and congenital rubella syndrome. The clinical presentation, laboratory examination, and treatment in these patients are similar to that of subvalvar pulmonic stenosis.

Peripheral Pulmonary Artery Stenosis

Pathologic branch PA stenosis (PAS) occurs in 3% to 6% of patients with congenital heart lesions predominantly as a postoperative complication. Many neonates, particularly those born prematurely, display the murmur of benign peripheral PAS, which usually resolves within 6 months.

Clinical Presentation

Patients with mild or moderate bilateral PAS usually are asymptomatic and are diagnosed on murmur evaluation. In severe cases, the following symptoms may be seen: dyspnea on exertion, easy fatigability, and right-sided heart failure.

Physical Examination

Typically, the systolic ejection murmur is heard best in the axilla and the back, although with severe stenoses the murmurs may appear more continuous.

Testing

The majority of patients maintain a normal ECG and CXR. Echocardiography aids in defining the size and relative flow patterns to each PA as well as right ventricular hemodynamics. Stenoses within the parenchymal vessels may be better delineated by other noninvasive testing such as magnetic resonance imaging. Cardiac catheterization is used to confirm and define the precise location of stenoses within the larger vessel. Hemodynamic tracings can differentiate patients with significant branch PAS from those with PA hypertension.

Therapy

In the majority of patients with mild to moderate isolated PA disease, no therapy is indicated. The need for intervention is based on symptoms of right ventricular hypertension or hypertrophy, diminished pulmonary blood flow, or poor exercise tolerance. Initial treatment tends to be transcatheter balloon angioplasty of the branch PASs (50%–70% success rates), which has improved with the addition of endovascular stent therapy (>85% success). Intraparenchymal stenoses are most difficult to treat effectively.

Left Ventricular Outflow Tract Obstruction

Aortic Stenosis

Isolated significant aortic valve stenosis occurs in 3% to 6% of patients with CHD. Abnormalities of the valve leaflets (unicuspid to tricuspid) and hypoplasia of the valve annulus may combine as components of the outflow tract disease. The incidence of mild abnormalities of the aortic valve such as a bicuspid aortic valve is 1% to 2% of the entire population. Associated cardiac lesions may occur in 20% of patients (e.g., PDA or coarctation of the aorta). The stenosis frequently progresses through life, but the rate of progression is variable (i.e., more rapid during growth spurts).

Clinical Presentation and Physical Examination

Neonates with significant outflow tract obstruction may present with severe CHF, whereas patients with mild or moderate valvar disease may simply present in infancy or later with a systolic ejection click and an asymptomatic harsh systolic ejection ("crescendo-decrescendo") murmur at the base of the heart. Rarely, patients present with anginal symptoms of diaphoresis or with chest or abdominal pain. Approximately 25% of patients also have an early diastolic murmur from aortic insufficiency. The cardiac examination may or may not correlate with the degree of obstruction to ventricular outflow, depending on cardiac output. A left ventricular heave or thrill (particularly in the suprasternal notch) usually is palpable with more severe obstruction.

Testing

The majority of patients demonstrate left ventricular and/or left atrial hypertrophy augmented by ST segment depression and T wave inversion; however, the correlation between ECG findings and transvalvar pressure gradings generally is poor. CXR does little to help define the severity of stenosis. Rounding of the left ventricular apex in the frontal plane may indicate concentric left ventricular hypertrophy. The echocardiogram is valuable for distinguishing valvar from subvalvar or supravalvar stenosis, for defining associated lesions, and for gauging ventricular chamber sizes and thickness of the ventricular wall or septum. Bicycle or treadmill exercise testing frequently is used in the evaluation of patients with aortic valve disease: it helps show abnormal ECG changes, symptoms, or hemodynamic instability. Cardiac catheterization is important for establishing the site and severity of the obstruction to left ventricular outflow.

Therapy

Although the original criteria for transcatheter or surgical intervention included a systolic gradient of at least 60 mm Hg, interventional catheterization can now be performed for lower gradients in the presence of symptoms or significant ventricular dysfunction. In most patients, technically adequate balloon valvulotomy is achieved in 70% to 80% and results in reduction of the systolic gradient to 25 to 35 mm Hg. Postintervention complications include dysrhythmias, restenosis (30%–40% within 10 years), ventricular dysfunction, or aortic insufficiency.

Subaortic Stenosis

Subvalvar aortic stenosis (membranous or fibrous) accounts for 8% to 10% of all cases of congenital aortic stenosis, may occur in conjunction with valvar aortic stenosis, and occurs more frequently in males than in females.

Clinical Presentation

Clinical history of patients with subvalvar aortic stenosis is similar to that of those who have valvar aortic stenosis.

Physical Examination

The presence (valvar) or absence (subvalvar) of a systolic ejection click may differentiate valvar and subvalvar aortic stenosis. The systolic murmurs tend to be similar.

Testing

The ECG is similar to that of patients with valvar aortic stenosis of a similar degree. CXR shows variable dilation of the ascending aorta with an otherwise normal cardiac silhouette. Echocardiography is valuable in confirming the clinical diagnosis, defining the degree of subvalvar stenosis and its etiology, and identifying subclinical degrees of aortic insufficiency.

Therapy

A gradient greater than 40 mm Hg between ventricle and ascending aorta or lesser gradients with associated aortic insufficiency are indications for intervention. The membranous or fibrous muscular ridge is surgically resected, although more extensive myomectomy of the ventricular septum and/or valve repair or replacement may be necessary. In 20% to 40% of patients, stenosis may recur within 10 years.

Supravalvar Aortic Stenosis

Supravalvar aortic stenosis (localized or diffuse narrowing of the aorta above the level of the coronary arteries) can present either in isolation or in association with idiopathic infantile hypercalcemia (Williams syndrome). Prolonged supravalvar stenosis occurring distal to the origins of the coronary arteries may lead to thickened coronary artery media and intima with associated premature coronary arteriosclerosis.

Clinical Presentation

In most patients without Williams syndrome, discovery of a systolic ejection murmur on physical examination and findings on echocardiography may lead to the diagnosis.

Physical Examination

Physical examination in patients who have isolated supravalvar aortic stenosis differs little from that of those who have subvalvar aortic stenosis.

Testing

Angiography has value in defining the ascending aortic anatomy as well as screening for coronary abnormalities.

Therapy

Balloon angioplasty of the supravalvar region has reported limited success. Surgical intervention involves patch angioplasty of the ascending aorta, creating an enlarged aortic outflow tract.

COARCTATION OF THE AORTA

Isolated coarctation of the aorta (membranous or long-segment hypoplasia) is among the most common congenital heart lesions and constitutes 7.5% of congenital heart defects in infants younger than 1 year of age in the New England Regional Study of Congenital Heart Defects. Associated congenital cardiac abnormalities include bicuspid aortic valve (in up to 85% of patients), PDA, VSD, mitral valve abnormalities, and berry aneurysms of the cerebral circulation. Coarctation is the most common congenital cardiovascular abnormality found in patients who have Turner syndrome.

Clinical Presentation

Neonates with significant coarctation may have differential oxygen saturations, blood pressure, and pulses between the upper and lower extremities and cyanosis of the feet. In contrast, in children, adolescents, and adults, the coarctation may not be discovered until murmur evaluation or systemic systolic hypertension is diagnosed.

Physical Examination

The diagnosis of coarctation of the aorta is made principally by noting differential blood pressures and pulses between upper and lower extremities. The systolic ejection murmur usually is heard in the left hemithorax, localized to the left axilla and the infrascapular areas. A systolic ejection click may be heard when there is associated aortic stenosis.

Testing

In the neonate and young infant who have aortic coarctation, the ECG may indicate right ventricular hypertrophy with or without strain in a right-axis deviation pattern. In older patients, left ventricular hypertrophy is more commonly diagnosed. A characteristic "3 sign" or rib notching may be noted on CXR. The echocardiogram is useful in confirming the diagnosis and determining associated abnormalities. In some older and larger patients, magnetic resonance imaging may be necessary to delineate the complete aortic anatomy.

Therapy

In the neonate who has severe left and/or right ventricular failure, attempts to reopen the ductus arteriosus using standard infusions of prostaglandin E_1 (alprostadil [Prostin VR Pediatric]) are necessary to increase descending aortic flow and to reverse metabolic acidosis and cardiogenic shock. Stabilization of the patients with inotropic support, if necessary, is crucial. In the neonate or infant who demonstrates clear evidence of CHF, intervention becomes more critical. Indications for intervention in the older child include systemic systolic hypertension unmanageable by medical therapy, systolic pressure gradients greater than 25 mm Hg, or significant ventricular dysfunction.

Transcatheter interventions for coarctation of the aorta can be performed in the cardiac catheterization laboratory by isolated balloon angioplasty and, more recently, by balloon angioplasty with associated endovascular stent implantation. Overall, the procedure successfully reduces systolic gradients in 65% to 75% of patients. In patients who have gradients of more than 50 mm Hg, success rates dropped to below 50%. Surgical repair of coarctation was first reported in the late 1930s and has included end-to-end anastomosis, patch aortoplasty, or subclavian flap angioplasty. Surgical repairs of these lesions have been complicated by restenosis rates as high as 40% and by aneurysm formation. Postoperative complications include postcoarctectomy syndrome (acute onset of severe systolic and diastolic hypertension). Long-term evidence exists for rebound hypertension during adolescence or young adult life in patients treated beyond 5 years of age even with excellent surgical or interventional repairs.

CYANOTIC HEART DISEASE

Fifteen percent to 20% of infants and children who have CHD will present with cyanosis secondary to right-to-left shunts (i.e., systemic venous blood bypasses the lungs and mixes with the systemic arterial circulation), obstruction to inflow to the right ventricle (i.e., tricuspid atresia), severe right ventricular outflow tract obstruction (i.e., tetralogy of Fallot), or abnormally configured great vessels. The most common form of cyanotic heart disease in the neonate is D-transposition of the great arteries, whereas tetralogy of Fallot is the most common cyanotic lesion beyond the neonatal period. In the majority of neonates with cyanotic heart disease, the Pa_{O_2} is less than 50 mm Hg in room air with little increase in supplemental oxygen and normal or decreased carbon dioxide levels. Other syndromes (i.e., mechanical interference with lung function, hematologic abnormalities, hypoglycemia, or sepsis) must be excluded in the differential diagnosis of cyanosis in the neonate.

Distribution of cyanosis is crucial. Peripheral cyanosis (*acrocyanosis*) involving only the hands and feet is common in the neonate and is usually benign. True central cyanosis involves superficial capillary-rich beds (lips, mucous membranes, and nail beds). CXR defines the cardiac silhouette and pulmonary vascular markings and rules out other causes for cyanosis. Clinical cyanosis associated with increased pulmonary vascularity on CXR is suggestive of complete transposition of the great arteries, total anomalous pulmonary venous return, truncus arteriosus, some forms of tricuspid atresia, and some forms of single ventricular anatomy. CXR demonstrating decreased pulmonary blood flow raises suspicion for critical pulmonary valve stenosis, tetralogy of Fallot, pulmonary atresia, tricuspid atresia, single ventricle anatomy, and Ebstein anomaly. In some patients who have cyanotic heart disease, characteristic ECG changes of the specific anomaly may be noted. The ultimate test in most cases will be either 2-D and Doppler echocardiography or cardiac catheterization. Initial management of the cyanotic newborn should include oxygen supplementation and, if indicated, stabilization of the airway with endotracheal intubation. Acidosis, hypoglycemia, anemia, or sepsis should be treated aggressively. When suspicion of congenital cyanotic heart disease is high, prostaglandin E_1 therapy should be initiated to maintain patency of the ductus arteriosus.

SPECIFIC LESIONS

Tetralogy of Fallot

Tetralogy of Fallot is composed of four components, including a malaligned VSD, pulmonary outflow tract obstruction, concomitant right ventricular hypertrophy, and an overriding aorta. In many patients, a right aortic arch is identified. In addition, in 5% to 15% of patients, the left anterior descending coronary artery arises directly from the right coronary artery, which may have significant technical implications at the time of surgical repair.

Clinical Presentation

Many patients with this lesion present in the neonatal period for evaluation of a systolic ejection murmur. Significant cyanosis is rare in the neonate. The classic presentation of the infant with tetralogy of Fallot is a "hyperpneic spell" or tetralogy spell ascribed to infundibular spasm.

Physical Examination

Physical examination may be dominated by significant generalized or localized cyanosis. The first heart sound is normal but consistent with severe pulmonary stenosis; the second sound may be either narrowly split or single. In the presence of significant pulmonary valvar disease, there may be a soft systolic ejection click. During a hypercyanotic spell, the loud systolic ejection murmur usually decreases in both intensity and frequency. In a patient who has tetralogy of Fallot and no pulmonary valve, a "to-fro" murmur may be heard.

Testing

Common findings on the ECG include right-axis deviation of the QRS complexes and right ventricular hypertrophy. Varying degrees of right bundle branch block also can be seen before and after surgical repair. The classic CXR reveals a *coeur en sabot* (boot-shaped heart) cardiac silhouette. Approximately 20% of patients who have tetralogy of Fallot will have a right aortic arch. Pulmonary vascular markings usually are normal or decreased. Echocardiography is valuable for confirming the diagnosis, identifying the level of outflow tract obstruction, defining the location and number of VSDs, and revealing associated anomalies. Angiography further defines the branch and hilar/parenchymal PAs and defects in the ventricular septum. In some patients, aortography also reveals the presence of aortopulmonary collaterals and coronary anatomy.

Therapy

Treatment of hypercyanotic spells is a medical emergency. The majority of spells respond to conservative measures such as calming of the child, administration of fluid boluses, and bending the knees to the chest. Oxygen should be administered. In more severe spells, sodium bicarbonate boluses (1–2 mEq/kg), intravenous sedation (morphine sulfate,* lorazepam [Ativan]*), and/or intravenous administration of β-blocking agents may be necessary. Intravenous or intramuscular ketamine (Ketalar), 1 to 2 mg/kg, or general anesthesia followed by emergency surgical intervention may be indicated in the most severe cases.

In the presence of increasing cyanosis, hemoglobin levels must be monitored carefully to avoid polycythemia, which may lead to brain abscesses in up to 2% of patients. Medical management in stable patients may include oral β-blockade to reduce infundibular spasm but is only preparatory for eventual surgery. Surgical intervention can be either palliative (Blalock-Taussig aortopulmonary shunt to increase pulmonary blood flow) or complete intracardiac repair. Surgical mortality is low, ranging in most centers from 2% to 4%, but residual hemodynamic abnormalities are common and may include outflow tract obstruction or a VSD. More data are accumulating about long-term consequences of tetralogy of Fallot repair pertaining to significant ventricular dysrhythmias and sudden unexpected death.

---

*Not FDA approved for this indication.

Pulmonary Valve Atresia With Ventricular Septal Defect

Pulmonary valve atresia with VSD is considered to be the most extreme tetralogy of Fallot and accounts for approximately 2% of patients with CHD. In some patients, aortopulmonary collateral flow and/or flow from the PDA may supply all of the lung tissue, but only rarely do both sources of pulmonary blood flow coexist in the same lung. Pulmonary valve atresia with VSD is frequently associated with a right aortic arch and a secundum atrial septal defect.

Clinical Presentation

The majority of patients present during the neonatal period. Because many who have this lesion have significant aortopulmonary collaterals, cyanosis may not be severe because of adequate pulmonary blood flow. The natural history of these collaterals, however, is to become more stenotic with advancing age, leading to worsening cyanosis.

Physical Examination

Common presenting signs beyond the neonatal period are mild cyanosis and/or multiple continuous murmurs heard throughout the chest, back, and axillae. The large run-off lesions from the collaterals or ductus arteriosus may lead to widened pulse pressures and fuller pulses. Patients usually demonstrate normal first heart sounds and single second heart sounds. Systolic murmurs may represent VSD flow or concomitant atrioventricular valve insufficiency.

Testing

The ECG pattern is consistent with significant right ventricular outflow tract obstruction. The boot-shaped heart is the most classic radiographic presentation in this lesion, similar to that in patients who have tetralogy of Fallot. Likewise, CXR is valuable in identifying sidedness of the aortic arch. Echocardiography may confirm the diagnosis but may not fully delineate the extent of the aortopulmonary collaterals, which may be better delineated by aortography. Confluence of the proximal native PAs must be defined before surgery.

Therapy

Therapy is primarily surgical. An initial systemic-to-PA shunt (i.e., Blalock-Taussig shunt) may be indicated either in the immediate neonatal period or in infancy. Eventual repair includes creation of a conduit from the right ventricle to the PA. When pulmonary blood flow from the right ventricle to the lungs is sufficient, the VSD can be closed surgically. A significant proportion of patients eventually will require replacement of their conduits because they either outgrow them or develop conduit stenosis and/or insufficiency.

Pulmonary Atresia With Intact Ventricular Septum

Pulmonary atresia with intact ventricular septum is a complex of significant right-sided heart abnormalities that in many cases has poor long-term outcomes. Although uncommon overall (3% of all congenital defects), about 25% of cyanotic newborns have such lesions. Right ventricular and tricuspid anomalies are common. Many patients develop moderate to severe tricuspid insufficiency and significant right atrial dilation in utero.

Clinical Presentation

The initial clinical symptom is significant cyanosis within hours or days after birth. Development of severe cyanosis usually is rapid and may be accompanied by progressive hypoxemia, metabolic acidosis, and worsening right ventricular failure. Neonates presenting with severe intrauterine tricuspid valve insufficiency may also manifest CHF.

Physical Examination

Cyanosis and the regurgitant murmur of tricuspid insufficiency dominate physical examination. There is a single second heart sound in most patients.

Testing

The most striking findings on ECG are severe right ventricular hypertrophy with strain, right atrial enlargement, and a somewhat leftward axis. The majority of patients who have pulmonary atresia with intact ventricular septum present with a normal to small cardiac silhouette and diminished pulmonary vascular markings. Patients who have associated severe tricuspid insufficiency may manifest severe cardiomegaly and right atrial enlargement. 2-D echocardiography is diagnostic. Determining the size of the tricuspid valve and right ventricular mass is important in deciding which surgical procedures are necessary. Color Doppler flow studies are invaluable in determining presence and degree of coronary sinusoidal flow. In many patients, cardiac catheterization and angiography become crucial in defining the presence of coronary artery fistulas and sinusoids between the right ventricle and coronary arteries. Significant coronary stenoses may be found where the abnormal sinusoid meets with the normal coronary artery.

Therapy

Initial therapy involves initiation of prostaglandin E_1 infusion to maintain ductal patency. Supportive measures should be performed as necessary. Systemic-to-PA shunts, pulmonary valvotomy, or combinations of these interventions have all been proposed as initial palliations, depending on the degree of right-sided heart hypoplasia. A significant factor in long-term survival is the presence or absence of the stenotic coronary sinusoidal connections. In many centers, patients with severely stenotic coronary fistulas are listed for primary orthotopic cardiac transplantation.

Tricuspid Atresia

Tricuspid atresia occurs in approximately 2.7% of patients. Three different types of tricuspid atresia have been broadly categorized. In approximately 70% of patients, tricuspid atresia exists concomitantly with normally related great vessels, in 20% to 30% of patients, with D-transposition of the great arteries and in 3% to 7% of patients, with L-transposition of the great arteries.

Clinical Presentation

More than 40% of patients present with cyanosis within the first day of life; the remainder present within 1 month with symptoms varying from low cardiac output and diminished pulmonary blood flow to CHF from pulmonary overcirculation (uncommon). Some patients who have severe cyanosis and concomitant polycythemia may present with cerebrovascular accidents or brain abscesses, particularly after acute febrile illnesses. In general, patients tend to have cyanosis, delayed growth, and clubbing.

Physical Examination

Physical examination depends on associated anomalies such as VSDs or pulmonary stenosis. The first heart sound tends to be single and may be accentuated, whereas the second heart sound may be single or normally split.

Testing

In more than 95% of patients, the ECG demonstrates a leftward and superior axis (0 to −90 degrees). In patients who have normal right ventricular mass, normal right-sided voltages may be noted. CXR varies depending on the constellation of anatomic abnormalities. Echocardiography provides data concerning size of the right ventricle, the relationship of the great vessels, the presence and size of ASDs and VSDs, and ventricular systolic function. Cardiac catheterization and angiography are valuable in further definition of the anatomy and physiology. If necessary, either blade or balloon atrial septostomies can be performed at the time of angiography to increase interatrial blood flow.

Therapy

Initial management includes maintaining ductal patency with prostaglandin E_1 infusion. Standard medical management for CHF (diuretic therapy, afterload reduction, inotropic support) should be initiated. In the presence of diminished pulmonary blood flow, many patients undergo palliative procedures, including aortopulmonary shunts. Single ventricle repairs including anastomosis of the superior vena cava to the PA and inferior vena cava anastomosis to the PA can be performed in children between 12 and 36 months of age. Long-term, patients need to be followed for significant atrial dysrhythmias and complications of systemic venous hypertension, including liver dysfunction and protein-losing enteropathy.

Complete Transposition of the Great Arteries

Complete transposition of the great arteries occurs in 5% to 7% of all children with congenital cardiac malformations. Morphologically, the aorta arises from the right ventricle and the PA from the left ventricle. Patients with this diagnosis have two circulations in parallel and little mixing of oxygenated and deoxygenated blood. Without any form of treatment, approximately 30% of neonates die within the first week of life, 50% within the first month, and 90% within the first year. Other associated anomalies include atrial septal defect (5%), VSD (30%–35%), and coronary abnormalities (30%).

Clinical Presentation

Neonates with transposition of the great arteries are usually born to multiparous women at full term and are well developed but present with significant cyanosis unresponsive to supplemental oxygen therapy.

Physical Examination

Auscultation in these patients may reveal a normal first heart sound and in the majority of patients, a single or loud second heart sound. No murmur is heard in about 40% of patients.

Testing

The ECG findings are variable from normal to significant ventricular hypertrophy. Other ECG findings may be present when there are associated lesions. The classic cardiac silhouette in patients who have transposed great arteries is described as an "egg on a string." Echocardiography plays an important diagnostic role. In the majority of cases, the proximal coronary anatomy can be fully delineated by 2-D imaging. Cardiac catheterization is indicated when better definition of coronary artery anatomy is needed but in most cases is performed for emergent transcatheter intervention (e.g., balloon atrial septostomy, a procedure in which a hole is created in the interatrial septum). Balloon atrial septostomy has improved 1-month survival in this condition from 50% to more than 95%.

Therapy

Initiation of prostaglandin E_1 therapy to preserve patency of the ductus arteriosus is indicated. Acidosis, hypoglycemia, pulmonary overcirculation, and CHF should be managed with standard medical therapy. With marked improvement in noninvasive imaging, many patients can undergo complete surgical repair based solely on echocardiographic anatomic evaluation. Senning and Mustard developed the atrial switch operation as the definitive surgical repair. Longer follow-up (>10 years) studies have indicated worsening right ventricular function and the eventual need for cardiac transplantation in many patients. Sinus and atrioventricular nodal disease and significant atrial and ventricular dysrhythmias have developed in a large minority of patients, necessitating pacemaker or automatic implantable cardioverter-defibrillator implantation. Since the late 1970s and early 1980s, the surgical preference in most centers has been an arterial switch operation.

With improving techniques, significant operative morbidity and mortality is 5% or less. The major complication after arterial switch surgery involves coronary kinking or tension on the anastomotic line of the coronary vessels, which may lead to acute myocardial ischemia in the immediate postoperative period.

Truncus Arteriosus

Persistence of the truncus arteriosus (progenitor of the aorta and PA) and large VSD is an uncommon cardiac malformation (1%–4% of cardiac deformities). Its primary association has been in patients who have DiGeorge syndrome. The single truncal valve may be deformed or functionally insufficient, and significant associated aortic arch abnormalities have been reported. PA anatomy has also been subcategorized in this condition, depending on the presence or absence of a main PA (48%–68%) and/or contiguity of the branch PAs (29%–48%).

Clinical Presentation

Patients usually present with mild cyanosis (oxygen saturations of 80%–85%). Over the first 4 to 6 weeks of life, cyanosis may disappear and be replaced by signs and symptoms of pulmonary overcirculation and CHF.

Physical Examination

Peripheral pulses usually are accentuated, and pulse pressure is increased. The first heart sound is normal and frequently is followed by a loud ejection click from the single, redundant truncal valve. The second heart sound usually is single and loud. Patients who have truncal valve insufficiency may present with a high-pitched diastolic murmur heard along the left sternal border.

Testing

The ECG demonstrates a normal QRS axis with variations in voltages depending on the degree of pulmonary overcirculation. Typically, the CXR demonstrates moderate cardiomegaly with variable pulmonary vascular markings depending on flow patterns. Echocardiography best defines the cardiac anatomy and great vessel abnormalities. Doppler techniques are useful in assessing pressure gradients and degrees of truncal valve stenosis and insufficiency. Angiography and pulmonary hemodynamic study may be valuable in delineating coronary and PA anatomy and pressures not well defined by noninvasive imaging.

Therapy

Standard anticongestive medications may be necessary. Without surgical intervention, outcomes are poor, with a mean age at death of 5 weeks and only 15% to 30% survival beyond 1 year of age. Most centers have advocated complete repair in early infancy consisting of closure of the VSD and a right ventricle to PA conduit repair. Additional operations become necessary over the course of the patient's life to replace these conduits because they either fail or are outgrown. Early studies of operative mortality in single center reports were 25% but have now fallen to below 10%. Severe incompetence of the truncal valve adds significantly to the overall surgical risk.

HYPOPLASTIC LEFT HEART SYNDROME

Hypoplastic left heart syndrome constitutes a continuum of left ventricular, atrial, and aortic hypoplasia. This malformation occurs in 7% to 9% of patients who have CHD with a 2:1 male predominance.

Clinical Presentation

Nearly 40% of infants with hypoplastic left heart syndrome present within the first 2 days of life, and an additional 35% present within 2 to 7 days. Cyanosis may be the initial presenting symptom, although patients also can present in cardiogenic shock.

Physical Examination

The physical examination reveals tachycardia, tachypnea, and hepatosplenomegaly in the patient in cardiogenic shock. The first and second heart sounds tend to be single; third and fourth heart sounds may be present.

Testing

The ECG may demonstrate decreased left-sided forces or apparent "increased" left-sided forces generated by right ventricular rotation toward the apex of the heart. Large P waves, indicative of right atrial enlargement, may also be noted. Coronary insufficiency from ductal restriction and inadequate aortic flow may yield ST-segment and T-wave abnormalities. There is no diagnostic radiographic pattern for this syndrome. Cardiac catheterization and angiography have become less common with improvements in noninvasive imaging studies.

Therapy

Institution of prostaglandin E_1 therapy is mandatory to maintain systemic cardiac output. Reversal of shock is crucial. When interatrial flow is restricted causing increasing pulmonary edema, balloon atrial septostomy, blade septostomy, or static balloon dilation of the interatrial communication has sometimes proven valuable. Without surgical treatment, nearly 95% of all infants will die by the first month. The two major surgical approaches at present are single ventricle three-stage palliative therapy (Norwood operation) and orthotopic heart transplantation. Survival after the first stage of the three-staged repair varies between 65% and 90%; survival through the second stage decreases to 60% to 85% and after the third stage varies from 50% to 75%. Initial survival after orthotopic heart transplantation is more than 90%. Issues of acute rejection and the increased incidence of leukemias, lymphomas, and infections still limit 5-year survival to 75%.

ANOMALOUS PULMONARY VENOUS RETURN

Almost any connection between the embryologic pulmonary veins, common pulmonary vein, and the other neonatal systemic venous circuits (e.g., superior and inferior vena cava) can occur, yielding the four major categories of anomalous pulmonary venous drainage:

Supracardiac (connections to the superior vena cava)
Cardiac (directly to right atrium or coronary sinus)
Infracardiac (connecting to inferior vena cava)
Mixed form that combines two of these categories

Associated complex cardiac anomalies are found in approximately 30% of patients (e.g., transposition of the great arteries, pulmonary atresia).

Clinical Presentation

Patients who have partial anomalous pulmonary venous return may have a presentation similar to that of patients with an atrial septal defect. Clinical presentation depends on the degree of pulmonary venous obstruction (varying from cyanosis to significant CHF).

Physical Examination

The first heart sound is increased and distinct, followed by a systolic ejection click caused by increased pulmonary blood flow. The second heart sound is widely split and does not vary with respiration. Loud "hums" that do not change with variation in position may also be found in patients who have supracardiac disease.

Testing

Some degree of right atrial enlargement (enlarged P waves) is identified on the ECG. Patients with partial anomalous pulmonary venous return or unobstructed total anomalous pulmonary venous return usually display a radiographic picture of right ventricular volume overload. Significant pulmonary venous obstruction may manifest by marked pulmonary venous congestion and a prominent innominate vein yielding the "snowman" sign. 2-D echocardiography is invaluable in defining the drainage patterns of the pulmonary veins. Selective pulmonary arteriography is undertaken when questions arise from noninvasive studies.

Therapy

In patients with partial anomalous pulmonary venous return or total anomalous pulmonary venous return without obstruction, intervention depends on the degree of symptomatology. Surgical intervention depends on the entry location of the anomalous veins and the presence or absence of an atrial septal defect. In patients with total anomalous pulmonary venous return and pulmonary venous obstruction, emergent surgical intervention is required. Surgery should be delayed only long enough to optimize the patient's clinical condition. Postoperative mortality in the 1970s was as high as 50%; subsequently, mortality has dropped to 27%. Long-term prognosis depends on the amount of preoperative pulmonary vascular injury. Postoperative stenoses at the anastomosis site to the left atrium requiring later intervention occur in 5% to 10% of patients.

HYPERTROPHIC CARDIOMYOPATHY

method of
PAOLO SPIRITO, M.D., and
MARCO PICCININNO, M.D.
Ente Ospedaliero Ospedali Galliera
Genoa, Italy

Hypertrophic cardiomyopathy (HCM) is a primary and usually familial cardiac disorder characterized by a clinical and pathophysiologic complexity that has challenged researchers and physicians since its modern description in the late 1950s. Much of the difficulty in the investigation and management of this disease comes from its extremely heterogeneous clinical presentation and prognosis, relatively low prevalence, and difficulty in enrolling large study populations not influenced by tertiary referral bias.

In recent years, rapid progress in the identification of the molecular causes of HCM and results of clinical studies based on large patient populations have greatly advanced our understanding of this disorder and identified new approaches in prognosis and treatment. Also, newly proposed interventional procedures have generated some debate and uncertainties regarding the optimal therapeutic strategies for patients with the obstructive form of the disease. This article examines our present knowledge of HCM and discusses patient treatment.

PREVALENCE AND DIAGNOSIS

Systematic screening of large study populations with echocardiography or electrocardiography has recently shown that the prevalence of HCM in the general population is higher than previously thought, ranging from 1 in 500 to 1 in 1000. Clinical and genetic screening of HCM pedigrees has confirmed these observations, showing that many affected family members are asymptomatic and unaware of the disease. Therefore, HCM is a frequent genetic disorder of the heart.

A hypertrophied and nondilated left ventricle is the characteristic morphologic marker of HCM. Wall thickening is usually asymmetric and varies greatly, ranging from 13 to more than 40 mm, with an average of 20 to 22 mm. In most patients, left ventricular hypertrophy first develops or progresses during childhood or adolescence, often in the absence of symptoms. The frequency of first development of hypertrophy in adulthood cannot be estimated at present, but it is likely to occur in a minority of patients and appears to be associated with the presence of molecular defects in the myosin-binding protein-C gene.

MOLECULAR FEATURES

During the past decade, molecular biology has shown that HCM can be caused by mutations in nine genes, providing further insights into the heterogeneity of this disorder. Each of these genes encodes a protein of the cardiac sarcomere: the β-myosin heavy chain gene, cardiac troponin T and I, α-tropomyosin, myosin-binding protein-C, cardiac actin, titin, and the cardiac myosin light chain genes. At present, the β-myosin heavy chain and myosin binding protein-C mutations appear to be the most common molecular defects. Other genes that cause HCM may be found in the future and are likely to encode sarcomeric proteins.

This genetic complexity of the disease is further increased by intragenic heterogeneity. More than 200 HCM-causing mutations have been identified in these genes of the sarcomere. Therefore, the molecular defect responsible for HCM in unrelated individuals is usually different. Some mutations would appear to be associated with a particularly unfavorable prognosis (e.g., Arg403Gln in the β-myosin heavy chain gene). Although these observations suggest that identification of the mutation in the individual patient could improve assessment of prognosis, genetic characterization remains complex and time-consuming because of both the number of genes involved and the high degree of intragenic heterogeneity. Also, the disease varies greatly in its clinical presentation within HCM families, suggesting that other factors such as modifier genes may play an important role in the phenotypic expression of the disorder.

PATHOPHYSIOLOGY AND NATURAL HISTORY

The pathophysiology of HCM is particularly complex. Diastolic function is abnormal with prolonged isovolumic relaxation, impaired rapid filling, and reduced compliance. Myocardial ischemia and altered vasodilator reserve (in the absence of coronary atherosclerosis) have been documented. Dynamic obstruction to left ventricular outflow is present in about 20% of patients. Malignant ventricular tachyarrhythmias and atrial fibrillation also play an important role in the clinical course of the disease.

Because the magnitude of hypertrophy and severity of functional alterations differ greatly in the individual patient, the natural history of HCM is extremely heterogeneous. Many patients have few or no symptoms and a normal longevity, some develop severe symptoms of heart failure, and others die suddenly, often at a young age and in the absence of previous symptoms. This diversity in clinical course identifies two distinct issues in the management of the disease: treatment of symptoms for improvement of quality of life and identification of those asymptomatic or mildly symptomatic patients who are at high risk of sudden death and deserve aggressive treatment. These two issues must be confronted by largely independent strategies and are addressed separately.

TREATMENT OF SYMPTOMS

Medical Treatment

β-Blockers (either propranolol [Inderal], 120–360 mg/d or long-acting and cardioselective β-blockers at comparative doses) are traditionally used as the initial treatment in patients with exertional dyspnea and fatigue (Figure 1). Verapamil (Calan, Isoptin), 240 to 460 mg/d appears to be more effective than β-blockers and is the drug of first choice when chest pain is the main symptom. In patients with an important outflow gradient, verapamil should be initiated at low doses (40 mg every 8 hours) because its vasodilatory effects may lead to deleterious hemodynamic responses. In patients with heart failure despite treatment with β-blockers or verapamil, the addition of diuretics in low doses usually is effective in improving symptoms.

In the 1980s, disopyramide (Norpace) was introduced as an alternative treatment for patients with obstructive HCM and severe symptoms unresponsive to standard medical therapy. This drug has the potential to reduce the outflow gradient and symptoms through its negative inotropic properties; however, the hemodynamic and clinical benefits often decrease with time. The possible proarrhythmic effects of disopyramide are of concern and have limited the use of this drug in HCM.

There is no evidence that β-blockers or verapamil administered prophylactically in asymptomatic patients prevents or delays the onset of symptoms and disease progression or reduces the risk of sudden death. Also relevant to this issue is the growing awareness that an important proportion of patients with HCM remain asymptomatic throughout life and have a normal longevity. Therefore, prophylactic drug treatment would not appear justified in many patients. However, a relationship has been recently identified between the presence of an outflow gradient and the risk of death due to heart failure in HCM. On the basis of these results, it may be advisable to use β-blockers in asymptomatic children or young adults with a marked outflow gradient, with

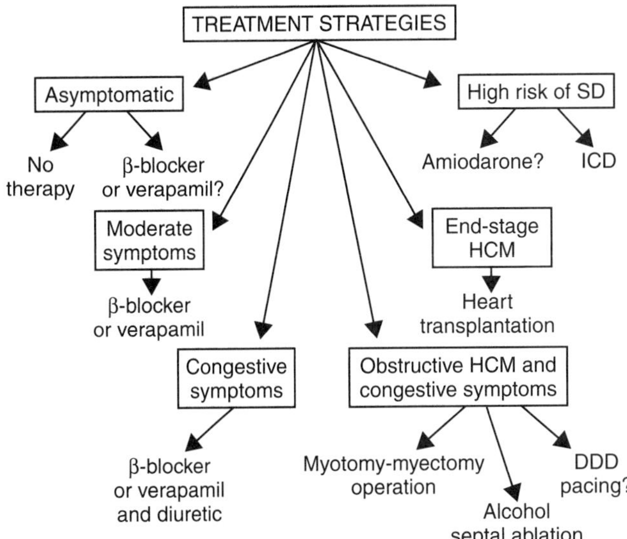

Figure 1. Treatment strategies for different clinical presentations of hypertrophic cardiomyopathy. Question marks indicate therapeutic approaches that remain uncertain.

the expectation that treatment could possibly improve prognosis. At present, there is no evidence that, in the absence of severe symptoms, invasive strategies aimed at reducing or abolishing the gradient are justified in this patient subgroup because of the acute complications and still undefined long-term risks of these procedures.

A small proportion of cases of HCM evolve to end-stage disease, characterized by left ventricular wall thinning, cavity enlargement, systolic dysfunction, and severe symptoms of congestive heart failure. The standard therapy for heart failure associated with systolic dysfunction is indicated in these patients, including diuretics, acetylcholinesterase inhibitors, and digitalis. Often, however, heart transplantation becomes the only therapeutic option.

Atrial fibrillation develops in an important minority of adult patients with HCM. Not infrequently, paroxysmal atrial fibrillation is associated with rapid clinical deterioration due to a high ventricular rate and impaired diastolic filling. Amiodarone appears to be the most effective drug for prevention of recurrent episodes; the doses used in HCM for this purpose are 1 to 2 g/week. β-Blockers or verapamil, alone or in combination, are usually effective in controlling heart rate in patients with chronic atrial fibrillation. Anticoagulation therapy is indicated in patients with either paroxysmal or chronic atrial fibrillation.

Invasive Treatment

Not uncommonly, the presence of a left ventricular outflow gradient is compatible with normal or near normal longevity in the absence of significant symptoms. Therefore, the gradient should not be identified with the disease nor become the sole or main justification for invasive treatment. Because it is unknown whether surgery or invasive alternatives to surgery prolong survival or reduce the risk of sudden death, invasive therapy is only indicated in the small subgroup of HCM patients (probably <5%) who have a marked outflow gradient under basal conditions and severe symptoms (New York Heart Association functional class III–IV) refractory to drug therapy (see Figure 1).

Data assembled over 30 years show that surgery (ventricular septal myotomy-myectomy) is associated with a substantial and long-term (>5 years) symptomatic improvement in about 70% of patients, and abolishes or greatly reduces the basal outflow gradient in more than 90% of patients. However, a particular expertise with this operation is required to achieve a low operative mortality (<3%), which is available only at a few centers in North America and Europe. Therefore, in recent years, there has been growing interest in potential alternatives to surgery.

Dual-chamber pacing has been used in HCM in an attempt to relieve the outflow gradient and improve symptoms. However, the effects of this technique on the gradient are extremely variable. In addition, three recent randomized, double-blind, crossover studies could not find objective evidence of improved functional capacity (e.g., an increase in exercise time or peak oxygen consumption) with pacing. Therefore, at present, dual-chamber pacing does not appear to be a valid alternative to surgery in most patients.

Percutaneous alcohol septal ablation has also been proposed as an alternative to surgery in patients with HCM. In brief, an angioplasty catheter is introduced into a septal perforator branch of the anterior descending artery. The balloon is then inflated to prevent spilling of alcohol into the artery. Alcohol is injected through the catheter into the myocardium to cause a localized necrosis at the level of the basal, anterior interventricular septum. The purpose of the procedure is to decrease septal thickness in the area of systolic contact between septum and mitral valve and, by this mechanism, increase left ventricular outflow tract size, reduce or abolish mitral-septal contact and the outflow gradient, and alleviate symptoms.

During the past 5 years, alcohol septal ablation has been performed in a rapidly increasing number of patients with HCM at a few centers in Europe and the United States. The experience reported by these centers has been positive regarding short- to mid-term results and reassuring about the potential risks. However, a note of caution is warranted because the septal perforator branches of the anterior descending artery interconnect among themselves and with similar septal branches from the right coronary artery, to produce a network of collateral channels. Therefore, alcohol injected into a septal perforator branch of the anterior descending artery may reach areas of myocardium far from its anatomic territory and cause a larger than expected necrosis. To assess the distribution of flow in the myocardium and reduce the risk of extensive damage, most centers inject an echocontrast agent into the selected septal perforator under echocardiographic monitoring, before injecting the alcohol.

Complications include complete atrioventricular block necessitating a permanent pacemaker (7%–30% of patients), dissection of the left anterior descending artery, extensive left ventricular infarction, papillary muscle infarction with acute mitral valve regurgitation, and ventricular fibrillation within days after the procedure. Also, the potential for increased long-term arrhythmogenicity in or around the infarcted area remains unknown. At centers with a particularly large experience with alcohol septal ablation, the mortality rate is 2% to 4%, not lower than that reported for surgery.

Stratification of Risk of Sudden Death

Sudden and unexpected cardiac death may occur at any age in HCM and this devastating event remains the most common modality of death in children and young patients. The available data suggest that ventricular tachyarrhythmias are the cause of sudden death in most patients, either as a primary event related to the arrhythmogenic myocardial substrate or as a secondary phenomenon triggered by myocardial ischemia, diastolic dysfunction, outflow obstruction, systemic arterial hypotension, or paroxysmal supraventricular tachyarrhythmias.

Despite intense investigation, risk stratification remains a major challenge. However, several strong indicators of high risk are known in HCM, such as a previous cardiac arrest with documented ventricular fibrillation, sustained ventricular tachycardia, or a malignant family history of sudden death (generally defined as two or more sudden deaths in young first-degree relatives) (Figure 2). Recently, the magnitude of left ventricular hypertrophy has been shown to be an independent predictor of the risk of sudden death. Adolescents and young patients with extreme hypertrophy (maximal wall thickness ≥30 mm) appear to be at a high long-term risk (~20% at 10 years and 40% at 20 years).

Other indicators of increased risk, such as abnormal blood pressure response during exercise or brief and sporadic episodes of nonsustained ventricular tachycardia on Holter monitoring, have low positive predictive accuracy. However, it is reasonable to infer that either frequent or prolonged episodes of nonsustained ventricular tachycardia may convey more malignant prognostic implications and justify treatment for the prevention of sudden death.

The capability of electrophysiologic testing to identify patients at high risk of sudden death in HCM remains uncertain. Particularly aggressive stimulation protocols frequently trigger nonspecific responses also in patients at low risk, while standard protocols seldom induce specific responses even in those who have survived a cardiac arrest. Therefore, programmed electrical stimulation would not appear helpful in making management decisions in this disorder.

Syncope is one of the most challenging clinical features in HCM because of the diversity of the mechanisms potentially responsible for this symptom. The prognostic significance of syncope also remains undetermined. However, isolated and remote episodes of syncope are not uncommon in HCM. Therefore, patients with such a clinical presentation should be treated conservatively, including prolonged Holter monitoring, assessment of blood pressure response during exercise, and implantation of electrocardiogram recorder systems. Conversely, a recent history of recurrent syncope, particularly in young patients and during exercise, is more alarming and may justify aggressive treatment for the prevention of sudden death.

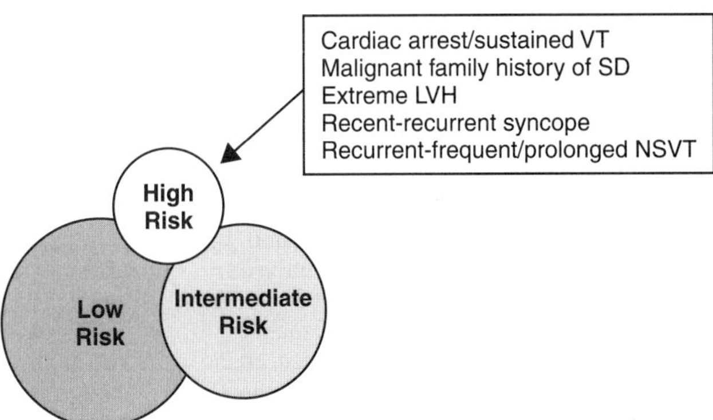

Figure 2. Summary of the indicators of high risk of sudden death in hypertrophic cardiomyopathy.

TREATMENT FOR PREVENTION OF SUDDEN DEATH

Amiodarone and the implantable cardiac defibrillator are the only two available options for the prevention of sudden death in high-risk patients with HCM. Evidence that amiodarone may be effective in preventing sudden death in this disease relies, however, on a single retrospective study published in the early 1980s. In recent investigations conducted in large HCM populations, 20% to 30% of sudden deaths occurred in patients who were taking amiodarone at the time of the event. These observations have raised doubts about the efficacy of this drug in preventing sudden death in this disease. Also, the long-term toxic effects of amiodarone limit its use in young patients.

Recently, the implantable cardiac defibrillator has been shown to be highly effective in terminating ventricular tachycardia/fibrillation in patients with HCM. Therefore, the device is warranted in patients known to be definitely at high risk of sudden death, such as those with a previous cardiac arrest, sustained ventricular tachycardia, malignant family history of sudden death, or adolescents and young patients with a left ventricular wall thickness that is at the extreme of the morphologic spectrum of the disease. In patients with a less-defined risk profile, management decisions should be based on the overall evaluation of risk, as well as the clinical judgment of the physician.

ACKNOWLEDGMENTS

We are indebted to Enrica Bagnato for her precious secretarial assistance.

MITRAL VALVE PROLAPSE

method of
GABRIEL A. ADELMANN, M.D., and
NEIL J. WEISSMAN, M.D.
Washington Hospital Center
Washington, D.C.

Mitral valve prolapse (MVP) is the systolic displacement of one or both mitral valve leaflets across the anular plane into the left atrium, with or without associated mitral regurgitation.

Although systolic clicks and late systolic murmurs were described in the late 19th century, their association with MVP was first established in the early 1960s by using left ventriculography. This complex was originally termed Barlow's syndrome, after the investigator who first described it. Other designations (mitral valve prolapse, click-systolic murmur syndrome, billowing mitral leaflet syndrome, floppy mitral valve syndrome, myxomatous mitral leaflet syndrome, or "hooding" mitral leaflets) are based on clinical, echocardiographic, or pathologic observations.

Mitral valve prolapse has been a controversial finding since it was first described almost 40 years ago. Many of the entities that identify an abnormality, such as prevalance of disease, associated findings, natural history, complications, and recommended treatment, are in a state of flux. At varying times, the prevalence was felt to be as high as 40% or as low as 1%. A variety of cardiovascular and psychiatric symptoms have been attributed to this valvular finding. Some have stated that MVP is the most common reason for mitral valve replacement, but others describe it as an interesting echocardiographic finding without clinical relevance.

Most of the controversy surrounding this finding has been due to the changing criteria for the diagnosis of MVP. Originally, MVP was diagnosed by the classic findings of a late systolic murmur and a midsystolic click, but this introduced patients with a wide assortment of other types of valvular disease. Later, M-mode echocardiographic criteria included various degrees of posterior leaflet prolapse, ranging from 1.5 to 3 mm, as diagnostic, criteria. However, there are several intrinsic limitations in the ability of M-mode echocardiography to diagnose MVP. The superiorly directed, apex-to-base leaflet bulging is perpendicular to the M-mode axis and thus cannot always be recorded. Moreover, the presence of M-mode findings consistent with MVP is strongly dependent on the direction of the interrogating beam. In the Framingham offspring cohort, M-mode findings of prolapse could be "brought out" in 5% to 55% of subjects, depending on beam angulation. Thus, M-mode echocardiography, in isolation, is no longer used for the diagnosis of MVP.

Two-dimensional (2-D) echocardiography has emerged as the diagnostic method of choice. Two-dimensional echocardiography allows visualization of the leaflets and of the anulus throughout the cardiac cycle, allowing proper identification of cases in which the mitral leaflets prolapse beyond the anular plane into the left atrium. Although it originally appeared that 2-D echocardiography would eliminate the confusion about the diagnosis of MVP, it inadvertently added to years of misdiagnosis!

Only after years of diagnosing MVP from multiple echocardiographic views did investigators at the Massachusetts General Hospital, using three-dimensional echocardiography, recognize that the mitral anulus is not planar but is instead saddle shaped. Parts of the anulus were higher than other parts (Figure 1). This led to the appearance of mitral leaflet prolapse into the left atrium in some views (the apical four-chamber view) but not in others (parasternal long-axis view). In fact, the displacement of the leaflets beyond the anular plane in the apical four-chamber view was very common in normal patients and added to the overdiagnosis of MVP. Currently, the diagnosis of MVP should be made from 2-D echocardiography on the parasternal long-axis view and should never be established solely on the basis of four-chamber views. (See later for details.)

CLASSIFICATION

Prolapse of the mitral leaflets can occur as a primary abnormality of the mitral valve or secondary to functional or structural changes in the mitral valve apparatus (mitral valve anulus, leaflets, chordae tendineae, papillary muscle, and adjacent aortic, left atrial, and left ventricular walls). MVP usually refers to the primary form of mitral valve prolapse but is occasionally misused to refer to secondary causes of leaflet prolapse. Because it can sometimes be difficult to classify a case of MVP as primary or secondary, it is worthwhile to be familiar with all the common secondary causes.

Secondary Mitral Valve Prolapse

Mitral valve prolapse can result from different conditions affecting the anatomy of the mitral valve and the myocardium. In some of these conditions, such as rheumatic fever causing distorted mitral leaflet morphology, there is anatomic involvement of the mitral valve and the subvalvular apparatus. In other conditions (hypertrophic cardiomyopathy, atrial septal defect), the leaflet morphology is histologically normal, but leaflet function is impaired by distortion of the surrounding cardiac anatomy.

Altered Geometry of the Papillary Muscles and the Mitral Valve. Papillary muscle dysfunction and relative papillary muscle displacement due to coronary ischemia can cause prolapsing of the mitral valve leaflets, with or without associated mitral regurgitation. Such changes have been demonstrated in animal models and have been observed in patients after an inferior myocardial infarction. Geometric changes affecting the function of the mitral valve and the subvalvular apparatus have also been noted in patients with cardiomyopathies. Hypertrophic cardiomyopathy may be associated with a distorted alignment of the papillary muscles, and dilated cardiomyopathy often causes mitral valve anulus dilation. All these abnormalities can result in prolapse of the mitral valve leaflets despite histologically normal mitral tissue.

Decreased Left Ventricular Cavity Size. When the left ventricular cavity is too small to accommodate the mitral valve, systolic prolapse may ensue. This is occasionally observed in patients with hypertrophic obstructive cardiomyopathy, as well as in those with conditions leading to a decrease in left ventricular filling (anorexia nervosa with associated decreased blood volume or atrial septal defect with a left-to-right shunt).

Distorted Mitral Valve Morphology Secondary to Systemic Disease. The histologic changes seen with rheumatic fever include fibrotic and inflammatory changes of the mitral valve leaflets and the subvalvular apparatus. The resulting geometric distortion may occasionally lead to leaflet prolapse.

Flail Mitral Leaflet. A closely related entity to mitral valve leaflet prolapse is a flail mitral valve. This is diagnosed when the leaflet tip is pointing toward the left atrial cavity in systole (as compared with MVP, in which the leaflet tips continue to point toward the left ventricle in systole). A flail mitral leaflet implies chordal or papillary muscle rupture. This can occur owing to subvalvular involvement resulting from primary MVP, myocardial ischemia, subvalvular trauma, or endocarditis.

Primary Mitral Valve Prolapse

Myxomatous valvular degeneration is the hallmark of the primary form of MVP. The valvular abnormality can occur in isolation or as part of a clinical spectrum of multisystem connective tissue disease.

The mitral valve leaflets are composed of three layers: (1) the atrialis, formed of thick collagen and elastic tissue on the atrial side of the leaflet; (2) the spongiosa, a thin, intermediate layer rich in mucopolysaccharides; and (3) the fibrosa, a fibrous layer on the ventricular aspect. In

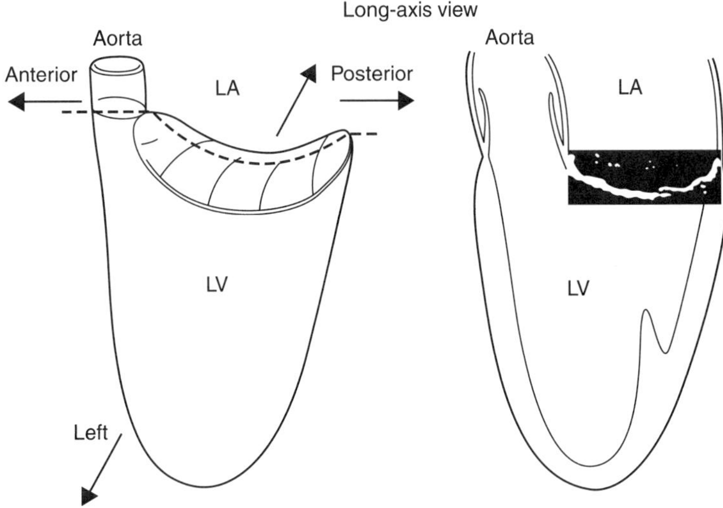

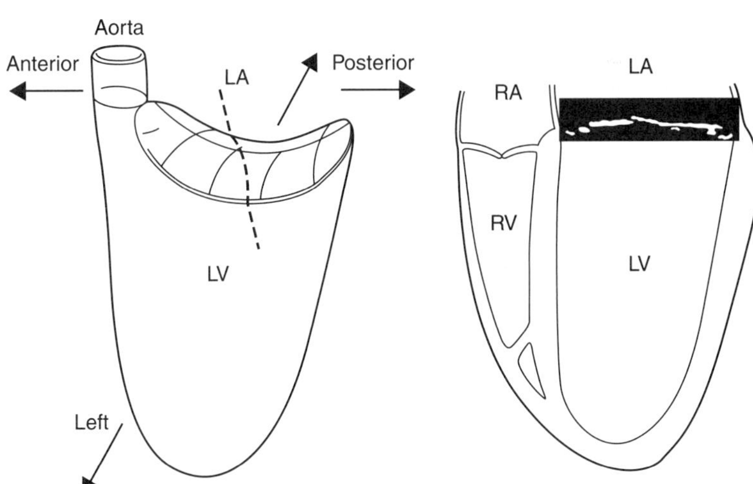

Figure 1. Discrepancy in leaflet-anular relationships in echocardiographic views of a saddle-shaped model structure. From Levine RA, Triulzi MO, Harrigan P, Weyman AE. The relationship of mitral anular shape to the diagnosis of mitral valve prolapse. Circulation 75:756–767, 1987.

primary MVP, there is excessive proliferation of the intermediary layer, causing disruption of the fibrosa and interchordal "hooding" of the valve leaflets with variable leaflet thickening. This proliferative process is often termed *myxomatous degeneration of the mitral valve*. Additional findings include secondary fibrosis of the mitral leaflets, thinning and elongation of the chordae tendineae, and associated ventricular friction lesions. These structural and functional abnormalities may predispose the affected valve to excessive trauma due to daily mechanical stress, resulting in mitral regurgitation.

The primary form of MVP usually occurs in isolation. The abnormal connective tissue is probably inherited via an autosomal dominant gene with variable penetrance. It may have a prevalence of 30% to 50% in first-degree relatives. Because MVP is a disorder of connective tissue, it is not surprising that there is an association between MVP and Marfan syndrome, Ehlers-Danlos syndrome, pseudoxanthoma elasticum, osteogenesis imperfecta, and skeletal abnormalities (pectus excavatum and straight thoracic spine). These diseases may result from defective embryogenesis in the mesenchymal layer, a theory supported by the association of primary MVP with hypomastia and with several coagulopathies, including von Willebrand disease.

SYMPTOMS

The multitude of symptoms classically reported in association with MVP have been collectively termed the *MVP syndrome*. This entity was initially considered to include chest pain, palpitation, dizziness, syncope, dyspnea, and exercise intolerance. In assessing the prevalence of these symptoms, it is essential to take into consideration how (and when) the diagnosis of MVP was made and any possible selection bias. Furthermore, all secondary causes of mitral valve leaflet prolapse (which themselves are associated with cardiovascular symptoms) must be excluded.

When strict diagnostic criteria are used and selection bias is avoided (using a community-based population such as the Framingham Study), the notion of an MVP syndrome is dismantled. The prevalence of atypical chest pain, dyspnea, exercise intolerance, syncope, anxiety, and panic attacks in patients with MVP is similar to that seen in the general population. Palpitation, an additional component of a presumed MVP syndrome, is highly prevalent in the general population, and its association with MVP has persisted in some studies but is felt to be coincidental in others. Overall, patients with primary MVP without any other underlying cardiovascular condition are relatively asymptomatic.

PHYSICAL FINDINGS

The physical findings in MVP reflect the abnormal valvular motion, the associated mitral regurgitation, and, infrequently, abnormalities typical of a coexistent connective tissue disease. These clinical manifestations lack both sensitivity and specificity and may vary between examinations and according to hemodynamic conditions. (See discussion of dynamic auscultation.) Thus, it is not uncommon to see patients being alternately diagnosed as having and not having this syndrome if the diagnosis is based solely on physical examination. The detection of suggestive clinical findings should prompt echocardiographic confirmation of the presence of MVP.

In the Framingham offspring cohort, subjects with mitral valve prolapse were leaner than those without prolapse. In the rare patient with a co-existent connective tissue disease (e.g., Marfan syndrome) the typical features of this condition may be evident on inspection.

The typical auscultatory finding in MVP is a midsystolic click, frequently followed by a late systolic murmur of mitral regurgitation. The reported incidence of these findings is widely variable among published studies, being as low as 10% or as high as 90%, depending on the degree of expertise of the examining physician and the hemodynamic conditions. The setting in which the diagnosis is made also plays an important role.

The single most frequent auscultatory finding in MVP, the apical midsystolic nonejection click, is thought to result from a sudden tensing of the mitral apparatus at the time of systolic billowing of the mitral valve. There may be multiple clicks, owing to prolapse of different portions of the mitral or the tricuspid valve at different times during systole. These clicks must be carefully differentiated from aortic or pulmonic ejection clicks as well as from other cardiac auscultatory findings, such as those associated with atrial septal aneurysms, atrial myxomas, or sounds originating in the pericardium. As opposed to nonejection clicks, semilunar valve ejection clicks do not change in timing or intensity with respiration or changes in body posture. Additionally, they are louder, are closer to the first heart sound, and occur before the upstroke of the carotid pulse. Also of note, a hyperdynamic state or dehydration can mimic a systolic click even in otherwise normal subjects. Conversely, volume overload (as in pregnancy) can prevent a mitral valve from prolapsing in a patient who previously had MVP.

Maneuvers decreasing the left ventricular end-diastolic volume, increasing left ventricular contraction, or decreasing the resistance to left ventricular ejection of blood cause the click or the murmur to occur earlier in systole. These include standing up from the supine position, isometric handgripping, the Valsalva maneuver, and amyl nitrite inhalation. Bradycardia or sudden squatting will exert the opposite effect.

ECHOCARDIOGRAPHIC RISK STRATIFICATION

As previously discussed, 2-D echocardiography is the most sensitive method of detecting MVP. Echocardiography also allows measurement of the degree of leaflet prolapse and valve thickness, assessment of the degree of associated mitral regurgitation, and identification of complications, such as chordal rupture and flail mitral valve.

American Heart Association class I recommendations for echocardiography in MVP include diagnosis and severity assessment in patients with suggestive clinical signs, as well as exclusion of the diagnosis in patients who have been told that they have the disorder but in whom there is no current supportive clinical evidence of it. Exclusion of MVP in the first-degree relatives of subjects with known myxomatous valve disease, as well as risk stratification in patients with an established diagnosis, are class IIa indications (suggestive of being helpful).

Echocardiography has been used to differentiate between patients with classic and those with nonclassic MVP, primarily by measuring mitral leaflet thickness (Table 1). The normal mitral leaflet is less than 5 mm in thickness (from the parasternal long-axis view) during diastasis. Patients with thickened leaflets are considered to have classic MVP, whereas prolapse is termed *nonclassic* in those with normal leaflet thickness. In a retrospective study of echocardiograms from the Massachusetts General Hospital, investigators found that patients with classic MVP as compared with those with nonclassic disease, had a higher rate of severe mitral regurgitation (12% versus 0% respectively), infective endocarditis (3.5% versus 0%), or mitral valve replacement (6.6% versus 0.7%). The Framingham offspring cohort study has also underscored the importance of this classification. The vast majority of MVP patients with severe mitral regurgitation had classic disease. The patients with mild billowing of morphologically normal valves carried a very low risk of subsequent mitral regurgitation. In that study of more than 3400 subjects, the prevalence of MVP was 2.4%, of which 1.3% was classic MVP.

TREATMENT

Mitral regurgitation and infective endocarditis are the only complications found to be clearly associated with primary MVP in large population-based studies. Both are especially common in older men, a group with increased prevalence of mitral leaflet thickening and dilation of the left heart chamber.

The most important initial step in the management of MVP is identifying high-risk patients, as described previously. Management of these high-risk patients includes yearly echocardiographic follow-up, endocarditis prophylaxis, and treatment of complications. In asymptomatic patients without significant mitral regurgitation (mild or less), clinical evaluation is indicated every 3 to 5 years, and no echocardiographic follow-up is necessary.

Mitral Regurgitation

In a surgical referral study, MVP was the most frequent cause of mitral regurgitation in developed countries. It is estimated that more than 50% of mitral valve replacements were due to primary MVP; 90% of these patients had ruptured chords. Mitral regurgitation was also due to the altered geometry and motion of the prolapsing leaflet, with or without associated anular dilation. Progressively worsening regurgitation and prolapse cause increased chordal tension and thinning, which can ultimately lead to chordal rupture and a flail mitral valve.

TABLE 1. **Use of Echocardiography for Risk Stratification in Mitral Valve Prolapse**

Study (Year)	N	Features Examined	Outcome	P Value
Nishimura (1985)	237	MV leaflet ≥5 mm	↑ Sum of sudden death, endocarditis, and cerebral embolus	P<.02
		LVID ≥60 mm	↑ MVR (26% vs. 3.1%)	P<.001
Zuppiroli (1994)	119	MV leaflet >5 mm	↑ Complex ventricular arrhythmia	P<.001
Babuty (1994)	58	Undefined MV thickening	No relation to complex ventricular arrhythmias	NS
Takamoto (1991)	142	MV leaflet ≥3 mm, redundant, low echo density	↑ Ruptured chordae (48% vs. 5%)	
Marks (1989)	456	MV leaflet ≥5 mm	↑ Endocarditis (3.5% vs. 0%)	P<.02
			↑ Moderate to severe MR (11.9% vs. 0%)	P<.001
			↑ MVR (6.6% vs. 0.7%)	P<.02
			↑ Stroke (7.5% vs. 5.8%)	NS
Chandraratna (1984)	86	MV leaflet >5.1 mm	↑ Cardiovascular abnormalities (60% vs. 6%) (Marfan syndrome, TVP, MR, dilated ascending aorta)	P<.001

Abbreviations: LVID = left ventricular internal diameter; MR = mitral regurgitation; MV = mitral valve; MVR = mitral valve replacement; TVP = tricuspid valve prolapse.

In the offspring cohort of the Framingham Heart Study, MVP was associated with a greater degree of regurgitation than was seen in subjects without MVP. In most subjects, however, mitral regurgitation was mild and mostly limited to those with the classic form of the syndrome. Severe regurgitation was seen in 7% of subjects with classic prolapse, as compared with 0.5% of those with nonclassic prolapse, and was virtually absent among subjects without prolapse. Therefore, in highly selected surgical patients, most cases of severe mitral regurgitation are associated with MVP, but the prevalence of severe mitral regurgitation related to MVP in an unselected population is very low.

Management of Mitral Regurgitation. Asymptomatic patients with mitral regurgitation, a normal left ventricle, and a left ventricular ejection fraction of greater than 60% should be treated conservatively with afterload-reducing agents (e.g., angiotension-converting enzyme inhibitors) and antibiotic prophylaxis. Patients with an ejection fraction of less than 60% or left ventricular dilation (left ventricular end-systolic diameter greater than 45 mm) should undergo mitral valve surgery, regardless of the symptomatic status. Up to 90% of these patients can undergo mitral valve repair, especially if the posterior leaflet is predominantly affected and there is minimal anular calcification. The decision to operate on a patient with severe mitral regurgitation and a severely decreased left ventricular fraction (<30%) must be individualized, taking into account the increased operative risk, the age of the patient, and the comorbid status, such as coexisting coronary artery disease.

Infective Endocarditis

The risk of infective endocarditis is considered to be increased fivefold in an unselected population of patients with MVP, as compared with the general population; however, this complication is seen mainly in high-risk patients with mitral regurgitation. Thus, in patients who do not exhibit a systolic murmur, the incidence of infective endocarditis is almost the same as in the general population (approximately 1 in 20,000). In elderly males with MVP and moderate or severe mitral regurgitation, however, the risk of endocarditis can be as high as 7% per year.

Endocarditis Prophylaxis. According to the American Heart Association guidelines (Table 2), there is a class I indication for endocarditis prophylaxis in the setting of procedures associated with bacteremia, in patients with a systolic click on auscultation and an associated systolic murmur, and in nthose with echocardiographic evidence of MVP and mitral regurgitation. The frequency of bacteremia is highest with dental and oral procedures, lowest with gastrointestinal diagnostic procedures, and intermediate with genitourinary procedures. Patients with an isolated systolic click (without a late systolic murmur) and echocardiographic evidence of high-risk MVP (thickened, redundant mitral valve leaflets) without mitral regurgitation have a class II indication for endocarditis prophylaxis. For patients with

TABLE 2. **Recommendations for Antibiotic Endocarditis Prophylaxis for Patients With Mitral Valve Prolapse Undergoing Procedures Associated With Bacteremia**

Indication	Class
Characteristic systolic click-murmur complex	I
Isolated systolic click and echocardiographic evidence of MVP and MR	I
Isolated systolic click, echocardiographic evidence of high-risk MVP	IIa
Isolated systolic click and equivocal or no evidence of MVP	III

an isolated systolic click and equivocal or absent evidence of MVP, the risk of adverse reactions to antibiotics probably outweighs the potential protective benefits, because the risk of endocarditis in these patients is extremely low.

Arrhythmia and Sudden Death

Supraventricular and ventricular arrhythmias have classically been associated with MVP. Despite numerous reports to this effect, however, it is still uncertain whether these findings are more common than in controls. This is at variance with the results of older studies, which reported a prevalence of atrial and ventricular ectopy of up to 90% in patients with MVP. This major discrepancy may reflect the use of nonuniform diagnostic criteria and selection bias (discussed earlier). Patients with significant mitral regurgitation, who are at higher risk of ectopy, may be overrepresented in some of the older series. It is important to note that the Framingham study did not include Holter monitoring and thus does not allow a definitive conclusion to be drawn concerning the association between arrhythmia and MVP.

Although sudden death is infrequent in patients with MVP without mitral regurgitation, the risk of this complication can be as high as 0.9% to 1.9% per year in the setting of significant mitral regurgitation. Additional risk factors include ischemic ST-T wave changes, documented ventricular ectopia, prolonged QT interval, or a history of syncope.

Because there is no conclusive evidence of an increased risk of arrhythmia in patients with uncomplicated MVP, Holter monitoring, electrophysiologic studies, and specific antiarrhythmic therapy should not be prescribed routinely for patients with asymptomatic MVP. Treatment of arrhythmias should be based on the clinical situation, regardless of the presence of MVP.

Neurohumoral, Neurologic, and Neuropsychiatic Symptoms

A variety of autonomic nervous system abnormalities have been described in patients with primary MVP, including an increase in either vagal or sympathetic tone. The clinical relevance of these findings is challenged by the results of the Framingham offspring study, which failed to demonstrate an increased prevalence of arrhythmia, hypotension, or syncope in patients with MVP as compared with matched controls.

Several reports have also described an association between MVP and stroke, especially in young patients. The neurologic events were postulated to occur as a result of fibrin and platelet clot embolization from the surface of the myxomatous mitral valve. A recent study, using strict echocardiographic diagnostic criteria, has not found significant association between MVP and stroke. Similarly, panic attacks and panic disorder have not been shown to be associated with MVP, once referral bias has been removed and strict diagnostic criteria have been applied.

Because there is no clear association between stroke and MVP, stroke prophylaxis should be given for the generally accepted indications (past history of embolic neurologic events, atrial fibrillation) regardless of the presence of MVP. The American Heart Association considers aspirin prophylaxis in patients in sinus rhythm with echocardiographic evidence of high-risk MVP to be a class IIa recommendation. In light of the results of a recent large study that failed to demonstrate an association between MVP and stroke, however, the true value of this strategy is uncertain.

In the four decades since MVP was first described, the appreciation of the true prevalence and spectrum of manifestations of this syndrome has evolved dramatically. MVP has been transformed from a benign physical examination finding to a perceived "epidemic" affecting almost 40% of otherwise healthy young women, with an impressive array of potential complications. The final understanding may be that it is a common (2% to 4%) connective tissue abnormality of the mitral leaflets that rarely develops significant complications.

CONGESTIVE HEART FAILURE

method of
ROBIN J. TRUPP, M.S.N., R.N., and
WILLIAM T. ABRAHAM, M.D.
University of Kentucky Chandler Medical Center
Lexington, Kentucky

Heart failure represents the most rapidly growing form of cardiovascular disease in the United States and in many other developed countries. Over the past 3 decades, both the incidence and prevalence of heart failure have increased at a near exponential rate. Currently, there are about 5 million Americans with heart failure, with 400,000 to 700,000 new cases diagnosed annually. Heart failure is a particularly important problem in the elderly population, where its prevalence is approaching 10%. In fact, more than 75% of patients with heart failure are older than 65 years of age. With the continued aging of the population, both the incidence and prevalence of heart failure are expected to continue to increase in the new millennium.

Heart failure is associated with high rates of morbidity, mortality, and economic cost. At any given time, approximately 30% of the heart failure population may be considered to have advanced disease, defined by a New York Heart Association (NYHA) Class III or IV impairment in functional capacity. Moreover, heart failure as a primary diagnosis accounts for approximately 1 million hospitalizations, or more than 6.5 million hospital days per year in the United States. Heart failure is the most frequent cause of hospitalization in those older than the age of 65 years. Despite recent advances in pharmacologic therapy, the 1- to 2-year mortality rate is on the order of 35% to 50% for advanced heart failure and the 4- to 5-year mortality rate ranges from 15% to 40% for those with asymptomatic left ventricular (LV) dysfunction or only mild to moderate symptoms. Finally, the total direct cost of heart failure care in the United States is estimated at $56.6 billion per year. This staggering figure represents approximately 5% of total health care costs in the United States.

SYSTOLIC VERSUS DIASTOLIC HEART FAILURE

There are two major forms of heart failure: (1) that associated with primary myocardial failure, called *systolic heart failure*, in which the key abnormality is seen during systole as impaired ventricular contractility; and (2) that related to impaired ventricular filling, called *diastolic heart failure*, in which the primary defect occurs during diastole and is manifested as a fall in ventricular compliance or relaxation. The hallmark of systolic dysfunction is a decrease in the LV ejection fraction substantially below its normal value of about 55%. Diastolic dysfunction may coexist with systolic heart failure; however, by definition, pure diastolic heart failure is associated with a normal LV ejection fraction. Thus, this latter form of the disease is also known as heart failure with preserved LV ejection fraction. Approximately 70% of patients with heart failure have primarily systolic dysfunction, and roughly 30% have diastolic dysfunction alone.

The most common primary cause of systolic heart failure is ischemic heart disease, which accounts for about 68% of cases, followed by idiopathic or familial dilated cardiomyopathy (≈13%), hypertension (≈7%), and other miscellaneous causes (e.g., myocarditis, valvular heart disease, postpartum state, drug- or toxin-induced cardiomyopathies). Risk factors for diastolic heart failure include ischemic heart disease, hypertension, diabetes mellitus, LV hypertrophy, and aging. Hypertension remains a major risk for both forms of the disease, antedating the onset of clinical heart failure in up to 91% of cases.

Because systolic and diastolic heart failure differ in pathophysiology, treatment goals and therapeutic approaches may differ as well. A thorough evaluation of the patient with suspected heart failure must include an assessment of ventricular systolic function to make the proper diagnosis and management decisions. As elaborated on later, systolic heart failure is managed by aggressively treating the neurohormonal aspects of the disease with angiotensin-converting enzyme (ACE) inhibition and β-blockade while balancing the hemodynamic disturbances with diuretics and digoxin. Optimal treatment of diastolic heart failure remains unclear because clinical studies of the disease are lacking.

Thus, the pharmacologic management of diastolic heart failure is largely empirical and directed at reducing symptoms. The goals of therapy for diastolic heart failure are to treat congestive symptoms, manage the underlying or aggravating disorder, and prevent ischemia. Treatment options include diuretics, nitrates, calcium channel blockers, and β-blockers. Symptoms caused by increased ventricular filling pressures may be treated with diuretics and long-acting nitrates. Some calcium channel antagonists and most β-blockers prolong diastolic filling time by slowing heart rate, thereby potentially improving the symptoms of diastolic heart failure. Calcium antagonists, β-blockers, diuretics, and ACE inhibitors may also promote regression of left ventricular hypertrophy and thus improve ventricular compliance, possibly preventing the development of diastolic heart failure in the first place. Because randomized controlled trials of diastolic heart failure are lacking, the remainder of this review focuses on the conventional evaluation and management of systolic heart failure.

PATHOPHYSIOLOGY OF SYSTOLIC HEART FAILURE

A conceptual model for systolic heart failure has evolved over the past several decades. Systolic heart failure is a cellular disorder characterized by altered gene expression, activation of cytokines, and cell loss from necrosis or apoptosis. A neurohormonal model explains the circulatory and renal abnormalities, the progression of the disease, and the high morbidity and mortality associated with heart failure (Figure 1). According to this model, myocardial injury leads to a fall in LV performance that activates various neurohormonal vasoconstrictor systems early in the course of LV dysfunction. Activation of these systems—namely, the sympathetic nervous system (SNS), the renin-angiotensin-aldosterone system (RAAS), the nonosmotic release of vasopressin (AVP), and the circulating endothelins—may initially produce compensatory effects, enabling the failing myocardium to function adequately for a period of months to years. However, they also cause a variety of hemodynamic abnormalities that ultimately produce the symptoms of heart failure. In particular, pe-

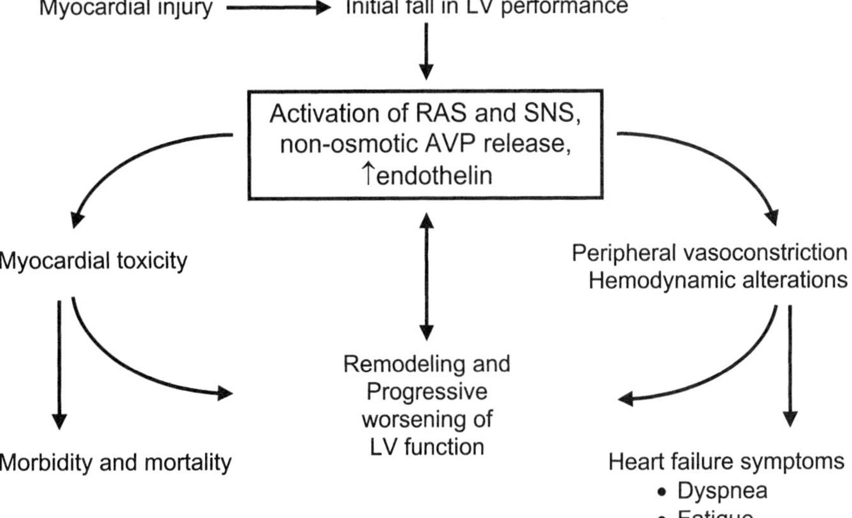

Figure 1. Central role for neurohormonal activation in the pathophysiology of heart failure. A decrease in cardiac performance, in response to some myocardial injury, activates the various neurohormonal vasoconstrictor systems implicated in heart failure disease progression, morbidity and mortality, and symptoms. *Abbreviations:* AVP = arginine vasopressin; LV = left ventricular; RAAS = renin-angiotensin-aldosterone system; SNS = sympathetic nervous system.

ripheral vasoconstriction and renal sodium and water retention lead to increased ventricular filling pressures and diminished cardiac output that cause the cardinal symptoms of heart failure, shortness of breath, and fatigue. The ultimate clinical consequence of these hemodynamic abnormalities and their symptoms is a decrease in functional or exercise capacity. In addition, these neurohormonal vasoconstrictor systems exert a direct adverse effect on the myocardium, contributing to ventricular hypertrophy and remodeling and thus to disease progression. These concepts underlie the contemporary management of systolic heart failure, which is directed at improving the myocardial, hemodynamic, and neurohormonal aspects of the disease.

CLINICAL EVALUATION OF HEART FAILURE

The first step in evaluating heart failure is to determine the severity and type of cardiac dysfunction by measuring ejection fraction through two-dimensional echocardiography and/or radionuclide ventriculography (Table 1). As mentioned earlier, measurement of ejection fraction is the gold standard for differentiating between the two forms of heart failure. Second, identification of reversible contributory factors is essential. These include valvular disease, myocardial ischemia, pericardial disease, supraventricular arrhythmias, bradycardia/heart block, metabolic abnormalities, alcohol/drug consumption, various systemic diseases, and noncompliance with medications or diet. Last, the physical examination should include assessment of symptoms, functional capacity, and fluid status.

Common symptoms of heart failure are dyspnea on exertion, orthopnea, paroxysmal nocturnal dyspnea, lower extremity edema, cough (usually worse at night), abdominal problems (nausea, vomiting, right upper quadrant tenderness, ascites), fatigue, nocturia, sleep disorders, and anorexia. Common physical findings include elevated jugular venous pressure, hepatojugular reflux, pulmonary crackles, sustained and displaced apical impulse, S3 gallop, hepatomegaly, ascites, and peripheral edema.

Functional capacity is measured through history taking or preferably an exercise test. Analysis of expired air during exercise offers a precise measure of the patient's physical limitations. The NYHA has classified heart failure into four stages: Class I, no limitations of physical activity, no symptoms (fatigue, dyspnea, palpitations, or angina) with ordinary activities; Class II, slight limitation, symptoms with ordinary activities; Class III, marked limitation, symptoms with less than ordinary activities; and Class IV, severe limitation, symptoms of heart failure at rest. For example, patients who can walk several blocks without symptoms but have difficulty climbing two flights of stairs may have Class II heart failure, whereas those who cannot walk several blocks easily or become winded while walking up a short flight of stairs might be considered as having Class III heart failure.

Assessment of fluid status through measurement of jugular venous pressure, auscultation of the lungs, and examination for peripheral edema is central to the physical examination of heart failure patients. The physical examination alone, however, is relatively insensitive for measuring extracellular fluid volume excess. A thorough appraisal of symptoms is therefore essential. Even in the absence of perceptible volume excess by physical examination, mild congestive symptoms can indicate volume excess. In addition, the chest radiograph, particularly in a patient with relatively new-onset heart failure, is a relatively sensitive measure of volume overload.

MANAGEMENT OF SYSTOLIC HEART FAILURE

The goals of therapy for systolic heart failure are to slow disease progression, thereby reducing the risk of morbidity and mortality, and to improve quality of life and clinical status through alleviation of symptoms. Treatment of heart failure is therefore a balance of managing symptoms while addressing the progression of the disease through approaches that block neurohormonal stimulation.

The nonpharmacologic treatment of heart failure includes reduced sodium intake, reduced physical (particularly isometric) exertion, and weight loss in obese patients. In general, sodium intake should be

TABLE 1. **Early Recognition, Diagnosis, and Management of Heart Failure**

		Management	
Early Recognition	**Diagnosis**	*Systolic Heart Failure*	*Diastolic Heart Failure*
Identify patients at risk, e.g., patients with Coronary artery disease Hypertension Diabetes mellitus Left ventricular hypertrophy Alcoholism Family history	Measure ejection fraction Echocardiography and/or Radionuclide ventriculography Identify reversible contributory factors Assess symptoms, functional capacity, fluid retention	Ejection fraction ≤40% Manage symptoms (diuretics ± digoxin) Reduce progression (ACE inhibitors, β-blockers) Additional therapies in selected patients (e.g., spironolactone, anticoagulants)	Ejection fraction >40% Diuretics Nitrates Calcium channel blockers β-blockers ACE inhibitors Suppression of AV conduction for atrial fibrillation Anticoagulation (selected indications)

Abbreviations: ACE = angiotensin-converting enzyme; AV = atrioventricular.

limited to about 2 g/d. In advanced heart failure, further dietary sodium restriction may be necessary to attenuate expansion of extracellular fluid volume and the development of edema. Hyponatremia should not discourage compliance with a restricted sodium diet, because the hyponatremia is usually dilutional and associated with total body sodium and water excess. Sodium repletion, therefore, should be considered only in overt cases of severe, excessive diuresis or dehydration. Salt substitutes may be used to improve the palatability of food. However, some of these agents substitute potassium chloride for sodium chloride and should be used in moderation, given the potential risk of hyperkalemia. Although dietary sodium restriction may attenuate the development of edema, it cannot prevent it because the kidneys are capable of reducing urinary sodium excretion to less than 10 mmol/d.

Although vigorous isometric exercise has been poorly evaluated in chronic heart failure, it is currently discouraged in symptomatic patients, given the marked increase in myocardial work seen with heavy weight training. Increased LV wall stress during isometric exercise would be expected to have an unfavorable influence on ventricular remodeling. On the other hand, a role has emerged for monitored cardiac rehabilitation and aerobic exercise training in patients with stable compensated chronic heart failure. In these patients, aerobic exercise training has been shown to consistently improve functional capacity while inconsistently improving LV function, suggesting that the benefits of aerobic training in chronic heart failure are mostly peripheral.

Although many patients with chronic heart failure have normal or low blood pressures, a sizable subset of patients remain substantially hypertensive. Because elevated blood pressure increases the workload of the heart, hypertension should be treated vigorously in patients with chronic heart failure. Blood pressure should probably be lowered into the low-normal range of systolic and diastolic blood pressures. Some patients with cardiomyopathy on the basis of hypertensive heart disease may recognize a marked improvement with treatment of the hypertension alone. This may be accomplished with standard heart failure treatment such as an ACE inhibitor or β-blocker.

Pharmacologic Agents

Diuretics. In addition to sodium restriction, diuretic agents are used to reduce volume overload. Because the majority of patients have some degree of sodium and water retention, diuretics are useful for most patients, even those with mild symptoms. The effect of diuretics on clinical outcomes is not known because clinical outcome trials have not been conducted with these agents. However, diuretics have been shown to decrease end-diastolic volume (cardiac preload), increase stroke volume and cardiac output, improve exercise treadmill time, and diminish heart failure symptoms in patients with systolic heart failure. Although diuretics can stimulate neurohormonal activation and may precipitate other adverse effects when used in excess (hypotension, renal insufficiency, and electrolyte disturbances), they are nevertheless an important component of therapy, as they relieve congestive symptoms.

Three classes of diuretics are commonly used in heart failure management: the loop diuretics, distal tubular agents, and the potassium-sparing diuretics (Table 2). Loop diuretics (furosemide, torsemide, bumetanide, and ethacrynic acid) are the most potent diuretic agents available for use in clinical medicine. This is not surprising, because several times more sodium chloride is reabsorbed in the loop of Henle than in the distal convoluted tubule. Because of their potency, the loop diuretics are generally effective in patients with advanced renal insufficiency (glomerular filtration rates <25 mL/min). Distal tubular diuretics (thiazides and metolazone [Zaroxolyn]) are generally less potent than the loop diuretics and thus reserved for patients with mild extracellular fluid volume excess. These agents, with the exception of metolazone, are six to eight times less potent than the loop diuretics. Thus, the distal tubular diuretics become ineffective as the glomerular filtration rate falls below 25 to 30 mL/min. Clinically available potassium-sparing diuretics include triamterene (Dyrenium), amiloride (Midamor), and the specific aldo-

TABLE 2. **Diuretics Used in the Management of Heart Failure**

Agent	Site of Action	Total Daily Dose (mg)	Frequency
Amiloride (Midamore)	Distal tubule (potassium-sparing)	5–20	Once or twice daily
Bumetanide (Bumex)	Loop of Henle	0.5–10	Once to thrice daily
Chlorothiazide (Diurel)*	Distal tubule (potassium-wasting)	500–1500	Once or twice daily
Ethacrynic Acid (Edecrin)*	Loop of Henle	50–200	Once or twice daily
Furosemide (Lasix)	Loop of Henle	20–500	Once to thrice daily
Hydrochlorothiazide (HydroDIURIL)*	Distal tubule (potassium-wasting)	25–100	Once or twice daily
Metolazone (Zaroxolyn)*	Distal tubule (potassium-wasting)	2.5–20	Once or twice daily
Spironolactone (Aldactone)*	Distal tubule (potassium-sparing)	25–200	Once to thrice daily
Torsemide (Demadex)	Loop of Henle	10–200	Once or twice daily
Triamterene (Dyrenium)*	Distal tubule (potassium-sparing)	100–300	Once or twice daily

*FDA approved for use in peripheral edema.

sterone antagonist spironolactone (Aldactone). The action of this last potassium-sparing diuretic depends on the presence of the adrenal cortex and circulating aldosterone. In contrast, the ability of triamterene and amiloride to block potassium secretion is independent of adrenal function. Often, these diuretics are not potent enough when used alone, but they may be used to avoid the potassium-wasting effects of diuretics that act at more proximal nephron sites. Importantly, it is now known that the combined use of moderate doses of two or more agents from different diuretic classes may promote a greater diuresis compared with the use of high doses of any single agent.

General guidelines for the use of diuretics in heart failure are as follows:

1. Initiate therapy with a loop or thiazide-type diuretic, depending on the severity of the heart failure. For mild heart failure, a thiazide diuretic will often suffice. For more advanced heart failure, particularly with overt fluid retention, the more potent loop diuretics should be used.
2. If a loop diuretic given twice daily in doses equivalent to about 200 mg/d of furosemide is inadequate for diuresis, add a thiazide diuretic or metolazone. This often results in a synergistic effect on solute and water excretion. This combination also results in substantial renal potassium and possibly magnesium wasting, so an increased need for electrolyte supplementation should be anticipated.
3. To conserve potassium or to further enhance the diuresis, a potassium-sparing diuretic may be added. However, triamterene should not be combined with furosemide because triamterene blocks the tubular secretion of furosemide, thus diminishing the delivery of furosemide to its tubular sites of action.
4. In mild-to-moderate heart failure, the goal of diuretic therapy is alleviation of congestive signs and symptoms, that is, those caused by pulmonary and/or peripheral edema. Once this goal has been met, the diuretic dose should be adjusted to maintain a euvolemic state.

With specifically tailored guidelines, patients may be instructed to alter their diuretic regimen on a "prn" basis to maintain a well-compensated state.

Digoxin. The ability of digoxin to improve physical function and symptoms in patients with systolic heart failure has been confirmed by studies of digoxin withdrawal. Overall, the beneficial effects of digoxin in patients with chronic heart failure include reduction in heart failure symptoms, improved NYHA functional class, increased maximal treadmill exercise time, modestly increased LV ejection fraction, enhanced cardiac performance (e.g., increased cardiac output and stroke work index), and decreased heart failure hospitalizations (when added to a regimen of ACE inhibition and diuretics). Despite these favorable clinical effects, digoxin does not improve survival in chronic heart failure. These clinical benefits of digoxin in heart failure may be due to its mildly positive inotropic effect owing to its apparent ability to diminish sympathetic activation in chronic heart failure or to a combination of these and other mechanisms.

Given its lack of effect on mortality, digoxin is often used as an add-on therapy in symptomatic patients. It should be used within recommended doses (usually 0.125–0.25 mg daily with adjustments made for renal dysfunction) and digoxin levels should be maintained in the low therapeutic range between 0.5 and 1.1 ng/mL to minimize toxicity. Although digoxin has been considered a mainstay of therapy for heart failure, its usefulness continues to be questioned as agents with greater beneficial effects on outcomes and with better safety profiles are developed. Thus, digoxin should be considered for patients with chronic heart failure who remain symptomatic on a diuretic, ACE inhibitor, and β-blocker and in patients with advanced (NYHA Class IV) heart failure.

As previously mentioned, the renin-angiotensin and sympathetic nervous systems play critical roles in the vicious cycle of heart failure. Stimulation of the renin-angiotensin system contributes to vasoconstriction, renal sodium and water retention, stimulation of aldosterone, vascular and myocardial hypertrophy and remodeling, activation of the sympathetic nervous system, and increased thirst. Manifestations of sympathetic nervous system stimulation in heart failure include vasoconstriction, renal sodium and water retention, tachycardia, stimulation of ventricular arrhythmias, induction of β-adrenergic receptor signal transduction abnormalities, stimulation of vasopressin (another vasoconstrictor hormone active in heart failure), and direct myocardial toxicity by means of calcium overload and/or induction of apoptosis (programmed cell death). Thus, ACE inhibitors and β-blockers represent two therapeutic approaches to inhibit these two systems and improve outcomes in heart failure.

ACE Inhibitors. ACE inhibitors are a critical component of heart failure management in that they not only reduce symptoms and improve exercise tolerance but also inhibit the renin-angiotensin system and favorably affect ventricular remodeling and dilation. Moreover, in addition to the reduction of circulating and tissue angiotensin II, ACE inhibitors may increase plasma concentrations of bradykinin, nitric oxide, and vasodilating prostaglandins and diminish activation of the adrenergic nervous system. ACE inhibitors have a role in reducing mortality in all classes of heart failure. The Survival and Ventricular Enlargement (SAVE) trial was conducted in Class I patients after myocardial infarction and the Studies of Left Ventricular Dysfunction (SOLVD) prevention study enrolled Classes I and II patients with chronic LV dysfunction. ACE inhibition significantly reduced mortality and/or morbidity in both trials. Among Class II to III patients in the SOLVD treatment trial, a significant reduction in all-cause mortality was observed; similarly, in Class IV patients in the Cooperative North Scandinavian Enalapril Survival Study (CONSENSUS), ACE inhibition significantly decreased all-cause mortality.

Over more than 15 years of clinical experience, the tolerability of ACE inhibitors has proven to be excellent. During open-label therapy in the SOLVD trial, reported side effects included symptomatic hypotension (2.2%), altered taste (1.1%), rash (0.7%), angioneurotic edema (0.04%), cough (0.14%), and hyperkalemia greater than 5.5 mmol/L (0.97%). The incidence of these reported side effects has been higher in some series, but at least 85% of patients with heart failure should be expected to tolerate therapy with an ACE inhibitor. Unfortunately, only 50% to 60% of patients with heart failure are receiving ACE inhibitors.

Moreover, the doses of ACE inhibitors used in clinical practice often fall short of those demonstrated to be of benefit in randomized controlled trials. The aforementioned advantages of ACE inhibitors in clinical trials in patients with heart failure were seen with the moderate-to-high doses mandated by these investigations. The recently reported Assessment of Treatment With Lisinopril and Survival (ATLAS) study confirmed the modest superiority of high doses versus low doses of lisinopril in patients with systolic heart failure. Compared with the low-dose regimen, the high doses of lisinopril produced a significant reduction in the combined endpoint of death or hospitalization for any reason. In addition, high-dose lisinopril significantly reduced heart failure hospitalizations.

Thus, ACE inhibitors should be used as first-line therapy for symptomatic heart failure and in patients with asymptomatic LV dysfunction. In nonedematous patients with low LV ejection fractions, ACE inhibitors (with or without a β-blocker) may constitute the sole pharmacologic therapy for the LV dysfunction. However, it is our practice to always combine an ACE inhibitor and β-blocker, regardless of the NYHA class of the patient, for complementary inhibition of these deleterious neurohormonal systems. Because most patients with heart failure manifest signs and/or symptoms of fluid overload, ACE inhibitors are often combined with diuretic therapy. The patient is begun on a low dose of an ACE inhibitor and the dose is titrated to the maximal tolerated dose within the usual dose range for survival advantage. Table 3 lists the ACE inhibitors that are FDA approved for heart failure and the usual dose ranges used in chronic heart failure management.

TABLE 3. **FDA-Approved Angiotensin-Converting Enzyme Inhibitors for Heart Failure**

Agent	Initial Dose (mg)	Target Dose (mg)
Captopril (Capoten)	6.25–12.5 tid	25–50 tid
Enalapril (Vasotec)	2.5 bid	5–20 bid
Enalaprilat (IV) (Vasotec)	1.25 q6h	2.5–10 q6h
Fosinopril (Monopril)	5–10 qd	10–40 qd
Lisinopril (Prinivil)	5–10 qd	10–40 qd
Quinapril (Accupril)	5 bid	5–20 bid
Ramipril (Altace)	1.25–2.5 bid	2.5–5 bid

β-Blockers. Although it was conventionally thought that short-term effects of β-blockers might have detrimental effects in heart failure, early studies in Sweden suggested that this class of agents might have long-term benefits, including favorable hemodynamic effects. A number of long-term clinical trials, including the Metoprolol in Dilated Cardiomyopathy (MDC) trial and Cardiac Insufficiency Bisoprolol Study (CIBIS), have suggested promising effects of β-blockers on morbidity of heart failure. However, neither of these trials conclusively supported the use of the β-blockers in heart failure.

Carvedilol, a nonselective vasodilating β-blocker with α_1-blocking activity, has been studied extensively in patients with mild, moderate, and severe heart failure (Classes II–IV). This agent has been shown to slow disease progression, improve ejection fraction and functional class, and reduce the combined risk of heart failure mortality, hospitalization for heart failure, and need for sustained increase in heart failure medications. In stable patients with advanced Classes III and IV disease, carvedilol also significantly reduced all-cause mortality in the Carvedilol Prospective Randomized Cumulative Survival (COPERNICUS) trial. The Second Cardiac Insufficiency Bisoprolol Study (CIBIS II) and Metoprolol Randomized Intervention Trial in Heart Failure (MERIT-HF) have extended these favorable observations to the β_1-selective agents bisoprolol and metoprolol CR/XL, whereas trials of other β-blockers (e.g., bucindolol*) have produced negative results.

Although definitive outcome data are lacking, combined α/β-blockade (carvedilol [Coreg]) appears to have several advantages over β_1-selective antagonism alone, particularly in promoting reverse remodeling of the failing heart. Carvedilol blocks all three adrenergic receptors implicated in heart failure disease progression (α_1, β_1, and β_2), decreases adrenergic activation, and does not up-regulate β_1 receptors in the heart. Moreover, the doses of β_1-selective agents shown to be effective in heart failure have been high (metoprolol CR/XL [Toprol XL],* 150–200 mg/d; bisoprolol [Zebeta],* 7.5–10 mg/d), whereas the MOCHA trial demonstrated the effectiveness of carvedilol at low doses beginning at 6.25 mg twice daily as well as at higher doses up to 25 mg twice daily. If these differing effects of β-blockers translate into improved survival, one might expect the results of the ongoing Carvedilol or Metoprolol European Trial (COMET) to favor improved outcomes in patients randomized to carvedilol versus metoprolol.

Thus, β-blockers are indicated for all stable (euvolemic) NYHA II through IV heart failure patients with systolic LV dysfunction. As stated earlier, we also favor their early use in patients with asymptomatic LV dysfunction. These agents should be used along with an ACE inhibitor to optimize outcomes and to slow disease progression. Given the heterogeneity of the β-blocker class, only drugs shown to improve outcomes in large-scale clinical trials should

*Not FDA approved for this indication.

TABLE 4. β-Blockers Used in the Treatment of Heart Failure

Agent	Initial Dose (mg)	Target Dose (mg)
Carvedilol (Coreg)	3.125 bid	6.25–25 bid
Metoprolol CR/XL (Lopressor)	12.5–25 qd	200 qd
Bisoprolol* (Zebeta)	1.25 qd	10 qd

*Not FDA approved for use in heart failure.

be used. These include carvedilol, metoprolol CR/XL, and bisoprolol. Carvedilol may be preferred, given its more extensive adrenergic blockade and superior effects on underlying mechanisms of disease progression. Initial and target doses for these agents are reviewed in Table 4.

Other Agents. Various other pharmacologic agents have been used in heart failure management. Some have proven to be beneficial adjuncts to treatment, whereas others have not. The beneficial effects of long-acting nitrates used alone or in conjunction with hydralazine in heart failure include increased exercise capacity, improved hemodynamics, decreased mitral regurgitation, improved endothelium-dependent vasodilation, modestly increased LV ejection fraction, and prolonged survival. These latter two effects have been observed only when long-acting nitrates are used in combination with hydralazine. Together or used alone, these agents decrease ventricular preload and afterload, improve cardiac output, and increase exercise capacity in patients with chronic heart failure. We use long-acting nitrates to treat residual heart failure symptoms (especially dyspnea) in patients on a diuretic, ACE inhibitor, β-blocker, and digoxin and to treat ischemia in patients with underlying coronary heart disease. Hydralazine is sometimes added for the further reduction of afterload in patients with hypertensive heart failure and/or persistently elevated systemic vascular resistance.

Calcium channel blockers are not efficacious in heart failure management. The first-generation agents (verapamil [Calan],* diltiazem [Cardizem],* and nifedipine [Adalat]*) exert a negative inotropic effect in the failing heart and should never be used in patients with reduced LV ejection fractions. The newer vascular selective agents, amlodipine (Norvasc),* and felodipine (Plendil),* appear to be safe for use in patients with heart failure but have no impact on heart failure mortality. Therefore, at the present time, calcium channel antagonists are not recommended for the treatment of heart failure. The vascular-selective agents may be considered for the management of hypertension or angina in patients with LV systolic dysfunction who are also receiving standard heart failure therapy.

In patients with mild-to-moderate heart failure, the effects of angiotensin II receptor antagonists on symptoms, exercise capacity, and systemic hemodynamics appear to be similar to those observed with ACE inhibitors. However, their effects on morbidity and mortality have not yet been shown to be superior to ACE inhibitors. Angiotensin receptor blockers (ARBs) may be used as an ACE inhibitor alternative in patients who have demonstrated intolerance to the latter class of agents. They may add additional small benefit when added to an ACE inhibitor–based heart failure regimen; however, this possibility requires further study. Finally, the ARBs appear to add no benefit, and may add potential harm, when combined with an ACE inhibitor and β-blocker.

Ventricular ectopic activity is common in patients with systolic heart failure, and sudden cardiac death (frequently from ventricular tachyarrhythmias) accounts for 40% to 50% of the mortality associated with this disease syndrome. Unfortunately, empirical antiarrhythmic drug therapy is of no proven benefit in patients with heart failure. Moreover, antiarrhythmic drug therapy is less effective and has been associated with a higher incidence of proarrhythmic complications in patients with LV systolic dysfunction. Of the antiarrhythmic agents studied in patients with heart failure, only amiodarone (Cordarone)* appears to be safe; in some patients it may be efficacious. Its role in heart failure management remains ill defined. Thus, antiarrhythmic drug therapy should probably be reserved for patients with documented ventricular tachycardia or fibrillation, syncope when it is likely due to ventricular tachyarrhythmia, or a history of sudden cardiac death. The suppression of nonsustained ventricular tachycardia or frequent ventricular ectopic activity in these patients requires further study. Although of great promise for reducing the incidence of sudden cardiac death in mild-to-moderate heart failure, the efficacy of prophylactic placement of an implantable cardioverter-defibrillator also remains unclear. This relates in part to the difficulty encountered in trying to identify patients with heart failure at the highest risk for sudden death. The utility of both invasive and noninvasive arrhythmia testing appears to be limited in this patient population. Ongoing trials of implantable cardioverter-defibrillator devices in systolic heart failure may better define their therapeutic role in this patient population.

Despite the risk of arterial thromboembolism (especially stroke), the routine use of anticoagulant therapy for LV systolic dysfunction is disputed. This controversy exists because there have been no randomized controlled trials of chronic anticoagulation in heart failure and there are obvious risks to anticoagulant therapy. All clinical practice guidelines agree that patients with heart failure who have chronic atrial fibrillation, a history of systemic or pulmonary embolism, or a documented mobile LV thrombus should receive chronic anticoagulant therapy. It is the practice of many specialized heart failure centers, including ours, to also use warfarin in patients with ejection fractions less than 25% to 30%. The goal is

*Not FDA approved for this indication.

*Not FDA approved for this indication.

to maintain the international normalized ratio around 2.0 to minimize the bleeding risk while offering some potential protection against thromboembolic events. Two ongoing randomized clinical trials should better define the role of chronic anticoagulant therapy in heart failure.

The continuous use of nonglycoside positive inotropic agents in the management of chronic heart failure remains controversial, because clinical studies of such therapy in heart failure have consistently demonstrated increased mortality. These agents certainly continue to play an important role in the management of acutely decompensated heart failure, where dobutamine (Dobutrex) and milrinone (Primacor) appear to be the positive inotropic drugs of choice. Alternatively, intravenous vasodilators may be used in the management of the decompensated patient. We tailor the regimen to the hemodynamic situation, preferring vasodilators for those with adequate or elevated blood pressures and congestive signs/symptoms and positive inotropic agents for those with a moderate-to-severe reduction in cardiac output.

FUTURE THERAPIES

Substantial development of new drugs, devices, surgical procedures, and gene therapies is ongoing in the arena of heart failure. Promising investigational therapies include endothelin receptor antagonists, vasopressin receptor antagonists, vasopeptidase inhibitors (combined neutral endopeptidase/ACE inhibitors), cytokine inhibitors/antagonists, adenosine receptor antagonists, partial fatty oxidase inhibitors, oral phosphodiesterase inhibitors, the natriuretic peptides, biventricular pacing, ventricular assist devices, totally implantable artificial hearts, cardiac constraint or remodeling devices, various other surgical techniques, and a variety of myocyte/gene-based therapies. Of these, the natriuretic peptides appear to be closest to widespread clinical availability. Based on its demonstrated efficacy in the treatment of decompensated heart failure, human B-type natriuretic peptide (Nesiritide)* is expected to gain FDA approval in 2001. Likewise, biventricular pacing or cardiac resynchronization therapy may become commercially available late in 2001.

*Investigational drug in the United States.

INFECTIVE ENDOCARDITIS

method of
DONALD P. LEVINE, M.D.
Wayne State University
Detroit, Michigan

It has been almost 120 years since Osler described "malignant endocarditis" in the Gulstonian Lectures. Much of what he described would be familiar to today's clinicians; yet we now have a much better understanding of the pathophysiology, clinical appearance, and, most importantly, the treatment of this fascinating disease.

TABLE 1. **Epidemiology of Infective Endocarditis**

Prevalence	Approximately 1 case per 1000 hospital admissions
Age	50% >50 years
Men:women	1.7:1
Valve	
Mitral	28%–45%
Aortic	5%–36%
Mitral and aortic	0%–35%
Tricuspid	0%–6%
Pulmonic	<1%

Classically, endocarditis was classified as either acute or subacute. Acute infection was characterized by a fulminant course with high fever, systemic toxicity, and rapid onset of complications and death within days to weeks. Subacute endocarditis was recognized in patients with known underlying valve disease and was characterized by an indolent course with progressive constitutional signs and symptoms and gradual deterioration, leading over weeks or months to death. Although this classification is descriptive, it has given way to a system based on the etiologic agent. This is preferable because it provides more useful information regarding the anticipated course of disease, the likelihood of underlying heart disease, and the optimal therapeutic regimen.

Infective endocarditis (IE) implies infection of the endocardial surface of the heart or its related structures. Such infection accounts for approximately 1 case per 1000 hospital admissions (Table 1). Until recently, rheumatic heart disease was the most common preexisting condition leading to IE. Because rheumatic fever occurred most frequently in children, IE was seen in a young population. Currently, more than 50% of patients are older than 50 years of age, largely because of the decrease in the population with rheumatic heart disease. Men are affected almost twice as often as women, and patients with left-sided infection far exceed those with involvement of the tricuspid or pulmonic valve. Table 2 details the common cardiac lesions that predispose to endocarditis. Each of these conditions leads to abnormal blood flow that causes formation of a platelet-fibrin clot that, in turn, becomes a nonbacterial thrombotic vegetation. When the patient develops bacter-

TABLE 2. **Cardiac Lesions Associated With Infective Endocarditis**

Congenital Heart Disease
Patent ductus arteriosus
Ventricular septal defect
Coarctation of aorta
Tetralogy of Fallot
Mitral valve prolapse (with murmur)
Idiopatic hypertrophic subaortic stenosis
Acquired Valve Disease
Rheumatic heart disease (25%; mitral predominates)
Degenerative cardiac lesions (30%–40% without underlying heart disease)
Prior endocarditis
?Injection drug use
Prosthetic Valve
Early (<60 d from surgery)
Late (>60 d from surgery)

emia with an organism capable of adhering to the vegetation, infective endocarditis may result. Lesions that are associated with low-pressure flow states, such as atrial secundum defects, are not associated with the development of nonbacterial thrombotic vegetation, whereas prosthetic valves or other foreign bodies carry an exagerated risk. Injection drug use is unique in that it is more likely than other risk factors to lead to right-sided infection despite apparently normal underlying cardiac valves. Why this occurs is not entirely clear, but it is possibly related to microscopic damage to the valves by impurities injected along with the illicit substances.

The common pathway for development of IE, regardless of the underlying pathology, is transient bacteremia. This may occur when a mucosal surface that is heavily colonized with bacteria is traumatized, such as during a dental or surgical procedure. In the case of injection drug use, studies failed to demonstrate bacteria in either the contraband drugs or the injection paraphernalia. The initial bacteremia is most likely the consequence of high-grade colonization of superficial cutaneous abscesses or injection into an area with established infection. Alternatively, bacteremia may result from a lesion that is remote from an injection site. Under most circumstances the bloodstream is cleared of bacteria within 15 to 30 minutes. In the presence of underlying valve disease, that is sufficient time for bacteria to adhere to the nonbacterial thrombotic vegetation and to transform it into an infected vegetation. Different organisms vary in their ability to adhere to a vegetation, but once they do they proliferate, initiating a process of further platelet-fibrin deposition. Within the vegetation the bacteria are sequestered from the circulation, living in a localized environment of impaired host resistance wherein bacteria multiply to enormous numbers, achieving concentrations as high as 10^{11}/g of tissue. As the disease evolves, the vegetation continuously fragments, exposing the bacteria to the circulation and leading to the most consistent feature of IE, continuous bacteremia. Ultimately, this sustained level of bacteremia stimulates both humoral and cellular immunity. Typically, rheumatoid factor is positive and antinuclear antibodies and circulating immune complexes are present.

MICROBIOLOGY

Most patients are infected with either streptococci or staphylococci, although the former predominate. Among the streptococci, the viridans group is responsible for the majority of cases, typically producing disease with an indolent course (Table 3). Most are part of the normal mouth flora and are classically associated with endocarditis after dental procedures. However, the association between routine dental procedures, such as teeth cleaning, and endocarditis is somewhat more tenuous than in the past. It is not unusual for endocarditis to occur in the absence of any such history. There does appear to be a link between certain procedures, such as extraction or deep scaling, and endocarditis, and prophylactic regimens are designed to prevent IE when these are performed in patients with known predisposing cardiac conditions. *Streptococcus bovis* is associated with underlying carcinoma of the colon, for which patients should be assessed when IE is caused by that organism. Enterococci similiarly inhabit the bowel but are more likely to result in endocarditis as a complication of urinary tract infection.

Coagulase-negative staphylococci rarely infect native valves, although they do cause disease in the setting of congenital or acquired valve disease. More commonly, infection due to coagulase-negative staphylococci occurs in the setting of a foreign body, such as a prosthetic valve or pacemaker wire. The HACEK group of organisms (see Table 3) consists of fastidious gram-negative bacilli that are very slow growing in usual culture media. Cases of "culture-negative" endocarditis may actually be due to these or other organisms that have unique growth requirements. In such cases, the microbiology laboratory should be alerted to the possibility of slow-growing organisms so that blood specimens can be cultured with special media and observed over an extended period of time. In contrast, *Staphylococcus aureus* almost always causes a fulminant course and is readily isolated from routine blood cultures. This organism is the most common cause of IE in injection drug users. In addicts, *S. aureus* is just as likely to produce disease on the tricuspid valve as on either the aortic or mitral valve. In those who do not use drugs, it is still associated with fulminant infection but almost always affects the mitral or aortic valve. Negative blood cultures in an injection drug user with suspected endocarditis may be due to the self-administration of antibiotics. Repeating blood cultures after a period of several antibiotic-free days will frequently lead to isolation of *S. aureus* or another typical pathogen. Groups A, B, and G streptococci also usually cause acute infection. IE caused by these organisms occurs most often in injection drug users, but even in this population it is almost always associated with left-sided infection. Enteric gram-negative bacilli and *Pseudomonas* are very uncommon causes of endocarditis. Endocarditis due to these organisms may be the result of injection drug use; other patients have antecedent urinary tract infections or underlying gastrointestinal pathology. Fungal endocarditis is confined almost entirely to injection drug users or patients with prosthetic valves. Among the fungi, *Candida* species are the most common cause, and of these, most are non–*C. albicans*. *Aspergillus* species present unique problems in that they typically infect recently inserted prosthetic valves and blood cultures are almost always negative.

TABLE 3. **Microbiology of Infective Endocarditis**

Organisms Usually Associated With Subacute/Chronic Infection

Streptococcus viridans
- *Streptococcus mutans*
- *Streptococcus mitis*
- *Streptococcus mitior*
- *Streptococcus sanguis*
- Others

Streptococcus bovis

Enterococcus
- *Enterococcus faecalis*
- *Enterococcus faecium*

Coagulase-negative staphylococci

HACEK group
- *Haemophilus* species
- *Actinobacillus actinomycetemcomitans*
- *Cardiobacterium hominis*
- *Eikenella corrodens*
- *Kingella* species

Organisms Usually Associated With Acute Infection

Staphylococcus aureus

Streptococcus Groups A, B, and G

Streptococcus pneumoniae

Fungi
- *Candida* species
- *Aspergillus* species

CLINICAL MANIFESTATIONS

In most cases, IE is an indolent infection. There is a variable "incubation period" of approximately 2 weeks from the time of inoculation to the onset of symptoms, although when the etiologic agent is *S. aureus* or another of the organisms that produces acute disease, the time to onset of symptoms is probably much shorter. The nature of the presentation depends on the pathologic process. In patients with less virulent pathogens, the time from onset of symptoms to diagnosis averages 5 weeks. In such cases, the presenting complaint is frequently related to a complication of the illness, such as sudden onset of paralysis due to a septic embolus to the cerebral circulation. Indeed, a stroke accompanied by fever should alert the clinician to the possibility of underlying IE. The history in most cases will almost always reveal a history of days to weeks of constitutional signs and symptoms. In some cases, the local destructive cardiac lesion leads to congestive heart failure. In others, emboli to either the pulmonary or the systemic circulation bring the patient to medical attention, with either pleuritic chest pain in the case of right-sided involvement or stroke or another ischemic complication dominating the clinical picture in patients with aortic or mitral valve disease. In others, the continuous bacteremia and seeding of metastatic foci and circulating immune complexes cause progressive ill-defined and nonspecific symptoms.

Table 4 lists the most common signs and symptoms of IE. Fever is almost always a feature, but it may be depressed in patients who are given empirical antibiotics, as well as those with renal failure, congestive heart failure, advanced age, or terminal illness. The other typical symptoms of endocarditis are so nonspecific that they rarely point to the correct diagnosis. It is rather the diffuse symptom complex indicating involvement of every organ that suggests the diagnosis.

Any patient with unexplained fever should be evaluated for IE. In addition, recent evidence demonstrates that patients with nosocomial *S. aureus* bacteremia have a high incidence of IE even without obvious signs or symptoms and some authors advocate the use of transesophageal echocardiography in those cases to assess for endocarditis. The clinical features of endocarditis are also difficult to distinguish from other causes of sepsis and bacteremia in injection drug users, although the diagnosis is likely in addicts presenting with fever, pleuritic chest pain, and radiographic evidence of multiple septic pulmonary emboli.

TABLE 4. **Signs and Symptoms of Infective Endocarditis**

Constitutional	**Local**
Fever (80%)	Neurologic
Chills (40%)	Confusion
Weakness	Delirium
Headache*	Focal deficits
Malaise*	Meningitis
Anorexia*	Respiratory
Weight loss*	Chest pain (pleuritic)
Nausea and vomiting*	Hemoptysis
	Cardiac
	Congestive heart failure
	Gastrointestinal
	Abdominal pain
	Musculoskeletal
	Arthralgia
	Myalgia

*Much more common in patients with subacute course (20%–40%).

TABLE 5. **Physical Findings in Patients With Infective Endocarditis**

Fever (90%)	Cardiac
Neurologic	Murmur (80%)
Delirium or confusion	Pericardial friction rub
Focal deficits	Abdomen
Aphasia	Splenomegaly
Hemiparesis or hemiplegia	Musculoskeletal
Ataxia	Myalgia
Meningitis	Arthralgia or arthritis
Ophthalmic	Skin/integument
Roth spots	Splinter hemorrhages
Conjunctival hemorrhages	Osler nodes
Respiratory	Janeway lesions
Crackles	
Pleural friction rub	

The diffuse organ involvement associated with endocarditis is also reflected in the physical examination (Table 5). The combination of sustained bacteremia, infected emboli, and immune complexes results in dysfunction of practically every organ, leading to several characteristic physical findings. In addition to fever and tachycardia, in patients with significant aortic valve insufficiency there may be a wide pulse pressure. The neurologic examination may reveal global or local abnormalities because patients may present with diffuse cerebritis, focal paralysis, or both. Conjunctival hemorrhages are common and Roth spots, although less frequent, are highly supportive of the diagnosis. There may be evidence of bilateral pulmonary involvement in patients with right-sided infection as manifested by splinting or signs of effusion or consolidation or by diffuse crackles in those with congestive heart failure (CHF). A heart murmur is detected in most patients and characteristically changes as the valve is remodeled by the disease or by alteration of blood flow as the vegetation changes shape. Evidence of heart failure is common in patients with significant aortic or mitral valve incompetence. A pericardial effusion is occasionally detected secondary to pericarditis, myocarditis, or rupture of the sinus of Valsalva with hemorrhage into the pericardial sac. Findings indicative of tamponade are rare, but they constitute a medical emergency.

Splenomegaly is unusual in patients with right-sided involvement but is frequently detected in those with mitral or aortic infection. In such cases splenic abscess should be considered. The musculoskeletal system may be infected by emboli, metastatic infection, immune complex disease, or all of these, leading to myalgia, arthralgia, or arthritis. Splinter hemorrhages are common but frequently are the result of local trauma and may be unrelated to IE. Osler nodes and Janeway lesions are much more specific but are also much less frequently found. Fingernail clubbing was described frequently in the past and may still be seen in 10% to 20% of patients, primarily in those with subacute endocarditis or congenital heart disease.

COMPLICATIONS

Complications of endocarditis are common events, and often is the trigger that brings the patient to medical attention (Table 6). As noted previously, manifestations of central nervous system involvement, most often stroke secondary to an infected embolus, are typical initial mani-

TABLE 6. **Major Complications of Endocarditis**

Central Nervous System
Stroke
Mycotic aneurysm
Seizures
Cranial nerve palsy
Toxic encephalopathy
Respiratory
Secondary pneumonia
Lung abscess
Empyema
Adult respiratory distress syndrome
Cardiac
Congestive heart failure
Valvular insufficiency or stenosis
Perivalvular abscess
Myocardial abscess
Myocardial infarction
Renal
Renal failure
Abscess
Immune complex glomerulonephritis
Intra-Abdominal
Splenic abscess
Mesenteric artery mycotic aneurysm
Ischemia or infarction
Musculoskeletal
Septic arthritis
Myositis

festations of disease. Seizures may also be the result of septic emboli, as are mycotic aneurysms. These aneurysms tend to be in the peripheral cerebral circulation, are difficult to detect, and, when they rupture, are associated with a very high mortality rate. Any patient with endocarditis who develops changes in neurologic function, particularly sudden onset of severe headache, should be evaluated for a mycotic aneurysm. Patients with right-sided endocarditis usually present with evidence of septic pulmonary embolism. Rarely, severe respiratory failure or adult respiratory distress syndrome may result from these repeated insults to the lung; however, these emboli are small and do not lead to major hemodynamic problems.

Aside from central nervous system effects, the most significant complications of IE are associated with cardiac damage. CHF results from valve damage, myocardial abscesses arising from emboli to the cardiac circulation, or disruption of the conducting system. Valve leaflet rupture may lead to sudden onset of CHF and is an indication for immediate surgical intervention. Perivalvular abscess formation may be responsible for arrhythmia, valve leaflet rupture, or continued sepsis and is another indication for early surgical intervention. Renal failure occurs in 25% to 35% from either septic emboli or immune complex glomerulonephritis or both. Fortunately, renal function usually recovers, but considerable time may be required and occasional patients need temporary dialysis support.

Less common complications of IE are splenic abscess and involvement of the gastrointestinal tract by emboli, which may lead to ischemia, infarction, or mycotic aneurysm formation.

DIAGNOSIS

The clinical presentation of endocarditis may be abrupt or insidious, depending on the infecting organism. Patients with an acute presentation tend to be injection drug users, diabetics, or elderly patients who are infected by *S. aureus*. In the case of addicts, acute onset of chest pain is typically due to septic pulmonary emboli. It should be noted, however, that drug addicts also develop left-sided infection, either alone or in combination with tricuspid or, more rarely, pulmonic valve infection. Patients with pulmonary artery catheters are also at risk for pulmonic valve involvement. Indwelling venous catheters also carry a risk of causing endocarditis as a complication of catheter infection and bacteremia. Frequently, these patients develop generalized sepsis that may mask the underlying cardiac infection. In such cases, disease progression may be swift and the mortality rate is high.

More commonly, patients have an indolent course. The onset of disease may be difficult to pinpoint. Usually there is a history of malaise, intermittent fevers, myalgia, or arthralgia. Many have previously seen a physician for nonspecific illness, and often will have received an empirical course of antibiotics that arrests the symptoms temporarily. In other cases, as noted earlier, patients present after suffering a catastrophic complication, such as embolic stroke or ruptured mycotic aneurysm. Even in these cases, the history will usually reveal a constellation of nonspecific symptoms that have been present for days to weeks.

Because virtually every organ is affected in some way, it is not surprising that multiple laboratory abnormalities are a feature of endocarditis (Table 7). The hallmark of endocarditis and the most consistent feature is persistently positive blood cultures. A myriad of additional abnormalities are routinely detected, none of which are specific or diagnostic. Anemia and elevated sedimentation rates are almost always found; leukocytosis and thrombocytopenia occur less often. Proteinuria and microscopic hematuria reflect glomerular damage. Pyuria may indicate pyogenic involvement of the renal parenchyma. Abnormal liver enzymes, elevated globulin, and decreased albumin are also routine findings. Patients with right-sided involvement have multiple nodular densities on chest radiographs, representing septic pulmonary emboli.

Given the nonspecific nature of both the clinical and laboratory features of endocarditis, confirming the diagnosis presents a challenge. Various approaches have been suggested, each with advantages and disadvantages. A team of investigators at Duke University devised a set of major and minor criteria that are now widely accepted. This schema considers the history and physical findings, a

TABLE 7. **Common Laboratory Abnormalities in Patients with Infective Endocarditis**

Blood Culture
Positive in >90%
Hematology
Anemia (70%–90%)
Thrombocytopenia (5%–15%)
Leukocytosis (20%–35%)
Elevated erythrocyte sedimentation rate (90%–100%)
Urinalysis
Proteinuria (50%–65%)
Microscopic hematuria (30%–60%)
Red blood cell casts (12%)
Hematuria (gross)
Pyuria
White blood cell casts
Bacteriuria

set of pathologic and laboratory abnormalities, and echocardiographic results to assign patients to different diagnostic categories. Recently, the criteria were revised to improve the specificity (Table 8). Although designed primarily as a tool for investigators they serve well to assist clinicians in confirming the diagnosis, especially when dealing with diagnostic dilemmas.

TREATMENT

Before the development of antibiotics, IE was a uniformly fatal disease. With antibiotics the prognosis is generally favorable, but it places special demands on the treating physician. Because the organisms within a vegetation are shielded from the host immune system, eradication depends on antibiotic activity alone. Hence, antibiotic selection must be based on carefully performed susceptibility testing. Only antibiotics with bactericidal activity should be selected. In some cases, such as in enterococcal endocarditis, a synergistic combination is required to achieve bactericidal activity. Parenteral therapy is required to obtain serum concentrations sufficient to induce an adequate antibiotic concentration at the core of the vegetation. Vancomycin (Vancocin), because of its poor bactericidal activity, should be reserved for situations when there is no acceptable alternative. In cases of enterococcal infection, consideration should be given to desensitizing patients with penicillin allergy, rather than using vancomycin. This is especially true when synergistic activity is not achievable by combination therapy. An additional

TABLE 8. **Definition of Infective Endocarditis According to the Proposed Modified Dukes Criteria**

Definite Infective Endocarditis

Pathologic Criteria

(1) Microorganisms demonstrated by culture or histologic examination of a vegetation or a vegetation that has embolized, or in an intracardiac abscess specimen; *or*
(2) Pathologic lesions, vegetation, or intracardiac abscess confirmed by histologic examination showing active endocarditis

*Clinical Criteria**

(1) Two major criteria, *or*
(2) One major criterion and 3 minor criteria; *or*
(3) Five minor criteria

Possible Infective Endocarditis

(1) One major criterion and one minor criterion; *or*
(2) Three minor criteria

Rejected

(1) Firm alternate diagnosis explaining evidence of IE; *or*
(2) Resolution of IE syndrome with antibiotic therapy for ≤4 days; *or*
(3) No pathologic evidence of IE at surgery or autopsy, with antibiotic therapy for ≤4 days; *or*
(4) Does not meet criteria for possible IE, as above

Definitions of Terms

Major Criteria

Blood culture positive for IE
- Typical microorganism consistent with IE from two separate blood cultures:
  - Viridans streptococci, *Streptococcus bovis,* HACEK group, *Staphylococcus aureus;*
    or
  - Community-acquired enterococci, in the absence of a primary focus; *or*
- Microorganisms consistent with IE from persistently positive blood cultures, defined as follows:
  - At least two positive cultures of blood samples drawn >12 hr apart; *or*
  - All of three or a majority of four or more separate cultures of blood (with first and last samples drawn at least 1 hr apart)
- Single positive blood culture for *Coxiella burnetii* or anti–phase I IgG antibody titer >1:800

Evidence of endocardial involvement
- Echocardiogram positive for IE (TEE recommended in patients with prosthetic valves, rated at least "possible IE" by clinical criteria, or complicated IE [paravalvular abscess]; TTE as first test in other patients), defined as follows:
  - Oscillating intracardiac mass on valve or supporting structures, in the path of regurgitant jets, or on implanted material in the absence of an alternative anatomic explanation; *or*
  - Abscess; *or*
  - New partial dehiscence of prosthetic valve

New valvular regurgitation (worsening or changing of preexisting murmur not sufficient)

Minor Criteria

Predisposition: predisposing heart condition or intravenous drug use

Fever: temperature >38°C

Vascular phenomena: major arterial emboli, septic pulmonary infarcts, mycotic aneurysm, intracranial hemorrhage, conjunctival hemorrhages, and Janeway lesions

Immunologic phenomena: glomerulonephritis, Osler nodes, Roth spots, and rheumatoid factor

Microbiologic evidence: positive blood culture but does not meet a major criterion as noted above* or serologic evidence of active infection with organism consistent with IE

Echocardiographic minor criteria eliminated

*Excludes single positive cultures for coagulase-negative staphylococci and organisms that do not cause endocarditis.

Abbreviations: IE = infective endocarditis; TEE, transesophageal echocardiography; TTE, transthoracic echocardiography.

Modified from Li JS, Sexton DJ, Mick N, et al: Proposed modifications to the Dukes criteria. Clin Infect Dis 30:633–638, 2000.

concern is the previously described enormous colony count of organisms within a vegetation. Many antibiotics suffer from an "inoculum effect"—that is, their activity is diminished in the presence of large numbers of organisms. Thus, only antibiotics that have been carefully studied in patients with endocarditis should be used. Finally, the treatment duration must be sufficiently long to ensure eradication of the in-

TABLE 9. **Therapy for Native Valve Infective Endocarditis**

Organism	Antibiotic	Dosage and Route	Duration (wk)
Penicillin-susceptible viridans streptococci and *Streptococcus bovis* (MIC ≤0.1 μg/mL)	Penicillin G	12 million U/d IV either continuously or in six equally divided doses	4
	or		
	Ceftriaxone (Rocephin)	2 g IV or IM q24h	4
	or		
	Penicillin G	12–18 million U/d IV either continuously or in six equally divided doses	2
	with gentamicin (Garamycin)	1 mg/kg IM or IV q8h	2
	or		
	Vancomycin (Vancocin)	30 mg/kg/d IV in two equally divided doses (do not exceed 2 g/24h)	4
Relatively penicillin-resistant viridans streptococci and *Streptococcus bovis* (MIC >0–1 μg/mL and <0.5 μg/mL)	Penicillin G	12–18 million U/d either continuously or in six equally divided doses	4
	with gentamicin	1 mg/kg IM or IV q8h	2
	or		
	Vancomycin	(as above)	4
Enterococci and viridans streptococci (MIC >0.5 μg/mL)	Penicillin G	18–30 million U/d IV either continuously or in six equally divided doses	4–6
	with gentamicin*	1 mg/kg IM or IV q8h	4–6
	or		
	Ampicillin	12 g/d IV either continuously or in six equally divided doses	4–6
	with gentamicin	1 mg/kg IM or IV q8h	4–6
	or		
	Vancomycin	(as above)	4–6
	with gentamicin	(as above)	4–6
Staphylococci	Nafcillin (Nallpen) or	2 g IV q4h	4–6
Methicillin sensitive	Oxacillin (Bactocill) with optional gentamicin	1 mg/kg IM or IV q8h	3–5 days
	or		
	Cefazolin (Ancef) (for β-lactam–allergic patients)	2 g IVq8h	4–6
	with optional gentamicin	1 mg/kg/d IV in two equally divided doses	3–5 days
	or		
	Vancomycin*	30 mg/kg/d IV in two equally divided doses (do not exceed 2 g/24h)	4–6
Methicillin resistant	Vancomycin	30 mg/kg/d IV in two equally divided doses (do not exceed 2 g/24h)	4–6
HACEK group	Ceftriaxone	2 g IV or IM once daily	4
	or		
	Ampicillin	12 g/d IV either continously or in six equally divided doses	4
	with gentamicin	1.0 mg/kg IM or IV q8h	4

*Use for enterococci demonstrated to have gentamicin synergy.
†Penicillin G preferred for penicillin-susceptible staphylococci (MIC ≤ 0.1 μg/mL) for penicillin-susceptible viridans streptococci.
‡Recommended only for patients allergic to penicillin.
Abbreviation: MIC = minimal inhibitory concentration.
Modified from Wilson WR, Karchmer AW, Dajani AS, et al. Antibiotic treatment of adults with infective endocarditis due to streptococci, enterococci, staphylococci, and HACEK microorganisms. JAMA 274:1706–1713, 1995. Copyright 1995, American Medical Association.

TABLE 10. **Therapy for Prosthetic Valve Infective Endocarditis**

Organism	Antibiotic	Dosage and Route	Duration (wk)
Staphylococci			
Methicillin sensitive	Nafcillin (Nallpen) with	2 g IV q4h	≥6
	rifampin (Rifadin)* and	300 mg orally q8h	≥6
	with gentamicin (Garamycin)	1.0 mg/kg IM or IV q8h	Initial 2 weeks
Methicillin resistant	Vancomycin (Vancocin)	30 mg/kg/d IV in two or four equally divided doses, not to exceed 2 g/24h	≥6
	with rifampin* and with	300 mg orally q8h	≥6
	gentamicin	1.0 mg/kg IM or IV q8h	Initial 2 weeks
Viridans streptococci or *Streptococcus bovis*	Same therapy as for native valve endocarditis due to enterococci		

*Not FDA approved for this indication.
Modified from Wilson WR, Karchmer AW, Dajani AS, et al: Antibiotic treatment of adults with endocarditis due to streptococci, enterococci, staphylococci, and HACEK microorganisms. JAMA 274:1706–1713, 1995. Copyright 1995, American Medical Association.

fecting organisms. In most cases this will be a minimum of 4 weeks.

The American Heart Association developed guidelines for the treatment of IE, for both native valve (Table 9) and prosthetic valve disease (Table 10). Because of insufficient published data, the committee was unable to suggest treatment recommendations for IE caused by unusual organisms, such as gram-negative bacilli and fungi. Clinicians treating such patients would most often benefit by consultation with an expert. Regardless of the treatment regimen, blood cultures should be repeated several times to verify that bacteremia has been eradicated. Rarely, patients appear well despite persistent bacteremia.

Most patients will respond to medical management. However, surgery may be life saving in selected cases. The most urgent indication for surgery is congestive heart failure that is unresponsive to medical management. This complication usually results from rupture of a valve leaflet or connecting structure. Persistent bacteremia is another indication for surgery; but in a stable patient, multidrug combinations are frequently effective at clearing the bloodstream and surgery can be avoided. Repeated major systemic embolization is another indication for surgery. Perivalvular abscess, even in the absence of CHF, is almost never curable without surgery.

IE due to organisms for which antibiotic therapy usually fails, such as fungi, is another indication for surgery. It has also been proposed that certain echocardiographic features should be an indication for surgery; however, these remain controversial. Among them are the finding of vegetations that persist after a major systemic embolic episode, anterior mitral valve leaflet vegetations more than 1 cm in diameter, vegetation size that increases after 4 weeks of treatment, acute aortic or mitral valve insufficiency, valve perforation or rupture, and perivalvular extension of infection. Most important, the decision to operate is based on hemodynamic factors rather than on the activity of the infection. Fortunately, a prosthetic valve can be implanted safely, even during the acute phase of endocarditis. The risk of subsequent prosthetic valve infection is only slightly greater than in patients who do not have active infection at the time of operation. Before performing surgery, a distant focus of infection, such as a splenic abscess, should be sought, so as to prevent secondary infection of the prosthetic valve by bacteremia arising from another source.

HYPERTENSION

method of
MUNAVVAR IZHAR, M.D., D.M., and
GEORGE BAKRIS, M.D.
Rush-Presbyterian-St. Luke's Medical Center
Chicago, Illinois

Persistent elevation in arterial pressure (AP), hypertension, is one of the most important public health problems in the world. An estimated 690 million people around the globe have hypertension, as defined by an AP of greater than 140/90 mm Hg. It is currently among the leading causes of morbidity and mortality in the world. In addition to the morbidity and mortality directly attributable to hypertension, it is recognized worldwide as a major cardiovascular risk factor that accounts for one third of the world's deaths. The linear relationship between cardiovascular risk and systemic AP is well established.

The prevalence of hypertension increases with age and is higher in African Americans than Mexican-Americans or non-Hispanic whites. Yet, with the aging of America, the National Health and Nutrition Examination Survey (NHANES-III) noted a reduction in the number of estimated individuals with hypertension in the United States in the decade of the 1990s compared with the 1980s. Widespread improvements in lifestyle over the past 10 to 15 years, improved public awareness and patient education, as well as greater physician efforts are responsible for the decrease in prevalence of hypertension.

An overview is presented of the definition and diagnosis of hypertension followed by emphasis on its treatment in a variety of circumstances. The focus is on a meaningful, yet simplified approach to treatment, integrating concepts from both the Sixth Joint National Committee Report on Prevention, Detection, Evaluation and Treatment of High Blood Pressure (JNC VI) and the National Kidney Foundation (NKF) Report.

DEFINITION

Over the past several decades, the levels that define hypertension for the general population have been reduced from more than 160/95 mm Hg to 140/90 mm Hg or higher. Moreover, most authorities now agree on several important principles:

- Hypertension should be defined by both systolic and diastolic AP levels.
- Simply defining and consequently categorizing individuals as hypertensive, based only on their AP level, neglects the value of using the presence or absence of other risk factors, co-morbidity, and target organ damage to assess prognosis and ultimately to guide therapy.
- The definitions of hypertension for home or ambulatory measurements are different. AP greater than 135/85 mm Hg for 24-hour ambulatory monitoring or home monitoring is the usual level that defines hypertension.
- The treatment approach for individuals with an AP beyond the accepted upper limits should not be simply focused on the AP level, which assesses the relative risk imparted by that AP, but also the remainder of the cardiovascular risk profile, which estimates the absolute risk of events at a particular AP. In the JNC VI classification and stratification of hypertension, stages 1 to 3 represent increasing relative risk as AP rises, whereas risk groups A through C denote increasing absolute risk as other risk factors and target organ damage are superimposed on the level of AP (Table 1).

MEASUREMENT OF ARTERIAL PRESSURE

Many expert panels have made recommendations regarding methodology of AP measurement, and these frequently do not agree in all details. However, several general principles can be distilled:

- There are six sizes of commonly available AP cuffs. Using a smaller-than-recommended cuff on a larger arm typically results in an overestimation of casual AP. In obese or muscular persons, the large adult-sized cuff is required for all those with an arm circumference at the mid-humerus over 38 cm. In very large individuals, use of the "thigh" cuff is often necessary.
- When accurately measuring AP, the deflation rate of the column of mercury should be 2 to 3 mm Hg/s; the lower rate of deflation should be used for persons with a heart rate less than 72 beats per minute; the more rapid deflation is appropriate only for those with resting tachycardia. If the precision of measurement is to be at least 2 mm Hg, the observer should have the opportunity to hear at least one Korotkoff sound at each 2 mm Hg gradation of the mercury column.
- It is unusual for a single AP measurement to be an accurate indicator of future cardiovascular risk; multiple measurements made on different occasions are more likely to be helpful in deciding if a particular person should have his or her AP lowered. It is traditional to average the second and third of a series of AP measurements in a single position (e.g., supine, seated, or standing) and record this as the "average AP" at a given visit.
- Physicians and patients are often more interested and impressed by AP readings taken in other settings (e.g., home monitors or ambulatory AP monitoring devices, both of which are discussed further later).

AP is subject to a large degree of intrinsic variability. Several steps can be taken to minimize this variability:

1. Take multiple measurements, especially when the pulse is irregular (e.g., atrial fibrillation). This is necessary because ventricular filling pressures vary considerably, because of variability of diastolic filling time. AP variability is prevalent particularly in older persons, with primarily or exclusively systolic AP evaluations.
2. Center the bladder of the cuff over the brachial artery, with its lower edge within 2.5 cm of the antecubital fossa. This leaves enough space so that the stethoscope head can be applied inferiorly without touching the cuff.
3. Have the subject rest silently and comfortably (with back support if seated) for at least 5 minutes before the measurement.
4. Question the patient as to whether he or she has abstained from drinking caffeine or alcohol-containing beverages or from tobacco use for 30 minutes before an AP measurement.
5. Ensure that the arm is supported at the level of the heart. Both muscular work (of tensed muscles around the elbow) and hydrostatic pressure due to a "dangling arm" increase the pressure necessary to obliterate the pulse and lead to overestimates of systolic AP.
6. Listen over the brachial artery using the bell of the stethoscope with minimal pressure exerted on the skin.
7. Determine the "peak inflation level" of the mercury column, using palpation of the radial artery before the

TABLE 1. **Stratification of Cardiovascular Risk and Links to Initial Treatment Strategy, According to JNC-VI**

	Risk Group		
BP Stage	*A* *(0 Risk Factors)*	*B* *(1 [not DM]) Risk Factor*	*C* *(≥2 [or DM]) Risk Factors*
	Target organ damage absent Cardiovascular disease absent	Target organ damage absent Cardiovascular disease absent	Target organ damage present Cardiovascular disease present
High Normal (130–139/85–89)	LM only	LM only	LM + drug therapy
Stage 1 (140–159/90–99)	LM × 12 months	LM × 6 months	LM + drug therapy
Stage 2 (160–179/100–109)	LM + drug therapy	LM + drug therapy	LM + drug therapy
Stage 3 (≥180/110)	LM + drug therapy	LM + drug therapy	LM + drug therapy

Abbreviations: DM = diabetes mellitus; LM = lifestyle modifications.

stethoscope is applied. For all subsequent AP measurements, the cuff should typically be inflated 20 mm Hg higher than the pressure at which the palpable pulse at the radial artery disappears. Important prognostic information may be missed if the "auscultatory gap" is not detected; this risk is minimized by determining the peak inflation level by palpation before the stethoscope is applied.

8. Attempt to avoid "terminal digit preference." Traditionally, AP measurements are rounded to the nearest 2 mm Hg (the typical markings on a mercury sphygmomanometer). Theoretically, in a large collection of systolic and diastolic AP measurements, there should be an equal number of readings ending in 0, 2, 4, 6, or 8 mm Hg.

9. Measurements of AP in both arms are typically obtained at the initial visit, and the arm with the higher AP is used thereafter if the difference is greater than 10/5 mm Hg. In such situations, there is often concern about coarctation of the aorta or Takayasu arteritis or moyamoya disease.

White-Coat Hypertension

The name "white-coat hypertension" is given to the situation in which AP measurements outside the office are considerably lower than those measured in the office. Careful studies originally done in Italy (and now corroborated in other countries) show that AP rises in response to an approaching physician who is not previously known to the subject. This apparently does not happen if the subject is approached by a nurse, even if she or he is wearing a white coat.

In general, this type of hypertension has an intermediate cardiovascular risk profile and requires that intervention focus on behavioral rather than pharmacologic means.

ROUTINE EVALUATION

The history, physical examination, and initial laboratory evaluation are the cornerstones in evaluating patients with hypertension. Six key issues must be addressed during the initial office evaluation of a person with elevated AP readings:

1. Documenting an accurate diagnosis of hypertension (see earlier)
2. Defining the presence or absence of target organ damage related to hypertension
3. Screening for other cardiovascular risk factors that often accompany hypertension
4. Stratifying risk for cardiovascular disease (according to risk group A, B, or C in JNC VI) (see Table 1)
5. Assessing whether the person is likely to have an identifiable cause of hypertension (secondary hypertension) and should have further diagnostic testing to confirm or exclude the diagnosis
6. Obtaining data that may be helpful in initial and subsequent choice of therapy

There are many diagnostic possibilities for explaining a single set of elevated AP readings. Aside from those who take one of several types of drugs known to elevate AP, many persons with only one elevated AP reading will have their AP decline and return to the normal range. This is the reason for recommending multiple encounters (at least two to three) before a diagnosis of hypertension can be firmly established.

History

Most patients with hyp rtension have no specific symptoms; hence, appropriately it is designated as a "silent killer." Headache is characteristic of stage 3 hypertension; such headaches are often localized to the occipital region and are often present on awakening in the morning. Patients with hypertension also complain of dizziness and palpitations. If severe, hypertension can manifest as chest pain and dyspnea due to cardiac failure. Pain from dissection of the aorta or to a leaking aneurysm may be a rare presenting symptom.

A strong family history of hypertension favors diagnosis of essential hypertension. The onset of hypertension before 30 and after 55 years of age may be a clue to presence of secondary hypertension. However, the number of people with essential hypertension being detected at 15 to 20 years of age is increasing. Finally, aspects of a patient's lifestyle that could contribute to hypertension or its treatment should be assessed, including diet, physical activity, work, and stress level. Symptoms of polyuria, polydipsia, and muscle weakness may suggest primary aldosteronism. History of weight gain may suggest Cushing disease; and a history of headaches, palpitations, diaphoresis, dizziness, and weight loss may suggest pheochromocytoma.

Physical Examination

The physical examination starts with the patient's general appearance. For instance, are the round face and truncal obesity of Cushing syndrome present? Is the muscular development in upper extremities out of proportion to that in the lower extremities, suggesting coarctation of aorta. The equality of heart rate and APs should be noted in the upper extremities. Palpation and auscultation of carotid arteries is important, because carotid artery disease might be a manifestation of hypertensive vascular disease. In cardiac and respiratory examinations one should look for left ventricular heave, presence of third or fourth heart sound, and pulmonary rales. Their presence suggests ventricular dysfunction and its sequelae. The abdominal examination should focus on detecting renal bruits, best heard above the umbilicus in the right or left of midline or in the flanks. The abdomen should also be palpated for presence of polycystic kidney disease. If the femoral pulse is delayed or decreased compared with the radial pulse, AP in lower extremities should be measured. AP in the lower extremities should be recorded at least once in patients in whom hypertension is discovered before the age of 30 years.

Proper examination of the optic fundus is an often neglected although valuable tool for evaluating the hypertensive patients. The optic fundus is the only site in the entire body where blood vessels can be directly examined. Very few patients with a recent onset of hypertension have Keith-Wagener-Barker grade III or VI fundi. Arteriosclerosis can be directly recognized, and the severity and duration of previous hypertension can be estimated by appreciation of abnormalities of the retinal arteries. The normal yellowish white color of the retinal arteries gradually changes to a reddish brown tone ("copper wire") and the ratio of artery-to-vein diameters is reduced from the normal 2:3 to less than 1:3. Over time, the column of blood within the artery gradually diminishes and the artery is reduced to a whitish thread ("silver wire"), despite a persistent (albeit reduced) flow of blood. "Arteriovenous nicking" is perhaps the most easily recognized ocular abnormality in hypertension. When the thickened artery containing blood at elevated pressure compresses a low-pressure, thin-walled vein within the shared adventitial sheath, the vein disappears from view. Hypertension is, therefore, an epidemiologic and pathophysiologic risk factor for retinal vein occlusion, although this is not a common occurrence.

When arterial blood flow is reduced sufficiently to cause infarction of underlying retinal tissue, round to oval white patches with fluffy borders are formed ("cytoid bodies," or "cotton-wool spots"). When there is breakdown in the blood-retinal barrier (due to a ruptured aneurysm, neovascularization—typically in diabetics—or "blowout" hemorrhages due to hypertension), intraretinal "flame-shaped" hemorrhages can be recognized on direct ophthalmoscopy. Grade IV retinopathy (papilledema), the hallmark of either retinal vein occlusion or a hypertensive emergency, is usually caused by ischemia in the optic nerve circulation, due to either increased intraocular or intracranial pressure and diminished axoplasmic flow in the optic nerve fibers. Papilledema without other evidence of hypertensive retinopathy is generally due to another cause.

Laboratory Assessment

Routine laboratory assessment recommended by both the JNC-VI and the NKF includes measurement of serum chemistries determination of glucose, potassium, and creatinine values, urinalysis, and an electrocardiogram. These basic laboratory studies should be performed in all patients with sustained hypertension.

TREATMENT

The length of time that the clinician should rely on lifestyle modifications before starting drug therapy has been clarified in JNC-VI and is based on risk estimates, not just on the level of AP (see Table 1). Those with stage 1 hypertension (systolic 140–159 mm Hg and/or diastolic 90–99 mm Hg) who have no other risk factors or end-organ damage (so-called risk group A) can be treated only with lifestyle modification for up to 1 year, even if goal AP is not reached, before drug therapy should be considered to be necessary. Patients with stage 1 hypertension who are in risk group B (other cardiovascular risk factors but no target organ damage or diabetes mellitus) should receive pharmacologic therapy after only a 6-month trial of lifestyle modification, unless goal AP is achieved without drugs. Those in risk group C (target organ damage, clinical cardiovascular disease and/or diabetes mellitus) should be treated with pharmacologic agents *and* lifestyle modification even if they have high normal AP (systolic 130–139 mm Hg and/or diastolic 85–89 mm Hg).

Lifestyle Modification

A summary of lifestyle modifications shown to reduce AP is listed in Table 2. The JNC-VI recommends weight loss for obese hypertensive patients, modification of dietary sodium intake to 100 mmol/d or less, and modification of alcohol intake to no more than two drinks per day. It also recommends an increase in physical activity for all patients with hypertension who have no specific condition that would make such a recommendation not applicable or safe.

There is little doubt that lifestyle factors such as diet, exercise, and stress can affect AP. There is a strong positive correlation between the level of body weight and body mass index (weight/height) and level of AP. The relationship of dietary sodium and AP is equally clear, especially at low and modest intakes of sodium and in those deemed to be salt sensitive. This is evident from the results of the DASH-sodium trial. This trial demonstrated as much as a 14-mm Hg reduction in systolic pressure among normotensive African-American women on a low-salt/high-potassium diet. Other nutrients such as potassium, omega-3 fatty acids such as present in fish oil, and possibly calcium and magnesium are inversely related to AP level.

Sedentary individuals who do little, if any, aerobic exercise, usually have higher APs than do appropriately matched controls, even when controlling for other confounding variables. The relationship of stress to AP is somewhat less clear. Physical or mental stress will raise AP temporarily, but the relationship of chronic anxiety and stress has been more difficult to demonstrate.

TABLE 2. **Lifestyle Modifications That Lower Blood Pressure**

1. Reduction of body weight (5 kg threshold, 10 kg reduces BP ~10/8 mm Hg)
2. Reduction in dietary salt consumption (target 100 mmol/d; can lower BP ~12/10 mm Hg, but individual responses vary)
3. Increase in physical activity to 30 to 45 minutes, four times a week (can lower BP 8/4 mm Hg and often helps control weight)
4. Increased consumption of fruits and vegetables (at least 4 servings/day, can lower BP ~6/3 mm Hg and often helps reduce salt consumption)—this increases potassium intake
5. Moderation of alcohol consumption (target 10–20 g ethanol for women, 20–30 g ethanol for men; can lower BP by up to 8/5 mm Hg in those who drink more than 5 drinks/day)
6. Stress management (randomized clinical trials outside the workplace have been unconvincing, but many psychologists still recommend the approach, despite a lack of detailed protocols that uniformly lower BP)

Other Lifestyle Modifications That Are Routinely Recommended

1. Tobacco avoidance (lowers cardiovascular risk independently of any effect on BP)
2. Fish consumption (improves lipid profiles and cardiovascular risk, more than expected if just BP effect alone was operative)
3. Increasing dietary fiber (improves lipid profiles and cancer risk, independently of effect on BP)

Lifestyle Modifications That Are *Not Routinely* Recommended

1. Biofeedback
2. Dietary calcium supplementation
3. Dietary magnesium supplementation
4. Micronutrient supplements

Pharmacologic Therapy

The primary goal of AP reduction is to achieve the recommended goal AP using the *least intrusive means possible.* "Intrusive" has several interpretations and can relate to economic effects, number of office visits, adverse effects, and convenience. The choice of the drug with which to begin therapy is probably the most important decision the clinician must make when treating hypertensive patients.

Individualizing Therapy

In view of the many effective options available, we must pay very close attention to each patient's needs and plan his or her regimen accordingly. We must treat each patient as an individual, not as a member of a population, and so the drug that we choose must be compatible with that individual patient's preferences, lifestyle, and job requirements. Whatever we select, it must be affordable. No amount of therapeutic wisdom will be effective if our patient does not have the funds to purchase our choice.

Achievement of Goal Pressure

We must strive to reduce systolic blood pressure to below 140 mm Hg and to reduce diastolic blood pressure to below 90 mm Hg, the goal currently articulated by several guidelines committees. In diabetics, the recommended goal is lower (systolic <130 mm Hg and diastolic <85 mm Hg). The JNC-VI recommended these more stringent goals for those with diabetes without proof from a clinical trial to support this aggressive approach. The subsequent publication of the Hypertension Optimal Treatment (HOT) trial and the United Kingdom Diabetes Prevention Study (UKDPS) provided the solid evidence that was needed to support this recommendation. These trials have led several organizations such as the NKF and the Canadian Hypertension Society to recommend achievement of an even lower goal arterial pressure of 130/80 mm Hg or less for those with diabetes.

In patients with renal disease and at least 1 g/d of proteinuria, the JNC-VI recommended an even lower goal (systolic <125 mm Hg and diastolic <75 mm Hg). This recommendation was based on one clinical trial; however, a randomized blinded clinical trial will soon be completed that may confirm this recommendation. A retrospective analysis of many clinical trials shows a crisp relationship between the rate of decline in renal function and the level of AP achieved (Figure 1).

The NKF has produced a consensus approach for achievement of AP goals with a focus on cardiovascular and renal risk reduction. The paradigm is shown in Figure 2. It incorporates a strategy of drug selection with a focus on antihypertensive additive and risk reduction. This NKF approach, however, is designed for those with lower AP goals, such as those with diabetes or renal insufficiency, and not for the general population.

Strategies of Drug Therapy

Most patients with established hypertension should be started with only one drug at a low to moderate dose. In elderly patients, physicians should "start low and go slow." Of course, some patients may need immediate and drastic reduction of blood pressure in the presence of impending cardiovascular catastrophes. However, the number of such hypertensive urgencies and emergencies is very small.

The AP goal for subgroups of people with renal disease or with diabetes and perhaps those of certain ethnic and racial groups should be less than 130/80 mm Hg. Data from clinical trials indicate that it takes an average of 3.2 different antihypertensive medications to come close to achieving such goals (Figure 3). Therefore, agents shown to reduce cardiovascular and renal risk should always be part of an antihypertensive "cocktail." The impact of antihypertensive agents on renal and cardiovascular morbidity is shown in Table 3.

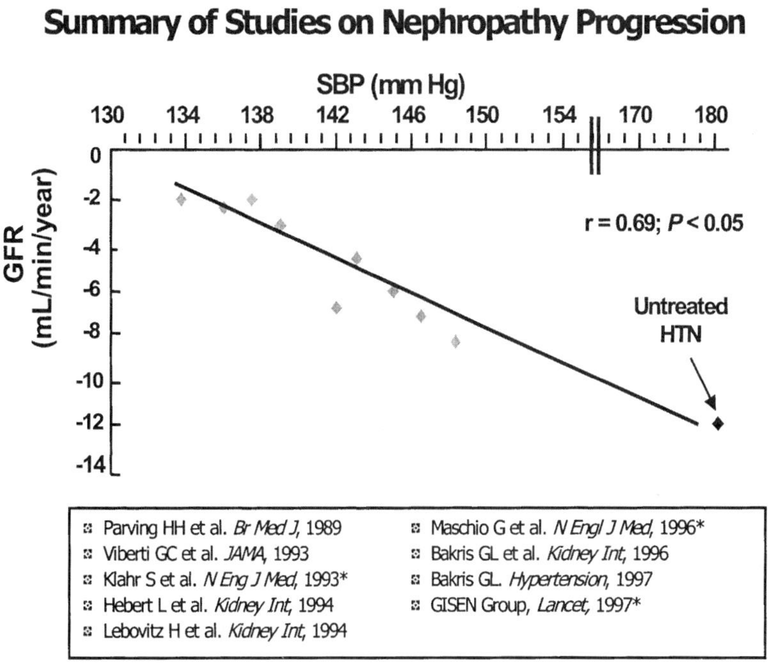

Figure 1. Association between level of systolic blood pressure (SBP) reduction achieved in clinical trials with renal endpoints and rate of decline in glomerular filtration rate (GFR). Note the moderately strong correlation between level of arterial pressure achieved and slowed rate of renal disease decline.

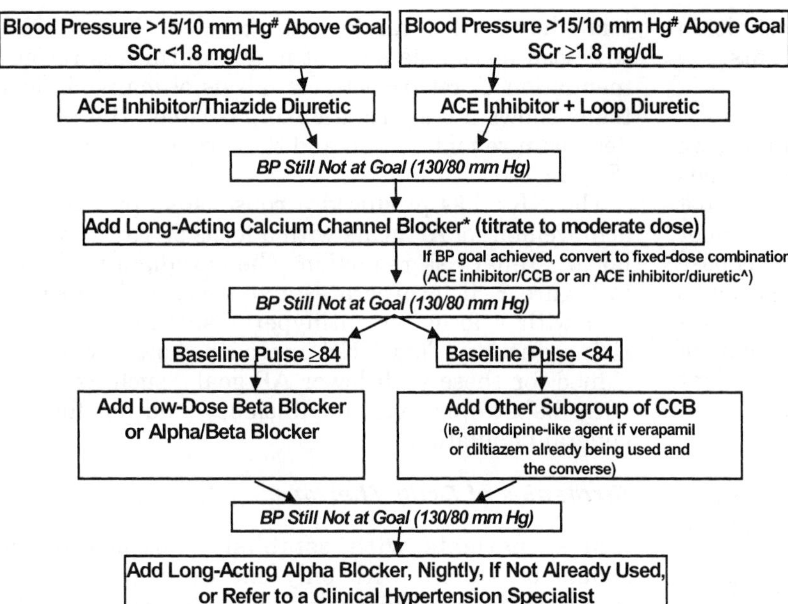

Figure 2. A suggested paradigm by which blood pressure (BP) goals in people with renal insufficiency and/or diabetes can be achieved by the least intrusive means possible. Everyone with diabetes and/or renal insufficiency should be instructed on lifestyle modifications as per the JNC-VI. Everyone, however, should be started on therapy if BP is greater than 130/80 mm Hg.* If BP is <15/10 mm Hg above goal (130/80 mm Hg), then an angiotensin converting enzyme (ACE) inhibitor alone may be used. The ACE inhibitor should be the same if two different fixed-dose combinations are used.† Non-dihydropyridine calcium channel blockers (CCBs) (verapamil, diltiazem) are preferred because they have been shown to reduce both cardiovascular mortality and progression of diabetic nephropathy independent of an ACE inhibitor. SCr = serum creatinine.

Factors Influencing Choice of Initial Drug Monotherapy

The factors in the choice of initial antihypertensive agents for a given patient should include a minimal side effect profile with little to no metabolic effects and evidence for reduced morbidity or mortality. Additionally, the agent should be affordable by a given patient. Table 4 outlines the factors to consider when selecting an antihypertensive regimen. The compelling and favorable indications for certain classes of antihypertensive drugs in particular disease states are summarized in Table 5. Likewise, the metabolic and renal effects of various antihypertensive drug classes are shown in Table 6.

Monotherapy, when titrated to appropriate doses, will achieve an AP goal of less than 140/90 mm Hg in 40% to 50% of all patients. Thus, in many cases, more than two drugs are needed to achieve the AP goal; drugs with additive or synergistic effects should be used. Table 7 lists the available fixed-dose combination agents shown to have additive AP-lowering capabilities. These agents are very helpful for improvement of medication adherence if two or more agents are required to achieve goal AP.

In clinical practice, more than 30% of the patients do not have the expected antihypertensive response or experience bothersome side effects from whatever drug is chosen. Therefore, drug substitution is needed in a sizable number of patients. It often takes

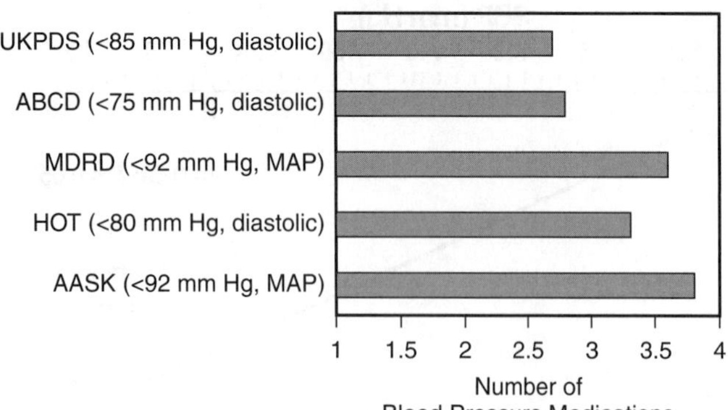

Figure 3. Average number of different antihypertensive agents needed to achieve lower blood pressure goals in all available trials that randomized for different levels of blood pressure control. AASK = African American Study of Kidney Disease in Hypertension; ABCD = Appropriate Blood Pressure Control in Diabetes; HOT = Hypertension Optimal Treatment trial; MAP = mean arterial pressure; MDRD = Modification of Dietary Protein in Renal Disease trial; UKPDS = United Kingdom Prospective Diabetes Study.

TABLE 3. **A Summary of Effects on Cardiovascular and Renal Events/Outcomes/Mortality by Different Classes of Antihypertensive Agents Among Those With Diabetic Renal Disease**

Antihypertensive Drug Classes	Cardiovascular Events	Renal Disease Progression
α-Blockers	→	→*
β-Blockers	↓	↓†
Diuretics	↓	↓
Angiotensin-converting enzyme inhibitors	↓	↓
Angiotensin receptor blockers	↓?	?
Calcium channel blockers		
Non-dihydropyridine	↓	↓
Dihydropyridine	→↑?	→
Potassium channel openers (hydralazine/minoxidil)	→	→

*Based on only one randomized trial with 2-year follow-up looking at rate of decline in glomerular filtration rate.

†Although β-blockers clearly slow progression of nephropathy, the degree of slowing is not as significant as either angiotensin converting enzyme inhibitors or non-dihydropyridine calcium channel blockers at blood pressure levels between 135–140/84–88 mm Hg.

TABLE 4. **Steps Recommended for Choosing an Antihypertensive Regimen and Then Altering It Until Goal Is Reached**

1. Deal first with cost. If the patient is unable to afford any but the least expensive drugs or cannot pay for the one that is selected, price becomes the primary issue.
2. Ascertain whether other risk factors or co-morbidity is present. Avoid drugs that may worsen these factors or conditions, and choose the ones that might tend to improve them.
3. Find out what clinical adverse reactions the patient whom you are treating would find the most troublesome, and avoid agents that are more likely to cause or exacerbate these problems.
4. Start with the lowest effective dose and plan to see the patient within 2 to 4 weeks unless the severity of the patient's hypertension or another problem warrants an earlier visit. Carry out appropriate biochemical monitoring when necessary. In some patients, start with a fixed-dose combination when it appears appropriate.
5. Increase the dose if goal blood pressure has not been reached, even if there has been only a minimal response. Do not increase the first dose, or any dose, prematurely. Give each dose adequate time to be fully effective. If intolerable side effects occur and are likely to be drug related, or if there has been no response, only then switch to another appropriate agent for monotherapy.
6. Continue the process of dose titration and monitoring until the maximum recommended dose has been reached. Stopping before the full dose has been reached leads to a situation in which the patient is treated with multiple agents at subtherapeutic doses when only one or two drugs is necessary.
7. If the drug of first choice fails to reduce blood pressure to goal, add a second agent that has a different mechanism of action and that is known to have additive antihypertensive effects to the first-choice agent. A fixed-dose combination that combines two drugs in the desired doses could also be used at this time.
8. The JNC-VI, World Health Organization, and International Society of Hematology support the concept of titrating with one, two, or even three medications plus lifestyle modifications until goal APs are reached.
9. Plan to see the patient who is at goal AP at least once every 3 months to be sure that AP control is sustained.
10. Reinforce the need for adherence to the regimen and always question each patient carefully about adverse reactions.
11. Long-term management of hypertension with the agents presently available will reduce deaths due to strokes, myocardial infarctions, and coronary heart disease.
12. Lowering APs to levels of 130/80 mm Hg is important in those with diabetes to retard progression to renal failure.
13. Concerns about reducing AP too much and possibly increasing the risk of myocardial infarction have largely been put to rest by the results of the HOT trial in which diastolic APs were reduced to levels as low as 70 mm Hg in subjects with ischemic heart disease without any ill effects. In the SHEP study, also diastolic APs were reduced to below 70 mm Hg with a decrease in cardiovascular events in patients with abnormal baseline electrocardiograms.
14. Patient education and awareness together with a physician's aggressiveness in achieving goal APs with adequate governmental support will help tackle the enormous problem of hypertension.

Abbreviations: HOT = Hypertension Optimal Treatment trial; JNC-VI = Sixth Joint National Committee Report on Prevention, Detection, Evaluation and Treatment of High Blood Pressure; SHEP = Systolic Hypertension in the Elderly Program.

TABLE 5. **Use of Antihypertensive Agents in Specific Clinical Conditions**

Indication	Drug Therapy	Indication	Drug Therapy
Compelling Indications Unless Contraindicated		Dyslipidemia	α-Blockers
Diabetes mellitus (type 1) with proteinuria	ACE I	Essential tremor	β-Blockers
Heart failure (systolic)	ACE I, diuretics, β-blockers, aldosterone receptor blockers	Hyperthyroidism	β-Blockers
Isolated systolic hypertension (older patients)	Diuretics (preferred), Ca^{2+} antagonists (dihydropyridines)	Migraine	β-Blockers (noncardioselective), Ca^{2+} antagonists (non-dihydropyridine)
Myocardial infarction	β-Blockers (non-ISA), ACE-I (systolic dysfunction)	Myocardial infarction	β-Blockers (cardioselective)
May Have Favorable *Effects on Co-Morbid Conditions*		Osteoporosis	Thiazide diuretics
Angina	β-Blockers, Ca^{2+} antagonists	Preoperative hypertension	β-Blockers
Atrial tachycardia and fibrillation	β-Blockers, Ca^{2+} antagonists (non-dihydropyridines)	Prostatism (benign prostatic hyperplasia)	α-Blockers
Cyclosporine-induced hypertension	Ca^{2+} antagonists (caution with the dose of cyclosporine)	Renal insufficiency (caution in renovascular disease)	ACE I, ARBs, K^+-sparing agents hypertension and creatinine (>3 mg/dL)
Diabetes mellitus (types I and 2) with proteinuria	ACE I (preferred), Ca^{2+} antagonists (non-dihydropyridines), low-dose diuretics	*May Have* Unfavorable *Effects on Co-Morbid Conditions*	
Heart failure	ACE I, losartan potassium, β-blockers	Bronchospastic disease	β-Blockers
Liver disease	β-Blockers	Depression	β-Blockers, central α-agonists, reserpine
Peripheral vascular disease	α-Blockers, Ca^{2+} antagonists	Diabetes mellitus (types 1 and 2)	β-Blockers, high-dose diuretics
Pregnancy	Labetolol, methyldopa	Dyslipidemia	β-Blockers (non-ISA), diuretics (high-dose)
Diabetes mellitus (type 2)	ACE I	Gout	Diuretics
		Second- or third-degree heart block	β-Blockers, Ca^{2+} antagonists (non-dihydropyridine)
		Renal insufficiency, renovascular disease	ACE I, ARBs

Abbreviations: ACE I = angiotensin-converting enzyme inhibitor; ARBs = angiotensin II receptor blockers; ISA = intrinsic sympathomimetic activity.
Adapted from the JNC-VI report.

TABLE 6. **Pharmacological Effects of Different Classes of Antihypertensive Agents on Surrogate Markers of Cardiovascular Disease**

	Central Agonists	α-Blockers	α, β-Blockers	Vasodilator	β-Blockers	ACEI	ARBs	Ca²+ Antagonists	Diuretics
Metabolic									
Cholesterol									
LDL	→	→	→	→	→* ↑	→	→	→	→ ↑
HDL	→	↑	→	→	→ ↓	→	→	→	→
Insulin resistance	→	↓	→ ↑	→ ↑	→ ↑	→ ↓	→ ↓	→	→ ↑
Glucose control	→	→	→	→	→ ↓	→ ↑	→	↓ →†	→ ↓
Cardiovascular									
Left ventricular hypertrophy	↓	↓	↓	→ ↑	↓	↓	↓	↓	→ ↓
Renal									
Microalbuminuria	→	→	→ ↓	→ ↑	→ ↓	↓ ↓	↓ ↓	↓ →‡	→ ↓

*Only β-blockers with intrinsic sympathomimetic activity.
†Only when used in high doses (e.g., 480 mg/d diltiazem, 480 mg/d verapamil, 90 mg/d nifedipine).
‡Only non-dihydropyridine calcium antagonists (verapamil, diltiazem).
→, no effect; ↑, increase; ↓, decrease.
Abbreviations: ACEI = angiotensin-converting enzyme inhibitor; ARBs = angiotensin II (ATI) receptor blockers; HDL = high-density lipoprotein; LDL = low-density lipoprotein.
Note: This table summarizes the general trends in the literature.

three or more antihypertensive medications to achieve goal AP. The common rationale for combining antihypertensive medications is enhanced efficacy (if properly chosen they would act on two different physiologic systems), limiting side effects and enhancing salutary effects on target organ by combination therapy over and above the effect expected from the fall in arterial pressure alone.

TABLE 7. **Combination Drugs for Hypertension**

Drug	Trade Name
β-Adrenergic Blockers and Diuretics	
Atenolol, 50 or 100 mg/chlorthalidone, 25 mg	Tenoretic
Bisoprolol fumarate, 2.5, 5, or 10 mg/hydrochlorothiazide, 6.25 mg	Ziac*
Metoprolol tartrate, 50 or 100 mg/hydrochlorothiazide, 25 or 50 mg	Lopressor HCT
Nadolol, 40 or 80 mg/bendroflumethiazide, 5 mg	Corzide
Propranolol hydrochloride, 40 or 80 mg/hydrochlorothiazide, 25 mg	Inderide
Propranolol hydrochloride (extended release), 80, 120, or 160 mg/hydrochlorothiazide, 50 mg	Inderide LA
Timolol maleate, 10 mg/hydrochlorothiazide, 25 mg	Timolide
Angiotensin-Converting Enzyme Inhibitors and Diuretics	
Benazepril hydrochloride, 5, 10, or 20 mg/hydrochlorothiazide, 6.25, 12.5, or 25 mg	Lotensin HCT
Captopril, 25 or 50 mg/hydrochlorothiazide, 15 or 25 mg	Capozide*
Enalapril maleate, 5 or 10 mg/hydrochlorothiazide, 12.5 or 25 mg	Vaseretic
Lisinopril, 10 or 20 mg/hydrochlorothiazide, 12.5 or 25 mg	Prinzide, Zestoretic
Angiotensin II Receptor Antagonists and Diuretics	
Losartan potassium, 50 mg/hydrochlorothiazide, 12.5 mg	Hyzaar
Calcium Antagonists and Angiotensin-Converting Enzyme Inhibitors	
Amlodipine besylate, 2.5 or 5 mg/benazepril hydrochloride, 10 or 20 mg	Lotrel
Verapamil hydrochloride (extended release), 180 or 240 mg/trandolapril, 1, 2, or 4 mg	Tarka
Felodipine, 5 mg/enalapril maleate, 5 mg	Lexxel
Other Combinations	
Triamterene, 37.5, 50, or 75 mg/hydrochlorothiazide, 25 or 50 mg	Dyazide, Maxide
Spironolactone, 25 or 50 mg/hydrochlorothiazide, 25 or 50 mg	Aldactazide
Amiloride hydrochloride, 5 mg/hydrochlorothiazide, 50 mg	Moduretic
Guanethidine monosulfate, 10 mg/hydrochlorothiazide, 25 mg	Esimil
Hydralazine hydrochloride, 25, 50, or 100 mg/hydrochlorothiazide, 25 or 50 mg	Apresazide
Methyldopa, 250 or 500 mg/hydrochlorothiazide, 12.5, 25, or 50 mg	Aldoril
Reserpine, 0.125 mg/hydrochlorothiazide, 25 or 50 mg	Hydropres
Reserpine, 0.10 mg/hydralazine hydrochloride, 25 mg/hydrochlorothiazide, 15 mg	Ser-Ap-Es
Clonidine hydrochloride, 0.1, 0.2, or 0.3 mg/chlorthalidone, 15 mg	Combipres
Methyldopa, 250 mg/chlorothiazide, 150 or 250 mg	Aldoclor
Reserpine, 0.125 or 0.25 mg/chlorthalidone, 25 or 50 mg	Demi-Regroton
Reserpine, 0.125 or 0.25 mg/chlorothiazide, 250 or 500 mg	Diupres
Prazosin hydrochloride, 1, 2, or 5 mg/polythiazide, 0.5 mg	Minizide

*Approved as first-line therapy for hypertension by the FDA.

Safety (Adverse Reactions and Side Effects)

The two primary types of adverse reactions and side effects that occur with antihypertensive therapy are clinical and biochemical. Clinical side effects are directly evident to the patient and are perceived by the patient or the clinician to be related to the drug. Cough and angioedema with angiotensin-converting enzyme (ACE) inhibitors are examples of the same. An additional factor that has contributed to the avoidance of ACE inhibitors in many patients who would benefit from them is a rise in serum creatinine concentration. A retrospective analysis of trials extending 4 or more years indicated that in any patient with a pre-existing serum creatinine value up to 3 mg/dL, a rise in serum creatinine level of up to 30% within the first 4 months of therapy initiation correlated with slower rates of decline in renal function, given the AP goal was achieved. Thus, a small limited rise in serum creatinine concentration should not limit their use.

Biochemical side effects may lead to clinically evident adverse reactions (e.g., hypokalemia from thiazide diuretics causing muscle weakness, palpitations, nocturia, or polyuria) (see Table 6). Usually the biochemical problems that occur with antihypertensive agents are often more troublesome to the clinician than they are to the patient.

At the now recommended lower doses, these changes and the electrolyte disturbances noted with thiazide diuretics are modest. It is still possible, however, that at high doses these agents could reduce serum potassium sufficiently, particularly in those with high sodium intake, to increase the rate of sudden cardiac death. Whether the increases in insulin resistance that are seen with thiazide diuretics and β-blockers or the hypokalemia that is seen with thiazide diuretics has precipitated diabetes sooner, or in patients who would not otherwise have become diabetic, also remains to be proved. Although it is not certain that these metabolic adverse reactions are clinically relevant, it may be prudent to select another option for patients with diabetes or a dyslipidemia, as long as AP is successfully reduced to goal.

Certain types of dual therapy may also ameliorate biochemical adverse reactions. ACE inhibitors and angiotensin II (ATI) receptor blockers and thiazides when given together produce few if any of the metabolic abnormalities associated with thiazides alone. Such combinations also exist in a single pill (see Table 7).

Specific Populations

African Americans and Other Ethnic Minorities

At lower doses, some classes of antihypertensive agents reduce AP more effectively in certain ethnic groups. Thiazide diuretics and calcium channel blockers, for example, are more effective in African Americans than whites, whereas ACE inhibitors, ARBs, and β-blockers are more effective at lower doses in whites. Many African Americans will respond to agents that block the renin-angiotensin system, but they often need higher doses than whites or Asians. Recent studies in African Americans demonstrate that starting with higher doses of an ACE inhibitor makes this class quite efficacious for lowering AP in this population. Trial data indicate that in African Americans with hypertension, ACE inhibitors confer a greater impact on the slowing of renal disease progression compared with dihydropyridine calcium channel blockers such as amlodipine. This difference was noted at the same level of AP control.

In general, the response rates to antihypertensive agents in Hispanics is intermediate between that seen in whites and African Americans, whereas East Asians, but not necessarily South Asians (patients from the Indian subcontinent), often need smaller doses than whites.

The Elderly

Although all classes of antihypertensive agents lower AP effectively in older persons, the doses needed to reach goal are often lower than the doses necessary in young and middle-aged hypertensive patients. Diuretics and dihydropyridine calcium blockers have both been shown to reduce morbidity and mortality in older persons with stage 2 or 3 isolated systolic hypertension, making them excellent choices in such patients.

Certain drug classes, however, should be avoided or used with caution in older hypertensive patients. Such drug classes include peripheral α-blockers that can exacerbate the postural fall in AP. This fall in AP is seen more frequently in older individuals with baroreceptor dysfunction. Other agents include nondihydropyridine calcium channel blockers and β-blockers; these may aggravate subtle or subclinical conduction defects or precipitate systolic dysfunction and heart failure. Verapamil (Calan) may not be well tolerated in some older persons who are already bothered by constipation. Cough that results from ACE inhibitors may be more common in older women.

Pregnancy

Hypertension is found in about 10% of pregnancies and is the major cause of perinatal morbidity and mortality in most developed countries. Hypertension in pregnancy is defined as either AP greater than 140/90 mm Hg on two measurements at least 4 hours apart or a diastolic AP greater than 110 mm Hg at any time during pregnancy or up to 6 weeks post partum.

The classification of hypertension in pregnancy typically requires some knowledge of AP status before conception. If there was pre-existing hypertension, the patient is said to have "chronic hypertension," which can be diagnosed before 20 weeks' gestation and persists at least 42 days post partum. Preeclampsia is hypertension appearing after 20 weeks' gestation, associated with proteinuria (at least 300 mg/24-hour collection or 2+ on a random dipstick), which typically resolves within 42 days after delivery. Hypertension with superimposed preeclampsia is a combination of the two.

Elevated AP (stage 1 hypertension) during pregnancy has traditionally been treated with nonpharmacologic approaches, including bed rest. However, if target organ disease is present or AP is greater than 150/100 mm Hg, antihypertensive treatment with methyldopa should be started. Most of the increased risk associated with chronic hypertension is due to superimposed preeclampsia.

For stage 2 hypertension (AP > 160 or 169/109 mm Hg) in outpatients that is not controlled with these measures to a diastolic AP between 90 and 100 mm Hg, hydralazine, labetolol, and nifedipine are routinely added in succession. Diuretics may also be used as additive treatment except in cases of reduced uteroplacental perfusion. ACE inhibitors and ARBs are contraindicated because of renal abnormalities in the fetus. For intrapartum management, until delivery can be achieved, intravenous magnesium sulfate has been a mainstay for the prevention of progression of preeclampsia to seizures and other more serious complications. If renal insufficiency is present, however, doses of magnesium sulfate should be reduced. Phenytoin may also be used as an alternative. No data are available for calcium channel blockers in this clinical setting.

Treatment of Secondary Causes

Renal Artery Stenosis

Stenosis of the renal artery does not necessarily translate into markedly elevated difficult-to-control hypertension. The renal artery needs to be at least 75% to 80% narrowed to cause clinical problems with marked AP elevations. Even with that degree of stenosis cases have been reported of hypertension not being significantly improved after treatment.

The treatment of renal artery stenosis is as much dependent on the pre-existing conditions and clinical status of the patient as much as anything else. In general, with the advent of stents, surgical treatment of this problem has been markedly reduced. Clearly, medical treatment of this condition is limited, because the rise in AP will escape any particular antihypertensive regimen after a period of 3 to 6 months. Thus, increasingly, antihypertensive medications with high doses will be needed over time to control pressure.

It is quite common to use agents such as ACE inhibitors if unilateral disease is present, yet these agents are contraindicated in those with bilateral disease. On average, five to six medications, including minoxidil (Loniten), will be needed in such patients to keep AP levels under 140/90 mm Hg.

Primary Hyperaldosteronism

The long-standing experience has been that the hypertension associated with primary aldosteronism is salt and water dependent and is best treated by sustained salt and water depletion. The usual doses of diuretic agents are hydrochlorothiazide, 12.5 to 25 mg/d, or furosemide (Lasix), 40 to 80 mg in divided doses twice daily in combination with either spironolactone (Aldactone), 100 to 200 mg/d, or amiloride (Midamor), 10 to 20 mg/d. These combinations usually result in prompt correction of hypokalemia and normalization of AP within 2 to 4 weeks.

In the majority of patients, surgical excision of an aldosterone-producing adenoma leads to normal tension as well as reversal of the biochemical defects. One year postoperatively, about 70% of patients are normotensive; but 5 years postoperatively, only 53% remain normotensive.

Hypertensive Crisis

Hypertensive crises include hypertensive *urgencies* and hypertensive *emergencies.* In hypertensive emergencies there is acute target organ damage.

Hypertensive crises occur in a variety of clinical settings. The most common is the chronic and often untreated patient with stage 3 essential hypertension (i.e., usual AP ≥ 180/110 mm Hg), whose AP rises above the autoregulatory range, triggering the pathophysiologic sequence involving the alteration of autoregulation in certain vascular beds (especially cerebral and renal), which is often followed by frank arteritis and ischemia in vital organs. Autoregulation is the ability of blood vessels to dilate or constrict to maintain normal organ perfusion. Normal arteries from normotensive individuals can maintain flow over a wide range of mean arterial pressures, usually 60 to 150 mm Hg. Chronic elevations of AP cause compensatory functional and structural changes in the arterial circulation and shift the autoregulatory curve to the right, which allows hypertensive patients to maintain normal perfusion and avoid excessive blood flow at higher AP levels. When AP increases above the autoregulatory range, tissue damage occurs.

Hypertensive Urgency. Hypertensive urgencies are situations in which acute target organ disease is *not* present; these require somewhat less aggressive management and nearly always can be handled with oral antihypertensive agents without admission to hospital. Nifedipine (Adalat), clonidine (Catapres), captopril (Capoten), labetolol (Trandate), and several other short-acting antihypertensive drugs have been used for this problem. Nifedipine has been reported to cause precipitous hypotension, stroke, myocardial infarction, and death (according to the U.S. Food and Drug Administration). Thus, if sublingual nifedipine is used, it "should be with the greatest caution, if at all." Otherwise, none seems to have a major advantage over all the others, and all are effective in most patients. *The most important aspect of managing a hypertensive urgency is to ensure compliance with antihypertensive therapy during long-term follow-up.*

Hypertensive Emergencies. Patients presenting with a hypertensive emergency should be quickly diagnosed and promptly started on effective parental therapy (often nitroprusside [Nitropress], 0.5 μg/kg/min) in an intensive care unit. AP should be reduced about 25% gradually over 2 to 3 hours. Oral antihypertensive therapy (usually requiring four or more different classes of antihypertensive medications) can be instituted after 6 to 12 hours of parenteral therapy; evaluation for secondary causes of hypertension may be considered after transfer from the intensive care unit. Because of advances in antihypertensive therapy and management, "malignant hypertension" should be malignant no longer.

The treatment of the different presentations of hypertensive emergencies is summarized in Table 8. There are several different types of common clinical presentations of hypertensive emergencies:

- Neurologic crises, namely, hypertensive encephalopathy is typically a diagnosis of exclusion; hemorrhagic and thrombotic strokes are usually diagnosed after focal neurologic deficits are corroborated by computed tomography. Subarachnoid hemorrhage is diagnosed by the typical findings on lumbar puncture. The management of each of these conditions is somewhat different, in that nimodipine may be the drug of choice for most neurologic crises, because of its antihypertensive and anti-ischemic effects. Many physicians still prefer nitroprusside or another intravenous vasodilator because it can be discontinued rapidly if the AP goes too low. Goal AP also depends on the presenting diagnosis and is usually lower for encephalopathy than for acute stroke in evolution.
- Cardiac crises include ischemia/infarction or pulmonary edema and can be managed with either nitroglycerin or nitroprusside, although typically a combination of drugs (including an ACE inhibitor when there is heart failure) is used in these settings.
- Aortic dissection is managed in a somewhat different fashion. A β-blocker is added to the intravenous vasodilator, and the goal AP is much lower: typically, 120 mm Hg systolic is recommended, but 100 mm Hg systolic may be even better.
- A *kidney crisis* is commonly followed by a further deterioration in renal function, even when AP is properly lowered. Some physicians prefer fenoldopam (Corlopam) to nicardipine (Cardene) or nitroprusside in this setting because of its freedom from toxic metabolites and specific renal vasodilating effects. AP should be reduced about 10% during the first hour, with a further 10% to 15% during the next 1 to 3 hours. The need for acute dialysis is often precipitated by AP reduction, but many patients are able to avoid dialysis in the long-term if AP is carefully and well controlled during follow-up.
- Hypertensive crises due to *catecholamine excess states* (e.g., pheochromocytoma, monoamine oxidase inhibitor crisis, cocaine intoxication) are best managed with an intravenous α-blocker (phentolamine [Regitine]), with the β-blocker being added later, if necessary. Many patients with severe hypertension due to sudden withdrawal of antihypertensive agents (e.g., clonidine) are easily managed by reinstituting such therapy.
- Hypertensive crises during *pregnancy* must be managed in a more careful and more conservative manner because of the presence of the fetus. Magnesium sulfate, methyldopa (Aldomet), and hydralazine (Apresoline) are the drugs of choice, with oral labetolol (Trandate) or nifedipine (Adalat) being drugs of second choice in the United States. Delivery of the infant will often assist in the man-

TABLE 8. **Types of Hypertension Crises, With Suggested Drug Therapy and Blood Pressure Targets**

Type of Crisis	Drug of Choice	Blood Pressure Target
Neurologic		
Hypertensive encephalopathy	Nitroprusside (Nitropress)*	25% reduction in MAP over 2–3 hours
Intracranial hemorrhage or acute stoke in evolution	Nitroprusside (controversial)*	0–25% reduction in MAP over 6–12 hours (controversial)
Acute head injury/trauma	Nitroprusside*	0–25% reduction in MAP over 2–3 hours (controversial)
Subarachnoid hemorrhage	Nimodipine (Nimotop)	Up to 25% reduction in MAP in previously hypertensive patients, 130–160 systolic in normotensive patients
Cardiac		
Ischemia/infarction	Nitroglycerin or nicardipine (Cardene)	Reduction in ischemia
Heart failure	Nitroprusside* or nitroglycerin	Improvement in failure (typically 10%–15% decrease in BP)
Aortic dissection	β-Blocker + nitroprusside*	120 mm Hg systolic in 30 minutes (if possible)
Renal		
Hematuria or acute renal impairment	Fenoldopam (Corlopam)	0–25% reduction in MAP over 1–12 hours
Catecholamine Excess States		
Pheochromocytoma	Phentolamine (Regitine)	To control paroxysms
Drug withdrawal	Drug withdrawn	Typically only one dose necessary
Pregnancy Related		
Eclampsia	$MgSO_4$, methyldopa, hydralazine	Typically <90 mm Hg diastolic, but often lower

*Some physicians prefer an intravenous infusion or either fenoldopam or nicardipine, neither of which has potentially toxic metabolites, over nitroprusside. Recent studies have also shown improvements in renal function during therapy with the former, as compared with nitroprusside.

Abbreviation: MAP = mean arterial pressure.

agement of hypertension in pregnancy and is often hastened by the obstetrician under these conditions.

CONCLUSIONS

The clinician should never lose sight of the goal blood pressure trying to be achieved in a particular setting. Clearly, the AP goals in people with certain pre-existing conditions such as diabetes and/or renal disease must be lower than those of the general population. Many times physicians will need to use three or four different antihypertensive medications in moderate doses to achieve such recommended goals. Antihypertensive agents should be selected based on a variety of factors, but the message of achieving an AP goal by the "least intrusive means possible" should be operative. Thus, physicians need to be critical of their own behavior and not give up until the recommended AP goals are achieved.

ACUTE MYOCARDIAL INFARCTION

method of
KENT DAUTERMAN, M.D., and
TONY M. CHOU, M.D.
University of California, San Francisco
San Francisco, California

It is estimated that 900,000 people in the United States have an acute myocardial infarction (AMI) each year. As a result, about 225,000 people die, many due to arrhythmia-induced sudden death, and many others are crippled by heart failure. Advances in patient education, emergency medical system response time, continuous electrocardiographic (ECG) monitoring with rapid defibrillation and arrhythmia treatment, hemodynamic medications, and early reperfusion strategies have all contributed to a substantial decrease in mortality and improvement in left ventricular systolic function.

PATHOPHYSIOLOGY

Myocardial infarction (MI) results from loss of coronary blood flow, which is precipitated in most cases by the formation of an acute occlusive coronary thrombus at the site of a vulnerable although not necessarily severely stenotic atherosclerotic plaque. A prolonged imbalance between myocardial oxygen supply and demand can also be due to four additional nonexclusive causes:

1. Vasospasm
2. Progressive atherosclerotic narrowing not due to thrombus or spasm
3. Inflammation
4. Factors external to the coronary arteries such as fever, tachycardia, thyrotoxicosis, hypotension, anemia, and hypoxemia

CORONARY ANATOMY

The location and extent of infarction depend on the anatomic distribution of the occluded vessel and the adequacy of the collateral circulation. Thrombosis in the left anterior descending coronary artery typically results in infarction of the anterior wall of the left ventricle and interventricular septum (ECG leads I, aVL, V_1–V_6). Occlusion of the left circumflex coronary artery produces a left ventricular lateral infarct (leads I, aVL, V_5–V_6). Right coronary thrombosis leads to infarction of the posteroinferior wall of the left ventricle and interventricular septum as well as right ventricle (ECG leads II, III; aVF; V_5–V_6; right precordial leads; and posterior leads V_1–V_2 or V_7–V_9).

DIAGNOSIS

The World Health Organization criteria for MI require two of the following three items: (1) prolonged anterior chest discomfort often associated with dyspnea, diaphoresis, nausea, emesis, and/or anxiety; (2) ST-segment elevation or depression, T-wave changes, or new Q waves; and (3) elevation in serum cardiac enzyme levels (i.e., creatinine kinase [CK]) or proteins (i.e., troponin). Given the very high sensitivity and specificity of serum troponin levels for detecting myocardial necrosis, there is a movement toward calling any elevation in troponin levels a myocardial infarction because these patients have a higher risk of death.

DEFINITION OF TERMS

AMI typically invokes images of a patient with crushing substernal chest pain and ST-segment elevation due to an occlusive coronary thrombus that will evolve into a Q wave or transmural MI unless early reperfusion is initiated. However, approximately 50% of patients with MI present with ST depression or T-wave inversions on ECG and are found to have nonocclusive yet high-grade and high-risk coronary stenoses that are associated with increased mortality and reinfarction rates.

Acute coronary syndrome refers to symptoms, signs, and/or ECG findings that are compatible with acute myocardial ischemia and encompass AMI (ST-segment elevation and depression, Q wave and non–Q wave) and unstable angina. When first seeing a patient, it is very important to determine whether he or she is having an ST-segment elevation MI or a non–ST-segment elevation MI/unstable angina because the early reperfusion strategy will depend on this stratification. The only distinction between non–ST-segment elevation MI and unstable angina is whether the serum troponin, CK, and myocardial creatinine kinase (CK-MB) levels become elevated. The determination of Q wave versus non–Q wave and transmural infarct versus nontransmural infarct typically occurs many hours later and has little effect on patient care.

CLINICAL FINDINGS

Symptoms

Only 25% of patients have typical angina associated with AMI. Twenty-five percent of patients have symptoms similar to reflux esophagitis; 25% have clinically silent disease; and 25% have very atypical symptoms such as jaw, neck, arm, or back pain. Women, elderly, and patients with diabetes mellitus are the most likely to have atypical symptoms. These symptoms typically occur at rest, build to a maximum intensity over a few minutes, and last more than 30 minutes. If they had angina in the past, the discomfort is usually similar in nature but more severe. Nitroglycerin may have little effect. Possible associated symptoms are dyspnea, diaphoresis, apprehension, nausea, emesis, or syncope.

Signs

Patients often appear anxious and diaphoretic. Tachypnea, inspiratory crackles, and an S3 gallop indicate heart failure. Tachycardia, hypotension, pulsus alternans, and cool extremities may indicate cardiogenic shock. Bradycardia may point to heart block, whereas elevated jugular venous pressure suggests right ventricular MI or heart failure.

Electrocardiography

ST-segment elevation of 0.1 mV or more has a specificity of 90% and a sensitivity of 50% for the diagnosis of AMI. The leads with ST-segment elevation are quite accurate in determining the cardiac region of injury, whereas ST-segment depression is less reliable in predicting the area of myocardial ischemia. Twenty percent of patients with cardiac enzyme/protein-proven MI will have ECG criteria for infarction. In AMI, both right and left bundle branch blocks (new and old) are associated with up to a 25% mortality rate. The ST segments and Q waves can be read somewhat reliably in right bundle branch blocks whereas little can be determined in patients with left bundle branch blocks.

Serum Enzymes / Proteins

CK is found in all muscle cells. The myocardial isoform (CK-MB) is highly expressed in cardiac myocytes, although it can be found in low levels throughout the body. For diagnosing AMI, an elevated CK-MB value provides a sensitivity of 70% at 6 to 9 hours and 97% at 9 to 12 hours. The CK-MB value begins to increase 6 to 10 hours after the onset of myocardial necrosis and returns to baseline after 48 to 72 hours. It is the chosen enzyme for reinfarction, but it is difficult to interpret in the setting of skeletal muscle injury such as surgery or trauma.

Troponin I and troponin T are cardiac-specific contractile proteins that are released 4 to 8 hours after the onset of myocardial necrosis, peak at 24 to 48 hours (similar to CK-MB), and decrease after 10 days, making them useful markers of late MI (>24 hours old). Clinically, troponin measurements are replacing lactate dehydrogenase as a late MI indicator. Troponin is more sensitive and specific for AMI than CK-MB. Thirty percent of patients who present with rest pain without ST-segment elevation who would otherwise be labeled as having unstable angina because of a lack of CK-MB elevation actually have non–ST-segment elevation MI when assessed with cardiac-specific troponin assays. However, troponin levels are not useful for reinfarction, and troponin T has been reported to be elevated in patients with acute muscle injury or chronic renal failure.

The optimal use of cardiac enzymes/proteins is not yet clear and there are wide variations in clinical practice. Most institutions obtain serial measurements ranging from every 3 hours for 4 samples to every 6 hours for 2 samples after the onset of chest pain in order to detect an MI as soon as possible. Note that the last measurement of CK-MB and/or troponin should be made at least 12 hours after the onset of chest pain.

PROGNOSIS

A patient's prognosis can be rapidly assessed at the initial presentation and is directly related to the amount of myocardium at risk. Five variables associated with an increased risk of death in the GUSTO trial were age, anterior MI, heart rate greater than 100 beats/minute, systolic blood pressure less than 100 mm Hg, and female gender. The Killip classification (Class I–IV) is determined by the degree of congestive heart failure and presence of cardiogenic shock (i.e., height of rales, presence/absence of an S_3 gallop, and presence of hypotension). Cardiogenic shock was shown in the SHOCK trial to have a mortality rate of approximately 50% regardless of treatment. Right ventricular infarction has a significant mortality rate if reperfusion is unsuccessful. Among ECG presentations in the GUSTO trial, left bundle branch block had the highest mortality rate at 25%.

CONDITIONS THAT MAY MIMIC ACUTE MYOCARDIAL INFARCTION

The following conditions may mimic ST-segment elevation MI: aortic dissection, pericarditis, myocarditis, pulmonary embolism, trauma, and anomalous coronary arteries, to name a few. Embarking on potent antiplatelet, antithrombin, and fibrinolytic therapy in patients with aortic dissection, pericarditis, and trauma can be lethal.

TREATMENT

The following statement is taken from the American Heart Association (AHA)/American College of Cardiology Guidelines for AMI: "The underlying principle of the early in-hospital evaluation of patients with suspected myocardial infarction is that the loss of time equals the loss of myocardial cells." Therefore, the patient should be seen and evaluated immediately upon arrival at the hospital. A 12-lead ECG should be obtained at the same time and continuous ECG monitoring begun. Table 1 outlines the AMI treatment principles. Table 2 is a quick reference in regard to AMI therapies. Table 3 provides a practical approach to the treatment of patients with AMI.

Analgesia

Morphine

Relieving a patient's suffering is a physician's foremost goal. In the case of AMI, it is also beneficial because it reduces a patient's catecholamine levels. Morphine also causes venodilation, which reduces preload and pulmonary edema.

TABLE 1. **Acute Myocardial Infarction Treatment Principles**

Time delay = myocyte loss
Rapid evaluation
Analgesia
Reperfusion
Rhythm monitoring/arrhythmia treatment
Neurohormonal and hemodynamic optimization (reduce myocardial oxygen demand and increase supply)

TABLE 2. **Recommendations for Acute Myocardial Infarction Treatment**

Treatment	ST Elevation MI/ New LBBB	Non-ST Elevation MI/ Unstable Angina
Analgesia		
Morphine	Yes	Yes
Reperfusion		
Antiplatelet agents		
Aspirin	Yes	Yes
Glycoprotein IIb/IIIa inhibitor	Studies ongoing	Yes
Clopidogrel/ticlopidine	Unknown	Studies ongoing
Antithrombin agents		
Unfractionated heparin	Yes	Yes
Low molecular weight heparin	Studies ongoing	Yes
Fibrinolytic (thrombolytic)	Yes	No
Primary PTCA	Yes	No clear benefit
Arrhythmia		
Continuous ECG monitoring	Yes	Yes
Prophylactic lidocaine	No	No
Type Ic antiarrhythmics	No	No.
Reperfusion	Yes	Yes
Beta-blocker	Yes	Yes
Potassium/magnesium repletion	Yes	Yes
Temporary pacemaker	For heart block	For heart block
IV lidocaine or IV amiodarone	For VF or >20 beat run of VT	For VF or >20 beat run of VT
Intra-aortic balloon pump	For refractory VT	For refractory VT
Hemodynamic / Adjunctive Medications		
Oxygen	Yes	Yes
Nitroglycerin	Yes, reasonable for first 48 h and especially for hypertension, CHF, and refractory angina	Yes, reasonable for first 48 h and especially for hypertension, CHF, and refractory angina
β-Blocker	Yes	Yes
ACE inhibitor	Yes	Yes
HMG CoA reductase inhibitor	Yes	Yes
Angiotensin II receptor blocker	Second-line therapy after ACE inhibitors	Second-line therapy after ACE inhibitors
Calcium channel blockers	Second-line therapy after β-blockers/ nitrates	Second-line therapy after β-blockers/ nitrates
Magnesium	Unclear	Unknown
Treat extrinsic stressors (e.g. fever, anemia, hypoxemia, etc.)	Yes	Yes
Invasive hemodynamic monitoring	Reasonable for cardiogenic shock	Reasonable for cardiogenic shock
Intra-aortic balloon pump	Yes for cardiogenic shock, severe MR and VSD	Yes for cardiogenic shock, severe MR and VSD
Nitroprusside	Reasonable for hypertension and CHF	Reasonable for hypertension and CHF
Inotropes	Try to avoid	Try to avoid
Nursing Care	CCU	CCU or intermediate care telemetry unit
Echocardiogram	Reasonable	Reasonable
Cardiology Consultation	Reasonable	Reasonable

Abbreviations: ACE = angiotensin converting enzyme; CCU = cardiac care unit; CHF = congestive heart failure; ECG = electrocardiogram; LBBB = left bundle branch block; MR = mitral regurgitation; VSD = ventricular septal defect; VT = ventricular tachycardia.

Reperfusion (Antiplatelet Agents, Antithrombin Agents, Fibrinolytics, and Primary Percutaneous Transluminal Coronary Angioplasty)

Aspirin

Aspirin irreversibly inhibits cyclooxygenase, which decreases the production of thromboxane A2. Based on International Study of Infarct Survival (ISIS)-2, aspirin provides a 22% reduction in mortality that was equivalent to the 22% reduction in mortality provided by streptokinase. Together, mortality was reduced by 44%, making their effects additive. Keep in mind that giving a 325-mg chewable aspirin is as important as giving a thrombolytic.

Glycoprotein IIb/IIIa Inhibitor

The small-molecule glycoprotein IIb/IIIa inhibitors, eptifibatide (Integrilin) and tirofiban (Aggrastat), have been shown to reduce the combined endpoint of death and MI in patients with prolonged angina and ST-segment depression, deep T-wave inversion, or CK-MB elevation (PURSUIT, PRISM, PRISM-PLUS). Abciximab (Reopro) was not found to be beneficial in this patient population (GUSTO IV ACS). Patients with ST-segment elevation MI were

TABLE 3. **Practical Strategy for the Treatment of Acute Myocardial Infarction**

1. Immediate ER evaluation with 12-lead ECG, continuous ECG monitoring, and bedrest
2. Aspirin 325 mg po (chew), can give pr if intubated
3. Supplemental oxygen
4. Two intravenous lines and send electrolytes, BUN, creatinine, glucose, CBC with platelets, PTT, troponin and/or CK and CK-MB, lipid panel, and urine toxicology screen if recreational drug use is suspected
5. Determine reperfusion strategy if ST segment elevation or new left bundle branch block is noted (emergency PTCA versus thrombolysis). Be aware of thrombolytic contraindications.
6. Low molecular weight heparin SQ or unfractionated heparin IV with initial bolus 60–70 U/kg (maximum 5000 U) followed by 12–15 U/kg/h (maximum 1000 U/h). Goal PTT is 50–75 seconds.
7. IV metoprolol (Lopressor), 5 mg q 5 min (typical maximum dose is 15–30 mg) until HR 50–60 bpm and systolic blood pressure 110–130 mm Hg. Do not use in patients with bradycardia, hypotension, or heart failure.
8. If chest pain persists, give nitroglycerin 0.4 mg sl q 5 min. Start IV nitroglycerin if the patient has pulmonary edema or severe hypertension.
9. If chest pain persists, give morphine sulfate 1–4 mg IV as needed.
10. Treat extrinsic stressors such as fever, anemia, hypoxemia, etc.
11. Transfer to CCU or intermediate care telemetry unit.
12. Keep serum magnesium and potassium repleted.
13. Start HMG CoA reductase inhibitor and ACE inhibitor on day 1.
14. Obtain transthoracic echocardiogram.

Abbreviations: ACE = angiotensin converting enzyme; BUN = blood urea nitrogen; CBC = complete blood cell count; CCU = cardiac care unit; CK = creatinine kinase; CK-MB = myocardial CK; ECG = electrocardiogram; PTCA = percutaneous transluminal coronary angioplasty; PTT = partial thromboplastin time.

excluded from these four studies. However, combined glycoprotein IIb/IIIa inhibitor and reduced-dose fibrinolytic pilot studies have shown a 90% patency rate at 90 minutes in patients with ST-segment elevation MI (TIMI 14). Large-scale trials are in progress.

Clopidogrel (Plavix)/Ticlopidine (Ticlid)

These thienopyridines inhibit adenosine diphosphate (ADP)–induced platelet aggregation but take several hours to attain their antiplatelet effects after ingestion, and they have not yet been studied in AMI. They are both used in intracoronary stent patients to prevent in-stent thrombosis, and clopidogrel has been shown to be superior to aspirin in patients with history of recent MI, recent stroke, and/or symptomatic peripheral vascular disease (CAPRIE). If a patient is allergic to aspirin, give clopidogrel 300 mg orally followed by 75 mg orally daily. Clopidogrel is generally preferred over ticlopidine because of its better safety profile.

Unfractionated Heparin

Heparin exerts its anticoagulant effect by accelerating the action of circulating antithrombin, a proteolytic enzyme that inactivates factor IIa (thrombin), factor IXa, and factor Xa. It prevents thrombus propagation but does not lyse existing thrombus. For ST-segment elevation MI, all thrombolytic studies used unfractionated heparin (intravenously [IV] or subcutaneously). Two meta-analyses for unstable angina and non–ST-segment elevation MI showed a reduction in clinically adverse events. Weight-based dosing is recommended. The bolus should be 60 to 70 U/kg (maximum 5000 U) followed by a maintenance infusion of 12 to 15 U/kg/min (maximum 1000 U/hour). The partial thromboplastin time should be maintained between 50 and 70 seconds.

Low Molecular Weight Heparins

Compared with unfractionated heparin, these agents (e.g., enoxaparin [Lovenox] and dalteparin [Fragmin]) inactivate factor Xa but not thrombin (factor IIa), have higher biovariability, and provide more reliable anticoagulation, thereby not requiring laboratory monitoring of activity (i.e., no need to monitor the partial thromboplastin time). In patients with non–ST-segment elevation MI and unstable angina, two trials with enoxaparin have shown a moderate benefit over unfractionated heparin (ESSENCE, TIMI 11B) and two trials (one with dalteparin and one with nadroparin) showed neutral and unfavorable trends (ESSENCE, FRAXIS). Enoxaparin is given 1 mg/kg subcutaneously every 12 hours with (TIMI 11B) or without (ESSENCE) an initial 30 mg IV bolus. Their effectiveness in ST-segment elevation MI is presently being studied. In patients who are obese or who are in renal failure, these agents may be contraindicated due to unpredictable factor Xa inhibition.

Fibrinolytic Agents (Thrombolytics)

The endogenous fibrinolytic system can spontaneously lyse an occlusive intracoronary thrombus, which results in 20% of patients having a patent vessel at 90 minutes. Fibrinolytic agents increase the patency rate (TIMI 2 or 3 flow) from 59% (streptokinase) to 81% (tissue plasminogen activator [TPA]) at 90 minutes and have been shown to decrease mortality in patients presenting within 12 hours from the onset of chest pain and ST elevation (≥0.1 mV) or new left bundle-branch block pattern (GUSTO-1). In patients with ST-depression or non–ST-elevation MI, thrombolytic agents increase the mortality rate and should not be used. The risk of intracranial hemorrhage is approximately 1%. Contraindications to use include active internal bleeding, history of cerebrovascular accident, intracranial or intraspinal surgery or trauma within 2 months, intracranial neoplasm, arteriovenous malformation, aneurysm, known bleeding diathesis, and severe uncontrolled hypertension (≥180/110 mm Hg). The commonly used fibrinolytic agents are streptokinase (Streptase), alteplase (TPA, Activase), tenecteplase (TNKase), and reteplase (Retevase).

Streptokinase

Streptokinase is a purified bacterial protein made by group C β-hemolytic streptococci that has been shown to reduce mortality by 22% in ST-segment elevation MI patients (ISIS-2). Compared with TPA, streptokinase may be the preferred fibrinolytic agent in the elderly given its reduced incidence of intracranial hemorrhage (GUSTO-1). The dose is 1,500,000 IU over 60 minutes. Streptokinase is cleared by antibodies and its half-life is about 23 minutes. Due to antibody formation, repeated usage may not be effective and anaphylactic reactions are rare. Aspirin 325 mg orally and unfractionated subcutaneous (12,500 U every 12 hours) or IV heparin is given as well.

ALTEPLASE (TISSUE PLASMINOGEN ACTIVATOR)

Alteplase is a TPA made by recombinant DNA technology. Compared with streptokinase, TPA reduced the absolute mortality by an additional 1% and appeared to be superior in patients with anterior MI presenting fewer than 4 hours after symptom onset or in patients younger than 75 years of age despite a slightly increased rate of intracranial hemorrhage (GUSTO-1). The weight-based, accelerated infusion regimen is as follows: 15 mg IV bolus followed by 0.75 mg/kg (maximum 50 mg) over next 30 minutes followed by 0.50 mg/kg (maximum 35 mg) over the next 60 minutes (see package insert). It is metabolized by the liver and has a half-life of 5 minutes. Aspirin 325 mg orally and IV heparin (5000 U bolus followed by 1000 U/hour maintenance infusion with goal partial thromboplastin time of 50–75 seconds) are typically given as well.

TENECTEPLASE

Tenecteplase is a mutated form of naturally occurring TPA that can be given by one simple injection, thereby avoiding the errors in administration occasionally seen with complicated accelerated TPA dosing regimens. In ASSENT-2, tenecteplase had similar outcomes to an accelerated TPA regimen (alteplase). The recommended total dose should not exceed 50 mg and is based upon patient weight. It is metabolized by the liver and has a terminal phase half-life of 90 to 130 minutes. Aspirin 325 mg orally and IV heparin (4000–5000 U bolus followed by 800–1000 U maintenance infusion with goal prothrombin time of 50–75 seconds) are given as well.

RETEPLASE

Reteplase is a mutated form of naturally occurring TPA that has been shown to provide similar clinical outcomes with alteplase (GUSTO-3). It is a non–weight-based medication given in two simple injections (10 U bolus followed 30 minutes later by another 10 U bolus) and cleared primarily by the kidneys with a half-life of 11 to 19 minutes. It is also given with aspirin and IV heparin.

Primary Percutaneous Transluminal Coronary Angioplasty

Compared to thrombolytic therapy, several studies have shown that primary percutaneous transluminal coronary angioplasty (PTCA) provides a lower mortality rate, improved efficacy (normal coronary flow: thrombolysis 60% versus PTCA 90%), a better safety profile (i.e., no intracranial hemorrhage), better preservation of left ventricular function, shorter hospital stay, and lower overall cost (PAMI, Mayo Clinic Study, Netherlands Trial, GUSTO-IIb, PAMI-II, C-PORT). There are also many patients with contraindications to thrombolysis (up to 40%) and thrombolytic efficacy is low in cardiogenic shock. However, an effective primary PTCA program requires a 24-hour on-call team, an experienced operator, well-trained catheter laboratory personnel, and minimal time delay (optimal time for emergency department arrival to coronary artery opening is <90 minutes).

Arrhythmia

Continuous Electrocardiographic Monitoring

Up until 30 years ago, most in-hospital AMI deaths were due to ventricular fibrillation and other arrhythmias. The implementation of continuous ECG monitoring and the availability of rapid electrical cardioversion have decreased the mortality rate by 50%.

Prophylactic Lidocaine

A meta-analysis of many small studies showed that prophylactic lidocaine causes a slight trend toward increased mortality. Therefore, it is not recommended.

Type Ic Antiarrhythmics

In patients with frequent premature ventricular contractions, the use of encainide and flecainide increased mortality (CAST Study).

Reperfusion

The best treatment for refractory ventricular arrhythmias is coronary reperfusion.

β-Blockade

β-Blocker use has been shown to prevent ventricular arrhythmias and decrease the arrhythmic mortality rate. If the patient has ventricular fibrillation or a greater than 20-beat run of ventricular tachycardia, then IV lidocaine or IV amiodarone (Cordarone) will be needed as well.

Potassium/Magnesium Repletion

Serum potassium levels less than 3.5 mmol/L increase the risk of ventricular tachyarrhythmias. There is concern that hypomagnesemia may increase the risk of ventricular arrhythmias as well. IV magnesium sulfate 1 to 2 g has proven to be useful in the treatment of torsade de pointes, which is not usually associated with AMI. It is unclear whether empiric magnesium use in all AMI patients is beneficial based on two large studies (LIMIT-2 and ISIS-4).

Temporary Pacemaker

Indications include asystole, third-degree block, Mobitz II second-degree block, prolonged sinus pauses (>3 seconds), symptomatic bradycardia (sinus, atrial fibrillation with slow ventricular response, idioventricular rhythm <40 beats/minute). Until a temporary transvenous pacemaker is placed, life-threatening bradyarrhythmias can be treated with atropine, dopamine, and/or transcutaneous pacing.

Intravenous Lidocaine or Intravenous Amiodarone

These medications can be used in the event of ventricular fibrillation or a greater than 20 beat run of ventricular tachycardia. Amiodarone has just been added to the 2000 advanced cardiac life support algorithm.

Neurohormonal and Hemodynamic Optimization/Adjunctive Medications

Oxygen

Supplemental oxygen is safe, inexpensive, and increases the myocardial oxygen delivery.

Nitrates

In the reperfusion era, nitroglycerin has not been shown to reduce mortality (ISIS-4 and GISSI-3 with >70,000 randomized patients). Nitroglycerin's vasodilatory effects are helpful in alleviating pain and treating coronary vasospasm, pulmonary edema, and hypertension.

β-Blockade

β-Blockers decrease myocardial oxygen consumption by reducing the double-product (i.e., heart rate and blood pressure). These medications decrease infarct size, decrease arrhythmic death, modestly decrease all-cause mortality, and act as anti-anginal agents (BHAT, Norwegian Timolol Study, TIMI-2B). Either oral or IV metoprolol is a good choice with a goal heart rate of 50 to 60 beats/minute and systolic blood pressure of 110 to 120 mm Hg. Do not use β-blockers in patients with significant pulmonary edema, hypotension, or bradyarrhythmias. Be wary of their use in patients with moderate to severely reduced left ventricular systolic function.

Angiotensin-Converting Enzyme Inhibitors

There is a significant reduction in mortality rate regardless of left ventricular systolic function and time of administration (SAVE, AIRE, SMILE, TRACE, GISSI-3, ISIS-4). The proposed mechanism of action is inhibition of post-infarct ventricular remodeling. However, angiotensin-converting enzyme (ACE) inhibitors reduce angiotensin II levels and may protect the vasculature as evidenced by the HOPE trial where patients with angina, stroke, or peripheral vascular disease and no history of MI or congestive heart failure had a significant reduction in mortality and all clinical outcomes with ACE inhibitors. Any ACE inhibitor is probably beneficial (i.e., drug class effect). Try to start during the hospitalization unless the patient is hypotensive or has renal failure. Monitor serum potassium level and renal function.

HMG CoA Reductase Inhibitor

The 4S, CARE, and LIPID studies showed that statins reduced the mortality rate of post-MI patients by 33% when started several months after the index event. Present NCEP guidelines recommend statins for post-MI patients if the lactate dehydrogenase level is greater than 100 mg/dL. However, these recommendations may change based on the recently announced MIRACL study reported at the AHA National Meeting in November 2000, which showed a reduction in adverse clinical outcomes when atorvastatin was started in-hospital in patients with acute coronary syndrome and a normal cholesterol level. There is speculation that statins have a "plaque stabilizing effect." We recommend checking a patient's fasting lipid panel as soon as possible during admission and starting an HMG CoA reductase inhibitor (simvastatin [Zocor] 20 mg every night, pravastatin [Pravachol] 20 mg every night, atorvastatin [Lipitor] 20 mg every night) if the lactate dehydrogenase level is greater than 100 mg/dL (assuming no liver disease). The classic teaching is that stress situations such as AMI reduce cholesterol levels (acute phase reactant produced by the liver) and can therefore be misleadingly low. However, a physician risks not identifying a patient with hyperlipidemia if he or she is lost to follow-up, thereby not starting a mortality-reducing medication. A fasting lipid level, liver function tests, and CK should be checked at follow-up in 4 weeks.

Angiotensin II Receptor Blockade

ACE inhibitors remain first-line therapy because no clinical trials have examined the effects of angiotensin II receptor blockers in AMI patients. However, if a patient cannot take an ACE inhibitor, then it is reasonable to prescribe an angiotensin II receptor blocker.

Calcium Channel Blockade

β-Blockers remain first-line therapy, given the wealth of data supporting their use. Dihydropyridines such as nifedipine (Adalat), especially the short-acting form, may be harmful and should not be used. For the heart rate–slowing drugs (verapamil [Calan] and diltiazem [Cardizem]), there is no controlled trial evidence for harm and they may even be beneficial unless a patient has reduced left ventricular systolic function or congestive heart failure. Calcium channel blockers can be considered in patients with refractory angina or atrial fibrillation with rapid ventricular response that is difficult to control. In general, these drugs are used too frequently at the expense of β-blocker, nitrate, and ACE inhibitor use.

Treat Extrinsic Stressors

Extrinsic coronary stressors such as supraventricular tachycardia, fever, sepsis, anemia, hypoxemia, thyrotoxicosis, hypotension, and so on should be corrected as soon as possible because these conditions either diminish myocardial oxygen delivery or increase myocardial oxygen consumption. Because the coronary artery oxygen extraction is so high, the hematocrit should be maintained at greater than 30% to 35% to maximize oxygen delivery.

Invasive Hemodynamic Monitoring

Arterial pressure monitoring and right heart catheterization (i.e., Swan-Ganz catheter, pulmonary artery catheter) can be incredibly helpful in managing critically ill patients with cardiogenic shock, low cardiac output, and/or pulmonary edema. Routine use in all patients with AMI in the cardiac care unit is not typically necessary.

Intra-Aortic Balloon Pump

The intra-aortic balloon pump is a useful mechanical device in the descending aorta that inflates during diastole (increases coronary perfusion) and deflates during systole (decreases ventricular afterload or workload), which can result in a 10% to 40% increase in cardiac output. This device is particularly useful in cardiogenic shock, severe mitral regurgitation, ventricular septal defect, and refractory ventricular tachycardia. Severe aortic regurgitation is a contraindication and peripheral vascular disease is a relative contraindication.

Nitroprusside

This arterial vasodilator is very useful in patients with severe hypertension and low cardiac output failure. Invasive arterial pressure monitoring is required. Cyanosis is typically not a concern the first 24 to 48 hours unless exceptionally high doses are being used.

Inotropes

Inotropic agents such as dopamine, dobutamine, milrinone, and norepinephrine typically increase contractility, heart rate, afterload, and therefore myocardial oxygen consumption. These medications are associated with increased infarct size and mortality. However, these medications are used in severe cardiogenic shock as a bridge to intra-aortic balloon pumping or simply because there is no other method of maintaining cardiac output and blood pressure.

Ventricular Assist Device

These devices are often used in patients with severe cardiac failure and serve as a bridge to cardiac transplantation. These devices require consultation with both cardiology and cardiothoracic surgery units.

NURSING CARE

Patients with ST-segment elevation, cardiac arrest, pulmonary edema, cardiogenic shock, arrhythmias, or greater than mild elevation in troponin or CK-MB should be admitted to the cardiac care unit. Patients who have no symptoms, have good hemodynamics and rhythm, a largely unremarkable ECG, and normal to mildly elevated troponin or CK-MB serum levels may be admitted to an intermediate care telemetry unit. All patients with an AMI should have continuous ECG monitoring.

TRANSTHORACIC ECHOCARDIOGRAM

A transthoracic echocardiogram provides a noninvasive assessment of left ventricular systolic function and valvular function as well as determining whether a patient has a ventricular thrombus or other structural abnormality.

CARDIOLOGY CONSULTATION

Several studies have shown that patients with AMI have significantly better outcomes when cardiologists are involved in their care. Another study by Frances showed that the proper use of evidence-based medications regardless of specialty provided similar clinical outcomes. We think that cardiology consultation in patients with AMI is certainly reasonable, especially in patients who are quite ill. However, the most important factors are that physicians are well-trained (i.e., knowledgeable regarding evidence-based medicine) and care for patients with AMI on a regular basis.

MECHANICAL COMPLICATIONS

Approximately 3 to 10 days after MI, the infarcted and increasingly necrotic myocardium is not yet fibrotic and is at risk for rupture of the septum (ventricular septal defect), papillary muscle (mitral regurgitation), and free wall (pericardial tamponade). Each of these conditions is life-threatening and requires immediate cardiothoracic surgery. An intra-aortic balloon pump may be indicated in ventricular septal defect and mitral regurgitation. Pericardiocentesis may be indicated in free wall rupture. In the patient with a new murmur or unexplained hypotension in the days following AMI, we recommend echocardiography to exclude mechanical complications.

PERICARDIAL DISEASE

method of
BRIAN D. HOIT, M.D.
Case Western Reserve University
Cleveland, Ohio

The pericardium consists of (1) a mesothelial monolayer that is firmly adherent to the epicardium and reflects over the origin of the great vessels (visceral pericardium), (2) a tough outer fibrous layer (parietal pericardium), and (3) a "potential" space between the two. Although the pericardium serves many important functions (Table 1), many are subtle and poorly understood.

Pericardial heart disease comprises pericarditis and its complications, tamponade and constriction. A resurgence of interest in pericardial heart disease is largely the result of an increase in the prevalence of pericarditis, owing to the greater use of cardiovascular surgery, hemodialysis, and immunosuppressive therapy; the longer survival of many cancer patients; and the emergence of AIDS.

Although the treatment of pericardial disease is often simple and rewarding, unexpected challenges and frustrations may emerge. Pericardial heart disease is often clinically silent, being detected only during the evaluation of unrelated complaints. In addition, there is a paucity of placebo-controlled trials from which appropriate therapy may be selected, and guidelines that assist in important clinical decisions are lacking. As a result, the physician often must rely heavily on data from small, uncontrolled trials and anecdotal experience. Finally, therapeutic options in most cases are limited to nonspecific anti-inflammatory agents, drainage of pericardial fluid, and pericardiectomy.

ACUTE PERICARDITIS

Pericarditis may be seen as an isolated phenomenon or may complicate variety of systemic disorders or the use of certain drugs. The major definable causes of pericardial heart disease are listed in Table 2; however, in many cases, the underlying cause of pericardial heart disease is never identified.

The majority of cases encountered in the outpatient setting are idiopathic or viral pericarditis. Acute fibrinous ("dry") pericarditis is a syndrome characterized by typical chest pain, a pathognomonic pericardial friction rub, and specific electrocardiographic changes. Hospitalization is warranted for most patients who present with an initial episode of acute pericarditis to determine an etiology and to observe for the development of cardiac tamponade. Acute pericarditis usually responds to oral nonsteroidal anti-inflammatory agents (NSAIDs), such as aspirin, 650 mg every 3 to 4 hours, or ibuprofen (Motrin, Advil), 600 to 800 mg every 6 hours for 1 to 4 days. Indomethacin (Indocin) reduces coronary blood flow and should be avoided. Selective COX-2 inhibitors are nonsteroidal anti-inflammatory drugs (NSAIDs) with few adverse gastrointestinal effects but have not been tested in acute pericarditis. Anecdotal data suggest that colchicine* (1 mg/d) is effective for the acute episode, is well tolerated, and may prevent recurrences. Narcotics may be required for severe pain, and some cases necessitate corticosteroid therapy to control pain (e.g., prednisone, 60–80 mg/d for a week, with the dosage tapered rapidly thereafter). Corticosteroids are also useful in acute pericarditis associated with uremic pericarditis and connective tissue diseases; tuberculous and pyogenic pericarditis should be excluded before corticosteroid therapy is initiated. Specific therapy should be directed toward the primary disorder in those patients in whom pericarditis represents one manifestation of systemic illness.

Recurrent or relapsing acute pericarditis is one of the most distressing disorders of the pericardium for both patient and physician. Recurrences occur with highly variable frequency over a course of many years, and although they may be spontaneous, they are more commonly associated with either discontinuation or tapering of anti-inflammatory drugs. Painful recurrences of pericarditis may respond to NSAIDs but commonly require corticosteroids. When these agents are necessary, the risks associated with long-term corticosteroid use should be minimized by using the lowest possible dose, alternate-day therapy, or combinations with NSAIDs. Colchicine* is both efficacious and safe for the prevention of recurrences; most authors recommend 1 mg/d orally for at least 1 year. Azathioprine (Imuran)* and cyclophosphamide (Cytoxan)* have been used to prevent recurrent episodes in patients who fail to respond to high-dose corticosteroids or who experience severe corticosteroid side effects. Pericardiectomy should be considered only when repeated attempts at medical treatment have clearly failed, especially when there is evidence of corticosteroid-induced complications.

TABLE 1. **Functions of the Pericardium**

Mechanical/protective
Facilitation of cardiac chamber interaction and coupling
Effects on atrial and ventricular filling, ventricular diastolic function, oxygen delivery, and cardiac output (during exercise)
Limitation of acute cardiac distention
Equalization of gravitational, inertial, and hydrostatic forces
Immunologic, vasomotor, and fibrinolytic activity
Modulation of myocyte structure, function, and gene expression by epicardial mesothelial cells
Potential route for gene delivery

TABLE 2. **Etiology of Pericardial Heart Disease**

Idiopathic
Infectious (viral, bacterial, mycobacterial, fungal, protozoal, AIDS)
Neoplastic (breast, lung, melanoma, lymphoma, leukemia, mesothelioma)
Post-myocardial infarction
Radiation induced
Nephrogenic (dialytic and uremic)
Traumatic (blunt and penetrating injuries, chylopericardium)
Connective tissue diseases and arteritides (rheumatoid arthritis, systemic lupus erythematosus, scleroderma, polyarteritis nodosa, Takayasu arteritis, Wegener granulomatosis)
Myxedema
Iatrogenic (diagnostic and therapeutic procedures, drugs)
Miscellaneous (sarcoidosis, amyloidosis, Whipple disease, dissecting aortic aneurysm)

*Not FDA approved for this indication.

PERICARDIAL EFFUSION

Indications for pericardial drainage include tamponade and suspected purulent pericarditis; persistent (>3 months), large, and unexplained effusions may warrant pericardiocentesis, and occasionally suspected malignancy or systemic disease may necessitate pericardial drainage and biopsy. However, routine drainage of large effusions (20-mm echo-free space in diastole) has a very low diagnostic yield and no therapeutic benefit.

Removal of small amounts of pericardial fluid (~50 mL) produces considerable symptomatic and hemodynamic improvement because of the steep pericardial pressure-volume relation. Unless there is concomitant cardiac disease or coexisting constriction (i.e., effusive-constrictive pericarditis), removal of all of the pericardial fluid normalizes pericardial, atrial, ventricular diastolic, and arterial pressures and cardiac output.

Unless the situation is immediately life threatening, pericardiocentesis should be performed (a subxiphoid approach is preferred because of its extrapleural and relatively avascular location) using a short (5–8 cm) beveled needle, by experienced staff in a facility equipped with radiographic, echocardiographic, and hemodynamic monitoring. For monitoring the needle tip electrocardiogram, it is essential that the apparatus have equipotential grounding. Using two-dimensional (2-D) echocardiographic guidance has increased the safety of the pericardiocentesis. A No. 6 to No. 8 French catheter may be placed using Seldinger technique and left in place for continued drainage (using only slight negative pressure). Drainage of the pericardial fluid using a catheter minimizes trauma, allows measurement of pericardial pressure and instillation of drugs into the pericardium, and helps prevent (but does not guarantee) reaccumulation of pericardial fluid. Patients should be monitored for recurrent tamponade, particularly those with hemorrhagic effusions, which may occur despite the presence of an intrapericardial catheter. Dilute heparin or fibrinolytic agents (see later) may be instilled in the catheter to prevent clotting.

Although pericardiocentesis may provide effective relief, percutaneous balloon pericardiotomy, subxiphoid pericardiotomy, or the surgical creation of a pleuropericardial or a peritoneal-pericardial window may be required. Needle pericardiocentesis is often the best option when the cause is known and/or the diagnosis of tamponade is in question, and surgical drainage is optimal when the presence of tamponade is certain but the cause is unclear. Pericardiocentesis is ill advised when there is less than 1 cm of effusion, loculation, or evidence of fibrin and adhesion.

Repeat pericardiocentesis, sclerotherapy with tetracycline, surgical creation of a pericardial window, or pericardiectomy may treat recurrent effusions. Subtotal pericardiectomy is preferred when the patient is expected to survive more than 1 year. A pleuropericardial window provides a large area for fluid reabsorption and is often performed in patients with malignant effusions. Pericardiectomy may be required for recurrent effusions in dialysis patients. In critically ill patients, a pericardial window may be created percutaneously with a balloon catheter.

CONSTRICTIVE PERICARDITIS

Constrictive pericarditis is a condition in which a thickened, scarred, and often calcified pericardium limits diastolic filling of the ventricles. Although acute pericarditis from most causes may eventuate in constrictive pericarditis, the most common antecedents are idiopathic factors, cardiac trauma and surgery, mediastinal irradiation, tuberculosis (particularly common in nonindustrialized countries) and other infectious diseases, neoplasms (particularly lung and breast), renal failure, and connective tissue diseases.

Pericardiectomy is the definitive treatment for constrictive pericarditis, but it is unwarranted either in very early constriction (occult and functional class I) or in severe, advanced disease (functional class IV), when the risk of surgery is excessive and the benefits are diminished. In asymptomatic patients, increasing jugular venous pressure, the need for diuretic therapy, evidence of hepatic insufficiency, and reduced exercise tolerance indicate the need for surgery. Operation should be delayed until it is clear that the constrictive process is transitory.

Medical therapy for constrictive pericarditis has a small but important role. In some patients, constrictive pericarditis resolves either spontaneously or in response to various combinations of NSAIDs, corticosteroids, and antibiotics; in the remaining patients, medical therapy is adjunctive. Specific antibiotic (e.g., antituberculous) therapy should be initiated before surgery and continued afterward. Preoperative diuretics should be used sparingly with the goal of reducing, not eliminating, elevated jugular pressure, edema, and ascites. Postoperatively, diuretics should be given if spontaneous diuresis does not occur; the central venous pressure may take weeks to months to return to normal after pericardiectomy. Diuretics and digoxin (in the presence of atrial fibrillation) are useful in those patients who are not candidates for pericardiectomy because of their high surgical risk.

Prevention of pericardial constriction consists of appropriate therapy for acute pericarditis and adequate pericardial drainage. Although instillation of fibrinolytics (urokinase, 400,000 U per instillation to 1.6 million U; streptokinase, 250,000 IU per instillation to 1 million IU) is promising, corticosteroid instillation is often ineffective.

TREATMENT OF SPECIFIC CAUSES OF PERICARDITIS

Infectious Pericarditis

Bacterial pericarditis is treated with surgical exploration and drainage (pericardiectomy is preferable) and appropriate systemic antibiotics, which should be considered adjuvant. Whenever purulent pericarditis is suspected, the pericardial space should be explored. Fibrinolytics may be used to lyse fibrous adhesions and prevent constrictive pericarditis.

In effusive tuberculous pericarditis, the fluid collection is often voluminous and hemodynamically significant. An adhesive phase follows resolution of the effusion and may eventuate in dense, calcific adhesions. Patients with tuberculous pericarditis should receive triple-drug therapy (isoniazid, 5 mg/kg to a maximum of 300 mg; rifampin [Rifadin], 10 mg/kg to a maximum of 600 mg; and either streptomycin, 15 mg/kg to a maximum of 1 g, or ethambutol [Myambutol], 5–25 mg/kg to a maximum of 2.5 g) for a minimum of 9 months. Corticosteroids may be useful if pericardial effusion persists or recurs during therapy and are beneficial acutely in reducing morbidity and mortality, but data supporting their use to prevent constriction in primary pericardial effusion are lacking. Early pericardiectomy has been recommended by some in all cases of tuberculosis pericarditis, but the long-term prognosis of patients without cardiac compression during the acute illness who are treated with medical therapy alone is excellent. Pericardiectomy may be necessary for recurrent cardiac tamponade. Patients should be observed for constriction because up to half of patients will require pericardiectomy. Failure to improve or worsening over 1 to 2 months, pericardial thickening, or evidence of constriction requires urgent pericardiectomy. Atypical mycobacterial infections (especially those due to *Mycobacterium avium-intracellulare*) may be resistant to treatment.

Pericarditis complicating deep fungal infection with *Histoplasma* or *Coccidioides* may be immunologic, resolve spontaneously, and not require specific therapy. Amphotericin B (Fungizone), up to 2.5 g total, itraconazole (Sporanox), 200–400 mg/d, ketoconazole (Nizoral),* 200–400 mg/d,* and fluconazole (Diflucan), 200–400 mg/d, are rarely required. Tamponading effusion and constriction require decompression. Surgical decompression and specific antifungal or antimicrobial therapy may be necessary for disseminated infection with *Candida, Aspergillus, Actinomyces*, and *Nocardia*.

Neoplastic Pericarditis

Metastatic neoplasia is the leading cause of pericardial disease in hospitalized patients. Although many cases are asymptomatic and found only incidentally at autopsy, others progress to cardiac tamponade. In almost every case, fluid should be removed if large effusions are refractory or if tamponade ensues. The specific approach depends on the patient's expected longevity and medical condition. Sclerosing agents, such as tetracycline* (500–1000 mg in 20 mL of sterile saline), reduce recurrences and can be considered for patients with a poor prognosis. However, sclerosis is painful, does not improve prognosis, and may not be superior to an indwelling catheter alone. Subtotal pericardiectomy is most effective but should only be performed in carefully selected patients. Balloon pericardiotomy avoids the discomfort and risk of surgery and will likely replace surgical subxiphoid pericardiotomy.

Post–Myocardial Infarction Pericarditis

Pericarditis is common in the first few days after myocardial infarction, occurring in as many as one fourth to one half of fatal infarctions but clinically apparent in far fewer. A pericardial friction rub occurring in the first 2 or 3 days without an associated pericardial effusion should not influence decisions regarding anticoagulant use, but pericarditis occurring later in the course or accompanied by pericardial effusion or tamponade is a contraindication to anticoagulant therapy.

Infarct pericarditis responds to aspirin (up to 650 mg every 4 hours for 5–10 days); corticosteroids should be avoided because of concerns of impaired infarct healing, corticosteroid dependency, and toxic side effects. Thrombolytic therapy almost invariably precedes the development of pericarditis; therefore, clinical decision-making is not usually affected. In fact, thrombolytic therapy reduces the incidence of postinfarction pericarditis by approximately one half and, for reasons not entirely clear, has helped render post–myocardial infarction pericarditis nearly obsolete. However, when acute pericarditis is mistaken for acute myocardial infarction, thrombolytic therapy can have catastrophic consequences.

Radiation-Induced Pericardial Disease

Acute radiation-induced pericarditis occurs after a highly variable (usually <1 year) delay and can be managed symptomatically as acute idiopathic pericarditis. Hemodynamically insignificant pericardial effusion can also be managed conservatively because spontaneous resolution is the rule; however, pericardiectomy should be offered to symptomatic patients with large, recurrent pericardial effusions. Acute pericarditis occurring early during radiation therapy is uncommon, most likely the result of the radiation-induced effects on the tumor rather than a direct toxic effect of the radiation on the pericardium, and should not disrupt radiation therapy (although a reduction in dose may be necessary). Constrictive pericarditis requires pericardiectomy unless a biopsy reveals significant endomyocardial fibrosis.

Nephrogenic Pericardial Disease

Intensification of dialysis is an accepted treatment modality for hemodynamically insignificant disease; however, considerable controversy exists regarding the optimal management of large, persistent, or recurrent pericardial effusion and tamponade. Severe tamponade is an indication for pericardial drainage, but a conservative approach (i.e., intensification of

*Not FDA approved for this indication.

dialysis and NSAIDs) may suffice in less severe cases. The instillation of nonabsorbable corticosteroids directly into the pericardial space has been advocated, but randomized controlled data are absent. If needle drainage is necessary, an indwelling catheter should be left in the pericardial space for at least 2 to 3 days. Dialysis-associated effusive pericarditis usually responds to intensification of dialysis and regional heparinization or to changing to peritoneal dialysis. Pericardiectomy may be necessary for intractable effusions.

Traumatic Pericardial Disease

Chronic constrictive pericarditis, recurrent pericardial effusion, and recurrent acute pericarditis are well-recognized complications of blunt and penetrating trauma. Chylous pericardial effusions generally follow traumatic or surgical injury to the thoracic duct but may result from neoplastic obstruction of the thoracic duct or they may be idiopathic. Failure to respond either to ligation of the thoracic duct and partial pericardiectomy or to a diet rich in medium-chain triglycerides warrants implantation of a valved pericardioperitoneal conduit.

Other Causes of Pericardial Disease

Pericarditis may accompany virtually any connective tissue disease and may present as either acute or chronic pericarditis with or without an effusion. However, most cases are subclinical and in many instances are recognized only at autopsy. In the absence of tamponading or secondarily infected effusions, NSAIDs and corticosteroids are useful. Myxedema-associated effusions develop slowly and may grow very large; slow resolution usually follows institution of thyroid replacement therapy.

Iatrogenic pericardial disease results from both the calculated complications and the unanticipated misadventures of diagnostic and therapeutic procedures. Importantly, a wide variety of drugs and toxins may cause pericardial heart disease, by producing either drug-induced lupus (e.g., procainamide [Pronestyl], hydralazine [Apresoline], isoniazid), a hypersensitivity or idiosyncratic reaction (e.g., penicillins, thiazides, anthracyclines), pericardial irritation, or hemorrhage (e.g., anticoagulants).

PERIPHERAL ARTERIAL DISEASE

method of
JOSEPH L. MILLS, Sr., M.D.
University of Arizona Health Sciences Center
Tucson, Arizona

Peripheral arterial disease (PAD) is a major cause of disability and death and is responsible for substantial health care expenditures in the United States. If one pauses to consider the extended lifespan of our society, then the diagnosis and treatment of patients with PAD will inevitably assume increasing importance early in the 21st century because the condition primarily affects the elderly population.

The term *PAD* has traditionally been applied to all arterial diseases excluding those involving the intracranial and cardiac vessels. PAD, therefore, encompasses conditions such as acute and chronic mesenteric ischemia, renovascular hypertension, peripheral aneurysms, upper extremity arterial diseases, nonatherosclerotic conditions (e.g., thromboangiitis obliterans), and vasospastic disease. Despite their significance, however, these latter entities are beyond the scope of this review. The following discussion is limited to consideration of the three most common peripheral arterial conditions the primary care or specialist physician is likely to regularly encounter in clinical practice: (1) lower extremity arterial occlusive disease, (2) abdominal aortic aneurysm (AAA), and (3) carotid artery disease.

CHRONIC LOWER EXTREMITY ARTERIAL OCCLUSIVE DISEASE

Atherosclerosis is the most common cause of chronic lower limb occlusive disease. Its precursor, the fatty streak, is frequently present in the arteries of many individuals in their early twenties. Genetic predisposition, as well as certain risk factors (Table 1), increase the likelihood that clinically important atherosclerotic disease will develop. The most important risk factors for the development and progression of atherosclerosis are smoking, hypertension, diabetes mellitus, and hyperlipidemia. Recent evidence suggests that hyperhomocysteinemia may also be important, particularly in patients with premature atherosclerosis.

Symptomatic lower limb arterial disease most commonly affects patients in the sixth and seventh decades of life. The presenting symptoms, in order of increasing severity and risk of limb loss, are intermittent claudication, ischemic rest pain, ischemic ulceration, and tissue necrosis or gangrene. A thorough history and physical examination, supplemented by appropriate noninvasive diagnostic tests, usually suffice to establish the presence and severity of the disease, locate the anatomic site of arterial obstruction, and suggest an appropriate treatment plan.

Intermittent claudication is defined as muscular pain in the buttock, hip, or calf, induced by exercise and relieved by rest. Vasculogenic claudication is typically highly reproducible; that is, it tends to occur in the same muscle groups each time the patient walks, at the same distance, with the same degree of exertion. If the patient walks at a more rapid pace or uphill, however, the symptoms will occur sooner. The symptoms, usually described as muscular cramps or fatigue, resolve with rest alone and do not require a change in position. The main condition from which it must be differentiated is *pseudoclaudication* or *neurogenic claudication,* which develops due to lumbar spinal stenosis. A careful history will usually differentiate the

TABLE 1. **Risk Factors for Peripheral Arterial Disease**

Cigarette smoking	Diabetes mellitus
Homocysteine	Obesity
Hypertension	Family history
Sedentary lifestyle	Hyperlipidemia

two entities; symptoms of neurogenic claudication are often more variable in onset and duration, may occur both at rest and with exercise, are frequently provoked and relieved by positional changes such as bending over, and often include sensory complaints such as paresthesias or numbness rather than just pain or cramping.

Most patients with intermittent claudication have abnormal peripheral pulses; the location of the pulse deficit suggests the anatomic site of disease. Femoral, popliteal, posterior tibial, and dorsal pedal pulses should be palpated in each patient with possible PAD. A diminished femoral pulse with or without a bruit suggests significant iliac artery occlusive disease. A normal femoral pulse with weak or absent distal pulses would indicate obstruction of the superficial femoral or popliteal arteries. Patients with diabetes mellitus frequently present with chronic limb ischemia and palpable femoral and popliteal pulses, but with absent foot pulses. These findings are due not to microvascular disease but to the propensity of diabetes mellitus to result in atherosclerotic stenosis or occlusion of the proximal tibial and peroneal arteries.

The vascular laboratory provides important diagnostic and prognostic information in patients with intermittent claudication, rest pain, or ischemic ulceration (Table 2). The most commonly performed test is a Doppler-derived ankle/brachial index (ABI). The ankle pressure is compared to the higher of the two brachial artery pressures. Both brachial pressures should be measured because of the propensity of atherosclerosis to asymptomatically involve the subclavian arteries, especially the origin of the left subclavian artery. A normal ABI is 1.0 or greater, and any value less than 0.9 is suspicious. The ABI generally correlates with the degree of ischemia and also long-term mortality. The presence and magnitude of a reduced ABI are markers of systemic atherosclerosis; the increased mortality in patients with PAD is not due to limb ischemia but rather associated coronary and cerebrovascular disease; the 5-year mortality for patients with claudication approximates 25% to 30%, whereas that for patients with ischemic tissue loss approaches 50%. Even asymptomatic patients with abnormal ABIs demonstrate an increased mortality compared to an age-matched population, and the more severe the ABI reduction, the greater the long-term mortality.

A lower extremity treadmill test is also extremely useful in the differential diagnosis of patients with atypical claudication. The usual protocol has the patient walk at 1.5 mph on a 10% to 11% grade (*incline*) for up to 5 minutes or until symptoms develop. A normal response is maintenance or an increase in the ABI after exercise. If the patient has vasculogenic claudication, pain onset and cessation of exercise will be associated with a significant decrease in the ABI after exercise. Patients in whom pain or weakness develops during the treadmill test without a corresponding ABI drop should be suspected of having neurogenic claudication. A lumbar computed tomography scan or magnetic resonance imaging might then be useful to evaluate the patient for lumbar spinal stenosis.

TABLE 2. **Correlation Between Ankle/Brachial Index and Degree of Arterial Ischemia**

Ankle/Brachial Index	Clinical Condition
1.1 ± 0.1	Normal
0.6 ± 0.2	Intermittent claudication
0.3 ± 0.1	Ischemic rest pain
0.1 ± 0.1	Impending tissue necrosis

Patients with ischemic rest pain and ulceration nearly always demonstrate obvious abnormalities on physical examination. Ischemic rest pain typically occurs in the toes or forefoot and is worsened when the patient is supine, often preventing the patient from falling asleep or waking him up from sleep. The pain is relieved by dependency; the patient must hang his foot over the edge of the bed; sleep sitting up in a chair; or stand, walk, or shake the affected foot. All these maneuvers restore the slight positive gravitational effect on ankle blood pressure, which may be sufficient to relieve ischemic rest pain. All patients with true ischemic rest pain have absent pedal pulses, and frequently demonstrate dependent rubor. This finding should not be confused with cellulitis. With leg elevation, the ruborous, chronically ischemic foot will become pale. ABIs in patients with rest pain are less than 0.3 to 0.4.

Patients with intermittent claudication should be counseled to stop smoking and begin an exercise program (walking); 70% to 75% of patients with claudication will stabilize or improve with such a regimen. Other risk factors should be addressed. Selected patients may benefit from oral cilostazol (Pletal) or pentoxifylline (Trental), but tobacco abstinence and exercise are by far the best initial and long-term treatment options. Patients who fail to improve or who worsen with a 3- to 6-month trial of conservative treatment should be referred to a vascular surgeon if the symptoms significantly affect the patient's job or lifestyle. Extensive disease is best treated with bypass; prosthetic grafts are suitable for reconstruction of aorto-iliac occlusive disease, but autogenous vein grafts are superior for infra-inguinal bypass. Short focal lesions, especially involving the common iliac artery, are effectively treated with percutaneous transluminal angioplasty, with or without a stent. Conservatism in the treatment of patients with claudication is suggested by the natural history of the disease. The risk of limb loss over 5 years in patients with claudication is only in the range of 3% to 7%, in stark contrast to the 30% 5-year mortality from myocardial infarction and stroke. Strong consideration should therefore be given to evaluating the coronary and carotid arteries in such patients.

Ambulatory, functional patients with suspected ischemic rest pain, ulceration, or gangrene are at significantly increased risk of limb loss without intervention and should be referred to a vascular surgeon for revascularization. Patients with diabetes mellitus also frequently have foot ulceration and are at significantly increased risk of limb loss. Lower extremity gangrene is 60 times more common in diabetics than nondiabetics.

The most common cause of foot lesions in diabetics is neuropathy: motor, sensory, and autonomic. Neuropathic ulceration frequently leads to infection. Recognition of infection, prompt antibiotic administration, and open surgical débridement are often required. In an important subset of diabetic patients, nonhealing ulcers develop due to the predilection of atherosclerosis to obstruct the tibioperoneal arteries. Absent foot pulses in such patients are not due to microvascular disease; well-performed angiography will nearly always demonstrate suitable target arteries for bypass. These patients are usually amenable to tibial or pedal artery bypass with autogenous saphenous vein. Bypass graft patency in diabetics is equal or superior to that obtained in nondiabetic patients.

ABDOMINAL AORTIC ANEURYSM

An *aneurysm* is defined as a localized enlargement of an artery such that its diameter is more than 1.5 times its normal caliber. The infrarenal abdominal aorta is the most common location of peripheral arterial aneurysm. AAAs are three to eight times more common in men than women and increase in frequency with age. Approximately 20% of AAAs are familial (i.e., there is a genetic component), but the vast majority of abdominal aneurysms are considered to be degenerative in nature and are associated with incompletely understood abnormalities in the metabolism of elastase and other enzymes.

Rupture is the chief concern in patients with an AAA. Aortic aneurysm rupture is the 13th leading cause of death in the United States, and overall mortality for ruptured AAA exceeds 75%. At least 40% of patients die before reaching the hospital, and the mortality remains 45% to 50% in those patients arriving at the hospital alive who undergo repair.

The prevalence of AAA has increased over the past 30 years. Major risk factors associated with AAA include cigarette smoking, hypertension, male gender, increasing age, and previous vascular surgery. The cost-effectiveness of screening large populations of patients for the presence of AAA has not been established; however, it would seem prudent to recommend ultrasound (US) screening of patients with a positive family history of AAA. A strong case can be made for screening men over 60 years of age, particularly in the presence of associated risk factors such as smoking, hypertension, or previous vascular surgery.

Physical examination is essential in evaluating all patients with risk factors for atherosclerosis and AAA. In addition to palpation of peripheral pulses and auscultation for carotid, abdominal, and femoral bruits, a careful, thorough abdominal examination is necessary. Most aneurysms of surgical importance (>5 cm) can be palpated on careful physical examination if the patient's abdominal girth is less than 100 cm. It has been recommended that patients with a family history of AAA and men over 60 years of age, particularly in the presence of risk factors, be screened with US. This technique is more sensitive than physical examination and allows detection of smaller aneurysms that can then be serially evaluated for expansion. Previous studies suggest that AAAs, on average, enlarge at the rate of 0.2 to 0.4 cm per year.

The major factor associated with AAA rupture is the maximal aortic diameter. Other risk factors for rupture include smoking, chronic obstructive pulmonary disease, and hypertension. Aortic aneurysms exceeding 6 cm in diameter are considered large; the estimated annual rupture risk is 9% per year (6–6.9 cm) and 25% per year (>7 cm). Repair should be offered to nearly all such patients with large AAAs barring the presence of severe co-morbidities or conditions associated with poor short-term survival (advanced malignancy). Aneurysms less than 4 cm generally are observed with serial US surveillance and monitored for expansion. Controversy persists with regard to the treatment of intermediate-diameter AAAs (4–6 cm). Most experienced vascular surgeons in North America recommend repair of AAAs over 5 cm in reasonable risk patients. In patients with 4 to 5 cm aneurysms, the decision depends on the presence or absence of other risk factors for rupture and on the patient's overall medical condition.

In addition to risk of AAA expansion and rupture, as well as medical co-morbidities, a key factor in determining when to recommend AAA repair is the operative mortality rate. Although some centers have reported mortality rates of 2% or less for AAA repair, most large population-based studies in Europe and North America report mortalities from conventional AAA repair in the range of 4% to 7%.

Conventional open surgical repair has been performed for nearly 50 years and requires an abdominal or flank incision through which the aneurysm is exposed, the proximal infrarenal aorta is cross-clamped, and a graft is sewn within the aneurysm sac to normal caliber vessels at the proximal and distal extent of the aneurysm. The main disadvantages of this procedure are a relatively prolonged hospital stay (5–7 days) and delayed return to normal activity and energy levels. Open surgical repair is extremely durable, however, and late reoperations are distinctly uncommon.

In 1999, the Food and Drug Administration approved two aortic endograft devices that can be inserted via endoluminal techniques through the femoral arteries exposed by means of short groin incisions. The principal advantages are decreased patient discomfort, more rapid recuperation, and shortened hospital stay. However, the mortality of endovascular AAA repair is not demonstrably lower than open repair. There appears to be an ongoing need for computed tomography surveillance following endovascular AAA repair, and reintervention to treat graft migration, leak, or graft limb kinking/thrombosis, is required in as many as 30% of patients. Because the endografts are held in place with stents or small metal hooks and are not sutured in place, there is concern over endograft durability and its reliability in preventing AAA rupture. In fact, ruptures have occurred following apparently adequate endoluminal graft placement. Until we have better data, many surgeons believe endovascular AAA repair should be restricted to high-risk patients.

CAROTID ARTERY DISEASE

Stroke remains one of the five leading causes of death in American adults. Despite its decline in frequency over the past decade, stroke remains relatively common, with an annual incidence of 195 per 100,000 population. Like lower extremity occlusive disease and AAA, the incidence of stroke increases with age; the incidence of stroke in men 75 to 84 years of age is 1440 per 100,000. About two thirds of individuals who survive a stroke are permanently disabled to some degree. Half of stroke victims surviving 30 days following the event will be alive at 5 years, and one third of survivors will require prolonged inpatient rehabilitation.

Stroke prevalence studies have identified about 2 million surviving stroke victims; 30% to 40% of strokes in the United States appear to be related to atherosclerotic carotid bifurcation disease. The plaque usually occurs within 3 cm of the carotid bifurcation and is therefore surgically accessible.

Carotid endarterectomy (CEA) has been a controversial operation since it was first performed in the early 1950s; however, to a greater extent than any other peripheral vascular disease, sound data are available from at least three large, prospective randomized trials on which to base treatment recommendations.

For patients with hemispheric symptoms, two trials (NASCET [North American Symptomatic Carotid Endarterectomy Trial], ECST [European Carotid Surgery Trial]) showed benefit for CEA in patients with carotid stenoses exceeding 70% diameter reduction. Each study, however, used different criteria for stenosis measurement. The relative stroke risk reductions in these two trials were 65% to 80% for CEA compared to aspirin and medical treatment. In the NASCET Trial, selected patients with greater than 50% stenosis also benefitted from CEA.

The Asymptomatic Carotid Atherosclerosis Study (ACAS) documented a 55% stroke reduction for asymptomatic good risk patients for CEA if the stenosis was greater than 60% (measurement based on angiography comparing the residual lumen diameter at the site of the stenosis with normal caliber distal internal carotid artery). Duplicating these excellent results in the community outside of prospective, randomized trials in centers of surgical excellence requires that the referring physician know the surgical complication rates (death and stroke) of the surgeons who will be performing CEA. Target stroke and death rates in asymptomatic patients should be less than 2% to 3% and should not exceed 5% to 8% in symptomatic individuals. Higher complication rates may negate the potential benefit of surgery.

Duplex scanning has become the most reliable and cost-effective noninvasive means of diagnosing significant carotid bifurcation disease. Duplex combines two-dimensional B-mode imaging with pulsed Doppler US, thus providing both anatomic and hemodynamic information regarding the presence and severity of carotid bifurcation stenosis. The most common indications for carotid duplex scanning are asymptomatic cervical bruit, amaurosis fugax (transient monocular blindness), focal hemispheric transient ischemic attacks (hemiparesis, aphasia), and nonhemispheric neurologic symptoms. The presence and characteristics of plaque can be identified and the degree of stenosis determined with results that correlate well with conventional angiography. In many experienced centers, evaluation of potential candidates for CEA is being performed with duplex alone, sometimes supplemented by magnetic resonance angiography with conventional arteriography reserved for only a small percentage of cases in which the results of the less invasive studies are equivocal or nondiagnostic. Angiography is invasive, expensive, and is associated with a small, but significant risk of stroke (0.4%–1.2%).

Carotid angioplasty and stenting are being performed in some centers, but the techniques have not been standardized and controlled, and prospective trials against standard CEA have not been carried out. Surgical CEA remains the standard of care for most patients requiring carotid artery intervention for high-grade bifurcation disease.

Individuals with lower extremity ischemia, AAA, and advanced carotid bifurcation atherosclerosis comprise primarily an elderly population with systemic atherosclerosis, frequently including significant coronary artery disease. Patients with significant risk factors for PAD deserve a thorough history and physical examination to uncover potentially life- and limb-threatening atherosclerotic lesions. Evidence-based screening criteria and improved noninvasive diagnostic techniques are rapidly evolving to improve screening, evaluation, and treatment of the aging population with advanced PAD.

VENOUS THROMBOSIS

method of
EDWARD N. LIBBY, M.D.
University of New Mexico Health Sciences Center
Albuquerque, New Mexico

Venous thromboembolism (VTE) is a common problem in primary care. The incidence of clinically evident VTE of the extremities and pulmonary embolism (PE) has been estimated to be 398,000 cases per year in the United States. A review of the diseases present on any hospital primary care ward will reveal that a significant percentage of admitted patients are in the hospital for VTE. In addition to the acute morbidity and mortality and cost associated with VTE and PE, postphlebitic syndrome of the legs causes significant chronic disability in 10% to 30% of VTE patients. Goals of physician intervention in VTE are to prevent extension, recurrence, and embolization of VTE.

RISK FACTORS

The risk of VTE is increased with secondary risk factors such as pregnancy, trauma, immobility, surgery, oral contraceptive usage, estrogen replacement therapy, myocardial infarction, stroke, cancer, and obesity. Inherited conditions that predispose patients to VTE include protein C and protein S deficiencies, antithrombin III deficiency, activated protein C resistance (factor V Leiden), the prothrombin gene G20210A mutation, antiphospholipid antibody syndrome, and hyperhomocysteinemia.

DIAGNOSIS

Venous Ultrasound and Contrast Venography

The gold standard test for diagnosis of VTE (Figure 1) is contrast venography, but this is uncommonly performed. The most common technique in the United States is real-time B-mode compression ultrasonography (US), in which the lack of compressibility of a venous segment documents thrombosis. Venous US is 89% sensitive and 97% specific for proximal deep vein thrombosis. Sensitivity for pelvic VTE is 71%. US is inadequate in the evaluation of the calf, where sensitivity is 50% to 87%. Patients whose clinical presentation strongly suggests calf VTE but who have a negative US evaluation should return for repeat US evaluation in 5 to 7 days. If the second test is negative, VTE is unlikely. Upper extremity VTE is important, representing 4% to 13% of all cases of VTE. US is a moderately useful technique for the diagnosis of upper extremity VTE, with a sensitivity of 78% to 100% in symptomatic patients.

The Superficial Femoral Vein

Clinicians should be aware that the vein inferior to the common femoral vein may be referred to as the *superficial femoral vein* by the vascular laboratory. This vein *is* part of the deep venous system; therefore, thrombosis in this location should be treated. Many centers now refer to this venous segment as the *femoral vein* to avoid confusion.

Recurrent Venous Thrombosis

Recurrent VTE is difficult to diagnose and can be easily confused with the postphlebitic syndrome. Only 50% of patients have a normal US evaluation 1 year after a VTE. Therefore, an abnormal US in a patient with previous VTE does not document recurrence unless the study can be compared with a normal study performed after resolution of the initial VTE. Clot echogenicity and venous distention are useful tools to differentiate chronic from recurrent clot but are neither specific nor sensitive in recurrence. With US, lack of compressibility at a new venous site or extension of a previous thrombosis documents recurrence but may not be detected. Contrast venography (CV) is specific and sensitive for recurrence but is generally not used. Clinicians should review the US results with their local experts and weigh the clinical and laboratory data carefully before concluding that recurrence has occurred. Anti-

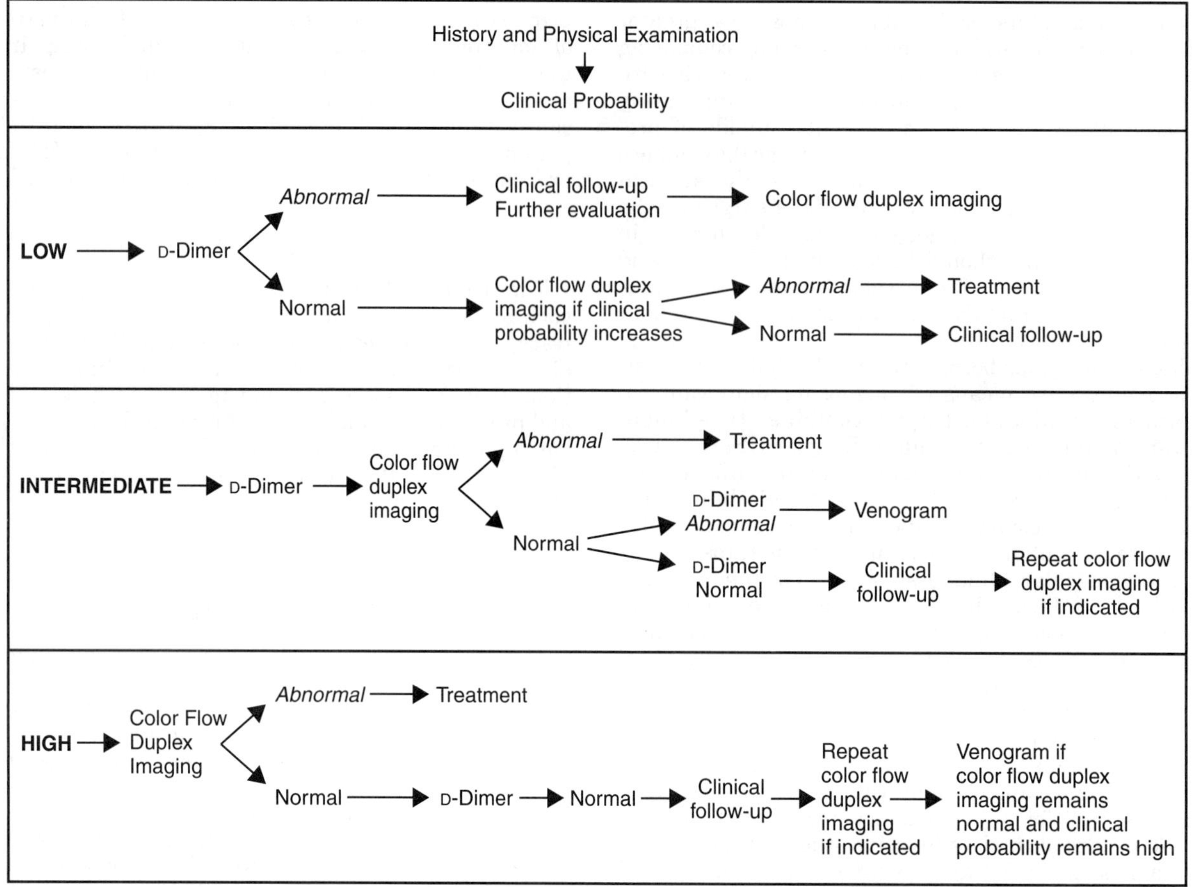

Figure 1. Diagnostic evaluation for suspected deep vein thrombosis. (From Baker WF: Diagnosis of deep vein thrombosis and pulmonary embolism. Med Clin North Am 82:459–476, 1998.)

coagulating patients without establishing the diagnosis of recurrent VTE should be avoided.

Computed Tomography and Magnetic Resonance Imaging

CT and magnetic resonance imaging (MRI) are not routinely used to diagnose VTE of the extremities but are valuable for evaluation of vena caval clots (CT) and pelvic thrombosis (MRI).

D-dimer

D-dimer, a degradation product of cross-linked fibrin, is an important new tool to evaluate for VTE. Sensitivity and specificity have been reported to be 95% to 100%, with negative predictive values (NPVs) of 98% for proximal VTE. Although the NPV of D-dimer is excellent, the positive predictive value (PPV) is poor. D-dimer has been studied successfully among patients in whom the suspicion is low for VTE. As a result, D-dimer has been incorporated into the VTE management strategy of many hospitals. D-dimer can help in situations in which there is a high clinical suspicion of VTE but US screening is equivocal or negative.

Many clinical situations can elevate D-dimer levels, lowering their specificity. Stress, infections, renal failure, severe illness, surgery, cirrhosis, hemorrhage, cancer, and disseminated intravascular coagulation have all been shown to increase D-dimer levels. Because of the lack of specificity, the PPV of D-dimer is poor, making the test unsatisfactory for confirming VTE. Conventional enzyme-linked immunosorbent assay (ELISA) for D-dimer is the gold standard test but is technically difficult to perform and unavailable at many institutions. Rapid ELISA testing is available, but lack of standardization between manufacturers limits reliability. Results of studies of traditional latex tests and whole-blood agglutination assays to rule out VTE have been disappointing. Latex or agglutination tests are not sufficiently sensitive to exclude a diagnosis of VTE.

Limitations of D-dimer

Studies have shown interobserver variability in D-dimer results between different laboratories using the same test methodology. Standardization of D-dimer testing will be critical if it is to gain wide acceptance and have clinical value. Currently, there is disagreement as to what are normal versus abnormal values, units of measurement, and definition of standard reference assays.

Usage of D-dimer

To prevent discharging patients home due to false-negative testing, the chosen technique should have a sensitivity as close to 100% as possible. Each hospital considering using D-dimer as part of their routine evaluation of VTE must rigorously test the methodology chosen. Use of D-dimer as a screening tool should be confined to outpatients because the likelihood of VTE is low in this population. ELISA testing for D-dimer *can* be used to rule out VTE in low-probability populations (see Figure 1). High-probability cases should not be routinely evaluated using D-dimer.

Subclinical Pulmonary Embolism

Asymptomatic PE can be found in 40% to 50% of patients who present with VTE of the extremities. Ventilation-perfusion scanning or pulmonary angiography is necessary only in patients with symptoms of PE and should not be routinely performed in VTE of the extremities.

TREATMENT

Treatment of acute VTE is important to prevent extension, recurrence, embolism, the postphlebitic syndrome, and death. The postphlebitic syndrome is associated with heaviness, edema, pain, hyperpigmentation, ulceration, cellulitis, and disability in the affected leg. Because the risk of these complications is highest in the acute thrombotic period, it is imperative to accomplish therapeutic anticoagulation quickly and safely.

An initial history and physical examination with attention to risk factors for bleeding are mandatory initial steps. Surgery within 2 weeks; recent cardiopulmonary resuscitation; recent hemorrhagic stroke; active peptic ulcer disease; and rectal, urinary, or vaginal bleeding all may preclude the use of anticoagulants or warrant rapid evaluation and therapy for the underlying condition before their use. All patients should have baseline laboratory studies including a blood cell count with platelets, prothrombin time (PT), activated partial thromboplastin time (APTT), and rectal examination with stool guaiac *before* the initiation of anticoagulation. Use of these screening tests is important to rule out preexisting anemia, thrombocytopenia, or underlying coagulopathy. Initiating anticoagulation in unscreened patients is dangerous. After performing the history and physical examination, obtaining screening laboratory test results, and making the diagnosis of VTE with US, anticoagulation can be started.

The treatment of VTE requires the use of heparin to stop the clotting process and the vitamin K antagonist warfarin (Coumadin) to prevent further clotting. For decades, intravenous unfractionated heparin (UFH) has been the drug of choice for rapid anticoagulation. Recently, the fractionated or low molecular weight heparins (LMWHs) have arrived in the United States and gained approval from the Food and Drug Administration (FDA) for a multitude of thrombotic indications (Table 1). Whether UFH or LMWH is chosen, the physician must understand that the primary role of these agents is to "bridge" the patient to warfarin and not to replace it.

Thrombolysis

For the vast majority of patients, thrombolysis is not necessary. Patients with PE and hypotension or massive iliofemoral thrombosis are candidates for thrombolytic therapy. The risk of intracranial hemorrhage with thrombolysis is 2% to 3%. Thrombolytics have not been shown to improve survival when compared with routine anticoagulation with heparin and warfarin.

The Heparins

Unfractionated Heparin

The use of a dosing adjustment normogram for intravenous UFH is strongly recommended. Dosing normograms allow the physician to achieve a therapeutic APTT in 80% of patients by 24 hours and 90% of patients by 48 hours. The ability to achieve therapeutic anticoagulation with UFH in patients who are dosed without normograms is less satisfactory. Failure to achieve therapeutic anticoagulation in the first 24 hours will increase the risk of recurrence or extension of VTE significantly. After starting intravenous heparin, APTT testing should be performed 4 to 6 hours after beginning the heparin drip and then every 6 hours until therapeutic. Once a therapeutic APTT has been achieved, all patients should be tested at least daily.

It is important for each hospital to establish its own therapeutic APTT range for UFH. This is necessary because of differences in reagents and techniques for measuring the APTT (similar to the problems that require the use of the International Normalized Ratio [INR] rather than the PT). Therapeutic APTT values should be equivalent to plasma heparin concentrations of 0.2 to 0.4 U/mL by protamine titration assay. Clinicians should be familiar with the specified therapeutic range for heparin in their hospital. The use of fixed APTT ratios to guide UFH dosing (i.e., 1.5–2.5 times control) may not reflect therapeutic heparin levels. The therapeutic range for the APTT may vary from hospital to hospital and can change when a laboratory obtains new reagents.

TABLE 1. **FDA-Approved Indications for Low Molecular Weight Heparin in Venous Thromboembolism Treatment and Prophylaxis***

Indication	Dalteparin (Fragmin)	Enoxaparin (Lovenox)	Tinzaparin (Innohep)
Venous thromboembolism treatment	No	Yes	Yes
Hip replacement	Yes	Yes	No
Knee replacement	No	Yes	No
Abdominal surgery	Yes	Yes	No

*As of 12/2000.

TABLE 2. **Comparison of Low Molecular Weight Heparin and Unfractionated Heparin**

	LMWH	UFH
Duration of Action	Prolonged, 4–6 hours SQ	Short, minutes IV
Dosing	Predictable dose response, qd or bid SQ	Unpredictable dose response, IV
Laboratory Monitoring	Unnecessary	Required
Heparin-Induced Thrombocytopenia	Rare	Up to 3% of patients
Osteoporosis	Rare	Up to 5% of patients
Bleeding in Venous Thromboembolism	Major bleeding: 0–3% Fatal bleeding: 0–0.8%	Major bleeding: 0–7% Fatal bleeding: 0–2%
Reversibility With Protamine	Poor	Good
Cost	High, 10–20 times UFH in the United States	Inexpensive

Abbreviations: LMWH = low molecular weight heparin; UFH = unfractionated heparin.

Low Molecular Weight Heparins

LMWHs have been used routinely in Europe and Canada for the last decade to treat VTE but have only recently begun being used in the United States. In 1996, Levine and Koopman each published separate studies in the *New England Journal of Medicine* that examined the use of LMWH to treat VTE on an outpatient basis. Each study used a different LMWH (enoxaparin [Lovenox] and nadroparin) and compared them with UFH. Recurrent VTE and major bleeding were the major endpoints analyzed. Collectively, 900 patients were randomized to either UFH in the hospital or outpatient LMWH therapy. The conclusion of these studies was that *LMWH is as safe and efficacious as UFH in the treatment of VTE* even when LMWH is used on an outpatient basis. The impact of these articles has resulted in dramatic changes in the way many physicians treat VTE. Prescriptions for LMWHs have increased, and the sales of LMWH have grown from 150 million dollars in 1997 to almost 1 billion dollars in 2000. Some authorities have predicted that UFH may disappear from the physician's armamentarium.

Advantages and Disadvantages of Low Molecular Weight Heparins. To use LMWHs one should have a basic understanding of the differences between UFH and LMWH (Table 2). The LMWHs have excellent bioavailability compared with UFH, allowing them to be given on a weight basis once or twice per day subcutaneously to achieve full anticoagulation. Unlike UFH, LMWHs do not interact significantly with plasma proteins, endothelial cells, or macrophages. These properties contribute to the simplified dosing regimen and predictable anticoagulant response of LMWH. In general, LMWHs do not require monitoring of the anticoagulant response. Disadvantages of LMWH include high cost, prolonged half-life (current treatments for bleeding complications in patients on LMWH are not satisfactory), poor reversibility with protamine, decreased renal clearance (patients with renal insufficiency/failure should be monitored with anti-Xa levels and/or expert consultation sought), and uncertainty regarding dosing in obesity (>300 lb). Many experts believe that each LMWH preparation has different clinical properties. Research is underway to define what the clinical differences among LMWHs are, if any.

Selection Criteria for Outpatient Treatment With Low Molecular Weight Heparin. Patients who were analyzed in the LMWH trials were carefully screened and followed rigorously with an algorithm for their care. In the outpatient trials mentioned previously, from 31% to 67% of patients were excluded from treatment with LMWH. Practicing clinicians will have similar difficulties in finding candidates for outpatient therapy, depending on their patients and the resources of their hospital. One should expect that from 35% to 70% of patients can be treated partially or completely as outpatients with LMWH. Physicians and hospitals would be wise to develop algorithms and care plans for management of patients with LMWH to ensure that patients are appropriate for outpatient care and receive adequate support as outpatients.

Patients with active bleeding, active peptic ulcer, or familial bleeding disorders should be excluded from outpatient LMWH treatment. The presence of concomitant conditions that suggest a need for hospitalization such as stroke, infection, cancer, or a high likelihood of noncompliance also warrant inpatient therapy with UFH or LMWH.

Patient Monitoring and Follow-Up. Patients on LMWH should be monitored carefully during their outpatient treatment (Table 3). Excellent doctor-patient-hospital-clinic communication is key to success-

TABLE 3. **Monitoring of Outpatient Management of Venous Thromboembolism**

	Day							
Management Method	*0*	*1*	*2*	*3*	*4*	*5*	*6*	*7*
History and physical examination	•							
Complete blood cell count	•							
Platelets	•				•			•
PT/PTT	•							
INR	•		•	•	•	•	•	•
Creatinine	•							
Warfarin and LMWH education	•							
Clinic visit or phone call	•		•	•	•	•	•	•

Abbreviations: INR = International Normalized Ratio; LMWH = low-molecular weight heparin; PT/PTT = prothrombin time/partial thromboplastin time.

ful outpatient therapy. Outpatient therapy for VTE should be avoided unless a system of care is in place. The LMWH management team should supervise the patient's management from diagnosis until discontinuation of LMWH and transfer of care to the primary physician.

The INR should be measured daily for the first 1 to 2 weeks and platelet counts checked twice weekly. We recommend having the patient visit the office or an anticoagulation clinic daily or every other day during LMWH therapy to check for bleeding or VTE recurrence, to reinforce the treatment regimen, and to confirm that the patient has adequate supplies of warfarin and LMWH. All patients should be treated for at least 5 days with concomitant UFH/LMWH and warfarin. Monitoring of LMWH with anti-Xa levels is generally unnecessary and not recommended except in children and those with cachexia, obesity (>300 lb), pregnancy, and renal insufficiency (creatinine ≥2.0 mg/dL or creatinine clearance <30 mL/min). Monitoring of LMWH is accomplished by measuring the anti-Xa level in blood. Most authorities believe that the anti-Xa level is an imperfect method of monitoring the anticoagulant effect of LMWH, but it is the only available test at this time. The therapeutic range for LMWH in VTE has not been definitively described. Many major centers report the therapeutic range of anti-Xa levels to be 0.5 to 1.0 IU/mL, measured 4 to 6 hours after the last injection.

Dosing of Low Molecular Weight Heparin in Renal Insufficiency. LMWH is cleared primarily by the kidney. Anti-Xa levels can rise dangerously in patients with renal dysfunction. In general, one should avoid treating patients who have renal insufficiency/failure with LMWH. If LMWH therapy is required in patients with renal compromise, expert consultation should be obtained to ensure appropriate dosage and monitoring.

Osteoporosis and Unfractionated Heparin/ Low Molecular Weight Heparin

Long-term use of UFH should be avoided due to the 30% risk of loss of bone density that has been described after greater than 1 month of UFH. Symptomatic osteoporosis probably occurs in less than 5% of patients on long-term UFH/LMWH. Long-term use of LMWH for VTE has not been widely studied, but the risk of osteopenia appears to be significantly lower than with UFH. In a study of patients comparing prophylactic doses of UFH with LMWH, the incidence of osteoporosis was 17.6% for UFH and 2.6% for LMWH.

Economic Considerations in Outpatient Management of Venous Thromboembolism

Analysis of cost savings using LMWH on an outpatient basis has shown that the average number of hospital days can be decreased by 40% to 83%. Medical costs may be reduced up to 64%. Many patients will require brief hospital admission to determine the severity of their illness and co-morbidity, accomplish anticoagulation education, guarantee a source for LMWH, and schedule adequate follow-up.

Reimbursement for LMWH can pose a problem because some insurance plans will not pay for outpatient drug therapy (Medicare). Patients should never be discharged from the hospital until resources for LMWH are ensured. The cost of LMWH is roughly 10 to 20 times the cost of UFH in the United States. Few patients can afford to pay for 1 week of LMWH at retail price. Cost savings and decreased hospital days will vary depending on the hospital and the population. Hospitalization is indicated if administration of injections, visits to the outpatient clinic, regular INR measurements, on-call service for emergencies, and good patient education cannot be performed in the outpatient setting.

Complications of Fractionated and Unfractionated Heparins

Bleeding With Unfractionated Heparin/ Low Molecular Weight Heparin

In a review of 10 studies comparing UFH to LMWH for treatment of VTE major bleeding was reported in 0 to 7% of patients on UFH and fatal bleeding occurred in 0 to 2%. In the same comparison, rates of major bleeding with LMWH were from 0 to 3% of patients and fatal bleeding was 0 to 0.8%. Most authorities believe that the risk of bleeding with LMWH is similar to that of UFH. The risks of bleeding with LMWH may be harder to appreciate clinically because patients do not have intravenous lines and are often treated outside the hospital. Careful screening of patients, appropriate dosing, and close follow-up will help to minimize complications of LMWH therapy.

Reversal of Unfractionated Heparin or Low Molecular Weight Heparin

Unfractionated heparin is relatively easy to manage in the event of bleeding and excessive anticoagulation. Its half-life is approximately 60 minutes, and therefore discontinuing the intravenous drip will allow its effects to wear off rapidly. Protamine can be used in clinical situations where rapid reversal of UFH is necessary, such as bypass surgery or uncontrollable hemorrhage. Bleeding with LMWH is problematic because its anticoagulant effects can last for 12 to 24 hours after the last injection. In addition, LMWH is incompletely neutralized with protamine. Unfortunately, there is no satisfactory treatment for excessive anticoagulation with LMWH at this time, and protamine is the only recourse.

Heparin-Induced Thrombocytopenia

The Heparin-Induced Thrombocytopenia (HIT) syndrome is an immune disease in which antibodies develop against heparin-platelet factor 4 (PF4) complexes. Complications of HIT include thrombocytopenia and thrombosis. HIT can be precipitated by therapeutic or prophylactic doses of UFH/LMWH and even from heparin flushes. HIT can be a very serious clinical complication, with a 25% to 30% mortality rate. Venous or arterial thrombosis is seen in 35% of patients. Up to 25% of patients with thrombosis require limb amputation.

HIT should be suspected whenever the platelet count falls or thrombosis occurs in spite of therapeutic anticoagulation. All patients on UFH or LMWH should be monitored for HIT by checking the platelet count two to three times per week for the first 3 weeks and then monthly for the duration of treatment. The frequency of HIT with UFH is 1% to 3%. The risk of HIT with LMWH is considerably lower at 0.1% to 0.3%. A fall in the platelet count of 30% to 50% from baseline or occurrence of thrombosis in spite of therapeutic anticoagulation with UFH or LMWH suggests HIT and should prompt a hematology consultation. Rarely, HIT without a fall in the platelet count has been described in patients. If HIT is suspected, UFH or LMWH should be discontinued immediately and a different form of anticoagulation substituted. The platelet count should rise within 5 to 7 days once heparin is discontinued. *LMWH cannot be substituted for UFH in the HIT syndrome* because there is a high incidence of antibody cross-reactivity. Direct thrombin inhibitors such as lepirudin (ReFludan) or argatroban (Acova) are acceptable alternative agents to substitute for UFH or LMWH in patients with HIT who require continued anticoagulation. Both drugs have been approved by the FDA for this indication. Danaparoid (Orgaran) is another potential replacement for UFH or LMWH in HIT.

Warfarin

The transition from UFH or LMWH to warfarin (Coumadin) requires a minimum of 4 to 5 days for patients to become fully anticoagulated with warfarin. The delay for complete warfarin anticoagulation occurs because the coagulation proteins affected by warfarin (VII, IX, X, II, protein C, and protein S) have different half-lives. Factor VII and protein C (an endogenous anticoagulant) fall within hours, but factor II (thought to be primarily responsible for the antithrombotic effect of warfarin) is not fully suppressed until days 4 to 5. Warfarin can safely be given on the first day of UFH or LMWH. The use of loading doses is discouraged because higher doses will not shorten the amount of time it takes for a patient to become fully anticoagulated (minimum of 4–5 days). In addition, the use of loading doses increases the incidence of excessive anticoagulation and may cause a hypercoagulable state from a rapid decline in protein C.

The INR is the appropriate test to use for warfarin monitoring. The PT and PT ratio are not dependable measurements of warfarin anticoagulation. *The therapeutic INR for VTE is 2.0 to 3.0.* The target INR should therefore be 2.5. The practice of maintaining INR values at less than the therapeutic range in VTE to avoid bleeding cannot be recommended. Subtherapeutic INR values increase the risk of VTE recurrence. In the antiphospholipid antibody syndrome, the therapeutic INR range is 2.5 to 3.5.

Average warfarin dosage to achieve therapeutic anticoagulation for VTE in patients younger than 60 is 5 mg/d. Elderly patients require a lower dose because of decreased liver metabolism. In practice, it will often require 7 to 10 days to achieve therapeutic oral anticoagulation with warfarin.

The INR should be therapeutic for 2 consecutive days before stopping UFH or LMWH therapy. Heparin or LMWH should not be discontinued early in the event that the INR becomes "therapeutic" on days 2 to 5. This is because the anticoagulant effect of warfarin precedes the antithrombotic effect and can deceive the clinician observing an early increase in the INR. The INR primarily reflects factor VII inactivation (i.e., the anticoagulant response) and therefore may increase long before levels of factors IX, X, and II have fallen. Failure to maintain anticoagulation with UFH or LMWH for 4 to 5 days concomitantly with warfarin will increase the patient's risk for extension, recurrence, PE, and death.

Warfarin can safely be given on the same day that heparin or LMWH therapy is begun. Delaying initiation of warfarin can prolong hospitalization or increase the number of days that a patient requires LMWH.

Risk of Bleeding With Warfarin

Bleeding is the most common and feared side effect of warfarin. Reports of major bleeding risk in VTE vary from 3% to 5% per year in modern studies. Risk is dependent on the anticoagulation intensity, quality of anticoagulation monitoring, physician/patient education, and patient characteristics such as age and co-morbidity. The number of drugs that interact with warfarin is staggering. The most common drugs that increase the INR are antibiotics. However, many other drugs interact with warfarin; therefore, physicians should always consult the literature before adding new agents to warfarin therapy. Whenever drugs that interact with warfarin are added or removed from a patient's regimen, the INR should be monitored more closely for several weeks. *The risk of bleeding increases significantly when the INR exceeds 4 to 5.* Patients whose INR has risen above 4 to 5 should be reevaluated every 24 to 72 hours and have their dosage adjusted carefully. Oral vitamin K in small doses (1.0 to 5.0 mg) safely and effectively reverses warfarin without complicating reestablishment of anticoagulation.

Duration of Warfarin Anticoagulation

Duration of anticoagulation therapy with warfarin (Table 4) is dictated by the presence or absence of reversible risk factors, such as surgery or trauma, and risk factors that are chronic, such as previous history of VTE or thrombophilia. Patients whose thrombosis occurred after trauma or surgery should be anticoagulated for 3 months with warfarin. In patients with an initial episode of idiopathic VTE, warfarin anticoagulation should be maintained for 6

TABLE 4. **Duration of Warfarin Anticoagulation in Venous Thromboembolism**

First episode of idiopathic VTE	6 months
Reversible or time-limited risk factors such as surgery or trauma	3–6 months
Recurrent VTE or continuing risk factors such as cancer, inhibitor deficiency states, or antiphospholipid antibody syndrome	Indefinite/lifelong
Homozygous factor V Leiden *or* heterozygous factor V Leiden with additional thrombophilic conditions	Indefinite/lifelong
Calf vein thrombosis	3 months

Abbreviation: VTE = venous thromboembolism.

months. Recurrent VTE should be treated indefinitely or throughout the patient's life. The presence of underlying, chronic risk factors complicating an initial VTE such as ongoing cancer, antiphospholipid antibody syndrome, or homozygous factor V Leiden, antithrombin III, protein C, or protein S deficiency requires indefinite or lifelong anticoagulation. A first episode of VTE in patients with heterozygous factor V Leiden deficiency *and* additional thrombophilic conditions also should be treated indefinitely or throughout the patient's life. Until recently, calf vein thrombosis was not treated with anticoagulation, but the recognition that 20% to 30% of calf VTE propagate to proximal veins has led to the recommendation that calf vein thrombosis should be treated for 3 months.

The use of follow-up US studies to determine or adjust the duration of anticoagulation is not supported by the literature and is costly.

Vascular Support Stockings

The majority of patients with VTE will benefit from vascular support stockings after hospital discharge and improvement of the initial edema. The stockings should be fitted when the edema is at its least severe (early in the morning when the patient has ambulated minimally). Patients should use these stockings during waking hours as long as they have symptoms of the postphlebitic syndrome.

PRECAUTIONS IN THERAPY OF VENOUS THROMBOEMBOLISM

Use of Nonsteroidal Anti-inflammatory Drugs or Acetylsalicylic Acid With Anticoagulants

In general, the use of acetylsalicylic acid (ASA) and nonsteroidal anti-inflammatory drugs (NSAIDs) is strongly discouraged during therapy with UFH, LMWH, or warfarin because of increased bleeding risk. These agents should be avoided except ASA in patients with documented coronary artery disease. The cyclooxygenase (COX)-2 inhibitors (celecoxib [Celebrex] and rofecoxib [Vioxx]) may possess a higher degree of safety, but this issue has not been studied.

Spinal/Epidural Anesthesia

Epidural or spinal hematoma resulting in paralysis is a devastating complication of neuraxial anesthesia/analgesia and anticoagulant therapy. The risk of neuraxial bleeding is increased with neuraxial instrumentation and anticoagulants, NSAIDs, platelet inhibitors, and traumatic or repeated epidural/spinal puncture. Clinicians should keep this caution in mind whenever patients undergo anticoagulation to avoid preventable injury to patients. Physicians can refer to the American Society of Regional Anesthesia (ASRA) 1998 consensus statement for guidance in the safe use of anticoagulants and neuraxial anesthesia.

Inferior Vena Cava Filters

The efficacy of introducing a filter in the inferior vena cava (IVC) to prevent embolism is uncertain. Only one randomized, controlled trial has been performed to define the utility of this therapy. This report compared the incidence of PE in 400 patients with VTE who were treated with anticoagulation and randomized to filter or no filter. The study showed that although PE was decreased in the first 2 weeks after the initial event, the overall mortality was unchanged and recurrent VTE was increased in the filter group after 2 years. In the absence of evidence-based data to guide the use of these devices, our suggestion is to use them only in patients with absolute contraindications to anticoagulation or in patients who have failed therapeutic anticoagulation. If possible, patients who receive filters should be anticoagulated afterward for the standard recommended duration for their respective thromboembolic event to prevent recurrence and postphlebitic syndrome in the extremities (filters do not prevent recurrence). Lifelong anticoagulation of patients with IVC filters is not required simply on the basis of the filter itself.

VENOUS THROMBOEMBOLISM IN PREGNANCY

Warfarin is contraindicated during pregnancy because it can induce fetal abnormalities. Active metabolites of warfarin are not expressed in mother's milk; therefore, warfarin can be used in nursing mothers (not FDA approved). LMWH is increasingly being used in pregnancy because of its ease of administration and decreased need for monitoring compared with UFH. However, LMWH is not FDA approved for use during pregnancy. LMWH does not cross the placenta, does not enter the fetal circulation, has no teratogenic effects, and is safe during breast feeding. The need for monitoring of anti-Xa levels during pregnancy is uncertain. During pregnancy, body mass and glomerular filtration rate increase. Studies have shown conflicting results regarding the need for monitoring. Until this controversy can be resolved, it is prudent to check the anti-Xa level at the beginning of therapy and at monthly intervals thereafter. Anti-Xa levels should be drawn 4 to 6 hours after subcutaneous injection of LMWH. Platelet counts should be checked twice a week for the first 3 weeks and then at monthly intervals during pregnancy to monitor for HIT. Ideally, LMWH should be stopped 24 to 48 hours before delivery and the patient switched to UFH until 12 to 24 hours before she gives birth. The use of protamine to reverse anticoagulation if delivery is emergent is a consideration, but the drug can have serious side effects, such as hypotension and allergic reactions. In addition, protamine does not reliably reverse LMWH. After delivery, patients should be treated with UFH or LMWH and converted to warfarin for a final 6 weeks of anticoagulation. Prolonging anticoagulation for more than 6 weeks after delivery may be indicated if the VTE occurred in the second or third trimester or was life threatening.

EVALUATION FOR THROMBOPHILIA

Thrombophilia is an inherited disposition to venous or arterial thrombosis. The most common changes include (1) structural changes in the coagulation proteins or changes in serum levels of the proteins (protein C and protein S, antithrombin III deficiency, factor V Leiden), (2) antibodies to phospholipid surfaces on which thrombi are assembled (antiphospholipid antibody syndrome), and (3) alteration in the levels of intrinsic vitamin cofactors that affect vascular endothelium (hyperhomocysteinemia). Fifty percent of VTE can now be explained on the basis of these inherited risk factors. Heterozygous factor V Leiden (activated protein C resistance) is the most common inherited defect.

Our recommendation is to test all patients younger than the age of 50 with unexplained thrombosis, recurrent thrombosis, or thrombosis in unusual sites (e.g., cerebral, mesenteric, renal) and anyone with a strong family history of VTE. Protein C or protein S and antithrombin III testing should not be performed in the perithrombotic period because these factors are consumed in acute VTE and laboratory assays can be altered with anticoagulation. Levels obtained during an acute VTE or while patients are anticoagulated may be low but not representative of deficiency. In general, testing should be performed 2 to 4 weeks after the patient has finished treatment with warfarin. If levels obtained at presentation (before initiating anticoagulation) are normal, then factor deficiency has been excluded.

PROPHYLAXIS OF VENOUS THROMBOEMBOLISM

The risk of VTE from many surgical procedures and medical illnesses varies from minimal to high. Prophylactic therapy is relatively safe, easy to administer, and inexpensive, so the benefit is high. Use of anticoagulant prophylaxis is dictated by the risk category of the patient (Table 5).

TABLE 5. **Prophylaxis of Venous Thromboembolism**

Orthopedic Surgery	
Knee replacement	Warfarin INR 2–3 or LMWH
Hip replacement	Warfarin INR 2–3 or LMWH
Hip fracture	Warfarin INR 2–3 or LMWH
General Surgery	
Selected very high-risk general surgery	Consider postdischarge LMWH or perioperative warfarin (INR 2.0–3.0)
Very high-risk general surgery with multiple risk factors	LDUH or LMWH combined with ES or IPC
Higher risk general surgery in patients with greater than usual risk of bleeding	Mechanical prophylaxis with ES or IPC
Higher risk general surgery*	LDUH, LMWH, or IPC
Moderate-risk general surgery patients†	LDUH, LMWH, ES, or IPC
Low-risk general surgery patients‡	Early ambulation
Trauma	LMWH
Neurosurgery	
High risk	IPC and/or ES with LMWH or LDUH
Acute spinal cord injury	LMWH
General neurosurgery	IPC with or without ES
Urologic Surgery	
Highest risk	ES plus or minus IPC, with LDUH or LMWH
Major open procedures	LDUH, ES, IPC, or LMWH
Transurethral or other low-risk procedure	Early ambulation
Gynecologic Surgery	
Extensive surgery for malignancy	LDUH TID
Major procedures for benign disease, without additional risk factors for thrombosis	LDUH BID
Brief procedures for benign disease	Early ambulation
Medical Patients	
General medical patients with risk factors for VTE (cancer, bedrest, CHF, or severe lung disease)	LDUH or LMWH
Acute myocardial infarction	LDUH or therapeutic IV UFH
Ischemic stroke	LDUH, LMWH, or danaparoid

*Higher-risk general surgery patients are those having nonmajor surgery over the age of 60 years or with additional risk factors or patients undergoing major surgery over the age of 40 years or with additional risk factors.

†Moderate-risk general surgery patients are those undergoing minor procedures but have additional thrombosis risk factors, those having nonmajor surgery between the ages of 40 and 60 years with no additional risk factors, or those undergoing major operations who are younger than 40 years with no additional clinical risk factors.

‡Low-risk general surgery patients are those undergoing minor surgery in patients <40 y with no additional risk factors.

Abbreviations: CHF = congestive heart failure; ES = elastic stockings; IPC = intermittent pneumatic compression; LDUH = low dose unfractionated heparin (5000 U SQ q8–12h); LMWH = low molecular weight heparin; UFH = unfractionated heparin; VTE = venous thromboembolism.

RESOURCES

The American College of Chest Physicians Consensus on Anticoagulation Therapy is published every 2 to 3 years (Chest, 119[1 suppl], 2001) and is a superior source of state-of-the-art and evidence-based recommendations on anticoagulation.

Section 5

The Blood and Spleen

APLASTIC ANEMIA

method of
ADRIANNA VLACHOS, M.D., and
JEFFREY M. LIPTON, M.D., PH.D.
Albert Einstein College of Medicine at the Long Island Jewish Medical Center
New Hyde Park, New York

Aplastic anemia, broadly defined as tri-lineage bone marrow failure, may be either acquired or constitutional. The appropriate treatment requires the distinction between and within these two broad nosologic groups (Table 1). Over the past decade, sophisticated immunologic and molecular techniques have greatly expanded our knowledge of the pathophysiology of bone marrow failure, but these disorders are still only incompletely understood.

ACQUIRED APLASTIC ANEMIA

Definition

Severe aplastic anemia is defined as peripheral pancytopenia with two of three of the following values:

1. Absolute neutrophil count (ANC) less than 500/mm^3
2. Platelet count less than 20,000/mm^3
3. Reticulocyte count less than 1% (corrected for the degree of anemia)

accompanied by a bone marrow cellularity, as determined by bone marrow biopsy, of less than 25% of normal.

The extent of peripheral neutropenia further defines the severity of the disease. Thus, severe aplastic anemia (SAA) has been subcategorized, acknowledging the particularly poor prognosis of patients with an ANC less than 200/mm^3, to include "very severe aplastic anemia." The range from "mild" to "moderate" aplastic anemia has been less precisely defined but generally refers to less severe degrees of hematopoietic cytopenias and marrow hypoplasia.

Pathophysiology

The pathophysiology of acquired aplastic anemia is complex and incompletely understood. Exposure to environmental toxins such as drugs and chemicals as well as some viral infections may exert a direct deleterious effect on hematopoietic stem cells, resulting in marrow failure, or rather these agents may alter the stem cell surface, rendering them vulnerable to immune attack and hematopoietic failure. Even clonal hematopoietic disorders such as paroxysmal nocturnal hemoglobinuria and hypoplastic myelodysplastic syndrome (MDS) may respond to immunosuppressive therapy, suggesting that immune mechanisms may also play an important role in aplastic anemia associated with these disorders.

Differential Diagnosis and Evaluation

Table 1 provides a generally accepted classification of severe aplastic anemia. Although the list of secondary causes of SAA is rather extensive, the majority of cases, particularly in children, appear to be idiopathic. As mentioned, every effort should be made to distinguish acquired SAA from the constitutional or genetic disorders because treatment options as well as the necessity for genetic counseling will vary considerably.

The evaluation of a patient with marrow failure is initiated by a complete blood cell count (CBC) to demonstrate tri- or bi-lineage cytopenias. Macrocytosis, as well as other signs of stress hematopoiesis (elevated fetal hemoglobin and erythrocyte i antigen), is common, and the platelets are generally small. Patients with macrocytosis should be evaluated for folate or vitamin B_{12} deficiency. A careful history and physical examination may reveal environmental exposures, a genetic disorder, or an infectious or noninfectious systemic disease. The findings of hemorrhage; fever, oral lesions, and infection; and pallor, fatigue, tachypnea, and tachycardia as a consequence of thrombocytopenia, neutropenia, and anemia, vary based on the severity of each cytopenia. A bone marrow aspirate and biopsy, indicated when two cell lines are depressed, will rule out most infiltrative disorders, malignant and nonmalignant, as well as infectious and noninfectious systemic disorders associated with peripheral pancytopenia in the presence of a cellular marrow. The marrow must also be evaluated for cytogenetic abnormalities consistent with MDS. Bacterial and viral cultures as well as serologic and molecular techniques may be used to detect infections associated with marrow hypoplasia. Elevated serum transaminase levels may implicate non-A, non-B, and non-C hepatitis. A sedimentation rate, immunoglobulin levels, and measures of T and B cell number and function, as suggested by the history and physical examination, will rule out most immune disorders. Specific evaluation of glycosylphosphatidylinositol (GPI)-linked surface proteins (CD55 and CD59) using flow cytometry has replaced the Ham test to diagnose paroxysmal nocturnal hemoglobinuria. The physical examination, specific tests, and/or a mutation analysis of known Fanconi anemia (FA), Shwachman-Diamond syndrome (SDS), and dyskeratosis congenita genes permit the diagnosis of these constitutional aplasias, described later.

Treatment

The treatment of choice for children and young adults with acquired SAA who have a human leukocyte antigen (HLA)-matched related donor is hematopoietic stem cell transplantation (HSCT). For those patients older than 50 years of age, those with medical problems or other circumstances precluding transplantation, or those lacking an appropriately matched related donor, the treatment is immuno-

TABLE 1. **Classification of Aplastic Anemia**

Acquired Aplastic Anemia

Secondary Aplastic Anemia

Radiation
Drugs and chemicals
  Regular effects
    Cytotoxic agents
    Benzene
  Idiosyncratic reactions
    Chloramphenicol
    Nonsteroidal anti-inflammatory drugs
    Antiepileptics
    Gold
    Others
Viruses
  Epstein-Barr virus (infectious mononucleosis)
  Hepatitis (non-A, non-B, non-C hepatitis)
  Parvovirus (rare; usually transient aplastic crisis, pure red cell aplasia)
  Human immunodeficiency virus (rare; more commonly dysplasia, multifactorial marrow failure)
Immune diseases
  Eosinophilic fasciitis
  Hypoimmunoglobulinemia
  Thymoma and thymic carcinoma
  Graft-versus-host disease in immunodeficiency
Paroxysmal nocturnal hemoglobinuria
Pregnancy
Mitochondrial cytopathies

Idiopathic Aplastic Anemia

Inherited Aplastic Anemia

Fanconi anemia
Dyskeratosis congenita
Shwachman-Diamond syndrome
Reticular dysgenesis
Amegakaryocytic thrombocytopenia
Diamond-Blackfan anemia
Familial aplastic anemias
  Preleukemia (monosomy 7, etc.)
  Nonhematologic syndromes (Down, Dubowitz, Seckel)

Adapted from Young NS: Bone Marrow Failure Syndromes. Philadelphia, WB Saunders, 2000.

modulation. Patients with mild to moderate aplastic anemia should be observed for spontaneous improvement or complete resolution. Those patients who progress to SAA need to be treated accordingly. The definitive treatment of SAA should follow diagnosis as rapidly as possible.

Hematopoietic Stem Cell Transplantation

As soon as the diagnosis of SAA is suspected, patients younger than age 50 years, with potential donors, should proceed to HLA typing. Those patients with related histocompatible donors (complete HLA match or a mismatch at a single HLA-A or -B locus) should go on to HSCT as soon as possible because the risk of transplant-related morbidity and mortality increases not only with advancing age but also with a longer interval from diagnosis to transplant, multiple transfusions, and occurrence of serious infections.

Because graft rejection is the major cause of morbidity and mortality in HSCT for SAA, the pretransplant preparative regimen of cyclophosphamide (Cytoxan)* and antithymocyte globulin (Atgam/Thymoglobulin) with inclusion of cyclosporine (Sandimmune)* in the graft-versus-host-disease (GVHD) prophylaxis regimen (Table 2) is designed to be highly immunosuppressive. Even when an identical twin donor is used, a similar preparatory regimen is recommended. Long-term survival in the range of 90% can be expected with HSCT done appropriately, using histocompatible related donors. The overall risk of alternative donor transplantation precludes its use as front-line therapy for SAA at this time. However, as improved HLA typing, preparative regimens, and GVHD prophylaxis are exploited, HSCT will, no doubt, become available to a wider group of patients with SAA.

Immunomodulatory (Immunosuppressive) Therapy

Those not undergoing HSCT should proceed to immunomodulatory therapy. In the past 2 decades, since the observation that treatment with antithymocyte or antilymphocyte globulin (ATG/ALG) is effective in over half of patients with SAA, immunomodulatory (immunosuppressive) therapy based on ATG and cyclosporine* has become the treatment of choice for patients unable to undergo HSCT. The term *immunomodulatory* indicates that the action of these agents may not be strictly immunosuppressive. In addition to ATG and cyclosporine, corticosteroids, methylprednisolone (Solu-Medrol)/prednisone (Prednisone), are added to prevent serum sickness. Granulocyte-macrophage colony-stimulating factor (GM-CSF [Leukine]) or granulocyte colony-simulating factor (G-CSF [Neupogen]) is used to achieve a more rapid increment in the granulocyte counts (Table 3). Short term, the survival using this approach is in the range of 85%.

Treatment Choices and Long-Term Follow-Up

Although the short-term outcome with immunosuppressive therapy is comparable to that obtained

*Not FDA approved for this indication.

TABLE 2. **Hematopoietic Stem Cell Transplant Preparative Regimen for Severe Aplastic Anemia**

Day −5	Morning: Cyclophosphamide, 50 mg/kg IV over 1 h Afternoon: ATG, 30 mg/kg IV. First dose of ATG is given over 8 h; subsequent doses are given over 4 h.
Day −4	Morning: Cyclophosphamide, 50 mg/kg IV over 1 h Afternoon: ATG, 30 mg/kg IV. First dose of ATG is given over 8 h; subsequent doses are given over 4 h.
Day −3	Morning: Cyclophosphamide, 50 mg/kg IV over 1 h Afternoon: ATG, 30 mg/kg IV. First dose of ATG is given over 8 h; subsequent doses are given over 4 h.
Day −2	Morning: Cyclophosphamide, 50 mg/kg IV over 1 h
Day −1	Rest, cyclosporine, 10 mg/kg/d PO daily adjusted for serum levels
Day 0	Marrow infusion

Abbreviation: ATG = antithymocyte globulin.

TABLE 3. **Immunomodulatory Therapy for Severe Aplastic Anemia**

1. Antithymocyte globulin, Atgam, 20 mg/kg/d IV, or thymoglobulin, 2.0 mg/kg/d IV once daily days 1 to 8.
2. Methylprednisolone, 2 mg/kg/d IV days 1 to 8. Divide into 0.5 mg/kg/dose IV every 6 hours.
3. Prednisone taper following an 8-day course of IV methylprednisolone. On days 9 and 10, prednisone, 1.5 mg/kg/d PO to be divided into two equal daily doses. On days 11 and 12, prednisone, 1 mg/kg/d PO to be divided into two equal daily doses. On days 13 and 14, prednisone, 0.5 mg/kg/d PO to be divided into two equal daily doses. On day 15, prednisone, 0.25 mg/kg/d PO to be given in one dose.
4. GM-CSF, 250 μg/m²/d SC once daily before bedtime starting on day 5. GM-CSF is to be continued until patient has been transfusion independent for 2 months, absolute neutrophil count > 1.0×10^9/L, hematocrit ≥ 25, and platelet count ≥ 40×10^9/L. At that point, taper GM-CSF by decreasing daily dose by 50 μg/m² every 2 weeks.
5. CsA, 10 mg/kg/d PO initially starting on day 1. Divide into two equal daily doses. Serum drug levels should be monitored as needed with the first level at 72 hours post initiation of therapy. CsA dose to be adjusted to keep serum trough levels between 100 and 300 ng/mL. CsA should be continued until patient is transfusion independent and GM-CSF has been discontinued; then decrease the dose by 2.0 mg/kg every 2 weeks.

Abbreviations: CsA = cyclosporine (formerly cyclosporin A); GM-CSF = granulocyte-macrophage colony-stimulating factor.

with HLA-matched related HSCT, the decision to choose HSCT for younger patients who have a histocompatible donor is based on the result of long-term follow-up. Although there is some late mortality, due to chronic GVHD and therapy-related cancer, in patients undergoing HSCT for SAA the survival curves are relatively flat. Improved GVHD prophylaxis and safer preparative regimens should further improve these results. In contrast, the risk of clonal hematopoietic disorders—MDS, acute myeloid leukemia (AML), and paroxysmal nocturnal hemoglobinuria—is unacceptably high relative to both the short- and long-term risks of HSCT in appropriately selected patients. Those undergoing immunomodulation must be closely followed for the development of clonal disorders. In terms of alternative donor HSCT, current risks favor the use of immunomodulatory therapy in those patients with SAA who cannot receive a matched related HSCT.

Salvage Therapy

For the patient who fails HSCT, has a partial response (ANC >500/mm³, but still is red cell– and platelet transfusion–dependent) or relapses after immunomodulatory therapy, management choices include alternative donor HSCT and further immunosuppressive therapy. These choices are under evaluation. Children and teenagers for whom a fully HLA-matched unrelated donor, determined by high-resolution typing, exists are good candidates for an alternative donor HSCT. A delay in transplantation, along with the associated risk of infection and additional transfusions attendant to a second course of immune therapy, seems unwarranted in this setting. For older patients and those without a good alternative donor, preliminary data suggest that high-dose cyclophosphamide* (Table 4) may be more effective than a second course of ATG/cyclosporine/G-CSF. Androgens† and alternative cytokines† are being evaluated and should be considered experimental.

Transfusion Therapy

The risk of bleeding and symptomatic anemia must be balanced against the risk of transfusion sensitization and iron overload. Unless patients are symptomatic, transfusions of red cells and platelets should be reserved for patients with hemoglobin levels and platelet counts of 7 g/dL and 10,000/mm³, respectively. Proceeding to transplantation as rapidly as possible minimizes transfusions in patients undergoing histocompatible HSCT. To avoid sensitization to transplant antigens there should be no transfusions from blood relatives. In all patients, blood products should be leukocyte-depleted to reduce the risk of sensitization and cytomegalovirus infection. Those patients receiving chronic red cell transfusion should be followed for evidence of iron overload and chelated appropriately. The use of single-donor platelets, when available, is recommended.

Supportive Care

The antifibrinolytic agent aminocaproic acid (Amicar) can be used to reduce mucosal bleeding in thrombocytopenic patients with good hepatic and renal function. A dose of 100/mg/kg every 6 hours is used. The maximum daily dose is 24 g.

Patients receiving immunosuppressive therapy should receive *Pneumocystis carinii* prophylaxis with trimethoprim-sulfamethoxazole (Bactrim, Septra). No antibacterial prophylaxis should be administered to afebrile, neutropenic patients. Patients with fever and neutropenia should be treated with broad-spectrum antibiotic coverage. The specific therapy depends on clinical status of the patient, presence of indwelling vascular access devices, and knowledge of the local flora pending specific culture results and antibiotic sensitivities. In patients who remain febrile for from 4 to 7 days, in the presence of broad antibacterial coverage, antifungal therapy with am-

*Not FDA approved for this indication.
†Investigational drug in the United States.

TABLE 4. **High-Dose Cyclosphosphamide Salvage Therapy for Severe Aplastic Anemia**

1. Cyclosphamide,* 45 mg/kg/d IV × 4 days
2. Mesna (Mesnex),* 360 mg/m²/dose IV with cyclophosphamide, as a 3-h infusion after cyclosphosphamide, and as bolus at h 6, h 9, and h 12 following cyclophosphamide
3. GM-CSF, 250 μg/m²/d SC starting 24 h after fourth dose of cyclophosphamide and to continue until absolute neutrophil count > 10×10^9/L

*Not FDA approved for this indication.
Abbreviation: GM-CSF = granulocyte-macrophage colony-stimulating factor.

photericin B should be started empirically. Therapy should be continued until the patient is afebrile and cultures are negative or a specific organism is identified. An appropriate course of therapy is administered if an organism is identified.

FANCONI ANEMIA

FA is an autosomal recessive disorder resulting from a presumed DNA repair defect. Eight complementation groups have been identified, and thus far six FA genes have been cloned. In addition to aplastic anemia, FA patients are predisposed to MDS and AML. A variety of congenital abnormalities have been noted in 75% to 85% of FA patients. These include skeletal abnormalities, particularly upper limb, urogenital, and renal anomalies, as well as abnormal skin pigmentation and short stature.

Diagnosis

Bone marrow failure is evident by 10 years of age in over 70% of patients. Most patients have characteristic congenital anomalies or other stigmata of FA. In addition, FA patients are predisposed to AML and nonhematologic malignancies, with the risk of MDS and AML approaching 50% in patients reaching adulthood. The diagnosis of FA should be pursued in all patients with SAA because FA-associated stigmata are not always apparent. Currently, the diagnosis of FA is made by the demonstration of increased chromosomal breaks, gaps, and rearrangements in FA lymphocytes in response to exposure to a DNA cross-linking agent such as diepoxybutane or mitomycin C. Cell cycle analysis by flow cytometry, demonstrating a G_2/M phase arrest of FA lymphocytes exposed to such agents is an excellent screening tool.

The age at onset of bone marrow failure in FA varies; thus, the CBC must be followed closely. When a diagnosis is made before the onset of significant cytopenias, a CBC should be done every 4 months and more often as marrow function deteriorates. A bone marrow aspirate and biopsy are necessary to evaluate cellularity, morphology, surface markers, and cytogenetics to establish a baseline and ultimately to differentiate among SAA, MDS, and AML. A bone marrow examination should be performed approximately yearly, or more frequently as clinically indicated, to detect evolution from aplasia to MDS or AML. Treatment of aplastic anemia, based on the peripheral blood cell counts, should begin when any of the following levels are reached (earlier treatment will not prevent the development of pancytopenia): ANC less than 500/mm^3, platelet count less than 30,000/mm^3, and a hemoglobin value less than 8 g/dL. Those patients with an HLA-matched sibling donor should undergo HSCT. Those patients with no suitable donor and pancytopenia should be managed with androgens and G-CSF.

Treatment

Hematopoietic Stem Cell Transplantation

Initially, stem cell transplantation in FA patients was complicated by systemic toxicity from "standard" preparative regimens. The recognition that patients with FA are intolerant of the usual transplant doses of alkylating agents and ionizing radiation has significantly improved survival for FA patients undergoing HLA-matched related marrow or cord blood HSCT. The overall survival is 65%, with children younger than 10 years of age having a disease-free survival, with full engraftment and manageable GVHD, of approximately 85%. Most approaches use low-dose cyclophosphamide, reduced-dose thoracoabdominal radiation, and ATG. Patients with MDS or AML are given higher, yet still significantly reduced, doses of the same agents. The results, however, are poor. Patients without a suitable donor are managed medically and undergo transplant only when this treatment fails to maintain blood cell counts at the previously mentioned levels or if MDS or AML intervenes. Advances in HLA typing and donor selection, preparative regimens, supportive care, and GVHD prophylaxis have improved survival for alternative donor HSCT in FA. Successful outcome is in the range of 35% with failures due to graft rejection and increased regimen-related toxicity. New approaches using nonmyeloablative, more immunoablative preparative regimens may be beneficial and increase survival in all patients undergoing HSCT. The outcome for alternative donor HSCT will no doubt change as safer and more effective approaches are developed. Patients with FA should be enrolled in appropriate research studies whenever possible.

Medical Management

The medical management of bone marrow failure in FA consists of androgens and hematopoietic growth factors. Medical management results in hematopoietic improvement is obtained in approximately half the patients, but this is frequently short lived. The treatment of anemia is the androgen oxymetholone (Anadrol). The concomitant use of corticosteroids is not recommended. Transfusions should be minimized. The initial dose of oxymetholone is 2 mg/kg/d rounded off to the nearest half tablet (25 mg). If there is a response, the dose should be tapered to the lowest effective dose after 3 months. If after approximately 4 months there is no response, the drug should be discontinued. The main side effects are virilization, growth acceleration with premature closure of bony epiphyses, and liver abnormalities, including the development of adenomas. Liver function tests should be monitored every 2 to 3 months. A liver ultrasound and α-fetoprotein determination should be done yearly. Similar therapy is recommended for thrombocytopenia; however, it may take up to 6 months for some patients to respond. Neutropenia usually does not respond to androgen therapy. With chronic neutropenia (an ANC less than 500/mm^3), or if there are infections at higher counts, the treatment is G-CSF at an initial dose of 5 μg/kg/d. Unless a response is detected within 8 weeks the drug should be discontinued; otherwise, the dose should be tapered to the lowest effective dose on an every-other-day to biweekly schedule. Cytokine treatment should be stopped if a clonal cytogenetic abnormality is detected. Transfusion and supportive care guidelines are the same as those described for acquired SAA.

SHWACHMAN-DIAMOND SYNDROME

SDS is a rare, autosomal recessive inherited disorder characterized by exocrine pancreatic insufficiency leading to malabsorption and chronic, cyclic, or intermittent neutropenia. Other associated findings include metaphyseal dysostosis (30%), mental retardation (15%), immune dysfunction, liver disease, growth failure, renal tubular defects, insulin-dependent diabetes mellitus, myocardial fibrosis, and other rare abnormalities. Approximately 25% of patients with SDS will develop aplastic anemia, with malignant transformation in perhaps as many as 30%. The SDS gene has been mapped to 7p12–q11.

Malabsorption is treated with pancreatic enzyme replacement. However, hematopoietic sequelae are the overwhelming causes of morbidity and mortality. The treatment of the marrow failure in SDS includes growth factors, transfusions, and bone marrow transplantation. Some patients may have a transient improvement with corticosteroids. G-CSF has been used with a good response in over 90% of patients with severe chronic neutropenia, including SDS, particularly in patients with recurrent serious infections. It has also been used in cases in which the degree of neutropenia and its side effects have limited normal daily activity. The actual risk of MDS and AML in SDS, as well as the incremental risk from G-CSF, are not known. Therefore, G-CSF should be used cautiously. Close monitoring of the bone marrow status with cytogenetic analysis is imperative and should be done on a semi-annual to annual basis especially for G-CSF–treated patients. Essential information regarding the risks and benefits of G-CSF in SDS patients is being analyzed. HSCT must be approached cautiously in patients with SDS and should be done in the context of a research study.

DYSKERATOSIS CONGENITA

Dyskeratosis congenita is an X-linked or less often autosomal recessive or dominant inherited disorder characterized by the triad of abnormal skin pigmentation, nail dystrophy, and leukoplakia. Other noncutaneous congenital anomalies are commonly found. The X-linked *DKC1* gene has been cloned.

The actuarial probability of developing bone marrow failure as defined by a single or by multiple cytopenias is over 90% by 40 years of age. There is also a predisposition to MDS and AML. Two thirds of all deaths in patients with dyskeratosis congenita are a consequence of bone marrow failure. The treatment of bone marrow failure is problematic. Transient responses have been noted with oxymetholone, G-CSF and GM-CSF, and even erythropoietin (Epogen, Procrit). The only curative approach to SAA in patients with dyskeratosis congenita is HSCT. The results, in the few transplanted patients, have been poor, predominantly owing to the pulmonary complications to which patients with dyskeratosis congenita are predisposed. This is another setting in which less toxic HSCT preparative regimens are being explored.

IRON DEFICIENCY

method of
GORDON D. McLAREN, M.D.
University of California, Irvine
Irvine, California

and

VICTOR R. GORDEUK, M.D.
Howard University School of Medicine
Washington, D.C.

Iron deficiency is the most common nutritional deficiency around the world. The condition is also prevalent in the United States, particularly in women of childbearing age, as well as infants and adolescents, whose rapid growth requires an enhanced iron supply to support a concomitant increase in red cell mass. Iron deficiency occurring in men or nonmenstruating women is usually the result of blood loss, most often from the gastrointestinal tract, and the specific site and cause must be sought.

IRON METABOLISM

Most of the body's iron (which totals about 4 g in adult males and somewhat less—a little over 3 g—in adult females) is present in hemoglobin, some is in myoglobin and iron-containing enzymes, and the remainder is mainly in storage form. Under normal circumstances, storage iron amounts to 1000 mg for men and 300 mg for women, and approximately 30 to 35 mg of iron is incorporated into the hemoglobin of developing erythrocytes daily. Body iron is highly conserved in a unidirectional metabolic cycle. Iron is incorporated into hemoglobin within erythroid precursors in the bone marrow, which are subsequently released into the bloodstream as erythrocytes that circulate for about 120 days. Senescent erythrocytes are removed from the circulation at the end of their life span by cells of the mononuclear phagocyte system within the spleen, bone marrow, and liver. Iron is then liberated from hemoglobin within the macrophages, and most of this iron is released to plasma transferrin, each molecule of which can bind up to two atoms of iron. Some of the iron may be retained as ferritin and hemosiderin within macrophages, which contain most of the body's storage iron. Iron carried in the plasma as monoferric or diferric transferrin is taken up by erythroid precursors in the bone marrow via specific plasma membrane transferrin receptors for reincorporation into hemoglobin. Most of the iron required for hemoglobin production is normally provided through this recycling mechanism. Iron absorbed from the gastrointestinal tract also appears in the circulation as transferrin-bound iron and is delivered to erythroid precursors in the same way. A small amount of plasma transferrin-bound iron is transported to nonerythroid cells for incorporation into essential heme-containing proteins and other iron-dependent enzymes.

Iron Absorption

Iron is essential for the growth and homeostasis of all cells, yet free iron is oxygen reactive and is highly toxic when present in excessive amounts. Although the earth's crust contains high levels of iron, its tendency to form insoluble compounds at physiologic pH makes it difficult for organisms to acquire. The iron content of a typical diet is small, and much of it is of limited bioavailability. Even so, the amount of iron in the diet exceeds requirements, and absorption of only 5% to 10% is sufficient to replace small, normal daily losses. The two forms of dietary iron are (1) *heme iron*, contained in meat, fish, and liver, and (2) ionic *nonheme iron* in other foods. Heme iron is much more readily absorbed than nonheme iron. Vitamin C and amino acids promote the absorption of nonheme iron, whereas tea and vegetable fiber inhibit its uptake. Iron is absorbed maximally in the duodenum and upper part of the jejunum, and the presence of gastric acid helps keep nonheme iron in the soluble, ferrous (Fe^{+2}) form that is taken up better by the intestinal brush border.

Iron absorption is inversely related to both body iron stores and the rate of erythropoiesis, so absorption increases with declining stores or with elevated levels of erythropoiesis and *vice versa*. Because the body does not have an active excretory pathway for iron, this mechanism also provides a means of maintaining iron balance by limiting absorption across the mucosa. Under normal circumstances, small obligatory losses of about 1.0 mg/d occur in men mainly through desquamation of epithelial cells from the gastrointestinal tract. Obligatory loss is higher in women of childbearing age secondary to menstrual blood loss and averages about 1.5 mg/d. If iron requirements are increased over basal losses, as in the setting of rapid growth or gastrointestinal blood loss, absorption tends to increase appropriately. The mechanism of this regulation is not fully understood, but it has been demonstrated that uptake of nonheme iron across the mucosal brush border is dependent on a divalent metal transporter (DMT1), and expression of this protein is increased in iron deficiency anemia.

CAUSES AND CONSEQUENCES OF IRON DEFICIENCY

When iron requirements or iron losses exceed the quantity of iron absorbed, the individual experiences a state of negative iron balance. With this negative balance, iron stores decrease progressively and synthesis of hemoglobin is impaired after storage iron is exhausted. Lack of body iron can be divided into two categories. (1) In *iron deficiency without anemia*, storage iron is absent but the deficit in iron is not sufficiently large to decrease hemoglobin below the normal level. (2) In *iron deficiency anemia*, the deficit in iron is so severe that stores are absent and hemoglobin is below the normal range.

Infants, adolescents, and women of childbearing age may become iron deficient because of inadequate dietary iron to meet high physiologic needs. Infants 1 to 2 years of age and adolescents have increased iron requirements from the demands of rapid growth. Women need more iron as a result of the loss of hemoglobin with menstruation and the high iron demands of pregnancy. In other settings, the finding of iron deficiency almost always signifies pathologic blood loss of some sort. Populations with hookworm infestation have an increased incidence of iron deficiency because of chronic intestinal blood loss. Individuals with gastrointestinal bleeding from ulceration, tumors, diverticula, polyps, and vascular malformations are prone to iron deficiency. Both women and men who are frequent blood donors have a high prevalence of iron deficiency. Iron deficiency develops in about 50% of hemodialysis patients as a result of blood loss during the procedure and frequent blood diagnostic tests. The finding of iron deficiency should always prompt the consideration that the patient may have a gastrointestinal cancer (esophageal, gastric, and colorectal are the most common), and intensive efforts should be made to find a curable malignancy. Hemoptysis or bleeding from a bladder tumor may also lead to iron deficiency.

Iron deficiency may occur in patients with defective absorption of food iron because of tropical or nontropical sprue and other tropical enteropathies, achlorhydria, and gastric resection. The condition may develop in the setting of intravascular hemolysis with associated hemoglobinuria; paroxysmal nocturnal hemoglobinuria and anemia in long-distance runners are examples. In pulmonary hemosiderosis, alveolar hemorrhage leads to iron loading of pulmonary macrophages; because this iron cannot be used for hemoglobin synthesis, the process can result in iron deficiency anemia.

Symptoms of iron deficiency anemia include fatigue, weakness, irritability, headaches, dizziness, and dyspnea. Pica, an unusual craving for and ingestion of certain substances, is common in iron deficiency and may include consumption of ice, starch, or clay; paradoxically, starch and clay are inhibitors of iron absorption and can aggravate the deficiency. The condition is also associated with reduced worker productivity, increased maternal and fetal morbidity and mortality, and growth retardation. Even in the absence of anemia, *iron deficiency* may have adverse effects. Nonanemic children with prolonged iron deficiency in the second year of life have impaired mental and motor development at 5 years of age. In pregnancy, maternal iron deficiency may be associated with low fetal birth weight and increased prematurity. In adults with iron deficiency, a reduced capacity for strenuous work and exercise has been reported.

Physical findings of iron deficiency anemia may include pallor, koilonychia, glossitis, and angular stomatitis, and it may be possible to demonstrate the presence of an esophageal web, achlorhydria, or gastritis. Other than pallor, however, these classic manifestations of severe, long-standing iron deficiency anemia are seen less often in current practice because the diagnosis tends to be established at earlier stages of the disease, often on the basis of laboratory tests performed as part of routine health maintenance. Slight splenic enlargement of unknown etiology occurs in about 10% of patients. Alert physicians will also be on the lookout for a rectal mass, hemorrhoids, or guaiac-positive stool.

DIAGNOSIS

In iron deficiency anemia, the automated complete blood count typically reveals a decreased hematocrit and hemoglobin concentration, a low red blood cell count, and a decreased mean corpuscular volume, as well as an increased red-cell distribution width. The diagnosis of iron

TABLE 1. **Typical Changes in the Complete Blood Count With Iron Deficiency Anemia and the Anemia of Inflammation**

Condition	Degree of Anemia	Mean Corpuscular Volume	Red-Cell Distribution Width	White Blood Cells	Platelets
Iron deficiency anemia	Mild to severe	Decreased	Increased	Normal	Normal to increased
Inflammation	Mild	Normal to decreased	Normal	Normal to increased	Normal to increased

deficiency anemia is also suggested by the presence of microcytic, hypochromic erythrocytes on the peripheral blood film. In addition, the reticulocyte count is low or normal. It must be kept in mind that these indices of fully developed iron deficiency may not all be present in the early stages. The first sign of iron deficiency that becomes apparent in the automated complete blood count is an increased red-cell distribution width, a finding that reflects the onset of iron-deficient erythropoiesis, which begins even before the hemoglobin concentration has fallen below the reference range. Further evidence in support of iron deficiency is decreased serum transferrin saturation (the ratio of serum iron to total serum iron-binding capacity). Measurement of the serum ferritin concentration is the best single test for iron deficiency, and a low value is diagnostic of the condition. Iron deficiency in the absence of anemia is characterized by a low serum ferritin concentration alone.

The differential diagnosis of microcytic anemia includes iron deficiency anemia, thalassemia minor, and anemia of inflammation (the anemia of chronic disease). Thalassemia trait is common in populations that originated in the Mediterranean, Middle East, Southeast Asia, and Africa. It is important to make the distinction between thalassemia trait and iron deficiency because iron therapy should not be given if iron deficiency is not present. Other causes of microcytic hypochromic anemia include lead poisoning and hereditary sideroblastic anemia. It is commonly necessary to distinguish between iron deficiency and the anemia of inflammation, which is often seen in association with chronic infection, disseminated neoplasia, or collagen vascular diseases such as rheumatoid arthritis. Table 1 summarizes changes in the complete blood count in the two conditions.

Transferrin saturation is not a reliable test for iron deficiency in the presence of acute and chronic inflammation because serum iron may be decreased in these circumstances, even when iron stores are replete. Transferrin saturation is also affected by diurnal variation in that it is higher in the morning and lower in the evening, so measurements performed on blood samples obtained later in the day may provide spuriously low values. The diagnostic problem can be further complicated by the fact that serum ferritin is a positive acute and chronic phase reactant and may be elevated into the normal range in patients having both iron deficiency and an inflammatory process or hepatic damage. In such situations, bone marrow examination may be necessary to assess iron stores directly. An absence of stainable iron establishes the diagnosis of iron deficiency. The serum transferrin receptor concentration can also be useful in diagnosing iron deficiency in patients with inflammatory disorders. The expression of transferrin receptors on the surface of red blood cells is inversely proportional to the intracellular iron concentration, and a portion of the receptor is proteolytically cleaved and released to the plasma. The production of transferrin receptors is not influenced by inflammation, and an increased serum level is an early indicator of iron depletion. Determination of the transferrin receptor level (or the receptor-ferritin ratio) can thus be used to detect iron deficiency even in the presence of inflammation and may obviate the need for bone marrow examination in this setting. Changes in indirect measures of iron status in iron deficiency and inflammation are summarized in Table 2.

TREATMENT

In the management of iron deficiency, it is critical that the cause be identified and corrected. Iron deficiency in men or nonmenstruating women is most often the result of gastrointestinal blood loss, and an occult malignancy may be identified and treated while curable if the first step in the management of iron deficiency is to identify the cause of the lack of iron. The treatment of choice for iron deficiency is almost always an oral iron preparation, which effectively replenishes iron stores in the vast majority of cases. A parenteral iron preparation is rarely indicated except in certain special situations. Correction of anemia is not usually urgent, and blood transfusion should be avoided unless the anemia is so severe that it causes cardiorespiratory embarrassment. If necessary, packed red blood cells should be adminis-

TABLE 2. **Typical Changes in Measures of Iron Status in Iron Deficiency and Inflammation**

Condition	Serum Iron	Total Iron-Binding Capacity	Transferrin Saturation	Serum Ferritin	Transferrin Receptors
Iron deficiency	Decreased	Increased	Decreased	Decreased	Increased
Inflammation	Decreased	Decreased	Decreased	Normal to increased	Normal

tered cautiously with appropriate monitoring of hemodynamic status and use of a potent diuretic.

Oral Iron Therapy

For many years, the most widely recommended oral iron agent has been ferrous sulfate, which is inexpensive, well absorbed, and generally well tolerated. However, many patients do suffer side effects, including nausea and epigastric pain occurring 30 minutes to an hour after ingestion, presumably related to the amount of ionic iron in the upper gastrointestinal tract, as well as constipation and diarrhea, although the latter are not dose related. All tablets containing iron salts such as ferrous sulfate must be kept out of the reach of young children because iron ingestion is a common cause of poisoning. In fact, iron-containing supplements are the leading cause of pediatric poisoning deaths in the United States. As few as 10 adult-sized ferrous sulfate tablets can prove fatal for an infant. For these reasons, we prefer to instead treat iron deficiency with *carbonyl iron*, a safer type of iron preparation than iron salts, as described later. Because many physicians use iron salts to treat iron deficiency, the approach to therapy with ferrous sulfate is reviewed here.

Iron Salts

In the treatment of iron deficiency anemia with ferrous sulfate, the usual adult dose is one 300-mg tablet three to four times daily (300 mg ferrous sulfate = 60 mg elemental iron). The pediatric dose is 5 mg/kg of elemental iron per day, in tablet or elixir form, in three divided doses. Iron is best absorbed when taken on an empty stomach. Iron absorption is enhanced in patients with iron deficiency anemia, and this condition initially facilitates the assimilation of medicinal iron, although absorption declines with correction of the anemia and reaccumulation of iron stores. Oral iron therapy usually raises the hemoglobin concentration to normal levels within 4 to 8 weeks at the rate of about 1 g/dL per week. Treatment should be continued for an additional 3 to 6 months to replenish iron stores, as indicated by a return of the serum ferritin concentration to a normal range (50 to 100 μg/L), at which time iron therapy should be discontinued. If upper gastrointestinal symptoms limit compliance, the medication can be administered with food or the dose reduced. One 300-mg ferrous sulfate tablet nightly at bedtime is effective therapy, although it may be necessary to continue treatment for two to three times as long to achieve the same effect as with full doses. The addition of ascorbic acid to the regimen enhances absorption but also increases the side effects. A large number of other types of iron salts have been studied and developed to identify preparations that are better absorbed or associated with fewer side effects, but these products generally do not offer significant improvement and are often more expensive. Patients who are not severely anemic can be treated with ferrous gluconate, which contains somewhat less elemental iron and is therefore less likely to cause side effects.

Carbonyl Iron

More recently, a new approach to iron repletion has become available with the identification of carbonyl iron as an effective therapy for iron deficiency. This iron preparation is a bioavailable form of elemental iron that has long been used for iron fortification of foods. It has a considerable advantage over iron salts in terms of safety because it is markedly less toxic and carries a much lower risk of poisoning in children. For these reasons, carbonyl iron is our first choice for oral iron therapy. We recommend the administration of 150 mg daily in three divided doses of 50 mg each. Carbonyl iron has an efficacy similar to that of other oral iron preparations in correcting iron deficiency, and the same principles outlined earlier for evaluating the response to therapy with iron salts are applicable to treatment with carbonyl iron. Some patients notice a metallic taste during carbonyl iron therapy. Iron deficiency anemia can be treated effectively with lower total daily doses of carbonyl iron (50 to 100 mg), but a longer duration of therapy may be needed at these doses to achieve iron repletion.

Parenteral Iron Therapy

In patients who fail to respond to oral iron therapy, the most common reason is poor compliance as a result of gastrointestinal side effects, which may cause the patient to refuse further treatment. In many cases, iron therapy can be resumed after discussion with the patient about ways to minimize symptoms by reducing the dose and taking the medication with food, as noted before. Rarely, patients may have a true inability to absorb iron, most often as a result of previous gastrectomy or celiac disease.

Until recently, the only parenteral iron preparation available in the United States has been iron dextran (InFeD). Iron dextran, whether given intramuscularly or intravenously, does not lead to a more rapid hematologic response than oral iron and carries the risk of anaphylactic reactions. The presence of iron deficiency must be rigorously proved before embarking on parenteral iron therapy, for its administration to patients with other forms of anemia can lead to iron overload. Two forms of parenteral iron are now available in the United States, iron dextran and sodium ferric gluconate complex. Each of these preparations will be considered separately.

Iron Dextran

Each 1 mL of iron dextran injection, U.S. Pharmacopeial Convention (USP), contains the equivalent of 50 mg of elemental iron (as an iron dextran complex). Some patients receiving parenteral iron dextran therapy experience severe allergic reactions, including anaphylaxis, and all patients should be monitored carefully. The manufacturer recommends that the maximum daily dose of iron dextran not exceed

2.0 mL of undiluted iron dextran (100 mg of elemental iron). The preparation should be used with extreme care in patients with serious impairment in liver function, and it should not be given during acute infection of the kidney. Before administering iron dextran, the total dose needed to both correct anemia and replace storage iron should be calculated according to the following formula:

Iron to Be Injected (mg) = (15 − Patient's Hemoglobin [g/dL]) × Body Weight (kg) × 3

For adults, this total amount of iron should be divided into 100-mg (2.0-mL) increments and administered daily either intramuscularly or intravenously until the total calculated amount is given. For children, smaller daily doses are used. Before starting therapy, a small test dose of 0.5 mL (25 mg) should be given to exclude the possibility of an allergic response. Although anaphylactic reactions after iron dextran administration are known to occur within a few minutes or sooner, it is recommended that at least 1 hour be allowed to elapse before the remainder of the initial therapeutic dose is given. The physician must be immediately available during this observation period, and means of resuscitation (including parenteral steroids and epinephrine) must be near at hand. When administered intravenously, iron dextran should be given undiluted at a slow, gradual rate not to exceed 50 mg (1 mL) per minute. When administered intramuscularly, iron dextran should be injected only into the muscle mass of the upper outer quadrant of the buttock and injected deeply with a 2- or 3-inch, 19- or 20-gauge needle by a Z-track technique to minimize the chance of subcutaneous leakage and discoloration. Side effects include arthalgias or myalgias the day after injection, but this pain usually responds to a mild analgesic such as acetaminophen. Often, physicians consider it impractical to administer iron dextran in divided doses and instead prefer total dose infusion; however, this practice is not recommended by the manufacturer. For parenteral iron administration, many physicians now favor using ferric gluconate complex rather than iron dextran, as discussed in the next section.

Sodium Ferric Gluconate Complex

In 1999, sodium ferric gluconate (iron gluconate, Ferrlecit) received Food and Drug Administration approval for iron replacement therapy by parenteral administration. This form of iron has been available outside the United States, principally in Europe, for several decades. Most of the recent reported experience has been in combination with erythropoietin for maintenance of an adequate blood hemoglobin level in patients receiving long-term hemodialysis for end-stage renal disease. Recent clinical trials in the United States have confirmed the safety and efficacy of this approach. Iron gluconate may similarly be considered for other applications requiring parenteral iron therapy that have traditionally been treated with iron dextran. The risk of allergic reactions, including full-blown anaphylaxis, is much lower with iron gluconate than iron dextran. In a typical course of treatment for patients undergoing hemodialysis who are receiving recombinant human erythropoietin therapy, sodium ferric gluconate complex in sucrose is administered in a dose of 125 mg/dose (62.5 mg/dose in children under 40 kg) by slow intravenous infusion on 8 consecutive days for a total dose of 1.0 g (0.5 g in children). In other contexts, it is appropriate to calculate the total dose of iron to be given in the same way as outlined earlier for iron dextran. For example, an adult with a calculated deficit of 2.0 g who is to be treated with ferric gluconate complex would require 16 infusions at 125 mg/dose to deliver the required amount of iron. Such a regimen is more practical for patients being treated by maintenance hemodialysis, for whom access to the circulation is a more frequent event than it is for patients requiring iron repletion in other settings. Unfortunately, higher doses or more rapid infusion rates may be associated with side effects (hypotension, malaise) accompanied by high serum iron concentrations and transferrin saturations above 100%, thus raising the concern of possible iron toxicity. Additional clinical experience should help clarify the role for this new product in specific clinical situations.

AUTOIMMUNE HEMOLYTIC ANEMIA

method of
YORIKO SAITO, M.D.
Dana-Farber/Partners Cancer Care and
Harvard Medical School
Boston, Massachusetts

and

W. HALLOWELL CHURCHILL, M.D.
Brigham & Women's Hospital and
Harvard Medical School
Boston, Massachusetts

Autoimmune hemolytic anemias (AIHAs) are a group of disorders in which autoantibodies against antigens on the red blood cell (RBC) membrane result in diminished RBC survival in the peripheral circulation. These disorders are traditionally subdivided into warm AIHA (WAIHA) and cold AIHA (CAIHA). In the case of WAIHA, the autoantibody optimally binds to the RBC membrane at 37°C. In CAIHA, the optimal binding occurs at temperatures lower than 37°C, commonly at 0°C to 5°C. This subtype includes cold hemagglutinin disease (CHD) and paroxysmal cold hemoglobinuria (PCH).

The incidence of AIHA is estimated to be approximately 10 cases per million, with a female preponderance. Thirty percent to 50% of AIHAs are idiopathic, whereas another 30% consists of AIHAs associated with lymphoproliferative disorders, immunodeficiency states, certain solid tumors, or connective tissue disorders. AIHA associated with infectious diseases such as mycoplasma and viral and parasitic infections makes up approximately 10%. The remainder consists of drug-induced hemolytic anemia (DIHA).

The characteristics of WAIHA and CAIHA are summarized in Table 1.

The pathophysiology of DIHA involves at least four known mechanisms:

1. Hapten-induced, in which immunogenic drug binds to RBCs, which then generate antibody against the drug
2. Immune complex formation, in which an immunogenic conjugate of the drug and plasma protein forms an immune complex, which binds to RBCs
3. Formation of immunogenic drug–RBC complexes, which induce antibodies with specificities both to the drug and to RBC antigens
4. True autoantibody induction

Common drugs associated with DIHA are listed in Table 2.

PRESENTING SYMPTOMS AND PHYSICAL FINDINGS

The severity of presenting symptoms is related to the time course of the hemolysis process. Those patients with low-grade hemolysis tend to be well-adjusted to a relative anemia, and they commonly present with weakness, dizziness, jaundice, and fever, which develop over weeks to months. Less frequently, patients present with more brisk hemolysis resulting in severe symptoms related to rapidly developing anemia such as progressive fatigue, dyspnea on exertion, and, in some cases, angina. On physical examination, hepatosplenomegaly, jaundice, and lymphadenopathy can be appreciated, whereas pallor, thyromegaly, edema, and other signs of heart failure are found less commonly. It is also important to search for evidence of associated illness such as lymphoma or chronic lymphocytic leukemia because treatment of associated illness is an essential part of AIHA management.

Patients with CHD commonly present with acute or chronic manifestations of intravascular agglutination rather than that of anemia. The acute symptoms include acrocyanosis, numbness, and pain in areas exposed to lower temperatures. Symptoms may include jaundice associated with bouts of intravascular hemolysis. Chronic manifestations include atrophic skin changes and, in rare cases, severe gangrene.

Patients with PCH typically present with malaise, fatigue, myalgias, muscle cramping, headache, nausea/vomiting, diarrhea, fever/chills, and hemoglobinuria, which develop minutes to hours after exposure to cold. On physical examination, jaundice, scleral icterus, hepatosplenomegaly, and pallor are commonly found. PCH must be differentiated from paroxysmal nocturnal hemoglobinuria (PNH), which has a similar presentation. PNH is a clonal disorder of the hematopoietic stem cell resulting in a biosynthetic defect of the glycosylphosphatidylinositol (GPI) anchor. The GPI anchor links a number of membrane proteins, including complement regulatory proteins such as decay accelerating factor (DAF, CD55) and membrane inhibitor of reactive lysis (MIRL, CD59). This renders the RBCs susceptible to complement-mediated lysis, characterized by intravascular hemolysis, hemoglobinemia, and hemoglobinuria. Venous thrombotic events and the presence of variable levels of bone marrow failure also characterize this disorder.

TABLE 1. **Autoimmune Hemolytic Anemias: Classification and Characteristics**

		Cold Antibody Type/CAIHA	
	Warm Antibody Type/WAIHA (60%–70%)	*Cold Hemagglutinin Disease (15%–25%)*	*Paroxysmal Cold Hemaglobinuria (<5%)*
Etiology	Primary/idiopathic (30%–50%) Secondary to (50%–70%): Collagen vascular diseases (SLE, RA, Sjögrens, scleroderma) Lymphoproliferative disorders and neoplasms of the immune system (NHL, HD, CLL, MM, WM, thymomas) Immunodeficiency states (hypo- and dysgammaglobulinemia, Wiskott-Aldrich syndrome) Infectious diseases (post-viral syndrome, EBV, CMV, HIV, babesiosis) Post–ABO-incompatible bone marrow transplantation Others (ovarian tumors, pregnancy, ulcerative colitis)	Primary/idiopathic Secondary to: Lymphoproliferative disorders (NHL, CLL, MGUS, WM) Infectious diseases (*Mycoplasma pneumoniae*, EBV)	Primary/idiopathic Secondary to: Infectious diseases (*Escherichia coli*, *Klebsiella pneumoniae*, *Haemophilus influenzae*, *Mycoplasma pneumoniae*, influenza, chickenpox, measles, mumps, EBV, CMV, syphilis, smallpox vaccination)
Incidence	1:50,000–80,000	1:100,000–200,000	1:600,000–800,000
Antibody characteristics	polyclonal>>monoclonal IgG>>IgA, IgM	polyclonal in post-infectious CHD, otherwise monoclonal IgM>>IgG	polyclonal IgG
Antibody specificity	Rh, Kell, Kidd, phospholipids	I, I, Pr	P
Direct antiglobulin test results	40%–50% IgG alone 45%–60% IgG and C3 0%–15% C3 alone 2%–4% negative	90% C3 alone 10% IgG and C3	90% C3 alone 10% IgG and C3

Abbreviations: CAIHA = cold autoimmune hemolytic anemia; CLL = chronic lymphocytic leukemia; CMV = cytomegalovirus; EBV = Epstein-Barr virus; HD = Hodgkin's disease; MGUS = monoclonal gammopathy of undetermined significance; MM = multiple myeloma; NHL = non–Hodgkin's lymphoma; RA = rheumatoid arthritis; SLE = systemic lupus erythematosus; WAIHA = warm autoimmune hemolytic anemia; WM = Waldenstrom's macroglobulinemia.

TABLE 2. **Common Medications That Can Cause Drug-Induced Immune Hemolytic Anemia**

Hapten	Immune Complex/Antibody Against Drug–Red Blood Cell Complex	True Autoantibody Induction	Unknown Mechanism
Penicillins	Quinine	Cephalosporins	Thiazides
Cephalosporins	Quinidine	Levodopa	Erythromycin
Streptomycin	Cephalosporins (cefotetan, cefotaxime, ceftriaxone, ceftazidime)	Methyldopa	Omeprazole
Tetracyclines	Chlorpropamide	Mefenamic acid	
Tolbutamide	Nitrofurantoin	Procainamide	
	Diclofenac	Ibuprofen	
	Phenacetin	Thioridazine	
	Hydrocholorothiazide	Diclofenac	
	Rifampin		
	Sulfonamides		
	Isoniazid		
	Insulin		
	Hydralazine		
	Acetaminophen		

Patients with DIHA can present with a wide range of symptoms, corresponding with severity and rapidity of hemolysis. Drug-dependent antibody-induced hemolysis tends to be severe and abrupt intravascular and extravascular hemolysis, resulting in a more acute presentation. In some cases, a history of new medication or recent change in medication can be obtained; however, lack of such recent changes does not preclude DIHA because some medications such as methyldopa cause hemolysis after a prolonged intake.

LABORATORY DIAGNOSIS

Hematology and chemistry test results reflect those of hemolytic anemia, including hemoglobin as low as 4 to 5 g/dL in all subtypes. Peripheral blood smear shows reticulocytosis, microspherocytosis, and nucleated RBCs. Other hematopoietic lineages tend to remain normal except in cases with underlying disease affecting those lineages, such as Evans' syndrome and lymphoproliferative disorders. A bone marrow examination may be warranted when lymphoproliferative process is suspected.

Although reticulocytosis is a hallmark of hemolytic processes, some patients present with inadequate reticulocytosis due to infection, nutritional deficiency, or other causes of delayed bone marrow response to decreased RBC mass. Because the combination of ongoing hemolysis with an inappropriate bone marrow production can lead to rapid development of life-threatening anemia, patients with inadequate reticulocytosis or with reticulocytopenia should be evaluated for potential immediate RBC transfusion.

Other laboratory abnormalities include signs of both intravascular and extravascular hemolysis. Serum total bilirubin level is usually below 5 mg/dL, most of which is unconjugated (or direct) bilirubin. Serum lactate dehydrogenase levels are usually elevated. Serum haptoglobin levels are commonly significantly lower than normal. In patients who experience acute episodes of hemolysis, hemoglobinuria can occur. In severe cases, this can precipitate acute renal failure which can be complicated by disseminated intravascular coagulation (DIC)/shock.

Serologic tests are a critical element in the laboratory diagnosis of AIHA. This includes the direct antiglobulin test (DAT or direct Coombs' test) as well as tests for the presence of direct agglutinins or hemolysin in the serum of the patient. The DAT is performed by incubating the patient's RBCs with a poly-specific antiglobulin reagent that recognizes IgG, C3b, and C3d. If the RBCs are coated with autoantibodies or complement components, the addition of DAT reagent will cause the RBCs to agglutinate and or lyse, resulting in a positive test.

In addition, the eluate from the patient's RBCs may help classify the type of hemolytic anemia. The presence of complement but not immunoglobulins in the eluate suggests either CAIHA or an immune complex–mediated disease, in addition to PNH. IgG on the RBC with no specificity in the eluate can be caused by nonspecific increase in γ-globulin (i.e., in multiple myeloma or prior use of intravenous immune globulin) or by hapten-induced hemolytic anemia. The latter is extremely rare and results from not using drug-coated RBCs in testing the eluate. IgG on RBCs with specificity for a red cell antigen is usually a delayed transfusion reaction and rarely an autoantibody mimicking alloantibody specificity. These two possibilities can be distinguished by phenotyping the recipient's RBCs. The presence of IgG on the RBCs with an eluate that reacts with all RBCs almost always indicates WAIHA.

In WAIHA, affected RBCs are coated with nonagglutinating autoantibodies (IgG $\gg$ IgA, IgM) and/or complement (C3b, C3d). The positive DAT confirms the presence of antibodies and complement bound to the RBCs. However, in less than 4% of patients with WAIHA, DAT can be negative, reflecting the fact that a minority of cases involve IgA or IgM antibodies, which cannot be detected by DAT.

In some cases of WAIHA, free unbound fraction of the autoantibodies can be detected in the patient's serum by the indirect antiglobulin test (IAT or indirect Coombs' test), resulting in positive IAT as well as positive DAT. In cases where only the IAT is positive with the DAT being negative, it is likely that an alloantibody, rather than autoantibody, is causing the hemolysis.

In CHD, the causal immunoglobulins are direct agglutinins of IgM subtype, which optimally agglutinate autologous RBCs at temperatures of 0 to 5°C. The serum agglutinin titers can be as high as 1:1 million in severe cases. The DAT is positive for complement only because the cold agglutinins dissociate from the RBCs during the washing steps of DAT while the complement components remain covalently attached to the RBC cell membrane.

In PCH, the causal immunoglobulins are of an IgG subtype that binds to autologous RBCs with cold-induced complement activation, which continues at higher temperatures leading to hemolysis. These autoantibodies are called *biphasic hemolysins* or *Donath-Landsteiner antibodies.* In this case, DAT is positive for complement during a brief period following the hemolytic episode. To test for the presence of biphasic hemolysins directly, normal RBCs are mixed with the patient's serum at 4°C then warmed to 37°C and checked for hemolysis (biphasic Donath-Landsteiner test).

In PNH, the hemolysis is caused by complement activation. The demonstration of RBCs and/or granulocytes lacking DAF (CD55) and/or MIRL (CD59) by flow cytometry provides strong evidence for the diagnosis.

In DIHA, the serologic detection of causal antibodies depends on the suspected mechanism involved. In medications causing DIHA via hapten-drug adsorption, the antibody binds only to RBCs coated with the drug, usually leading to negative DAT when the drug has been discontinued and drug-coated cells are no longer present in vivo. On the other hand, IAT done using the drug-coated RBCs as test RBCs will be positive. In medications causing immune complex–mediated hemolysis, the DAT will be positive for complement but eluate will be negative. In medications causing DIHA by autoantibody induction, the DAT will be positive for IgG but not for complement. DAT, in this case, can remain positive for over a year after discontinuation of the drug, even though hemolysis usually resolves promptly.

TREATMENT

Warm Autoimmune Hemolytic Anemia

Transfusion

RBC transfusion may be considered if the hemolytic anemia is severe and life-threatening, especially with patients with underlying cardiopulmonary conditions or with potential for cerebrovascular ischemia. In life-threatening anemia, RBC transfusion can help patients survive through an acute phase of the disease; however, the life span of the transfused RBCs are no longer than the patient's own RBCs. RBC transfusion should never be withheld in a life-threatening situation while appropriate tests are in progress. In such cases, the blood bank should assist in selecting the least incompatible RBCs to use as a temporizing transfusion.

Selection of RBCs for transfusion in WAIHA can be extremely challenging due to the difficulty in cross matching blood. Because of the autoantibody present in the patient's serum, antibody screens will be positive and cross-matching can result in apparent incompatibility. Autoantibodies with broad specificity for RBC antigens will cause a majority of available donor units to be cross-match incompatible. The priority for the blood bank in this situation is to rule out the presence of any alloantibodies that can be masked by the autoantibodies. Once alloantibodies have been excluded, the blood bank can issue units that are least incompatible with the recipient's serum and be confident that the residual incompatibility is only from the autoantibodies. Obtaining the pretransfusion specimen from the patient is essential. Phenotyping the patient's RBC at the time of initial diagnosis is also important in treating future episodes of hemolysis because it will help in identification of potential alloantibodies and in selection of phenotypically matched RBCs for transfusion, if available. Transfusions should be administered slowly under close monitoring for signs of acute hemolysis.

Glucocorticoids

Glucocorticoids have been the mainstay of treatment for WAIHA for more than 4 decades, with dramatically increased survival rates. Complete remission can be obtained in about 20% of the patients, and 10% show minimal or no response. Oral prednisone at 60 to 100 mg/d for 10 to 14 days with a rapid taper to 30 mg/d following stabilization or rise in hematocrit is a standard approach. With continued improvement, the prednisone dose can be further tapered at a rate of 5 mg/d every week to a dose of 15 to 20 mg/d. This should be maintained for 8 to 12 weeks after the resolution of the acute hemolytic episode. If the patient remains in complete remission, prednisone can be further tapered off over the following 4 to 8 weeks. Patients must be closely monitored after discontinuation of steroids for several years because relapses may occur.

When a patient presents acutely ill with a brisk hemolysis, treatment with intravenous methylprednisolone at 100 to 200 mg over the first 24 hours is warranted. This can be followed with conversion to oral prednisone as the acute severe hemolysis improves.

Splenectomy

Approximately one third of patients with WAIHA do not respond to the initial treatment with corticosteroids or require chronic prednisone treatment at doses higher than 15 mg/d. These patients may be candidates for splenectomy, which is thought to affect the disease process by the removal of the primary site of RBC destruction. The response rates can be as high as 66% with either a partial or complete remission; however, relapse rate is relatively high. Because it is difficult to predict which patients will respond to splenectomy, a careful consideration of short- and long-term risks and benefits should be undertaken. In general, the immediate morbidity and mortality from splenectomy is low, with higher rates of complications in patients with more severe disease and co-morbidities. The major long-term risk of splenectomy is the increased risk of infections by encapsulated organisms. Before splenectomy, pneumococcal vaccination is required. Patient education regarding signs of serious infections is critical.

Immunosuppression

In patients who are unresponsive to corticosteroids and splenectomy or for those who are poor surgical candidates, cytotoxic therapy has been used with some success. The most commonly used cytotoxic agents are azathioprine (Imuran)* at 1 to 2 mg/kg/d

*Not FDA approved for this indication.

and cyclophosphamide (Cytoxan)* at 1 to 2 mg/kg/d. When using cytotoxic agents, white blood cell count must be monitored closely because these agents are bone marrow suppressive. In addition, monitoring the reticulocyte count is important to assess the suppressive effect on RBC precursors. Because the prolonged use of these agents is associated with an increased risk of neoplasia, they should be tapered and discontinued after 4 to 6 months if there is no significant response. More recently, use of high-dose cyclophosphamide at 50 mg/kg/d for 4 days followed by granulocyte colony–stimulating factor rescue has been reported in a small number of selected patients to be effective in highly refractory WAIHA patients.

Women of childbearing age receiving cytotoxic agents should avoid pregnancy because of the risk of birth defects.

Other immunosuppressive agents such as lymphocyte immune globulin, antithymocyte or antileukocyte globulins, vincristine, vinblastine-loaded platelets, and/or thymectomy have been used with variable results. Cyclosporine (Sandimmune) has also been used at 4 to 5 mg/kg/d. When using cyclosporine, renal function should be closely monitored, and infection prophylaxis should be considered. In a recent report of patients treated concurrently with prednisone and cyclosporine, a major cause of mortality was severe infections.

Anti-CD20 monoclonal antibody, rituximab, has been reported to be effective in both patients with primary WAIHA and with WAIHA secondary to lymphoproliferative diseases. Long-term effects and response rates are yet to be determined.

Other

Danazol (Danocrine)* is a synthetic androgen that has been used in WAIHA with some success. The treatment schedule has been an initial dose of 600 to 800 mg/d followed by a taper down to 400 mg/d after response has been observed. Side effects include mild masculinization and cholestasis.

Intravenous γ-globulin (IVIg)* at 0.4 mg/kg/d for 5 days has also been reported effective in a number of patients, with additional single doses given as required. Some refractory patients may respond to total doses larger than 2 g/kg. In administration of IVIg, it is essential to closely monitor the renal function, especially in patients with diabetes or other causes of renal insufficiency.

Plasmapheresis alone is not indicated in the treatment of WAIHA, although in combination with other treatment modalities, it may be of some benefit in highly selected acutely ill patients.

Cold Autoimmune Hemolytic Anemia

Many patients with both CHD and PCH can be effectively managed by avoiding exposure to cold. Patients with mild chronic hemolysis are particularly benefited from this approach and typically have a benign disease course. Neither corticosteroids nor splenectomy are particularly effective in treating CHD or PCH. Both CHD and PCH associated with viral infections are typically self-limited and resolve without any specific treatment.

In both CHD and PCH, resolution of hemolysis following successful treatment of underlying disease process has been reported. Secondary CHD associated with lymphoproliferative disorders usually responds to the treatment of the primary disease with alkylating agents such as cyclophosphamide, chlorambucil, nucleoside analogues, or rituximab. Similarly, PCH has been successfully treated by treating the underlying disease such as lymphoma or syphilis.

As with WAIHA, RBC transfusions should be reserved for those patients who have severe anemia with potential for cardiopulmonary or CNS compromise. Washed RBCs may be required for patients with very active hemolysis and concurrent complement depletion. Plasmapheresis may be of use in conjunction with other therapies. This intervention may modify the rate of hemolysis acutely but will not produce a sustained remission without treatment of associated illness or the addition of immunosuppression.

Drug-Induced Hemolytic Anemia

The critical steps in the treatment of DIHA are the identification of the offending drug and its discontinuation. Withdrawal of the offending drug should lead to the resolution of hemolysis. The additional therapies in managing DIHA are supportive in nature. In patients with DIHA associated with medications acting through immune complex formation, hemolysis can be severe. In these patients, hemoglobinuria may lead to acute renal failure requiring renal hemodialysis. Transfusion of RBCs may be required in life-threatening anemia. Steroids may modify the rate of hemolysis of IgG-coated RBCs, but definitive therapy requires identification and removal of offending drug.

NONIMMUNE HEMOLYTIC ANEMIAS

method of
JINGXUAN LIU, M.D., PH.D.,
LIBERTO PECHET, M.D., and
L. MICHAEL SNYDER, M.D.
UMass Memorial Health Care
Worcester, Massachusetts

Nonimmune hemolytic anemias are the result of lysis or destruction of red blood cells (RBCs) by nonimmunologic mechanisms. Nonimmune hemolytic anemias are either congenital or acquired and are due to either endogenous or exogenous causes. Thus, abnormalities of the membrane, hemoglobin, or RBC enzymes may predispose RBCs to lysis, whereas a turbulent external environment as a result of endothelial or cardiac valvular alteration in surfaces

*Not FDA approved for this indication.

may also cause hemolysis. Because nonimmune hemolytic anemia is such an extensive topic, the focus here is only on common conditions. Hemoglobinopathies, although common, are discussed elsewhere in this book.

ACQUIRED NONIMMUNE HEMOLYTIC ANEMIAS

Anemias Caused by Destruction of Red Blood Cells by Mechanical Forces (Shearing Force and Entrapment)

The hemolysis occurs in either the heart and large vessels (macroangiopathic hemolytic anemia) or small vessels (microangiopathic hemolytic anemia).

Macroangiopathic Hemolytic Anemia

Clinical Manifestations. Microangiopathic hemolytic anemia is the result of increased shearing forces produced by high flow rate and turbulence in the cardiovascular system. The RBCs are torn, resulting in hemolysis. This phenomenon is observed occasionally in congenital heart disease. Infants with ventricular septal defects and patent ductus arteriosus can present with hemolytic anemia. Patients with congenital heart disease without anemia may develop hemolysis after surgical repair. The hemolysis can be so severe that patients require transfusion. Hemolysis sometimes resolves after replacement of the prosthetic valves. In contrast to cardiac valve pathology or after repair with residual defects, abnormalities in arteries and veins are unlikely causes for hemolysis. The transient hemolysis seen after venous stent placement is probably due to the slower blood flow rate in these locations compared with that in the heart.

Laboratory Diagnosis. The peripheral blood smear reveals increase in *schistocytes* (broken, deformed RBCs) to more than 5 per 1000 red cells. Occasionally, thrombocytopenia may also be present. Indirect bilirubin level is increased and serum haptoglobin is usually low.

Treatment. Management consists basically of diagnosing the underlying disease. With its eradication, the hemolytic anemia abates as well. Transfusion of RBCs is occasionally necessary.

Microangiopathic Hemolytic Anemia

Clinical Manifestations. Microangiopathic hemolytic anemias are seen in three conditions: disseminated intravascular coagulation, carcinomatosis (especially with tumors of the stomach, breast, prostate, and lung), and thrombotic thrombocytopenic purpura/hemolytic-uremic syndrome. In all, the basic mechanism is similar: the entrapment and destruction of RBCs in small vessels, with local thrombosis. To be noted, neoplasia may cause a hypercoagulable state by itself or through metastatic lesions. Other causes of microangiopathic hemolytic anemia include dialysis, non–immune-mediated processes in connective tissue diseases, viral infections, and specific drugs.

Laboratory Diagnosis. The diagnosis is similar to that of macroangiopathic anemia.

Treatment. The management is also similar to that of macroangiopathic anemia, with emphasis on eliminating the underlying cause.

Paroxysmal Nocturnal Hemoglobinuria

Clinical Manifestations. Paroxysmal nocturnal hemoglobinuria (PNH) is due to acquired abnormalities in the cell membrane of hematopoietic lineage cells. The clinical hallmarks are paroxysmal hemolytic episodes and hemoglobinuria, thrombocytopenia, venous thrombosis, and neutropenia. Anemia is the most common presentation with a median hemoglobin level of 8.0 g/dL. Only 25% to 50% of patients actually present with nocturnal hematuria. The median age at onset is between 30 and 40 years, but it may develop as early as age 10 years or younger or as late as age 80 years or older, occasionally as a variant of, or preceding, a myelodysplastic syndrome. It may also transform into acute leukemia. A frequent complication of PNH is thrombosis, which affects 40% of patients. It may occur in the inferior vena cava, hepatic vein (often presenting as the Budd-Chiari syndrome), cerebral and mesenteric veins, and other venous sites. When PNH related, the causes of death include thrombosis and hemorrhage. A small fraction of patients experience spontaneous remission.

Molecular and Cellular Bases of the Disease. Two cell surface molecules responsible for inactivation of complement, CD55 and CD59, are not expressed or are expressed at low levels on the RBCs, platelets, and white cells of patients with PNH. Therefore, the clinical manifestations of PNH are the results of uninhibited activation of the complement system. The unchecked complement activation may also be accountable for the thrombotic complications, possibly owing to the increased conversion rate of prothrombin to thrombin by the complement system in the absence of CD55 and CD59. It should be noted that distinct RBC populations coexist in a PNH patient: cells expressing normal levels of CD55 and CD59, expressing low levels of CD55 and CD59, and expressing very low levels of CD55 and CD59. The relative proportion of the severely affected RBCs determines the severity of the disease.

Laboratory Diagnosis. Traditionally, the Ham and the sugar-water tests have been used to demonstrate the susceptibility of RBCs to lysis in an acidified medium. Because of their lack of specificity, direct assessment of expression levels of CD55 and CD59 on RBC surface by flow cytometry is now recommended for specific diagnosis.

Treatment. The management of patients with PNH is dual: it consists first of symptomatic relief, such as transfusions when indicated by the severity of anemia and anticoagulation for the treatment of thrombosis, which may be an urgent necessity. Administration of fibrinolytic agents, similar to their use in acute myocardial infarction, may be life saving in acute thrombotic episodes, such as the Budd-Chiari syndrome. The second level of management is an effort to eradicate the disease. This may be accomplished by bone marrow transplantation. Although experience is limited, some excellent results have been reported. Obviously, the choice of bone marrow transplantation must be a cautious one.

CONGENITAL NONIMMUNE HEMOLYTIC ANEMIAS

Hemolytic Anemia Caused by Red Blood Cell Enzyme Defects

Although many enzyme defects have been described in RBCs, genetic defects of two enzymes account for most cases of hemolytic anemia in this category: glucose-6-phosphate dehydrogenase (G6PD) and pyruvate kinase (PK). G6PD is a pivotal enzyme for oxidative glycolysis in the pentose phosphate pathway. This pathway generates a chemical, glutathione (GSH), which reduces hydrogen peroxide and other reactive oxygen groups. A G6PD defect makes the RBCs prone to lysis when they face oxidative challenges. This enzyme defect affects a population of 400 million worldwide. PK is an enzyme in the anaerobic glycolytic pathway, the Embden-Meyerhof pathway. A defect in PK results in insufficient energy generation for RBCs and makes them prone to lysis. So far only about 400 patients with defective PK have been described.

G6PD Deficiency

Clinical Manifestations. Hemolytic anemia is the hallmark of G6PD deficiency, being severe and continuous in the Mediterranean variant of the disease but mild and interspersed with acute hemolysis in the African variety. The hemolytic crises occur after exposure to oxidant drugs (e.g., sulfa drugs), after ingestion of fava beans (favism), and during acute infections; it may also accompany diabetes. G6PD deficiency was discovered in the 1950s by the search for causes of hemolytic anemia in patients who took the antimalarial premaquine.* Although drug and food attract more attention as the cause of hemolysis, some authors believe that infections are the more common cause of hemolysis. Jaundice at birth is a clinically important manifestation of the Mediterranean variant of G6PD deficiency. It may be complicated by kernicterus, in the absence of obvious anemia.

Molecular and Cellular Bases of the Disease. The enzyme G6PD is a protein encoded by a gene linked to the X chromosome. Therefore, G6PD deficiency is an X-linked disease. More than 400 defects of this gene, such as point mutations and deletions, have been characterized. These genetic defects cause reduced enzyme activity of G6PD.

Laboratory Diagnosis. The diagnosis of G6PD deficiency is made by quantitative measurement of G6PD enzyme activity of red blood cells. Immediately after an episode of acute hemolysis the result can be falsely negative in the African variant because immediately after an acute hemolytic episode, most old RBCs are hemolyzed and young RBCs dominate. They have relatively normal G6PD activity. Therefore, 2 to 3 weeks of waiting is recommended before ordering the tests after an acute hemolytic episode. Further studies can be obtained to characterize the genetic defect in a patient with G6PD deficiency, but this is rarely necessary in clinical practice.

Treatment. Avoidance of medications and food known to result in oxidative insults is the most important step, once the diagnosis of G6PD deficiency has been established. RBC transfusion may be necessary in severely anemic patients. Splenectomy may be beneficial in cases with chronic, severe anemia. For severe jaundice in G6PD-deficient neonates, phototherapy and exchange transfusion are used.

Pyruvate Kinase Deficiency

PK deficiency leads to moderate to severe hemolytic anemia. It is an autosomal recessive disorder and hence clinically expressed only in homozygotes. The diagnosis of PK deficiency depends on the quantitative measurement of PK activity in RBCs. Genetic studies of PK-deficient patients are possible. Therapy is supportive, and transfusions may be necessary, depending on the severity of anemia. Splenectomy increases the hemoglobin level by 1 to 3 g/dL.

Hemolytic Anemias Caused by Abnormalities of Red Cell Membranes

Red cell membrane abnormalities are a group of hemolytic disorders characterized morphologically by abnormal RBC shapes due to defects of genes encoding red cell membrane skeletal proteins. The hemolytic diseases in this category are divided into four different subtypes according to the morphology of the red cells: (1) hereditary spherocytosis, (2) hereditary elliptocytosis and pyropoikilocytosis, (3) Southeast Asian ovalocytosis, and (4) hereditary stomatocytosis. Because the first and second subtypes are more common and better characterized, the focus of this discussion is on these two subtypes.

Hereditary Spherocytosis

Clinical Manifestations. One of every 4000 to 5000 whites is affected by hereditary spherocytosis (HS) in the United States. The prevalence is lower in the African American population. Anemia, jaundice, and splenomegaly are the most common clinical presentations. Bilirubin gallstones affect many patients, and quite early in life.

Molecular and Cellular Bases of the Disease. The list of the genetic defects is a long one and includes genetic changes affecting the RBC membrane proteins ankyrin (band 2.1), anion exchanger (band 3), protein 4.2, and spectrins (bands 1 and 2). In about two thirds of the cases, HS is transmitted in the dominant form, and in one third, recessively.

*Not available in the United States.

Laboratory Diagnosis. RBCs appear on peripheral blood smears as round, uniformly dark cells (spherocytes). Osmotic fragility testing with hypotonic solutions is a confirmatory study. Analysis of membrane skeletal proteins with electrophoresis can be done in research laboratories. Characterization of the genetic defects is rarely necessary.

Treatment. When the anemia is severe, especially after aplastic crises due to suppression of marrow erythropoiesis by viral infections, RBC transfusions become necessary. Splenectomy is an effective treatment modality for HS because it generally controls the anemia. To reduce the risk of overwhelming sepsis, a rare but potentially fatal complication after splenectomy, vaccinations (anti-pneumococcus, anti–*Haemophilus influenzae,* and anti-meningococcus) are administered before the procedure. Long-term penicillin administration is recommended after splenectomy, particularly during childhood. Splenectomy should not be performed before age 6. Partial splenectomy has been proposed, because this procedure preserves immune functions and reduces hemolysis in the spleen. Treatment of gallstones frequently requires cholecystectomy. Genetic counseling of family members is advisable.

Hereditary Elliptocytosis

Clinical Manifestations. In the United States, hereditary elliptocytosis (HE) affects mainly African Americans and people of Mediterranean origin. It is estimated that 1 of 2000 to 4000 subjects has HE. The prevalence could be higher because only a small proportion of HE patients are symptomatic. Anemia, when present, ranges from mild to severe.

Molecular and Cellular Bases of the Disease. Genes of several RBC skeletal protein molecules, spectrins α and β, protein 4.1, and glycophorin C, are affected in different families. Both autosomal dominant and recessive transmissions have been reported.

Laboratory Diagnosis. Peripheral blood smear reveals elliptocytes. In some cases all the RBCs may appear elliptocytic and still the patient may be asymptomatic.

Treatment. The management of patients with severe HE is similar to that of patients with HS, including splenectomy for the most severe cases.

PERNICIOUS ANEMIA AND OTHER MEGALOBLASTIC ANEMIAS

method of
RONALD A. SACHER, M.D.
University of Cincinnati College of Medicine
Cincinnati, Ohio

The megaloblastic anemias are a group of disorders characterized by the presence of hypersegmented neutrophils and oval macrocytes in the blood or the presence of megaloblasts in the bone marrow. The word *megaloblast* is a descriptive term referring to the abnormal red cell precursors found in the bone marrow of patients with these anemias. Appropriate therapy for megaloblastic anemia requires an understanding of the differential diagnosis and laboratory evaluation of other causes of anemia with macrocytic red blood cells. The most common cause of megaloblastic anemia is deficiency of either cobalamin (vitamin B_{12}) or folate.

Cobalamin deficiency is almost always due to malabsorption. Pernicious anemia is the usual cause and is likely due to a lack of intrinsic factor, the essential cofactor needed for cobalamin absorption in the terminal ileum. Intrinsic factor is normally produced by the parietal cells of the gastric mucosa and is deficient in any condition depleting this production, such as autoimmune atrophic gastritis or gastrectomy. Occasionally, dietary deficiency (veganism) and malabsorption states or bacterial overgrowth with organisms requiring intestinal vitamin B_{12} for their metabolism may produce cobalamin deficiency.

In contrast, deficiency of folic acid is nearly always due to a dietary deficiency. Stores of folic acid are only sufficient for 3 months. These can be rapidly depleted in conditions of increased folate demand (e.g., pregnancy, rapid growth, rapid cell turnover [hemolytic anemias]), poor folate intake, and alcoholism. Occasionally, folic acid deficiency may occur with other malabsorption states or with selective interference by drugs such as birth control pills and anticonvulsants.

CLINICAL FEATURES

Clinical features, though not specific, are often helpful in differentiating pernicious anemia from folic acid deficiency. Table 1 lists the seven clinical P's of pernicious anemia helpful with this distinction. Macrocytic anemia occurring with alcoholism or in a postpartum state is more likely to be due to folic acid deficiency. Ultimately, however, cobalamin (vitamin B_{12}) deficiency and folate deficiency are confirmed only by laboratory assay.

LABORATORY FINDINGS

Macrocytosis occurs when the mean cell volume (MCV) is greater than 100 fL. Erythrocytic macrocytosis can easily be determined with the aid of an automatic electronic particle counter, which gives an accurate and reproducible value for the MCV. The finding of macrocytic indices does not automatically imply megaloblastic anemia, as can be seen from Table 2. An elevated MCV, however, is an abnormal finding and may precede by months or years the onset of a megaloblastic anemia. Megaloblastic anemia may be masked in the presence of complicating infections, inflammatory disease, or iron deficiency.

Spurious macrocytosis can occur, and an elevated MCV must be corroborated by examination of the peripheral blood smear. The peripheral blood smear findings are in-

TABLE 1. **Seven Clinical P's of Pernicious Anemia**

Pancytopenia
Peripheral neuropathy
Posterior spinal column neuropathy
Pyramidal tract signs
Papillary (tongue) atrophy
pH elevation
Psychosis

TABLE 2. **Differential Diagnosis of Macrocytosis**

Actual
Megaloblastic anemias
Liver disease
Reticulocytosis
Myeloproliferative diseases (leukemia, myelofibrosis)
Multiple myeloma
Metastatic disease of bone marrow
Hypothyroidism
Aplastic anemia
Drugs (post chemotherapy, alcohol)
Spurious
Autoagglutination/cold agglutination disease

valuable in differential diagnosis. The earliest sign of megaloblastic anemia reflected in the peripheral blood is hypersegmentation of the polymorphonuclear leukocytes. Red cell morphology can help distinguish the macrocytosis of liver disease (round macrocytes), megaloblastic anemia (oval macrocytes), reticulocytosis (basophilic round macrocytes), and acute leukemias. A bone marrow examination is useful in cases in which the peripheral blood findings are equivocal. However, the bone marrow examination cannot distinguish vitamin B_{12} deficiency from folic acid deficiency.

DIAGNOSTIC WORKUP

The initial laboratory evaluation for cobalamin deficiency always includes a complete blood cell count with examination of the peripheral smear. Cobalamin and serum folate levels are then obtained. The diagnosis of cobalamin deficiency is usually made from the finding of low serum cobalamin and normal serum folate levels. A bone marrow examination can be useful if the peripheral blood finding is equivocal and shows megaloblastic maturation. If vitamin B_{12} deficiency is documented, a Schilling test should be done to demonstrate the lack of intrinsic factor versus other malabsorptive states. This test determines cobalamin absorption using the urinary excretion of radiolabeled cobalamin after an oral dose given with or without intrinsic factor. Initially, a parenteral loading dose of cobalamin (vitamin B_{12}), 1000 μg, is administered so that when cobalamin is absorbed a significant amount is subsequently excreted in the urine. This loading dose can, however, correct the laboratory and hematologic evidence of megaloblastosis. Measurement of serum levels of methylmalonic acid and total homocysteine may also be useful in equivocal cases. These amino acids are increased in cobalamin-deficient states because enzymes responsible for their conversion are cobalamin dependent. These amino acid levels may be elevated before the falling cobalamin levels and diagnostic bone marrow morphologic findings are recognized.

TREATMENT

Immune-Mediated Cobalamin Deficiency (Pernicious Anemia)

Therapeutic aims are directed at reversing the immediate sequelae of the disorder, such as the anemia and neurologic abnormalities (initial treatment), toward maintenance of the remission and prevention of relapse (maintenance treatment). Without treatment, the patient develops pancytopenia or a progressive neurologic disease (peripheral neuritis and subacute combined degeneration of the spinal cord).

Initial Treatment

The aim is to correct the deficiency and to replenish the stores. Because the disorder is caused by cobalamin malabsorption in most cases, parenteral cobalamin supplementation is given, using preferentially the intramuscular or subcutaneous routes. After injection, significant amounts of the vitamin (up to 80%) are excreted in the urine; therefore, initial therapy should be several large doses (100 to 1000 μg) of cobalamin. Injections given a day apart replenish stores more rapidly than daily injections, although no established regimen works better then the others. My approach is to administer a series of seven 100-μg injections of cobalamin every other day over a period of 2 weeks. Patients or family members can be taught to inject the vitamin themselves. After this, I usually continue with weekly injections over the next 4 weeks to ensure replacement of the vitamin stores and then monthly for life.

Administration of cobalamin is complete therapy for uncomplicated disease. Because the underlying cause of the cobalamin deficiency cannot be corrected, therapy is lifelong and the patient should be informed that therapy must never be stopped.

It is not clear whether large and more frequent doses of cobalamin are needed in patients with neurologic damage; however, in these patients, I give the same schedule of cobalamin as aforementioned, but, after a 2-month period of weekly injections, I continue giving therapy every 2 weeks for a period of 6 months and, from that point on, one injection every month for the lifetime of the patient. There are, of course, no hard data on duration of initial therapy, but one tends to administer more aggressive treatment to patients with neurologic dysfunction.

The clinical response to initial therapy is often dramatic. Rapid reversal of pancytopenia and mucosal changes can occur with even minimal doses (as low as 1 μg). The patients often describe an immediate sense of well-being, and within a week the mucosal changes reverse. Hematologic response is frequently noted after 3 days, with improvement in the hemoglobin 5 to 7 days after treatment. Disappearance of macrocytic red cells and correction of the MCV may take several weeks. During initial therapy, it is advisable to monitor daily serum potassium levels for at least 4 days because rejuvenation of new cells may produce hypokalemia owing to movement of plasma potassium into the rapidly proliferating hematopoietic cells. Patients who are on diuretic therapy and have an initial hypokalemia, patients with a history of cardiac disease, and those on digitalis therapy should be especially carefully monitored. Potassium, in a dose of 40 mEq/d, should be administered promptly to patients manifesting hypokalemia.

Coexistent iron deficiency or marginal bone marrow iron stores can limit the recovery and should be treated with 300 mg of ferrous sulfate three times a day.

The second aim of vitamin replacement therapy is to maintain the vitamin stores so that relapse does not occur. Good clinical remission can be maintained even with partial repletion of the stores. After repletion of the stores and in situations in which the underlying disease is irreversible as in pernicious anemia, lifelong maintenance therapy is then administered. My program for maintenance is to administer monthly injections of 1000 μg of cobalamin. Cyanocobalamin is the most widely used and inexpensive form of vitamin B_{12} available in the United States. Another preparation, hydroxocobalamin, is more physiologic and has a longer biologic half-life than cyanocobalamin and if available may be given by intramuscular injection every 3 months. It is more expensive but does have the advantage of being retained longer after injection than cyanocobalamin.

Although patients may be instructed in self-administration of the injections, they should be followed at least once or twice a year by a physician. I see my patients at least annually, at which time they have a general examination and complete blood cell count. Clinical evaluation includes three serial stool guaiac determinations because there is a 2% to 3% incidence of gastric carcinoma and a higher incidence of gastric carcinoid tumors (usually benign) in patients with pernicious anemia. Evaluation of thyroid studies in patients with suggestive symptoms is also performed because there is an association between pernicious anemia and autoimmune thyroid disorders.

The need for continuous monitoring should be stressed to these patients because the requirement of lifelong therapy is essential. Proper patient education requires reinforcement of this fact, inasmuch as relapse in pernicious anemia is not uncommonly seen.

Other Cobalamin Deficiency States

Treatment of nonpernicious vitamin B_{12} deficiency anemia obviously depends on the underlying cause. Patients who have had their source of intrinsic factor removed, such as those who have had a gastrectomy, also require lifelong therapy. My program for these patients and for those who have had an ileal resection is identical to the management of patients with pernicious anemia. Vegans who are deficient in vitamin B_{12} because of negligible intake can be supplemented by small amounts of oral cyanocobalamin. Doses of 25 μg daily may be sufficient. Alternatively, these patients may be given injections of cyanocobalamin every 6 months or even high doses of oral cobalamin with follow-up of serum levels.

Folic Acid Deficiency

The clinical findings of pure folic acid deficiency are similar to those found with pernicious anemia, except for the important observation that these patients lack any neurologic symptoms. The laboratory findings are also similar to those found in pernicious anemia, with the complete blood cell count, peripheral blood smear, and bone marrow examination being indistinguishable from those in cobalamin deficient states. The diagnosis is usually made after determination of a low serum folate level. This test should be interpreted with caution. Serum folate levels can be normal in the presence of low folate stores, especially immediately after folate intake. A red blood cell folate level can be obtained and is more sensitive to assessing folic acid deficiency in these circumstances.

Treatment of folic acid deficiency, which usually occurs as a result of decreased dietary intake, is aimed at reversal of the initial effects of the deficiency, replenishment of folate stores, and maintenance of sufficient dietary intake to ensure adequate folate nutrition.

Folate absorption occurs throughout the small intestine. Megaloblastic anemia from folic acid deficiency responds readily to oral folate doses as low as 100 to 200 μg. In general, however, larger doses are administered and are usually sufficient to correct deficiency even in malabsorption states. Most available preparations contain 1 mg of folic acid. My general approach is to give 1 mg of folic acid daily except in situations of severe malabsorption, when I administer 2 to 5 mg daily. In these cases, I ensure that cobalamin deficiency is not coexistent and may initially administer 1000 μg of cobalamin monthly until such time as the malabsorption state is corrected. Replenishment of folate stores can be achieved within several weeks of oral therapy. If the underlying cause can be reversed, maintenance therapy is not indicated.

No significant primary toxicity from folate treatment has been reported. Its use in cobalamin-deficient patients can, however, precipitate subacute combined degeneration of the spinal cord; thus, one must exclude vitamin B_{12} deficiency in patients with folate deficiency.

In any patient with nutritional deficiency, a good understanding as to the need for folate replacement must be emphasized. Patients should be educated about foods containing the best source of folate, such as green leafy vegetables, and about the fact that folic acid is a labile vitamin and can easily be destroyed by overcooking or boiling.

In pregnancy, relative folic acid deficiency can occur despite apparently adequate normal blood levels when there is an enhanced requirement for both mother and fetus. Prevention and treatment of megaloblastic anemia of pregnancy can be accomplished with 1 mg of folic acid daily administered throughout pregnancy and during the period of lactation. In alcoholics, poor nutrition is compounded by poor compliance and by the fact that alcohol per se is an antagonist to biologic folate cofactors. I treat these patients with higher doses, such as 5 mg of folate daily, inasmuch as compliance is the major limiting factor and the potential for side effects of megavitamin therapy is remote.

Other individuals requiring folate supplementation include patients requiring long-term hemodialysis and those with disorders of increased cellular turnover, such as chronic hemolytic states. These patients are indoctrinated as to the necessity of receiving 1 mg of folate daily as lifelong therapy.

Patients taking drugs that decrease normal folate absorption (birth control pills, phenytoin [Dilantin]) may require folate supplementation (1 mg/d) if they develop evidence of folate deficiency. Folinic acid (citrovorum factor) is a reduced form of folic acid that bypasses the antifolate activity of the chemotherapeutic agent methotrexate. It is usually administered parenterally to "rescue" systemic antifolate effects of the drug, enabling higher "antimitotic" doses to be given.

Severe Megaloblastic Anemia

Acute Management

Transfusion therapy is rarely indicated because many patients do not exhibit overt hemodynamic decompensation (inasmuch as anemia is slowly progressive) and because response to the appropriate vitamin replacement is usually rapid and symptoms can be controlled by bed rest. Furthermore, "shotgun" therapy with cobalamin and folate pending diagnostic laboratory studies is usually unnecessary. However, patients with deteriorating neurologic signs or altered mental status should receive 1000 μg of intramuscular cobalamin immediately.

In the severely anemic patient with circulatory distress or in the elderly patient with cardiac or neurologic dysfunction, transfusion may be essential. These patients invariably have an increased plasma volume. Therefore, red cell concentrate transfusions should be administered slowly (3 hours per unit) with intravenous diuretics (e.g., furosemide [Lasix]) and potassium supplementation. Hypokalemia during the initial recovery phase after vitamin replacement therapy is particularly serious and these patients should receive empirical potassium replacement with 40 mEq/d.

THALASSEMIA

method of
ALAN R. COHEN, M.D.
*University of Pennsylvania School of Medicine
Philadelphia, Pennsylvania*

PATHOPHYSIOLOGY

The thalassemias are a group of disorders characterized by deficient or absent production of globin. This quantitative defect leads to an impairment of hemoglobin synthesis and an excess of the unaffected globins; both of these effects contribute to the pathophysiology of the disease. The thalassemias are distinctly different from most of the purely qualitative disorders of globin, such as sickle cell disease in which normal amounts of globin are made but the resulting hemoglobin molecule behaves abnormally. However, in some instances (e.g., Hb E) a globin mutation resulting in an abnormal hemoglobin may most closely resemble a thalassemic defect. In this situation, the structural change causes no harm but the underproduction of the abnormal globin may cause a clinically important form of thalassemia.

Thalassemic disorders are generally identified by the affected globin chain. Thus, β-thalassemia refers to disorders in which mutations in one or both β-globin genes cause decreased production of β-globin. α-Thalassemia refers to quantitative disorders of one or more of the four α-globin genes. The second level of definition describes whether the production of the affected globin chain is reduced or absent. In β-thalassemia, for example, the former is called a β plus (β^+) mutation and the latter is a β zero (β^0) mutation. The third level of definition refers to the clinical severity of the disorder. Patients who have thalassemia major require regular red cell transfusions because of severe anemia and other clinical manifestations (see later). This group most often includes individuals with β-thalassemia but may also include patients with Hb E β-thalassemia or patients with severe α-thalassemia. Patients with thalassemia intermedia are less anemic than those with thalassemia major and do not need regular transfusions. This group most often includes individuals with homozygous β-thalassemia but at least one β^+ mutation, with Hb E β-thalassemia, or with abnormalities of three of the four α-globin genes. The distinction between thalassemia major and thalassemia intermedia is sometimes in the eyes of the treating physician. The hemoglobin levels and other signs and symptoms may lead one physician to initiate a regular transfusion program while another physician may decide that transfusions are unnecessary. Thalassemia trait refers to mutations in one of two β-globin genes or two of four α-globin genes. Individuals with thalassemia trait have only a mild microcytic anemia.

Many features of thalassemia may contribute to the chronic anemia that is the hallmark of this group of disorders. The diminished production of globin impairs hemoglobin synthesis. The inheritance of two β^0-thalassemia genes prohibits the production of normal adult hemoglobin (α_2, β_2). Production of alternative hemoglobins such as fetal hemoglobin (α_2, γ_2) can only partially compensate for the total loss of adult hemoglobin. An equally or more important mechanism of anemia is the relative excess of the normally produced globin. When β-globin is reduced or absent, excess α-globin forms aggregates on red cell membranes. These structurally compromised erythrocytes are readily destroyed in the bone marrow, causing intensely ineffective erythropoiesis. The compensatory attempts are remarkably destructive. Bone marrow expansion causes abnormal facies and cortical thinning and easy fractures of the long bones. Extramedullary erythropoiesis causes massive enlargement of the liver and spleen. A third contributor to the pathophysiology of thalassemia lies in the altered function of abnormal hemoglobins that form as a result of the missing globin. For example, the hemoglobin H (β_4) and hemoglobin Barts (γ_4) that form in the α-thalassemia syndromes are unstable and unload oxygen poorly. Ineffective erythropoiesis is the dominant pathophysiologic mechanism in most thalassemic disorders. The relative contribution of the other factors varies with the specific type of thalassemia.

DEMOGRAPHICS

The demographics of thalassemia in North America have changed considerably in the past decade. Once thought to be primarily a disease of people of Italian or Greek ethnic background, thalassemia in the United States and Canada today is most commonly newly identified in individuals of ethnic backgrounds that include the Middle East countries, India, Pakistan, Southeast Asia, and Southern China. Among Southeast Asians, the high frequency of thalassemia intermedia makes it particularly important to consider this disease in the evaluation of unexplained anemia, even in older patients.

DIAGNOSIS AND CLINICAL FINDINGS

Children with thalassemia major usually develop signs and symptoms of severe anemia in the latter part of the first year of life when normal hemoglobin synthesis becomes increasingly dependent on β-globin. Affected children are usually pale and lethargic. Their appetites begin to wane, and they are often irritable. Extramedullary hematopoiesis causes enlargement of the liver and spleen. The peripheral smear is usually diagnostic. The red cells are markedly hypochromic. Variation in red cell size is dramatic, but small and large red cells alike contain little hemoglobin. The reticulocyte count is modestly to markedly elevated, and nucleated red cells are often present in the peripheral blood. In homozygous β^0 thalassemia, the hemoglobin electrophoresis shows only fetal hemoglobin. In compound heterozygotes (β^0/β^+), some hemoglobin A is present. In syndromes such as Hb E β-thalassemia or Hb Lepore β-thalassemia, the electrophoresis shows the abnormal hemoglobin. Parental studies reveal the mild anemia and microcytosis typical of thalassemia trait. In some centers, molecular diagnosis is employed to help predict the clinical course based on the particular mutations. Given the wide variation between genotype and phenotype, other centers use molecular diagnosis primarily to unravel difficult diagnostic problems or to assist in later prenatal diagnosis.

Patients with thalassemia intermedia may be identified throughout childhood and even during adulthood. Milder forms may first become apparent during an acute illness or during pregnancy. The anemia is associated with poor exercise tolerance, jaundice, and splenomegaly. The red cell morphology resembles that found in thalassemia major, although the abnormalities may be less severe. Hemoglobin electrophoresis demonstrates increased levels of fetal hemoglobin or the presence of an abnormal hemoglobin such as Hb E or Hb H.

Ideally, the diagnosis of thalassemia should be made at or before birth, based on the identification of the parents as carriers. In particular, the finding of a non–iron-responsive microcytic anemia in the pregnant woman should prompt a careful evaluation for thalassemia trait that, if present, should lead to a similar evaluation of the father. This approach permits the family to consider in utero diagnosis. In some states, the newborn screening programs for hemoglobinopathies, designed primarily to identify sickle cell anemia, also notify the family or physician when the electrophoresis shows an absence of hemoglobin A that strongly suggests thalassemia. However, this pattern is limited to infants with two β^0 mutations; therefore, many infants with clinically important thalassemia disorders will escape detection.

MANAGEMENT OF THALASSEMIA MAJOR

Transfusion Therapy

Transfusion therapy is the cornerstone of the treatment of patients with thalassemia major. Table 1 presents general guidelines for the use of transfusion therapy in thalassemia. The initiation of regular red cell transfusions follows the identification of the thalassemic disorder and the determination that the hemoglobin remains unacceptably low in the absence of other causes such as acute illnesses. No specific hemoglobin level separates those children who do or do not need transfusion therapy, but levels below 6 to 7 g/dL usually are associated with unacceptable symptoms such as disfiguring bone changes or impaired growth. The goal of transfusion therapy is to maintain the hemoglobin level greater than 9 to 10 g/dL at all times. This target is usually associated with the suppression of ineffective erythropoiesis, thus reducing bone marrow expansion and extramedullary hematopoiesis. Hemoglobin levels greater than 9 to 10 g/dL also allow normal levels of activity. Lower pretransfusion hemoglobin levels should be avoided because they often fail to achieve the benefits of transfusion therapy but still carry all of the same risks.

TABLE 1. **Guidelines for Transfusion Therapy in Thalassemia Major**

Blood Product
Leukoreduced red cells
Storage time <2 weeks
Volume and Duration of Transfusion
10–20 mL/kg over 2–4 hours
Smaller volumes for young children and patients with impaired cardiac function
Interval Between Transfusions
2–4 weeks
Target Pretransfusion Hemoglobin Level
9–10 g/dL

The usual volume of transfused red cells is 10 to 15 mL/kg. Assuming a hematocrit of 75% for the donor cells, this volume of transfused red cells will raise the hemoglobin by 3 to 4 g/dL. The subsequent rate of fall in the hemoglobin level is approximately 1 g/dL per week, giving a transfusion interval of 3 to 4 weeks. Smaller volumes of blood can be given more frequently but may interfere with the patient's school activities or work. Larger volumes of blood would theoretically increase the interval between transfusions but should be avoided because of the possibility of volume overload and complications associated with sudden, large increases in the hemoglobin level.

Newer additive solutions such as AS-1 and AS-3 extend the storage time of donor red cells but reduce the hematocrit of the transfusion product to approximately 60%. As a result, larger volumes are required to achieve the same post-transfusion hemoglobin level. For most older children and adults, the one or two units administered with each transfusion will contain 300 to 600 mL and can be given over 2 to 4 hours without difficulty. Patients with impaired cardiac function may require smaller aliquots or slower infusion rates, and they may also need a diuretic such as furosemide. Younger children may need to receive a fraction of a unit to avoid post-transfusion hemoglobin levels that are too high or too low.

Donor red cells should undergo leukoreduction to decrease the likelihood of febrile transfusion reactions and to reduce the risk of HLA sensitization, a possible impediment to stem cell transplantation. The importance of storage time of donor red cells remains uncertain. Red cell recovery 24 hours after transfusion remains greater than 70% to 75% after as long as 42 to 48 days of storage in some additive solutions, but the subsequent half-life is less well studied. Small changes in the recovery and half-life of donor red cells may have a significant impact on the overall blood requirements of patients on chronic transfusion programs. Therefore, the conventional practice is to use red cells that are less than 2 weeks old.

Patients who have repeated allergic reactions should receive an antihistamine before transfusion. Although rare, acute hemolytic transfusion reactions still occur and may be life threatening. These reactions are characterized by hypotension, back pain, and a sense of impending doom. Acute hemolytic transfusion reactions are usually the result of mislabeling the blood sample for crossmatching, administering the wrong unit to a patient, or failing to detect a red cell antibody. The risk of such problems may increase when patients with thalassemia receive transfusions in centers that are not familiar with their care.

Before the first transfusion, the blood bank should characterize the full antigen profile of the red cells of the patient. Red cell alloantibodies will develop in 5% to 20% of patients with thalassemia, and some patients will also develop red cell autoantibodies. Knowledge of the patient's own red cell antigens will help to identify the specificity of a new alloantibody and will also help to distinguish alloantibodies from autoantibodies.

Splenectomy

Although current transfusion programs usually prevent massive splenomegaly, lesser degrees of splenic enlargement may increase transfusion requirements and therefore the rate of iron loading. Regular monitoring of blood usage will help to identify those patients who will benefit from removal of the spleen. Annual transfusion requirements in patients who have undergone splenectomy usually do not exceed 150 mL/kg of packed cells with a hematocrit of 75%. Thus, a patient whose annual transfusion requirement exceeds 220 mL/kg, in the absence of other causes such as red cell alloantibodies, is likely to have a reduction of at least 30% in blood usage after splenectomy. The rate of transfusional iron loading will fall proportionately. The decision regarding splenectomy in this situation must weigh the benefits of slowing the rate of iron accumulation against the risk of surgical complications, which are uncommon, and the risk of postsplenectomy sepsis, which can be devastating. In general, patients who are having difficulty managing iron overload (see later) will benefit considerably from splenectomy when transfusion requirements are excessive. However, such patients should receive preoperative immunizations against *Haemophilus influenzae*, pneumococcus, and meningococcus, and they should receive penicillin, 250 mg twice daily, after surgery. Immediate evaluation of febrile illnesses, usually including blood cultures and administration of parenteral antibiotics, is an extremely important part of the prevention of overwhelming sepsis. Because the risk of this complication is particularly high in young children, splenectomy should be avoided before 5 years of age. Fortunately, hypersplenism is distinctly unusual before this age when the hemoglobin level is maintained above 9 to 10 g/dL.

Iron Overload

The accumulation of excessive iron from repeated red cell transfusions is the most common complication of thalassemia major and the cause of major morbidity and mortality. Each unit of red cells contains approximately 200 mg of iron. A patient with thalassemia major who receives 2 units of red cells every 3 weeks will accumulate almost 7 g of iron annually. In the absence of a physiologic mechanism for the excretion of excessive iron, the metal is deposited in the liver, heart, endocrine glands, and other sites. When the total iron accumulation exceeds 1 g/kg, the risk of iron-induced cardiac failure or arrhythmia is high. Lesser degrees of iron overload also cause heart disease as well as liver fibrosis, diabetes mellitus, impaired growth and sexual development, and other endocrinopathies. Before the introduction of iron chelation therapy, most patients with thalassemia major died by age 20 as a result of iron-related organ damage.

Deferoxamine

Deferoxamine (Desferal),* licensed as an iron chelator in the 1960s, remains the only drug available in North America for the treatment of iron overload. Deferoxamine-induced urine and stool iron excretion exceeds the rate of transfusional iron loading in most patients, establishing negative iron balance. The removal of excessive iron and the prevention of new iron accumulation are associated with numerous clinical benefits. Regular therapy with deferoxamine decreases the risk of liver fibrosis, increases the likelihood of normal growth and sexual development, and lowers the risk of cardiac disease. Most importantly, retrospective analyses of large cohorts have demonstrated that chelation therapy markedly extends the life span of patients with thalassemia major.

Table 2 presents general guidelines for the use of deferoxamine. Because of its short half-life and limited gastrointestinal absorption, deferoxamine must be administered by continuous parenteral infusion.

*Not FDA approved for this indication.

TABLE 2. **Guidelines for Chelation Therapy With Deferoxamine**

Initiation of Therapy
After 20 transfusions
Ferritin >1000–2000 ng/mL
Liver iron concentration >3.2 mg/g dry weight
Dose
25–50 mg/kg/d
Lower doses for young children and patients with mild to moderate iron overload
Higher doses for older children and adults with moderate to severe iron overload
Administration
Subcutaneous or intravenous infusion over 8–24 hours
Monitoring Effectiveness
Serum ferritin level every 3–6 months
Liver iron concentration (see text)
Monitoring Safety
Annual audiologic and ophthalmologic examinations
Annual radiographs of legs/vertebral column until age 5 years
Measurement of standing and sitting heights every 3–6 months

Doses range from 25 to 50 mg/kg/d, infused subcutaneously over 8 to 12 hours 5 to 7 days per week. The lower doses are often used in children younger than 5 years of age because of concern regarding drug-induced bone changes and impaired growth. In older children and adults, the dose is usually selected according to the degree of iron overload. Such an approach takes into account two counterbalancing factors. First, deferoxamine-induced iron excretion increases as the dose of the chelator is raised, although the relationship may not be linear. Second, the toxicity of deferoxamine increases when the dose of the drug is high in relationship to the degree of iron overload. Thus, it is essential to carefully evaluate the iron load of each patient to maximize the effectiveness of iron removal and to minimize the risk of side effects. One approach is to adjust the dose of deferoxamine so that the ratio of the dose (mg/kg) to the ferritin level (ng/mL) is maintained below 0.025. Using this formula, patients receiving deferoxamine at a dose of 50 mg/kg should have a ferritin level of at least 2000 ng/mL.

Ideally, chelation therapy should be initiated with sufficient time to prevent irreversible damage from iron overload. Unfortunately, this point cannot be identified by clinical or laboratory findings. Many clinicians wait until the patient has received 20 transfusions. Some use a serum ferritin level of 1000 to 2000 ng/mL, others are guided by a liver iron concentration greater than 3.2 mg/g dry weight, and still others wait until 3 to 4 years of age to avoid deferoxamine-related bone changes. The overall success of chelation therapy probably relies less on which of these approaches is used to begin treatment than on the regular use of deferoxamine over the many years that follow.

Continuous intravenous infusions of deferoxamine may be useful in the management of patients with severe iron overload and patients with serious iron-induced heart disease. The benefits of this approach are probably related to the prevention of toxicity from non–transferrin-bound iron that would otherwise be present between infusions and the ability to administer higher doses of deferoxamine than can be given subcutaneously. This approach to iron chelation therapy may also be helpful in rapidly reducing iron stores before treatment of hepatitis C in patients with thalassemia, thereby enhancing the success of the antiviral treatment. Because most clinicians choose to discontinue deferoxamine for at least the first two trimesters of pregnancy, women with thalassemia and iron overload may also benefit from intensive, intravenous chelation therapy before attempting to become pregnant. For patients with very large iron stores or evidence of deteriorating cardiac function, doses greater than 50 mg/kg/d may increase the rate of iron removal and may halt or reverse heart disease. However, the toxicity of deferoxamine increases at higher doses, and patients should be monitored carefully. At present, it is not clear whether conventional doses of deferoxamine given 24 hours a day or high doses given over 8 to 24 hours is the preferable method of administering deferoxamine intravenously.

Vitamin C levels may be low in patients with iron overload, and the administration of vitamin C may increase deferoxamine-induced iron excretion in such patients. Because vitamin C may enhance the toxicity of iron, it should not be administered except during the infusion of deferoxamine, and the dose should not exceed 100 mg. Before adding vitamin C to a patient's chelation regimen, it is helpful to document that it increases deferoxamine-induced iron excretion by measuring 24-hour urinary iron levels.

Monitoring Chelation Therapy

Serum ferritin levels and liver iron concentrations are the two methods used most successfully to monitor the effectiveness of iron chelation therapy in patients with thalassemia. Maintenance of ferritin levels below 2500 ng/mL is associated with a high likelihood of survival free of cardiac disease. Maintenance of liver iron concentrations below 15 mg/g dry weight is associated with improved survival. The serum ferritin level has the advantage of being easily and inexpensively measured. However, it may be elevated by liver disease and depressed by vitamin C deficiency, both of which are common in thalassemia. In addition, the correlation between ferritin levels and liver iron concentrations is imperfect, raising doubt as to how well ferritin levels reflect total body iron stores. Nonetheless, measurement of serum ferritin levels every 3 to 6 months is a long-standing method for monitoring the effectiveness of therapy with deferoxamine, determining the safety of a particular dose of the chelator, and estimating the risk of the critical outcome of iron-induced cardiac disease.

The liver iron concentration is viewed by most clinicians as the best reflection of the total body iron load. At present, the measurement of liver iron concentration requires a liver biopsy for most patients. Accurate biochemical determination of hepatic iron levels requires a sample that weighs at least 1 mg and that is free of extensive cirrhotic nodules. Because of the discomfort and risk associated with liver biopsy, some clinicians prefer to use this approach primarily when the ferritin level does not seem commensurate with the patient's chelation history or clinical condition. Others measure the liver iron concentration annually as the main guide to adjusting the dose of deferoxamine and determining the risk of iron-related complications. Most patients should undergo liver biopsy at least occasionally to be certain that the chelation program is appropriate and effective. Unfortunately, the guidelines for dose adjustment and risk of clinical complications that are based on liver iron concentration are broad and derived largely from data from heterozygotes for genetic hemochromatosis, a disease with a different type of iron loading. More data are needed to characterize the optimal levels of both serum ferritin and liver iron during chelation therapy.

The assessment of liver iron by magnetic susceptometry is a noninvasive alternative to liver biopsy. Measurements with this technique correlate well with biochemical determinations, but only four such instruments are currently available worldwide. Determination of liver iron by magnetic resonance imaging and susceptibility with conventional instruments remains semi-quantitative and requires further development to replace biopsy.

Complications of Deferoxamine

The major complications associated with deferoxamine include high-frequency hearing loss, impaired visual acuity and night blindness, rickets-like bone changes, growth retardation, pneumonitis, unusual bacterial or fungal infections, and allergic reactions (Table 3). The hearing and vision changes occur most commonly when the dose of deferoxamine is inappropriately high for the level of iron overload. Skeletal abnormalities occur predominantly in children younger than 5 years of age and also may be related to the dose of the chelator. Lung disease is a rare but sometimes fatal complication that develops during infusions of deferoxamine that exceed 150 to 200 mg/kg/d. *Yersinia enterocolitica* and, less commonly, other gram-negative and fungal infections may occur during treatment with deferoxamine, presumably as a result of enhanced availability of iron to the pathogen. Allergic reactions range from urticaria to anaphylaxis. Therapy with deferoxamine should be stopped when any of these complications is suggested. The chelator can be reintroduced at the previous dose after resolution of bacterial or fungal infection or after successful desensitization for allergic reactions. For other complications, the dose of deferoxamine should be reduced with careful monitoring for recurrence of the problem.

The most common side effect of deferoxamine is the presence of painful or pruritic swelling at the site of the subcutaneous infusion. Even with regular rotation of the infusion site around the abdominal wall, the patient may have significant discomfort. Some clinicians recommend the addition of small amounts of hydrocortisone to the infusion to reduce local reactions, but the effectiveness of this approach is unproven.

Poor compliance remains the most important obstacle to successful chelation therapy. Under study conditions, patients administered fewer than 70% of their prescribed doses. In routine use, compliance is often even poorer, especially among teenagers, despite intensive counseling. Because a markedly increased risk of death is associated with administration of fewer than four to five infusions per week, it is not surprising that many patients with thalassemia continue to die of iron overload despite the availability of deferoxamine.

Other Chelators

The orally available iron chelator deferiprone (Ferriprox)* is licensed in Europe for patients with thalassemia for whom deferoxamine therapy is contraindicated or who have serious toxicity with deferoxamine therapy. Although this chelator, when administered at a dose of 75 mg/kg/d, induces less iron excretion than deferoxamine at a dose of 50 mg/kg/d, the higher compliance that is likely with an oral rather than a parenteral agent may increase its therapeutic effectiveness. In general, deferiprone reduces iron stores in heavily iron overloaded patients and stabilizes iron stores in patients with lesser degrees of iron overload. However, individuals vary widely in their response to deferiprone, and careful monitoring of the iron load is important. Higher doses of deferiprone (80–100 mg/kg/d) have been effective in patients who excreted insufficient iron in response to

*Not available in the United States.

TABLE 3. **Complications of Iron Chelation Therapy**

Complication	Monitoring	Response
Sensorineural hearing loss	Audiogram	Stop or reduce dose
Visual changes	Ophthalmologic examination	Stop or reduce dose
Bone changes	Skeletal radiographs	Stop or reduce dose
Growth impairment	Sitting and standing height	Stop or reduce dose
Allergic reactions	Clinical observation	Desensitization
Pneumonitis	Clinical observation	Stop therapy
Infection	Clinical observation	Interrupt therapy

75 mg/kg/d. Agranulocytosis occurs in less than 1% of patients receiving deferiprone at a dose of 75 mg/kg/d when the blood cell count is monitored weekly and the drug is stopped if the absolute neutrophil count falls below 1500 cells/mm^3. The frequency of agranulocytosis at higher doses of the chelator or with less rigorous monitoring is uncertain. Concerns about accelerated liver fibrosis during deferiprone therapy have not been substantiated by subsequent studies. At present, deferiprone appears to have a valuable role in the management of patients with thalassemia who fail treatment with deferoxamine because of intolerable side effects or inadequate compliance despite intensive counseling.

Late Complications

As patients with thalassemia major live longer because of improved transfusion and chelation therapy, they are encountering new problems, including diabetes mellitus, osteoporosis, hypothyroidism and hypoparathyroidism, impaired fertility and sexual function, and chronic hepatitis C. The management of the endocrinopathies generally focuses on hormonal replacement therapy. Bone marrow expansion and iron overload may both contribute to osteoporosis, a potentially crippling complication of thalassemia. Supplementation with calcium and vitamin D should be initiated for patients with decreased bone mineral density. The role of bisphosphonates in the management of osteoporosis in thalassemia is under investigation. Hepatitis C is very common in patients with thalassemia major who received transfusions before 1990. Two important factors distinguish the treatment of hepatitis C in these patients from the treatment of other patients. First, increased iron stores may reduce the effectiveness of antiviral therapy. As described earlier, reduction of iron stores with intensive chelation therapy before initiation of specific treatment for hepatitis C may increase the likelihood of eradicating the virus. Second, when ribavirin is used in combination with interferon, transfusion requirements may increase because of hemolysis. Except in very heavily iron overloaded patients, the antiviral benefits of ribavirin outweigh the increased transfusional iron loading that accompanies its use.

THALASSEMIA INTERMEDIA

The clinical spectrum of thalassemia intermedia ranges from a mild hemolytic anemia to more severe red cell destruction accompanied by severely ineffective erythropoiesis. Splenectomy usually raises the hemoglobin level by at least 1 to 2 g/dL and reduces the erythropoietic drive. Red cell transfusions may be necessary if the hemoglobin level falls during infections, during pregnancy, or at other times. Some patients with thalassemia intermedia become increasingly anemic or symptomatic in adult life and require regular transfusion therapy.

Patients with more severe forms of thalassemia intermedia may have facial changes and thinning of the cortices of the long bones due to bone marrow expansion. Because the facial changes are usually irreversible after the first 5 to 10 years of life, the clinician must carefully consider the benefits of regular transfusions for such patients. Some patients may also develop serious neurologic problems if the expanded marrow extends outside the vertebral bodies and impinges on the spinal cord. Early diagnosis is important to prevent permanent neurologic damage. These masses of extramedullary hematopoiesis shrink readily with radiation therapy and resolve more slowly with transfusion therapy to suppress erythropoiesis.

Patients with thalassemia intermedia have an increased need for folic acid and should receive 1 mg daily to prevent megaloblastic anemia. The gastrointestinal absorption of dietary iron is increased and may eventually lead to iron overload, especially if the patient receives red cell transfusions intermittently. Assessment of iron overload is especially difficult in thalassemia intermedia because the serum ferritin level may markedly underestimate the total iron stores. Measurement of liver iron should be strongly considered in all patients with elevated ferritin levels. The need for chelation therapy with deferoxamine should be based on the severity of iron overload. As a less expensive and safer alternative to chelation therapy, some patients may be able to undergo regular phlebotomy despite their anemia. Patients with thalassemia intermedia should drink tea with meals to reduce iron absorption, and they should avoid iron-fortified foods such as some cereals.

α-THALASSEMIA SYNDROMES

Most patients who have three of four alpha genes that are missing or nonfunctional (Hb H disease or Hb H-Constant Spring) will have a clinical syndrome that most closely resembles thalassemia intermedia, and their management is generally similar to that of patients with β-thalassemia intermedia. However, the Hb H that is found in these disorders has two properties that affect clinical management. First, its increased susceptibility to oxidant stress causes exacerbations of anemia during febrile illnesses or exposure to oxidant drugs, and patients may require transfusions at such times. Second, because Hb H has no Bohr effect and therefore has a reduced rate of oxygen unloading, the actual oxygen delivery to the tissues may be considerably less than the total hemoglobin concentration suggests. Therefore, the need for transfusion should be based on clinical signs such as tachycardia and tachypnea rather than on hemoglobin level alone.

Although homozygous α-thalassemia, in which all α genes are missing or nonfunctional, is usually lethal to the fetus, a few affected infants have been saved by transfusions in utero or by early delivery and intensive resuscitation. These patients will have a clinical picture of thalassemia major and will need regular red cell transfusions.

STEM CELL TRANSPLANTATION

More than 1500 patients with thalassemia have undergone stem cell transplantation, usually receiving bone marrow from a human leukocyte antigen–identical sibling. The best outcomes have occurred in children 16 years of age or younger who have been compliant with chelation therapy and who have no hepatic enlargement or fibrosis. Data from the largest center identify the probability of disease-free survival in such patients as 91%. For children of similar age who have been noncompliant with chelation therapy and who have evidence of hepatic involvement, the probability of disease-free survival falls to 58% to 83%. Patients older than 16 years of age have a 62% probability of disease-free survival. Stem cell transplantation using umbilical cord blood has been successfully applied to thalassemia, but experience is limited in comparison with bone marrow cells. Results with alternative donor transplants, such as those using matched, unrelated donors, have generally been unsatisfactory. Successful hematologic recovery in some patients with partial chimerism has increased interest in transplants using less intensive preparatory therapy.

Many patients with thalassemia major who have undergone successful stem cell transplantation will still have increased iron stores. To prevent iron-related complications that may occur even in the absence of further transfusions, these patients should begin regular phlebotomies and continue with this therapy until iron stores are reduced to normal levels.

The role of stem cell transplantation in the management of a patient with thalassemia major who has an HLA-identical sibling requires careful comparison of the risks and benefits of this approach versus conventional transfusion and chelation therapy. Ongoing improvements in both approaches add to the difficulty of this comparison. Parents of a child with thalassemia major should strongly consider saving umbilical cord blood from future infants to determine its suitability as a source of stem cells.

OTHER APPROACHES

Drugs such as 5-azacitidine*, hydroxyurea, and butyric acid derivatives increase fetal hemoglobin levels by promoting synthesis of gamma globin. Their role in the treatment of the β-thalassemias remains unclear. Although hemoglobin levels have increased in a few patients treated with intravenously administered arginine butyrate or orally administered sodium phenylbutyrate, the overall response rate is very low. Current studies are evaluating new dosing schedules for the butyrates and also therapy combining two or more agents that enhance fetal hemoglobin production. Stimulation of red cell production with recombinant erythropoietin raises the hemoglobin level in some patients with thalassemia intermedia, but the long-term benefits of a small improvement in the anemia accomplished by further stimulation of an already overactive bone marrow are uncertain.

*Investigational drug in the United States.

SICKLE CELL DISEASE AND HEMOGLOBINOPATHIES

method of
ERNEST A. TURNER, M.D.
Cook County Children's Hospital
Chicago, Illinois

In 1972 the National Sickle Cell Anemia Control Act (Public Law No. 92–294, 86 Statute 138, May 16, 1972) was passed. Although a tremendous amount of progress has been made toward understanding the pathophysiology of sickle cell anemia, today a cure is possible only with a bone marrow transplant. However, it is available only to a limited number of individuals with sickle cell anemia who meet the criteria for transplantation. Nevertheless, the overall impact has been to improve the quality of life and life expectancy for those individuals with sickle cell anemia and sickle cell disease (SCD). The overall result has been to increase the median survival from approximately 17 years in 1972 to 46 years today.

In 1910 the first report of SCD appeared in the United States medical literature. Since that time enormous progress has been made toward the understanding of a group of genetic disorders known as SCD, of which sickle cell anemia is the prototype. In 1925, Thomas Cooley and Pearl Lee described a form of severe anemia in children of Italian origin that was characterized by splenomegaly and specific bone changes. The disorder reported was later termed *thalassemia* from the Greek word for "sea," *thalassa*. The genetic disorder described was realized to be a recessive mendelian disorder not confined to those of Mediterranean descent but occurring widely throughout tropical countries. The two important forms of this disorder, α- and β-thalassemia, are the result of the defective synthesis of α- and β-globin chains of hemoglobin. Besides the prevalent α- and β-thalassemia, there are the rarer disorders of γβ-, δ-, γ-, and δβ-thalassemia (also called F-thalassemia), with variable clinical importance. A related condition that is harmless in either the heterozygote or homozygote form is hereditary persistence of fetal hemoglobin (HPFH).

HEMOGLOBIN

For the practitioner to treat SCD effectively, it is important to understand the structure and function of both normal and abnormal hemoglobin.

Normal Hemoglobin

Hemoglobin is a heterodimeric tetramer composed of two α-like globin chains and two non–α-globin chains (β, γ, or δ) that are conjugated to four heme moieties. The globin gene clusters are located on chromosomes 16 and 11. The different globin chains are synthesized independently and then combined with each other to produce different hemoglobin that are highly regulated through the embryo, fetal, and adult periods. The production of the complex hemoglobin molecules Hb A and the fetal hemoglobin Hb F is a delicate process in which the synthesis of the α chains is carefully balanced with that of the β and δ chains in the adult and with that of the γ chains in the fetus and the newborn. After birth, the γ chain synthesis is gradually replaced by β and γ chain synthesis, but the balance between the production of the α chains and non–α chains is maintained. The presence of duplicated genes, such as two α chain genes on chromosome no. 16, and two γ chain genes, one β chain gene, and one δ chain gene on each chromosome no. 11 greatly aids in this balanced equilibrium.

Abnormal Hemoglobin

Abnormal hemoglobin variants are formed by additions, deletions, substitutions, or inversions of one or more amino acids in one or more of the genes for the globin chains.

Currently, 800 hemoglobin variants and a nearly equal number of thalassemias have been described. In general, the majority of the hemoglobin variants described are harmless, having neither clinical nor hematologic manifestations. However, one should be concerned and investigate the possibility of a hemoglobin variant if there exists an unexplained cause for abnormal complete blood cell morphology and/or hematologic data such as microcytosis, anemia, or erythrocytosis (Table 1). In Hb S the α-globin chain is the same as in Hb A, but the β-globin chain differs from the normal by the substitution of valine for glutamic acid at the sixth position, a neutral-charged amino acid with a negative-charged amino acid. The globin gene clusters are located on chromosomes 16 and 11. The different globin chains are synthesized independently and then combined with each other to produce the different hemoglobins that are highly regulated through the embryonic, fetal, and adult periods of the human. As a result of the associated ontogeny in the normal person older than 6 months of age, hemoglobin A makes up 97% and fetal hemoglobin less than 1% of the total hemoglobin that is sequestered in a small minority of erythrocytes called F cells. These latter concepts have become important in the development of management strategies for sickle cell disease.

PATHOPHYSIOLOGY

The biochemical basis of sickle cell anemia is due to the substitution of thymine for adenine in the glutamic acid DNA codon (GAG→GTG) that results in substitution of β6 valine for glutamic acid. Hemoglobin exists in two conformations, the oxy (relaxed, R) and deoxy (tense, T) states. Molecules of deoxy-Hb S have a strong tendency to aggregate. The aggregate hemoglobin solution turns into a gel. The distorted sickle red cell is the end result of this molecular aggregation. This process is time dependent. Initially, there is a rate-limiting nucleation process. After a few molecules of sickle hemoglobin aggregate to form a "seed," the process of more aggregation occurs rapidly. The sickling process is characterized by a long delay that is strongly dependent on temperature and hemoglobin concentration and other factors (Table 2).

TABLE 1. **Hematologic Manifestation of Hemoglobin Variants**

Sickle cell formation
Microcytosis
Target cells
Heinz body formation
Increased-decreased oxygen affinity
Methemoglobin formation
Erythrocytosis
Basophilic stippling

TABLE 2. **Factors Modifying Polymerization of Hb S**

Factor	Increases	Decreases
O_2 saturation	Deoxyhemoglobin	Oxyhemoglobin
Hb S concentration	High % S	High % F
	High MCHC	Low MCHC
	Dehydration	Hyponatremia
Temperature	Fever	Euthermia
Blood pH	Acidosis	Alkalosis

Abbreviation: MCHC = mean corpuscular hemoglobin concentration.

When a cell sickles and unsickles repeatedly, the membrane is affected and the cell becomes irreversibly sickled. If oxygen at high pressures is increased, the cells remain sickled. An irreversibly sickled cell has a high hemoglobin concentration, high calcium content, low potassium content, and is adenosine triphosphate depleted.

The thalassemias are defined as disorders in which there is primarily a diminution in hemoglobin formation. They are classically defined as β^+ and β^0, which is representative of the presence or absence of messenger RNA production. Classic thalassemias manifest erythrocytic microcytosis. Thalassemias are classified according to which globin gene is affected, such as α-thalassemia when one or more of the α-globin genes is affected or β-thalassemia when one or more of the β-globin genes is affected.

The α-thalassemias occur widely throughout Africa, the Mediterranean countries, the Middle East, and Southeast Asia. The β-thalassemias are widespread throughout Africa, Myanmar, southern China, the Indian subcontinent, Indonesia, the Malay peninsula, and the Middle East. The clinical pictures of α- and β-thalassemia vary widely, and knowledge of the phenotypes as genetic modifiers is being amassed.

DIAGNOSIS

In human beings there are six different globin chains: alpha (α), beta (β), delta (δ), epsilon (ε), and zeta (ζ). Each of these chains has different numbers of amino acids, oxygen affinity, and electrical charge, which accounts for the variation in electrophoretic mobility.

Traditionally, the diagnoses of sickle cell disease and hemoglobinopathies have been made by the laboratory techniques of acid and alkaline electrophoresis (Figure 1). These hemoglobin electrophoresis methods have proved to be reliable for confirming the presence of a variety of hemoglobins. Although not absolute, the tests require only minute samples. The limitation of such procedures is that almost invariably only variants that are characterized by differences in charge can be detected. Newer methods involve isoelectric-focusing (IEF), polyacrylamide gel electrophoresis (PAGE), and different types of high-pressure liquid chromatography (HPLC).

IEF is electrophoresis in a pH gradient. It is a separation method that resolves proteins on the basis of their isoelectric points. Over the past years, ultramicro-column chromatographic procedures have been developed. These columns are filled with a special cation or anion exchanger and are developed in 10 to 120 minutes at high pressure

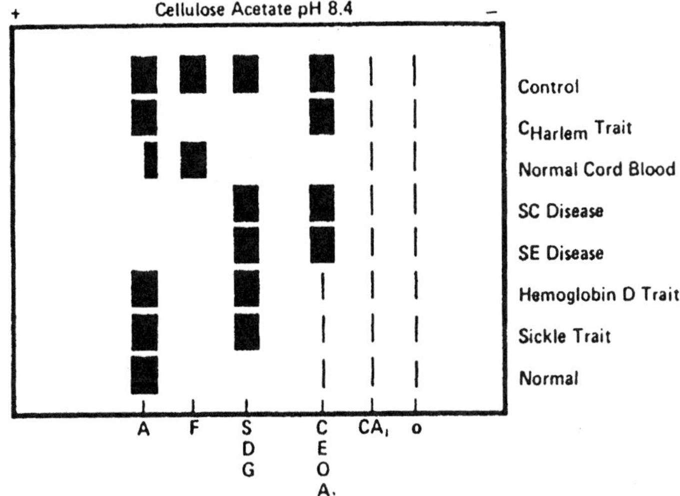

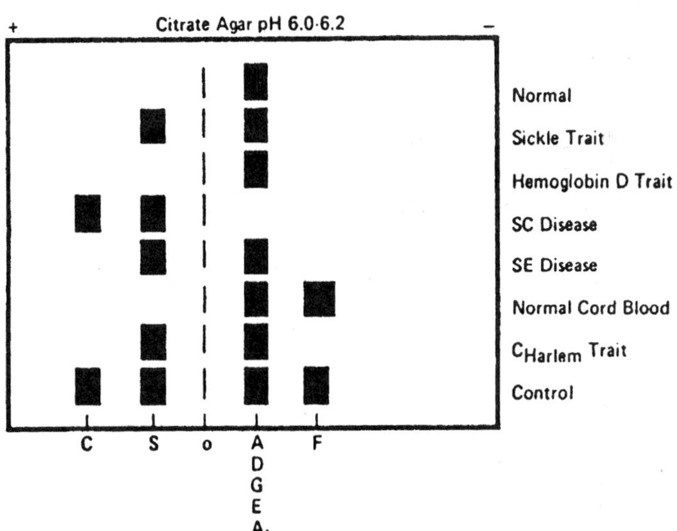

Figure 1. Comparison of various hemoglobin samples on cellulose acetate and citrate agar.

and high flow rate, thus the name HPLC. Each of these procedures has its own sensitivity and specificity.

CLINICAL MANIFESTATIONS

Sickle cell anemia can be considered the prototype of the SCDs, and in general the clinical features, and currently the treatment, of all the SCDs is the same.

The SCDs vary widely in their clinical severity. The clinical manifestations and hematologic features of sickle cell anemia are apparent by 12 to 16 weeks of age. The newborn is protected by the high level of fetal hemoglobin in the red cells during the first weeks of life.

Currently, no fully satisfactory specific treatment of SCD has yet become available for all individuals, although it is recognized that there are genetic modifiers (Table 3). Thus, physicians and other health care providers must focus their therapeutic efforts on continuous and effective general medical care and appropriate management of complications as they arise.

TABLE 3. **Genetic Modifiers of Sickle Cell Disease**

Alpha haplotypes	Hb F levels
Beta haplotypes	Gender

Acute Chest Syndrome

Acute chest syndrome (ACS) is characterized by fever, tachypnea, chest pain, leukocytosis, and a new pulmonary infiltrate(s). Pulmonary crises are the number one cause of hospitalization in patients suffering from sickle cell anemia. Before the development of the pneumococcal vaccine and routine use of penicillin prophylaxis, pulmonary crises in children were primarily caused by community-acquired pneumonia. The most common organisms involved were *Streptococcus pneumoniae*, *Mycoplasma pneumoniae*, *Haemophilus influenzae*, *Salmonella*, and *Escherichia coli*. Since then, infection with pulmonary crisis has been the cause of one third of the cases. An infectious cause of the pulmonary consolidation in the adult was not frequently proven, and until recently, antibiotics were not recommended when ACS was suggested. In adults, common causes of pulmonary crisis include in situ vaso-occlusion secondary to erythrocyte stasis, deep vein thrombi, and fat from infarcted bone marrow. ACS is characterized by a precipitous decrease in hemoglobin concentration and increase in the number of platelets and leukocytes. The most common presenting symptoms of ACS are fever, cough, and chest pain.

Less common presenting symptoms include dyspnea, wheezing, hemoptysis, chills, and productive cough. The frequency of presenting symptoms is age dependent. Fever and cough more commonly present in children aged 2 to 4. The incidence of chest pain, dyspnea, chills, productive cough, and hemoptysis increases with increasing age. There is no difference in frequency of presenting symptoms between patients with Hb SS and Hb SC disease except for severe pain, which presents more often in patients with Hb SS disease. Vital signs at the time of hospitalization are found to be age dependent, with children experiencing higher temperatures, pulse rates, and respiratory rates than adults. The most frequent findings on physical examination are rales and dullness to percussion. The second most common physical finding is a normal result on lung examination. Another common physical finding is lower extremity pain. Radiographic findings are also age dependent. In young children, isolated upper lobe disease and middle lobe disease are more common than lower lobe disease. Adults present with multilobe disease and pleural effusions. The incidence of ACS is related to the season of the year. Seasonal variation is noted most often in young children. Children experience a lower incidence of ACS in the summer and an increasing rate in the winter. Adults experience a similar trend, but it is less pronounced. The treatment of ACS includes prompt recognition of the disease, appropriate antibiotics, and the proper respiratory support; sometimes the patient will require transfer to the intensive care unit and intubation with ventilatory support. The treatment of choice for ACS is exchange transfusion. Exchange transfusion replaces the entire blood volume using an apheresis machine. The therapeutic objective is to reduce the Hb S to under 30%. Patients clinically improve within hours of the exchange. Hemoglobin electrophoresis should be done before and after the transfusion. Increasing oxygen saturation and decreasing shortness of breath indicate clinical recovery. Interval improvement in the chest radiograph usually lags behind the clinical improvement. One of the most frightening clinical manifestations of SCD is ACS. The patient can quickly progress to respiratory failure and death if ACS is not properly recognized.

Large Vessel Disease

The cardiovascular system is stressed by chronic anemia, recurrent small pulmonary artery occlusions, and myocardial hemosiderosis. Because of the anemia that sickle cell patients experience, they have an increase in cardiac output. The increase in cardiac output causes an enlargement of the heart in early childhood. Clinically, there is an increased incidence of murmurs created by the increase in blood flow through normal heart valves. There may be a holosystolic murmur that mimics the murmur of mitral regurgitation. There may be an ejection click. There can also be a systolic impulse in the second left intercostal space. This results from the transmission of pulmonary artery pulsations to the chest wall. This is suggestive of pulmonary hypertension, but usually the pulmonary artery pressure is normal. Other factors serve as a source of cardiac embarrassment secondary to the chronic anemia. The shunting of blood through infarcted, nonoxygenated portions of the lung compromises the arterial oxygen saturation. Pulmonary hypertension results from sludging of sickled red blood cells through small pulmonary vessels. Myocardial hemosiderosis is the result of chronic transfusion therapy. Hemosiderosis predisposes to intractable heart failure. Intermittent hypertension occurs during sickle cell crisis, and associated elevations in the renin activity are attributed to the reversible sludging of erythrocytes in the renal microvasculature.

Other Complications

Hepatomegaly manifests usually after the first year of life. Histologically, erythrocytes distend the sinusoids. Kupffer cells that line the hepatic sinusoids phagocytize sickled red blood cells. There are deposits of hemosiderin pigment and periportal fibrosis. As adults, sickle cell patients suffer from diffuse nodular cirrhosis. Acute enlargement of the liver occurs with subcapsular infarction or hepatic vein thrombosis. Intrahepatic infarcts may be complicated by abscess formation. Another histologic finding is bile stasis. The severity of hepatic disease is age dependent. In children, the only physical findings are hepatomegaly and splenomegaly. In children, liver function is only moderately impaired. In adults with SCD, fulminant hepatic failure is not uncommon. Another ailment common to SCD is hyperbilirubinemia. It can be caused by infectious hepatitis, intrahepatic sickling, or choledocholithiasis. With viral hepatitis the serum bilirubin level can reach 100 mg/dL. The hyperbilirubinemia is caused by several factors, including increased heme catabolism and glucose-6-pyruvate dehydrogenase deficiency. The increase in heme catabolism causes an increase in pigmentary gallstones. Both radiolucent and radiopaque gallstones have been documented in children as young as 5 years of age. The incidence of gallstones increases with age. The incidence in the 2 to 4-year age-group is 12%. In teenagers 15 to 18 years of age the incidence is 42%. In adults the incidence is 60%. The pain of choledocholithiasis can be hard to distinguish from that of abdominal vaso-occlusive crisis. After cholecystectomy, the patient may experience less abdominal crisis.

Renal Pathology

A number of renal pathologic processes are associated with SCD. Even in the absence of clinical disease, there is histologic evidence of small cortical infarctions and hemosiderin deposits in the epithelium of the nephron. There is also hypertrophy and sclerosis of the nephron. Symmetric enlargement of the kidneys is common, and distortion of the collecting system is a common finding on the intravenous pyelogram. Papillary necrosis may also occur. Hyposthenuria and limited hydrogen ion excretion start to manifest at 6 to 12 months of age. Hyposthenuria is defined as the production of urine with low specific gravity due to the inability of the renal tubules to produce concentrated urine. Because of the large amounts of fluid required, the patient experiences nocturia or enuresis. The cause of the concentrating defect in the urine is thought to be the sludging of cells in the collecting tubules, which acts to disrupt the countercurrent mechanism of the kidneys. The accompanied destruction of the vasa rectae is consistent with this hypothesis.

Hematuria is another common renal manifestation of SCD. The duration of the hematuria can be brisk or prolonged. The most common defect is an ulcer in the renal pelvis at the site of a papillary infarction. Chronic hemolysis can cause urate nephropathy, which can lead to microscopic hematuria. There can also be painless hematuria caused by poststreptococcal glomerulonephritis. Nephrotic syndrome is another well-documented complication of SCD that occurs in both adolescents and adults. The syndrome is often characterized by hematuria, hypertension, and progressive renal insuffiency, leading eventually to renal failure. Histologically, the lesion is a membranoproliferative glomerulonephritis with significant reduplication of the basement membranes, mesangial proliferation, fusion of foot processes, dense deposits in glomeruli, interstitial fibrosis, tubular atrophy, and deposits of hemosiderin. The development of nephrotic syndrome is thought to be caused by the accumulation of autoimmune complexes. Immunoglobulins, complement particles, and renal tubular epithelial antigens have been found in a granular pattern on the glomerular basement membrane. Anti–renal tubular antigen antibodies have also been found circulating in the blood. It is thought that renal ischemia and tubular damage produced by erythrocyte sickling are associated with the release of renal tubular epithelium antigen. Immune complexes formed by the antigen and specific antibody are deposited on the glomerular basement membrane, giving rise to the nephrotic syndrome.

Leg Ulcers

Cutaneous leg ulcers are common manifestations of SCD. The breakdown of skin over the malleoli and in the distal portions of the legs is a common problem in adults with SCD. Minor abrasions are unable to heal because of blood stasis in small blood vessels. These ulcers then become secondarily infected by bacterial pathogens. Leg ulcers are found in 25% of patients 10 years of age and older. In patients older than 20, leg ulcers are found more often in men than in women. There is a positive correlation with low steady-state hemoglobin concentration and with a low level of Hb F. The healing of the ulcers can take a long time, and the ulcers often recur.

THERAPEUTIC APPROACHES

There are no specific inhibitors of Hb S polymerization. One of the most important ways to decrease the intracellular concentration of Hb S is by using blood transfusion. Blood transfusion improves both blood and tissue oxygenation. It temporarily suppresses the production of erythrocytes containing Hb S. Blood transfusion also decreases the amount of sickling by diluting the patient's amount of diseased red blood cells with normal red blood cells. By adding normal red blood cells, the increased viscosity of the sickled, deoxygenated blood cells would be reduced. Just adding one fourth of Hb A to three fourths of Hb S decreases the viscosity of deoxygenated blood by 50%. To prevent vaso-occlusive crisis, the amount of erythrocytes containing Hb S should be reduced by 60%. Blood transfusion therapy can be given two ways. Exchange transfusion removes a portion of the patient's blood and replaces it with normal packed red blood cells. Simple blood transfusions are also equally effective in replacing deoxygenated blood. Packed erythrocytes given every 3 weeks will keep the amount of donor cells above 50%. The amount of donor erythrocytes can be monitored by quantitative electrophoresis. Chronic blood transfusions do have a downside; they increase the chances of exposure to infectious pathogens such as hepatitis, HIV, alloimmunization, and the accumulation of hemosiderin. Approximately 30% of patients with sickle cell disease become alloimmunized. The greater risk of alloimmunization is the result of racial differences because of the donor and recipient populations.

Another mechanism of treatment against sickle cell disease is the induction of Hb F. Hb F is the predominant hemoglobin during fetal life. It is the predominant hemoglobin in the newborn. In normal adults Hb F makes up only 1% of hemoglobin. Although Hb F is the predominant hemoglobin, there are no clinical manifestations of SCD. Drugs such as hydroxyurea (Hydrea) and butyrate compounds function to increase the amount of Hb F. Hydroxyurea is a cytotoxic drug that increases the production of Hb F. It has no effect on DNA methylation. It arrests the development of more mature red blood cell precursors. This shifts hematopoiesis to earlier red blood cell precursors with a greater capacity to create Hb F. Hydroxyurea is believed to change globin synthesis by erythroid precursors. An increase of Hb F is noticed within 2 to 3 days after hydroxyurea administration. This is sooner than would be expected if the rise were due to bone marrow suppression. F-reticulocyte response to hydroxyurea is inversely proportional to the suppression of colony-forming unit–erythroid. It is thought that hydroxyurea via multiple mechanisms alters γ-globulin gene expression and acts to augment γ-globulin synthesis. On a cellular level, hydroxyurea inhibits ribonucleotide reductase, stopping DNA synthesis and cell division. Hematologically, hydroxyurea increases the mean corpuscular volume, decreases the number of dense cells, and reduces the amount of sickled cells in the circulation. Clinically, hydroxyurea decreases the amount of hemolysis in some sickle cell anemia patients and ameliorates symptoms in some patients with SCD.

In general, patients treated with hydroxyurea have half the number of painful crises, have longer periods between the crises, have fewer attacks of ACS, are hospitalized less often, and have fewer transfusions. Patients treated with hydroxyurea should meet certain criteria: they should be 18 or older, they should have had more than three severe vaso-occlusive crises, and they should be using birth control while on hydroxyurea. Certain contraindications to the use of hydroxyurea are pregnancy, drug allergy, and either thrombocytopenia or neutropenia. Initially, bimonthly blood cell counts are required for people using the drug, after which the frequency is adjusted to meet the clinical situation. Hydroxyurea is started at 15 mg/kg/d. After a period of 8 weeks it may be increased. The usual maintenance regimen is between 1000 and 2000 mg/d, or a maximum dose of 35 mg/kg/d. A rising mean corpuscular volume is a good indication of rising HbF levels. The drug has been shown to be teratogenic in mice embryos; however, teratogenicity for humans has yet to be proven. Erythropoietin is another valuable weapon in the arsenal against SCD. It acts to potentiate the effects of hydroxyurea. Arginine butyrate is a byproduct of hyperglycemia. It has been observed that diabetic mothers with poor glucose control produce large amounts of Hb F. A group of investigators studied this effect in relation to sickle cell anemia and found, when given intravenously, that arginine butyrate has a half-life of only 5 minutes and increased the Hb F levels. Arginine butyrate also caused mild alterations of liver functions, nausea, vomiting, and anorexia.

Health Maintenance

Individuals with SCD are predisposed to increased amounts of infection; thus, vaccinations are a necessary part of the management of SCD. The reason the patients are more susceptible to infection is because of the dysfunction of the spleen. Enlargement of the spleen takes place during the first years. By the teenage years the patient's spleen has suffered recurrent infarctions. These multiple infarctions cause splenic atrophy. Because of the lack of splenic function, blood-borne particulates fail to elicit the proper antigenic response and immune protection. Because of the increased susceptibility of children with SCD, pneumococcal vaccination and the use of penicillin prophylaxis are required. Primary prevention and prompt medical intervention help to prevent the development of serious complications such as meningitis and reduce the mortality of the illness overall. It is recommended that all children with SCD be fully immunized by 2 years of age and that they receive a booster every 5 years. The booster is well tolerated and produces a major antibody response. The vaccine being used today is effective in children younger than 2 years of age. Chemoprophylaxis decreases pharyngeal colonization and reduces septicemia and death from infection. It is recommended that they receive penicillin starting by 2 months of age and that it should be continued to 5 years of age. Individuals with SCD should also be immunized with influenza virus vaccine annually.

Pain Management

The management of a painful crisis is one of the most important clinical aspects of treating patients with SCD. It is the painful crisis that causes frequent visits to the emergency department and hospital admissions. There is no specific description of the pain that is pathognomonic for painful crises. The pain can involve the chest, abdomen, and the extremities. Of great importance in the treatment of the painful crisis is fluid management. There is a three-step treatment regimen recommended by the World Health Organization. Patients with mild pain can be treated at home with non-narcotic medications and oral fluids. Acetaminophen, ibuprofen, and naproxen are some of the other non-narcotic analgesics that can be used. For moderate to severe pain, narcotic analgesics should be used. The clinician can start by using oral narcotic agents such as codeine and oxycodone. Intravenous agents should be employed if the oral agents are not effective in controlling the pain or if they cannot be used because of severe nausea and vomiting. For severe pain the treatment of choice is morphine. Meperidine (Demerol) has side effects that make it less attractive, and it has been associated with seizures in people with impaired renal function and in high doses. It has a short half-life, requiring more frequent dosing. It may also cause fibrosis, infection, and abscess formation at the injection site if it is given intramuscularly. Antihistamines and antiemetics are also very helpful in the management of the painful crisis. They help to sedate the patient and minimize the emetic episodes, thus making the patient more comfortable. Laxatives such as docusate (Colace), senna (Senokot), and magnesium citrate will maintain bowel function, which can be impaired by the opioids that are being used for pain control.

PROGNOSIS

The life expectancy in people with sickle cell anemia is decreased when compared with the average population. The average life span for men with sickle cell anemia is 42 years, and for women it is 48 years. The most common cause of death from SCD is renal failure. A large percentage of patients die of ACS. A high level of Hb F predicts improved survival.

NEUTROPENIA

method of
MELVIN H. FREEDMAN, M.D.
Hospital for Sick Children and Research Institute
Toronto, Ontario, Canada

An absolute neutrophil count (ANC) is equal to the total white blood cell count per microliter multiplied by the combined percentage of neutrophils and bands. Neutropenia is defined as an ANC more than 2 standard deviations less than the normal mean. Normal neutrophil levels can be stratified for age and race. For whites beyond infancy, the lower limit for normal neutrophil counts is 1500/μL. Blacks have somewhat lower neutrophil counts; the lower limit of normal is approximately 1200/μL. Individual patients may be characterized as having mild neutropenia with cell counts of 1000 to 1500/μL, moderate neutropenia with cell counts of 500 to 1000/μL, or severe neutropenia with cell counts less than 500/μL. This stratification is useful for predicting risk because only patients with severe neutropenia have increased susceptibility to life-threatening infections.

CLASSIFICATION

Table 1 is a classification for formulating an informative clinical and laboratory assessment that leads to a specific diagnosis of neutropenia. There are some general points to consider when using this table. Unlike anemia and thrombocytopenia, which can be confidently categorized as being due to decreased production or increased destruction because of marrow morphology and specific laboratory indicators, neutropenia is much more complex to define kinet-

TABLE 1. **Classification of Neutropenia**

Acquired or Extracellular Causes
Viral-induced marrow suppression
Nonviral infection or sepsis
Drug-induced
Chemotherapy
Other drugs
Immune-mediated
Autoimmune disease at all ages
Neonatal isoimmune
Neonatal neutropenia/maternal hypertension
Neonatal neutropenia/organic acid disorders
Hypersplenism
Nutritional deficiencies (vitamin B_{12}, folate, copper)
Pure white cell aplasia
Congenital, Inherited, or Intracellular Causes
Congenital neutropenia (agranulocytosis)/Kostmann syndrome
Cyclic neutropenia
Autosomal dominant familial neutropenia
Dysgamma-/agammaglobulinemia
Shwachman-Diamond syndrome
Glycogen storage disease type 1b
Other causes
Fanconi aplastic anemia
Myelokathexis
Lazy leukocyte syndrome
Reticular dysgenesis
Cartilage-hair hypoplasia
Dyskeratosis congenita
Pseudoneutropenia

ically and laboratory testing is not as refined. Thus, for practical reasons, the classification in Table 1 is based on the *cellular basis* for neutropenia, either an acquired extracellular cause or a congenital, inherited, or intracellular disorder.

Many of the diagnoses are age related. Most of the congenital or inherited diagnoses are detected early in infancy or childhood. In adolescence and adulthood, most of the disorders are acquired, but there is obviously some overlap. Some neutropenic conditions are common, others are rare. Viral-induced marrow suppression is the most common cause of childhood neutropenia, whereas the congenital or inherited disorders are very rare. Drug-induced, autoimmune, and nutritional deficiency neutropenias are encountered more frequently in adult patients. There is also a clinical distinction between acute-onset and severe chronic neutropenia. Acute neutropenia often develops when there is rapid neutrophil use coupled with impaired production.

Drugs used for chemotherapy are particularly likely to induce neutropenia because of the high proliferative rate of neutrophil precursors and relatively short half-life of blood neutrophils. Other non-chemotherapeutic drugs can induce severe neutropenia by idiosyncratic or hypersensitivity reactions. These drugs include analgesics, antipsychotic drugs, anticonvulsants, antithyroid drugs, cardiovascular drugs, sulfa drugs, and antibiotics.

Severe chronic neutropenia is a general term that has crept into the hematologic lexicon and is used to describe conditions with regular ANCs less than 500/μL. Because neutrophils are crucial in protecting the body against invasion by bacteria, severe chronic neutropenia regularly predisposes a patient to pyogenic infections. Chronic neutropenia is caused by a variety of hematologic disorders as well as immunologic, metabolic, and infectious diseases. Congenital neutropenia, cyclic neutropenia, and idiopathic neutropenia are three major diagnostic categories of severe chronic neutropenia that respond to granulocyte colony-stimulating factor (G-CSF) therapy (see later).

Some neutropenias are serious with overt symptomatology, whereas others are clinically silent and are discovered in the context of a routine medical examination. Most severe forms of neutropenia ultimately present with one or more of the following: fever of unknown origin (so-called fever-neutropenia), chronic oropharyngeal ulcers, gingivitis, periodontal disease, bacterial or fungal septicemia, cellulitis of the skin or perirectal area, abscesses despite the absence of true pus, and other life-threatening infections.

CLINICAL AND LABORATORY EVALUATION

A complete medical history is an essential first step. Key historical information about previous blood cell counts may require some detective work. These counts are routinely performed in other physicians' offices for evaluation of other medical problems; this information can provide immediate confirmation that an episode of neutropenia is acquired or of recent onset. By using Table 1, other useful historical data can be generated. A detailed evaluation of infections is needed to determine the type, severity, duration, and recurrences, as well as the age at onset of symptoms to document whether the disorder is congenital or acquired. Antecedent viral infection should be noted; this is by far the most common explanation for neutropenia in young children. Medication usage, including that of nonprescription drugs, should be elicited. Symptoms of other systemic disorders such as autoimmune disease or chronic liver dysfunction that could produce splenomegaly must also be reviewed. The nutritional history should include symptomatology of vitamin B_{12} or folic acid deficiency.

For infants and children with neutropenia, the historical questions are more specific. In neonatal neutropenia, failure to thrive is suggestive of a metabolic disorder. A maternal history of hypertension is an important explanation for neonatal neutropenia. Similarly, in neonates, a family history of previously affected siblings with the same problem suggests an autosomal recessive inheritance pattern as seen in Kostmann syndrome, some immune deficiency disorders, Shwachman-Diamond syndrome, glycogen storage disease type 1b, and metabolic disorders. A history of a parent as well as one or more offspring with neutropenia implies an autosomal dominant mode of transmission as seen in one form of cyclic neutropenia and in a type of noncyclic severe chronic neutropenia. The history for classic cyclic neutropenia is that of mouth ulcers, periodontal complaints, fever, malaise, or infections every 21 days.

The physical examination is directed to sites of current or recent infection, especially the oral cavity, skin, perineum, and perirectal area. In adults, the focus should also be on signs of nutritional deficiency, collagen vascular disease, and splenomegaly, as well as pallor, bruises, or petechiae, which suggest a more generalized marrow disorder owing to replacement or a myelodysplastic syndrome. In infants and children, particular attention is paid to growth and developmental parameters. A detailed evaluation is also performed for the presence of phenotypic abnormalities and skeletal anomalies, which are seen in Shwachman-Diamond syndrome, in Fanconi anemia, and in some of the other syndromes listed in Table 1.

In infants and young children, the workup also includes blood cell counts on parents and siblings to unmask an inherited cause; testing for antineutrophil antibodies to diagnose autoimmune neutropenia of infancy; serologic studies for collagen vascular disorders; immunoglobulin quantitation and cellular immunity screening for diagnosis of an immunodeficiency syndrome; serial blood cell counts three times a week for 4 to 8 weeks to determine a predictable cyclic pattern; bone marrow aspiration and biopsy for diagnostic morphology, cytogenetic studies to exclude a malignant clonal change, and a polymerase chain reaction molecular analysis of the cells for Epstein-Barr virus, cytomegalovirus, and herpes simplex virus. The marrow morphology can be very specific in diagnosing congenital neutropenia/Kostmann syndrome (maturation arrest at the myelocyte stage) and myelokathexis (myeloid hypercellularity with degenerative, pyknotic granulocytes).

Specific syndromes listed in Table 1 such as Shwachman-Diamond syndrome, glycogen storage disease type 1b, neutropenia associated with metabolic disorders, and Fanconi anemia require highly specialized diagnostic testing and usually require referral to a subspecialty center. Many of the investigations for infants and younger children are also pertinent for older children and adults. Additional testing for older patients, however, should include determination of serum copper, serum vitamin B_{12}, and red blood cell folate levels; an HIV detection study in the appropriate clinical setting; and, if hypersplenism is present, imaging and other diagnostic testing to determine the cause.

THERAPY

General Measures

Management depends on the degree of the neutropenia, its etiology, and the patient's previous history of infections. In healthy-appearing, asymptomatic adults and older children with isolated neutropenia, and with cell counts greater than 750/μL, clinical observation only without further diagnostic study may be warranted. Medications that may account for the neutropenia should be stopped, if possible. Serial blood cell counts will determine if the neutropenia is transient or persistent. If it persists longer than 4 to 8 weeks, additional workup is needed. If anemia or thrombocytopenia is present at any time, however, bone marrow aspiration or biopsy is the next diagnostic test. Infants, younger children, and patients of all ages with a history of chronic, recurrent, or severe infection with neutrophil counts less than 750/μL, especially less than 500/μL, require further diagnostic testing and a decision about medical intervention.

General preventive measures should include good hand washing, meticulous skin care, and good oral hygiene with regular dental checkups and professional cleaning. For neutropenic mouth ulcers, a "magic mouthwash" can be prepared by a pharmacist containing equal parts of 2% viscous lidocaine (Xylocaine) and diphenhydramine (Benadryl) in normal saline. A peroxide-based mouthwash can also be used for oral hygiene. Rectal examinations and rectal temperature taking, as well as suppositories and enemas, should be avoided if possible.

Patients who are neutropenic but with ANCs greater than 1000/μL generally exhibit normal defense against infection and can be regarded in the same manner as non-neutropenic patients. For patients with ANCs greater than 500/μL but less than 1000/μL who have recurrent infections, preventive medical therapy is an option. Before the cytokine era, prophylactic antibiotics were sometimes used. The most popular agents were the penicillins and trimethoprim-sulfamethoxazole (Bactrim, Septra). These antibiotics may be effective in diminishing the frequency of infections and can be tried, but there may be significant problems associated with their continuous use. These include gastrointestinal complaints, "selection" and then overgrowth of antibiotic-resistant organisms, and allergic reactions.

Patients whose ANC is less than 500/μL are at serious risk of bacterial infection, particularly from pathogens such as *Staphylococcus aureus* and gram-negative organisms. These are often of endogenous origin in the neutropenic host. The onset of fever of greater than 38.5°C (101.3°F) in these patients should be regarded as a medical emergency. By virtue of the low neutrophil counts, they may have few signs of inflammation but they must be hospitalized and empirically treated with antibiotics while awaiting culture results. In my clinic and emergency department, we immediately activate a treatment protocol before admission to avoid any delay in antibiotic therapy. The protocol was developed in our institution for management of patients on chemotherapy who developed fever-neutropenia, but it is equally suitable for any patient with a neutrophil count of less than 500/μL.

Emergency Department Management

Stop all medications. Start an intravenous line and give standard fluids at 1.5 times maintenance. Order a chest film, a serum creatinine study, and urinalysis, and obtain cultures of blood and urine and from any apparent focus of infection. When selecting antibiotics, always consider the patient's past history regarding resistance patterns of previously cultured organisms as well as the patient's clinical stability. Standard initial antibiotics for the stable patient as described next may not be appropriate for a patient who has had previous serious infection due to an antibiotic-resistant organism.

Administer the following antibiotics stat (i.e., they should be given before patient transfer to any other area and before administration of any blood product):

- Piperacillin (Pipracil): children: 50 mg/kg intravenously every 6 hours; adults: 2 to 4 g intravenously every 4 to 6 hours (maximum: 24 g/d)
- Tobramycin (Nebcin): children: 2.5 mg/kg intravenously every 8 hours; adults: 150 mg intravenously every 8 hours. (Tobramycin requires therapeutic drug monitoring.)

If a significant β-lactam allergy exists, give

- Tobramycin, as before
- Ciprofloxacin (Cipro): children: 10 mg/kg intravenously every 12 hours; adults: 400 mg intravenously every 12 hours
- Clindamycin (Cleocin): children: 8 mg/kg intravenously every 8 hours; adults: 600 mg intravenously every 8 hours

If the patient is unstable or in septic shock, give

- Tobramycin, as before
- Meropenem (Merrem IV): children: 20 mg/kg intravenously every 8 hours; adults: 1 g intravenously every 8 hours
- Vancomycin (Vancocin): children: 15 mg/kg intravenously every 6 hours; adults: 1 g/dose intravenously every 6 hours. (Vancomycin requires therapeutic drug monitoring.)

If a significant β-lactam allergy exists, give

- Ciprofloxacin, as before
- Vancomycin, as before
- Amikacin (Amikin): children: 10 to 15 mg/kg/dose intravenously every 8 hours; adults: 500 mg/dose intravenously every 8 hours

Management After Admission

Vital signs are measured hourly until the patient's condition stabilizes and then every 4 hours or as indicated, and the patient is admitted as soon as possible. If blood cultures are subsequently positive, repeat cultures should be drawn when this result becomes known. Antibiotics specifically directed toward the identified organism should be added to the broad-spectrum therapy if the initial antibiotics do not provide adequate coverage. Broad-spectrum coverage must not be replaced by specific antibiotics alone in the neutropenic patient.

For therapeutic drug monitoring, before and after levels should be ordered with the third dose of tobramycin. An after level of 7 to 9 mg/L should be targeted. Subsequently, a prelevel should be ordered once weekly to detect tobramycin accumulation. If the patient is receiving concurrent nephrotoxic drugs (e.g., amphotericin, acyclovir) or has unstable renal function, twice-weekly prelevels are warranted. For patients who become afebrile, with a neutrophil count greater than 500/μL and with negative cultures, antibiotics can be stopped. For patients who become afebrile and with negative cultures but with neutrophils less than 500/μL, antibiotics can usually be stopped after a duration of 48 hours of therapy.

Patients who are persistently febrile but stable should continue to receive the initial empirical antibiotic regimen as described. If the patient's condition indicates an evolving infection at a particular site (e.g., abdominal pain, severe mucositis, pneumonia), antibiotics directed toward possible causative organisms should be added to the broad-spectrum coverage. After 5 to 7 days of persistent fever, consider the addition of amphotericin.

Specific and Growth Factor Treatment

Referring to Table 1, there are several diagnoses of acquired neutropenia that respond to specific treatment. Excluding chemotherapy-induced neutropenia, when a drug is suspected as causing the problem, the product should be stopped and general supportive measures instituted. If neutropenia is severe, administration of growth factor (cytokine therapy) should be started (see later). Autoimmune neutropenia of infancy occurring in the first 3 years of life is clinically benign and self-limited, but the spontaneous resolution may take months to years; no therapy is needed unless a bacterial infection ensues, at which point cytokine therapy is initiated in combination with antibiotics.

Treatment of chronic autoimmune neutropenia in older children and adults is usually supportive if the neutropenia is an isolated manifestation. Cytokine therapy and antibiotics should be used, however, if infection is a problem. A more generalized multisystem autoimmune disorder usually requires specialized management, conventionally starting with corticosteroids. One of these disorders, Felty syndrome (rheumatoid arthritis, splenomegaly, and neutropenia), is managed with options ranging from splenectomy, antirheumatic therapy, immunosuppression, plasmapheresis, intravenous immunoglobulin, and cytokine therapy.

Isoimmune neonatal neutropenia is the neutrophil equivalent of Rh hemolytic disease of the newborn and lasts an average of 7 weeks postnatally. Therapy is supportive with antibiotics as necessary, but in life-threatening infections, plasma exchange to remove antineutrophil antibodies, transfusion of maternal neutrophils that lack the immunogenetic antigen, intravenous immunoglobulin, and cytokine therapy can be used individually or in combination. In neutropenic neonates born to mothers with pregnancy-induced hypertension, the condition is characteristically limited to the first 72 hours of life and seldom requires treatment.

"Hypersplenic" neutropenia is seldom severe enough to cause serious infection. Therapy should be directed at correcting the underlying cause of the splenomegaly if possible; splenectomy is a last resort. Replacement therapy for nutritional deficiencies of vitamin B_{12} and folic acid will specifically and promptly correct the associated neutropenia. Pure white cell aplasia, in which the bone marrow morphology shows absence of myeloid precursors, occurs in most cases with a thymoma, and occasionally with ibuprofen therapy. Thymectomy may be effective in the former situation but usually also requires immunosuppression and/or intravenous immunoglobulin. With ibuprofen-induced neutropenia, stopping the drug corrects the problem.

For many of the congenital or inherited neutropenias, cytokine therapy is extremely effective in reversing the abnormal hematology. Severe chronic neutropenia was targeted in 1987 for clinical trials with G-CSF (filgrastim [Neupogen]), and more than 95% of patients with congenital, cyclic, and idiopathic forms of neutropenia responded completely. Based on data compiled by the Severe Chronic Neutropenia International Registry (University of Washington, Seattle), G-CSF is now considered the standard, first-line treatment for these conditions. A second product, granulocyte-macrophage colony-stimulating factor

(GM-CSF, sargramostim [Leukine]), is currently believed to be second-line therapy for severe chronic neutropenia in North America because of less predictable neutrophilic responses.

For patients with a neutrophil count of less than 500/μL with congenital neutropenia (encompassing Kostmann syndrome, Shwachman-Diamond syndrome, glycogen storage disease type 1b, and Fanconi anemia), and for the cyclic and idiopathic forms, G-CSF is started at 5 μg/kg/d subcutaneously. If the neutrophil count rises to 1000 to 5000/μL and plateaus, the same G-CSF dosage is maintained. If the count exceeds 5000/μL, the dose is reduced to 3 μg/kg/d to bring the count to 1000 to 5000/μL. If the neutrophil count still exceeds 5000/μL with 3 μg/kg, the dose is lowered further to 1 μg/kg/d or to alternate-day dosing, for example, 1 to 2 μg/kg every second day.

If there is no response to the starting dose, the G-CSF is increased to 10 μg/kg/d. If there is still no effect, increments are continued every 2 to 4 weeks to 20 μg/kg/d, then 30 μg/kg/d, and so on up to a maximum of 120 μg/kg/d (which would require a twice-daily administration or multiple subcutaneous injections at the same time). A patient who fails to respond to 120 μg/kg/d is defined as being refractory to G-CSF treatment. A trial of GM-CSF would then be warranted using a starting dose of 3 to 15 μg/kg/d (250 μg/m²/d) subcutaneously.

G-CSF, 5 to 10 μg/kg/d, either intravenously or subcutaneously, is also indicated for other forms of severe neutropenia, especially those associated with chemotherapy, using the following guidelines that we at the Hospital for Sick Children developed:

- For febrile neutropenic patients who have positive blood cultures, have an identified focus of infection, and/or whose vital signs are unstable
- For patients receiving chemotherapy protocols that predictably induce severe neutropenia to increase safety and to ensure that the full course of chemotherapy is given and given on time; G-CSF should be administered after the first and subsequent cycles of chemotherapy in these patients
- With antineoplastic dose-escalation protocols that predictably induce severe neutropenia
- For patients enrolled in multicenter chemotherapy protocols that specify the use of G-CSF
- For patients receiving antineoplastic agents in conjunction with large-volume irradiation involving the bone marrow

In this setting as a preventive agent, G-CSF can be stopped when neutrophils are more than 1500/μL for 2 consecutive days. When G-CSF is given for fever-neutropenia, or to patients whose condition is unstable or who have a focus of infection or a positive culture, it can be stopped when neutrophils are greater than 1000/μL for 2 days if the patient is clinically improved, the focus has resolved, and the cultures are negative.

HEMOLYTIC DISEASE OF THE FETUS AND NEWBORN*

method of
SHAWN S. OSTERHOLT, M.D.
Blanchfield Army Community Hospital
Ft. Campbell, Kentucky

and

MICHAEL K. YANCEY, M.D.
Tripler Army Medical Center
Honolulu, Hawaii

A French midwife first reported hemolytic disease of the newborn in a set of twins in 1609. The first twin appeared hydropic and was stillborn, whereas the second twin became extremely jaundiced in the first few days of life, developed kernicterus, and died several days later. Hemolytic disease of the newborn and fetus continued to be a frequent cause of perinatal morbidity and mortality until approximately 3 decades ago, when effective primary preventive strategies were introduced.

Any anemia in which the lifespan of the erythrocyte is shortened is referred to as a *hemolytic anemia*. The normal lifespan of the erythrocyte is 120 days. However, in the newborn, the lifespan of the erythrocyte is reduced to 70 to 90 days. Hemolytic disease of the fetus and newborn is associated with a heterogeneous array of problems both in the fetus and neonate. Red blood cell destruction begins in the fetus and can lead to hydrops fetalis and intrauterine death. The neonate is born with anemia and jaundice that can worsen in the first few days of life, leading to kernicterus with the possibility of permanent brain dysfunction and death. The causes of hemolytic anemia can be divided into four general classifications:

1. Immune-mediated disorders
2. Hemoglobinopathies
3. Erythrocyte enzyme deficiencies
4. Defective erythrocyte membrane disorders (Table 1)

Hematopoiesis in the embryo begins in the yolk sac by the fourth week of gestation. In the second trimester, fetal erythropoiesis is transferred from the yolk sac and occurs predominantly in the liver and spleen; and finally, fetal erythropoiesis shifts predominately to the bone marrow in the third trimester. In the fetus, the predominant hemoglobin is composed of two α chains and two γ chains, which is referred to as *fetal hemoglobin* or *hemoglobin F.* Before term, the fetus begins to synthesize adult hemoglobin composed of two α and two β chains, referred to as *hemoglobin A.* At term, hemoglobin F represents 60% to 90% of the newborn's hemoglobin, which drops to less than 5% by 4 months of age, the typical amount of fetal hemoglobin found in a healthy adult. Erythropoiesis in the fetus is responsive to erythropoietin, a glycosylated 165-amino acid protein produced by real cortical interstitial cells that stimulates the production and maturation of erythrocytes. With the erythrocyte destruction that occurs with hemolytic anemia, erythropoietin levels are increased. When the production of erythrocytes in the bone marrow is unable to keep up with red blood cell destruction, extramedullary sites of

*The opinions and assertions contained herein are the expressed views of the authors and are not to be construed as official or reflecting the opinions of the Department of Defense or the Department of the Army.

TABLE 1. **Etiology of Hemolytic Anemia in the Fetus and Newborn**

Isoimmunization
Rh incompatibility
Minor groups of antigens
ABO incompatibility
Hemoglobinopathies
Homozygous α-thalassemia—Bart hemoglobin (γ^4)
Erythrocyte Enzyme Deficiencies
Glucose-6-phosphate dehydrogenase deficiency
Pyruvate kinase deficiency
Hexose monophosphate shunt defects
Embden-Meyerhof pathway defects
Defective Red Blood Cell Membrane
Hereditary spherocytosis
Hereditary elliptocytosis

red blood cell production are stimulated, primarily in the liver and spleen with smaller amounts in the kidney and adrenal gland. When extramedullary hematopoiesis occurs, there is poor control of red blood cell production, with many immature erythrocytes appearing in the fetal circulation. These immature fetal red blood cells are referred to as erythroblasts; thus, the synonym for hemolytic disease of the newborn is *erythroblastosis fetalis*.

ISOIMMUNIZATION

More than 400 red blood cell antigens have been described in the literature. Fortunately, only a few of the erythrocyte antigens are clinically important causes of isoimmunization leading to hemolysis of fetal and newborn erythrocytes. The most common cause of hemolytic disease of the fetus and newborn is due to anti-D IgG. Accordingly, we first examine Rh isoimmunization in detail followed by a short discussion of ABO incompatibility and minor blood group antigen isoimmunization that can lead to fetal and neonatal hemolytic anemia in rare instances.

Rh Isoimmunization

In 1932, Diamond and associates reported that hydrops fetalis, neonatal jaundice, and newborn anemia were all due to the same disease process and associated with circulating erythroblasts. Landsteiner and Wiener, in 1940, discovered the rhesus (Rh) factor when they detected an agglutinable factor in human blood using serum of rabbits previously immunized with blood from rhesus monkeys. In 1941, Levine and colleagues reported that hemolytic disease of the newborn was closely associated with Rh antibodies in women whose blood type was Rh negative.

Since this early work, many details of the Rh blood group system have been elucidated. The Rh system is composed of three basic pairs of antigens: Cc, Dd, and Ee. The CDE antigens are located on the short arm of chromosome 1 in two homologous genes. The presence of D determines whether an individual is Rh positive. Because d, the reciprocal of D, has not been discovered, it is the absence of D that makes an individual Rh(D) negative. The Rh antigens are inherited in two sets of three pairs of homologous genes, with one set being contributed by each parent. The D antigen is much more immunogenic than C, c, E, e; thus, production of anti-D in Rh(D)-negative women is the primary cause of hemolytic disease in fetuses who are Rh(D) positive. Because the d antigen has not been found, the zygosity for D of an Rh(D)-positive person can only be established for certain by having an Rh-negative offspring. The zygosity of the father is of extreme importance because if the father is homozygous for the D antigen (DD), all of his children will be Rh(D) positive and thus can be afflicted with Rh hemolytic disease if a mother is Rh(D) negative and produces anti-D antibody. In contrast, if the father is homozygous for the D antigen (Dd), then only 50% of the children he fathers will be Rh(D) positive and at risk for hemolytic disease of the newborn.

INCIDENCE

The incidence of the Rh(D)-negative blood type does not differ by gender but does differ according to race (Table 2). Many factors are associated with incidence and degree of Rh isoimmunization in exposed pregnancies. These include the density of red cell antigens on the fetal erythrocyte, the variable antigenicity of these sites on the fetal membrane, the variability of the maternal response to the antigen in her bloodstream, the degree of transplacental passage of the antibody, and the protection of ABO incompatibility against isoimmunization. Before the introduction of anti-D immunoglobulin for the prevention of anti-D isoimmunization, the incidence of D isoimmunization was reported to be 16% for a term Rh(D)-negative woman who gave birth to an infant who is Rh(D) positive with ABO-compatible blood type. Anti-D IgG antibody could be detected in 8% of such women 6 months after delivery and in the remaining 8% at the onset of a subsequent pregnancy. In contrast, if an Rh(D)-negative woman gave birth to an infant who is Rh(D) positive with ABO-incompatible blood type, the incidence of Rh isoimmunization was 1.5% to 2.0%. First trimester abortion, elective terminations of pregnancy, threatened abortion, chorionic villus sampling, amniocentesis (regardless of whether the needle traverses the placenta), external cephalic version, blunt abdominal trauma, and ectopic pregnancy have all been associated with fetal-maternal hemorrhage and isoimmunization. In the absence of immunoprophylaxis with anti-D immunoglobulin, first trimester spontaneous abortion is associated with a 2% incidence of isoimmunization, whereas elective termination of pregnancy is associated with a 5% incidence of isoimmunization.

PATHOPHYSIOLOGY

The Rh(D) antigen sites are found on the erythrocyte membrane in a lattice-like pattern. Fetal erythrocyte production occurs by 4 weeks after conception, whereas the Rh(D) antigen has been reported on the surface of the fetal red blood cell by 38 days after conception. For Rh isoimmunization to occur, three circumstances must exist: (1) the fetal blood type must be Rh(D) positive and the maternal blood type Rh(D) negative; (2) the mother must

TABLE 2. **Incidence of Rh-Negativity Among Different Populations**

Race	Percentage Rh-Negative
Basque population in Spain	30%–35%
White	15%
African American	8%
Native American	1%–2%
African	4%

have had prior exposure to the Rh(D)-positive blood type and, thus, have the immunogenic capacity to produce antibody directed against the D antigen; and (3) a sufficient number of fetal red blood cells must gain access to the maternal circulation to stimulate an immune response.

There are three proposed causes of sensitization to the Rh(D) antigen in an Rh(D)-negative person. The most common mechanism is a fetal-maternal hemorrhage. With the use of flow cytometry, microscopic fetal-maternal hemorrhage has been found to be virtually universal. There is a graded dose-dependent response for the initial isoimmunization, with 15% of volunteers sensitized after 1 mL of Rh-positive erythrocytes, 33% after 40 mL, and 65% to 70% after 250 mL. With the use of serial assessment of the volume of fetal erythrocytes in the maternal circulation, only 3% of Rh-negative women will become sensitized if the maximal volume of Rh(D)-positive fetal erythrocytes is less than 0.1 mL. However, the secondary immune response in a previously sensitized woman has been associated with as little as 0.1 mL of fetal blood in the maternal circulation. A second potential etiology of Rh(D) isoimmunization is transfusion of Rh(D)-positive blood to an Rh(D)-negative woman. In contemporary practice, blood transfusion is an uncommon cause of Rh isoimmunization because blood is crossmatched for Rh type; however, blood transfusions are the most common cause of atypical (non-D) isoimmunization because blood is not crossmatched for many minor antigens. The third proposed mechanism is that of the "grandmother theory." This theory suggests that a fetus is immunized at birth from her mother's Rh-positive cells during the birth process. Thus, the fetus's maternal grandmother is the source of Rh(D)-positive erythrocytes, which causes maternal isoimmunization.

In general, an Rh(D)-negative individual must have two exposures to the D antigen to produce a significant immune response. With the first exposure, primary sensitization occurs. This primary response is mostly IgM anti-D, which has a large molecular weight and thus cannot cross the placenta. After this initial IgM production, most women convert to IgG production, which has a low molecular weight and thus can cross the placenta; however, the amount of IgG antibody produced during the primary response is relatively low. Therefore, the fetus carried by an Rh(D)-negative woman who has mounted a primary immunogenic is generally unaffected. The secondary response occurs with subsequent exposure to Rh(D) antigen, typically with fetal erythrocytes gaining access to the maternal circulation during a subsequent pregnancy. This is an anamnestic response, leading to rapid increase in the IgG anti-D level.

The exact mechanism of fetal red blood cell destruction is unclear, but it is likely mediated through immune mechanisms other than complement. The basic pathophysiology is the binding of maternal IgG anti-D antibodies to the fetal erythrocyte membrane. This leads to chemotaxis in which the antibody-antigen complex is bound to fetal macrophages. Macrophages surrounded by a ring of erythrocytes are called *rosettes*, which are trapped in spleen and the erythrocytes are subsequently lysed. Once destruction of fetal erythrocytes exceeds production, the fetus becomes anemic, which stimulates extramedullary production of erythrocytes in the liver, kidney, spleen, adrenal gland, and placenta. In the liver, the hypertrophy of the erythropoietic cells leads to compression and destruction of normal hepatic cells. The destruction of normal hepatic cells leads to decreased synthesis of albumin, which lowers the intravascular colloid oncotic pressure, leading to fluid shifts into the extravascular compartment and ultimately resulting in hydrops fetalis.

PREVENTION

There is currently a prevention strategy only targeted for Rh(D) isoimmunization. There is no prevention strategy for ABO incompatibility or for any of the minor blood group antigens. The immunology principle that passively administered antibodies can prevent active immunization to its specific antigen has been known for decades before its use for the prevention of Rh isoimmunization. In 1968, the Food and Drug Administration approved anti-D immunoglobin (Rh immunoglobin) for the prevention of Rh isoimmunization after its efficacy was proven in male prisoner volunteers. Today, failure to administer anti-D immunoglobin to pregnant or recently delivered women at risk is the most common cause of hemolytic disease in the newborn. Anti-D immunoglobin is extracted by cold alcohol fractionation of plasma donated by individuals with high anti-D titers. Because anti-D immunoglobin is a derivative of blood products, there is a concern for the passage of infectious diseases; however, it is thought that infectious diseases, such as HIV and hepatitis, are inactivated in the processing, and there have been no substantiated cases of infectious diseases secondary to anti-D immunoglobin administration.

The precise mechanism by which anti-D immunoglobin prevents isoimmunization remains unclear. The most likely mechanism of action is that of central inhibition because the circulating anti-D immunoglobulin immediately binds D antigen on the surface of fetal erythrocytes, thus suppressing the primary immune response by interrupting B-cell recognition of the foreign antigen and subsequent plasma cell transformation. This blocking of the primary immune response effectively prevents endogenous immunoglobulin production. To be effective, there must be sufficient amounts of available anti-D immunoglobulin to bind all available D antigens.

Before the introduction of anti-D immunoglobin, 9% to 10% of susceptible pregnancies were affected by hemolytic disease of the fetus and newborn. Approximately 90% of cases of isoimmunization occur secondary to fetal-maternal hemorrhage at term. Initially, anti-D immunoglobin was given within 72 hours postpartum, which reduced the incidence of Rh isoimmunization from 16% to 2% (a 90% decrease) in susceptible women. Subsequently, it was shown that an additional antenatal administration at 28 to 29 weeks reduced the incidence from 2% to 0.1% in susceptible women. The recommendation that anti-D immunoglobin be given within 72 hours of birth is due to the design of the initial studies on prisoners in which investigators were permitted to visit the prisoners at 72-hour intervals. Anti-D immunoglobin has been proven to prevent isoimmunization if given up to 13 days postpartum. If anti-D immunoglobin is missed in the early postpartum period, many authorities recommend administration up to 28 days postpartum.

The current recommendations from the American College of Obstetrics and Gynecology are to administer a standard 300-μg dose of anti-D immunoglobin at 28 to 29 weeks and again within 72 hours postpartum to at-risk women. When the risk of fetal-maternal hemorrhage occurs in the first trimester, such as in spontaneous abortion, threatened abortion, ectopic pregnancy, and elective termination of pregnancy, a 50-μg prophylactic dose of anti-D immunoglobin should be given to those women at risk. In the second and third trimester, additional 300-μg doses of anti-

D immunoglobin should be administered when risk factors for fetal-maternal hemorrhage are present, such as amniocentesis, chorionic villus sampling, blunt abdominal trauma, and antenatal hemorrhage. If the time from the last dose of anti-D immunoglobin and delivery is less than 21 days, then the postpartum dose of anti-D immunoglobin can be withheld as long as the passively acquired antibodies are still present in the maternal blood and no excess maternal fetal hemorrhage has occurred. If anti-D IgG is present in the serum of a woman who has not recently received anti-D IgG, the prophylactic use of anti-D immunoglobin is contraindicated because it is not beneficial in a patient who is already sensitized.

Anti-D immunoglobin has a half-life of 24 days, with a standard dose generally providing protection for approximately 12 weeks. The 300-μg standard prophylactic dose of anti-D immunoglobin can prevent isoimmunization after exposure of up to 30 mL of Rh(D)-positive fetal blood or 15 mL of fetal erythrocytes. If the mother is exposed to greater than 30 mL of fetal blood, a larger dose of anti-D immunoglobin is required. It is estimated that 1 in 1250 pregnancies are associated with a fetal-maternal hemorrhage in excess of 30 mL. There are certain risk factors for excessive maternal-fetal hemorrhage such as placental abruption, abdominal trauma, intrauterine manipulation, placenta previa, fetal demise, multiple gestation, and manual removal of the placenta; however, risk factors only identify 50% of patients with fetal-maternal hemorrhage in excess of 30 mL. Thus, after delivery all patients should be screened with a rosette test that will identify fetal-maternal hemorrhage in excess of 10 mL. If the rosette test is positive, the mother should then be screened with a Kleihauer-Betke test. The Kleihauer-Betke test relies on the fact that adult hemoglobin is more readily lysed in the presence of acid then fetal hemoglobin. The test uses citrate phosphate buffer to remove adult hemoglobin. Maternal blood is fixed on a slide with 80% ethanol and treated with citrate phosphate buffer, followed by staining with hematoxylin and eosin. The extent of maternal fetal hemorrhage is estimated based on the following formula:

$$\text{Number of Fetal Cells/Number of Maternal Cells} = \times/\text{Estimated Maternal Blood Volume in mL (85 mL/kg)}$$

Where $\times$ = mL of Fetal Maternal Hemorrhage

DETECTION AND MANAGEMENT OF THE Rh(D) ISOIMMUNIZED PREGNANCY

At the initial prenatal visit, the patient's blood should be tested for ABO type and Rh(D) type, as well as be screened with an indirect Coombs test for erythrocyte antibodies (antibody screen). In a patient who is Rh(D) negative and has no demonstrable erythrocyte antibody detected on the initial prenatal antibody screen, a repeat antibody screen is performed at 28 weeks along with the administration of 300 μg of anti-D globulin at this time. The antibody screen should be repeated during labor and then the administration of 300 μg of anti-D immunoglobin should be administered within 72 hours of delivery. If the father is known to be Rh(D) negative and there is no question of paternity, the prophylactic doses of anti-D immunoglobin can be eliminated.

If the antibody screen demonstrates anti-D IgG, which is not secondary to administration of prophylactic anti-D immunoglobin, the fetus is at risk for hemolytic disease if the fetal blood type is Rh(D) positive. Again, if the father is Rh(D) negative (and there is no question of paternity), then the fetus is not at risk for hemolytic disease because the anti-D IgG demonstrable in the maternal plasma may be secondary to prior pregnancy conceived with a different partner or a prior blood transfusion.

The goal of the Rh-sensitized pregnancy is to minimize fetal morbidity and mortality by identifying infants at risk for significant hemolytic disease both in utero and during the newborn period. First, in the patient with demonstrable anti-D IgG in her circulation and when the father is determined to be Rh(D) positive, an estimation of his zygosity for the D antigen can be made. There are no readily available tests to determine the zygosity of an Rh(D)-positive individual because no d antiserum has been identified. By determining the C, c, E, and e status of the paternal blood type, an estimation of the paternal zygosity can be made by the blood bank according to established tables because certain combinations of antigens are more common than others. If a husband is homozygous for the D antigen, then all of his children will be Rh(D) positive; if he is heterozygous, then only 50% of his children will be Rh(D) positive and at risk.

Next, a thorough obstetric history is important in the management of the sensitized pregnancy. As a general rule, if a mother had a prior fetus with hemolytic disease, subsequent pregnancies are associated with hemolytic disease as severe as or more severe than previous pregnancies. If a pregnant patient has a fetus that developed hydrops, there is a 90% chance that hydrops fetalis will develop in a subsequent pregnancy at the same or an earlier gestational age.

In the first pregnancy sensitized by anti-D IgG, the level of anti-D antibody is of some value in predicting the severity of Rh hemolytic disease if carried out by experienced personnel in a reliable laboratory. Each laboratory should establish a critical value, which is the value below which severe hemolytic disease does not occur. This value will vary among laboratories, depending on techniques used. The dilutional titer below which severe hemolytic disease and hydrops fetalis does not occur generally will be between 1:8 and 1:32. In a patient's first sensitized pregnancy, this titer should be determined on a monthly basis. Once the critical titer is reached, the patient should undergo amniocentesis. In patients with a prior pregnancy complicated by hemolytic disease of the newborn, antibody titers are not needed and fetal evaluation with amniocentesis or cordocentesis should be undertaken. The gestational age at onset of hemolytic disease as well as the severity of hemolytic disease should be used as a guide as to when to initiate invasive testing. The fetal Rh(D) status can be determined by polymerase chain reaction analysis of the amniocytes, thus determining if the fetus is at risk for hemolytic disease.

With fetal hemolysis, there is an increased production of bilirubin. Because amniotic fluid is essentially a fetal byproduct, the bilirubin is excreted into the amniotic fluid primarily by means of fetal tracheal and pulmonary secretions. It has been shown that the spectrophotometric absorption of amniotic fluid bilirubin correlates with the severity of fetal hemolysis. With the use of a semi-logarithmic graph, normal amniotic fluid has a linear curve between wavelengths of 525 to 375 nm; however, bilirubin causes a shift in the optical density at 450 nm. The amount of shift of the observed absorption of amniotic fluid bilirubin at 450 nm from the expected absorption of normal amniotic fluid is referred to as ΔOD_{450}. Results are plotted on a graph based on gestational age described by Liley in 1961, referred to as a Liley curve. This plot then indicates the risk for severe hemolytic disease for a given ΔOD_{450}. Liley's original data studied pregnancies of between 27 and 41 weeks. This curve has been modified at earlier gestational ages by many authors without universal agreement on the accuracy before 27 weeks.

Because single ΔOD_{450} values are rarely helpful unless they are very high or very low, serial evaluation of ΔOD_{450} is often indicated to establish a trend. The Liley curve is divided into three zones. If the ΔOD_{450} is in zone III, the fetus is at high risk for severe hemolytic disease and fetal death within 7 to 10 days; thus, intrauterine transfusion or delivery is indicated based on gestational age. If serial ΔOD_{450} values remain in zone I, the fetus is either Rh(D) negative or is mildly affected and can be delivered at term. If the ΔOD_{450} is in zone II, the fetus is at moderate to severe risk for deterioration in utero and early delivery is indicated. The management of a pregnancy in zone II depends on many factors, such as gestational age, serial ΔOD_{450} values for trend, assessment of fetal lung maturity, biophysical assessment of fetal well-being, and past obstetric history to determine whether delivery, in utero transfusion, or repeat analysis in 1 to 2 weeks is indicated.

Direct fetal blood sampling should be carried out for fetuses at risk for hydrops before 34 weeks' gestation. With direct fetal blood sampling, the Rh status, hematocrit level, reticulocyte count, and bilirubin level of the fetus can be determined. If the hematocrit level is less than 30% or there is ultrasonographic evidence of hydrops, then intrauterine fetal transfusion should be performed with group O, Rh(D)-negative, cytomegalovirus-negative, irradiated, densely packed erythrocytes (ideally packed to a hematocrit of 85% to 90%). The volume of packed red blood cells required is 30 to 100 mL with the endpoint of transfusion being a fetal hematocrit of 45% to 55%. In general, for isoimmunized fetuses requiring transfusion, the initial transfusion volume is approximately 50 mL/kg estimated nonhydropic fetal weight. Occasionally, in the severely anemic fetus, several transfusions may be required over a span of a week to attain the target post-transfusion hematocrit level to avoid hypervolemia. The goal for transfusion therapy is to achieve a hemoglobin level that results in cessation of endogenous hematopoiesis and production of Rh(D)-positive erythrocytes. A decline of the post-transfusion hematocrit level can be estimated at approximately 1% per day, with subsequent transfusion scheduled when the fetal hematocrit level is predicted to be less than 30%. With intrauterine fetal transfusion, the perinatal survival rate has been reported to be 84% (75% in fetuses with hydrops and 90% if the fetus does not suffer from hydrops).

There are two methods of intrauterine fetal transfusion currently in use. *Intraperitoneal transfusions* deposit erythrocytes into the fetal peritoneal cavity under direct ultrasonographic visualization. These erythrocytes then enter the circulation through the subdiaphragmatic lymphatics. This method should be avoided if the fetus is hydropic because the erythrocytes are not readily absorbed in such circumstances. An alternative, and more popular, technique is *direct intravascular transfusion* by means of cordocentesis, in which a needle is guided into the umbilical vein with the aid of real-time ultrasonography and packed erythrocytes are inserted directly into the fetal vasculature. Complications of fetal transfusion include fetal fluid overload with overt cardiac failure and circulatory collapse, infection, premature rupture of membranes, placental abruption, preterm labor, fetal-maternal hemorrhage, umbilical cord laceration or thrombosis, umbilical artery spasm with fetal bradycardia, graft-versus-host disease, and a 1% to 2% incidence of fetal demise.

Other modalities used to assess fetal well-being in sensitized pregnancies include ultrasound and fetal nonstress testing. Serial ultrasound examinations are used to assess fetal growth and search for signs of fetal hemolytic disease; however, in the absence of hydrops fetalis, ultrasound cannot reliably distinguish mild from severe hemolytic disease. Ultrasonographic signs of worsening fetal anemia include increased liver size, increased placental thickness (>4 cm), pericardial effusion, dilated right atrium, thickened bowel wall, abnormalities on pulsed Doppler-flow velocity waveforms, and ascites. In the future, fetal middle cerebral artery peak systolic velocity as determined by Doppler ultrasound may be an alternative to amniocentesis and cordocentesis. This modality has been found to correlate well with fetal hematocrit level, as assessed by fetal blood sampling; however, there have not yet been published series using noninvasive methods such as middle cerebral Doppler velocimetry as the primary fetal assessment method in isoimmunized pregnancies.

TREATMENT OF THE NEONATE

Of infants born with hemolytic disease, 50% will have mild disease and no treatment is necessary. These infants are born with hemoglobin concentrations of more than 12 to 13 g/dL and bilirubin levels that do not exceed 16 to 20 mg/dL. No postnatal treatment is needed.

Moderate disease is present in 25% of affected infants. These infants are born in good condition but have risk of severe jaundice, death from kernicterus, or sequelae of bilirubin encephalopathy such as neurosensory deafness, spastic choreoathetosis, and some degree of mental retardation unless treated after birth. These sequelae are secondary to elevated levels of indirect bilirubin that is lipid soluble and neurotoxic as it gains access to neurons that have high lipid membrane content.

The final 25% of infants are born with hydrops fetalis (anasarca and ascites). This is no longer thought to be secondary to heart failure but rather to hepatic dysfunction and decreased albumin production.

The severely affected infant with severe hyperbilirubinemia should be managed with exchange transfusion. A randomized controlled trial reported a neonatal mortality rate of 33% with simple transfusion compared with a mortality rate of 13% with exchange transfusion. However, exchange transfusions are not without risk because they may predispose to oxygen toxicity, and thus retinopathy of prematurity. Hyperbilirubinemia should be treated with phototherapy that converts native bilirubin to a more water-soluble form by photo-isomerization.

ABO INCOMPATIBILITY

Although ABO incompatibility is the cause of mild to moderate anemia and hyperbilirubinemia in the neonate, moderate-to-severe hemolytic disease in the fetus and hydrops fetalis are not generally caused by ABO incompatibility. Anti-A and anti-B antibodies are predominantly IgM and thus do not readily cross the placenta. Additionally, there are relatively few A and B antigen sites on the fetal erythrocyte as compared with the adult erythrocyte. Phototherapy is the first line of therapy for the affected neonate. Exchange transfusion is required in fewer than 1% of cases.

MINOR BLOOD GROUP ANTIGENS

There are hundreds of non-D antigens that exist on the erythrocyte membrane, and many of these have been reported to cause hemolytic disease of the newborn. The most common minor antigens associated with hemolytic disease of the fetus and newborn are Kell, Kidd, and Duffy. Blood transfusion is the most common cause of isoimmunization from atypical antibodies, with 1% to 2% of recipients developing antibodies after transfusion. Although a commonly identified antibody in antenatal populations, anti-Lewis is not associated with hemolytic disease of the fetus and newborn because these antibodies are predominantly IgM and the Lewis antigen is poorly expressed on the fetal erythrocyte. A number of these minor antigens can result in production of IgG in the maternal circulation and thus can lead to fetal hemolytic anemia and hydrops. These pregnancies are managed in the same manner noted earlier for Rh(D) isoimmunized pregnancies, with the exception of Kell sensitization. With Kell sensitization, there have been reported cases of severe anemia in fetuses of women with relatively low antibody titers and amniotic fluid ΔOD_{450} values in Liley zone II. It has been postulated that anti-Kell antibodies may bind and damage fetal erythroprogenitor cells, resulting in a more severe anemia without evidence of hemolysis relative to anti-Rh(D) isoimmunization.

RARE CAUSES OF HEMOLYTIC DISEASE OF THE FETUS AND NEWBORN

Hemoglobinopathies

Disorders of hemoglobin structure and synthesis are referred to as *hemoglobinopathies*. These are very rare causes of hemolytic anemia of the fetus and newborn. Hemoglobinopathies that result in qualitative defects in the production of α- and β-globin chains are referred to as thalassemias. Bart disease, the most severe form of α-thalassemia in which all four α-globin genes are deleted, can lead to hydrops fetalis. Intrauterine blood transfusion has been attempted and has led to fetal survival; however, these fetuses require chronic blood transfusions postnatally. Hemoglobin H disease, a form of α-thalassemia, is due to the deletion of three α-globin genes. This disease leads to an accumulation of β chains, which form β^4 tetramers (termed *hemoglobin H*) within the erythrocyte and lead to decreased survival of the red blood cell. These infants suffer from varying degrees of hemolytic anemia at birth. Other hemoglobinopathies, such as β-thalassemia and sickle cell anemia, do not result in symptoms in utero or at birth, owing to the protective effects of fetal hemoglobin.

Defective Erythrocyte Membrane Disorders

Red cell membrane defects are another rare cause of hemolytic disease in the newborn. The most common congenital red blood cell disorder is hereditary spherocytosis. This disorder is due to instability of spectrin, a membrane protein responsible for the stability of the RBC membrane. Hereditary elliptocytosis, hereditary pyropoikilocytosis, and hereditary stomatocytosis are other rare inherited erythrocyte membrane defects that occasionally can cause hemolytic anemia in the newborn.

Erythrocyte Enzyme Deficiencies

Erythrocyte enzyme abnormalities are a rare cause of hemolytic disease in the newborn. There are two major metabolic pathways within the red blood cell: the Embden-Meyerhof pathway and the hexose monophosphate shunt. Defects in the enzymes within these pathways lead to decreased erythrocyte survival. Glucose-6-phosphate dehydrogenase (G6PD) deficiency is the most common erythrocyte enzyme deficiency. It is sex linked with partial expression in females and full expression in males. Its prevalence is highest in Africans, those of Mediterranean origin,

Southeast Asians, and Native Americans. G6PD deficiency can lead to severe hemolytic disease and hyperbilirubinemia with oxidant stress. Many other erythrocyte enzyme deficiencies exist that are rare and may occasionally lead to hemolytic disease of the newborn. The treatment of these neonates is generally directed toward management of postnatal hyperbilirubinemia.

HEMOPHILIA AND RELATED DISORDERS

method of
WING-YEN WONG, M.D.
Children's Hospital Los Angeles
Los Angeles, California

Hemophilia A and B and von Willebrand disease (vWD) are the most common causes of bleeding. However, there are diverse groups of less common bleeding disorders that need to be considered in the orderly workup of any coagulopathy. Often, a heightened index of suspicion toward the possible existence of such disorders and persistence in the diagnostic workup are needed. Approximately 5% of neonates with severe coagulopathy present with intracranial hemorrhage at delivery. The newborn with prolonged bleeding after circumcision, the toddler with bruises not only on the shins and arms but also on areas not usually subject to direct trauma, such as the torso and neck, and the teenager with more than 5 to 7 days of heavy menstrual bleeding all deserve attention. The axiom that joint bleeding is usual for the hemophilias and that mucosal bleeding is typical for vWD tends to hold true. However, severe vWD can have joint bleeding, and extreme lyonization can result in female carriers of hemophilia presenting with moderate menorrhagia. The one important criterion for diagnosis is the patient's medical and family history augmented by age-appropriate interpretation of laboratory tests. The following focuses on a practical approach to diagnosis and treatment choices for hemophilia A and B and vWD.

EPIDEMIOLOGY AND GENETIC TRANSMISSION

Inheritance patterns are divided into three main groups: (1) hemophilia A and B are X-linked recessive, (2) vWD is usually autosomal dominant, although (3) some vWD and other factor deficiencies are autosomal recessive. Approximately 30% of hemophilia patients present with new mutations and have a negative family history. Incidence of hemophilia A is estimated at 1:5,000 male births and that for hemophilia B at 1:30,000.

There are no geographic or racial differences. Mild hemophilia is often misdiagnosed and therefore may be underrepresented. Carrier and prenatal testing from blood and amniotic samples has more than 90% accuracy if performed at established laboratories, particularly if blood samples from various affected family members are available for DNA linkage studies. An inversion within intron 22 of the factor VIII gene has been found in over 45% of severely affected hemophilia A patients. Molecular genetic testing by DNA analysis for this and other mutations is available at certain research laboratories. Testing from chorionic villus sampling can be done at 10 to 12 weeks' gestation if the specific genetic mutation is known, but sampling of fetal blood for factor VIII activity cannot be done before 16 weeks' gestation.

The incidence of vWD is unknown and estimates can vary from 0.2% to 2.0%, because a large number of affected individuals are not diagnosed. There are no gender or racial differences. The complexity of the various vWD subtypes and the generally mild nature of vWD have not lent vWD to easy prenatal testing; thus, this testing is not usually performed. A large number of vWD molecular gene defects have been identified, and the information can be obtained from online databank sites. DNA testing can be helpful for certain vWD subtypes such as type 2N, which can be misdiagnosed as hemophilia A, because both disorders have low levels of factor VIII. Factor XI deficiency is the most common hereditary coagulopathy in the Jewish population.

DISEASE CLASSIFICATION AND LABORATORY TESTING

The partial thromboplastin time (PTT) measures most of the clotting factor abnormalities associated with bleeding diatheses except for those involving factor VII and factor XIII. Some causes of a prolonged PTT not associated with significant bleeding even with major trauma or surgery include deficiencies of high molecular weight kininogen (HMWK), prekallikrein, and factor XII. Exclusion of an inhibitor such as antiphospholipid antibody should also be considered in the presence of a prolonged PTT and relative benign bleeding history. The mechanism of disease in the coagulopathies may involve failure of synthesis of the necessary coagulation factor or synthesis of abnormal proteins with impaired activity. Hence, the functional protein activity may differ from the antigen or protein measured.

Hemophilia A and B result in inadequate generation of thrombin for clot formation. The degree of disease severity and onset of symptoms vary with plasma factor VIII or factor IX activity levels. Boys with less than 1% factor activity have severe disease with early onset of joint and muscle hemorrhage. Those with hemophilia A have bleeding symptoms earlier in life, usually within the first year, compared with hemophilia B. Moderate and mild disease correlate to factor activity levels of greater than or equal to 1% to 5% and more than 5%, respectively. Carrier females may have factor levels ranging from 30% to 70%.

In vWD, the mechanism of disease is associated with failure to form an effective primary platelet plug. There are three main types of vWD and numerous subtypes. Type 1 vWd is due to a partial quantitative deficiency of von Willebrand factor (vWF), type 2 has qualitative variants, and type 3 has a marked, sometimes complete, deficiency of vWF. Overall, patients with type 1 and type 2 tend to have mild to moderate severity of bleeding, whereas the patient with the rarer type 3 vWD tends to have severe disease. Type 2N has a defective affinity for factor VIII, and both factor VIII and vWF are markedly decreased. It is critical that physicians, especially gynecologists and obstetricians, consider the workup and diagnosis for vWD in any female with complaints of excessive menstrual bleeding.

The main characteristics of hemophilia A and vWD are outlined in Table 1.

TREATMENT OPTIONS

Hemophilia A and B

The hallmark of effective treatment remains replacement of the deficient or abnormal factor as early

TABLE 1. **Comparison of Hemophilia A and von Willebrand Disease**

	Hemophilia A	vWD*
Inheritance	X-linked	Autosomal
Bleeding pattern	Mainly joint, muscle bleeding	Mainly mucous membrane bleeding (e.g., epistaxis, menorrhagia)
Partial thromboplastin time	↑	Nl or ↑
Factor VIIIa	↓	Nl or ↓
Von Willebrand factor antigen (vWF:Ag)	Nl	↓ or Nl
Ristocetin cofactor (RcoF)	Nl	↓ or Nl
Ivy bleeding time	Nl	↑

*Modifying factors include blood type (type O has decreased vWF), stress, physical activity, estrogen use, and pregnancy. Normal values do not definitively exclude diagnosis of vWD and can vary from time to time within the same individual.
Abbreviation: Nl = normal.

and promptly as possible, at the appropriate dosage and frequency. The ability to self-infuse or have a caregiver administer the factor at home at the first sign of any bleeding has had a positive impact on disease outcome. For this approach to be effective, early recognition of bleeding is required. Early symptoms for joint or muscle bleeding include increased warmth, tingling sensations, and a vague feeling at the affected or target joint. Increased irritability in the infant or young child often heralds the onset of bleeding. Patients should not wait for swelling or discoloration to infuse.

Another step contributing to a significant improvement in disease outcome has been a close association with a specialty hemostasis/hemophilia treatment center. These facilities have the necessary expertise in coordination of all aspects of diagnosis and care, acute and chronic, as well as a multifaceted team approach. Close telephone contact should be maintained between the family and treatment center personnel in the event of any bleeding episode, even when home therapy has been initiated successfully.

For mild hemophilia A, Stimate, a concentrated form of desmopressin, can be used without exposure to blood products. This is particularly helpful in persons avoiding blood products for religious reasons as well as decreasing the risk of infectious transmissions. Details of this treatment option are covered in the later section on the treatment of vWD.

The current treatment of choice for newly diagnosed severely affected individuals with hemophilia A or B is recombinant factor VIII or factor IX, preferably free of any protein associated with animal or human blood sources such as calf serum or albumin. New products within this category are being added to our armamentarium. Choice of treatment product for previously treated patients is largely dependent on patient preference and prior rating of clinical efficacy. Studies have shown that infusion of ultra-high-purity products have been associated with preservation of CD4+ counts in HIV-infected individuals.

Replacement factor choices for hemophilia A and B are listed in Table 2 in categories of purity. With established efficacy, random changes are not advisable unless otherwise clinically indicated. However, owing to intermittent product shortages, physicians and patients are sometimes required to substitute proprietary factor concentrates. I attempt to keep within a similar category if at all possible. A product may have two different brand names but can be interchangeable (e.g., Helixate and KoGENate).

Treatment Dosage and Frequency

Dosing regimens are targeted to maintain replacement plasma factor at certain levels based on the severity and site of bleeding. Factor VIII has a shorter half-life than factor IX and should be infused every 8 to 12 hours for an acute hemorrhage, compared with every 12 to 24 hours for factor IX. Factor XIII has the longest half-life and can be replaced on a monthly basis for most patients. Mild muscle and soft tissue hemorrhages require 30% factor plasma level for 1 to 2 days. Major hemorrhage, surgeries, gastrointestinal, or central nervous system hemorrhages require maintenance of more than 90% to 100% levels for at least 72 hours. Continuous infusions are often employed for major surgeries or severe hemorrhages to achieve consistent plasma factor levels. Calculations to achieve these targeted levels are listed below:

Factor VIII Infusions

Number of Units Required per Dose =
Weight (kg) × % Factor Level Desired × 0.5

TABLE 2. **Factor VIII and Factor IX Concentrates**

Factor Type	Factor VIII	Factor IX
Recombinant	KoGENate-FS ReFacto Helixate/KoGENate Recombinate/Bioclate	Benefix
Ultra-high-purity Plasma-derived	Hemophil M Monarc M Monoclate P	AlphaNine SD Mononine
Other plasma-derived	Alphanate* Humate-P* Koāte-HP* Profilate SD*	Bebulin VM Konyne-SD Profilnine SD Proplex T

*Contains varying amounts of vWF.

For example, to achieve 100% in a 50-kg person,

Number of Units Required per Dose =
$$50 \times 100 \times 0.5 = 2500 \text{ Units}$$

However, wastage of extra factor above the calculated range is discouraged. Hence, the amount actually given is often "rounded up" to the closest vial size.

Factor IX Infusions

Number of Units Required per Dose =
Weight (kg) × % Factor Level Desired × 1

Benefix Infusions

Number of Units Required per Dose =
Weight (kg) × % Factor Level Desired × 1.2

Monitoring of plasma levels (at 1 hour post infusion) with initial infusions and at times of dosage change will guide adjustment of the amount needed.

Treatment in the Presence of Inhibitors

Inhibitory antibodies to factor VIII arise in 30% of severely affected children with hemophilia A and in 3% to 5% children with hemophilia B during the first 15 to 30 infusion exposures. These antibodies develop after exposure to the exogenous protein and, therefore, tend to occur in those with large gene deletions and severe disease. The presence of inhibitors should be suspected when failure to achieve adequate hemostasis with routine replacement therapy is observed. Inhibitors are measured by the Bethesda assay in Bethesda units (BU). Values for high-titer or high-responding inhibitors are greater than 10 BU. The level of inhibitor activity determines the choice of appropriate management options. Low-titer or low-responding factor VIII inhibitors can be managed by using higher doses of factor concentrate. For mild to moderate bleeding, a dose of twice the routine amount usually suffices. For major hemorrhages, a bolus of 100 to 150 units/kg followed by continuous infusion at 15 to 20 units/kg/h for 3 to 4 days may be required. Inhibitor titers may rise sharply owing to an anamnestic response and need to be monitored for optimum care.

High-responding inhibitors pose a difficult therapeutic challenge. Often, continuous infusions fail to achieve and maintain hemostasis, particularly in major hemorrhages or during surgery. Porcine factor VIII at 100 to 150 units/kg starting dose has been successfully used for hemophilia A inhibitor patients. Monitoring for antiporcine factor VIII should be performed because antibodies do develop. Prothrombin complex concentrates (PCCs), a pool of factors II, IX, X, and VII, can be used at 75 to 100 units/kg of factor IX for minor hemorrhages. The dose can be repeated once or twice every 12 hours. If bleeding is not controlled within two to three doses, alternate treatment should be used. Heparin should be added at 5 to 10 units/mL of the reconstituted PCC. The mechanism of action is unclear.

Activated prothrombin complexes (aPCCs) can be similarly applied at 50 to 75 units/kg of factor IX. Both PCCs and aPCCs have increased thrombogenic potential, and myocardial infarcts have been reported with their use. However, frequent, routine monitoring of fibrin-split products or D-dimers as signals of thrombosis is of questionable value. The PCCs and aPCCs are plasma-derived pooled concentrates. They had been the mainstay of inhibitor therapy and had demonstrated good efficacy. A new alternative, recombinant factor VIIa, is currently available with less thrombogenic effect. Thrombin generation with recombinant factor VIIa is reported to be localized at the site of endothelial injury. Dosage for recombinant factor VIIa is recommended at 90 μg/kg every 2 to 4 hours, but optimum dosing is not currently known. Recombinant factor VIIa can be used in either the home or the hospital setting. PCCs or aPCCs should not be administered in close temporal proximity to recombinant factor VIIa because that would potentiate the danger of thrombosis.

A specific group of factor IX inhibitor patients develop anaphylactoid reactions on infusion of concentrates containing any amount of factor IX. The reactions vary from feeling flushed with chest discomfort to coughing, wheezing, and frank hypotension and shock requiring intubation and resuscitative efforts. Vigilance for possible anaphylactoid reactions in hemophilia B patients should be exercised, and PCCs and aPCCs should be avoided when such reactions are detected. The use of recombinant factor VIIa has proven a safe and effective recourse for these patients.

Long-term management of hemophilia A and B inhibitor patients includes consideration of immune tolerance induction (ITI) to eradicate the antibody completely. There are numerous approaches involving the use of an immunosuppressant and daily high doses of factor VIII. These methods vary with the dose of factor VIII, use of intravenous immunoglobulin (IVIG) and/or cyclophosphamide (Cytoxan),* antibody adsorption column, or corticosteroids. The decision to initiate such therapy should be taken only after serious consideration of the risks of failure (10%–30%), intercurrent bleeding, and the enormous commitment required for such an undertaking. Low pre-ITI inhibitor titer and early intervention are associated with a higher success rate. Immune tolerance induction should be performed under the care of a specialty hemophilia treatment center experienced with ITI. As such, specific protocols are not outlined in this article.

Acquired Hemophilia

Acquired inhibitors arise later in life and are autoantibodies, predominantly to factor VIII. Risk factors include diseases such as systemic lupus erythemato-

*Not FDA approved for this indication.

sus (SLE), rheumatoid arthritis, malignancies, inflammatory bowel disease, and the postpartum period. Over 50% of cases have no identifiable cause. Thirty percent to 40% remit spontaneously, and heroic interventions may not be necessary. When needed, the management of such patients can be difficult, with mortality rates exceeding 20%. A similar approach as outlined earlier for congenital hemophilia patients can be used, including ITI. Recombinant factor FVIIa has had greater than 90% efficacy in the surgery setting for this high-risk group.

Preventive Measures

The primary focus of early intervention is to prevent the onset of chronic sequelae associated with bleeding. To that aim, primary and secondary prophylaxis have been advocated. The success of prophylaxis is evidenced by the marked decline in arthropathies and hospitalizations in the past 5 years. Factor infusion at 20 to 40 units/kg two to three times a week, particularly before organized sports or physical activity, helps reduce hemorrhages. Plasma factor level should be kept within the 1% to 2% range for effective prophylaxis, although beneficial effects can be seen even when these levels are not strictly enforced. In the infant and young child, primary prophylaxis is started before onset of chronic arthropathy or co-morbidities. This requires central venous access with associated risks of infection and line thrombosis. Secondary prophylaxis should be encouraged in the older child or teenager and adult because the benefits of decreased hemorrhages, increased school or work attendance, and general quality of life have been well documented.

Routine well-child immunizations, including the hepatitis A and B vaccines, should be given to each affected child. Regular exercise and development of good muscle tone and strength decrease joint and muscle hemorrhages, not to mention optimizing the development of self-esteem and social interaction. Affected children are encouraged to participate in activities such as swimming and group sports with the proviso of consistent use of protective gear (e.g., helmets and knee and elbow pads).

Adjunctive Therapy

ε-Aminocaproic acid (EACA) or tranexamic acid has been used frequently to decrease clot lysis. EACA is available in liquid, tablet, and intravenous forms. The liquid preparation comes in 250 mg/mL, and 50 mg/kg can be used four times a day for 5 to 7 days. It should be used with extreme caution, if at all, in patients with gastrointestinal or renal bleeding as well as with the concomitant use of PCCs and aPCCs. Antifibrinolytics can be used in conjunction with recombinant factor VIIa. Other agents include fibrin sealants, topical thrombin, and microfibrillar collagen, especially in the presence of mucosal hemorrhage. Adequate analgesia (e.g., acetaminophen [Tylenol] with codeine or morphine) may be necessary for pain relief. Anti-inflammatory medications such as corticosteroids have been used in some cases to reduce the edema in cases of acute hemorrhage or synovitis. However, medications affecting platelet function such as aspirin or ibuprofen should be avoided. The mnemonic RICE—rest, ice, compression, elevation—summarizes the management of joint hemorrhages, although ice is often difficult to maintain on an irritable child. Oral contraceptives with estrogen/progesterone combinations may reduce menorrhagia and also increase plasma factor VIII and factor IX levels.

Gene Transfer

Preliminary clinical trials of various factor VIII and factor IX gene transfer modalities appear promising, but a detailed discussion is beyond the scope of this article.

von Willebrand Disease

Desmopressin has been effective in raising factor VIII and vWF levels three to four times that of baseline levels in most individuals with mild to moderate disease. It can be used for dental extractions and minor procedures in these individuals. Desmopressin does not raise the level in severely affected individuals adequately to achieve hemostasis; for example, a 1% baseline level would increase to only 3% to 4% after administration. Desmopressin can be administered intravenously or intranasally. Intravenous dosage is 0.3 μg/kg. Intranasal dosage is 1 squirt (~75 μg) for those weighing less than 50 kg and 2 squirts for patients heavier than 50 kg. Intranasal administration is more convenient for most patients with faster access to treatment because they can carry the dispenser with them at all times.

Side effects include facial flushing, transient blood pressure increases, and fluid retention. Fluid restriction is required to decrease the risk of hypertension, hyponatremia, and seizures. Stimate is contraindicated in neonates. Average time to peak level of factor VII and vWF is 45 minutes after intravenous administration and 90 minutes after intranasal administration. Because of the rapid response, it is most likely that the mechanism of action of desmopressin is release of the premanufactured factor VIII and vWF from storage sites. Due to depletion of stores from frequent use, desmopressin should be given only one to two times a day for a maximum of 3 days consecutively. A trial dose is given at the treatment center and predose and postdose levels are measured to document an adequate response before prescription of the drug for use. A few patients may respond to the intravenous route of administration after failing the intranasal trial.

Key points in the use of desmopressin for mild hemophilia A and type 1 vWD include the following:

1. Only the concentrated form (1.5 mg/mL) of desmopressin should be used. The trade name is Sti-

mate. Reference should be made only to Stimate as the appropriate medication to avoid prescription and dispensing errors. The preparation used for enuresis is ineffective in achieving hemostatic control.

2. Fluid restriction is begun just before and continued for 12 to 24 hours after administration.

3. The treating physician should be notified if hemostasis is not achieved after the first two doses. Tachyphylaxis and concomitant side effects should be considered.

Treatment of patients with type 2 and 3 vWF requires intravenous factor concentrate replacements containing adequate amounts of vWF. These preparations are listed in Table 2 and include Humate-P and Alphanate. Dosage for Humate-P can be calculated based on the vWF activity expressed as ristocetin cofactor (vWF:RcoF) units. For minor procedures and bleeding, 40 to 50 IU/kg every 8 to 12 hours for one or two doses is usually sufficient. However, major surgeries and hemorrhages, including suspected intracranial hemorrhage, would require a loading dose of 60 to 80 IU/kg, then 40 to 60 IU/kg every 8 to 12 hours for a minimum of 5 to 10 days, keeping the vWF:RcoF activity at greater than 50%. Stimate has been used as adjunctive therapy in type 3 vWD, but its use should be avoided by most type 2 and platelet-type vWD patients. Recombinant and high-purity factor VIII and factor IX concentrates should NOT be used for vWD.

Recombinant vWF is available only at a research level and is being developed for future clinical trials. Adjunctive therapy as listed for hemophilia applies generally to vWD as well, including oral progesterone-containing contraceptives.

Other Related Disorders

Deficiencies of the other factors are often diagnosed by the screening tests of the PTT, prothrombin time (PT), and thromboplastin time (TT). There are rare cases of familial combined factor deficiencies (e.g., factor V + factor VIII; factor VIII + factor IX; factor II + factor VII + factor IX + factor X). In the last case, high doses of vitamin K may be helpful.

Severe factor VII deficiency (prolonged PT, <1% factor VII) can vary in presentation, although most neonates succumb to intracranial hemorrhage. It would seem rational that the principle of replacing the deficient factor applies in this disease as in hemophilia A and B. Recombinant factor VII has been efficacious in maintaining hemostasis at 20 to 30 μg/kg every 6 to 12 hours but is currently not listed for Food and Drug Administration–approved use in the United States. For the rest of the factor deficiencies that present with bleeding, fresh frozen plasma (FFP) is often effective. Specific factor replacement is usually not available in this country. Fibrinogen (factor I) abnormalities require cryoprecipitate for effective hemostasis. Factor XIII deficiency can be treated with FFP or cryoprecipitate. Prophylactic treatment with FFP uses 10 mL/kg, or 1 to 2 units, in adults every 4 to 6 weeks, or cryoprecipitate, 1 bag/10 kg of body weight. Plasma-derived factor XIII concentrate is available only through clinical trials. The amount of each factor in FFP and cryoprecipitate varies according to the donor pool. Dosage varies according to severity of hemorrhages and the half-life of the plasma factor involved. It would be advisable for the overall treatment of any patient with a bleeding diathesis to be carried out in cooperation with or under the guidance of a specialty center.

PLATELET-MEDIATED BLEEDING DISORDERS

method of
LOUIS M. ALEDORT, M.D.
The Mount Sinai School of Medicine
New York, New York

From the early observation by the pathologist Zahn, platelets have been implicated in the production of a clot. Their role in lining blood vessels to prevent oozing and, when inadequate, in leading to petechiae, purpura, and bleeding, gave another dimension to their role in hemostasis. These observations led to substantial investigation to better understand the physical and biochemical aspects of the platelet to define its function.

The clinical symptoms of abnormal platelet function prompted significant discoveries of the major loci of defects of congenital qualitative platelet disorders. These studies have defined the key elements of platelet function.

The platelet glycoprotein Ib/IX/V is important for adherence to von Willebrand factor, which, in turn, is necessary for adhesion to subendothelial collagen. Glycoprotein IIb/IIIa is responsible for association with fibrinogen. This adherence leads to the platelet release phenomenon, which aids platelet aggregation, producing the primary hemostatic plug that produces hemostasis. Each element of the process has been identified to have either an inherited abnormality or an acquired defect.

Abnormalities of platelets (either quantitative or qualitative changes) lead to similar clinical syndromes. Hemarthrosis is the hallmark of deficiencies of clotting factors in the hemophiliac. In contrast, platelet abnormalities lead to mucocutaneous bleeding. This may manifest as petechiae, bruises, or purpura. Gastrointestinal, genitourinary, and pulmonary bleeding and epistaxis are all common manifestations of either abnormal numbers or functional defects. Although oral cavity bleeding is common in hemophilia, gingival bleeding is more often a manifestation of abnormal platelet function.

One cannot overestimate the importance of a careful history and physical examination aided by laboratory studies in arriving at an appropriate diagnosis. A family history, length of time symptoms have persisted, menorrhagia, peripartum bleeding, careful medication elaboration, acquired diseases, and past surgical experience are pivotal in unraveling the etiology. Laboratory evaluation includes platelet count, peripheral blood smear to assess number and size of platelets, bleeding time, platelet aggregation, and platelet membrane glycoproteins.

GENERAL ISSUES RELATED TO REPLACEMENT WITH BLOOD OR BLOOD DERIVATIVES

Many patients who experience platelet-mediated bleeding require replacement with either platelet transfusions or red cells. There are some important principles to follow. If the patient is known to have an inherited disorder, it behooves the clinician to prevent transfusion-transmitted diseases when possible. Vaccines to prevent hepatitis A and B are now available. Although hepatitis A is rarely transfusable, it has been reported. Despite markedly increased testing after donor screening, hepatitis B is not totally eliminated. Three timed vaccinations over 6 months will protect subsequent blood recipients from contracting hepatitis B. With blood donations being tested for HIV, hepatitis B antigen, hepatitis C antibody, syphilis, and liver function abnormalities, the transmission of these agents has been almost completely eliminated. The current study of the impact of hepatitis C and HIV polymerase chain reaction as a screening technique may result in its implementation soon. The use of leukocyte depletion filters has decreased the risk of alloimmunization. For some patients who require immune modulation, intravenous immunoglobulin (IVIG) is a frequently used treatment. Because there have been outbreaks of hepatitis C from IVIG in the past, in addition to donor screening, viral inactivation techniques have been added to virtually eliminate hepatitis C transmission. Fibrin glues, recently licensed in the United States, when applied to a bleeding surface, have been successful in producing hemostasis. The biologics used in these glues have also undergone viral inactivation.

TABLE 1. **Quantitative Platelet Disorders: Thrombocytopenia**

Decreased Production
Bone marrow failure
Infiltration—fibrosis, granuloma, cancer
Drugs
Chemotherapy
Radiation
Vitamin deficiency—B_{12}, folate
Splenic Sequestration
Hypersplenism
Portal hypertension
Splenomegaly—primary, infiltrative portal hypertension
Thrombotic
Disseminated intravascular coagulation
Thrombotic thrombocytopenic purpura—primary or drug induced
Hemolytic-uremic syndrome–primary or drug induced
Dilutional
Immune
Immune thrombocytopenia
Disease related
Vasculitis
Infection—HIV, Epstein-Barr virus
Drug
Post-transfusion
Neonatal
Thrombocythemia
Myeloproliferative disease

QUANTITATIVE PLATELET DISORDERS

The quantitative platelet disorders are easily divided into two groups: in one production is impaired; in the second there is normal to increased production and either consumption or destruction (Table 1). The bleeding manifestations are similar in both situations, but the management is quite different for each. Although the platelet count, no matter what the cause, is frequently a predictor of bleeding, there is a wide range of variation in clinical manifestations. Most agree, however, that bleeding is likely to occur with platelet counts under 10,000/mm^3. Whether the cause is lack of production or destruction, one is usually comfortable with counts above 30,000/mm^3. In patients not producing platelets, central nervous system and pulmonary hemorrhage is more common than in those whose etiology is peripheral destruction. Patients presenting with platelet counts of 60,000 to 100,000/mm^3 frequently represent those with splenic sequestration due to portal hypertension or mild drug toxicity. Bleeding in patients with thrombocytopenia is potentiated with the use of medication that produces a qualitative platelet defect such as aspirin or nonsteroidal anti-inflammatory drugs.

Therapy

The approach to therapy includes assessment of the etiology of the platelet disorder, as well as the extent of the hemorrhagic diathesis. In platelet destructive disorders, for example, when platelet survival is minimal, platelet transfusions are of little help, except in life-threatening situations. In consumptive coagulopathies, platelet transfusion should be cautiously administered because it may perpetuate the consumption or neutralize the heparin that might be used to stop the clotting process but is effective if the patient is bleeding. Trauma or surgical intervention, leading to bleeding in either quantitative or qualitative disorders, requires replacement therapy. When needed, single donor apheresis platelets or 6 to 8 units of pooled platelets are given. Filtered blood reduces alloimmunization, which is frequently an issue for patients who require continued platelet transfusion. Occasionally, human leukocyte antigen–matched platelets are required.

QUALITATIVE PLATELET DISORDERS

Whether congenital or acquired, oral cavity and mucous membrane bleeding may be persistent (Table 2). In addition to platelet transfusions, adjunctive therapies have been very useful.

Therapy

In addition to the genitourinary tract, the saliva has a large amount of fibrinolytic activity. ε-Aminocaproic acid (Amicar) is an effective antifibrinolytic agent. It is particularly effective in the oral cavity and can be administered by mouth up to 6 g every 6

TABLE 2. **Qualitative Platelet Disorders**

Type

Congenital

Bernard-Soulier syndrome—cannot bind von Willebrand factor (glycoprotein Ib deficiency)
Glanzmann's thrombasthenia—cannot bind to fibrinogen (GPIIb/IIIa deficiency)
Storage pool disease
Release abnormalities

Acquired

Uremia
Myelodysplastic syndromes
Paraprotein disorders
Liver disease
Drug induced (e.g., acetylsalicylic acid)
Fibrinogen (fibrin degradation products)

Treatment Approach

Thrombocytopenia

Decreased production—platelet transfusion
Splenic sequestration—eliminate primary issue
Thrombotic
Disseminated intravascular coagulation—eliminate underlying cause
Thrombotic thrombocytopenic purpura, hemolytic-uremic syndrome—pheresis with or without plasma
Immune—immunomodulation, splenectomy

hours. Side effects can be nausea, lightheadedness, and retrograde ejaculation. A liquid form can be used to rinse the mouth without swallowing, especially with gum bleeding.

Extractions or gum surgery can result in a good deal of bleeding in these settings. Avitene (microcrystalline collagen) either alone or with Gelfoam or topical thrombin is useful. Bovine thrombin has the problem of rare immunization to factor V with an associated additional bleeding diathesis.

Fibrin glues are combinations of fibrinogen, thrombin, and calcium, with or without aprotinins. When applied locally they are very effective.

Desmopressin (1-deamino-8-D-arginine vasopressin [DDAVP]) has become an important agent in the management of qualitative platelet disorders. In patients with hereditary disorders, it is particularly useful in those with difficulty with release abnormalities. Its role in acquired qualitative disorders has been well characterized. In patients who have had aspirin, desmopressin will reverse the abnormal bleeding time without altering the inhibition of cyclooxygenase activity. In uremia, particularly in those patients with anemia, desmopressin will correct the bleeding time approximately 50% of the time. For patients with liver disease, as in those with uremia, tissue samples are frequently needed for diagnosis. The prolonged bleeding time often precludes biopsy, and desmopressin is particularly useful in providing hemostasis and correcting the bleeding time. Given intravenously, the dose is 0.3 μg/kg over 15 minutes in 50-mL saline and its effect is maximal at 30 minutes to 1 hour. A new nasal spray preparation (Stimate), equivalent to 0.2 μg/kg intravenously, is effective in 95% of patients who respond to the intravenous preparation. For an adult, one spray into each nostril is the optimal dose; for children, it is one spray into one nostril. Side effects are flushing and/or hypotension.

Factor VIIa (NovoSeven) hemostasis by means of coagulation factors is triggered by the interaction of tissue factor and factor VIIa. A newly licensed recombinant factor VIIa has been shown to be effective in producing hemostasis in hemophiliacs with inhibitors to factor VIII. Case reports have now produced anecdotal evidence for its usefulness in patients who are bleeding with Glanzmann's thrombasthenia, one of the hereditary platelet membrane defects. Rates for the prevalence of the adverse reactions disseminated intravascular coagulation and thrombosis are not known, and the drug is not indicated for this.

Erythropoietin (EPO, Procrit),* has been useful in elevating the hematocrit of persons with renal failure. Its mechanism for enhancing platelet function was believed to be due to normalizing the hematocrit. Although this agent is not indicated for improving platelet function, studies affirm that it has an independent ability to do so.

Thrombocythemia is a common hematologic issue. It is most often reactive secondary to either iron deficiency, inflammatory disease, or tumors, or occurs after splenectomy. In those circumstances, the elevated platelet count rarely causes symptoms. However, the thrombocythemia associated with myeloproliferative diseases is fraught with either bleeding or clotting, which can occur separately or concomitantly. The reversal of the bleeding diathesis is related to reversing the platelet count to normal. Treatment modalities are hydroxyurea (Hydrea),* the dose varying with the patient's response, or anagrelide (Agrylin), with similar dose requirements. It is unusual that treatment can be stopped or that remissions are self-sustained.

IMMUNE THROMBOCYTOPENIA

Medications have notoriously been involved in producing thrombocytopenia. Their mechanisms differ substantially. Procainamide (Pronestyl) and hydralazine (Apresoline) produce a lupus-like syndrome with an antibody that produces platelet sequestration. Cessation of drug stops the process. Quinidine and quinine act as antigens to which an antibody is formed, and this antigen-antibody complex attacks platelets, leading to sequestration. The thrombocytopenia is usually profound with major oral bleeding. After stopping the drug, it takes at least 7 to 10 days to clear the medication so thrombocytopenia will abate. Immune modulation (i.e., with corticosteroids) may be required before the counts begin to rise. These are rare occurrences.

On the other hand, 3% to 5% of all patients exposed to heparin more than once develop immune-mediated heparin-induced thrombocytopenia. Intravenous, in-

*Not FDA approved for this indication.

termittent, and continuous, as well as subcutaneous, flushes have been associated with this phenomenon. The counts slowly drift downward but can reach clinically significant levels. If so, and if continued anticoagulation is required, low molecular weight heparins (LMWHs) do not always cross over; and if one is concerned or if LMWH perpetuates the problem, antithrombin agents such as danaproid (Orgaran) or hirudin (Refludan) can be used.

Post-transfusion purpura, from either pregnancy or transfusion, rarely results in a platelet surface antigen incompatibility. Recognition of this disorder is important because the PL^{A1} antigen is most often implicated. The antibody produced destroys not only PL^{A1}-positive platelets but also the patient's platelets. Treatment with corticosteroids or IVIG can reverse the situation.

Idiopathic thrombocytopenia purpura, an autoimune thrombocytopenia, is the most common type of isolated thrombocytopenia. The disease in children is frequently self-limited, often needing no therapy, and is not covered here. The autoantibody, not easily measured, is directed against the major platelet surface glycoproteins (GPIb/IV/V or GPIIb/IIIa). These antibodies lead to rapid destruction in the reticuloendothelial system. The goal of therapy is to stop acute hemorrhagic symptoms and/or cure the disease. Although most patients present as if they had acute thrombocytopenia, the large majority of patients have chronic disease.

When patients present with platelet counts below $30{,}000/mm^3$, several approaches have been used. One is to prescribe 1 mg/kg of prednisone orally until the platelet count reaches normal levels and then slowly taper the dose in hopes of a cure. Another approach is to prescribe dexamethasone (Decadron), 40 mg for 4 days every 4 weeks, for up to six cycles in an attempt at a cure. This approach has not yet been shown to be equivalent to the 60% to 70% cure rate of prednisone. For those patients who either have resisted the possibility of splenectomy or are not good candidates for splenectomy, the use of IVIG (1 g/kg/d × 2) or anti-D (WinRho), 75 μg/kg (for patients who are Rh+), is used. The response in platelet count is in 5 to 10 days and either may be short lived (days) or may last 1 to 2 months. IVIG is costly, can produce meningitis, and requires a lengthy infusion time. Anti-D is less costly and has a short infusion time but can produce significant hemolysis with renal consequences.

Patients who present with severe thrombocytopenia are often treated with corticosteroids and either IVIG or anti-D. If life-threatening bleeding occurs, platelet transfusions are indicated.

For those patients who fail attempts to cure the disease and cannot maintain a platelet count of more than $30{,}000/mm^3$, or whose lifestyle demands a more secure platelet count, splenectomy is recommended.

Splenectomy can now be carried out via laparoscopic techniques. The patient should be vaccinated before splenectomy with pneumococcal and *Haemophilus influenzae* vaccine. This is necessary because patients who have had splenectomy are susceptible to sepsis with encapulated bacteria. Some treaters also vaccinate against meningococcus.

Of those requiring splenectomy, 25% to 30% fail. Attempts at response include the following armamentarium: immunosuppressive therapy with azathioprine (Imuran), cyclophosphamide (Cytoxan), long-term corticosteroids, intermittent IVIG or anti-D, or danazol (Danacrine) at 600 mg/d. All of these treatments have the side effects of the individual therapies. Danazol has liver toxicity and is also masculinizing and should not be used in premenopausal women. Fortunately, only a small proportion of those presenting with immune thrombocytopenia have intracranial hemorrhage as a cause of serious morbidity or mortality.

ACKNOWLEDGMENT

This study was supported in part by Health Services Administration Grant MCB-360001; Health and Human Services Grant HS-30567; the Regional Comprehensive Hemophilia Diagnostic and Treatment Center; the Margie Boas Fund; the International Hemophilia Training Center of the World Federation of Hemophilia; the Polly Annenberg Levee Hematology Center, Department of Medicine, Mount Sinai School of Medicine of the City University of New York; and grant 5MO1RR00071 for the Mount Sinai General Clinical Research Center from the National Center for Research Resources, National Institutes of Health.

DISSEMINATED INTRAVASCULAR COAGULATION

method of
MARGARETA BLOMBÄCK, M.D., Ph.D., and
SIXTEN S. E. BREDBACKA, M.D., Ph.D.
Karolinska Institutet/Karolinska Hospital
Stockholm, Sweden

Disseminated intravascular coagulation (DIC) is intravascular coagulation with loss of localization of response arising from different causes and structures. It can originate from and cause damage to the microvasculature, which, if sufficiently severe, can produce organ dysfunction (opinion of Subcommittee DIC, SSC/International Society on Thrombosis and Haemostasis). It occurs in many different conditions and to different degrees, from chronic compensated DIC to fulminant thrombohemorrhagic conditions.

DIC usually starts with a hypercoagulative state causing microembolism from fibrin complexes, platelets, and leukocytes. The microembolism leads to occlusion of small vessels in different organs and systems such as the lungs, kidneys, central nervous system, and skin, resulting in organ failure.

Microembolization is considered to be part of the multiple organ failure syndrome. It occurs in many different conditions, as shown in Table 1.

TABLE 1. **Examples of Triggering Events for Disseminated Intravascular Coagulation**

Factors Contributing to Development of DIC
Shock
Hypoxia/ischemia
Acidosis
Decreased immune defense
Kidney and liver failure
Factors Contributing to Worsening of DIC
Inherited thrombogenic defects (e.g., deficiency of coagulation inhibitors: antithrombin, protein S, protein C)
Activated protein C–resistance
Lupus anticoagulant
Cardiolipin antibodies
Acquired high tissue plasminogen activator inhibitor-1 levels
Conditions Triggering DIC
Sepsis
Trauma (including burns and heat stroke)
Obstetric complications
Malignancies
Toxins (e.g., snake venom)
Immunologic/allergic disorders
Vascular disorders

Abbreviation: DIC = disseminated intravascular coagulation.

Hypercoagulation causes consumption of coagulation factors, inhibitors, and platelets. Thromboplastin or other tissue factor is considered to be the main trigger for coagulation activation and is released from tissue damage or exposition on perturbed monocytes or endothelium (e.g., in sepsis).

Tissue factor binds and activates coagulation factor VII, and the coagulation cascade is activated "downstream" involving coagulation factors IX, X, VIII, and V, resulting in thrombin formation. Thrombin is the key substance in coagulation. It converts fibrinogen to fibrin monomers, which polymerize and finally crossbind into a fibrin mesh.

Thrombin has multiple effects on its own formation, platelet activity, and the endothelium. Through feedback it increases its own formation in low concentrations. But at higher concentrations, it inhibits its formation through thrombomodulin, which activates protein C (APC) to degrade activated coagulation factors V and VIII. Quantitatively, the most important coagulation inhibitor is antithrombin (AT), which not only binds and inhibits thrombin but also binds, to varying degrees, all other activated coagulation factors. Heparin accelerates the effect 100 to 1000 times. Another important inhibitor is protein C.

Secondary to the normal (and local) coagulation activity, a reactive enzymatic degradation (*fibrinolysis*) of fibrin occurs, caused by plasmin in the presence of fibrin. Plasmin is activated by tissue plasminogen activator released from damaged endothelium or subendothelial structures. It may also degrade fibrinogen and other coagulation factors. Plasmin release is balanced by tissue plasminogen activator inhibitor-1 (PAI-1), which is also released from the endothelium. If plasmin should occur free in plasma, normally it is immediately inactivated by plasmin inhibitor (previously called *α_2-antiplasmin*). Thus, fibrinolysis normally only occurs on fibrin clots. Extended fibrinolysis results in an increase in fibrinogen-fibrin degradation products (e.g., D-dimers), which inhibit fibrin polymerization and platelet activation leading to bleeding.

If this delicate system becomes unbalanced, accelerated coagulation with occult or overt clotting will occur and consumption of coagulation factors and inhibitors may eventually lead to consumptive hemorrhage. This may be amplified by unbalanced fibrinolysis.

Depending on the stage of the disorder, both clotting and bleeding can be seen at the same time.

Furthermore, there is a "cross-talk" between the coagulation systems and kallikrein and inflammatory systems, which probably has important therapeutic implications.

In a few conditions, there is a primary activation of the fibrinolytic system without simultaneous activation of the coagulation, as is the case in promyelocytic leukemia.

THE CLINICAL PICTURE

Typical symptoms occur and are caused by microclotting and hemorrhage in the most perfused organs, central nervous system, kidneys, lungs, skin, and mucous membranes. Symptoms range from small organ disturbances to fulminant multiple organ failure.

DIAGNOSIS DEPENDS ON THE STAGE OF THE PROCESS

The most important first step in diagnosis is to suspect DIC and identify the patient at risk (see Table 1). Second,

TABLE 2. **Simplified Initial Treatment Scheme**

Condition	Antithrombin	Soluble Fibrin	D-Dimers	Suggested Treatment
Non-overt DIC	Normal	Normal	Normal	LMWH SC or IV in thromboprophylactic dose
In between stage, nonbleeding	Normal or decreasing	Increasing or high	Increasing or high	LMWH SC or IV in thromboprophylactic dose and/or plasma
Overt DIC *without* bleeding	Low	High	High	LMWH SC or IV in thromboprophylactic dose and/or plasma. Consider addition of antithrombin concentrate.
Overt DIC *with* bleeding	Low	High	High	Plasma. Consider factor concentrates, platelet concentrate, tranexamic acid (see text).

Purified FVIII, FVIII/von Willebrand factor, fibrinogen concentrates or cryoprecipitate* as well as prothrombin complex concentrates† are often available and can be used in severe DIC, when factor deficiency is present. However, concentrates should not be given unless bleeding caused by factor deficiency occurs.

*Contains FVIII, FVIII/von Willebrand factor, fibrinogen, and fibronectin.

†Contains FII, VII, IX, X, protein C, and protein S.

Abbreviations: DIC = disseminated intravascular coagulation; LMWH = low molecular weight heparin.

identify the subtle organ dysfunction that may herald DIC. Third, do repeated laboratory analyses such as activated partial thromboplastin (APT)-time, prothrombin time (INR), and platelet count. These tests usually do not confirm the diagnosis until relatively late in the course when a pronounced consumption of coagulation factors and inhibitors has occurred. This is the reason why DIC very often has been associated with bleeding and not primarily with pathologically increased coagulation.

Early diagnosis—at the hypercoagulative state—is emphasized because with early diagnosis, treatment has a chance for success. Except for clinical signs, a battery of repeated tests should be conducted on high-risk patients because trends are more important than isolated tests.

Although tests that measure fibrin D-dimer, platelet count, fibrinogen level, and prothrombin time (INR) are globally useful in establishing DIC diagnosis, other more sophisticated tests such as AT and soluble fibrin complexes should be performed, if feasible.

TREATMENT

In acute situations, diagnosis and treatment must be prompt and adequate for the best results (Table 2). First, the cause of DIC must be eliminated or blunted (e.g., sepsis, major tissue trauma, extensive fractures, necrotic tissue or abscesses, retained fetus). Also, intensive care treatment with stabilization of circulation, ventilation, renal function, and pain relief must be provided. At this point, DIC usually resolves itself, but sometimes more specific therapy against the disordered coagulation system must be instituted.

The specific treatment for the coagulation disturbance is still being debated because the pathophysiology is complex and there is a lack of sufficient studies. The primary hypercoagulation and early DIC at the stage at which coagulation dominates (non-overt DIC) may be treated with low molecular weight heparin (LMWH) in thromboprophylactic doses. Non-overt DIC is primarily a laboratory diagnosis, but it may lead to a diagnosis of overt DIC. For overt DIC, inhibitors need to be substituted and this may be achieved by giving leukocyte and platelet-poor stored (fresh) or fresh-frozen plasma. The content of factors in plasma is not considered to "feed the fuel" as was formerly believed. If the patient is bleeding, there may well be a need to substitute factors and (rarely) platelets.

Laboratory tests should be repeatedly evaluated during treatment. Once the bleeding situation is under control, reinstitution of LMWH must be considered because the patient once again may become hypercoagulable. If plasma treatment has not been successful or the patient does not tolerate a high-volume load, substitution treatment with AT concentrates should be considered. LMWH with increasing AT levels may, however, amplify the anticoagulative effect, resulting in risk of bleeding. Low levels of AT must be combined with other pathologic hypercoagulation parameters to indicate consumption because low AT levels can also be seen after dilution from fluid resuscitation or liver failure, but in a dilution situation, the albumin level is also low and the prothrombin time (INR) increased. There is still a balance, although more delicate, among factors and inhibitors of coagulation in the latter cases. The dosage of AT should aim at "above normal" levels of AT as indicated from some sepsis studies.

Substitution with purified factor concentrates, fibrinogen, or platelet transfusion should only be done if the level of fibrinogen is very low (<0.5 g/L) or if the platelet count is very low ($<20 \times 10^9$/L) and the patient is bleeding.

In some situations in which there is an almost pure fibrinolysis, tranexamic acid (Cyklokapron),* or aprotinin (Trasylol),* may be considered. Epoprostenol (Flolan)* treatment (in low dose) can be considered for a patient with, for example, sepsis and gangrenous (from microemboli) fingers and toes.

*Not FDA approved for this indication.

THROMBOTIC THROMBOCYTOPENIC PURPURA

method of
MARIAN PETRIDES, M.D.
University of Mississippi Medical Center
Jackson, Mississippi

Thrombotic thrombocytopenic purpura (TTP) is a disorder characterized by the formation of platelet-rich thrombi in the microvasculature. Classically, TTP presents as a pentad of signs and symptoms: microangiopathic hemolytic anemia (with schistocytes on peripheral blood smear), thrombocytopenia, fluctuating neurologic impairment, renal dysfunction, and fever. However, it is not uncommon for patients to lack one or more of these findings, particularly at initial presentation. Untreated TTP is fatal in more than 90% of patients, but treatment with plasma exchange has reduced the fatality rate to 10% to 15%, although a significant percentage of responders (30%–40%) will have one or more relapses.

ETIOLOGY AND PATHOGENESIS

The cause of TTP appears to be the presence of unusually large von Willebrand factor (vWF) multimers, which are not found in normal plasma, in the circulation of affected patients. These multimers bind to damaged endothelium and result in platelet adhesion and, particularly in areas of high shear stress, in platelet aggregation. The microthrombi that result are rich in platelets but lack fibrin because the soluble coagulation system is not involved.

Major strides have been made recently in elucidating the mechanism underlying the presence of these unusually large vWF multimers in TTP. Chronic relapsing TTP is often familial and is characterized by absence of the metalloprotease that cleaves vWF. Acute TTP, however, tends not to be familial but rather occurs in response to transient development of autoantibodies that inhibit the activity vWF-cleaving protease. Patients with hemolytic-uremic syndrome (HUS), whose clinical presentation is often similar to that of TTP but whose response to plasma exchange is less consistent, have normal levels of vWF-cleaving protease and no evidence of inhibitory autoantibody (Table 1). At the moment, testing for vWF-cleaving protease and for autoantibodies directed against this protease are research procedures but the prospect exists that these assays may some day become clinically applicable.

Although TTP is most often idiopathic, some cases are associated with drug therapy or with connective tissue disease, malignancy, or infection. Indeed, TTP has been observed, albeit rarely, as the first presenting sign of HIV infection. There have also been reports of refractoriness to plasma exchange therapy in patients with TTP and occult bacterial infection. Drugs that have been linked to TTP include a variety of chemotherapeutic agents; cyclosporine (Sandimmune); quinine; and the antiplatelet drugs ticlopidine (Ticlid) and clopidogrel (Plavix).

DIFFERENTIAL DIAGNOSIS

Because there is currently no single definitive test to establish the diagnosis of TTP, the diagnosis of TTP must be considered whenever microangiopathic hemolytic anemia with schistocytosis is accompanied by thrombocytopenia in the absence of another disease entity that explains these findings—even when neurologic abnormalities and renal dysfunction are not present.

A negative direct antiglobulin test (direct Coombs test) helps differentiate TTP from Evans syndrome—autoimmune hemolytic anemia accompanied by autoimmune thrombocytopenia. Because TTP does not involve the soluble coagulation system, one can usually differentiate TTP from disseminated intravascular coagulation (DIC) based on the coagulation profile. TTP is characterized by normal or near-normal coagulation profile (prothrombin time [PT], partial thromboplastin time [PTT], and fibrinogen level) and the absence of D-dimer, whereas in DIC elevation of PT, PTT, and D-dimer is accompanied by a drop in fibrinogen. Note, however, that in rare cases, TTP may occur concomitantly with DIC.

TREATMENT

Therapeutic plasma exchange is the mainstay of treatment for TTP, presumably functioning to remove the pathogenic unusually large vWF multimers and/or the inhibitory autoantibody while at the same time replacing the missing protease. Because prompt inception of plasma exchange can be lifesaving, one should maintain a high index of suspicion for TTP whenever a patient presents with acute-onset thrombocytopenia and hemolytic anemia accompanied by schistocytes. When the diagnosis of TTP cannot be excluded, even if it is not definitively established, emergent treatment with plasma exchange should be initiated. When plasma exchange is not readily available, simple infusion of fresh frozen plasma (FFP) should be started until plasma exchange can be arranged. In most cases, high-dose corticosteroid therapy should accompany plasma exchange.

Generally, a daily exchange of one plasma volume using allogeneic FFP as the replacement fluid is sufficient. In patients who fail to respond to exchange with FFP, either plasma from which cryoprecipitate has been removed (cryoprecipitate-reduced plasma) or solvent-detergent (SD) plasma, which also has reduced levels of vWF, may be effective. Beyond the obvious consideration that SD plasma is virally inactivated whereas FFP and cryoprecipitate-reduced plasma are not, there is no definitive evidence for a therapeutic advantage to either of these more costly alternatives over FFP.

Because failure to respond to plasma exchange therapy has been reported in association with occult bacterial infections, evidence of infection should be sought when patients either fail to respond to plasma exchange or experience an exacerbation while being treated. In this setting, empirical broad-spectrum antibiotic treatments may also be appropriate.

During plasma exchange therapy, the patient should be monitored clinically for signs of neurologic impairment. Because microthrombi can also occur in the heart, particularly in the conducting system, one must also be alert to the presence of cardiac involvement, especially arrhythmia.

TABLE 1. **Differentiation Between Thrombocytopenic Purpura and Hemolytic-Uremic Syndrome**

Entity	Clinical Presentation	Proposed Mechanism
Acute TTP	Classic pentad Microangiopathic hemolytic anemia Thrombocytopenia Rising BUN and creatinine Neurologic dysfunction Fever (May be missing one or more sign, especially at the outset) Responds well to plasma exchange in most cases	Autoantibodies to vWF-cleaving protease
Chronic, recurrent TTP	Recurrent episodes with signs as above Responds well to plasma exchange in most cases	Deficiency of vWF-cleaving protease
HUS	Microangiopathic hemolytic anemia Thrombocytopenia	No deficiency of vWF-cleaving protease No autoantibodies to vWF-cleaving protease
	Rising BUN and creatinine Response to plasma exchange less consistent	

Abbreviations: BUN = blood urea nitrogen; HUS = hemolytic-uremic syndrome; TTP = thrombocytopenic purpura; vWF = von Willebrand factor.

Daily laboratory monitoring should include measurement of hemoglobin/hematocrit, platelet count, and renal function tests (blood urea nitrogen and creatinine). Daily lactate dehydrogenase (LDH) levels should also be followed, although recent isoenzyme studies have suggested that the rise in LDH in TTP, which was once attributed directly to hemolysis, may instead derive from ischemic tissue damage to muscle and liver. In any event, because the enzyme is removed by the apheresis procedure itself, it is best to measure LDH levels on the morning after a procedure rather than immediately after exchange.

A patient who is responding to therapy would be expected to show stabilization and then a rise in platelet count, accompanied by a decrease in both LDH and in the number of schistocytes visible on the peripheral blood smear. The time course to complete response is highly variable, ranging from a few days to several weeks. Daily plasma exchanges should be continued at least until the platelet count normalizes, and anecdotal evidence suggests it may be prudent to continue exchanges for 1 or 2 days beyond this point. Patients who show signs of recurrence when plasma exchange is discontinued may benefit from tapering of therapy after normalization of platelet counts—alternating plasma exchange one day with plasma infusion the next.

Although plasma exchange is the standard of care for treatment of TTP, a number of other measures, of which high-dose corticosteroid therapy is but one, have also been employed in conjunction with plasma exchange. Antiplatelet agents such as dipyridamole (Persantine)* and aspirin*; intravenous immunoglobulin (IVIG, Sandoglobulin)*; chemotherapeutic agents such as vincristine (Oncovin)*; immunosorbent column apheresis; and even splenectomy have all been tried, with varying success, in the treatment of patients refractory to plasma exchange.

One final caveat is that platelets are contraindicated in all but the most exceptional cases of TTP. Rather than being beneficial, transfused platelets simply provide more substrate from which platelet-rich thrombi can be formed, resulting in thrombotic episodes—most notably strokes—and even in death.

*Not FDA approved for this indication.

HEMOCHROMATOSIS

method of
PAUL ADAMS, M.D.
University of Western Ontario
London, Ontario, Canada

Hemochromatosis is the most common genetic disease in people of European ancestry. The diagnosis can be elusive because of the nonspecific nature of the symptoms. With the discovery of the hemochromatosis gene in 1996 (*HFE*) comes new insights into the pathogenesis of the disease and new diagnostic strategies.

A fundamental issue that has arisen since the discovery of the *HFE* gene is whether the disease *hemochromatosis* should be defined strictly on phenotypic criteria such as the degree of iron overload (transferrin saturation, ferritin, liver biopsy, hepatic iron concentration, iron removed by venesection therapy) or whether the *condition* should be defined as a familial disease in Europeans most commonly associated with the C282Y mutation of the *HFE* gene and varying degrees of iron overload. Because the genetic test has increasingly been used as a diagnostic tool, most studies now use a combination of phenotypic and genotypic criteria for the diagnosis of hemochromatosis.

CLINICAL FEATURES OF HEMOCHROMATOSIS

Liver Disease

Although hemochromatosis is often classified as a liver disease, it is a systemic genetic disease with multisystem involvement. The liver is central in both the diagnosis and prognosis of hemochromatosis. Hepatomegaly remains one of the more common physical signs in hemochromatosis but may not be present in the young (younger than 40 years) asymptomatic homozygote. In a study of 410 homozygotes from Canada and France, 22% had cirrhosis of the liver at the time of diagnosis. The prevalence of cirrhosis in asymptomatic or screened patients is much lower. The mean aspartate transaminase (AST) and alanine transaminase (ALT) were within the normal range in these 410 patients. Cirrhotic patients and patients with concomitant alcohol abuse were more likely to have abnormal liver enzymes. It seems likely that there are factors other than iron overload that contribute to cirrhosis in hemochromatosis. The effect of iron depletion therapy has usually been stabilization of the liver disease. This may account for the relatively small number of C282Y homozygotes that have required liver transplantation. The other common clinical manifestations are arthralgias, pigmentation, diabetes, congestive heart failure, impotence, and fatigue.

DIAGNOSIS OF HEMOCHROMATOSIS

A paradox of genetic hemochromatosis is that the disease is underdiagnosed in the general population, yet it is overdiagnosed in patients with secondary iron overload.

Underdiagnosis of Hemochromatosis

Preliminary population studies using genetic testing have demonstrated a prevalence of homozygotes of approximately 1 in 200 in whites. The fact that many physicians consider hemochromatosis to be rare implies either a lack of penetrance of the gene (nonexpressing homozygote) or a large number of patients that remain undiagnosed in the community.

Diagnostic Tests for Hemochromatosis

TRANSFERRIN SATURATION

An elevated transferrin saturation has a sensitivity of greater than 90% for hemochromatosis in family studies. The sensitivity of transferrin saturation is lower in population screening studies designed to detect C282Y homozygotes (genotypic case definition) and may be in the normal range in young female homozygotes.

UNSATURATED IRON-BINDING CAPACITY

The unsaturated iron-binding capacity is a one-step colorimetric assay that has been used in many reference labo-

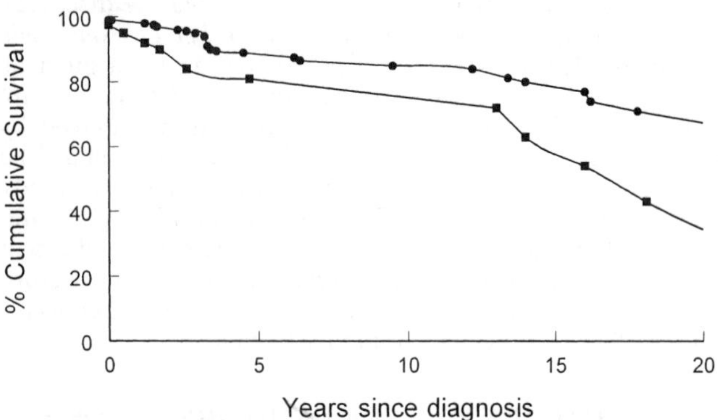

Figure 1. Actuarial survival of C282Y homozygotes in cirrhotic (□) and noncirrhotic patients (○) (n = 277, P = 0.04, log-rank test).

ratories to calculate the transferrin saturation. It is an inexpensive test compared with transferrin saturation and has been demonstrated to be a promising initial screening test for hemochromatosis.

SERUM FERRITIN

The relationship between serum ferritin and total body iron stores has been clearly established by strong correlations with hepatic iron concentration and amount of iron removed by venesection. However, ferritin can be elevated secondary to chronic inflammation and histiocytic neoplasms. A major diagnostic dilemma in the past was whether the serum ferritin is related to hemochromatosis or another underlying liver disease such as alcoholic liver disease, chronic viral hepatitis, or nonalcoholic steatohepatitis. It is likely that most of these difficult cases will now be resolved by genetic testing.

LIVER BIOPSY

Liver biopsy has previously been the gold standard diagnostic test for hemochromatosis. Liver biopsy has shifted from a major diagnostic tool to a method of estimating prognosis and concomitant disease. The need for liver biopsy seems less clear now in the young asymptomatic C282Y homozygote in whom there is a low clinical suspicion of cirrhosis based on history, physical examination, and liver biochemistry. A large study conducted in France and Canada suggested that C282Y homozygotes with a serum ferritin of less than 1000 μg/L, a normal AST, and without hepatomegaly have a very low risk of cirrhosis.

Patients with cirrhosis have a 5.5-fold relative risk of death compared with the noncirrhotic hemochromatosis patients (Figure 1). Cirrhotic patients are also at increased risk of hepatocellular carcinoma. Although early detection has been clearly demonstrated by serial ultrasound and α-fetoprotein determination, curative treatment options remain limited.

Liver biopsy is considered in typical C282Y homozygotes with liver dysfunction and in iron overloaded patients without the typical C282Y mutation. Simple C282Y heterozygotes, compound heterozygotes (C282Y/H63D) and patients with other risk factors (alcohol abuse, chronic viral hepatitis) with moderate-to-severe iron overload (ferritin >1000 μg/L) may be considered for liver biopsy.

Before genetic testing, hepatic iron concentration was useful in the diagnosis of hemochromatosis. The hepatic iron index is calculated as follows:

$$\frac{\text{Hepatic Iron Concentration } (\mu\text{mol/g})}{\text{Age (years)}}$$

The hepatic iron index will become less useful with the advent of genetic testing. It will remain a tool to aid the clinician with his or her clinical judgment about an individual case. It may be most useful in the unusual hemochromatosis patient who is negative by conventional genetic testing but clinically seems to have genetic hemochromatosis.

Genetic Testing for Hemochromatosis

A major advance that stems from the discovery of the hemochromatosis gene is the use of a diagnostic genetic test. Most studies report that greater than 90% of typical hemochromatosis patients were homozygotes for the C282Y mutation. A second minor mutation, H63D, was also described in the original report. Compound heterozygotes (C282Y/H63D) and less commonly H63D homozygotes may resemble C282Y homozygotes with mild-to-moderate iron overload. It is likely that more mutations will be found but they will only be relevant to a minority of patients. There will be patients with a clinical picture indistinguishable from genetic hemochromatosis that will be negative for the C282Y mutation. Most of these patients will be isolated cases, although a few cases of familial iron overload have been reported with negative C282Y testing.

A negative C282Y test should alert the physician to question the diagnosis of genetic hemochromatosis and reconsider secondary iron overload related to cirrhosis, alcohol, viral hepatitis or iron-loading anemias. If no other risk factors are found, the patient should begin venesection treatment similar to any other hemochromatosis patient. The interpretation of the genetic test in several settings is shown in Table 1. Genetic discrimination is a concern with the widespread use of genetic testing. In the case of hemochromatosis, the advantages of early diagnosis of a treatable disease outweigh the disadvantages of genetic discrimination.

Family Studies in Hemochromatosis

Once the proband case is identified and confirmed with the genetic test for the C282Y mutation, family testing is imperative. Siblings have a one in four chance of carrying the gene and should be screened with the genetic test (C282Y and H63D mutation), transferrin saturation, and serum ferritin. A cost-effective strategy now possible with the genetic test is to test the spouse for the C282Y mutation to assess the risk in the children. If the spouse is not a C282Y heterozygote or homozygote, the children will be obligate heterozygotes. This assumes paternity and excludes another gene or mutation causing hemochromatosis. This strategy is particularly advantageous where the children are geographically separated or may be under a different health care system.

TREATMENT OF HEMOCHROMATOSIS

The therapy of hemochromatosis continues to use the medieval therapy of periodic bleeding. At my center, patients attend an ambulatory care facility, and the venesections are performed by a nurse using a kit containing a 16-gauge straight needle and a collection bag (Blood Pack MR6102, Baxter, Deerfield, Illinois). Blood is removed while the patient is in the reclining position over 15 to 30 minutes. A hemoglobin level is taken at the time of each venesection. If the hemoglobin decreased to less than 10 g/

TABLE 1. **Interpretation of Genetic Testing for Hemochromatosis**

C282Y Homozygote

This is the classic genetic pattern that is seen in more than 90% of typical cases. Expression of disease ranges from no evidence of iron overload to massive iron overload with organ dysfunction. Siblings have a one in four chance of being affected and should have genetic testing. For children to be affected, the other parent must be at least a heterozygote. If iron studies are normal, false-positive genetic testing or a nonexpressing homozygote should be considered.

C282Y/H63D—Compound Heterozygote

This patient carries one copy of the major mutation and one copy of the minor mutation. Most patients with this genetic pattern have normal iron studies. A small percentage of compound heterozygotes have been found to have mild-to-moderate iron overload. Severe iron overload is usually seen in the setting of another concomitant risk factor (alcoholism, viral hepatitis).

C282Y Heterozygote

This patient carries one copy of the major mutation. This pattern is seen in about 10% of the white population and is usually associated with normal iron studies. In rare cases, the iron studies are high, in the range expected in a homozygote rather than a heterozygote. These patients may carry an unknown hemochromatosis mutation, and liver biopsy is helpful to determine the need for venesection therapy.

H63D Homozygote

This patient carries two copies of the minor mutation. Most patients with this genetic pattern have normal iron studies. A small percentage of these patients has been found to have mild-to-moderate iron overload. Severe iron overload is usually seen in the setting of another concomitant risk factor (alcoholism, viral hepatitis).

H63D Heterozygote

This patient carries one copy of the minor mutation. This pattern is seen in about 20% of the white population and is usually associated with normal iron studies. This pattern is so common in the general population that the presence of iron overload may be related to another risk factor. Liver biopsy may be required to determine the cause of the iron overload and the need for treatment in these patients.

No *HFE* Mutations

There will likely be other hemochromatosis mutations discovered in the future. If iron overload is present without any *HFE* mutations, a careful history for other risk factors must be reviewed, and liver biopsy may be useful to determine the cause of the iron overload and the need for treatment. Most of these cases are isolated and nonfamilial.

dL, the venesection schedule is modified to 500 mL every other week.

Venesections are continued until the serum ferritin is approximately 50 g/L. The concomitant administration of a salt-containing sport beverage (e.g., Gatorade) is a simple method of maintaining plasma volume during the venesection. Three to four maintenance venesections per year are performed after iron depletion in most patients, although the rate of iron reaccumulation is highly variable. The transferrin saturation will remain elevated in many treated patients and will not normalize unless the patient becomes iron deficient. Patients with mild iron abnormalities can be encouraged in some countries to become voluntary blood donors.

Chelation therapy with deferoxamine (Desferal),* is not recommended for hemochromatosis. Patients are advised to avoid oral iron therapy and alcohol abuse, but there are no dietary restrictions. Patient support groups are discouraged by the practice of iron fortification of foods, but much of this iron is in an inexpensive form with poor bioavailability.

POPULATION SCREENING FOR HEMOCHROMATOSIS

Early diagnosis and treatment of hemochromatosis leads to a long-term survival similar to the general population. Screening tests are available and inexpensive. Large scale population screening projects are underway in 15 countries. These studies should answer some of the critical questions such as the percentage of C282Y homozygotes with iron overload or symptoms and the optimal screening protocol.

Hemochromatosis is a common and often underdiagnosed disease. Early diagnosis and treatment results in an excellent long-term prognosis. The development of a diagnostic genetic test has improved the feasibility of prevention of morbidity and mortality from hemochromatosis.

*Not FDA approved for this indication.

HODGKIN'S DISEASE

method of
CLAIRE S. BARLOW, M.B.B.S., and
T. ANDREW LISTER, M.D.
St. Bartholomew's Hospital
West Smithfield, London, England

It was in 1832 that Thomas Hodgkin first recognized a distinct lymphoid neoplasm from his postmortem observations of the lymph nodes and spleen. The disease was described in more detail later in the century by Sir Samuel Wilks, who named it *Hodgkin's disease*. After the invention of the microscope, the unique cell characterizing this disease was described first by Sternberg and then by Dorothy Reed. Although the Reed-Sternberg cell is diagnostic of Hodgkin's disease, it is found only in the minority in any given lymphoid mass. Successful treatment was initiated at the beginning of the 20th century, and it is now not only a highly curable malignancy but also a disease from which we have learned much by following patients for many years after completion of therapy. Figure 1 shows the overall survival of Hodgkin's disease over 30 years, and remission duration can be seen in Figure 2.

The incidence of Hodgkin's disease is 25 per million per year. It is more common in men than in women and in certain geographic regions and racial groups. There is a bimodal age distribution. The most common peak by far is in adolescents and young adults. The disease seems to be diminishing in the over-55 age group, in which it also carries a less favorable prognosis.

There has been much speculation as to the etiology of Hodgkin's disease. It was for a long time thought to be an infectious illness, and many infectious agents have been

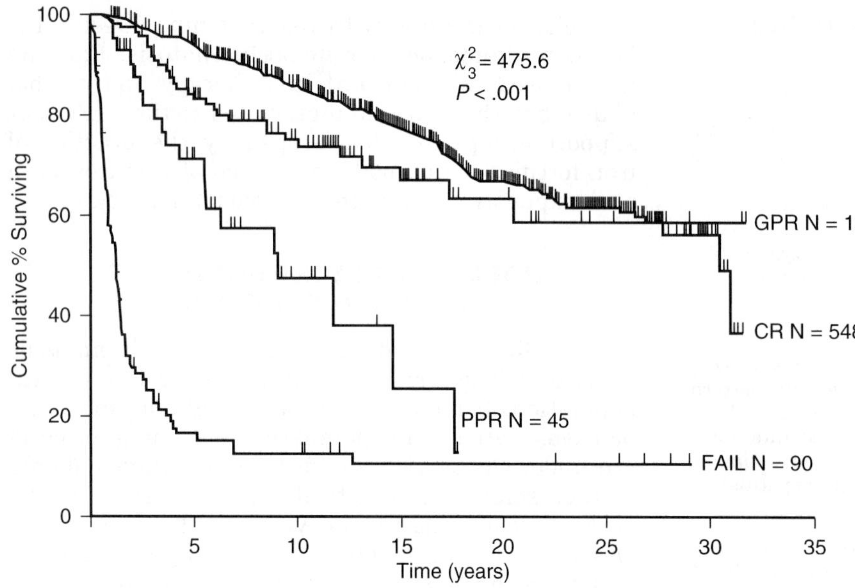

Figure 1. Overall survival of Hodgkin's disease by outcome to treatment.

found to be associated with it, including Epstein-Barr virus, human herpes virus 6, and HIV, but without actual proof of cause. At the molecular level, most Reed-Sternberg cells are late/postgerminal B cells that are no longer able to express immunoglobulin. Cells such as these would normally be eliminated by apoptosis. In Hodgkin's disease, it seems that apoptosis is prevented. It is conceivable that the viruses found to be associated may somehow be involved in this mechanism.

In 1966, at the Rye conference, four histological subtypes of Hodgkin's disease were recognized: lymphocyte predominant, nodular sclerosis (the most common subtype), mixed cellularity, and lymphocyte depletion (very rare). It is now known that nodular lymphocyte predominant disease differs from other classical Hodgkin's disease, both in immunophenotype and behavior (see later). The new World Health Organization (WHO) classification of Hodgkin's lymphoma is shown in Table 1.

The most common presentation is enlarging painless lymphadenopathy, often of the cervical glands. Currently, staging is carried out by computed tomography (CT) scanning of the chest, abdomen, and pelvis. The original Ann Arbor Classification was devised in the early 1970s. In 1989, with increasing use of CT, the Cotswold Modification was applied in order to further take into account the volume of lymph node masses involved. The stages are further subclassified according to the presence or absence of so-called B-symptoms: fever, drenching night sweats, and weight loss of more than 10% of body weight.

Laparotomy with splenectomy was previously used as a staging tool. The routine use of this procedure was abandoned in 1994 because it was believed that the reduction in survival from laparotomy-related deaths outweighed the marginal benefit in progression-free survival.

Lymph node biopsy is mandatory in order to confirm the diagnosis histologically. Bone marrow aspiration and trephine are performed for all but stage IA and IIA disease. The initial serum LDH is also of prognostic importance.

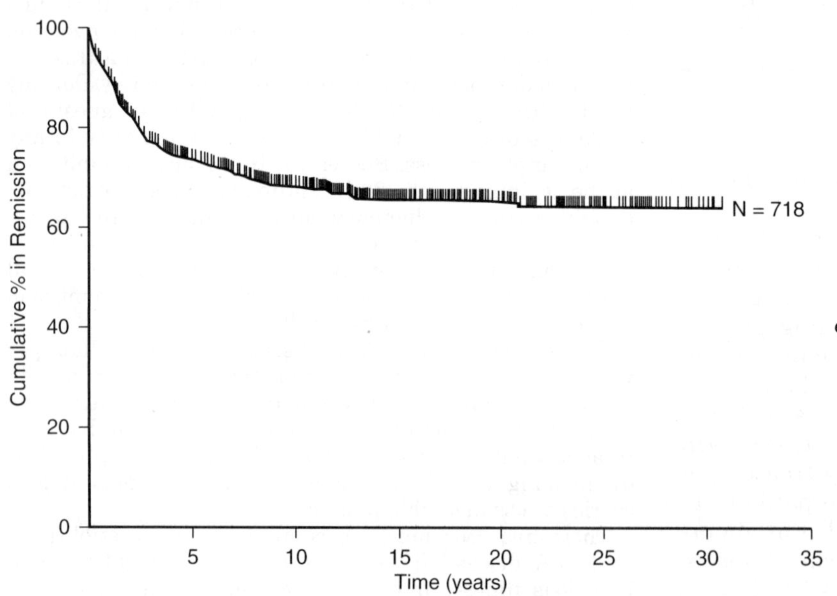

Figure 2. Remission duration of Hodgkin's disease.

TABLE 1. **WHO Classification of Hodgkin's Lymphoma**

Lymphocyte Predominant Lymphoma
Nodular
Diffuse (very rare)
Classical Hodgkin's Lymphoma
Nodular sclerosis (grades 1 and 2)
Lymphocyte-rich classical Hodgkin's lymphoma
Mixed cellularity
Lymphocyte depleted

Abbreviation: WHO = World Health Organization.

CHEMOTHERAPY

Historically, radiotherapy was the first treatment modality used for patients with Hodgkin's disease, being the only treatment available at the start of the 20th century.

Extended field irradiation was found to be highly effective in early stage disease and was associated with an excellent overall survival. Radiation therapy developed as an adjunct to chemotherapy in the context of advanced and bulky disease and also as a palliative treatment for patients without curable disease.

More recently, practices have been changing with regard to the use of radiotherapy. Follow-up has shown that some of the most important long-term complications of treatment, in particular heart disease, pulmonary toxicity, and second cancers, are associated with both the dose and extent of irradiation. New treatments are developed with the aim of improving/maintaining efficacy while reducing toxicity. Attention has therefore focused on reducing radiotherapy doses and field size wherever possible. This, coupled with the introduction of newer, less toxic chemotherapy agents, has broadened the use of this treatment modality in current (and likely future) practice.

Advanced Stage Disease

With the advent of effective anticancer agents in the 1960s, a chemotherapeutic approach was developed initially for the treatment of advanced stage Hodgkin's disease (Table 2). Single agent therapy served to palliate, but not cure, leading to the concept of *combination chemotherapy.* The original principles defining combination chemotherapy remain; that is, the individual drugs must be clinically effective, combinations of drugs are given in cycles, and treatment is given over a prolonged period. In practice, this is usually six to eight cycles of therapy.

In 1963, the first four-drug combination to be used was MOMP (nitrogen mustard, vincristine [Oncovin], methotrexate, and prednisolone). This was shortly to be succeeded by MOPP; methotrexate was replaced by procarbazine (Matulane). Response rates increased to 80% with an overall disease-free survival at 5 years of approximately 50%. Combination chemotherapy having been shown to effectively cure Hodgkin's disease, attention was drawn to maintaining efficacy while reducing both short- and long-term side effects. Initial side effects of MOPP included nausea and vomiting, myelosuppression, and neurotoxicity. MVPP and ChlVPP were shown to be better tolerated and equally efficacious. The long-term data concerning these agents show that overall median survival from presentation is about 14 years and that for those entering a complete remission, disease-free survival is two in three at 10 to 15 years.

TABLE 2. **Combination Chemotherapy Regimens**

MOPP		
Nitrogen mustard	6 mg/m² IV	Days 1, 8
Vincristine	1.4 mg/m² IV	Days 1, 8
Procarbazine	100 mg/m² po	Days 1–14
Prednisolone	40 mg/m² po	Days 1–14
Cycle repeated day 28.		
MVPP		
Nitrogen mustard	6 mg/m² IV	Days 1, 8
Vinblastine	6 mg/m² IV	Days 1, 8
Procarbazine	100 mg/m² po	Days 1–14
Prednisolone	40 mg/m² po	Days 1–14
Cycle repeated days 28–42.		
ChlVPP		
Chlorambucil	6 mg/m² po	Days 1–14
Vinblastine	1.4 mg/m² IV	Days 1,8
Procarbazine	100 mg/m² po	Days 1–14
Prednisolone	40 mg/m² po	Days 1–14
Cycle repeated day 28.		
ABVD		
Adriamycin	25 mg/m² IV	Day 1
Bleomycin	10,000 U/m² IV	Day 1
Vinblastine	6 mg/m² IV	Day 1
Dacarbazine	375 mg/m² IV	Day 1
Cycle repeated day 15.		
ChlVPP/EVA		
ChlVPP	*(Vinblastine day 8 only)*	
Etoposide	100 mg/m² po	Days 1–5
Vincristine	1.4 mg/m² IV	Day 1
Adriamycin	50 mg/m² IV	Day 8
Cycle repeated day 28.		
COPP		
Cyclophosphamide	650 mg/m² IV	Days 1, 8
Vincristine	1.4 mg/m² IV	Days 1, 8
Procarbazine	100 mg/m² po	Days 1–14
Prednisolone	40 mg/m² po	Days 1–14
Cycle repeated day 28.		
Stanford V		
Doxorubicin	25 mg/m² IV	Days 1, 15
Vinblastine	6 mg/m² IV	Days 1, 15
Mechlorethamine	6 mg/m² IV	Day 1
Vincristine	1.4 mg/m² IV	Days 8, 22
Bleomycin	5000 U/m² IV	Days 8, 22
Etoposide	60 mg/m² IV	Day 15
Prednisolone	40 mg/m² po	Days 1–28
Cycle repeated every 28 days.		

BEACOPP	*Basic*	*Escalated*	
Bleomycin	10,000 U/m² IV	10,000 U/m² IV	Day 8
Etoposide	100 mg/m² IV	200 mg/m² IV	Days 1–3
Doxorubicin	25 mg/m² IV	35 mg/m² IV	Day 1
Cyclophosphamide	650 mg/m² IV	1250 mg/m² IV	Day 1
Vincristine	1.4 mg/m² IV	1.4 mg/m² IV	Day 1
Procarbazine	100 mg/m² po	100 mg/m² po	Days 1–7
Prednisolone	40 mg/m² po	40 mg/m² po	Days 1–14
Cycle repeated day 22.			

In 1973, ABVD was developed by the Milan Group in order to reduce the main long-term effects noted with use of the earlier regimens, namely infertility, leukemia, and secondary myelodysplasia. These effects are clearly of particular importance when treating young people. Trials have compared MOPP with ABVD and also with MOPP/ABVD in alternating cycles. Both ABVD regimens were noted to be superior with regard to complete response rates, disease-free survival, and overall survival at 5 years. In addition, ABVD has been found to be less myelotoxic, necessitating fewer dose reductions. For these reasons, it has been adopted as the standard treatment for advanced stage Hodgkin's disease in many centers. "Hybrid" regimens such as Ch1VPP/EVA and COPP (the German variant of MOPP/ABVD) were developed with the intention of reducing cross-resistance to chemotherapy.

Two notable newer regimens have been developed. Both show promising early results, although mature data with regard to efficacy and toxicity are awaited. These are the Stanford V and the German BEACOPP (basic and escalated) regimens. In Stanford V, the drugs are administered weekly, alternating myelosuppressive and nonmyelosuppressive agents. A substantial dose of radiotherapy is also incorporated in both.

The role of radiotherapy in the treatment of advanced disease is not satisfactorily defined. Most clinicians feel that radiotherapy has a role as an adjunctive treatment in advanced disease, particularly in treating sites of initial bulk. This decision is based on the observation that most patients who relapse will relapse in the sites of previous disease. Whether or not radiotherapy is in fact an essential component of treatment is not entirely clear, and as concern grows over the negative long-term effects of radiotherapy, its role is questionable.

Early Stage Disease

As extended field megavoltage irradiation is an extremely effective method of eradicating early stage disease, and those patients who relapse following such treatment, for the most part, are salvaged with combination chemotherapy; this has been the traditional approach. The role of chemotherapy in early disease is to eradicate subclinical disease. Treatment can therefore be of shorter duration than in advanced disease, with consequent reduced toxicity.

In light of the data concerning the long-term effects of irradiation, shorter courses of chemotherapy known to be effective in advanced stage disease have been combined with various radiation strategies. The published data so far suggest that both the dose intensity and field size may be safely reduced with the addition of brief chemotherapy.

Special Situations

Bulky Disease

Bulky disease is defined as a mass greater than 10 cm in diameter or, in the case of an anterior mediastinal mass, occupying more than a third of the intrathoracic diameter. In staging, the suffix "x" denotes disease bulk. Patients with Hodgkin's disease commonly present with an anterior mediastinal mass. Although this should be considered to be early stage if there are no other sites of disease, it is known that single modality therapy is insufficient treatment in this situation. The best approach is to downstage the size of the mass using chemotherapy in the first instance, consolidating with radiotherapy, which would thus encompass a smaller field and result in less toxicity to the mediastinal structures.

Lymphocyte Predominant Hodgkin's Disease

Lymphocyte predominant Hodgkin's disease (LPHD) was first described by Jackson in 1937. It has more recently become apparent that at both the clinical and molecular levels this is actually a separate entity from other cases of Hodgkin's disease, which are termed *classical Hodgkin's disease*. The cells in LPHD express CD20 and do not express CD30 and CD15 seen in classical disease. A nodular pattern is seen in almost all cases; diffuse LPHD is extremely rare. Clinically LPHD behaves as an indolent B-cell lymphoma but with a propensity to transform to diffuse large B-cell lymphoma at a later stage. This must be distinguished both from a lymphocyte-rich form of classical Hodgkin's disease (LRCHD) and also from T-cell rich large B-cell lymphoma. Currently, LPHD is either treated with involved field radiotherapy (most) or managed expectantly. Treatment with monoclonal anti-CD 20 (rituximab) [Rituxan] is also an interesting strategy in this group of patients.

Relapsed and Refractory Disease and the Role of High-Dose Therapy

Although long-term remission can be induced in the majority of patients with Hodgkin's disease, there remains a definitive population in whom the disease is refractory to therapy or will recur. There is no doubt that this is a difficult situation, and the outlook, even for those who achieve a second remission, remains poor, with a median survival following first recurrence of 4 years. One of the most important prognostic indicators appears to be the duration of the first remission. It has been reported that for those in whom this is less than 1 year, the prognosis is notably worse.

Salvage therapy is more effective with non–cross-resistant chemotherapy. High-dose therapy with autologous bone marrow–peripheral blood stem cell support has been used for selected patients over a number of years and is currently being evaluated. Several factors favor this approach to consolidation therapy. First, Hodgkin's disease is known to be a highly chemosensitive condition, hence dose escalation is an attractive concept. Second, the patients themselves are, for the vast majority, young and able to withstand intensive therapy. Third, in practical terms, stem cell–bone marrow collection is usually feasible because the bone marrow itself is only infrequently involved.

It is, however, difficult to compare the results of patients treated with and without high-dose chemotherapy because pretreatment schedules, transplant techniques, and the use of adjuvant radiotherapy vary widely among high-dose patients.

It is feasible to proceed directly to high-dose therapy at recurrence if the disease volume is small, although usually one to three cycles of chemotherapy are given in an attempt to induce disease remission while the plan for high-dose therapy is instigated. Some use induction chemotherapy to test sensitivity and would not transplant nonresponders because intrinsic resistance cannot be overcome simply by dose escalation. However, there is still some evidence of benefit even in resistant patients. Total body irradiation (TBI) is given infrequently with high-dose therapy because many patients have been previously irradiated. Typical regimens include BEAM, CBV, and high-dose melphalan (Alnkeran) (Table 3).

Only one randomized trial has demonstrated a favorable outcome to high-dose compared with conventional chemotherapy, but encouraging results have also been obtained from numerous phase II studies. The 2-year disease-free survival following autologous transplant for relapsed/refractory disease has been found to be 50% to 60%. The use of tandem transplants is currently under investigation. Complete response and PFS rates may be improved, although toxicity is considerable.

Generally speaking, inferior outcomes are observed if high-dose therapy is used in second or subsequent relapse, mostly due to increased transplant-related mortality. It is important to consider the heavy pretreatment of these patients, making it difficult to mobilize stem cells and making the cytogenetic changes of myelodysplasia more likely.

LONG-TERM EFFECTS OF TREATMENT

The excellent cure rates associated with the treatment of Hodgkin's disease give us an insight into the long-term effects of therapy. This is information that is not available with regard to the treatment of most other malignancies. It is true to say that treatment is justified because it is impossible to suffer the long-term consequences of therapy if one has died from the original illness. However, certain important observations from long-term follow-up have encouraged the modification of therapy in order to improve the long-term outlook of the young population we are exposing to toxic treatment.

Fertility

Early chemotherapy regimens resulted in the inevitable sterilization of patients undergoing therapy. If it is known that treatment is certain or even likely to result in loss of fertility, a variety of techniques for sperm and egg storage are now widely available (although their benefit is not yet known) and should be offered to all except those requiring emergency treatment. Newer regimens, such as ABVD, are favored where preservation of fertility is desirable.

Cardiac and Pulmonary Toxicity

Anthracyclines are well known to cause occasional long-term cardiac complications, usually in the form of cardiomyopathy and usually 10 to 15 years posttreatment. As a precautionary measure, baseline investigations should be carried out, certainly with an electrocardiograph (ECG) and preferably with some measure of left ventricular function (e.g., echocardiography, MUGA scanning). It is important to bear in mind the recommended lifetime doses of anthracycline drugs. More recently, cardioprotection drugs have become available and are used in some circumstances.

Several chemotherapeutic agents are known to cause pulmonary toxicity, the most notable in the treatment of Hodgkin's disease being pulmonary fibrosis caused by bleomycin. Lung function tests are a mandatory investigation for any patient with respiratory disease and for all patients before high-dose therapy.

Additional cardiopulmonary toxicity also undoubtedly occurs from mediastinal irradiation.

Second Malignancies

The occurrence of second cancers is felt to be the most serious long-term consequence of the treatment of Hodgkin's disease and has been found to be associated with both radiotherapy and chemotherapy (particularly the use of alkylating agents).

TABLE 3. **Examples of High Dose Regimens**

BEAM	BCNU	300 mg/m² IV	Day 6
	Etoposide	200 mg/m² IV	Days 5 to 2
	Cytosine arabinoside	200 mg/m² IV bd	Days 5 to 2
	Melphalan	140 mg/m² IV	Day 1
CBV	Cyclophosphamide	1500 mg/m² IV	Days 5 to 2
	BCNU	300 mg/m² IV	Day 6
	Etoposide	125 mg/m² IV	Days 5 to 2
M	Melphalan	200 mg/m² IV	Day 1
CY/TBI	Cyclophosphamide	60 mg/kg	Days 1–2 then radiotherapy
	Total body irradiation		

Myelodysplasia and leukemia generally occur within the first 10 years following treatment, relative risks being significantly higher after chemotherapy and combined modality treatment. The use of alkylating agents is associated with −5 and −7 cytogenetic abnormalities, resulting in MDS leading to frank AML in 3 to 5 years. Topoisomerase II inhibitors, such as etoposide, can result in explosive AML within 2 years of the original treatment.

Solid tumors generally arise more gradually, often 10 to 20 years following initial treatment. Most common tumors have been noted after treatment with either or both modalities; however, an increased risk of breast cancer has been noted only after radiotherapy. There is no consensus regarding the screening of young women for breast cancer; however, most units recognize the need for vigilance and have adopted a local policy.

Age at initial treatment has been shown to affect risk. The younger the age at initial treatment, the greater the relative risk of leukemia and solid tumors. Absolute excess risk, however, remains greater at older rather than younger ages.

OTHER APPROACHES TO TREATMENT

Hodgkin's disease is a highly curable malignancy. Nevertheless, for a proportion of individuals, treatment will fail, necessitating fresh approaches to therapy.

High-dose therapy with autologous transplantation is now supported by some randomized data to be consolidation therapy in difficult disease and is becoming a standard treatment.

Allogeneic transplantation has not generally been considered as a treatment for Hodgkin's disease, mostly due to the high associated treatment-related mortality. Some success has been achieved, however, and it will be interesting to explore the graft-versus-lymphoma effect in these patients.

Non-myeloablative transplant techniques are currently being developed, enabling the treatment of older patients and patients with premorbid states precluding a full transplant.

Immunomodulatory treatments, such as monoclonal antibody therapy with rituximab in CD20 positive disease, add a further dimension to the treatment of Hodgkin's disease either alone or in combination with chemotherapy.

HODGKIN'S DISEASE: RADIATION THERAPY

method of
PELAYO C. BESA, M.D.
Pontificia Universidad Catolica de Chile
Santiago, Chile

Hodgkin's disease is a malignancy of lymph nodes with a predictable pattern of spread. Advances in treatment have made Hodgkin's disease a highly curable cancer with a long-term survival rate of more than 90%. *Cure rate,* defined as 10-year freedom from relapse, for early stage disease is in the range of 80% to 90%; for intermediate stage disease, 70% to 80%; and for advanced disease, 30% to 50%.

Radiation therapy plays a major role in the management of Hodgkin's disease. Treatment planning and patient selection are based on thorough clinical staging and review of the pathology. Most patients afflicted with Hodgkin's disease are young and will be cured; therefore, they will be at risk of late toxicity from treatment. Ideal therapy should provide the highest cure rate with minimal long-term toxicity. With this goal, treatment programs have gradually adjusted therapy to the different clinical settings.

Adequate radiation therapy requires pretreatment simulation and therapy with a linear accelerator with a minimal photon beam energy of 6 MV through parallel opposed fields that deliver a tumoricidal dose in a fractionated fashion. Treatment reproducibility is verified periodically with portal films. After completion of therapy, the patient is observed regularly to detect early relapse and evaluate treatment-related toxicity.

PATIENT EVALUATION AND STAGING

To determine the best treatment approach, the patient needs to undergo disease staging. A complete medical history is obtained with special attention to the tumor history, presence of B symptoms (unexplained fever, drenching night sweats, and unexplained weight loss), and general performance status. The physical examination should be thorough, with special attention to all nodal areas, Waldeyer ring, liver, and spleen. When a single nodal site is involved, the low neck or supraclavicular area is involved in 60% of the cases, the mediastinum in 15%, axillae in 10%, and the inguinal-femoral regions in 10%. The disease progresses with involvement of contiguous nodal regions. Upper abdominal nodes are considered contiguous to the supraclavicular nodes through the thoracic duct. A biopsy must be performed, preferably with sampling from the most clinically suspicious node.

The hematologic assessment should include complete blood cell and platelet counts, erythrocyte sedimentation rate, and screen chemistries, including lactate dehydrogenase and thyroid function studies. An elevated erythrocyte sedimentation rate has been associated with high risk of subclinical disease in the abdomen. An abnormal blood cell count and an elevated lactic dehydrogenase level suggest bone marrow involvement. Thyroid function testing must be done as a follow-up study because of a substantial risk of later dysfunction caused by radiation therapy.

Routine imaging studies include chest radiographs and computed tomography (CT) of the chest, abdomen, and pelvis. Magnetic resonance imaging (MRI) is used occasionally to better delineate hilar adenopathy and chest wall and pericardial extension and, in the abdomen, to distinguish unfilled bowel and vessels from adenopathy. Gallium scans are most useful for distinguishing between active disease and fibrosis in a residual mediastinal mass. Gallium sensitivity is low, limiting its value for initial diagnosis.

Bone marrow biopsies are performed in all patients except those with early stage (stage I or II) disease and no B symptoms. The overall frequency of bone marrow involvement in Hodgkin's disease is only 5%. Hodgkin's disease is staged according to the Ann Arbor staging classification system (Table 1). The lymphoid regions used in this system are shown in Figure 1. Note that the supraclavicular, cervical, occipital, and preauricular areas are a single region.

RADIATION TREATMENT TECHNIQUE

Treatment planning starts by reviewing the staging evaluation and pathology report. Clinical and radiologic studies are used to outline the extent of disease. The treatment fields include the known disease areas and adjacent nodal regions. Treatment volume varies according to the treatment plan. The *treatment volumes* are defined as involved field, extended field, and subtotal nodal irradiation. *Involved field irradiation* includes the entire nodal area in which nodes with Hodgkin's disease are noted; for example, if a low neck node is involved, the entire neck and supraclavicular areas are treated. *Extended field irradiation* treats the entire nodal region. *Subtotal nodal irradiation* includes all the regions at risk: the supradiaphragmatic area, including neck, supraclavicular, infraclavicular, axillary, mediastinal, and hilar nodes, and the infradiaphragmatic area, including para-aortic nodes, spleen, pelvic, and inguinal-femoral nodes. The nodal areas not included are mesenteric, presacral, popliteal, brachial, and epitrochlear nodes, because they are only rarely involved with Hodgkin's disease. These regions are treated in three areas: (1) the mantle for the supradiaphragmatic region, (2) the abdomen, and (3) the pelvis, including inguinal and femoral nodes (Figure 2). The junction between the fields must be placed away from the tumor to prevent underdosing, and normal tissue tolerance must be considered to avoid organ toxicity.

After the treatment plan has been determined, the radiation field is simulated and marked on the patient. The simulator is a diagnostic radiography unit that reproduces the geometry of the therapy machine and takes verification films of the treatment fields. To optimize reproducibility of the daily setup, patient immobilization devices are used; for example, a face mask of low-temperature thermal plastic (polycarbolactone) or vacuum body mold can be used for the mantle. Treatment fields are determined by anatomic body landmarks on the patient and fluoroscopic examination during simulation. Contrast material can be used to better localize some organs, such as the kidneys and bowel. Treatment fields include lymphoid regions, and to encompass all these areas, large and irregular fields are necessary.

The simulation radiographic films are used to outline the field to be treated and to design the blocks for the areas to be protected from irradiation. Divergent blocks are constructed from the drawings on the films using a low-melting-point alloy such as Lipowitz metal (Cerrobend). Typically, the dose is prescribed to be delivered along the central axis at the mid

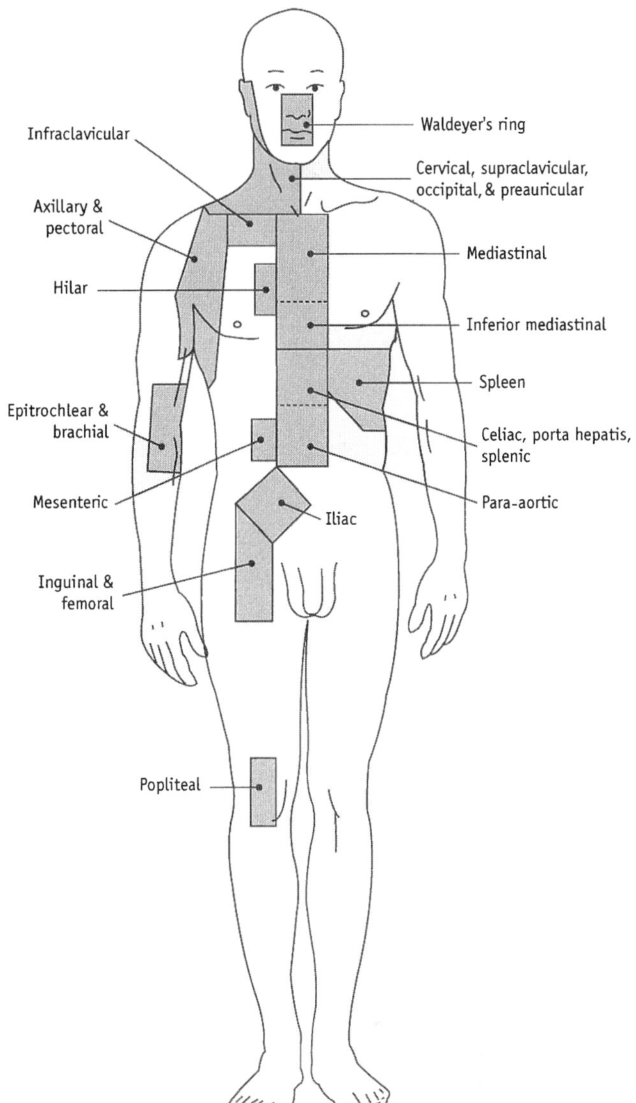

Figure 1. Lymphoid regions for Ann Arbor staging of Hodgkin's disease.

TABLE 1. **Ann Arbor Staging Classification System**

Stage I

Involvement of a single lymph node region (I) or localized involvement of an extralymphatic organ or site (IE)

Stage II

Involvement of two or more lymph node regions on the same side of the diaphragm (II) or localized involvement of an extralymphatic organ or site and one or more nodal regions on the same side of the diaphragm (IIE)

Stage III

Involvement of lymph node regions on both sides of the diaphragm (III), which may be accompanied by localized involvement of an extralymphatic organ or site (IIIE)

Stage IV

Diffuse involvement of one or more extralymphatic organs with or without associated lymph node involvement

Systemic Symptoms

A: Absence of systemic symptoms defined as B

B: Unexplained fever with temperatures above 38°C, unexplained weight loss >10% body weight, or drenching night sweats

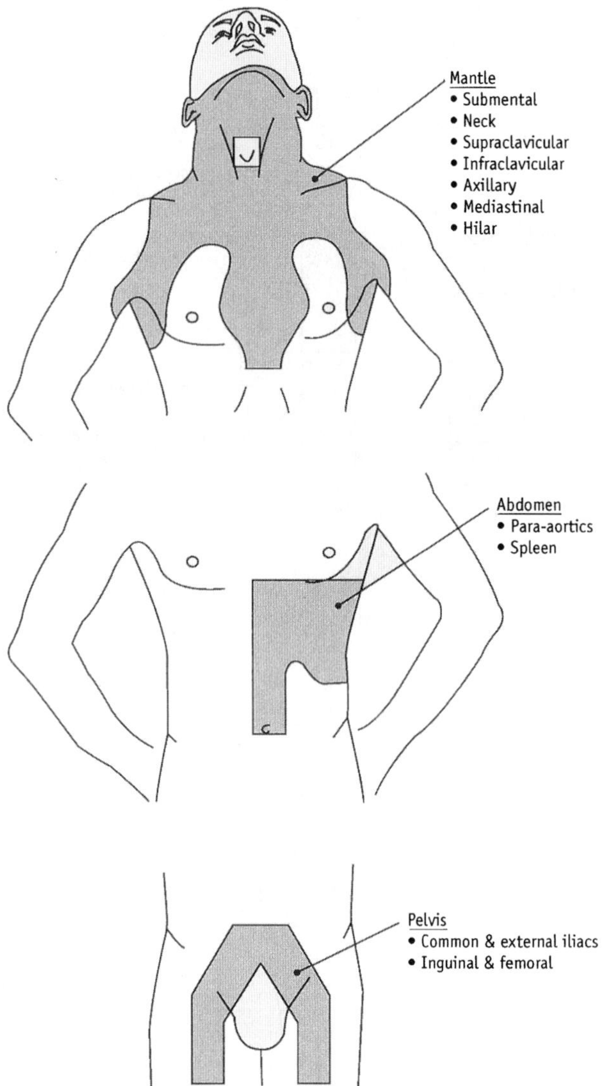

Figure 2. Radiation therapy extended fields: supradiaphragmatic: mantle; infradiaphragmatic: abdomen and pelvis.

plane. The dose is higher for thin areas where diameters are small. To calculate the dose in the different areas, planning CT is done and a three-dimensional reconstruction and dose distribution is obtained. Partial transmission blocks or shrinking field technique are used to compensate for the difference in the diameters and to make the dose homogeneous throughout the treatment field.

Patients are treated on a linear accelerator at a 100-cm source-to-surface distance, usually using 6-MV photons for the upper torso and 20-MV photons for the abdomen and pelvis. The patient is seen on the treatment table by the radiation oncologist to verify the proper location of the fields. Machine portal films for verification are taken at the beginning of treatment and weekly thereafter. The dose delivered to the visible tumor areas is 39.6 Gy in 22 fractions over 4½ weeks. The nodal areas treated prophylactically receive 30.6 Gy in 17 fractions over 3½ weeks. In general, the treatment field is arranged with parallel opposed fields, using even-weighted beams, and all fields are treated daily. When two fields are matched (e.g., mantle and abdomen), special gap calculations are used to avoid overlap. If the adjacent fields overlie the spinal cord, a CT scan is taken and computer-generated isodose calculations are made to determine the dose at the cord.

MANTLE FIELD IRRADIATION

Radiation to the mantle field treats the supradiaphragmatic nodal regions. The mantle field extends from the mastoid and base of the mandible to the diaphragm and encompasses the submental, occipital, cervical, supraclavicular, infraclavicular, axillary, mediastinal, and hilar nodes. The patient is treated using parallel opposed anteroposterior fields, with individually contoured lung and heart blocks. Usually, the cervical spine is blocked posteriorly, the larynx anteriorly, and both humeral heads anteriorly and posteriorly. The mantle is treated with equally loaded beams to a dose of 30.6 Gy in 17 fractions. At this point, treatment is stopped for the areas of prophylactic irradiation and continues only for the areas of gross involvement to a dose of 39.6 Gy. Low-dose lung irradiation is given when hilar nodes or lung are involved. The lungs receive 15 Gy in 15 fractions to decrease the risk of disease relapse in the lungs. Obese patients have a wide mediastinum when they lie on their back and can be treated sitting in a specially designed chair to decrease the amount of normal lung treated.

SUBDIAPHRAGMATIC IRRADIATION

Subdiaphragmatic nodal areas are usually divided into two treatment fields: (1) the abdomen, which includes the para-aortic nodes and spleen, with or without the liver, and (2) the pelvis, which includes the common and external iliac nodes and the inguinal-femoral regions. If the pelvic field is treated concurrently with the para-aortic field, the term *inverted Y* is used.

The field encompassing the para-aortic and spleen areas extends from the diaphragm to the bottom of the fourth lumbar vertebra; field edges are matched with those of the mantle with an appropriate skin gap; to encompass the para-aortic nodes, the field is drawn to the width of the transverse processes of the lumbar vertebral bodies, provided that the abdominal CT scan does not show nodes in a more lateral position. Radiation is delivered using parallel opposed anteroposterior fields with equally loaded beams that deliver a dose of 30.6 Gy in 17 fractions. An additional 9-Gy boost in 5 fractions is given to areas with tumor involvement. Individually contoured blocks are made to protect kidneys and bowel.

Often, it is not necessary to treat the pelvic lymph nodes and the radiation treatment stops at the level of the fourth lumbar vertebra. If needed, pelvic treatment is given through parallel opposed anteroposterior fields with 6-MV photons from the front (because the inguinal-femoral nodes are superficial) and 20-MV photons from the back. The pelvic field matches the abdomen field at the level of the fourth lumbar vertebra and extends to encompass the femoral lymph nodes. The nodal areas must be evaluated on the CT scan.

Careful blocking is used to spare the bone marrow as much as possible and, in young females, the ovaries. The ovaries are transposed medially and placed as low as possible behind the uterus to avoid radiation-induced amenorrhea and sterility. The ovaries are marked with radiopaque clips to aid in the placement of a double-thickness block. At a distance of 2 cm from the edge of the block the ovaries receive approximately 8% of the pelvic dose.

TABLE 2. **Treatment Results for Hodgkin's Disease**

Series	Stage	Treatment	Survival % (y)	Freedom From Relapse % (y)
MDACC	I–IIA favorable	XRT	92 (4)	78 (4)
MDACC	I–II unfavorable	2-MOPP-XRT	100 (4)	79 (4)
MDACC	I–II large mediastinal mass	2-MOPP-XRT	84 (4)	66 (4)
MDACC	III (except III_3)	2-MOPP-XRT	87 (10)	83 (10)
Yale University	IIIB–IV	CMT XRT	66 (10)	69 (10)

Abbreviations: CMT = combined modality therapy (3 regimens—MVVPP [mechlorethamine/vincristine/vinblastine/procarbazine/prednisone], MOPP, and MOPP-ABVD [MOPP-Doxorubicin/Bleomycin/Vinblastine/Dacarbazine]); MDACC = M.D. Anderson Cancer Center; MOPP = mechlorethamine/vincristine/procarbazine/prednisone combination; XRT = radiotherapy.

COMBINED MODALITY THERAPY

Many patients with intermediate or advanced Hodgkin's disease benefit from combined chemotherapy and radiation therapy. To reduce the toxicity from the combined modality approach, treatment must be tailored to the extent of disease and the risk of normal tissue injury. Special attention must be paid to the chemotherapy drugs, the number of cycles, the total dose, the time frequency between cycles or intensity, the radiation fields, the volume of tissue irradiated, and doses. Both the medical oncologist and the radiation oncologist must work together from the beginning to tailor the treatment plan.

Most patients with Hodgkin's disease treated with combined modality receive initially two cycles of a combination of doxorubicin (Adriamycin), bleomycin (Blenoxane), vinblastine (Velban), and dacarbazine (DTIC) (the ABVD regimen), followed by radiation therapy to the tumor and areas at risk of subclinical disease. For supradiaphragmatic presentations the mantle and para-aortic and spleen areas are treated. For patients with advanced Hodgkin's disease (stage IIIB or IV) or mediastinal masses larger than 15 cm, six cycles of chemotherapy are given, followed by radiation therapy to the involved sites.

Gallium scan is used to evaluate the treatment response to chemotherapy. The test is done before chemotherapy begins and, if positive, repeated before radiation is delivered. Patients who become negative have a lower relapse rate.

TREATMENT RECOMMENDATIONS AND RESULTS

Supradiaphragmatic Favorable Stages I and IIA

Upper torso presentation in patients younger than 40 years of age, with three or fewer sites of involvement and no B symptoms should be treated with radiation therapy alone. Radiation is given to the mantle field and the para-aortic and spleen areas. (see Figure 2). Patients with mediastinal disease are excluded because they benefit from induction chemotherapy, which reduces the mediastinal mass and decreases radiation to normal lung. Freedom from relapse for this group of patients is 80% to 90% (Table 2).

Patients with stage IA nodular lymphocyte predominant Hodgkin's disease are a special subgroup who tend to have disease localized and have a late relapse pattern similar to low-grade nodular lymphomas. These patients must be treated to the involved field (Figure 3).

Supradiaphragmatic Unfavorable Stages I Through IIA and IIB

This group includes all patients with stages I and II disease who do not meet the "favorable" criteria. These patients have an increased risk of abdominal involvement, approaching 30% according to the laparotomy data. Treatment is with combined modality therapy. Chemotherapy (two cycles of ABVD) is given first, followed by radiation therapy to the mantle, the para-aortics, and the spleen. Patients in this group, treated with two cycles of mechlorethamine (Mustargen), vincristine, procarbazine, and prednisone (the MOPP regimen) followed by radiation therapy have a disease-free survival of 79% and a 100% survival rate at 4 years. Preliminary results with ABVD instead of MOPP are equivalent.

Stages I and II With Mediastinal Involvement

Mediastinal involvement is very common in Hodgkin's disease and presents a special challenge to the radiation oncologist because toxicity to the lungs and heart must be avoided. The extent of mediastinal tumor involvement is determined by measuring the maximum single horizontal width of the mediastinum on a standing posteroanterior chest radiograph. Three categories are defined: tumors less than 7.5 cm are small, those larger than 7.5 cm to less than

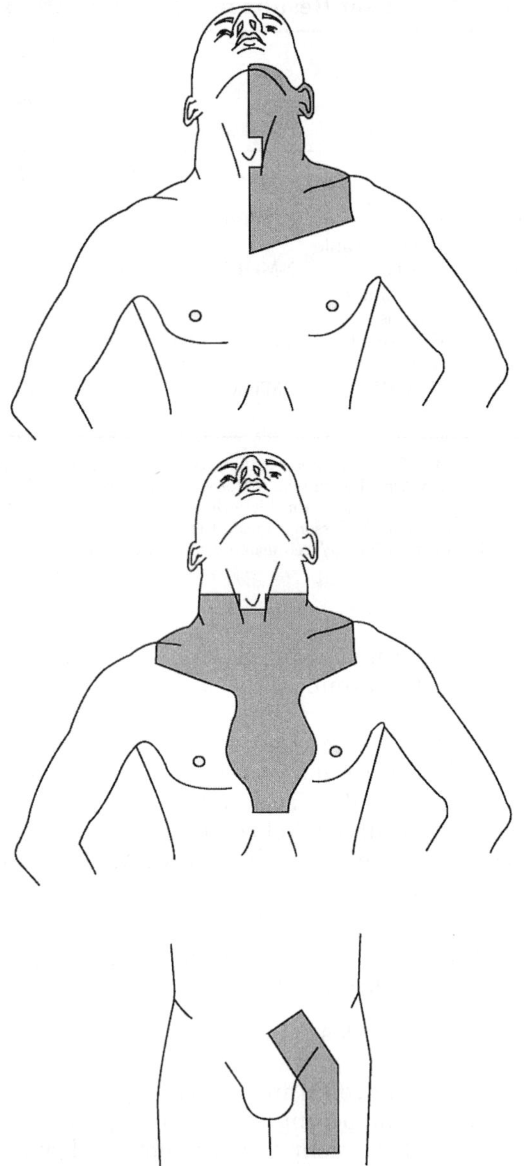

Figure 3. Radiation therapy involved field examples: neck, mediastinum, and inguinal-femoral.

15 cm are large or bulky, and those larger than 15 cm are massive.

Most of these patients are treated with combined modality therapy. Chemotherapy is administered first to decrease the size of the mediastinal tumor. Patients with small mediastinal tumors receive two cycles of chemotherapy followed by radiation to the mantle field and para-aortic and spleen areas. Patients with bulky tumors or hilar involvement receive six cycles of combination chemotherapy followed by radiation therapy to the involved field.

Stages I and II: Subdiaphragmatic Involvement

Fewer than 10% of patients with stage I or II Hodgkin's disease present with disease limited to the subdiaphragmatic areas. CT of the abdomen and pelvis is used to evaluate nodal and spleen involvement, and treatment is adjusted to the extent of tumor involvement.

For stage IA inguinal presentation, radiation is delivered to the involved field. More advanced cases receive combined modality therapy. Radiation therapy fields include the para-aortic nodes, the spleen, the common and external iliac nodes, and the inguinal-femoral regions. Treatment results for these patients are similar to those with supradiaphragmatic presentations.

Stage III

Nodal involvement in patients with stage III disease varies greatly. This heterogeneous group of patients is divided into subgroups according to extent of abdominal disease. Stage III_1 includes patients with disease limited to the upper abdomen (involving the celiac region, splenic hilum, and spleen). When the disease extends to the para-aortic region, it is classified as stage III_2; and if the pelvis or inguinal region is involved, the classification is stage III_3.

With the exception of patients presenting with stage III_3 disease, all patients with stage III receive two cycles of combination chemotherapy, followed by radiation therapy to the mantle, abdomen, and pelvic fields (see Figure 2). The relapse-free rate for this group is 85%, with a cause-specific survival of 89% at 5 years. The few patients who present with stage III_3 are treated with the advanced disease regimen.

Stages III_3 and IV

The majority of patients with stage III_3 and many with stage IV receive combined modality therapy. Only about 35% of patients with advanced-stage disease treated with chemotherapy alone are alive and well at 10 years. Patterns of failure after chemotherapy show that recurrence overwhelmingly occurs in previously involved areas. Patients with stage III_3 and IV Hodgkin's disease are treated initially with six cycles of combination chemotherapy (doxorubicin, bleomycin, vinblastine and dacarbazine—ABVD), followed by irradiation to the involved sites. Bleomycin is stopped after the fourth cycle if mantle irradiation is planned. With combined modality therapy, relapse-free survival of 69% and overall survival of 66% at 10 years have been reported (see Table 2).

COMPLICATIONS

Complications are classified as acute or late. Acute complications occur during or shortly after the course of radiation therapy; they are treated symptomatically and resolve quickly after the completion of treatment. *Acute complications* include mild skin reactions and hair loss in the irradiated areas, dysphasia, dry cough, nausea, and diarrhea. These complications are treated symptomatically with skin ointments, analgesics, cough suppressants, and antinausea and antidiarrheal agents.

Late complications occur after treatment has been completed, months or years later, and tend to be permanent. *Late complications* include pneumonitis, pericarditis, hypothyroidism, dental caries, and second malignancies. These reported toxicities observed in long-term survivors are clearly associated with treatment techniques that are different from the ones used today; therefore, in the future a decrease in these toxicities is expected.

Radiation pneumonitis occurs infrequently, and its risk is proportional to the volume of lung irradiated, the total dose, and the fraction size. The patient typically presents 6 to 12 weeks after the completion of the radiation therapy with dry cough, shortness of breath, pleuritic chest pain, and fever. The chest radiograph reveals interstitial infiltrates. Severe cases require treatment with high doses of corticosteroids for 4 to 6 weeks, with gradual tapering to avoid recurrence of symptoms.

Pericarditis is rare, occurring 6 to 12 months after treatment and usually after irradiation of the entire heart. Pericarditis presents as an acute episode of chest pain, fatigue, fever, and friction rubs or sometimes with decreased heart sounds due to pericardial effusion. Patients with mild pericarditis are managed with nonsteroidal anti-inflammatory agents, and for severe cases corticosteroids are used. Constrictive pericarditis and pericardial tamponade are rare complications that require surgical correction.

Subclinical hypothyroidism develops in one third of patients treated with mantle field irradiation. Patients are asymptomatic, and the physician is alerted by the elevation in the thyroid-stimulating hormone seen on the routine yearly blood measurement. Thyroid hormone replacement is necessary to avoid development of symptomatic hypothyroidism with weight gain, lethargy, temperature intolerance, irritability, and changes in skin and hair.

Xerostomia (mouth dryness) develops during irradiation of the mantle field that treats a portion of the salivary glands. There is minimal risk of clinically significant xerostomia, but partial decrease in saliva produces a favorable environment for dental caries. This complication can be prevented with pretreatment dental evaluation, careful dental care, and the daily use of fluoride.

Serious abdominal complications are extremely rare. An occasional gastric ulcer may occur. Bowel obstruction is related to prior laparotomy. In men, pelvic irradiation with adequate testicular shielding produces only temporary azoospermia. In women, ovariopexy is needed before pelvic irradiation to preserve fertility. The ovaries are meticulously shielded, but even this may not preserve ovarian function, especially in women older than age 30.

The improved survival of patients with Hodgkin's disease has been associated with an increase in the frequency of second malignancies. Leukemias have been associated with the use of alkylating agents, and solid tumors have been associated with radiation therapy. The most common cancers seen are breast cancer that occurs at a younger age, lung cancer in smokers, thyroid cancer, and non-Hodgkin's lymphoma. Workup for early detection of cancer must be included in the yearly follow-up and recommendations to avoid smoking given to all patients.

ACUTE LEUKEMIA IN ADULTS

method of
HARRY P. ERBA, M.D., Ph.D.
University of Michigan
Ann Arbor, Michigan

Acute leukemia is defined as the malignant accumulation of a transformed hematopoietic progenitor cell. The leukemic blast cell retains the capability of self-renewal but, unlike normal hematopoietic stem cells, has limited (if not completely absent) potential for terminal differentiation. Leukemic infiltration of the marrow space ultimately leads to bone marrow failure so that the majority of patients will present with cytopenia. The acute leukemias can be classified based on morphology, histochemical staining, and immunophenotype into two broad categories: acute myelogenous leukemia (AML) and acute lymphoblastic leukemia (ALL). The distinction between the two acute leukemias is clinically important because the etiology, treatment, and prognosis of AML and ALL differ.

CLINICAL PRESENTATION

Patients with acute leukemia most often present with constitutional symptoms and consequences of bone marrow failure. Fatigue and weakness are due to both symptomatic anemia and a hypermetabolic state. However, occasional patients are not anemic at presentation, owing to the explosive onset of acute leukemia and the relatively long survival of red blood cells (RBCs). Thrombocytopenic hemorrhage most often is manifest by petechiae and atraumatic ecchymoses. Neutropenic infections are potentially life-threatening complications of acute leukemia. Typically, patients will present with pneumonia, cellulitis, or sepsis. The most common causative agents are staphylococcal, streptococcal, and enteric gram-negative bacteria and a variety of fungal species. Opportunistic infections with *Pneumocystis carinii, Toxoplasma gondii,* and cytomegalovirus are rare. Finally, bone marrow infiltration may result in severe bone pain.

Although a minority of patients will be leukopenic at presentation and may not have significant numbers of circulating malignant blasts, the majority of patients with acute leukemia present with leukocytosis. Stasis of blood flow may occur in the cerebral and pulmonary vasculature when the blast count is above 50,000 cells/μL. Leukostasis is more common in AML than in ALL, likely due to the larger size of the blasts and the presence of cell surface adhesion proteins. Patients with cerebral leukostasis will complain of headache, confusion, and visual disturbance but may progress quickly to coma or a variety of stroke syndromes. Pulmonary leukostasis can cause dyspnea at rest, tachypnea, inspiratory rales, and pulmonary infiltrates.

Both disseminated intravascular coagulation (DIC) and primary fibrinolysis contribute to the hemorrhagic diathesis of acute leukemia. Induction chemotherapy for any acute leukemia can precipitate DIC. However, patients with acute promyelocytic leukemia (see later) typically present with DIC and/or fibrinolysis that can result in either intracranial or gastrointestinal hemorrhage before any treatment. Although the prothrombin and partial thromboplastin times are elevated and the fibrinogen level is low in DIC, patients with fibrinolysis may only have an elevation of fibrin degradation products such as the D-dimer.

Leukemic blasts can infiltrate any organ. Patients with ALL are more likely to present with adenopathy and splenomegaly, owing to infiltration of these lymphoid organs. AML with monocytic differentiation is most often associated with extramedullary disease. Cutaneous infiltration (leukemia cutis) and gingival hypertrophy are frequently seen in patients with acute monoblastic leukemias. Leukemic involvement of the skin usually appears as violaceous, nontender, subcutaneous nodules or plaques. Leukemia cutis must, however, be distinguished from hematomas, cutaneous infections such as ecthyma gangrenosum, and Sweet's syndrome, a noninfectious acute febrile neutrophilic dermatosis.

Leukemic meningitis is unusual at presentation of either acute leukemia (<5% of adult patients) but is more common during the subsequent course of patients with ALL, especially if prophylactic central nervous system (CNS) therapy is not administered. Rarely, patients may present with extramedullary leukemia without involvement of the peripheral blood or bone marrow. These solid tumors of leukemic myeloblasts (known as *chloromas, granulocytic sarcomas,* or *myeloblastomas*) are often mistaken for non-Hodgkin's lymphoma unless careful pathologic examination is performed. Without systemic therapy, these patients will usually develop medullary disease within weeks to months.

A number of metabolic abnormalities are found in patients with acute leukemia at presentation. Manifestations of tumor lysis may be present before any therapy, especially in ALL. Hyperuricemia and hyperphosphatemia can lead to renal insufficiency due to urate nephropathy and nephrocalcinosis. Although patients with tumor lysis syndrome may develop life-threatening hyperkalemia, many acute leukemia patients are actually hypokalemic at presentation, possibly due to renal tubular injury by lysozyme released from blasts. Elevation of serum hepatic transaminases is common. Finally, artifactual hypoglycemia or hypoxia may result from the metabolic activity of the leukemic blasts, if blood samples are not kept cold after diagnostic phlebotomy.

DIAGNOSIS AND CLASSIFICATION

Accurate diagnosis and classification of acute leukemia is critically important for selection of appropriate therapy. Classically, blasts must account for more than 30% of the nucleated cells in a bone marrow aspirate to make a diagnosis of acute leukemia. More recently, the World Health Organization has suggested that the threshold for diagnosis of AML be lowered to 20% blasts. Unless Auer rods, which are only present in the cytoplasm of myeloblasts, are identified, the morphologic distinction between AML and ALL can at times be difficult. However, cytochemical stains and immunophenotype are now commonly used to distinguish eight morphologic subtypes of AML and three immunologic subtypes of ALL.

AML is classically divided into subtypes by the French-American-British (FAB) classification system based on apparent level of differentiation: undifferentiated (M0), granulocytic (M1–2), progranulocytic (M3), monoblastic (M4–5), erythroblastic (M6), and megakaryoblastic (M7). Myeloperoxidase can be detected in AML blasts using cytochemical stains; the presence of nonspecific esterase helps to define monoblastic differentiation. Flow cytometric analysis of myeloblasts will typically demonstrate cell surface expression of CD13, CD33, and CD117. Other immunophenotypic markers help to define subtypes of AML: CD14 in M4–5, glycophorin A expression in M6, and von Willebrand factor and CD41 (gpIIb/IIIa) in M7. Recognition of acute progranulocytic leukemia (APL or M3 AML) is critical, because therapy differs for this subtype of AML (see later).

ALL is divided into three morphologic classes by the FAB system (L1–L3), but it is most commonly subclassified by immunophenotype. Seventy percent of adult ALL is leukemia of precursor B cells. There is rearrangement of the immunoglobulin heavy-chain genes in precursor B lymphoblasts. These blasts may express CD10, CD19, cytoplasmic CD22, cytoplasmic μ heavy chain, and nuclear terminal deoxynucleotidyl transferase (TdT). Twenty-five percent of adult ALL has a T-cell phenotype, expressing a subset of the following antigens: CD1a, CD3, CD4, CD5, CD7, CD8, and TdT. There is monoclonal T-cell receptor gene rearrangement in the malignant T lymphoblasts. Patients with T-cell ALL often present with a mediastinal mass. Finally, 5% of adult ALL patients have lymphoblasts with a mature B-cell immunophenotype. These blasts are characteristically larger, with deeply basophilic cytoplasm and cytoplasmic vacuolization (L3 blasts). They express surface immunoglobulin but lack expression of TdT.

Nonrandom chromosomal translocations, deletions, and additions are found in the leukemic blasts (but not in germ cells or other somatic cells) in over 50% of adult acute leukemia patients. A few cytogenetic changes are pathognomonic for various subtypes of acute leukemia and are helpful diagnostically. For example, the translocation t(15;17)(q22;q21) is only found in APL and is due to a fusion of the *PML* gene on chromosome 15 with the retinoic acid receptor α *(RARα)* gene on chromosome 17. The translocations t(8;14), t(2;8), and t(8;22) are only found in mature B-cell ALL and Burkitt's lymphoma. These chromosomal rearrangements result in dysregulation and overexpression of the c-*myc* gene on chromosome 8 by juxtaposition to the enhancer elements of the immunoglobulin heavy- or light-chain gene loci. On the other hand, the Philadelphia chromosome, t(9;22)(q34;q11), can be found in less than 5% of adult AML and 25% to 30% of adult ALL blasts. Likewise, translocations involving the *MLL* gene located at chromosome band 11q23 are found in both acute monoblastic leukemia [e.g., t(9;11)(p21;q23)] and precursor B-cell ALL [e.g., t(4;11)(q21;q23)]. Identification of cytogenetic abnormalities in leukemic blasts is important for determination of prognosis and selection of post-remission therapy (see later).

INITIAL MANAGEMENT AND SUPPORTIVE CARE

Curative therapy for acute leukemia depends on effective transfusion support. The threshold for RBC transfusion will depend on the patient's physiologic state; younger patients will generally tolerate a lower hemoglobin level than an elderly patient with cardiopulmonary disease. Recent studies of patients with acute leukemia have established a platelet count of

10,000/μL as a reasonable threshold for prophylactic platelet transfusion, except for patients with fever, chemotherapy-induced mucositis, and DIC, in whom more than 20,000/μL is more appropriate. Patients with acute leukemia should receive leukocyte-depleted RBC and platelet transfusions to prevent transmission of cytomegalovirus, alloimmunization, febrile transfusion reactions, and refractoriness to platelet transfusion therapy. Irradiated blood products are often prescribed to prevent transfusion-associated graft-versus-host disease (GVHD), especially for patients undergoing allogeneic hematopoietic stem cell transplantation (HSCT). GVHD is a rare, but uniformly fatal, complication of transfusion.

Leukostasis is a medical emergency. Patients with leukocytosis and circulating blasts should be referred for emergency evaluation by a hematologist because the rate of increase in white blood cells or the development of leukostasis cannot be accurately predicted. Intravenous hydration and leukapheresis are used for urgent reduction of the peripheral blood blast count. Hydroxyurea (Hydrea), 1 to 2 g/m^2/d orally, may be used for rapid cytoreduction before definitive diagnosis. If the blasts have a lymphoid morphology, then the addition of high doses of corticosteroids may be helpful. Alternatively, if the diagnosis has been confirmed, appropriate induction chemotherapy can be initiated. Arbitrary RBC transfusion should be avoided in patients with extreme leukocytosis, because it may acutely raise whole blood viscosity and precipitate leukostasis.

Management of DIC is controversial. Replacement of plasma coagulation factors and platelets is obviously important: fresh frozen plasma to maintain the prothrombin time less than 15 seconds, cryoprecipitate to maintain the fibrinogen level greater than 100 mg/dL, and platelet concentrate to maintain the platelet count greater than 50,000/μL. The role of heparin and antifibrinolytic agents is less clear. Although low-dose heparin will slow the consumptive process, monitoring therapy is difficult. In a large retrospective analysis of patients with acute promyelocytic leukemia with DIC, heparin or antifibrinolytic agents did not appear to add benefit to factor replacement alone.

Tumor lysis syndrome should be anticipated. Intravenous hydration should be prescribed to ensure a brisk saline diuresis. Allopurinol (Zyloprim), 300 mg/d, will usually prevent the accumulation of uric acid. Urine alkalinization will increase the solubility of uric acid and help prevent urate nephropathy, especially if the serum uric acid concentration is elevated at diagnosis. Uric acid oxidase, which catalyzes the conversion of uric acid to the more soluble allantoin, may soon be commercially available. Despite these maneuvers, acute renal failure may result during induction chemotherapy for acute leukemia, and hemodialysis is rarely necessary.

Placement of a tunneled central venous catheter (e.g., Hickman catheter) is advisable before beginning induction chemotherapy. Assessment of cardiac function (e.g., radionuclide ventriculogram) is also typically performed in anticipation of administration of an anthracycline chemotherapy agent, especially in older patients and those with pre-existing cardiac disease. Patients who may be eligible for subsequent allogeneic HSCT should have tissue typing performed on a sample of peripheral blood.

TREATMENT OF ACUTE MYELOGENOUS LEUKEMIA

Induction Chemotherapy

Curative therapy of AML can be divided into two phases: induction chemotherapy and post-remission therapy. The goal of induction chemotherapy is to obtain a complete remission (CR). *CR* is specifically defined: less than 5% blasts in a bone marrow sample, no peripheral blood blasts, transfusion independence, normal hematopoiesis (absolute neutrophil count >1500/μl, platelet count >100,000/μL, and hemoglobin >9 g/dL), and resolution of all extramedullary leukemic infiltrates.

The anthracycline daunorubicin (Daunomycin), 45 to 60 mg/m^2 by intravenous push each day for 3 days, plus cytarabine (Cytosar, Ara-C), 100 to 200 mg/m^2 by continuous intravenous infusion each day for 7 days (3 + 7 regimen), has remained the standard induction chemotherapy regimen since its introduction nearly 30 years ago. Fourteen days after induction chemotherapy, bone marrow biopsy and aspirate are repeated. If marrow aplasia has been attained and there is no morphologic evidence of residual leukemia, the patient is supported until marrow recovery occurs. If the marrow is not aplastic but there is evidence of significant cytoreduction, an abbreviated schedule of induction chemotherapy is administered (2 + 5 regimen). If there is no evidence of cytoreduction, the patient is typically treated with a high-dose cytarabine-based regimen or enrolled in a clinical trial. If patients do not attain CR with induction chemotherapy, their prognosis is grim. Allogeneic HSCT can salvage 10% to 20% of patients with primary refractory AML and result in long-term disease-free survival (DFS).

Patients require intensive supportive care during induction chemotherapy. Chemotherapy-induced emesis can usually be prevented with a serotonin antagonist, such as granisetron (Kytril), 2 mg orally each day. Patients often complain of painful ulceration of the oral mucosa, dysphagia, dyspepsia, and diarrhea due to mucositis. Narcotic analgesics and topical anesthetics are usually prescribed. Topical (nystatin) or systemic (fluconazole) antifungal agents will help prevent oropharyngeal candidiasis.

Patients who demonstrate evidence of previous exposure to herpes simplex virus (HSV IgG positive) should receive prophylactic acyclovir (Zovirax). Induction chemotherapy causes predictable grade 4 myelosuppression lasting 21 to 28 days. Most patients develop febrile neutropenia. In the absence of a positive microbiologic culture, empirical antibiotics are needed to treat infection by enteric gram-negative bacteria (especially *Pseudomonas* species), cutaneous gram-positive cocci (*Staphylococcus, Streptococcus* species), and fungi (*Candida, Aspergillus*). Neutropenic enterocolitis (typhlitis) is an especially severe complication of induction chemotherapy. Patients experience abdominal tenderness (usually in the right lower quadrant) often with signs of peritoneal irritation. Computed tomography of the abdomen will demonstrate thickening of the colonic wall (most notably in the cecum) and infiltration of the mesenteric fat. Treatment is primarily supportive, with bowel rest, parenteral nutrition, narcotic analgesia, and antibiotic suppression of colonic flora (both enteric gram-negative bacilli and anaerobes such as *Clostridium* species). Surgical intervention is reserved for patients who develop colonic perforation, obstruction, or hypotension. Unfortunately, 10% to 25% of patients will succumb to the toxicities of induction chemotherapy.

Induction chemotherapy with daunorubicin and cytarabine will result in CR in 50% to 75% of adult AML patients. Several different approaches have been investigated in an effort to increase the response rate. Other anthracycline drugs have been substituted for daunorubicin. Doxorubicin (Adriamycin) caused more typhlitis than daunorubicin. On the other hand, idarubicin (Idamycin), 12 to 13 mg/m^2/d by intravenous injection for 3 days in combination with cytarabine resulted in higher CR rates (70%–80%) when compared with daunorubicin. However, the idarubicin/cytarabine combination caused more prolonged myelosuppression, suggesting that the two anthracyclines were not compared at biologically equivalent doses. A recent randomized trial in AML patients older than 55 years failed to demonstrate any benefit of either idarubicin or mitoxantrone over daunorubicin in terms of CR rate and DFS.

High doses of cytarabine can overcome chemotherapy resistance of AML blasts. Therefore, the role of high-dose cytarabine (HiDAC) has been investigated in AML induction therapy. The Australian Leukemia Study Group compared standard-dose (100 mg/m^2/d for 7 days) with high-dose (3 g/m^2 for 8 doses) cytarabine in combination with daunorubicin plus etoposide (VePesid)* for AML induction therapy. Although the CR rates were not significantly different in the two arms of this study, the relapse-free survival was improved with HiDAC. Unfortunately, the toxicity was also greater with HiDAC during induction therapy. When cytarabine, 2 g/m^2 every 12 hours, was added on days 8 through 10 to a 3 + 7 regimen, the CR rate was 90% in one study. However, in two large multicenter trials using this induction regimen, the CR rate was much lower and the toxicity was considerable, including an increased incidence of typhlitis.

Adult patients with AML fail to enter CR for two reasons: (1) resistance of the leukemic blasts to induction chemotherapy, and (2) mortality during chemotherapy-induced marrow aplasia due to neutropenic infections and, less commonly, thrombocytopenic hemorrhage. Therefore, decreasing the length of chemotherapy-induced myelosuppression by administration of hematopoietic growth factors seemed to be a rational approach to increase the CR rate in AML. Several randomized trials evaluated the addition of the myeloid colony-stimulating factors (CSF)—granulocyte CSF (G-CSF) and granulocyte-macrophage CSF (GM-CSF)—versus placebo after completion of induction chemotherapy in patients with newly diagnosed AML. Both G-CSF and GM-CSF shortened the length of chemotherapy-induced neutropenia by several days. Randomized trials have also demonstrated a significant clinical benefit from G-CSF (Neupogen), in terms of length of hospitalization, parenteral antibiotic use, duration of fever, and requirement for antifungal therapy. Yeast-derived GM-CSF (Leukine) treatment was associated with an improvement in overall survival. Unfortunately, addition of myeloid CSF to standard induction chemotherapy did not improve the CR rate in any of these studies. Recombinant human megakaryocyte growth and development factor (rHu-MGDF) not only failed to increase the CR rate in adult AML patients undergoing induction chemotherapy but also did not shorten the length of thrombocytopenia or decrease the platelet transfusion requirement.

*Not FDA approved for this indication.

Post-Remission Therapy

Induction chemotherapy only results in a 1000-fold reduction in the number of leukemic blasts. Because there are approximately 10^{12} blasts present at the time of diagnosis, a significant leukemic burden remains after successful remission induction, and post-remission therapy is necessary. Prolonged maintenance chemotherapy with subcutaneous cytarabine in combination with antimetabolite drugs such as mercaptopurine, thioguanine, and methotrexate can prolong the duration of remission. This therapy is well tolerated and not significantly myelosuppressive. However, chemotherapy of similar intensity to induction therapy (consolidation chemotherapy) has been shown to be more effective than maintenance treatment. Typically, patients receive several (2–4) monthly cycles of an anthracycline* for 2 days and standard dose cytarabine by continuous intravenous infusion for 5 days. A minority of patients achieves long-term DFS (10% of patients in first CR) with standard consolidation chemotherapy.

Intensification of post-remission therapy cures more patients with AML in first remission than standard consolidation or maintenance chemotherapy. There are three choices for intensive post-remission therapy in AML patients: high-dose cytarabine (HiDAC)–based regimens, allogeneic HSCT, and autologous HSCT. Forty-five percent of AML patients younger than 60 years in first remission are alive and disease-free 4 years after up to four monthly cycles of cytarabine, 3 g/m^2 every 12 hours for 6 doses on days 1, 3, and 5. In an Eastern Cooperative

*Not FDA approved for this indication.

Oncology Group study a single course of cytarabine, 3 g/m^2 every 12 hours for 12 doses, with amsacrine (Amsidyl),* also resulted in improved DFS when compared with standard consolidation chemotherapy. The major reason for treatment failure is relapse. Unfortunately, one third of patients older than 60 years experienced severe cerebellar toxicity from HiDAC in a large cooperative group trial. HiDAC did not improve DFS in elderly patients with AML in first remission.

Single institution phase II trials of allogeneic HSCT for adult patients with AML in first remission consistently reported DFS rates of 60%. Only one third of patients will have an HLA-matched family member donor available. The predominant reason for treatment failure is treatment-related mortality. Graft-versus-host disease, hepatic veno-occlusive disease, and opportunistic infections account for the majority of treatment-related mortality. Likewise, single institution studies of autologous HSCT have demonstrated high rates of prolonged DFS (60%–70%). Hematopoietic stem cell harvest (either by multiple bone marrow aspirations or leukapheresis) is performed once the patient is in remission. Unfortunately, some patients have inadequate hematopoietic stem cell collections and cannot proceed to autologous HSCT. The benefit of in vitro purging of leukemic blasts from the hematopoietic stem cell harvest using cytotoxic drugs (e.g., 4-hydroxyperoxycyclophosphamide†) has not been proven. Most reports of HSCT suffer from an inherent reporting bias: only patients who survive in first remission and maintain a good performance status will actually undergo HSCT. Because it may take as long as 3 months to arrange either allogeneic or autologous HSCT, patients with more resistant AML may relapse before HSCT and not be reported.

Three randomized trials have compared these three forms of intensification therapy in adult AML patients in first CR. The conclusions of these studies are remarkably similar. In the United States Intergroup trial, adult AML patients up to age 55 received induction chemotherapy with idarubicin and cytarabine, and 70% of patients entered CR. After a single cycle of standard consolidation therapy, patients with a human leukocyte antigen (HLA)–matched family member donor were allocated to receive an allogeneic HSCT. Otherwise, patients were randomized to receive either a single cycle of HiDAC (12 doses) or purged autologous HSCT. A median of 14 weeks elapsed between attaining CR and either autologous or allogeneic HSCT. Only 54% of patients actually received the autologous HSCT due to either refusal or inadequate stem cell harvest.

The DFS at 4 years was higher (not significant) in the allogeneic HSCT group compared with either autologous HSCT or HiDAC (43% versus 35% versus 35%, respectively). However, there was no significant difference in overall survival at 4 years (46% versus 43% versus 52%, respectively). There are two major reasons for this observation. Although the relapse rate was higher after HiDAC compared with allogeneic HSCT (61% versus 25%), the treatment-related mortality was higher with allogeneic HSCT (25% versus 3%). Patients who relapse after HiDAC intensification can be salvaged with HSCT. Studies in both France and the United Kingdom have also failed to demonstrate a survival advantage with allogeneic HSCT compared with HiDAC intensification.

*Not FDA approved for this indication.
†Not yet approved for use in the United States.

PROGNOSTIC FACTORS IN ADULT AML

The probability of achieving CR and long-term DFS is influenced by a number of factors. Advanced age is an important negative prognostic factor. The incidence of AML increases with age; the median age at diagnosis is 65 years. Only 45% to 50% of AML patients older than 60 years achieve CR, and overall survival from diagnosis in this population is only 5% to 10%. Conversely, the CR rate is 75%, and overall survival at 4 years is 35% to 40% in patients younger than 40 years. The outcome for elderly patients is so poor that the value of intensive induction and consolidation chemotherapy in these patients has been questioned. However, a European randomized control trial completed in 1987 demonstrated improved survival with 3+7 induction and consolidation chemotherapy compared with palliative therapy with hydroxyurea and low doses of cytarabine. Only patients who received intensive chemotherapy were alive more than 2 years after diagnosis.

There are several explanations of the worse outcome for elderly AML patients. Elderly patients cannot tolerate the treatment-related toxicity of HiDAC and HSCT and therefore are not typically offered these potentially curative approaches. Co-morbid illnesses complicate the management of AML in the elderly. For example, patients with cardiomyopathy cannot be safely treated with anthracycline-based chemotherapy. Elderly patients are more likely to have a poor performance status or nutritional state (low albumin), two factors that are associated with a worse prognosis in many cancers, including AML. Because there is less bone marrow reserve with advancing age, the period of marrow aplasia is longer and complications of myelosuppression are more likely to occur. Elderly patients do not tolerate neutropenic infections as well as younger patients. But the biology of AML is also distinctive in elderly patients (see later).

The prognosis of adult AML patients varies with specific cytogenetic changes found in the leukemic blasts at diagnosis. Two important translocations, each found in 5% to 10% of adult AML patients, affect the genes encoding subunits of the heterodimeric transcription factor, core binding factor (CBF). CBF regulates expression of many genes involved in hematopoietic stem cell differentiation. The translocation, t(8;21)(q22;q22), results from fusion of the *AML1* gene on chromosome 21 (encoding a CBFα subunit) with the *ETO* gene on chromosome 8.

The pericentric inversion of chromosome 16, inv(16)(p13;q22), results from fusion of the genes for *CBF*β and the smooth muscle myosin heavy chain *(MYH11)*. Although loss of CBF function during embryogenesis is known to cause embryonic death due to failure of normal hematopoiesis, the mechanism by which these alterations of the CBF subunits contribute to the malignant transformation of hematopoietic stem cells remains unclear.

The t(8;21) and inv(16) are usually found in FAB types M2 and M4eo AML, respectively. Leukemic blasts with t(8;21) often demonstrate aberrant expression of the B cell marker CD19, and the karyotype may also show loss of the sex chromosome. The incidence of extramedullary leukemia including leukemic meningitis is higher in patients with the t(8;21) translocation and inv(16). These two translocations have been associated with an excellent prognosis. AML patients with t(8;21) and inv(16) (now referred to as CBF AML) have a 90% probability of entering CR with a single cycle of induction chemotherapy. Furthermore, 70% to 80% of patients with CBF AML are alive and disease-free at 5 years after HiDAC consolidation therapy. Unfortunately, elderly patients are much less likely to have these relatively good-risk cytogenetic changes.

Many other chromosomal translocations and deletions, however, result in a worse outcome for adult AML patients. Deletion of the long arm of either chromosome 5 or 7, monosomy 5 or 7, the Philadelphia chromosome t(9;22), most deletions or translocations involving chromosome band 11q23, inv(3)(q21;q26), as well as karyotypes with multiple chromosomal abnormalities, have all been individually associated with lower CR rates and decreased probability of DFS. For example, AML patients in first remission with poor-risk cytogenetic changes have only a 20% chance of DFS at 5 years with HiDAC intensification. These same cytogenetic changes are also known to be predictive of outcome after allogeneic HSCT performed during first remission. In a retrospective review of data from the International Bone Marrow Transplant Registry, the DFS of AML patients with poor-risk cytogenetic changes was only 24%. Nevertheless, the North American Intergroup trial demonstrated an improved DFS for AML patients with poor-risk cytogenetics in first CR who received an allogeneic HSCT compared with HiDAC intensification or autologous HSCT.

Patients with a preceding history of a bone marrow disorder also fair poorly. Elderly AML patients are more likely to have an antecedent myelodysplastic syndrome (MDS). The risk of progression from MDS to AML is related to older age, number of cytopenias, the presence of specific cytogenetic abnormalities, such as monosomy 7, del(7)(q), complex karyotypic changes, and percentage of bone marrow myeloblasts. Patients with myeloproliferative disorders may also develop AML. The risk is highest in patients with chronic myelogenous leukemia (CML), but patients with polycythemia vera, myeloid metaplasia, and essential thrombocythemia have a less than 10% risk of AML. AML will develop in 5% to 10% of patients with aplastic anemia in remission after immunosuppressive therapy. These secondary leukemias tend to be more resistant to cytotoxic chemotherapy.

AML can be a devastating complication of curative chemotherapy for another malignancy. Two classes of cytotoxic agents have been associated with secondary AML. The alkylating agents, such as cyclophosphamide (Cytoxan), chlorambucil (Leukeran), melphalan (Alkeran), nitrogen mustard, and busulfan (Myleran), can cause MDS or AML usually 3 to 5 years after treatment. The first observation of this complication was in Hodgkin's disease patients in prolonged remission after MOPP chemotherapy. Deletions of chromosomes 5/5q or 7/7q and multiple cytogenetic changes characterize alkylating agent–induced AML. Topoisomerase II inhibitors such as the epipodophyllotoxins (etoposide [VePesid], teniposide [Vumon]) and doxorubicin (Adriamycin) can lead to acute monoblastic leukemia without a preceding MDS. The latency is typically shorter than alkylating agent–induced AML. Translocations or deletions involving the *MLL* gene at chromosome band 11q23 are common in epipodophyllotoxin-associated AML. Treatment-related AML is highly resistant to chemotherapy; the prognosis, even with allogeneic HSCT, remains poor.

AML blasts often demonstrate multidrug resistance (MDR) at presentation. The *MDR1* gene encodes the 170-kd transmembrane protein P-glycoprotein (P-gp). P-gp is an adenosine triphosphate–dependent drug efflux pump that is normally expressed in hematopoietic stem cells, in the hepatocyte membrane of the bile canaliculus, in the capillary endothelial cells of the brain, and in renal tubular cells. P-gp expression is more common in the AML blasts of elderly patients, in whom it has been associated with a lower CR rate. Theoretically, inhibition of P-gp may increase intracellular concentrations of anthracyclines and result in higher CR rates. Unfortunately, in randomized clinical trials the addition of the P-gp inhibitors cyclosporine and valspodar (PSC-833) to induction chemotherapy has not improved the CR rate of adult AML patients. Because P-gp inhibitors affect the pharmacokinetics of anthracyclines and etoposide, the doses of these drugs needed to be reduced to decrease nonhematologic toxicity.

There are other factors that are predictive of AML relapse: failure to attain CR with a single cycle of induction chemotherapy, hyperleukocytosis at presentation (WBC >100,000/μL), and expression of the hematopoietic stem cell marker CD34. All of these prognostic factors are used to select post-remission therapy for young patients with non-M3 AML in first CR. Patients with CBF AML are typically treated with HiDAC intensification. Patients with "poor risk" features such as high-risk cytogenetic changes, history of MDS, history of previous chemotherapy, and failure to achieve CR with a ingle cycle of induction therapy are referred for allogeneic HSCT. Patients in first CR without good-risk or poor-risk features are offered either HiDAC or allogeneic HSCT. Because elderly patients cannot tolerate treatment intensification, prognostic factors typically do not influence the choice of standard post-remission consolidation therapy.

TREATMENT OF ACUTE PROMYELOCYTIC LEUKEMIA

The therapeutic approach to adults with acute promyelocytic leukemia (APL, M3 AML) is very different from that for other AML patients. Therefore, APL must be recognized at presentation. APL accounts for 5% to 15% of adult AML. The blasts are characterized by abundant primary cytoplasmic granules, at times obscuring the nucleus, and frequent Auer rods. The nucleus is often bilobed or displays "sliding plate" morphology. The cytoplasm demonstrates intense cytochemical staining for myeloperoxidase. The nuclear features and myeloperoxidase content are diagnostically helpful for recognition of the microgranular variant of APL. Patients with APL have a younger median age (30–40 years), often present with leukopenia, and have evidence of DIC and/or fibrinolysis at diagnosis. The diagnosis of APL depends on either cytogenetic or molecular genetic detection of the PML/RARα fusion. Less than 1% of APL patients will have variant translocations that involve the *RAR*α gene, such as t(11;17) due to fusion of the *PLZF* gene with the *RAR*α gene.

All-*trans*-retinoic acid (ATRA, tretinoin, Vesanoid) is a vitamin A analogue that will induce complete remissions in the majority (>85%) of newly diagnosed APL patients. The usual dose of ATRA is 45 mg/m^2/d in two divided oral doses with meals. ATRA does not cause blast lysis or marrow aplasia but instead induces the differentiation of the APL blasts. Resolution of DIC occurs rapidly. Mucocutaneous dryness, headache, pseudotumor cerebri, hypertriglyceridemia, and abnormal liver function tests are common adverse effects from high-dose vitamin A therapy. However, patients with active APL treated with ATRA can also develop a capillary leak syndrome characterized by weight gain, edema, fever, hypoxia, pulmonary infiltrates, and pleuropericarditis. The retinoic acid or APL differentiation syndrome occurs within a few days to 3 weeks of ATRA initiation and is often associated with a rapidly rising peripheral blood WBC count. Unless recognized early and treated with corticosteroids (dexamethasone [Decadron], 10 mg intravenously twice daily), the APL differentiation syndrome can be rapidly fatal. It is not clear that ATRA has to be discontinued in this situation, as long as corticosteroids are administered. Co-administration of ATRA with induction chemotherapy will decrease the incidence of the APL differentiation syndrome from 25% to less than 5%.

Without either concomitant induction chemotherapy or subsequent consolidation chemotherapy, ATRA-induced remissions are not durable. Although some ATRA-resistant APL blasts will have acquired mutations of the retinoic acid–binding site of the *PML/RAR*α fusion protein, the APL blasts of most ATRA-resistant patients will retain sensitivity in vitro to retinoic acids. A likely explanation for this observation is that ATRA induces the hepatic P450 cytochrome system and its own catabolism. The French APL 91 trial compared ATRA with standard 3 + 7 induction therapy followed by daunorubicin plus cytarabine consolidation. The trial was stopped early owing to a significant advantage of ATRA in terms of event-free survival (62% versus 15% estimated at 4 years) and overall survival (76% versus 49% estimated at 4 years). In the North American Intergroup trial, APL patients who were treated with ATRA induction alone, two cycles of daunorubicin plus cytarabine consolidation, and 1 year of daily ATRA maintenance therapy had a 74% DFS. The simultaneous administration of ATRA with daunorubicin,* 60 mg/m^2 by intravenous injection each day for 3 days, and cytarabine, 200 mg/m^2 by continuous intravenous infusion each day for 7 days, results in an identical CR rate but lower relapse rate compared with sequential ATRA followed by chemotherapy.

A new agent has been added to our armamentarium against APL. In October 2000, the U.S. Food and Drug Administration (FDA) approved arsenic trioxide (ATO) for the treatment of APL in relapse. ATO induces apoptosis in APL cells. The reason for the sensitivity of APL blasts to ATO is unclear. Patients are usually treated with ATO, 0.15 mg/kg by intravenous infusion over 2 hours daily, until remission. The CR rate is 85%, with the majority of patients attaining molecular remission (i.e., no evidence of the *PML/RAR*α fusion by reverse transcriptase-polymerase chain reaction [RT-PCR] amplification) after ATO consolidation therapy. The toxicities of ATO include nausea, emesis, diarrhea, rash, cardiac toxicity (prolongation of the QT interval, atrioventricular block, torsades de pointes), neurotoxicity, and serum hepatic enzyme elevations. ATO has also been associated with hyperleukocytosis and the APL differentiation syndrome. The treatment of choice for APL patients who experience relapse after ATRA/anthracycline-based therapy is ATO followed by either allogeneic HSCT or autologous HSCT (especially if the patient has attained a molecular remission).

TREATMENT OF ACUTE MYELOGENOUS LEUKEMIA IN RELAPSE

Relapse after CR continues to be a major problem in the care of adult AML patients. High-dose chemotherapy followed by HSCT is considered the only treatment that is likely to result in long-term DFS (i.e., cure). Whether a patient must first attain a second remission or can proceed directly to HSCT is debatable. However, unless a family member HLA-matched donor has already been identified or an autologous hematopoietic stem cell collection has been

*Not FDA approved for this indication.

stored, most patients will require salvage chemotherapy before HSCT. Because elderly patients are currently not eligible for high-dose chemotherapy and HSCT, the treatment of relapsed AML in this population is palliative.

The single most important factor predictive of attaining a second CR is the length of the first remission: The longer the first CR, the greater the chance of attaining a second remission. If the first remission has been more than 2 years, then it is reasonable to prescribe standard induction chemotherapy (3 + 7). Various combinations of mitoxantrone and etoposide have been used in patients with relapsed AML. However, patients with shorter first remissions are usually treated with salvage chemotherapy containing intermediate- to high-dose cytarabine. The Southwest Oncology Group treated adult AML patients in first relapse with cytarabine, 3 g/m^2 (2 g/m^2 for patients older than 50 years) every 12 hours for 6 days, with or without mitoxantrone (Novantrone), 10 mg/m^2 intravenously each day for the next 3 days. The second CR rate was 44% or 32%, respectively. A 6-day regimen of daily intravenous etoposide, 80 mg/m^2, cytarabine, 1000 mg/m^2, and mitoxantrone, 6 mg/m^2, (MEC) is also effective salvage therapy. Unfortunately, these regimens are fairly intensive, causing prolonged myelosuppression and significant mucositis.

In May 2000, a novel immunoconjugate was approved by the FDA for treatment of relapsed AML in patients older than 60 years. Gemtuzumab ozogamicin (Mylotarg) is a humanized murine anti-CD33 monoclonal antibody that is covalently coupled to the potent antitumor antibiotic calicheamicin. The CD33 glycoprotein is expressed on the leukemic blasts of 80% to 90% of AML patients but not on nonhematopoietic tissues or hematopoietic stem cells. Interaction of CD33 with the monoclonal antibody results in internalization of the complex. Calicheamicin is released from the monoclonal antibody by acid hydrolysis of the linker in the lysosome. After activation, calicheamicin binds in the minor groove of DNA and causes double-strand DNA breaks and cell death.

The efficacy and safety of gemtuzumab ozogamicin in adult patients with CD33-positive AML in first relapse were tested in three concurrent phase II trials. Gemtuzumab ozogamicin, 9 mg/m^2, was administered intravenously over 2 hours; a second dose was given 14 to 28 days later. Thirty percent of patients attained a remission. Despite pretreatment with acetaminophen and diphenhydramine, the majority of patients experienced fever and chills within 6 hours that resolved within 24 hours of the infusion. Greater than 95% of patients developed severe neutropenia and thrombocytopenia, likely due to expression of CD33 on committed hematopoietic progenitor cells. The median time to recovery of the neutrophil and platelet counts in responding patients was 40 days. One fourth of treated patients had transient elevations of the serum hepatic transaminases and/or bilirubin. Hepatic veno-occlusive disease has also been observed in patients treated with gemtuzumab ozogamicin. However, severe mucositis, alopecia, cardiotoxicity, and renal failure were not seen after therapy with gemtuzumab ozogamicin. Many patients received this therapy as outpatients, and 4% never required hospitalization. Therefore, the toxicity profile of gemtuzumab ozogamicin suggests it will be useful in the treatment of elderly patients and possibly patients eligible for HSCT to reduce pretransplantation morbidity.

TREATMENT OF ACUTE LYMPHOBLASTIC LEUKEMIA IN ADULTS

The remarkable successes that have been realized in the treatment of ALL in children over the past 40 years have only partially been achieved in adults. Many drugs are active in ALL, including the antimetabolites (thioguanine,* mercaptopurine, and methotrexate), anthracyclines (daunorubicin, doxorubicin), glucocorticosteroids, vincristine, cytarabine, cyclophosphamide, L-asparaginase, and the epipodophyllotoxins (etoposide,* teniposide). Standard therapy consists of a 2-year program of induction chemotherapy with four or five drugs, early and late intensification therapy, CNS prophylaxis with intrathecal methotrexate ± cranial irradiation, and prolonged maintenance chemotherapy. The minor differences between the numerous ALL treatment protocols are not as important as the comfort with which an oncologist prescribes a particular one. The CR rate with anthracycline, glucocorticosteroids, and vincristine (Oncovin)–based induction chemotherapy is 80% to 90% in most recent studies. Unfortunately, the relapse rate remains high in adult patients.

As in AML, certain factors have been associated with increased risk of relapse in adults with ALL. The most important of these prognostic factors are age, cytogenetics, and immunophenotype. In contrast to the excellent prognosis of children ages 2 to 9 years, adults older than 60 years have less than a 10% chance of DFS after CR. The presence of the Philadelphia chromosome and translocations involving chromosome band 11q23 are associated with a very high risk of relapse with standard chemotherapy. The translocation t(12;21)(p12;q22) that is due to fusion of the *TEL* and *AML1* genes is found in 25% of childhood ALL cases and is associated with an excellent prognosis. Unfortunately, this genetic event is not typically found in adults with ALL. Adult patients with T-cell ALL fair better than those with the precursor B-cell type. Although co-expression of one or two myeloid antigens can be frequently detected in ALL blasts, recent studies have failed to demonstrate any effect on prognosis. Mature B-cell (FAB L3) ALL has previously been associated with a poor prognosis. However, intensive chemotherapy regimens that include fractionated cyclophosphamide, intermediate- to high-dose methotrexate, and

*Not FDA approved for this indication.

CNS prophylaxis have resulted in improved survival rates (70%–80%). A number of other negative prognostic factors have been identified, including hyperleukocytosis at presentation, failure to achieve CR within 4 weeks of beginning induction therapy, and high LDH levels.

A randomized trial conducted in France beginning in 1987 investigated the role of allogeneic and autologous HSCT as post-remission therapy for adult patients with ALL in first CR. Patients received a four-drug induction followed by consolidation chemotherapy. Patients (15–40 years old) in first CR with an HLA-matched family member donor were assigned to allogeneic HSCT. All others were randomized to standard therapy versus autologous HSCT. The autologous hematopoietic stem cell harvest was purged of residual leukemic cells in vitro with a cocktail of anti–B-cell or anti–T-cell antibodies. There was no difference in outcome for patients treated with either standard therapy or autologous HSCT, regardless of prognostic factors for relapse. There was also no significant difference in DFS for patients at standard risk of relapse treated with allogeneic HSCT compared with those receiving standard therapy or autologous HSCT (43% versus 31% at 10 years). However, for patients at high risk of relapse (e.g., presence of the Philadelphia chromosome, WBC count >30,000/μL, >4 weeks to attain CR), the overall survival was significantly better after allogeneic HSCT (44% verus 11% at 10 years). Therefore, family member donor allogeneic HSCT is considered the treatment of choice for adult ALL patients who are at increased risk of relapse.

FUTURE DIRECTIONS IN THE TREATMENT OF ADULTS WITH ACUTE LEUKEMIA

We need to remember that the majority of AML patients are elderly. They have a high mortality rate during induction chemotherapy and are not eligible for currently available intensive post-remission therapies. Decreasing the toxicities of these therapies is clearly important. Standard chemotherapy is being studied in combination with a chemoprotectant agent, amifostine (Ethyol). Gemtuzumab ozogamicin will be studied either alone or with cytarabine as initial induction therapy for elderly patients. Because calicheamicin is a substrate for *MDR1,* P-gp inhibitors will likely be used in combination with gemtuzumab ozogamicin. Because the pharmacokinetics of this immunoconjugate should not be affected by inhibition of P-gp, the toxicity should not increase. Finally, nonmyeloablative conditioning regimens for allogeneic HSCT are being studied in elderly patients with acute leukemia. These regimens allow engraftment of donor stem cells but cause less systemic toxicity such as mucositis. Whether nonmyeloablative allogeneic HSCT will improve the overall survival and decrease the relapse rate of elderly patients with AML remains to be proven.

In the past 3 decades, we have seen remarkable advances in our knowledge of the molecular pathogenesis of leukemia. However, improvement in the clinical outcome of adult patients with acute leukemia has been more modest. Nonetheless, at the close of the 20th century we have witnessed the successful clinical application of our understanding of the pathogenesis of two types of leukemia, APL and CML. Pharmacologic targeting of the novel fusion proteins in these two diseases (ATRA in APL and the abl tyrosine kinase inhibitor STI571 [Gleevec] in CML) has resulted in clinical responses without the usual toxicities of cytotoxic chemotherapy. ATRA must be used in combination with chemotherapy in APL patients to prevent retinoic acid resistance. Although responses have been seen in patients with Philadelphia chromosome–positive acute leukemia, the responses have been brief. Therefore, it is likely that STI571 will also be combined with other agents to improve the duration of response in *bcr/abl*-positive acute leukemias. Major advances in the treatment of acute leukemias will only be realized as our understanding of the genetic events underlying these illnesses improves. Because the majority of adults with acute leukemia continue to have a poor prognosis and because samples of human acute leukemia cells will be needed for laboratory-based investigation, these patients should be treated on investigational protocols whenever possible.

ACUTE LEUKEMIA IN CHILDHOOD

method of
GARY V. DAHL, M.D.
Stanford University Medical School
Stanford, California

There are two primary types of acute leukemia: acute lymphocytic leukemia (ALL) and acute nonlymphocytic leukemia (ANLL). In children younger than 15 years of age, approximately 2500 cases of acute leukemia are diagnosed in the United States each year. Leukemia cells are classified according to a morphologic scheme called the *FAB* (French American British) classification. Using morphologic, cytochemical, immunologic, cytogenetic, and molecular genetic criteria, approximately 80% of cases are ALL and 20% are ANLL.

Currently, laboratory investigators are identifying biologic differences in leukemic cells not previously appreciated with microscopy. New genetic and molecular information is helping investigators explain the differences in cure rates and form the basis for new therapy development. Eventually, treatment will be not only designed for different subtypes of leukemia but also directed toward specific abnormalities of the leukemic cells in individual patients.

The treatment and cure rate for ALL in childhood has improved greatly over the past 30 years. Presently, nearly 80% of children are cured. For ANLL, therapy leads to cure approximately 50% of the time. This remarkable result has been accompanied by advances in the classification of acute leukemia, improvements in the use of chemotherapeutic agents, new and improved antibiotics for infectious complications, and safer supportive care with blood products.

For ALL, risk-specific schemata have been developed based on the patient's clinical and biological characteristics. Criteria at diagnosis such as age, leukocyte count, central nervous system (CNS) involvement, leukemia cell immunophenotype, ploidy group, karyotype, and specific genetic abnormalities identified by molecular techniques, are used to select appropriate therapy. For ANLL, similar characteristics are important.

The Pediatric Oncology Group (POG) has elected to use clinical and biologic characteristics to guide the selection of therapy for ALL. Separate treatment protocols are used for patients with B-precursor disease (~85% of ALL), T-cell disease (~12% of ALL), B-cell ALL (1%–2% of ALL), infant ALL (~3% of ALL), and ANLL. This approach is based on the differences in drug sensitivities, relapse risk, and proliferation rate of the leukemic cells in these different phenotypes.

PRESENTATION OF LEUKEMIA

Acute leukemia commonly presents with signs and symptoms caused by replacement of normal bone marrow with up to 10^{12} leukemic cells. Clinically, pallor, petechiae (or signs of bleeding), and fever, along with hepatosplenomegaly and adenopathy are the most frequent findings on physical examination. Laboratory findings usually include anemia, thrombocytopenia, and an elevated white blood cell count with neutropenia. Additionally, elevated uric acid and lactate dehydrogenase levels are frequently noted. At diagnosis, it is most common to find quantitative abnormalities in at least two of the three bone marrow–derived cell types (anemia, leukocytosis, and thrombocytopenia), with blast cells identified in the peripheral blood smear. Suspicion of a diagnosis of leukemia warrants a prompt referral to a center with experience in pediatric oncology because the evaluation of a new patient includes quantitative and qualitative tests for biologic features that are of prognostic importance.

DIAGNOSTIC WORKUP

The diagnostic workup (Table 1) starts with a review of the medical history and a thorough examination. The blood smear is promptly reviewed for the identification of circulating blasts. Chest radiographs (posteroanterior and lateral views) are obtained as part of the initial evaluation to look for a mediastinal mass and possible airway compromise. An abdominal flat plate or ultrasound is optional; however, nephromegaly at diagnosis is usually due to leukemic infiltration and an increased risk of renal failure with tumor lysis when therapy is begun.

A bone marrow aspirate specimen and frequently a bone marrow biopsy specimen are obtained to determine cell morphology, cytochemical staining characteristics, immunophenotype, cytogenetics, and DNA ploidy. From the initial bone marrow specimen, the leukemia cell karyotype is of utmost importance for diagnosis and follow-up of acute leukemia.

At least 80% to 90% of acute leukemia cases in childhood are found to exhibit clonal chromosome abnormalities. Lumbar puncture must be performed before starting treatment. The presence of leukemia cells in the spinal fluid is a negative prognostic factor. Because these abnormalities dictate treatment, immediate referral of the child to a specialized center where critical information can be obtained is crucial.

A diagnosis can usually be made within 24 hours. During the period of evaluation, before the diagnosis is certain, it is important to address psychosocial issues and offer the family support from the medical, nursing, and social work staff. The family should be reassured that acute leukemia is most frequently curable and that almost all patients go into remission.

TABLE 1. **Diagnostic Workup**

Medical history and physical examination
Blood smear review
Hemoglobin, WBC and differential count, platelets
Electrolytes, uric acid, phosphorus, calcium, creatinine, ALT, total bilirubin, alkaline phosphatase, LDH, glucose, amylase
Urinalysis
PT, PTT, fibrinogen
Immunoglobulins, Varicella titer
Chest radiograph (PA and lateral) and KUB or renal ultrasound if specifically indicated
Bone marrow aspirate; cell morphology with cytochemical stains, immunophenotype, DNA ploidy, cytogenetics, and storage for future studies

Abbreviations: ALT = alanine aminotransferase; KUB = kidneys, ureter, and bladder; LDH = lactate dehydrogenase; PA = posteroanterior; PT = prothrombin time; PTT = partial thromboplastin time; WBC = white blood cell count.

TABLE 2. **Initial Management**

Anemia	Transfuse if in high output heart failure with 5 mL/kg of packed red blood cells.
Bleeding	Transfuse 0.2 U/kg of platelets. Evaluate for disseminated intravascular coagulation.
Hyperleukocytosis	Hydration 2.4–3 L/m^2. Allopurinol, alkalinization. Leukopheresis if respiratory or CNS symptoms. Intravenous contrast material should never be given prior to IV hydration and diagnostic studies.
Fever	Blood cultures. Careful examination for source. Antibiotics to cover gram-negative and gram-positive organisms.
Hyperkalemia	Kayexalate, sodium bicarbonate, calcium gluconate, insulin, and glucose.
Hyperuricemia	Allopurinol 100 mg/m^2 TID.
Hyperphosphatemia	Aluminium hydroxide 100–150 mg/kg/day.
Hypocalcemia	Calcium gluconate 100–200 mg/kg/dose, if symptomatic.
Renal failure	Hemodialysis.

COMPLICATIONS AND INITIAL TREATMENT

Infection, metabolic abnormalities, hyperleukocytosis, anemia, and bleeding are the most common serious problems complicating the initial treatment of the newly diagnosed child with acute leukemia. These clinical problems are most often the result of leukemic infiltration of the bone marrow and other organs. The greater the leukemic burden—manifested by high white blood cell count; enlarged liver, spleen, kidneys, or lymph nodes—the greater the degree of clinical difficulty in treating the patient during the initial phases of therapy (Table 2).

FEVER

Over 50% of patients with acute leukemia present with a fever greater than 38.5°C. Fever caused by leukemia is rare and likely indicates the presence of a potentially serious infection.

Nevertheless, fever should be considered due to infection until proved otherwise. Untreated infection may progress quickly and terminate fatally. If severe neutropenia exists (<500 neutrophils/mm^3), it is necessary to identify sites of infection. If none are found, blood and urine cultures are obtained and antibiotic therapy is initiated empirically with broad-spectrum coverage for gram-negative and gram-positive organisms. A lumbar puncture is performed only with the clinical suspicion of meningitis. At our institution, ceftazidime 50 mg/kg (maximum 2 g/dose) is given intravenously (IV) every 8 hours. If the patient appears ill (toxic or with hypotension or tachypnea), we add gentamicin to the initial antibiotic regimen to provide coverage for gram-negative organisms. If the patient is allergic to ceftazidime, aztreonam (Azactam) +/− gentamicin (Garamycin) is considered. Cultures are performed periodically if the fever persists. No change in coverage is made if the patient is stable and results of culture are not positive. If still febrile after 72 hours, vancomycin (Vancocin), 10 mg/kg, IV every 6 hours is added. Vancomycin levels must be monitored to prevent renal toxicity. Other medical centers may use two or three antibiotic regimens as initial therapy for fever and neutropenia. Resistant bacteria and disseminated fungal infections need to be considered if the patient does not improve clinically. Antibiotic use varies among institutions based on their experience with patterns of resistance. Early institution of antifungal therapy may be necessary for patients who continue to be febrile from 5 to 7 days on adequate antibiotic coverage.

Prophylactic therapy with trimethoprim-sulfamethoxazole (Bactrim), 150 mg/m^2 of trimethoprim divided twice a day for 3 consecutive days per week is initiated during induction to prevent *Pneumocystis carinii* pneumonia, a frequently fatal interstitial pneumonitis. This is continued in all patients with acute leukemia while they are undergoing chemotherapy.

TUMOR LYSIS SYNDROME

Uric acid obstructive nephropathy, manifested by elevated uric acid and creatinine levels with low urine flow, can occur before chemotherapy is given and/or develop once chemotherapy is started. It may be life-threatening. Hyperuricemia can lead to renal failure by precipitation of uric acid in renal tubules. Patients with large tumor burdens at diagnosis are more likely to have this complication. As therapy is started, biochemical abnormalities develop that can also lead to renal failure. This constellation of problems is referred to as *acute tumor lysis syndrome.* Lysis of blast cells will release potassium, purines, and phosphorus, resulting in hyperkalemia, hyperuricemia, and hyperphosphatemia with secondary hypocalcemia.

To prevent these complications, creatinine, blood urea nitrogen, uric acid, electrolytes, calcium, and phosphorus levels are measured on admission and then every 6 hours once therapy is begun until the risk of tumor lysis has subsided. Vigorous hydration at 2.5 to 3 L/m^2/d with 5% dextrose and 0.25 normal saline with sodium bicarbonate ($NaHCO_3$) 20 to 40 mEq/L is used to keep urine pH greater than 6.0. If the urine output is less than 2 to 3 mL/kg/hour, diuretics (i.e., furosemide) may be needed. Hydration will ensure good urine output and kaliuresis when therapy is begun. Allopurinol (Zyloprim) is started at 100 mg/m^2 three times a day to prevent hyperuricemia. A new agent, recombinant urate oxidase (Rasburicase)* converts uric acid to allantoin, which is readily excreted in the urine and is 5- to 10-fold more soluble than uric acid. This agent, when commercially available, will largely eliminate the problems caused by hyperuricemia.

Mild hyperkalemia can be treated with sodium polystyrene sulfonate (Kayexalate), 1 g/kg administered orally and mixed with sorbitol. Renal failure may result in increasingly worse hyperkalemia, which in turn can cause cardiac arrhythmias. Severe hyperkalemia, with a serum potassium level greater than 7.0 to 7.5 mEq/L, should be treated with $NaHCO_3$, calcium gluconate, and insulin with glucose. If these methods fail, hemodialysis is indicated to prevent cardiac arrhythmias.

Additional metabolic abnormalities develop once therapy is initiated. The release of phosphorus from lysis of leukemic blasts causes hyperphosphatemia. When the phosphate or calcium levels exceed the calcium and phosphorus solubility, calcium phosphate can precipitate and cause hypocalcemia and may further worsen renal damage. In the case of severe hyperphosphatemia, alkalinization should be discontinued and the use of aluminum hydroxide 100 to 200 mg/kg/d* in four divided doses should be considered. Diamox 5 mg/kg per dose repeated two to three times over 24 hours can be used to keep urine pH greater than 7 if $NaHCO_3$ needs to be discontinued. Severe symptomatic hypocalcemia can be treated with IV calcium gluconate 100 to 200 mg/kg per dose.

HYPERLEUKOCYTOSIS

Complications from hyperleukocytosis are rare and more common in ANLL than ALL. Stasis can develop with white blood cell counts greater than 100,000 cells/mm^3. The increased viscosity of blood and poor deformability of blast cells impairs the microcirculation, greatly increasing the risk of primary thrombotic and secondary hemorrhagic complications. Hyperleukocytosis in acute leukemia is associated with a risk of intracranial hemorrhage. CNS leukemic involvement can result in visual blurring, papilledema, and headache. Hyperleukocytosis can affect pulmonary function and often, tachypnea, dyspnea, and hypoxia can be seen.

Once the diagnosis is confirmed, our approach to hyperleukocytosis is hydration with greater than or equal to 3 L/m^2/d of IV fluid administered with $NaHCO_3$ for alkalinization, and allopurinol daily before and during the first few days of induction. Leukopheresis can be used to reduce the cell count if renal compromise develops; however, its effect is temporary and may not prevent sludging in the microcirculation.

ANEMIA

The degree of anemia depends on the duration and type of disease. The growing leukemia cell population gradually crowds out normal hematopoietic bone marrow precursors leading insidiously to severe anemia. T-cell leukemia, characterized by more bulky extramedullary disease, may present with mild anemia because many times the thymus is the site of origin with later spread to the marrow. If there is any evidence of cardiac failure or respiratory compromise not secondary to hyperleukocytosis, the patient undergoes transfusion with 10 mL/kg of irradiated, cytomegalovirus-negative, packed red blood cells over 4 hours. All blood products are irradiated to prevent rare cases of graft vs host disease caused by the infusion of immunocompetent lymphocytes from the donor. If the patient presents with

*Investigational drug in the United States.

*Exceeds dosage recommended by the manufacturer.

severe anemia (hemoglobin <6 g/dL), red cell transfusions with 5 mL/kg packed red blood cells can be given over 4 hours every 6 to 8 hours until the hemoglobin level approaches 8 g/dL. The majority of patients are promptly referred to oncology centers and usually do not undergo transfusion before referral.

BLEEDING

Bleeding is usually a result of thrombocytopenia, a coagulopathy due to infection, or leukemia-associated disseminated intravascular coagulopathy. If thrombocytopenia is the cause, transfusion of 0.2 U of irradiated, cytomegalovirus-negative platelets per kilogram (4–6 U/m^2) should increase the platelet count by 75,000/mm^3. It is common practice to transfuse platelets when the platelet count is below 10,000/mm^3 or if bleeding is a problem. Patients with ANLL are at higher risk of hemorrhagic complications. Disseminated intravascular coagulation is frequently associated with promyelocytic (FAB M3) and monocytic (FAB M5) leukemia. Initial therapy of M3 ANLL with all-*trans*-retinoic acid (ATRA, Vesanoid) may abrogate the bleeding problem. Frequent transfusions with platelets and fresh frozen plasma may help control the disseminated intravascular coagulopathy–related bleeding until specific therapy has a chance to work.

DRUG TOXICITY

Chemotherapeutic agents can cause organ toxicity; often, it is reversible. Schedules and doses of chemotherapeutic agents may have to be modified or held depending on bone marrow, renal, and hepatic function. Adverse reactions to chemotherapeutic agents are listed in Table 3, and the management of chemotherapy extravasation is listed in Table 4.

TABLE 3. **Drugs Used to Treat Acute Leukemia**

Drug	Adverse Reactions
Vincristine (Oncovin)	Alopecia, neuritic pain, constipation, difficulty in walking, peripheral neuropathy, leukopenia, severe cellulitis if extravasated
Dexamethasone	Immunosuppression, increased appetite and weight gain, Cushing's syndrome, myopathy, mood changes, hyperglycemia, relative adrenocortical insufficiency in times of stress
L-Asparaginase (Elspar)	Anaphylactic reactions, decreased protein synthesis (including coagulation factors), pancreatitis, hyperglycemia
6-Mercaptopurine	Myelosuppression, hematotoxicity, immunosuppression
Methotrexate	Stomatitis, myelosuppression, immunosuppression, photosensitivity, hepatic fibrosis
Daunorubicin (Cerubidine)	Myelosuppression, cardiac toxicity, alopecia, nausea and vomiting, stomatitis, gastrointestinal ulceration, severe cellulitis if extravasated, hypersensitivity reactions
Cytarabine (Cytosar-U)	Myelosuppression, nausea and vomiting, stomatitis, ocular toxicity with high doses, cerebellar dysfunction
Etoposide (VePesid) teniposide (Vumon)	Nausea and vomiting, diarrhea, fever, hypotension, allergic reactions, alopecia, peripheral neuropathy, mucositis, hepatic damage with high doses
Thioguanine	Nausea and vomiting, bone marrow depression, hepatic damage, stomatitis
Amsacrine (Amsidyl)	Leukopenia, phlebitis, nausea, vomiting, diarrhea, arrhythmias, alopecia, allergic reactions
Mitoxantrone (Novantrone)	Myelosuppression, nausea, vomiting, stomatitis, cardiac toxicity
Arsenic trioxide	Acute promyelocytic leukemia differentiation syndrome (fever, dyspnea, weight gain, abnormal chest auscultatory findings), QT prolongation and other ECG abnormalities, hyperleukocytosis, nausea, vomiting, diarrhea, cough, rash

Abbreviation: ECG = electrocardiogram.

ACUTE LYMPHOCYTIC LEUKEMIA TREATMENT

In general, there are several criteria that can be used to identify patients who will have a good outcome with minimal therapy and patients who should receive more aggressive and therefore toxic therapy. The clinical criteria used to identify a child with B-cell precursor ALL at low risk of recurrent disease are 1 to 9 years old and a leukocyte count less than 50,000/mm^3. Patients in other age groups or those with higher leukocyte counts are considered to be at higher risk. This grouping can be explained largely by the presence of specific leukemia cell genetic abnormalities. Other factors including immunophenotype, genotype, CNS involvement at diagnosis, and early response to therapy have been added to this simple clinical risk classification system. Ongoing trials are exploring the importance of these clinical and biologic features.

The treatment for ALL is divided into three components: induction, consolidation/intensification, and maintenance. Throughout these three components, the CNS is treated with intrathecal chemotherapy because most children with leukemia have subclinical CNS involvement at diagnosis. Occasionally, cranial irradiation may be necessary for some patients, particularly those with initial high white blood cell counts or with CNS involvement at diagnosis.

With current therapy, high-risk patients can expect greater than 65% event-free survival (EFS), whereas low-risk patients have an EFS of 80% to 90%. Current results for 6 months of therapy indicate an EFS of 85% for B-cell (Burkitt's) leukemia patients.

Induction

To obtain a complete remission and allow for the return of normal hematopoiesis, the present POG protocols include administering vincristine (Oncovin), asparaginase (Elspar), and dexamethasone to low-risk and standard-risk patients over a 4-week period; daunorubicin (Cerubidine) is included for high-risk patients. With this therapy, greater than 97% of patients achieve remission. Dexamethasone has replaced prednisone during induction in the three-drug regimen because it appears to provide better CNS protection. In the four-drug regimen for high-risk patients, prednisone is still used owing to early toxicity noted when dexamethasone replaced

TABLE 4. **Prevention and Treatment of Chemotherapy Extravasation**

Vesicants should not be administered in areas of flexion. Avoid the antecubital fossa. The dorsum of the hand should be the first choice. The forearm is acceptable.
Stop infusion immediately if extravasation is suspected. Keep the needle in place.
Using a 3 mL syringe, aspirate as much of the infiltrated drug as possible.
Elevate the extremity.
Cleanse site with hospital-approved antiseptic.
Inject a specific antidote if one is available. For vincristine, etoposide, and teniposide, use hyaluronidase (150 U/mL). Inject 3–5 syringes of 0.2 mL with a 27G needle around the leading edge of the extravasation. Dose will depend on the size of the infiltrate. Apply warm compresses for 30–60 min and then alternate on/off every 15 min for 24 h. For all other vesicants and irritants (i.e., doxorubicin, daunorubicin, and mitoxantrone) use cold compresses. For doxorubicin, daunorubicin, idarubicin, and amsacrine, apply DMSO 50% 1.5 mL to site every 6 h. Allow to dry; do not cover. Elevate limb for at least 2 h up to 48 h if possible.
Tissue necrosis may not be evident for 1–2 wk. Arrange for follow-up in 7–10 d.
If an open wound develops, apply silver sulfadiazine cream TID.

prednisone. For some very high-risk patients, additional agents are used to intensify induction. At the end of induction, patients in remission have normal blood cell counts and physical examinations and no evidence of leukemia in blood or bone marrow (i.e., <5% blast cells).

Consolidation/Intensification

Once remission is achieved, a period of therapy begins with intermediate-dose methotrexate (>1 g/m^2), 6-mercaptopurine (Purinethol), steroid and vincristine pulses, standard dose methotrexate, and, often, re-induction given over several months. CNS prophylaxis with intrathecal methotrexate used during induction is continued and given periodically over the first 2 years of therapy.

The most recent EFS improvements in ALL have been attributed to the intensity of this phase of therapy. Randomizations in the present clinical trials involve differences in the intensity and drug combinations used during consolidation/intensification.

Maintenance

Prolonged therapy is required for ALL. This maintenance treatment is less intensive and is given to eliminate residual, slowly dividing leukemia cells or to suppress their growth and let apoptosis occur. The backbone of ALL maintenance therapy is daily oral 6-mercaptopurine and weekly oral or intramuscular methotrexate. Intermittent pulses of vincristine and a glucocorticoid seem to offer an additional effect. There appears to be no advantage to prolonging this phase of therapy beyond 2.5 to 3 years. Attempts to shorten therapy to less that 2.5 years from diagnosis have been unsuccessful.

SPECIAL CATEGORIES

Infants with ALL tend to have high white blood cell counts, CNS involvement, and high-risk chromosome translocations (70% have 11q23 rearrangements) at diagnosis. With the addition of multiple courses of marrow hypoplasia–inducing drug combinations, the EFS for infants is improving. Therapy-associated mortality can be high and early relapse is frequent. Bone marrow transplantation (BMT) should be considered in first remission for those with a human leukocyte antigen (HLA) identical sibling donor or a closely matched unrelated donor.

The diagnosis of leukemia in the first 3 months of life can be complicated. During this period, children with Down syndrome can present with a transient myeloproliferative syndrome or pseudoleukemia. Thrombocytopenia, leukocytosis, and circulating blast cells can be identified along with hepatosplenomegaly. In most instances, these physical and hematologic findings will resolve within a few months and not need therapy other than occasional blood product transfusions. It is estimated that frank ANLL will develop in one third of these patients 12 to 36 months later, which will require therapy. Occasionally, this transient disorder can develop in normal-appearing newborns without the stigmata of Down syndrome. Consequently, the diagnosis of true congenital leukemia (presents in the first 3 months of life) can be quite a problem.

RELAPSE

Recurrent leukemia can occur in the marrow, extramedullary sites (testis, CNS, eye), or a combination of sites. Patients who experience relapse in the bone marrow while on therapy or within 6 months following therapy are likely to experience relapse again if treated with chemotherapy alone even though a second remission can usually be obtained. Bone marrow transplantation offers a cure for 35% to 60% of these children. Isolated extramedullary relapses or bone marrow relapses over 36 months from diagnosis can be treated successfully with chemotherapy alone. The use of bone marrow transplantation for these isolated extramedullary or late bone marrow relapses is controversial.

BONE MARROW TRANSPLANTATION

Children likely to fail standard therapy can be identified by certain characteristics at diagnosis. The Philadelphia (Ph) chromosome t(9;22) (q34;q11), identified in the leukemia cells of 3% to 4% of children with ALL, is the worst prognostic feature. Transplantation of bone marrow from HLA-matched related donors is superior to other types of transplantation and to intensive chemotherapy alone. Early BMT in first remission should also be considered for infants with ALL and the 11q23 translocation. Patients who fail to achieve complete remission with initial induction agents should also be considered for BMT once they achieve remission. The fact that most children do not have a matched related donor available has led to the use of a matched unrelated BMT for patients who relapse or have a particularly bad prognosis. Unrelated donor transplants are associated with increased morbidity and graft versus host disease.

ACUTE NONLYMPHOCYTIC LEUKEMIA

Although up to 85% of children with ANLL will achieve remission, EFS with chemotherapy is approximately 50% effective. Intensive induction regimens including daunorubicin, cytosine arabinoside, 6-thioguanine, etoposide,* and dexamethasone given with intensive timing or similar intensive therapy utilizing additional mitoxantrone (Novantrone),* and amsacrine (Amsidyl)† give the best results to date. Five percent to 10% of children have resistant disease and 10% to 15% die from infection or complications during induction. Patients who relapse usually do so during the first year of therapy and patients who remain in remission for over 2 years are usually cured. Thus, the current approach to treatment of ANLL is to prolong the duration of initial remission with early intensification using chemotherapy or with BMT only for those with HLA-identical related bone marrow donors.

A number of biologically important factors indicating a better prognosis have been recently identified in children with ANLL. Acute promyelocytic leukemia is best treated with a combination of all-*trans*-retinoic acid in addition to an anthracycline regimen, plus or minus cytosine arabinoside. Pediatric patients are currently being admitted to a national protocol that will test whether arsenic trioxide (Trisenox), a newly identified differentiating agent, and/or continuing doses of all-*trans*-retinoic acid will improve the outlook for this subgroup of patients who now have a 70% EFS. Children with Down syndrome and ANLL can be treated with a somewhat less aggressive chemotherapy regimen resulting in an 80% EFS. Two chromosomal abnormalities associated with a more favorable outcome are t(8;21), or inv(16) plus or minus additional abnormalities.

Induction

Remission is achieved in over 80% of children with ANLL when two consecutive courses of intensive chemotherapy are given. Idarubicin may be used in place of daunorubicin, but it may be associated with increased toxicity.

Consolidation/Maintenance

Once remission is achieved, repetitive courses of intensive chemotherapy are given. These courses are similar to the induction therapy but additional agents are used in an attempt to overcome cross resistance. Following this 4- to 5-month period, depending on the protocol, patients may continue on a less toxic maintenance regimen for up to a year or more. There is no proven role for maintenance therapy at this time although this is an area of investigation.

Once a patient achieves a complete remission he or she may go on to an allogeneic-BMT if there is an HLA-matched family member. At present, there is no role for autologous-BMT or matched unrelated BMT in children with ANLL in first remission. With the advent of genetic testing to monitor for minimal residual disease, early relapse can be identified before morphologic changes are noted in the bone marrow. This detection of relapse, while the population of leukemia cells is small, can be used to help one decide whether alternative treatments such as reinduction, differentiating agents, or BMTs from matched unrelated donors should be considered before obvious relapse occurs.

Late Effects

Successful treatment strategies have led to increasing numbers of patients cured of acute leukemia. Many hazards remain for patients who have completed therapy. Second cancers have been identified in excess of what would be predicted based on age and gender alone. Cardiomyopathies from cardiotoxic drugs are being identified, and effects on growth are noted in those who required cranial irradiation as part of their therapy. Interference with growth and development by therapy directed at malignancies is a well-recognized long-term effect that requires vigilance and long-term follow-up.

*Not FDA approved for this indication.
†Investigational drug in the United States.

CHRONIC LEUKEMIAS

method of
NIZAR M. TANNIR, M.D., and
SUSAN O'BRIEN, M.D.
MD Anderson Cancer Center
Houston, Texas

Chronic lymphocytic leukemia (CLL) is a lymphoproliferative disorder characterized by a progressive accumulation of small, mature-appearing, long-lived, and functionally defective lymphocytes in the blood and bone marrow, lymph nodes, and spleen. It is the most common leukemia in the western world and accounts for 30% of all adult leukemias. About 8000 new cases are diagnosed in the United States each year; the median age of the patients is 65 years, and the male:female ratio is 1.3:1. Among leukemias, CLL has the strongest familial aggregation. The cause of CLL is not known; it is the only leukemia not associated with exposure to radiation. Population studies have not shown any evidence linking CLL to known occupational or environmental risk factors.

BIOLOGY

The normal counterpart of the typical CLL cell is the CD5+ B-lymphocyte, which is present in the mantle zone of the secondary lymphoid follicle and in the peripheral blood in small numbers. CD5+ B cells are the predominant B-cell population in fetal spleen and peripheral blood and constitute 10% to 25% of normal adult B cells. CLL cells have a very low proliferative index and accumulation of these cells is related to defects in apoptosis.

The most common genetic abnormality in CLL is on the long arm of chromosome 13 and involves the site of a presumed tumor suppressor gene D13S25. Rearrangements at this site have been associated with improved survival when patients are compared to those with other genetic abnormalities or a normal karyotype. Trisomy 12 is the second most common cytogenetic abnormality and is typically associated with variant morphology. Translocations involving chromosome 14 exhibit breakpoints at band q32, the site of the Ig heavy chain gene locus, with the donor chromosome most commonly being chromosome 11. Structural abnormalities of chromosome 11 are the fourth most common abnormality. In general, abnormal karyotypes confer a worse prognosis than normal cytogenetics, and the prognosis is worst for those with multiple clonal abnormalities.

CLINICAL MANIFESTATIONS AND LABORATORY FINDINGS

With the use of routine blood testing, the number of CLL patients who are asymptomatic at diagnosis has increased to about 40%. When constitutional symptoms are present, the most common complaint is fatigue or malaise. Less often, enlarged lymph nodes or the development of an infection is the initial manifestation. An exaggerated reaction to insect bites is also common. In contrast to lymphoma, fever in the absence of infection is rare in CLL.

Lymphocytosis may be severe, but unlike in acute leukemia, leukostasis is uncommon. Prolymphocytes may be seen but constitute less than 10% of cells. Ruptured lymphocytes or "smudge" cells reflect cell fragility during the preparation of the peripheral smear.

Anemia (hemoglobin <11.0 g/dL) or thrombocytopenia (platelets $<100 \times 10^9$/L) is noted at diagnosis in about 20% of patients. These cytopenias can occur as a result of bone marrow failure due to bone marrow packed by CLL, as a result of an immune-mediated process, or as a result of hypersplenism. A positive result on direct antiglobulin test is seen in 25% of patients, but overt autoimmune hemolytic anemia (AIHA) occurs less frequently. Autoimmune thrombocytopenia and pure red cell aplasia may also be encountered. Hypogammaglobulinemia occurs in about 50% of patients with CLL, and the incidence increases significantly with disease progression. Significant hypogammaglobulinemia and neutropenia result in increased susceptibility of patients to major bacterial infections.

DIFFERENTIAL DIAGNOSIS

Several B-cell malignancies in which there are increased numbers of small lymphoid cells in the peripheral blood have overlapping clinical manifestations and should be differentiated from CLL. The disorders most likely to be confused with CLL are prolymphocytic leukemia, and the leukemic phase of non-Hodgkin's lymphoma (usually mantle-cell lymphoma, follicular lymphoma, or splenic lymphoma with circulating villous lymphocytes). CLL cells express the B-cell markers CD19, CD20, and CD23. The hallmark of CLL is coexpression of a common T-cell marker, CD5. Mantle cell lymphoma expresses CD5, but CD23 should be negative. Follicular lymphoma cells typically express CD10, an antigen not present on CLL cells. Immunophenotyping is helpful in differentiating these disorders.

STAGING

The natural history of CLL is extremely variable, with survival times ranging from 2 to more than 20 years from initial diagnosis. In 1975, Rai and associates proposed a staging system consisting of five stages (Rai 0–IV) that was later modified into a three-stage system (Table 1). A similar staging system was developed in Europe by Binet and associates. Both staging systems are recognized as simple and accurate prognostic indicators of survival (see Table 1).

Although patients in the high-risk group usually have a progressive clinical course, the course of the disease is not uniform in the other risk groups. Patients in the low- and intermediate-risk groups may have indolent disease over many years or even decades, or the course may be progressive and associated with a short survival time.

Several prognostic factors have been found to be associated with inferior survival in CLL. These include a short lymphocyte doubling time (<12 months), a diffuse pattern of bone marrow infiltration, advanced age and male gender, abnormal karyotype, and high serum levels of β_2-microglobulin and soluble CD23. Newer prognostic factors in CLL include the mutational status of Ig genes and CD38 expression on CLL lymphocytes. A recent report suggested that IgV gene mutations within CLL lymphocytes correlate with a significantly longer survival time. Although controversial, some investigators have suggested that mutated IgV genes correlate with low expression of CD38 (<30%) on CLL lymphocytes. Although this correlation may not be exact, data examining CD38 expression on CLL lymphocytes clearly show a strong correlation between increased expression of CD38 and inferior survival.

TABLE 1. **Staging Systems for Chronic Lymphocytic Leukemia**

Rai *Original Five-Stage System*	*Modified Three-Stage System*	*Clinical Features*	*Median Survival (y)*
0	Low risk	Lymphocytosis	12.5
I		Lymphadenopathy	
II	Intermediate risk	Splenomegaly or hepatomegaly	7
III		Anemia (Hb <11.0 g/dL)	
IV	High risk	Thrombocytopenia (platelets $<100 \times 10^9$/L)	1.5

Binet *Stage*	*Clinical Features*	*Median Survival (y)*
A	<3 areas* of clinical adenopathy, no anemia or thrombocytopenia	12
B	≥3 involved node areas; no anemia or thrombocytopenia	7
C	Hb <10 g/dL and/or platelets $<100 \times 10^9$/L	2

*Lymphoid-bearing areas: cervical nodes, axillary nodes, inguinofemoral nodes, spleen, and liver.

TREATMENT

The first decision to be made in CLL is whether the patient requires treatment at initial diagnosis. This cautionary approach is based on the older age of the patient, the heterogeneity of the disease course, and lack of evidence that early treatment affects long-term survival. Given these vagaries, the National Cancer Institute Working Group has devised guidelines for the initiation of treatment for CLL. These include constitutional symptoms, progressive bone marrow failure, AIHA and autoimmune thrombocytopenia poorly responsive to corticosteroid therapy, massive or progressive lymphadenopathy or splenomegaly, progressive lymphocytosis, or a lymphocyte doubling time less than 6 months. Hypogammaglobulinemia or the development of a monoclonal protein alone are not sufficient criteria to initiate therapy.

Chemotherapy

For several decades, the backbone of chemotherapy in CLL has been two alkylating agents: chlorambucil (CLB; Leukeran) or cyclophosphamide (CTX; Cytoxan), with or without the addition of corticosteroids. Both agents are rapidly absorbed from the gastrointestinal tract and can be administered orally. Dose and schedules of CLB vary significantly. Commonly used schedules include a daily dose of 0.08 mg/kg (4–8 mg total dose/d), or an intermittently pulsed schedule of 0.8 mg/kg (30–40 mg/m^2) given in a single day every 3 to 4 weeks, or half this dose given every 2 weeks. The dose is adjusted to avoid serious myelosuppression, which is more common with the daily schedule. CLB is administered for several weeks until a maximal clinical response is reached. Maintenance chemotherapy is usually not given but CLB may be restarted if disease recurrence is noted. CTX is given at a daily dose of 1 to 2 mg/kg. The overall response (OR) rate with either CLB or CTX is about 40% to 60%, with about 3% to 5% complete remission (CR).

Prednisone has been administered as a single agent, usually at a dose of 100 mg with gradual tapering. The major indication for the use of single agent prednisone in CLL is the treatment of AIHA and autoimmune thrombocytopenia. In an attempt to improve response rates, alkylating agents have been combined with steroids. Higher response rates were reported in two series, but with the small number of patients, these differences were not statistically significant; no survival differences were noted. Two clinical trials conducted by the French Cooperative Group on CLL in Binet stage A disease compared immediate treatment with CLB (first trial) or CLB plus prednisone (second trial) versus delayed treatment until evidence of progression was noted. Patients on the delayed treatment arm had a somewhat superior survival compared to those on the immediate treatment arm due to higher incidence of second malignancies with prolonged CLB exposure.

Nonrandomized trials initially reported excellent responses using intermittent CTX, vincristine (Oncovin),* and prednisone (CVP or COP) in patients with advanced CLL with 44% of patients achieving a CR. However, two large randomized studies comparing CLB versus COP reported no differences in response or survival rate.

Several purine analogues have demonstrated clinical activity in CLL; these include fludarabine monophosphate (Fludara), 2-chlorodeoxyadenosine/2-CdA (cladribine; Leustatin),* and deoxycoformycin (DCF; Pentostatin).

Fludarabine administered at 30 mg/m^2 daily for 5 days produces response rates of 40% to 60% in previously treated patients with CLL, with 15% achieving CR. Addition of prednisone to fludarabine did not increase the response rate but was associated with an increased incidence of *Pneumocystis carinii* and *Listeria monocytogenes* infections.

When used in previously untreated patients, fludarabine produces OR rates of 80% with 30% CR. Fludarabine has been compared to CLB in previously untreated patients with CLL. This Intergroup trial enrolled 500 patients who received fludarabine 25 mg/m^2/d for 5 days every 4 weeks or CLB as a single 40 mg/m^2 dose every 4 weeks. A third arm administering fludarabine 20 mg/m^2/d for 5 days plus CLB at 20 mg/m^2 on day 1 every 4 weeks was closed early because of toxicity. Crossover was permitted for nonresponse or early relapse. The OR rate with fludarabine was 63% with a 20% CR rate, whereas the OR rate with CLB was 33% with 3% CR rate. A longer duration of response and an improved progression-free survival were noted in patients treated with fludarabine, but median overall survival was not statistically different between the two groups. Half of the patients who failed to respond to CLB responded to fludarabine, including 14% CR. This was in contrast to a 7% partial remission rate with CLB in patients who failed to respond to fludarabine. The incidence of neutropenia, thrombocytopenia, and infections was similar.

2-CdA* has also been evaluated in CLL and has similar anti-tumor activity but may be more likely to produce thrombocytopenia. Like fludarabine, 2-CdA is immunosuppressive, with infections being the major toxicity. Although preliminary data suggested that patients resistant to fludarabine might respond to 2-CdA, this finding was not confirmed. In a trial of 28 patients who had disease resistant to fludarabine, only 2 patients had a PR with 2-CdA. Pentostatin has been less extensively evaluated in CLL. The OR rate for pentostatin is approximately 16% to 35% with rare CRs.

Although response rates to fludarabine are high, particularly in previously untreated patients, residual disease is usually detectable and all patients will experience relapse. Thus, strategies to improve on the single agent efficacy are needed. One approach is the use of fludarabine and alkylating agents. In vitro

*Not FDA approved for this indication.

synergy has been observed with fludarabine, resulting in inhibition of repair of DNA crosslinks induced by alkylating agents.

Flinn and associates administered fludarabine 20 mg/m^2 daily for 5 days together with CTX 600 mg/m^2 on day 1 to 60 previously untreated patients with low-grade lymphomas or CLL. The OR rate among the 17 patients with CLL was 100% with 47% CR. The use of growth factor support and prophylactic antibiotics resulted in a low incidence of myelosuppression/infections. O'Brien and coworkers used fludarabine 30 mg/m^2 and CTX 300 mg/m^2 for 3 days in 128 patients with CLL. Patients refractory to fludarabine had an OR rate of 38%, whereas all other patients had an OR rate greater than 80%. Comparison of fludarabine to fludarabine and CTX is being evaluated in randomized trials by the Eastern Cooperative Oncology Group (ECOG) and the German CLL Study Group.

Monoclonal Antibodies

Monoclonal antibodies are an exciting new therapeutic modality in lymphoid malignancies. Rituximab (Rituxan)* is a chimeric monoclonal antibody that binds to the B-cell antigen CD20 and received Food and Drug Administration (FDA) approval for the treatment of relapsed low-grade lymphoma. Winkler and associates treated 10 patients with CLL at the standard dose of 375 mg/m^2/week for 4 weeks and only 1 patient responded. Two groups have explored escalated doses of rituximab in the treatment of CLL. Byrd and associates administered the standard 375 mg/m^2 dose thrice weekly for 4 weeks and reported a 45% response rate in 33 patients. In a dose-escalation trial of 40 patients with previously treated CLL, O'Brien and associates administered rituximab 375 mg/m^2 the first week, then increased the dose from 500 mg to 2250 mg/m^2 weekly for 3 weeks. The OR rate in CLL was 36% and a dose response was observed. Trials combining rituximab with chemotherapy are ongoing in CLL.

Alemtuzumab (Campath-1H)† is another chimeric monoclonal antibody that binds to CD52, a pan-lymphocyte antigen present on both B and T lymphocytes. A recent pivotal trial in fludarabine-refractory patients showed a response rate of 33%. Alemtuzumab was particularly effective in clearing the blood, bone marrow, and spleen of CLL but was less effective in bulky lymph nodes sites. Alemtuzumab is an immunosuppressive antibody, which may be associated with infections and viral reactivation. Thus, all patients receiving this antibody should receive prophylaxis against *P. carinii* pneumonia and herpesvirus. This antibody was recently approved by the FDA for the treatment of patients with CLL refractory to fludarabine.

*Not FDA approved for this indication.
†Investigational drug in the United States.

Bone Marrow Transplantation

Several studies have reported on the feasibility of allogeneic bone marrow transplantation (alloBMT) and autologous bone marrow transplantation (autoBMT) in CLL. However, the impact of transplantation on survival is not known. A large study reported the results of 54 CLL patients younger than 60 years old from 30 centers worldwide. The majority of patients received chemotherapy and total body irradiation followed by bone marrow from HLA-matched siblings. The 3-year probability of survival was 46% with a projected survival at 5 years of 30% to 40%. Recently, with the advent of minitransplantation that uses nonmyeloablative regimens, and relies on harnessing the graft-versus-leukemia (GVL) effect, the option of stem cell transplantation (SCT) has been expanded to patients up to 70 years old. Patients transplanted with sensitive disease achieve a better outcome than those with resistant disease. Because 60% of CLL patients younger than 55 years old eventually develop progressive disease, and have a median survival probability of only 5 years after treatments, innovative therapies with curative intent, including the use of SCT, will play an increasing role in the future.

CHRONIC MYELOGENOUS LEUKEMIA

Chronic myelogenous leukemia (CML) is a clonal myeloproliferative disorder that arises in a pluripotent hematopoietic progenitor cell leading to excessive proliferation of marrow granulocytes, erythroid precursors, and megakaryocytes. These cells harbor a distinctive cytogenetic abnormality, the Philadelphia (Ph) chromosome, which serves as a disease marker and results from a translocation between the long arms of chromosomes 9 and 22.

Epidemiology

CML is diagnosed in approximately 4000 to 5000 patients in the United States yearly, representing an incidence of 1 to 2 per 100,000 with a male to female preponderance of 1.4 to 2.2:1. CML accounts for 7% to 15% of leukemias among adults, with a median age at presentation between 45 and 55 years. One third of patients are older than 60 years. CML is uncommon in children and adolescents.

Etiology

The etiology of CML is unknown. No familial aggregation has been noted. Radiation exposure, as evidenced following the atomic bomb explosions in Hiroshima and Nagasaki and the Chernobyl nuclear reactor accident, has been implicated as a causative agent. Effects of therapeutic doses of radiation on the development of CML are disputed. No association with infectious agents has been reported.

Molecular Pathogenesis

Ninety-five percent of patients with the clinical picture of CML demonstrate the Ph chromosome in

95% to 100% of marrow metaphases. A reciprocal translocation between the long arms of chromosomes 9 and 22 results in a large 3' segment of the ABL gene on chromosome 9q34 fusing to a 5' segment of the BCR gene (on chromosome 22q11); this creates a hybrid BCR-ABL gene on 22q11. In about two thirds of patients, a reciprocal ABL-BCR gene rearrangement can be detected on the derivative chromosome 9q+; the pathogenetic role of this gene in CML is uncertain but its presence has no effect on survival. Most of the time, the ABL exons 2 to 11 are transposed to the major breakpoint cluster region (M-bcr) of BCR between exons 13 and 14. The BCR-ABL fusion mRNA extends over 8.5 kb and is translated into a chimeric protein of 210 kDa termed p210. The native ABL gene encodes a nonreceptor tyrosine kinase (p145) and its activity is rigorously controlled. It is also involved in signal transduction and regulation of cell growth. In contrast, p210 shows increased and uncontrolled kinase activity. The constitutive activation of this kinase results in upregulation of transcription of genes affecting proliferation and transformation of hematopoietic progenitor cells. A core element of BCR-ABL signaling is Ras. Activation of Ras-mediated pathways leads to upregulation of antiapoptotic pathways and may result in growth factor independence.

Using transgenic mice and retrovirus-mediated gene transfer into murine hematopoietic cells, in vitro and in vivo animal experiments have demonstrated that expression of BCR-ABL can initiate the clinical manifestations of CML. Progression of disease is thought to result from additional molecular abnormalities. Consonant with this is the fact that 70% to 80% of patients demonstrate additional karyotypic abnormalities at the time of progression into blastic phase. Genes shown to be altered in the progression of CML include p53, RB1, c-myc, $p16^{inkya}$, ras, and AML/EVI-1.

Clinical Manifestations

CML is a triphasic disease that can progress through chronic, accelerated, and blastic phases. At diagnosis, more than 90% of patients are in chronic phase. Symptoms at diagnosis may reflect the expanded myeloid pool and increased turnover of hematopoietic cells. Patients may complain of weakness, night sweats, and weight loss. Splenomegaly is noted in up to 50% of patients and is the most common finding on physical examination; this may result in increased abdominal girth and discomfort. Lymphadenopathy and fever are uncommon in chronic phase but may herald an accelerated phase. Approximately one half of patients in recent studies are asymptomatic at presentation and are diagnosed by results on routine blood tests. Occasionally, easy bruisability and bleeding are noted due to platelet dysfunction. Thrombotic events may occur as a result of thrombocytosis. Rarely the initial presentation may be related to manifestations of hyperleukocytosis such as strokes, priapism, and digital ischemia.

Laboratory Tests

Leukocytosis, thrombocytosis, and basophilia in the peripheral blood are typical laboratory features of CML in chronic phase. A white blood cell count (WBC) greater than 100×10^9/L may be seen in 70% to 90% of patients. Anemia is frequent, but usually mild. Examination of the bone marrow reveals hypercellularity with a myeloid:erythroid ratio between 10:1 and 15:1. All stages of myeloid maturation are seen with a preponderance of myelocytes and promyelocytes. Megakaryocytes are frequently increased. Approximately 50% of patients display increased collagen in bone marrow reticulin stains. However, marrow fibrosis is usually focal in early stage disease but may progress to a more diffuse pattern with disease progression. Additional laboratory findings include a decreased leukocyte alkaline phosphatase score and elevated serum B12 level, B12 binding protein, lactate dehydrogenase, and uric acid levels.

Cytogenetic analysis demonstrates the presence of the Ph chromosome as well as other chromosomal abnormalities that develop with disease progression (clonal evolution). In about 10% of patients, no t(9;22) is detected by karyotypic analysis. However, molecular studies may detect BCR-ABL rearrangements in one third to one half of such patients. Patients who are both Ph and BCR-ABL negative have a worse prognosis and need to be distinguished from typical CML.

Molecular assays are used in the diagnosis of CML and the assessment of response to therapy. Results of therapy can be monitored by polymerase chain reaction and fluorescence in situ hybridization (FISH). FISH allows analysis of metaphases as well as nondividing interphase cells, is easily quantifiable, and can be performed on peripheral blood specimens. However, it overestimates the cytogenetic response at high Ph-positive percent values and has a false-positive rate of 10%. The use of dual color probes for FISH may produce superior sensitivity and specificity. Hypermetaphase FISH is as time-efficient as interphase FISH, does not generate false-positive results, but must be performed on bone marrow samples.

Progression of Chronic Myeloid Leukemia

When treatment does not lead to partial or complete suppression of the Ph clone, such as with hydroxyurea (HU; Hydrea) or busulfan (Myleran), CML invariably progresses to an accelerated phase, which is followed 3 to 18 months later by blast crisis. The likelihood of entering blast crisis is initially about 10% per year, with the risk starting to rise sharply by the third year from diagnosis. Before the advent of therapeutic modalities that suppressed or eradicated the Ph clone, the median time to blast crisis

TABLE 2. **Criteria for the Definition of Accelerated and Blastic Phase Chronic Myelogenous Leukemia**

Accelerated Phase	Blastic Phase
MD Anderson	≥30% blasts in peripheral blood and/or bone marrow
Peripheral blood blasts ≥15%	Extramedullary infiltrates of leukemic cells
Peripheral blood blasts and promyelocytes ≥30%	Blastic phase is:
Peripheral blood basophils ≥20%	Lymphoid in one third of patients (TdT+, CD10+, CD19+, CD20+, frequent coexpression of myeloid markers)
Platelet count <100 × 10⁹/L unrelated to therapy	Myeloblastic or undifferentiated in two thirds of patients.
Karyotypic evolution	
International Bone Marrow Transplant Registry	
WBC difficult to control with use of busulfan or hydroxyurea	
Rapid doubling time of WBC count (<5 d)	
≥10% blasts in peripheral blood/bone marrow	
≥20% blasts and promyelocytes in peripheral blood/bone marrow	
≥20% basophils and eosinophils in peripheral blood	
Anemia or thrombocytopenia unresponsive to busulfan or hydroxyurea	
Persistent thrombocytosis	
Karyotypic evolution	
Progressive splenomegaly	
Development of chloromas or myelofibrosis	

Abbreviation: WBC = white blood cell count.

ranged between 3 and 4 years. Criteria for the definition of accelerated and blastic phases have been proposed (Table 2).

Several prognostic models have been developed in CML (Table 3). These models have been helpful in assigning patients to good, intermediate, and poor risk groups with median survivals of 6, 3 to 4, and 2 years, respectively, for patients receiving conventional therapy. The median survival of patients with CML was historically 3 years with less than 20% of patients alive 5 years from diagnosis. In recent times, patients in chronic phase have a median survival of 5 to 7 years, with a 10-year survival rate of 30% to 40%. Earlier diagnosis, better supportive care, and more effective therapies account for this improvement.

HISTORICAL AND CONVENTIONAL THERAPY

Response criteria in CML are summarized in Table 4. The first chemotherapy agent used in the treatment of CML was the alkylating agent busulfan. This agent is oral, inexpensive, and maintains reduction in the WBC for prolonged periods. However, because of its toxicities, which include severe and/or irreversible myelosuppression, pulmonary fibrosis, Addison's disease–like syndrome, and cutaneous hyperpigmentation, busulfan was replaced by HU in the 1970s. HU is a cell cycle–specific inhibitor of DNA synthesis. It is also an oral agent that is well tolerated and allows rapid hematologic control. Side effects are uncommon but include nausea at high doses and, rarely, cutaneous ulcers. Both drugs produce complete hematologic remissions (CHR) in 80% of patients. Cytogenetic remissions occur but are rare, and neither HU nor busulfan alters the natural course of the disease. In a large randomized study, both median duration of chronic phase (47 versus 37 months) and median survival (56 versus 44 months) were significantly longer in patients treated with HU compared to busulfan. The use of busulfan prior to allogeneic treatment had an adverse effect on post-transplant survival (3-year disease-free survival of 61% for patients treated with HU versus 45% for patients treated with busulfan). Doses of HU ranging between 500 mg and 4 g given as a single daily dose are used to control WBCs, with higher doses being used for higher WBCs. Allopurinol is frequently used until the WBC is less than 20 × 10^9/L. HU is usually continued until the WBC decreases to less than 10 × 10^9/L and then discontinued. It is then reinstated when the WBC climbs to greater than 25 × 10^9/L. Thrombocytosis that is not controlled with HU may respond to anagrelide (Agrylin),* the addition of interferon-alfa (IFA) or intermittent therapy with thiotepa (Thioplex*; 75 mg/m^2 intravenously every 3 weeks).

Patients with persistent and symptomatic splenomegaly and refractory cytopenias may benefit from splenectomy. Splenectomy performed prior to allogeneic transplant decreases the time to marrow recovery but does not affect long-term outcome. Busulfan and HU have little effect on the natural history of CML. This is likely related to the fact that cytogenetic responses are rare. Thus, the CML clone is not eradicated and further molecular events occurring in dividing cells may result in dedifferentiation and disease evolution to a more lethal stage (blast crisis). This led to interest in developing therapies that would eliminate the malignant clone (as evidenced clinically by a cytogenetic response). Combination chemotherapy (similar to that used to treat acute leukemia) has been shown to induce cytogenetic remissions. However, these remissions are short-lived and cells bearing the Ph chromosome inevitably recur. The first therapy (other than BMT) to cause cytogenetic remissions that were durable was interferon (IFN).

Interferon-Alfa With or Without Cytosine Arabinoside

IFNs are a group of naturally occurring proteins that have pleiotropic biologic activities. The mechanism of action of IFN is unknown. Although antiproliferation may be important, restoration of cytoadhe-

*Not FDA approved for this indication.

TABLE 3. **Prognostic Models in Chronic Myelogenous Leukemia**

	Sokal Model		Synthesis Model (MD Anderson)
Characteristics	Age		POOR-PROGNOSIS CHARACTERISTICS
	Platelet count		Age ≥60 y
	Spleen size		Spleen ≥10 cm below costal margin
	% Blood blasts		Blasts ≥3% in peripheral blood or ≥5% in bone marrow
			Basophils ≥7% in peripheral blood or ≥3% in bone marrow
			Platelets ≥700 × 10^9/L
			ACCELERATED-PHASE CHARACTERISTICS
			Karyotypic evolution
			Peripheral blood blasts ≥15%
			Peripheral blood blasts and promyelocytes ≥30%
			Peripheral blood basophils ≥20%
			Platelets <100 × 10^9/L
*Risk Group**	Low risk	(<0.8)	1 0–1 poor-prognosis criteria
	Intermediate risk	(0.8 –1.2)	2 2 poor-prognosis criteria
	High risk	(>1.2)	3 ≥3 poor-prognosis criteria
			4 ≥1 accelerated-phase criteria (regardless of number of poor-prognosis criteria)

*Risk is based on hazard ratio values in Sokal model and on summation of poor-prognosis factors in Synthesis model.

$$\lambda_1/\lambda_0(t) = EXP\ 0.0255\ (Spin - 8.14) + 0.0324\ (Blasts - 2.22)$$

$$+0.1025\left[\left(\frac{Plt}{700}\right)^2 - 0.627\right] - 0.0173\ (Hct - 34.2) - 0.2683\ (Sex - 1.40)$$

(Platelets: 10^9/L. Gender: male = 1.0, female = 2).

sion of hematopoietic cells to bone marrow stroma, immunomodulation, and antiangiogenesis represent other possible mechanisms.

In the original studies of IFN at MD Anderson Cancer Center (MDACC), patients received IFN at 5 MU/m² or the maximally tolerated lower dose (MTD) daily. CHR was seen in 80% and cytogenetic response in 58% with an estimated median survival of 89 months. Achieving a cytogenetic response after 1 year of therapy produced a significant survival benefit in landmark analysis: 5-year survival rates from 1 year into treatment were 90% with a complete cytogenetic response, 88% with a partial cytogenetic response, 76% with a minor cytogenetic response, and 38% in other response categories ($P < 0.001$). The benefit of cytogenetic response was observed within each risk group. Other trials have reported similar results. In four randomized trials from Japan, the United Kingdom, Italy, and Germany, patients treated with IFN achieved higher rates of major and complete cytogenetic response than those treated with conventional chemotherapy. Achievement of cytogenetic response was associated with prolonged survival in the Italian and Japanese trials; this was also true in a recent report from the Medical Research Council in the United Kingdom. A meta-analysis compared IFN with chemotherapy in CML and confirmed improved survival with IFN (57% at 5 years) compared to that seen with either HU ($P = 0.001$) or busulfan ($P = 0.00007$). Recently, two randomized trials have shown superiority of the combination of IFN plus low-dose ara-C over IFN alone. In a large French trial, the CHR and major cytogenetic response rates were significantly higher with the combination. Survival was also superior for the combination (86% versus 79% at 3 years, $P = 0.02$). Patients achieving a cytogenetic response with either IFN alone ($P < 0.001$) or with the combination of IFN plus ara-C ($P < 0.001$) had a significantly longer survival compared to patients who did not achieve a cytogenetic response. In this French trial, cytarabine (ara-C, Cytosar-U) was administered at 20 mg/m² for 10 days per month. In an Italian trial that randomized patients to IFN (median dose, 3.65 MU/m² /d) versus IFN (median dose, 3.8 MU/m²/d) plus low-dose ara-C (40 mg/kg/d subcutaneously for 10 days per month) the rates of major and complete cytogenetic response were significantly higher in the combined treatment arm.

Up to 50% of patients treated with IFN require dose reductions, and discontinuation of treatment

TABLE 4. **Criteria for Cytogenetic and Hematologic Remissions in Chronic Myelogenous Leukemia**

Response	Parameters	
Complete hematologic response	Complete normalization of peripheral counts (WBC <10 × 10^9/L, platelets <450 × 10^9/L, no immature cells like blasts, promyelocytes, metamyelocytes)	
	No signs and symptoms of disease, disappearance of palpable splenomegaly	
Partial hematologic response	As for complete hematologic response, except	
	1. Persistence of immature cells	
	2. Platelets <50% of pretreatment level but >450 × 10^9/L *or*	
	3. Persistent splenomegaly but <50% of pretreatment	
Cytogenetic response (in patients in complete hematologic response)		
Complete	No Ph-positive cells	Major
Partial	1%–34% Ph-positive cells	Major
Minor	35%–90% Ph-positive cells	

Abbreviation: WBC = white blood cell count.

due to toxicity occurs in 20%. To reduce the magnitude of early toxicity, principally fever, chills, anorexia, nausea, vomiting, flulike syndrome and myalgias, initial cytoreduction with HU to decrease the WBC to less than 20×10^9/L should be used. Subsequently IFN can be initiated at a lower dose and increased gradually (3 MU daily for 3–7 days, then 5 MU daily for 3–7 days, then 5 MU/m^2 or MTD). The dose of IFN is not reduced unless the WBC is less than 2×10^9/L or the platelets drop to less than 50×10^9/L. Common chronic side effects are fatigue, depression, insomnia, weight loss, decreased libido, and impotence. Neurotoxicity (lack of concentration, depression, psychosis) is more common in patients with psychiatric problems and those older than 60 years.

Stem Cell Transplantation

Matched related allogeneic SCT can cure a proportion of carefully selected patients with suitable donors. In most studies of chronic phase CML, projected 3-year to 5-year survival rates range between 50% and 60% and up to 80% at large centers. Relapses occur in 15% to 30% of patients, usually within 5 years; however, late relapses after transplant can occur. Transplant-related mortality (TRM) ranges between 10% and 40% but can be as high as 70% in older patients who receive bone marrow from mismatched or unrelated donors. Several factors influence transplant outcome. These include age, CML phase, pretransplant chemotherapy, preparative regimen, and graft-versus-host disease (GVHD) prophylaxis. Younger patients have the best outcome, with older patients experiencing increased TRM and graft-versus-host disease (GVHD). Disease-free survival rates decrease from 40% to 60% in chronic phase to less than 15% in blastic phase.

Timing of transplantation in chronic phase is controversial. Some centers propose transplantation within 1 year of diagnosis. However, recent data suggest similar rates of 5-year disease-free survival for transplants performed within 12 to 24 months from diagnosis. Prior therapy with IFN does not appear to affect outcome of matched related SCT if it is discontinued more than 3 months before transplantation. The influence of IFN on matched unrelated donor transplantation is more controversial. T-cell depletion before transplantation improves tolerance and reduces TRM. However, this advantage is offset by increased leukemia relapse, indicating the importance of GVL-effect in maintaining remission in CML. IFN may induce durable cytogenetic remissions in 20% to 40% of patients with cytogenetic relapse after allogeneic SCT. Donor lymphocyte infusions (DLI) have generated CHR and cytogenetic responses in approximately 75% of patients. Disease-free survival at 3 years is between 40% and 85%. Responses are considerably less frequent and short-lived in transformed CML phases. DLI toxicity includes myelosuppression and induction of GVHD.

MANAGEMENT OF ACCELERATED AND BLASTIC PHASE CML

The treatment outcome of the transformed phases of CML remains unsatisfactory. IFN has no role in this phase of the disease and outcome with SCT is poor. In one third of CML patients who develop blastic phase disease, the blasts have a lymphoid phenotype, although myeloid markers may be coexpressed. Other patients have a myeloid or undifferentiated phenotype. Patients with lymphoid blastic phase respond to regimens active in acute lymphocytic leukemia (ALL). The CR rate is 60%, with half of the patients achieving a cytogenetic response; remission duration is 9 to 12 months. Patients with myeloid blastic phase have a CR rate of only 20% to 30% when treated with AML-type regimens. Recently, decitabine, a hypomethylating agent, and the BCR-ABL tyrosine kinase inhibitor (STI)-571, have shown activity in advanced phase disease.

New Agents and Modalities

The plant alkaloid Homoharringtonine* (HHT) has produced significant CHR and cytogenetic response rates in CML. To avoid the cardiovascular side effects of bolus administration, the drug is given by continuous infusion for 5 to 14 days at a dose of 2.5 mg/m^2. A CHR rate of 92% and a cytogenetic response rate of 68% were achieved in patients given six cycles of HHT for remission induction followed by IFN maintenance. Trials evaluating the combinations of HHT plus IFN and ara-C are underway with promising early results. Modifying IFN by attaching it to polyethylene glycol (PEG) results in a longer half-life. This agent can be given once a week (subcutaneously) instead of daily and may have less toxicity and the potential for overcoming resistance to the parent compound.

The most recent progress made in the treatment of CML is with the use of a specific tyrosine kinase inhibitor. Based on promising preclinical studies of signal transduction inhibitor (STI)-571* that showed inhibition of BCR-ABL in vitro, phase I clinical studies have been conducted in patients with CML in chronic and transformed phases. At daily oral doses of 300 mg and higher, STI-571 yielded a CHR rate of 96% and a cytogenetic response rate of 33% in patients with chronic phase CML who had failed IFN therapy. STI-571 was well tolerated with no dose-limiting toxicity except for myelosuppression at doses of greater than 300 mg. Recently, a multicenter phase II trial confirmed this significant activity of STI-571 in chronic phase CML. Among 532 patients refractory to or intolerant of IFN, STI-571 at 400 mg daily yielded a CHR rate of 90% and a major cytogenetic response rate of 56% in patients completing 6 months of therapy. A randomized clinical trial comparing STI-571 with IFA plus low-dose ara-C in patients with early chronic phase CML is ongoing. Although

*Investigational drug in the United States.

STI-571 has yielded hematologic and cytogenetic responses in blastic phase CML, these responses have been transient, underscoring the need for continued efforts to find effective therapy for transformed CML.

NON-HODGKIN'S LYMPHOMA

method of
JOHN P. LEONARD, M.D., and
MORTON COLEMAN, M.D.
*Weill Medical College of Cornell University and New York Presbyterian Hospital
New York, New York*

The non-Hodgkin's lymphomas (NHLs) are a heterogeneous group of tumors arising from lymph nodes and extranodal lymph tissue. These malignancies have traditionally been classified by morphology; however, more recently, immunophenotypic and molecular analysis have been recognized as critical to accurate diagnosis. Although staging is of some importance, precise classification of the NHL subtype is key in establishing the prognosis and appropriate therapy for a given setting. Some types of NHL have an indolent, but slowly progressive and incurable course. Aggressive tumors generally have a more rapid growth pattern but may often be cured with chemotherapy and/or radiotherapy. Lymphoma has been in the forefront in the development of biologic therapy for cancer, the most prominent of which is monoclonal antibody therapy. The addition of radioisotopes to antibodies (radioimmunotherapy) and vaccine therapy are promising new modalities currently under evaluation. The incidence of NHL has been on the rise over recent years. Although viruses (such as HIV) and environmental exposure (such as pesticides) may play a role, most patients affected with NHL have no definable cause of their disease. Unfortunately, most patients with NHL are not cured of their disease, and these malignancies remain a significant challenge to oncologists at the present time.

CLASSIFICATION

Adequate tissue for evaluation is of critical importance for the accurate diagnosis and classification of NHL. If at all possible, adequate tissue should be provided through an excisional lymph node biopsy. In some cases, a core needle biopsy (under computed tomographic guidance) is all that is practical (such as with abdominal lymphadenopathy only), although such a biopsy may be suboptimal. Fine-needle aspirates are usually inadequate because they do not allow assessment of lymph node architecture. Pathology review generally includes histologic analysis, as well as immunophenotyping by flow cytometry or immunohistochemistry. Immunophenotyping allows more precise diagnosis by providing characterization of the antigens expressed on the malignant cells. These markers allow more definitive classification as B-cell or T-cell NHL, as well as further subtyping. Molecular studies for genetic translocations or to establish clonality (such as through analysis of immunoglobulin gene rearrangements) may also be helpful in some cases. At the present time, the most widely used classification system is the Revised European and American Lymphoma (REAL) classification (Table 1), which has generally replaced several older schema. The REAL classification separates NHL into B-cell (roughly 90%) and T-cell or natural killer cell types, with further subclassification within these groups based on morphology and immunophenotype. A newer classification system, the World Health Organization system, has recently been developed but is quite similar to the REAL system in most instances.

TABLE 1. **Summary of the WHO Classification of Some Tumors of Hematopoietic and Lymphoid Tissues**

B-Cell Neoplasms	
Precursor B-Cell Neoplasm	
Precursor B-lymphoblastic leukemia[1]/lymphoma[2]	9835/3[1] 9728/3[2]
Mature B-Cell Neoplasms	
Chronic lymphocytic leukemia[1]/small lymphocytic lymphoma[2]	9823/3[1] 9670/3[2]
B-cell prolymphocytic leukemia	9833/3
Lymphoplasmacytic lymphoma	9671/3
Splenic marginal zone lymphoma	9689/3
Hairy cell leukemia	9940/3
Plasma cell myeloma	9732/3
Solitary plasmacytoma of bone	9731/3
Extraosseous plasmacytoma	9734/3
Extranodal marginal zone B-cell lymphoma of mucosa-associated lymphoid tissue (MALT-lymphoma)	9699/3
Nodal marginal zone B-cell lymphoma	9699/3
Follicular lymphoma	9690/3
Mantle cell lymphoma	9673/3
Diffuse large B-cell lymphoma	9680/3
Mediastinal (thymic) large B-cell lymphoma	9679/3
Intravascular large B-cell lymphoma	9680/3
Primary effusion lymphoma	9678/3
Burkitt lymphoma[1]/leukemia[2]	9687/3[1] 9826/3[2]
B-Cell Proliferations of Uncertain Malignant Potential	
Lymphomatoid granulomatosis	9766/1
Post-transplant lymphoproliferative disorder, polymorphic	9970/1
T-Cell and NK-Cell Neoplasms	
Precursor T-Cell Neoplasms	
Precursor T lymphoblastic leukemia[1]/lymphoma[2]	9837/3[1] 9729/3[2]
Blastic NK cell lymphoma†	9727/3
Mature T-Cell and NK-Cell Neoplasms	
T-cell prolymphocytic leukemia	9834/3
T-cell large granular lymphocytic leukemia	9831/3
Aggressive NK cell leukemia	9948/3
Adult T-cell leukemia/lymphoma	9827/3
Extranodal NK/T cell lymphoma, nasal type	9719/3
Enteropathy-type T-cell lymphoma	9717/3
Hepatosplenic T-cell lymphoma	9716/3
Subcutaneous panniculitis-like T-cell lymphoma	9708/3
Mycosis fungoides	9700/3
Sezary syndrome	9701/3
Primary cutaneous anaplastic large cell lymphoma	9718/3
Peripheral T-cell lymphoma, unspecified	9702/3
Angiomimmunoblastic T-cell lymphoma	9705/3
Anaplastic large cell lymphoma	9714/3
T-Cell Proliferation of Uncertain Malignant Potential	
Lymphomatoid papulosis	9718/1

*Morphology code of the International Classification of Diseases (ICD-O), third edition. Behavior is coded /3 for malignant tumors and /1 for lesions of low or uncertain malignant potential.

†Neoplasm of uncertain lineage and stage of differentiation.

From Jaffe ES, Harris NL, Stein H, Vardiman JW (eds): World Health Organization Classification of Tumours. Pathology and Genetics of Tumours of Haematopoietic and Lymphoid Tissues. France, IARC Press, Lyon, 2001.

STAGING AND PROGNOSTIC FACTOR ASSESSMENT

A number of staging procedures (Table 2) are generally performed to assess the extent of disease in patients with NHL, and several of these tests may be repeated at various times throughout the course of the disease to determine response to therapy.

Table 2. **Staging Workup**

History of B symptoms: fever, sweats, weight loss
Detailed physical examination
Adequate node biopsy
Blood work: complete blood count, biochemical profile including serum LDH and β-2M, serum protein electrophoresis, ESR, HIV serology
Bone marrow aspirate and biopsy (bilateral in indolent lymphoma)
Chest radiograph
CT scans of chest, abdomen, and pelvis
Lymphangiogram
Gallium scan
PET scan
± Bone scan, GI workup, CSF examination

Abbreviations: CBC = complete blood count; CSF = cerebrospinal fluid; CT = computed tomography; ESR = erythrocyte sedimentation rate; GI = gastrointestinal; LDH = lactate dehydrogenase; β-2M = β_2-microglobulin; PET = positron emission tomography.

Once the disease burden has been fully assessed, patients are described as ranging from stage I through stage IV in the most widely used Ann Arbor staging system (Table 3). Staging in NHL is less important than in most other cancers because most lymphomas are not localized, and the histologic classification becomes the critical factor in determining prognosis and treatment. For example, advanced-stage patients (such as stage IV) with NHL can still be cured if they have an aggressive type of disease, whereas those with stage IV indolent NHL are generally considered incurable. However, staging can provide some prognostic information, if only by directly reflecting tumor burden, and can be important in guiding appropriate therapy. Several important findings in a staging evaluation can prompt more specific investigation and therapies. For instance, NHL involvement of the Waldeyer ring area is commonly associated with gastrointestinal tract involvement and may suggest that endoscopic evaluation is indicated. Bone marrow involvement of aggressive lymphomas is associated with central nervous system (CNS) involvement in roughly 20% of cases, and thus cerebrospinal fluid evaluation and prophylactic intrathecal chemotherapy may be warranted.

The most valuable prognostic information in NHL is provided by the "International Prognostic Index," which was developed through an extensive analysis of patients with aggressive NHL in the International Non-Hodgkin's Prognostic Factor Project. This index has provided four separate risk categories as defined by five characteristics present at the time of diagnosis (Table 4).

Table 3. **Ann Arbor Staging System**

Stage I	One lymph node (LN) region or one extranodal organ or site (IE)
Stage II	Two or more LN regions on the same side of the diaphragm or one localized extranodal organ or site (IIE) and one or more LN regions on the same side of the diaphragm
Stage III	LN regions on both sides of the diaphragm
Stage IIIE	Stage III plus localized involvement of one extranodal organ or site or the spleen (IIIS) or both (IIISE)
Stage IV	One or more extranodal organs with or without associated LN involvement (diffuse or disseminated)

Table 4. **Alternative Prognosticating Systems for Non-Hodgkin's Lymphoma**

International Index		
Parameter	*Criteria*	*Score*
Age	<60 y	0
	>60 y	1
Ann Arbor stage	I–II	0
	III–IV	1
Serum LDH level	Normal	0
	Higher than normal	1
Performance status	0–1	0
	>1	1
Extranodal sites	0–1	0
	>1	1

Score	**Risk**
0, 1	Low
2	Low-intermediate
3	High-intermediate
4, 5	High

These factors take into account features that reflect the characteristics of tumor biology and extent (lactate dehydrogenase, stage, and extranodal disease) and the ability of the patient to successfully tolerate therapy (age and performance status). This score is widely used in the assessment of patients with aggressive NHL and may be of some utility for patients with more indolent histologies. More sophisticated pathologic evaluations (including cytogenetic analysis and expression of protein products of genetic translocations, such as the bcl-2 protein derived from the translocation of chromosomes 14 and 18) are gaining more widespread use and may potentially be helpful in establishing the prognosis. Very recently, computer chip analysis of gene expression in NHL samples has been studied and has established genetic "signatures" that may correlate with prognosis. After further study in the near future, this "lymphochip" analysis may rapidly provide detailed information that may ultimately specifically define the prognosis and guide therapy based on genetic profiling.

MANAGEMENT

For the purposes of treatment, with some exceptions, lymphomas are generally categorized broadly as clinically indolent, aggressive, and highly aggressive entities.

Indolent B-Cell Lymphomas

Indolent lymphomas constitute approximately 40% to 50% of cases of NHL and consist of a number of entities in the REAL classification, including small cell lymphocytic lymphoma/chronic lymphocytic leukemia; follicle center lymphoma, follicular grades 1 and 2 (small cleaved and mixed small cell and large cell); and marginal zone lymphoma. The clinical features and course of these disorders generally include advanced stage at diagnosis, long median survival (at least 8 to 10 years), relatively slow disease progression, high initial response rates to treatment with recurrences and treatment resistance developing over time, possibility of transformation to a more aggressive NHL subtype, and low chance of ultimate cure. The clinical course of patients with these entities may be quite variable, and prognostic scores have been of little value in predicting an individual patient's ultimate course. Some patients may be refractory to even their initial course of chemotherapy, whereas others may have an initial remission lasting decades. This variability in conjunction with the usual slow pace of disease makes clinical trials to assess treatments more complicated, and relatively fewer randomized studies have been performed. Hence, a number of different treatment regimens are available that can induce a response in the disease, but a clear standard chemotherapy program has not been established for the indolent lymphomas.

Management of Localized Disease

A relatively small group of patients will initially be seen with localized indolent lymphoma. These patients are generally treated with involved-field radiation therapy (doses of 30 to 40 cGy), which can induce significant long-term responses in most patients. The idea of cure is a controversial one for this patient population. Given the propensity for disease dissemination in low-grade lymphoma, most patients with apparently localized disease actually have microscopic tumor elsewhere that is not detectable by conventional means. When these patients have recurrent disease, it typically occurs outside the radiation field, thus suggesting that the disease was truly of undetected advanced stage at initial diagnosis. Nevertheless, the observation of long-term remissions (even lasting decades) in some individuals suggests that local radiation therapy can be quite effective. The addition of chemotherapy to radiation treatment is of uncertain benefit because of the limitations of this modality in low-grade NHL, and it is not usually included.

Management of Disseminated Disease

Understanding an individual patient's symptoms and overall situation is critical in the determination of therapy for advanced-stage indolent NHL. Options range from no therapy (if asymptomatic) to single-agent chemotherapy, multiagent treatment, and high-dose chemotherapy with autologous or allogeneic stem cell transplantation. More recently, monoclonal antibody therapy (with rituximab [Rituxan], a chimeric antibody directed against the CD20 B-cell antigen) has been established as a safe and effective modality in this setting. Other biologic agents such as interferon may convey an antilymphoma effect. Exciting investigational agents include other monoclonal antibodies targeting different antigens, radiolabeled monoclonal antibodies that augment the immunotherapy with targeted irradiation, tumor-specific vaccines and antisense molecules, and "mini-allogeneic" transplants (conveying less toxicity than a conventional allotransplant). This array of options for this generally incurable, but indolent malignancy can be quite confusing for patients and clinicians. A conservative approach is followed in some settings because early institution of treatment has not been demonstrated to convey a survival advantage in asymptomatic patients. The "watch and wait" approach is commonly used for the group of patients with no symptoms and minimal disease burden, with the institution of therapy delayed until symptoms or evidence of significant disease progression occurs. This approach is appealing to some individuals who wish to avoid treatment, and it minimizes therapy-associated toxicity. Other approaches for asymptomatic patients, such as early institution of chemotherapy, more intense treatments, or the application of new agents such as those described previously, are of uncertain benefit but hold great promise and are under intense investigation. Symptomatic patients (or those with rapidly progressive or bulky disease) can clearly benefit from institution of therapy, although comparative data between different regimens are limited. Whereas certain patients (and clinicians) prefer programs that intervene as little as possible, others find the "minimalist" approach more difficult psychologically and wish to be more aggressive in their management. Optimism about the potential for newer treatments must be balanced with realism about treatment limitations and the possibility of long-term toxicity. Given the limited comparative information available about different therapeutic regimens, choices are usually guided by patient and clinician expectations and individual preferences. For this group of patients in particular, enrollment in clinical trials that are assessing new regimens or comparing them with older ones is especially encouraged.

Single-agent therapy has traditionally included oral chlorambucil (Leukeran) or cyclophosphamide (Cytoxan), administered on an outpatient basis. This approach remains quite reasonable for many settings and is more widely used in elderly patients. Combinations, particularly the more commonly used CVP (cyclophosphamide/vincristine/prednisone), have not been shown to have a clear advantage over single agents (Table 5). The CHOP regimen (cyclophosphamide/doxorubicin/vincristine/prednisone), long the standard therapy for aggressive NHL, is also widely used. The addition of doxorubicin, an anthracycline, may contribute to a more rapid response and has been shown to be of benefit in one study of follicular, mixed NHL, although it can add toxicity. Purine analogues have emerged as another treatment option, including fludarabine* (Fludara) and 2-chlorodeoxyadenosine. These agents have a slightly different toxicity profile (predominantly cytopenia and immunosuppression) and also result in a high response rate. Combination regimens have been developed (including FND—fludarabine/mitoxantrone*/dexamethasone—and fludarabine/cyclophosphamide), but any potential advantages have yet to be conclusively proven. In all of these chemotherapy-based treatments, it appears that initial overall response rates are high (complete response rates ranging in the

*Not FDA approved for this indication.

TABLE 5. **Chemotherapy for Indolent Lymphomas**

Regimen	Dose
Single Agent	
Chlorambucil (Leukeran)	14–16 mg/m² daily × 5 d PO q21–28d or 0.1–0.2 mg/kg daily for 4–6 wk
Cyclophosphamide (Cytoxan)	500–1000 mg/m² IV q21–28d or 60–100 mg/m² PO qd
Combination	
CVP (21-d cycle)	
Cyclophosphamide	400 mg/m² daily PO d 1–5
Vincristine (Oncovin)	1.4 mg/m² IV d 1
Prednisone	100 mg/m² daily PO d 1–5
CHOP (21-d cycle)	
Cyclophosphamide	750 mg/m² IV d 1
Doxorubicin* (Adriamycin)	50 mg/m² IV d 1 or infused over 72 h
Vincristine	1.4 mg/m² IV d 1
Prednisone	100 mg/m² daily PO d 1–5
Purine Analogues	
Fludarabine (Fludara) (4-wk cycle)	25 mg/m² daily IV d 1–5
Cladribine† (Leustatin)	0.14 mg/kg daily IV d 1–5

*Formerly hydroxydaunomycin.
†Cladribine is 2-chlorodeoxyadenosine (2-CDA).

10% to 50% range), with response durations lasting months to several years. However, virtually all patients relapse. Second-line and subsequent courses of treatment are generally associated with lower response rates and shorter remissions.

Rituximab (anti-CD20) monoclonal antibody therapy was first developed for indolent lymphoma. This antibody has the potential to mediate an antilymphoma effect through antibody-dependent cellular cytotoxicity, complement-mediated cytotoxicity, induction of apoptosis of tumor cells, and other potential mechanisms. In relapsed indolent NHL, approximately 50% of patients receiving a course of four weekly infusions achieve an objective response, with roughly 5% complete responders. Activity is greater in the follicular subtypes, with less effect in the small lymphocytic lymphoma/chronic lymphocytic leukemia group of patients. This treatment is generally well tolerated, has non-overlapping toxicity with chemotherapy, and is a useful option for many patients. Efforts to capitalize on the possibility of synergy between rituximab and chemotherapy have led to its combination with virtually every regimen. Additional toxicity can be seen but is unusual, and assessment of additional antitumor effects is under evaluation in randomized trials. Other antibodies, such as epratuzumab (directed against the CD22 antigen) and Hu1D10 (against HLA-DR), appear to be promising new agents and are under evaluation in clinical trials. Radioimmunoconjugates, which incorporate radioactive iodine 131 or yttrium 90 with a monoclonal antibody, seem to have augmented activity over the unlabeled antibodies because they include the antitumor modality of target irradiation. Two compounds in clinical trials that also target the CD20 antigen include iodine I 131 tositumomab* (Bexxar) and yttrium Y90 ibritumomab tiuxetan* (Zevalin). Radioimmunotherapy has been predominantly assessed as a single agent in indolent NHL, and combination regimens with chemotherapy appear to hold significant promise.

Interferon-alfa is used in some centers as part of the treatment regimen for indolent NHL. Some evidence has suggested that interferon may prolong remission duration after chemotherapy and may improve overall survival when used in this setting. Other studies have not demonstrated this benefit. The uncertain clinical benefit and toxicity profile of the agent have limited its widespread use for NHL in the United States, although interferon is more commonly used in Europe.

High-dose chemotherapy with peripheral blood stem cell rescue has been evaluated as therapy for indolent NHL. The rationale is justified because chemotherapy can induce a disease response and higher doses of treatment (which require previous stem cell collection, cryopreservation, and later reinfusion) may result in better efficacy. Some studies have also incorporated a variety of stem cell "purging" methods including monoclonal antibodies to remove tumor cells from the stem cell product. Although long-term remissions have been observed and are more common when the procedure is performed early in the course of disease (such as in "first remission") rather than later, it is not clear that the procedure can be curative. Allogeneic transplantation, which is without risk of tumor cell contamination in the stem cell infusate and conveys the potential added immunotherapy of a "graft-versus-lymphoma" effect, has also been associated with long-term remissions and possible cure. The toxicity of this procedure has been reduced by using mini-allogeneic transplants, which incorporate less intensive chemotherapy but keep the immunologic component intact. Follow-up is short in this newer technique, but early results are encouraging. Optimal timing for the use of these more intensive (and toxic), though possibly curative treatments is unclear, particularly in light of the generally indolent nature of the underlying disease and the array of novel treatment options under development.

Aggressive Lymphomas

Patients with aggressive lymphoma are generally treated with curative intent with combination chemotherapy (Table 6) at the time of diagnosis. These entities in the REAL classification include diffuse large B-cell lymphoma (most common), primary mediastinal large B-cell lymphoma, anaplastic large cell lymphoma of T-cell and null cell types, and peripheral T-cell lymphoma. Although a number of treatment regimens have been developed and continue to be assessed, randomized trials have resulted in the generally accepted standard being CHOP for most clinical situations. Given the goal of treatment in this

*Investigational drug in the United States.

TABLE 6. **Chemotherapy for Aggressive Lymphomas**

Regimen	Dose
CHOP	
Cyclophosphamide (Cytoxan)	750 mg/m² IV d 1
Doxorubicin (Adriamycin)	50 mg/m² IV d 1 or infused over 72 h
Vincristine (Oncovin)	1.4 mg/m² IV d 1
Prednisone	100 mg/m² daily PO d 1–5

patient population, maintenance of dose intensity is paramount to avoid compromise of the chance for cure.

Management of Localized Disease

Early-stage (I or II) disease is more commonly found in the aggressive lymphomas than in the indolent subtypes. The standard of care for this group of patients is CHOP for three cycles and involved-field radiotherapy. This combination therapy has been established in a randomized trial to be superior to a full course (eight cycles) of chemotherapy alone. Three quarters of patients with limited disease treated in this fashion will ultimately be cured of their disease. Certain individuals with poor prognostic features, such as elevated serum lactate dehydrogenase or bulky disease, despite their limited stage, may be considered for more intensive approaches.

Management of Disseminated Disease

The standard approach for patients with disseminated aggressive lymphoma is six to eight cycles of multiagent chemotherapy with the CHOP regimen. Although other regimens have been evaluated with promising results, little evidence has been found in randomized trials to currently suggest any superiority. These programs have incorporated continuous infusion rather than bolus schedules, alternating regimens of different drugs, or various other agents. The recent availability of rituximab monoclonal antibody therapy has led to the development of combinations with CHOP. A recent French study has suggested an advantage of CHOP plus rituximab over CHOP alone in patients older than 60 years with respect to response rates and 1-year survival. Follow-up is ongoing in this and another randomized multicenter study in the United States that is also evaluating this issue. One important scenario in aggressive lymphoma is that involving bone marrow infiltration with malignant lymphocytes, which occurs roughly 10% of the time. This finding is associated with a risk of CNS involvement, and these patients often receive additional intrathecal chemotherapy and/or radiation therapy as part of their treatment regimen. Treatment of patients with bulky disease, primarily in the mediastinum, is often augmented with radiotherapy after chemotherapy. This addition has been demonstrated to improve disease-free survival in some patients.

Response rates and overall survival in aggressive lymphomas have been correlated with the International Prognostic Index (see Table 4). Given the poor overall prognosis of individuals falling into the higher risk groups, attempts have been made to intensify therapy to improve the ultimate outcome. Some studies have suggested a benefit with the incorporation of high-dose chemotherapy and stem cell transplantation as first-line treatment after initial CHOP chemotherapy. This issue is being actively investigated in an ongoing randomized U.S. multicenter study.

Salvage chemotherapy regimens for patients who are either refractory to or have relapsed from initial therapy generally incorporate a number of chemotherapy agents different from those in CHOP, commonly including ifosfamide* (Ifex), cisplatin* (Platinol) or carboplatin* (Paraplatin), etoposide* (Toposar), and cytarabine* (Cytosar). The prognosis is better in patients with a longer duration of first remission, but efficacy is poor for those who are refractory to their initial regimen of chemotherapy. Although patients may occasionally be cured with standard doses of second-line agents, the best long-term results are observed when chemotherapy-sensitive patients in second response receive high-dose chemotherapy and stem cell transplantation. This more intensive type of program is generally limited to patients with a reasonably good performance status that will allow them to withstand the rigors of the therapy. Allogeneic stem cell transplantation is less commonly performed. The potential role of mini-allogeneic transplants is under active investigation.

Immunotherapy with single-agent rituximab has demonstrated less activity in the aggressive lymphomas in both the up-front and relapsed setting. Rituximab has been combined with a number of salvage regimens, including stem cell transplantation, and the role of the antibody in these settings is presently unclear. Other investigational antibodies, including epratuzumab† have demonstrated activity as single agents in this patient population. Radioimmunoconjugates have been less extensively evaluated in relapsed aggressive NHL, although yttrium 90–labeled epratuzumab has shown encouraging initial results, and the CD20-based radioimmunoconjugates and iodine 131 Lym-1 (targeting HLA-DR) also appear to have antitumor effects. With more widespread use of these therapeutic modalities, it is anticipated that their roles will be more clearly defined.

Mantle cell lymphoma is a distinct entity in the REAL classification that combines the worst features of the indolent and aggressive lymphomas. The pace of the disease can be more rapid, with a median survival of 36 months or less, and it is incurable in the vast majority of cases. CVP, CHOP, intensive hyper-CVAD, or other multiagent chemotherapy regimens seem to result in temporary remissions, and high-dose chemotherapy with stem cell transplantation is of uncertain benefit. Some investigators have

*Not FDA approved for this indication.
†Investigational drug in the United States.

advocated allogeneic stem cell transplantation for eligible patients.

Highly Aggressive Lymphomas

The highly aggressive lymphomas are less common in adults and include Burkitt's lymphoma, Burkitt's-like lymphoma, and lymphoblastic lymphoma. More commonly found in patients with HIV infection and in children or young adults, these tumors are characterized by a rapid growth rate, high risk of tumor lysis, and a propensity for CNS involvement. Treatment regimens consist of multiple agents and include CNS prophylaxis (intrathecal chemotherapy or radiotherapy). Lymphoblastic lymphoma therapies are comparable to those used in acute lymphocytic leukemia. Commonly incorporated drugs include cyclophosphamide, vincristine, corticosteroids, doxorubicin, methotrexate and cytarabine. Reported cure rates have been very high, although treatment-associated toxicity can be significant in certain individuals, particularly the elderly. Autologous and allogeneic stem cell transplants are frequently used in high-risk or relapsed settings.

AIDS-Related Lymphomas

The incidence of lymphoma is significantly increased in HIV-positive individuals in comparison to the general population. Tumors are predominantly of the aggressive NHL subtypes and are characterized by rapid growth rates with more frequent CNS or extranodal site involvement. Toxicities may be compounded by reduced bone marrow reserve and the development of opportunistic infections. Response rates to chemotherapy and overall survival are generally diminished in this group of patients. CHOP chemotherapy is commonly administered, but other regimens such as reduced-dose m-BACOD (methotrexate with leucovorin [Wellcovorin] rescue, bleomycin, doxorubicin, cyclophosphamide, vincristine, dexamethasone) have been used as well. Hematopoietic growth factor support, antiretroviral agents, and infection prophylaxis for opportunistic pathogens are important adjuncts to therapy. Primary CNS lymphomas occur at an increased frequency in AIDS patients relative to others and account for up to one third of lymphomas in this population. Because the diagnosis can be confused with opportunistic infections such as toxoplasmosis, a brain biopsy, if feasible, may be very helpful in determining pathology. Radiation therapy is generally administered in this setting with palliative intent, although survival is usually measured in months. In contrast, primary CNS lymphomas are rare in non-immunocompromised patients, although with significantly better results, including some cures noted with multiagent chemotherapy alone or in combination with radiotherapy.

Gastrointestinal Lymphomas

The most common site of extranodal involvement of NHL is the gastrointestinal tract, with most of these lymphomas being gastric. A number of different histologic subtypes are frequently observed in this region, including the indolent mucosa-associated lymphoid tissue (MALT), diffuse large B-cell, and mantle cell types. Gastric MALTomas have been associated with *Helicobacter pylori* infection, and antibiotic therapy can often result in cure in selected patients. These individuals can be monitored endoscopically for response and receive either chemotherapy, radiotherapy, or surgery if initial treatment fails. Except in selected cases, given that comparable or greater response rates are obtained with less morbidity, chemotherapeutic approaches have largely supplanted surgery for more aggressive histologies. The role of radiotherapy is unclear, but it is often applied in localized or bulky disease settings. Mantle cell lymphoma is most commonly associated with disseminated disease, including the gastrointestinal tract, and is usually treated with systemic chemotherapy with limited long-term results. Overall, treatment goals for lymphomas include minimizing morbidity in the curative setting while preventing obstruction in palliative situations.

MULTIPLE MYELOMA

method of
CHRISTINE I. CHEN, M.D., and
A. KEITH STEWART, M.D.
Princess Margaret Hospital
Toronto, Ontario, Canada

Multiple myeloma is a malignancy arising from a single clone of malignant plasma cells that proliferate and accumulate in the bone marrow. These plasma cells typically produce an immunoglobulin, also referred to as a *monoclonal protein* (M protein), which can be detected in blood, urine, or both. Myeloma is not a common disease (incidence of 3 to 4 per 100,000/y) and mainly affects older individuals (median age, 65 years). Because myeloma is a relatively slow-growing malignancy, many patients will have had the disease for months or even years before diagnosis and may continue to follow an indolent course. The pathogenesis is poorly understood, but triggers for malignant transformation of plasma cells (radiation or toxin exposure, viral infections such as human herpesvirus-8, and acquired or inherited genetic mutations) have been hypothesized.

CLINICAL FEATURES

Characteristic clinical features of multiple myeloma are anemia, renal failure, bony lesions with pathologic fractures and associated pain, hypercalcemia, and recurrent infections (Table 1). These features may result directly from mass accumulations of plasma cells in tissues (plasmacytomas) or indirectly from effects of the M protein and/or cytokines secreted by plasma cells. Many patients, however, will present with asymptomatic anemia or monoclonal gammopathy discovered on incidental laboratory testing.

TABLE 1. **Clinical Features of Multiple Myeloma**

Skeletal

"Punched out" lytic bone lesions (skull, long bones common)
Generalized osteoporosis
Pathologic fractures and bone pain

Renal

Renal dysfunction due to light-chain toxicity and/or deposition, hypercalcemia, amyloid deposition

Hematologic

Cytopenias (anemia common) due to plasma cell infiltration of bone marrow, renal failure, anemia of chronic disease
Bleeding tendency—mostly due to interference of coagulation by M protein or thrombocytopenia from marrow infiltration
Hyperviscosity syndrome—visual changes, headache, confusion, bleeding, coma, "sausage veins" on fundoscopy

Neurologic

Cord compression from vertebral collapse and/or plasmacytoma
Mental changes (may be due to hyperviscosity, hypercalcemia)
Peripheral neuropathy due to M protein, amyloidosis

Metabolic

Hypercalcemia—confusion, polyuria, polydipsia, constipation, weakness, fatigue

Immunologic

Predisposition to recurrent infections due to suppression and dysfunction of normal immunoglobulins or neutropenia from chemotheraphy

LABORATORY FEATURES

The vast majority (99%) of patients with myeloma will have a serum M protein measurable by serum protein electrophoresis and/or a urine M protein with excreted light chains (Bence Jones protein) detectable by electrophoresis of a 24-hour urine collection. The heavy- and light-chain components of the M protein can be identified by immunoelectrophoresis or immunofixation. The most common immunoglobulin subtype is IgG (60%), followed by IgA (20%), light chains alone (10%), and, less commonly, IgD, IgE, and IgM (<10%). In approximately 1% of patients, no M protein in either serum or urine can be detected. A bone marrow aspirate and biopsy will show an increase of plasma cells (>10%) that often have immature morphologic features. Other characteristic but less specific laboratory findings include a normocytic, normochromic anemia, *rouleaux* ("stacked coin" appearance) of red blood cells on peripheral film analysis, and an elevated sedimentation rate. Presence of one of these nonspecific findings that is not otherwise explained clinically should trigger an investigation for multiple myeloma.

RADIOLOGIC FINDINGS

A skeletal survey that includes plain radiographs of the skull, ribs, spine, pelvis, shoulders, and long bones of the limbs is used to identify osteopenia or typical "punched out" lesions of myeloma. Because myeloma lesions are osteolytic in nature, a bone scan that best detects osteoblastic lesions is not generally useful. Computed tomography (CT) or magnetic resonance imaging (MRI) may be used to delineate plasmacytomas, particularly in areas of cord compression requiring urgent treatment. MRI of the spine is sensitive in detecting patchy plasma cell involvement of the bone marrow and may be used for this purpose when a skeletal survey is negative but the index of suspicion for myeloma is high.

DIAGNOSIS

The diagnosis of multiple myeloma requires a greater than 10% bone marrow plasmacytosis plus one of the following (Table 2):

1. A serum M protein level
2. A urine M protein level
3. Lytic bone lesions or generalized osteoporosis as seen on skeletal survey
4. Presence of a soft tissue plasmacytoma

Patients with greater than 10% bone marrow plasmacytosis *without* bone lesions or other clinical manifestations of myeloma are considered to have *smoldering myeloma.* Asymptomatic patients with less than 10% bone marrow plasmacytosis, low concentrations of M protein in urine or blood, and absent bone lesions or cytopenias have a *monoclonal gammopathy of uncertain significance* (MGUS). MGUS may be difficult to distinguish from smoldering or early-stage myeloma. Features that may help to support a diagnosis of myeloma include reciprocal depression of the normal immunoglobulin levels, high paraprotein concentration (>30 g/L in serum or 1 g/d urinary M protein), and abnormal plasma cell morphology (e.g., immature forms, multinuclearity). Although neither MGUS nor smoldering myeloma requires immediate therapy, it is nevertheless important to distinguish between the two because prognoses differ.

Amyloidosis is a complication of myeloma whereby amyloid fibrils composed of components of the M protein deposit in tissues and cause organ dysfunction. This disorder should be suspected in myeloma patients with progressive neuropathy, cardiac dysfunction with hypotension, enlarged tongue, swollen joints, hepatomegaly, or nephrotic syndrome. A needle biopsy of involved tissue for special staining is most likely to yield a diagnosis, but if the area is inaccessible, blind abdominal fat pad needle aspirates may be helpful.

STAGING AND PROGNOSTIC FACTORS

Staging systems (such as the Salmon-Durie system) use a variety of clinical factors that correlate with tumor cell mass and survival. These systems tend to be less reliable than objective prognostic testing. Bone marrow cytogenetics, serum β_2-microglobulin and C-reactive protein in combination, and plasma cell labeling index are powerful prognostic factors but are not always widely available.

TABLE 2. **Investigations in Multiple Myeloma**

1. Serum protein electrophoresis
2. 24-Hour urine collection for total protein quantitation
3. Immunoelectrophoresis or immunofixation of serum and urine
4. Complete blood cell count with differential and reticulocyte counts
5. Serum creatinine, calcium, uric acid, electrolytes, lactate dehydrogenase, and alkaline phosphatase determinations
6. Bone marrow aspirate and biopsy for plasma cell percentage; cytogenetics recommended
7. Skeletal survey
8. If indicated, biopsy of soft tissue masses
9. If available, β_2-microglobulin, C-reactive protein, plasma cell labeling index
10. If suspect hyperviscosity, serum viscosity test
11. If clinically indicated, cryoglobulins, magnetic resonance imaging or computed tomography of affected areas, staining for amyloidosis

TREATMENT

Although there are many treatment options for patients with multiple myeloma, there is presently no cure for the disease. The disease may remain indolent for years in many patients, particularly in those with low level M protein (<30 g/L) and absent bony lesions. Because there is no evidence that early treatment prolongs survival, therapy should be reserved for patients with symptoms. Those with smoldering myeloma should not be treated except on clinical trial. Treatment should be initiated, however, in patients with impending complications (such as bony lytic lesions predisposing to pathologic fractures) even if not yet symptomatic. Because myeloma is a systemic disorder from the onset, the primary treatment modality is chemotherapy.

Management of Complications

Renal Failure

Approximately 20% of patients with myeloma will have renal dysfunction. Prompt chemotherapy and adequate hydration are keys to management and can reverse mild dysfunction in half of the patients. Severe renal failure may require hemodialysis support to administer chemotherapy. In patients without renal failure and particularly in those with Bence Jones proteinuria, preventive hydration (3000 mL of fluid per day) is recommended. Plasmapheresis may be useful in clearing nephrotoxic light chains from the blood, but long-term benefit to renal function is not confirmed. Nonsteroidal anti-inflammatory drugs and antibiotics that may exacerbate renal dysfunction should be avoided.

Hypercalcemia

Aggressive hydration with normal saline (150–200 mL/h) and corticosteroid therapy (prednisone, 100 mg/d) generally leads to rapid resolution of hypercalcemia. Treatment directed at the myeloma should then be instituted. Intravenous bisphosphonates such as pamidronate (Aredia, 60–90 mg intravenously in a single dose) are now also commonly employed.

Anemia

Anemia is present in most patients with myeloma and is often multifactorial in etiology. Recombinant erythropoietin (Epogen) may be beneficial in severe anemia (hemoglobin ≤80 g/L), even in the absence of renal failure, because myeloma patients may have decreased levels and/or impaired response to endogenous erythropoietin. Erythropoietin doses of 300 to 450 U/kg/wk in three times weekly subcutaneous injections have led to reported hematologic responses and improved performance status in up to 70% of patients. Lower doses may be effective in patients with renal failure.

Hyperviscosity

M protein in high concentrations, particularly subtypes IgM and IgA, which are most likely to polymerize, can lead to the hyperviscosity syndrome. A serum viscosity of greater than 4 Cp (viscosity of water = 1 Cp) indicates an elevated risk of hyperviscosity. Plasmapheresis is used to acutely reduce the plasma levels of M protein and relieve symptoms, but myeloma chemotherapy should be instituted as soon as possible to decrease paraprotein production.

Bone Pain and Fractures

Bone pain may be generalized from diffuse osteoporosis or may be localized to sites of lytic bone lesions or pathologic fractures. Adequate analgesia, often requiring narcotics, is vital. Prophylactic stool softeners to avoid constipation are recommended. Painful bony lesions inadequately controlled with analgesia are best managed with localized radiation (20–30 Gy). For compression fractures of the spine, vertebroplasty is a new and effective treatment used to decrease pain and stabilize the vertebrae. In this outpatient technique, a mineral bone cement is injected percutaneously into the affected vertebral body under radiologic guidance.

Bisphosphonates are a class of drugs with antiresorptive activity in bone. Both pamidronate (Aredia) and clodronate (Bonefos or Ostac)*† have been shown to reduce the risk of skeletal events such as bone pain, pathologic fractures, and need for bone surgery or irradiation. Myeloma patients with osteoporosis or bone lesions should receive monthly infusions of pamidronate (90 mg) or oral clodronate (1600 mg/d orally) as adjuncts to chemotherapy.

Spinal Cord or Nerve Root Compression

Compression of the spinal cord or nerve roots may result from bony vertebral collapse or extradural impingement from a soft tissue plasmacytoma. Lower back pain with dermatomal radiation is a typical presenting symptom. Worrisome clinical features such as leg weakness, urinary incontinence, or obstipation indicate impending cord damage. Urgent MRI or CT is indicated to identify the site of compression. To avoid permanent paraplegia, temporizing therapy using high-dose corticosteroids (dexamethasone, 16–96 mg/d) to reduce cord edema should be initiated while arranging irradiation (25–30 Gy) to the site of impingement. This approach has now supplanted surgical laminectomy as the primary modality for decompression.

Conventional Chemotherapy

For elderly patients or those who either do not want or cannot tolerate aggressive therapy, various oral chemotherapy regimens may be used. Traditionally, combined therapy with oral melphalan (Alkeran), 9 mg/m^2, and prednisone, 100 mg (MP regimen) daily for 4 days given at 4- to 6-week intervals, has been most frequently used. Because melphalan has erratic gastrointestinal absorption, it should be

*Not approved for this indication.
†Not available in the United States.

given in the morning on an empty stomach and doses must be titrated to the mid-cycle blood cell counts. A nadir of mild neutropenia (1000–1500/μL) and/or thrombocytopenia (<100,000/μL) is recommended to ensure maximal efficacy. Severe cytopenias requiring cycle delays or transfusion support should be avoided by reducing the dose of melphalan by 2- to 4-mg/d decrements. Treatment is continued until maximal reduction in the M protein has occurred and a plateau reached for a minimum of 4 months (generally, 1 year of treatment). At this point, treatment is stopped, although recent studies have suggested a survival benefit to maintenance with prednisone (50 mg orally alternate days) with or without α-interferon (3 mU subcutaneously three times weekly). α-Interferon (Inferon) alone for maintenance therapy has been reported to prolong the duration of remission but does not generally alter overall survival. Cyclophosphamide (Cytoxan) at doses of 400 to 500 mg orally or intravenously weekly can be used in place of melphalan in selected patients. Cyclophosphamide is less likely to suppress thrombopoiesis and, unlike melphalan, has less myelosuppressive potentiation in renal failure. It is often administered in conjunction with prednisone, 100 mg orally on alternate days.

When the standard MP regimen is used, 50% to 60% of patients will respond with a greater than 50% drop in the M protein, but fewer than 5% will attain a *complete remission,* defined as complete clearing of M protein and bone marrow and no other evidence of disease. Median overall survival is 3 to 4 years. Advantages to this regimen include ease of administration and minimal toxicity. Unfortunately, alkylating agents such as melphalan predispose to late development of myelodysplasia and leukemia.

Multidrug regimens using combinations of vincristine, anthracyclines, melphalan, BCNU, cyclophosphamide, and prednisone or dexamethasone may provide a faster onset of action than melphalan and prednisone and thus may be useful in patients with high tumor loads and acute renal failure. The most common of these regimens is VAD (intravenous vincristine [Oncovin], 0.4 mg; doxorubicin [Adriamycin], 9 mg/m^2 by continuous infusion, and oral dexamethasone [Decadron], 20 mg/m^2/d for 4 days starting on days 1, 9, and 17 of each month). The VAD regimen is easily administered, is well tolerated, and has minimal myelosuppressive effect. Combination chemotherapy regimens such as VAD do not, however, improve response or survival rates over standard MP. Nevertheless, they have gained in popularity, particularly for use in induction before high-dose therapy and transplantation.

Dexamethasone, when used as a single agent (usually given in a similar dosing schedule as in VAD), is also effective in treatment of myeloma. Although unproved, it is generally considered as effective as VAD. Complications such as osteoporosis, avascular necrosis of bone, diabetes, cataracts, hypertension, and recurrent infections may limit long-term use.

Relapse After Conventional Chemotherapy

Generally, within 1 to 2 years of discontinuation of therapy, disease will recur. Half of those patients who have relapsed after a first course of the MP regimen will respond to its reinstitution starting at previously effective doses. Development of drug resistance, however, will eventually limit repeated cycles. At this point, a switch to the VAD regimen or dexamethasone alone may be efficacious. The latter is particularly useful in patients with cytopenias and in those reluctant to continue intravenous therapy. If recurrence is localized to a single bony lesion, palliative localized radiation as a single agent may be appropriate.

High-Dose Therapy With Autologous Stem Cell Transplantation

This approach is presently the standard of care in patients with symptomatic myeloma who are younger than age 65. If very high doses of chemotherapy are used alone to ablate myeloma cells, concurrent damage to normal bone marrow cells will lead to death from bleeding or infections. With autologous stem cell transplantation, intensive chemotherapy is followed by infusion of the patient's own blood stem cells, which can repopulate a normal bone marrow and support a return of normal hematopoiesis.

In preparation for the transplant, patients generally first receive four to six cycles of conventional chemotherapy for induction. Induction regimens using nonalkylating agents (e.g., the VAD regimen) are specifically chosen to avoid damage to stem cells. The stem cells are then collected from the patient by means of a cell separator (apheresis) and are frozen until the time of reinfusion after high-dose chemotherapy. High-dose melphalan, 200 mg/m^2, is the most common transplant agent used. Mortality from transplant toxicity is low at 1% to 3%; hence, it is relatively safe. In a landmark, randomized trial in myeloma patients younger than age 65, the transplant procedure led to improved overall survival of 52% at 5 years versus 12% in patients treated with conventional chemotherapy alone. Unfortunately, after transplantation, most patients will continue to have evidence of the disease and all will eventually relapse. Maintenance therapies with various agents (e.g., α-interferon, corticosteroids, combination chemotherapy) after high-dose therapy have been used in clinical trials in an attempt to improve on these results. Another approach is to intensify high-dose therapy with double (or tandem) transplants, but again this has not yet proven to be superior to standard single autologous transplantation.

Relapse After High-Dose Therapy and Autologous Transplant

There is no clear standard of treatment after relapse after high-dose therapy and autologous transplant, but repeat autotransplantation, allotransplantation, or experimental agents such as thalidomide are under investigation. Although most centers use some form of maintenance therapy post transplant (the most frequently used regimen is α-interferon alone), there is no evidence supporting improved survival with this approach.

Allogeneic Transplantation

An allogeneic transplant uses stem cells obtained from a human leukocyte antigen (HLA)-matched donor, usually a sibling, rather than the patient's own cells for regenerating the bone marrow. There is evidence that an immunologic reaction mounted by the infused donor lymphocytes against the patient's myeloma cells (graft-versus-myeloma) can help control the disease. This proposed reaction is comparable to that proven in leukemia patients undergoing allogeneic transplantation (graft-versus-leukemia). Allotransplantation in myeloma can lead to significant reduction in tumor mass with high response rates (complete remissions ~40%). Unfortunately, toxic deaths are common (>20%), and this mode of treatment is infrequently used.

Refractory Myeloma

Only 10% of myeloma patients not responsive to induction chemotherapy (primary refractory) will respond to an alternate regimen. The most effective regimen to salvage disease refractory to alkylating agents is VAD. Alternatives include high-dose dexamethasone, cyclophosphamide intravenously, and other chemotherapy combinations such as VBAP (vincristine, BCNU, doxorubicin, and prednisone).

Myeloma Variants

Monoclonal Gammopathy of Unknown Significance

Patients with MGUS have less than 10% bone marrow plasmacytosis, low concentration M protein in urine or blood, and absent bone lesions or cytopenias and are asymptomatic. The frequency of MGUS increases with age, affecting 5% of individuals older than age 70 and 10% of those older than age 80. One third will ultimately progress to either myeloma, lymphoma, or macroglobulinemia over 15 years (conversion rate 1%–2%/year). Patients with MGUS, therefore, should have their M proteins monitored initially every 3 to 6 months and then, if no progression, yearly. No treatment is needed unless progression is noted.

Isolated Plasmacytoma of Bone

Patients with a solitary lytic bone lesion do not have bone marrow plasmacytosis and are otherwise asymptomatic. The diagnosis is made on needle biopsy of the bone lesion itself. Half of the patients will have a detectable serum M protein level that usually resolves with radiation therapy. Local radiation to the lesion (35–45 Gy) will lead to a greater than 50% survival over 10 years, significantly better than in myeloma. Two thirds of patients, however, will eventually progress to myeloma and require systemic treatment. There is no evidence, to date, that initiating chemotherapy early at the solitary bone lesion stage changes the rate of conversion to myeloma.

Extramedullary Plasmacytoma

Plasmacytomas may also present as soft tissue tumors, most commonly in tonsils, nasopharynx, and paranasal sinuses, without evidence of bony disease or marrow plasma cell infiltration. As with solitary bone plasmacytomas, radiation therapy is the primary mode of treatment. A wider radiation field than with bone plasmacytomas is used, however, because the pattern of spread is through regional lymph nodes. Surgical resection can also be used but should be followed by adjunctive radiation therapy. An associated serum M protein found in one third of patients usually disappears with adequate treatment. Persistence or a recurrence of a previously resolved M protein should warn of disease progression. Myeloma will eventually develop over 15 years in approximately 20% of patients, at which point systemic chemotherapy is indicated.

POEMS Syndrome

Patients with POEMS syndrome have an osteosclerotic myeloma (versus osteolytic in typical myeloma) with any one or more of the following:

P—polyneuropathy: demyelinating
O—organomegaly: hepatosplenomegaly, lymphadenopathy
E—endocrinopathy: hypogonadism, hypothyroidism
M—M protein in blood or urine
S—skin abnormalities: hyperpigmentation, hypertrichosis

Bone marrow plasmacytosis is usually less than 5%. Renal failure and hypercalcemia are rare. Survival for patients with POEMS syndrome (median, 96 months) appears improved over that for myeloma patients (median, 30 months). Treatment is anecdotal, with responses reported to standard melphalan and prednisone, radiation therapy, corticosteroids alone, and plasmapheresis. Plasmapheresis has been used to decrease the M protein presumed to cause neuropathy, but responses are variable and usually transient.

POLYCYTHEMIA VERA

method of
ANDREW I. SCHAFER, M.D.
Baylor College of Medicine and The Methodist Hospital
Houston, Texas

Polycythemia vera (PV) is one of the chronic myeloproliferative disorders. It involves a clonal abnormality of the pluripotent hematopoietic stem cells of the bone marrow. Therefore, although PV manifests primarily with erythrocytosis, many patients also have thrombocytosis and leukocytosis.

DIAGNOSIS AND CLINICAL FEATURES

The diagnosis of PV requires its differentiation from the two other major causes of elevated hemoglobin and hematocrit: (1) relative polycythemia and (2) secondary polycythemia.

Relative polycythemia is caused by contraction of the circulating plasma volume, and it can be readily distinguished from PV and secondary polycythemia by the finding of a normal red cell mass (RCM). However, measurement of the RCM is usually unnecessary in men with hemoglobin values more than 18.5 g/dL and in women with hemoglobin values more than 16.5 g/dL because these degrees of polycythemia are almost always associated with an increased RCM.

Secondary polycythemia is caused by increased erythropoietin, which may be physiologically appropriate (e.g., high altitude, smoking, hypoxic lung disease) or physiologically inappropriate (e.g., erythropoietin-secreting renal cell carcinoma). In addition to evaluation for underlying diseases that might cause secondary polycythemia, measurement of the serum erythropoietin level can be useful in the differential diagnosis. In PV, erythropoietin production is down-regulated by a negative feedback mechanism and serum levels are usually low or normal. In contrast, the secondary polycythemias are driven by elevated erythropoietin levels. Other findings supporting the diagnosis of PV are splenomegaly, persistent leukocytosis and/or thrombocytosis, and the laboratory finding of endogenous erythroid colony growth.

Bleeding and thrombosis (both venous and arterial) are the major causes of morbidity and mortality in PV. Other clinical manifestations include vasomotor disturbances (erythromelalgia, cerebrovascular symptoms) and pruritus after bathing. Some patients with PV undergo transformation to acute leukemia or myeloid metaplasia.

TREATMENT

In general, secondary polycythemia per se does not require treatment. In these cases, management should be directed at identification and correction of the underlying disorder causing polycythemia, if possible (e.g., hypoxic lung disease, renal cell carcinoma, other tumors, congenital cyanotic heart disease). Although phlebotomy often leads to symptomatic improvement in breathing ability and mental acuity in patients with polycythemia secondary to hypoxic lung disease, it is not associated with objective improvement in pulmonary function or exercise tolerance.

Patients with PV do poorly without treatment. Historically, about 50% of untreated patients died within 18 months after onset of symptoms, mainly due to thrombosis. However, life expectancy in effectively treated PV patients approaches that of the general population, at least among older patients in whom the disorder is most common. Therefore, the importance of making a correct diagnosis of PV and promptly initiating therapeutic control of the disease is indisputable.

The only potentially curative therapy is stem cell transplantation. However, this is considered only in exceptionally rare cases of PV, such as in younger patients who develop postpolycythemic myeloid metaplasia with myelofibrosis. All other treatment modalities discussed later must be considered palliative.

Palliative therapy for PV includes (1) phlebotomy, (2) myelosuppression and cytoreduction, and (3) antiplatelet agents. The major goal of treatment is to maintain the hematocrit below 45% in men and 42% in women. Thrombotic complications in patients with PV increase markedly when the hematocrit is above this level. In occasional patients, cerebrovascular symptoms may occur despite good control of the hematocrit, necessitating a further lowering of the target hematocrit on an individualized basis. Thrombocytosis in PV, particularly when it develops in association with phlebotomy therapy, likewise requires cytoreduction in most cases to prevent thromboembolic problems.

In patients whose PV cannot be controlled with only phlebotomy, the variable leukemogenic potential of some of the myelosuppressive agents must be weighed against their benefits. PV can be considered a preleukemic disease in that it may spontaneously transform to acute leukemia in a small number of patients. Therefore, the additional leukemic risk of some treatments (radiophosphorus, alkylating agents, and possibly hydroxyurea) must be carefully considered, particularly in prescribing them for long-term use in younger patients. The consideration of adjunctive antiplatelet therapy should be individualized because PV patients are at risk of not only thrombotic but also serious bleeding complications.

Figure 1 displays an algorithm for treatment of PV. It is based on risk for thrombotic and vascular complications, age, and the presence or absence of thrombocytosis. Each treatment modality is described in detail next.

Phlebotomy

Phlebotomy has long been considered the mainstay of management of PV because it permits rapid reduction of the hematocrit and its readily controlled maintenance at target levels. Phlebotomy of 1 unit of blood can be performed as frequently as twice weekly when necessary at the initiation of treatment, usually with isovolemic intravenous fluid replacement. The long-term goal of phlebotomy therapy is to actually attain iron deficiency, which will inhibit erythropoiesis sufficiently to reduce or even eliminate the requirement for further phlebotomy. Therefore, oral iron-containing supplements should be avoided.

Patients treated with phlebotomy alone are at increased risk of thrombotic and vascular complications, especially early in the course and if they also have thrombocytosis. The concomitant use of aspirin or other antiplatelet drugs may not prevent thrombotic complications and may actually precipitate se-

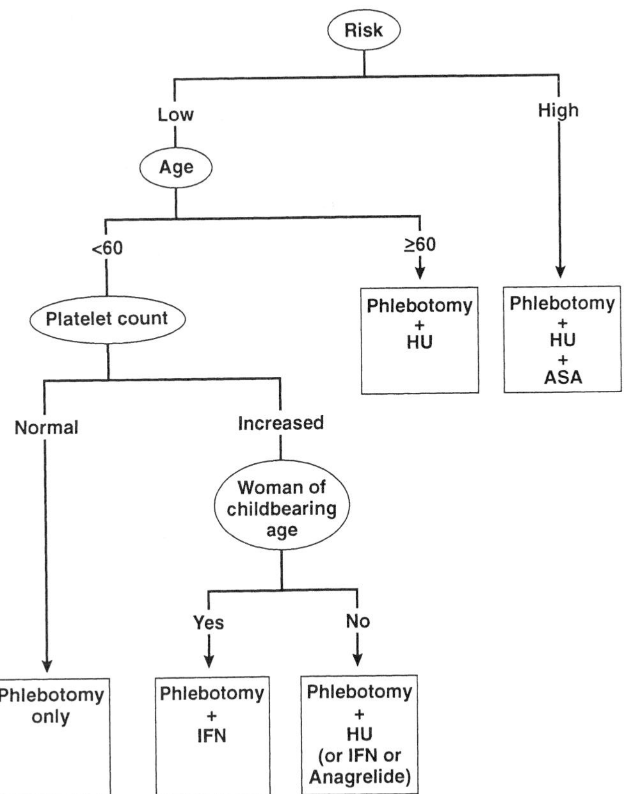

Figure 1. Treatment algorithm for polycythemia vera. High risk patients are those with a history of thrombosis and/or vascular disease.

Abbreviations: ASA = aspirin*; HU = hydroxyurea*; IFN = interferon.*

*Not FDA approved for this indication.

vere bleeding, so their indiscriminate use as antithrombotic prophylaxis cannot be recommended. Repeated phlebotomies may also increase the risk of transformation of PV to myelofibrosis. Finally, in some patients the severe iron deficiency that develops with phlebotomies may impair quality of life and even cause incapacitating symptoms. The lack of leukemogenic and teratogenic effects of phlebotomy continues to make it the treatment of choice in younger patients, particularly women of childbearing age. However, older patients with PV, those with thrombocytosis, and those who have had or are at high risk for thrombotic and vascular events should be treated with myelosuppression in addition to or instead of phlebotomy.

Myelosuppression and Cytoreduction

Because of their clearly demonstrated leukemogenic potential, radiophosphorus (^{32}P) and alkylating agents (e.g., chlorambucil,* busulfan*) have been largely abandoned in the treatment of PV. Today, these agents are used only in exceptional cases that are refractory to other, safer therapy or involve poor patient compliance.

*Not FDA approved for this indication.

Hydroxyurea (Hydrea)* is presently the most commonly used first-line myelosuppressive drug in the treatment of patients with PV. This nonalkylating agent causes myelosuppression by blocking ribonucleotide diphosphate reductase and thereby inhibiting DNA synthesis. It is administered orally at an initial dose of 15 mg/kg/d. The dose is subsequently titrated, based on frequent (initially weekly) blood cell counts, to control the hematocrit without causing leukopenia or thrombocytopenia. About 80% of patients achieve normal hematocrit values within 12 weeks. Phlebotomy should be used liberally while a stable dose of hydroxyurea is determined. The average effective maintenance dose of hydroxyurea is 500 to 1000 mg/d, although there is wide individual variability in sensitivity to the drug. Even after a stable dose of hydroxyurea has been established, patients should have blood cell counts every 6 to 8 weeks. If the drug is discontinued, relapse of the elevated blood cell counts occurs within 7 to 10 days.

Although hydroxyurea is a highly effective, relatively easily administered and well-tolerated oral agent, the dose of which can be readily adjusted based on blood counts in most patients, it does have adverse effects. Side effects are unusual and mild, including gastrointestinal symptoms, rashes, and nail changes. A small number of patients develop painful leg ulcers that resolve with discontinuation of the drug. Although the causal relationship is not as conclusively proven as with radiophosphorus and alkylating agents, recent studies suggest that hydroxyurea may also be leukemogenic.

Recombinant interferon alfa-2a (Roferon A),* is broadly effective for treatment of the chronic myeloproliferative disorders, including PV. Interferon alfa is a biologic response modifier that causes myelosuppression through its antiproliferative actions. Like hydroxyurea, it affects all hematopoietic cell lines. In PV, the drug controls the polycythemia in over 75% of patients. It is also highly effective in reducing the platelet count, spleen size, and constitutional symptoms, especially pruritus. The usual initial dose is 3 million units subcutaneously three times a week, but upward or downward dose modifications may be required. An alternative initial regimen, aimed at minimizing side effects, is 1 million units subcutaneously three times a week, followed by dose escalation by 0.5 million units every 2 to 4 weeks until the target dose of 3 million units three times a week is reached. Full response to interferon alfa usually requires 6 months to 1 year of treatment.

Cost and toxicity of interferon alfa are major limitations to its use in PV. Severe influenza-like symptoms can be controlled with acetaminophen or aspirin but sometimes require discontinuation of the drug. Other toxicity of interferon alfa includes liver function abnormalities and depression. The efficacy of interferon alfa in the treatment of PV has yet to be studied in a randomized trial, and theoretical concerns have been raised about the long-term conse-

*Not FDA approved for this indication.

quences of using this immunomodulatory agent. At this time, interferon alfa should be considered in PV as treatment of women of childbearing age or when symptoms cannot be controlled by other therapy.

Anagrelide (Agrylin) is an orally active quinazoline derivative that controls thrombocytosis in more than 80% of patients. Its mechanism of action is to inhibit platelet production by interfering with megakaryocyte maturation in the bone marrow. Because of its relatively selective effects on platelets, anagrelide has been used primarily in essential thrombocythemia. It could also be used in conjunction with phlebotomy to control thrombocytosis in PV. However, the role of this drug in the management of PV has not been established. In patients with myeloproliferative disorders, anagrelide at a dose of 0.5 to 1.0 mg orally four times daily controls thrombocytosis within 2 to 4 weeks. Thrombocytosis recurs rapidly after discontinuation of the drug. Toxicity includes gastrointestinal symptoms, headache, palpitations, and fluid retention that are related to the drug's vasodilatory and inotropic effects.

Antiplatelet Agents

An early prospective randomized trial showed that higher doses of aspirin* (325 mg three times a day) did not reduce life-threatening thrombotic complications and actually increased the frequency of bleeding problems in PV. Therefore, antiplatelet therapy should be used on an individualized basis in this disease.

The risk of thrombosis in PV increases with advancing age and past history of thrombosis. In patients at high risk (see Figure 1), low-dose aspirin* (75–300 mg/d) should be administered in conjunction with cytoreductive treatment unless there are clear contraindications to antiplatelet therapy. In patients with PV who continue to have thrombotic or vascular symptoms despite aspirin and good control of the hematocrit and platelet count, a thienopyridine antiplatelet agent (clopidogrel [Plavix],* 75 mg/d orally, or ticlopidine [Ticlid],* 250 mg orally twice daily) should be considered. A clearer understanding of the risk-benefit profile of long-term low-dose aspirin therapy in PV awaits the results of large-scale clinical trials.

*Not FDA approved for this indication.

THE PORPHYRIAS

method of
ELISABETH I. MINDER, M.D., and
XIAOYE SCHNEIDER-YIN, PH.D.
Municipal Hospital Triemli
Zurich, Switzerland

The porphyrias are a group of inherited metabolic disorders caused by impaired function of one of the seven enzymes of heme biosynthesis (Table 1). Their symptoms are caused by either toxicity of accumulating intermediary products of the porphyrin precursors and the porphyrins or eventually by lack of the end product heme. Each specific enzyme deficiency leads to a disease entity. It has, however, proved useful for clinical and therapeutic purposes to group these diseases according to their clinical picture and the therapeutic strategies applied to them.

Two main symptoms characterize the porphyrias: neurovisceral damage and photosensitivity. Depending on the specific disorder (or enzyme deficiency), either one, the other, or both symptoms may be present (see Table 1). Despite the fact that heme biosynthesis is affected, no anemia is present in most of the porphyrias.

THE ACUTE PORPHYRIAS

The four so-called acute (hepatic) porphyrias are characterized by neurovisceral manifestations. They include acute intermittent porphyria (AIP), corresponding in our experience to about two thirds of all cases; porphyria variegata (PV), corresponding to about one third; hereditary coproporphyria (HC), which is comparably infrequent; and the very rare aminolevulinic acid dehydratase (ALAD) deficiency. The first three disorders are autosomal dominant, whereas the last is autosomal recessive.

DIAGNOSIS OF ACUTE PORPHYRIAS

Clinical Symptomatology

The leading symptoms of these four porphyrias are acute, mostly self-limiting attacks of several days' duration of severe, colicky abdominal pain, nausea, constipation, vomiting, tachycardia, and hypertension, eventually combined with hyperesthesia, seizures, and psychic disturbances, such as nervousness and sleeplessness. A dark, reddish brown urine is often noted by the patients during symptomatic phases. If not properly diagnosed and managed, the attacks may progress to motor palsy, coma, and eventually death.

Acute porphyrias rarely cause symptoms before puberty. In most patients, clinical manifestations begin when they are young adults. In some patients, however, the first symptoms can appear later, even in senescence. Females are more often symptomatic than males. ALAD deficiency may be symptomatic from early infancy.

Laboratory Diagnosis

The diagnosis of acute porphyria in a *symptomatic* patient is proved by a significant increase of the two porphyrin precursors aminolevulinic acid (ALA) and porphobilinogen (PBG) in a 24-hour urine sample, whereby *significant* means more than 5 times, usually 10 to 20 times, above the upper limit of normal. Only ALA, not PBG, is significantly elevated in the rare ALAD deficiency and in lead intoxication, with the latter showing a symptomatology comparable to an acute porphyria and being in effect an acquired porphyrinopathy.

Readers interested in more clinical details are referred to the books in Suggested Readings.

TREATMENT OF THE ACUTE PORPHYRIAS

Initial Measures in an Acute Attack

If a diagnosis of an acute attack is established, the first measure is to *remove any precipitating factor*

TABLE 1. **The Porphyrias: Synopsis of Biochemistry and Symptomatology**

Affected Enzyme	Name of Disease	Acute Neurovisceral Symptoms	Cutaneous Symptomatology
ALA dehydratase	ALAD deficiency	Present	None
PBG deaminase	Acute intermittent porphyria (AIP)	Present	None
Uroporphyrinogen cosynthase	Congenital erythropoietic porphyria (CEP)	None	Severe mutilating disease, anemia
Uroporphyrinogen decarboxylase	Porphyria cutanea tarda (PCT)	None	Blisters of 1–2 cm diameter, scarring, skin fragility
	Homozygous form: hepatoerythropoietic porphyria (HEP)	None	HEP: severe mutilating disease
Coproporphyrinogen oxidase	Hereditary coproporphyria (HC)	Present	Blisters as PCT
Protoporphyrinogen oxidase	Porphyria variegata (PV)	Present	Blisters as PCT
Ferrochelatase	Erythropoietic protoporphyia	None	Acute painful photodermatosis, vesicles only after mechanical traumatization of affected skin

Abbreviations: ALA = aminolevulinic acid; ALAD = aminolevulinate dehydratase deficiency; PBG = porphobilinogen.

such as alcohol overconsumption, drug consumption (including nonprescription ones if not vitally required), hormone intake, and starvation. It must be emphasized that drug sensitivity in acute porphyria does not mean an acute reaction occurring within minutes but symptoms appearing within several days after exposure.

The severe pain attacks are mostly opiate demanding (e.g., pethidin,* 50 mg/d). A combination with chlorpromazine (Thorazine), 75 mg/d in a saline infusion over 24 hours improves analgesic efficacy.

Adequate glucose supplementation (300–500 g/d) is thought to inhibit the rate-limiting enzyme ALA-synthase (ALAS). Because nausea and vomiting are symptoms of acute attacks, often oral substitution is not possible, but glucose infusions are required.

The most efficacious treatment is intravenous heme application, leading to a negative feedback inhibition of the rate-limiting enzyme ALAS. Conventionally, heme is instituted if glucose supplementation for 48 hours is without improvement or if muscular weakness is noted. Several European porphyria specialists tend to begin immediately with heme treatment together with glucose infusions instead of observing its effect for 48 hours, when the severity of an attack necessitates hospitalization. Heme arginate (Normosang)* (available in Europe) and, alternatively, panhematin (Hemin) (in the United States/Canada) are infused both in a dosage of 3 to 4 mg/kg/d during 4 to 5 days. Both substances may cause phlebitis. Panhematin, but not heme arginate, may induce coagulation disturbance (thrombocytopenia and intravascular consumption of coagulation factors). Hence, monitoring of appropriate laboratory test parameters is necessary. If panhematin is dissolved in an albumin solution in an equimolar ratio (e.g., 10 mg panhematin per gram of albumin), or if the ordinarily used daily dose of 250 mg panhematin is dissolved in 250 mL of 10% albumin solution, its adverse effects are reduced. Heme treatment is not grounded on evidence-based guidelines because its efficacy has been proved by small, neither double-blind nor placebo-controlled studies only because of the scarcity of the disease. The convincing clinical experience from 30 years of heme application renders any placebo-controlled study unethical nowadays as judged by expert porphyria specialists.

Abdominal symptomatology of patients usually ameliorates within 2 to 3 days after initiation of heme therapy. An impressive drop in the urinary excretion of porphyrin precursors (ALA, PBG) even precedes the clinical improvement and is noticeable within the first 24 hours.

Labile hypertension often presents during acute attacks and eventually requires treatment. β-blocking agents are suitable, and in severe hypertension even α/β-blockers can be used. Orthostasis primarily caused by the acute attack is aggravated by these drugs. Furthermore, these substances have been blamed for inducing severe bradycardia in a few porphyria cases. Therefore, careful monitoring of possible cardiovascular complications is strongly recommended.

Surveillance During the Course of an Attack

Hyponatremia is frequently either due to the syndrome of inappropriate secretion of antidiuretic hormone (SIADH) or to a decreased intravascular volume requiring correction of fluid and electrolyte losses. Epileptic seizures may be precipitated by electrolyte imbalance, including a possible hypomagnesemia. An epileptic seizure is treated by 10 mg of diazepam (Valium) given intravenously followed immediately by a regimen with bromides or magnesium sulfate to prevent further seizures. It is controversial as to whether high doses of diazepam impair a porphyric attack.

Respiratory insufficiency caused by impaired mus-

*Not available in the United States.

cle function demands artificial ventilation. Established neurologic damage with motor paresis is reversible but only slowly, the restitution requiring months and years. Prompt institution of the very effective heme application is indicated in any proved acute porphyria attack if the patient develops signs of motor paralysis to prevent both severe acute as well as long-term sequelae.

Long-Term Management of Acute Porphyria

Preventive Strategies

Prophylaxis is of utmost importance to improve the lifetime course of this genetic disorder: the patient has to be instructed to avoid precipitating factors. Oral information should be supplemented by a leaflet with a list of safe drugs (Table 2) and a certificate stating his or her genetic predisposition.

Because 50% of direct relatives of an index patient are carriers of the defective gene in these autosomal dominant diseases, family screening—if possible by the most sensitive technique of DNA-mutation analysis—is endorsed. Mutation carriers need the same instructions as patients because they are as susceptible to drug reactions and other offending agents as are patients with overt disease.

Chronic or Frequently Recurrent Attacks

Some patients develop chronic or frequently recurrent attacks. Most of them are female, and often regular exacerbations occur in the premenstrual days. Although these patients require repeated administration of narcotic analgesics, only a small minority of them develop opiate dependency; therefore, these efficient analgesics should not be withheld from patients with severe pain.

Patients with frequent recurrent attacks are best referred to a porphyria specialist for optimal management. Some further therapeutic measures are listed below:

- The "minipill" (low estrogen-progestagen preparation) is helpful in some patients with premenstrual attacks, whereas others have adverse reactions.
- Luteinizing hormone releasing hormone (LH-RH) antagonists are most effective but carry the long-term risk for osteoporosis. A low-estrogen substitution should be added to reduce the risk of this complication but carries the risk of exacerbating the porphyria.
- Other patients with chronic disease profit from one to two doses of heme arginate* in the beginning of recurrent exacerbations, eventually by means of a Port-a-Cath device and in an ambulatory setting. Heme may be needed as frequently as every week.

A decrease of disease activity is observed in female patients when they reach menopause. Induction of artificial menopause by ovariectomy does not improve the course of chronic disease and is discouraged.

*Not FDA approved for this indication.

TABLE 2. **Drugs Known To Be Safe in Acute Porphyrias**

Symptom Disorder	Drug
Allergy	Diphenhydramine (Benocten)
Epileptic seizures	Diazepam (Valium) IV, 10 mg once only Magnesium sulfate
Nausea, vomiting	Droperidol (Inapsine) Chlorpromazine (Thorazine) Promazine (Sparine) Promethazine (Phenergan)
Hypertension, tachycardia	Propranolol (Inderal) Atenolol (Tenormin) Labetalol (Trandate)
Diuretics	Amiloride (Midamor) Furosemide (Lasix)
Cardiac disease	Atropine Digoxin Procainamide (Pronestyl) Adrenalin Nitroglycerine
Obstipation, ileus	Neostigmine (Prostigmin)
Psychosis, panic attacks	Chlorpromazine (Thorazine) Promazine (Sparine) Triazolam (Halcion) Temazepam (Restoril)
Bacterial infections	Penicillin Ciprofloxacin (Cipro) Amoxycillin (Amoxil) Gentamicin (Garamycin) Ampicillin (Omnipen)
Pain	Acetylsalicylic acid (Aspirin) Naproxen (Naprosyn) Buprenorphine (Buprenex) Codeine Pethidin Morphine and derivatives
Sleeplessness	Midazolam (Versed) Chlorpromazine (Thorazine)
Local anesthesia	Bupivacaine (Marcaine) Procaine (Novocain)
Vaccination	All available
Antidepressant	Maprotilin (Ludiomil) Nortriptyline (Aventyl, Pamelor) Lithium salt
Anticoagulation	Coumarin derivatives Heparin, incl. low molecular weight heparin
Nutrition	Vitamins
Hormones	Dexamethasone (Decadron) and other corticoids ACTH (Acthar) Insulin Metformin (Glucophage)

Current as of October 2000. See also web sites http://www.uq.edu.au/porphyria and http://www.porphyries.com.fr.

Acute Porphyria and Gravidity

A diagnosis of acute porphyria is not a contraindication for pregnancy. Most patients improve during pregnancy, but their susceptibility for an acute attack is increased in the postpuerperal phase. The risk of transmission to the baby is 50%, but only 10% to 20% of affected offspring became symptomatic later.

Treatment of Intercurrent Disorders in Latent or Overt Acute Porphyria

Because intercurrent diseases may be a precipitating factor, they should be consequently treated. Only drugs proved to be safe are to be used. In acute life-threatening situations, however, necessary treatment should never be withheld. As soon as possible, the emergency treatment is to be replaced by "safe drugs," and any eventually induced attack requires application of carbohydrates or heme, as outlined earlier. A list of drugs safely used in acute porphyrias is given in Table 2, and more exhaustive lists are found on the Internet at http://www.uq.edu.au/porphyria and http://www.porphyries.com.fr/.

Acute Porphyria and Liver Cancer

Carriers of acute porphyria have an increased risk of liver carcinoma; it should be carefully searched for when symptoms are suggestive.

Acute Porphyria and Depression

Some patients develop severe depression that eventually is partly refractive to antidepressant treatment, and suicide is a cause of premature death. Different agents known to be innocuous in acute porphyria should be tested for their effectiveness. Heme is not operative in this situation.

THE CUTANEOUS PORPHYRIAS

The second main symptom of the porphyrias is *photosensitivity*, with manifestations being restricted to sun-exposed skin areas (back of hands, face, feet). Clinically, two different forms are distinguished: either skin blisters of 1- to 2-cm diameter and skin fragility or an acute, severely painful photodermatosis often with relatively unimpressive objective signs.

Specific treatment strategies are outlined later, but, as a general principle, protection of the skin from sunlight is a priority. Because light in the visible, not in the ultraviolet (UV), range is damaging, even sunshine passing through window glass induces symptoms. UV-absorbing sunscreens are futile, but reflecting ones containing titanium oxide may be beneficial. The most effective measure is to wear hats, gloves, long sleeves, dense socks, and long trousers.

Porphyrias With Skin Blisters

Porphyric skin blisters in adulthood are caused by either porphyria cutanea tarda (PCT), a chronic disorder, or by PV and HC, both diseases belonging to the acute porphyrias. Differentiating between these disease entities is only possible by biochemistry, not by histology. The pattern of porphyrins in a 24-hour urine specimen and in feces is diagnostic.

Porphyria Cutanea Tarda

PCT is characterized by urinary uroporphyrin excretion surpassing at least five times the upper limit of normal and 50% to 70% as much heptacarboxyporphyrin. ALA and PBG levels are normal or less than two times elevated. PCT is induced by diverse liver afflictions, predominantly by liver hemosiderosis due to alcohol overconsumption eventually in combination with a mutated *HFE* gene (hemochromatosis gene), by chronic hepatitis, or by estrogen therapy. Removal of offending agents is advisable, if possible. Hemosiderosis of the liver, evident by increased ferritinemia and hyperferremia, is a causative factor that may be treated by weekly or twice-weekly phlebotomies of 400 to 500 mL of blood until the disappearance of skin symptoms or until appearance of a slight iron-deficient anemia. Urinary porphyrins may or may not normalize. Eventually, a combination with low dose hydroxychloroquine (Plaquenil)* (100 mg two times a week until symptoms disappear) is more effective in severe cases. If phlebotomies are contraindicated, hydroxychloroquine can be used alone. Symptoms may reappear several years after successful treatment and eventually must be repeated. Treatment of hepatitis C with interferon has not yet been proved effective on porphyric skin lesions.

Skin Blisters in Chronic Dialysis. Skin blisters in patients on chronic dialysis may be caused by two different diseases: PCT or pseudoporphyria. PCT will be confirmed by a typical porphyrin pattern in plasma or feces. Phlebotomies are not suitable because these patients suffer from renal anemia. Hydroxychloroquine, which works by increasing urinary porphyrin excretion, stops operating in renal failure. Instead, erythropoietin supplementation, in a gradually increased dosage, is given to increase erythropoiesis and thereby depleting excessive body iron stores.

Variegate Porphyria and Hereditary Coproporphyria

As emphasized earlier, skin manifestations in these two disorders may be neither clinically nor histologically different from PCT, and patients may never suffer from any neurovisceral symptoms. Treatment of skin manifestation by phlebotomies or hydroxychloroquine is not helpful or even contraindicated. Instead, removal of precipitating factors, as outlined under the section The Acute Porphyrias, is recommended, and protection of the skin from sunlight and from any trauma is the only remedial possibility. Counseling the patient about his or her drug sensitivity and examining his or her family members to find out if they are carrying a predisposition for porphyria is mandatory, as outlined under The Acute Porphyrias.

Neonatal Porphyria

Skin blisters in the neonatal period or in early infancy may be caused by two autosomal rare recessive porphyrias: congenital erythropoietic porphyria (CEP) or hepatoerythropoietic porphyria (HEP). Both are serious, chronic progressive, and mutilating dis-

*Not FDA approved for this indication.

eases, but there is a more benign variant called *late onset* CEP that begins after puberty.

Urine has a reddish brown color from the first day of life and exhibits a purple fluorescence under long UV light. The diagnosis is confirmed by a characteristic porphyrin pattern in urine and other body fluids.

Any strong light, including phototherapy of the newborn, is to be avoided. Oral beta carotene and application of reflecting sunscreen improve symptomatology, although progressive and mutilating damage of the light-exposed skin is inevitable in the severe neonatal forms. High doses of oral charcoal or cholestyramine (Questran),* despite its published efficacy, are ineffective in our experience. An early referral to a porphyria specialist is recommended to discuss bone marrow transplantation as a curative treatment.

Porphyria With Acute Photoreactions

Erythropoietic Protoporphyria

Clinical manifestation of erythropoietic protoporphyria (EPP) begins in infancy or in childhood with acute and severely painful photosensitivity within a few minutes of excess light exposure and lasting for several days. Exposed skin shows a pale swelling and, characteristically, the face and dorsum of hands are most strongly affected.

Urine porphyrin levels are normal, but a significantly elevated erythrocytic protoporphyrin level confirms the diagnosis. Patients often exhibit a slight microcytic, hypochromic anemia and display low to decreased serum iron and ferritin levels, suggesting iron deficiency. Two percent to 5% of patients may develop acute or subacute liver failure by intrahepatic accumulation of protoporphyrin.

Acute burning pain is ameliorated by application of cold water, but in severe cases, strong analgesics are indicated. Beta carotene (75–100 mg/d orally; optimal blood concentration of 11–15 μmol/L carotene) improves light tolerance in about one third of patients but leads to a reddish orange discoloration of the skin. A reflecting sunscreen and protective clothing are beneficial. Light tolerance may be increased by very short amounts (a few minutes) and by slowly increasing exposure to light in the UVA spectrum. Cysteine* has been shown to be effective in a small group of patients, but there is no approved drug on the market.

Supplementation of iron to correct any deficiency should only be prescribed under careful monitoring because both photosensitivity and liver function may deteriorate under its substitution.

Patients with EPP should be monitored at least annually because of the risk of liver failure. Exogenous factors, especially excess alcohol consumption and viral hepatitis, as well as a hereditary factor called a *null allele mutation,* increase the risk for this fatal complication. None of the different measures proposed to prevent or to halt deterioration of liver function is efficacious. Liver transplantation saves the life of the patient, but it does not correct the disease, and even recurrent protoporphyrin accumulation in the graft has been noted in some patients. Bone marrow transplantation apparently is curative but too hazardous in uncomplicated cases.

*Not FDA approved for this indication.

SUGGESTED READINGS

Kappas A, Sassa S, Galbraigth RA, Nordmann Y: The porphyrias. In Scriver CR, Beaudet AL, Sly WS, Valle D (eds): The Metabolic and Molecular Bases of Inherited Disease, 7th ed. New York, McGraw-Hill, 1995.

Minder E, Schneider-Yin X: The porphyrias. In Blau N, Duran M, Gibson KM, Blaskovics ME (eds): Physician's Guide to the Laboratory Diagnosis of Metabolic Diseases, 2nd ed. Heidelberg, Germany, Springer, 2001.

THERAPEUTIC USE OF BLOOD COMPONENTS

method of
THOMAS J. RAIFE, M.D., and
KENNETH D. FRIEDMAN, M.D.
The Blood Center
Milwaukee, Wisconsin

In the United States, blood products are considered "biological products" and are regulated by the Food and Drug Administration (FDA) much like pharmaceuticals. This similarity suggests a framework for managing their use: the benefits of blood administration must be weighed against the risks of adverse events. Accordingly, appropriate use of blood products depends on knowledge of each product's benefits and risks and experience applying that knowledge to patient care.

GLOBAL RISKS OF TRANSFUSION

As with pharmaceutical agents, adverse events from blood transfusion arise from production and distribution problems and from idiosyncratic patient reactions. *Production and distribution problems* include pathogen contamination, mislabeling, mishandling, and misidentification of recipient. *Idiosyncratic reactions* range from unpleasant to fatal. Despite increasing rarity, *pathogen transmission,* especially HIV, continues to be the greatest worry to many patients. In practical terms, however, idiosyncratic reactions are far more frequent and a greater cause of morbidity.

Estimates of the incidence of viral disease transmission from blood products in the United States range from about 1 per 1.5 million unit exposures for HIV, to 1 per 220,000 for hepatitis C, and 1 per 135,000 for hepatitis B. By contrast, febrile and allergic transfusion reactions occur in 1% to 30% of transfusions. Other dangerous reactions include hemolysis, anaphylaxis, transfusion-associated acute lung injury, transfusion-associated graft-versus-host disease, and posttransfusion purpura. Collectively, transfusion reactions are more frequent than transmission of viral diseases, and they can be equally serious.

In recognition of the disproportionate concern among

patients about viral transmission from blood, clinicians do well to counsel patients about transfusion risks in a manner that is accurate and balanced. This is increasingly accomplished through informed consent for which the time investment may be well rewarded. When doubt arises about the risks and benefits of blood transfusion, it is advisable to consult the medical director of the blood bank or transfusion service.

RED BLOOD CELL TRANSFUSION

With few exceptions, red blood cell (RBC) transfusions are used to increase the oxygen-carrying capacity of blood. Additional factors that determine oxygen perfusion of tissues include the capacity of the cardiopulmonary system to oxygenate and circulate blood, the metabolic state of tissues, and the condition of the vasculature. These parameters vary widely among patients, as do transfusion requirements.

Anemia is a physiologic condition. Healthy people have a variance of up to 40% in hemoglobin levels and can tolerate markedly decreased hemoglobin concentrations for brief periods. Tolerance of anemia depends on the rate of hemoglobin decline, the metabolic requirements of the patient, and the physiologic support provided. A gradual decline in hemoglobin allows compensatory mechanisms to develop. Acute blood loss poses a much greater physiologic challenge. Maintenance of intravascular volume, oxygen support, and the physical demands of the patient all are important determinants of blood needs. There is no laboratory definition of when transfusion is needed; transfusion decisions must be based on a combination of laboratory and physiologic data (Figure 1).

Indications

Physical assessment of the patient is the first step in determining the need for RBC transfusions. Signs and symptoms that indicate possible need for transfusion include fatigue, anxiety, tachycardia, dyspnea, angina, and stupor. Hemoglobin (or hematocrit) values provide important correlative data to guide RBC transfusion therapy. Critical data include both current and recent changes in laboratory values. In stable patients, transfusion decisions can be made with careful consideration of laboratory values. In cases of massive hemorrhage, laboratory data may not be sufficiently timely or accurate to guide transfusion.

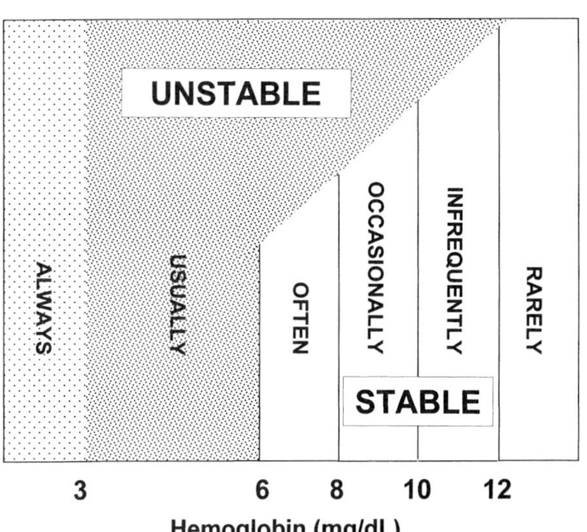

Figure 1. Red blood cell transfusion guidelines. The frequency of the need for red blood cell transfusion is presented in relation to hemoglobin concentration and patient stability. Unstable patients (bleeding or physiologically unstable) are more likely to require transfusion than stable patients.

Guidelines

A 1988 National Institutes of Health consensus panel on transfusion provided a widely cited benchmark for transfusion trigger in stable patients. In stable perioperative patients without evidence of tissue hypoxia, a transfusion trigger of less than 7 g/dL of hemoglobin was recommended. In current practice, most hospital transfusion committees regard a hemoglobin value of 7 to 8 g/dL as a threshold that requires no justification for transfusion.

In bleeding patients, the loss of greater than 25% of blood volume is a common transfusion trigger. As previously noted, blood requirements in massive hemorrhage must be anticipated primarily on the basis of clinical assessments rather than hemoglobin levels, and transfusion at higher thresholds is often necessary to keep pace with ongoing blood loss.

Red Blood Cell Products and Dosages

Most RBC products are manufactured as packed RBCs (PRBCs), made by centrifugation of whole blood with replacement of the plasma by anticoagulant solutions. PRBCs contain total volumes of 250 mL to 350 mL with a hematocrit of approximately 65%. In an average adult, one transfused unit of PRBCs should increase the hemoglobin concentration approximately 1 g/dL. Because such a modest increase is usually not worth the cost and risk of transfusion, it is common to defer transfusion until two or more units are needed.

Additional Considerations

The tissue-oxygenating capacity of blood and the cardiopulmonary system is highly dependent on intravascular volume. Animal experiments demonstrate that temporary reduction of hemoglobin levels to 2 g/dL is tolerated when intravascular volume is maintained. Replacement of intravascular volume with colloid and crystalloid solutions is a critical adjunct to RBC transfusions.

Chronic anemia associated with nutritional deficiency warrants consideration of hematinic therapy, including iron, folate, and vitamin B_{12}. In some patients with anemia of chronic disease or renal disease, recombinant erythropoietin can reduce or replace the need for transfusion. Erythropoietin may also be an alternative to autologous blood donation before elective surgery.

In rare emergencies in which RBCs cannot be used because of religious beliefs or other obstacles, oxygen-carrying blood alternatives may be available. Although none are licensed at this writing, products that have been available for compassionate use include PolyHeme by Northfield Laboratories, Hemopure by Biopure, Hemosol by Hemosol, and Oxygent by Alliance Pharmaceutical. Information is available for these products on the Internet.

PLATELET TRANSFUSIONS

Platelet transfusions are administered to prevent or treat bleeding in thrombocytopenic patients and patients with inherited platelet defects. Current trends in platelet supply and demand indicate that occasional shortages will occur at many hospitals. For this reason, judicious use of platelets is of paramount importance, and consultation with transfusion medicine specialists is highly recommended.

Prophylactic Platelet Transfusion

Platelet transfusion is used preoperatively to minimize hemorrhage in thrombocytopenic patients. The degree of thrombocytopenia that warrants prophylactic platelet transfusion depends on the extent and anatomic site of the procedure. In surgical procedures with moderate expected blood loss, a platelet count of 50,000/μL is usually adequate (Figure 2). In extensive procedures and those with risk of hemorrhage into closed spaces, a preoperative platelet count of 100,000/μL is sometimes required.

The majority of platelet transfusions in the United States are administered to oncology patients as prophylaxis for bleeding. Because spontaneous bleeding increases when platelet counts fall below 20,000/μL, this value has been a widely used transfusion trigger. However, prophylactic transfusion thresholds have evolved downward in recent years, and many institutions currently use 10,000/μL as a transfusion trigger. In view of this shift, it should be recognized that at platelet counts below 20,000/μL, the likelihood of bleeding is increased by complications such as fever, infection, renal failure, and other coagulation defects. It is therefore important to consider the entire clinical picture (as well as the limited supply of platelets) to determine appropriate thresholds for prophylactic platelet transfusions.

Treatment of Bleeding

Complicating factors are often present in patients who bleed with platelet counts above 50,000/μL. Common factors include large vessel bleeding, platelet dysfunction from drugs or uremia, and clotting factor deficiencies from liver disease, disseminated intravascular coagulation (DIC), and massive transfusion. Infrequent factors include acquired clotting inhibitors and congenital defects such as hemophilia, von Willebrand disease, congenital platelet defects, and inherited vascular abnormalities.

Bleeding time does not correlate reliably with clinical bleeding and its use for guiding platelet transfusion therapy is not recommended. Whenever considered, it is advisable to consult an experienced hematologist or transfusion medicine specialist.

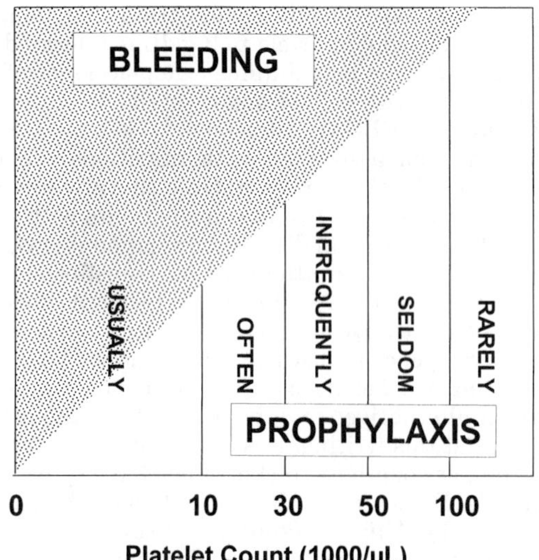

Figure 2. Platelet transfusion guidelines. The frequency of platelet transfusion is presented in relation to the platelet count and bleeding status. Most prophylactic transfusions are for counts less than 30,000/μL. Bleeding patients may be transfused at platelet counts up to 100,000/μL.

Contraindications

Platelet transfusions are generally unnecessary in massive transfusion and routine cardiac surgery. Transfusion should be avoided unless bleeding is excessive after adequate surgical control. In immune thrombocytopenic purpura, prophylactic platelet transfusions are seldom effective and should be reserved for significant bleeding episodes. In thrombotic thrombocytopenic purpura and the hemolytic-uremic syndrome, platelets are consumed in microvascular thrombosis. It is widely held that platelet transfusions exacerbate these pathologic conditions and should be avoided except to treat critical hemorrhage. Immunization against platelet or human leukocyte antigens may occur following repeated exposures to platelets. Alloimmunization can make future use of platelet transfusions difficult. Leukoreduction reduces this likelihood, and judicious use of platelet transfusions may help.

Products and Dosages

Platelets for transfusion are provided as apheresis products or pooled concentrates derived from processed whole blood units. The platelet content of a single dose averages 4×10^{11} platelets but may vary between about 3×10^{11} and 6×10^{11}. One apheresis unit (one dose) is usually equivalent to about six pooled concentrates.

Platelet transfusions are ordinarily given one dose at a time followed by assessment of efficacy, as described later. In exceptionally large patients or in patients with uncontrolled bleeding, two consecutive dosages may be warranted. Multiple dosages over a short time are generally unwarranted. When multiple dosages are considered, attention to complicating factors and other possible treatments are recommended.

Efficacy

Platelet count increments are the primary indicators of successful prophylactic platelet transfusions. When there are no mitigating factors, each standard dose of 4×10^{11} platelets should increase the platelet count of a 75-kg patient by 40,000 to 60,000/μL. The posttransfusion platelet count should be obtained within 1 hour.

There are multiple reasons for a poor platelet count response in very ill patients, including drugs, hypersplenism, fever, and platelet consumption from hemorrhage or DIC. When the platelet count increase from transfusion is disappointing, clinical assessment of hemostatic improvement is important. Sometimes hemostasis can improve when no practical amount of transfused platelets will satisfactorily increase the platelet count. Clinical evidence of improvement may include reduced oozing from venipuncture sites, catheters, drains and surgical wounds, reduced urine or fecal blood content, reduced epistaxis or menstrual blood loss, and stabilized hemoglobin levels.

Alternatives

Platelet-dependent hemostasis involves many factors including platelet concentration, platelet function, and soluble factors including fibrinogen and von Willebrand factor (vWF). Therefore, in bleeding patients, it is critical to consider all possible treatment options. In addition to platelet transfusions, adequate dosages of plasma, cryoprecipitate, and other hemostatic agents may be helpful. Treatment of complicating factors such as DIC and surgical control of gross bleeding are essential.

Bleeding associated with uremia or mild von Willebrand disease can often be effectively treated by administration of desmopressin acetate (DDAVP), which causes release of stored vWF and factor VIII. Unremitting life-threatening bleeding despite adequate surgical control and transfusion support may improve with antifibrinolytic drugs such as ϵ-aminocaproic acid (EACA). EACA can have serious thrombotic consequences and should be used with the advice of an experienced consultant.

PLASMA PRODUCTS

Plasma is separated from whole blood by centrifugation. It is stored frozen and thawed for transfusion without modification (fresh-frozen plasma, FFP) or used for fractionation into purified concentrates of albumin, immunoglobulin, and coagulation factors. By definition, 1 U of coagulation factor concentrate is the amount present in 1 mL of pooled normal plasma. Standard units of FFP contain 200 to 250 mL of FFP and therefore 200 to 250 U of each coagulation factor.

Indications for Plasma Transfusion

FFP is most frequently transfused to replenish multiple coagulation factors in patients with documented coagulation abnormalities who are bleeding or at risk of bleeding during surgery. Prophylaxis in nonbleeding patients in whom interventions are not planned is usually unwarranted. Laboratory evidence of coagulopathy is generally regarded as a 1.5-fold prolongation of either the prothrombin time or activated partial thromboplastin time, but the correlation between bleeding risk and these indices of coagulation is imprecise. Excessive bleeding with less prolonged coagulation times may involve mechanisms other than multiple coagulation factor deficit. The efficacy of FFP transfusions in this setting is unreliable.

Acquired coagulopathies in which FFP transfusion should be considered include liver disease, dilutional coagulopathy from massive transfusion, and oral anticoagulant effect or vitamin K deficiency when immediate correction is required (vitamin K replacement is effective in 12–24 hours). FFP is also used for replacement of individual coagulation factors that are not available as concentrates (factors II, V, X, XI). FFP is occasionally used to replace hemostatic regulatory proteins such as antithrombin III, protein C, or protein S. Indications for FFP transfusion to replace these regulatory proteins are not well defined, and anticoagulation therapy is more frequently used.

Although albumin solutions are typically used as replacement fluid for patients undergoing therapeutic plasma exchange, empiric evidence has made FFP the standard replacement therapy in management of thrombotic thrombocytopenic purpura. FFP is also occasionally used near the termination of other therapeutic apheresis procedures in patients with increased risk of bleeding from dilutional coagulopathy. FFP should not be used for plasma volume expansion, nutritional support, treatment of hypogammaglobulinemia, or the treatment of disorders that are better managed with a factor concentrate (e.g., factor VIII, factor IX, antithrombin III, vWF, or immunoglobulin).

Plasma Products, Dosage, and Monitoring

There are currently three types of plasma products available in the United States. Regional preference plays a strong role in product availability. Most of the plasma transfused is the standard FFP product that has been used for more than 3 decades but with much added testing. Some centers provide "donor-retested" plasma (FFP-DR) in which FFP is quarantined for several months until the donor returns and has negative results for bloodborne pathogens. This measure adds yet another increment of safety to FFP. Some centers provide solvent/detergent (S/D) treated plasma. This product is made from pooled plasma that is treated to disrupt viral envelopes and packaged into 200-mL bags. S/D treatment inactivates lipid-enveloped viruses (including HIV, hepatitis C virus, and hepatitis B virus). S/D plasma has adequate levels of procoagulant factors, but is deficient in some control proteins including antiplasmin, protein S, and protein C.

The dose of FFP for treatment of coagulation disorders depends on the expected rate of consumption or depletion of the transfused factors and individual patient factors. A common starting dose is 15 to 20 mL/kg. Follow-up doses of FFP should be determined by assessment of bleeding risk and results of coagulation laboratory monitoring.

Cryoprecipitate Indications, Dosage, and Monitoring

Cryoprecipitate is a cold-insoluble protein fraction derived from FFP. Each unit of cryoprecipitate contains approximately 225 mg of fibrinogen and 80 U of factor VIII and vWF in a volume of 20 to 50 mL.

Cryoprecipitate is the only form of concentrated fibrinogen available for transfusion. It is mainly used to augment fibrinogen concentration in bleeding patients with a fibrinogen level under 100 mg/dL. These may include patients with severe liver disease, DIC, and dilutional coagulopathy. Although dosages can be calculated from the plasma volume of the patient and the desired increment in fibrinogen, empiric therapy monitored by fibrinogen level is often chosen. Accordingly, one bag of cryoprecipitate per every 5 kg will increase fibrinogen by approximately 75 mg/dL. Ongoing consumption or dilution often shortens the posttransfusion fibrinogen half-life below the normal 3 to 5 days.

Cryoprecipitate is an emergency source of factor VIII or vWF for patients who are unresponsive to DDAVP, but virally attenuated factor concentrates are the products of choice, if available. The dosage of cryoprecipitate for this purpose assumes 1 U of cryoprecipitate will raise the factor level by 40 U/dL for each 10 kg of body weight. The posttransfusion factor levels should be monitored with appropriate laboratory assays.

Plasma Derivatives

Plasma-derived purified factor VIII, factor IX, prothrombin-complex and antithrombin concentrates are available, in addition to recombinant protein concentrates of factor VIII, factor IX, α_1-antiproteinase, and an expanding list of other proteins. Use of plasma derivatives in the treatment of hemophilia is described in other sections.

Albumin and plasma protein fraction are pooled, pasteurized products derived from human plasma. Intravascular volume expansion with albumin is controversial. Although much more expensive than crystalloid, albumin does not dilute the patient's protein concentration, and thus limits edema. The volume of albumin required is about one third the volume of crystalloid required for the same effect. For these reasons, albumin is frequently used as replacement fluid in therapeutic apheresis. Albumin solutions contain at least 96% albumin protein and are available in concentrations of 25% and 5%. Twenty-five percent solutions may be diluted to 5% using isotonic saline. Plasma protein fraction is a less expensive product that contains at least 83% albumin protein and is used for many of the same purposes as albumin.

Immunoglobulins

Pooled, concentrated, virally attenuated immunoglobulin preparations for intravenous infusion are available from several manufacturers. Virally attenuated immunoglobulin preparations for intravenous infusion solutions contain at least 90% IgG. Labeled indications include HIV, immune thrombocytopenia, and Kawasaki disease. Unlabeled uses include an array of autoimmune and immunologic disorders. Dosage and administration schedules vary depending on disease indication. Laboratory monitoring of virally attenuated immunoglobulin preparations for intravenous infusion therapy is generally not required. Adverse reactions include rare anaphylaxis, febrile reactions, headache, and renal failure.

SPECIAL TOPICS

Blood Volume

It may be useful to calculate total blood volume (TBV) when determining dosages of certain blood products. The adult TBV is derived from the approximate value of 70 mL/kg of ideal body weight. Plasma volume and RBC volume are easily derived from TBV and hematocrit.

Platelet Corrected Count Increment

The corrected count increment (CCI) is an index of platelet transfusion efficacy that accounts for patient size and platelet dosage. The calculation is as follows:

$$\text{CCI} = \text{Platelet Count Increment (Platelets/}\mu\text{L)} \times \text{Body Surface Area (in m}^2\text{)/ Platelet Dose (in multiples of }10^{11}\text{ platelets)}$$

For example, 15,000 (increment) $\times$ 1.2 (m^2) $\div$ 4.4 ($\times 10^{11}$ platelets) = 4090. CCI values less than 5000 can indicate a condition of refractoriness to platelet transfusions. The CCI calculation requires knowledge or estimate of the platelet dosage, which can be obtained from the blood bank.

Leukocyte Reduced Blood

Current indications for leukoreduced blood products are controversial and local practices vary. Accepted indications include reduced risk of febrile transfusion reactions, human leukocyte antigen alloimmunization, and cytomegalovirus transmission. Less clear indications include reduction of immunomodulation and transmission of other leukotropic pathogens. Because of established and theoretical benefits, many institutions have adopted broad or universal use of leukoreduced blood products. This may soon be a regulatory requirement.

Irradiation of Blood Components

Transfusion-associated graft-versus-host disease is a rare but often fatal transfusion complication caused by viable transfused T lymphocytes. Patients at risk include recipients of blood donated by first-degree relatives, and many immunocompromised patients. Susceptible patients should receive gamma-irradiated blood products. Leukoreduction has not been proven to prevent transfusion-associated graft-versus-host disease.

Washed Blood Products

Platelets and RBCs can be washed to remove noncellular constituents that cause immunologic or allergic transfusion reactions. Washing is most often used to remove potentially harmful antibodies or plasma allergens when anaphylaxis is a concern. Careful consideration of the need for washed blood products is important because washing is resource-intensive and availability may be limited.

WEBSITES

http://www.nhlbi.nih.gov/health/prof/blood/transfusion
http://www.cma.ca/cmaj/vol-156/issue-11/blood

ADVERSE REACTIONS TO BLOOD TRANSFUSIONS

method of
CHARLES J. PARKER, M.D.
University of Utah School of Medicine and VA Medical Center
Salt Lake City, Utah

The blood supply in the United States is safe for the following two reasons.

1. Blood is collected from volunteer donors whose medical history and physical health are carefully scrutinized. In addition, potential donors are screened for possible contact with transfusion-transmissible diseases based on questioning about sexual behavior, drug use, and travel to areas of endemic disease.
2. The donated blood products are tested for compatibility and for the presence of markers of transmissible infectious agents (Table 1).

Despite the care with which donors are selected and the thoroughness with which the blood products are screened for transmissible diseases and compatibility, adverse reactions to blood transfusion still occur, albeit infrequently. Most of the untoward consequences of blood transfusion fall into the category of minor transfusion reactions (e.g., febrile or allergic reactions). Although these adverse reactions are disconcerting to the patient, significant morbidity is uncommon, and mortality is rare. In most instances, minor reactions can be prevented, but because these events occur infrequently and because morbidity is relatively low, it is fiscally unsound to institute measures aimed at preventing all minor transfusion reactions. For example, using leukodepleted blood could prevent most febrile nonhemolytic transfusion reactions. However, because these reactions occur only 1 time per 200 transfusions (at most) and because the consequences are relatively minor, there is

TABLE 1. **Mandatory Testing on All Units of Blood Collected for Transfusion**

ABO group and Rh type
Screening for blood-group antibodies
Serologic test for syphilis
The following serologic test for HIV:
- HIV-1 antibody
- HIV p24 antigen
- HIV-2 antibody
- HTLV I antibodies

The following serologic tests for hepatitis:
- HBV surface antigen
- HBV core antibody
- HCV antibody

Nucleic acid amplification test for HCV and HIV is undergoing pilot testing. This testing is expected to reduce the window phase for HCV from 70–80 days to 10–30 days and for HIV from 16 days to 10 days.

Abbreviations: HBV = hepatitis B virus; HCV = hepatitis C virus; HTLV = human T-cell lymphotrophic.

little support for leukoreducing all red cell and platelet products before infusion for the sole purpose of preventing febrile transfusion reactions.

The emphasis of this article is on the recognition and treatment of adverse reactions to blood transfusion that occur during or soon after the infusion. Although transfusion-transmitted diseases are discussed briefly, their management is omitted because treatment is the same as it would be if the disease were contracted outside the setting of blood transfusion. Due to space limitations, this article does not include a review of platelet alloimmunization or posttransfusion purpura. In this review, adverse reactions are discussed under the following headings: (1) Transfusion Transmitted Diseases; (2) Transfusion Reactions; (3) Alloimmunization; and (4) Transfusion-Associated Graft-Versus-Host Disease (TA-GVHD).

TRANSFUSION TRANSMITTED DISEASES

Hepatitis B Virus

Hepatitis B virus (HBV) is transmitted through parenteral and sexual routes. The incubation time is a mean of 90 days with a range of 30 to 180 days. As noted in Table 1, donor blood is routinely screened for HBV surface antigen (HBsAG) and HBV core antibody (HB_cAb). Those who have received the HBV vaccination are not eliminated from blood donations by this analysis because they have HBV surface antibody (HB_sAb) present but not HBsAG or HB_cAb, thus distinguishing them from patients with a prior infection. The risk of transmission of HBV per unit of blood transfused is 1 in 30,000 to 1 in 150,000. Blood recipients can also be infected with hepatitis delta, a defective RNA virus that needs a coexistent HBV infection to replicate.

Hepatitis C Virus

Hepatitis C virus (HCV) is transmitted primarily via parenteral routes with the incidence of sexual transmission being lower than initially thought (presumably because the viral load is usually relatively low). The incubation period is 6 to 8 weeks. Blood bank testing for HCV began in 1990. Currently, blood is tested only for HCV antibody, but pilot studies are underway that test the efficacy of nucleic acid amplification as a method for increasing sensitivity and reducing the window for detecting recent infections from 70 to 80 days to 10 to 30 days (see Table 1). The risk of transmission of HCV is similar to that of HBV (1 in 30,000 to 1 in 150,000).

AIDS

The first cases of AIDS contracted from blood or blood components were reported in 1982, although the cause was unknown at that time. In 1983, changes in donor criteria were made to exclude those at high risk for transmission of HIV. The first testing for HIV was initiated in 1985. That test detects the presence of HIV antibody in donor serum (see Table 1). In 1996, testing for the p24 antigen of HIV became mandatory (see Table 1). Nucleic acid amplification testing for HIV is undergoing pilot studies. This very sensitive analysis is expected to reduce the window for detecting recent HIV infection from 16 days to 10 days. Currently, the risk of transmission of HIV is estimated to be between 1 in 200,000 and 1 in 2 million.

Human T-Cell Lymphotrophic Virus-1

Human T-cell lymphotrophic virus-1 (HTLV-1) is a retrovirus (as is HIV) that is endemic in Japan and the Caribbean. The virus has been implicated as causing adult T-cell leukemia/lymphoma and a neurologic disorder similar to multiple sclerosis. Blood is routinely screened for antibodies to HTLV-1 (see Table 1). The risk of transmission of HTLV-1 is 1 in 250,000 to 1 in 2 million; however, disease develops in only 1% to 3% of seropositive individuals.

Cytomegalovirus

Depending on geographic location, the prevalence of cytomegalovirus (CMV) antibodies in the population ranges from 50% to 80%. Donor blood is not routinely tested for CMV. Blood contaminated with CMV, however, can result in significant morbidity and mortality in premature infants and in immunocompromised hosts who are CMV seronegative and who receive blood products infected with the virus. In immunocompromised patients, CMV infection can lead to pneumonitis, hepatitis, and gastroenteritis. Congenital CMV infection is associated with jaundice, hepatosplenomegaly, microencephaly, and thrombocytopenia, with mortality rates approaching 20%. Premature infants (1200-g birth weight) who are born to CMV-seronegative mothers but who become infected with the virus as a result of blood transfusion are at risk for hemolytic anemia as well as the other abnormalities previously noted. Here is a list of indications for use of CMV-seronegative blood products:

1. Premature infants (<1200 g) born to CMV-seronegative mothers
2. CMV-seronegative allogeneic and autologous hematopoietic stem cell transplant recipients
3. CMV-seronegative HIV-positive patients
4. CMV-seronegative recipients of solid organs (kidney, liver, heart) from CMV-seronegative donors
5. CMV-seronegative patients who are potential stem cell transplant recipients
6. CMV-seronegative pregnant women

CMV resides intracellularly in leukocytes. Thus, blood components containing white blood cells are the source of transmission, and CMV is not transmitted by acellular blood components such as plasma and cryoprecipitate. Although there is still some debate, most transfusion medicine specialists consider leukofiltration (using third-generation filters that reduce the leukocyte count in the final component to $<5 \times 10^6$) to be equivalent to transfusion of seronegative blood as a means of preventing CMV infection. Frozen, deglycerolized red blood cells (RBCs) can also be used.

Other Diseases

RBC products rarely transmit malaria, although the number of transfusion-associated cases of malaria is at an all-time high. There are no practical laboratory tests available to screen donor blood for malarial infection. Therefore, donors who have traveled to areas where malaria is endemic are excluded from donating blood for 6 months. Other diseases that are rarely transmitted by blood products include the following: babesiosis, Lyme disease, and Chagas disease. There are no cost-effective laboratory tests available for screening blood donors for these diseases.

TRANSFUSION REACTIONS

Allergic Transfusion Reactions

The most common adverse reaction to blood transfusion is the allergic transfusion reaction, occurring at a risk rate of 1 in 100 to 1 in 500 (Table 2). The clinical manifestations vary but involve one or more of the following signs and symptoms: erythema, pruritus, urticaria (mild, moderate, or severe), vasomotor instability, bronchospasm, and anaphylaxis. The pathophysiologic process that underlies these clinical manifestations is poorly understood but appears to involve the interaction of recipient antibodies (usually IgG, but IgM has also been implicated) with donor plasma proteins. The immune complexes subsequently evoke the cellular response that initiates the allergic reaction.

TABLE 2. **Types of Transfusion Reactions***

Allergic Reaction
Allergic reaction to donor plasma proteins
Allergic reaction to IgA in IgA-deficient recipients
Febrile Reaction
Transfusion-associated lung injury (TRALI)
Bacterial contamination
Circulatory overload

*Hemolytic transfusion reactions due to ABO incompatibility and delayed transfusion reactions are discussed under the heading Alloimmunization.

Treatment consists of stopping the infusion and giving 25 to 50 mg of diphenhydramine. If the initial clinical symptoms are relatively mild (i.e., absence of hypotension, bronchospasm, or tachycardia), and if there is evidence that the patient has responded to this treatment, the infusion of the blood product can be restarted.

Allergic reactions are rarely serious and usually do not recur. Thus, attempts to prevent recurrences by using washed RBCs is not justified unless the patient has had more than one allergic reaction or the first event is clinically severe (e.g., hypotension, bronchospasm). Leukodepletion is of no value in preventing allergic reactions because the filtration process does not exclude the plasma proteins. In general, washed RBCs should be used to prevent allergic reactions only if a patient has a history of severe or recurrent episodes. Premedication with diphenhydramine is usually sufficient to prevent symptoms in patients who have had relatively mild reactions.

Anti-IgA antibodies in recipients who are IgA deficient may cause allergic reactions with symptoms of anaphylaxis. The antibodies react with IgA in the donor blood component, resulting in hypertension followed by profound hypotension, bronchospasm, and gastrointestinal symptoms in the absence of fever. Immediate treatment with epinephrine may be required to prevent complete cardiovascular collapse and death.

Febrile Nonhemolytic Transfusion Reactions

A temperature rise of 1°C or greater, usually accompanied by shaking chills, that occurs during or soon after a transfusion is consistent with a febrile nonhemolytic transfusion reaction (FNHTR). The fever is cytokine-mediated (interleukin 1B [IL-1β], IL-6, tumor necrosis factor α [TNF-α]). Antibodies present in recipient plasma bind to antigen on donor lymphocytes, granulocytes, or platelets. The antibodies are usually human leukocyte antigen (HLA) specific, although antibodies specific for neutrophil or platelet antigens are also observed. The antigen-antibody complex is recognized by IgG Fc receptors on macrophages, monocytes, and neutrophils, resulting in prostaglandin synthesis stimulated by IL-1. As a consequence, the thermoregulatory center of the hypothalamus is stimulated and fever ensues. FNHTRs are usually observed in patients who have received frequent transfusions and in multiparous women. The estimated frequency of FNHTR ranges from 1 in 200 to 1 in 10,000 events.

FNHTR is characterized clinically by fever and chills occurring shortly after the transfusion has begun, although symptoms can also occur several hours after conclusion of the infusion. Patients often complain initially of feeling uncomfortable or chilly, but symptoms frequently progress from a slight tremor to frank rigors. FNHTRs are usually self-limited with symptoms lasting 8 to 10 hours if untreated. Although febrile reactions are usually not life-threatening, they can often produce significant anxiety in the patient. In elderly patients or those with debilitating co-morbid conditions, FNHTRs can result in cardiovascular collapse and death.

If an FNHTR is suspected, the transfusion should be stopped and the intravenous line should be used to infuse saline or a suitable crystalloid. The patient should be reassured because the anxiety associated with FNHTR can be extremely disconcerting. The laboratory evaluation should begin immediately. The workup consists of eliminating the possibility of a hemolytic reaction by reconfirming the ABO type of the patient and the donor unit. In addition, the crossmatch should be repeated to confirm compatibility, and direct antiglobulin testing on the pretransfusion and posttransfusion samples should be performed. Plasma should be analyzed for the presence of free hemoglobin, and the paperwork must be rechecked for accuracy. Blood culture specimens from the patient and culture specimens of the transfused products should be obtained to exclude the possibility of infusion of bacterially contaminated blood.

Treatment consists of antipyretics (aspirin, nonsteroidal anti-inflammatory agents, and acetaminophen are all effective). In the absence of signs and symptoms of an allergic component to the reaction (e.g., flushing, hives, or pruritus), diphenhydramine should not be prescribed. Severe shaking chills can be ameliorated almost immediately by using meperidine (Demerol).* Patients who experience cardiovascular collapse as a result of a severe FNHTR require blood pressure support and monitoring in the setting of an intensive care unit.

Studies suggest that the probability that a patient will experience a second FNHTR is one in eight. Thus, an argument can be made that pretreatment to prevent FNHTR is not indicated unless the patient has experienced two or more febrile reactions. Premedication approximately 30 minutes before the infusion with antipyretics can reduce symptoms associated with FNHTR, and patients with a history of multiple febrile transfusion reactions should receive leukoreduced blood products.

Transfusion-Related Acute Lung Injury

The onset of respiratory insufficiency with decreased O_2 saturation occurring within 4 hours of starting a transfusion should alert the clinician to the possibility of transfusion-related acute lung injury (TRALI). The chest radiograph reveals diffuse pulmonary infiltrates consistent with pulmonary edema, but when measured, left-sided cardiac pressure is normal. Thus, the findings are consistent with noncardiogenic pulmonary edema. The patient may also develop fever, chills, cyanosis, or hypotension. HLA- or granulocyte-specific antibodies of donor origin underlie the disease process. In this case, the antibodies activate neutrophil adhesion molecules resulting in adherence of the cells to the endothelial surface of pulmonary capillaries, followed by diapedesis, and eventually capillary leak syndrome.

If TRALI is suspected, the transfusion should be stopped immediately. Conclusively distinguishing cardiogenic from noncardiogenic pulmonary edema requires measurement of pulmonary artery wedge pressure. Ventilatory assistance (including intubation if indicated) should be provided along with blood pressure support. Steroids (the equivalent of 60–100 mg of prednisone) should be administered. Diuretics are of no value, and there is some evidence that they may be detrimental.

In many cases, it appears that the HLA/neutrophil antigen-antibody reactions are idiosyncratic and do not recur in association with subsequent transfusion. For patients who have experienced an episode of TRALI, however, it seems prudent to use leukodepleted blood products when transfusions are required.

Bacterial Contamination

Blood products can be contaminated with bacteria during collection, and the bacteria can grow both during storage at room temperature and during refrigeration. The most common bacterial contaminants of blood products are psychrophilic organisms (e.g., *Yersinia enterocolitica*). The contamination rate in the United States is less than 1 U/million. Patients receiving blood products contaminated with bacteria can experience sepsis and die. The possibility of bacterial contamination must be considered and investigated when fever, tachycardia, and hypotension develop in association with a transfusion event.

Circulatory Overload

Administration of blood products can result in circulatory overload, particularly in patients with cardiac dysfunction.

ALLOIMMUNIZATION

The development of alloantibodies requires exposure to foreign antigens. Individuals who have the O blood group phenotype develop anti-A and anti-B antibodies because these blood group antigens are polysaccharides that are present on a number of substances found in the environment. Allosensitization can also occur as a result of pregnancy or transfusion. In the case of pregnancy, the mother may become

*Not FDA approved for this indication.

sensitized because of exposure to "foreign" antigens (primarily Rh) present on the small amounts of fetal RBCs that cross the placenta at parturition. Because of the large number of different membrane constituents, transfusion recipients are exposed to many foreign antigens. The relatively low incidence of alloimmunization after transfusion is due to the fact that most RBC constituents are not strongly immunogenic. An exception is the Rh antigen, but in this case, allosensitization is eliminated by the crossmatching process that ensures that only Rh-compatible blood is transfused.

Major Transfusion Reactions

Acute, major transfusion reactions are almost always due to infusion of ABO-incompatible blood, and transfusion of ABO-incompatible blood is almost always the result of clerical rather than technical errors in compatibility testing. Major transfusion reactions are rare, having an incidence of 1 in 250,000 to 1 in 1 million.

The potentially devastating consequences of transfusion of ABO-incompatible blood are the result of massive, complement-mediated intravascular hemolysis. The pathophysiologic processes that accompany the reaction are due primarily to formation of immune complexes and to complement activation rather than to release of hemoglobin. As a consequence of complement activation, C3a and C5a are generated, and these vasoactive peptides appear to be responsible for the vascular instability that underlies the clinical consequences of major transfusion reactions.

In some cases, symptoms may be relatively subtle, but major transfusion reactions are usually associated with sudden, dramatic clinical deterioration of the recipient. Patients complain of chest pain (frequently substernal), back pain (frequently paravertebral), leg pain, dyspnea, anxiety, flushing, chills, and diaphoresis. Hypotension and renal failure are frequently observed, and evidence of intravascular hemolysis (hemoglobinuria and serum-free hemoglobin) is apparent.

When a hemolytic reaction is suspected, the transfusion should be stopped immediately because the severity of the injury is in part related to the volume of blood infused. Plasma and urine should be examined for evidence of hemoglobin, and the blood from the transfusion set along with that of the recipient should undergo compatibility testing.

Treatment of major acute hemolytic transfusion reactions is primarily supportive. Once the diagnosis is established, or if there is a high degree of suspicion, the recipient should receive furosemide (80–120 mg intravenously) and urine output should be maintained at more than 100 mL/h. Nonblood volume expanders (e.g., colloid or crystalloid) can be used to help maintain renal perfusion (the use of mannitol in this setting is controversial), but patients must be closely monitored for signs of volume overload. Based on the observation that hemoglobin is more soluble in alkaline solutions, it has been suggested that alkalinization of the urine may ameliorate the renal damage associated with a major transfusion reaction. Evidence supporting this hypothesis, however, is not compelling. Vasopressors may be required to maintain blood pressure, but agents that have the attendant feature of restricting renal blood flow are contraindicated. In patients in whom renal failure develops, short-term dialysis may be required while waiting for the damaged kidneys to recover.

The diffuse intravascular coagulation that arises as part of a major transfusion reaction is usually self-limited. Accordingly, overzealous treatment should be avoided and therapeutic intervention should be reserved for patients who exhibit evidence of uncompensated disease (clinically significant bleeding or thrombosis). Platelet transfusion and fresh frozen plasma as sources of coagulation factors may be beneficial, but the use of heparin (either low dose or therapeutic amounts) is controversial. Moderate-to-severe hypofibrinogenemia can be treated by using cryoprecipitate.

Delayed Transfusion Reactions

Delayed transfusion reactions (those occurring 3–21 days after infusion of the blood) are usually the result of an anamnestic immune response. In these cases, the initial allosensitization most likely occurred as a result of pregnancy or prior transfusion, but at the time the compatibility testing is done, the presence of the alloantibody is not observed because the titer is too low. Thus, unlike major transfusion reactions, which are almost always the result of human error, delayed transfusion reactions are usually unavoidable.

The transfused cells bearing the alloantigen stimulate an anamnestic immune response that generates a marked increase in the titer of the alloantibody. As a consequence, the donor cells become sensitized and subsequently undergo immune destruction. The time required for the anamnestic response to occur accounts for the delay in the onset of clinical signs and symptoms. Depending on the characteristics of the antibody and antigen, either intravascular or extravascular hemolysis may be the predominant process. Symptoms are usually mild (often low-grade fever only, but chills, pallor, and jaundice may be observed). In rare instances, renal failure and diffuse intravascular coagulation have been observed in association with delayed transfusion reactions.

The diagnosis is made by demonstrating an alloantibody in the patient's serum. Results of the indirect Coombs test are usually strongly positive because the antibody must be present in relatively high concentrations for clinically significant hemolysis to be apparent. The need to distinguish a delayed transfusion reaction from autoimmune hemolytic anemia (AIHA), however, may create a dilemma. The problem is complicated by the observation that transfusion can stimulate development of AIHA.

Standard laboratory tests (lactate dehydrogenase,

indirect bilirubin, and haptoglobin) document hemolysis but do not differentiate between AIHA and delayed transfusion reaction. Results of the direct Coombs' test are positive in the case of both AIHA and delayed transfusion reaction. Results of the indirect Coombs' test are almost invariably positive in delayed transfusion reactions. Although the test results are also positive in approximately 50% of the cases of AIHA, it may be informative to compare the relative strength of the direct and indirect test results. In AIHA, results of the direct test are usually stronger. In contrast, results of the indirect test are usually stronger in cases of delayed transfusion reaction. Determination of antibody specificity differentiates AIHA from delayed transfusion reactions. Autoantibodies are panagglutinins. In contrast, alloantibodies are truly specific in that they fail to react with cells that lack the antigen.

Delayed transfusion reactions usually require only minimal symptomatic and supportive treatment. If the anemia is severe, however, transfusion may be necessary. Kidney function should be monitored. In the unusual circumstance in which there is evidence of renal impairment, treatment should be initiated using the management guidelines provided earlier for acute major transfusion reactions.

TRANSFUSION-ASSOCIATED GRAFT-VERSUS-HOST DISEASE

TA-GVHD results when immunologically competent donor lymphocytes are infused into a recipient whose immune system does not recognize the transfused lymphocytes as foreign. Under these circumstances, the donor lymphocytes can proliferate and subsequently mount an attack on the recipient. The result is devastating; more than 90% of patients with TA-GVHD die, usually as a result of immunologically mediated bone marrow aplasia.

Failure of the recipient's system to recognize transfused lymphocytes as foreign is usually the result of an incompetent or immature immune system. The process can also occur, however, in immunocompetent recipients. In this case, the transfused lymphocytes are antigenetically similar enough to the recipient to avoid immune surveillance. For example, a directed blood donation from a first-degree relative may result in TA-GVHD if the donor and recipient share the same HLA haplotype. The clinical manifestations of TA-GVHD (fever, rash, watery or bloody diarrhea, elevated liver enzyme levels, and hyperbilirubinemia) are similar to those of GVHD observed in the setting of bone marrow transplant with one major exception. With TA-GVHD, marrow aplasia is the characteristic terminal event in the disease process because the bone marrow of the recipient is seen as foreign by the donor lymphocytes. In transplant-associated GVHD, immune-mediated marrow aplasia is not observed because the bone marrow and the immunocompetent lymphocytes are both of donor origin.

TA-GVDH is refractory to treatment, but it is preventable. The key to preventing TA-GVHD is to be aware of the patients who are at risk for developing the disease and to provide them with irradiated blood when transfusion is required. The groups with a well-defined risk follow:

1. Bone marrow transplant recipients
2. Patients with congenital immunodeficiency syndromes
3. Recipients of intrauterine transfusion
4. Recipients of transfusions from first-degree relatives
5. Patients with Hodgkin's disease

Patients in these categories should receive blood products that have been irradiated sufficiently to completely inactivate T lymphocytes. In vitro studies suggest that doses of 2500 to 3000 cGy may be required for complete inactivation of T cells in transfused cellular products. Currently, it is unclear if leukodepletion is adequate to prevent TA-GVHD.

Other groups that may be at risk for developing TA-GVHD include the following:

1. Premature newborns
2. Patients with hematologic malignancies other than Hodgkin's disease
3. Patients with some solid tumors (including neuroblastoma, glioblastoma, rhabdomyosarcoma) treated with chemotherapy or radiation
4. Solid organ transplant recipients

The risk of TA-GVHD for this group is less well defined, but consideration should be given to the use of irradiated cellular blood products in these patients. On the other hand, there is no clearly defined risk for full-term newborns, patients with AIDS, or nontransplant patients receiving standard immunosuppressive therapy.

Section 6

The Digestive System

CHOLELITHIASIS AND CHOLECYSTITIS

method of
JAY B. PRYSTOWSKY, M.D.
Northwestern University Medical School
Chicago, Illinois

CHOLELITHIASIS

Twenty to 30 million people in the United States have cholelithiasis (gallstones in the gallbladder). The prevalence of gallstones is higher in women than men and increases with aging. Other risk factors for the development of gallstones include class III obesity, diabetes mellitus, exogenous estrogen administration, pregnancy, rapid weight loss, hemolytic disorders, biliary infection, alcoholic cirrhosis, truncal vagotomy (a common feature of peptic ulcer surgery), and long-term total parenteral nutrition. Hereditary and ethnic factors also have a role in the pathogenesis of gallstones. A frequently cited study of Pima Indian women in the southwestern United States demonstrated a 73% incidence of gallstones between the ages of 25 and 34 years.

Gallstones are classified as cholesterol, pigment, or mixed type. In fact, all gallstones contain cholesterol, phospholipids, bile pigments, and calcium salts. The classification of gallstones depends on their predominant component. In the United States, cholesterol gallstones are the most common type, whereas pigment gallstones are the most common type worldwide.

The pathogenesis of cholesterol gallstones is not entirely clear, but most researchers point to four factors in their development:

1. Cholesterol supersaturation of bile
2. Mucus hypersecretion of the gallbladder
3. Nucleation (the formation and agglomeration of cholesterol crystals)
4. Gallbladder stasis

The pathogenesis of pigment gallstones is also unclear, although the final common pathway is altered solubilization of unconjugated bilirubin with precipitation of calcium bilirubinate and insoluble salts.

Gallstones are primarily discovered in one of two situations. First, a patient may complain of symptoms suggestive of cholecystitis. Ultrasonography (US) of the abdomen is done to determine the presence of gallstones. This procedure is highly accurate for gallstone detection, and, considering that it is a relatively low-cost, noninvasive imaging technique, it is the test of choice for detecting gallstones.

Alternatively, unsuspected gallstones may be detected by US, computed tomography, magnetic resonance imaging, and even plain radiography during the evaluation of patients for some other intra-abdominal problem. In these circumstances, the patient may seek the advice of a physician for incidentally discovered gallstones. Regardless of the mode of discovery, proper management of the patient with gallstones requires familiarity with the natural history of gallstones and the symptoms they may elicit.

In past decades, many believed the presence of gallstones alone was an indication for cholecystectomy. More recently, several important studies have reported the natural history of gallstone disease. Collectively, these studies suggest that the incidence of the development of symptoms in patients with gallstones ranges from 10% to 30% over a period of 2 to 15 years. Also, once a patient develops symptomatic gallstones, the incidence of recurrent symptoms is very high. These studies are the foundation of an important principle in the management of gallstones: observation alone is warranted for patients with asymptomatic cholelithiasis, whereas intervention is indicated for patients with symptomatic gallstones. Thus, the first objective of a physician in the evaluation of a patient with gallstones is to determine if the patient has symptoms consistent with cholecystitis.

CHRONIC CHOLECYSTITIS

Chronic cholecystitis is a clinical and pathologic diagnosis. For the pathologist, chronic inflammatory cells and frequently fibrosis are observed in the gallbladder wall. For the clinician, patients often present with complaints of recurrent epigastric or right upper quadrant abdominal pain. The pain is usually more severe than pain associated with peptic ulcer or gastroesophageal reflux disease. The pain increases gradually in severity, plateaus in intensity, and then gradually resolves. It usually lasts for hours per episode and frequently follows ingestion of a fatty meal or awakens patients from sleep at night. The pain often radiates to the right subscapular region and there is associated nausea and vomiting. Most patients report more than one episode. The pain of chronic cholecystitis is often referred to as *biliary colic*. In fact, the pain is not colicky but constant. *Biliary colic* is a misnomer, but the term is often used to describe the pain of chronic cholecystitis.

Patients with chronic cholecystitis most commonly present to their physician in the outpatient setting with mild to moderate recurrent symptoms. A complete history, physical examination, complete blood cell count, and liver enzyme test should be performed. In the presence of patient symptoms that are suggestive of chronic cholecystitis, US of the gallbladder is recommended to detect gallstones. In addition, gallbladder wall thickening (suggestive of gallbladder inflammation) and bile duct dilation (suggestive of gallstones passing into the bile duct) can be assessed. Other tests may be needed depending on the differential diagnosis and the patient's co-morbid conditions. Biliary colic along with documented gallstones suggests the clinical diagnosis of chronic cholecystitis. There is no test per se that confirms the diagnosis; rather, the diagnosis is primarily based on the patient's history and US findings of gallstones. Because of the recurrent nature of this disease, intervention is warranted once the diagnosis is established; the patient should be referred to a surgeon for elective cholecystectomy.

ACUTE CHOLECYSTITIS

Ten percent to 20% of patients with symptomatic cholelithiasis will present with *acute cholecystitis.* These patients complain of severe abdominal pain consistent with biliary colic. In addition, they manifest fever, right quadrant abdominal tenderness, and leukocytosis. The classic physical finding of acute cholecystitis is the Murphy sign—arrest of inspiration with palpation of the right upper quadrant abdominal wall. Many of these patients have previously undergone gallbladder US for minor symptoms and may report the presence of gallstones. For some, this may be their first attack and US of the gallbladder should be performed to detect gallstones.

Characteristic symptoms and active inflammatory signs along with documented gallstones establish the clinical diagnosis of acute cholecystitis. In some cases, the history and physical findings are suggestive but not characteristic of acute cholecystitis. Because the pathogenesis of acute cholecystitis is cystic duct obstruction, biliary scintigraphy is particularly useful in confirming the diagnosis of acute cholecystitis.

An organic anion (iminodiacetic acid or related compound) that is labeled with technetium-99m is injected intravenously. The anion can be seen with nuclear scanning as it is taken up by the liver and excreted into the biliary tract. In patients without acute cholecystitis, the cystic duct is patent and the anion passes into the gallbladder. Nuclear scanning demonstrates gallbladder visualization. In patients with cystic duct obstruction, the anion does not pass into the gallbladder and nuclear scanning demonstrates gallbladder "nonvisualization." Biliary scintigraphy provides accurate assessment of cystic duct patency or obstruction and is therefore very helpful in establishing the diagnosis of acute cholecystitis.

Most patients with acute cholecystitis present to a local emergency department. Hospital admission is appropriate once the diagnosis is established. These patients should receive intravenous fluids, be given nothing orally, and take broad-spectrum intravenous antibiotics effective against the most common biliary tract organisms (i.e., *Escherichia coli, Klebsiella, Proteus,* and enterococcus). Other co-morbid illnesses should be addressed. There is controversy regarding the timing of surgery in those patients with acute cholecystitis who respond favorably to initial medical measures. Some favor a "cooling-off" period of at least 6 weeks before operation, whereas other surgeons favor early surgery (within 2–3 days of hospital admission). Regardless of timing, all would agree that these patients will suffer recurrent attacks and surgery should not be delayed indefinitely.

A small percentage of patients with acute cholecystitis do not respond favorably to initial medical treatment. Often, these patients are elderly with high fever and markedly elevated white blood cell counts. The clinician should have a strong index of suspicion for gallbladder gangrene; in such circumstances, cholecystectomy should be performed promptly. Some patients may have co-morbid illnesses that place them at very high risk for surgery. Percutaneous cholecystostomy should be performed in these patients to decompress the gallbladder. This procedure is usually performed by an interventional radiologist under US guidance using local anesthesia. It is frequently successful at ameliorating gallbladder inflammation and can be used as a temporizing measure until the patient can be properly prepared for surgery.

A small percentage of patients will develop acute cholecystitis in the absence of gallstones. Acute acalculous cholecystitis is unusual but should be considered in critically ill patients who manifest inflammatory signs in the right upper quadrant of the abdomen or who manifest sepsis of uncertain etiology. Depending on the severity of co-morbid conditions, cholecystectomy or percutaneous cholecystostomy should be performed.

It is important to emphasize that the diagnosis of chronic and acute cholecystitis is largely based on an accurate history of the patient's symptoms. Millions of patients experience abdominal pain; many of them harbor gallstones. However, the two entities, abdominal pain and gallstones, may not always be related. The discriminating clinician should not be biased to the diagnosis of cholecystitis just because of the presence of gallstones. Nonetheless, once the clinician is satisfied with the diagnosis of cholecystitis, intervention is warranted to ameliorate current symptoms and prevent recurrent symptoms.

CHOLEDOCHOLITHIASIS

An important consideration in patients with gallstones is the possibility that gallstones may pass into the bile duct. Choledocholithiasis or bile duct stones may be discovered incidentally with preoperative or intraoperative imaging techniques. Alternatively, patients may develop symptoms such as jaundice, cholangitis, or pancreatitis secondary to obstructing bile duct stones. In general, bile duct stones should be removed when discovered. Endoscopic retrograde cholangiopancreatography (ERCP) with stone extraction and sphincterotomy is the most common method for bile duct stone removal and is an excellent adjunct to cholecystectomy.

TREATMENT

Multiple nonoperative methods have been used for the treatment of cholelithiasis. In the past 15 years, two methods have received significant attention: oral dissolution agents and gallbladder lithotripsy (alone or in combination). Both techniques appear to be safe but are applicable to a relatively small number of patients with a small burden of noncalcified stones. Even for this select group of patients, these treatments are not reliable in rendering the gallbladder free of gallstones. Perhaps the greatest disadvantage of these treatments is that even if a patient is effectively treated and the gallbladder becomes free of stones, the recurrence rate of gallstones is approximately 50% within 5 years. In short, nonoperative therapy for cholecystitis is ineffective in terms of providing a long-term cure.

Surgical extirpation of the gallbladder, namely cholecystectomy, is the treatment of choice for both chronic and acute cholecystitis. The preferred surgical procedure is laparoscopic cholecystectomy. The laparoscopic approach requires general anesthesia. Typically, four small incisions (1–2 cm in length; one at the umbilicus and three along the right costal margin) are used. Insufflation of carbon dioxide into the peritoneal cavity is accomplished to separate the abdominal wall from underlying organs. A telescope is inserted through the abdominal wall to view the intra-abdominal contents. The telescope is connected to a camera that, in turn, is connected to a monitor for viewing by the surgical team. Specialized instruments are placed into the abdomen through the other incisions. The gallbladder is dissected and removed through one of the small incisions.

Laparoscopic cholecystectomy is not pain free, but most patients are discharged from the hospital within 24 hours of the procedure and continue their convalescence at home. Most patients comfortably resume pervious activities within 7 to 14 days of their operation. Complications of surgery include (but are not limited to) bleeding, infection, bile leak from the gallbladder fossa or cystic duct stump, and bile duct injury. Bile duct injury occurs in approximately 0.4% of patients undergoing cholecystectomy. Although uncommon, it is a serious injury that often requires reoperation and bile duct reconstruction. Bile duct injury is the most common cause of litigation surrounding cholecystectomy in the United States.

In 2% to 5% of patients with chronic cholecystitis and 5% to 25% of patients with acute cholecystitis, it may be necessary for the surgeon to convert a laparoscopic procedure to an open operation. The open technique employs a 10- to 18-cm right subcostal incision and permits greater exposure of the biliary tract. In patients with severe inflammatory changes around the gallbladder or cystic duct, excessive bleeding, or biliary tract anomalies, conversion to an open procedure is an option that the surgeon may exercise. Using the open technique produces a need for a longer hospital stay and a longer time for return to normal activity for the patient (bigger incision equals more pain equals longer recovery). However, the decision to convert to an open technique may facilitate a safer operation, which is the first surgical priority. Although disappointing to the patient, conversion to an open procedure should not be considered a surgical complication. More accurately, it comprises sound surgical judgment to prevent operative complications. Patients should be properly informed before surgery of this possibility.

Many patients ask how their lives will change without a gallbladder. Because the gallbladder does not manufacture any substance that is important for digestion, most patients will perceive no difference in their lifestyle or diet after cholecystectomy. Eight percent to 10% of patients will experience postcholecystectomy diarrhea. These patients experience a strong sense of rectal urgency after surgery and complain of 3 to 5 loose stools per day. In most of these patients, these symptoms resolve gradually within 4 to 6 weeks of surgery. Some patients may experience diarrhea beyond this period and require treatment with cholestyramine (Questran, a bile-salt binding agent, 4 g/d) to resolve their symptoms.

Approximately 5% of patients who undergo cholecystectomy will continue to have the symptoms that prompted surgery in the first place. These patients are classified as having the *postcholecystectomy syndrome*. A thorough evaluation of other possible causes of their symptoms should begin and include an ERCP. In performing this test, the gastrointestinal endoscopist is able to view the distal esophagus (for reflux disease), the stomach (for gastritis or ulcers), and the duodenum (for ulcers) and can obtain a contrast study of the bile duct (for bile duct stones or injuries). In addition, biliary manometry may be performed to assess spasm of the distal bile duct or sphincter of Oddi. Endoscopic sphincterotomy can be performed if distal bile duct spasm is suspected. Despite a complete evaluation, the cause of some patients' pain is never identified.

CIRRHOSIS

method of
H. FRANKLIN HERLONG, M.D., and
MEGAN RIST HAYMART, B.A.
The Johns Hopkins University School of Medicine
Baltimore, Maryland

Characterized histologically by irreversible fibrosis and nodular regeneration, cirrhosis results from the wound-healing response of the liver to chronic injury from toxins, viruses, cholestasis, or metabolic disorders. Patients with cirrhosis may be asymptomatic or present with palmar erythema, caput medusae, gynecomastia, jaundice, spider angiomas, splenomegaly, hematemesis, or other findings associated with portal hypertension. Although radiographic studies or biochemical abnormalities may suggest cirrhosis, a definitive diagnosis often requires a liver biopsy. The Child-Pugh Staging Score can be used to assess prognosis and evaluate risk of surgery. Class A patients have a mean survival rate of 40 months compared with 32 months for Class B and 8 months for Class C (Table 1).

The treatment of cirrhosis can be divided into three categories. One category is *etiology-specific treatment*. This involves identifying the potential cause of cirrhosis and limiting further disease progression. Another category of treatment is addressing *complications associated with portal hypertension*. Distortion of liver architecture by cirrhosis can increase portal pressure greater than 5 mm Hg above inferior vena cava pressure. Increased dependence on systemic circulation and decline in toxin filtration via the liver can lead to ascites, spontaneous bacterial peritonitis (SBP), hepatic encephalopathy (HE), esophageal varices, and hepatorenal syndrome (HRS). The third treatment category focuses on *complications of cirrhosis not associated with portal hypertension*. Hematologic abnormalities, hepatic osteodystrophy, altered drug metabolism, and hepatocellular carcinoma are other such complications of cirrhosis.

TABLE 1. **Child-Pugh Score**

Parameter	Points		
	1	*2*	*3*
Encephalopathy (grade)	None	1–2	3–4
Ascites	Absent	Slight	Moderate
Bilirubin (mg/dL)	<2.0	2.0–3.0	>3.0
Albumin (g/dL)	>3.5	2.8–3.5	<2.8
Prothrombin time (s prolonged)	1.0–4.0	4.0–6.0	>6.0

Class A = 5–6 points; Class B = 7–9 points; Class C = 10–15 points.

ETIOLOGY-SPECIFIC TREATMENT

The incidence of cirrhosis is estimated to be 360 in 100,000 people, with hepatitis C virus (HCV) and excess alcohol consumption accounting for most of the cases. Other less common causes include hepatotoxicity from medications such as isoniazid, methotrexate, or amiodarone; metabolic diseases such as hemochromatosis, Wilson disease, and α_1-antitrypsin deficiency; autoimmune liver disease; and nonalcoholic steatohepatitis (NASH).

Alcoholic Cirrhosis

The estimated average total intake required to develop cirrhosis is 80 g of ethanol per day for 20 years, but doses less than 80 g can still increase the risk of cirrhosis. In addition, women have a greater likelihood than men of developing cirrhosis when ingesting the same amount of alcohol. Abstinence from alcohol consumption is the most important factor in the treatment of alcoholic cirrhosis. Progression of liver disease and accelerated mortality are likely in patients who continue to drink. Many alcoholic patients also have specific nutritional needs to address. They may need supplements of thiamine (vitamin B_1) 50 to 100 mg/d, pyridoxine (vitamin B_6) 100 mg/d, and folic acid 1 mg/d. Supplementation with magnesium, phosphorus, and potassium is also necessary if serum levels are low.

Viral Hepatitis

Viral hepatitis has surpassed alcohol as the primary cause of cirrhosis in the United States. Immune-mediated injury to infected hepatocytes contributes to hepatocellular injury and fibrosis. Ideally, treatment of viral hepatitis should be started before the development of cirrhosis to retard progression. However, the same treatment options still have some efficacy even if cirrhosis is already present. The likelihood of a desirable response to antiviral therapy is influenced by both the genotype of the virus and the viral load as measured by polymerase chain reaction. Patients with genotype 1B and a viral load greater than 2 million copies/mL are less likely to respond.

Interferon alfa-2b (Intron A) 3 million U three times a week combined with ribavirin (Virazole) 600 mg two times a day (as Rebetron) is the standard treatment for chronic HCV. Side effects of interferon alfa include fatigue, depression, nausea, vomiting, diarrhea, dry mouth, anemia, flulike symptoms, fever, and weight loss. Ribavirin can be associated with adverse reactions such as hemolysis, dizziness, and ocular irritation.

Interferon alfa is also first-line therapy for hepatitis B virus (HBV). Patients should be treated with 10 million U three times a week or 5 million U six times a week for a total of 4 months. Another therapeutic option for HBV is lamivudine (3TC or Epivir) 100 mg/d for 3 months. Lamivudine can decrease HBV DNA, increase loss of hepatitis B early antigen (HB_eAg), increase the development of hepatitis B early antibody (HB_eAb), decrease progression to cirrhosis, and lead to normalization of alanine transaminase (ALT) levels. Lamivudine is better tolerated than interferon alfa but emerging resistance to the drug is a problem.

Autoimmune Liver Diseases

The cholestatic autoimmune liver diseases include primary biliary cirrhosis (PBC) and primary sclerosing cholangitis (PSC). PBC is an autoimmune-mediated disorder characterized by progressive destruction of intrahepatic bile ducts and the presence of antimitochondrial antibodies. The patient is usually a middle-aged woman who presents with fatigue, pruritus, and serum alkaline phosphatase elevation. Ursodiol (Actigall)* 13 to 15 mg/kg/d decreases the progression of PBC and delays the need for liver transplantation. Ursodiol is safe, well tolerated, and believed to function by counteracting the effects of toxic bile acids on the hepatocytes. Immunosupressants such as prednisone, azathioprine (Imuran), and methotrexate have questionable benefits and often undesirable side effects in patients with PBC.

Pruritus is often associated with PBC and other forms of cholestasis and is related to the effects of endogenous opioid production. Mild pruritus is treated with the ionic-binding agent, cholestyramine (Questran)* 16 g/d. This drug should be divided into two 8-g doses, with the first dose before breakfast when puritogen concentrations in the intestinal lumen are greatest. Antihistamines such as hydroxyzine (Atarax), have little effect on pruritus but can act as a sedative and may be used in the evening to alleviate pruritus-induced insomnia. Rifampin (Rimactane)* 10 mg/kg orally once a day or phenobarbital* 100 mg/d is considered second-line therapy. Opioid antagonists, such as naloxone (Narcan)* 0.4 mg intravenous (IV) bolus, followed by 0.2 μg/kg/min IV infusion, can offer transient relief to refractory pruritus.

Malabsorption of fat and the fat-soluble vitamins D, A, K, and E is another complication of PBC. Because there is a decline in concentration of bile salts entering the intestinal lumen, there is a reduction in micelle formation resulting in steatorrhea and associated vitamin malabsorption. If a patient has diarrhea from steatorrhea, fat can be restricted to less than 40 g/d. If fat calories are insufficient, medium chain triglycerides (MCT oil 1 tablespoon three or four times a day, or Portagen three to four 8-oz servings), which do not require bile salts for absorption, can be administered. Treat vitamin deficiencies with 25,000 U of vitamin A (Aquasol A) daily, 5 mg a day of vitamin K (AquaMEPHYTON), 400 IU of vitamin E daily, and 2000 IU/d of vitamin D (then reduce to 400 IU/d for maintenance).

PSC is caused by autoimmune injury to extrahepatic and intrahepatic ducts and is associated with

*Not FDA approved for this indication.

inflammatory bowel disease, typically ulcerative colitis, in up to 90% of patients. PSC patients also have an increased risk of cholangiocarcinoma, and they may have serum antinuclear antibodies or anticytoplasmic neutrophil antibodies. Treatment for secondary biliary cirrhosis from PSC is the same as that for PBC except biliary decompression via endoscopic stent placement may relieve obstruction from strictures. Although ursodeoxycholic acid is the recommended medical treatment for PSC, the long-term outcome of ursodeoxycholic acid therapy in patients with PSC is less clear.

Autoimmune hepatitis primarily affects women and is characterized by elevated gamma globulin levels, antinuclear antibodies, and antismooth muscle antibodies. Patients respond well to immunosuppressive therapy, especially if the therapy is started when the disease is first recognized. Therapy is initiated with 40 mg of prednisone daily. As the transaminase levels fall below 100 IU/dL, the patient can be started on a maintenance dose of 10 to 15 mg of prednisone per day. The addition of azathioprine (Imuran) 50 to 100 mg/d often allows the dose of prednisone to be reduced further. Azathioprine 100 mg/d can be used alone for maintenance in some patients, thus avoiding the risks of long-term corticosteroid therapy. Immunosuppression must be used for several years in most patients. Patients frequently relapse once immunosuppressive therapy is withdrawn. In these patients, therapy must be reinstituted promptly.

Metabolic Liver Disease

Decreasing the mineral or metabolite in excess can retard progression to cirrhosis in diseases such as hemochromatosis and Wilson's disease. Primary hemochromatosis is an autosomal recessive disorder resulting in increased intestinal absorption of iron and iron deposition in multiple organs. Repeated phlebotomy should be used with the removal of 500 mL of blood weekly until transferrin saturation is less than 50%, ferritin is less than 50 ng/mL, or hemoglobin falls below 10 mg/dL. Even if the patient with hemochromatosis already has cirrhosis, iron depletion via phlebotomy can alleviate some of the hepatic and extrahepatic manifestations of the disease. Therapy with an iron chelator, deferoxamine (Desferal), can be initiated if phlebotomy is not well tolerated.

Wilson's disease is an autosomal recessive disease resulting in copper accumulation in the liver, kidneys, and central nervous system. Patients have serum ceruloplasmin levels less than 20 mg/dL, elevated urinary copper excretion, elevated liver copper on biopsy specimen, and may have Kayser-Fleisher rings in the cornea. Penicillamine (Cuprimine) 1 to 2 g/d divided into four doses can retard copper accumulation, but the side effects of penicillamine, including skin reactions, arthralgias, proteinuria, and a systemic lupus–like syndrome, limit its usefulness. An alternative therapy is oral zinc sulfate 250 mg or zinc acetate 50 mg three times a day. Zinc prevents copper absorption in the gastrointestinal tract.

Nonalcoholic Steatohepatitis

The histologic appearance of NASH is identical to that seen in alcoholic liver. The profile of a patient with NASH is typically an obese middle-aged woman with type II diabetes mellitus and hyperlipidemia who does not have a history of excess alcohol consumption. However, NASH can also occur in younger, leaner individuals who do not have a history of diabetes mellitus or dyslipidemia. Ten percent to 15% of patients with NASH progress to cirrhosis. In addition, recent studies have suggested that patients with cryptogenic cirrhosis have characteristics compatible with NASH (obesity and type II diabetes mellitus), suggesting NASH may be an important cause of cryptogenic cirrhosis.

Potential treatment options for NASH include weight loss, gemfibrozil (Lopid)* 600 mg twice a day, and ursodiol. Weight loss and lifestyle modifications are difficult to maintain but can result in a reduction in aminotransferase levels and in some cases an improvement in histologic appearance. A trial of 4 weeks of gemfibrozil therapy decreased ALT and aspartate transaminase levels in patients with NASH. One year of ursodiol therapy decreased ALT and alkaline phosphatase levels in patients with NASH but did not change histologic appearance.

Multiple Etiologies

Coexisting liver diseases (e.g., HCV and alcoholism) can increase the rate of progression of cirrhosis. For this reason, patients with cirrhosis from any cause should receive recombinant HBV vaccine as well as hepatitis A vaccine to prevent superimposed liver disease. In addition, all individuals with cirrhosis should limit alcohol consumption.

TREATMENT OF COMPLICATIONS ASSOCIATED WITH PORTAL HYPERTENSION

Ascites

Ascites is caused by cirrhosis in most patients, with a combination of portal hypertension, hypoalbuminemia, splanchnic arteriolar dilation, and increased sodium absorption by the kidneys contributing to its formation. Ascites carries an ominous prognosis for patients with cirrhosis with fewer than 40% of patients with ascites alive 2 years after it is first recognized. The physical examination alone is unreliable in the detection of ascites. If there are doubts about ascites' existence, an abdominal sonogram can confirm its presence and identify an appropriate site for a diagnostic paracentesis.

Fifty milliliters of fluid should be removed via

*Not FDA approved for this indication.

paracentesis for analysis of protein and glucose content, blood cell count with differential analysis, albumin, amylase, Gram stain of a fluid sample, bacterial culture, and mycobacterial culture. The serum-ascites albumin gradient (SAAG) should be calculated by subtracting the ascites albumin concentration from the serum albumin concentration. If SAAG is greater than or equal to 1.1 g/dL, portal hypertension–induced ascites is likely. If SAAG is less than 1.1 g/dL, neoplasm, tuberculosis, pancreatitis, and other nonhepatic origins of ascites are more likely. Similarly, if the ascites fluid is transudative (protein content <2 g/dL), ascites due to cirrhosis is probable.

Sodium restriction and diuretic therapy are the cornerstones of ascites management. Sodium restriction to 40 to 60 mEq/d combined with spironolactone (Aldactone) 50 to 100 mg/d (with the maximum dose of 400 mg/d) is first-line therapy. Furosemide (Lasix) 40 mg/d has a greater risk of azotemia than spironolactone, but can be added if spironolactone and salt reduction are ineffective or if potassium levels are elevated with spironolactone use. The maximum dose of furosemide is 160 mg/d. Patients can safely lose up to 2 lb of fluid a day without intravascular volume depletion. If the patient has both peripheral edema and ascites, a greater weight loss is acceptable.

When maximum diuretic doses and sodium restriction result in urine sodium excretion of less than 10 mEq/d, the ascites is considered refractory to medical treatment. Therapeutic paracentesis with 4 to 6 L removed per visit is acceptable treatment for these patients. Six to 8 g of albumin can be infused per liter of fluid removed to reduce the risk of azotemia. Therapeutic paracentesis is not recommended as initial therapy because repeated paracentesis can increase the risk of bacterial peritonitis.

Transplantation should be considered when ascites is refractory to medical therapy. However, if a patient is not an acceptable transplant candidate, transjugular intrahepatic portosystemic shunting (TIPS) is another option.

Spontaneous Bacterial Peritonitis

SBP occurs in 10% to 30% of cirrhotic patients with ascites. Signs of SBP include fever, abdominal pain, HE, hypotension, or worsening hepatic function. The diagnosis is confirmed by ascitic fluid analysis. If the ascitic fluid has more than 250 polymorphonuclear neutrophils per mm^3, a presumptive diagnosis of SBP is made and empiric antibiotic therapy initiated with a third-generation cephalosporin such as cefotaxime (Claforan) 1 to 2 g IV every 6 to 8 hours or ceftriaxone (Rocephin) 500 to 1000 mg IV every 12 hours. The antibiotic should be continued for 5 to 7 days. Aminoglycosides should be avoided because they are associated with a high prevalence of ototoxicity and nephrotoxicity in cirrhotic patients.

One third of patients with SBP have a decline in renal function, which is inversely related to mortality. The renal impairment associated with SBP is presumed to be due to infection, further decreasing renal blood flow and glomerular filtration rate leading to activation of the renin-angiotensin system. Albumin infusion plus cefotaxime significantly decrease renal impairment and in-hospital mortality compared to cefotaxime alone.

Hepatic Encephalopathy

HE is a particularly disabling complication of cirrhosis. HE has two main components: motor disturbances and altered consciousness. The motor disturbances include hyperreflexia, positive Babinski sign, cogwheel rigidity, asterixis, fine tremor, decline in motor coordination, monotone speech, slow pupil responses, ocular saccades, and immobile facies. The altered consciousness can vary from confusion to coma. Before the development of confusion, patients may have a change in their sleep-wake cycles or exhibit abnormal behavior. The onset of HE may be gradual or rapid and patients may have single or multiple attacks.

The first step in the treatment of HE is to exclude other causes of motor disturbances and mental status changes. For example, hypercapnia, salicylate poisoning, drug intoxication, and brainstem lesions can cause asterixis. Hypoxia, hyperglycemia or hypoglycemia, metabolic acidosis, delirium tremens, and central nervous system infection can all cause mental status changes in patients with cirrhosis.

The second step in the therapy of HE is to eliminate precipitants. Uremia, increased protein intake, gastrointestinal hemorrhage, constipation, hypokalemia, alkalosis, sedative drugs, and infections can precipitate HE.

HE is caused by the shunting of portal blood around a poorly functioning liver, leading to the accumulation of toxins in the blood and central nervous system. To decrease toxins such as ammonia and other nitrogen-containing compounds, the patient should receive a protein-restricted diet (0.5 g/kg body weight) for a few days. Because malnutrition is undesirable, protein restriction can be liberalized when symptoms improve.

Initially, water or lactulose enemas can be used to cleanse the gastrointestinal tract and identify a possible gastrointestinal hemorrhage, followed by oral lactulose (Cephulac) 30 mL every 6 to 12 hours. The dose of oral lactulose is titrated until the patient has two to four loose stools a day. Lactulose induces an osmotic diarrhea and creates an acidic environment that decreases bacterial generation of ammonia. Oral antibiotics can also be used to reduce bacterial ammonia production. Neomycin 6 g/d is frequently used but because of the risk of ototoxicity, metronidazole (Flagyl) 250 to 500 mg orally three times a day is another option. Another alternative to lactulose is oral sodium benzoate 5 g twice a day. Sodium benzoate increases nitrogen excretion and appears to be efficacious in treating HE. Sodium benzoate is less expensive than lactulose but can cause gastrointestinal intolerance in some patients.

Hepatorenal Syndrome

HRS is a disorder in which intrinsically normal kidneys fail in the setting of advanced liver disease. HRS is characterized by decreased renal blood flow, decreased glomerular filtration rate, and decreased cortical perfusion. Patients typically have a normal urine osmolality but urinary sodium excretion is low (<10 mEq/L). The prognosis is poor when HRS develops in a patient with cirrhosis. Nephrotoxic drugs, such as nonsteroidal anti-inflammatory drugs, should be avoided and intravascular volume maintained. In most patients, reversal of HRS requires correcting the liver disease with transplantation. Dialysis can be used if a patient is awaiting transplant, but there is little long-term benefit in the patients who are not transplant candidates. TIPS has been reported to improve HRS but randomized control trials have not been performed.

TREATMENT OF COMPLICATIONS NOT DIRECTLY RELATED TO PORTAL HYPERTENSION

Hematologic Abnormalities

Several conditions contribute to coagulation abnormalities in patients with cirrhosis. Malabsorption of vitamin K in patients with steatorrhea leads to deficits in factors II, VII, IX, and X. Therefore, patients with a prolonged prothrombin time should receive 10 mg of vitamin K subcutaneously. Impaired hepatic synthesis of all coagulation factors (except VIII and von Willebrand) contributes to coagulation abnormalities. If a cirrhotic patient has active bleeding and impaired coagulation, fresh frozen plasma (2 U every 6 hours until bleeding ceases) should be administered.

Splenic sequestration of platelets in a patient with portal hypertension can result in thrombocytopenia. In addition, a reduction in platelet count can be caused by immune-mediated thrombocytopenia in patients with autoimmune hepatitis or HCV. Chronic alcohol consumption can cause folate deficiency and impair bone marrow production. Low-grade disseminated intravascular coagulation (DIC) can also cause thrombocytopenia. Platelet transfusions before invasive procedures are required when the platelet count is less than 50,000/mm^3.

Anemia is another common hematologic abnormality seen in patients with cirrhosis. Decreased production of red blood cells because of folic acid, iron, or vitamin B_{12} deficiency along with increased destruction associated with hypersplenism can be seen in some patients. Anemia of chronic disease and relative anemia secondary to increased plasma volume are other explanations for a low hematocrit level. Correcting anemia depends on appropriately identifying the cause. If serum folic acid levels are low, the patient should receive folate 1.0 mg orally once a day. Iron deficiency can be treated with 325 mg of ferrous sulfate (Feosol) orally three times a day.

Hepatic Osteodystrophy

Hepatic osteodystrophy refers to the metabolic bone disease that occurs in patients with chronic liver disease. It is especially common in patients with cholestatic liver disease. Patients with PBC and PSC lose two times more bone mass per year than the general population. Although hepatic osteodystrophy includes both osteoporosis and osteomalacia, osteoporosis is the most frequent cause of osteopenia.

To prevent hepatic osteodystrophy, serum calcium, phosphate, and 25-hydroxyvitamin D should be measured in all patients. Bone mineral density should be assessed with dual-energy x-ray absorptiometry (DEXA). The level of osteopenia and fracture risk can be evaluated with DEXA. Depending on dietary calcium consumption, patients should be started on 0.5 to 2.0 g/d of calcium carbonate or calcium citrate. Vitamin D intake should be 400 to 2000 IU/d, depending upon the degree of vitamin deficiency. Tobacco use and alcohol consumption should be eliminated. Postmenopausal women should be offered hormone replacement therapy to improve lumbar bone mineral density.

The decreased bone mass associated with osteoporosis causes fractures of vertebrae, hips, and forearms. In patients with autoimmune hepatitis, long-term corticosteroid use stimulates osteoclast activity, decreases calcium absorption, and increases calcium excretion, therefore elevating patients' risk of osteoporosis. Decreased estrogen production in postmenopausal women further contributes to the risk of osteoporosis.

Therapy for osteoporosis includes 1.0 to 2.0 g of calcium a day plus vitamin D 400 to 2000 IU a day, and 100 IU of calcitonin a day. Hormone replacement therapy and a bisphosphonate such as etidronate (Didronel) 5 to 10 mg/kg/d or alendronate (Fosamax) 5 to 10 mg a day can also be administered. Progression of osteoporosis can be monitored with DEXA.

Osteomalacia is characterized by decreased mineralization of the bone matrix and is frequently associated with bone pain, fractures, and proximal muscle weakness. The two most probable causes of osteomalacia in patients with cirrhosis are vitamin D malabsorption and defective hepatic 25-hydroxylation of vitamin D. Patients with PBC and PSC may malabsorb fat-soluble vitamin D and have decreased absorption of calcium due to low vitamin D levels.

In patients with low serum levels of vitamin D, 1000 to 4000 IU of oral vitamin D can be initiated. If a patient's vitamin D level is deficient due to impaired hepatocellular 25-hydroxylation of vitamin D, the patient can take the more expensive calcidiol (25OHD) or calcitriol (1,25OHD). If serum calcium is low, 1 to 2 g of calcium a day can be added to the regimen. Excess vitamin D can cause hypercalcemia and hypercalciuria; urinary calcium excretion or serum calcium should be monitored to determine the appropriate level of vitamin D supplementation.

Unlike other complications of cirrhosis, hepatic osteodystrophy often persists after transplantation.

Pre-existing osteopenic bone, poor nutrition, immobilization, steroid use, and cyclosporine use can all contribute to osteodystrophy after transplant.

Drug Metabolism

Drug metabolism is altered in a cirrhotic liver. Drugs eliminated by phase I oxidative reactions are primarily affected by changes in hepatic blood flow whereas drugs eliminated by phase II reactions are sensitive to hepatocyte dysfunction. Medications that normally have a short half-life may accumulate in patients with end-stage liver disease. Therefore, patients with cirrhosis may need smaller and less frequent doses of these medications. Because many drugs are protein bound, decreased albumin production by the liver can lead to an increase in the volume of distribution of certain drugs. For example, when a patient is hypoalbuminic, sedatives, which are a known precipitant of HE, have a higher proportion unbound, which subsequently leads to increased bioavailability and a higher proportion of sedatives reaching the brain. Drug elimination also varies with the cause of cirrhosis. For example, nafcillin is primarily excreted via the biliary route and is more affected by PBC than by alcoholic hepatitis.

Hepatocellular Carcinoma

The risk of hepatocellular carcinoma is increased in patients with cirrhosis. Cirrhosis due to hemochromatosis and viral hepatitis carries the greatest risk of hepatocellular carcinoma and warrants surveillance. Every 6 months, these patients should have serum α-fetoprotein levels measured and an abdominal ultrasound performed. If a suspicious lesion is identified with ultrasound or computed tomography, gadolinium-enhanced magnetic resonance imaging has greater specificity and can be used. A definitive diagnosis can be made with ultrasound-guided or computed tomography–guided biopsy. Early diagnosis of hepatocellular carcinoma offers the best chance of cure because the average survival time once hepatocellular carcinoma is clinically apparent is less than 6 months. The treatment options once hepatocellular carcinoma is detected include resection, liver transplantation, percutaneous ethanol injection, and chemoembolization via the hepatic artery. Chemoembolization is primarily palliative and ethanol injection is recommended for individuals who are not surgical candidates. Outcome is poor if the tumor is multifocal, invades blood vessels, or is greater than 5 cm.

Liver Transplantation

Liver transplantation is the only "cure" for cirrhosis with 85% of transplant recipients alive 5 years after their surgery. Patients should be referred to a transplant center when they have their first complication associated with cirrhosis. Due to the limited number of donor organs, patients are carefully screened for other conditions that would decrease the likelihood of success. Six months of alcohol abstinence is routinely required before transplantation will be performed in an individual with alcoholic cirrhosis.

BLEEDING ESOPHAGEAL VARICES

method of
BRIAN L. BLEAU, M.D.
Tacoma Digestive Disease Center
Tacoma, Washington

In patients with upper gastrointestinal (GI) bleeding, about 10% of bleeding episodes are secondary to varices. Patients with variceal hemorrhage tend to have more rapid bleeding and more complications than other types of upper GI hemorrhage. Most esophageal varices occur as a result of portal hypertension. Damage to the liver parenchyma results in increased resistance to blood flow through the portal veins of the liver. As a result of this pressure increase, less blood is able to flow through the liver and collateral channels are opened that allow some of the blood to bypass the liver. The most common area in which these enlarged vessels form is the lower esophagus, where the vessels have little supporting tissue but they can form anywhere along the GI tract. As the varices dilate, the tension on the vessel wall increases; as a result, the risk of rupture increases. The amount of bleeding depends on the size of the varices, the size of the tear, the portal pressure, and the degree of coagulopathy. Approximately one third of patients with varices will bleed from their varices, and hemorrhage from bleeding gastroesophageal varices will ultimately result in death in about half of the patients affected.

PATIENT ASSESSMENT AND RESUSCITATION

Patients with variceal bleeding require urgent management. The magnitude of blood loss can be massive and potentially fatal. Patients with known portal hypertension are at greatest risk for variceal bleeding, but they also can bleed from other lesions in up to 50% of bleeding episodes. In patients with variceal bleeding, there is often associated nausea and hematemesis of fresh blood and clots. Blood passes rapidly through the GI tract and maroon stools or melena may occur. Depending on the degree of bleeding, the patient may be hemodynamically unstable. Rapid assessment is required. Blood needs to be drawn (complete blood cell count, electrolytes, international normalized ratio [INR]), two large-bore intravenous catheters placed, and a type and crossmatch done. Intravenous resuscitation should be limited to reversing hypotension while awaiting blood and fresh frozen plasma. Caution needs to be taken not to fluid overload the patient. Red blood cells, fresh frozen plasma, and platelets are initiated as required for correction of anemia, elevated INR (>1.5), and thrombocytopenia (<20,000). Nasogastric tube placement increases the risk of inducing further variceal damage and should be limited to those patients with active hematemesis or in whom endoscopic intervention is likely to be delayed. If the patient has a high risk for aspiration, endotracheal intubation should be considered. Early endoscopy is preferable to determine the site of bleeding and to provide therapy.

The Sengstaken-Blakemore tube and Minnesota tube can be useful in temporarily controlling variceal hemorrhage. These tubes have gastric and esophageal balloons and a gastric suction lumen. The Minnesota tube has a modification that allows suction above the esophageal balloon to decrease the risk of aspiration. Proper placement is essential. The gastric balloon is inflated and snugged up against the gastroesophageal junction, and the esophageal balloon is then inflated. Initial hemostasis is achieved in about 90% of patients. Rebleeding is frequent when the balloons are deflated. Complications occur in up to 30% of patients, including mucosal injury that may result in esophageal perforation, aspiration, and chest pain. Use of balloon tamponade should likely be reserved for patients with known variceal bleeding in whom endoscopic therapy will be delayed and for patients in whom endoscopy has failed to control bleeding.

Pharmacologic therapy reduces variceal bleeding by decreasing the portal pressure gradient. Vasopressin (Pitressin)* has been shown to control active variceal bleeding in more than 50% of patients. Vasopressin alone is associated with significant complications, including cardiac arrhythmias, peripheral ischemia, and myocardial infarction. Adding a nitroglycerin infusion decreases the morbidity of vasopressin and increases the efficiency in the control of acute variceal hemorrhage. Somatostatin and octreotide (Sandostatin) reduce portal pressure and acute variceal bleeding similar to vasopressin, although studies have been inconsistent. Despite the lack of well-proven efficacy, pharmacologic therapy is widely used in North America. Acute pharmacologic therapy should likely be reserved for patients with acute bleeding who are at high risk for variceal bleeding in whom endoscopic therapy will be delayed and those patients with ongoing bleeding despite endoscopic therapy.

ENDOSCOPIC MANAGEMENT OF THE ACUTE VARICEAL BLEEDING EVENT

Endoscopic sclerotherapy and, more recently, banding therapy provide immediate control of hemorrhage and eradication of varices and rebleeding in about 90% of patients. Sclerotherapy results in hemostasis through the induction of thrombosis or by external compression of the vessel. Band ligation achieves hemostasis by physical constriction of the varices.

Endoscopic treatment of esophageal varices was first described in 1939 with a rigid endoscope used under general anesthesia. By the late 1970s, studies demonstrated the efficacy of endoscopic sclerotherapy. In early studies there were a wide variety of endoscopic methods used, including different types and amounts of sclerosant, different needles, different areas of injection (paravariceal versus intravariceal), and different frequencies of treatment. Flexible endoscopy has replaced rigid endoscopy because it is much easier to perform and has fewer complications. In patients with active bleeding, the use of an overtube may be helpful to protect the airway and allow large volume lavages but is associated with an increased risk of esophageal perforation.

Endoscopy is performed with the aid of conscious sedation when possible. Patients who cannot be adequately sedated may require intubation and general anesthesia to allow endoscopy to be safely accomplished. A quick but complete endoscopic examination is performed in a search for the bleeding site. If an actively bleeding varix is identified, treatment is directed at the active lesion first and then the rest of the varices can be visualized and treated more easily.

*Not FDA approved for this indication.

SCLEROTHERAPY FOR ACTIVE VARICEAL BLEEDING

Sclerotherapy results in hemostasis through the induction of thrombosis or by external compression of the vessel. The most common sclerosants include sodium tetradecyl sulfate (Sotradecol),* ethanolamine oleate (Ethamolin), polidocanol,† and alcohol. Variceal injections are started at the gastroesophageal junction. Injection of 1 to 5 mL of sclerosant is placed intravariceal or paravariceal. Injections are then performed circumferentially as the endoscope is withdrawn.

Sclerosants have been compared in a number of studies. Overall, there is not a clearly optimal sclerosant. Alcohol, although least expensive, may have higher rates of complications, and ethanolamine appears to have the lowest complication rates. As to the timing of treatment, emergency sclerotherapy appears to have a higher risk of complications but decreases rebleeding and mortality when compared with medical management and delayed endoscopy.

Sclerotherapy has been compared with sham sclerotherapy in patients with active bleeding from esophageal varices. Sclerotherapy was significantly better in stopping bleeding (91% versus 60%), reducing death during hospitalization (25% versus 49%), rebleeding (20% versus 51%), and transfusion requirements (4 versus 8 units). A number of studies have compared sclerotherapy with noninvasive therapy. Overall, sclerotherapy results in better control of initial bleeding, less rebleeding, and lower mortality when compared with conservative therapy.

ENDOSCOPIC VARICEAL LIGATION FOR ACTIVE VARICEAL BLEEDING

The variceal endoscopic ligation device was developed from an instrument used to band hemorrhoids. The varices are aspirated by suction into the cap placed on the distal end of the endoscope. A rubber band is then released, leading to strangulation and obliteration of the vascular channels. Ligation results in replacement of submucosal structures, including varices, with scar tissue resulting in eradication of varices. When the results of a number of studies comparing sclerotherapy with band ligation are combined, initial control of active bleeding was obtained in 91% of the ligation group versus 77% of the sclerotherapy group. Rebleeding occurred in 24% with banding and 47% with sclerotherapy. Survival

*Not FDA approved for this indication.
†Investigational drug in the United States.

was higher and complication rates were significantly lower in patients undergoing banding. Complications include esophageal perforation and strictures, esophageal dysmotility, ulcerations, and infectious sequelae. The first banding devices required an overtube and reloading after each band was fired; this increased the time required to perform banding. Currently, many devices are available that deliver multiple bands and do not require the use of an overtube. This reduces the risk of esophageal rupture and allows many bands to be placed relatively quickly.

The addition of sclerotherapy along with banding has failed to demonstrate any benefit over ligation alone, and the complication rates with combination therapy are higher. Endoscopic band ligation of esophageal varices has proved to be a useful tool in the control of acute variceal bleeding and the prevention of recurrent bleeding. This endoscopic technique is faster than sclerotherapy in obliterating esophageal varices and appears superior to sclerotherapy in control of bleeding, decreasing rebleeding, and increasing survival. On this basis, ligation should be considered the endoscopic treatment of choice for patients with esophageal variceal bleeding.

OTHER ENDOSCOPIC MODALITIES

Although the Nd:YAG laser has been used in the management of variceal bleeding, it does not appear to offer any benefit over other less costly and more portable modalities. Endoscopic injection of tissue adhesives has been described for the treatment of both esophageal and gastric varices. These gluelike agents solidify instantly when they come into contact with blood or tissue. A cast forms almost immediately within the varix, obstructing blood flow. In a few weeks, the overlying mucosa sloughs and the cast is extruded. *N*-Butyl-2-cyanoacrylate (Histoacryl)* is the most commonly used agent in Canada and Europe. Injection therapy with polymers involves a significant risk of the glue's causing damage to the endoscope. Cyanoacrylate is an effective sclerosant, but the added risks involved with its use do not justify its use for esophageal varices, when other methods are as effective. It does appear to be an ideal agent for the management of gastric varices, which are otherwise very difficult to manage endoscopically. Fibrin glue, thrombin, and detachable snares have all been used in the management of acute variceal bleeding and show promise, but further evaluation and randomized studies are required to confirm their benefit.

INTERVENTIONAL RADIOLOGIC MANAGEMENT

Varices can be thrombosed percutaneously with cannulation of the portal vein and embolization by radiologists. Complications are higher and success rates are not improved compared with endoscopic therapy.

Transjugular intrahepatic portosystemic shunt (TIPS) has become an important tool when endoscopic therapy is unsuccessful in controlling variceal bleeding. A shunt is placed by an interventional radiologist between the hepatic and portal veins to bypass the increased resistance to blood flow through the portal veins. The resultant reduction in portal pressure to less than 12 mm Hg reduces variceal rebleeding, provided the shunt maintains patency. Patients have an increased risk of developing encephalopathy after shunt placement. The TIPS should be followed on a regular basis to be certain it maintains patency, and balloon angioplasty of the stent lumen may be required to maintain flow. Trials suggest that TIPS is more effective than endoscopic treatment in the prevention of variceal rebleeding, although no difference in survival has been observed. Long-term follow-up is needed to see if TIPS retains its advantage over time, as well as to address issues of cost effectiveness.

SURGICAL THERAPY FOR VARICEAL BLEEDING

A variety of surgical procedures have been employed for management of variceal hemorrhage. These include various portosystemic shunts, esophageal transection, and devascularization procedures. Although surgically treated patients have less rebleeding, survival is not improved, encephalopathy is increased, and total health care costs are higher. The initial cost savings of sclerotherapy do disappear because patients treated with sclerotherapy rebleed. Liver transplantation is also an option for patients who qualify.

GASTRIC VARICES

After obliteration of esophageal varices, gastric varices will develop in about 10% of patients. Gastric varices can be classified as gastroesophageal varices and isolated gastric varices. Gastroesophageal varices at the cardia behave more like esophageal varices and can be managed with endoscopic sclerotherapy and banding. The drainage of isolated gastric varices is more diffuse and presents a more difficult management problem. In comparison with esophageal varices, gastric varices bleed significantly less often but more severely. Sclerotherapy and banding are not particularly effective in the management of isolated gastric varices. Overall, cyanoacrylate appears to be the best endoscopic agent in terms of immediate efficacy, low volume requirement, time required for hemostasis, and reduction of variceal size. Currently, TIPS should be considered the treatment of choice for bleeding isolated gastric varices.

PREVENTION OF RECURRENT VARICEAL BLEEDING

Approximately one third of patients with a variceal hemorrhage will rebleed in the first 6 weeks. Endo-

*Not available in the United States.

scopic sclerotherapy or banding repeated every few weeks until varices are eradicated reduces rebleeding and improves survival. Endoscopy does need to be repeated on an ongoing basis to treat any recurrent varices. Depending on the patient, this could be every few months to yearly. β-Blocker therapy given twice daily to reduce the resting heart rate by 25% has been shown to decrease the risk of rebleeding. Adding isosorbide to β blockers may improve efficiency. In selected patients, surgical options discussed earlier should also be considered.

DYSPHAGIA

method of
WILLIAM J. RAVICH, M.D.
The Johns Hopkins University School of Medicine
Baltimore, Maryland

The term *dysphagia,* as used in clinical practice, has two distinct, but related, meanings. On the one hand, it refers to a symptom—the patient's complaint of a sensation of delayed transit of food or liquid. On the other hand, it is often used to represent a group of disorders unified by their propensity to cause swallowing problems. Although commonly presenting with the symptom of dysphagia, patients with swallowing disorders may have a variety of other complaints and occasionally deny the presence of the dysphagia altogether. Although a nonspecific symptom, coughing, especially when reproducibly associated with swallowing of food or liquid (including saliva), suggests aspiration. Other symptoms that suggest the presence of a swallowing disorder are regurgitation (the return of pharyngeal or esophageal contents to the nose, pharynx, or mouth) and reflux (return of gastric contents to the pharynx or mouth).

CLASSIFICATION

Classification by Location

Pharyngeal dysphagia (more inclusively, *oropharyngeal dysphagia*) refers to a set of disorders that causes dysphagia as a result of abnormal structure or function of the oral cavity or pharynx (Table 1). Cancer, neurologic or myogenic dysfunction, deformity due to prior surgery of the head and neck, and hypopharyngeal diverticula are among the most common. *Esophageal dysphagia* refers to those swallowing disorders that affect the esophagus (Table 2). Esophageal motor disorders, gastroesophageal reflux disease, benign esophageal stricture, and esophageal cancer are most often responsible.

Although it is often stated that patients with dysphagia accurately localize symptoms to the level of obstruction, studies suggest that this is not true. About one third of patients who point to the upper chest or neck as the location of food hold-up are found to have pathology restricted to the distal esophagus or esophagogastric junction. The opposite does not appear to be true. Esophageal localization is virtually always associated with esophageal disorders. Any pharyngeal abnormalities detected are most likely incidental or secondary phenomena.

TABLE 1. **Causes of Pharyngeal Dysphagia**

Central Nervous System Disease

Cerebrovascular accident (especially, but not exclusively, brainstem strokes)
Amyotrophic lateral sclerosis
Dyskinesia (including drug-induced tardive dyskinesias)
Dystonia
Huntington disease
Parkinson disease
Poliomyelitis
Supranuclear palsy
Multiple sclerosis
Myoclonus
Traumatic brain injury
Central nervous system neoplasms
Chronic meningitis
Guillain-Barré syndrome

Neuromuscular or Myogenic Processes

Myasthenia
Polymyositis
Mitochochondrial cytopathies (including inclusion-body myositis)
Myotonic dystrophies
Oculopharyngeal dystrophies
Hyperthyroidism
Hypothyroidism
Isolated upper esophageal sphincter dysfunction

Structural Disorders of Head and Neck

Pharyngeal or hypopharyngeal webs
Cervical osteophytes
Head and neck malignancy
Hypopharyngeal (Zenker's) diverticulum
Radiation changes
Prior head and neck surgery
Prior radiation therapy

Local Inflammatory Conditions

Acute pharyngitis
Cicatricial pemphigoid
Pemphigus
Sarcoid
Eosinophilic-myalgia syndrome

Classification by Mechanism

Alternatively, dysphagia can be divided into two groups: structural abnormalities and motility disorders. Structural disorders include luminal stenosis and diverticula. Motor

TABLE 2. **Causes of Esophageal Dysphagia**

Motor Disorders

Paretic disorders (including the "sclerodermatous esophagus")
Spastic disorders (e.g., esophageal spasm, the "nutcracker esophagus")
Lower esophageal sphincter dysfunction (e.g., achalasia, isolated lower esophageal sphincter dysfunction)

Structural Disorders

Webs and rings (including Schatzki rings)
Congenital strictures
Inflammatory stricture (e.g., reflux-related, infectious, drug-induced, anastomotic)
Esophageal malignancy (e.g., squamous cell cancer, adenocarcinoma, metastatic cancer, leiomyosarcoma)
Extrinsic masses
Vascular compression (e.g., aberrant subclavian artery, double aortic arch, tortuous aorta, cardiomegaly)
Diverticula (primarily pulsion diverticula)

disorders include paresis, dysmotility, or sphincteric dysfunction.

STRUCTURAL DISORDERS

Luminal stenosis typically presents as solid food dysphagia. Dysphagia is often bolus-size related (i.e., symptoms are minimized by the patient carefully cutting and chewing solid food and by avoidance of foods recognized as causing difficulty). Although often occurring with foods that are difficult to chew, such as tough meat and raw vegetables, pasta and bread, which tend to absorb saliva and are often swallowed as large cohesive boluses, may also cause particular difficulty for some patients. A diverticulum is a saclike protrusion from the normal lumen. It characteristically causes regurgitation of recognizable food and liquid, often long after the meal is finished. Most diverticula are consequences of chronically increased intraluminal pressure resulting from stenotic lesions or motor abnormalities distal to the diverticulum itself. Treatment of the underlying obstructive process may improve or eradicate symptoms, especially when the diverticulum is small. Recurrence after surgical treatment is common unless the obstructive lesion is treated.

MOTOR DISORDERS

The swallowed bolus is normally propelled by the muscular activity of the tongue, pharyngeal constrictor, and esophageal circular muscles. Paretic or uncoordinated muscular contractions can cause swallowing problems. Both typically cause dysphagia for liquids and solids. Sphincters are zones of tonically elevated pressure, which serve to partition segments of the alimentary tract. There are two sphincters that regulate flow of the swallowed bolus. The upper esophageal sphincter (UES) separates the pharynx from the esophagus and prevents esophageal distention during inspiration and esophagopharyngeal regurgitation. The lower esophageal sphincter (LES) separates the esophagus from the stomach, forming part of the antireflux barrier. These sphincters normally relax during swallowing to allow ready passage of the swallowed bolus. Failure of sphincteric relaxation may cause obstruction. As with other motor disorders, symptoms usually occur with both liquids and solids.

DIAGNOSTIC EVALUATION

The diagnostic evaluation begins with a clinical assessment. By analyzing the patient's symptoms a reasonable guess can be made about the site of obstruction and the type of testing that might be required. An algorithm for the diagnostic evaluation of swallowing disorders is offered (Figure 1). The following discusses specific advantages and limitations associated with the various studies available.

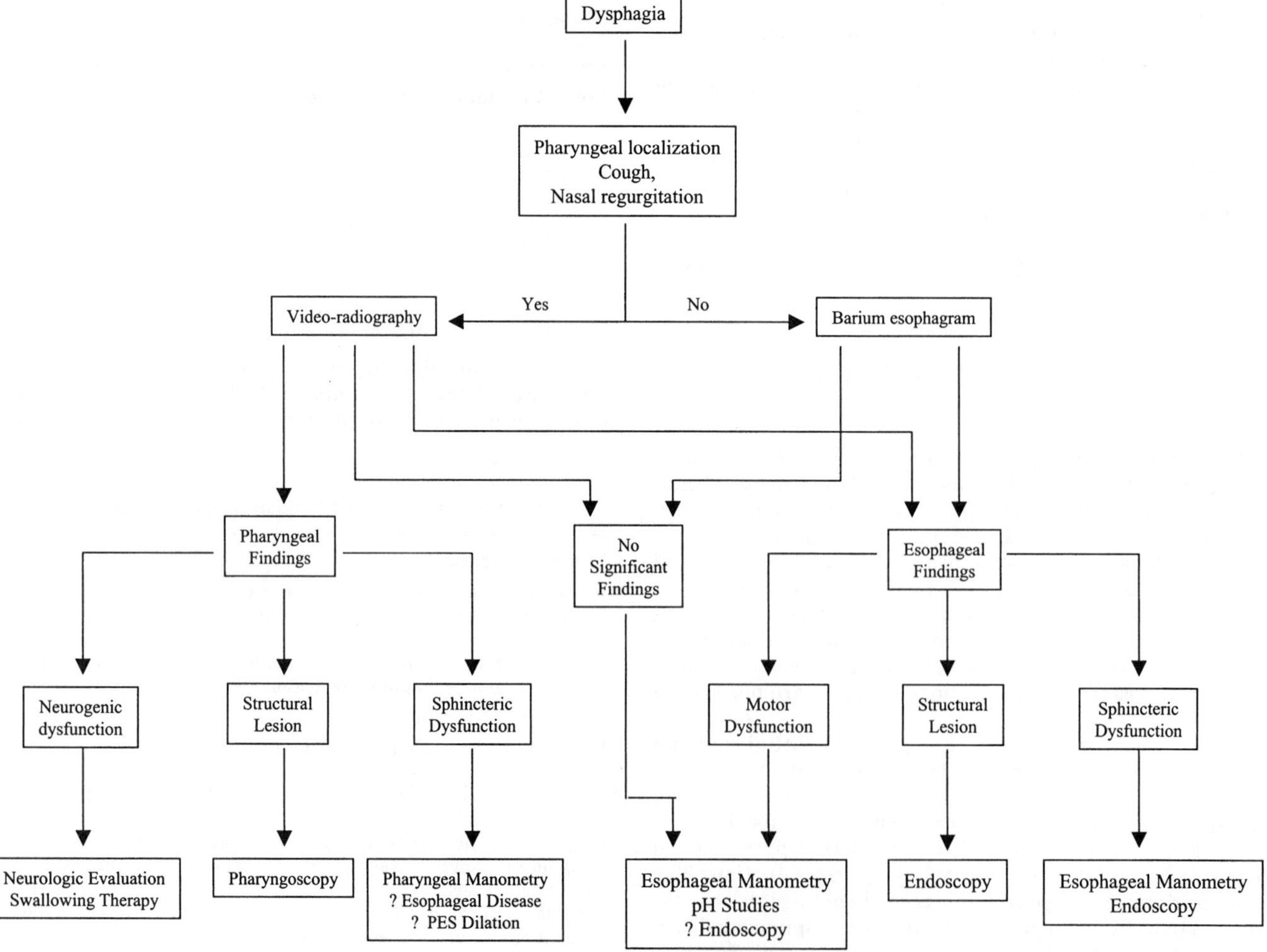

Figure 1. Algorithm for the evaluation of dysphagia.

Rakel and Bope: Conn's Current Therapy 2002. Copyright 2002 by W.B. Saunders Company.

Barium Studies

Radiographic contrast study should almost always be the first test in the evaluation of swallowing disorders. Barium studies provide the best balance between detecting both structural and motor disorders. In the experience of the Johns Hopkins Swallowing Center, more mistakes are made by skipping the barium study in a patient with dysphagia than any other reason.

The type of barium study requires some comment. The standard barium esophagogram, often performed as part of an upper gastrointestinal series, is satisfactory when the location of the swallowing problem is known to be the esophagus. However, whenever there is concern about the possibility of pharyngeal pathology or dysfunction, the standard barium esophagogram is inadequate. Bolus transit through the pharynx is too fast for the radiologist to see or document with spot films. When pharyngeal function needs to be assessed, a videoradiographic barium study is required.

A few caveats are in order. First, because patients *do not* always accurately localize their symptoms to the region of pathology, it is essential to evaluate the esophagus at some point in the evaluation of almost all patients with swallowing disorders. Second, if swallowing problems occur primarily with the ingestion of solids, the radiographic examination should include evaluation of transit of a solid bolus unless an explanation for the patient's symptoms is clearly revealed on the initial liquid phase study. Finally, in many hospitals, when a videoradiographic study of swallowing is requested, a modified barium swallow—a test developed to assess the impact of maneuvers used in swallowing rehabilitation therapy on swallowing efficiency—is performed, rather than a full assessment of pharynx and esophagus. In general, the modified barium swallow should be used only after a complete radiographic evaluation of both pharynx and esophagus has been performed by a properly trained radiologist.

Endoscopic Studies

Although appropriately applied to either pharyngoscopy and esophagoscopy, the term *endoscopy* is commonly assumed to mean the latter. Endoscopy is a poor test for the evaluation of motility disorders. It is a good test for detecting strictures and permits dilation in a single session; however, it can miss mildly tight strictures. Although endoscopy is an excellent test for mucosal inflammation and for detecting mass lesions, the vast majority of patients with swallowing disorders have neither inflammation nor a mass.

It is frequently stated that esophagoscopy is essential in all patients with dysphagia. This reflects the prejudice of the gastroenterologic perspective, which focuses on the esophagus exclusively. There are many patients, for example, those with symptoms and radiographic findings consistent with neurogenic dysphagia and nothing to suggest significant esophageal pathology, for whom routine esophagoscopy is unwarranted. Perhaps a better rule of thumb would be that esophagoscopy should be performed unless radiographic findings clearly explain the patient's clinical presentation.

Pharyngoscopy is commonly performed by otolaryngologists as part of their initial clinical examination. On the grounds of efficiency, safety, and common practice, it would seem ill advised to interfere with initial pharyngoscopy. However, it should be pointed out that, all swallowing patients considered, a large number of examinations are unrevealing. Extensions of the pharyngoscopic examination include fiberoptic endoscopic evaluation of swallowing for assessment of pharyngeal retention and laryngeal penetration during ingestion of liquids and foods of various consistency. More recently, endoscopic evaluation of pharyngeal sensation using air pulses directed at the arytenoid processes has been advocated for an assessment as a measure of the risk of aspiration pneumonia. The clinical value of these tests, as compared with videoradiography, has not been adequately studied.

Manometric Studies

Esophageal manometry evaluates the strength and coordination of esophageal peristalsis and the resting pressure and relaxation function of the LES. It is most often used as part of the workup of patients with chest pain or dysphagia when radiographic studies are negative or suggest that symptoms result from a disorder of esophageal motility. Manometry can confirm the diagnosis of esophageal spasm, achalasia, and isolated LES dysfunction. Manometry is also used to properly position the acid-sensitive probe for continuous pH monitor studies. The value of esophageal manometry when radiographic studies are abnormal, for example, when radiographs show esophageal dysmotility or achalasia, is uncertain. Pharyngeal manometry is only occasionally used in clinical practice. Its major clinical value may be to confirm UES dysfunction in patients with pharyngeal dysphagia and evidence of a narrowed pharyngoesophageal segment on videoradiographic study.

pH Probe Studies

Gastroesophageal reflux may present with swallowing symptoms such as dysphagia and coughing. In the absence of these typical reflux symptoms, or when symptoms do not respond to antireflux therapy, a continuous pH monitor (CpHM) may be used to confirm gastroesophageal reflux disease (GERD). In this study, an acid-sensitive probe, attached to a small computer or tape recorder, is placed through the nose into the distal esophagus and worn for up to 24 hours to monitor the frequency and duration of acid reflux events. Because a majority of normal volunteers are found to reflux acid during CpHM, a diagnosis of GERD requires documentation of an abnormal amount or pattern of acid reflux. CpHM appears to have few false-positive results, but there is a significant false-negative rate of perhaps 10% to 20%. This may result in part from the fact that patients do not eat or behave normally with a tube in their nose. A negative pH probe test in a patient with convincing symptoms does not rule out GERD.

Radionuclide Studies

Radionuclide studies for swallowing disorders have been used primarily for research purposes. The only radionuclide test commonly used for clinical purposes is a solid-phase esophageal clearance study, most often using cornflakes soaked in milk containing a small amount of radioactive technetium ("esophageal cornflake study"). The cornflake study is used primarily to assess the response to therapy directed at lowering LES pressure. Its advantage over barium contrast studies is that it provides quantitative information about esophageal clearance with much lower radiation exposure than the doses required for barium esophagrams.

SPECIFIC DISORDERS

The treatment of swallowing problems depends completely on the diagnosis. A detailed discussion of treatment for specific conditions is beyond the scope of this brief summary. The intention here is to provide an overview of therapeutic approaches.

Neurogenic Dysphagia

The term *neurogenic dysphagia* is used to describe a set of radiographic findings on barium contrast studies believed to be suggestive of a neurologic, neuromuscular, or myogenic disease. The sensitivity and specificity of the radiographic interpretation of neurogenic dysphagia has not been adequately studied. Nonetheless, clinical experience suggests that most patients with multiple compatible abnormalities of moderate to marked severity on radiographic studies do have a "neurogenic" process. Typical findings include poor control of the barium bolus with premature or post-swallow leakage of oral contents into the pharynx, abnormal motion of the tongue or weak tongue thrust against the posterior pharynx, weak contraction of the pharyngeal constrictor muscles, poor elevation of the larynx with incomplete closure of the larynx, pharyngeal retention after the swallow is complete, poor epiglottic tilt, and poor opening of the pharyngoesophageal segment. It is not always possible to determine the precise disorder involved, even after a thorough neurologic examination.

Strokes, amyotrophic lateral sclerosis, and myopathies are among the more common causes of neurogenic dysphagia. It is critical to look for treatable causes of neurogenic dysphagia, such as polymyositis, myasthenia gravis, Parkinson disease, and both hypothyroidism and hyperthyroidism, because these conditions should respond to specific drug therapy. Occasionally patients have been reported in whom psychotropic drugs have impaired swallowing function, with improvement after drug withdrawal. Isolated or mild findings suggesting oral or pharyngeal dysfunction are not uncommon, especially in the elderly.

Not unexpectedly, many causes of neurogenic dysphagia have no direct specific therapy. Treatment of these forms of neurogenic dysphagia focuses on swallowing therapy, in which the therapist introduces a variety of modifications in the size and type of bolus swallowed, the position of head and neck, and the timing of respiration in relation to swallowing in an attempt to improve swallowing efficiency and minimize aspiration. Clinical, radiographic (modified barium swallow), and endoscopic means are used to determine the effect of these maneuvers. Recently there has been an interest in the impact of exercises on improving pharyngeal function (e.g., the Shaker exercises). Although the pharyngoesophageal segment often fails to open normally on radiographic studies, this usually results from pharyngeal weakness and impaired laryngeal elevation, rather than from cricopharyngeal dysfunction. Selected patients may respond to UES dilation or myotomy, but most do not respond to treatment directed at the UES.

Isolated UES Dysfunction

The large majority of patients with the radiographic finding of a prominent pharyngoesophageal segment (PES), often referred to as a hypopharyngeal bar, have associated pharyngeal or esophageal disorders that may be responsible for symptoms. As described earlier, impaired PES opening is commonly seen in neurogenic dysphagia and treatment directed at weakening the UES is often unsuccessful. When associated with esophageal disorders, the prominent PES may reflect a physiologic response of the UES intended to prevent esophagopharyngeal regurgitation.

Incomplete PES opening is only rarely found as an isolated phenomenon. Under these circumstances, treatment directed at the UES is more likely to be effective. Traditionally, treatment of UES dysfunction involves surgical myotomy. More recently, dilation has been found to be effective in some patients. There have been reports of using botulinum toxin for PES dysfunction. However, the technique and dosage have not been established and the duration of effect is relatively short (3–4 months). Furthermore, the use of botulinum toxin for a variety of cervical muscular disorders has been associated with dysphagia that can be severe. This potential complication limits the appeal of this drug for UES dysfunction.

LES Dysfunction

In achalasia, incomplete LES relaxation, in combination with the complete absence of progressive peristalsis in the distal two thirds of the esophageal body, causes retention of swallowed secretions, food, and liquid in the esophagus. Late regurgitation of recognizable food is a characteristic symptom. The radiographic findings of achalasia include a dilated esophagus, esophageal retention with a column of barium ending in an air-fluid level, and a long smooth symmetric narrowing at the esophagogastric junction. Upper endoscopy is necessary to rule out a benign or malignant stricture. Failure of LES relaxation is confirmed by esophageal manometry that also reveals complete absence of contractile activity, referred to as aperistalsis ("classic achalasia") or persistent spastic contractions ("vigorous achalasia"). In the presence of typical radiographic and endoscopic findings, manometry rarely alters the diagnosis or treatment of achalasia.

All treatment options are directed toward weakening the nonrelaxing LES, permitting food to pass into the stomach under the influence of gravity. Although smooth muscle relaxants lower LES pressure, their effect on symptoms is generally partial and of limited duration. For many years the primary choice was between brusque dilation with a large-diameter balloon or surgical myotomy of the LES. Dilation is successful in 70% to 80% of patients, although a second dilation is often required to achieve this response rate. Many patients have long-term relief of symptoms. The major risk of dilation is perforation.

Surgery produces a higher response rate of 80% to 90%. However, a substantial proportion of patients develop clinically significant reflux disease postoperatively. To avoid reflux, most surgeons perform an antireflux operation at the time of myotomy. Laparoscopic and thoracoscopic approaches to myotomy decrease the recovery period, increasing the appeal of surgical intervention to many patients. In the early 1990s, intrasphincteric injection of the LES with botulinum toxin was introduced as an alternative therapeutic modality. Some studies indicate a response comparable to that for dilation, with very low risk of side effects. However, the duration of response averages about 1 year. Periodic re-treatment is therefore required, and not all patients who respond initially continue to respond to re-injection.

Isolated abnormality of LES pressure and function are much less common causes of dysphagia than achalasia. They can theoretically be handled in the same way as achalasia, but information on the efficacy of therapy is limited.

Diverticulum

Diverticula of either the pharynx or esophagus may cause swallowing problems. Because diverticula usually result from increased intraluminal pressure, which is in turn a consequence of increased resistance to flow, it is important to look for an obstructive process downstream to the diverticulum, such as a nonrelaxing sphincter, spasm, or a stricture. Diverticula often produce typical symptoms that include dysphagia and regurgitation of undigested food, often hours after ingestion. Small diverticula are generally asymptomatic. Treatment of the obstructive process alone often results in improvement or even eradication of symptoms. Surgical removal (diverticulectomy) or suspension (diverticulopexy) is usually required for larger diverticula. Failure to recognize and treat the obstructive process will lead to a high rate of postoperative recurrence of the diverticulum.

Because radiographic evidence of UES dysfunction is always present and considered to be the most common cause of downstream resistance in patients with a Zenker's diverticulum, a surgical myotomy of the UES is usually performed at the time of diverticulectomy or diverticulopexy. Endoscopic techniques in which the posterior wall of the sphincter is cut, thereby removing the resistance to flow and allowing the diverticulum to drain directly into the cervical esophagus have been developed. Whether these endoscopic approaches are superior to the percutaneous surgical approach has not been established.

Spastic Disorders of the Esophagus

Although esophageal dysmotility may be a primary motor disorder (idiopathic diffuse esophageal spasm), clinically significant esophageal spasm is often a secondary condition, with GERD the most common cause. Intensive treatment of GERD, without the use of smooth muscle relaxants that can aggravate reflux, should be the first line of treatment for anyone in whom GERD is considered likely. Esophageal irritation due to drug-induced esophagitis (especially from nonsteroidal anti-inflammatory drugs, tetracycline, iron or potassium supplements, quinidine, or alendronate [Fosamax]) or infection in the immunocompromised host (primarily from cytomegalovirus, herpes virus, or *Candida*) should also be considered. Treatment involves withdrawal of the offending medications for the former and initiation of appropriate antiviral or antifungal agents for the latter.

Patients with symptomatic esophageal spasm are often concerned about the possibility of cancer (when dysphagia dominates) or heart disease (when chest pain dominates). Reassurance is an important therapeutic modality. Smooth muscle relaxant therapy (either nitrates or calcium channel blockers) may be helpful but are often associated with uncomfortable side effects (headache, dizziness, weakness), especially in the nonhypertensive patient. The drugs should be started at low doses and increased slowly. Long-acting formulations may be helpful in improving tolerance to the drugs.

Stenotic Lesions

Stenosis refers to luminal narrowing by some form of structural lesions. Webs, rings, extrinsic compression, and both inflammatory and malignant strictures all would fit into this category. Benign stenotic lesions are usually treated by dilation, which is often performed at the time of endoscopy. The normal esophageal wall is quite elastic; a 3.0-cm balloon can be fully distended in the normal channel without producing any evidence of trauma or discomfort. The lumen must be compromised by about 50% before symptoms of dysphagia for solids are likely to occur. Even at this stage the presence and severity of symptoms vary considerably. Dilation to 18 mm usually eradicates symptoms due to benign strictures; dilation to a larger diameter is rarely required. In inflammatory stricture, it is important to look for the underlying cause for stricture formation, because effective treatment of the underlying cause is critical if symptom recurrence is to be delayed or prevented. Dilation alone is rarely satisfactory for malignant strictures. Malignant strictures may be treated by surgical resection (especially when cure is possible), irradiation often combined with chemotherapy, laser therapy (either with Nd:YAG laser or photodynamic therapy), or stent placement. The choice of techniques often reflects local experience and availability of equipment.

DIVERTICULA OF THE GASTROINTESTINAL TRACT

method of
EDWIN J. ZARLING, M.D.
Loyola University Medical Center
Maywood, Illinois

and

FARID U. AHMAD, M.D.
Roseburg VA Hospital
Eugene, Oregon

A *diverticulum* is a pouch or sac that originates from a hollow organ. It is lined with epithelium and contains normal mucosal folds. A false diverticulum does not have a muscular layer but is formed by herniation of mucosa and submucosa through a defect in the muscular wall, generally at the site of a nutrient artery. The term *pseudodiverticulum* is often used interchangeably with false diverticulum. In the gastrointestinal (GI) tract, the colon is the most common location for diverticula. Most patients with uncomplicated diverticulosis have either no symptoms or have symptoms that are minor in nature. Diverticular complications are common and can manifest with pain, bleeding, infection, or perforation.

ESOPHAGUS

Zenker's Diverticulum

This common diverticulum of the esophagus is located in the hypopharyngeal region. It results when mucosa protrudes posteriorly and to the left between the fibers of pharyngeal inferior constrictor muscle and cricopharyngeus muscle. Zenker's diverticulum usually occurs in patients who are in the seventh or eighth decade of life. It is found in 2% of patients with dysphagia.

The most common symptom of Zenker's diverticulum is dysphagia for both solids and liquids. The patient often presents with regurgitation of retained food eaten hours earlier, which can also cause halitosis. Other symptoms include cough, hoarseness, bronchitis, fullness in the throat, and gurgling noises during eating. Complications associated with Zenker's diverticulum include aspiration pneumonia, chronic pneumonia, and lung abscess. Accidental perforation of Zenker's diverticulum can occur during passage of a nasogastric tube or endoscope, and during intubation for anesthesia. Ulceration of Zenker's diverticulum can occur secondary to aspirin or nonsteroidal anti-inflammatory drug incarceration. Cancer, hemorrhage, and fistulization to the trachea are rare. The diagnosis should be suspected in elderly patients with a history of dysphagia and regurgitation. Barium-contrast radiography is the primary method for detecting Zenker's diverticulum. Lateral views should be obtained, as most diverticula are located posteriorly.

Treatment

Patients with a symptomatic Zenker's diverticulum require treatment. Treatment options are surgical and include (1) excision of the diverticulum, (2) cricopharyngeal myotomy, and (3) *diverticulopexy* (lifting the diverticulum). Successful endoscopic excision has been reported with both a rigid and a flexible fiberoptic instrument and involves the resection of the wall between the diverticulum and esophagus. An endoscopic approach with stapling of the diverticulum has also been reported.

Diverticula of the Esophageal Body

A midesophageal diverticulum is typically found at the level of the tracheal bifurcation (T4-5) and is found most often on the right side. These are very rare in the developed countries. Current theories suggest that these diverticula of the esophageal body develop either as a consequence of a motility disorder or secondary to the deformation or pulling of the esophagus by chronic mediastinal inflammatory disease such as tuberculosis and histoplasmosis. Midesophageal diverticula are almost always asymptomatic.

A distal esophageal diverticulum, also called an *epiphrenic diverticulum,* occurs several centimeters above the gastric cardia. It may be single or multiple and is usually found on the right side. These diverticula likely are related to motility disorders such as diffuse esophageal spasms. Most patients with epiphrenic diverticula are asymptomatic. Potential symptoms include dysphagia, cough, bronchitis, chest pain, and regurgitation leading to aspiration pneumonia. Ulceration and bleeding occur rarely. Esophageal diverticula can be diagnosed with barium-contrast studies or endoscopy.

Treatment

Asymptomatic or minimally symptomatic diverticula require no treatment. Patients with significant dysphagia and regurgitation require surgical treatment. A careful preoperative evaluation with endoscopy and motility studies is required. If an associated motility disorder is present, it should be addressed first. Surgical treatment requires excision of the diverticulum, usually with myotomy of the distal esophagus along with fundoplication. Most patients report long-term relief.

Pseudodiverticula of the Esophageal Body

Esophageal intramural pseudodiverticulosis is a rare condition. These pseudodiverticula are characterized by 1- to 4-mm flask-shaped outpouchings that protrude from the lumen into the esophageal wall. These are usually multiple and may be present diffusely or in a segment of esophagus. Pathologically, they represent dilated excretory ducts of esophageal submucosal glands. Blockage of intramural ducts by inflammatory debris leads to their dilation. Esophageal intramural pseudodiverticulosis is an acquired condition and is seen mainly in middle-aged patients. A history of gastroesophageal reflux and candidiasis infection is common, and most of the patients have stricture formation. An antecedent erosive injury to the esophagus may increase susceptibility to this condition. The majority of patients present with chronic dysphagia due to a stricture. The diagnosis is often made with barium-contrast studies. Endoscopy shows tiny pinpoint openings.

Treatment

Treatment of esophageal intramural pseudodiverticulosis is directed toward the underlying condition. Significant strictures should be dilated to relieve dysphagia. Reflux esophagitis and candidiasis should be treated if present.

STOMACH

Gastric diverticula are outpouchings of the stomach that may involve all (*true diverticula*) layers or some (*pseudodiverticula*) layers of the stomach wall. Approximately 75% of true gastric diverticula are located on the posterior wall of the cardia near the lesser curvature. Pseudodiverticula are associated with tumors, healing ulcers, or prior surgical repairs.

A gastric diverticulum can present at any age and is usually asymptomatic. Rarely, it can present with pain or fullness in the epigastric area. Ulceration, bleeding, perforation, and torsion of these diverticula have also been reported. Most of the gastric diverticula are diagnosed incidentally by endoscopy or barium-contrast study.

Treatment

Asymptomatic diverticula do not require any treatment. When indicated, definitive treatment is diverticulectomy.

SMALL INTESTINE

Duodenal Diverticula

Duodenal diverticula are acquired and their incidence increases with age. They range from a few millimeters to several centimeters in diameter. They occur at the entrance site of large vessels or pancreaticobiliary ducts and are commonly identified in the periampullary region. Duodenal diverticula are usually asymptomatic and are generally seen during endoscopy, endoscopic retrograde cholangiopancreatography, or barium-contrast study. Symptoms, when present, include vague epigastric pain, fever, and nausea. Computed tomography may show thickening with inflammatory changes. Bacterial overgrowth can also occur in these diverticula. Duodenal diverticula are associated with increased incidence of gallstones and common bile duct stones. Intraluminal diverticula are rare, occupying half or full lumen, and can extend from the second portion to the fourth portion of the duodenum.

Treatment

Duodenal diverticula rarely require treatment. In cases of complications, they are treated with antibiotics or surgery.

Jejunal and Ileal Diverticula

Diverticula of the jejunum and ileum are rare. They occur most commonly on the antimesenteric border of the proximal jejunum. These diverticula are acquired and are frequently associated with motility disorders such as scleroderma, pseudo-obstruction, neuropathy, and myopathy. Most jejunal diverticula are asymptomatic. Symptoms are the result of bacterial overgrowth causing malabsorption symptoms such as steatorrhea, bloating, weight loss, and fat-soluble vitamin deficiencies. These diverticula are usually diagnosed with barium-contrast study.

Treatment

Diverticulitis and bleeding may necessitate surgery with resection of the involved portion of small bowel. Patients with bacterial overgrowth usually respond to broad-spectrum antibiotics given as chronic therapy (1–2 weeks/month). Tetracycline* 250 mg four times daily or metronidazole (Flagyl)* 250 mg twice daily are usually effective. Fat-soluble vitamins and vitamin B_{12}* and folic acid* should be supplemented.

Meckel's Diverticulum

Meckel's diverticulum is the most common congenital anomaly of the GI tract. The incidence in autopsy series is 2% to 3% of the population. Meckel's diverticulum results from failure of the vitelline duct to close. It arises on the antimesenteric border of the distal ileum, and contains all layers of the intestine. Most of these diverticula are located within 100 cm of the ileocecal valve and range from 1 to 10 cm in size. Half of these diverticula are lined by ileal mucosa, and the remainder have mucosa from stomach, pancreas, duodenum, or colon.

Acid production by gastric mucosa within a Meckel's diverticulum can result in intestinal ulceration. Painless bleeding (currant jelly stools) is the most common presenting symptom of the Meckel's diverticulum. It usually presents in children less than 2 years of age. Other complications may include intestinal obstruction, diverticulitis simulating appendicitis, perforation, and carcinoma.

The diagnosis of Meckel's diverticulum can be suggested by findings on small-bowel radiology. The presence of gastric mucosa is established by technetium 99m scan using pentagastrin, which is selectively taken up by the gastric mucosa.

Treatment

Laparotomy with diverticulectomy is the treatment of choice for symptomatic Meckel's diverticulum.

COLON

In the Western World, the colon is the most common GI site for the development of diverticula. Colonic diverticulosis is present in one third of people by age 50, and in two thirds of people by age 80. The most common anatomic site of diverticulosis is the sigmoid colon. Factors involved in the pathogenesis include disordered motility and high intraluminal

*Not FDA approved for this indication.

pressure. Low fiber diets yield small-volume stools, which in turn cause increased intraluminal pressure. This increased pressure eventually causes herniation of the mucosa and submucosa through the muscle layer at the point where the blood vessel penetrates from serosa through the muscularis mucosa into submucosa. Thus, colonic diverticula are pseudodiverticula, as they do not involve all layers of the colonic wall. The diagnosis of diverticulosis is most often established with barium-contrast enema examination, which determines the extent and severity of diverticulosis. Colonoscopy can also confirm the diagnosis and rule out concomitant lesions such as neoplasm.

The majority of patients with diverticula in the colon are asymptomatic. Clinical sequelae of diverticulosis can consist of pain, bleeding, and diverticulitis. Painful diverticular disease presents with intermittent abdominal discomfort associated with altered bowel habits, bloating, and flatulence. Bleeding is typically abrupt, painless, and large in volume with maroon or red color. Most episodes of diverticular bleeding cease spontaneously.

The incidence of bleeding from diverticula of the colon may be lower than previously thought because it is distinctly uncommon to find blood issuing from a diverticulum during colonoscopy. Diverticulitis is the most common complication of diverticulosis. By definition, in *diverticulitis* there is a microperforation at the base of the inflamed diverticulum. It usually occurs in the sigmoid area but can involve any segment of the colon. The most common symptom of diverticulitis is left lower quadrant abdominal pain, which is frequently associated with a change in bowel habits, either constipation or diarrhea, and fever. Anorexia with nausea and vomiting can also occur. Due to the proximity of the urinary bladder, patients have also reported dysuria and urinary frequency. Physical examination shows tenderness in the involved area with guarding and rebound tenderness. A phlegmon may also be palpable. Leukocytosis may be present. The diagnosis is usually made on clinical grounds. When the diagnosis is in doubt, computed tomography should be performed. Endoscopy adds little information to the acute diagnosis and may be hazardous.

Treatment

The treatment of painful diverticular disease is to increase fiber through diet or medicinal supplementation. Antispasmodic medications may be reserved for patients unresponsive to fiber therapy.

As with any other case of GI bleeding, patients with diverticular bleeding should first receive supportive care with hemodynamic stabilization. An upper source of GI bleeding should be ruled out. For brisk bleeding, angiography should be done to localize the site. In patients with less active bleeding, colonoscopy should be done to identify the bleeding site. Surgery is reserved for patients who fail medical, angiographic, or endoscopic treatment. Segmental colectomy is the procedure of choice if the bleeding site can be identified. Subtotal colectomy may be required in some patients if the bleeding site cannot be localized.

Mild attacks of acute uncomplicated diverticulitis can often be treated on an outpatient basis. Clear liquid diet and ciprofloxacin (Cipro)* 500 mg twice daily plus metronidazole* 500 mg twice daily are the cornerstone of outpatient treatment. Hospitalization can be considered for patients who are elderly, have severe disease, are immunocompromised, or have comorbidities. These patients should receive either a clear liquid diet or bowel rest, and intravenous fluids and antibiotics. Most patients improve in 3 to 4 days.

Patients with diverticulitis that is complicated by abscess formation warrant additional therapy. A small abscess can be managed with aggressive medical management. A large abscess requires drainage either by computed tomography–guided percutaneous approach or surgery. Fistula formation can occur when a diverticular abscess extends into an adjacent organ. Fistula into the urinary bladder is most common and presents with pneumaturia and urinary tract infection. Other sites of fistulization could be the vagina, skin, or intestines. Treatment is resection of the involved bowel and fistulous tract. Generalized peritonitis can result from free perforation of the diverticulum, which results in devastating purulent or feculent peritonitis. These complications are rare but require urgent surgical intervention with resection of the involved segment. A temporary colostomy is usually needed.

After the diverticulitis has resolved, a decision is necessary regarding resection of a portion of the colon. Factors leading toward surgical resection include severe disease, complicated disease, presence of colonic stricture, or two to three episodes of recurrent diverticulitis. In immunosuppressed patients, the signs and symptoms of diverticulitis may be subtle. Such patients have higher rates of perforations and failure on medical therapy. Due to these factors, elective resection should be considered after one documented attack.

*Not FDA approved for this indication.

INFLAMMATORY BOWEL DISEASE

method of
ALAIN BITTON, M.D.
McGill University Health Center
Montreal, Quebec, Canada

Inflammatory bowel disease (IBD) is a chronic gastrointestinal disorder that encompasses two main disorders: Crohn's disease and ulcerative colitis. *Crohn's disease* is characterized by transmural inflammation affecting any gastrointestinal site but with predilection for the ileum and/or colon. *Ulcerative colitis* is characterized by colonic inflammation limited to the mucosa and submucosa. Patients with these conditions present with abdominal pain, diarrhea, and weight loss. Because of its transmural nature, patients with Crohn's disease can also present with fistulas, abscesses, and gastrointestinal obstruction. The natural history of IBD is subject to great individual variability but most often is characterized by a chronic intermittently relapsing course.

The aim of therapy in IBD is to induce and maintain remission while preserving an excellent health-related quality of life. Therapy also aims at reducing the risk of long-term complications such as malnutrition, osteoporosis, and colon cancer. In recent years, the therapeutic armamentarium in IBD has expanded significantly. Agents that allow for targeted delivery of drugs to specific sites of active intestinal inflammation have been formulated. With increased insight into the immunopathogenesis of IBD, therapeutic agents that target specific immune processes or mediators are being evaluated.

DRUG THERAPY

Aminosalicylates

Sulfasalazine

Sulfasalazine (Azulfidine) is composed of a sulfonamide, sulfapyridine, linked to a 5-aminosalicylic acid (5-ASA) by an azo bond. It is effective for treating mild-to-moderately active ulcerative colitis and for maintaining remission. The evidence supporting the use of sulfasalazine in Crohn's disease is not as compelling as for ulcerative colitis; nonetheless, sulfasalazine* can be used to induce remission in patients with Crohn's disease primarily involving the colon. Sulfasalazine has not been shown in clinical trials to maintain medically or surgically induced remissions of Crohn's disease. However, patients who have achieved medical remission with this agent may benefit from its long-term use.

5-Aminosalicylates

Studies that demonstrated that the active ingredient in sulfasalazine was the 5-ASA led to the development of various formulations that deliver 5-ASA to the ileum and colon. These include acrylic-coated 5-ASA (mesalamine; Asacol, Salofalk,† and Claversal†) that is released in a pH-dependent manner, or a slow-release form (Pentasa), which consists of 5-ASA encapsulated in ethylcellulose microgranules that dissolve in the small and large bowel in a time- and pH-dependent manner. There is also a 5-ASA preparation that binds 5-ASA via an azo bond to itself, olsalazine (Dipentum), or to an inert carrier molecule, balsalazide (Colazal).*

Oral and rectal 5-ASA formulations are known generically as mesalamine. Oral 5-ASA agents are effective in treating mild-to-moderately active ulcerative colitis and for maintaining remission. Mesalamine enemas and suppositories (Rowasa) are effective in active and quiescent distal colitis (involving the rectum and/or sigmoid). There is a modest benefit to using oral mesalamine* to treat active Crohn's disease and to maintain medically or surgically induced remission, and the benefit is dose-dependent.

*Not FDA approved for this indication.
†Not available in the United States.

The sulfapyridine moiety of sulfasalazine is responsible for many of the drug's side effects. Dose-dependent side effects with sulfasalazine include headaches, nausea, and vomiting. Azoospermia, a side effect with sulfasalazine, is reversible and does not occur with the 5-ASA drugs. Neutropenia, agranulocytosis, and hemolytic anemia have occurred with sulfasalazine but are rarely seen with the 5-ASA agents. Hypersensitivity reactions have been reported with both agents and include serum sickness, skin rashes, pneumonitis, pericarditis, myocarditis, hepatitis, and pancreatitis. Interstitial nephritis is rare and is associated mainly with the oral 5-ASA agents. Watery diarrhea is a common side effect with olsalazine. Exacerbation of ulcerative colitis has also been reported with both drugs.

Topical 5-ASA agents seem to have minimal side effects. Anal irritation or pruritus can be seen with these agents. Although over 80% of patients who are intolerant or allergic to sulfasalazine will tolerate 5-ASA, caution is warranted in patients who have had a severe hypersensitivity reaction with sulfasalazine and are switched to a 5-ASA preparation. Patients on sulfasalazine should be on folate supplements of 1 mg/d. Sulfasalazine can be used safely in pregnancy. A recent study has reported the safe use of oral mesalamine 2 g/d or less during pregnancy.

Corticosteroids

Standard steroid preparations are highly effective in treating active IBD, but their prolonged use is associated with significant toxicity. Hydrocortisone enemas (Cortenema) and foams (Cortifoam) are effective in treating distal ulcerative colitis; the foam is better tolerated. Their use in Crohn's disease of the distal colon as well as their efficacy in maintaining remission have not been assessed. Oral prednisone or prednisolone is effective in moderately severe ulcerative colitis and Crohn's disease but are ineffective as maintenance agents. Parenteral steroids, in the form of prednisolone, methylprednisolone (Solu-Medrol), or hydrocortisone (Solu-Cortef), are indicated in hospitalized patients with severe IBD. Adrenocorticotropic hormone administered intravenously is used by some physicians instead of parenteral steroids.

The serious adverse effects associated with conventional steroids have provided the incentive to develop steroid analogues with similar potency but with fewer endocrine side effects. Budesonide* controlled ileal release is one such steroid, which is delivered to the distal ileum and proximal colon. It has a high affinity for the glucocorticoid receptor and once absorbed it has a high first-pass hepatic metabolism so that it has reduced systemic effects. Budesonide controlled ileal release is effective in active Crohn's disease involving the ileum and/or right colon but does not appear to be effective for maintenance of

*Not available in the United States.

remission. Budesonide* enemas are also available for use in distal colitis.

Antibiotics

There is evidence that luminal bacteria are important in the pathogenesis of IBD. Antibiotics are emerging as primary therapy for Crohn's disease. Metronidazole (Flagyl)† is useful in treating patients with active Crohn's disease of the colon with or without ileal involvement. It is effective in treating perianal fistula. It may also delay the recurrence of Crohn's disease following ileocolonic resection. Side effects of metronidazole include nausea, a metallic taste, and paresthesias. Ciprofloxacin (Cipro)† alone or in combination with metronidazole† may be beneficial in patients with active intestinal Crohn's disease or in those with perianal fistula. Multidrug antimycobacterial therapies have shown some efficacy in Crohn's disease. Antibiotics do not seem to be effective as primary therapy in ulcerative colitis.

Immunomodulators

Azathioprine and 6-Mercaptopurine

Azathioprine (Imuran)† and its metabolite 6-mercaptopurine (6-MP, Purinethol)† are purine analogues that inhibit ribonucleotide synthesis. These agents have been shown to induce and maintain remission and allow for steroid withdrawal in patients with Crohn's disease or ulcerative colitis refractory to standard medical therapies.

In published series, toxicity of the antimetabolites in well-monitored patients is generally mild and reversible although severe complications can occur. Toxicity includes infections, pancreatitis, bone marrow suppression, allergic reactions, and hepatitis. There has been the concern of lymphoma complicating 6-MP or azathioprine treatment in patients with IBD. Large series, however, have reported either no increased risk or a very low incidence of lymphoma in these patients. The potential risk of fetal abnormalities has also been a great concern for many physicians who discontinue these agents prior to conception. Preliminary data on 6-MP or azathioprine use during pregnancy in patients with IBD suggest that the risk of fetal abnormalities may not be increased.

Cyclosporine

Cyclosporine is a cyclic polypeptide that has an inhibitory effect on T-cell function and proliferation. Placebo-controlled trials have shown no benefit of oral cyclosporine in chronically active Crohn's disease. Intravenous cyclosporine† may be helpful in treating fistulizing Crohn's disease. Intravenous cyclosporine† is effective in averting colectomy in hospitalized patients with severe colitis who have not responded to steroid treatment. Cyclosporine toxicity includes nephrotoxicity, which may be irreversible; paresthesias; hypertension; hypertrichosis; opportunistic infections; and malignancy.

*Not available in the United States.
†Not FDA approved for this indication.

Methotrexate

Methotrexate is a folic acid antagonist that inhibits enzymes important in the synthesis of DNA. Methotrexate* has been shown to induce and maintain remission in chronic active Crohn's disease while allowing for steroid reduction. Toxicity includes interstitial pneumonitis and leukopenia. Although hepatotoxicity can occur with methotrexate, it remains controversial whether patients with IBD should be monitored with liver biopsy after a cumulative dose of 1.5 g. Patients taking methotrexate should receive folic acid 1 mg/d. To date, there is no strong evidence supporting the use of methotrexate in ulcerative colitis.

Other Agents

Nicotine

Epidemiologic observations that smokers have a decreased risk of ulcerative colitis and that the risk increases in those who stop smoking have led to therapeutic trials of nicotine* in treating ulcerative colitis. Nicotine seems beneficial in mild-to-moderate ulcerative colitis, but its use is limited by its side effects of nausea and headache. It may be useful in the patient with a colitis exacerbation who has recently stopped smoking.

Heparin

Heparin* has antithrombotic and anti-inflammatory properties that may be useful in the treatment of IBD. Open-labeled studies have shown a benefit of this agent in active ulcerative colitis.

Newer Immunomodulator Therapies

Anti–Tumor Necrosis Factor-α Chimeric Monoclonal Antibody

Tumor necrosis factor-α (TNF-α) is a potent proinflammatory cytokine that has a wide range of effects that are pivotal in the immunopathogenesis of IBD. A chimeric (mouse/human) monoclonal antibody (infliximab) that neutralizes TNF-α has been developed and is being used in Crohn's disease. Placebo-controlled trials have demonstrated the efficacy of infliximab in patients with medically refractory Crohn's disease or in patients with perianal or enterocutaneous fistulas. Infliximab (Remicade) is administered as an infusion. Its onset of action is rapid (within 2–4 weeks) and in general it is well tolerated. Long-term side effects of infliximab, including the potential risk of lymphoma, remain to be determined.

Interleukin-10

Interleukin 10† (IL-10) is a cytokine with anti-inflammatory properties. A large multicenter trial in

*Not FDA approved for this indication.
†Investigational drug in the United States.

chronic active Crohn's disease yielded disappointing results with no difference in remission rates in patients receiving IL-10 compared with placebo. A smaller study in mild-to-moderate Crohn's disease showed superiority of IL-10 compared with placebo in achieving remission. The role of IL-10 in IBD therapy remains to be defined.

Other Newer Immunomodulators

Tacrolimus (Prograf),* Mycophenolate Mofetil (CellCept),* thalidomide,* interleukin 11,† humanized anti-TNF-α (CDP571),† anti-α4β7 antibodies are other immunomodulatory agents being evaluated as therapies in Crohn's disease.

MEDICAL MANAGEMENT

The anatomic site, extent, and clinical activity of disease as well as drug side effects dictate what medical therapies should be considered in patients with IBD (Tables 1 and 2). Clinical activity may be defined as mild to moderate (symptomatic with no overt systemic signs or symptoms) or severe (symptoms associated with fever, weight loss, anemia, hypoalbuminemia).

*Not FDA approved for this indication.
†Investigational drug in the United States.

TABLE 1. **Medical Therapy for Ulcerative Colitis**

Active Disease	Medication
Mild to moderate	
Distal colitis	Mesalamine suppositories/enemas Steroid foams/enemas Mesalamine, olsalazine, or balsalazide Sulfasalazine Oral 5-ASA + rectal mesalamine/rectal steroids
Left-sided colitis and pancolitis	Mesalamine, olsalazine, or balsalazide Sulfasalazine Oral 5-ASA + rectal mesalamine/rectal steroids
Moderately severe	Prednisone
Severe	IV methylprednisolone IV hydrocortisone IV cyclosporine (refractory patients)
Maintenance of Remission	
Distal colitis	Mesalamine suppositories/enemas Mesalamine, olsalazine, or balsalazide Sulfasalazine Oral 5-ASA + rectal mesalamine
Left-sided colitis and pancolitis	Mesalamine, olsalazine, or balsalazide Sulfasalazine Oral 5-ASA + rectal mesalamine
Refractory Disease	6-MP or azathioprine

Abbreviation: 5-ASA = 5 aminosalicylic acid.

TABLE 2. **Medical Therapy for Crohn's Disease**

Active Disease	Medication
Mild to moderate	
Ileitis +/− proximal colitis	Mesalamine Ciprofloxacin +/− metronidazole
Colitis	Mesalamine Sulfasalazine Metronidazole
Moderately severe	Budesonide* Prednisone
Severe	IV methylprednisolone IV hydrocortisone IV cyclosporine (refractory patients)
Maintenance of Remission	
Ileitis +/− proximal colitis	Mesalamine
Colitis	Mesalamine Sulfasalazine
Postoperative	Mesalamine
Refractory Disease	
Active	6-MP/azathioprine Methotrexate Infliximab
Maintenance	6-MP/azathioprine Methotrexate Infliximab
Fistula	Metronidazole +/− ciprofloxacin† Infliximab 6-MP/azathioprine Cyclosporine

*For patients with ileitis +/− proximal colitis.
†For perianal fistula.

Ulcerative Colitis

Distal Colitis (Proctitis/Proctosigmoiditis)

Patients with proctitis (rectal inflammation) and proctosigmoiditis (rectosigmoid inflammation) usually present with urgency, tenesmus, and mucus and blood in the stool and rarely have systemic symptoms. First-line therapy for ulcerative proctitis and proctosigmoiditis should be twice daily mesalamine suppositories (Rowasa), 500 mg per suppository, or a nightly mesalamine enema (4 g), respectively. Treatment should continue for at least 2 to 3 weeks to evaluate efficacy. If there is no response, a second topical mesalamine preparation or a rectal steroid such as a foam, budesonide enema (2 mg), or hydrocortisone enema (100 mg) can be added. In patients who remain symptomatic, an oral 5-ASA agent or sulfasalazine should be added to the regimen. Uncommonly, optimal oral 5-ASA and rectal therapy do not control symptoms, in which case prednisone is needed. Patients achieving remission should be offered long-term therapy with mesalamine suppositories or enemas, which can be used as little as every third night. Individuals in remission who cannot tolerate rectal preparations can be switched to oral 5-ASA agents or sulfasalazine. Patients who required combination oral and topical preparations to induce a remission may require this combination for maintenance. The long-term use of steroid enemas is discouraged because of the potential for corticosteroid-related adverse effects.

Left-Sided Colitis and Pancolitis

For mild-to-moderately active left-sided colitis or pancolitis sulfasalazine (2 g/d), oral mesalamine (Asacol, 2–2.4 g/d), or olsalazine (Dipentum), 1 g/d can be initiated and the dose escalated until resolution of symptoms. Therapeutic response should be achieved within 4 weeks and may only occur at maximal doses of sulfasalazine (6 g/d),* oral mesalamine (4–4.8 g/d),* or olsalazine (3 g/d)*. In patients with left-sided colitis, the combination of oral and topical mesalamine may induce more rapid improvement in symptoms than either agent alone. Once remission is induced with an oral 5-ASA drug, maintenance therapy is recommended with the same agent. Maintenance doses for sulfasalazine are 2 to 4* g/d, oral mesalamine 1.2 to 2.4* g/d, and olsalazine 1 to 2* g/d. The efficacy of these agents for maintenance treatment is dose-dependent with some patients requiring doses similar to those used for induction. In addition, some patients may require dual therapy with oral and rectal 5-ASA agents to maintain remission. Although sulfasalazine is much less expensive, its dose is limited by adverse effects. Patients who are on long-term sulfasalazine or 5-ASA should have periodic measurement of serum urea nitrogen and creatinine and a urinalysis to monitor for the remote possibility of nephrotoxicity.

Oral corticosteroids should be considered in patients who are either unresponsive to 5-ASA drugs or those with a degree of severity that will not allow for the gradual response usually seen with 5-ASA drugs. Prednisone 40 to 60 mg/d should be initiated. Improvement should occur within 48 hours. Once remission is attained, the prednisone dosage should be reduced by 10 mg every 7 to 10 days until a dosage of 20 mg/d at which time it can be tapered by 5 mg/week until discontinuation. It is important to maintain oral 5-ASA (4–4.8 g/d)* or sulfasalazine (4–6 g/d)* at maximal dosages while the steroid is being reduced. Oral steroids are not recommended for long-term maintenance treatment.

Severe Colitis

Patients who have not responded to oral steroids or who have severe exacerbations manifested by weight loss, more than six bloody bowel movements per day, tachycardia, fever, anemia, and hypoalbuminemia should be admitted to the hospital for parenteral corticosteroids. In general, methylprednisolone (48–60 mg/d), which has fewer mineralocorticoid side effects than hydrocortisone, is used. It may be administered as bolus therapy every 8 hours or as a continuous infusion. If tolerated, rectal mesalamine or steroid preparations may help improve symptoms. Patients whose symptoms worsen with oral feeding should be on bowel rest. Peripheral parenteral nutrition can be initiated. Total parenteral nutrition is reserved for the severely malnourished patient and is not used as primary therapy. Adjunctive therapy includes intravenous rehydration, correction of electrolyte imbalance, and blood transfusions if necessary.

Narcotics or any agents that may predispose to toxic megacolon are contraindicated. Broad-spectrum antibiotics in combination with metronidazole should be given to patients with fever, leukocytosis (with bands), or who appear toxic with or without megacolon. In the patient with toxic megacolon, a nasogastric tube as well as rolling from supine to prone position for 15 to 20 minutes every 2 to 3 hours may help decompress the colon. A surgeon should evaluate and observe the patient from the beginning of hospitalization. Frequent physical examinations along with abdominal series should be done to monitor for colonic dilatation or perforation.

Patients with severe colitis who have a therapeutic response with formed, non-bloody stools, absence of abdominal pain, and who tolerate oral feedings may be switched to oral prednisone 40 to 60 mg/d. Patients with toxic colitis with or without megacolon who do not improve within 48 to 72 hours should undergo colectomy. Patients without toxicity or megacolon who have partial or no response after 7 days of parenteral steroids are candidates for surgery or intravenous cyclosporine (Sandimmune).* Both of these options including their risks and benefits must be discussed in detail with the patient. The decision to use cyclosporine with its potential serious adverse effects must be weighed against the fact that this disease is curable with surgery. A low cholesterol level predisposes to seizures and is a relative contraindication to cyclosporine use. Once the decision is made, cyclosporine 2 to 4 mg/kg/d can be initiated and the dosage is adjusted according to whole blood levels. Patients should be monitored carefully for hypertension, hypomagnesemia, nephrotoxicity, and infection. Patients usually improve within 3 to 5 days and once in remission are switched to oral cyclosporine (Neoral).* Azathioprine (Imuran)* or 6-MP is initiated. Steroid withdrawal followed by cyclosporine tapering is done over 3 to 6 months allowing for 6-MP or azathioprine to exert their therapeutic effect. Vigilant monitoring of cyclosporine levels and side effects is important. Of great concern are isolated reports of *Pneumocystis carinii* pneumonia (PCP) with or without fatality in patients with IBD treated with cyclosporine. PCP prophylaxis with sulfamethoxazole/trimethoprim (Septra) is advocated.

Crohn's Disease

Gastroduodenal

Gastroduodenal involvement with Crohn's disease occurs in less than 5% of cases. Patients can present with symptoms similar to peptic ulcer disease includ-

*Exceeds dosage recommended by manufacturer.

*Not FDA approved for this indication.

ing epigastric pain and postprandial nausea and vomiting. Proton pump inhibitors such as omeprazole (Prilosec) or histamine 2 (H_2) receptor antagonists may help improve symptoms. Persistent symptoms will usually respond to oral steroid therapy.

Ileitis/Ileitis and Proximal Colitis

A large percentage of patients with Crohn's disease have involvement of the terminal ileum alone or in combination with the right colon. Patients can present with nausea, abdominal pain, diarrhea, and weight loss. For mild-to-moderately active disease, oral mesalamine (Pentasa, Asacol) 3 to 4.8 g/d can be used as first-line therapy. Patients who do not respond after 3 to 4 weeks of maximal mesalamine may benefit from the addition of ciprofloxacin (Cipro) 500 mg twice daily alone or in combination with metronidazole (Flagyl) 10 to 20 mg/kg/d. A therapeutic response should be obtained within 2 to 3 weeks. Patients are maintained on the antibiotics for 3 to 4 months. Oral corticosteroids are indicated in patients who do not improve or worsen after mesalamine and antibiotic therapy. If available, budesonide controlled ileal release* 9 mg/d can be initiated. Otherwise prednisone 40 to 60 mg/d is prescribed until symptoms resolve and is the dosage is tapered over 2 months. Patients who have achieved medical or surgical remission should be considered for long-term therapy with mesalamine 3 to 4.8 g/d.

Occasionally a patient may present with fever, leukocytosis, and right lower quadrant tenderness mimicking appendicitis. These patients have localized peritonitis due to contained microperforation. Computed tomography of the abdomen should be performed to rule out an intra-abdominal abscess, which will require drainage. Broad-spectrum antibiotics in combination with metronidazole should be the initial treatment. Steroids in general are withheld.

Colitis

For mild-to-moderately active Crohn's colitis, sulfasalazine 4 to 6 g/d or oral mesalamine 3 to 4.8 g/d can be used. In patients who do not improve after 3 to 4 weeks, metronidazole 10 to 20 mg/kg/d should be added. Prednisone 40 to 60 mg/d should be initiated in patients who remain symptomatic or who worsen. Once remission is achieved, the steroid dosage is tapered and a maintenance regimen of sulfasalazine 3 to 4 g/d or oral mesalamine 3 to 4.8 g/d is recommended. The approach and therapy of hospitalized patients with severe Crohn's colitis is similar to that described for patients with ulcerative colitis. Patients with active distal Crohn's colitis will benefit from mesalamine or hydrocortisone enemas.

Fistula

Antibiotics are first-line therapy for draining perianal fistula. Metronidazole 10 to 20 mg/kg/d can be used with or without ciprofloxacin 500 mg twice daily. For those intolerant to metronidazole, ciprofloxacin can be used alone. Response is usually seen within 3 to 4 weeks. Some patients may have chronically draining fistula, requiring chronic intermittent antibiotic treatment. In these patients, azathioprine or 6-MP may be beneficial. Alternatively, infliximab given as an infusion of 5 mg/kg and repeated at 2 and 6 weeks later is very effective in healing active fistula. The effect, however, is often transient and patients may require repeated infusions. Cyclosporine* may be useful in fistulas unresponsive to other medical therapy.

Medically Refractory Disease

A subgroup of patients with IBD are refractory to maximal standard medical therapy with 5-ASA, antibiotics, and corticosteroids. These patients may be chronically symptomatic despite corticosteroids (steroid-refractory) or are controlled on steroids but become symptomatic as the steroids are tapered (steroid-dependent). Azathioprine* or 6-MP* is a therapeutic alternative to surgery in this situation. Azathioprine* or 6-MP* can be initiated at a dose of 50 mg/d. If after 2 weeks these drugs are well tolerated, the dosages can be increased to a maximum of 2.5 mg/kg/d for azathioprine* or 1.5 mg/kg/d for 6-MP.* Treatment must be continued for 3 to 6 months to fully evaluate therapeutic efficacy. Patients remain on corticosteroids until these agents exert their therapeutic effect. A complete blood cell count and liver profile should be monitored every 1 to 2 weeks initially for 1 month. Leukopenia and transaminitis respond to dose reduction. If blood tests are stable, these parameters can then be monitored on a monthly basis for 3 months and then every 3 months. Measurements of 6-MP metabolites are now available and can be used to optimize therapeutic response while minimizing drug toxicity. The optimal duration of therapy with azathioprine* or 6-MP* remains controversial, although there are some data suggesting that patients with Crohn's disease do better if they stop the drug after being in remission for at least 4 years.

In patients with Crohn's disease who do not respond to 6-MP* or azathioprine* and who want to avoid surgery, methotrexate is an alternative. A dosage of 25 mg/week intramuscularly is initiated. A complete blood cell count and liver profile should be monitored regularly. A response should be observed by 6 to 12 weeks. Methotrexate* should be discontinued if there is no therapeutic gain by week 16. Patients who achieve remission with methotrexate can be placed on a maintenance dosage of 15 mg/week intramuscularly. For patients with Crohn's disease who do not respond to immunosuppressive therapy, a single infusion of infliximab (5 mg/kg) is effective in improving symptoms and inducing remission.

*Not FDA approved for this indication.

*Not FDA approved for this indication.

Readministration of infliximab* is often necessary to maintain a therapeutic response.

SURGERY

Colectomy in ulcerative colitis is indicated in patients with chronic symptomatic disease that is refractory to medical therapy and in hospitalized patients with severe colitis who do not respond to intensive medical therapy. Urgent indications for colectomy include massive hemorrhage, toxic megacolon, and perforation. The finding of dysplasia, colonic strictures, or carcinoma on colonoscopy are indications for surgery. Colectomy with the construction of an ileo-anal pouch that acts as a reservoir is now the standard surgical procedure. Symptomatic inflammation of the pouch (pouchitis) can occur but usually responds well to antibiotic therapy such as metronidazole.

Indications for surgery in Crohn's disease include chronic symptomatic disease with or without nonhealing enteric fistula unresponsive to medical therapy. Occasionally perianal fistulas are best treated by surgery. Complications such as abscess, perforation, massive hemorrhage, toxic megacolon, and bowel obstruction that does not respond to medical treatment are urgent indications for surgery. In patients with recurrent obstructive symptoms due to small-bowel strictures, strictureplasties can be performed to improve symptoms while conserving bowel length. Unlike ulcerative colitis, surgery in Crohn's disease is not curative. Postoperative recurrence will occur in many patients.

NUTRITIONAL SUPPORT AND THERAPY

Nutritional support in IBD is important to maintain an adequate caloric and nutrient intake. In active Crohn's disease enteral or parenteral nutrition may improve symptoms whereas in ulcerative colitis these have no value as primary therapy. The benefit of specific dietary modifications including elimination diets has not been clearly proven. However, particular foods that trigger intestinal symptoms should be avoided by patients. Lactose intolerance should be considered in patients with IBD since this may contribute to symptoms. Patients with iron deficiency anemia will require iron supplements. Oral iron preparations may be difficult to tolerate and may occasionally worsen patients' symptoms, in which case parenteral iron is required.

In ulcerative colitis, parenteral nutrition has a supportive role. Hospitalized patients with severe colitis receiving maximal medical therapy who cannot tolerate oral intake or who are severely malnourished may benefit from parenteral nutrition. Short-chain fatty acids (SCFA), which appear to be an essential nutrient for the colonic epithelial cell, in enema form, may be useful in distal ulcerative colitis.

*Not FDA approved for this indication.

Eicosapentaenoic acid is an omega-3 fatty acid found in fish oil. It serves as an alternative substrate to arachidonic acid in the 5-lipoxygenase pathway resulting in the decreased production of the pro-inflammatory mediator leukotriene B4. It may be helpful as adjunctive therapy in ulcerative colitis.

Patients with active Crohn's disease who are malnourished and who want to avoid corticosteroids may benefit from a course of enteral nutrition (elemental or polymeric formulations). Parenteral nutrition with bowel rest may be helpful in patients with medically refractory Crohn's disease particularly if they are severely malnourished. Closure of fistulas may be induced by parenteral nutrition but this beneficial response is often lost once patients resume oral feeding. An enteric-coated fish oil (Purepa)* preparation may be useful in maintaining remission in Crohn's disease. Patients with small-bowel strictures should be advised to follow a low-residue diet and should avoid particular foods that may cause obstruction such as nuts, seeds, or corn. Vitamin B_{12} may be needed in patients with bacterial overgrowth or those with extensive ileal disease or ileal resection. Patients with fat malabsorption will likely require calcium and fat-soluble vitamins. These patients will benefit from dietary fat restriction. Patients with calcium oxalate nephrolithiasis resulting from hyperoxaluria secondary to fat malabsorption should be advised to follow a low-oxalate diet. Periodic monitoring with appropriate supplementation of potassium, magnesium, and zinc is necessary in patients with chronic diarrhea or extensive small-bowel disease or resection.

SUPPORTIVE MEDICAL AND PSYCHOSOCIAL MEASURES

Patients with IBD and ongoing chronic diarrhea may benefit from the use of antidiarrheal agents such as loperamide (Imodium). Antidiarrheal medications are contraindicated in acute IBD since these may precipitate small-bowel ileus or toxic megacolon. In patients with ileal resections, diarrhea may be induced by malabsorbed bile salts. Cholestyramine (Questran)† is a bile acid–binding resin useful in controlling diarrhea. One packet (4 g) can be initiated and titrated up to 4 packets a day until diarrhea is controlled. Cholestyramine should not be given to patients with steatorrhea. Patients with IBD can have superimposed irritable bowel syndrome so that antispasmodic agents such as hyoscyamine sulfate (Levsin) or dicyclomine (Bentyl) can be helpful at times when there is no overt clinical evidence of active disease.

The role of psychosocial stress as a potential cause of IBD has not been established. There is, however, evidence in animal models linking stress to gut inflammation. Psychological stress can impact the course of IBD. Physicians should be aware and sensi-

*Not available in the United States.
†Not FDA approved for this indication.

tive to the psychological impact a chronic illness such as IBD may have on a patient. Patients face many disease-related issues that they may have difficulty coping with. Chronic pain, change in body image, fear of future surgery or cancer risk, and loss of job due to illness may provoke anxiety and depression. A supportive and encouraging approach from the physician and family is important. The Crohn's and Colitis Foundation of America has local resources that can help in patient education and can provide social support groups.

OSTEOPOROSIS

Osteoporosis, which may lead to long-term fractures and debilitating symptoms, is an important complication associated with IBD. Possible contributing factors to bone loss in IBD include corticosteroid use, calcium and vitamin D malabsorption, and proinflammatory mediators. Corticosteroid-induced bone loss is dependent on the dose and duration of steroid use. It can occur as early as within the first 3 months of steroid use. In IBD patients receiving corticosteroids, a baseline bone densitometry study by dual-energy x-ray absorptiometry should be obtained and repeated every year steroids are given. In patients with normal densitometry studies, preventive therapy with vitamin D and calcium supplements is necessary. Avoidance of future corticosteroids if possible is recommended. Patients with an abnormal dual-energy x-ray absorptiometry scan should be treated with biphosphonates such as etidronate (Didronel) or alendronate (Fosamax). Calcium and vitamin D supplements are required along with biphosphonates.

COLON CANCER SURVEILLANCE

The most important determinants of colon cancer risk for patients with ulcerative colitis are the duration and extent of disease. Hospital- and population-based studies have reported cumulative risks of colon cancer of approximately 5% after 8 to 10 years of ulcerative colitis. Thereafter the risk seems to be 1% per year and does not appear to plateau. Primary sclerosing cholangitis increases the risk of colon cancer in ulcerative colitis. Patients with proctitis have a risk that is comparable to that of the general population. Colonoscopic surveillance after 8 to 10 years of extensive colitis and 12 years of left-sided colitis is recommended. Mucosal biopsy specimens of the entire colon at 10-cm intervals are taken. Biopsy of nodular areas and sessile masses must be performed. The finding of dysplasia on a biopsy specimen is significant and is an indication for colectomy. Dysplasia occasionally may be difficult to distinguish from reactive cellular changes due to inflammation so that slides should always be reviewed by more than one pathologist. Patients with negative biopsy results should have subsequent surveillance colonoscopies every 1 to 2 years. There are preliminary data in the form of a case-control study suggesting that long-term mesalamine greater than or equal to 1.2 g/d may reduce the risk of colon cancer. Crohn's disease of the colon is also associated with an increased risk of colon cancer. This is particularly true if colonic involvement is extensive. Patients with Crohn's colitis should undergo surveillance colonoscopy in the same manner as that in ulcerative colitis.

IRRITABLE BOWEL SYNDROME

method of
KEVIN W. OLDEN, M.D.
Mayo Clinic Scottsdale
Scottsdale, Arizona

Irritable bowel syndrome (IBS) is a chronic disorder characterized by abdominal discomfort or pain associated with changes in stool frequency and/or stool form. IBS is considered a *functional* gastrointestinal (GI) disorder in that it is manifested as a disorder of GI motility, characterized by slow gut transit (constipation), fast gut transit (diarrhea), or spastic nonperistaltic colonic contractions (pain). IBS is not associated with any known anatomic or biochemical abnormality. Despite being characterized as a disorder of GI motility, no specific pattern of gut dysmotility has ever been definitively associated with IBS. Like other symptom-defined syndromes, such as fibromyalgia, a diagnosis is made based on clinical as opposed to anatomic or biochemical grounds. The diagnostic criteria for IBS, as defined by the Rome International Working Teams on functional gastrointestinal disorders, are outlined in Table 1. It is clear that symptoms of abdominal pain, diarrhea, or constipation can represent a wide spectrum of GI disorders. The key to effectively using the Rome criteria for the diagnosis of IBS is to first exclude the presence of so-called alarm symptoms and to confirm that the patient presents with the epidemiologic factors that are commonly seen with IBS. IBS is unaccompanied by inflammation of the GI tract and has no systemic manifestations. Therefore, the presence of obvious or occult GI bleeding, fevers, weight loss, laboratory abnormalities such as anemia, or elevated nonspecific inflammatory markers such as erythrocyte sedimentation rate (ESR) are all inconsistent with the diagnosis of IBS. These symptoms may suggest other diseases that can present as abdominal pain, constipation, or diarrhea.

IBS tends to present in early adult life. It is uncommon for IBS to present de novo in patients after the age of 50. Patients in that age group with symptoms of new-onset diarrhea, constipation, or abdominal pain should be thoroughly investigated for causes of their symptoms. In a patient younger than 50 years of age and in the absence of alarm symptoms, the Rome diagnostic criteria have good

TABLE 1. **Rome II Criteria for Irritable Bowel Syndrome**

At least 12 weeks, which need not be consecutive, in the preceding 12 months the patient has experienced abdominal discomfort or pain that has two of three features:
1. Relieved with defecation; and/or
2. Onset associated with a change in frequency of stool; and/or
3. Onset associated with a change in form (appearance) of stool.

positive predictive value. Recent studies have suggested a sensitivity of over 65% and a specificity of 100% for the Rome criteria in patients without alarm symptoms.

EPIDEMIOLOGY

IBS is an extremely common disorder in North American and European populations. Studies performed in Africa and Asia have also suggested a remarkably similar prevalence of IBS across national and ethnic boundaries. By and large, IBS tends to be more common in women. The male-to-female ratio found in most studies is 1.2 to 2.0:1.0. However, these data may overstate the prevalence in that they many times reflect individuals presenting to treatment settings as opposed to community samples. Likewise, in western cultures, women are generally more likely to seek medical care than men, which may account for the higher prevalence of IBS reported in women.

IBS is the most common disorder seen in gastroenterologic practice, accounting for 40% of all visits. It is also an extremely common disorder seen in primary care practice, accounting for 20% to 25% of all visits to primary care physicians for GI complaints. Approximately 70% of people with symptoms of IBS do not seek medical care. There is evidence to suggest that patients who seek treatment for IBS are more psychosocially distressed than patients who meet the diagnostic criteria for IBS but who choose not to seek medical care. This is an important modulating fact that the physician needs to be aware of to maximize the effectiveness of the doctor-patient interaction. The average age at presentation is between 30 and 50 years. The incidence of IBS decreases with age.

PSYCHOSOCIAL FACTORS

Numerous studies have shown that patients with IBS have excess levels of anxiety and mood disorders. In particular, panic disorder has been studied in patients with diarrhea-prominent IBS. The presence of a concomitant psychiatric disorder can have significant implications for the treatment of patients with IBS because it can modulate and, many times, intensify the distress generated by IBS symptoms. Consequently, the ability to diagnose and properly treat a concomitant psychiatric disorder can lead to significant improvement in the patient's overall sense of well-being above and beyond the relief of GI symptoms per se. Reciprocally, the failure to effectively identify a concomitant psychiatric diagnosis can lead to less than optimal response to medical management of patients with IBS symptoms.

In addition to psychiatric disorders, a number of psychosocial states have also been associated with IBS. Numerous studies have documented the finding that patients who have suffered physical or sexual abuse either in childhood or in adult life are much more likely to have IBS. Additional studies have suggested that the severity of the abuse history can predict the severity of IBS symptoms as well as the patients' overall level of functional impairment due to their GI symptoms. However, no studies to date have suggested a *causal* relationship between either psychiatric disorders or abuse history and subsequent development of IBS. Psychosocial factors should be regarded as important modulating variables that can influence treatment strategies and outcome. Screening for psychiatric disorders and abuse history can facilitate the identification of factors that drive so-called refractory IBS symptoms. In addition, early identification of psychosocial factors can avoid unnecessary, costly, and, in many cases, redundant diagnostic medical testing.

TABLE 2. **Causes of Chronic Diarrhea**

Medication-Induced Diarrhea/Constipation
Infection
Bacterial
Salmonella species
Clostridium difficile
Campylobacter jejuni
Yersinia enterocolitica
Parasitic
Giardia lamblia
Entamoeba histolytica
Inflammatory Bowel Disease
Crohn's disease
Ulcerative colitis
Microscopic/collagenous colitis
Malabsorptive Disorders
Sprue
Lactose intolerance
Pancreatic insufficiency
Postgastrectomy syndromes
Bacterial overgrowth
Pancreatic insufficiency
HIV-Associated Diarrhea
Neuroendocrine Tumors
Gastrinoma
VIPoma
Medullary thyroid carcinoma (calcitonin)
Carcinoid

DIFFERENTIAL DIAGNOSIS

It is best to conceptualize patients with IBS-like symptoms into three groups: (1) patients with predominant diarrhea, (2) patients with predominant constipation, and (3) patients with a pattern of alternating constipation and diarrhea and abdominal pain. Patients who present with a chronic diarrheal illness, particularly those with painless diarrhea, need to be approached somewhat differently from patients who meet the classic diagnostic criteria for IBS. Painless, chronic diarrhea is a highly nonspecific symptom that has a wide differential diagnosis. The possible causes of chronic diarrhea are numerous, but the more common ones are outlined in Table 2. Likewise, a predominant history of either acute or chronic constipation demands its own workup. This is particularly true if other symptoms of IBS such as abdominal pain are absent and alarm symptoms such as weight loss, anemia, or rapid onset/older age at onset are present. Causes of constipation are outlined in Table 3.

One important form of constipation not uncommonly as-

TABLE 3. **Causes of Chronic Constipation**

Drug-induced constipation
Colonic motility disorder (slow transit constipation)
Rectal outlet constipation
Partial colonic obstruction
Neoplasm
Diverticular stricture
Eating disorders
Laxative abuse
Endocrine causes
Hypothyroidism
Diabetes mellitus
Addison's disease

sociated with IBS is so-called outlet constipation. This disorder does not result from changes in colonic motility, but rather from incoordination of the muscles of the pelvic floor. This dysfunction, in turn, impedes the passage of stool through the rectum and anal canal. Patients with this disorder will frequently report that they cannot "push" stool out at the time of a bowel movement. These patients will also not uncommonly report the need to manually disimpact themselves in order to move stool. As in IBS, patients with outlet constipation tend to be psychosocially distressed and, in some cases, may also have a history of physical or sexual abuse. This disorder is recognized by its typical history—difficulty in pushing stool with a bowel movement and the need to resort to manual disimpaction to remove stool from the rectal vault. Outlet constipation is diagnosed by the use of anorectal manometry testing that can identify changes in the function of the internal and external anal sphincters that detect changes in rectal sensitivity to distention. Outlet constipation is effectively treated with anorectal biofeedback, which can be accomplished by nurses or physical therapists trained in this modality. Success rates up to 85% have been reported using anorectal biofeedback for outlet constipation.

PATHOPHYSIOLOGY

To date, no pathognomonic abnormality has been identified to fully explain the symptoms of IBS. Over the past 3 decades, a number of different areas of investigation have been undertaken with varying degrees of success. Numerous studies over the past 30 years have demonstrated abnormalities of both small bowel and colonic motility in patients with IBS. Patients with IBS tend to have more high-amplitude peristaltic contractions than controls. Although this would seem to explain the symptoms of IBS, correlation between actual motility abnormalities as measured by ambulatory motility testing and the patient's reported symptoms is quite poor. Agents used to affect GI motility such as anticholinergics, prokinetics, and smooth muscle relaxants all have shown only minimal benefit in relieving IBS symptoms.

More recently, researchers have demonstrated abnormal visceral sensation in patients with IBS. Studies of balloon distention in the sigmoid, ileum, and colon have demonstrated lower pain thresholds in patients with IBS when compared with non-IBS controls. Further studies have demonstrated decreased thresholds for painful stimulation of the colon in patients with IBS, suggesting that the hyperalgesia is localized to the viscera. Other studies have also shown an increased awareness of normal GI motility function in patients with IBS. Abnormal central processing of pain may also play a role in the visceral hyperalgesia in IBS patients.

Because nearly one third of patients with IBS report the onset of symptoms after an episode of GI infection, theories of possible infectious and inflammatory causes for IBS have been proposed. The mechanism involved in these cases remains unknown. Some studies have demonstrated an increased number of inflammatory cells in such patients (i.e., mast cells in patients with "postinfectious" IBS) compared with that in controls. These theories remain controversial, however.

BRAIN-GUT INTERACTIONS

In studying IBS, increasing interest has been devoted to the concept of the enteric nervous system. This refers to the combination of sensory and motor nerve connecting the gut to the spinal cord and brain. This so-called visceral hypersensitivity has been discussed previously. Studies have demonstrated changes in brain processing of visceral sensations in patients with IBS. A number of recent studies have also demonstrated increased activity in the anterior cortex in patients with IBS compared with controls.

DIAGNOSIS

In IBS, the concept of a "positive," diagnostic approach is advocated. The diagnosis should be based on the presence of Rome II criteria for IBS, the patient's presenting symptom complex (i.e., diarrhea or constipation), the patient's history and physical examination, and focused diagnostic testing. Limited laboratory studies, including a complete blood cell count, routine chemistry studies, thyroid-stimulating hormone determination, and an erythrocyte sedimentation rate or test for C-reactive protein should be performed. Although the diagnostic yield is low, stool studies checking for fecal hemoglobin and/or fecal leukocytes can be performed. Routine screening for ova and parasites should not be performed unless there is a travel history to support this concern. Screening in the form of colonoscopy is indicated in patients older than the age of 50, patients with diarrhea-predominant symptoms, and patients with a family history of colon cancer. Routine abdominal ultrasonography is considered unnecessary in diagnosing IBS and can even be counterproductive, owing to detection of minor, unrelated abnormalities that could lead to further testing and diagnostic dilemmas. Rectal biopsy is not considered useful unless the patient has chronic diarrhea as the predominant complaint. Testing for lactose intolerance should be limited to patients from high-risk populations.

The presence of alarm features, such as weight loss, nocturnal symptoms, blood mixed in the stools, recent antibiotic use, family history of colon cancer, and abnormalities on abdominal examination, would prompt more extensive evaluation. A chronic diarrheal illness demands a colonoscopy with biopsies to rule out inflammatory bowel disease or microscopic or collagenous colitis. Likewise, biopsies of the upper small bowel to rule out celiac disease and aspiration of the small bowel to rule out the presence of bacterial overgrowth should be performed, particularly in patients who have signs of malabsorption. Likewise, a change in the clinical picture or symptom pattern over time may also warrant further investigation.

TREATMENT

An effective physician-patient relationship is an invaluable component of treatment in IBS. It is important to obtain a thorough history, including an abuse history using a nonjudgmental, patient-centered approach. A complete physical examination in conjuction with a cost-effective evaluation is important to build patient confidence in the diagnosis. The physician should provide a thorough explanation of the diagnosis and reassure the patient using terminology the patient can understand. The physician should give the patient realistic expectations regarding prognosis. It is important for patients with IBS to have an ongoing relationship with their physician. Together, these measures can have a significant impact on patient acceptance and understanding of the diagnosis and may prevent unnecessary diagnostic testing in the future. An effective physician-patient relationship has also been shown to positively influence patient outcome.

SYMPTOM STRATIFICATION

Approximately 70% of patients with IBS have mild symptoms that can be managed with measures such as patient education, reassurance, and lifestyle modification. Dietary modification to reduce intake of lactose, fat, alcohol, and caffeine and increase fiber can be helpful for these patients.

Approximately 25% of patients have moderate symptoms. Although these patients may have increased levels of psychological distress, they do not tend to have severe psychosocial or psychiatric disturbances. Pharmacotherapy in these patients should be symptom focused. The use of agents such as loperamide (Imodium) or diphenoxylate/atropine (Lomotil) for the control of diarrhea and the use of antispasmodics such as dicyclomine (Bentyl) or hyoscyamine (Levsin) for the control of cramping may benefit these patients. The use of fiber supplementation to increase bulk and to avoid constipation can also be helpful. However, the physician is cautioned to counsel patients on overuse of fiber, which in itself can produce additional bloating, diarrhea, and cramping. These patients may also benefit from psychological treatment, including individual or group therapy and relaxation training.

Less than 5% of patients with IBS can be classified as having severe symptoms. These patients commonly have pain as a predominant symptom and present with significant levels of impairment in their activities of daily living and overall function. These patients are more likely to have a psychiatric disorder and to have suffered physical or sexual abuse. Treatment of these patients should include modification of lifestyle, discretion as to diet, use of antispasmodics and antidiarrheal agents as indicated, and use of antidepressants. Antidepressants, particularly tricyclic antidepressants, have been shown to be beneficial for patients with moderate to severe IBS independent of any other antidepressant effect. The high levels of anxiety and depressive disorders in these patients further justify the use of antidepressants in this population. The dosages of commonly used antidepressants are outlined in Table 4. A number of studies in the past 5 years have demonstrated significant benefit from the use of psychotherapy for the treatment of patients with refractory or severe IBS. The use of interpersonal psychotherapy and, increasingly, cognitive behavioral therapy has been shown to be particularly effective in patients who have failed medical management. The goal of cognitive behavioral treatment is to help these patients reconceptualize their illness, identify positive attributes that they possess, mobilize these attributes in addressing their illness, and support and encourage positive progression for the patients' clinical course in response to these efforts. Finally, new agents are in development that modulate serotonergic activity in the gut. These new agents, such as tegaserod, a $5HT_4$ agonist, hold promise for the treatment of IBS.

TABLE 4. **Antidepressant Dosing Guidelines**

Antidepressant	Dosage (mg)	Range (mg/d)
Amitriptyline (Elavil)	10–150	50–300
Desipramine (Norpramin)	10–100	50–300
Doxepin (Sinequan)	10–150	75–300
Fluoxetine (Prozac)	10–20	20–80
Imipramine (Tofranil)	10–150	50–300
Paroxetine (Paxil)	10–20	20–50
Sertraline (Zoloft)	25–50	50–150
Trazodone (Deseryl)	25–50	150–450

The most important aspect of treating a patient with IBS is for the physician to adopt a positive and supportive approach. Studies have demonstrated that patients whose physicians listen to complaints, explore areas of psychosocial distress or trauma, and commit themselves to an ongoing relationship with each patient tend to have better outcomes than patients whose physicians provide only diagnostic services and medical intervention. The broadening of the physician's horizon in the care of these patients to include social, psychological, as well as medical issues, the so-called biopsychosocial model, increasingly has been shown to produce good outcomes in these patients.

PROGNOSIS

The prognosis for IBS is quite good. A number of long-term prospective cohort studies have shown that patients with IBS have no excess mortality from any cause and no excess incidence of cancer or inflammatory bowel disease. Their symptoms of IBS tend to remit over time. Informing patients of the positive prognosis at initial presentation when their levels of anxiety about the disease tends to be quite high is of critical importance. The ability to reassure patients with ongoing medical and emotional care seems to be the optimal treatment for patients with this common and often disabling disorder.

HEMORRHOIDS, ANAL FISSURE, AND ANORECTAL ABSCESS AND FISTULA

method of
THOMAS E. READ, M.D.
Washington University School of Medicine
St. Louis, Missouri

HEMORRHOIDS

Signs and symptoms of anorectal disease—bleeding, itching, burning, tissue prolapse, pain—are frequently attributed to "hemorrhoids" by both patients and physicians without an adequate search for other causes. Unfortunately, these symptoms are as likely to be caused by anal fissure, fistula, abscess, rectal adenocarcinoma, anal epidermoid carcinoma, condylomata, pruritus ani, proctalgia fugax, and rectal prolapse as they are to be a consequence of hemorrhoidal disease. The multimillion dollar industry of over-the-counter hemorrhoidal remedies serves to reinforce this misconception in the public, and the natural aversion to performing anorectal examination contributes to the ease of making the diagnosis of hemorrhoids by physicians without an adequate investigation for other causes of the patient's symptoms.

For patients misdiagnosed with hemorrhoids who have another benign cause of their anorectal symptoms, this misguided practice results in a delay in diagnosis and appropriate treatment. For patients with cancer of the anus or rectum, such a delay can be fatal.

Symptomatic hemorrhoids, however, are a significant cause of morbidity in our society. Hemorrhoids are vascular cushions located in the distal rectum and anal canal, whose exact function is unknown, although they may play a role in discrimination of rectal contents and fecal continence. Despite popular misconceptions, hemorrhoids are normal anatomic structures. They consist of a network of arterioles and dilated venules in a supporting matrix of fibroelastic connective tissue and smooth muscle. This network helps to anchor the hemorrhoid to the underlying circular smooth muscle of the distal rectum and anal canal. Internal hemorrhoids arise proximal to the dentate line and are usually painless, owing to the lack of somatic innervation. External hemorrhoids consist of the subcutaneous venous plexus distal to the dentate line and can produce acute pain when they thrombose and produce acute swelling of the overlying skin.

The pathogenesis of symptomatic internal hemorrhoids is uncertain, but it appears to be related to repeated straining in the squatting position during defecation. Consumption of a high-fat, low-fiber diet without adequate fluid intake may contribute by causing constipation. The internal hemorrhoidal complexes are progressively displaced distally through the anal canal and enlarge as the underlying connective tissue network is disrupted.

On physical examination, *prolapsing internal hemorrhoids* appear as submucosal cushions, typically in the left lateral, right anterior, and right posterior positions. The folds of the mucosa are aligned radially, which helps to differentiate prolapsing hemorrhoids from *full-thickness rectal prolapse,* in which the mucosal folds appear in a circular orientation. Trauma to the engorged vascular cushions can cause rectal bleeding, which is usually painless. The blood is typically bright red, which is understandable given that disruption of the mucosa overlying the arteriovenous plexus will result in the most rapid bleeding from the high-pressure, arterial side of the plexus. Patients may also complain of prolapse of tissue, which sometimes requires manual reduction after bowel movements. Persistent prolapse of mucosa leads to chronic mucus drainage, which can be confused with true anal incontinence. Patients typically also complain of perianal irritation and pruritus.

Internal hemorrhoids are classified by their degree of prolapse; this classification can aid in the selection of appropriate therapy. *First-degree hemorrhoids* bleed but do not prolapse. *Second-degree hemorrhoids* prolapse during defecation and reduce spontaneously. *Third-degree hemorrhoids* prolapse and require manual reduction. *Fourth-degree hemorrhoids* are those that cannot be effectively reduced. Usually, patients with fourth-degree hemorrhoids have mixed hemorrhoids (with both an internal and external component) that are chronically prolapsed and nontender. However, some patients suffer from acutely prolapsed hemorrhoids that become incarcerated and their vascular supply compromised. These patients have severe pain and need urgent attention because ischemic necrosis can result.

Before ascribing anorectal symptoms to hemorrhoids, it is necessary to perform a detailed anorectal examination, which should include proctoscopy and anoscopy. Examination of the proximal colon with flexible sigmoidoscopy, colonoscopy, or air-contrast barium enema should be performed in patients whose symptoms are atypical or whose age, medical history, or family history of colorectal neoplasia places them at risk of developing colorectal carcinoma.

Treatment of Internal Hemorrhoids

The selection of the various treatment options for symptomatic hemorrhoids depends on the severity of symptoms and the degree of prolapse. Regardless, increasing fiber consumption concomitant with increasing fluid consumption is the mainstay of treatment. This regimen will bulk the stool and reduce straining at defecation. Caffeine and alcohol should be avoided because they are diuretics. Patients should be counseled to avoid prolonged periods of straining at stool; reading material and other distractions should be removed from the bathroom. Topical corticosteroids, such as hydrocortisone suppositories, may help reduce inflammation and swelling. The vast majority of other over-the-counter remedies have no therapeutic value.

Symptomatic first-, second-, and third-degree hemorrhoids may be treated in the office by elastic ligation (banding), sclerotherapy, and infrared photocoagulation. Each of these procedures produces a focal area of inflammation and subsequent fibrosis at the proximal apex of the hemorrhoid that restores fixation of the hemorrhoid to the muscular layer of the distal rectum and reduces vascular engorgement. Elastic ligation has been shown to be the most effective and least expensive of these methods. If care is exercised to place the band proximal to the dentate line and to avoid incorporation of the muscular wall of the rectum, the procedure is well tolerated without anesthesia. Postprocedure discomfort is usually mild, and complications are rare. Delayed hemorrhage and thrombosis of external hemorrhoids occur in less than 3% of patients. Although the serious complication of perineal sepsis is extremely rare, any patient with severe anal pain, fever, or urinary retention after elastic ligation warrants immediate evaluation.

Other outpatient treatment methods such as bipolar diathermy, direct-current electrocoagulation, and cryotherapy have been advocated by some practitioners but are not recommended because of lack of proven efficacy and/or higher complication rate. Anal dilation has also been used as a treatment of symptomatic hemorrhoids, primarily based on the finding that some patients with hemorrhoidal disease have elevated anal sphincter resting pressures as measured by anal manometry. Although dilation may improve hemorrhoidal symptoms in some patients, most colon and rectal surgeons have avoided this technique because of the risk of sphincter disruption and anal incontinence.

Excisional hemorrhoidectomy is reserved for patients with a large external component of their disease, for patients who fail elastic ligation, or for patients with acutely prolapsed, incarcerated hemorrhoids. The procedure is usually performed on an outpatient or short-stay basis under local or regional anesthesia. Urinary retention occurs in up to 10% of patients, and most patients report discomfort for several weeks after the procedure. Hemorrhage and anal stenosis occur in 1% to 2% of patients. Excisional hemorrhoidectomy is an effective treatment for symptomatic hemorrhoids, with excellent long-term patient satisfaction. However, patients who return to straining at stool because of their dietary or bathroom habits may eventually have recurrent symptoms.

Laser hemorrhoidectomy has been advertised by some practitioners as a less traumatic and less painful method of performing excisional hemorrhoidectomy. However, comparative trials have shown no benefit to laser hemorrhoidectomy versus standard hemorrhoidectomy, and the extra cost of the procedure is not warranted. A novel method of hemorrhoidectomy, circular stapled hemorrhoidectomy, is now undergoing clinical testing. This new technique may reduce the postoperative discomfort associated with traditional excisional hemorrhoidectomy.

Hemorrhoidal disease in patients with inflammatory bowel disease should be approached with caution. Although hemorrhoids are usually considered to be unrelated to inflammatory bowel disease, patients with Crohn disease who are undergoing hemorrhoidectomy may develop fistulas and nonhealing wounds. Some patients have even required proctectomy for complications related to hemorrhoidectomy performed in the setting of active proctitis.

Treatment of External Hemorrhoids

Thrombosis of an external hemorrhoid is one of the most common causes of acute anal discomfort. The patient will often report the acute onset of pain and a palpable lump at the anal verge after straining at defecation or vigorous physical activity. Patients who present with severe discomfort are best managed by excision of the clot and overlying skin under local anesthesia. Simple incision and evacuation of the clot is associated with early rethrombosis and is not recommended. Most patients, however, are seen several days after the onset of symptoms, when their severe pain is subsiding. They are best managed with sitz baths, analgesics, fiber supplements, and reassurance. The thrombosis will resolve within 4 to 6 weeks. Some patients will have a residual skin tag at the site of the thrombosed external hemorrhoid, but most are asymptomatic.

ANAL FISSURE

Anal fissure is the most common cause of painful anal bleeding. Fissures begin as acute linear tears in the anoderm, extending from the dentate line to the anal verge. They develop after trauma to the anoderm, usually following a hard stool. Acute fissures can progress to become chronic nonhealing ulcers, with exposed internal sphincter fibers, an overhanging sentinel skin tag, and a hypertrophied anal papilla at the base of the fissure. Hypertonicity of the internal anal sphincter with poor arterial inflow to the area of the fissure, combined with repetitive trauma, results in nonhealing.

Fissures are found in the posterior midline of the anal canal in approximately 90% of patients. The anterior midline is the second most common site. Fissures located in eccentric positions should raise the possibility of Crohn disease, carcinoma, or syphilis. Pain with defecation and a small amount of anal bleeding, usually bright red, are the most common symptoms. Because of severe patient discomfort, it may be difficult to perform a detailed examination of the anorectum when the patient is evaluated initially. However, gentle separation of the buttocks usually is adequate to expose the anal margin and see the ulcer and/or overhanging sentinel skin tag. Occasionally, it is necessary to perform examination with the patient under anesthesia to determine the cause of severe anal pain in a patient who cannot be adequately examined in the office.

Treatment

Initial therapeutic measures include fiber bulking agents and fluid, laxatives if necessary, and soaks in warm water. The goal is to interrupt the cycle of constipation, hard stool, repetitive traumatic injury, pain, spasm, and nonhealing. Topical corticosteroids in the form of suppositories or ointments are sometimes effective. Anesthetic ointment applied immediately before bowel movements can be helpful by lessening the discomfort of defecation. Narcotic analgesics should be avoided because they can exacerbate constipation.

In the past several years, alternative pharmacologic treatments have been developed that may be efficacious in the treatment of patients with acute and chronic anal fissures. Most of these therapies have been directed at relaxation or temporary paralysis of the internal anal sphincter muscle in an attempt to transiently decrease resting tone, increase arterial blood flow to the fissure, and promote healing. Relaxation of the internal anal sphincter is mediated by release of nitric oxide, and investigators found that topical application of nitrates to the anal canal produced a decrease in anal canal resting pressure by 20% to 25%. Topical nitroglycerin* ointment, 0.2% to 0.4%, applied two to four times per day has been used to treat patients with both acute and chronic fissures. Initial clinical trials of nitroglycerin ointment were encouraging, although more recent studies have reported mixed results. The major side effect is headache, which occurs in 10% to 50% of

*Not FDA approved for this indication.

patients. Injection of botulinum toxin into the internal anal sphincter causes chemical denervation of the muscle that persists for 3 to 4 months. Most published series are from Europe, where investigators report healing of anal fissures in 60% to 80% of patients. The side effect of temporary incontinence occurs in a small number of patients. Experience with this agent in the United States is limited.

Patients with symptomatic fissures who fail medical management should be considered for lateral internal sphincterotomy, with expectation of healing in greater than 90%. The procedure entails division of the distal portion of the internal sphincter muscle through a small incision. Mucosal perfusion is improved, and healing of the fissure usually occurs within 4 weeks. Complications such as hematoma and abscess formation are rare. Continence status should be carefully assessed preoperatively because some minor change in continence is reported in 10% to 15% of patients. Women with prior obstetrical injury or patients with chronic diarrhea or irritable bowel syndrome should be approached with caution.

Every attempt should be made to manage patients with anal fissures nonoperatively if they have impaired anal continence. Nonhealing ulcers should be sampled to rule out malignancy. Anal dilation under anesthesia is an alternative to sphincterotomy; however, this procedure produces an uncontrolled tearing of the sphincter complex. Dilation is associated with a higher fissure recurrence rate and an increased risk of fecal incontinence and thus should be avoided.

Anal ulcers secondary to Crohn disease can be confused with idiopathic anal fissures. Although most anal fissures in Crohn disease occur in the midline, there is a higher incidence of lateral location and multiplicity than in the general population. They are often less painful than one would guess based on their appearance. These ulcers typically have a benign course and respond to nonoperative measures aimed at reducing symptoms. In patients with Crohn disease, sphincterotomy should be performed only in carefully selected patients because of the risks of poor healing and impaired continence should the patient develop other anorectal complications of the disease.

ANORECTAL ABSCESS AND FISTULA

The vast majority of anorectal abscesses and fistulas are cryptoglandular in origin. Obstruction of an anal gland located in the crypts at the dentate line causes an infection that extends from the intersphincteric space in a variety of directions. Cephalad spread in the intersphincteric plane results in an intersphincteric abscess; caudad spread results in a perianal abscess; lateral spread through the external sphincter muscle results in an ischiorectal space abscess. Spontaneous or surgical drainage of the abscess will relieve the acute symptoms. In approximately 60% of patients, however, a chronic fistula tract will persist from the involved anal gland at the dentate line to the external drainage site.

Patients with an anorectal abscess complain of progressive, throbbing perianal pain, sometimes associated with fever, constipation, or difficulty voiding. Physical examination reveals a tender, erythematous, fluctuant area at the anal verge (perianal abscess) or over the ischiorectal space (ischiorectal abscess). Patients with an intersphincteric or postanal space abscess may present with deep-seated anorectal pain with no external signs of infection. Digital rectal examination in these patients often reveals a tender, fluctuant area proximal to the sphincter complex. Examination under anesthesia may be necessary to confirm the diagnosis.

Patients with a fistula-in-ano typically complain of persistent purulent drainage from an external opening on the perineum. Intermittent closure of the overlying skin may produce a cycle of abscess formation, increased pressure, and spontaneous drainage. The external opening is usually apparent on physical examination and is often associated with a palpable cord extending toward the anal verge. Digital rectal examination and anoscopy may reveal the internal opening at the dentate line.

Another cause of anorectal abscess and fistula is Crohn's disease. Proctoscopy should be performed before operation in any patient with anorectal fistula to exclude proctitis because treatment for a fistula arising from anorectal Crohn's disease may be markedly different from that for a cryptoglandular fistula. Hidradenitis suppurativa may cause superficial abscesses in the perianal region, secondary to infection of the apocrine sweat glands of the skin, which are sometimes confused with cryptoglandular abscesses. Patients with hidradenitis will not have fistulous communication to the anal canal or rectum and will often have disease in the axilla and groin.

Treatment

The treatment of cryptoglandular abscess and fistula is surgical. Prolonged antibiotic therapy alone is virtually never successful at effecting healing. Abscesses require incision and drainage, which can occasionally be performed under local anesthetic in an outpatient setting if the abscess is small and superficial. However, patient comfort is improved and adequate drainage ensured when the procedure is performed in the operating room under more controlled conditions. Local anesthesia with intravenous sedation, regional anesthesia, or general anesthesia may be used, depending on the complexity of the abscess and co-morbid conditions of the patient.

Many surgical texts advocate making a large cruciate incision over the maximal point of fluctuance, excising skin, and packing the abscess cavity with gauze. This technique is unnecessarily morbid and should be avoided. Rather, the abscess should be drained as close as possible to the anal verge because this will result in the shortest possible fistula tract. A small (10–14 French) mushroom catheter is placed into the abscess cavity through a small stab incision after pus has been evacuated. The catheter may be removed in the office several weeks after the inflammation has subsided and the cavity has collapsed. Malecot catheters should not be used for this purpose because the side holes are large enough to permit tissue ingrowth, which makes subsequent removal difficult. Perioperative antibiotics should be considered if patients have associated cellulitis, diabetes, or immune suppression.

Approximately 60% of patients will have a residual fistula identified after the abscess has resolved. Treatment depends on the amount of external sphincter muscle encompassed by the fistula tract. Intersphincteric and superficial transphincteric fistulas can usually be treated by fistulotomy, without significant alteration of continence. The fistula tract is clearly identified from internal to external opening, unroofed, and débrided. Continence status should always be assessed before division of any portion of the anal sphincter complex because women with prior obstetrical injury or patients who have had prior anorectal surgery may be at risk for fecal incontinence after fistulotomy.

High transphincteric or suprasphincteric fistulas should not be treated by fistulotomy because division of the majority of the external sphincter muscle will result in fecal incontinence. Several treatment options are available. Many experienced surgeons favor endoanal sliding advancement flap, in which a tongue of mucosa and circular smooth muscle is mobilized and sutured so as to obliterate the internal opening of the fistula. Although more technically complex than other techniques, the endoanal advancement flap has the advantage of leaving the sphincter muscle intact and preserving continence. Slow-cutting setons, in which a suture or Silastic loop is placed through the fistula tract and slowly tightened over 4 to 12 weeks, are used with the intention of causing fibrosis and scarring to prevent wide separation of the external sphincter muscle as it is slowly divided. However, many patients will report some change in continence after the procedure.

Injection of autologous or commercially prepared fibrin glue into the fistula after débriding the tract in the operating room has been effective in the treatment of some patients with complex fistulas unresponsive to other treatments. Fibrin glue injection has the advantage of preserving the sphincter muscle, causing minimal morbidity, and can be repeated without difficulty. The only major drawback is cost. Recurrent abscesses and fistulas are most often the result of improper identification of the internal opening of the fistula at the dentate line or misdiagnosis of perianal Crohn's disease or hidradenitis suppurativa.

GASTRITIS AND PEPTIC ULCER DISEASE

method of
DUANE T. SMOOT, M.D.
Howard University
Washington, D.C.

Peptic ulcer disease is a common gastrointestinal disease whose management and treatment have changed dramatically over the past 25 years. Treatment of peptic ulcer disease has evolved from dietary modifications and antacids to gastric acid suppression with H_2-receptor antagonists and proton pump inhibitors and then to eradication of *Helicobacter pylori* infection. Before the development of H_2-receptor antagonists, patients with peptic ulcers were frequently managed as inpatients and surgery for complicated ulcer disease was commonplace. Surgery for complicated ulcer disease has dramatically declined over the past 2 to 3 decades with use of H_2-receptor antagonists and proton pump inhibitors; management of peptic ulcers has changed from an in-hospital to a largely outpatient setting. In the late 1980s, it became clear that the majority of peptic ulcers were etiologically related to the gram-negative bacterium *H. pylori.* The incidence of peptic ulcer disease is now on the decline, which is at least in part related to the eradication of *H. pylori.*

Gastritis usually refers to abdominal pain centered in the upper abdomen (also known as *dyspepsia*) that may be aggravated or relieved by food, in the absence of ulcer disease. This is better known as *nonulcer dyspepsia. Gastritis* is a pathologic term to describe histologic inflammation of the stomach; however, the relationship between abdominal pain or dyspepsia and gastritis is not well understood. Many patients will have dyspepsia in the absence of gastritis, whereas documented gastritis frequently occurs in persons who do not have dyspepsia, including many people with *H. pylori*–associated gastritis.

GASTRITIS

Gastritis should be considered in persons who complain of upper midabdominal pain. In most cases the pain will either be relieved or aggravated by food, although not always. Although it is important to take a good history to try to determine the type and character of the abdominal pain, it is often difficult for the patient to accurately describe his or her pain or discomfort to the physician. To help physicians, many attempts have been made to classify upper abdominal pain into specific categories to identify the underlying cause, such as reflux-like dyspepsia, ulcer-like dyspepsia, and motility-like dyspepsia. These categories may be useful for research studies but have not been very helpful to physicians in day-to-day patient care. Findings on physical examination are usually limited, and significant disease can be present with only mild tenderness on abdominal examination. Therefore, the medical history plays a very important role. Severe symptoms that prevent a person from working or doing normal activities and pain that awakens a person from sleep or prevents a person from eating to the point that he or she loses

TABLE 1. **Alarm Signs/Symptoms in Patients Presenting With Dyspepsia**

Anorexia	Early satiety
Anemia	Hematemesis
Weight loss	Melena or blood in stool

weight are given a lot of significance. In addition, there are so-called alarm symptoms that if present may signify a more serious disease than gastritis (Table 1). When alarm symptoms or signs are present, immediate evaluation of the gastrointestinal tract with endoscopy is indicated. Also, older patients (older than age 50) who present with moderate to severe pain in the absence of alarm symptoms should also undergo early endoscopic evaluation of the gastrointestinal tract because of their higher risk of having ulcer disease or cancer.

Management of a person who presents with abdominal pain without alarm symptoms or other absolute need for immediate endoscopy would include (1) empirical trial of acid suppression therapy, (2) further diagnostic evaluation with upper gastrointestinal endoscopy and ultrasonography to rule out gallstones, and (3) testing for *H. pylori* infection and treating with antibiotics if positive. For persons with alarm symptoms or older patients when there is a suspicion for significant disease, one should immediately proceed with upper gastrointestinal endoscopy.

Acid Suppression Therapy

Acid suppression to treat nonspecific upper abdominal pain or dyspepsia can begin with H_2-receptor antagonists. Ranitidine (Zantac) or nizatidine (Axid) can be given 150 mg twice daily or 300 mg/d; famotidine (Pepcid) can be given 20 mg twice daily or 40 mg/d; and cimetidine (Tagamet) can be given 400 mg twice daily. Many patients will have already tried over-the-counter H_2-receptor antagonists with limited or no relief. Depending on the severity of symptoms or the lack of response with over-the-counter H_2-receptor antagonists, one may elect initially to treat symptoms with a proton pump inhibitor. Five proton pump inhibitors are available for use, including omeprazole (Prilosec), 20 mg/d; lansoprazole (Prevacid), 15 mg/d; rabeprazole (Aciphex), 20 mg/d; pantoprazole (Protonix), 40 mg/d; and esomeprazole (Nexium), 40 mg/d. Treatment should be given for 4 to 8 weeks. If the symptoms still continue without relief from the medication, a diagnostic workup is indicated. If there is partial relief, one can increase the dose of the medication; however, this may indicate more severe disease and a diagnostic workup should be considered at this time. If there is resolution of symptoms, the medication should be discontinued and the patient followed to see if symptoms recur. In many patients symptoms will recur, at which time the medication can be restarted; however, a diagnostic workup should be considered. In this situation persons may have undiagnosed gastroesophageal reflux disease or *H. pylori*–associated peptic ulcer disease, both of which will respond to acid suppression therapy.

Diagnostic Evaluation

Evaluation of upper abdominal pain is best done with upper gastrointestinal endoscopy. Barium upper gastrointestinal series is not a good test to evaluate persons with upper abdominal pain (this test should be reserved for patients with dysphagia). Upper gastrointestinal endoscopy can diagnose gastritis, peptic ulcer disease, and esophagitis, as well as rule out gastric or esophageal cancer. Diagnosis of *H. pylori* infection can also be made at the time of upper endoscopy (Table 2). Gastric biopsy specimens can be taken for bacterial culture, rapid urease assays, or histology with specific staining for this bacterium. It is important to consider gallstone disease in these patients. If no diagnoses to explain the abdominal pain are made on upper endoscopy, then abdominal ultrasonography should be performed.

Diagnosis and Treatment of *H. pylori* Infection

Treatment of *H. pylori* infection in persons with abdominal pain who do not have documented peptic ulcer disease or who are not at increased risk of stomach cancer is controversial. Patients who have or have had an ulcer clearly need to be treated for *H. pylori* infection if present. Several studies have been conducted to evaluate the effectiveness of treating *H. pylori* infection in persons with abdominal pain who do not have ulcer disease (nonulcer dyspepsia). The majority of these studies have not shown that the antibiotic therapy is any better than placebo in relieving abdominal pain. In several of these studies treating *H. pylori* infection resulted in resolution of abdominal pain in 20% to 25% of subjects, but the placebo response rate was as high as 20%, resulting in no significant difference. Although there cannot be a uniform recommendation to test and treat persons with abdominal pain without ulcers for *H. pylori* infection, this should be considered on a case-by-case basis. It is important to know that when evaluating patients with abdominal pain before diagnostic workup (uninvestigated dyspepsia), deciding

TABLE 2. **Diagnostic Tests for *Helicobacter pylori***

Diagnostic Tests	Sensitivity (%)	Specificity (%)
Office whole blood tests	70–88	75–90
Laboratory serology tests	85–94	80–95
^{13}C & ^{14}C urea breath tests	90–96	90–98
Stool antigen test	88–98	90–98
Rapid urease assays	88–95	95–99
Histology (Genta, Giemsa, silver stains)	93–96	97–99
Bacterial culture	80–94	100

whether or not to test and treat for *H. pylori* depends on the prevalence of peptic ulcers in the population that you are serving. If ulcer disease is relatively common in your patient population, then it would be useful to test and treat *H. pylori* infection in your patients with abdominal pain because many of these patients will have underlying peptic ulcer disease. But if ulcer disease is rare in your patient population, you are not likely to find any benefit in testing and treating *H. pylori* infection in your patients with upper abdominal pain as the initial management. *H. pylori* infection is still very common in developing countries, along with peptic disease. Immigrants from countries with a high prevalence of *H. pylori* and peptic ulcer disease should be considered candidates for testing and treating *H. pylori* before an expensive diagnostic workup.

H. pylori is the most common cause of gastritis; therefore, it is important to consider diagnosis of this infection in persons with dyspepsia. There are numerous diagnostic tests available to determine if patients are infected with this bacterium (see Table 2). Overall, the sensitivity and specificity of most of these tests are excellent. The most frequently used diagnostic tests are antibody assays that use serum or whole blood. These tests indicate prior exposure to *H. pylori* and do not indicate whether infection is currently present. The advantages of serology are the relatively low cost and the noninvasiveness. If a patient has not been previously treated, blood antibody tests are very reliable, with sensitivity and specificity of about 85%. The major disadvantage of the antibody-based assays is the likelihood of false-positive results in patients previously treated with antibiotics, because *H. pylori* antibody titers are slow to fall and may remain positive in some people after successful treatment. Other frequently used noninvasive diagnostic tests include urea breath tests and the stool antigen test. Both of these tests detect current *H. pylori* infection and can be used for initial diagnosis of this infection and for evaluating treatment success when performed 4 to 6 weeks after the completion of antibiotic therapy. Two carbon-labeled urea breath tests (^{13}C and ^{14}C) have been developed that make use of *H. pylori's* urease enzyme that is produced in great abundance. The urea breath tests can be administered in the office as either a liquid (^{13}C-labeled urea) or capsule (^{14}C-labeled urea) followed by collecting a breath sample with a balloon 10 to 20 minutes later. Breath samples can then be analyzed by the laboratory for excess production of $^{13}CO_2$ or $^{14}CO_2$, which confirms the presence of *H. pylori* infection. The stool antigen test (Premier Platinum HpSA) is performed on a spontaneously passed stool that can be evaluated for the presence of *H. pylori* antigens. The accuracy of the urea breath test and the stool antigen test is about 95% both before antibiotic treatment and to confirm successful eradication. The noninvasive diagnostic tests have not been well evaluated in children; therefore, one needs to be careful in using these tests in this population.

Specific antibiotic therapy for *H. pylori* infection is given in Table 3.

PEPTIC ULCER DISEASE

The causes of peptic ulcer disease can be divided into four major categories: *H. pylori*–induced ulcers, nonsteroidal anti-inflammatory drugs (NSAIDs), acid hypersecretory conditions (e.g., Zollinger-Ellison syndrome), and idiopathic ulcers. In addition, gastric and duodenal ulcers can be caused infrequently by chronic disease states (e.g., Crohn disease, systemic mastocytosis), chronic alcoholism, malignancy, and viral infections (from herpes simplex virus, cytomegalovirus). Stress in specific circumstances has also been implicated in ulcer disease. Experimental stress has been shown to cause gastric but not duodenal ulcers in rats. In humans, stress associated with severe illnesses, such as extensive skin burns and admission to an intensive care unit, are associated with gastric ulcers. Life stresses in otherwise healthy people in the past were believed to be a cause of ulcers; however, stress has not been shown in nonhospitalized patients to be an actual cause of ulcers, even though it may be associated with stomach discomfort/pain and increased acid secretion.

H. pylori–Induced Ulcers

In initial studies, *H. pylori* was identified in over 90% of adult patients with chronic gastritis and 85% to 90% of adult patients with peptic ulcer disease. However, more recent studies have shown that the prevalence of *H. pylori* in peptic ulcer disease is gradually decreasing to 60% to 75%. The decline in preva-

TABLE 3. **Recommended Antibiotic Regimens for *Helicobacter pylori***

Antimicrobial Regimens*	Duration
Bismuth subsalicylate (Pepto-Bismol), 525 mg (2 tabs) qid, + metronidazole (Flagyl), 250 mg qid, + tetracyline, 500 mg qid, + H_2receptor antagonist†	Antibiotics for 2 weeks H_2 antagonist for 4 weeks
Lansoprazole (Prevacid), 30 mg, or omeprazole (Prilosec), 20 mg bid, + clarithromycin (Biaxin), 500 mg bid, + metronidazole (Flagyl), 500 mg bid	2 Weeks
Lansoprazole (Prevacid), 30 mg or omeprazole (Prilosec), 20 mg bid, + clarithromycin (Biaxin), 500 mg bid, + amoxicillin, 1 g bid	2 Weeks
Bismuth subsalicylate (Pepto-Bismol), 525 mg (2 tabs) qid, + metronidazole (Flagyl), 250 mg qid, + tetracyline, 500 mg qid + omeprazole (Prilosec), 20 mg, or lansoprazole (Prevacid), 30 mg q AM	2 Weeks

*Antibiotics are believed to work best when taken with food, and proton pump inhibitors work best when taken before breakfast.

†To be taken in the dosage and frequency indicated by manufacturer for the treatment of ulcers.

lence of *H. pylori* in patients with peptic ulcers is likely due to a decrease in the prevalence of *H. pylori* infection in this country, which is a consequence of both the aging of the population and the eradication of the infection in persons with ulcers. The reduction in *H. pylori*–associated ulcers with no change in idiopathic ulcers will cause a reduction in the percentage of ulcers overall that are associated with *H. pylori* infection. *H. pylori*–infected patients have higher meal-stimulated acid secretion and higher serum gastrin levels in response to a meal than do noninfected controls. Gastric acid secretion is increased sixfold in infected patients with duodenal ulcer compared with normal individuals. However, acid secretion in persons infected with *H. pylori,* but without ulcer disease, is frequently within the normal range. Although everyone infected has increased gastrin secretion, there is a wide variability in acid secretion, which may in part depend on a person's sensitivity to gastrin. In addition, infection with *H. pylori* has been shown to decrease duodenal mucosal bicarbonate secretion. The combination of increased acid secretion and reduced mucosal protection is believed to be responsible for the increased risk of ulcer disease in patients infected with this organism. Duodenal ulcer patients have been shown to develop gastric metaplasia in the duodenum. This metaplastic tissue can then be colonized by *H. pylori* and when directly present in the duodenum greatly increases one's risk of mucosal ulceration.

Treatment of peptic ulcers in persons infected with *H. pylori* can be best accomplished with antibiotic therapy. By treating *H. pylori,* one is able to heal ulcers, but more importantly, the natural history of peptic ulcer disease is changed by reducing ulcer recurrence from 75% in 1 year to less than 10% within a year. Several therapies have received U.S. Food and Drug Administration (FDA) approval. The best treatment regimens include two to three antibiotics plus a proton pump inhibitor or an H_2-receptor antagonist. The most frequently used regimen is omeprazole, 20 mg, or lansoprazole, 30 mg, plus clarithromycin (Biaxin), 500 mg, and amoxicillin, 1 g, all taken twice a day (see Table 3). Treatment should be prescribed for 10 or 14 days. Studies from Europe have shown excellent results with 7 days of therapy, but these same rates of eradication have not been achieved in the United States with only 7 days of therapy. Antibiotic therapies are fairly well tolerated; the main reasons for lack of response to therapy are antibiotic resistance, lack of compliance by the patient, and the physician incorrectly prescribing the medication and/or dosage. Antibiotic resistance with metronidazole (Flagyl) ranges between 30% and 48%, and resistance to clarithromycin has continued to increase and is now over 10% (Table 4). Antibiotic resistance to amoxicillin and tetracycline is uncommon. No resistance to bismuth (Pepto-Bismol) appears to develop. Because of the concern with resistance, persons who need to be treated a second time should be treated using different antibiotics. If a third treatment is needed, then endoscopy with biopsy would be justified to culture *H. pylori* and conduct antibiotic sensitivity testing to identify an appropriate antibiotic regimen.

TABLE 4. ***Helicobacter pylori* Resistance With Antibiotics***

Antibiotic	Primary Resistance
Clarithromycin (Biaxin)	8%
Metronidazole (Flagyl)	43%
Tetracycline	<1%
Amoxicillin	3%

*Sensitivity numbers from Centers for Disease Control and Prevention.

Now that the FDA has approved various treatment regimens for eradication of *H. pylori* infection, the question of whom to treat has come to the forefront. Widespread use of antibiotics to eradicate this bacterium is not without risk, including the possibility of accelerating the emergence of resistant strains of the organism. Studies demonstrating the association of *H. pylori* and duodenal ulcer have been generated observing patients with active (acute) duodenal ulcers. In these patients, the benefits of eradication therapy are clear. Patients with a documented history of duodenal ulcer who do not have an ulcer crater at the time of presentation have not been well studied in controlled trials. If they are at similar risk for recurrence and complications, it follows that they, too, should be candidates for *H. pylori* testing and treatment. However, if, as some believe, peptic ulcer disease becomes "inactive" or "burns out" with time, an argument could be made for not treating this subgroup of patients. However, analysis of the data shows little support for the phenomenon of peptic ulcer disease "burn out" and that, in fact, peptic ulcer disease resulting from *H. pylori* infection is a chronic, relapsing condition, lasting for decades, if not a lifetime. The literature is compatible with the view that, in the majority of patients, duodenal ulcers occur on a background of an "ulcer diathesis" that is fueled by *H. pylori* infection and "burn on, not out" until and unless the infection is eradicated.

NSAID-Induced Ulcers

NSAIDs are only second to *H. pylori* as the most common cause of gastric and duodenal ulcers. NSAIDs have been known to be a major factor in gastric ulcers, especially in elderly patients. Studies have shown that NSAIDs can also cause duodenal ulcers. Approximately 33 million Americans commonly use NSAIDs. Upper endoscopy in long-term NSAID users will find ulcers up to 10% of the time. The risk of developing serious gastrointestinal complications from ulcers (perforation, bleeding, obstruction) due to NSAIDs is 0.5% to 4.0% per year. Risk factors for serious gastrointestinal complications from NSAIDs include age older than 75, concurrent corticosteroid use, prior history of ulcer disease or upper gastrointestinal bleeding, and history of car-

TABLE 5. **Patients at Risk for Developing Ulcers From NSAIDs**

History of ulcer disease or upper gastrointestinal bleeding
Age>60 years
Concomitant use of corticosteroids
Concomitant use of anticoagulants
Chronic major organ impairment
High doses or use of multiple NSAIDs

diovascular disease (Table 5). The risk of gastrointestinal complications increases directly with increasing the NSAID dose. Approximately 10% of persons taking NSAIDs will develop abdominal discomfort. In the absence of risk factors, it is difficult to identify persons taking NSAIDs who may go on to develop gastrointestinal complications, because most people who develop serious gastrointestinal complications have no abdominal discomfort.

NSAIDs are particularly harmful to the gastric and duodenal mucosa because they can cause acute mucosal injury (submucosal hemorrhages and erosions with gross bleeding); chronic administration leads to ulcerations from a systemic effect of the NSAIDs, which are frequently complicated by bleeding. NSAIDs, however, do not cause a diffuse gastritis as is seen with *H. pylori.* The use of enteric-coated aspirin does not cause acute mucosal injury (topically induced) but may still cause ulcers and gastrointestinal bleeding with chronic use (due to the systemic effects). Other NSAIDs have been shown to cause both gastric and duodenal ulcers, which are due to the systemic effects of the NSAID. Prostaglandins are fatty acids produced by almost all cells in the body, and they protect against injury in the gastrointestinal tract. NSAIDs inhibit cyclooxygenase (COX), the rate-limiting enzyme in prostaglandin synthesis. Therefore, suppression of prostaglandins is a major factor involved in the development of ulcers from NSAIDs because prostaglandins protect the gastric mucosa through stimulation of mucus and bicarbonate secretion and by increasing mucosal blood flow. NSAID-induced ulcers are prevented just as well by administering prostaglandins as by inhibiting acid secretion.

NSAID-induced ulcers are directly due to toxicity from the medication; therefore, eliminating or reducing the dosage is the first step in treatment. Misoprostol (Cytotec) is approved for the prevention of NSAID-induced ulcers in persons at high risk of developing ulcers. Ulcer healing can be accomplished by using full-dose H_2-receptor antagonists or proton pump inhibitors. If the NSAID cannot be stopped, then a proton pump inhibitor is preferred to heal the ulcer; however, the lowest dose possible of the NSAID should be used. In a large randomized, double-blind treatment study on subjects taking NSAIDs with ulcers, omeprazole was found to heal and prevent ulcers more effectively than ranitidine. Misoprostol and omeprazole are both good in preventing NSAID-associated ulcers in subjects who have had a prior ulcer from an NSAID. Omeprazole should be administered at a dose of 20 mg/d. Misoprostol (Cytotec) is most effective when administered at 200 μg three times a day, but this dose frequently causes side effects; a dose of 200 μg twice daily can also be used (Table 6). Because *H. pylori* also causes ulcers, one should check and treat for *H. pylori* infection in persons who develop ulcers while taking NSAIDs. It is not recommended, however, that a person be checked for *H. pylori* before starting NSAIDs if he or she has no history of peptic ulcer disease.

Patients who are at high risk for developing NSAID-induced ulcers (see Table 5), because of previous history of ulcers (either on or off of NSAIDs), on anticoagulants or corticosteroids, or older age, should be considered for treatment with one of the new cyclooxygenase-2 (COX-2) inhibitors: celecoxib (Celebrex) or rofecoxib (Vioxx). COX-2 inhibitors have a reduced risk of ulcers and gastrointestinal bleeding than the conventional NSAIDs. If patients get better relief with a conventional NSAID, then co-treatment with misoprostol or a proton pump inhibitor can be used to reduce the risk of ulcers. Proton pump inhibitors are better at preventing duodenal ulcers and are similar to misoprostol in preventing gastric ulcers.

ACID-INDUCED ULCERS

Idiopathic

Studies have shown that as we treat *H. pylori*-associated ulcers the percentage of idiopathic ulcers is increasing. Currently, it appears that 30% to 40% of peptic ulcers have no obvious cause and fall into the idiopathic category. Analysis of gastric acid secretion in ulcer patients who are not taking NSAIDs and are negative for *H. pylori* with apparent idiopathic ulcers shows the same abnormalities that have historically been associated with peptic ulcer disease. People infected with *H. pylori* who develop ulcers also have these same abnormalities in acid secretion. Because the acid secretion abnormalities are the same regardless of *H. pylori* infection, it is impossible to tell if the abnormalities in acid secretion are due to *H. pylori* infection before treatment with antibiotics. People who continue to have ulcers after successful treatment of their *H. pylori* infection show no change in acid secretion, whereas the acid secretion returns to normal in people who have no further ulcers after eradication of *H. pylori* infection.

Idiopathic ulcers should be treated in the same way that ulcers had been treated before the discovery

TABLE 6. **Treatment Options for Persons at Increased Risk of Gastrointestinal Complications From NSAIDs**

Ulcer prophylaxis
A proton pump inhibitor (standard dose)
Misoprostol (Cytotec), 200 μg PO bid or tid
Use a COX-2 Selective NSAID
Celecoxib (Celebrex) or rofecoxib (Vioxx)

of *H. pylori.* Either proton pump inhibitors or H_2-receptor antagonists may be used. As in the past, there is a high risk of ulcer recurrence after discontinuing antisecretory therapy. Whereas only acute therapy is indicated for 6 to 8 weeks, these persons should be followed closely and with recurrent symptoms be restarted on antisecretory therapy and considered for maintenance therapy. Proton pump inhibitors are preferred for maintenance therapy, because they have been shown to be superior to H_2-receptor antagonists in preventing the development of recurrent ulcers. For maintenance therapy lansoprazole can be given at 15 mg/d and omeprazole at 10 or 20 mg/d; rabeprazole (Aciphex) and pantoprazole (Protonix) are only available at 20 mg and 40 mg, respectively, and would be administered once daily.

CONCLUSIONS

Overall, peptic ulcer disease is declining in the United States. However, the incidence of peptic ulcers will vary throughout the country. Immigrants and low-income populations continue to have a relatively high prevalence of peptic ulcers, mostly due to infection with *H. pylori.* Physicians will continue to find that a higher proportion of ulcers are either due to NSAIDs or have no clear etiology (idiopathic); these ulcers are likely related to increased acid secretion, and these subjects will need to be treated with acid suppressive medications, as was done before the discovery of *H. pylori.* With continued widespread use of NSAIDs, primary care physicians will continue to be confronted with gastrointestinal bleeding and gastric/duodenal ulcers, which occur in up to 10% of patients taking these medications on a daily basis. The use of proton pump inhibitors or the new COX-2–specific NSAIDs will help to reduce serious gastrointestinal side effects from conventional NSAIDs.

ACUTE AND CHRONIC VIRAL HEPATITIS

method of
ADRIAN REUBEN, MBBS
Medical University of South Carolina
Charleston, South Carolina

Viral hepatitis is the most common cause of liver disease in the United States and worldwide. Whereas many severe systemic viral infections can affect the liver, viral hepatitis is usually caused by one of five human hepatotropic viruses that are labeled A through E and named *hepatitis A virus (HAV), hepatitis B virus (HBV),* and so on (Table 1). These viruses were discovered 11 to 30 years ago. Before adoption of the current alphabetic nomenclature, the illnesses caused by these hepatitis viruses were known as *infectious hepatitis (HAV); serum hepatitis (HBV); non-A, non-B hepatitis (HCV);* and *epidemic or enterically transmitted non-A, non-B hepatitis (HEV),* respectively. HDV was originally called the *delta agent.* As yet, there is no hepatitis F because a putative virus originally given this name proved to be an artifact.

Recently, additional hepatotropic viruses have been discovered, namely, hepatitis G virus (HGV) and a transfusion-associated agent called *TT virus (TTV)* and its many variants. HGV is identical to one of the so-called GB viral agents, GBV-C. The initials GB and TT were derived from the names of patients in whom these viruses were identified. HGV and TTV are prevalent in the general population (2%–4% for HGV and 10%–12% for TTV), but because the association of these newer viruses with liver disease is still unclear, HGV and TTV will not be discussed further in any detail.

After the specific hepatotropic viruses, viral hepatitis is caused next most commonly by members of the herpesvirus family. When Epstein-Barr virus causes acute hepatitis, it is usually one of the manifestations of infectious mononucleosis that commonly occurs in children and young adults. Herpes simplex virus has occasionally caused devastating acute hepatitis in pregnancy. For the most part, acute hepatitis caused by Epstein-Barr virus, herpes simplex virus, or other herpes family viruses (cytomegalovirus, varicella-zoster, and human herpesviruses) is a serious opportunistic infection in immunosuppressed individuals, such as transplant recipients and HIV-infected patients.

The hepatitis viruses HAV through HEV have been well characterized physically and biologically (see Table 1), and reliable laboratory methods are readily available for their diagnosis (Table 2). HBV is a double-stranded DNA virus that replicates in a manner similar to retroviruses, through an RNA intermediate using a viral-encoded reverse transcriptase. TTV is a DNA virus too. HAV, HCV, HDV, HEV, and HGV are all single-stranded RNA viruses. HAV and HEV are nonenveloped viruses that are transmitted by the fecal-oral route and cause acute self-limited but not chronic infection; HAV has occasionally been transmitted parenterally. HBV, HCV, and HDV are enveloped viruses that are spread parenterally (including sexually and perinatally, especially HBV) and can cause acute self-limited as well as chronic infection with chronicity rates of 3% to 5% for HBV, 85% for HCV, and greater than 50% for HDV in non-immunosuppressed adults.

Liver disease is a significant cause of morbidity, mortality, and economic loss in the United States and elsewhere. In the United States, liver disease ranks as the 10th most frequent cause of death overall and seventh in the 25- to 64-year-old age group. Fifty-four percent of liver deaths are due to viral hepatitis, of which three quarters are hepatitis C and one quarter hepatitis B. In comparison, alcohol alone accounts for one quarter of liver disease deaths. The Centers for Disease Control and Prevention (CDC) has estimated that HAV, HBV, and HCV combined cost the United States a total of $1.5 billion annually (in 1991 dollars) in medical expenses and work loss, excluding transplantation.

Current information about viral hepatitis including recommendations for treatment and vaccination can be found on the CDC hepatitis website and related links on the Internet, such as *www.cdc.gov/ncidod/diseases/hepatitis/index.htm.*

ACUTE VIRAL HEPATITIS

The term *acute hepatitis* refers to an illness caused by liver injury of recent onset, whose duration is limited to 6 months from the beginning of symptoms and/or liver test abnormalities to resolution. Although acute viral hepatitis is usually caused by one of the five specific hepatotropic

TABLE 1. **The Common Hepatitis Viruses***

Features	HAV	HBV	HCV	HDV	HEV
Nucleic acid	ss RNA	ds DNA	ss RNA	ss RNA	ss RNA
Virus family	Picornaviridae	Hepadnaviridae	Flaviviridae	Deltaviridae	Unclassified†
Discovery	1973	1970	1989	1977	1980
Transmission	fecal-oral‡	parenteral, sexual, perinatal	parenteral, sexual, perinatal	parenteral, sexual, perinatal (rare)	fecal-oral
Incubation period (d)	15–50	45–180	14–180	21–140	15–60
Incidence§					
Acute infections	179,000	185,000	38,000	5000	unknown
Acute cases	90,000	39,000	6000	1000	very rare
Deaths (%)	300 (0.3)	400 (1)	rare	80 (8)	0‖
Chronic disease#					
Prevalence	n/a	1.25 million	2.7 million	70,000	n/a
Annual mortality	n/a	5000	8000–10,000	1000	n/a

*Severe systemic viral infections can also cause viral hepatitis, especially herpes family viruses in immunosuppressed patients. HGV and TTV are human hepatotropic viruses of doubtful clinical importance.
†Formerly classified in Calciviridae family.
‡Occasional parenteral spread.
§United States, CDC 1997 data.
‖10%–25% case-fatality rate in pregnancy in the Third World.
#CDC and NHANES III estimates, 2000.
Abbreviations: CDC = Centers for Disease Control and Prevention; ds = double stranded; HAV = hepatitis A virus; HBV = hepatitis B virus; HCV = hepatitis C virus; HDV = hepatitis D virus; HEV = hepatitis E virus; HGV = hepatitis G virus; n/a = not applicable; NHANES III = Third National Health and Nutrition Examination Survey; ss = single stranded; TTV = TT virus.

TABLE 2. **Guide to the Laboratory Diagnosis of Viral Hepatitis**

Hepatitis A	
IgM anti-HAV	New and recent (<6 mo) exposure to HAV, i.e., acute HAV infection
Total anti-HAV	Prior (distant) exposure to HAV; "total" includes IgG and IgM • Use IgM anti-HAV *positivity* to distinguish acute exposure from immunity
Hepatitis B	
HBsAg	Indicates infection with HBV *but not its duration*, i.e., HBsAg is positive in *both* acute and chronic infection • May be negative in acute infection *when viral clearance is rapid* (often preceded by rapid HBeAg loss too)
IgM anti-HBc	Best indicator of acute HBV infection (*occasionally* positive in chronic infection exacerbations)
Total anti-HBc	Indicates exposure to HBV, recent or distant, acute or chronic; total includes IgG and IgM • Use IgM anti-HBc *positivity* to distinguish recent acute from distant exposure
Anti-HBs	Usually indicates immunity after resolved infection or vaccination • May be artifactually positive in 30% of chronically infected patients in whom it *does not* indicate immunity
HBeAg	Indicates high viral replication • Early disappearance of HBeAg heralds recovery from acute HBV infection • Negative in active infection with so-called "pre-core mutant" *that cannot make* the *e* antigen
Anti-HBe	Indicates transition from high to low viral replication state • May be positive in active infection with so-called "pre-core mutant" that cannot make the *e* antigen
HBV DNA	Used occasionally to confirm HBV infection but mostly *to assess viral load* and response to antiviral treatment • Several assays with different sensitivities are commercially available (see text)
Hepatitis C	
Anti-HCV	Indicates exposure to HCV and usually ongoing infection too • *False-positive* results occur, especially in low-prevalence populations and patients with high globulins • *False-negative* results occur in hemodialysis patients
RIBA	*Supplementary test* for HCV exposure that usually "confirms" positivity of anti-HCV • Uses same reagents as in anti-HCV EIA but *visualizes* antibodies in serum against individual recombinant viral proteins (see text)
HCV RNA	Used to confirm HCV infection, quantify viral load, and monitor response to treatment; can determine genotype too • Several assays are commercially available (see text)
Hepatitis D	
HDV antigen	Indicates infection with HDV, *but not its duration,* i.e., HDV antigen is positive in 25% of acute and all chronic infections
IgM anti-HDV	Positive in acute co-infection, acute superinfection, and chronic infection
IgG anti-HDV	Positive in acute co-infection, acute superinfection, and chronic infection
Hepatitis E	
IgM anti-HEV	Indicates *recent* acute exposure to HEV and likely current infection
IgG anti-HEV	Indicates *distant* exposure to HEV, i.e., resolved infection

viruses or herpes family viruses, on rare occasions it may be caused by one of many other viruses.* Other organisms can also cause acute hepatitis, such as Q fever, Rocky Mountain spotted fever, mycobacteria, spirochetes, and protozoa.

Although the majority of cases of acute viral hepatitis conform to the time course definition previously given, occasionally a seemingly acute presentation of hepatitis may actually be a flare-up of unrecognized chronic liver disease. Acute-on-chronic hepatitis is well recognized with HBV infection (and with the nonviral liver disease, autoimmune hepatitis). Patients with chronic liver disease are also susceptible to intercurrent acute hepatitis due to a new viral infection or an adverse reaction to a drug, alcohol, environmental toxin, and so on. Thus, any patient with acute viral hepatitis, especially that due to HBV (± HDV) or HCV, should be observed for complete resolution of infection and to detect underlying or evolving chronic liver disease. Furthermore, vaccination against HAV and/or HBV is advocated for patients with chronic liver disease who are not immune to both of these viruses.

The diagnosis of acute viral hepatitis and an indication of its cause are based on the history, physical examination, and standard and specific laboratory testing (see Table 2). Liver biopsy is rarely necessary, except to differentiate viral hepatitis from other causes of liver injury and to seek co-existing or chronic disease. Acute viral hepatitis must be distinguished from other causes of acute hepatic injury such as ischemia, biliary obstruction, rejection in liver transplant recipients, and toxic damage.

The spectrum of clinical presentations of acute viral hepatitis ranges from asymptomatic elevations of liver enzyme levels in the serum (notably aminotransferases) to fulminant hepatic failure and death. Following an asymptomatic incubation period, patients may have a viral prodrome of flulike symptoms, malaise, anorexia, low-grade fever, nausea, and loose stools. A relatively small proportion of patients with acute viral hepatitis become jaundiced (icteric), which varies with the viral agent and the age of the patient. Jaundice is more common in adults than in children, and is more likely with HAV, HBV, and HEV than with HCV. Elevations of aminotransferase levels, namely, aspartate aminotransferase (AST, formerly called *SGOT*) and alanine aminotransferase (ALT, formerly called *SGPT*), are variable but are usually in the 10- to 200-fold range, with less than 3-fold elevations of alkaline phosphatase. Bilirubin level may rise 2- to 30-fold. Coagulopathy and a decrease in serum albumin level occur in patients with the most severe liver injury. Patients may remain jaundiced for 1 to 4 weeks, during which time symptoms usually resolve and laboratory abnormalities begin to return to normal. In a minority of patients with acute viral hepatitis, especially that due to HAV, recovery may be temporarily delayed by minor relapses or late cholestasis that eventually resolves spontaneously.

Although viral hepatitis infrequently progresses to fulminant hepatic failure and death (see Table 1), it accounts for up to 10% of all reported cases of fulminant hepatic failure in the United States and the United Kingdom. In other countries from which series of fulminant hepatic failure have been collected, such as France, India, and Denmark, approximately 30% of cases were due to HBV. In the Third World, HEV infection has a case-fatality rate of up to 25% among pregnant women.

Contrary to earlier belief, no special diet is necessary in patients with acute viral hepatitis. Rather, patients should avoid foods that they cannot tolerate, which often means adhering to a carbohydrate-rich, low-fat diet. Nausea and vomiting should be treated with antiemetics such as promethazine (Phenergan), prochlorperazine (Compazine), or metoclopramide (Reglan). An adequate fluid intake must be assured, using intravenous infusion where necessary in patients with protracted vomiting. Because hepatic metabolism may be impaired at the height of the illness, alcohol should be avoided and drug use kept to a minimum. Except with recent or continuing heavy alcohol use, acetaminophen (Tylenol) may be prescribed and is preferable to nonsteroidal anti-inflammatory drugs for analgesia. Once recovery is in progress, there is no prohibition of alcohol in moderation, and patients can exercise as tolerated.

No specific antiviral therapy is recommended for acute viral hepatitis except perhaps for acute HCV hepatitis because preliminary studies in this illness suggest that interferon in combination with ribavirin may reduce the likelihood of HCV chronicity. However, the true benefit of interferon/ribavirin therapy for acute HCV hepatitis is yet to be proven by extensive prospective randomized controlled clinical trials and should not yet be considered the standard of practice.

CHRONIC HEPATITIS

Of the viral hepatitis agents known, only HBV (±HDV) and HCV cause chronic hepatitis. It follows from the definition of acute hepatitis that chronic hepatitis is present when liver injury and inflammation continue for more than 6 months. Chronic hepatitis can be recognized histologically if significant fibrosis is seen, even if the duration of illness is unknown. However, without knowing the duration of illness and without finding fibrosis or cirrhosis, it may be premature or erroneous to diagnose chronic hepatitis histologically. The inflammatory histologic features of chronic hepatitis may also be seen in resolving acute viral hepatitis, when a biopsy specimen is obtained early in recovery.

Patients with chronic viral hepatitis are often asymptomatic in the early years of infection, before cirrhosis and its complications supervene. When symptoms occur, they are generally nonspecific, such as fatigue, malaise, anorexia, right upper quadrant ache or discomfort, pruritus, and arthralgias. The physical examination may be normal or simply show right upper quadrant tenderness and/or mild hepatomegaly. Extrahepatic manifestations of chronic viral hepatitis are more common with HCV than HBV and are often immune-mediated. Obviously, the finding of jaundice, palmar erythema, spider nevi, palpable splenomegaly, ascites, or encephalopathy will indicate the presence of advanced liver disease, namely, cirrhosis, and possibly hepatic decompensation.

Laboratory abnormalities in chronic hepatitis vary with the cause and state of liver injury. Aminotransferase levels may be normal repeatedly, especially in asymptomatic HBV carriers and about a quarter of chronic HCV cases. Otherwise, AST and ALT elevations are common but are usually far lower than those in acute viral hepatitis; there is a poor correlation with necroinflammatory change histologically and none with fibrosis. Elevations of bilirubin level, depression of albumin level, and prolongation of prothrombin time usually indicate progression to cirrhosis with decompensation, or exuberant necroinflammatory change at least. The viral etiology of chronic hepatitis is

*For example, reovirus, mumps, yellow fever, Coxsackie B, syncytial giant-cell virus, echovirus, Marburg virus, Rift Valley fever virus, adenovirus, rubella, and Lassa fever virus.

easily diagnosed by specific serologic and/or nucleic acid testing (see Table 2).

The natural history of chronic viral hepatitis is variable and is governed by both host and viral factors, and will be influenced adversely by co-infection with another hepatitis virus or HIV. Disease progression in chronic hepatitis C is accelerated by heavy alcohol ingestion. In addition to the risk of decompensation, patients with cirrhosis are also at risk for the development of hepatocellular carcinoma, as are long-term HBV carriers even in the absence of cirrhosis.

HEPATITIS A

HAV is a picornavirus that is distantly related to both polio and the common cold. The 7.5-kb RNA genome codes for viral capsid proteins and nonstructural proteins that are involved in viral replication. Unlike other hepatitis viruses, HAV can be grown in cell culture giving a source of viral antigen for use in inactivated vaccines. The viral capsid proteins together form a single serotype so that immunity induced by natural infection or vaccination is universal.

HAV appears to infect intestinal cells during the early stages of viral infection. However, most of the virus shed in the stools is replicated in the liver and reaches the small intestine via the bile. This is the major source of virus for the transmission of infection that occurs via contaminated food, water, or seafood such as oysters. It is often unappreciated that there is significant viremia in infected persons that persists during the prodromal and early clinical phases of the disease. This viremia is the likely source of transmission among injection drug users and rare contamination in certain lots of blood products. Although viral antigens and viral RNA can be detected in feces after the onset of symptoms, the infectivity of feces falls precipitously following resolution of acute liver injury; chronic fecal shedding does not occur.

HAV prevalence varies geographically, being highest in North Africa and the Middle East and moderately prevalent in Central and South America, southern Africa, and the Indian subcontinent. In the United States, HAV disease rates are highest in the western and southwestern regions. Low standards of sanitation favor viral spread. Among racial and ethnic groups, rates of infection are highest among Native Americans and Alaskan natives and less so among Hispanics. Almost 30% of cases are in children younger than 15 years of age, with the highest rates in the 5- to 15-year-old age group. The common sources for infection are household or sexual contact with an infected individual, children and adults connected with daycare centers, international travel, and food or waterborne outbreaks. Almost half of patients with HAV have no recognized source of infection. Overall approximately 33% of Americans have evidence of prior infection with HAV.

The incubation period for HAV is usually about 4 weeks (15–45 days). The frequency of icteric hepatitis rises with age from less than 10% in children younger than 6, to 40% to 50% in older children, and 70% to 80% in adults. Asymptomatic infected children probably represent the major reservoir for HAV transmission. The incidence of infection in the United States is 125,000 to 200,000 (most recently 179,000 [1977]) annually, of which approximately half are symptomatic. The severity of disease varies with age, being greatest in persons above the age of 40. Mortality is low, 0.3% recently, with the highest case-fatality rates in adults over the age of 50 (7 in 1000) and in children younger than 5 years old (1.5 in 1000). Acute hepatitis may be more severe in patients with underlying chronic hepatitis B and C, underscoring the need for vaccination in persons with chronic liver disease. Aside from acute hepatitis that may occasionally relapse or have a prolonged cholestatic phase, there are other unusual manifestations of hepatitis A. Skin rashes, acute neurologic disease, renal failure, and red cell aplasia have been described. Recently cases of acute pancreatitis have been reported with HAV. The diagnosis of acute hepatitis A is readily made by finding serum IgM anti-HAV positivity [+]. Total anti-HAV[+] does not distinguish between recent acute and distant exposure, the latter being diagnosed by finding total anti-HAV[+] and IgM anti-HAV[−]. The treatment of hepatitis A is supportive. Late cholestasis usually resolves spontaneously but may be treated with a short course of corticosteroids. Fulminant hepatic failure may require liver transplantation.

HAV vaccination is safe and effective. The Advisory Committee on Immunization Practice (ACIP) recommends pre-exposure hepatitis A vaccination for people at increased risk. Two inactivated vaccines are licensed in the United States, namely, Havrix and Vaqta. The recommended intramuscular doses are 720 ELU or 25 U, respectively, for children 2 to 18 years, and 1440 ELU or 50 U, respectively, for adults, followed by a second injection 6 to 12 months later. Individuals for whom pre-exposure vaccination is recommended include travelers to countries with moderate or high HAV endemic rates, men who have sex with men, illegal drug users (injection and noninjection), recipients of clotting factor concentrates, patients with chronic liver disease, children age 2 and older living in communities with elevated rates of hepatitis A, and persons with an occupational risk of infection. For prophylaxis following exposure, immunoglobulin 0.02 mL/kg body weight should be given intramuscularly within 2 weeks of exposure. Immunoglobulin should also be given to travelers in addition to hepatitis A vaccine, if the latter cannot be given earlier then 4 weeks before travel. Travelers whose travel period exceeds 2 months should be administered immunoglobulin at 0.06 mL/kg, which must be repeated if the travel period exceeds 5 months.

HEPATITIS B

HBV is a small doubled-shelled virus of the Hepadnaviridae family that includes morphologically similar DNA viruses of mammalian and avian species such as woodchucks and squirrels, and ducks, respectively. Three particulate forms are associated with HBV, namely, 42-nm complete virions (Dane particles) and DNA-free 22-nm diameter spheres and tubules. The 3.2-kb HBV DNA genome encodes four genes: hepatitis B surface antigen (HBsAg), hepatitis B core antigen (HBcAg), DNA polymerase (pol, which is also a reverse transcriptase) and the so-called X protein (HBX). HBsAg, the protein of the virion lipoprotein envelope, also forms the 22-nm spheres and tubules that result from vastly excessive synthesis and secretion of free HBsAg by infected hepatocytes.

Multiple HBsAg antigenic subdeterminants have been defined, but induction of neutralizing antibody directed against a common group determinant ensures universal immunity (except against certain HBsAg-mutant strains). HBcAg, the nucleocapsid protein of the virion nucleic acid core, is derived from a precursor protein by cleaving off a small soluble fragment termed the "e" antigen (HBeAg) that is then released from the liver into the circulation. HBeAg gives a clinical index of viral replication, infectivity, severity of disease, and response to therapy, except during infection with a so-called pre-core mutant (which is a variant HBV mutant that cannot cleave and secrete HBeAg). HBV pol, synthesized intracellularly during infection, is packed in the virion core filling in the gap formed by the incomplete strand of the DNA pair. The biological function of HBX protein is poorly understood but it appears to have an accessory role in the cellular replication of HBV DNA.

HBV is distributed worldwide, with highest prevalence in southeastern Asia and some countries of southern Africa. Prevalence is moderate in the South Pacific, the Mediterranean littoral, and sub-Saharan Africa. In the United States and other developed nations, carriers comprise 0.1% to 0.9% of the population. Carrier rates up to 10 times greater occur in African Americans, Asian Americans, injection drug users, men who have sex with men, and certain institutionalized and immunosuppressed individuals. Other risk factors for HBV acquisition include hemodialysis, sexual contact with an infected person, extensive heterosexual practice, prior treatment of a sexually transmitted disease, blood transfusion before 1992, receipt of a clotting factor concentrate before 1987, health care work, and birth by an HBV-infected mother. Among adults, sexual exposure and injection drug use account for most cases of acute HBV infection.

The incubation period for HBV is usually about 12 weeks (45–180 days). Acute HBV infection is icteric in 10% of children and 30% to 50% of adults. HBV infection becomes chronic in 90% of those infected at birth, 25% to 50% of children infected at 1 to 5 years of age, and about 2% to 6% of persons infected as older children or adults. Annually there are about 140,000 to 320,000 acute HBV infections in the United States, of which approximately half are symptomatic, resulting in 8400 to 19,000 hospitalizations and 0.2% deaths annually (1% in 1997). There are 5000 to 6000 deaths annually from chronic HBV liver disease, including primary liver cancer.

Icteric HBV cases present clinically with typical acute hepatitis. Extrahepatic manifestations of HBV may present in the prodrome and during the acute illness, as polyarthritis, rashes, angioneurotic edema, and transient glomerulonephritis. Polyarteritis nodosa and chronic glomerulonephritis are rare complications of HBV infection, although HBV is a cause of up to 50% of cases of polyarteritis nodosa.

In the interpretation of HBV serologic test results, certain principles apply (see Table 2). HBsAg[+] denotes HBV infection that can be diagnosed as acute with IgM anti-HBc[+] or chronic with total anti-HBc[+] and IgM anti-HBc[−] (because total anti-HBc includes both IgG and IgM antibodies). In HBV infection, HBeAg[+] indicates high replication rates and infectivity, whereas HBeAg[−] and anti-HBe[+] denote reduction in viral replication and often herald clearance of viremia. An exception occurs in patients with the HBV pre-core mutant that cannot make and secrete HBeAg; infected patients will be HBeAg[−] and anti-HBe[+]. When patients are HBsAg[−], in the presence of anti-HBs[+] and/or anti-HBc[+], this usually indicates clearance of HBV infection and likely immunity. An isolated anti-HBs[+] is also the immune response of successful vaccination. However, up to 30% of patients with chronic HBV infection are also anti-HBs[+], but this does not indicate immunity. Isolated anti-HBc[+] may indicate prior exposure to HBV and latent immunity that may be confirmed by eliciting an exuberant anti-HBs response with vaccination. Isolated anti-HBc[+] may also be a false-positive artifact in an HBV-naive individual. Some anti-HBc[+] individuals do harbor latent HBV (with HBsAg below the limit of detection) because use of an isolated anti-HBc[+] liver for transplantation can cause *de novo* HBV infection in the recipient.

DNA testing is rarely necessary to diagnose HBV infection but it is useful in accessing viral load before antiviral therapy and for gauging the therapeutic response. HBV DNA assays vary in sensitivity and accuracy and, to date, none are FDA-approved. Polymerase chain reaction (PCR)-based methods are extremely sensitive. Quantitative PCR assays can give reliable titers where the viral load is modest but can be too sensitive and detect HBV nucleic acid in patients otherwise considered to have resolved infection. Assays based on hybridization, such as the branched DNA (bDNA) assay are accurate and reliable for high viral loads, but may be too insensitive to confirm HBV infection in all cases. Thus the choice of an HBV DNA assay depends on the clinical setting and need.

Prevention of HBV infection is now achievable with safe and effective vaccination. In the United States there are three FDA-approved HBV vaccines, produced by recombinant DNA technology, namely, Recombivax HB, Engerix B, and Comvax (hepatitis B vaccine combined with an Haemophilus influenza B vaccine). A combined hepatitis A/hepatitis B vaccine, Twinrix, is likely to be licensed soon. Currently ACIP recommends HBsAg testing of all pregnant women and, regardless of the result, HBV vaccination is recommended for all newborn infants. Infants born to HBsAg[+] mothers should also be given 0.5 mL HBIG within 12 hours of birth. ACIP has recommended that hepatitis B vaccination be done as part of a routine adolescent vaccination visit at age 11 to 12 years. Vaccination should also be given to persons at high risk of HBV infection, namely, adolescents who inject drugs or have multiple sexual partners, persons with occupational hazards, clients and clinic staff of institutions for the mentally disabled, hemodialysis patients, recipients of clotting factor concentrates, household and sexual partners of HBV carriers, adoptees from countries in which HBV is endemic, international travelers to endemic areas, inmates of long-term correctional facilities, injection drug users, sexually active homosexual and bisexual men, and heterosexual men and women with multiple partners or a recently diagnosed sexually transmitted disease.

In a three-dose regimen for adults, Recombivax HB 10 μg or Engerix-B 20 μg is given intramuscularly followed by a second dose after 4 weeks and the third at 6 months. Reduced doses (one quarter to one half) are recommended for infants and increased doses for dialysis patients and other immunocompromised persons. A series of three injections of vaccine induces protective levels of anti-HBs (>10 mIU/mL) in more than 95% of infants and children and 90% of healthy adults. Smoking, obesity, immunodeficiency, and advancing age are associated with lower rates of response. A repeat series of three injections is recommended for nonresponders. Two-dose and four-dose regimens are also described.

Postvaccination testing for anti-HBs is not necessary except for high-risk groups, such as health care workers and immunosuppressed persons. Routine booster vaccination is not recommended except for hemodialysis patients. When exposure to HBV occurs in nonimmune individuals, HBIG should be given (0.06 mL/kg intramuscularly) within 48 hours of exposure, followed by active vaccination.

Two medications have been improved in the United States for treatment of chronic hepatitis B, namely, the immunostimulatory antiviral protein interferon alpha-2b (IFNα-2b [Intron A]) and the antiviral nucleoside lamivudine (Epivir). Antiviral treatment for acute hepatitis B is not recommended. IFNα-2b therapy should be considered in patients with chronic hepatitis B who have replicative infection (HBeAg[+], HBV DNA [+]) and active liver disease (elevated ALT and chronic hepatitis on biopsy). It can also be used in patients with well-compensated cirrhosis. IFNα-2b is far less effective in patients with very high viral loads and those without liver inflammation, as is usually the case in Asians many of whom were infected perinatally. In patients with clinically apparent cirrhosis, there is a risk of serious infection or provocation of hepatic failure with IFNα-2b therapy. Children with replicative infection and elevated ALT levels tolerate IFNα-2b well and do respond to therapy. IFNα is usually given as subcutaneous injections of 5 million U daily or 10 million U three times a week for 16 weeks. IFNα causes many side effects such as flulike symptoms, fatigue, anorexia, weight loss, and mild-to-severe emotional disturbance. IFNα-2b can also cause neutropenia and thrombocytopenia. IFNα-2b suppresses HBV replication and stimulates a flare of hepatitis due to an immune response against infected hepatocytes. Clearance of HBeAg occurs in only 20% to 30% of treated patients. Most responders (80%–90%) maintain their response long term but complete eradication of HBV is rare. Delayed clearance of HBsAg occurs in 25% to 65% of responders in North America and Europe but not in Asia. Lamivudine (Epivir), a cytodine analogue reverse transcriptase inhibitor, is as effective as IFNα-2b in the treatment of chronic hepatitis B. Lamivudine is also effective in some patients who do not respond to IFNα-2b. Lamivudine 100 mg orally daily for 12 months almost universally suppresses viremia. Lamivudine leads to HBeAg loss in approximately 30% of treated patients, anti-HBe[+] seroconversion in 16% to 18%, and sustained ALT normalization and improvement in liver histologic findings in approximately 50% of treated patients. HBeAg loss is durable in 70% to 80% of responders. Lamivudine has few side effects, and although minor flareups of ALT can occur during therapy, they are clinically insignificant. In patients who lose HBeAg, lamuvidine can be discontinued after 12 months of therapy, as long as they are monitored for reactivation that would necessitate resumption of therapy. Patients who have not achieved HBeAg[−] are recommended to continue treatment. Unfortunately, resistance to lamivudine may occur within 6 months of starting therapy, affecting up to 30% of patients treated for 1 year and up to 50% after 3 years of treatment, rendering the therapy ineffective. Nonetheless, lamivudine treatment should be continued because the lamivudine-resistant mutant is not particularly virulent, whereas return of the original HBV can cause a severe flareup of hepatitis. As yet there is no clear consensus whether IFNα-2b or lamivudine should be considered first-line therapy because of differences in convenience, duration of treatment, side effects, and potential long-term risks and benefits. Many other antiviral agents are being evaluated. It is likely that eventually combination antiviral therapy will be devised for HBV similar to current treatment of HIV.

HEPATITIS C

HCV is accorded its own genus in the flavivirus family, which it shares with the flavivirus genus that includes dengue and yellow fever, and with pestiviruses that infect cattle and pigs. The HCV RNA genome is distinguished by marked genetic heterogeneity, yielding six major genotypes and over 100 subtypes. All genotypes are represented worldwide but there are marked regional differences. Genotypes 1a, 1b, 2a, 2b, 2c, and 3a account for about 90% of HCV infections in the Americas, Europe, Russia, China, Japan, and Australasia. In all of these regions genotype 1 dominates, accounting for 70% or more of infections in North and South America, Europe, Russia, Australia, and New Zealand. Within infected individuals, HCV circulates as *quasispecies,* which are mixtures of closely related but distinct genomes that differ from each other by 1% to 2% and result from viral mutation. The 9.6-kb HCV RNA genome codes for a large polyprotein precursor that is cleaved to yield proteins of the viral envelope and non-structural proteins that participate in viral processing, RNA replication, and viral assembly. Viral-encoded enzymes, such as protease and helicase, are obvious targets for antiviral drug development. The marked heterogeneity of the viral envelope proteins means that it will be very difficult to develop a universal vaccine.

Approximately 170 million people worldwide are chronically infected with HCV. HCV prevalence varies widely geographically, from as low as 0.5% in the Scandinavian countries to greater than 20% in Egypt. Three to 4 million people have been infected with HCV in the United States but in recent years there have been marked changes in incidence and routes of transmission. The incidence of HCV rose from 18 per 100,000 before 1965 to peak at 130 per 100,000 in the 1980s. Since 1989, the incidence of new HCV infections has fallen more than 80%. Blood transfusion, which previously accounted for 20% to 40% of acute infections, now is virtually unknown as a cause of HCV acquisition (current risk is 0.001% per unit transfused). Injection drug use currently accounts for 60% of HCV transmission in the United States. Approximately 20% of persons with HCV infection report sexual exposure in the absence of a percutaneous risk factor, even though sexual transmission is inefficient. Other risk factors include health care work, hemodialysis, household exposure, and perinatal transmission (especially in HIV infected mother-infant pairs). None of these routes of transmission are efficient and it should be noted that HCV prevalence among health care workers is no higher then in the general population. All told, a risk factor can usually be accounted for in all but 10% of HCV infections. Contrary to expectation, case-controlled and population-based studies do not implicate medical, surgical, or dental procedures, intranasal cocaine use, tattooing, acupuncture, body piercing, military service, or foreign travel in the absence of another recognized exposure risk. The highest incidence of acute HCV infection is found in the 20- to 39-year age group with male predominance. Whereas whites and African Americans have similar incidences of acute disease, prevalence is substantially higher among African Americans from 30 years of age upwards. Thus the CDC recommends routine HCV testing for any person who has ever injected illegal drugs or has received clotting factor concentrates before 1987, has a persistent ALT elevation, or a person who has received a blood transfusion or organ transplant before 1992. Individuals exposed to HCV by needlestick or other injury and children born to HCV-positive mothers should be tested, but not all health care workers, pregnant women, household contacts of HCV-positive persons, or the general population.

The incubation period for HCV is 6 to 7 weeks (14–180 days). Persons with acute HCV infection typically either are asymptomatic or have mild clinical illness. Although less than 20% of acutely infected patients become jaundiced, the clinical illness of those who seek medical care is similar to that of other forms of viral hepatitis even though enzyme elevations tend to be lower. Fulminant hepatic failure is very rare.

It is widely accepted that only in 15% of patients, acute hepatitis C infection resolves spontaneously, but emerging data suggest that 25% to 45% may be a more accurate recovery rate for HCV acquisition at a young age, especially for young women. Of chronically infected patients, it is estimated that approximately one third are at risk of progression to end-stage liver disease over a lifetime. The basis for disease progression is not fully understood, but determinants include male gender, older age at time of acquisition, and heavy alcohol consumption. In patients with well-compensated cirrhosis, it has been estimated that approximately one third will decompensate and require transplantation within 10 to 12 years, and perhaps as many as 1% to 5% per year will develop hepatocellular carcinoma. In decompensated cirrhosis, survival is only 50% at 5 years. Chronic hepatitis C infection is typified by low-level fluctuating aminotransferase elevations that are often within the normal range. Extrahepatic manifestations are more common than those with chronic hepatitis B and include arthralgias, cryoglobulinemia with symptomatic vasculitis, membranoproliferative glomerulonephritis, and porphyria cutanea tarda. The association of other extrahepatic manifestations, such as lichen planus, diabetes mellitus, pulmonary fibrosis, and non-Hodgkin's lymphoma, has not been well established.

The diagnosis of HCV infection is suggested initially by EIA anti-HCV antibody screening, which is positive in greater than 97% of infected patients 6 to 12 weeks after infection. In patients with risk factors for HCV and elevated ALT level, EIA anti-HCV positivity is more than 95% reliable in the diagnosis of active HCV infection. False-positive results are prevalent when there is a low probability of HCV infection with normal ALT, but can also occur in patients with chronic antigenic stimulation or other causes of high globulins. False-negative EIA anti-HCV results occur in patients with advanced chronic renal failure and in some immunosuppressed individuals. EIA positivity can be supported by the recombinant immunoblot assay (RIBA) in which antibody reaction to the same recombinant viral proteins that are used in the EIA, is visualized directly. RIBA testing is useful for excluding false-positive EIA results. However, neither EIA nor RIBA positivity distinguishes between resolved and ongoing infection. The latter is best confirmed nowadays by HCV RNA testing. Several HCV RNA tests are available commercially, none of which are licensed. Both reverse transcriptase (RT)-PCR-based (quantitative and qualitative) and hybridization-based assays are available. Standardization of testing and reporting of HCV RNA titers has been introduced, so that results should now be reported universally in international units using an internationally agreed standard. Some RNA assays suffer from insensitivity to low viral loads and may give misleadingly negative results. Assays that are inaccurate at high viral titers may underestimate the true viral load. Thus results must be interpreted with caution. There are also commercially available assays to determine the genotype of HCV infection because this useful information is required when treating HCV infection. However, at present, quasispecies remain a research investigation.

Treatment is recommended for patients with chronic hepatitis C who have established cirrhosis and who are at greatest risk for progression to cirrhosis, as characterized by persistently elevated ALT levels, detectable HCV RNA, and a liver biopsy indicating either portal or bridging fibrosis and/or a moderate degree of inflammation and necrosis. It is less clear whether to treat patients with mild histologic disease or patients younger than 18 years and older than 60 years. Treatment is generally not recommended for patients with persistently normal ALT values, decompensated cirrhosis, major depressive illness, active chemical dependency, renal transplantation, hyperthyroidism, autoimmune disease, or pregnancy. Three forms of IFNα are licensed for HCV treatment, namely Intron A, Roferon, and Infergen. IFNα-2b (Intron A) in combination with oral ribavirin (Rebetol), a guanosine nucleoside analogue, is the treatment of choice now because it is more efficacious than IFNα-2b alone. Combination interferon/ribavirin therapy (Rebetron) gives sustained remission rates following completion of therapy of approximately 30% for HCV genotype 1 patients (with 12 months of therapy) and approximately 60% for HCV genotypes 2 and 3 (with only 6 months of therapy). Generally, genotypes 1 and 4 are relatively resistant to treatment, whereas types 2 and 3 are responsive. In addition to the side effects of IFNα, ribavirin causes hemolysis and can also give rashes and a nonproductive cough. Ribavirin must be avoided in patients with vascular compromise, like coronary artery disease, because of the risk posed by drug-induced anemia. Ribavirin is teratogenic; both men and women of childbearing potential must use effective contraception during treatment and for at least 6 months afterward.

Currently clinical trials are underway with many other antiviral agents alone and in combination. The drug most likely to be approved next for HCV treatment is a long-acting so-called pegylated form of interferon (Pegasys and PEG-Intron*) that is twice as effective as short-acting IFNα alone and approximately 10% to 15% more effective than Rebetron when combined with ribavirin.

HEPATITIS D

HDV is a defective virus that requires HBV for synthesis of its envelope protein composed of HBsAg, which is used to encapsulate the HDV genome. This is the only helper function provided by HBV. HDV has been suggested to be related to the plant viroids, simple infectious RNAs. At 1.7-kb RNA, the HDV genome is the smallest known to infect humans. HDV RNA encodes two antigens that play competing yet complementary roles in RNA synthesis and packaging. There are three distinct HDV genotypes with different geographic distributions and associated disease patterns.

HDV follows HBV distribution globally, with some distinct features. Where there is low prevalence of HBV (such as in the United States, Europe, and Australia), HDV infection is restricted to injection drug users and hemophiliacs. In countries with moderate-to-high HBV prevalence, HDV prevalence is highly variable ranging from high penetration among all HBV-infected individuals (as a result of direct contact with family members and intimate contacts) to relative rarity as occurs in Southeast Asia and China. Epidemics of severe HDV leading to fulminant hepatic failure and death (10%–20% case-fatality rates) have occurred in isolated regions of some South American countries and in the Amazon River Basin.

Two patterns of HDV infection occur, namely co-infection with HBV, or superinfection of an HBV carrier. The modes of HDV transmission are similar to those for HBV, with percutaneous exposure being more effective than sexual exposure. Perinatal transmission of HDV is rare. Persons with HBV-HDV co-infection may have more severe acute disease and a higher risk fulminant hepatitis (2%–20%) compared to those infected with HBV alone. Chronic HBV carriers who acquire HDV superinfection have greater than a 70% chance of developing HDV chronicity and 70%

*FDA approved 1/19/01.

to 80% of developing cirrhosis compared to a 15% to 30% chance of cirrhosis with HBV alone. The HBV-HDV co-infection incubation period is the same as that of HBV, and HDV viremia follows the appearance of HBsAg in serum. In the majority of cases, co-infection is self-limiting as it is in HBV infection alone. Both IgM and IgG anti-HDV are present in most cases of HBV-HDV co-infection whereas HDsAg is detectable in only 25% of such patients. In about 15% of patients, only IgM anti-HDV is detected in the early stages or IgG anti-HDV is detected during recovery. When there is viral clearance, no markers persist to indicate previous exposure to HDV. With HDV superinfection of an HBV carrier, the incubation period is about 8 weeks (21–140 days). Several characteristic serologic events happen. HBV replication falls transiently and HBsAg declines and may even disappear from the serum transiently when HDAg appears. Testing during this interval may give the misleading impression that the patient is not an HBsAg carrier. HDAg persists indefinitely because chronic HDV infection is the rule. Both IgM and IgG anti-HDV are present and also persist indefinitely. Thus the diagnosis of HDV may be made by finding HDsAg or anti-HDV antibodies in the serum but distinguishing acute from chronic infection is best done clinically.

There is no specific treatment for acute HDV co-infection or superinfection. Because HDV is dependent on HBV for replication, HBV-HDV co-infection can be prevented by HBV vaccination. HDV superinfection can only be prevented by avoidance. IFN∞ is less effective in the treatment of chronic HBV-HDV infection compared to the treatment of HBV alone. Lamivudine is not effective in the treatment of HDV because reduced HBV viremia is rarely accompanied by HBsAg loss. Interestingly, liver transplantation for chronic HBV-HDV cirrhosis has a better outcome than transplantation for HBV alone and there is less likelihood of graft infection with HBV and HDV after transplantation. In the immediate post-transplant setting, there is the unusual circumstance that HDV reappears before HBV and seems capable of infecting the new liver in the absence of HBsAg.

HEPATITIS E

HEV was the fifth of the human hepatitis viruses to be discovered and it is yet to be classified. It was originally grouped with the Norwalk agent and other gastroenteritis viruses, but genetically it appears closer to rubella. HEV may be amenable to cell culture but thus far this has not yielded a vaccine nor helped to characterize the virus.

HEV is a virus of the developing world, exhibiting four major genotypes that seem to have geographic predilection. HEV is especially prevalent in tropical and subtropical regions where it principally infects older children and young adults. HEV is endemic in the developing world from where travelers bring it back into the developed world. A small number of cases have been reported from North America and Europe, without antecedent travel to an endemic area. HEV may be zoonotic, that is, infection may be acquired directly or from contaminated water from domestic and wild animals (such as monkeys, swine, sheep, cattle, and rats).

The incubation period for HEV is approximately 6 weeks (15–60 days). Clinical symptoms and signs of acute hepatitis E are similar to those of other types of viral hepatitis. Overall the case-fatality rate is 1% to 3% with 15% to 25% death rates in pregnancy. Mortality in pregnancy appears to increase with each succeeding trimester.

The diagnosis of HEV is made by finding IgM anti-HEV positivity in serum up to 3 to 4 months after infection. IgG anti-HEV is usually present too and may rise to high titers during early convalescence. IgG anti-HEV diminishes with time but usually can be detected for up to several years after the infection and it appears to lend some degree of protection against re-infection. There is no specific treatment yet for HEV. Prevention relies primarily on the provision of clean water supplies and instituting hygienic practices. There is no prophylactic immunotherapy yet available. Immunoglobulin from plasma collected in non-endemic areas is not effective in preventing disease whereas the efficacy of locally prepared plasma is still unclear. Experimental hepatitis E vaccines consisting of recombinant viral proteins appeared efficacious in preclinical trials and are currently undergoing clinical evaluation.

MALABSORPTION

method of
RICHARD NEIL FEDORAK, M.D., and
CYRUS P. TAMBOI, M.D.
University of Alberta
Edmonton, Alberta, Canada

Malabsorption syndrome is a term applied to any situation in which disease of the intestine adversely interferes with the extraction of energy and nutrients from orally ingested food. Malabsorption includes disorders of intraluminal mixing and digestion, in addition to disorders of intramural transport and absorption. It is thus conceptually useful to classify this syndrome into disorders causing impaired intraluminal digestion and/or impaired intramural absorption (Table 1).

Although nonspecific treatments are available for the diarrheal symptoms associated with malabsorption, appropriate therapy and management of the malabsorption depends on the underlying physiologic defect being recognized and addressed. Because many diverse conditions (see Table 1) are capable of leading to clinical malabsorption, an understanding of pertinent intestinal physiology is useful to develop an appropriate therapeutic plan.

CARBOHYDRATE DIGESTION AND ABSORPTION

The orally ingested monosaccharide and disaccharide carbohydrates maltose, glucose, fructose, sucrose, and lactose are key sources of food energy. Starch is the only polysaccharide significantly utilized by humans. In the mouth, salivary α-amylase begins digesting starch, but it is rapidly inhibited in the acid milieu of the stomach. In the small intestine, pancreatic α-amylases continue to digest starch to produce oligosaccharides, maltose, maltotriose, glucose polymers, and α-limit dextrins. These molecules, along with ingested disaccharides, are subsequently further digested into monosaccharides by brush border disaccharidases, maltase, lactase, α-limit dextrinase, and sucrase-isomaltase into glucose, galactose, and fructose. All monosaccharides are then transported across the gastrointestinal epithelium via a series of active transporters located in the brush border.

From these physiologic considerations, carbohydrate malabsorption can occur in the following circumstances: (1) pancreatic insufficiency, (2) deficiencies of brush border disaccharidases (i.e., lactase deficiency), (3) generalized impairment of brush border and enterocyte function (i.e.,

TABLE 1. **Classification of Malabsorption Syndromes**

Defective Intraluminal Digestion

Gastric Mixing Disorders

Postgastrectomy

Pancreatic Insufficiency

Primary
- Cystic fibrosis

Secondary
- Chronic pancreatitis
- Pancreatic carcinoma
- Pancreatic resection

Reduced Intestinal Bile Salt Concentration

Liver and biliary disease
- Hepatocellular disease
- Cholestasis (intrahepatic or extrahepatic)

Abnormal small-bowel bacterial proliferation
- Afferent loop stasis
- Strictures
- Fistulas
- Ileocecal valve resection
- Blind loop(s)
- Multiple diverticula of the small bowel
- Hypomotility states (i.e., diabetes, scleroderma, intestinal pseudo-obstruction)
- Hypochlorhydria

Interrupted enterohepatic circulation of bile salts
- Ileal surgical resection
- Ileal inflammatory disease (Crohn's disease)
- Primary bile acid malabsorption
- Postcholecystectomy and truncal vagotomy

Drugs (by sequestration or precipitation of bile salts)
- Neomycin
- Calcium carbonate
- Cholestyramine

Defective Intramural Absorption

Inadequate Absorptive Surface

Intestinal resection or bypass
- Mesenteric vascular disease with massive intestinal resection
- Crohn's disease with multiple bowel resections
- Jejunoileal bypass

Mucosal Absorptive Defects

Biochemical or genetic abnormalities
- Celiac disease
- Disaccharidase deficiency
- Hypogammaglobulinemia
- Abetalipoproteinemia
- Hartnup disease
- Cystinuria
- Monosaccharide malassimilation

Inflammatory or infiltrative disorders
- Crohn's disease
- Amyloidosis
- Scleroderma
- Lymphoma
- Radiation enteritis
- Eosinophilic enteritis
- Tropical sprue
- Infectious enteritis (e.g., salmonellosis)
- Collagenous sprue
- Nonspecific ulcerative jejunoileitis
- Mastocytosis
- Dermatologic disorders (e.g., dermatitis herpetiformis)

Lymphatic obstruction
- Intestinal lymphangiectasia
- Whipple's disease
- Lymphoma

celiac disease), and (4) loss of mucosal surface area (i.e., short-bowel syndrome).

Carbohydrate malabsorption leads to residual unhydrolyzed carbohydrates in the lumen of the intestine, which augments intraluminal fluid accumulation and diarrhea, by virtue of its osmotic effect. Furthermore, bacterial fermentation of malabsorbed carbohydrates that reach the colon produces short chain fatty acids (which aggravates diarrhea) and hydrogen and carbon dioxide gases (which cause flatulence and bloating).

PROTEIN DIGESTION AND ABSORPTION

Pepsin, liberated from the stomach, is active and cleaves ingested proteins in the presence of an acidic pH. Once it enters the duodenum, gastric pepsin is rapidly inactivated by duodenal bicarbonate, and pancreatic proteases (trypsin, chymotrypsin, elastase, DNAse, RNAse, and carboxypeptidases A and B) and brush border dipeptidases complete the intraluminal protein digestion. The resultant individual amino acids are then transported across the enterocyte via sodium-dependent and sodium-independent amino acid and oligopeptide cotransporters.

From these physiologic considerations, protein malabsorption would be expected in diseases causing (1) pancreatic insufficiency, (2) generalized impaired enterocyte function (i.e., celiac disease), and (3) loss of mucosal surface area (i.e., short-bowel syndrome).

Protein malabsorption is much less common than carbohydrate or fat malabsorption. When protein malabsorption does occur, protein-losing enteropathy ensues with subsequent hypoproteinemia and weight loss.

LIPID DIGESTION AND ABSORPTION

Although the process of fat digestion and absorption yields the highest caloric value per gram ingested, it is also the most complex and therefore vulnerable to dysfunction from a variety of causes. Lingual lipase can digest up to 30% of ingested lipids, whereas gastric lipase activity becomes significant only in the presence of pancreatic lipase insufficiency. The overall process of fat digestion and absorption consists of four distinct phases related to the respective functions of the pancreas, liver, intestinal mucosa, and lymphatics. Physiologically, these functions respectively involve (1) lipolysis of dietary triglyceride to fatty acid and β-monoglyceride; (2) micellar solubilization with bile acid; (3) uptake into the mucosal cell, with reesterification and assembly of the monoglyceride and fatty acid to form triglycerides, as well as chylomicron formation in the presence of cholesterol, cholesterol esters, phospholipids, and protein; and (4) delivery of chylomicrons in lymphatics to the body for utilization of fat.

From these physiologic considerations, malabsorption of fat caused by impaired lipolysis or micellar solubilization would be expected to occur in the following circumstances: (1) rapid gastric emptying and improper mixing, (2) altered duodenal pH, (3) pancreatic insufficiency, (4) chlolestasis, and (5) an interrupted enterohepatic circulation. Fat malabsorption from impaired mucosal uptake, assembly, or delivery would be expected to occur after (1) generalized impaired enterocyte function, (2) failure of the repackaging process, (3) disorders of lymphatics, and (4) loss of mucosal surface area.

Failure to digest or absorb fat results in both fat malabsorption and a deficiency in fat-soluble vitamins. Loss of fat into the colon results in the hydroxylation of long chain fatty acids into hydroxyl-fatty acids, which cause diarrhea by stimulating the colon to secrete fluid and by virtue of their osmotic effect.

HISTORY AND PHYSICAL EXAMINATION

A malabsorption syndrome may be suspected after a thorough medical history and physical examination. The patient may have one or more manifestations of the underlying disease or resultant nutrient deficiencies. These signs and symptoms are variable and may be subtle (Table 2). Classic textbook descriptions of florid nutrient deficiencies are rarely encountered in clinical practice in developed countries. Nevertheless, all patients with significant malabsorption will have some degree of abdominal pain, bloating, diarrhea, flatulence, or weight loss. Increased delivery to the colon of osmotically active particles, especially carbohydrates and lipids, leads to colonic secretion of water and electrolytes and resultant chronic diarrhea. Fat malabsorption may cause foul-smelling, pale, greasy stools that are difficult to flush. Floating stools are caused by increased fecal gas content from increased bacterial fermentation of carbohydrates. The patient may complain of fatigue and weakness, often associated with anemia. Protein-calorie malnutrition may cause edema. Deficiencies of fat-soluble vitamins (A, D, E, and K) may be manifested as night blindness, bone pain and osteomalacia, neurologic symptoms, or easy bruising, respectively. Skin and mucosal disorders, such as seborrheic dermatitis, hyperkeratosis, xerosis, cheilosis, and alopecia, are commonly due to one or more water-soluble vitamin deficiencies such as vitamin B_6, niacin, or vitamin C. Intensely pruritic erythematous papules over the extensor surfaces is typical of *dermatitis herpetiformis*, which is associated with gluten sensitivity in 10% to 20% of cases. Peripheral neuropathy occurs with vitamin B_{12} deficiency and is manifested as loss of position or vibration sensation. A past medical history of previous abdominal surgery may suggest mixing disorders, pancreatic insufficiency, small-bowel bacterial overgrowth, bile salt wastage, or loss of intestinal mucosal surface area.

TABLE 2. **Clinical Signs and Symptoms of Malabsorption**

Clinical Sign or Symptom	Deficient Nutrient
General	
Weight loss, decreased libido, anorexia, fatigue, amenorrhea	Protein-calorie
Skin, Hair, and Nails	
Psoriasiform rash, eczema	Zinc
Pallor	Folate, iron, vitamin B_{12}
Follicular hyperkeratosis	Vitamin A
Perifollicular petechiae	Vitamin C
Flaking dermatitis	Protein-calorie, niacin, riboflavin, zinc
Bruising	Vitamin K
Thick, dry skin	Linoleic acid
Pigmentation changes	Niacin, protein-calorie
Sparse thin hair, alopecia	Protein
Flat brittle nails, leukonychia	Iron, protein
Eyes	
Night blindness	Vitamin A
Xerosis, Bitot's spots	Vitamin A
Keratomalacia	Vitamin A
Corneal vascularization	Riboflavin
Mouth	
Glossitis	Riboflavin, niacin, folic acid
Tongue atrophy	Riboflavin, niacin, iron
Angular stomatitis	Riboflavin, iron
Cheilosis	Riboflavin
Hypogeusia	Zinc
Bleeding gums	Riboflavin, vitamin C
Scarlet, raw, fissured tongue	Niacin
Head and Neck	
Muscle wasting	Protein-calorie
Extremities	
Muscle wasting, edema	Protein-calorie
Neurologic	
Tetany	Calcium, magnesium
Paresthesias	Vitamin B_{12}, thiamine
Hyporeflexia, wristdrop/footdrop	Thiamine
Ataxia, proprioception defects	Vitamin B_{12}, folate
Dementia, disorientation	Niacin

SYMPTOMATIC ANTIDIARRHEAL THERAPY

Effective therapy for malabsorption syndromes depends on identifying and treating the underlying disease, correcting nutritional imbalances, and providing symptomatic relief.

Oral Rehydration Therapy. Oral rehydration therapy is used to prevent dehydration and electrolyte loss. It works by enhancing sodium, and thus water, absorption through cotransport of sodium and glucose. Oral rehydration preparations should have a balanced sodium-to-glucose ratio (see Table 4). Solutions that have excess glucose may aggravate existing diarrhea as a consequence of their osmotic effect.

Hydrophilic Bulking Agents. Dietary fiber supplementation may be useful in the management of diarrhea. The ultimate effectiveness of a fiber depends not only on its water-holding capacity but also on its ability to hydrolyze fatty and bile acids, which if not hydrolyzed, directly stimulate intestinal secretion. Bulking agents also increase chyme viscosity and thereby delay gastric emptying and reduce colonic transit times. Psyllium (5–7.5 g every 12 hours) is a hydrophilic agent that increases fecal water-holding capacity and may reduce diarrheal symptoms. Many psyllium-containing products are mixed with laxatives; these products must be avoided in patients with malabsorption and diarrhea.

Opioids. Opioids reduce diarrhea by decreasing intestinal secretion and/or promoting intestinal absorption, reducing intestinal motility, and increasing anal tone. Available opioids include naturally occurring preparations (paregoric and opium alkaloids) and synthetic preparations (codeine, diphenoxylate, and loperamide). These agents are very effective for symptomatic use in acute and chronic diarrhea caused by malabsorption; however, side effects limit their acute use and tolerance usually occurs with chronic use. Diphenoxylate (Lomotil), (5 mg initially and then 2.5 mg after each loose bowel movement to a maximum of 20 mg/d), and loperamide (Imodium)

4 mg initially and then 2 mg after each loose bowel movement to a maximum of 16 mg/d have fewer central nervous system (CNS) side effects than noted with other opioids. Diphenoxylate has been combined with atropine to limit its potential for abuse. Loperamide, which has the least number of side effects or abuse potential, is available without prescription. Codeine (30–60 mg every 4 hours as needed) is the most effective antidiarrheal opiate, but it also has the greatest side effect profile.

DEFECTIVE INTRALUMINAL DIGESTION

Gastric Mixing Disorders

Surgical alterations in gastric innervation, pyloric structure, and gastric capacity may have significant effects on nutrition. Nutritional disturbances and chronic weight loss occur predominantly in patients who have had a subtotal gastrectomy in the past. These patients may have disorders of calcium homeostasis or anemia secondary to iron and, less frequently, vitamin B_{12} deficiency and require appropriate nutritional supplementation. Extensive gastrectomy can also be associated with symptoms of a small gastric reservoir. Patients typically complain of early satiety and a sensation of epigastric postprandial discomfort, which can be prevented by eating small, frequent meals.

Pancreatic Insufficiency

Pancreatic insufficiency may be primary and due to cystic fibrosis or secondary and due to chronic pancreatitis, pancreatic resection, or rarely, pancreatic carcinoma. Of these causes, chronic pancreatitis is by far the most common and leads to weight loss because of anorexia or because of fear that eating will initiate pain by activating the pancreatitis. Only after 90% of the exocrine secretory capacity of the pancreas is lost does chronic pancreatic exocrine insufficiency occur and result in malabsorption and weight loss. During pancreatic insufficiency, fat malabsorption is dominant, perhaps because of a limited capacity to up-regulate lipase production. Cystic fibrosis is a childhood equivalent of chronic pancreatic insufficiency, but the weight loss in this disease is probably caused as much by the anorexia of chronic infection as it is by the malabsorption induced by pancreatic enzyme and bile acid deficiencies.

Because of insufficient quantities of pancreatic enzyme in commercial oral supplements and because of acid pepsin inactivation of orally administered pancreatic enzymes, complete correction of the fat malabsorption resulting from pancreatic insufficiency is rarely accomplished. The postprandial delivery of pancreatic lipase is approximately 560,000 IU during the 4 hours after a meal. Malabsorption does not occur if approximately 5% (28,000 IU over a 4-hour period) is delivered to the duodenum with each meal. Pancreatic supplements are highly variable in enzyme activity (Table 3), with the lipase content ranging from 4000 to 25,000 IU per capsule. Therefore, it is important to know the lipase content of the preparation prescribed and ensure that sufficient amounts (at least 28,000 IU per meal) are being delivered to the duodenum.

Another important factor to consider in the management of pancreatic insufficiency is acid and pepsin inactivation of orally administered pancreatic enzymes. Less than 8% of ingested lipase and less than 22% of ingested trypsin successfully pass through the stomach and remain active in the duodenum. Preventing acid peptic neutralization of enzyme supplements by coating capsules with acid-resistant and alkali-sensitive materials or by using antacids has resulted in little improvement in the delivery of lipase to the duodenum. Antacids increase gastric se-

TABLE 3. **Pancreatic Enzyme Preparations**

		Enzyme Content (Units per Capsule)		
Therapeutic Agent	**Type**	*Lipase*	*Amylase*	*Protease*
Cotazym	C	8,000	30,000	30,000
Cotazym ECS-4	ECMS	4,000	11,000	11,000
Cotazym ECS-8	ECMS	8,000	30,000	30,000
Cotazym ECS-20	ECMS	20,000	55,000	55,000
Creon 10	ECMS	10,000	33,200	37,500
Creon 25	ECMS	25,000	74,700	62,500
Pancrease	ECMS	4,000	20,000	25,000
Pancrease MT 4	ECMT	4,000	12,000	12,000
Pancrease MT 10	ECMT	10,000	30,000	30,000
Pancrease MT 16	ECMT	16,000	48,000	48,000
Ultrase	ECMS	4,500	20,000	25,000
Ultrase MT 12	ECMT	12,000	39,000	39,000
Ultrase MT 20	ECMT	20,000	65,000	65,000
Viokase	UCT	8,000	30,000	30,000
Viokase	P	16,800	70,000	70,000
Zymase	ECMS	12,000	24,000	24,000

Abbreviations: C = capsule; ECMS = enteric-coated microspheres encased in a cellulose capsule; ECMT = enteric-coated microtablets encased in a cellulose capsule; P = powder; UCT = uncoated tablet.

cretion, and dilution of enzyme concentrations below critical levels may explain the relative ineffectiveness of antacids. Enteric coating is effective only if pancreatic enzymes are delivered into the duodenum at the same time as ingested food and if adequate intraduodenal dissolution occurs.

Recently, pancreatic enzyme preparations coated with a pH-dependent polymer were developed to be stable at gastric pH (<4) and dissolve at a pH greater than 5 in the duodenum. This pH dissolution profile theoretically delivers pancreatic enzymes to the upper part of the small bowel intact. However, if gastric and duodenal pH remains low (<4) throughout the postprandial period, the enteric coat will not dissolve and the pancreatic enzyme supplement will traverse the upper gastrointestinal tract and not assist in digestion and absorption. A major criterion for determining the efficacy of enteric-coated enzyme preparations is the size of the microspheres. These microspheres influence the timing of enzyme delivery to the small intestine. It has been shown that microspheres with a diameter of approximately 1.4 mm appear to mix with chyme most thoroughly and are emptied from the stomach at the same rate as food.

Therefore, an ideal enteric-coated pancreatic enzyme capsule preparation should contain a high concentration of lipase to maximize fat digestion, be enteric coated to avoid destruction by gastric acid, and contain microspheres approximately 1.4 mm in diameter to allow efficient delivery of enzyme to the small bowel. In addition, H_2-receptor antagonists and proton pump inhibitors decrease acid production and pepsin activity and can be used to optimize pancreatic enzyme concentrations in the duodenum. Additional therapeutic maneuvers include smaller and more frequent meals, each with pancreatic enzyme replacement, and reduction of the amount of fat in the diet to 50 to 75 g/d.

Finally, deficiencies of the fat-soluble vitamins A, D, E, and K and the respective clinical signs of deficiency have all been demonstrated with pancreatic insufficiency. Supplemental vitamins should be provided. The water-soluble vitamins are readily absorbed with the exception of B_{12}, whose absorption depends on pancreatic enzymes to cleave B_{12} from R protein to allow B_{12} to be absorbed in the ileum. With adequate pancreatic enzyme replacement, supplemental B_{12} is usually unnecessary.

Reduced Intestinal Bile Salt Concentration

Liver and Biliary Disease

Severe hepatocellular dysfunction and/or bile duct obstruction can cause steatorrhea. Indeed, the incidence of mild steatorrhea is 25% to 50% in patients with cirrhosis alone. Steatorrhea in these patients occurs as a consequence of inadequate micelle formation from bile salt insufficiency; however, secondary factors, including malnutrition, portal hypertension, bacterial overgrowth, and drugs (i.e., neomycin) may also play a role. In both biliary obstruction and severe liver disease, nutrient malabsorption is not often a significant clinical problem, and the weight loss is usually multifactorial.

Abnormal Small-Bowel Bacterial Proliferation

Small-bowel bacterial overgrowth is a syndrome characterized by nutrient malabsorption associated with excessive numbers of bacteria in the small intestine. In addition to intraluminal bacterial metabolism, evidence indicates that bacteria-induced mucosal injury also results in the malabsorption of fats, carbohydrates, and proteins; however, there is no evidence that bacterial invasion into the mucosal wall is involved in the malabsorption process.

Bacterial deconjugation of bile acids is the primary mechanism for malabsorption of fats and fat-soluble vitamins during abnormal small-bowel bacterial proliferation. Normal fat absorption requires a critical concentration of conjugated bile acids for the assembly of mixed micelles. Bacterial deconjugation of bile acids by luminal bacteria, particularly anaerobic organisms, reduces the level of conjugated bile acids below the critical micellar concentration and leads to fat malabsorption. Clinical vitamin D, A, and E deficiencies can occur, but the synthesis of vitamin K by luminal bacteria accounts for the absence of coagulopathy in patients with bacterial overgrowth. In addition, deconjugated bile acids and bacteria-hydroxylated fatty acids have a direct toxic effect on the intestinal mucosa that results in further malabsorption of fats. Finally, both deconjugated bile acids and hydroxylated fatty acids are direct secretagogues that contribute to the development of rapid intestinal transit and diarrhea.

Bacterial overgrowth results in carbohydrate malabsorption secondary to its direct toxic effect on intestinal mucosa and the subsequent reduction of brush border disaccharidases and decreased uptake of monosaccharides. Lactase activity is the first to be reduced and is the last disaccharidase activity to recover after antibiotic therapy has been administered.

Hypoproteinemia is common in bacterial overgrowth, although severe protein malabsorption is rarely seen. Disruption of normal protein assimilation is caused by multiple factors: bacteria compete with the host for protein substrates, decreased amino acid and peptide uptake occurs as a result of mucosal injury, decreased levels of enterokinase impair the activation of pancreatic proteases, and finally, a protein-losing enteropathy can ensue.

The association of macrocytic anemia with bacterial overgrowth is the result of direct competition between the anerobic intestinal flora and the host for vitamin B_{12}. When bacteria take up the vitamin, not only does it become unavailable to the host, but inactive metabolites are also produced that compete with normal vitamin B_{12} binding and absorption. Thiamine and nicotinamide are two other water-soluble vitamins that have been reported to be low in patients with bacterial overgrowth. Although iron deficiency anemia has not been clearly associated with bacterial overgrowth in humans, increased intestinal losses of iron and blood have been seen in severe cases. Mineral and trace element deficiencies have not been reported in patients with bacterial overgrowth.

Initial management of bacterial overgrowth consists of fluid and nutritional support, including the replacement of vitamin deficiencies. After diagnosing bacterial overgrowth, an attempt to identify an underlying cause should be made and surgical correction of anatomic causes of intestinal stasis considered. Bacterial overgrowth resulting from severe motility disorders is more difficult to manage. Prokinetic agents have been shown to normalize gastric motility in patients with motor disorders; however, their role in treating small intestinal bacterial overgrowth remains limited because of the absence of a potent small intestinal prokinetic.

Often, the underlying lesion is not correctable, and primary treatment is directed at suppressing the bacterial overgrowth with antibiotics. Numerous antibiotics have been reported to be effective, including tetracycline, ampicillin, erythromycin, clindamycin (Cleocin), ciprofloxacin (Cipro), metronidazole (Flagyl), and oral aminoglycosides. Many patients experience a remission after a single 7- to 10-day course of therapy with tetracycline or metronidazole. In patients with repeated recurrence of bacterial overgrowth, a repeating and rotating antibiotic regimen can be tried, such as 2 weeks of metronidazole followed by 2 weeks of ciprofloxacin.

Interrupted Enterohepatic Circulation of Bile Salts

Three types of bile acid–induced malabsorption occur and may result from (1) severe disease, resection, or bypass of the distal ileum; (2) primary bile acid malabsorption; and (3) truncal vagotomy or cholecystectomy.

Ileal disease, resection, and bypass (i.e., Crohn's disease) permits dihydroxy bile salts to escape ileal absorption and enter the colon. If concentrations higher than 2 mmol/L are attained in the colon, diarrhea ensues as a consequence of a direct secretory effect of bile acids on the colon. Bile acid diarrhea must be differentiated from fatty acid diarrhea, which occurs if ileal disease or resection involves such a large segment of ileum (>100 cm) that hepatic synthesis cannot maintain an adequate intraluminal bile salt pool. Under these circumstances, steatorrhea ensues, and fatty acid–induced intestinal secretion complicates the picture. It is important to differentiate these two related syndromes because bile acid diarrhea responds to bile salt binders such as cholestyramine* (Questran) (4 g every 12 hours) but the diarrhea of fatty acid malabsorption does not, and indeed, bile salt binders may worsen the symptoms. Therapy for fatty acid diarrhea is a low-fat diet supplemented with medium chain triglycerides (which are absorbed directly into the portal vein without the need for digestion) to prevent severe weight loss.

Primary bile acid malabsorption is characterized by excessive bile acid loss, which is responsive to cholestyramine, but is not associated with histologic or macroscopic ileal disease. Increased fecal bile acids in patients with postcholecystectomy diarrhea suggest that cholecystectomy can lead to bile acid malabsorption syndromes. It is unclear why interruption of gallbladder storage would lead to increased bile acid malabsoprtion. Although many patients respond to cholestyramine, some do not, which raises the question of whether other pathophysiologic mechanisms are involved in this form of diarrhea. Neither primary bile acid malabsorption nor the postcholecystectomy syndrome results in significant enough bile loss to overwhelm the liver's ability to up-regulate synthesis, and thus steatorrhea does not occur.

Drugs That Affect Digestion and Absorption

Drugs that interfere with nutrient absorption by direct interaction include tetracycline, which chelates calcium ions; cholestyramine, which binds to iron and vitamin B_{12}; and aluminum and magnesium hydroxide, which precipitate calcium and phosphate ions. Mucosal injury resulting in diminished nutrient absorption can occur with colchicine, neomycin, and methotrexate. Neomycin, 6 to 12 g/d, causes brush border damage by inhibiting enterocyte protein synthesis. Neomycin is also thought to impair micellar solubilization of bile salts, cholesterol, fatty acids, and fat-soluble vitamins by directly binding to bile salts. Methotrexate decreases the height of intestinal microvilli, as well as brush border membrane protein and lipid content. Drugs that produce histologic flattening in jejunal mucosa and that have been reported to cause fat malabsorption include methyldopa (Aldomet), allopurinol (Zyloprim), and mefenamic acid (Ponstel).

DEFECTIVE INTRAMURAL ABSORPTION

Inadequate Absorptive Surface

Short-bowel syndrome is a term that covers the symptoms and pathophysiologic disorders associated with a malabsorptive state resulting from the removal of a large portion of the small or large intestine. The extent of intestinal resection that will produce this syndrome varies from one person to another. In children, survival without enteral supplements or total parenteral nutrition is generally possible if more than 40 cm (i.e., 20% of normal length) of small intestine remains. In adults, survival without enteral or parenteral nutrition is generally possible if the residual length of small intestine is more than 150 cm (i.e., 25% of normal length). In general, if the ileocecal valve is removed, longer lengths of residual bowel may not prevent short-bowel syndrome.

*Not FDA approved for this indication.

Short-bowel syndrome refers only to a well-organized clinical pattern sometimes seen in patients with intestinal resection and is not necessarily related to the length of intestine removed. The clinical consequences of removing a portion of the small intestine are extremely variable and depend on a number of factors, including the extent of resection, site of resection, and subsequent adaptive processes.

Nutritional management of short-bowel syndrome is a dynamic process that follows the evolution of the clinical and adapted state of the bowel. Depending on the length of resection and the postsurgical adaptation, the process will result in one of four nutritional outcomes: maintenance of balanced nutritional status on a normal or modified oral diet, maintenance through the use of defined enteral formula diets, maintenance through enteral intake with parenteral electrolyte and fluid supplementation, or maintenance through total or partial parenteral nutrition supplemented by variable amounts of enteral intake. Whatever the source of nutrition, caloric intake should be increased slowly and progressively until it reaches a target of about 32 kcal/kg ideal body weight per day. This caloric intake goal, in general, will meet the increased losses that result from inefficient and inadequate absorption.

Parenteral Therapy. In the immediate postoperative period, all patients with extensive small intestinal resection require total parenteral nutrition. As the amount of enteral nutrition is gradually increased, the duration and intensity of the parenteral nutrition infusion can be reduced. If more than 25% of a person's intestine remains, it should be possible for the patient to stop total parenteral nutrition completely.

Oral Therapy. A balanced solution containing carbohydrates and electrolytes can be given orally once stool output is less than 2 L daily. Clear fluid diets are not useful because they are inadequate in nutritional value; they are also severely hyperosmolar and likely to provoke osmotic diarrhea. Full fluid diets are also poorly tolerated because they contain lactose and most patients with short-bowel syndrome are lactose intolerant. To optimize oral fluid and electrolyte absorption, a balanced oral replacement solution is necessary. A solution that contains an iso-osmotic sodium and glucose mixture takes advantage of the small intestinal sodium glucose cotransport carrier to enhance salt and water absorption (Table 4). Sport drinks such as Gatorade are too low in sodium to be of much use in patients with short-bowel syndrome.

Patients with more than 60 to 80 cm of small bowel should approach the reintroduction of oral feeding slowly until a normal or modified oral diet level is reached. Because gastric emptying is slower for solids, these patients should eat dry solids at a meal and take only isotonic fluids 1 hour later because this regimen improves the absorption of nutrients. Diarrhea that occurs as a consequence of oral feeding can usually be managed by using an antidiarrheal agent, which should be taken on a regular basis 1 hour before meals and snacks. Waiting to take the antidiarrheal agent after the meal has started and the diarrhea has occurred is not effective.

Divalent cations, including calcium, magnesium, zinc, and copper, may bind to fatty acids in the stool, and excessive fecal losses of these minerals have been documented in patients with steatorrhea. Steatorrhea will also accentuate the malabsorption of fat-soluble vitamins (A, D, E, and K). Increased fecal fat losses also enhance dietary oxalate absorption, oxaluria, and renal stone formation. Recommendations based on dietary fat therefore need to be responsive to the individual patient's symptoms after bowel resection. In addition, it is important to balance the beneficial effects of fat restriction against the limitations on food palatability and caloric intake imposed by low-fat diets. A low-fat and low-oxalate diet, for instance, is likely to be completely unpalatable.

Medium chain triglycerides can be used as caloric supplements for patients with short-bowel syndrome. Medium chain triglycerides are hydrolyzed in the intestinal lumen to water-soluble components, which are absorbed in the absence of bile salts. Medium chain triglycerides have an unpleasant taste, however, and sometimes produce diarrhea because of their osmotic load in the proximal part of the small intestine (when given in a dose of more than 35 g/d) and thus do not provide essential fatty acids.

Enteral Therapy. Patients who cannot tolerate a normal oral diet and those with a short bowel (<60–80 cm) can often benefit from an enteral formula. If a chemically defined formula is used, it is important to control the rate of infusion to match osmotic inflow with osmolar absorption. Rates of full-strength infusion usually begin at 25 mL/h and gradually increase to 125 mL/h. The rate is modulated according to the tolerance displayed by the small intestine. If a polymeric formula is used, it should be lactose-free because most patients with massive

TABLE 4. **Oral Replacement Solutions**

Solution	Glucose (mmol/L)	Sodium (mmol/L)	Potassium (mmol/L)	Chloride (mmol/L)	Base (mmol/L)	Osmolality (mOsm/L)
WHO	111	90	20	80	30	331
Pedialyte	139	45	20	35	30	269
Gastrolyte	100	50	20	52	18	240
Gatorade	227	22	3	27	0	333

Abbreviation: WHO = World Health Organization.

small intestinal resections do not have an adequate lactase reserve.

Vitamin and Mineral Supplementation. Enteral and parenteral solutions are supplemented with vitamins and minerals. As patients are weaned from these solutions and once the patient has stopped enteral or parenteral solutions completely, vitamin and mineral deficiencies may slowly occur because of inadequate intake (as the patient tries to prevent diarrhea), excess nutrient losses (from the short bowel), or a combination of both. Liquid vitamin and mineral oral supplementation regimens can be considered in some patients as they are weaned off parenterally supplied vitamins and minerals (Table 5). Liquid supplements are preferable to solid pills because hard outside matrices are often not dissolved during their rapid transit through a short bowel.

Mucosal Absorptive Defects

Celiac Disease

Celiac disease is treated with a gluten-free diet that involves avoiding all food products containing wheat, rye, barley, and oats. Because a gluten-free diet has a low roughage and fiber content, patients may require fiber supplementation. Specific nutrient deficiencies, including iron, folic acid, and calcium deficiency, should be corrected. It is important to note that many of the vitamin supplements contain gluten in the capsules, so a gluten-free vitamin pill needs to be identified for these patients.

Should the patient's symptoms persist or the jejunal biopsy findings remain grossly abnormal after 3 to 4 months of ingesting a gluten-free diet, the initial diagnosis should be questioned. However, the most common reason for inadequate response is a lack of patient compliance or inadvertent gluten ingestion. Corticosteroids can be used in cases of refractory sprue that does not respond to gluten withdrawal. The initial dose is 40 to 60 mg of prednisone daily, tapered off over a period of 1 to 2 months.

TABLE 5. **Sample Short-Bowel Oral Multivitamin/Mineral Routine**

ADEKs Multiple Vitamin

2 to 4 tablets daily (chewed or crushed thoroughly)
Each tablet contains vitamin A, 4000 IU; beta carotene, 3 mg; vitamin D, 400 IU; vitamin E, 150 IU; vitamin K, 0.15 mg; vitamin C, 60 mg; folic acid, 0.2 mg; thiamine, 1.2 mg; riboflavin, 1.3 mg; niacin, 10 mg; vitamin B_6, 1.5 mg; vitamin B_{12}, 12 μg; biotin, 50 μg; pantothenic acid, 10 mg; zinc, 7.5 mg

Calcium Gluconate Liquid

400 mg PO twice daily = 400 mg elemental calcium twice daily

Ferrous Sulfate Liquid

300 mg PO twice daily = 60 mg elemental iron twice daily

Osto-Forte (vitamin D_2) Capsule

50,000 IU once per week

Phosphate-Novartis (tablet dissolved)

500 mg PO twice daily = 500 mg elemental phosphorus twice daily

K-10 Potassium Liquid

60 mL PO twice daily = 40 mEq KCl twice daily

Magnesium Glucoheptonate Liquid

30 mL PO twice daily = 150 mg magnesium twice daily

Disaccharidase Deficiency

The clinical symptoms associated with lactose or sucrose malabsorption are caused by low levels of the microvillus membrane disaccharidases required for their hydrolysis: lactase and sucrase-isomaltase, respectively. These reduced levels may be due to genetic alterations in expression of the enzymes or to reductions in enzyme activity as a consequence of intestinal injury. The clinical features and symptoms are those of malabsorption of carbohydrates.

Treatment of lactose intolerance includes (1) restriction of dietary lactose, (2) substitution of alternative nutrients to avoid reductions in energy and protein intake, (3) supplemental calcium intake, and (4) the use of commercially available enzyme substitutes. When lactose restriction is necessary, patients must be instructed to read labels of commercially prepared foods to identify hidden lactose. Calcium is supplemented in the form of calcium carbonate, 1000 mg/d. Commercially available lactase preparations are bacterial or yeast β-galactosidases. These products are not capable of completely hydrolyzing all dietary lactose, so patients must still restrict dietary lactose intake.

Isomaltase deficiency is a rare disorder caused by impaired synthesis of the intestinal enzyme sucrase-isomaltase. Patients are initially seen in childhood or, occasionally, adolescence. The primary approach to the treatment of sucrase-isomaltase deficiency is elimination or restriction of dietary sucrose.

Abetalipoproteinemia

After lipid digestion, fatty acids and monoglycerides are taken up by enterocytes and rearranged into apolipoprotein B–containing particles necessary for their transfer into the lymphatic circulation. Abetalipoproteinemia is an autosomal recessive disease characterized by the absence of apolipoprotein B. Triglycerides cannot be packaged for transfer and thus accumulate in the cytoplasm of enterocytes. This accumulation of fat in enterocytes results in malabsorption of fat because the fat-engorged enterocytes are incapable of processing or transporting any more lipid.

Fat restriction, in particular, long chain fatty acids, will alleviate the malabsorption. Medium chain fatty acids may be used temporarily if severe malnutrition is present, but routine use should be avoided because it can worsen hepatic steatosis. The inability to form chylomicrons also leads to a deficiency in fat-soluble vitamins, and vitamin replacement therapy is necessary in all patients.

Lymphatic Obstruction

Intestinal Lymphangiectasia

Intestinal lymphangiectasia is a disease that can be either congenital or acquired in association with trauma, lymphoma, carcinoma, or Whipple's disease, and it causes protein-losing enteropathy and steatorrhea. It is the classic form of post–intramural obstruction malabsorption. The unique combination of malabsorption of fat, protein, and lymphocytes but normal absorption of carbohydrates relates to the obstructed lymphatic channels, which are the route of absorption for fat, protein, and lymphocytes. Absorption of carbohydrates takes place by way of the portal circulation and remains unaffected. Treatment involves surgical repair of the underlying trauma or neoplasia.

Whipple's Disease

Whipple's disease represents infiltration of the intestine and lymphatics with *Tropheryma whippelii.* The histopathologic appearance of the small-bowel mucosa in Whipple's disease is diagnostic. The lamina propria is infiltrated by large foamy macrophages, which grossly distorts normal villous architecture and gives the villi a blunted, clublike appearance. The cytoplasm of these macrophages is filled with large periodic acid–Schiff–positive glycoprotein granules. The lymphatic channels in the mucosa and submucosa are dilated, and fat droplets may be seen in the extracellular spaces within the lamina propria as a result of lymphatic obstruction by enlarged mesenteric lymph nodes. The gastrointestinal symptoms are thus those of clinical malabsorption. Similar histologic findings can be seen in any organ in the body because Whipple's disease is a diffuse process. Given the concern with CNS involvement and relapses, it is reasonable to assume that all patients may have CNS involvement and to treat initially with an antibiotic that readily crosses the blood-brain barrier. Trimethoprim-sulfamethoxazole (Bactrim),* one double-strength tablet (trimethoprim, 160 mg–sulfamethoxazole, 800 mg) given twice daily for 1 year, is the best long-term option.

*Not FDA approved for this indication.

ACUTE PANCREATITIS

method of
JOHN S. MINASI, M.D.
Zassi Medical Evolutions, Inc.
Fernandina Beach, Florida

Acute pancreatitis is an inflammatory disorder of the pancreas that has both local and systemic manifestations. Gallstones and alcohol abuse account for approximately 80% of all cases, with other causes accounting for 10% and the remaining 10% being idiopathic. Improved intensive care unit management has decreased mortality over the years, and about 5% mortality is now seen in cases of acute pancreatitis. Any reading about pancreatitis, however, can be confusing because of variations in nomenclature. An international symposium held in Atlanta in 1992 reached a consensus on terminology for describing various conditions associated with pancreatitis. This terminology is based on computed tomography (CT) and clinical findings and includes: (1) acute interstitial pancreatitis, (2) necrotizing pancreatitis, (3) sterile necrosis, (4) infected necrosis, (5) acute fluid collections, (6) pancreatic pseudocyst, and (7) pancreatic abscess.

PATHOPHYSIOLOGY

The causes of acute pancreatitis are many and varied, and it has a fairly uniform clinical picture. Common causes are listed in Table 1. The inciting events remain unclear, but autodigestion of the pancreas by various proteolytic enzymes within the organ is known to cause necrosis and intraglandular vascular damage. However, the specific role of exposure to alcohol, duct obstruction or overdistention, hypertriglyceridemia, hypercalcemia, and hyperstimulation of the gland is unclear. In addition, the contribution of the immune response to the pathophysiology of pancreatitis is under intensive study. Immunocyte cytokine release probably plays a role in the systemic manifestations of severe pancreatitis, including respiratory failure, increased capillary permeability, and shock.

CLINICAL FEATURES

In most patients with acute pancreatitis, the predominant symptom is abdominal pain. It is usually excruciatingly severe and appears as an acute abdominal emergency. Occasionally, the pain may be less severe and localized in the midepigastrium, the right or left upper quadrant, or the back. The attack may occur after a heavy meal or an alcoholic binge. In biliary pancreatitis, the patient may report a history of less severe attacks and finally seek medical assistance after a severe episode. The pain is typically persistent and constant, which distinguishes it from peptic ulcer or biliary colic. The severity of the pain tends to exceed the findings on examination. Acute pancreatitis and acute mesenteric ischemia are two diseases in which severe pain may be associated with a paucity of abdominal signs. Nausea and vomiting frequently accompany the pain, but vomiting does not alleviate the pain.

On physical examination, patients in the hospital are

TABLE 1. **Causes of Acute Pancreatitis**

Biliary tract disease	Viral infection
Alcohol	Scorpion venom
Hyperlipidemia	Idiopathic
Hypercalcemia	Drugs
Familial	Azathioprine (Imuran)
Trauma	Estrogens
External	Thiazide diuretics
Operative	Furosemide (Lasix)
Retrograde pancreatography	Ethacrynic acid (Edecrin)
Ischemia	Sulfonamides
Hypotension	Tetracycline
Cardiopulmonary bypass	L-Asparaginase
Atheroembolism	Corticosteroids
Vasculitis	Phenformin*
Pancreatic duct obstruction	Procainamide
Tumor	Valproic acid (Depakote, Depakene)
Pancreas divisum	Clonidine (Catapres)
Ampullary stenosis	
Ascaris infestation	
Duodenal obstruction	
Congenital web	
Periampullary diverticulum	

*Not available in the United States.

usually found lying still in bed because movement exacerbates pain. Some patients will lean forward to suspend the viscera off the inflamed pancreas. Low-grade fever is typically present at the onset of the attack, but high fever may be seen after a few days of severe pancreatitis, even without infection. Tachycardia, oliguria, and other signs of volume depletion are commonly noted. The abdomen is mildly distended, tender, and characterized by guarding. These signs can be seen in the upper portion of the abdomen or diffusely, but they typically do not have the boardlike quality of a perforated duodenal ulcer. Though uncommon, severe necrotizing pancreatitis with a hemorrhagic component can be accompanied by ecchymoses in the flanks (Grey Turner sign), the periumbilical area (Cullen sign), or the inguinal region (Fox sign).

In severe cases, hypotension, hypoperfusion, and obtundation may be observed. Jaundice may be present as a result of choledocholithiasis in gallstone-associated pancreatitis or swelling of pancreatic tissue surrounding the bile duct.

DIAGNOSIS

The single most useful test in establishing a diagnosis of pancreatitis in a patient with acute abdominal pain is the serum amylase level. It is elevated early in the course of the disease and returns to normal levels over a few days, with an improving clinical course in uncomplicated cases. Hyperamylasemia is not specific to pancreatitis. Other causes may need to be considered, such as acute cholecystitis, small-bowel obstruction, small-bowel infarction, acute appendicitis, ruptured ectopic pregnancy, acute salpingitis, ovarian cysts and tumors, or ruptured abdominal aortic aneurysm. The serum lipase concentration can be helpful as an adjunct to determination of amylase levels. Lipase is more specific to the pancreas and remains elevated longer than amylase does. The combination of elevations in serum amylase and serum lipase more reliably differentiates a pancreatic source for hyperamylasemia. Results of assays for lipase in patients in the hospital can be confusing, especially in the absence of hyperamylasemia, and modest elevations can be seen with heparin use and intravenous intralipid administration.

Imaging studies are necessary to exclude other causes of hyperamylasemia, look for an etiology for the gallstones, or assess the severity of the pancreatitis. Plain radiographs can support the diagnosis with findings of left pleural effusion, the "sentinel loop sign," the "colon cutoff sign," cholelithiasis, nonspecific ileus, or pancreatic calcifications. Radiographs are most useful in ruling out small-bowel obstruction or free air from a perforated viscus.

Right upper quadrant ultrasound is absolutely necessary to search for gallstones, detection of which has an extremely high positive predictive value for gallstones as the etiology. CT scans give excellent correlation with the severity of the disease. Rapid-bolus spiral scans are extremely accurate in rating areas of hypoperfusion or necrosis in severe pancreatitis. Magnetic resonance imaging or magnetic resonance cholangiopancreatography and endoscopic retrograde cholangiopancreatography (ERCP) are not recommended for the routine diagnosis of acute pancreatitis, but they are extremely useful in the assessment of patients who have recurrent attacks from other causes, such as tumors, duct strictures, or pancreas divisum.

Patients should be adequately resuscitated before embarking on any imaging studies. Patients with severe pancreatitis should be in the intensive care unit and not the radiology or endoscopy suites.

ASSESSMENT OF SEVERITY

The severity of pancreatitis can be estimated by both clinical and radiographic criteria. Every third-year medical student on the surgical service can recite Ranson's criteria (Table 2) for estimating severity. These 11 criteria were found to predict survival in patients with acute pancreatitis; more than 3 criteria signified severe disease. These criteria can be useful reminders to check calcium levels and to be aware of the massive fluid requirements that can be seen with acute pancreatitis. The Acute Physiology and Chronic Health Enquiry (APACHE-II) Severity of Disease Classification System has also been used to predict outcome in acute pancreatitis; however, because it is far more complex than Ranson's criteria, it is less commonly used.

In view of the importance of necrosis in determining the patient's outcome, disease severity can also be assessed by CT. Greater than 50% necrosis of the gland, the presence of extensive peripancreatic fluid collections, and the presence of gas within the pancreas or adjacent soft tissue are all markers predicting poor outcome.

MANAGEMENT

Mild Acute Pancreatitis

This category accounts for 90% of patients with acute pancreatitis and therefore requires emphasis. The disease is usually relatively mild and self-limited if recognized and managed properly. Amylase measurement should be a routine test in the initial evaluation of individuals with biliary symptoms. Their first episode of gallstone pancreatitis may be the event that gets their attention and brings them to the physician. This diagnosis should also be suspected in a patient with multiple gallstones seen on ultrasound who reports attacks that last several hours to a day, especially with vomiting.

In the acute setting, the patient should be admitted to the hospital and supported with intravenous hydration and analgesics. The adequacy of volume replacement should be closely monitored, and these patients should ingest nothing by mouth. Dehydration and pancreatic stimulation by food have been shown to convert otherwise mild pancreatitis into a more severe form. Prophylactic antibiotics are of no

TABLE 2. **Ranson's Early Prognostic Signs of Acute Pancreatitis**

At Admission
Age older than 55 y
WBC >16,000 cells/mm³
Blood glucose level >200 mg/dL
Serum lactate dehydrogenase level >350 IU/L
Aspartate aminotransferase level >250 U/dL
During Initial 48 h
Hematocrit fall >10%
BUN level elevation >5 mg/dL
Serum calcium level fall to <8 mg/dL
Arterial P_{O_2} <60 mm Hg
Base deficit >4 mEq/L
Estimated fluid sequestration >6 L

Abbreviations: BUN = blood urea nitrogen; WBC = white blood cell count.

benefit. CT is unnecessary if the clinical picture is clear and resolving progressively. Not only are ERCP and sphincterotomy unnecessary, but pancreatography can also introduce infection into an otherwise sterile, inflamed gland and lead to complications. The serum amylase level will typically fall by 50% or more per day, and the patient will become pain free. Persistent elevation of amylase and continued pain are signs of more complicated pancreatitis. Mild elevations in bilirubin should also be monitored with ERC reserved for those with rising bilirubin levels or signs of cholangitis. Surgical consultation should be obtained early in the course, and laparoscopic cholecystectomy should be performed at a convenient time before discharge from the hospital and institution of an oral diet. An intraoperative cholangiogram should be obtained during cholecystectomy. Cholangiography adds little cost and risk to the patient in this situation, and if laboratory values are normal at the time of surgery, choledocholithiasis will be found in only 10% to 15% of cases. Laparoscopic common bile duct exploration or postoperative ERC with endoscopic sphincterotomy and stone extraction should be performed. Pancreatography should be avoided in this acute setting as it may exacerbate the pancreatitis. The outcome with this strategy is excellent.

Immediate cholecystectomy (within 24 hours) should also be avoided because this procedure will greatly increase the number of common bile duct explorations needed and has an unacceptably high morbidity rate.

Mild alcohol-induced pancreatitis resolves more slowly than gallstone pancreatitis but entails the same supportive approach. Counseling is recommended. Other etiologies of pancreatitis may require more extensive evaluation once resolved to rule out tumor or other anatomic features. CT, magnetic resonance imaging/cholangiopancreatography, ERCP, and tumor markers are all useful.

Moderate to Severe Acute Pancreatitis

Patients with moderate or severe pancreatitis should be managed in the intensive care unit. Aggressive support is mandatory. Resuscitation, resuscitation, resuscitation! Sequestration of fluid can be massive in this group and needs to be closely assessed with urinary catheters, determination of central venous pressure, pulmonary artery catheters, echocardiography, or arterial lines. Organ support such as mechanical ventilation, inotropic agents, blood transfusion, and hemodialysis may be necessary. Such individuals will not be well resuscitated by transport to the radiology or endoscopy suite and should remain in the unit. CT scans are much more useful 72 hours after admission. The prerenal elevation of blood urea nitrogen and creatinine may have normalized and allow the use of intravenous contrast, which may find a viable pancreas in a bed of peripancreatic edema, areas of nonperfusion, or potential infected necrosis.

Intensive Care Unit Management

The overall mortality in severe acute pancreatitis is approximately 30%. Deaths occur in two phases. Early deaths within the first 2 weeks of onset are related to multisystem organ failure caused by the release of inflammatory mediators and cytokines. Late deaths are secondary to local or systemic infections. Sterile necrosis carries only a 10% mortality, but infected necrosis can increase the mortality to 40% to 50%. Early management of acute necrotizing pancreatitis consists of a combination of intensive medical care and prevention of infection with prophylactic antibiotics. Late management involves adequate débridement of local infectious complications.

The use of imipenem/cilastatin (Primaxin), 500 mg intravenously every 8 hours for 2 to 4 weeks, has been shown to reduce the rate of infectious complications. Other antibiotics, including the quinilones, have not proved effective to date. Superinfection with *Candida* species can be seen with use of this broad-spectrum antibiotic. It is prudent to treat patients with an antifungal agent such as fluconazole (Diflucan). The use of enteral nutrition may preserve the gut barrier and decrease infectious complications.

Nutritional Support

A trend away from parenteral nutrition to enteral nutrition is finding its way in the management of severe acute pancreatitis. Recent randomized trials have shown that enteral nutrition initiated beyond the ligament of Treitz within 48 hours of the onset of illness is well tolerated, has no adverse clinical effects, and results in significantly fewer total and infectious complications. It has been my practice over the last several years to obtain enteral access by bedside endoscopy or bedside fluoroscopy early in the course of illness. Standard formula Feedings with the addition of ½ to 1 tsp of pancrelipase powder per can of formula or low-fat–containing formulas may be used. Overfeeding and hyperglycemia should be avoided. If poorly tolerated, supplemental parenteral nutrition can be used to balance delivery. Studies have shown that 10% to 20% of the protein needs delivered enterally can maintain the gut barrier and immunologic function of the gastrointestinal tract. Care should be taken to not deliver full enteral feedings to an under-resuscitated patient or a patient receiving vasoconstrictive inotropic support because of the possibility of intestinal necrosis. Carbohydrate intolerance has been linked to mortality. Enteral carbohydrates are much better tolerated than parenteral ones; in addition, enteral nutrition appears to attenuate the acute phase response in acute severe pancreatitis.

Management of Necrosis

Aggressive pancreatic necrosectomy remains the standard of care for infected necrosis. There is little evidence that débridement of sterile necrosis is of benefit, and recent studies have shown increased morbidity and mortality in this setting. The use of CT-directed fine-needle aspiration of suspected areas of necrosis has been extremely helpful in differentiating these two groups because their clinical picture may be identical and other sites of infection that do not require operative débridement may be better delineated (urinary tract, invasive lines, lungs). Insertion of CT-guided percutaneous drains can be extremely useful when placed posteriorly as a guide to the surgeon when using unilateral or bilateral flank approaches to necrosectomy. Complications in the abdominal cavity can be lessened and management of the ensuing pancreatic fistula can be simplified.

Endoscopic Intervention

Patients with a high likelihood of choledocholithiasis as determined by a rising bilirubin or alkaline phosphatase concentration or evidence of cholangitis should have urgent ERC with sphincterotomy and stone extraction. In complicated necrosis, ERCP should be avoided early to prevent conversion of sterile to infected necrosis. ERCP with pancreatic stenting or pseudocyst drainage can be very useful in expert hands to control fistulas. It can prevent or delay the need for surgical intervention until a time that is more suitable in the course of recovery. The pancreatic duct and biliary tree can then be addressed more definitively during an elective surgical procedure.

Other Complications

The most common complication associated with acute pancreatitis is an acute fluid collection, but the nomenclature of these fluid collections has spawned great controversy. The nomenclature was clarified in the International Consensus Conference in Atlanta in 1992, but confusion still exists in the literature. Acute fluid collections occur in nearly 60% of episodes of acute pancreatitis. Most of them resolve spontaneously and are related to edema and minor duct disruption without abnormalities in the major ducts. Asymptomatic collections should be monitored. Symptomatic collections can be drained by percutaneous, endoscopic, or surgical techniques. Before any surgical procedure, the status of the pancreatic duct should be investigated and any strictures or obstruction corrected during the procedure to provide long-lasting drainage. Infected fluid collections should be percutaneously drained if possible.

Pancreatic ascites is usually well managed with ERCP and pancreatic duct stenting. Surgical intervention may be necessary to rule out perforation of the gastrointestinal tract as the cause of amylase-rich ascites.

Bleeding may occur from erosion of pseudocysts into vessels, false aneurysms, or gastric varices from splenic vein thrombosis. Interventional radiologic or surgical techniques, including splenectomy, may be necessary.

Gastrointestinal complications can be classified as compressions, strictures, or erosions. The most common sites are the duodenum, transverse colon, and splenic flexure of the colon. Surgical bypass, diversion, or resection is often necessary. Biliary strictures may be treated with endoscopic or percutaneous transhepatic stenting or with surgery.

Summary

Most cases of pancreatitis are mild. Gallstones and alcohol are the most common causes. Proper management is necessary to prevent complications. Intensive care management is crucial in managing severe acute pancreatitis. Pancreatitis of unclear etiology should always be investigated to rule out other causes, especially tumors.

CHRONIC PANCREATITIS

method of
CRISTINA FERRONE, M.D., and
DAVID W. RATTNER, M.D.
Harvard Medical School
Boston, Massachusetts

Chronic pancreatitis is a condition caused by a variety of different diseases that result in progressive destruction of pancreatic parenchyma, loss of exocrine and endocrine function, and diminished life expectancy. Because inflammation is a prominent pathologic feature of this condition, pain is the most common complaint. Most of the interaction between patients with chronic pancreatitis and their physicians centers around therapy to relieve pain. As such, these patients are often viewed as "difficult patients," and physicians frequently see the condition as hopeless or at best hard to treat. In fact, many patients can be relieved of pain by appropriate surgical, endoscopic, or neurolytic therapies. This chapter presents the pathophysiology of chronic pancreatitis and its complications and highlights the opportunities for successful intervention.

INCIDENCE AND ETIOLOGY

The annual incidence worldwide of chronic pancreatitis is about 4 per 100,000 people. The exact U.S. prevalence is not known, but autopsy series report a prevalence of about 0.5%. Diabetes mellitus will develop in over half of the patients and nearly half will eventually require surgery for pain or complications.

The hallmarks of the disease are abdominal pain, weight loss, steatorrhea, and pancreatic calcification. The median age of onset for chronic pancreatitis is 44 years. The median time from onset of symptoms to calcification is 9 years. Surprisingly, only 56% of all patients with chronic pancreatitis develop pain severe enough to come to medical attention. Approximately one quarter of all patients with chronic pancreatitis die within 20 years of the diagnosis, a much higher number than in an age-matched healthy population.

Among American adults, alcohol abuse accounts for about 70% of cases. These patients usually have an alcohol intake of 150 g/d or more for more than 5 years before the disease develops. The type of alcohol (i.e., beer, wine, or spirits) seems to have no bearing on the development of the disease. A large group of adult patients, perhaps as high as 25%, have no identifiable etiology for chronic pancreatitis. In these patients with idiopathic chronic pancreatitis, pain is universally present and the progression to calcification is slow, with a median time to calcification of 20 to 25 years. This subgroup has a bimodal age distribution with peak onset of symptoms at median ages of 19 and 56 years.

In younger adults and adolescents, diagnoses include tropical pancreatitis, hereditary pancreatitis, and obstructive pancreatitis. *Hereditary pancreatitis* is a rare, dominantly inherited condition with 80% penetrance, which is due to a mutation of the trypsinogen gene. Identification of the gene is the gold standard for the diagnosis in this small subset of patients. *Tropical pancreatitis* occurs in developing countries within 30 degrees of the equator. The disease usually affects young adults and is characterized by large intraductal calculi, marked dilation of the pancreatic ducts, atrophy, and fibrosis. The cause of tropical pancreatitis is unclear, but possibilities include protein malnutrition, micronutrient deficiencies, and cassava consumption.

Obstructive pancreatitis occurs due to congenital or acquired obstruction of the pancreatic duct. Congenital narrowing most commonly is caused by stenosis of the minor ampulla in patients with pancreas divisum. If the condition is recognized early, sphincteroplasty of the minor ampulla can alleviate obstruction and prevent development of chronic pancreatitis. Acquired narrowing or stricture of the pancreatic duct can occur from trauma, tumors, or healing after necrotizing pancreatitis. It is important to realize that in the absence of ductal strictures, acute pancreatitis does not lead to chronic pancreatitis. However, when changes of chronic pancreatitis are seen in the absence of a clear etiologic agent, an obstructing tumor or intraductal papillary mucinous tumors must be excluded.

Because time is required for the changes of chronic pancreatitis to develop, this entity is rarely seen in children. In children, cystic fibrosis is the most common cause. Tenacious secretions in these children are believed to cause obstruction of the pancreatic duct with subsequent scarring, atrophy, and loss of function. The common causes of chronic pancreatitis are listed in Table 1.

PATHOLOGY

On a macroscopic level, chronic pancreatitis is characterized by a firm, fibrotic gland with or without gross dilation of the pancreatic duct. Although the disease process usually affects the entire gland, the morphologic changes can be nonuniform. Some patients may have diffuse atrophy of the gland whereas others may have asymmetric changes with localized inflammatory masses mimicking tumors. The earliest detectable clinical changes are the appearance of prominent secondary branches of the pancreatic duct.

The histopathologic findings in chronic pancreatitis include loss of acini, glandular shrinkage, calcification, and ductal stricturing. As the disease progresses, parenchymal loss is more pronounced and, in late stages, one can see destruction of islets as well as exocrine structures. Dense collagen and fibroblastic proliferation in the parenchyma also becomes more prominent as the disease progresses. Although most of the parenchymal inflammatory changes are chronic, elements of acute pancreatitis including edema, acute inflammation, and even necrosis may be superimposed. Recently attention has focused on perineural changes and attempts have been made to correlate histologic finding with pain syndromes. Lymphocytes and plasma cells are frequently present in areas of fibrosis and around nerve bundles. Neuronal changes include an increase in nerve number, enlargement of the pancreatic nerve diameters, and visible destruction of the perineurium best seen by electron microscopy. Theoretically, the destruction of the perineurium indicates a loss in the barrier between nerve fibers and bioactive material in the perineural space.

TABLE 1. **Etiology of Chronic Pancreatitis**

Alcohol
Cystic fibrosis
Idiopathic pancreatitis
Hereditary pancreatitis
Tropical with severe protein-calorie malnutrition
Obstruction
Pancreatic divisum
Congenital or acquired strictures
Post-inflammatory
Trauma
Neoplasm
Pancreatic adenocarcinoma
Periampullary
Intraductal papillary tumors

PATHOPHYSIOLOGY

There are many theories regarding the events that initiate the inflammatory process of chronic pancreatitis. Particular attention has been paid to the pathophysiology of alcohol-induced chronic pancreatitis. The toxic metabolic theory suggests that ethanol or one of its metabolites has a direct injurious effect by distorting the sorting function of the Golgi complex, which results in premature activation of enzymes. This enzymatic autodigestion results in progressive intrapancreatic lipid deposition with inflammatory and fibrotic changes. In animal models alcohol seems to reduce regional pancreatic blood flow. Foitzig and associates suggest that relative pancreatic ischemia is due to reduced capillary flow resulting in chronic hypoxia. Reduced capillary flow may be due to alcohol-induced acinar injury resulting in edema and capillary compression or due to red cell aggregation. Ethanol-provoked pancreatic hypoxia provides a possible mechanism by which alcohol contributes to pancreatic injury.

The oxidative stress hypothesis proposes that excess free radicals ultimately result in peroxidation of the lipid components of the membrane within the pancreatic acinar cell, leading to mast cell degranulation, platelet activation, and an inflammatory response. Other theories include disturbance of acinar and ductal function resulting in protein leakage with subsequent development of protein plugs. These plugs then cause ductal obstruction resulting in inflammation and scarring. Obstructive pancreatitis from acquired and congenital ductal obstruction is associated with uniform inflammatory changes and rare protein plugs. These patients tend not to develop pancreatic stones. The differences between patients with congenital and acquired obstruction compared to those with ductal calculi without obstruction remain unexplained.

The mechanism of pain in chronic pancreatitis is multifactorial, although not fully understood. As the disease progresses, fibrotic encasement of sensory nerves and inflammatory injury to the nerve sheaths are observed. New pain theories include alterations in neurotrophic factors such as nerve growth factor and its receptor TrkA, as well as increases in neuronal growth–associated protein-43, a marker of neuronal plasticity. Aside from the perineural changes, it is likely that increased interstitial pressure in the pancreatic parenchyma creates a pancreatic compartment syndrome. This results in decreased capillary perfusion and some have postulated that pain in chronic pancreatitis may relate to tissue ischemia. According to this theory, when the capsule of the pancreas is incised longitudinally to perform a longitudinal pancreaticojejunostomy (see next) the compartment syndrome is released.

CLINICAL EVALUATION

The classic triad of chronic pancreatitis is pancreatic calcification, diabetes mellitus, and steatorrhea. This triad is seen, however, only when chronic inflammation has destroyed 90% of the pancreatic parenchyma. Most patients come to medical attention before reaching the end stage of their disease. Severe and persisting abdominal pain is the most common reason patients seek medical attention. The pain is typically in the epigastrium with radiation through to the back. Eating may aggravate the pain, but this feature is not always present. The pain can be quite variable in severity and there may be intervals during which the patient is pain-free. Pain is often difficult to quantify and assessment of its impact is often clouded by the patient's addiction to alcohol and/or narcotics, as well as a preponderance of psychiatric/personality disorders. There are no pathognomonic findings on physical examination. Most patients are thin due to anorexia and malabsorption. Epigastric tenderness is a common finding and mild jaundice may be present if the common bile duct is compressed by inflammation in the head of the gland.

The differential diagnosis of patients presenting with pain in the absence of the classic triad includes peptic ulcer disease, biliary tract disease, mesenteric vascular disease, and malignancy. A careful history and appropriate imaging studies can usually establish the diagnosis. In contrast to acute pancreatitis, hyperamylasemia is a nonspecific finding. During flareups of the disease in which an element of acute inflammation is present, the serum amylase level may be elevated, but a normal serum amylase level does not exclude the presence of chronic pancreatitis.

It can be extremely difficult to distinguish between chronic pancreatitis and pancreatic carcinoma because they have overlapping clinical, serologic, and imaging patterns. Furthermore, patients with chronic pancreatitis have an increased incidence of pancreatic adenocarcinoma compared to the general population. Patients with chronic pancreatitis generally have a longer duration of symptoms than patients with pancreatic carcinoma and are more likely to have abused alcohol. Serum markers, findings on pancreatography on computed tomography, and biopsy results are also helpful. Table 2 describes useful factors in differentiating pancreatic cancer from chronic pancreatitis. At times, however, it is impossible to exclude the possibility of carcinoma and surgical resection must be performed.

Serologic markers have been extensively studied to help distinguish chronic pancreatitis from pancreatic carcinoma. The CA 19-9 antigen is the most widely used marker for determining the prognosis and management of patients with pancreatic cancer. CA 19-9 serum levels correlate directly with tumor bulk in those tumors that release the antigen. However, CA 19-9 is not suitable for diagnosing pancreatic cancer because elevated levels of CA 19-9 have also been detected in patients with benign pancreatic disease. The overall sensitivity and specificity of CA 19-9 are 70% and 90%, respectively.

TABLE 2. **Factors That Differentiate Chronic Pancreatitis From Pancreatic Cancer**

Chronic Pancreatitis	Pancreatic Neoplasm
Long duration of symptoms	Short duration of symptoms
History of alcohol abuse	History of smoking
History of pancreatic trauma	New onset diabetes mellitus
Abdominal pain	Weight loss
Weight loss	Jaundice
Steatorrhea	Courvoisier's sign
Diabetes mellitus	
Pancreatic calcifications	Pancreatic mass
Diffuse morphologic changes	Peripancreatic lymph nodes
	Extrapancreatic spread
TPS<200 U/mL	TPS>200 U/L
CA 19–9<37 U/mL	CA 19–9>37 U/mL
Total bililrubin<10 mg/dL	Total bilirubin>20 mg/dL

Abbreviation: TPS = tissue polypeptide–specific antigen.

One of the newer serologic markers is tissue polypeptide–specific (TPS) antigen. TPS measures a specific epitope structure of soluble cytokeratin 18 fragments. In contrast to CA 19-9, TPS reflects the activity of tumor growth. Slesak and coworkers used immunoassays to measure TPS and CA 19-9 levels in 48 patients with pancreatic carcinoma and 74 patients with chronic pancreatitis. Neither marker had levels that correlated with TNM stage. However, a TPS value of greater than 200 U/L has a sensitivity of 97% and a specificity of 98% for differentiating pancreatic carcinoma from chronic pancreatitis.

PANCREATIC FUNCTION TESTS

Traditionally, the fecal fat assay has been used to assess steatorrhea. Quantitative stool fat collection (<7 g fat/24 hours on 100-g fat diet over 48–72 hours) is the gold standard for malabsorption, but is not specific for chronic pancreatitis. Steatorrhea develops only when greater than 90% of pancreatic exocrine function is lost. Assays of fecal exocrine proteins such as chymotrypsin have been used to help assess pancreatic output and function. Chymotrypsin is very stable in stool. Measurement of fecal chymotrypsin has a sensitivity of 90% in severe chronic pancreatitis, but loses its usefulness in patients with mild or moderate disease.

Fecal elastase 1 was reported to have a 93% specificity for all patients with pancreatic exocrine insufficiency. However, Lankisch and associates found it to be less than 50% sensitive for mild-to-moderate disease. The pancreolauryl test has the highest sensitivity in patients with moderate degrees of pancreatic dysfunction. The test is based on the hydrolysis of fluorescein dilaurate by pancreatic cholesterol esterase. Fluorescein dilaurate is taken by the patient with breakfast. The hydrolysis releases fluorescein, which is conjugated in the liver, and can then be measured in the urine or in the serum. The sensitivity is highest in severe pancreatic insufficiency and less in mild-to-moderate disease. False-positive results are observed with liver disease or small-bowel mucosal disease, resulting in specificities between 46% and 97%.

None of the pancreatic function tests is 100% specific for diagnosis. If the pancreatic duct is obstructed by a stone or tumor, these tests will show the same exocrine deficiency as in the case of massive parenchymal loss. In patients with known chronic pancreatitis, however, these tests can be used to assess the severity of the exocrine function deficit and be used to gauge the adequacy of enzyme replacement.

IMAGING STUDIES

Because many of the symptoms of chronic pancreatitis are nonspecific, imaging studies play an essential role in the diagnosis of chronic pancreatitis. Plain abdominal radiographs reveal pancreatic calcifications in 35% to 80% of patients when all causes of chronic pancreatitis are considered. These calcifications actually represent intraductal stones rather than true calcification of the parenchyma. The visualization of pancreatic stones is sufficient to establish the diagnosis of chronic pancreatitis. Even though this finding is pathognomonic, the number of stones correlates neither with the degree of endocrine or exocrine insufficiency nor the severity of abdominal pain.

Transabdominal ultrasonography (US) is often performed for the evaluation of upper abdominal pain. US is an appealing modality because it provides real-time images and does not expose the patient to ionizing radiation. It does not require intravenous contrast or a specialized room, making it particularly appealing for patients with renal failure or claustrophobia. A successful US can reveal calcification, ductal dilation, presence of a pseudocyst, changes in parenchymal echo texture, or variations in the size and shape of the gland. Unfortunately, US is very operator-dependent. Furthermore, the pancreas is difficult to visualize in patients who are obese or have overlying bowel gas. Thus US is less useful as a primary diagnostic modality than as a means to follow complications of chronic pancreatitis such as pseudocysts or bile duct dilation.

Many of the limitations of transabdominal US can be overcome by placing the transducer in proximity to the pancreas. Endoscopic US (EUS) combines upper gastrointestinal (GI) endoscopy with US to accomplish this purpose. The entire pancreas can be viewed through the duodenal and gastric walls. In experienced hands, EUS is the best modality to appreciate subtle changes in the pancreatic parenchymal texture, including hyperechogeneic foci, lobularity of the gland, and cysts. The pancreatic duct is also well visualized and ductal changes such as hyperechoic thickening, irregularity, dilation, and calcified duct stones are readily seen. This modality is ideal for precisely directed biopsies of suspicious areas or aspiration of cystic lesions. In spite of these advantages, EUS may not be able to establish the diagnosis of chronic pancreatitis in elderly patients or in patients with early stage disease. With aging, lobularity of the gland and echogenic foci are commonly seen and not necessarily indicative of chronic pancreatitis.

A further refinement of EUS is intraductal pancreatic sonography. This technique utilizes a rotating radial 20-MHz US transducer that can be passed through the biopsy channel of a side viewing endoscope and into the pancreatic duct. Preliminary data are promising, especially in differentiating chronic pancreatitis from pancreatic carcinoma, and for precise evaluation of pancreatic duct abnormalities.

Computed tomography (CT) is the gold standard for noninvasive imaging of the pancreas. CT scans are more sensitive than US at detecting pancreatic calcifications. Modern helical CT scans provide outstanding anatomic detail, can identify lesions as small as 2 mm, and are nearly universally available. Chronic pancreatitis is associated with a wide range of CT abnormalities. These include focal enlargement (particularly of the head of the gland), diffuse atrophy, calcifications, ductal dilation, and pseudocysts. It is unusual to have focal enlargement of the tail of the gland unless there is a known cause for mid-ductal obstruction.

To glean the most information from a CT scan, it is important to use adequate oral contrast material. This allows differentiation of the pancreas from the surrounding duodenum and stomach. Intravenous contrast material is helpful if pancreatic necrosis is suspected or if vascular compression/occlusion is a consideration. Conventional portal phase imaging is used for patients suspected of having pancreatitis, whereas dual phase scans (arterial and portal) are used for pancreatic neoplasms or when definition of arterial anatomy is required. During the portal phase, the peripancreatic veins and liver parenchyma show maximal contrast enhancement. The arterial phase optimizes contrast enhancement of the pancreatic parenchyma for detection of small hypodense pancreatic or islet cell masses.

Endoscopic retrograde cholangiopancreatography (ERCP) currently is the most sensitive imaging modality for the diagnosis of chronic pancreatitis because the earliest changes are prominence of the secondary branches of the main pancreatic duct. ERCP allows for direct visualization of the pancreatic duct and distal common bile duct, as well as the opportunity for therapeutic intervention. Complications of chronic pancreatitis such as stenosis of the common bile duct, strictures of the pancreatic duct, and ductal disruptions are easy to identify. In spite of these capabilities, ERCP is often not capable of providing direct evidence that distinguishes benign from malignant processes. A disadvantage of ERCP is that the pancreatic parenchyma cannot be directly visualized and that there is a finite risk of worsening an episode of pancreatitis due to the manipulation of the papilla or high-pressure injection into the pancreatic duct.

Magnetic resonance imaging is not widely used as a first-line imaging modality for pancreatic disease. At this time, the main strength of magnetic resonance imaging is the ability to noninvasively image the pancreatic and biliary duct via magnetic resonance cholangiopancreatography. Under optimal conditions, magnetic resonance imaging can produce images similar to those seen on ERCP. It has advantages over ERCP in that it is noninvasive and thus cannot cause postprocedure pancreatitis, and also has the ability to depict the ducts in an axial or three-dimensional format. When an abnormality is identified, however, ERCP is often required for confirmation as well as therapeutic intervention. Despite the potential advantages of magnetic resonance cholangiopancreatography, most centers currently use a combination of helical CT and ERCP for pancreatic imaging due to the lower cost, wide availability, ease of image interpretation, and ability to perform biopsies or deliver endoscopic therapy.

TREATMENT

There is no treatment that halts the inexorable fibrosis and parenchymal destruction of chronic pancreatitis. Therefore therapy is directed at managing complications of the disease. Although some have argued that watchful waiting will allow the inflammatory process to burn out, this nihilistic approach is not justifiable in an era when many surgical and nonsurgical options are both safe and effective at relieving complications of chronic pancreatitis.

Dietary Management

Total abstinence from alcohol should be encouraged in all patients. Studies regarding the resolution of pain or slowing of the progression of symptoms with total abstinence from alcohol have shown contradictory results. It is clear, however, that alcohol abuse can exacerbate inflammation and cause acute inflammation in the setting of chronic pancreatitis. Therefore, total abstinence should be recommended.

Because fat is a strong stimulant of pancreatic secretion and may worsen pain, fat should not exceed more than 30% to 40% of the patients' total daily calories. Medium-chain triglycerides have been recommended in certain circumstances because they require minimal digestion, but their use has been limited because they are unpalatable. Protein intake should be 1.0 to 1.5 g/kg/d. Vitamins and other micronutrients should also be replaced if a deficiency is detected.

Nutritional Supplementation/Enzymatic Replacement

Protein calorie malnutrition is common in patients with chronic pancreatitis for multiple reasons, including alcoholism with concomitant liver dysfunction, anorexia, steatorrhea, altered postprandial motility, and recurrent postprandial abdominal pain. Postprandial abdominal pain makes it difficult for patients to increase their caloric intake. Therefore, analgesics should be given 30 minutes before meals to prevent postprandial exacerbation of abdominal pain. Unfortunately, chronic pain and use of narcotics often lead to anorexia.

Steatorrhea and azotorrhea occur after lipase and trypsin secretions are reduced by 90%.

Pancreatic enzyme replacement can correct protein malabsorption and improve steatorrhea. The minimal dosage of lipase required per meal is 28,000 IU (eight 3500-IU tablets, Viokase), which needs to be taken with the meal, not before or after the meal. A low gastric or duodenal pH can inactivate lipase. Therefore, if there is no symptomatic improvement of diarrhea and a decrease in the 72-hour fecal fat excretion test, an H2 receptor antagonist, sodium bicarbonate, or a proton pump inhibitor can be added. Calcium-containing and magnesium-containing antacids should not be used. If the addition of these agents fails, enteric-coated preparations (pancreatin [Creon]) may be effective. Currently Suzuki and associates are developing a bacterial lipase from *Burkholderia plantarii*, which survives better in human gastric and duodenal juice than porcine lipase.

The most frequently reported adverse reactions to pancreatic enzymes include diarrhea, constipation, nausea, vomiting, bloating, cramping, allergic reactions, hyperuricemia, and hyperuricosuria. Colonic strictures (fibrosing colonopathy) have been seen in children with cystic fibrosis receiving high doses of pancreatic enzyme preparations containing large amounts of lipases and proteases. This complication has not been reported in adults.

Treatment of Pain

Pain is the most common reason patients with chronic pancreatitis seek medical attention. Because alcohol abuse is the most common cause of chronic pancreatitis, the psychological issues of dependency can make pain difficult to quantify and treat. Thus both physiologic and psychological approaches need to be used.

Amman and coworkers previously suggested that progressive glandular insufficiency and calcification would lead to burn-out of the pancreas and relief of the pain. However, no timeline for this has been established. Layer and associates looked at 315 patients observed for a median of 12 years and discovered that 64% to 77% of patients with either idiopathic or alcoholic pancreatitis had a decrease in the severity and frequency of pain. However, the decrease in pain was independent of calcification and exocrine or endocrine insufficiency. Spontaneous remission of pain is variable and unreliable; therefore, it is not a realistic option for most patients.

The medical palliation of pain utilizes analgesics of various classes. Because treatment is likely to be a long-term endeavor, narcotics must be used judiciously to prevent addiction. When narcotics must be used, long-acting agents should be chosen over short-acting drugs such as those frequently used in the treatment of postoperative pain or traumatic injury. Nonopioid analgesics that inhibit the production of prostaglandins by blocking the cyclooxygenase pathway should be a mainstay of therapy. Tramadol (Ultram) inhibits norepinepherine and serotonin re-uptake, and also has mild opioid receptor affinity. It is being currently studied due to its effectiveness in other chronic pain states. Antidepressants may be helpful adjuncts to opioid and non-opioid analgesics because they potentiate the effective concentrations of catecholamines and serotonin.

Medical treatment relies not only on analgesics, but also attempts to ameliorate pain by suppression of pancreatic secretions. Oral pancreatic enzymes are a mainstay of therapy. Not only do they help digest food in those patients with exocrine insufficiency, the orally administered enzymes cause a decrease in pancreatic secretion by negative feedback inhibition. The mechanism is indirect and is based on the denaturation of cholecystokinin, a potent stimulus for acinar secretion, in the duodenum. By administering oral pancreatic enzymes there is more complete denaturation of cholecystokinin, resulting in diminished secretion and therefore pain. Although diminished protein secretion may improve pain control, reducing bicarbonate secretion in the pancreatic duct by using octreotide has not proven to be efficacious.

Gastric acid suppression is also an important component of medical therapy. By blocking gastric acid secretion the duodenal pH is increased, reducing the stimulus for pancreatic secretion, which in theory should decrease pain. Furthermore, many pancreatic enzyme replacement preparations are inactivated at acid pH. For the enzyme replacement therapy to be effective, the enzymes must survive transit through the stomach to the duodenum and hence acid neutralization is important.

Recently there has been interest in antioxidant therapy. Experimental studies have implicated free radicals in the inflammatory process of chronic pancreatitis. Thus treatment using allopurinol (Zyloprim)* or a combination of selenium,* β-carotene,* vitamin E,* vitamin C,* and methionine* has been proposed. Antioxidants (selenium; vitamin A, C, E; and methionine) are benign and inexpensive, and can, for some patients, ameliorate the attacks of pancreatitis and pain.

Nerve Block

The pain pathway involves transmission of nociceptive information from the visceral afferent nerves. This information travels through the splanchnic nerves, the sympathetic nervous system (celiac plexus), the spinal cord, and, ultimately, to the brain. Therefore there are ample opportunities to disrupt transmission of nerve impulses either at the level of the celiac ganglion or splanchnic nerves. The appeal of these procedures is that they do not remove parenchyma and generally are perceived as less invasive than surgical procedures. The complication rates are low, but the efficacy seems to vary from one center to the next.

A celiac plexus block is performed by injecting a neurolytic agent (50% alcohol or 6% phenol), a local anesthetic (lidocaine or bupivacaine) or a depot of corticosteroid (methylprednisolone or triamcinolone) in proximity to the celiac plexus. A celiac plexus block is usually performed percutaneously with radiographic guidance to direct the needle anterior to the first lumbar vertebral body. Side effects of celiac plexus block include orthostatic hypotension, bowel hypermotility, or rare neurologic deficits due to spread of neurolytic solution. Neurolytic celiac plexus block usually provides short-term analgesia (weeks to months) in most patients, but long-term relief requires repeated procedures. There seems to be diminishing efficacy with each repeated procedure.

Thoracoscopic splanchnicectomy interrupts the splanchnic nerves to relieve pain due to chronic pancreatitis or pancreatic cancer. Sensory nerves from the pancreas run along the hepatic, splenic, and superior mesenteric arteries to the semilunar ganglion where they are incorporated in the greater and lesser splanchnic nerves (5th–11th ganglia on either side of the vertebra). This has little if any deleterious effect on GI tract function because parasympathetic innervation is supplied by the vagus nerves. Although the celiac plexus can be blocked percutaneously in an awake patient, thoracoscopic splanchnicectomy requires general anesthesia and involves a relatively simple surgical procedure. Using video-assisted thoracoscopy, the surgeon identifies the greater splanchnic nerves in the chest and transects them. Ihse and associates studied 44 patients, 21 with chronic pancreatitis and 23 with pancreatic cancer who underwent bilateral thoracoscopic splanchnicectomy for pain. Postoperatively a visual analogue scale was used, and consumption of narcotics was documented. Patients' pain scores were reduced by greater than 50%, with continued pain relief at 42 weeks. There were no signs of impaired pancreatic function when analyzed by the secretin test, insulin levels, and C peptide levels. There was a 9% postoperative minor complication rate related to bleeding from a vessel near the splanchnicectomy site or from a port site.

Endoscopic Treatment of Pain

There are very few circumstances in which endoscopic modalities should be used to treat pain caused by chronic pancreatitis. When the pancreatic duct is obstructed by stones proximal to a dominant stricture, extracorporeal shockwave lithotripsy can be used to fragment the calculi. It is then necessary to place a stent in the pancreatic duct traversing the stricture to allow egress of the stone fragments. Because pseudocysts are common in chronic pancreatitis, it is tempting to perform endoscopic cystogastrostomy or cystoduodenostomy with the hope of providing pain relief. However, most pseudocysts arising in the setting of chronic pancreatitis are small and asymptomatic. When the pseudocyst appears to be compressing the common bile duct, one must exclude a distal stricture before proceeding with decompression. Strictures of the pancreatic duct and bile duct are chronic in nature and do not respond well to long-term indwelling stents. Because these procedures risk introducing infection into the ductal system, and their benefits are questionable, they should be used judiciously.

Surgical Management of Pain

Intractable pain is the most common indication for surgical therapy. If pain control requires the continuous use of narcotics, investigations should be undertaken to identify if a surgically correctable lesion is present. When found, an operation should be offered to the patient before the development of narcotic dependence. Surgically correctable lesions are a focal inflammatory mass, usually in the head of the gland, and a dilated pancreatic duct. These may exist in isolation or in combination with other complications of chronic pancreatitis such as biliary or duodenal obstruction. Other indications for surgery include the inability to exclude pancreatic malignancy, pseudocyst, internal and external pancreatic fistulas, and splenic vein thrombosis (Table 3).

Surgical options include decompression/drainage procedures, denervation procedures, or pancreatic resections. Most recent series quote a 0% to 3% operative mortality rate. Decompressive procedures are easier to perform but seem to have a lower long-term success rate than resections of the head of the

*Not FDA approved for this indication.

TABLE 3. **Indications for Surgical Intervention in Patients With Chronic Pancreatitis**

Intractable pain (i.e., narcotic addiction of frequent relapses)
- Dilated pancreatic duct
- Mass in pancreatic head

Suspicion of malignancy
Complications of chronic pancreatitis
- Symptomatic pancreatic pseudocyst
- Internal fistulas
  - Pancreatic ascites
  - Pancreaticopleural fistulas
- Biliary or duodenal obstruction
- Infection

Splenic vein thrombosis

pancreas. However, the patient groups are often not comparable and there have been no good prospective randomized controlled trials comparing drainage versus resection (Table 4).

Decompression/Drainage Procedures

The first drainage procedure was proposed in the 1950s by DuVal. The operation included both a transduodenal sphincteroplasty and caudal pancreaticojejunostomy. The success rate has proved to be very low and this procedure is of only historical interest. In 1958 Peustow and Gillesby described a lateral pancreaticojejunostomy, which was later modified by Partington and Rochelle in 1960. The Partington-Rochelle modification of the Peustow procedure is the most commonly performed operation for chronic pancreatitis. The presumption is that when the pancreatic duct is dilated to greater than 5 to 6 mm, duct pressures are abnormally high, resulting in pain and further duct dilation. Therefore, opening the pancreatic duct longitudinally and decompressing it into the jejunum should lower intraductal pressure and relieve pain (Figure 1). We prefer to perform this operation when the duct diameter is greater than 7 mm because it is a safe operation, with good results, that does not further compromise pancreatic exocrine and endocrine function. Over the past 8 years, 39 of 134 (29%) patients at Massachusetts General Hospital undergoing surgical intervention received a lateral pancreaticojejunostomy. The average duration of chronic pancreatitis before surgery was 8.3 years.

TABLE 4. **Choosing a Surgical Procedure in Chronic Pancreatitis**

Peustow procedure if:
- Pancreatic duct dilated >7 mm
- ±Pseudocysts
- ±Dilated bile duct

Distal pancreatectomy only if:
- Inflammation confined to the tail
- Normal right-sided pancreas at laparotomy
- Isolated ductal stricture in body or tail

Pancreaticoduodenectomy (or variant) if:
- Mass in head of pancreas
- ±Dilated or non-dilated pancreatic duct
- ±Dilated bile duct

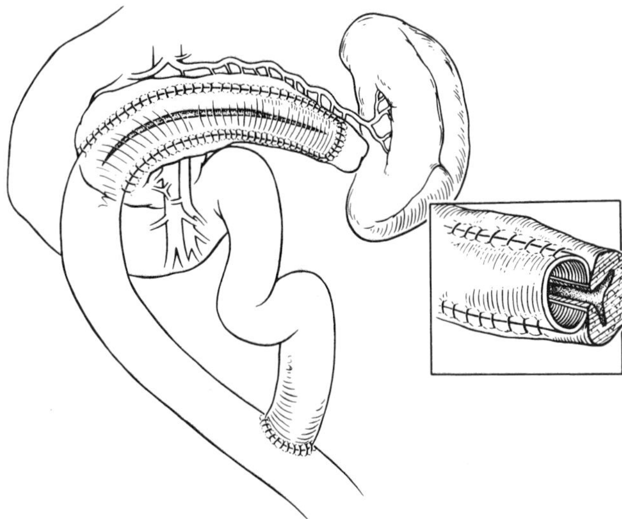

Figure 1. The Puestow procedure is a lateral pancreaticojejunostomy designed to decompress a dilated pancreatic duct. For optimal results, the diameter of the main pancreatic duct should be greater than 7 mm and the duct should be widely opened from the tail of the gland to the right of the gastroduodenal artery. (From Eckhauser FE, Turcotte JG: Current trends and new developments in chronic pancreatitis. In Zuidema GD [ed]: Shackelford's Surgery of the Alimentary Tract, 4th ed. Philadelphia, WB Saunders, 1996.)

Follow-up was available in 34 of the 39 patients (87%), for an average duration of 54 months. Good results were seen in 50% of the patients, and 24% and 26%, respectively, had fair and poor results. Of the nine patients with poor results, three had subsequent pancreatic resections and one was found to have pancreatic cancer and the other two were improved. In a separate study by the Massachusetts General Hospital group, 10 of 14 patients with failed Peustow procedures underwent a subsequent Whipple resection of the pancreatic head, with fair or good relief of pain.

Pancreatic Resection

Pancreaticoduodenectomy (Whipple procedure) is a very effective procedure to relieve pain in properly selected patients. The head of the pancreas is often the pacemaker of the disease process. Inflammatory pseudotumors often obstruct the pancreatic and biliary ducts and may cause duodenal narrowing. Hence surgical therapy directed at this region affords the opportunity to relieve both pain and obstruction as well as exclude malignancy. The procedure is technically more demanding than drainage procedures, but in experienced centers the mortality rate is extremely low. There is a higher potential for late morbidity due to exocrine and endocrine insufficiency because a pancreaticoduodenectomy removes approximately 40% of the pancreatic parenchyma. In a series from the Mayo Clinic, the mean time to onset of postoperative diabetes mellitus was 4.7 years in patients who were not diabetic preoperatively. Postoperative exocrine insufficiency manifested as steatorrhea was seen in 43% of patients. However, endocrine and exocrine insufficiency often develop in the absence of any surgical resection as a part of the natural course of the disease, so it is difficult to ascribe these complications solely to surgical resection. In patients without a dilated pancreatic duct, pancreaticoduodenectomy (PD) or one of its modifications is the procedure of choice.

The Mayo Clinic retrospectively reviewed the long-term results of PD for head-dominant, small duct chronic pancreatitis in 105 patients. All patients had failed medical management, including oral pancreatic enzymes, pancreatic stents, or chemical splanchnicectomy. Complete (67%) or substantial pain relief was achieved in 89% of patients for a mean follow-up period of 6.6 years. The mean duration of pain before surgery was 3.3 years, and patients who had a longer duration of symptoms were more likely to have unsatisfactory results. In another study, the Massachusetts General Hospital group performed 72 PDs for patients with chronic pancreatitis and intractable pain. Follow-up results were available in 90% of patients, over an average of 41 months. Good results were seen in 65% of patients. Lack of improvement of pain was seen in 23 of the 72 patients (32%), 6 of whom underwent completion pancreatectomy within a year of surgery.

The major objection to PD has been nutritional complications caused by loss of the duodenum and gastric antrum. Therefore several variations of PD have been devised to maintain GI tract continuity. Longmire and Traverso described the pylorus-preserving pancreaticoduodenectomy (PPPD) (Figure 2). This variation preserves the antrum and duodenal bulb with the intent of avoiding the dumping syndrome. We recently compared PD and PPPD at Massachusetts General Hospital to see if the purported advantages were realized. Delayed gastric emptying was seen in 33% of the PPPD group and in only 12% of the PD group (patients having the standard Whipple procedure have an antrectomy). Six months following surgery there was no difference in nutritional indices, need for pancreatic enzyme replacement, new onset diabetes mellitus, or pain relief. In the PPPD group there was a slightly higher, although not statistically significant, incidence of peptic ulcer and GI bleeding, and there was one patient with dumping and biliary gastritis in the antrectomy group. Hence we do not think that PPPD offers any advantage over standard PD.

Beger took the work of Longmire and Traverso a step further and devised a duodenum-preserving resection of the head of the pancreas. In this operation the pancreas is divided at its neck, and all of the head is removed except for the small portion of pancreas between the common bile duct and the medial wall of the duodenum. A Roux-en-Y loop is created and the end is sewn to the distal pancreas, while the remnant of the head is sewn to a proximal portion of the limb (Figure 3). Beger reported that 80% of his patients have had complete pain relief. Furthermore, he reports improved long-term survival compared with historical controls undergoing drainage procedures and standard PD. Although many European centers have adopted this procedure, it is not as popular in the United States. Some American surgeons have adopted the Frey procedure, which can be thought of as an intermediate step between the Peustow procedure and the Beger procedure. It combines a lateral pancreaticojejunostomy with limited resection of the pancreatic head leaving the gastroduodenal passage and common bile duct intact. In a highly selected series, approximately 87% of patients had relief of their pain at 37 months.

Some patients have predominantly left-sided inflammation. In specific circumstances, resection of the tail of the pancreas can be very effective. These

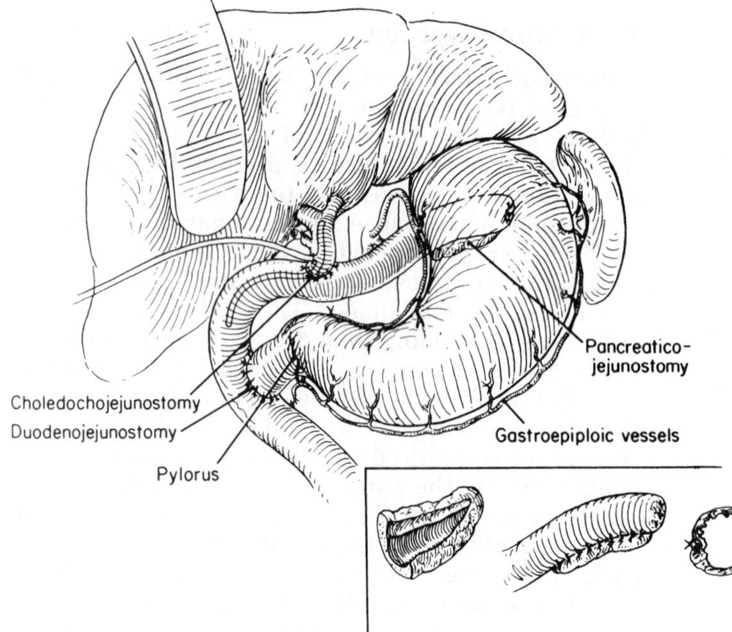

Figure 2. The pylorus-preserving pancreaticoduodenectomy does not include resection of the gastric antrum. In spite of the preservation of the distal stomach, most studies have failed to demonstrate a nutritional or functional benefit when compared to the classic Whipple procedure. (From Eckhauser FE, Turcotte JG: Current trends and new developments in chronic pancreatitis. In Zuidema GD [ed]: Shackelford's Surgery of the Alimentary Tract, 4th ed. Philadelphia, WB Saunders, 1996.)

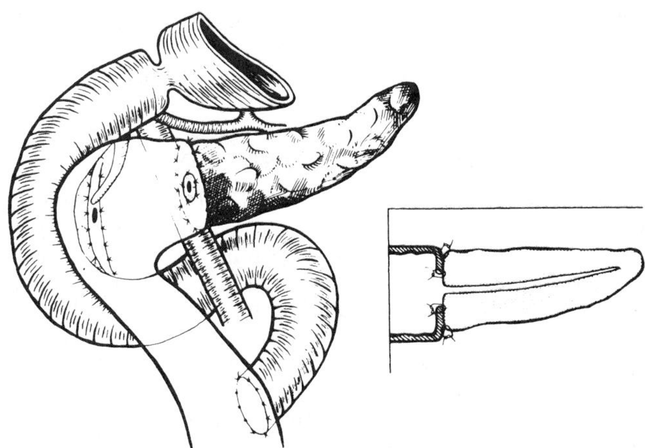

Figure 3. Duodenum-preserving resection of the pancreatic head, first described by Beger, is a popular operation for chronic pancreatitis in Europe, but it has not been widely adopted in the United States. It is purported to maintain better nutritional status than pancreaticoduodenectomy. (From Eckhauser FE, Turcotte JG: Current trends and new developments in chronic pancreatitis. In Zuidema GD [ed]: Shackelford's Surgery of the Alimentary Tract, 4th ed. Philadelphia, WB Saunders, 1996.)

include patients with a mid-duct stricture or a pseudocyst of the tail of the gland. In the absence of these anatomic findings, the results of distal pancreatectomy may be disappointing. In a recent study 20 patients underwent distal pancreatectomy for chronic pancreatitis involving primarily the tail of the pancreas. Of the 20 patients, 11 had good results, 3 had fair results, and 6 had poor results. There was no significant difference in outcomes based on age, alcohol history, prior pancreatic surgery, or preoperative narcotic use. The presence of a pseudocyst in the tail of the pancreas or complete occlusion of the mid-pancreatic duct with a history of surgical trauma or necrotizing pancreatitis were the main factors associated with successful relief of pain. Based on this study, distal pancreatectomy has a limited role in the management of pain secondary to chronic pancreatitis.

Total pancreatectomy should be performed only in patients who have had a failed segmental resection for chronic pancreatitis. The sequelae, including insulin-dependent diabetes mellitus and impaired GI function, are difficult to treat in patients who are often noncompliant. In some patients, abdominal pain persists even though there is no pancreatic parenchyma remaining.

OTHER COMPLICATIONS OF CHRONIC PANCREATITIS

Pancreatic Ascites and Pancreaticopleural Fistulas

Pancreatic pseudocysts are seen in 10% of patients with chronic pancreatitis. Although small cysts are usually asymptomatic, large cysts may cause symptoms by mass effect, erosion into adjacent structures, or rupture. Symptomatic pseudocyst should be treated by internal drainage procedures. Endoscopic cystogastrostomy and cystoduodenostomy should be performed only by experienced interventional gastroenterologists. Surgical drainage procedures are extremely safe and associated with excellent long-term results. Pseudocysts developing in conjunction with a dilated pancreatic duct afford the opportunity to drain both the pseudocyst and duct using the Peustow procedure with anticipation of long-term pain relief.

When chronic pancreatic pseudocysts rupture, pancreatic juice leaks either into the peritoneal cavity or retroperitoneum. Pancreatic ascites results from an anterior pancreatic duct disruption. Patients present with painless massive ascites, which may initially be confused with ascites due to cirrhosis. Paracentesis results that reveal fluid high in amylase and in albumin are usually diagnostic. Pancreaticopleural fistula is less common than pancreatic ascites. It results from posterior disruption of the pancreatic duct into the retroperitoneal space. The pancreatic juice tracks cephalad into the mediastinum and pleural space, resulting in a large pleural effusion, usually on the left side. Patients present with dyspnea or cough and the diagnosis is easily made by identifying elevated levels of amylase in the pleural fluid.

Due to the similar pathophysiology of pancreatic ascites and pancreaticopleural fistula, their management follows a similar algorithm. Initially, pancreatic secretion should be suppressed by administering octreotide and giving the patient nothing by mouth. Total parenteral nutrition is generally necessary for several weeks because these patients tend to be nutritionally depleted secondary to the large protein losses from the fistula. In patients with a pancreaticopleural fistula, a chest tube should be placed to drain the effusion and allow re-expansion of the lung. Furthermore the chest tube output allows monitoring of the fistula output to gauge the success of therapy. In patients with pancreatic ascites, large volume paracentesis should be performed. Medical therapy is successful in about 50% of patients. Patients who fail to resolve with 2 weeks of medical therapy should be considered for surgical closure of the fistula. Before surgery, it is useful to define the origin of the fistula. ERCP and CT are most commonly used to delineate the anatomy of the fistula; however, these tests are unnecessary if surgery is not being contemplated. If there is a distal duct disruption in the tail of the gland a distal pancreatectomy is usually performed. For more proximal duct disruptions a Roux-en-Y pancreaticojejunostomy is preferred because it preserves pancreatic parenchyma. It is also possible to place a pancreatic stent across the site of duct rupture endoscopically in some cases and allow healing to occur over the stent.

Biliary Obstruction

Approximately 3 cm of common bile duct passes through the pancreas, making it vulnerable to stricture or compression by pancreatic fibrosis, inflammation, or pseudocyst. The manifestations of periductal fibrosis are quite variable, ranging from asymptomatic bile duct dilation to jaundice and, rarely, cholangitis. Asymptomatic biliary dilation can often be observed if the patient is not jaundiced. However, monitoring these patients should include periodic measurement of serum alkaline phosphatase. Patients with greater than twofold elevation of alkaline phosphatase are at risk for the development of secondary biliary cirrhosis. Therefore patients with dilated bile ducts and a twofold elevation of alkaline phosphatase should have obstruction relieved. Treatment options include endoprosthesis, a biliary enteric bypass, or a pancreaticoduodenectomy. Endoprosthesis includes plastic stents and self-expanding metal stents. Barthet and associates treated 19 patients with 9-French to 12-French plastic stents, which were replaced every 4 months. After 10 months, only 10% had a complete response and 31% had no response. Deviere and associates achieved better results by placing 34-mm self-expanding metal stents in 20 patients with chronic pancreatitis–associated biliary strictures. After 33 months, 90% of patients had no further problems and 10% of patients developed stent occlusion due to epithelial hyperplasia. In the long run, however, most of these stents can be expected to occlude and therefore surgical decompression is the optimal choice for patients with a reasonable life expectancy. For isolated biliary obstruction, a simple choledochoduodenostomy will provide long-term relief, whereas more complex patients (i.e., mass in the pancreatic head and/or dilated pancreatic and biliary duct) may benefit from a more extensive surgical procedure.

GASTROESOPHAGEAL REFLUX DISEASE

method of
JOHN E. PANDOLFINO, M.D., and
PETER J. KAHRILAS, M.D.
Northwestern University Medical School
Chicago, Illinois

Gastroesophageal reflux disease (GERD) encompasses all clinical disorders resultant from gastroesophageal reflux. The clinical presentation may take the form of *reflux esophagitis* (visible lesions in the esophageal mucosa) or *endoscopy-negative GERD,* in which patients have reflux symptoms but no endoscopic esophagitis. The symptom burden that differentiates GERD from episodic heartburn is two or more episodes per week based on quality of life analyses. A U.S. survey found that 7% of adults experienced heartburn daily, 14% weekly, and 15% monthly.

Reflux disease is equally prevalent in both genders; however, there is a male preponderance of esophagitis (2:1–3:1) and of Barrett metaplasia (10:1). All forms of GERD affect whites more frequently than other races. Although it is established that peptic ulcer disease is linked to chronic *Helicobacter pylori* infections, this is *not* true of GERD. In fact, epidemiologic data reveal that GERD patients with esophagitis are *less* likely to harbor an *H. pylori* infection and recurrent esophagitis is *not* prevented by *H. pylori* eradication.

CLINICAL MANIFESTATIONS

The most common symptoms of GERD are heartburn, regurgitation, and dysphagia. Heartburn is a discomfort or burning sensation behind the sternum arising from the epigastrium and radiating upward. Heartburn is most commonly experienced within 60 minutes of eating, during exercise, and while lying recumbent. Regurgitation is the effortless return of esophageal or gastric contents into the pharynx without nausea or retching. Patients note a sour or burning fluid in the throat that may also contain food particles. Bending, belching, or maneuvers that increase intra-abdominal pressure can produce regurgitation. Dysphagia is also common with GERD, potentially caused by a stricture, impaired peristalsis, or simply by mucosal inflammation. Less common symptoms of reflux disease include water brash, globus sensation, and odynophagia.

Extraesophageal manifestations of GERD, encompassing a spectrum of pulmonary and otolaryngologic disorders, may be the primary (or only) manifestation. The implicated syndromes include posterior laryngitis, asthma, chronic cough, recurrent pneumonitis, chronic hoarseness, chest pain, pharyngitis, sinusitis, and dental erosions. Proposed mechanisms to explain how acid reflux causes extraesophageal syndromes include both direct irritation from regurgitation/aspiration and indirectly through esophagopulmonary/laryngeal reflexes.

COMPLICATIONS AND NATURAL HISTORY

Patients presenting with GERD typically report preexisting symptoms for 1 to 3 years. No consistent disease progression or correlation between symptom severity and disease severity is evident. With respect to esophagitis, especially severe esophagitis, the majority of cases are chronic and relapsing. After healing with medical therapy, recurrence can be anticipated in approximately 80% of patients, most within 3 months of discontinuing therapy.

Mortality associated with GERD (other than adenocarcinoma) is minimal, with estimates of 0.1 per 100,000 being typical. The prevalence of peptic stricture in patients with esophagitis ranges from 8% to 20% and that of ulceration is 5%, but recent data suggest that this is decreasing, most likely because of widespread use of proton pump inhibitors. Significant bleeding is uncommon, occurring in less than 2% of patients, and perforation is extremely rare.

The most severe histologic consequence of GERD is Barrett metaplasia with the associated risk of esophageal adenocarcinoma. The incidence of this cancer is rapidly increasing in Western societies, although it is still relatively rare. There were an estimated 5500 new cases in the United States in the year 2000, 90% of whom were white males. The prevalence of long-segment Barrett metaplasia in patients undergoing upper gastrointestinal endoscopy (a clearly identifiable risk for adenocarcinoma) is approximately 1%, and the prevalence increases as GERD becomes more severe. The average age of affected patients ranges from 55 to 65 years with a male:female ratio of 10:1 and a white:black ratio of 10:1.

PATHOPHYSIOLOGY

The pathophysiology of GERD is related to the balance between factors tending to erode the esophageal epithelium and those that preserve it. Esophagitis occurs when the constituents of acid reflux overwhelm esophageal acid clearance mechanisms and mucosal resistance. Reflux episodes are normally prevented by a physiologic barrier at the esophagogastric junction that can be compromised by transient lower esophageal sphincter relaxations, lower esophageal sphincter hypotension, or anatomic disruption secondary to hiatal hernia. Once reflux occurs, esophageal pH is restored by peristalsis and the buffering action of salivary bicarbonate. Acid clearance can be impaired by peristaltic dysfunction and/or hiatal hernia, both of which are common with esophagitis.

DIAGNOSTIC EVALUATION

The history is usually sufficient to diagnose GERD and institute appropriate treatment. Diagnostic studies are indicated when symptoms or response to therapy are atypical, when chronic heartburn raises the possibility of Barrett metaplasia, or when the so-called warning signs of dysphagia, odynophagia, gastrointestinal bleeding, or weight loss are present. Endoscopy should be the first diagnostic test because it provides a means for detecting esophagitis, managing complications, and excluding other diseases. However, only 30% to 40% of patients with GERD have esophagitis. Ambulatory 24-hour esophageal pH monitoring can be useful in this context. The principal indications for pH monitoring are to document excessive acid reflux in a patient without esophagitis or to evaluate the efficacy of medical or surgical treatment.

An alternative management strategy for a patient with suspected GERD is an empirical trial of proton pump inhibitor therapy. Although this is a very pragmatic approach to identifying patients with acid-related symptoms, it is impossible to attach a sensitivity or specificity to such a strategy in the absence of a gold standard for the diagnosis of GERD. Furthermore, empirical treatment may be associated with false-positive results by masking the symptoms of peptic ulcer disease or malignancy, and there is a failure to diagnose Barrett metaplasia.

TREATMENT

Of the estimated 36% of the adult U.S. population who suffer from occasional heartburn, few seek medical care. Consequently, as many as 27% of adult Americans take antacids at least twice a month and most of these are reflux sufferers. Along with antacids, nonprescription therapy for GERD often includes lifestyle modifications and on-demand use of over-the-counter histamine-2 (H_2) receptor antagonists. Lifestyle modifications include head-of-the-bed elevation, avoidance of tight-fitting garments, weight loss, dietary modification, restriction of alcohol, reduced coffee consumption, and elimination of smoking. These interventions are aimed at enhancing esophageal acid clearance, minimizing the occurrence of acid reflux, or both. Dietary modifications affecting GERD may be related to the type of food, the timing of meals, and the size of meals. Many foods such as chocolate and fried food have been shown to decrease lower esophageal sphincter pressure, and these should be avoided in individuals *in whom these foods cause heartburn.* Patients should also avoid assuming a supine position after meals and should not eat within 3 hours of bedtime. In general, minimal data exist on the efficacy of these nonpharmacologic therapies for GERD, making it unlikely that they will suffice for more than mild GERD cases.

Prescription Therapy

Despite the fact that hypersecretion of acid is rare in GERD, the most common and effective treatment of GERD is suppression of acid secretion with either H_2 receptor antagonists or proton pump inhibitors. The object of these therapies is to raise the intragastric pH above 4 during the periods of the day that reflux is likely to occur. The more extreme an individual's esophageal acid exposure, the greater the degree of acid suppression required.

There are four H_2 receptor antagonists (cimetidine [Tagamet], ranitidine [Zantac], famotidine [Pepcid], and nizatidine [Axid]) and five proton pump inhibitors (omeprazole [Prilosec], lansoprazole [Prevacid], rabeprazole [AcipHex], pantoprazole [Protonix], and esomeprazole*) currently in clinical use. The efficacy of H_2 receptor antagonists is limited by the rapid development of tachyphylaxis and the inability to effectively suppress meal-related acid secretion. Proton pump inhibitors suppress acid much more effectively than any dose of H_2 receptor antagonist because they act on the final common pathway of acid secretion rather than on one of the three classes of membrane receptors (histamine, acetylcholine, gastrin) as in the case of the H_2 receptor antagonists. This improved acid control also translates into improved clinical benefit; in a major therapeutic trial, all of the patients with refractory esophagitis were healed during 20 weeks of therapy with omeprazole, 40 to 60 mg/d.

Prokinetics

An ideal therapy for GERD would target the pathophysiologic abnormalities, obviating the need for acid suppression. Most recently, metoclopramide and cisapride have been used, but their utility is limited by associated side effects. Up to 25% of patients taking metoclopramide (Reglan) experience central nervous system side effects such as tremor, Parkinsonism, depression, or tardive dyskinesia. The clinical use of cisapride (Propulsid)† has been curtailed owing to its cardiotoxic effects, especially when used in combination with agents that are metabolized by the cytochrome P450 system. Prolongation of the QT interval, ventricular arrhythmia, and death have been reported.

Maintenance Therapy

Because esophagitis relapses, maintenance therapy is often necessary. Current evidence suggests that maintenance therapy with H_2 receptor antagonists is significantly less effective than that with

*Investigational drug in the United States.

†Not available in the United States.

proton pump inhibitors. A randomized prospective study on 175 patients with esophagitis healed with omeprazole revealed that remission was maintained for 12 months in 49% of the ranitidine group versus 80% of the omeprazole group. Very few data support the use of step-down therapy for maintenance treatment in esophagitis initially shown to require proton pump inhibitor therapy. In a large clinical study of 230 refractory esophagitis patients undergoing maintenance therapy with omeprazole for a mean period of 6.5 years, despite sporadic increases and decreases in the omeprazole dose for individual patients, the median dose required to maintain remission was at or near the healing dose.

As maintenance therapy has become the rule rather than the exception in GERD patients, drug safety becomes an important issue. For short-term use, proton pump inhibitors are quite safe, although they stimulate the cytochrome P450 system, sometimes necessitating dosage adjustment of warfarin (Coumadin), phenytoin (Dilantin), and diazepam (Valium). The most common side effects are headache (<5%) and diarrhea (<5%), both of which are reversible with cessation of therapy. Two safety issues raised regarding long-term treatment with proton pump inhibitors are the induction of hypergastrinemia with the potential occurrence of gastric carcinoid tumors and the occurrence of gastric atrophy associated with concomitant *H. pylori* infection. Currently, there is no evidence to suggest that long-term treatment is associated with any form of gastric malignancy or any significant difference in gastric histology in patients with or without *H. pylori* gastritis.

Nonerosive Gastroesophageal Reflux Disease

Although few studies have assessed the efficacy of antireflux therapy in patients with nonerosive GERD, available evidence reveals a hierarchy of efficacy for symptom control similar to that seen in esophagitis (proton pump inhibitors better than H_2 receptor antagonists). Furthermore, the data do not support the viewpoint that nonerosive GERD is more responsive to therapy than esophagitis. However, contrary to the observations on severe esophagitis, data on endoscopy-negative GERD support a less aggressive therapeutic approach to maintenance. More than half of nonerosive GERD patients maintained adequate symptom relief with on-demand therapy.

Antireflux Surgery

The most commonly performed surgical procedure for GERD is a laparoscopic Nissen fundoplication, which can produce excellent results in some hands. Unfortunately, although modern techniques have minimized risk, the nature of surgery is such that there will always be a finite mortality. In addition, fundoplication also has the potential to produce clinically significant dysphagia, bloating, and flatulence. Estimates of the frequency with which these complications occur vary among series, most of which are uncontrolled. How antireflux surgery compares with modern medical therapy is difficult to ascertain because there are currently no valid data comparing laparoscopic antireflux therapy with long-term proton pump inhibitor therapy. Thus, the decision to pursue medical or surgical therapy ultimately depends on a risk-benefit analysis that will usually favor medical therapy.

Summary of Management Principles

Most cases of GERD can be diagnosed on the basis of symptom assessment and empirical trials of antireflux medications, without resorting to diagnostic tests. Endoscopy should be performed if there is doubt regarding the diagnosis or when heartburn is extremely chronic (raising the possibility of Barrett metaplasia), refractory to treatment, or accompanied by the warning signs of dysphagia, odynophagia, gastrointestinal bleeding, or weight loss.

The need for pharmacologic therapy and the required doses are decided on the basis of symptom assessment (Table 1). Patients with intermittent mild GERD symptoms may be treated with nonprescription therapy and lifestyle modification. The most effective therapeutic agents for patients with esopha-

TABLE 1. **Hierarchy of Medical Therapies in the Management of Gastroesophageal Reflux Disease**

Therapy	Indication
Nonprescription therapy Lifestyle modification Over-the-counter antacids Over-the-counter histamine-2 receptor antagonists	Mild episodic GERD (heartburn less than twice a week)
Full-dose histamine-2 receptor antagonists Cimetidine, 400 mg bid Ranitidine, 150 mg bid Nizatidine, 150 mg bid Famotidine, 20 mg bid	Endoscopy-negative GERD in a cost-restrictive environment Intolerance of proton pump inhibitors
Full-dose proton pump inhibitors Omeprazole, 20 mg/d Lansoprazole, 30 mg/d Rabeprazole, 20 mg/d Pantoprazole, 40 mg/d Esomeprazole, 20–40 mg/d	Endoscopy-negative GERD Erosive esophagitis Inadequate response to lesser therapy
Twice-a-day proton pump inhibitors (full dose bid)	Patients not responding to daily full-dose therapy Patients initially diagnosed with severe erosive esophagitis
Increased dose proton pump inhibitors (more frequent dosing interval and/or higher dose depending on response pattern)	Refractory heartburn (positive pH study on therapy or failure to heal esophagitis with lesser therapies) Poorly responsive atypical symptoms

Abbreviation: GERD = gastroesophageal reflux disease.

gitis or nonerosive GERD are the proton pump inhibitors. These agents should be first-line therapy for most patients with reflux symptoms more than twice a week. Full-dose H_2 receptor antagonists may be substituted if cost is a major concern, but these agents are less effective than proton pump inhibitors and are ineffective in the setting of erosive esophagitis. When patients do not respond to full-dose proton pump inhibitor therapy, increasing the dose by using twice-a-day therapy is rational. Patients not responding to twice-a-day proton pump inhibitor therapy should be deemed refractory and reassessed with endoscopy and pH monitoring. Laparoscopic antireflux surgery is an alternative to maintenance therapy with proton pump inhibitors, but, in the absence of relevant trials comparing it with pharmacologic therapy, its place in the therapeutic algorithm remains controversial.

ACKNOWLEDGMENT

This work was supported by grant RO1 DC00646 (PJK) from the Public Health Service.

TUMORS OF THE STOMACH

method of
JAMES O. PARK, M.D., and
MITCHELL C. POSNER, M.D.
University of Chicago Hospitals
Chicago, Illinois

Gastric tumors can be classified as benign or malignant, with hyperplastic polyps and adenocarcinomas composing the overwhelming majority within each category. Benign gastric tumors are of little clinical significance, except for the necessity to distinguish them from malignant lesions. Although a wide variety of neoplastic entities may be encountered in the stomach, this review focuses on the more common and clinically pertinent tumors: adenomas, adenocarcinomas, lymphomas, carcinoid tumors, and stromal tumors.

ADENOMAS

Gastric polyps are divided into two categories based on their potential for malignant transformation: *hyperplastic* (no potential) and *adenomatous* (10%–25% risk). *Adenomas* are benign pedunculated or sessile lesions lined by dysplastic, pseudostratified epithelium. The peak incidence is in the fifth to seventh decades of life, with a high prevalence in patients with familial adenomatous polyposis or Gardner syndrome. Although adenomas can cause dyspepsia and hemorrhage, patients generally have few symptoms or physical findings, and a solitary, tubular or villous, antral lesion is usually found incidentally on barium study or endoscopy. Adenomas carry a distinct malignant potential that is proportional to size (significantly greater for polyps >2 cm), number, and degree of dysplasia. The presence of an adenoma also serves as a marker for increased risk of synchronous or metachronous carcinomas in the remaining gastric tissue.

Treatment

Adenomas are premalignant lesions that should be treated by polypectomy whenever clinically feasible. Pedunculated lesions are amenable to endoscopic removal, and this is sufficient therapy if no stalk invasion is found on histologic evaluation. Segmental resection is usually warranted for sessile lesions, or those with bleeding complications, and formal gastrectomy is recommended for invasive lesions, multiple polyposis, or multiple recurrent adenomas.

ADENOCARCINOMA

Incidence

Gastric adenocarcinoma, commonly referred to as *gastric carcinoma* or *stomach cancer,* accounts for 90% to 95% of all malignant tumors of the stomach. Worldwide, adenocarcinoma of the stomach remains the second most common cancer and cause of cancer death, with death rates measuring 50 to 78 per 100,000 in high-prevalence countries such as Costa Rica, Chile, Hungary, and Japan. The United States has seen a steady decrease in the incidence of gastric cancer over the past 6 decades, with intestinal-type antral tumors accounting for much of this decline. It is estimated that 13,400 men and 8,100 women in the United States alone were diagnosed with stomach cancer in 2000, with 7,600 men and 5,400 women dying of the disease.

The incidence and mortality increase with advancing age, with a peak incidence in the sixth to seventh decades. Higher rates of gastric cancer are observed in African, Asian, and Hispanic Americans and in lower socioeconomic groups. Studies of migrants from areas of high (Japan) to low (United States) risk suggest that environmental exposure in early life may influence the risk of developing gastric cancer but that other factors may continually affect the predisposition to cancer.

Types

Two distinct histologic subtypes of gastric cancer—intestinal and diffuse—are described by Lauren. *Intestinal-type tumors* have a glandular structure, arise from areas of gastric atrophy or intestinal metaplasia, occur more commonly in older men, and represent the dominant histologic type in regions with epidemics of stomach cancer, suggesting an environmental etiology. Ingestion of preserved foods containing nitrates and nitrites, cigarette smoking, and *Helicobacter pylori* infection are associated with an increased risk of developing intestinal-type cancer, whereas diets rich in fiber, beta carotene, and ascorbic acid are protective. A model for the pathogenesis of intestinal-type cancer proposes that chronic inflammation and atrophy of normal mucosa in association with hypochlorhydria or achlorhydria leads to subsequent bacterial overgrowth, resulting in chronic atrophic gastritis and free radical induced mucosal injury by bacterial conversion of nitrates and nitrites to nitrosamines. Continued epithelial injury can cause metaplasia, dysplasia, carcinoma in situ, and, ultimately, invasive carcinoma. Previous partial gastrectomy and vagotomy for benign conditions, pernicious anemia, Ménétrier disease, and familial polyposis all contribute to an increased risk through this model sequence.

Diffuse-type tumors are more widespread throughout the mucosa, do not typically arise from precancerous lesions, occur more frequently in younger women, and represent the major subtype in endemic areas with a familial occurrence, suggesting a genetic etiology. Although the overall decline in incidence of gastric cancer appears to reflect the reduction of the intestinal-type tumors, the diffuse subtype is seen with increasing frequency as the incidence of proximal gastric cancer has become more predominant in the past 15 to 20 years. This is a worrisome prospect because the diffuse-type lesions have a poorer prognosis stage for stage. Many other classifications based on gross morphology and histologic differentiation exist, although none are independent prognostic indicators (Table 1).

Clinical Manifestations

Most patients with gastric cancer present with advanced disease. This reflects the insidious nature of the disease and the fact that symptoms of early gastric cancer are vague and nonspecific. Patients may have anorexia with weight loss, nausea and vomiting, early satiety and dysphagia, or epigastric discomfort. These symptoms may mimic those of benign gastric ulcer disease and may be either ignored or treated medically without further evaluation. Dysphagia occurs with tumors in the cardia with extension through the gastroesophageal junction. Early satiety is indicative of diffusely infiltrative tumor with loss of gastric wall distensibility. Persistent vomiting can occur with antral tumors obstructing the pylorus. Approximately 10% of patients present with signs of disseminated disease, including supraclavicular (Virchow) or axillary (Irish) nodes; periumbilical (Sister Mary Joseph node), ovarian (Krukenburg tumor), or pelvic (Blumer shelf) metastasis; jaundice, hepatomegaly, or ascites.

TABLE 1. **Morphologic and Histologic Classifications of Gastric Adenocarcinoma**

Morphologic Categories
Fungating or polypoid
Ulcerating
Superficial spreading
Diffusely spreading (linitis plastica)
Borrmann Classification
Type I: circumscribed, polypoid
Type II: ulcerated with elevated borders
Type III: ulcerated, with partial infiltration
Type IV: diffusely infiltrative
Type V: unclassifiable
Ming Classification
Expanding-type tumors (favorable prognosis)
Infiltrative tumors (poor prognosis)
World Health Organization Histologic Classification
Tubular
Papillary
Mucinous
Signet-ring cell
Broder's Histologic Grade
I (well differentiated) to IV (anaplastic)

Diagnosis

A barium study or flexible upper endoscopy with tissue biopsy can be performed when gastric cancer is suspected. Double-contrast barium study is a sensitive, cost-effective test for detection of even small gastric lesions and is used for mass screening in Japan. Fiberoptic esophagogastroduodenoscopy is the diagnostic modality of choice for gastric cancer and should be performed in any patient with localized disease with anticipated surgical intervention. Accuracy of endoscopy is over 95% when biopsy samples are taken, and cytology obtained by fine-needle aspiration, lavage, or brushings yields a near 100% positive predictive value. Once a diagnosis is established, evaluation of the extent of disease involves clinical examination, routine blood tests (complete blood cell count, chemistries, liver profile), chest radiography, and abdominal and pelvic computed tomography. Endoscopic ultrasonography is a diagnostic adjunct that can provide highly accurate staging of the depth of primary tumor invasion and limited assessment of lymph node status. Laparoscopy and peritoneal lavage have been used as diagnostic tools to avoid open laparotomy and major resections in patients with disseminated disease not detectable by other modalities.

Staging

Depth of primary tumor penetration, presence of regional lymph node involvement, and spread to adjacent organs or distant sites remain the most important prognostic indicators for gastric cancer. Therefore, the American Joint Committee on Cancer (AJCC) staging classification, based on the TNM system, is currently used in the United States for staging of gastric cancer (Table 2). T stage has been demonstrated to be an independent prognostic indicator. *Early gastric cancer,* defined as disease confined to the mucosa or submucosa (Tis, T1) regardless of lymph node status, has a 5-year survival after resection of 70% to 95%, depending on the presence of nodal involvement. *Advanced gastric cancer* implies invasion of the muscularis propria, and these lesions are frequently associated with distant or contiguous spread, a higher stage, and poorer prognosis. Unfor-

TABLE 2. **American Joint Committee on Cancer Staging Classification for Gastric Adenocarcinoma**

Primary Tumor (T)

TX: Primary tumor cannot be assessed
T0: No evidence of primary tumor
Tis: Carcinoma in situ
T1: Invasion into lamina propria or submucosa
T2: Invasion into muscularis propria or subserosa
T3: Penetration of serosa without invasion of adjacent structures
T4: Invasion of adjacent structures

Regional Lymph Nodes (N)

The regional lymph nodes include perigastric nodes and nodes along the left gastric, common hepatic, splenic, and celiac arteries. Involvement of hepatoduodenal, retropancreatic, mesenteric, and para-aortic nodes is classified as distant metastasis.
NX: Regional lymph nodes cannot be assessed
N0: No regional lymph node metastasis
N1: 1–6 metastatic regional lymph nodes
N2: 7–15 metastatic regional lymph nodes
N3: >15 metastatic regional lymph nodes

Distant Metastasis (M)

MX: Distant metastasis cannot be assessed
M0: No distant metastasis
M1: Distant metastasis

AJCC Clinical Stage Groupings

Stage 0: TisN0M0
Stage IA: T1N0M0
Stage IB: T1N1M0, T2N0M0
Stage II: T1N2M0, T2N1M0, T3N0M0
Stage IIIA:T2N2M0, T3N1M0, T4NB0M0
Stage IIIB:T3N2M0
Stage IV: Any TN3M0, T4N1M0, T4N2M0, Any N, Any NM1

tunately, early gastric cancer represents only 10% to 15% of diagnosed cases in the United States. N stage is the single most significant determinant of recurrence and survival.

Treatment

Surgical resection remains the standard and only potentially curative therapy in localized gastric cancer. However, controversy persists regarding the extent of gastric resection (total versus subtotal gastrectomy), the extent of lymphadenectomy, and the role of adjuvant chemoradiotherapy. Retrospective Japanese series report survival rates of more than 95% with gastrectomy and perigastric lymphadenectomy for early gastric cancer. Gastric resection with regional lymphadenectomy is the treatment of choice for stage I, II, and III disease. Subtotal gastrectomy is the standard operative option for pyloric, antral, or body tumors. Subtotal resection provides survival equivalent to that of total gastrectomy if an adequate gross proximal margin is obtainable, with less associated morbidity. For proximal tumors involving the fundus or cardioesophageal junction, or for diffusely infiltrative lesions, total gastrectomy provides better functional results, with equivalent operative morbidity and mortality, when compared with proximal gastric resection. Standard regional lymphadenectomy involves removal of greater and lesser curvature perigastric lymph nodes.

Retrospective reports indicate that extended D2 lymphadenectomy for potentially curable gastric cancer can be performed safely, provides more staging information, and may result in improved survival compared with a more limited D1 resection. However, several more recent prospective randomized trials failed to demonstrate a survival advantage with D2 resections, bringing into question the therapeutic value of the routine application of D2 dissection. Routine prophylactic splenectomy is not advocated because it provides no survival benefit and leads to increased complications. Endoscopic treatment using cauterization, local injection, and laser therapy for protruding and depressed lesions without ulceration of less than 1 cm have been reported. Currently, these techniques are reserved for patients at high risk for conventional operations due to age or comorbidities. Dysphagia due to tumors of the cardia may be relieved by endoscopic destruction of the lesion obstructing the gastric inlet or by endoscopic placement of stents.

Results of a recent randomized intergroup trial demonstrated improved disease-free and overall survival in stage II and III cancer patients receiving postoperative adjuvant chemoradiation therapy. Preoperative induction chemoradiation therapy is under investigation. All patients with stage IV disease should be considered for clinical trials. Although neither cure nor prolongation of life is achieved with chemotherapy, substantial palliation and occasional durable remissions are possible in select patients. Palliative radiation therapy may also alleviate bleeding, pain, and obstruction. There is little benefit in performing palliative total gastrectomy in patients with metastatic disease, and this procedure should be reserved for patients with uncontrollable bleeding or obstruction. Because survival is poor with all available single and multimodal treatment strategies, patients with recurrent gastric cancer should be considered candidates for phase I and II clinical trials.

LYMPHOMA

Incidence

Lymphoma is the second most common gastric malignancy after gastric adenocarcinoma, constituting 3% to 5% of all malignant tumors of the stomach. More than 50% of patients with non-Hodgkin lymphoma have gastrointestinal (GI) involvement. The stomach is the most common extranodal site involved, accounting for more than half of all primary GI lymphomas. In the United States, the annual incidence is less than 1 in 100,000, although the numbers are increasing. More than 95% of gastric lymphomas are non-Hodgkin's lymphomas, and more than 90% are of intraepithelial B-cell origin, with 90% of the high-grade large cell type. Primary gastric lymphomas originate in the stomach without other solid organ or systemic involvement until very late in the disease, whereas secondary lymphomas are systemic nodal lymphomas with secondary gastric involvement. The peak incidence is in the sixth decade of life, with a male predominance of 1.7:1. A fivefold increased risk is seen in patients with AIDS.

Clinical Manifestations

Less than 20% of cases present asymptomatically; however, the signs and symptoms are often nonspecific and difficult to distinguish from those of gastric adenocarcinoma. Symptoms of systemic lymphoma, namely, weight loss, fever, and night sweats, can be present in up to 40%. Complications including bleeding, obstruction, perforation, and fistulization are not uncommon; and findings such as massive splenomegaly and palpable peripheral adenopathy may indicate diffuse lymphoma. Mucosa-associated lymphoid tissue (MALT) tumors are low-grade monoclonal B-cell variants noted in the setting of chronic gastritis that are associated with *H. pylori* infection, with more than 90% seropositivity. Reports suggest that antibiotic eradication of the *H. pylori* may lead to tumor regression.

Diagnosis

The diagnosis of primary gastric lymphoma can be confirmed after exclusion of palpable peripheral lymphadenopathy and hepatosplenomegaly on examination, an abnormal peripheral blood smear, mediastinal adenopathy on chest radiography, and systemic involvement on imaging studies. Gastric lymphoma is difficult to distinguish from adenocarcinoma by contrast radiography or even endoscopy. Radiographically, primary gastric lymphoma presents as ulcers, enlarged folds, or multiple nodules, whereas a diffusely infiltrating lesion with the appearance of linitis plastica is more suggestive of secondary lymphoma. Ten percent to 20% of patients have completely normal results of an upper GI series. Upper endoscopy with biopsy and cytologic evaluation, yielding an accuracy of nearly 90%, is usually required for diagnosis, although deep biopsies, occasionally full thickness, may be necessary. One distinguishing feature from adenocarcinoma is that peristalsis is often preserved in lymphoma.

Immunophenotyping by immunoperoxidase staining for lymphocyte markers may also be helpful in distinguishing malignant from benign disease. Endoscopic ultrasonography can define depth of tumor infiltration and abnormal perigastric lymph nodes with very high sensitivity and specificity and is a useful adjunct in diagnosis and staging. Computed tomography and magnetic resonance imaging are frequently used to detect distant metastases, including hepatic and splenic involvement.

Treatment

The Ann Arbor system is commonly used to stage primary gastric lymphoma (Table 3). Treatment of localized primary gastric lymphoma remains controversial because, unlike for other lymphocytic lymphomas, surgical resection has been traditionally recommended. For stage I and II disease limited to the stomach and regional nodes, attempted curative surgical resection followed by adjuvant radiation, chemotherapy, or both has been advocated. Postoperative radiation therapy for stage II disease has been shown to reduce local regional recurrence and improve 5-year survival. Therefore, radiation therapy has been advocated as an adjunct to surgery in patients with advanced but resectable disease, and combination chemotherapy and radiation therapy has been advocated in patients with unresectable disease or as second-line alternative therapy in poor surgical candidates.

TABLE 3. **Ann Arbor Staging System for Lymphoma**

Stage I: involvement of a single lymph node region (I) or a single localized extralymphatic site (IE)
Stage II: involvement of two or more lymph node regions on the same side of the diaphragm (II) or with localized involvement of a single associated extralymphatic site (IIE)
Stage III: involvement of lymph node regions on both sides of the diaphragm (III) or with localized involvement of an extralymphatic site (IIIE), the spleen (IIIS), or both (IIIS+E)
Stage IV: disease that is diffusely spread throughout an extranodal site
The stages can be subclassified into A and B categories; the B designation is given to patients with constitutional symptoms of weight loss, fever, and night sweats

Recent data suggest that nonoperative management with radiation and chemotherapy therapy alone may produce comparable outcomes to surgery in early stage primary gastric lymphoma with preservation of the stomach. The main theoretical disadvantage of radiation or chemotherapy as a primary treatment modality is increased GI complications, including bleeding or perforation, particularly in patients with advanced disease. However, these complications are rare. Patients with stage III and IV disease who present with complications of bleeding, obstruction, or perforation should also undergo attempted resection followed by adjuvant therapy. Patients without complications presenting with preoperative documentation of stage III or IV disease should be treated with radiation therapy and chemotherapy initially, and surgical resection should be reserved for persistent local disease of the stomach or for complications. For low-grade MALT lesions, data suggest that a trial of antibiotic eradication of *H. pylori* infection to induce regression of the tumor is warranted, although further follow-up is required to confirm its effectiveness.

CARCINOID TUMORS

Pathophysiology

Carcinoid tumors arise from enterochromaffin-like (ECL) cells of neural crest origin and are classified as neuroendocrine or amine precursor uptake and decarboxylation (APUD) tumors. Although carcinoid tumors constitute 55% of all gut endocrine tumors, merely 2% to 3% of carcinoid tumors are found in the stomach and account for only 0.3% of all gastric tumors. The peak incidence is in the sixth to seventh decades, with a slight male predilection. Gastric carcinoids have been found in association with long-standing conditions of hypergastrinemia, such as pernicious anemia, atrophic gastritis, and Zollinger-Ellison syndrome with multiple endocrine neoplasia syndrome type 1.

Histologically, solid nests of small monotonous cells with rare mitoses and acinar or rosette formation are found in these tumors, located in the glandular base or submucosa. The benign or malignant nature of carcinoid tumors cannot be determined histologically; only the presence of metastases or invasion of adjacent structures is a true indicator of malignancy. Many carcinoid tumors are slow-growing indolent tumors that can be treated and often cured, especially in early stages. The occurrence of metastasis from carcinoid tumor relates directly to the size of the primary tumor (lesions <1 cm rarely, whereas lesions >2 cm frequently metastasize). Even when carcinoid tumors are malignant, however, they may be compatible with long-term survival, with an average time from the onset of symptoms to death from the disease of 8 years. The 5-year survival for carcinoid tumors approaches 100% with noninvasive tumors less than 2 cm, 40% when the tumor diameter is more than 2 cm, and 20% to 40% with hepatic metastases.

Clinical Manifestations

Carcinoid tumors secrete a variety of neuroendocrine peptides such as serotonin (manifested by elevated urinary 5-hydroxyindoleacetic acid), prostaglandins, kallikreins, catecholamines, somatostatin, and gastrin. Gastric carcinoid tumors are usually asymptomatic; however, they may cause chronic, intermittent abdominal pain or bleeding, suggesting partial obstruction or intussusception. Malignant carcinoid tumors induce fibrosis, which by fibrous adhesions may cause mechanical obstruction even when the primary tumor is small. Diarrhea, weight loss, and a palpable abdominal mass may also be present. Patients with carcinoid tumor are at increased risk for synchronous or metachronous second noncarcinoid GI malignancies. Malignant carcinoid syndrome (flush, diarrhea, bronchoconstriction, cardiac valvular lesions, arthropathy, and telangiectasia) is encountered in less than 10% of patients with gastric carcinoid tumors.

Diagnosis

Endoscopy and biopsy are valuable for diagnosing primary gastric carcinoid tumors. Positive argentaffin and argyrophil stains suggest the carcinoid tumor, and neurosecretory granules seen on electron microscopy are confirmatory. Computed tomography is valuable for demonstrating the mesenteric fibrosis and can evaluate tumor extension in the mesentery, the retroperitoneal space, and the liver. Somatostatin receptor localization techniques, measurement of plasma substance P, neurotensin, neuron-specific enolase, and chromogranins may aid in the diagnosis.

Treatment

Resection is the standard curative modality of localized disease, although gastric carcinoids tend to be less localized than those in other GI sites. Gastric carcinoid tumors less than 1 cm may be amenable to endoscopic excision. If the primary tumor is localized and all visible disease is resectable, 5-year survival rates are 70% to 90%. However, long-term follow-up is warranted because late recurrences do occur. Even if the regional disease is deemed unresectable or distant metastases are present, the disease is usually indolent with median survivals of more than 2 years. Local complications, such as obstruction and intussusception, can be effectively palliated with either resection or bypass. In select patients with symptomatic hepatic lesions resection or hepatic artery infusion of chemotherapeutic agents, combined with embolization with collagen, Gelfoam or alcohol may provide palliation and decrease tumor bulk. The long-acting somatostatin analogue octreotide provides effective palliation in patients with carcinoid syndrome. Immunotherapy using low-dose interferon alfa has been described with limited efficacy in controlling flushing and diarrhea. The prognosis for patients with recurring or relapsing disease is poor, and these patients should be considered for clinical trials. Attempts at re-resection of slow-growing tumors recurring in any single site can reduce tumor volume and provide long-term palliation.

MESENCHYMAL TUMORS

Incidence

Tumors of mesenchymal origin account for 1% to 3% of all gastric malignancies. The median age at diagnosis is 55, with a slight male predominance.

Pathophysiology

These stromal tumors were previously designated as smooth muscle tumors or as leiomyomas and leiomyosarcomas owing to the muscle marker staining that was observed. Most have a spindle cell histology and are of mesenchymal origin. Based on characteristic findings seen on electron microscopy and the indistinct cell line of origin with varying differentiation patterns, the term *gastrointestinal stromal tumor* has been assigned to these tumors. Other less common tumors arising in the gastric mesenchyme include liposarcomas, fibrosarcomas, angiosarcomas, glomus tumors, and autonomic nerve tumors. Stromal tumors are indolent, slow-growing tumors found deep within the submucosa. Lesions smaller than 2 cm are generally clinically silent, whereas larger tumors have a tendency for ulceration and subsequent hemorrhage.

Clinical Manifestations and Diagnosis

Common symptoms include weight loss, abdominal pain, fullness, early satiety, GI bleeding, and abdominal mass. The initial diagnosis is by contrast radiography or endoscopy, followed by assessment of metastatic involvement of the liver and lung using liver profile, chest radiography, and computed tomography. These studies often demonstrate smooth, lobulated, intraluminal lesions or highly invasive ulcers that are extraluminal. They are usually located antrally (25%) or corporally (40%). Primary tumor size and depth of primary invasion are important prognostic factors, with lesions bigger than 5 cm in diameter having poorer survival. Mitotic index is the most reliable predictor of malignancy, and lesions with more than 10 mitotic figures per 10 high-power fields have increased risk of metastasis.

Treatment

Currently, there are no definitive guidelines for the management of stromal tumors, and many centers treat these tumors based on experience with other soft tissue sarcomas. Two thirds of the lesions are resectable at presentation. Complete resection with a grossly normal margin, using wedge resection for small lesions and formal gastrectomy for more involved lesions, is recommended. Routine regional lymphadenectomy is not indicated because lymph node metastases are rare except by direct extension and studies have not shown survival benefit. The 5-year survival rates vary from 80% for low-grade lesions to 32% for high-grade lesions after resection. Intra-abdominal recurrence is quite common, with high mitotic index lesions recurring in up to 90% of cases within 5 years. This propensity for recurrence has prompted evaluation of radiation and chemotherapeutic adjunctive regimens. Because of the slow-growing nature of these tumors, long-term follow-up is required, including frequent abdominal computed tomography and consideration of re-resection if deemed feasible.

TUMORS OF THE COLON AND RECTUM

method of
ALAN G. THORSON, M.D.
Creighton University School of Medicine and University of Nebraska College of Medicine
Omaha, Nebraska

Adenocarcinoma is the most common tumor of the colon and rectum. Other tumors, both benign and malignant, are relatively rare and together account for fewer than 5% of all colorectal tumors. These include but are not limited to carcinoid, neuroendocrine carcinoma, melanoma, squamous cell and adenosquamous carcinoma, lymphoma, the group of tumors known as gastrointestinal stromal tumors (leiomyoma, leiomyosarcoma), lipoma and liposarcoma, neurofibroma and other tumors of neural origin, endometriosis, colitis cystica profunda, and metastatic tumors. Because most tumors of the colon and rectum ultimately will present with bleeding, anemia, and/or features of bowel obstruction, the primary importance of being knowledgeable about these tumors lies in securing a proper diagnosis. A biopsy to confirm a histologic diagnosis is imperative to ensure appropriate treatment. The remainder of this discussion will focus on colorectal adenocarcinoma.

Adenocarcinoma represents the end result of the adenoma-carcinoma sequence. This well-documented pathway from adenomas (tubular, tubulovillous, and villous polyps) to adenocarcinoma is a slow process. It is generally accepted that on average it takes from 5 to 10 years for an adenoma to change into a carcinoma. This is the window of opportunity that we are afforded from which colorectal cancer (CRC) is best approached. The proper management of this long “dwell time” between the first onset of premalignant markers and the development of CRC makes CRC a truly preventable cancer and has earned it the name *the cancer no one needs to have.*

EPIDEMIOLOGY

CRC is the second leading cause of cancer death in the United States. Only carcinoma of the lung and bronchus is more deadly. It was estimated that in the United States in 2001 there would be 135,400 new cases of CRC and 56,700 deaths from CRC. This represents a lifetime risk of about 6% and translates into 1 of every 17 people having CRC at some point in their lifetime. Men have a slightly greater risk of rectal cancer and women have slightly greater risk of colon cancer. Overall, however, CRC is considered a gender-neutral cancer.

The risk for the average population begins rapidly accelerating following age 50 and peaks in the seventh and eighth decades. It is estimated that 5% to 10% of CRC is hereditary, another 10% to 15% familial, and roughly 80% sporadic. The current overall 5-year relative survival rate for CRC is approximately 60% for white men and women and 48% for black men and women. Mortality is low in Native Americans and high in native Alaskans. These differences may be partially but incompletely explained by differences in stage of disease at diagnosis, aggressiveness of therapy, and socioeconomic and cultural characteristics of the various groups.

ETIOLOGY

CRC results from a multifactorial process including genetic changes and environmental influences. The genetic alterations associated with CRC may be inherited or spontaneous. The two most prominent hereditary forms of CRC are familial adenomatous polyposis (FAP) and hereditary nonpolyposis CRC (HNPCC or Lynch syndrome). FAP accounts for about 1% of CRC and HNPCC for an estimated 5% to 10%. Both result in the onset of CRC at a much younger age than sporadic CRC.

Patients with hereditary CRC carry a germline genetic defect within all cells in their bodies. In a most simplistic explanation, hereditary patients already harbor at birth the first step in the multistep genetic process that must occur for colonic mucosa to change from normal to a polyp and then to a cancer. Patients with sporadic CRC harbor the necessary genetic changes only in the affected cells of the colon and must start the neoplastic change process from normal cells at the molecular level. This head start in patients with hereditary cancers may partially explain the younger age of onset.

Patients with familial CRC start with a genetic basis that leads to increased risk for CRC at an average age that is older than for hereditary forms but may be somewhat younger than that for sporadic cancers. An example of familial CRC may be the I1307K found in the Ashkenazi Jewish population. This defect in the APC gene does not actually lead to CRC in these patients as it does in FAP patients but seems to increase the susceptibility of the APC gene to further somatic mutation. The result is an 18% to 30% lifetime risk of developing CRC. This gene has been labeled as a minor colorectal susceptibility gene. It is theorized that similar genetic changes might be found in other familial clusterings of CRC in the future.

Family history has a very important role in CRC. All patients seeking an evaluation for CRC risk should start by developing a detailed analysis of their family history with particular attention to their first-degree relatives (parents, siblings, and offspring). Patients with first-degree relatives having a history of colon polyps or cancer at less than age 60 deserve special scrutiny. If there are any positive findings in this initial screen, an expansion of the pedigree to look at grandparents and aunts and uncles must be completed.

Numerous studies have looked at the effect of diet and other factors on the development of CRC. Although many dogmatic statements have been issued on these topics, there is little in the form of prospective trials to give credence to any recommendation. However, it is generally accepted that dietary measures that may be beneficial include increasing fiber and decreasing fat in the diet. Calcium has an important role in the maintenance of cell membranes and signal transmission, that is, in the maintenance of healthy cells. Low calcium intake may be associated with an increased incidence of CRC. People with sedentary lifestyles have a higher risk of developing CRC than their counterparts with physical work or active exercise programs.

The role of aspirin and nonsteroidal anti-inflammatory drugs in the development of CRC is still being evaluated. Generally, it is thought that both agents might have the potential for a significant impact on the course of CRC through inhibition of cyclooxygenase-mediated prostaglandin synthesis that could lead to a negative impact on polyp development. The cox-2 inhibitors are the newest pharmaceutical agents with some potential to limit neoplastic growth in the colon. However, with only a 28% to 32% response in recent clinical trials of patients with FAP, these agents are clearly not the complete answer to the problem of CRC.

It is clear, that for the near term, the most important preventive step we can take with regard to CRC is to educate the public and primary care physicians about colorectal screening. By identifying and removing premalignant polyps through screening, we are in fact preventing cancer. This approach is the most preferred by patients, who by large numbers would rather never have a cancer as opposed to having a cancer diagnosed at an early and treatable stage. Thus the most important role that physicians can play to ensure that patients have the best opportunity for prevention is to actively encourage patients to participate in CRC screening programs.

SCREENING PRINCIPLES

Basic Assumptions

Screening identifies individuals without signs or symptoms of disease who are more likely to have that disease. In the case of colorectal cancer, screening identifies those patients more likely to have cancer or adenomatous polyps.

The concept of colon and rectal cancer detection by testing for occult blood in the stool is based on the simple observation that cancers and polyps bleed more than normal mucosa. It is estimated that about two thirds of cancers will bleed in the course of any given week. Statistically, bleeding will increase as the size of a polyp or the stage of the cancer increases. The bleeding is not continuous so that blood may be distributed unevenly throughout the stool. Accordingly, it is known that the sensitivity of fecal occult blood testing (FOBT) increases with the number of samples per stool and the number of stool samples. Therefore the success of FOBT as a screening tool is based on the recommendation that a patient provide samples from several areas within a stool, that several consecutive stools be tested (usually over 3 days), and that the test be administered on an annual basis.

It is generally accepted that most colorectal cancers arise from preexisting adenomatous polyps. Adenomatous polyps are found in 25% to 60% of individuals by the time they are 50 years of age. The large discrepancy in these figures is dependent on the type of series being considered, clinical or autopsy, with the autopsy estimates much higher. It is estimated that only about 2.5 per 1000 polyps per year will progress to cancer. Indirect observations suggest that it takes an average of about 10 years for a polyp that is less than 1 cm to progress to an invasive malignancy.

This long dwell time is an important element in the concept of screening for colorectal cancer. Because sensitivity of FOBT for neoplasia is relatively low, the more times the test is repeated, the greater the opportunity to obtain a positive result. A single test is not accurate enough to be used as a screening method. FOBT is not a hit-and-miss proposition. However if done every year, there is a theoretical 10-year opportunity to find a polyp before malignant degeneration occurs. If done appropriately, an individual would have 30 stools tested during this period, significantly enhancing the potential that even intermittent bleeding will be detected.

Evidence for Effectiveness

Solid evidence demonstrating the effectiveness of FOBT in screening for colorectal cancer has previously been lacking. However, there have now been five prospective trials that have conclusively shown the efficacy of this simple test.

The first completed randomized trial was conducted in Minnesota and reported by Mandel in 1993. A total of 46,551 asymptomatic patients between the ages of 50 and 80 years were randomized to screening with FOBT alone done once every 2 years, annually, or not at all. All patients with positive FOBT tests (one or more of three) underwent colonoscopy. The 13-year cumulative mortality per 1000 patients was 5.88 for the group screened annually, 8.33 for the group screened biennially, and 8.83 for the control group. Overall, 13-year mortality was reduced by 33% in the group screened once a year.

A Danish study published in 1996 reported on a prospective controlled trial of 61,993 asymptomatic patients between the ages of 45 and 75 years randomized between screening every 2 years and no screening at all. Ten years following initiation of the study, an 18% reduction in colorectal cancer mortality was observed in the screened group.

An English study published in the same year reported on a prospective study of 150,251 asymptomatic patients between the ages of 45 and 74 years randomized to have screening every 2 years or not at all. After a mean follow-up of 7.8 years, investigators found a 15% reduction in colorectal mortality in the screened group. The screened group also had a higher proportion of early Dukes' A cancers.

Most clinical trials currently in effect or recently reported have used the Hemoccult-II (SmithKline Diagnostics, Sunnyvale, California) guaiac test for the detection of occult blood. Other tests have been developed but have not been prospectively evaluated. Currently available home test kits for use in the toilet bowl have not demonstrated enough of an advantage from increased compliance to offset their lower sensitivity, have not been tested in large randomized prospective trials, and therefore cannot be recommended as part of a screening program.

The other standard components of colorectal screening, that is, flexible sigmoidoscopy, barium enema, and colonoscopy, have not been studied in well-designed prospective randomized studies. The best available evidence on the effectiveness of sigmoidoscopy comes from case-control studies. Selby reported on the Kaiser experience in California. The screening history of patients dying of colorectal cancer was compared with age- and sex-matched controls. Only rigid sigmoidoscopy was studied; however, there was a 59% reduction in mortality from cancer in the rectosigmoid colon in those patients undergoing screening.

Only one controlled trial has studied the combination of FOBT with sigmoidoscopy in screening for colorectal cancer. There is certainly a theoretical basis to consider combining these two tests. Up to two thirds of cancers developing in patients being screened by FOBT are found in the rectosigmoid colon. In addition, sigmoidoscopy is more accurate than FOBT for detecting adenomatous polyps. It follows that sigmoidoscopy offers the possibility of detecting more polyps and detecting cancers at an earlier stage.

Colonoscopy offers several potential advantages as a screening tool. It is both diagnostic and potentially therapeutic. There is ample evidence that removing polyps reduces colorectal cancer incidence and that detecting colorectal cancer at an earlier stage lowers mortality. Colonoscopy will detect most polyps and most colorectal cancers.

Cost-Effectiveness

An effective screening program must provide potential benefits that outweigh the potential harm resulting from the program and the cost of the program. In an attempt to assess this cost-effectiveness in screening for colorectal cancer, the Office of Technology Assessment of the federal government developed a computer simulation model examining the use of FOBT, flexible sigmoidoscopy, double-contrast barium enema, and colonoscopy alone and in various combinations. The model used estimated costs for screening beginning at age 50 and continuing until age 85.

All strategies examined were found to cost less than $20,000 per life year saved, which is well within the acceptable range of cost-effectiveness that has been established by U.S. health standards and is considerably less than the cost of screening for breast cancer. The cost per person entered into the program beginning at age 50 years ranged from $250 to $1200, depending on the strategy selected. Finally, the returns on investment in terms of life-years saved were very high, ranging from 5000 to 7500 years per 100,000 persons screened.

THE NEW GUIDELINES

The American Cancer Society recommends screening guidelines that recognize the need to stratify screening recommendations based on varying genetic risks in the asymptomatic population. Average-risk patients are defined as those asymptomatic individuals aged 50 and older who have no additional risk factors. Approximately 70% to 80% of all colorectal cancer occurs among people of "average risk."

Moderate-risk patients include those with a history of polyps or cancer, those with colorectal neoplasia in first-degree relatives younger than age 60 years or in two or more first-degree relatives of any age, and those with colorectal cancer in other relatives. High-risk patients are defined as those with a family history of FAP or HNPCC or a personal history of inflammatory bowel disease. It is estimated that 15% to 20% of colorectal cancer occurs among people at moderate risk. Approximately 5% to 10% of colorectal cancer occurs among people at high risk.

Based on this stratification, screening recommendations for colorectal cancer for the average-risk patient who is asymptomatic and has obtained the age of 50 years includes the choice of annual FOBT or flexible sigmoidoscopy every 5 years or annual FOBT with flexible sigmoidoscopy every 5 years. As an alternative, an individual may select a double-contrast barium enema every 5 years or a colonoscopy once every 10 years. Screening recommendations for other risk groups can be found in Table 1.

Screening for colorectal cancer provides a greater opportunity for saving lives and reducing mortality than with any other cancer except possibly those related to tobacco control issues. Unfortunately, less than 30% of American adults currently participate in such screening. The number one reason given by patients for this failure to participate is the failure of their physician or managed care organization to recommend it. This should be a correctable situation that could well save thousands of lives per year.

TREATMENT

The treatment of colorectal cancer is fairly straightforward, although variations within a standard treatment approach are constantly changing as new chemotherapeutic agents and surgical techniques are introduced. For instance, the role of laparoscopic resection in the treatment of colorectal cancer is awaiting results of randomized trials. Preliminary results suggest survival will be similar between open and laparoscopic cases. The factor of cost has not been fully assessed. Most authorities continue to recommend that if the laparoscopic approach is used, it be done in the setting of a randomized trial.

Other surgical advances have minimized the use of stomas both for temporary and permanent fecal diversion. Obstructing colorectal cancer can now be managed with expandable metal stents that allow delayed single-stage procedures. The same stents can be used in the management of obstructing lesions in palliative situations in which life expectancy is limited. Obstructions can be relieved while avoiding surgery, thus decreasing length of hospital stay while enhancing quality of life.

Adjuvant therapy has become a standard of care for stage III (lymph node–positive) disease of the

TABLE 1. **American Cancer Society Guidelines on Screening and Surveillance for the Early Detection of Colorectal Adenomas and Cancer—Women and Men at Increased Risk or at High Risk**

Risk Category	Age to Begin	Recommendation	Comment
Increased Risk			
People with a single, small (<1 cm) adenoma	3–6 years after the initial polypectomy	Colonoscopy*	If the exam is normal, the patient can thereafter be screened as per average risk guidelines.
People with a large (1 cm +) adenoma, multiple adenomas, or adenomas with high-grade dysplasia or villous change	Within 3 years after the initial polypectomy	Colonoscopy*	If normal, repeat examination in 3 years; if normal then, the patient can thereafter be screened as per average risk guidelines.
Personal history of curative-intent resection of colorectal cancer	Within 1 year after cancer resection	Colonoscopy*	If normal, repeat examination in 3 years; if normal then, repeat examination every 5 years.
Either colorectal cancer or adenomatous polyps, in any first-degree relative before age 60, or in two or more first-degree relatives at any age (if not a hereditary syndrome)	Age 40, or 10 years before the youngest case in the immediate family	Colonoscopy*	Every 5–10 years. Colrectal cancer in relatives more distant than first-degree does not increase risk substantially above the average risk group.
High Risk			
Family history of familial adenomatous polyposis (FAP)	Puberty	Early surveillance with endoscopy, and counseling to consider genetic testing	If the genetic test is positive, colectomy is indicated. These patients are best referred to a center with experience in the management of FAP.
Family history of hereditary non-polyposis colon cancer (HNPCC)	Age 21	Colonscopy and counseling to consider genetic testing	If the genetic test is positive or if the patient has not had genetic testing, every 1–2 years until age 40, then annually. These patients are best referred to a center with experience in the management of HNPCC.
Inflammatory bowel disease Chronic ulcerative colitis Crohn's disease	Cancer risk begins to be significant 8 years after the onset of pancolitis, or 12–15 years after the onset of left-sided colitis	Colonoscopy with biopsies for dysplasia	Every 1–2 years. These patients are best referred to a center with experience in the surveillance and management of inflammatory bowel disease.

*If colonoscopy is unavailable, not feasible, or not desired by the patient, double contrast barium enema (DCBE) alone, or the combination of flexible sigmoidoscopy and DCBE are acceptable alternatives. Adding flexible sigmoidoscopy to DCBE may provide a more comprehensive diagnostic evaluation than DCBE alone in finding significant lesions. A supplementary DCBE may be needed if a colonoscopic exam fails to reach the cecum, and a supplementary colonoscopy may be needed if a DCBE identifies a possible lesion, or does not adequately visualize the entire colorectum.

From Guidelines for the early detection of cancer. CA Cancer J Clin 51:50, 2001.

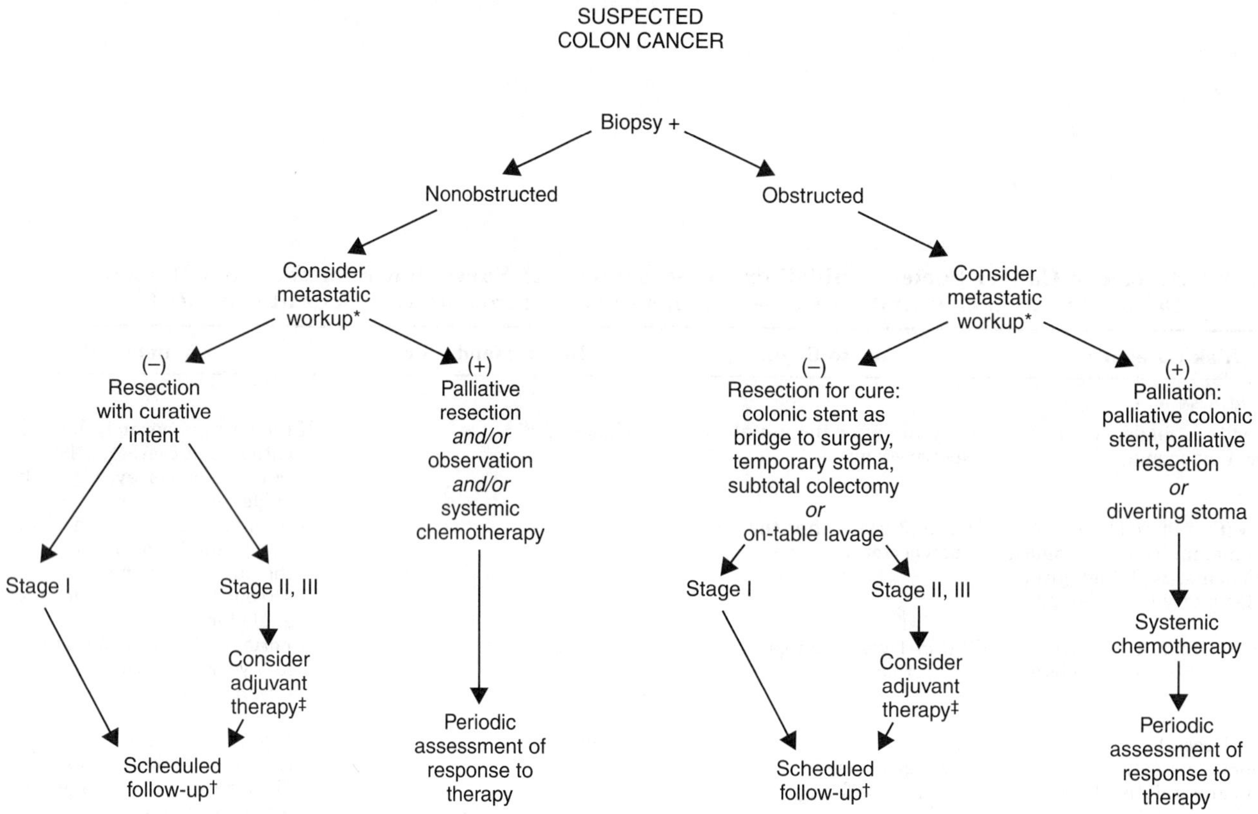

SUSPECTED
COLON CANCER

Biopsy +

Nonobstructed

Consider
metastatic
workup*

(–)
Resection
with curative
intent

Stage I

Scheduled
follow-up†

Stage II, III

Consider
adjuvant
therapy‡

Scheduled
follow-up†

(+)
Palliative
resection
and/or
observation
and/or
systemic
chemotherapy

Periodic
assessment of
response to
therapy

Obstructed

Consider
metastatic
workup*

(–)
Resection for cure:
colonic stent as
bridge to surgery,
temporary stoma,
subtotal colectomy
or
on-table lavage

Stage I

Scheduled
follow-up†

Stage II, III

Consider
adjuvant
therapy‡

Scheduled
follow-up†

(+)
Palliation:
palliative colonic
stent, palliative
resection
or
diverting stoma

Systemic
chemotherapy

Periodic
assessment of
response to
therapy

Figure 1. Management of colon cancer. (Resectable metastatic disease not considered in this algorithm.)

*Metastatic workup might include computed tomography (CT) scan of the abdomen, pelvis, or chest; chest radiograph; and carcinoembryonic antigen (CEA).

†Scheduled follow-up might include periodic physical examination, CEA if it is a CEA-producing tumor, CT scans for signs and symptoms suggesting recurrence including rising CEA and abnormal blood chemistries, and endoscopy per American Cancer Society guidelines.

‡Adjuvant therapy is indicated in Stage III, node-positive disease; many authorities recommend therapy in Stage II disease in selected individuals.

colon and stage II and III (full-thickness wall involvement or lymph node–positive) disease of the rectum. In the case of rectal cancer, radiation therapy is also often administered concomitantly with chemotherapy (most commonly 4500 to 5040 cGy). Although 5-fluorouracil (Adrucil) and leucovorin (Wellcovorin) remain the foundation of such therapy, newer agents, such as irinotecan (Camptosar) and oxaliplatin (Eloxatin)* are finding a distinct role.

There is a clear dichotomy that separates the treatment of and follow-up of colon cancer from rectal cancer (Figures 1 and 2). This separation is most prominent in the surgical management of CRC and results largely from attempts to maintain gastrointestinal continuity without sacrificing curative intent. The use of newer surgical techniques by experienced specialists maximizes this potential to safely avoid stomas.

The follow-up of CRC should be tailored to the individual and his or her cancer. Approximately 30% to 50% of patients with CRC will experience a recurrence. Almost 80% of these will occur within the first 2 years and in excess of 95% within 5 years. Generally there is not a defensible role for the routine use of computed tomography, blood chemistries, chest radiography, and endoscopy on an annual basis.

Endoscopic follow-up should follow guidelines presented earlier in this discussion. Endoscopy is geared mainly toward the detection of metachronous lesions, as most recurrences will not occur within the bowel lumen. The possible exception is the use of frequent proctoscopy in patients with a history of rectal cancer and a low anastomosis. Many centers recommend proctosigmoidoscopy every 3 months for the first 2 years in these patients and then every 6 months for another 3 years. Early detection of a local recurrence in this situation may provide an opportunity for a salvage resection. Most other tests should be based on the development of symptoms or an increasing carcinoembryonic antigen level in patients who have demonstrated a carcinoembryonic antigen–producing tumor.

SUMMARY

The best opportunity for reducing the incidence and mortality of colorectal cancer depends on the use of screening programs that have proven effective in

*Investigational drug in the United States.

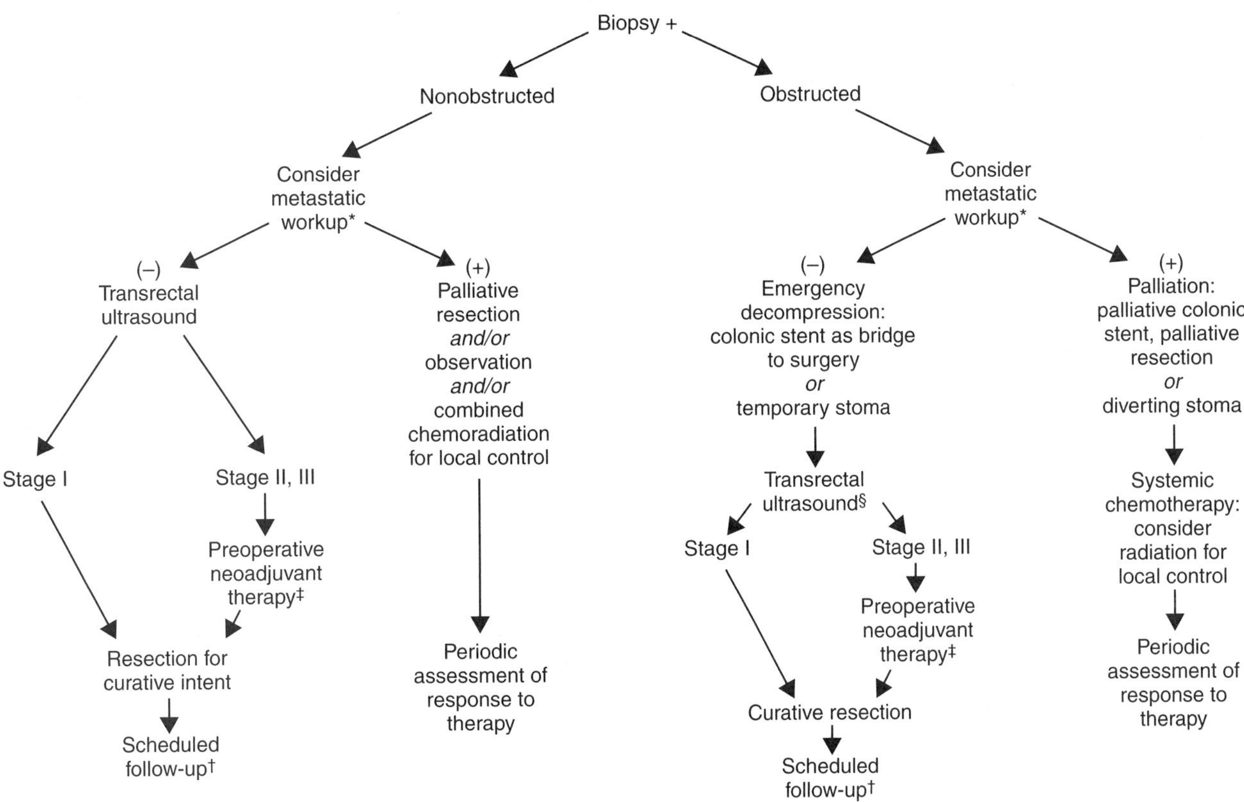

Figure 2. Management of rectal cancer. (Resectable metastatic disease not considered in this algorithm.)
*Metastatic workup might include computed tomography (CT) scan of the abdomen, pelvis, or chest; chest radiograph; and carcinoembryonic antigen (CEA).
†Scheduled follow-up might include periodic physical examination, CEA if it is a CEA-producing tumor, CT scans for signs and symptoms suggesting recurrence including rising CEA and abnormal blood chemistries, and endoscopy per American Cancer Society guidelines.
‡Adjuvant therapy is indicated in Stage II and III disease. Neoadjuvant therapy consists of combined radiation and chemotherapy.
§Transrectal ultrasound is performed if the extent of local involvement is in doubt.

prospective randomized trials. Data show that colorectal cancer screening is currently woefully underutilized. There is evidence that the most influential reason for this underutilization is the failure of physicians to recommend screening to their patients. The reversal of this pattern must become a primary goal of primary caregivers in the United States.

INTESTINAL PARASITES

method of
VERNON ANSDELL, M.D.
University of Hawaii
Honolulu, Hawaii

INTESTINAL PROTOZOA

Giardiasis occurs worldwide, and in many countries it is the most common intestinal parasite infection. *Giardia lamblia* is a protozoan that typically infects the upper portion of the small intestine. Many infections are asymptomatic, but acute or chronic diarrhea with pale greasy stools, abdominal cramps, bloating, fatigue, and weight loss may be encountered. Infection usually occurs after ingesting contaminated water or food. Individuals at increased risk of infection include children in daycare, travelers to developing countries and to St. Petersburg, Russia, patients with hypogammaglobulinemia, and hikers who drink inadequately treated surface water, particularly in mountainous regions of the United States.

Metronidazole* (Flagyl), 250 mg (adult dose) orally three times daily for 5 to 7 days, is the drug of choice in the United States for treating giardiasis. It is 85% to 95% effective. Side effects, even at this low dose, are relatively common and include nausea, dizziness, headache, and a metallic taste in the mouth. Much less common side effects include seizures, peripheral neuropathy, ataxia, and pancreatitis. Patients should not use alcohol while taking metronidazole because a disulfiram-like reaction can occur. Metronidazole is a Food and Drug Administration (FDA) pregnancy category B drug. It is probably safe to use in the second and third trimesters of pregnancy.

A related drug, tinidazole,* is very effective when given

*Not FDA approved for this indication.

in a single 2-g dose and has fewer side effects than metronidazole.

Quinacrine (Atabrine) given for 5 to 7 days has an efficacy of about 95%. Common side effects include nausea, vomiting, and temporary yellow staining of the skin, urine, and sclerae. Rarely, serious side effects such as toxic psychosis, exfoliative dermatitis, and corneal edema may occur. Quinacrine is contraindicated in patients with psoriasis and should be used with caution in patients with underlying liver disease. It is not available commercially in the United States but can be compounded by certain pharmacies (Table 1).

Furazolidone (Furoxone), a nitrofurantoin, given for 7 to 10 days has an efficacy of about 80%. It is available as a liquid suspension. Side effects include nausea, vomiting, and headache, and it may turn the urine a brown color. Patients who are deficient in glucose-6-phosphate dehydrogenase may have mild hemolysis, and a disulfiram-like reaction may occur in patients who drink alcohol while taking this drug. It is a monoamine oxidase inhibitor, so patients taking this drug should avoid tyramine-containing foods (e.g., broad beans, yeast extracts, beer, wine, pickled herring, and chicken livers), indirectly acting sympathomimetic amines (e.g., phenylephrine, ephedrine), anorectics (amphetamines), and other drugs that inhibit monoamine oxidase.

Paromomycin* (Humatin) is a nonabsorbable aminoglycoside. When taken for 5 to 10 days it has an efficacy of only about 60%. Because it is nonabsorbable, it is considered safe in pregnancy, including the first trimester.

Albendazole† (Albenza), 400 mg daily (adult dose) for 5 days, has an efficacy of about 90% in the treatment of giardiasis.

After successful treatment, diarrhea usually stops within 1 to 2 days and abnormalities of small intestinal function and morphology resolve in 1 to 2 months. Cyst excretion stops about 2 days after starting treatment.

Entamoeba Histolytica

Disease caused by *E. histolytica* includes asymptomatic cyst passage, intestinal amebiasis, and dysenteric colitis. It is important to differentiate between this pathogen and

*Not available in the United States.
†Not FDA approved for this indication.

TABLE 1. **Drugs for the Treatment of Protozoal Infections**

Infection	Drug	Adult Dosage	Pediatric Dosage
Amebiasis *(Entamoeba histolytica)*			
Asymptomatic			
Drug of choice	Iodoquinol (Yodoxin)	650 mg tid × 20 d	30–40 mg/kg/d (max 2 g) in 3 doses × 20 d
	or		
	Paromomycin (Humatin)	25–35 mg/kg/d in 3 doses × 7 d	25–35 mg/kg/d in 3 doses × 7 d
Alternative	Diloxanide furoate (Furamide)*	500 mg tid ×10 d	20 mg/kg/d in 3 doses × 10 d
Mild to moderate intestinal disease			
Drug of choice†	Metronidazole (Flagyl)	500–750 mg tid × 10 d	35–50 mg/kg/d in 3 doses × 10 d
	or		
	Tinidazole‡	2 g/d × 3 d	50 mg/kg (max 2 g) qd × 3 d
Severe intestinal disease and liver abscess			
Drug of choice†	Metronidazole	750 mg tid × 10 d	35–50 mg/kg/d in 3 doses × 10 d
	or		
	Tinidazole‡	600 mg bid or 800 mg tid × 5 d	50 mg/kg or 60 mg/kg (max 2 g) qd × 5 d
Balantidium coli			
Drug of choice	Tetracycline	500 mg qid × 10 d	40 mg/kg/d (max 2 g) in 4 doses × 10 d (not recommended in children <8 y)
Alternative	Iodoquinol	650 mg tid × 20 d	40 mg/kg/d (max 2 g) in 3 doses × 20 d
Blastocystis hominis infections§			
Cryptosporidiosis *(Cryptosporidium parvum)*			
Drug of choice‖	Paromomycin¶	500–750 mg qid	
Cyclospora species			
Drug of choice	Trimethoprim (TMP) sulfamethoxazole (SMZ; Bactrim, Septra)¶**	TMP 160 mg, SMZ 800 mg bid × 7 d	TMP 5 mg/kg, SMZ 25 mg/kg bid × 7 d
Dientamoeba fragilis infection			
Drug of choice	Iodoquinol	650 mg tid × 20 d	40 mg/kg/d (max 2 g) in 9 doses × 20 d
	or		
	Paromomycin¶	500 mg tid × 7 d	25–30 mg/kg/d in 3 doses × 7 d
	or		
	Tetracycline¶	500 mg qid × 10 d	40 mg/kg/d (max 2 g/d) in 4 doses × 10 d (not recommended in children <8 y)

TABLE 1. **Drugs for the Treatment of Protozoal Infections** *Continued*

Infection	Drug	Adult Dosage	Pediatric Dosage
Giardiasis *(Giardia lamblia)*			
Drug of choice			
Alternatives††			
Metronidazole¶	250 mg tid × 5 d	15 mg/kg/d in 3 doses × 5 d	
Tinidazole‡	2 g once	50 g/kg once (max 2 g)	
or			
Quinacrine‡‡	100 mg tid ×5–7 d	2 mg/kg tid × 5–7 d	
or			
Furazolidone (Furoxone)	100 mg qid × 7–10 d	6 mg/kg/d in 4 doses × 7–10 d	
or			
Paromomycin	500–750 mg tid × 5–10 d	25–35 mg/kg/d in 3 doses × 5–10 d	
Isosporiasis *(Isospora belli)*			
Drug of choice	Trimethoprim-sulfamethoxazole¶§§	160 mg TMP, 800 mg SMZ qid × 10 d, then bid × 3 wk	25–35 mg/kg/d in 3 doses × 5–10 d
Microsporidiosis			
Intestinal *Enterocytozoon bieneusi, Septata intestinalis)*			
Drug of choice‖ ‖	Albendazole (Albenza)¶	400 mg bid × 2–3 wk	

*Available from the CDC Drug Service, Centers for Disease Control and Prevention, Atlanta, Georgia; (404) 639-3670.

†Treatment should be followed by a course of iodoquinol or paromomycin in the dosage used to treat asymptomatic amebiasis.

‡Not available in the United States. The higher dosage listed is for amebic liver abscess.

§Clinical significance of *Blastocystis* is controversial, but metronidazole, 750 mg three times daily or iodoquinol 650 mg three times daily for 10 days, may be effective (as reported anecdotally) (Boreham PFL, Stenzel DJ: *Blastocystis* in humans and animals: Morphology, biology, and epizootiology. Adv Parasitol *32*:1–70, 1993; Keystone JS: *Blastocystis hominis* and traveler's diarrhea [editorial]. Clin Infect Dis *21*:102–105, 1995; Markell EK: Is there any reason to continue treating *Blastocystis* infections? [editorial]. Clin Infect Dis *21*:104–105, 1995).

‖Infection is self-limited in immunocompetent patients. Azithromycin in doses of 500 to 1000 mg initially and then 250 to 500 mg per day has been helpful in limited studies. Duration of treatment may need to be prolonged.

¶An approved drug but considered investigational for this condition by the U.S. FDA.

**AIDS patients may need a higher dose (1 double-strength tablet four times daily) and long-term maintenance therapy (Papa JW, Verdier RI, Boney M, et al: *Cyclospora* infection in adults infected with HIV. Clinical manifestations, treatment, and prophylaxis. Ann Intern Med *121*:654–657, 1994).

††Albendazole, 400 mg/d for 5 days, may be effective (Hall A, Nahar Q: Albendazole as a treatment for infections with *Giardia duodenalis* in children in Bangladesh. Trans R Soc Trop Med Hyg *87*:84–86, 1993).

‡‡No longer produced in the United States. May be obtained from Panorama Pharmacy, Panorama City, CA; (800) 247-9767.

§§In sulfonamide-sensitive patients, pyrimethamine, 50 to 75 mg daily, has been effective. AIDS patients may need long-term maintenance therapy.

‖ ‖Atovaquone, 750 mg three times daily for 1 month, may control symptoms in some patients. Ostreotide may also help to control the diarrhea.

Adapted from Drugs for parasitic infections. Med Lett Drug Ther *40*:1–12, 1998.

the morphologically indistinguishable but nonpathogenic *Entamoeba dispar,* which is often confused with *E. histolytica.* Extraintestinal spread of *E. histolytica* may occur to the liver, lungs, pericardium, brain, and skin. The diagnosis of significant intestinal amebiasis is made by detecting hematophagous trophozoites in the stool or material collected from colonic ulcers.

Serology is positive in about 80% of patients with intestinal disease and in over 95% of those with amebic liver abscess.

Noninvasive infection is treated with drugs that are active in the lumen of the gut. Effective luminal agents include iodoquinol, paromomycin, and diloxanide furoate. Side effects from iodoquinol include rash, diarrhea, optic neuritis, and peripheral neuropathy. Diloxanide furoate is poorly absorbed and usually well tolerated, but it may produce side effects such as flatulence, nausea, and diarrhea.

Metronidazole (Flagyl) is the drug of choice for treatment of intestinal or extraintestinal invasive disease. If available, tinidazole* is an even better alternative. After treatment with metronidazole or tinidazole, an effective luminal agent such iodoquinol (Yodoxin), paromomycin (Humatin), or diloxanide furoate† (Furamide) should be given. Amebic liver abscess is usually treated adequately with medical therapy. If multiple abscesses are present or the abscess is in danger of rupture, aspiration may be indicated.

*Not available in the United States.

†Not FDA approved for this indication.

Cryptosporidium

Cryptosporidium parvum is an intestinal coccidian parasite that may be an important cause of chronic diarrhea, particularly in an immunocompromised patient. It is typically water-borne and, in immunocompetent hosts, produces self-limited, watery, nonbloody diarrhea with nausea and abdominal pain. In immunocompromised hosts (e.g., AIDS), it causes severe dehydrating diarrhea, wasting, weight loss, and significant morbidity. The diagnosis is made by identification of 2- to 6-mm cysts in the stools.

No reliable treatment is available for cryptosporidiosis. In immunocompetent hosts, treatment is symptomatic and supportive because the infection is self-limited. In immunocompromised patients, treatment should be focused on correction of fluid and electrolyte abnormalities. In patients with AIDS, paromomycin (Humatin), with or without the addition of azithromycin* (Zithromax), has been shown to be of some benefit. If a response to paromomycin is noted, patients with AIDS may benefit from long-term "maintenance" therapy. Some evidence indicates that nitazoxanide† (Cryptaz) may be effective in some patients.

*Not FDA approved for this indication.

†Investigational drug in the United States.

Cyclospora

Cyclospora cayetanensis is a recently identified coccidian protozoan parasite that was first described in travelers and expatriates in Nepal. It is an unusual but important cause of chronic diarrhea in immunocompetent hosts. In the immunocompromised, symptoms may last for several months. Cases have been described in travelers to Asia, the Caribbean, Mexico, and Peru. Typical symptoms include diarrhea, marked fatigue, nausea, anorexia, abdominal pain, and weight loss. Fever is rare. Transmission is typically water-borne, but some outbreaks have been linked to contaminated raspberries from Guatemala and also lettuce and basil. The diagnosis should always be considered in patients with prolonged diarrhea, particularly travelers from high-risk areas, and a modified Kinyoun acid-fast stain test of the stool requested to detect the 8- to 10-mm cysts. Treatment with trimethoprim-sulfamethoxazole (Bactrim), twice daily for 1 week, has been shown to be effective in immunocompetent hosts. In immunocompromised patients (e.g., HIV), prolonged treatment may be necessary, followed by suppressive therapy three times weekly.

Isospora Belli

Isospora belli is a coccidian parasite that may be an important cause of diarrhea in immunocompromised patients, particularly those with HIV infection. Diagnosis is by demonstration of 13 × 28-mm oocysts on modified acid-fast stain. In immunocompetent hosts, treatment is with trimethoprim-sulfamethoxazole. If the patient is allergic to sulfonamides, pyrimethamine* (Daraprim) is an effective alternative. AIDS patients may require long-term prophylaxis with low-dose pyrimethamine* (25 mg) or trimethoprim-sulfamethoxazole.*

Microsporidia

Human microsporidiosis comprises a group of emerging infectious diseases associated with a wide range of clinical syndromes. *Enterocytozoon bieneusi* and *Encephalitozoon (Septata) intestinalis* cause intestinal symptoms. Most cases occur in immunosuppressed patients with AIDS or post-transplant immunosuppressed patients, although a few cases have been reported in immunocompetent individuals. Typical symptoms include chronic diarrhea, anorexia, weight loss, nausea, vomiting, and fever. *E. intestinalis* infection may be accompanied by colitis with blood in the stool. Disseminated infection involving the biliary tree, liver, muscle, central nervous system, and eye may occur. The diagnosis is made by identifying microsporidia in the stool by trichrome stain or in duodenal contents by light microscopy. In some situations, duodenal biopsy with electron microscopy may be necessary for diagnosis. Albendazole* (Albenza) is the drug of choice for treatment. Octreotide* (Sandostatin) may provide symptomatic relief in patients with large-volume diarrhea. Oral fumagillin has been effective in treating *E. bieneusi* infections. There is good evidence that highly active antiretroviral therapy (HAART) may produce a microbiologic and clinical response in HIV-infected patients with microsporidial diarrhea.

Less Common Protozoa

Dientamoeba fragilis is an ameba-like flagellate organism. It is usually transmitted from person to person, although some cases may be water-borne. Close correlation is seen between *Enterobius vermicularis* and *D. fragilis* infections, possibly because pinworm eggs or larvae may act as a transmitting agent for *D. fragilis*. Symptoms include intermittent diarrhea, abdominal pain, fatigue, and anorexia. Many cases are asymptomatic. Treatment is with paromomycin, iodoquinol,* or tetracycline.*

Balantidium coli is a large ciliated protozoan. Infection in humans is rare, with most cases being reported in areas of poor hygiene and sanitation where pigs and human beings are in close contact. Intermittent diarrhea, abdominal pain, and weight loss may be noted, as well as a dysenteric form with blood and mucus in the stool. Fulminating dysentery may lead to life-threatening hemorrhage and intestinal perforation. The treatment of choice is tetracycline. Alternatives include iodoquinol* and metronidazole.

Blastocystis hominis is a commonly identified protozoan organism, but it remains unclear whether it is pathogenic. Treatment may be indicated in symptomatic patients with heavy infections in the absence of other recognized pathogens. High-dose metronidazole for 10 days or iodoquinol* for 20 days can be given. Trimethoprim-sulfamethoxazole* is an alternative regimen.

Nonpathogenic Protozoa

Nonpathogenic protozoa include *Entamoeba hartmanni, Entamoeba coli, Endolimax nana, Iodameba butschlii, Chilomastix mesnili,* and *Trichomonas hominis*. Treatment is not indicated.

INTESTINAL HELMINTHS

Intestinal helminths are classified as nematodes (roundworms) or platyhelminths (flatworms). Flatworms are further subdivided into cestodes (tapeworms) and trematodes (flukes). In general, members of each group are usually susceptible to the same drugs or family of drugs. Nematodes that live in the gut lumen, such as *Ascaris* worms, hookworms, and *Trichuris* worms, are treated with drugs such as albendazole, mebendazole, or pyrantel pamoate. Tissue nematodes (e.g., *Strongyloides stercoralis*) are usually treated with albendazole or ivermectin. Intestinal cestodes (e.g., *Taenia saginata, Taenia solium, Hymenolepis nana, Diphyllobothrium latum*) are treated with praziquantel and the larval forms (e.g., cysticercosis, *Echinococcus*) with albendazole or praziquantel. Trematode infections are usually treated with praziquantel, although bithionol is the drug of choice for fascioliasis, and *Schistosoma mansoni* infections may also be treated with oxamniquine.

Mebendazole (Vermox) is a synthetic benzimidazole derivative with a broad spectrum of activity against a variety of intestinal and extraintestinal helminths. Cure rates of greater than 90% are often seen for hookworm infection, ascariasis, and enterobiasis. Only 2% to 10% of the drug is absorbed after an oral dose, which is not a concern when the drug is used for treating luminal worms. In standard doses, side effects are very rare but may include nausea, diarrhea, abdominal pain, headache, and dizziness. Mebendazole is not recommended during pregnancy because it is embryotoxic and teratogenic in rats. It should be used with caution in children younger than 2 years because of limited experience.

*Not FDA approved for this indication.

*Not FDA approved for this indication.

Albendazole, another synthetic benzimidazole derivative, has a broad spectrum of activity against a wide variety of intestinal and extraintestinal nematodes and cestodes. Single-dose therapy is effective against trichuriasis, enterobiasis, ascariasis, and hookworm infections. Once-daily therapy for 3 days is also effective in strongyloidiasis, taeniasis, and *H. nana* infections. Prolonged courses of up to 30 days or longer are used in treating cysticercosis and hydatid disease. It is rapidly but only partially absorbed after an oral dose, although absorption is enhanced by taking the drug with a fatty meal. Side effects are rare with single-dose or short-term therapy but may include epigastric discomfort, diarrhea, nausea, headache, and dizziness. In high-dose or long-term therapy (≥30 days), fever, alopecia, abnormal liver function, and transient leukopenia have been reported. Albendazole is teratogenic and embryotoxic in rats and rabbits and is contraindicated in pregnancy. It should be used with caution in children younger than 2 years or in patients with severe hepatocellular disease.

Pyrantel pamoate (Antiminth) is a pyrimidine derivative that is very effective against *Ascaris lumbricoides, E. vermicularis,* and *Ancylostoma duodenale.* It is moderately effective against *Necator americanus.* It is poorly absorbed, and side effects are mild and infrequent but include nausea, vomiting, diarrhea, abdominal pain, dizziness, photosensitization, and allergic reactions. Stools are stained bright red. The drug should be used with caution in patients with renal or hepatic disease.

Thiabendazole (Mintezol) is a benzimidazole compound with a broad spectrum of activity against a variety of intestinal and extraintestinal nematodes. It is rapidly absorbed after an oral dose. Side effects are common and often severe and include nausea, vomiting, anorexia, and dizziness, which limit its usefulness. Rare side effects include liver damage, angioneurotic edema, and Stevens-Johnson syndrome.

Ivermectin (Stromectol) is an avermectin derived from *Streptomyces avermitilis.* It has been used extensively in veterinary medicine and has a broad spectrum of activity against a wide variety of gastrointestinal and extraintestinal nematodes. Single doses are very effective in the treatment of strongyloidiasis, trichuriasis, and enterobiasis, but the drug is not effective for hookworm infections. Side effects are very rare when treating intestinal nematode infections in otherwise healthy patients. Headache has been reported, however. The drug should be avoided during pregnancy and lactation. If possible, it should not be given with other drugs that increase γ-aminobutyric acid activity such as barbiturates, benzodiazepines, and valproic acid.

Praziquantel (Biltricide) is a synthetic isoquinoline-pyrazine derivative unrelated to other anthelmintic agents. It is highly effective in treating a wide variety of trematode and cestode infections. Praziquantel is rapidly absorbed after oral administration, metabolized to inactive ingredients in the liver, and excreted mainly via the kidney. It crosses the blood-brain barrier and produces concentrations in cerebrospinal fluid approximately 20% of those in plasma. The drug is usually well tolerated but may cause side effects such as headache, dizziness, drowsiness, nausea, vomiting, anorexia, abdominal pain, diarrhea, fever, pruritus, and urticaria and other rashes. Side effects tend to be dose related. They are infrequent with single doses of 5 to 10 mg/kg but occur in up to 50% of patients who receive doses of 25 mg/kg. Because of inadequate data, praziquantel should be used in pregnancy only if clearly indicated. Lactating women should not nurse while taking praziquantel or for the following 72 hours. Safety in children younger than 4 years has not been established.

Bithionol (Bitin) is structurally related to hexacholorophene and is effective against a variety of trematode and cestode infections. It is the drug of choice for the treatment of fascioliasis. Side effects are relatively common, tend to be mild and transient, and include diarrhea, abdominal pain, nausea, vomiting, urticaria and other rashes, dizziness, headache, and excessive salivation. Rarely, leukopenia, proteinuria, and hepatitis may occur. The drug should be avoided in pregnancy and lactation unless very clearly indicated.

Oxamniquine (Vansil) is a tetrahydroquinolone that is an alternative to praziquantel for the treatment of *S. mansoni* infections. It is well absorbed orally and may produce an orange or red discoloration of urine. Side effects include neuropsychiatric disturbances, dizziness, rash, anorexia, abdominal pain, diarrhea, nausea, and vomiting. The drug may rarely cause seizures, and it is contraindicated in patients with a history of epilepsy. Electrocardiographic changes and abnormal liver function may occur. Oxamniquine should not be used in pregnancy.

NEMATODES (ROUNDWORMS)

Important intestinal roundworms include ascaris *(A. lumbricoides),* hookworms (*N. americanus* and *A. duodenale*), whipworms *(Trichuris trichiura),* pinworms or threadworms *(E. vermicularis),* and *S. stercoralis.* Ascaris and whipworm infections result from the ingestion of infective eggs via contaminated fingers, food (especially uncooked vegetables), or polluted water. Children are particularly likely to be infected and often have heavier infections than adults. Threadworm infections result from the ingestion of infective eggs that have contaminated fingers, food, or articles such as bedclothes, underwear, or even pet fur. Hookworm and *Strongyloides* infections occur when infective larvae penetrate intact skin, which typically occurs after walking barefoot or handling contaminated soil. With the exception of pinworm, infections are most frequent in developing countries. Infection with more than one parasite is common, and prevalence rates of over 50% may occur in countries with poor hygiene and sanitation.

A. lumbricoides, or the large intestinal roundworm, measures about 15 cm in length and closely resembles an earthworm in size and shape. Ingested eggs hatch in the intestine, and the larval form migrates through the lungs (sometimes causing cough, wheezing, dyspnea, and chest pain) before developing into the adult worm living in the small intestine. Treatment is with a single dose of albendazole* (Albenza) or pyrantel pamoate (Antiminth) or a 3-day course of mebendazole (Vermox). Albendazole and mebendazole have broad anthelmintic activity and are useful if multiple parasites are present.

Hookworm larvae penetrate intact skin, migrate through the lungs, and develop into adult worms in the small intestine. Most infections are light and do not produce significant symptoms. Heavy infections may cause abdominal pain, nausea, anorexia, diarrhea, iron deficiency anemia, and hypoalbuminemia. Treatment is with single-dose albendazole or a 3-day course of mebendazole or pyrantel pamoate. Iron supplements should be given for anemia. Larval forms of the dog hookworm *(Ancylostoma caninum)* or cat hookworm *(Ancylostoma braziliense)* may penetrate human skin, but because they are in the wrong host, they are unable to complete their life cycle. They migrate subcu-

*Not FDA approved for this indication.

taneously and produce an intensely pruritic localized reaction. Most lesions occur on the feet, but sometimes they are found in other areas such as the buttocks or hands. This illness is often referred to as cutaneous larva migrans or "creeping eruption." Treatment is with ivermectin* (Stromectol), 12 mg in a single dose, or albendazole, 400 mg daily for 1 to 3 days. Topical thiabendazole (Mintezol), 15% for 3 to 5 days, is an alternative to oral treatment. Oral thiabendazole is no longer recommended because of common side effects. Attempts at local excision or topical freezing are definitely not recommended.

Pinworm or threadworm infections cause pruritus ani, which may result in insomnia and irritability. Scratching may cause a local dermatitis and secondary bacterial infection. It is important to try to confirm the diagnosis by touching the perianal area with the adhesive side of transparent cellophane tape and examining it for eggs under a microscope. Treatment is with single-dose pyrantel pamoate, mebendazole, or albendazole, repeated after 2 weeks. It is important to treat other family members and launder and iron bedclothes, sheets, and towels to prevent reinfection.

S. stercoralis infection occurs when infective larvae burrow through intact skin, migrate through the lungs, and mature as adult worms in the upper part of the small intestine. Female worms produce eggs that hatch in the intestine, and sometimes the larvae mature sufficiently to reinfect the host rather than require a certain period in soil to mature and become infective. This autoinfection cycle accounts for persistent infection seen many years or even decades after the original infection. Most infections in immunocompetent hosts are asymptomatic. When they occur, symptoms include nausea, vomiting, diarrhea, and abdominal pain. An urticarial rash may be noted. External autoinfection may produce a very characteristic serpiginous, pruritic rash ("larva currens"). A life-threatening hyperinfection syndrome is associated with impaired cellular immunity and is characterized by a greatly increased worm burden and massive dissemination of larvae to the lungs, brain, and other tissues. Mortality is high even if diagnosed and treated promptly. Immunosuppressed states in which this syndrome may occur include chronic corticosteroid therapy (e.g., asthmatics), other immunosuppressive and chemotherapeutic drug treatment, lymphomas, leukemias, malnutrition, and post–organ transplant patients. Disseminated strongyloidiasis has been reported in AIDS patients but is not as common as might be expected, except in individuals co-infected with human T-cell lymphotropic virus type 1. In immunocompetent hosts, the diagnosis is made by identifying larvae in the stool or duodenal contents or by serologic testing (enzyme-linked immunosorbent assay). In disseminated strongyloidiasis, the larvae may also be present in sputum, peritoneal fluid, cerebrospinal fluid, urine, or pleural fluid. Eosinophilia is common in immunocompetent hosts but is often absent in disseminated infection. Ivermectin is the drug of choice for uncomplicated infection. Albendazole,* 400 mg daily for 3 days, is also effective. Thiabendazole is very effective but, because of side effects, is normally only used in disseminated infection, where a 5- to 10-day course is given. If infection cannot be cleared or immunosuppression reversed, monthly 2-day courses may be indicated to prevent dissemination. All diagnosed cases should be treated regardless of symptoms because of the possibility of hyperinfection if the host subsequently becomes immunosuppressed.

*Not FDA approved for this indication.

Trichinella spiralis infection (trichinosis) occurs as a result of eating infected, undercooked meat from domestically raised pigs, boars, wild bears, and other mammals. Ingested larvae invade the intestinal mucosa and mature to adult worms in the intestine. After mating, further larvae are produced and invade human muscle and occasionally the central nervous system. The first phase produces nausea, vomiting, abdominal pain, and diarrhea. During muscle invasion, myalgia, fever, facial edema, and occasionally mental status changes are encountered. Treatment is with albendazole* or mebendazole* plus steroids (prednisone, 40 to 60 mg daily) to reduce severe symptoms associated with larval invasion.

Capillaria philippinensis is a filamentous nematode that may infect people who have eaten raw freshwater fish. It is endemic in the Philippines and, less commonly, other countries in Southeast Asia. Symptoms include abdominal pain, diarrhea and malabsorption, and weight loss. Treatment is with albendazole* or mebendazole.

Anisakiasis occurs after eating raw marine fish such as mackerel, salmon, herring, or squid containing infective larvae. Raw seafood in the form of sashimi or sushi is a common source of infection. Symptoms include abdominal pain, nausea, vomiting, and diarrhea. Anthelmintic drugs are ineffective, and treatment is by endoscopic or surgical removal of the larvae.

Trichostrongylus is a zoonotic nematode that mainly infects cattle in parts of the Middle and Far East. Most infections are asymptomatic. Heavy infections produce gastrointestinal symptoms and are treated with a single dose of pyrantel pamoate or albendazole* or a 3-day course of mebendazole.*

Angiostrongylus costaricensis infection occurs in Latin America as a result of the inadvertent ingestion of raw slugs or the ingestion of infective larvae shed in slug secretions and contaminating food. Symptoms include abdominal pain, often in the right iliac fossa and mimicking appendicitis. Treatment is with mebendazole* or thiabendazole.*

CESTODES (TAPEWORMS)

When human beings are the definitive host for cestode infections, the adult tapeworm (e.g., *T. saginata, T. solium, D. latum,* and *H. nana*) lives in the lumen of the intestine. When people act as the intermediate host, however, larval forms of the cestodes develop in the tissues and often create a serious, potentially life-threatening situation (cysticercosis, echinococcosis). Tapeworm infections usually result from the ingestion of raw or inadequately cooked meat or fish containing encysted larvae. The adult tapeworm develops in the lumen of the intestine and may reach a length of 12 m or longer. Most tapeworm infections produce few symptoms or are totally asymptomatic. *D. latum* infection may cause a macrocytic anemia as a result of vitamin B_{12} deficiency. The drug of choice for treating human tapeworm infections is praziquantel. Higher doses are needed to treat *H. nana* infections.

Treatment of larval (tissue) cestodes is much more difficult. In cysticercosis, larval forms of *T. solium* invade tissues such as skeletal muscle, the brain, and the eye. A variety of serious neuropsychiatric symptoms may be produced. Human cysticercosis occurs as a result of ingesting material contaminated by human feces containing *T. solium* eggs. It does not result from eating infected pork

*Not FDA approved for this indication.

TABLE 2. **Drugs for the Treatment of Helminth Infections**

Infection	Drug	Adult Dosage	Pediatric Dosage
Angiostrongyliasis *(Angiostrongylus costaricensis)*			
Drug of choice	Mebendazole (Vermox)*	200–400 mg tid × 10 d	200–400 mg tid × 10 d
Alternative	Thiabendazole (Mintezol)†	75 mg/kg/d in 3 doses × 3 d (max 3 g/d); toxicity may require dosage reduction	75 mg/kg/d in 3 doses × 3 d (max 3 g/d); toxicity may require dosage reduction
Anisakiasis (*Anisakis* and other genera)			
Treatment of choice	Surgical or endoscopic removal		
Ascariasis *(Ascaris lumbricoides)*			
Drug of choice	Albendazole†	400 mg once	400 mg once
	or		
	Mebendazole	100 mg bid × 3 d	100 mg bid × 3 d
	or		
	Pyrantel pamoate (Antiminth)†	11 mg/kg once (max 1 g)	11 mg/kg once (max 1 g)
Capillariasis *(Capillaria philippinensis)*			
Drug of choice	Mebendazole†	200 mg bid × 20 d	200 mg bid × 20 d
Alternative	Albendazole†	400 mg daily	400 mg daily
Cysticercosis; see Tapeworm infection			
Enterobius vermicularis (pinworm) infection			
Drug of choice	Pyrantel pamoate	11 mg/kg once (max 1 g); repeat after 2 wk	11 mg/kg once (max 1 g); repeat after 2 wk
	or		
	Mebendazole	A single dose of 100 mg; repeat after 2 wk	A single dose of 100 mg; repeat after 2 wk
	or		
	Albendazole†	400 mg once; repeat in 2 wk	400 mg once, repeat in 2 wk
Flukes (intestinal infection)			
Fasciolopsis buski, Heterophyes heterophyes, Metagonimus yokogawai			
Drug of choice	Praziquantel†	75 mg/kg/d in 3 doses × 1 d	75 mg/kg/d in 3 doses × 1 d
Nanophyetus salmincola			
Drug of choice	Praziquantel†	60 mg/kg/d in 3 doses × 1 d	60 mg/kg/d in 3 doses × 1 d
Flukes (liver infection)			
Opisthorchis sinensis (Chinese liver fluke)			
Drug of choice	Praziquantel†	75 mg/kg/d in 3 doses × 1 d	75 mg/kg/d in 3 doses × 1 d
	or		
	Albendazole†	10 mg/kg × 7 d	
Fasciola hepatica (sheep liver fluke)			
Drug of choice‡	Bithionol (Lorothidol)§	30–50 mg/kg on alternate days × 10–15 doses	30–50 mg/kg on alternate days × 10–15 doses
Metorchis conjunctus (North American liver fluke)			
Drug of choice	Praziquantel†	75 mg/kg/d in 3 doses × 1 d	75 mg/kg/d in 3 doses × 1 d
Opisthorchis viverrini (SE Asian liver fluke)			
Drug of choice	Praziquantel†	75 mg/kg/d in 3 doses × 1 d	75 mg/kg/d in 3 doses × 1 d
Hookworm infection *(Ancylostoma duodenale, Necator americanus)*			
Drug of choice	Albendazole†	400 mg once	400 mg once
	or		
	Mebendazole	100 mg bid × 3 d	100 mg bid × 3 d
	or		
	Pyrantel pamoate†	11 mg/kg/d (max 1 g) × 3 d	11 mg/kg (max 1 g) × 3 d
Schistosomiasis (bilharziasis)			
Schistosoma haematobium			
Drug of choice	Praziquantel	40 mg/kg/d in 2 doses × 1 d	40 mg/kg/d in 2 doses × 1 d
Schistosoma japonicum			
Drug of choice	Praziquantel	60 mg/kg/d in 3 doses × 1 d	60 mg/kg/d in 3 doses × 1 d
Schistosoma mansoni			
Drug of choice	Praziquantel	40 mg/kg/d in 2 doses × 1 d	40 mg/kg/d in 2 doses × 1 d
Alternative	Oxamniquine (Vansil)‖	15 mg/kg once (higher doses are used in some areas)	20 mg/kg/d in 2 doses × 1 d

Table continued on following page

TABLE 2. **Drugs for the Treatment of Helminth Infections** *Continued*

Infection	Drug	Adult Dosage	Pediatric Dosage
Schistosoma mekongi			
Drug of choice	Praziquantel	60 mg/kg/d in 3 doses × 1 d	60 mg/kg/d in 3 doses × 1 d
Strongyloidiasis *(Strongyloides stercoralis)*			
Drug of choice¶	Ivermectin (Stromectol)	200 μg/kg/d ×1 d	200 μg/kg/d × 1 d
	or		
	Thiabendazole	50 mg/kg/d in 2 doses (max 3 g/d) × 2 d; ≥5 d for hyperinfection	50 mg/kg/d in 2 doses (max 3 g/d) × 2 d; ≥5 d for hyperinfection
Tapeworm infection—adult (intestinal stage)			
Diphyllobothrium latum (fish), *Taenia saginata* (beef), *Taenia solium* (pork), *Dipylidium caninum* (dog)			
Drug of choice	Praziquantel†	5–10 mg/kg once	5–10 mg/kg once
Hymenolepis nana (dwarf tapeworm)			
Drug of choice	Praziquantel†	25 mg/kg once	25 mg/kg once
Cysticercus cellulosae (cysticercosis)			
Treatment of choice**	Albendazole††	400 mg bid × 8–30 d, repeated as necessary	<60 kg, 15 mg/kg/d (max 800 mg) in 2 or 3 doses × 8–30 d, repeated as necessary
	or		
	Praziquantel†	50 mg/kg/d in 3 doses × 15 d	50 mg/kg/d in 3 doses × 15 d
Echinococcus granulosus (hydatid cyst)			
Treatment of choice‡‡	Albendazole	400 mg bid × 28 d, repeated as 1-mo courses as necessary	<60 kg, 15 mg/kg/d (max 800 mg) × 28 d, repeated as necessary
Echinococcus multilocularis			
Treatment of choice§§	Surgery		
Alternative	Albendazole for inoperable disease		
Trichinosis *(Trichinella spiralis)*			
Drug of choice	Mebendazole† plus steroids for severe symptoms	200–400 mg tid × 3 d, then 400–500 mg tid × 10 d	
Alternative	Albendazole†, ‖‖ plus steroids for severe symptoms	400 mg bid × 7–10 d	
Trichostrongylus infection			
Drug of choice	Pyrantel pamoate†	11 mg/kg once (max 1 g)	11 mg/kg once (max 1 g)
Alternative	Mebendazole†	100 mg bid × 3 d	100 mg bid × 3 d
	or		
	Albendazole†	400 mg once	400 mg once
Trichuriasis (*Trichuris trichiura,* whipworm)			
Drug of choice	Mebendazole	100 mg bid × 3 d	100 mg bid × 3 d
	or		
	Albendazole†	400 mg once; may require 3 d for heavy infection	400 mg once; may require 3 d for heavy infection

*Exceeds dosage recommended by the manufacturer.

†An approved drug but considered investigational for this condition by the U.S. FDA.

‡Tricalbendazole (Fasinex-Novartis), a veterinary fasciolicide, has been safe and effective (79%) after a single dose of 10 mg/kg (Apt W, Aguilera X, Vega F, et al: Treatment of human chronic fascioliasis with tricalbendazole: Drug efficacy and serologic response. Am J Trop Med Hyg 62:532–535, 1995).

§Available from the CDC Drug Service, Centers for Disease Control and Prevention, Atlanta, Georgia; (404) 639–3870.

‖Oxamniquine may be effective in areas where there is a decreased response to praziquantal (Stelma FF, Sall S, Daff B, et al: Oxamniquine cures *Schistosoma mansoni* infection in a focus in which cure rates with praziquantel are unusually low. J Infect Dis 176:304–307. 1997).

¶For disseminated infection, ivermectin is not FDA approved and thiabendazole may be preferred.

**Corticosteroids should be given for 2 to 3 days before therapy and then during treatment for neurocysticercosis. Any cysticercocidal drug may cause irreparable damage when used to treat ocular or spinal cysts, even when corticosteroids are used (White AC: Neurocysticercosis: A major cause of neurological disease worldwide. Clin Infect Dis 24:101–115, 1997). An ophthalmologic examination should be performed before treatment.

††Eight days of therapy with albendazole may be as effective as 30 days (Botero D, Uriba CS, Sanchez JL, et al: Short course albendazole treatment for neurocysticercosis in Colombia. Trans R Soc Trop Med Hyg 87:576–577, 1998).

‡‡Some patients will benefit from or require surgical resection of cysts. Praziquantel or albendazole may be used preoperatively or in case of spillage during surgery. Percutaneous drainage under ultrasound or CT guidance, with instillation of a protoscolicide, plus albendazole has been effective for management of hepatic hydatid cysts (see text) (Khuroo MS, Wani NA, Javid G, et al: Percutaneous drainage compared with surgery for hepatic hydatid cysts. N Engl J Med 3397:881–887, 1997).

§§Surgical excision is the only reliable means of therapy; however, some cases may be inoperable. In these situations, high-dose albendazole or mebendazole may be tried (Hao W, Pei-Fan Z, Wen-Guang Y, et al: Albendazole chemotherapy for human cystic and alveolar echinococcosis in north-western China. Trans R Soc Trop Med Hyg 88:340–343, 1994; World Health Organization (WHO) Informal Working Group on Echinococcosis: Guidelines for treatment of cystic and alveolar echinococcosis in humans. Bull World Health Org 74:231–242, 1996).

‖‖Information on albendazole efficacy is limited. (Cabié A, Bouchaud O, Houzé S, et al: Albendazole versus thiabendazole as therapy for trichinosis: A retrospective study. Clin Infect Dis 22:1033–1035, 1996).

containing cysticercal larvae. The eggs hatch in the intestine and develop into fluid-filled cysticerci in tissues such as skeletal muscle, the brain, and the eye.

Clinical features may include headache, vomiting, seizures, cranial nerve palsies, or psychiatric illness. It is important to emphasize that inactive cysticerci may not require anthelmintic treatment. Active lesions can be treated with albendazole or praziquantel. Dying larval worms often trigger a potentially harmful local inflammatory response, which can be decreased by giving corticosteroids for 2 to 3 days before starting anthelmintics and continuing throughout treatment. Praziquantel* levels may be reduced by steroid or anticonvulsant therapy. Albendazole* should be taken with a fatty meal to enhance absorption. A thorough eye examination is recommended before starting anthelmintic therapy because the inflammatory reaction from dying larvae may cause permanent eye damage. Neurosurgery is indicated in certain situations, such as for hydrocephalus or for lesions in critical areas of the brain and spinal cord.

Anticonvulsants are indicated for seizures. Ocular cysticercosis is usually treated surgically.

TREMATODES (FLUKES) SCHISTOSOMES

Schistosomiasis (bilharzia) is a very important trematode infection that is responsible for considerable morbidity and mortality in many developing countries. *S. mansoni* infection occurs in Africa, the Middle East, Latin America, and the Caribbean. *Schistosoma haematobium* infection (urinary schistosomiasis) occurs in Africa and the Middle East, and *Schistosoma japonicum* infection occurs in east Asia. Less common forms of human schistosomiasis are caused by *Schistosoma mekongi* in Southeast Asia and *Schistosoma intercalatum* in central Africa.

Freshwater snails are the intermediate host for schistosomiasis. Human infections occur when infective cercarial larvae burrow through intact skin during exposure to freshwater (rivers, lakes, and streams). Adult worms develop in the mesenteric veins (intestinal schistosomiasis) and vesical veins (urinary schistosomiasis). Schistosome eggs may become embedded and provoke an inflammatory response in organs such as the intestine, bladder, liver, lungs, and less commonly the spinal cord and brain. A wide range of clinical syndromes may result from infection, including periportal fibrosis, portal hypertension, ascites, esophageal varices, and splenomegaly (intestinal schistosomiasis), as well as hematuria, bladder calcification, obstructive uropathy, and pulmonary hypertension (urinary schistosomiasis).

*Not FDA approved for this indication.

Praziquantel is the drug of choice for all forms of schistosomiasis, but dosing depends on the species (Table 2). Cure rates vary from 60% to 100%. Oxamniquine (Vansil) is an alternative drug for the treatment of *S. mansoni* infections. Strains in South America and equatorial Africa appear to be more sensitive to oxamniquine than strains in northern and southern Africa.

OTHER INTESTINAL, LIVER, AND LUNG FLUKES

Other fluke infections are relatively rare, although in certain localized areas, prevalence rates of over 50% may be observed. Some flukes live in the intestine (e.g., *Fasciolopsis buski, Heterophyes heterophyes, Metagonimus yokogawai*), the liver (e.g., *Opisthorchis sinensis, Opisthorchis sinensis*), and the lung (e.g., *Paragonimus westermani*). Infection occurs after ingesting infective metacercarial larvae that are contaminating raw freshwater fish (e.g., *H. heterophyes, M. yokogawai, C. sinensis, Opisthorchis viverrini*), uncooked freshwater plants *(F. buski, Fasciola hepatica),* and raw crabs *(P. westermani).* The treatment of choice for these flukes is praziquantel,* except for *F. hepatica,* which responds better to bithionol* (Bitin).

*Not FDA approved for this indication.

Section 7

Metabolic Disorders

DIABETES MELLITUS IN ADULTS

(Type 2 Diabetes)

method of
SEYMOUR R. LEVIN, M.D.
West Los Angeles VA Medical Center and UCLA School of Medicine
Los Angeles, California

Table 1 depicts diabetes-oriented information obtained from the initial history and physical examination. Most of this initial information-gathering process can be obtained in 10 to 15 minutes. Many physicians who have passed through our training program have translated this into a form, which can be used to help obtain information at the initial visit. Because patients with diabetes can develop conditions not strictly related to diabetes, the information in Table 1 does not replace appropriate examination of all systems.

In terms of metabolic manifestations, most patients who have even a modest response to treatment do not have classic symptoms of hyperglycemia (polyuria, polyphagia, and polydipsia). Moreover, it is unlikely that patients can subjectively detect their glucose level unless it is at extremes greater than 350 mg/dL or less than 55 mg/dL. Blurred vision may be a symptom of hyperglycemia because glucose entering the lens causes swelling and consequent difficulty in altering the anterior-posterior lenticular diameter, which is necessary for visual accommodation. But some patients with hypoglycemia also note visual difficulty, including flashing lights or blurring. This might be due to glucose deprivation of the optic neural system. Patients with neuropathy may not sense when they are hypoglycemic. This hypoglycemic nonrecognition also may be present in patients without neuropathy who adhere to a tight glycemic control regimen as well. Thus, the presence of symptoms should not be the major guideline for clinical and laboratory assessment. Self-monitoring of blood glucose (SMBG), done properly, can be included in the overall assessment as a guideline for therapy.

TABLE 1. **History and Physical Examination: Diabetes Mellitus**

History

Manifestations
- Metabolic
- Anatomic

Onset circumstances
Medications (past and present) for diabetes and other conditions
Monitoring of glycemia: how learned and how often
Status of
- Exercise (versus sedentary life)
- Emotional impact
- Eating habits
- Education in self-care
- Eye visits
- Everything else (e.g., other diseases, smoking habits, erectile dysfunction, pregnancy history)

Physical Examination

Along with vital signs, perform the following:
Neurological and foot examination
Eye examination
Renal evaluation
Disease of the macrovasculature evaluation

ANATOMIC MANIFESTATIONS

The anatomic manifestations may include a presenting syndrome, such as chest pain, claudication, and ophthalmic symptoms. It is probable that many patients have had diabetes or a condition of increased risk for transition to type 2 diabetes called the *syndrome of insulin resistance* ("syndrome X"), with variable degrees of glucose tolerance, years before the diagnosis of *diabetes mellitus* (fasting glucose ≥126 mg/dL) is made.

Nevertheless, most patients have no symptoms at all. Thus, laboratory screening is essential for all individuals. Inquiry should be made regarding symptoms to address specific complications. Questions about renal status have been omitted from Table 1, not because they are less important but because symptoms of this complication early in the disease are rare. A history of nephrotic syndrome or end-stage renal disease reminds caregivers that it is wiser and more economical to prevent the complications of diabetes than to treat them.

ONSET

The mode of onset is an important factor in determining and maintaining therapy. For example, a patient in good glycemic control taking insulin since the onset of diabetes should not undergo a trial of oral agents if the initial symptoms included nausea, vomiting, weight loss, and admission to an intensive care unit. This history strongly suggests type 1 diabetes with absolute insulin dependence.

MEDICATION HISTORY

It is essential to know the patient's medication history. For example, some patients might have been changed from sulfonylurea drugs to insulin before the availability of metformin. With adequate monitoring, these patients may be tried on combinations of drugs that increase insulin secretion and enhance insulin action. Drugs for other conditions that are bound by albumin (e.g., warfarin-type drugs) can enhance the action of hypoglycemic agents or might be influenced by these agents. Nonsteroidal anti-inflammatory agents taken regularly and daily might cause deterioration of renal function. Alternative medicines, such as certain herbs, may have unpredictable effects on plasma glucose.

SELF-MONITORING OF BLOOD GLUCOSE

SMBG is a powerful adjunct to self-care if appropriate advice is given about values obtained. The patient must do the tests correctly. Bringing in a logbook and/or a computerized hardcopy recording indicates that the patient is concerned and cooperating and the log should be examined carefully by the caregiver. Additionally, there is some evidence that self-monitoring of blood pressure is of more value than the single measures taken at intervals in the clinic. It is certainly less costly than SMBG. Again, the patient must be trained and assurance of accuracy and proper usage must be obtained by matching with observations in the office.

EXERCISE

Exercise, even walking, may never have been part of many patients' habits. A sedentary lifestyle appears to be a risk factor for acquiring type 2 diabetes. Many patients cannot make running, swimming, or even long walks part of their lives because of time restrictions, because of arthritis, or because they are overweight. Therefore, we have developed a system of chair exercises (see Physical Activity).

EMOTIONS

Clinicians must determine their patient's motivation. If the patient feels that controlling the disease is preferable to letting the disease control him or her, then successful learning about self-care and lifestyle changes are more likely. If the patient is unwilling to take control, often feeling depressed with a sense of passive hopelessness, then a partnership between the patient, the clinician, and a counselor is indicated.

EATING HABITS

A daily nutritional history is often not dependable, but information about a typical breakfast, lunch, and dinner and a few questions about what the patient believes is a healthy diet is helpful. Most medical centers have trained, registered dietitians who are valuable partners in providing advice to patients. Dealing with obesity and adhering to suggested meal plans rank with practical exercise regimens as great challenges to the patient with type 2 diabetes.

EDUCATION IN SELF-CARE

Many patients have not had classes specifically addressing diabetes management in language and practices that they can understand. Absence of such knowledge can reduce chances of successful outcomes. Certified Diabetes Educators (CDEs) who have up-to-date knowledge and can explain all issues are essential parts of the team. Many centers, however, do not have CDEs. If not, others on the staff should be assigned to the task of education in self-care. Patients without such information should be told where they can obtain training. Many insurance plans now cover the cost of self-care education.

EYE EXAMINATIONS

Clinical Practice Recommendations of the American Diabetes Association (ADA) promote the annual comprehensive, dilated examination by an eye professional for patients who have had diabetes for 3 to 5 years. The ADA recommends that clinical judgment be applied regarding these recommendations. I require that patients receive annual examinations from the time of diagnosis and increased visit frequency as required. Despite these recommendations, many patients deny having a visit to an ophthalmologist or optometrist throughout the course of their disease.

KNOWLEDGE OF THE PATIENT

Knowledge about everything else in the patient's life is often necessary for optimal management. For example, a current smoker may want to stop. To this end, the caregiver can use further education, pharmacologic approaches, and motivational classes. If a patient does not wish to stop and enjoys the habit, then further education should be continued, but medication and motivational sessions are less likely to be successful or acceptable.

PHYSICAL EXAMINATION

Foot Examinations

Essential to the physical examination are the vital signs and blood pressure. Of equal importance are neurologic and general foot examinations. I rank foot examinations high because surveys have shown that this is a neglected area. A cool, pulseless foot, even without lesions, may be an indication that the patient should be seen by specialists in vascular surgery. Indications for podiatric referral include areas of redness or even minor ulcerations, toenail deformities, tinea, warts, calluses, excessive moisture, or excessive dryness. Defects in light-touch perception after examination with the 5.07/10-g monofilament also should prompt a podiatric referral.

While glycemia and other elements of the "Big Four" (Table 2) are being managed correctly, the podiatrist can prevent limb loss by early intervention with protective insoles, special shoes, and prosthetic devices that protect the foot from damage. Thus, examination of foot pulses, lesions, and sensation rank high as important tools for limb salvage. The ADA position statement recommends an annual foot examination to detect high-risk foot conditions and that those with high-risk factors be examined more frequently, with visual examination of the foot at each visit. I believe the foot examination should be done at each visit whether or not patients have risk factors.

Eye Examination

Retinopathy and microvascular lesions are not the only damage suffered by the diabetic eye. Glaucoma, cataracts, and macular lesions also are more frequent. I include an eye examination with the undilated pupil and am often able to detect gross lesions (e.g., cataracts and advanced retinopathy). I do not have any special eye examination instruments in the diabetes clinic. I rely on reports and therapy by eye care specialists.

Renal

There is not much to detect related to renal problems, but examination for generalized edema suggesting the increasingly rare nephrotic syndrome is reasonable. Assessing the general state of hydration is important in older patients with poor glycemic control. Such patients may have postural hypotension that is not necessarily the result

TABLE 2. **The "Big Four"**

Factor	Evaluation Recommended Frequency*	Recommended Goals
Glycemia	SMBG 1–4 or more times/day (see text); laboratory (see text)	Premeal: 80–120 mg/dL (whole blood)
Hb**A**$_{1c}$	Quarterly (twice a year if stable, i.e., in target range)	In 7% ranges, action indicated if >8%
Blood pressure	At each examination (weekly at home, if accuracy verified in clinic)	130/80 mm Hg
Cholesterol and other lipemic elements (fasting)	Annual (semiannually)	LDL <100 mg/dL Triglycerides <200 mg/dL HDL >45 mg/dL (55 mg/dL for females)
Discovery of the foot by clinician and patient	At each examination (daily at home)	Inspection, pulses, sensation: 5.07/10-g monofilament

*Modified from ADA Clinical Practice Recommendations. Diabetes 24(suppl 1) 2001.
Abbreviations: HDL = high-density lipoprotein; LDL = low-density lipoprotein.

of cardiovascular autonomic neuropathy as much as related to obligatory water loss and volume depletion.

Dehydration may raise the serum creatinine level secondary to prerenal azotemia, sometimes necessitating the halting of metformin in patients who are responding to this drug. Taking diuretics may add to this problem. Because it seems to occur most frequently in hot weather when increased insensible water loss adds to the dehydration, I have called it "summer syndrome." Intervention by instructing the patient to drink two to three glasses of water a day may bring the serum creatinine to normal.

Disease of the Macrovasculature

Examination of the foot and leg pulses has been discussed. Carotid examination for intensity of pulse and for bruits will help clarify whether studies of arterial patency are required. The history and physical examination may be abridged and modified in subsequent visits, but a complete initial inventory allows caregivers enough information to initiate therapy.

GOAL-ORIENTED TREATMENT OF TYPE 2 DIABETES

Table 2 lists the Big Four factors that need to be regulated in order to prevent or slow the evolution of complications. The Big Four should be controlled from the day diabetes is diagnosed. In general, when complications occur, their treatment involves greater effort, more staff, more complex treatment, and higher costs than when the majority of skill and energy is spent to prevent them. For example, an educator-physician team teaching 20 patients about overall care in 5 hours of classes costs less than $100 per patient. On the other hand, more than 20 caregivers are involved in the removal of a leg that today involves overall costs of more than $40,000 per patient. Two parameters of the Big Four are (1) laboratory data and (2) physical examination. Follow-up of the impact of regulating these elements is listed in Table 3. Although many reviews on therapy focus on glycemia, evidence-based literature indicates that reducing morbidity and mortality in diabetes requires attention to multiple factors.

Frequency of visits is a highly individual matter. If any of the elements are extremely out of control, visits for examination, education, and referral are important. Use of the telephone, fax machine, and mail are excellent cost- and time-saving adjuncts when compared with the cost of the visit.

Glycemia

In regulating glycemia in large clinics, focusing on communicating by phone with a few patients per week saves caregivers time. With information regarding glucose (weight, home blood pressure) and current medication dosage, patients will accept a brief response and instructions about the next indicated communication. Data about SMBG results and information about meals, snacks, and exercise are often helpful. To most clinicians, the resources and time required to regulate blood pressure, evaluate lipid disorders, and perform foot examinations are more available than regulating glycemia. The guidelines presented in the section, Specific Therapy for Type 2 Diabetes, should facilitate this essential component of the Big Four.

The ADA recommendations add that the goal for the average bedtime glucose should be 100 to 140 mg/dL. The lower level might be too low for some patients (see Prevention and Treatment of Hypoglycemia). Pre-exercise glucose levels should be somewhat higher than 100. Much attention is currently being paid to postprandial glucose values. At this time, I recommend an average glucose value of 170 mg/dL 2 hours after a mixed meal (700–850 calories).

Frequency of Self-Glucose Monitoring

This is a controversial area, especially for patients taking oral agents only or whose diabetes is managed solely with diet and exercise. The ADA has brought forth no clear recommendations. Several studies have compared matched patients taking oral agents, separating into frequently monitoring (3–4 times/d) and rarely monitoring groups. No difference in HbA_{1c} was observed after observation periods of up to 1

TABLE 3. **Following the Diabetic Patient**

Factor	Frequency	"Big Four" Determinant
Eye examination by eye care professional	Annually or more frequently, if pathology is present	Glucose, blood pressure, ?lipids
Function of the kidney Urinalysis Urine albumin Spot urine for microalbumin/creatinine ratio (if no gross albuminuria), serum creatinine, urine culture (if indicated)	2 to 3 times/y	Blood pressure, glucose
Good overall response to therapy Symptoms and side effects of medications Altered lifestyle (e.g., smoking, weight, exercise) Hypoglycemic or hyperglycemic episodes Infections and dental care Liver function tests (especially with patients taking certain medications, e.g., statins, thiazolidinediones) Evaluate self-care knowledge	As required	Glucose, blood pressure, lipids, foot inspection
Heart and large vessels Symptoms (claudication? central nervous system?) Electrocardiogram	1 to 3 times/y	Glucose, blood pressure, lipids

year. In most of the studies, the groups started with very high HbA_{1c}, suggesting that many in each group were no longer responding to oral agents and should have been taking insulin. There was little or no description of what actions were to be taken for each SMBG result (e.g., exercise at time of determination, food intake for the next meal). Thus, I have concluded that frequency of monitoring may have no relevance to glycemic control in patients who are not instructed about what to do with the data or who may not be oral-agent responsive.

Nevertheless, because of these experiments, many health care organizations have strictly limited the number of glucose strips a patient may receive as part of the care plan. In contrast, patients receiving insulin are often allowed to receive more strips than those on oral agents. The VA Cooperative Study showed that excellent glycemic control could be obtained in patients with type 2 diabetes with twice-daily testing. Thus, insulin-treated patients with stable diabetes whose glycemic control is at good levels may be offered too much testing, whereas patients taking oral agents are mandated too little testing. I believe all patients with diabetes should have the resources to self-test at least once daily. If necessary, *skip testing,* that is, testing at different preprandial and postprandial times in a single daily test, can be performed. In a month-long record, for example, this can provide caregivers with information about glycemic excursion throughout the day. Patients on tight control regimens require more frequent testing.

There has not been a long-term (5–10 years), large-scale study of elderly patients (beginning at age 70) to test whether harmful effects can occur in patients who adhere to the glycemic goals indicated in Table 2. Thus, individualization for every special circumstance must be made. *Good control* in elderly and other patients with co-morbidities can be defined as being as close as possible to the goals without harmful effects.

Finally, urine testing may be a reasonable alternative, in homeless patients and patients with very limited dexterity. Most patients can be given the name of a member of the diabetes team to contact if his or her urine tests always show high glucose.

Strategies for Treatment of Hypertension, Dyslipidemia, and Obesity

These strategies are discussed elsewhere in this text. Foot examination and interaction with others in the limb salvage team were discussed earlier in this article.

THE IMPACT OF REGULATING THE "BIG FOUR"

Table 3 indicates what is required for follow-up of the risks and benefits of interventions in the care of people with diabetes. The final portion of this article addresses therapy: education, exercise, diet, and medications. Each of these areas has certain risks and benefits, which also must be monitored.

Examination of the urine to evaluate kidney function is essential. The use of a spot urine test for evidence of early damage ("incipient nephropathy," or *microalbuminuria* [MA]) is essential because there is evidence that early intervention with glycemic control and angiotensin-converting enzyme inhibitors can slow or prevent renal damage even in patients who do not have hypertension. *MA* is defined as the presence of small amounts of albumin in the urine, which is negative for protein with the usual, qualitative "dipstick test": an albumin:creatinine ratio of 0.03 to 0.3 where each is reported in mg/dL.

In evaluating the overall response to therapy, issues such as infections and dental health can influence control. In the laboratory, the ADA also recommends an initial TSH in type 1 diabetic patients. I recommend this in type 2 patients as well, because hypothyroidism can promote hyperlipidemia. Glycemic control can influence the lipid profile, especially by lowering triglycerides and raising HDL. Thus, introducing lipid-lowering drugs for these values might be deferred while the effect of glycemic control is evaluated.

Hypoglycemia and episodes of severe hyperglycemia must be dealt with even in patients with HbA_{1c} in the ideal range.

SPECIFIC THERAPY FOR TYPE 2 DIABETES

Care of the patient with diabetes involves a team of professionals interacting with a patient, the family, and the socioeconomic environment. Special considerations always enter into decisions. For example, a homeless patient who requires insulin may not be able to get three meals a day, carry a month's worth of syringes and alcohol sponges, and monitor glucose with a meter. He or she may need to take small amounts of intermediate-acting insulin and/or short-acting insulin, the latter with meals when they are available; re-use syringes; and monitor for very high glucose levels with urine strips. Excellent glycemic control may be impossible, and the goal may be to simply avoid recurrent hospitalizations. Properly fitting shoes and resources for food may need to be obtained from outside agencies. Although this is an extreme example, the diabetes team must be able to deal with a variety of circumstances. One of the most difficult challenges is promoting lifestyle changes in patients who have had lifelong sedentary habits and unhealthy nutritional routines.

The four elements of therapy require that caregivers understand specific details about education in self-care, nutrition plans, exercise, and medication. The statement: "Make sure you eat right, take your medicine, and get some exercise" is not enough to start the patient on a path to optimal care.

Education About Self-Care

In many respects, education delivered by qualified individuals is as important as medication in preventing the complications of diabetes. Ensure that the educator is a Certified Diabetes Educator (CDE) or is preparing to become certified. My VA center offers a complete set of instruction in medications, stress management, basic facts, nutrition, and foot care. Patients are encouraged to ask questions, such as the following:

What is my A1? What should it be? How can we get it there?

What is my blood pressure? Can we get it to 130/80?

What is my "LDL" cholesterol? How can we get it to the proper level?

I'm about to leave and you haven't examined my feet. Can you do this? They look okay when I examine them.

Many excellent resources are available, including literature and the Internet (ADA website, www.diabetes.org). These should supplement but not replace educational classes.

The Value of Adhering to a Nutritional Plan

Adoption of an appropriate diet program is difficult for patients who are in the habit of eating too much or densely caloric, high-fat diets. However, what we often interpret as "noncompliance" may simply be lack of information. Registered dietitians are available at most centers to teach patients on a one-to-one basis or in class. The January 2001 ADA Nutrition Recommendations emphasize individualized treatment and a comprehensive approach to not only glucose values but to blood pressure, blood lipids, physical activity, weight, and renal function. The recommendations are evolving into statements about what is a reasonable, sound diet for people with or without diabetes. They take into consideration cultural styles and economic limitations. Many patients need repeated instruction about dietary modifications and evaluation of motivation and retention of facts and concepts.

Physical Activity

Many studies of exercise as a therapeutic tool in diabetes indicate that poor aerobic fitness enhances cardiovascular risk factors. Exercise is an important part of dealing with the *insulin resistance syndrome,* characterized by hypertension, central obesity, and dyslipidemia. With this syndrome, insulin levels are high, reflecting insulin resistance. However, I do not recommend insulin measurement to these patients. They may be hyperglycemic or at risk for diabetes. Exercise recommendations should take into account whether a patient has *insensate feet* (loss of protective sensation). The ADA position statement on exercise advises against patients with insensate feet using a treadmill, prolonged walking, jogging, or doing step exercises.

All of these activities are certainly contraindicated with foot ulceration. Swimming, bicycling, and rowing are recommended because of the reduced weight-bearing. I consider walking and jogging to be very difficult for heavy patients, even those without neu-

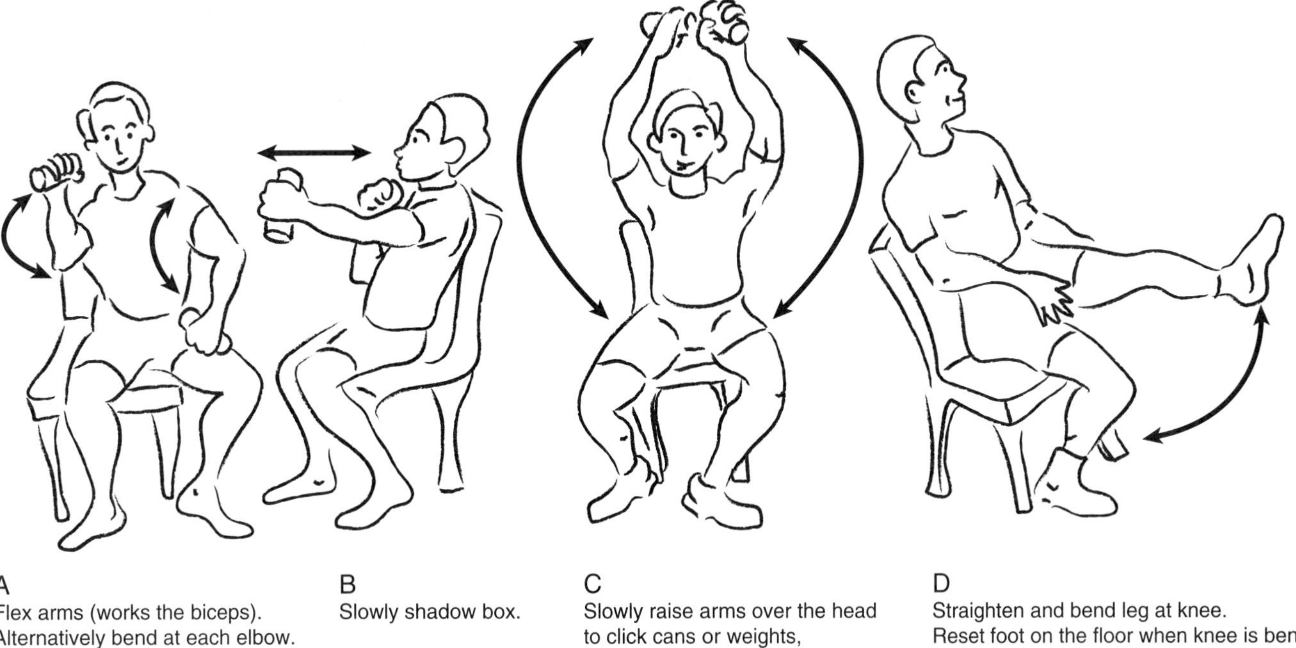

Figure 1. Chair exercises for the patient with diabetes mellitus. The patient sits back, relaxed, gently breathing throughout the exercise, holding a 1.5-lb food can in each hand. Later, when maximum repetitions are achieved, up to 5 lb in each hand can be used, if well tolerated. *Instructions to the patient:* Start with 4 to 5 repetitions of each exercise once a day. Then, at weekly intervals, go to 3 sessions a day if comfortable and if time, workplace, and other conditions permit. Next, increase by 1 repetition of each exercise each week. The sessions can be performed while watching television or reading. Stop if the exercise becomes painful or is overtaxing. *Final goal:* 10 to 15 repetitions of each exercise, 2 to 3 sessions a day. Working up to this goal should take 7 to 8 weeks or more. Do not do too much too soon. Make sure the back is well supported with a cushion or other device.

ropathy. Chair exercises are adaptable for all patients.

Figure 1 illustrates specific chair exercises because people who do not ordinarily exercise need a detailed description. Upper limb exercises may be enhanced by holding a can of food or small weights. I have no evidence that chair exercises lower the glucose as well as medication, but I believe that this form of exercise is better than any activity that patients will not accept over the long term.

Frequency and number of repetitions need to be gradually increased, and these increases should be limited so that the patient finds the exercise enjoyable. Ideally, over a number of weeks, repetitions can be increased from 2 to 3 once a day of each of the upper extremities and leg exercises to 15 to 20 repetitions, two to three times a day. The activity can be done before each meal and while watching television or reading. Physician advice related to other conditions (e.g., coronary heart disease) is always necessary, as with any exercise plan.

Pharmacologic Management of Type 2 Diabetes

How and When to Use Oral Hypoglycemic Agents

Type 2 diabetes is a metabolic disorder of nutrient metabolism resulting from the inability of the endocrine pancreas to maintain sufficient insulin secretion to overcome resistance to the action of this hormone. As the disease progresses, certain anatomic complications result. The objective of education, nutrition, and pharmacologic agents is to enhance insulin levels in the bloodstream, ideally at appropriate times, and/or to reduce insulin resistance.

Although diabetes is diagnosed when fasting glucose is 126 mg/dL or greater on several occasions, there is no definite glucose level at which to begin pharmacologic therapy. Symptoms cannot be used because many patients have no symptoms at glucose levels that clearly induce glycation of proteins (e.g., HbA_{1c}).

On the other hand, there are patients with "impaired fasting glucose" of 111 to 125 mg/dL who are not currently diagnosed as diabetic and who may be at increased risk for macrovascular events. As with diabetic patients these patients who have hypertension, obesity, and dyslipidemia require treatment. It is still not clear, however, whether physicians need to introduce oral hypoglycemic agents in this group. Partial answers will be forthcoming when the National Institutes of Health completes its type 2 diabetes prevention trial. At this time, I recommend oral hypoglycemic agents when education, diet, and exercise cannot get the fasting glucose to the ranges recommended in Table 2.

Table 4 indicates the currently used oral agents,

TABLE 4. **Oral Hypoglycemic Agents**

Mechanism	Minimum/Maximum Dosing
Enhance Insulin Secretion	
SULFONYLUREAS	
Glyburide (Micronase, DiaBeta)*	1.25/20 mg once (AM)
Glipizide (Glucotrol)*†	2.5/10 mg divided (bid)
Glimepiride (Amaryl)	0.5/8 mg once (AM)
MEGLITINIDES	
Repaglinide (Prandin)	0.5/8 mg indicated dose just before each meal (1–5 minutes)
Nateglinide (Starlix)	60/120 mg indicated dose just before each meal (1–5 minutes)
Enhance Insulin Action (sensitizers)	
METFORMIN (GLUCOPHAGE)†	500/2000 mg; start lowest dose in evening, then divide total (bid)
THIAZOLIDINEDIONES	
Rosiglitazone (Avandia)	2/4 mg bid
Pioglitazone (Actos)	15/45 mg once (AM)
Slow Gut Absorption of Complex Carbohydrates	
α-GLYCOSIDASE INHIBITORS	
Acarbose (Precose)	25/100 mg just before meals
Miglitol (Glyset)	25/100 mg just before meals

*Available as generic.
†Available in sustained-release form (once daily).

their descriptive mechanisms of action, and what I consider the minimum and maximum dosages. Table 5 indicates advantages and disadvantages of each. In general, the agents that enhance insulin secretion can cause hypoglycemia. If the patient misses meals or exercises he or she may be at greater risk for hypoglycemia. Also at risk for hypoglycemia are elderly patients who may miss meals, and patients who are losing weight intentionally. In these patients, dosage reduction may be indicated. As a rule, as monotherapy, the agents that enhance insulin action (metformin, thiazolidine diones), or those that reduce glucose absorption (the α-glycosidase inhibitors) do not cause hypoglycemia. When these agents are combined with other oral agents or with insulin, however, excessive glucose-lowering effects may be accentuated.

With metformin and α-glycosidase inhibitors, it is often best to introduce very small doses (half lowest effective dose) for 7 to 14 days, with gradual increases. This allows adjustment if the patient experiences gastrointestinal symptoms. These side effects seem to diminish with gradual introduction to effective dosage. If hypoglycemia were to occur in a patient taking an α-glycosidase inhibitor, it most likely would be reversed with glucose tablets or juice because sucrose (table sugar) or maltose breakdown would be slowed by this drug class.

How does the clinician choose which medication to use for initiation of therapy? Because of early evidence from the United Kingdom study, risk of macrovascular events can be reduced with metformin monotherapy in obese patients with diabetes, and I initiate metformin in this group. In patients who are not obese (body mass index <27 kg/m^2), I use sulfonylurea drugs as initial therapy.

TABLE 5. **Advantages and Disadvantages of the Oral Hypoglycemic Agents**

Advantages	Disadvantages and Cautions
Sulfonylureas	
Improve insulin secretion	Hypoglycemia may be prolonged or severe
Endogenous insulin delivered	Weight gain
Excellent and rapid response in "oral-agent-naive" patients	Caution with renal or hepatic dysfunction
May respond, at first, to very low dosages	Effect may wane after months or years
Meglitinides	
Same as sulfonylureas but...	Must be taken before each meal
Insulin high only around mealtime	Can cause weight gain or hypoglycemia
If meal missed, may also miss dose	Caution with renal or hepatic insufficiency
Biguanides	
Decrease insulin resistance (reduce hepatic glucose production)	Should not be used if serum creatinine >1.5 mg/dL (males) or >1.4 mg/dL (females); threat of lactic acidosis
Good initial glycemic response	Initial gastrointestinal side effects
Possible reduced macrovascular disease	Hold for 1 day before and after iodocontrast studies or surgery
Less or no weight gain than sulfonylureas	Do not use in patients with heart failure, excess alcohol, hepatic/renal insufficiency
Little hypoglycemia when used as monotherapy	May accentuate hypoglycemia when used with other agents
Thiazolidinediones	
No hypoglycemia	Weight gain and fluid retention (use caution in patients with heart failure)
Can be used for patients with renal insufficiency	May increase low-density lipoprotein cholesterol
Increases uptake of glucose by fat and muscle (also reduces hepatic glucose output)	Liver monitoring required (every 2 months for first year); do not use if values are >2.5 upper limits of normal
Increases high-density lipoprotein (reduces macrovascular risk)	Up to 10 to 12 weeks for maximum effect
α-Glycosidase Inhibitors	
Good safety record	Causes bloating and gas
Can be used to "fine tune" HbA_{1c}	Modest effect
	Less effect with low-carbohydrate diet

Effects on glycemia are usually excellent with any of the oral agents at the initiation of pharmacotherapy, and these drugs may lower HbA_{1c} as much as two to three percentage points. Achievement of optimal glucose reduction with thiazolidinediones in obese patients would be similar to metformin, but the latter drug class is less likely to be associated with weight gain and is less costly (~\$1–\$2/d versus \$4–\$6/d, respectively). The α-glycosidase inhibitors as initial monotherapy are unlikely to lower the HbA_{1c} more than 0.5% to 0.7%. They may have use in patients whose fasting glucose is near goal, but HbA_{1c} and postprandial glucose are elevated.

Each of the oral agents take time to reach optimal effectiveness because the dosage is being gradually adjusted. Thus, for all drugs, expect to wait up to 3 to 4 weeks before maximal effect on fasting glucose is reached. It will take 3 to 5 months before the HbA1c nadir is attained. Rapidity of response is generally sulfonylureas > metformin > α-glycosidase inhibitors > thiazolidinediones. If two drugs are in the same class, I recommend that clinicians become accustomed to finding their favorite and include cost as a criteria. Table 5 includes the advantages and disadvantages of the oral agents.

Combination Therapy With Oral Hypoglycemic Agents

A major principle is that in patients who have been on oral agents for some time, when the fasting glucose is consistently very high (>275 mg/dL), pancreatic B-cell function is greatly depleted; it is time to use exogenous insulin, alone or in combination with oral agents. When glucose levels are below the mid-200s (mg/dL), the advantage of combining oral agents is that a secretagogue can be used with an enhancer of insulin action or two enhancers of insulin sensitivity can be used with or without a secretagogue. In some cases, triple oral therapy has been carried out successfully to bring HbA_{1c} to goal, for a time.

The disadvantages of combined oral therapy are that the caregiver must survey for all the side effects and toxicities, be cautious about increased risk of adverse drug interactions among these agents, and look out for adverse drug interactions with other medications. I prefer a serious trial with two agents before adopting a third. I do not use a C-peptide measurement to decide whether a patient has enough endogenous insulin to continue oral agents; rather, I consider the current glucose and the response to another agent as a therapeutic test. Gradual introduction of the second agent seems wise. When a therapeutic response is noted, reducing the first agent is reasonable. It also seems wise to use less than maximal doses of each for most patients.

One combination to avoid is the α-glycosidase inhibitor plus meglitinides because the insulin response to ingested carbohydrate may be blunted when absorption is slowed. It is not clear if there is any advantage to combining meglitinides with sulfonylureas, and I do not use this combination.

A ready-made combination of glyburide and metformin is now marketed (Glucovance). This combination is safe and effective in lowering glucose with submaximal dosages in patients who have failed diet and exercise regimens but have not failed a course of oral agents. Whether early initiation of a combination of secretagogue and sensitizer will prolong the intactness of B-cell function and target organ response remains to be seen.

My favorite combinations include sulfonylurea-metformin, meglitinide-metformin, and metformin-thiazolidine, but virtually all combinations will lower HbA_{1c} toward goal *provided the patient has reasonable endogenous insulin reserve,* as reflected in the reduction of fasting glucose.

How and When to Use Insulin for the Patient With Type 2 Diabetes

The majority of insulin sold in this country is to patients who have type 2 diabetes. This is because these patients outnumber type 1 (ketosis prone) patients by 10:1. The old term, *non–insulin-dependent diabetes mellitus* (NIDDM), thus, was confusing to many clinicians. In patients with type 2 diabetes, I would rather use the term *insulin-requiring type 2 diabetes.* There are at least 30 variations of insulin regimens. Some are more adaptable to type 1 patients. Table 6 depicts the regimens I use most frequently.

There are three indications for using insulin in type 2 diabetic patients. The first and most frequent is when the oral agent or agents no longer maintain glycemia at goal. If the fasting glucose is consistently greater than 275 mg/dL (sometimes even less) on a maximum dose of a single oral agent or combination of two or three agents, insulin is required. Of course, if the patient is not on a reasonable diet and exercise regimen and adopts such a program, oral agent–responsiveness may return. I have been able to discontinue insulin, even high doses, by introducing oral agents in some patients who had insulin therapy initiated before the insulin sensitizers and combined oral agents were introduced.

The second indication for insulin therapy is when hyperglycemia supervenes in times of stress, such as infection, a hyperosmolar state, trauma, surgery, or introduction of glucocorticoids. Space does not permit discussion of management of these acute syndromes.

The last indication for insulin therapy is the rare appearance of ketosis proneness in the nonstarved patient who may have been managed as a type 2 diabetic for years. Often, there is involuntary weight loss. Management usually requires multiple injections of insulin.

The four methods in Table 6 are relatively simple. Some patients can follow self-management protocols using decision plans I have set for them. Most require interaction with staff. There is no need to admit a patient to the hospital to teach injection techniques.

TABLE 6. **Use of Insulin in Type 2 Diabetes**

Regimen	Advantages	Disadvantages
Bedtime injection of intermediate-acting insulin NPH, Lente	Reduces hepatic glucose output at night Single injection	Occasional nocturnal hypoglycemia Oscillations with meals not covered
Two-dose split and mixed (intermediate and regular)	Covers the eating hours Constant low levels of background insulin	Patient needs to mix insulins Regular and intermediate may produce hypoglycemia during the day
Three-dose split and mixed	Bedtime insulin reduces hepatic glucose output Covers eating hours	Requires injections three times/d
Insulin as above, combined with insulin sensitizers or secretagogues	Reducing insulin resistance is part of therapy, reducing total insulin dose	Side effects of oral agents, as well as insulin must be considered Secretagogues plus insulin not effective in lowering glucose during eating hours unless patient has some endogenous insulin

- For bedtime (h.s.) insulin, I recommend beginning with 15 to 20 units of NPH (or Lente). I usually withdrawn all or all but one of the prior oral agents. For heavier patients, I may begin with 20 to 25 units h.s. Every week or so, based on accurate SMBG, insulin h.s. can be increased 5 units until the fasting glucose goal is reached. By reducing fasting glucose, peak postprandial glucose is reduced, though the change from basal may remain the same. By introducing insulin secretagogues in the morning or just before meals (sulfonylureas or more physiologically, meglitinides), endogenous insulin secretion is encouraged.
- Two-dose split and mixed involves calculating insulin dose in terms of current body weight. I begin with 0.5 unit/kg, but nonobese patients will eventually require 0.7 to 0.8 units/kg, and obese patients will require 0.9 to 1.2 unit/kg if insulin monotherapy is used. Less insulin may be required if insulin is combined with drugs that enhance insulin action. The total dose is divided so that two thirds is given before breakfast and one third is given before supper. Two thirds of the morning dose is NPH or Lente (intermediate-acting insulin [INT]), and one third is regular. Half of the evening dose is INT.

SAMPLE PATIENT. 220 pounds (100 kg).

OBJECTIVE. Find a "permanent" dose that will get SMBG to preprandial levels of 80 to 120 mg/dL.

0.5 U/kg = 50 U/d. This is a conservative starting dose. (Doses are approximations calculated to nearest fraction.)

Total A.M. dose (⅔ daily) = 34 U	Total P.M. dose (⅓ daily) = 16 U
A.M. NPH (⅔ total A.M. dose) = 22 U	P.M. NPH (½ total P.M. dose) = 8 U
A.M. Regular (⅓ total A.M. dose) = 12 U	P.M. Regular (½ total P.M. dose) = 8 U
Thus, initial A.M. dose is: 22 U NPH 12 U Regular	Initial P.M. dose is: 8 U NPH 8 U Regular

If SMBG throughout the day is in the 200 range for 4 to 6 days, raise the dose by 0.1 unit/kg and repeat the fractional calculations until most of samples are between 160 and 200 mg/dL. Then, targeting of glucose can begin (i.e., add 2 to 5 units of presupper NPH to control morning glucose and 2 to 5 units of morning NPH to control presupper glucose). Morning regular can also be used to target prelunch glucose, and presupper regular can be used to target h.s. glucose. "Sliding scale" regular insulin is not usually given because this may mislead calculation of the dose. However, if glucose is greater than 300 mg/dL, patients may take 5 units regular, especially if symptomatic.

If, when regular insulin is given, hypoglycemia occurs before the next meal and yet when regular is reduced, preprandial hyperglycemia occurs, use of lispro insulin (Humalog) is recommended. This insulin is more rapid-acting than regular and of shorter duration (2 hours versus 6 hours), so it helps to metabolize the nutrients but is less elevated during the postabsorptive state.

Often, 70/30 insulin can be used in type 2 diabetes. This is a mixture of 70% NPH and 30% regular, premixed by the manufacturer. Advantages include freedom from need to mix and the ability to use in insulin "pens." Disadvantages include inability to subtract or add intermediate or regular insulins as required to target subsequent glucose levels to establish a "permanent" dosage.

The 70/30 insulin mixtures can thus be used for two-dose, split and mixed regimens.

- Three-dose split and mixed insulin. In this regimen, dosage calculation is similar to that applied in the two-dose split and mixed schedules. The difference between these two programs is that the calculated regular is given before supper, and the calculated intermediate-acting insulin (NPH or Lente) is given at bedtime, often with a small (200 calorie) snack. I recommend three-dose split and mixed insulin when the average prebreakfast glucose is the highest value throughout the day. Here, as with insulin h.s. alone, the bedtime NPH insulin is administered to target the fasting glucose.

- *Insulin combined with oral agents.* This regimen spares the dosage of both insulin and the oral agent. Any of the above regimens can be used with oral agents. The agent can be the secretion-activating agents or the insulin sensitizers. The insulin can be intermediate-acting or long-acting, such as, Ultralente at bedtime. We have many patients in our large clinic taking insulin-metformin. Currently, I have a number of patients on combined bedtime Ultralente (caution: do not use above 10 to 15 units to avoid overlap with the following day) and premeal repaglinide (Prandin). However, the possible combinations are numerous. The major principle is that insulin levels need to be sustained, as a background for sensitizers and/or insulin secretory enhancers.

A new, chemically engineered version of single injection, 24-hour-duration insulin has been approved: glargine (Lantus). Levels of this insulin are more sustained; therefore, a single injection (h.s. or prebreakfast) may be satisfactory, especially when superimposed on single or multiple oral agents.

It is probable that some patients with type 2 diabetes will respond to pumps, which infuse insulin subcutaneously. A VA Cooperative Study showed excellent results and sparing of insulin dosage in type 2 diabetes when the infusion tip was placed into the abdominal cavity. Pumps could be used with insulin sensitizers to spare dosage and avoid frequent need to fill the pump reservoir.

Prevention and Treatment of Hypoglycemia

Avoidance of hypoglycemia is a matter of both clinician and patient education. Some of these issues were discussed earlier. The VA study showed that type 2 patients undergoing intensive glycemic control had one-twentieth the serious hypoglycemia as seen with type 1 patients with similar degrees of control. Nevertheless, patients need to be aware that insulin and/or hypoglycemic agents must be matched with meals. Severe hypoglycemia can occur as a consequence of missing meals (alcohol will accentuate this), exercise without prior increase in food (or decrease of hypoglycemic agent), or overdose or wrong timing of medication. Some patients who are initially cooperative with programs lose weight only to encounter hypoglycemic reactions. This may discourage them and they may return to excessive food intake. Thus, as weight is lost, and even before, patients will require lower dosages of hypoglycemic medication. The degree of dosage reduction requires interaction with caregivers because this varies.

Patients who begin to exercise or go to bed with a blood glucose of less than 100 to 120 mg/dL may have hypoglycemia during the night. One can titrate up the glucose before an event with Lifesavers candy or glucose tablets (5–20 g). For each Lifesavers or 5-g glucose tablet, the blood glucose should rise 10 mg/dL in 20 minutes in a 70-kg patient. Thus, if, for example, before mowing the lawn the glucose is 80 mg, the patient may ingest a 20-g glucose tablet to raise the glucose to 120 mg/dL. Dosage will be higher for obese patients, and the effect lasts 20 to 30 minutes. Prevention of hypoglycemia is preferable to treatment, in which a patient must often take sufficient simple carbohydrates to raise blood glucose to very high levels.

Other Medications

Herbs and Alternative Medicine

Many herbs have hypoglycemic properties. Even biguanides are present in the French lilac. More work needs to be done, and separation of active components from inactive or even harmful components will be required before I routinely prescribe herbal therapy for my patients. Acupuncture is being studied as a modality for neuropathy, but glycemic control must not be ignored.

Antioxidants

Because hyperglycemia results in increased oxidation of a variety of circulating substances, especially lipoproteins, control of glucose is of utmost importance. Until trials are completed, I advise some antioxidants, such as vitamin E, 400 IU/d, and vitamin C, 250 mg/d.

Aspirin

Because studies have shown that there is a reduced risk of cardiovascular complications, the ADA recommends at least 81 mg of aspirin a day. At this dose, the drug does not exacerbate retinopathy, renal dysfunction, or ulcer disease. The antiplatelet drug clopidogrel (Plavix), 75 mg/d, is slightly more effective than aspirin 325 mg/d in reducing combined risk of stroke, myocardial infarction, and vascular death. In patients with a history of myocardial infarction, angina, or heart failure, aspirin can lessen the beneficial effects of angiotension-converting enzyme inhibitors. We are trying to institute low-dose aspirin in all type 2 patients who do not take anticoagulants or other antiplatelet drugs.

Treatment of hypertension, dyslipidemia, and other complications was discussed earlier or in other articles of this book.

DIABETES MELLITUS IN CHILDREN AND ADOLESCENTS

method of
DAVID W. COOKE, M.D., and
LESLIE PLOTNICK, M.D.
Johns Hopkins University School of Medicine
Baltimore, Maryland

Diabetes mellitus is a group of diseases that have in common a defect in the metabolic homeostasis that is controlled by insulin. This results in abnormalities of lipid and carbohydrate metabolism. Diabetes has been divided based on pathophysiology into four major groups: type 1, type 2, gestational, and a group encompassing "other specific types" of diabetes. Until very recently, virtually all of diabetes in the pediatric age range was due to type 1 diabetes. However, in the past decade, there has been a striking increase in the identification of adolescents newly diagnosed with diabetes who have type 2 diabetes mellitus, therefore, those caring for children must now be familiar with the diagnosis and treatment of all types of diabetes.

CLASSIFICATION

Type 1 Diabetes

Type 1 diabetes has previously been referred to as *type I, juvenile,* or *insulin-dependent diabetes mellitus (IDDM)* and has its highest incidence during childhood. It is caused by the autoimmune destruction of the insulin-producing β cells of the pancreatic islets of Langerhans. Autoantibodies directed against islet antigens develop in the majority of patients with type 1 diabetes; this finding can be helpful in categorizing diabetes in some pediatric patients. There is a clear genetic susceptibility for type 1 diabetes, with a well-defined, strong linkage to the human leukocyte antigen (HLA) D locus. Nonetheless, most patients diagnosed with type 1 diabetes do not have a family history of type 1 diabetes.

Type 2 Diabetes

Type 2 diabetes has been previously referred to as *type II, adult-onset,* or *non–insulin-dependent diabetes (NIDDM).* The prevalence of type 2 diabetes increases steadily with age. The pathology of type 2 diabetes is in some regards more complex than that of type 1 diabetes, in that two defects are present that combine to cause the disease. The first is a defect in the intracellular signaling of insulin, leading to a state of insulin resistance. This defect necessitates a higher concentration of insulin to induce the desired physiologic signal, that is, a higher fasting insulin level to suppress hepatic glucose production to maintain a normal fasting glucose level and higher postprandial insulin levels to stimulate peripheral glucose uptake to maintain normal postprandial glycemia.

Obesity is a major cause of insulin resistance in patients with type 2 diabetes. There is a strong genetic component to the risk of type 2 diabetes; most patients diagnosed with type 2 diabetes will have a family history of type 2 diabetes. Some of this risk can be attributable to the inheritance of a genetic risk for obesity as up to 70% of the variability of weight can be attributed to genetic risk, but there is also an inherited component of insulin resistance that is not due to obesity. Type 2 diabetes is due to more than just insulin resistance, however. Although all subjects who are obese are insulin resistant, most obese people do not develop diabetes. This is because their bodies compensate for the insulin resistance by increasing insulin secretion to meet the higher needs. The second defect that is present in type 2 diabetes is a defect in insulin secretion. With this second defect, the increased insulin requirements are not achieved. Although the relative contribution of the two defects, insulin resistance and an insulin secretory defect, may vary from patient to patient, both are present in the patient with type 2 diabetes.

Other Specific Types

The category of "other specific types" of diabetes includes a number of disorders that can occur during childhood, although they are all very rare, even when combined as a group. Some discussion of maturity-onset diabetes of the young (MODY) is warranted, however, because of potential confusion of type 2 diabetes that presents in childhood with MODY.

The underlying defects in MODY are now understood at the genetic level—these are autosomal dominant diseases caused by mutations in single genes. Each of these mutations (mutations in five different genes have been identified) in some way cause a defect in insulin secretion. There is variability in the clinical findings that occur with each form of MODY, with the age at presentation ranging from early childhood to early adulthood and the insulin deficiency varying from mild to more severe. In contrast to patients with type 2 diabetes, insulin resistance is not a part of MODY and these patients are generally not obese. Although it is reasonable to consider the diagnosis in a nonobese child with a non–insulin-requiring form of diabetes and a strong family history that indicates autosomal dominant inheritance of early-onset diabetes, MODY remains a rare cause of diabetes. The increased diagnosis of non–insulin-dependent diabetes in children is due to an increased incidence of type 2 diabetes, not MODY.

Treatment of patients with MODY is directed at their defect in insulin secretion and can be accomplished using insulin secretagogues, although some forms of MODY may progress to a degree of insulin deficiency requiring treatment with insulin to maintain metabolic control.

EPIDEMIOLOGY

Diabetes mellitus is the most common chronic disease afflicting children. Until recently, perhaps as recently as 10 years ago, virtually all of the diabetes that presented in children was type 1 diabetes. Type 1 diabetes can present at any age from infancy to adulthood. The overall prevalence of type 1 diabetes is 2 to 3 per 1000 children at 18 years of age. In adults, type 2 diabetes is much more common than type 1 diabetes, accounting for over 90% of cases. The prevalence increases steadily with increasing age, with an overall prevalence in the population of 5% to 10%. However, there is a very large difference in prevalence across racial and ethnic groups, with type 2 diabetes being much more common in minority populations, including African, Hispanic, and Native American populations, with the Native American populations having the highest prevalence.

The incidence of type 2 diabetes is increasing dramatically in the United States, coincident with the increased prevalence of obesity. Recently, it has been recognized that this rising epidemic is extending into pediatric populations. As expected from the adult epidemiology, type 2 diabetes in children affects predominantly, although not exclusively, minority populations, again including African, Hispanic, and Native Americans. The normal physiology of puberty includes an increase in insulin resistance with the onset of puberty that returns to normal insulin sensitivity at the end of puberty. This explains the finding that, with rare exceptions, type 2 diabetes is found in children only after the onset of puberty. This increase in incidence of type 2 diabetes is such that, in some reports, one third of the adolescents with newly diagnosed diabetes had type 2 diabetes.

DIAGNOSIS

The diagnosis of diabetes rests on the demonstration of hyperglycemia. The goal for patients with type 1 diabetes is to make this diagnosis before the deterioration into diabetic ketoacidosis. However, because overt type 1 diabetes develops over an acute to subacute time frame, screening is not useful. Timely diagnosis requires testing when there are symptoms caused by hyperglycemia: polydipsia and polyuria. At the time of diagnosis, there may also be a history of weight loss, in spite of a period of polyphagia. The symptoms, when elicited, will generally have been present for a defined time period of some weeks. The hyperglycemia is almost always elevated to a degree where the diagnosis is clear (e.g., >200 mg/dL). One caveat to keep in mind is that the metabolic stress response to illness can be quite vigorous, especially in the young child. Therefore, even marked hyperglycemia during a significant illness (including a viral illness with a high fever) in the absence of a preceding history of polydipsia and polyuria may not represent permanent diabetes mellitus.

The presence of type 2 diabetes in pediatric patients has complicated the diagnosis of diabetes in adolescents. First is the ability to differentiate type 1 from type 2 diabetes in the adolescent with newly diagnosed diabetes. Second is the ability to identify asymptomatic patients with type 2 diabetes. With regard to the second issue, most adolescents with type 2 diabetes have not been diagnosed based on the classic symptoms of hyperglycemia. Many have been asymptomatic, with the diagnosis made by the identification of hyperglycemia on "routine" screening laboratory studies (blood chemistries or urinalysis), with many girls identified during the evaluation for vaginal candidiasis. In large part because of this, the American Diabetes Association and the American Academy of Pediatrics issued a joint statement in 2000 that, for the first time, recommended a screening strategy for the diagnosis of type 2 diabetes in children. It is not recommended that all adolescents be screened for type 2 diabetes, only those characterized as being at high risk by the guidelines summarized in Table 1. The criteria for the diagnosis of diabetes are the same as those used in adults and are summarized in Table 2.

TABLE 1. **Screening for Type 2 Diabetes in Children**

Who: Children older than 10 years old (or younger children who have entered puberty) who are
- Obese
  - Plus have two of the following risk factors:
- Family history of type 2 diabetes in first- or second-degree relative
- Member of a minority population (Native American, African American, Hispanic, Asian/Pacific Islander)
- Signs of insulin resistance or conditions associated with insulin resistance (acanthosis nigricans, hypertension, dyslipidemia, polycystic ovary syndrome)

When: every 2 years

How: Fasting plasma glucose test

Adapted from type 2 diabetes in children and adolescents. Pediatrics 105:671–680, 2000.

TABLE 2. **Diabetes Mellitis: Diagnostic Criteria**

Symptoms of diabetes plus casual plasma glucose concentration ≥200 mg/dL (11.1 mmol/L).

or

Fasting plasma glucose ≥126 mg (dL (7.0 mmol/L).

or

Plasma glucose level ≥200 mg/dL (11.1 mmol/L) at the 2-hour point during an oral glucose tolerance test

In the absence of unequivocal hyperglycemia with acute metabolic decompensation, these criteria should be confirmed by repeat testing on a different day. "Casual" is defined as any time of day without regard to time since last meal. The classic symptoms of diabetes include polyuria, polydipsia, and unexplained weight loss. Fasting is defined as no caloric intake for at least 8 hours. The third measure, using the oral glucose tolerance test, is not recommended for routine clinical use.

Adapted from Report of the expert committee on the diagnosis and classification of diabetes mellitus. Diabetes Care 20:1183–1197, 1997.

The question of how to categorize adolescents who are newly diagnosed with diabetes is important so that an appropriate treatment plan can be prescribed. Patients with type 1 diabetes must be treated with insulin. Without insulin treatment they will develop ketoacidosis once their endogenous insulin production declines to a sufficient degree. In contrast, children with type 2 diabetes will respond to the same variety of agents with which adults with type 2 diabetes are treated. Type 2 diabetes is still extremely rare before the onset of puberty, so that except in very unusual circumstances, prepubertal children diagnosed with diabetes should be classified as having type 1 diabetes.

In the pubertal child diagnosed with diabetes, the following factors would suggest a diagnosis of type 1 diabetes:

1. Family history of type 1 diabetes
2. Thin body habitus
3. Subacute symptoms (polyuria and polydipsia easily dated to a number of weeks)
4. White race
5. Family history of other autoimmune diseases

The following factors would suggest a diagnosis of type 2 diabetes:

1. Family history of type 2 diabetes
2. Obesity (body mass index greater than the 85th percentile for age)
3. Acanthosis nigricans (the dark, thick, velvety skin on the nape of the neck and in the axilla and other intertriginous areas that is an indicator of insulin resistance)
4. Member of a minority population

For many pubertal children, it is not difficult to classify their diabetes. For example, a thin, white child with no family history of type 2 diabetes can be assumed to have type 1 diabetes without further testing. Similarly, an obese African American adolescent who has acanthosis nigricans and whose grandparents have type 2 diabetes can be assumed to have type 2 diabetes.

For other patients, however, it may be useful to measure autoantibodies to help guide classification of their diabetes. One must look for antibodies against insulin (this must be obtained before any insulin treatment), glutamic acid decarboxylase (GAD 65), the tyrosine phosphatases IA-2 and IA-2β, or whole islet cells. A diabetic patient with autoantibodies is classified as having type 1 diabetes and should be treated with insulin. Conversely, in the appropriate context, the absence of autoantibodies, particularly if two or more are looked for, suggests the patient has type 2 diabetes.

However, obesity does not "protect" a predisposed individual from developing type 1 diabetes; and given the high and rising prevalence of both obesity and type 2 diabetes in the general population, the occurrence of type 1 diabetes in an obese adolescent with a family history of type 2 diabetes will not be uncommon. In addition, a small but significant percentage of patients with type 1 diabetes will not have detectable autoantibodies at diagnosis. Consequently, the absence of autoantibodies, even when multiple antibodies are tested for, does not completely exclude the diagnosis of type 1 diabetes.

Whatever classification is initially considered, it should be considered a working classification, particularly if the patient is classified as type 2 and treated with oral agents. If these patients have been misclassified, their glucose control will deteriorate and they will develop ketosis as their endogenous insulin production wanes. Insulin and C-peptide levels are higher at diagnosis in patients with type 2 diabetes than in those with type 1 diabetes, but the difference is often not useful in the individual patient. However, significant C-peptide levels more than 2 years after diagnosis in a patient presumed to have type 1 diabetes would suggest that the patient may in fact have type 2 diabetes.

Ketoacidosis is relatively uncommon in adults with type 2 diabetes, particularly at the time of diagnosis or soon thereafter in the absence of confounding factors such as debility or intercurrent infections. Because of this, there may be a tendency to use the occurrence of ketoacidosis as an indicator that the patient has type 1 diabetes. However, it is now clear that ketoacidosis is not uncommon in children with type 2 diabetes and can be just as severe as that which occurs in type 1 diabetes. In addition, the goal is to diagnose patients with type 1 diabetes before they develop ketoacidosis. Therefore, the presence or absence of ketoacidosis is not of much use in classifying the type of diabetes that an adolescent has.

TREATMENT

Type 1 Diabetes

Since the Diabetes Control and Complication Trial (DCCT) data were published, starting in 1993, there has been firm rationale for tighter metabolic control in type 1 diabetes. To achieve this goal, the management regimens have become more complex, with multiple daily injections and insulin pumps being used for many children and adolescents with diabetes to attain satisfactory glycohemoglobin levels. With improved blood glucose monitoring equipment and new insulins with different timing of action, the means to achieve excellent control are available for many children and their families.

Education

Education of the child and family is fundamental to management success. Education begins at diagnosis and is life long. Patients and families learn about what causes type 1 diabetes and the need for insulin. They need to understand how insulin, food, and exercise interact and affect blood glucose levels. Many technical skills need to be taught. "Survival skills" are usually taught first. These are listed:

- Preparing and injecting insulin and understanding different types of insulin
- Monitoring blood glucose levels, checking urine ketone, and keeping records
- Planning meals, including food types and amounts and timing of eating
- Engaging in physical activity and exercise
- Recognizing and handling acute problems, especially hypoglycemia, including glucagon use

There are many excellent educational tools available to accomplish these tasks. Books and online sites are readily available.

At our hospital, we admit most newly diagnosed children and use a clinical pathway to facilitate the educational plan. This pathway is written for 3 days (and 2 nights) but can be accelerated or slowed depending on the receptivity of the individual child and family to learning.

Insulin

Most children and adolescents will be started on at least two injections per day of a combination of a short-acting insulin (regular or lispro [Humalog]) and an intermediate-acting insulin (NPH or Lente). If two doses are used, the doses of a combination of short- and intermediate-acting insulin are given at breakfast and dinner. If three doses are used, the breakfast dose is a combination of short- and intermediate-acting insulins; the dinner dose is short-acting insulin, and the bedtime dose is intermediate-acting insulin. Insulin requirements are generally 0.5 to 1.0 unit/kg/d but may be as high as 1.5 units/kg/d during adolescence. Initial doses are usually begun at the lower end of this range to avoid hypoglycemia and then increased as indicated by blood glucose levels. The initial dose is divided so that about two thirds is given at breakfast and one third in the evening (dinner or dinner plus bedtime). The ratio of short-acting to intermediate-acting insulin dosing is usually about 1:1 to 1:2.

In our clinic, we usually move to multiple injection regimens and pumps if and when the family is able to master the complexities needed for these more complicated regimens. For a multiple injection regimen, short-acting insulin is given at each meal and snack. The dose is based on the amount of carbohydrate to be eaten and is adjusted based on the blood glucose level. This is the same approach used to calculate meal bolus doses with an insulin pump (see later). An evening dose of long-acting insulin or twice-a-day doses of a small amount of intermediate-acting insulin are added to provide coverage for basal insulin needs. With the anticipated addition of glargine (Lantus), a newly approved long-acting insulin added to the insulin armamentarium, and as we gain experience with this insulin, more regimens may

TABLE 3. **Insulin Preparations**

	Onset	Peak	Duration
Short-acting			
Lispro	15 min	30–60 min	3–4 h
Regular	30–60 min	2–4 h	4–6 h
Intermediate-acting			
NPH (isophane)	2–4 h	6–10 h	10–16 h
Lente	2–4 h	8–12 h	12–20 h
Long-acting			
Ultralente	6–10 h	8–15 h	18–24 h
Glargine	Slower than NPH	None	24 h

shift to reliance on glargine as a basal insulin with coverage of meals and snacks with lispro.

Timing of action of various insulin preparations is shown in Table 3. The ranges are large for onset, peak, and duration and may lead to some of the variability and unpredictability seen with exogenous insulin use.

Example. A 10-year-old 40-kg prepubertal girl presents with new-onset type 1 diabetes. Estimating insulin needs at 0.75 unit/kg/d, her dose requirements will be about 30 units. A possible starting regimen is as follows:

Two thirds at breakfast = 20 units: 7 lispro + 13 NPH
One third at dinner = 10 units: 5 lispro + 5 NPH

Subsequent insulin doses are adjusted based on blood glucose levels.

Insulin Pumps

The number of children and adolescents using insulin pumps has increased recently with some centers now treating 50% or more of their patients with pumps. The pump only delivers insulin: the child and family still need to measure blood glucose levels and decide how much insulin to give (i.e., the pump is not a closed-loop system). Pumps use only short-acting insulin, delivering a slow infusion to provide for basal insulin needs (including overnight) with small boluses of insulin given when the child eats. The pump basal rate is set to keep the blood glucose level stable when the child is not eating and generally comprises approximately 50% of the total daily insulin dose.

A different basal rate may be needed for different times of the day; commonly, a higher basal rate is needed in the early morning, with a lower rate needed in the evening and first half of the night. The bolus doses given with meals and snacks are planned based on the amount of carbohydrates in the meal. The diabetes team helps the family find an insulin-to-carbohydrate ratio, which can range from 1 unit of insulin per 5 g of carbohydrate in some teenagers to 1 unit per 30 g of carbohydrate in prepubertal children. This ratio may also vary based on the time of day, for example, with a higher amount of insulin at breakfast (perhaps 1 unit per 10 g of carbohydrate) and a lower amount at dinner (perhaps 1 unit per 15 g) and may also differ for meals versus snacks. Finally, the meal bolus dose is adjusted with a correction factor (or sliding scale) based on the blood glucose level to bring the level back into the target range. Insulin pumps can be safe and effective in motivated families willing to do the work needed to achieve and maintain good control. They offer the advantage of increased flexibility in the timing and content of meals and snacks.

Example. A teenager may need 1 unit per each 8 carbohydrate grams consumed. Thus, for a meal with 80 g of carbohydrate, 10 units will be required. A preteen may need 1 unit per 20 g of carbohydrate and therefore would need only 4 units to cover an 80-g meal. When the blood glucose concentration is outside the target range (e.g., 80–120 mg/dL), a correction factor is added or subtracted. Based on an empirical rule of 1800, a child taking 30 units of lispro per day would need 1 unit to lower blood glucose by about 60 points (1800/30 = 60) or 0.5 unit to lower blood glucose by about 30 points. Therefore, for each 30 blood glucose points above 120 mg/dL, this child would add 0.5 unit to the premeal insulin dose.

Meal Planning

The timing and content (amount and types of foods) of meals and snacks are important in the management of diabetes. The nutritionist is an integral part of the diabetes management team. Individualized meal plans are needed for each child and family, and recommendations will of course change as the child gets older, grows, and has different schedule needs. Meal plans should meet all the nutrient and calorie requirements for the individual child's needs. Most recommended diets have a goal of 50% to 55% of calories from carbohydrates. The fat content should be less than 30% of total calories and should be mostly unsaturated. Meals should be eaten at about the same time each day and have similar content for time of day. In addition, between-meal (especially mid-afternoon when the morning NPH is usually peaking) and bedtime snacks are recommended.

The constancy of meal timing and content is more important in regimens that include intermediate-acting insulin (i.e., those regimens requiring two to three injections per day) because this produces a need for caloric intake to coincide with the insulin peaks. Meal timing is more flexible, with the regimens employing multiple short-acting doses of insulin with meals (either multiple injections or the insulin pump) in which basal insulin needs are met with a long-acting insulin or with the basal rate of the pump. In these cases, there is no insulin peak except for that from the meal dose of insulin. However, as noted earlier, when multiple injection and pump regimens are used, children and families need to learn carbohydrate counting and how to adjust insulin doses for the amount of carbohydrates to be consumed.

Physical Activity

Exercise is important for both physical and psychologic reasons. It has the effect of lowering the blood glucose quickly by increasing glucose utilization. In some people, exercise may at times produce a delayed effect, lowering the glucose level several hours later. Caloric intake and insulin doses need to be adjusted based on activity. Planned activity can be worked into the regimen in advance. However, the spontaneous, unplanned activity of children may require additional caloric intake to avoid hypoglycemia. This can be addressed by giving a snack before and/or during the activity, depending on its intensity and duration and the child's blood glucose level. For a planned activity, either decrease the insulin dose likely to be active at the time of the planned activity (e.g., morning NPH for an after-school sport) by 10% to 20% or add or increase the amount of a snack at the time of the activity to help avoid hypoglycemia.

When diabetes is poorly controlled, and especially when positive urine ketones are present, exercise can worsen the hyperglycemia and ketosis (probably through an increase in catecholamines) and care must be taken here: either improve control or avoid the activity at that time.

Monitoring and Record Keeping

Many systems of meters and strips are available for blood glucose monitoring. Currently, all require a drop of blood. However, faster meters, smaller blood drop size, and use of sites other than fingertips to obtain the blood sample (e.g., forearms) make this process easier than in the past. Ideally, blood glucose should be checked at least three to four times per day, before meals, and at bedtime. For patients using a multiple injection regimen or an insulin pump, this becomes a requirement because the meal insulin dose is based on the blood glucose level. In all cases, additional more frequent monitoring is needed at times of instability and illness. Overnight blood glucose levels need to be checked periodically to try to avoid nighttime hypoglycemia. In particular, times of decreased caloric intake, increased activity, or changes in insulin doses, especially in the evening, are times when overnight blood glucose levels need to be checked. The more information one can get about blood glucose patterns, the better the child's metabolic control is likely to be.

Urine ketones should be checked during any illness and when blood glucose levels are high, above 250 to 300 mg/dL. The presence of significant ketones indicates the need for additional insulin.

Record keeping is important. Although memory meters have been wonderful for data collection and storage, they can have a negative effect on keeping the kinds of records that allow for review of patterns and necessary dose adjustments. Either electronic printouts that contain insulin doses or written records should be kept and reviewed frequently to assess for patterns that may indicate need for modifications of the regimen. This is hard for many families to do but is necessary if good control is to be achieved.

Goals

Blood glucose and glycohemoglobin goals are important to discuss for each individual child and family. Infants and toddlers have higher blood glucose goals because of the real fear of severe hypoglycemia in this age group. Older children and adolescents may achieve lower blood glucose levels without unacceptably increasing the risk of hypoglycemia. Typical goals are in the 100- to 200-mg/dL range for infants and toddlers and 70 to 150 (or 180) mg/dL in older children and adolescents. In addition, overnight levels should have a minimum goal of 70 to 100 mg/dL depending on the child's age and his or her previous history of hypoglycemia.

Based on information from the DCCT, the goal for glycohemoglobin levels would be a hemoglobin A_{1c} (HbA_{1c}) level near 7%. If lower levels can be achieved without significant hypoglycemia, that is ideal. In the DCCT, only 5% of patients were able to achieve consistently normal glycohemoglobin levels, even with an intensity of clinician involvement not achievable in real life. HbA_{1c} levels under 8% can often be achieved in children and adolescents. Infants and toddlers may need higher goals to avoid hypoglycemia.

Long-Term Monitoring

It is generally recommended that people with type 1 diabetes have quarterly medical appointments with the diabetes team. For the first few months after diagnosis, patients are seen more frequently. Interim phone contact must be available as needed. At the onset, these calls may need to be daily. Education needs to be updated and made appropriate to the child's age and cognitive stage.

Visits need to include physical examinations and laboratory testing to assess overall control and monitor for complications as recommended by the American Diabetes Association (ADA) standards of care. Screening for lipids, nephropathy (with blood pressure, and urine microalbumin measurements), and retinopathy (with ophthalmologic examinations) continues lifelong. Associated autoimmune disease, particularly thyroid, is increased in type 1 diabetes. There also appears to be an increased incidence of celiac disease in patients with type 1 diabetes, which has led some diabetes experts to recommend screening all patients with type 1 diabetes for celiac disease. At a minimum, celiac disease should be considered in children with type 1 diabetes who demonstrate subnormal growth or who have gastrointestinal (GI) symptoms.

Assessment of the child's overall health status, psychological and social adjustment, and school success is important. Depression is not uncommon in diabetes, and depression can worsen metabolic control. Physical examinations need to include height, weight, blood pressure, pubertal status, thyroid gland and injection site inspection and palpation, eye and foot examination, as well as the other routine parts of the physical examination. Plotting growth curves and looking for deviations from normal patterns are important because this information can point to problems in the regimen.

Insulin doses are always changing. Requirements vary from day to day, and dose requirements increase as body size increases and as the child goes through puberty because pubertal hormones make the cells less sensitive to insulin. Regular medical visits are important also to reinforce the child's and parents' knowledge and understanding of all the tasks and skills needed for day-to-day management and to keep them up-to-date on new technology and new research advances and any new recommendations for management.

Complication Monitoring

The acute complications of hypoglycemia, ketosis, and diabetic ketoacidosis and prevention of these complications are discussed at diagnosis in the initial educational plan and are reviewed at each visit. Intermediate complications, like poor growth and lipodystrophy, are also evaluated frequently. Yearly formal ophthalmologic examinations after the first few years of diagnosis, yearly urine microalbumin levels to assess baseline urine protein spill and any changes over time, and serum lipid levels every few years, as recommended by the ADA, are part of ongoing and long-term care. Treatment of diabetic ketoacidosis is discussed elsewhere.

Life with diabetes is hard work for the child and family, and support and encouragement of the diabetes team is needed in the effort to keep hope alive for these families and help them through the difficult times, which inevitably occur for all families.

Type 2 Diabetes

As with type 1 diabetes, long-term studies, notably the United Kingdom Perspective Diabetes Study (UKPDS), have clearly demonstrated that the risk of microvascular complications in type 2 diabetes can be lowered by maintaining lower blood sugar levels. In contrast to type 1 diabetes, however, adolescents with type 2 diabetes can frequently be controlled to the degree that the HbA_{1c} is normalized, or very nearly so, and this should be the goal.

Diet and exercise are important components of the management of type 2 diabetes. Because obesity is a major contributor to the insulin resistance that plays such an important role in type 2 diabetes, weight loss improves insulin sensitivity. Exercise, in addition to aiding diet in achieving weight loss, also has a weight-loss independent effect to improve insulin sensitivity. If insulin sensitivity is improved sufficiently by diet and exercise, there may not be a need for medication. Unfortunately, studies in adults have found that less than 10% of diabetics will achieve normal glucose levels by means of diet alone, and there is no reason to expect better success in children with type 2 diabetes. However, success with diet and exercise may allow the patient to discontinue medication once control is achieved, so compliance with nutritional guidelines and an exercise program is to be encouraged. As for patients with type 1 diabetes, the diet should contain less than 30% of calories as fat, with a minimum of saturated fat. This is important because of the long-term risk of atherosclerotic vascular disease in patients with diabetes.

As is true for many diseases, many of the medications that are useful for treating type 2 diabetes have not been tested for safety and efficacy in children. In fact, the only diabetes medication that has been approved for use in children is insulin. Fortunately, with a mandate from the Food and Drug Administration, studies of oral diabetes drugs are being performed in pediatric patients. Until results from these studies are available, however, extrapolation of data from use in adults and anecdotal experience in children will have to be used to guide treatment.

The major categories of drugs that can be used to treat type 2 diabetes are insulin, insulin secretagogues, insulin sensitizers, and glucosidase inhibitors. Each of these has been shown to be effective in adults, and there is no information to indicate that they would not work similarly in children with type 2 diabetes.

In adults, the oral diabetes medications all have a certain incidence of primary treatment failure—the inability to achieve blood glucose control when the medication is begun—and a certain rate of secondary treatment failure—the inability to maintain control with that agent over time. Experience so far suggests that the rates of both primary and secondary treatment failure are low in pediatric patients, most of whom can be managed on a single oral agent. In adults, the oral agents each can improve glucose control to a degree that will decrease the HbA_{1c} by 1% to 2%. A patient presenting with an HbA_{1c} more than this amount above the normal range would therefore be unlikely to be well controlled on a single oral agent. As discussed later, these patients may benefit from the initial combined treatment with insulin plus an oral agent, with the possibility of discontinuation of the insulin once glucose levels are controlled.

Next, we briefly review the medications that can be used to treat type 2 diabetes in children and highlight those aspects that may have particular relevance to their use in these patients. More detailed discussion of the use of oral agents can be found in the article Diabetes Mellitus in Adults.

Insulin

Insulin must be used in the treatment of type 2 diabetes when ketoacidosis or marked hyperglycemia are present. In addition, in adults, type 2 diabetes generally progresses to the point that insulin must be added to the treatment regimen; how often and how quickly this will occur in children remains to be seen. Insulin can be used as initial treatment for type 2 diabetes. However, hypoglycemia is a risk with insulin treatment, which can limit the ability of insulin to normalize glucose control. Hypoglycemia is less common with treatment with insulin secretagogues than with insulin and is not a side effect of the other oral agents. In addition, adolescents may have a higher degree of compliance with oral agents compared with the injections required of insulin treatment. For these and other reasons, oral agents are generally preferable as initial therapy for type 2 diabetes.

Ketoacidosis is an indication of severe insulin deficiency; whether the underlying disease is type 1 or type 2 diabetes, ketoacidosis must be treated with insulin. High glucose levels impair insulin secretion from the pancreas—the so-called glucotoxic effect. This likely plays a role in the development of ketoacidosis in type 2 diabetes. In addition, patients whose fasting blood sugar level is above 200 to 250 mg/dL will generally not have adequate correction of their glucose levels if they are only begun on treatment with an oral agent, whether it be an insulin sensitizer or an insulin secretagogue. This is true whether this degree of hyperglycemia is detected at diagnosis or if it occurs after a period of good control with use of an oral agent, either because of noncompliance with the oral agent or because of progression of the disease. In many cases, even if the patient presented in ketoacidosis, the treatment with insulin may only need to be given for a brief period of a few weeks. With a decrease in the circulating glucose level and relief from the glucotoxicity, endogenous insulin secretion may improve to a level that allows continued metabolic control with an oral agent. (This is similar to the phenomenon that leads to the "honeymoon" period in patients newly diagnosed with type 1 diabetes.)

The approach to treating a child with type 2 diabetes with insulin is similar to that outlined for the treatment of a patient with type 1 diabetes, as outlined earlier. One difference, however, would be the use of a single night-time injection of an intermediate-acting insulin, such as NPH, beginning at a dose of 0.1 unit/kg and increased with a goal of a morning blood glucose level in the normal range. In adults, this is often added to the diabetes treatment after oral agents have stopped maintaining adequate control.

Insulin Sensitizers

Insulin sensitizers act to ameliorate one of the two primary defects present in type 2 diabetes, insulin resistance. Two classes of agents have been identified that increase insulin sensitivity: the biguanides and the thiazolidenediones (TZDs). By improving insulin sensitivity, circulating insulin levels decline in patients treated with either metformin (Glucophage) (the only biguanide now in use) or a TZD. This could theoretically decrease the risk of macrovascular complications. In addition, these agents do not cause hypoglycemia.

Metformin acts primarily to increase the insulin sensitivity of the liver, decreasing hepatic glucose production. In some studies, although not in all, patients treated with metformin lost weight. This is clearly of benefit in a disease in which obesity plays such a central role. Metformin is the only diabetes medication for which this is true; insulin, TZDs, and insulin secretagogues all have a tendency to promote weight gain. The advantages of metformin use resulted in a recommendation by the Consensus Development Conference on Type 2 Diabetes in Children and Adolescents that metformin be considered as the first-line therapy for pediatric patients with type 2 diabetes. If the patient requires initial treatment with insulin because of the degree of hyperglycemia, metformin can be started concurrently. If the patient presents in ketoacidosis, this should be corrected with insulin; metformin should only be started after there is complete resolution of the dehydration and the patient is metabolically stable.

Metformin has been in use in adults for more than 20 years. It can cause lactic acidosis, which in rare cases can be fatal. The major contraindications to metformin use are hepatic or renal disease or conditions impairing renal function (e.g., dehydration and use of radiographic contrast agents). However, in appropriate patients with the appropriate cautions, the use of metformin in adults has been very safe. As with all the other oral agents, there is no extensive experience with the use of metformin in children, but there is no evidence that metformin has a different safety profile in children compared with the experience in adults. Metformin has a high incidence of GI side effects, including diarrhea and abdominal cramps. These effects generally resolve with time, however, and can be minimized by starting with a lower dose and increasing it and by taking metformin with meals. Patients should be informed of the transient nature of the GI side effects to avoid discontinuation of metformin by the patient.

The TZDs bind to the nuclear hormone receptor PPARγ and act mainly to increase peripheral insulin sensitivity, correcting the abnormality in glucose uptake into muscle and fat cells, with higher doses also inhibiting hepatic glucose production. Two TZDs are currently available: pioglitizone (Actos) and rosiglitizone (Avandia). A third TZD, troglitazone (Rezulin),* was removed from the market because of an association of its use with liver dysfunction, in rare cases leading to fulminant liver failure causing death or requiring liver transplantation. Pioglitizone and rosiglitizone do not appear to have the same risk of liver toxicity that troglitizone had, although they both have only been available for widespread use for a few years. Although TZDs may ultimately be useful for the treatment of type 2 diabetes in children, there is too little safety data available at this time to support their widespread use in pediatric patients.

Insulin Secretagogues

Insulin secretagogues attack the second component of the pathophysiology of type 2 diabetes, the insulin secretory defect. They act on the β cells of the pancreas to increase insulin secretion. The sulfonylureas are the prototypic insulin secretagogues and were

*Not available in the United States.

the first oral agents used to treat type 2 diabetes as a class, having been used since the 1950s. Recently, repaglinide (Prandin), a new nonsulfonylurea secretagogue, was developed that has different pharmacodynamic properties compared with the available sulfonylureas. The sulfonylureas have a very long track record of safety and efficacy in the treatment of type 2 diabetes in adults. Although no formal studies of the use of these drugs in children have been published, experience has shown that they can be useful agents in children with type 2 diabetes.

The major risk with treatment with insulin secretagogues is of inducing hypoglycemia. This occurs because these drugs stimulate insulin secretion in the absence of a glucose stimulus. If the drugs are taken and caloric intake is decreased, the unregulated insulin secretion could lead to hypoglycemia. The well-known erratic eating habits of adolescents could theoretically make this a problem, but in practice this is rarely a problem. Decreased caloric intake with an illness, such as a viral gastroenteritis, however, could put a patient taking an insulin secretagogue at risk of hypoglycemia. This is particularly true of the sulfonylureas, which have a long half-life. Repaglinide, which has a very quick onset of action and brief duration of action, has a much lower risk of hypoglycemia. Repaglinide is taken just before meals; therefore, if a meal is missed because of convenience or illness, no drug is taken, thus there is little risk of hypoglycemia. However, repaglinide's advantage is also its disadvantage. The need for a dose with each meal is likely to make compliance more difficult—particularly for the adolescent who is eating many meals away from home. The sulfonylureas can often be taken once a day or at most on a twice-a-day schedule. For patients who could not tolerate the GI side effects of metformin, or for those for whom metformin is otherwise not a good choice, the insulin secretagogues are an appropriate alternative initial therapy.

Glucosidase Inhibitors

Acarbose (Precose) and miglitol (Glyset) inhibit the intestinal enzyme α-glucosidase. Given with meals, this will delay carbohydrate absorption, allowing endogenous insulin secretion a better chance at providing appropriate activity. These agents are primarily effective in reducing postprandial glucose. Because of the carbohydrate that passes into the colon with use of these drugs, GI side effects are common, although tolerance will develop if a low dose is begun and slowly increased. Because these drugs do not significantly affect fasting glucose levels, they are unlikely to be effective as single agent therapy. There is little experience with their use in children, and the GI effects are likely to make their use in children poorly accepted.

Education and Monitoring

For the newly diagnosed patient with type 2 diabetes who requires initial treatment with insulin, either because of ketoacidosis or because of a presentation with marked hyperglycemia, we will generally admit the child to the hospital to initiate treatment. The teaching of survival skills is outlined earlier in the section on the treatment of type 1 diabetes. For patients who do not require treatment with insulin, therapy may be initiated as an outpatient, but education remains an important element. Further details regarding education and monitoring can be found in the section on the treatment of type 1 diabetes in this article and in the article Diabetes Mellitus in Adults. However, one aspect should be highlighted in caring for children with type 2 diabetes. Because children with type 2 diabetes appear to be at a higher risk of ketoacidosis than adults with type 2 diabetes, and because of the possibility of misclassifying a patient who has type 1 diabetes as having type 2 diabetes, recommendations for urine ketone testing should be the same as those for children with type 1 diabetes. That is, urine should be tested for ketones during any illness or when the blood glucose level rises above 250 to 300 mg/dL. The presence of significant ketones may indicate the need for at least temporary addition of insulin to the treatment regimen.

DIABETIC KETOACIDOSIS

method of
DANIEL T. STEIN, M.D.
Albert Einstein College of Medicine
Bronx, New York

Diabetic ketoacidosis (DKA) is a potentially life-threatening metabolic disturbance. Mortality has remained steady in recent years at 2% to 10%, predominantly due to serious concurrent illness such as sepsis or myocardial infarction. Successful outcomes are best ensured by prompt diagnosis and treatment, along with awareness of the potential complications associated with therapy.

The metabolic derangements of DKA result from severe insulin deficiency in the context of elevated counter-regulatory (anti-insulin) hormones, including glucagon, cortisol, catecholamines, and growth hormone. The insulin deficiency is severe in the patient with newly diagnosed type 1 diabetes or in the patient whose insulin therapy has been omitted or interrupted. Under these circumstances, counter-regulatory hormones are elevated due to evolving stress. Insulin deficiency may be relative if the primary initiating event was a major physiologic stress—severe infection, vomiting, trauma, or dehydration—which led to elevated counter-regulatory hormones and cytokines that antagonize insulin action.

DKA in the setting of relative insulin deficiency is increasingly observed in adolescents, young adults with type 2 diabetes, particularly in the so-called atypical diabetes found often in the African Caribbean individual. Once the DKA has resolved, many will go on to recover enough β cell function not to require insulin therapy.

PATHOPHYSIOLOGY

Insulin is an anabolic hormone that is not only important for glucose utilization but also necessary for the synthesis of glycogen, protein, and lipids in liver, muscle,

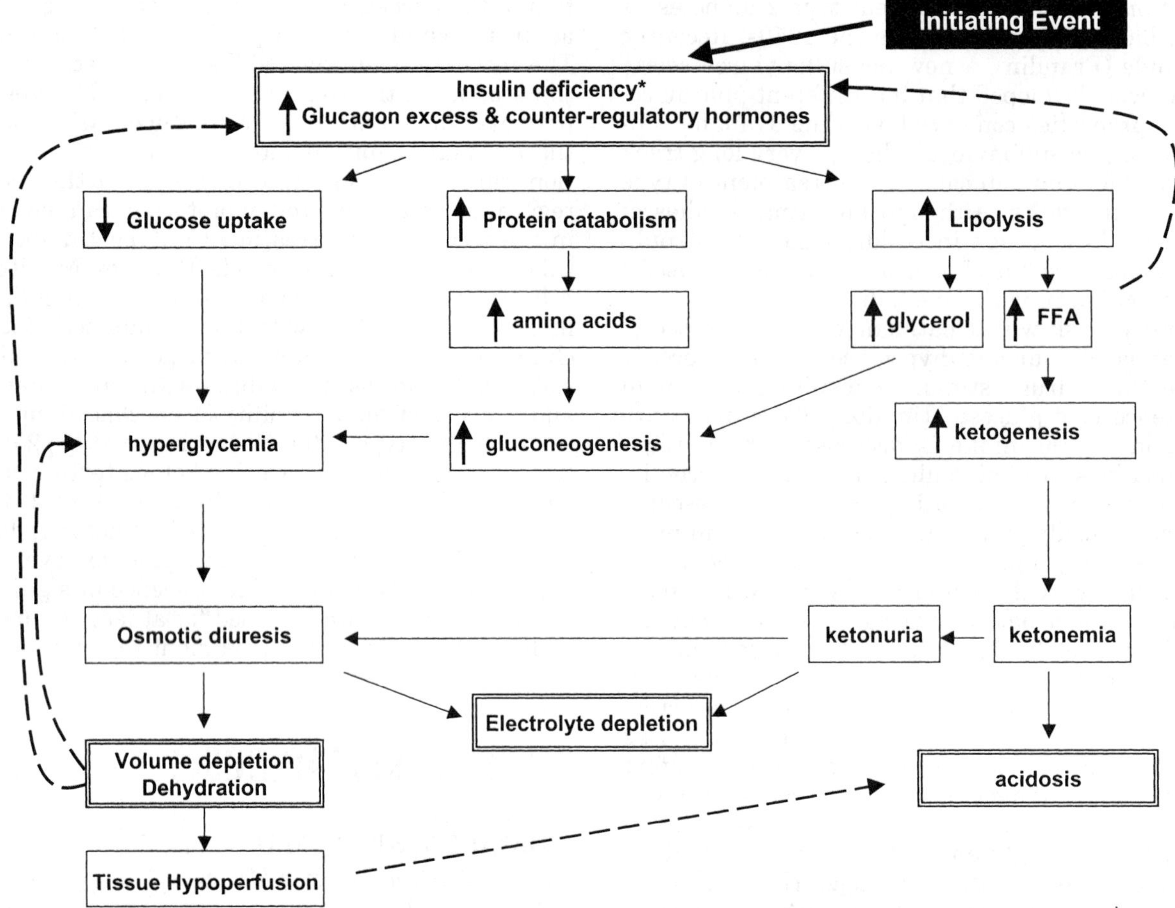

Figure 1. Unrestrained mobilization of tissue energy reserves in insulin deficiency, resulting in ketoacidosis and electrolyte and volume depletion.

and fat. Insulin inhibits glycogenolysis, gluconeogenesis, proteolysis, lipolysis, and ketogenesis. Conversely, insulin deficiency allows unrestrained mobilization of tissue energy reserves (Figure 1). Absolute or relative insulin deficiency in combination with counter-regulatory hormone excess results in severely impaired insulin action that results in the following:

1. Increased glucose production
2. Impaired glucose uptake and storage
3. Excessive adipose tissue lipolysis with delivery of free fatty acids to the liver
4. Accelerated ketogenesis and accumulation of serum ketoacids (betahydroxybutyrate and acetoacetate)
5. Increased muscle proteolysis with release of amino acids and intracellular ions

When hyperglycemia exceeds the renal threshold for reabsorption (~180 mg/dL), an osmotic diuresis ensues with loss of circulating electrolytes and free water in excess of sodium. Dehydration may reach 10% to 20%. Apparent hyponatremia is due to hyperglycemia and hypertriglyceridemia, and when corrected for these confounders, apparent hyponatremia often reveals true hyperosmolarity (Table 1). As hypovolemia progresses, glomerular filtration of glucose is decreased, exacerbating hyperglycemia. The stress of hypovolemia stimulates cortisol and catecholamine output, further antagonizing insulin action, the latter also directly inhibiting insulin secretion. β-Cell function in susceptible individuals, such as those with new onset diabetes, may also be depressed due to the "lipotoxic" effects of prolonged exposure to elevated free fatty acids.

Hepatic overproduction and impaired use of ketone bodies (acetoacetate and betahydroxybutyrate), which are strong acids, results in the excess formation of hydrogen ion. Bicarbonate is the main source of buffering capacity and is consumed, leading to an anion gap acidosis. The acidosis and insulin deficiency cause potassium and phosphate to move out of the cell into the extracellular compartment. As the ketone bodies are cleared by the kidneys, the resultant ketonuria not only contributes to the osmotic diuresis but also causes further urinary losses of cations (such as potassium, sodium, calcium, and magnesium), which are necessary to maintain electroneutrality. These significant electrolyte losses are frequently compounded

TABLE 1. **Useful Formulas**

Anion gap	$AG = ([Na^+] - [Cl^-] - [HCO_3^-])$. Normal = 12 ± 4
Effective serum osmolarity	$Posm = 2 \times ([Na^+] + [K^+]) + (glucose^*/18)$
Corrected serum sodium	$Na_{corr} = [Na^+] + 1.6 \times ([glucose^* - 100])/100$
PCO_2 in compensated metabolic acidosis	$PCO_2 = 1.5 \times [HCO_3^-] + 8 \pm 2$

*Glucose measured in mg/dL.

by vomiting or diarrhea. In the latter stages of severe dehydration with hypoperfusion, tissue hypoxia generates a degree of lactic acidosis. Once in motion, the process of DKA inexorably continues to accelerate out of control, with progressive acidosis, neurologic impairment, and shock. The outcome is ultimately coma then death unless urgent interventions are instituted to break the metabolic vicious cycle.

DIAGNOSIS

The diagnosis of DKA is straightforward with simple laboratory testing. The hallmarks of DKA are hyperglycemia (glucose >250 mg/dL), ketonemia (serum ketones + 1:2), and acidosis (pH <7.3, HCO_3^- <15 mEq/L), invariably accompanied by glycosuria and ketonuria. Glucose levels lower than 250 mg/dL may occasionally be seen in true DKA when associated with alcohol consumption, pregnancy, and prior insulin treatment with low carbohydrate intake. All patients without a known history of diabetes presenting with altered mental status, shock, dehydration, respiratory distress, or evidence of other major illness should be rapidly screened by urine test strips for glucose and ketones. The presence of hyperglycemia with dehydration and large ketonuria is sufficient to make a provisional diagnosis and to institute treatment pending the outcome of further confirmatory laboratory tests. For those familiar with their use, semiquantitative measures of plasma ketones may be made with crushed reagent tablets (Acetest). A deep purple color with a 1:2 dilution of plasma confirms the diagnosis in the setting of hyperglycemia.

Three quarters of all cases of DKA occur in patients with known diabetes. Therefore, any diabetic presenting with nausea/vomiting, abdominal pain, change in mental status, shortness of breath, fever, other signs of infection, or unexplained elevations in blood sugar above 250 mg/dL should be suspected to have DKA. Positive glycosuria with a negative urine strip, trace or small (1+) for ketones, virtually eliminates the diagnosis, whereas moderate or large ketones are supportive. Laboratory confirmation is obtained after demonstrating acidemia, anion gap acidosis, and ketonemia (see Table 1). Significant ketosis may occasionally be missed if the body redox potential is shifted dramatically in favor of betahydroxybutyrate instead of acetoacetate, for example, during acute alcohol intoxication or shock. Typical reagents for testing plasma and urine for ketones are based on the nitroprusside reaction and only detect acetoacetate. Autoanalyzer and bedside assays for betahydroxybutyrate are now available in some clinical laboratories in response to this need.

DKA and hyperglycemic hyperosmolar coma (HHC) are part of an overlap syndrome. In HHC, glucose levels are typically >500 mg/dL; however, there are no ketones in the blood or urine. Other hyperketotic states include starvation and ethanol, paraldehyde, or isopropyl alcohol intoxication. The conditions of intoxication should be apparent from the history, an osmolar gap, and screening for toxins, and all are distinguished by lack of hyperglycemia.

The potential for mixed acid–base disturbances due to coexisting respiratory and metabolic acid-base processes should be kept in mind, especially those due to vomiting and sepsis, which will result in superimposed alkalosis. Other laboratory abnormalities commonly found in DKA include urea nitrogen increased out of proportion to creatine, variable changes in sodium, potassium, and phosphorus despite depletion of total body stores (see later discussion of fluids), increases in amylase (typically of salivary origin), modest elevations in transaminases, hypertriglyceridemia, increases in Hgb/Hct due to hemoconcentration, and leukocytosis. Increased acetoacetate can cause spurious elevations in creatinine in some autoanalyzer assays.

CLINICAL ASSESSMENT

After emergency assessment of neurologic and cardiorespiratory function, initial evaluation should include thorough history and physical directed toward identifying precipitating causes (Table 2). In subjects with known diabetes, the most common precipitating causes of DKA are infection or interruption/inadequate insulin therapy. Less common but potentially catastrophic underlying illnesses that should be actively sought in older patients include myocardial infarction (which is often silent in long-standing diabetics), cerebrovascular accidents, or a major intraabdominal process such as pancreatitis or gastrointestinal bleeding.

Evidence of dehydration and acidosis includes poor skin turgor, dry mucous membranes, tachycardia, hypotension, and Kussmaul respirations. Hypotension and/or lack of supine jugular venous filling implies at least a 10% volume deficit. Pneumonia, urinary tract infection, and sepsis should be screened for by chest radiograph, urinalysis, and cultures, respectively. Abdominal pain along with vomiting is common and may mimic an acute abdomen. It is generally recommended that the response to treatment be monitored over 8 to 12 hours if the patient is stable before making a decision as to whether to proceed with exploratory laparotomy. Pelvic and rectal exams should not be deferred, and women of reproductive potential should be tested for pregnancy. Presence of fever is highly significant

TABLE 2. **Precipitating Factors in DKA**

- Diabetes
  - New onset
  - Poor control
  - Interruption of insulin therapy
    - Omission
    - Pump malfunction
      - Wrong/spoiled insulin
      - Catheter blockage
      - Electromechanical
- Infection
  - Respiratory, urinary, gastrointestinal, central nervous system, osteomyelitis, endocarditis, other
- Vascular thrombosis
  - Myocardial infarction
  - Cerebrovascular accident
  - Pulmonary embolus
- Acute abdominal process
  - Infection
  - Acute pancreatitis
  - Gastrointestinal retroperitoneal hemorrhage
- Severe emotional stress
- Trauma or burns
- Thyrotoxicosis or other endocrinopathies
  - Cushing's syndrome, pheochromocytoma, adrenal insufficiency, acromegaly
- Pregnancy
- Cancer
- Substance abuse (cocaine, alcohol)
- Drugs that interfere with insulin action or release
  - Glucocorticoids
  - Protease inhibitors
  - Pentamidine
  - Dobutamine, terbutaline

but its absence does not rule out infection because hypothermia may accompany DKA. Leukocytosis is common; however, unless it is accompanied by significant bandemia, it is not predictive of infection. Necrotic lesions in the nasal passages and/or upper palate suggest mucormycosis, a highly invasive fungi that thrives in acid environments. An initial electrocardiograph (ECG) is important to assess plasma potassium status and, in the appropriate age group, screen for coronary ischemia in conjunction with cardiac enzymes.

TREATMENT

Patients who are able to maintain oral fluid intake and are capable of monitoring glycemia and urine ketones may be allowed to treat their condition with increasing doses of subcutaneous insulin in close consultation with the diabetes health care team. Patients who are vomiting, or whose ketonuria has not responded to increased insulin over 2 to 3 hours should be hospitalized. All patients should be closely monitored by the medical staff who are implementing intensive treatment. Therapy should be initiated rapidly and focus on the management of fluid status, electrolytes, insulin, and concurrent diseases. A comprehensive flowsheet, such as in Figure 2, facilitates understanding of the patient's response to therapy and provides efficient transfer of medical care information when the responsible physician changes. Measures for monitoring patient progress are shown in Table 3.

Adequate (large bore) peripheral intravenous access should be established for both sampling and infusion of fluids, electrolytes, and insulin. If cannulation is difficult, a central line or cut down should be performed. Gastric decompression with a nasogastric tube may be helpful to avoid aspiration because severe gastric distention with large amounts of fluids can result in vomiting and aspiration pneumonia. Bladder catheterization is essential in the comatose patient in order to monitor fluid balance. For milder cases of DKA in which the patient is awake, voiding, and cooperating with frequent body weight measurements, we feel this unnecessary, particularly given the increased risk of iatrogenic infection.

Fluids

The first goal of fluid therapy is to restore effective intravascular volume, stabilize blood pressure, and

Name DOB Sex Height Weight Date

	VITAL SIGNS				FLUID BALANCE					BLOOD CHEMISTRY										CONSCIOUSNESS	EKG	TREATMENT							
TIME	Temp (F°) / Weight	BP	PULSE	RESP	INTAKE (ml) p.o.	I.V.	OUTPUT (ml) URINE	GASTRIC	URINE Glu / Ket	GLU mg/dl	BUN mg/dl	Na meq/L	K meq/L	Cl meq/L	CO_2 meq/L	ANION Gap	Osmo-lality	pH	Serum ketone	I Alert II Drowsy III Stupor IV Light Coma V Coma		INSULIN Reg. i.v.	s.c./i.m.	NPH or Lente	Na meq/L	K meq/L	Bicarb meq	Anti-biotic	Other
8a.m.																													
9																													
10																													
11																													
12																													
1p.m.																													
2																													
3																													
4																													
5																													
6																													
7																													
8																													
9																													
10																													
11																													
12																													
1a.m.																													
2																													
3																													
4																													
5																													
6																													
7																													
TOTAL:																													

Figure 2. Comprehensive flowsheet, designed to facilitate the understanding of the patient's response to therapy and provide efficient transfer of medical care information when the responsible physician changes.

TABLE 3. **Monitoring the Patient in DKA**

1. BP, pulse, RR, mental status (temperature q 8)	q 2–4 h×24, then q 8 h
2. Fluid intake/output	q 1–2 h
3. Weight–admission	q 24 h
4. Insulin therapy	Hourly and total
5. Electrolytes	Hourly and total
6. Glucose (either capillary blood or plasma*)	q 1 h until on s.q. insulin, then q.i.d.
7. Na, K, Cl	q 2–4 h, qh
8. Blood gas (arterial or venous)	Admission, then q 6 until pH >7.1
9. PO4, Mg, Ca	Admission, q 12; more frequent if low
10. Serum ketones, lactate	Admission
11. Urine ketones, glucose	q void
12. BUN/creatinine	q 12
13. CBC, urinalysis	Daily
14. CPK, troponin, lipase	Admission
15. Blood, urine, CSF cultures	As indicated
16. ECG	Admission, and prn if K abnormal

*Blood glucose levels above 400 or below 50 are unreliable and should be confirmed by plasma measurement.

All tests should be repeated until the patient is stable and acidosis is reversed.

Abbreviations: BP = blood pressure; BUN = blood urea nitrogen; CBC = Complete blood cell count; CPK = creatine phosphokinase; CSF = cerebrospinal fluid; ECG = electrocardiograph; RR = respiratory rate.

establish urine flow. This is best achieved by infusion of an isotonic fluid such as 0.9% saline or lactated Ringer's solution at a rate of 500 to 1000 mL/h for the first 2 hours (500 mL/m^2 in adolescents), followed by a third liter for persistent hypotension or when 10% dehydration is assessed on presentation. Shock is an indication for colloid.

The second goal is to restore 50% of water and sodium losses over the first 12 to 24 hours. Typical volume losses are 5 to 11 liters; however, fluid balance should be always adjusted for ongoing urinary, gastric, and insensible losses, particularly if there is fever. Because water losses are in excess of sodium, 0.45% saline is generally appropriate in this phase and should be infused at 150 to 500 mL/h, depending on the clinical status of the patient. When plasma glucose concentrations approach 250 mg/dL, glucose should be added as well to avoid an excessively fast drop in plasma osmolality and hypoglycemia (see later). Serum sodium concentrations are typically low on admission, but after correction for glycemia or hypertriglyceridemia (see Table 1), these concentrations are normal or even increased. It has been demonstrated that subclinical pulmonary and cerebral edema is common during the rehydration phase; this is thought to be due to water moving from the extracellular space into cells. This has been attributed to the relative hypotonicity of plasma as glucose declines, and the solvent drag effect of insulin on glucose and potassium uptake into cells.

Insulin

Insulin therapy is essential to reverse the course of DKA but should only be initiated in close time proximity to the initial fluid resuscitation and after ensuring potassium replacement in those with hypokalemia by laboratory tests or ECG. Insulin administration significantly before fluid therapy may precipitate vascular collapse by further depletion of intravascular water or hypokalemia-induced arrhythmia. Short-acting insulins (regular, insulin lispro [Humalog], insulin aspart [NovoLog]) are preferred owing to their rapid onset and ease of control, particularly when given intravenously. Although not essential, we give an initial bolus of insulin (0.1 U/kg, or 8 U) to immediately produce a therapeutic level, particularly if any delay is expected in the preparation of the insulin infusion. Insulin infusion is made up at a concentration of 0.5 U/mL by adding 250 U to a 500 mL bag of 0.9% saline. It is important to flush 30 to 50 mL of this solution through the intravenous tubing set to saturate insulin binding sites and therefore provide consistent insulin delivery. The insulin is piggybacked using an infusion pump into another infusion of saline or dextrose, with both controlled by infusion pumps. Initially insulin is infused at 0.1 U/kg/h (~6–10 U/h) and is subsequently adjusted based on a sliding scale as shown in Table 4. Subcutaneous or intramuscular injection of insulin at 10 U/h can also be effective but may provide erratic insulin absorption if peripheral and particularly external perfusion is poor due to severe volume contraction. It is therefore not recommended except in cases of very mild DKA or when adequate fluid intake has been maintained to prevent dehydration. An effective dose of insulin by either intravenous or alternative routes of administration is expected to cause plasma glucose to drop 50 to 100 mg/dL/h. If there is not a 10% change in glucose or improvement in the anion gap within 2 hours, insulin infusion rates should be doubled every 2 hours until a response is attained. Extreme degrees of insulin resistance are unusual and tend to be associated with critically ill patients in the intensive care unit receiving pressors or high-dose steroids. Rare cases due to insulin antibodies have been documented, which responded briskly to substituting an insulin analogue (e.g., insulin lispro). Urine strips

TABLE 4. **Insulin-Glucose Infusion* for DKA**

	Insulin Infusion		**D5W**	**D10W**	**D50W†**
Blood Glucose	*Units/h*	*mL/h*	*mL/h*	*mL/h*	*mL/h*
70‡	0.5	1.0	150	75	25
71–100	1.0	2.0	125	65	20
101–150	1.5	3.0	100	50	17
151–200	2.0	4.0	100	50	17
201–250	3.0	6.0	75	35	17
251–300	4.0	8.0	50	25	12
>300	10.0	20.0	0	0	10

*Rates are just a guide and may need to be changed based on individual responses.

†Use when volume restricted (e.g., congestive heart failure or renal failure).

‡Give 10 mL bolus D50 and repeat glucose measurement in 15 minutes.

only detect acetoacetate, and as the ketoacidosis is reversed, betahydroxybutyrate is converted to acetoacetate. The apparent increase in ketonuria does not necessarily indicate failure of therapy. Clearing of the gap acidosis should be the therapeutic yardstick.

When the plasma glucose concentration reaches approximately 250 mg/dL, 10% dextrose or the equivalent is added to the infusion fluids at a rate of about 25 mL/h. If the glucose level continues to drop, the insulin infusion is slowed and dextrose increased. Insulin infusion should never be discontinued owing to the potential for rapid return of ketoacidosis. An advantage of this type of protocol lies in the automatic addition of dextrose as plasma glucose concentrations approach 250 mg/dL. This is necessary because glycemia is corrected much faster than the acidosis. In addition to the risk of hypoglycemia with continued insulin therapy, over-rapid correction of plasma osmolality may risk causing cerebral or pulmonary edema. Another practical advantage is that maintenance amounts of glucose are infused after acidosis is reversed and glucose is finally normalized. This allows a reasonable estimate of basal insulin requirements once the patient is ready to start eating.

Conversion to a structured insulin regimen is best undertaken after acidosis has cleared and urinary ketones have totally or almost completely resolved. The first injection of subcutaneous insulin should overlap with the infusion by at least 30 minutes to avoid rebound ketoacidosis. I place known diabetics without a precipitating illness back on their regular regimen. For new onset diabetics or for those still stressed by illness, I use the calculated 24-hour dose of insulin from the last 12 hours of infusion as a basal requirement and administer it as a split dose of intermediate acting insulin: two thirds before breakfast and one third before supper or preferably at bedtime. Regular insulin in an amount equal to one half of the basal requirement is split into at least four doses daily, with a proactive approach guided by a sliding scale of preprandial and bedtime glucoses.

Potassium

Despite the invariably large deficit in total body potassium stores, serum concentrations are typically normal or elevated at presentation due to acidosis forcing the ion out of cells in exchange for hydrogen and lack of insulin-stimulated uptake. The institution of insulin can cause a rapid and profound shift of potassium intracellularly, resulting in life-threatening hypokalemia due to arrhythmia or respiratory muscle weakness.

Treatment, therefore, is geared toward always keeping serum potassium within the normal range while potassium stores are being replenished.

Potassium infusion should not commence until significant hyperkalemia has been ruled out either by ECG (flat P, peaked T waves) or lab testing and continued urine output has been documented. Potassium is typically infused at 10 to 30 mEq/h, initially. If the potassium level is below normal before insulin begins or if bicarbonate therapy is also given, the rate should be higher. In the event of developing hypokalemia with renal failure, potassium should still be given, albeit at a much reduced rate (5–15 mEq/h), in conjunction with careful blood and cardiac monitoring. Full repletion of potassium stores is not necessary during the acute phase of DKA and may be completed orally on recovery.

Bicarbonate

The use of bicarbonate to treat acidosis in DKA is controversial and has never been demonstrated to increase the rate of recovery from DKA or decrease mortality. The acidosis corrects spontaneously in response to insulin suppression of ketogenesis. In addition, bicarbonate therapy increases the risk of hypokalemia, and it may cause central nervous system acidosis, which suppresses the respiratory drive, worsens tissue oxygen delivery, and impairs respiratory compensation of the ongoing acidosis. During severe acidemia (pH <7.0, HCO_3 <5) associated with left ventricular pump failure, refractory hypotension, or severe hyperkalemia, bicarbonate replacement should be used by administering sodium bicarbonate (1–2 amps; 44–88 mEq) diluted into 0.45% saline to avoid making a hypertonic solution, and infused over 1 to 2 hours. Additional potassium should be given, unless hyperkalemia was the original indication for treatment. The endpoint for stopping therapy is a pH higher than 7.1.

Phosphate and Magnesium

Depletion of phosphate and magnesium also occur in DKA. Levels of phosphate initially increase and then drop as insulin activates phosphorylation of glycolytic intermediates within cells. Extreme phosphate deficiency states have rarely been described to cause neurologic disturbances and muscle weakness and theoretically can cause increased tissue hypoxia by inhibiting formation of 2.3 diphosphoglycerate and shifting the oxygen dissociation curve to the left. Nevertheless, controlled trials have never documented any benefit from phosphate repletion in DKA, even in severe cases of hypophosphatemia. In addition, phosphate infusion carries a risk of hypocalcemia and metastatic calcification. I do not routinely administer phosphate. It may be considered if (1) calcium levels are not low or high, and (2) phosphate has decreased to less than 1.0 to 1.5 mg/dL. Treatment consists of adding one 5 mL ampule of potassium phosphate consisting of 465 mg of phosphorus and 20 mEq of potassium to a bag of infusion fluids. Phosphate and calcium levels should be monitored every 4 to 6 hours. It is rarely necessary to infuse more than one vial.

Magnesium levels are not routinely measured because they do not represent intracellular magnesium stores. However, magnesium replacement may be necessary in patients with seizure disorders, prolonged QT intervals, and cardiac arrhythmias and in those with difficulty replacing potassium stores.

COMPLICATIONS OF DIABETIC KETOACIDOSIS

Hypotension and Shock

Hypotension and shock occur commonly in DKA, are usually due to intravascular volume depletion, and thus should be readily reversible with rapid fluid replacement. When hypotension remains unresponsive to therapy, other causes should be considered including severe acidosis, hypokalemia, occult bleeding, myocardial infarction, sepsis, and adrenal insufficiency.

Acute Renal Failure

Acute renal failure, although most commonly the result of severe volume depletion, may also be the result of postrenal obstruction. Acute papillary necrosis is associated with pyelonephritis, and oliguria may also be seen with the dilated atonic bladder seen in comatose patients and those with severe autonomic neuropathy.

Thrombosis

Thromboses, both pulmonary and venous, are well described in DKA, and frequently do not become manifest until the DKA is already well on the path to resolution. Prophylactic anticoagulation (subcutaneous heparin sodium 5000 U every 12 hours) may be considered in those at high risk for venous thrombosis or congestive heart failure, provided there is no evidence of active hemorrhage.

Cerebral Edema

Cerebral edema is one of the most feared complications of DKA, resulting in very high morbidity and mortality. For unclear reasons it affects children almost exclusively, particularly those younger than 5 years of age presenting for the first time with DKA. Risk factors in addition to age include severe bicarbonate deficit, high degree of azotemia, failure of the (calculated) serum sodium to rise with insulin treatment, and bicarbonate treatment itself. The etiology is thought to involve movement of water intracellularly during overly rapid rehydration or cerebral ischemia with thrombosis during the late pretreatment phase of DKA due to hypoperfusion. Subjects with the biochemical features just listed should be watched closely for changes in mental status or signs of increased intracranial pressure. The most effective treatment is mannitol (Osmitrol); some authorities also advocate limiting fluid input to less than 4.0 L/m^2/d; glucocorticoids may be useful as well.

Hyperchloremic Acidosis

This non-anion gap acidosis is commonly observed in the recovery phase of DKA, particularly in those receiving excessive amounts of sodium chloride. Hyperchloremic acidosis is due to the replacement of lost ketoacids with chloride anion, but it is of no consequence and resolves spontaneously.

Other Complications

Other known complications include acute respiratory distress syndrome and disseminated intravascular coagulation.

FOLLOW-UP

The best therapy for DKA is prevention. Recovery typically lasts a few days after diabetic coma, time that should be spent identifying precipitating factors and educating the patient about diabetes. Interruption or omission of insulin therapy is particularly common among young adults and adolescents with recurrent DKA. Insulin omission may be caused by a fear of gaining weight with tight metabolic control, fear of hypoglycemia, rebelliousness, substance abuse, or emotional stress. Young women with eating disorders are particularly at risk. The increased use of rapid acting insulins (e.g., insulin lispro, insulin aspart) by subcutaneous insulin pumps and even by multiple injection regimens has generally improved metabolic control and decreased the rate of recurrent DKA yet, ironically, due to the rapid absorption and short half-lives of these insulins, these same patients are at risk to slip rapidly (within 12 hours) into severe acidosis should the insulin delivery be interrupted or other major stressor intervene.

HYPERURICEMIA AND GOUT

method of
DAVID E. BLUMENTHAL, M.D.
Cleveland Clinic Foundation
Cleveland, Ohio

PATHOPHYSIOLOGY

In males, uric acid levels rise after puberty. In females, uric acid levels rise after menopause. In most patients, hyperuricemia is caused by underexcretion of urate by the kidneys. Underexcretion can be worsened by renal insufficiency, lead intoxication, ethanol, diuretics, pyrazinamide, ethambutol, cyclosporine, and low-dose aspirin. Only about 10% of gout patients are overproducers of uric acid. Hematopoietic malignancies, hemolytic anemia, psoriasis, glycogen storage diseases, alcoholism, HGPRTase deficiency, and PRPP synthetase superactivity can contribute to urate overproduction.

The maximum solubility of sodium urate at 37°C is 6.8 mg/dL, and at 35°C it is only 6.0 mg/dL. If the serum uric acid concentration exceeds these levels for a sustained period, monosodium urate will come out of solution and form crystals. Microtophi will begin to accumulate, particularly in the cooler parts of the body such as the distal extremities and the ears. Sustained hyperuricemia is a risk factor for acute gouty arthritis, tophaceous gout, and uric acid nephrolithiasis. However, most patients with asymptomatic hyperuricemia will never have an attack of gout and no treatment is required.

Typically, the first attack of acute gout occurs after 15 to 20 years of asymptomatic hyperuricemia. In males, attacks usually begin between age 35 and 50; in females, attacks begin 15 to 20 years after menopause. Attacks are usually monarticular and are more prevalent in the lower extremity, particularly in the first metatarsophalangeal joint (podagra), the midfoot, the ankle, and the knee. With time, upper extremity attacks become more frequent, including the wrist, the elbow, and the small joints of the hands. In the elderly, upper extremity attacks and polyarticular attacks are more common. Acute gouty arthritis is characterized by an abrupt appearance of redness, swelling, intense pain, and tenderness of the affected joint. Attacks can be precipitated by minor trauma, surgery, any illness requiring hospitalization, excessive ethanol intake, or any perturbation of the serum uric acid levels. The attacks usually resolve in 7 to 14 days even if untreated.

Clinically detectable tophi often appear between 10 and 20 years after the initial attack if the hyperuricemia is not corrected. They can occur anywhere in the body, but they are most common over the fingers and toes and the forearms or embedded in a chronically swollen olecranon bursa. Tophi can be identified by probing them with a needle and confirming the presence of monosodium urate crystals by polarized light microscopy. On plain radiographs, a tophus will appear as a periarticular soft tissue density with a rim of calcified bone.

DIAGNOSIS

The classic patient is a middle-aged man with a monarticular, lower extremity synovitis. Older patients are more likely to have upper extremity or polyarticular presentations. The differential diagnosis includes other types of crystalline arthritis (calcium pyrophosphate dihydrate, calcium apatite), infection, spondyloarthropathy, or (rarely) rheumatoid arthritis. Arthrocentesis for polarized light microscopy will usually reveal urate crystals and is the best way to confirm the diagnosis. Serum urate levels can be normal at the time of an attack and cannot be used to confirm or exclude gout. Gout and infection can coexist in the same joint, and the presence of typical urate crystals does not exclude the possibility of septic arthritis.

TREATMENT

Treatment is directed at aborting the attack of acute gouty arthritis and preventing future attacks.

Aborting the Acute Attack

Treatment options include nonsteroidal anti-inflammatory drugs (NSAIDs), oral colchicine, intra-articular corticosteroids, and systemic corticosteroids. In general, the best results are obtained when therapy is started shortly after the onset of symptoms.

Any NSAID will lessen the pain and swelling of gout if the dosage chosen is sufficiently high. Indomethacin (Indocin), 50 mg three to four times a day for 2 days with a subsequent taper, has been frequently used but is not a good choice in the elderly. Naproxen (Naprosyn), 500 mg three times a day, ibuprofen (Motrin),* 800 mg four times a day, or high doses of any of the conventional NSAIDs are acceptable alternatives. COX-2 selective NSAIDs (celecoxib [Celebrex], rofecoxib [Vioxx], or meloxicam [Mobic]) do not prolong the bleeding time and reduce the risk of NSAID gastropathy, but they may still have adverse renal and hepatic effects and their efficacy in gout is not established. NSAIDs should be avoided in patients with prior peptic ulcer disease or gastrointestinal bleeding, serum creatinine greater than 1.6 mg/dL, congestive heart failure, inflammatory bowel disease, or systemic anticoagulation with warfarin or heparin and should be used with caution in the elderly.

Colchicine is often prescribed as 0.6 mg orally every 1 to 2 hours until the gout attack is aborted or until nausea, vomiting, or diarrhea appears. However, this regimen is poorly tolerated. In a patient with normal renal function, 0.6 mg every 3 to 4 hours on day 1, followed by 0.6 mg daily to twice daily, is more realistic, although less effective. If the serum creatinine is greater than 1.6 mg/dL, the colchicine dose should not exceed 0.6 mg/d. Intravenous colchicine rarely has caused fatal bone marrow suppression, mainly in elderly patients with renal and/or hepatic insufficiency, and is not recommended.

Corticosteroids can provide relief rapidly and safely once infection has been ruled out. Intra-articular corticosteroids are ideal for monarticular attacks in a medium or large joint, such as a wrist, elbow, or knee. Methylprednisolone (Depo-Medrol), 80 mg into a knee or 40 mg into an ankle or wrist, can abort an attack of gouty arthritis with little risk of toxicity. Intra-articular injection can be safely performed in an anticoagulated patient if systemic therapy is undesirable. When the inflammation is polyarticular or the joint is difficult to inject, prednisone 35 mg/d (or equivalent) tapered to zero over 7 to 14 days is usually effective. Intramuscular adrenocorticotropic hormone offers no advantage when compared with systemic corticosteroids and is not recommended.

Prevention of Future Attacks

Future attacks can be prevented by interfering with neutrophil function or by lowering serum uric acid levels.

Colchicine, 0.6 mg/d given twice daily, impairs the ability of neutrophils to ingest urate crystals, thereby preventing attacks of acute gout. If the serum creatinine is greater than 1.6 mg/dL, the colchicine dose should not exceed 0.6 mg/d. Chronic colchicine therapy can cause bone marrow suppression, peripheral neuropathy, proximal myopathy, nausea, diarrhea, and abdominal cramping. Adverse effects are more likely to occur in patients with renal or hepatic insufficiency. Chronic use of NSAIDs can also prevent attacks of acute gout.

*Not FDA approved for this indication.

Uric acid–lowering therapy will be necessary if the patient is having gout attacks with unacceptable frequency or if tophi are present. Before starting a new medication, the patient should try abstinence from alcohol and discontinuation of medications that might decrease uric acid excretion. Starting allopurinol (Zyloprim) or a uricosuric can precipitate an attack of acute gout; one should wait for resolution of the current attack and institute prophylaxis with colchicine or an NSAID before initiating urate-lowering medications. Prophylaxis can be discontinued after the patient has normal urate levels and has been asymptomatic for at least 6 months. If acute gout occurs after starting urate-lowering therapy, the allopurinol or uricosuric should be continued while the acute attack is treated.

Uricosuric agents attempt to correct the underexcretion present in most patients with gout. Despite the logic of this strategy, they are seldom prescribed today. The ideal candidate for uricosuric therapy is described in Table 1. Treatment can begin with probenecid (Benemid), 250 mg twice daily, or sulfinpyrazone (Anturane), 50 mg twice daily. The dose is gradually increased to achieve a serum uric acid of less than 6.0 mg/dL. Liberal fluid intake and alkalinization of the urine can be used to decrease the risk of renal stones.

Allopurinol lowers serum uric acid by blocking xanthine oxidase. It is the medication of choice for patients with urate overproduction (urinary uric acid >600 mg/24 h), tophaceous gout, or any contraindication to uricosuric treatment. The starting dose is adjusted according to the patient's renal function (Table 2). If a 24-hour urine collection has not been obtained, the creatinine clearance can be estimated from the serum creatinine by the following formula:

$$\text{ClCr (mL/min)} = (140 - \text{Age})/\text{Serum Cr (mg/dL)}$$

Subsequently, the allopurinol dose should be adjusted until the serum uric acid level is consistently less than 6.0 mg/dL. Allopurinol doses as high as 800 mg/d may be required in occasional patients. Potential adverse effects of allopurinol include rash, fever, bone marrow suppression, dyspepsia, granulomatous hepatitis, vasculitis, and xanthine renal calculi. Rarely, patients will develop the potentially fatal allopurinol hypersensitivity syndrome of rash, eosinophilia, hepatitis with possible hepatic failure, and renal insufficiency. The hypersensitivity syndrome is more likely to occur if the allopurinol dose is inappropriately high for the patient's renal function.

TABLE 1. **The Ideal Candidate for Uricosuric Therapy**

No history of uric acid renal calculi
Urinary urate value <600 mg/24 h
No tophi
Normal renal function
Able to drink at least 2 L of fluid daily
No treatment with low dose aspirin

TABLE 2. **Dosing of Allopurinol According to Renal Function**

Creatinine Clearance (mL/min)	Allopurinol Dose
100	300 mg qd
80	250 mg qd
60	200 mg qd
40	150 mg qd
20	100 mg qd
10	100 mg qod
0	100 mg twice weekly

Allopurinol will potentiate the effect of warfarin (Coumadin) and theophylline and will decrease the metabolism of azathioprine (Imuran). If it becomes necessary to prescribe both azathioprine and allopurinol, the azathioprine dose should be reduced to 25% of its previous value and the peripheral blood counts monitored closely to screen for bone marrow toxicity.

SPECIAL CIRCUMSTANCES

Postoperative Patient

Postoperative patients are at increased risk for gout but may be unable to take medication by mouth and are at increased risk for gastrointestinal bleeding and renal failure. In this setting, intra-articular corticosteroids are the best option for acute gout. Intravenous corticosteroids may impair wound healing and increase the risk of infection but can be used safely if the exposure is brief. Methylprednisolone (Solumedrol), 30 mg intravenously, followed by a taper over 5 to 7 days is usually effective and safe. There is no published experience on the use of ketorolac (Toradol) intramuscularly or intravenously in gout.

Patient With Renal Insufficiency

If the serum creatinine concentration is greater than 1.6 mg/dL, intra-articular or systemic corticosteroids are preferred for terminating acute attacks. For prophylaxis, NSAIDs should be avoided and colchicine used with caution. The colchicine dose should not exceed 0.6 mg/d and should be avoided if the creatinine clearance is less than 10 mL/min. Probenecid and sulfinpyrazone will be less effective as the creatinine clearance falls. Benzbromarone* is a more potent uricosuric that remains effective in the presence of moderate renal insufficiency, but it is currently unavailable in the United States. Allopurinol dosing should initially be adjusted for the creatinine clearance, but it can be carefully increased until the goals for the serum uric acid are achieved.

Transplant Patient

Transplant patients may develop high serum urate levels, acute gout, and tophi within a few years of

*Not available in the United States.

transplantation. Many of the problems with urate excretion are caused by cyclosporine (Sandimmune). Patients may have concurrent renal insufficiency or azathioprine therapy that influences their gout treatment. Ideally, decisions about gout treatment should be made in collaboration with the transplant team. In the patient with normal renal function, acute attacks can be treated with colchicine, intra-articular injection, or systemic corticosteroids. NSAIDs are best avoided because of the potential for renal insufficiency or hyperkalemia in the cyclosporine-treated patient. Colchicine can be used for prophylaxis, with the dose adjusted for renal function and close observation for toxicity. Uric acid–lowering therapy is almost always necessary, given the more severe clinical course. Uricosuric agents may be used in the occasional patient with normal renal function and no contraindications. More often, allopurinol will be preferred, with the initial dose adjusted for renal function. If the patient is on azathioprine, the azathioprine dose should be reduced to 25% of its previous value or discontinued and replaced by mycophenolate mofetil (CellCept).

Patient With Allopurinol Intolerance

Rashes are seen in about 2% of patients treated with allopurinol and are more likely to occur if there has been co-administration with ampicillin. If simple allopurinol sensitivity occurs, not associated with toxic epidermal necrolysis or the acute hypersensitivity syndrome, the patient may be a candidate for desensitization with very low doses of oral allopurinol. Patients with more severe reactions to allopurinol should not be re-challenged and should be considered for uricosuric agents. Patients who appear to have no conventional options should be considered for research protocols, which might provide access to treatment with uricase,* oxypurinol,* or more potent uricosurics.

Patient With Large Tophi

To reduce the size of large tophi, it is necessary to lower the serum uric acid more aggressively. A serum urate level of less than 5.0 mg/dL is desirable. If it is not possible to achieve this with allopurinol alone, a uricosuric agent may be added. Allopurinol increases the biologic effect of probenecid, whereas probenecid shortens the half-life of the active metabolite of allopurinol, oxypurinol. Thus, combination therapy may require a lower than usual dose of probenecid with a higher dose of allopurinol. Prophylaxis with colchicine or NSAIDs should be continued until visible tophi are resorbed.

*Investigational drug in the United States.

HYPERLIPOPROTEINEMIAS

method of
CHRISTIE M. BALLANTYNE, M.D.
Baylor College of Medicine
Houston, Texas

Hyperlipoproteinemia, particularly elevated low-density lipoprotein cholesterol (LDLC), has been associated with increased risk of coronary heart disease (CHD) in numerous epidemiologic studies. Large randomized, placebo-controlled trials of therapy with HMG CoA reductase inhibitors (statins), which primarily reduce LDLC, have shown significant reductions in cardiovascular morbidity and mortality and all-cause mortality in patients with severely elevated or only mildly to moderately elevated LDLC and in patients with or without existing CHD. However, many patients with CHD do not have substantially elevated LDLC; instead, low high-density lipoprotein cholesterol (HDLC) is often the predominant lipid abnormality. Other lipid abnormalities that have been associated with CHD risk are elevations of triglyceride and lipoprotein(a) (Lp[a]) and a preponderance of small, dense LDL particles. The guidelines of the third Adult Treatment Panel (ATP III) of the National Cholesterol Education Program emphasize LDLC as the primary target of therapy while incorporating absolute risk assessment in determining the need for and intensity of treatment in each individual; triglyceride and HDLC are secondary considerations for treatment.

TREATMENT GUIDELINES

Based on the available clinical trial evidence, the ATP III guidelines continue to focus on LDLC in assessing and reducing CHD risk. Treatment initiation levels and goals reflect individual risk for a CHD event, with risk first stratified by category, defined by the presence or absence of known CHD and specified CHD risk factors, and then further refined by estimation of absolute risk for a CHD event during the next 10 years (Table 1).

Risk Assessment

The guidelines classify as secondary prevention, and therefore at highest risk, individuals with established CHD or other atherosclerotic diseases: peripheral vascular disease, abdominal aortic aneurysm, or carotid artery disease. However, also at high risk are patients with type 2 diabetes and patients with multiple risk factors whose absolute risk for a CHD event is greater than 20% for the next 10 years. Although clinical judgment may be required, in general, patients in either of these categories should be treated as aggressively as patients with known CHD.

Primary prevention patients are stratified according to whether they have fewer than two or two or more risk factors (see Table 1). High HDLC (≥60 mg/dL) is a negative risk factor that decreases by one the total number of risk factors. To refine risk assessment, a quantitative estimate of risk for a CHD event over the next 10 years is calculated by using a risk equation developed by investigators of the Framingham Heart Study that is based on age,

TABLE 1. **Low-Density Lipoprotein Cholesterol Goals and Cutpoints for Therapeutic Lifestyle Changes and Drug Therapy in Different Risk Categories**

	LDL Cholesterol (mg/dL)		
Risk Category	*Goal*	*Initiation Level for TLC*	*Consideration Level for Drug Therapy*
CHD or CHD risk equivalents* (10-y risk >20%)	<100	≥100	≥130 (100–129: drug optional)†
≥2 risk factors‡ (10-y risk ≤20%)	<130	≥130	10-y risk 10%–20%: ≥130 10-y risk <10%: ≥160
0–1 risk factors‡	<160	≥160	≥190 (160–189: LDL-lowering drug optional)

*CHD, other clinical forms of atherosclerotic disease (peripheral arterial disease, abdominal aortic aneurysm, and symptomatic carotid artery disease), diabetes, or multiple risk factors that confer a 10-year risk for CHD >20%.

†Some authorities recommend use of LDL-lowering drugs in this category if an LDL cholesterol level of <100 mg/dL cannot be achieved by TLC. Others prefer use of drugs that primarily modify triglycerides and high-density lipoprotein (HDL) cholesterol (e.g., nicotinic acid or fibrate). Clinical judgment also may call for deferring drug therapy in this subcategory.

‡Cigarette smoking, hypertension (blood pressure ≥140/90 mm Hg or on antihypertensive medication), low HDL cholesterol (<40 mg/dL), family history of premature coronary heart disease (male first-degree relative aged <55 years; female first-degree relative aged <65 years), age (men ≥45 years; women ≥55 years); HDL cholesterol ≥60 mg/dL is a negative risk factor, decreasing by 1 the total number of risk factors.

Abbreviations: CHD = coronary heart disease; LDL = low-density lipoprotein; TLC = therapeutic lifestyle changes.

total cholesterol, HDLC, blood pressure, and smoking and also accounting for the influence of gender.

Risk Reduction

LDLC treatment goals are determined by the risk of the patient (see Table 1). Diet and lifestyle modification is the initial therapy in all patients and should target not only atherogenic diet but also obesity and physical inactivity. Although the ATP III guidelines focus on LDLC as the primary target of therapy, efforts should be made to reduce all CHD risk factors, including smoking cessation, blood pressure normalization, and glucose control.

Patients at highest risk—those with known CHD or CHD equivalent (other atherosclerotic disease, diabetes mellitus, or 10-year absolute risk for a CHD event >20%)—have the most aggressive LDLC target: less than 100 mg/dL. Within this high-risk category, the recommended therapy for reducing LDLC is based on the LDLC level at baseline. In patients with an LDLC of 130 mg/dL or greater, therapy should include diet (Table 2) and concomitant initiation of drug therapy with an agent that primarily reduces LDLC, such as a statin. In patients with LDLC between 100 and 130 mg/dL, diet therapy should be initiated, and if LDLC remains greater than 100 mg/dL after 3 months of diet, the addition of a drug such as a statin and/or a fibrate should be considered.

For primary prevention, the initiation level and goal of therapy depend on the number of risk factors and the patient's 10-year absolute risk (see Table 1). As noted earlier, patients with a 10-year absolute risk greater than 20% should be treated as aggressively as patients with known CHD. Patients with a 10-year absolute risk of 10% to 20% should be considered for drug therapy if LDLC is 130 mg/dL or greater (see Table 1). In general, patients without known CHD should be treated first with diet therapy for at least 3 months, and if LDLC remains above target, drug therapy should be added to diet.

Although LDLC is the primary target of therapy in the ATP III guidelines, CHD risk is also greatly increased in individuals with the metabolic syndrome, a constellation of risk factors that include high triglyceride, low HDLC, small dense LDL particles, hypertension, glucose intolerance, a prothrombotic state, and a proinflammatory state (see Table 2). This syndrome appears to enhance the atherogenic effects of LDLC.

Hypertriglyceridemia is an independent risk factor for CHD but is often associated with low HDLC levels, insulin resistance, and hyperinsulinemia in patients. The ATP III definition of hypertriglyceridemia and recommended targets for therapy are presented in Table 3. Diet and lifestyle modification should include weight control, increased physical activity,

TABLE 2. **Clinical Identification of the Metabolic Syndrome**

Risk Factor	Defining Level
Abdominal obesity* (waist circumference)†	
Men	>40 in. (102 cm)
Women	>35 in. (88 cm)
Triglycerides	≥150 mg/dL
High-density lipoprotein cholesterol	
Men	<40 mg/dL
Women	<50 mg/dL
Blood pressure	≥130/≥85 mm Hg
Fasting glucose	≥110 mg/dL

*Overweight and obesity are associated with insulin resistance and the metabolic syndrome. However, the presence of abdominal obesity is more highly correlated with the metabolic risk factors than is an elevated body mass index. Therefore, the simple measure of waist circumference is recommended to identify the body weight component of the metabolic syndrome.

†Some male patients can develop multiple metabolic risk factors when the waist circumference is only marginally increased (e.g., 37–40 in. [94–102 cm]). Such patients may have strong genetic contribution to insulin resistance and they should benefit from changes in life habits, similar to men with categorical increases in waist circumference.

TABLE 3. **Adult Treatment Panel III Guidelines Definitions and Therapeutic Targets for Hypertriglyceridemia**

Category	Triglyceride Level (mg/dL)	Target of Therapy
Borderline high	150–199	Metabolic syndrome
High	200–500	VLDL remnants and non-HDLC
Very high	>500	Prevention of pancreatitis

Abbreviations: non-HDLC = non–high-density lipoprotein cholesterol; VLDL = very low density lipoprotein.

exercise, and a Mediterranean diet that replaces saturated fats with monounsaturated fats and decreases carbohydrate consumption. If drug therapy is required, the agent chosen depends on the patient's LDLC level; if LDLC is elevated, the primary goal of therapy is to lower LDLC, with the reduction of triglyceride by nicotinic acid or a fibrate being a secondary consideration. If the triglyceride level is 200 mg/dL or greater, non-HDLC is a secondary target of therapy, with goals 30 mg/dL higher than the corresponding LDLC goals.

Low HDLC increases CHD risk and is the primary lipid abnormality in many patients with CHD. The ATP III defines low HDLC as less than 40 mg/dL and recommends weight control and increased physical activity as therapeutic lifestyle changes. Drug therapy with nicotinic acid or a fibrate may be added, but the ATP III guidelines do not set a goal for HDLC-raising therapy because of insufficient clinical trial evidence. The primary target of therapy remains LDLC.

Diet Therapy

Diet and other lifestyle modifications are primary therapy in all patients with dyslipidemia. In patients who also require drug therapy, the drug should be added to, not substituted for, diet. Diet therapy consists of three integral components: diet modification, weight control, and increased physical activity.

Diet

The recommended diet for a desirable blood cholesterol and lipoprotein profile limits saturated fat and cholesterol and substitutes grains and unsaturated fats (see Table 2). Consultation with a dietitian is recommended at the initial prescription of a diet and at the 6-week and 3-month follow-ups.

Physical Activity

Regular exercise can increase HDLC levels, reduce weight, and improve hypertension and insulin resistance. Exercise of moderate intensity (30 to 60 minutes) should be performed three to four times weekly.

Weight Control

Obesity, particularly abdominal obesity, is associated with dyslipidemia and the metabolic syndrome. Caloric intake and expenditure should be adjusted to achieve and maintain a desirable body weight (body mass index, 21 to 25 kg/m^2).

Pharmacologic Therapy

All the available lipid-regulating agents affect multiple components of the lipid profile. Evidence from angiographic trials suggests that the beneficial effects of lipid-regulating therapy result from plaque stabilization more than from average changes in stenosis severity, which are generally modest and disproportionate to the reduction in clinical events. Lipid-regulating therapy also improves endothelial function by providing vasodilatory, antithrombotic, and anti-inflammatory effects.

HMG CoA Reductase Inhibitors (Statins)

The advent of the statins has dramatically improved the efficacy and tolerability of lipid-lowering therapy. Agents available in the United States are atorvastatin (Lipitor), cerivastatin (Baycol), fluvastatin (Lescol), lovastatin (Mevacor), pravastatin (Pravachol), and simvastatin (Zocor). Statin trials with clinical event endpoints have shown 25 to 35% reductions in clinical coronary events, 20 to 40% reductions in revascularization procedures, 20 to 30% reductions in stroke, and 20 to 30% reductions in all-cause mortality. Although benefits are greatest in high-risk patients, such as those with known CHD and severely elevated LDLC, benefit has also consistently been reported in primary prevention patients and in patients with mild to moderate LDLC elevations.

Mechanism of Action. Statins competitively inhibit hepatic HMG CoA reductase, the rate-limiting step in cholesterol biosynthesis, and thereby result in decreased hepatic intracellular cholesterol and therefore increased LDL-receptor activity. The predominant effect is on LDL particles, but the clearance of other apolipoprotein B (apo B)-containing particles—very low density lipoprotein (VLDL) and intermediate-density lipoprotein (IDL)—is also enhanced. Statins may improve endothelial function by increasing endothelial nitric oxide synthesis and promoting the antithrombotic and vasodilatory properties of the endothelium, and they may promote plaque stability by decreasing extracellular and macrophage lipid deposits, neointimal inflammation, and metalloproteinase-9 secretion.

Efficacy. LDLC is reduced by approximately 39 to 60% with atorvastatin (Lipitor), 10 to 80 mg/d; 28 to 42% with cerivastatin (Baycol), 0.3 to 0.8 mg/d; 22 to 36% with fluvastatin (Lescol), 20 to 80 mg/d; 24 to 40% with lovastatin (Mevacor), 20 to 80 mg/d; 25 to 31% with pravastatin (Pravachol), 20 to 40 mg/d; and 29 to 47% with simvastatin (Zocor), 10 to 80 mg/d. HDLC is increased by 5 to 15% and triglyceride is decreased by 10 to 30%; the triglyceride-lowering effect is more prominent with higher dosage atorvastatin and simvastatin. Statins do not appear to affect the Lp(a) level. Because the peak activity of

HMG CoA reductase occurs around midnight, efficacy is slightly better when the drugs are administered in the evening, except for atorvastatin, which has a long half-life. Maximal lipid effects are apparent by 2 to 4 weeks of therapy. After 4 to 6 weeks of statin therapy, a lipid profile should be reassessed, and if lipid levels are not optimal, the dose should be adjusted and a repeat profile obtained in another 4 to 6 weeks.

Side Effects and Drug Interactions. In widespread clinical use and in major clinical event trials enrolling a total of more than 30,000 patients monitored for approximately 5 years, statins have been shown to be safe and well tolerated, with infrequent and reversible adverse events. In large placebo-controlled studies, the frequency of adverse effects was similar to placebo (2 to 3%).

Persistent transaminase elevations of three times or more the upper limit of normal occur in approximately 1% of patients receiving statin therapy, but they are not generally associated with other signs or symptoms of hepatic dysfunction. When hepatic toxicity does occur in patients receiving statin therapy, associated factors such as concomitant hepatotoxins (high-dose niacin, excessive ethanol consumption) or viral illnesses are often present. Alanine transaminase and aspartate transaminase should be measured before statin therapy is initiated, 6 to 12 weeks after initiation of statin therapy or an increase in statin dosage, and every 6 to 12 months afterward. In patients with a history of hepatic disease or excessive alcohol consumption and patients receiving hepatotoxic medical therapy, transaminases should be monitored every 3 to 4 months for the first year or when symptoms occur. Minor transaminase elevations are usually transient and do not warrant discontinuation of statin therapy; transaminases should be remeasured in 2 to 6 weeks. For persistent elevations of three or more times the upper limit of normal, statin therapy should be discontinued until levels normalize, usually within 14 days, and then reinitiated at a reduced dosage or with a different statin.

Muscle toxicity is even less common; however, rare cases of rhabdomyolysis, characterized by creatine kinase (CK) elevations 10 or more times the upper limit of normal, have occurred in less than 0.1% of patients, usually with concomitant use of fibrates (fenofibrate [Tricor], gemfibrozil [Lopid]), azole antifungal agents (itraconazole [Sporanox], ketoconazole [Nizoral]), cyclosporine (Sandimmune), or erythromycin. Patients in whom serious muscle toxicity develops are usually ill at baseline; patients with immunosuppression, infection, long-standing diabetes, or renal failure should be closely monitored. Because CK is elevated in up to 30% of patients receiving placebo and serious myopathy is frequently associated with muscle pain, tenderness, and weakness, routine CK monitoring is not necessary in asymptomatic patients receiving statin monotherapy and may result in unwarranted interruption of statin therapy.

Nicotinic Acid (Niacin)

Nicotinic acid (niacin) has been used to treat dyslipidemia for 40 years. In addition to improving LDLC, HDLC, and triglyceride, niacin is one of the few agents known to reduce Lp(a). Niacin is especially effective in treating patients with mixed dyslipidemia.

Mechanism of Action. Niacin reduces the production and release of VLDL and thereby leads to a reduction in IDL and LDL. Niacin also decreases the release of free fatty acids, a substrate for triglyceride synthesis, from adipose tissue into the circulation. Although the niacin-induced increase in HDLC is largely due to the reduction in triglyceride, niacin may also decrease HDL catabolism. The mechanism by which niacin reduces Lp(a) is not known.

Efficacy. Niacin at a dosage of 1.5 to 6 g/d decreases LDLC by approximately 10 to 25%, increases HDLC by 15 to 35%, and decreases triglyceride by 20 to 50%; niacin at a dosage of 3 g/d or greater reduces Lp(a) by 25 to 40%. Immediate-release (crystalline) niacin is typically started at a dosage of 100 mg once or twice daily and gradually titrated up to 2 to 3 g/d over a period of 1 to 3 weeks, often with a schedule of 1 g two or three times daily. Niacin may be taken with meals to reduce side effects. A recently developed sustained-release formulation (Niaspan) that provides once-daily dosing is started at 500 mg at bedtime, after a low-fat snack, and titrated up to 1000 to 2000 mg/d at bedtime over a period of 2 to 6 weeks.

Side Effects and Drug Interactions. Cutaneous flushing and pruritis are virtually universal side effects of niacin. The flushing is prostaglandin mediated and may be blunted by concomitant administration of aspirin, 81 to 325 mg/d. Sustained-release formulations are associated with reduced flushing.

Niacin can adversely affect glucose metabolism, particularly in patients with underlying insulin resistance and at high dosages ($\geq$3 g/d). In patients with diabetes mellitus or impaired glucose tolerance, niacin should be used with caution and careful monitoring.

Increased hepatic transaminases occur in 1 to 2% of patients and can occasionally progress to irreversible chronic liver disease and, rarely, fulminant hepatic failure. Hepatic dysfunction occurs more often in patients taking earlier formulations of sustained-release niacin at high doses.

Combining niacin with a statin may increase the risk of hepatitis and myopathy.

Niacin can cause uric acid elevations and occasionally precipitates gout. Niacin may also activate peptic ulcers and should not be used in patients with untreated peptic ulcer disease.

Fibric Acid Derivatives (Fibrates)

Fibrates effectively reduce triglyceride and raise HDLC levels. The fibrates most commonly used in clinical practice are gemfibrozil (Lopid) and fenofibrate (Tricor). Clinical trial data on potential benefit with fibrate therapy have been mixed, with coronary benefit reported in the Helsinki Heart Study and the Veterans Affairs HDL Cholesterol Intervention Trial (both with gemfibrozil), but not in the Bezafibrate Infarction Prevention Study with bezafibrate.

Mechanism of Action. Fibrates decrease plasma triglyceride by increasing the activity of lipoprotein lipase, which hydrolyzes triglycerides from VLDL particles. Fibrates also decrease hepatic cholesterol synthesis and increase cholesterol excretion in bile. The increase in HDLC concentration seen with fibrates is mediated by peroxisome proliferator–activated receptor α through the transcriptional induction of apo A-I, apo A-II, and lipoprotein lipase synthesis and decreased hepatic transcription of apo C-III.

Efficacy. Gemfibrozil 1200 mg/d (administered in two divided doses 30 minutes before morning and evening meals), or fenofibrate, 200 mg/d given once daily, decreases triglyceride levels by approximately 20 to 50% and increases HDLC by 10 to 15%. LDLC typically decreases by 10 to 15% but in patients with hypertriglyceridemia, LDLC may increase; it is not clear whether this fibrate-mediated increase in LDLC is detrimental because fibrates shift the composition of small, dense LDL particles toward a less atherogenic phenotype. Fenofibrate may provide more effective LDLC lowering.

Side Effects and Drug Interactions. Fibrates are usually well tolerated, with generally mild side effects. Gastrointestinal disturbances (dyspepsia, nausea, vomiting, constipation, diarrhea) and rash are among the most common. Increased lithogenicity of bile has been reported with clofibrate but has not been clearly demonstrated with other fibrates.

In patients with severe hepatic or renal insufficiency, including primary biliary cirrhosis, fibrates should be used with extreme caution, if at all. In patients with renal insufficiency, fenofibrate should be initiated at a lower dose (67 mg/d). Pre-existing gallbladder disease is a contraindication to fibrate therapy because of increased risk for cholelithiasis and cholecystitis.

Fibrates may occasionally raise hepatic transaminase levels, which usually return to normal on discontinuation of drug therapy. Periodic monitoring of hepatic transaminases is recommended, and if elevations are persistent, fibrate use should be discontinued.

Myopathy may occasionally be seen with fibrate monotherapy, but rhabdomyolysis causing acute renal failure is uncommon but may occur in patients with pre-existing renal insufficiency. The risk for myositis, myopathy, and rhabdomyolysis is increased when fibrates are used in combination with statins. Patients should be instructed to promptly report muscle pain, tenderness, or weakness, especially if accompanied by malaise or fever. Fibrate therapy should be discontinued if myopathy is diagnosed or if CK is 10 or more times normal.

Fibrates potentiate the effect of warfarin and may increase the risk for bleeding. Prothrombin times should be monitored to optimize warfarin (Coumadin) dosing, which may need to be decreased by as much as 30%, and to prevent bleeding complications.

Bile Acid Sequestrants (Resins)

Bile acid sequestrants are anion exchange resins and are now used primarily in combination with statin therapy in patients requiring further reductions in LDLC. The available bile acid sequestrants are cholestyramine (Questran), colestipol (Colestid), and colesevelam (WelChol).

Mechanism of Action. Bile acid sequestrants interrupt the enterohepatic circulation of bile acids through nonspecific binding of bile acids, which increases fecal excretion of the cholesterol-rich bile acids. Decreased re-absorption of bile acids results in increased flux of intrahepatic cholesterol for the production of bile acids because the activity of 7α-dehydroxylase, the rate-limiting enzyme of bile acid synthesis, is increased. The subsequent decrease in intrahepatic cholesterol leads to up-regulation of LDL-receptor activity, which increases the removal of LDL, IDL, and VLDL particles from plasma. However, the decrease in intrahepatic cholesterol also increases the synthesis of cholesterol within hepatocytes through increased activity of HMG CoA reductase and thus results in diminished long-term efficacy with bile acid sequestrant monotherapy.

Efficacy. Cholestyramine is generally started at a daily dosage of 4 to 8 g and increased gradually as tolerated up to 12 to 24 g/d in two to three divided doses taken before or during meals. Colestipol is initiated at a daily dosage of 5 to 10 g and increased gradually as tolerated up to 15 to 30 g/d in two to three divided doses taken before or during meals. Colesevelam is initiated at 3750 mg/d once daily or in two divided doses with meals and can be increased up to 4375 mg/d. Bile acid sequestrants administered at these dosages typically reduce LDLC by 15 to 30% and may increase HDLC by 3 to 5%; the triglyceride level is not usually affected, but occasionally, primarily in patients with previous hypertriglyceridemia, the triglyceride level may be increased.

Side Effects and Drug Interactions. The most common side effect is constipation, which occurs in up to 30% of patients. To minimize constipation, resins should be initiated at a low dose with a gradual increase in dosage, and intake of fluid and dietary fiber should be increased; the use of stool softeners may be helpful but is typically not as useful as other measures. Other gastrointestinal side effects include abdominal discomfort, flatulence, hemorrhoids, and fecal impaction. Long-term compliance with high-dose resins (>12 g/d cholestyramine or >15 g/d colestipol) is often limited by gastrointestinal side effects; colesevelam appears to have a lower incidence of gastrointestinal side effects. Because resins are better tolerated at lower doses, they are useful as adjunctive therapy with other lipid-regulating agents.

Their nonspecific binding causes bile acid sequestrants to inhibit the intestinal absorption of coadministered drugs, including warfarin, digoxin, thiazide diuretics, β-blockers, penicillin G, tetracycline, phenobarbital, fat-soluble vitamins, and thyroxine. To prevent these interactions, bile acid sequestrants should be taken 1 hour after or 4 hours before susceptible agents.

Fish Oil

The omega-6 fatty acid docosahexaenoic acid (DHA) and the omega-3 fatty acid eicosapentaenoic acid (EPA) reduce elevated triglyceride levels when administered at high dosages. Even low-dose fish oil (1 g/d), however, was shown in the Gruppo Italiano per lo Studio della Sopravivenza nell'Infarto Miocardico (GISSI) Prevention Study to reduce the risk for death, nonfatal myocardial infarction, or stroke by 10% and significantly decreased total mortality by 14%. Fish oil may be used as monotherapy or combined with a fibrate or niacin.

Mechanism of Action. High doses of fish oil increase the intracellular degradation of apo B-100 and consequently lead to decreased VLDL production.

Efficacy. Approximately 1 g DHA and 2 g EPA (6 to 12 capsules, available as over-the-counter preparations) reduce triglyceride by approximately 20 to 50% and increase HDLC by 5 to 6%. LDLC often increases in hypertriglyceridemic patients, but this increase is thought to reflect a shift in LDL particle size to a larger, less atherogenic species. To improve compliance, therapy is generally initiated at a dosage of two capsules two to three times daily.

Side Effects and Drug Interactions. The most commonly reported side effects are gastrointestinal complaints and nausea. Although fish oils have an antithrombotic effect, increased risk of bleeding has not been found in clinical trials. Complaints about taste and odor may vary with the formulation.

Estrogen Replacement Therapy

Estrogen has been associated with a decreased risk of CHD events in observational studies, but in clinical intervention trials, no benefit on CHD events has been observed. In the Heart Estrogen/Progestin Replacement Study, estrogen plus progestin did not reduce the incidence of nonfatal myocardial infarction or CHD death and increased the risk for thromboembolic events and gallbladder disease; during the first year of treatment, more cardiovascular events occurred in women receiving hormone therapy than in those receiving placebo, but fewer events occurred with hormone therapy during the fourth and fifth years of the trial. Estrogen also failed to provide angiographic benefit in the Estrogen Replacement and Atherosclerosis trial. Until additional clinical trial results become available, the routine use of estrogen replacement therapy for the prevention of cardiovascular disease in women is not supported by the data; at the current time, estrogen replacement therapy is not indicated to treat dyslipidemia.

Combination Therapy

Patients whose lipid levels are not adequately improved with pharmacologic monotherapy and maximal diet therapy may require the addition of a second lipid-modifying agent.

Statin Plus Niacin. For many patients with severe mixed dyslipidemia characterized by elevated LDLC and triglyceride and low HDLC, the combination of niacin and a statin is the most effective means of normalizing all lipid parameters, including improvements in LDL particle size and reductions in Lp(a) levels. Lower dose niacin (1 to 2 g/day) combined with a statin is better tolerated than high-dose niacin, and the addition of niacin to a statin reduces LDLC by approximately 30 to 40%, reduces triglyceride by approximately 30%, and increases HDLC by approximately 30%. This combination may increase the risk for myopathy and hepatitis and should be avoided in patients with significant underlying hepatic or renal disease and in patients receiving concomitant medication that increases toxicity, such as cyclosporine, erythromycin, or itraconazole. Patients should be taught to recognize the symptoms of myopathy and to discontinue use of the medication if they become acutely ill or hospitalized.

Statin Plus Fibrate. Combining a statin with a fibrate may also be useful in treating mixed dyslipidemia. This combination reduces LDLC by approximately 35 to 40%, reduces triglyceride by approximately 20 to 40%, and increases HDLC by approximately 20%. In addition to these improvements in lipid levels, the addition of a fibrate to a statin may improve LDL particle size and decrease fibrinogen levels. Because this combination may increase the risk of myopathy, patients should be taught to recognize the symptoms and discontinue use of the medication if they become acutely ill or hospitalized. Patients with renal or hepatic dysfunction or those receiving immunosuppressive therapy should not receive this combination. Reducing the dose of fibrate or statin may also reduce the risk.

OBESITY

method of
DONALD D. HENSRUD, M.D., M.P.H.
Mayo Medical School and Mayo Clinic
Rochester, Minnesota

ETIOLOGY OF OBESITY

In simple terms, obesity results from chronic energy intake exceeding energy expenditure. However, reversing this seemingly simple equation and losing weight is extremely challenging, as demonstrated by the currently high and increasing prevalence of obesity in the United States and other countries. Although genetic factors may exert a predisposition to weight, environmental factors that ultimately affect diet and activity determine body weight. The increase in the prevalence of obesity in the United States by one third over the past 2 decades has resulted from environmental causes; genetic factors do not operate in such a relatively short time. In contrast to traditional societies, developed countries such as the United States permit limited physical activity and easy

TABLE 1. **Predisposing Factors to Obesity**

Factor	Comment
Decreased physical activity	
Activities throughout the day	Major contributor to increasing obesity in the United States
Exercise	The strongest effects of exercise are prevention of obesity and maintenance of weight loss
Increased energy intake	
Various factors	Increased portion size; high-energy–dense foods including fat, sugar, and processed food; decreased intake of vegetables and fruits
Alcohol	Increases abdominal weight gain
Smoking cessation	Mean increase of 6–10 lb
Medications	
Corticosteroids	
Tricyclic and other antidepressants	
Pregnancy	Mean increase of 4–6 lb after each pregnancy
Endocrine/metabolic	<1%–2% of all obesity
Hypothyroidism	Weight gain usually only in longstanding hypothyroidism
Cushing's syndrome	Characteristic fat deposition
Genetic conditions	Very rare
Prader-Willi syndrome	
Lawrence-Moon-Betel syndrome	
Other medical conditions	
Depression	
Physical limitations that limit activity	
Yo-yo dieting—gaining and losing weight multiple times	Does not result in sustained depression of metabolic rate and increased risk of weight gain despite popular belief

access for most people to large quantities of high-energy–dense food.

Table 1 lists various factors that predispose to obesity. Modifying the individual and societal factors that contribute to obesity can be challenging, but not impossible. At Mayo Clinic, we use an approach based on promoting lifestyle changes in eating patterns, physical activity, and other weight-related behaviors. Within these areas, we individualize the approach to each patient according to the factors that are contributing to their increased weight.

TABLE 2. **Health Co-Morbidities of Obesity**

- Increased overall mortality
- Glucose intolerance and type 2 diabetes mellitus
- Hypertension
- Dyslipidemia
  - Hypertriglyceridemia
  - Low HDL cholesterol
- Cancer
  - Endometrium
  - Breast
  - Possibly ovarian, colon, kidney, and prostate
- Degenerative arthritis
- Respiratory problems
  - Obstructive sleep apnea
  - Restrictive lung disease
- Hepatobiliary problems
  - Cholelithiasis
  - Hepatosteatosis

HEALTH RISKS OF OBESITY

Obesity is associated with a number of health co-morbidities (Table 2). In general, the greater the degree of obesity, the greater the health risks, including overall mortality. Body fat distribution can also have a large impact on the risk for morbidity and mortality. Compared to people with excess weight in the hips, thighs, and buttocks (lower body fat distribution or "pears"), people with predominantly abdominal obesity (upper body fat distribution or "apples") are at higher risk for type 2 diabetes mellitus, hypertension, dyslipidemia (high triglycerides and low high-density lipoprotein [HDL] cholesterol), coronary artery disease, and overall mortality.

CLASSIFICATION OF OVERWEIGHT AND OBESITY

Tables 3 and 4 outline the current risk classification of overweight and obesity. These guidelines classify people with a body mass index (BMI) of 25 to 29.9 kg/m² as overweight and those with a BMI of 30 kg/m² or greater as obese. Using these definitions, 61% of the U.S. adult population are at least overweight, and 26% are obese. Men with a waist measurement of more than 40 inches and women with a waist measurement of more than 35 inches, which reflect upper body fat distribution, are at increased health risks, as previously discussed.

The need for weight loss and weight management is greatest for people with established co-morbidities of obesity that will improve with weight loss, followed by individ-

TABLE 3. **Classification of Overweight and Obesity**

Variable	BMI (kg/m²)*	Obesity Class	Disease Risk: *Low Waist Circumference*	Disease Risk: *High Waist Circumference*†
Underweight	<18.5		—	—
Normal	18.5–24.9		—	—
Overweight	25.0–29.9		Increased	High
Obesity	30.0–34.9	I	High	Very high
	35.0–39.9	II	Very high	Very high
Extreme obesity	≥40	III	Extremely high	Extremely high

*Body mass index (BMI) can be calculated as wt(kg)/ht²(m), or wt(lb) × 703/ht²(in). Tables of weight, height, and BMI are also available.
†High waist circumference is defined as >40 in. in men and >35 in. in women.

TABLE 4. **Body Mass Index Table**

Height	Healthy		Overweight			Obese			
	BMI 18.5	*BMI 24.9*	*BMI 25*	*BMI 27*	*BMI 29.9*	*BMI 30*	*BMI 35*	*BMI 40*	*BMI 45*
	Weight in Pounds								
4′10″	89	119	120	129	143	144	167	191	215
4′11″	92	123	124	134	147	148	173	198	223
5′0″	95	127	128	138	153	154	179	205	230
5′1″	98	131	132	143	158	159	185	211	238
5′2″	101	136	137	148	163	164	191	218	246
5′3″	104	140	141	152	168	169	197	226	254
5′4″	108	145	146	157	174	175	204	233	262
5′5″	111	149	150	162	179	180	210	240	270
5′6″	115	154	155	167	185	186	217	247	278
5′7″	118	158	159	172	190	191	223	255	287
5′8″	122	163	164	177	196	197	230	263	296
5′9″	125	168	169	183	202	203	237	270	304
5′10″	129	173	174	188	208	209	244	278	313
5′11″	133	178	179	193	214	215	251	286	322
6′0″	136	183	184	199	220	221	258	294	331
6′1″	140	188	189	204	226	227	265	303	340
6′2″	144	193	194	210	232	233	272	311	350
6′3″	148	199	200	216	239	240	280	319	359
6′4″	152	204	205	221	245	246	287	328	369

uals with an upper body fat distribution who are at risk for many of these conditions, and finally lower body obese individuals. This stratification can be used to guide the intensity of treatment. For example, a patient who has a BMI of 42 kg/m^2 and has hypertension, type 2 diabetes mellitus, and obstructive sleep apnea may be a candidate for bariatric surgery. On the other hand, someone who is mildly overweight and otherwise healthy would certainly not want to resort to extreme measures for cosmetic weight loss.

EVALUATION OF THE OBESE PATIENT

The medical history is important for a number of reasons (Table 5). The patient's readiness to undertake weight loss should be assessed. If other life stresses are present, it may be difficult to institute lifestyle changes related to weight management. In this case it may be better to postpone efforts until a better time. A weight history can determine if obesity was present as a child or if weight gain occurred mainly during adult years.

TABLE 5. **Items to Assess in the Medical History for Obesity Evaluation**

Readiness/motivation to undertake weight loss
Reasons/expectations for weight loss
Available support
Previous methods of weight loss and results (including why results were not successful)
Potential barriers to weight loss and maintenance (time, finances, established habits)
High school graduation weight, minimum and maximum adult weight
Periods of increased weight gain (e.g., pregnancy, smoking cessation, stressful life periods)
Current (and past) diet
Triggers to eating
Current (and past) exercise/activity
Factors the patient believes are responsible for weight
Binge eating, purging, laxative or diuretic use
Family history of obesity
Medications

A diet history can give clues to adverse dietary practices that make it difficult to lose weight. A relatively quick question to assess diet is "What do you eat in a typical day for breakfast, lunch, dinner, and snacks?" It is important to determine what factors the patient believes are responsible for their weight. By doing this, specific issues can be addressed that may help promote more successful weight loss and maintenance. Previous efforts to lose weight, including treatment programs, should be inquired about and the reasons why these efforts were not successful should be discussed. Triggers that initiate habit eating and excessive energy intake should be assessed and addressed during treatment using problem-solving techniques.

Height and weight should be recorded and body fat distribution can be assessed by gross visual inspection, or preferably by waist measurement. Physical signs of Cushing's syndrome or hypothyroidism should be noted.

Laboratory studies should include a thyroid-stimulating hormone level; fasting blood glucose level; and serum total cholesterol, triglyceride, HDL cholesterol, and calculated low-density lipoprotein (LDL) cholesterol levels. Liver function tests can be considered to check for hepatosteatosis. Ultrasonography can be done if there is suspicion of gallstones. In patients with suspected Cushing's syndrome, a 24-hour urine cortisol measurement followed by a low-dose dexamethasone suppression test may be helpful. If there is a history of apneic spells (usually best obtained from a significant other) or excessive daytime somnolence, referral for an overnight sleep study or, at a minimum, overnight oximetry should be considered.

TREATMENT OPTIONS FOR OBESITY

Although there are virtually hundreds of different types of programs, the cornerstones of treatment for obesity remain diet and activity, instituted through modifying behavior. Specific treatment approaches are listed in Table 6. Whatever treatment method is

TABLE 6. **Summary of Various Treatments for Obesity**

Treatment	Approximate Target Body Weight	Comments
Low-calorie diets	BMI ≥25 kg/m²	Many different variations
Very-low–calorie liquid formula diets	BMI ≥30 kg/m²	Not practical long-term, rapid weight loss but generally more rapid weight regain after cessation compared to more conservative treatment
Behavioral modification	BMI ≥25 kg/m²	Modest weight loss ultimately results from changes in diet and activity
Pharmacologic treatment	BMI ≥30 kg/m², or ≥27 kg/m² with complications	Reasonable results as long as drugs are continued, usually weight regain after cessation
Bariatric surgery	BMI ≥40 kg/m² with complications	Best long-term results but greatest risks also
Exercise and physical activity	Any weight	Should be part of every weight loss program (in addition to being recommended for the general population: obese and nonobese)

used, the emphasis should be on improvement in health conditions and long-term weight maintenance in addition to initial weight loss.

Risks Associated With Weight Loss

The risk of gallstone formation increases exponentially with increasing rates of weight loss, particularly above 1.5 kg/week. Psychological dysfunction can result from dieting and this can become a vicious cycle. People can become extremely preoccupied with losing weight, which can lead to unhealthy dietary treatments, excessively restrictive dieting, obsession with food, and depression. Restrictive dieting can lead to the restrained eater phenomenon that may predispose to binge eating. These are not reasons to avoid weight loss. Rather, by being aware of these risks and using proper methods of weight loss, they can be avoided.

Dietary Treatment of Obesity

There are many different dietary programs that have been promoted as being effective in inducing weight loss. Dietary programs that are used to treat obesity should have a sound scientific rationale, be safe and nutritionally adequate, and practical enough to allow long-term compliance.

Popular Diets

Many popular diets espouse a program that leads to effortless weight loss. Any program that leads to weight loss must decrease energy intake relative to energy expenditure. If weight loss is achieved by following some popular diets, long-term health may not improve if less healthy foods are consumed. For example, eating foods high in saturated fat will lead to weight loss if overall calorie intake is reduced, but the risk of certain cancers, coronary heart disease, and other diseases may increase.

A major theory behind many of the currently popular diets is that insulin leads to increased weight gain and other health problems. Carbohydrate intake promotes insulin production; therefore, carbohydrate intake should be limited. The problem is the reasoning is backward—excess total calories (not just from carbohydrate) leads to obesity, which then leads to insulin resistance and increased insulin levels, not the reverse. Also, fasting (and sustained) insulin levels are a more important risk for disease compared to a temporary increase in insulin following consumption of carbohydrate. Insulin resistance and increased fasting insulin levels are associated with increased health risks, and play a central role in syndrome X (central obesity, hypertension, dyslipidemia, glucose intolerance). However, obesity, primarily abdominal obesity, is the basic predisposing factor in this condition, not increased carbohydrate intake.

In general, the negative aspects of these diets outweigh any potential benefits. There is little supportive evidence for most popular diets. People would be much better off investing their efforts in safe and scientifically sound programs. It may not lead to rapid weight loss but will lead to beneficial lifestyle habits that are more likely to sustain weight loss and, most importantly, improve long-term health.

Very Low Calorie Diets

Very low calorie diets (VLCDs), also referred to as *protein-sparing modified fasts,* provide 800 or less kcal/d. Restricting energy under 800 kcal/d does not seem to result in increased weight loss and is not recommended. VLCDs have shown large amounts of weight loss initially, up to 20 kg in 12 to 16 weeks. Early results of VLCDs showed rapid weight regain after stopping the program, often to levels above pretreatment weight. In recent years, in an attempt to improve long-term results, VLCDs have been used initially followed by a moderate calorie-restricted diet, behavior modification, or medications. Limited data have shown this to be slightly more effective, but long-term results remain no better than those with behavioral modification alone.

Liquid Meal Replacements

Liquid meal replacements have been promoted as an over-the-counter method to promote weight loss, and there is limited evidence they do so. They have the advantage of reduced cost and convenience. One liquid meal replacement, SlimFast, encourages healthful dietary modifications, including snacks of fruits and vegetables, along with their product. A German study reported increased weight loss and better long-term weight maintenance in subjects using SlimFast compared to standard dietary treatment over a 2-year period.

Low-Calorie Diets

Balanced hypocaloric diets prescribe a calorie deficit of usually 500 to 1000 kcal/d, and provide calories from protein, carbohydrate, and fat but in reduced amounts. Different types of implementation strategies are used such as counting calories, counting fat grams, keeping track of food by assigning points to a specific amount of each food, or prescribing servings similar to a diabetic exchange system. Theoretically, a calorie deficit of 500 to 1000 calories per day should promote a weight loss of 1 to 2 pounds a week. One problem with dietary programs based on caloric prescriptions is that people tend to underestimate the amount of calories they consume by at least 20% on average, and obese subjects may underestimate even more: up to almost 50% in one study.

Energy Density

Energy density is the number of calories in a given amount of food. Foods vary widely in energy density. Fats and sugar have a relatively large amount of calories in a small volume and, therefore, have a high energy density. For the same number of calories, vegetables occupy a much larger volume and have a low energy density. This is because of their large content of water and fiber that contributes weight and volume but not calories. For example, a tablespoon of butter and 10 cups of mixed greens contain the same amount of calories but the volume of food is quite different.

The way in which energy density affects calorie intake is that the weight and volume of food are important determinants of satiety and, therefore, the amount of calories consumed. By eating foods that have a low energy density, people can consume a large volume and weight of food and feel satisfied, yet ingest a lower amount of calories. Studies performed at the University of Alabama at Birmingham and Pennsylvania State University have supported this concept. Vegetables and fruits have a low energy density, carbohydrates (grains and other starches) higher energy density, and foods high in fat or sugar the highest energy density.

Mayo Clinic Healthy Weight Pyramid

Consuming low-energy–dense foods is one of the principles behind the Mayo Clinic Healthy Weight Pyramid (Figure 1). Another unique feature of the pyramid is that it emphasizes healthy choices within each category. Finally, daily physical activity is at the center of the pyramid, emphasizing the central role physical activity has in weight management and health.

Vegetables and fruits are on the bottom of the pyramid, and unlimited amounts of whole foods (not juice or dried fruit) from each of these groups are

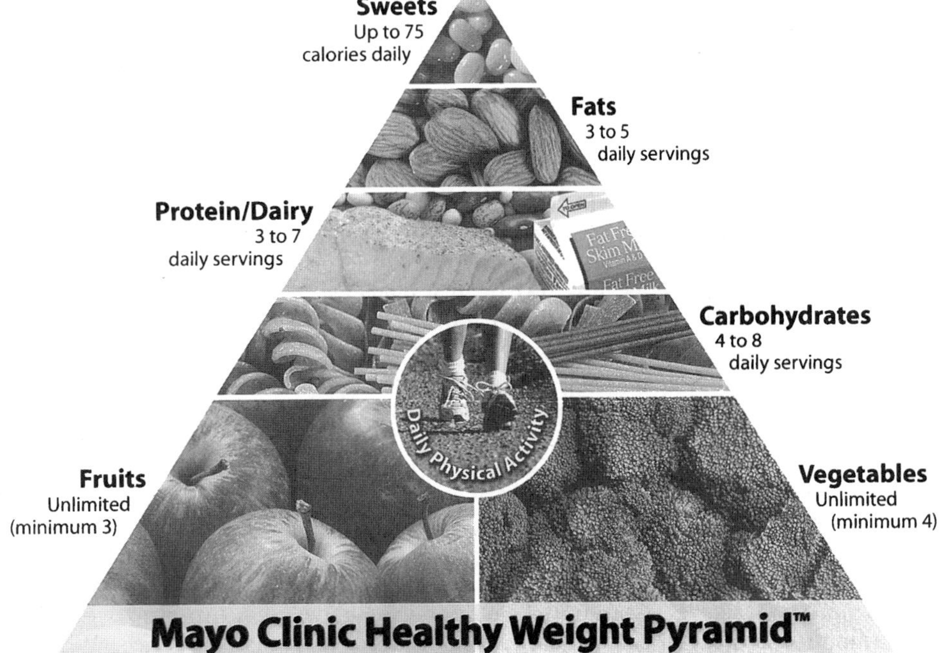

Figure 1. The Mayo Clinic Healthy Weight Pyramid encompasses several principles, emphasizing the consumption of low-energy–dense foods, the selection of healthy choices within each category, and the importance of daily physical activity in weight management and health. (By permission of Mayo Foundation for Medical Education and Research.)

TABLE 7. **Serving Recommendations for 1200 and 1400 Calorie Diets From the Mayo Clinic Healthy Weight Pyramid**

Food Group	1200*	1400†
Vegetables	Minimum of 4	Minimum of 4
Fruits	Minimum of 3	Minimum of 4
Carbohydrates	4	4
Protein/dairy	3	4
Fats	3	3
Sweets	Up to 75 kcal/d	Up to 75 kcal/d

*Recommended as an initial calorie goal to promote weight loss for most women under 250 pounds.

†Recommended as an initial calorie goal to promote weight loss for most men under 250 pounds.

encouraged. The number of servings from the other food groups is limited. For patients who are overweight but weigh less than 250 pounds, a dietary plan with an initial calorie goal of 1200 kcal/d is recommended for women and 1400 kcal/d for men. However, because the amounts of vegetable and fruit servings are unlimited, the actual calorie intake may be more than this, but should remain low enough to promote weight loss. Serving recommendations for 1200- and 1400-kcal diets are shown in Table 7. Lists of the serving sizes of various foods can be found in the book *Mayo Clinic on Healthy Weight*.

More important than losing weight is improving health. Within each food group, emphasis is placed on foods associated with greater health benefits using a "best foods" list. For example, in the carbohydrate group whole grains are emphasized over refined grains. Soybeans and other legumes, fish, and low-fat dairy products are emphasized in the protein/dairy group. Monounsaturated fats including olive oil, canola oil, and nuts are emphasized in the fat group. Sweets are limited to 75 kcal/d.

Physical Activity

Physical activity includes formal exercise and activities throughout the day. It's been suggested that a major factor related to the increased prevalence of obesity over the past 2 decades has been a decrease in daily activities. If one looks at traditional societies where obesity is uncommon, regular physical activity is common and incorporated within people's lifestyles. Because of the relatively sedentary lifestyle in developed countries, more effort needs to be directed toward formal exercise to increase energy expenditure. Yet many types of physical activity can be incorporated within a day's activities. For example, taking the stairs instead of an elevator, parking farther away from a destination, walking over the noon hour, and other activities can often be easily performed throughout the day. If performed consistently over time, these activities can result in a large amount of expended energy.

Formal exercise takes additional time out of the day to perform but has the advantage of burning more calories per unit time. Guidelines for exercise include the following:

Choose an exercise that is enjoyable
Make it a scheduling priority
Maintain it consistently over time

The greater the intensity, frequency, and duration, the greater the energy expenditure. People need to balance this with practical aspects, including the ability to maintain the activity consistently over time. People should start out with a moderate and sustainable program, and gradually increase intensity, frequency, and duration over time. The type of activity should be tailored to the person. Some people may have physical restrictions that limit certain activities. Most people, however, can find some activity to perform if they are willing to make a moderate effort. Eventually, all adults should try and obtain 30 minutes of moderately vigorous physical activity most days, which is the goal for the general population.

Regular physical activity is one of the most effective methods to promote long-term weight maintenance. To successfully maintain weight requires a commitment. People who have successfully lost weight and maintained that weight loss often exercise up to 1 hour a day. Keeping an exercise log may help with compliance.

Exercise can not only lead to weight loss but can improve health through improved cardiovascular conditioning, lower blood pressure, decreased serum lipid levels, decreased risk of colon cancer, and better glucose control in patients with glucose intolerance or type 2 diabetes mellitus. Regular exercise can also increase muscle mass and lead to less depression and an improved sense of well being.

The mindset toward making changes in exercise and daily activity is important. It is human nature to conserve energy and use step-saving activities. Instead, people should look for opportunities to obtain physical activity, such as walking to talk with a coworker instead of sending him or her an e-mail message. Focusing on the beneficial aspects of obtaining activity such as burning calories, feeling better, and improving health can help maintain a positive mindset.

Practical Aspects of Lifestyle Changes

Permanent changes in lifestyle habits related to diet and exercise are necessary to realize long-term results. Thus, the focus should be on the process and not on the end result. By contrast, many people focus primarily on the numbers on the scale without appropriate attention given to the methods used to change those numbers. By making changes in diet and exercise habits, weight loss should follow as a natural consequence. Whatever changes someone makes in diet and exercise habits should be comfortable and realistic enough to be sustained indefinitely to promote long-term weight management.

People who are making dietary changes to lose

weight commonly approach this as "going on a diet." Going on a diet implies eventually going off a diet, and therefore it is likely to fail. Indefinite changes in eating habits, instead of going on a diet, are more likely to lead to sustained weight loss. Like any behavioral change, adopting new nutritional patterns and getting rid of old ones can be difficult, but not impossible.

An individual approach should be used because of the variability in issues and problems among people trying to manage weight. For some people portion control may be difficult, whereas others may struggle with late-night eating, eating increased amounts of certain high-calorie foods, or many other habits and triggers that lead to increased calorie intake and weight gain. Keeping diet records can help by providing feedback on what is actually consumed compared to dietary goals. People who keep diet records are more successful at losing weight and maintaining weight loss.

A typical attitude about making dietary changes to lose and manage weight is that it is a negative experience. This negative outlook sets people up for failure. This may lead to restrained and restrictive eating patterns that may promote short-term weight loss but are difficult to continue long-term. After a short period, people may realize they cannot continue and then abandon all efforts and go back to previous unhealthy patterns. A positive attitude and focusing on consuming palatable low-energy–dense food rather than continuing to dwell on previous foods that are now limited may help maintain nutritional changes. Adopting healthy eating habits that are comfortable enough to be maintained indefinitely rather than overly restrictive eating patterns can help lessen feelings of restraint.

Dietary habits and specific foods that people eat tend to be repeated, that is, a certain recipe or meal is consumed regularly, perhaps every couple of weeks. To help establish new dietary habits, it is necessary to try new recipes or modify old ones. For example, instead of pasta with a cream sauce, substitute a marinara sauce with different vegetables. Cookbooks and other resources can help with ideas for this. New recipes should be palatable as well as healthy, and practical enough to fit in a busy lifestyle. In general, people underestimate their ability to adopt new taste preferences, but taste preferences can change. An example of this is changing from whole milk to low-fat milk, which many people have done.

Process Goals

Because the focus should be on the process and not the end result, process goals should be used instead of outcome goals. These goals should be specific, achievable, and measurable. For example, instead of using a nonspecific outcome goal such as "I'm going to lose some weight," an appropriate process goal would be "I'm going to start eating four servings of vegetables per day." This can be monitored with diet records and efforts can be adjusted, if necessary, to achieve that goal.

Problem-Solving Techniques

One way to tackle the barriers to changing lifestyle habits and managing weight is through problem-solving techniques. First, the problem is identified. Next, all the benefits to changing the behavior are written down. Then, all the barriers to changing the behavior are recorded. Finally, solutions to the barriers are determined. It is important to write these items down as this helps to clearly identify all related factors and potential solutions.

PHARMACOLOGIC TREATMENT

Sibutramine

Sibutramine (Meridia) is a reuptake inhibitor of both serotonin and noradrenaline, and both of these mechanisms acting synergistically are responsible for its effect on food intake. Sibutramine does not have a major effect on appetite. Rather, it increases satiety after the onset of eating.

Weight loss with sibutramine appears to be dose-related. A representative study of sibutramine showed weight loss of 3 to 5 kg with 10 mg and 4 to 6 kg with 15 mg of sibutramine compared to almost 2 kg with placebo.

The most common side effects observed during treatment with sibutramine are headache, dry mouth, constipation, and insomnia. The most concerning side effect with this drug is a tendency to increase blood pressure, which is also dose-related similar to treatment efficacy. Although the mean increase in blood pressure is only 2 mm Hg systolic and diastolic, 10% of people will experience an increase in diastolic blood pressure of at least 10 mm Hg. For these reasons, subjects started on sibutramine should have their blood pressure observed closely.

Health practitioners who prescribe sibutramine should be familiar with contraindications to treatment, including uncontrolled hypertension and established cardiovascular disease. Sibutramine is available in 5-, 10-, and 15-mg doses given once/day. The recommended starting dose is 10 mg/day. The 15-mg dose can be used in subjects who do not adequately respond to 10 mg, and the 5-mg dose can be used in those who do not tolerate the 10-mg dose.

Orlistat

Orlistat (Xenical) is a reversible lipase inhibitor that blocks the absorption, on average, of about 30% of ingested dietary fat. The drug is not absorbed and therefore has few systemic side effects. The main side effects are related to the gastrointestinal tract.

Pooled data from five clinical trials (some unpublished) indicated the overall mean weight loss after 1 year was 6.1 kg in patients treated with orlistat and 2.6 kg in placebo-treated patients, a difference of 3.5 kg. Studies lasting up to 2 years show that one fourth to one third of the weight lost during the first year is regained during the second year of treatment, but overall weight loss is still significantly, but modestly, greater than placebo. Improvements in serum lipid and glucose values have also been significantly greater in subjects taking orlistat compared to placebo in patients with diabetes mellitus and subjects without diabetes mellitus.

Adverse events that occurred in more than 20% of subjects during the first year of clinical trials included oily fecal spotting, flatus with discharge, fecal urgency, and fatty or oily stools. During the second year of treatment almost all gastrointestinal side effects occurred in 5% or less of subjects taking orlistat.

Orlistat is prescribed at 120 mg three times/day with meals (that contain fat). It is recommended that all patients taking orlistat also take a multivitamin at least 2 hours before or after taking orlistat. Orlistat is contraindicated in patients with chronic malabsorption, cholestasis, or hypersensitivity to orlistat or any of its components. It may be difficult to use in patients with chronic gastrointestinal conditions such as irritable bowel syndrome.

Issues Related to Pharmacotherapy for Obesity

Clinical indications for both sibutramine and orlistat are a BMI of greater than 30 kg/m^2, or greater than 27 kg/m^2 in the presence of obesity-associated co-morbidities. Because improvement in health is a primary goal in treating obesity, pharmacotherapy at Mayo Clinic is limited to patients with co-morbidities from their weight that will improve with weight loss (Table 8). Short-term use of pharmacotherapy does little good. Yet, it is not clear how long medications should be continued, and weight regain usually follows cessation of drug use.

Patients should be well informed about the use of drugs to promote weight loss. They need to have realistic expectations about the amount of weight loss that is likely. Weight loss has plateaued after about 6 months in almost all studies using pharmacotherapy. Patients should be clear that changes in diet and physical activity are the ultimate determinants of body weight, and efforts in these areas should be continued during drug treatment. Results will vary, and some patients will not lose any weight. In these situations, medications should be discontinued once this is clear.

TABLE 8. **Indications for Pharmacologic Treatment for Obesity in the Nutrition Clinic at Mayo Clinic***

Body mass index (BMI) >27 kg/m^2
One or more complications or conditions that are likely to improve with weight loss
Previous failure of conservative treatment with diet and exercise
Agree to a 2–4 week trial of making initial changes in diet and exercise before starting pharmacotherapy
Agree to continued treatment with diet, exercise, and behavioral modification while on pharmacologic treatment
Agree to periodic follow-up
Premenopausal females (able to have children) must use some form of contraception
Consider a pregnancy test when initiating treatment if there is any possibility of pregnancy
No contraindications to the specific drug used for pharmacologic treatment

*All of these variables should be present to qualify for pharmacologic treatment.

Bariatric Surgery

Bariatric surgery should, in general, be reserved for people who have a BMI greater than 40 kg/m^2 with complications from their obesity. In some cases, bariatric surgery may be acceptable for a patient with complications from their weight and a BMI between 35 and 40 kg/m^2. A strong effort at conservative treatment with diet, exercise, and behavioral modification should have been attempted prior to considering a surgical approach for weight loss.

Bariatric surgery should be done by an experienced team composed of a surgeon and other experts from medicine, nutrition, and psychology or psychiatry. It is extremely important to fully evaluate each potential candidate because the changes required in diet and lifestyle following bariatric surgery are considerable. Patients should be well informed about the potential complications, required changes, follow-up requirements, and expected results. In addition to operative complications, long-term complications include dumping syndrome, persistent vomiting, diarrhea, temporary hair loss, cholelithiasis, and deficiencies of vitamin B_{12} and iron. This procedure should be done cautiously in women of childbearing age because if pregnancy is subsequently undertaken there may be a risk of fetal damage secondary to nutritional deficiencies. Although it possesses more risks, bariatric surgery is more successful long-term compared to other treatments for weight loss.

EXPECTED RESULTS FROM OBESITY TREATMENT

Weight loss should occur at one to two pounds per week, which will eventually plateau and hopefully will be maintained. Unfortunately, past data do not reflect a favorable long-term outcome after weight loss treatment. Regardless of the approach, approximately 95% of people will regain their weight within 5 years. Bariatric surgery is one exception in that approximately 50% of excess weight is lost and maintained in the long term. However, the extreme nature of this approach makes it appropriate only for the select population described earlier.

One of the most favorable factors associated with long-term success is regular physical activity. Ongoing support from individuals (e.g., dietitians) or groups can help weight maintenance efforts. In addition, people who make a commitment to permanent changes in diet and other lifestyle habits are more

TABLE 9. **Measures of Success in Treatment of Obesity**

Weight loss
Long-term weight maintenance
Prevention of weight gain
Improvement in co-morbidities of obesity
Inches lost
Changes in body composition
Improved health habits
Feeling better

likely to achieve lasting weight maintenance. Success can be defined in ways other than weight change (Table 9). Even more important are improvements in health conditions associated with obesity such as hypertension, type 2 diabetes mellitus, and the other complications mentioned earlier. Subjective factors such as improved mood and healthier dietary habits can also define successful long-term treatment.

SUGGESTED READINGS

Brownell KD: The LEARN Program for Weight Control 2000. Dallas: American Health, 2000.

Hensrud DD (ed): Mayo Clinic on Healthy Weight. Rochester, Minn: Mayo Foundation for Medical Education and Research, 2000.

The Practical Guide to the Identification, Evaluation, and Treatment of Overweight and Obesity in Adults (NIH). Bethesda, Md: Publication No. 00-4084. National Heart, Lung, and Blood Institute, 2000.

VITAMIN K DEFICIENCY

method of
FRANK R. GREER, M.D., and
CAROL A. DIAMOND, M.D.
University of Wisconsin
Madison, Wisconsin

Vitamin K is a fat-soluble vitamin important for the formation of many vitamin K–dependent proteins including the plasma coagulation proteins (II, VII, IX, X) and the plasma proteins C, S, and Z. Other vitamin K–dependent proteins are found in bone (osteocalcin, matrix Gla protein), kidney (nephrocalcin), spleen, lung, uterus, placenta, pancreas, thyroid, thymus, and testes. All of the known vitamin K–dependent proteins have in common γ-carboxyglutamic acid (Gla), the unique amino acid formed by the postribosomal action of vitamin K–dependent carboxylase. Vitamin K is a necessary cofactor for the activity of this glutamyl carboxylase, located on the membrane of the endoplasmic reticulum. The Gla residues formed by the action of this carboxylase are located on the homologous aminoterminal domain of the protein, with a high degree of amino acid sequence identity common to all vitamin K–dependent proteins. They are required for the protein conformation that allows for calcium binding and the calcium-mediated interaction of these proteins with phospholipids.

The daily recommended intake for vitamin K is 1 μg per kg of body weight. The most important dietary form of this vitamin is vitamin K_1, or phylloquinone. Green leafy vegetables are the best dietary source (50–800 μg/100 g), but other foods contain significant amounts of vitamin K_1, including dairy products, meats, eggs, cereals, fruits, and other vegetables (1–50 μg/100 g). Although human milk is very low in vitamin K (2 μg/L), all infant formulas used in the United States have vitamin K_1 added (50 μg/L). Another potential source of vitamin K is the bacterial flora of the jejunum and ileum, which synthesize vitamin K_2, or menaquinone. The extent that this form of vitamin K can be used by human beings is unclear, and it is even possible that menaquinone may be converted to phylloquinone, as has recently been shown in rodents. From 40% to 70% of dietary vitamin K is absorbed from the small intestine, and the absorption via chylomicrons and the lymphatic system is dependent on bile, pancreatic secretions, and dietary fat.

CLINICAL FEATURES

Vitamin K deficiency results in a coagulopathy and a bleeding disorder. Specific signs of deficiency include bruising, epistaxis, bleeding from the gastrointestinal or genitourinary tracts, menometrorrhagia, retroperitoneal bleeding, and intracranial hemorrhage (particularly in infants). Bleeding may follow trauma, needle punctures, and surgery.

ETIOLOGY

Vitamin K deficiency may result from decreased intake or fat malabsorption. Antibiotic inhibition of vitamin K_2 synthesis by intestinal bacteria may also be a factor. Prolonged total parenteral nutrition without supplemental vitamin K has also been reported to cause deficiency. Causes of fat malabsorption that may be associated with vitamin K deficiency include short bowel syndrome, biliary atresia, cholestatic jaundice, α_1-antitrypsin deficiency, pancreatic insufficiency (e.g., cystic fibrosis), and diseases of the small intestine (e.g., nontropical sprue, regional enteritis).

Therapy with vitamin K antagonists such as warfarin may present as a coagulopathy identical to vitamin K deficiency. Warfarin (Coumadin), is an active ingredient of some rodenticides, although superwarfarins (e.g., brodifacoum, difenacoum, chlorophacinone, bromadiolone, diphacinone, pindone, valone, flocoumafen, coumatetralyl) are now preferred as rodenticides due to warfarin resistance in rats. Poisoning with these rodenticides occurs accidentally or by attempted suicide. Poisoning has been observed after smoking a mixture of marijuana and d-CON, a rodenticide containing brodifacoum.

Vitamin K deficiency causes hemorrhagic disease in infants. This may occur early (within the first week) or later (up to 3 months) in life. The late form, with an incidence of one in many thousands, has the most significant mortality and morbidity. Because vitamin K crosses the placenta poorly, vitamin K levels are nearly undetectable in umbilical cord blood. Human milk is also very low in vitamin K; therefore, breast-fed infants are particularly at risk for hemorrhagic disease. A bleeding diathesis in newborns attributed to vitamin K deficiency has also been associated with maternal administration of anticonvulsants (e.g., phenobarbital, phenytoin [Dilantin], primidone [Mysoline]).

β-Lactam antibiotics with an *N*-methyl-5-thiotetrazole side chain (cefamandole [Mandol], cefoperazone [Cefobid], cefoxitin [Mefoxin]) also contribute to the coagulopathy of vitamin K deficiency because they inhibit Gla synthesis in coagulation factors.

DIAGNOSIS

Prolongation of the prothrombin time (PT) and the activated partial thromboplastin time (aPTT) characterize a deficiency of vitamin K. Values for platelet counts, plasma fibrinogen level, thrombin time, fibrinogen degradation or split products, and D-dimer are normal. Because vitamin K blood levels are not readily available, other laboratory evaluations are not indicated. The diagnosis is confirmed by demonstration that vitamin K replacement restores PT and aPTT values to normal (within hours after parenteral vitamin K administration). Differential diagnosis includes disseminated intravascular coagulation (DIC) and liver disease (Table 1). PT and aPTT values in infants are notably higher than adult levels until at least 6 months of age.

FORMULATIONS OF VITAMIN K_1

Vitamin K_1 is available as a tablet (Mephyton, 5 mg) or a parenteral form for intramuscular or subcutaneous injection (AquaMEPHYTON, 10 mg/mL or 2.0 mg/mL). AquaMEPHYTON, when given intravenously, should be infused slowly at a rate of not more than 1 mg/min to minimize adverse reactions such as anaphylaxis and hypotension. It can be diluted (1 mg/mL) with a solution of 0.9% NaCl or 5% dextrose to facilitate the slow infusion rate.

TREATMENT

Parenteral vitamin K_1 should be given to patients with a suspected deficiency showing evidence of bleeding or extremely abnormal PT and aPTT values. The initial dose is 1.0 mg for newborns (0.5 mg for premature infants weighing ≤1000 g), 2 to 3 mg for children up to 12 months of age, and 5 to 10 mg for ages 1 year to the midteens. The usual adult dose is 10 to 20 mg. Subcutaneous injection is preferred to the intramuscular route, which may result in hematoma formation. Slow intravenous infusion (5%/min of the total dose diluted in saline or glucose) rarely causes hypotension or anaphylaxis. PT and aPTT should respond within 6 hours to a parenteral injection of vitamin K and within 24 hours of oral administration. When there is no response, another diagnosis should be considered.

For those poisoned with a superwarfarin preparation in whom rapid correction of coagulation status is necessary, the initial dose of vitamin K_1 in adults should be 10 mg given intravenously (5% of the total dose/min diluted in saline or glucose), followed by a daily oral dose of 50 mg for weeks or months until superwarfarin is no longer detected in blood and normal measurements of PT and aPTT persist.

For those with vitamin K deficiency with extremely severe bleeding manifestations (e.g., intracranial hemorrhage in an infant), treatment includes not only vitamin K replacement but also fresh-frozen plasma (10–20 mL/kg of body weight). Infusions of prothrombin-complex concentrates should be avoided because they carry a risk for thrombosis, especially in those patients who have associated liver disease. A risk of transmitting viral illnesses always exists whenever blood products are given.

TABLE 1. **Differential Diagnosis of Vitamin K Deficiency**

Test	Vitamin K Deficiency	Liver Disease	DIC
aPTT	Increased	Increased	Increased
PT	Increased	Increased	Increased
Platelets	Normal	Decreased	Decreased
Fibrinogen	Normal	Decreased	Decreased
D-Dimer/FDP/FSP	Normal	Normal or increased	Increased

Abbreviations: aPTT = activated partial thromboplastin time; DIC = disseminated intravascular coagulation; FDP/FSP = fibrin degradation products/fibrin split products; PT = prothrombin time.

PREVENTION

All newborns should receive 1.0 mg of vitamin K_1 intramuscularly within the first hour after birth (0.5 mg for premature infants ≤1000 g birth weight). It has been recommended that pregnant women on anticonvulsants should receive 10 to 20 mg of vitamin K_1 daily for 2 to 3 weeks before delivery.

Patients with a decreased intake of vitamin K or malabsorption of the vitamin should receive prophylactic supplements. Prophylaxis is especially needed for severely ill patients in intensive care units who are not taking vitamin K and may be receiving prolonged antibiotic therapy. Prophylactic treatment with vitamin K_1 may be given orally in doses of 2.5 mg/d, 5.0 mg thrice weekly, or 10 mg subcutaneously once a week.

OSTEOPOROSIS

method of
PAUL D. MILLER, M.D.
*University of Colorado Medical School, Denver, and Colorado Center for Bone Research
Lakewood, Colorado*

Throughout the past several years, the field of osteoporosis has been associated with the publication of numerous prospective, randomized, placebo-controlled clinical trials documenting the efficacy of several antiresorptive therapies on bone mineral density (BMD), biochemical markers of bone turnover, and fracture incidence in postmenopausal women. Now, registrations for male osteoporosis (alendronate) and glucocorticoid-induced osteoporosis (alendronate [Fosamax] and risedronate [Actonel]) have also been completed. In addition, alendronate has recently been approved for a once-a-week formulation (70 mg/wk).

Cyclical etidronate therapy for postmenopausal osteoporosis treatment has been registered in 27 other nations outside the United States. The U.S. Food and Drug Administration (FDA) requirement of 3-year vertebral fracture incidence reduction for treatment registration has been fullfilled by only four compounds: nasal calcitonin, alendronate, risedronate, and raloxifene. In this context, because estrogen replacement therapy (ERT) has not fulfilled this requirement, this chapter will focus on pharmacologic interventions that have satisfied this U.S. government requirement. In addition, this chapter will discuss alternative surrogate endpoints for antiresorptive efficacy—serial BMD changes and serial biomarker changes—because in the future, fracture endpoints may become unethical with the currently approved therapies now known to reduce fractures. Moreover, this chapter will address the issue of therapies that reduce the incidence of vertebral fracture versus hip fracture and other nonvertebral fractures. Hip fractures represent the greatest health economic consequence of osteoporosis. Certain antiresorptive therapies have prospectively demonstrated hip fracture reduction.

PREVENTION OF POSTMENOPAUSAL BONE LOSS

Before discussing the FDA-approved therapies for osteoporosis, a brief section should be given to strategies for preventing early postmenopausal bone loss. The FDA registration for prevention of postmenopausal bone loss does not require fracture outcomes, simply preservation of skeletal mass. This somewhat arbitrary division of separate FDA requirements for prevention versus treatment registration has to some degree polarized those who believe that earlier intervention at the initiation of menopause is more important than treatment in later menopausal women. Prevention advocates emphasize early intervention to reduce lifetime fracture risk, especially in women who enter menopause with low bone mass and have additional osteoporotic risk factors. In contrast, nonprevention advocates believe that interventions should be started later in life because of direct, prospective fracture (current or 5-year fracture risk) data showing current fracture reduction with certain interventions. Prevention is believed to be important for the following reasons:

1. Nearly all postmenopausal women will lose bone mass if not receiving specific therapy (estrogen, bisphosphonates, or selective estrogen receptor modulators [SERMs]) despite taking adequate calcium and vitamin D.
2. Women entering menopause with low bone mass and/or rapid rates of bone loss who are left untreated will have even lower BMD in their elderly years, a time of life when current fracture rates do increase, in part related to their low BMD and in part resulting from the effect of increasing age on bone fragility.
3. Early prevention of postmenopausal bone loss will help prevent fragility fractures later in life.

It is also believed that early prevention strategies will reduce the lifetime fracture risk (in contrast to the current or 5-year fracture risk), the risk that may occur over the lifetime of an untreated woman. Lifetime fracture risk models suggest that the lower the BMD at menopause, the greater the lifetime fracture risk. Although these models are intuitively correct, they have not been validated by direct fracture data; moreover, they may never be validated because it would now be unethical to monitor early menopausal women throughout their lifetime and allow them to remain untreated to calculate differential lifetime risks according to the level of BMD at menopause. A few long-term fracture trials do suggest that lifetime fracture risk models may closely approximate the projected lifetime fracture risk. In this regard the longest prospective (10-year) hip fracture data have just recently been published. These data, derived from Swedish white women and men of variable age, calculate the 10-year absolute fracture risk as a function of the T score at baseline derived from the National Health and Nutrition Examination Survey III (NHANES III) white female young normal database. The

TABLE 1. **Ten-Year Prospective Hip Fracture Risk in Swedish White Women and Men From Age 70 Years Calculated From the "T Score" at the Hip From the NHANES III Female Young Normal Reference Database**

	10-Year Absolute Risk		
T Score	*Age*	*Women*	*Men*
−2.5 SD	70y	24%	24%

Abbrevation: NHANES = National Health and Nutrition Examination Survey.

Swedish data show that the absolute risk is similar between women and men, even in the men when the T score is calculated from the female database (Table 1).

All of the current fracture risk data that validate the strong relationship between low BMD and current fracture risk have been obtained in women and men who are elderly. Early menopausal women have very low current fracture risk. Hence, critics of early prevention strategies point to the lack of current fracture benefit with prevention interventions in the early menopausal years. Nevertheless, for women who are concerned about osteoporosis and are proactive about prevention of disease, initiation of agents proven to prevent postmenopausal bone loss is an important option for the clinician to offer. For these reasons, the National Osteoporosis Foundation recommends that interventions for prevention be offered to postmenopausal women younger than 65 years with one or more risk factor for osteoporosis except menopause. Early prevention strategies seem logical, but critics point to the number needed to treat (NNT) to prevent the first fracture as a reason to oppose early prevention strategies. The NNT for early postmenopausal women may be high, but if the cost of therapy decreases and higher risk groups are more carefully selected, the NNT concept will be less important in terms of broad health economic issues, versus physician-patient issues. Both issues are necessary for all of us involved in patient and national policies. They often conflict, but each needs careful analysis.

Prevention options are shown in Table 2. Certainly, all postmenopausal women should be advised to take 1500 mg of calcium per day through natural calcium sources and/or calcium supplements, as well as 400 IU of vitamin D per day. It is important, however, to emphasize to these women that calcium and vitamin D alone *will not* prevent early postmenopausal bone loss. In all of the early prevention trials of ERT, alendronate, risedronate, and raloxifene (Evista), the "control" group actually received supplemental calcium and vitamin D, yet lost BMD. Therefore, for this early menopausal population, active BMD agents are required in addition to calcium and vitamin D. The osteoporosis field is being damaged by calcium marketers who claim that calcium alone is adequate. Over-the-counter product labeling needs to be tightened by the FDA for many of these issues to avoid misleading the public. This

TABLE 2. **Prevention Strategies for Osteoporosis**

Calcium (1500 mg/d)
Vitamin D (400–800 IU/d)
Modification of risk factors that can be changed
Pharmacologic interventions: full-dose estrogen, raloxifene, alendronate, risedronate

TABLE 3. **Risk Factors for Fracture**

Hip bone mineral density 1 SD below the mean population value
Noncarboxylated osteocalcin
Biochemical index of bone resorption above the premenopausal range
Previous fragility fracture after the age of 50 years
Body weight below 57.8 kg
Hip axis length 1 SD above the population mean value
First-degree relative aged 50 years or older with a history of fragility fractures
Maternal history of hip fracture
Current cigarette smoking
Poor visual acuity and/or depth perception
Low gait speed
Increased body sway

author is an advocate of tighter FDA regulation in this matter.

In addition, modifying risk factors that may be associated with bone loss should also be universally applied. Risk factors for osteoporosis (low BMD or fracture) are listed in Table 3. Some of these risk factors are modifiable and some are not. FDA-approved prevention options include ERT or, for women with intact uteri, hormonal replacement therapy because the addition of progesterone is needed to protect against uterine estrogen effects. Full-dose estrogen is often required in the early menopausal years and probably throughout life for estrogen to both protect against bone loss and reduce fracture rates. Several large population-based studies suggest that for elderly women who were previous estrogen users but had discontinued estrogen for over 5 years, both their BMD and fracture rates may differ little from those of women who had not previously taken estrogen. Furthermore, from the Study of Osteoporotic Fractures (SOF) and the National Osteoporotic Risk Assessment survey, many current estrogen users had low bone mass and/or fractures, which suggests that although estrogens are very capable of preventing early postmenopausal bone loss, the effect may not be sustained in later years. Because of previous observations surrounding the uncertainty of the protective effect of estrogen on the aged skeleton and the lack of strong or consistent prospective fracture reduction as yet reported for estrogen, the National Osteoporosis Foundation recommends performing BMD tests in women 65 years or older, even those receiving ERT. A much larger clinical problem than the lack of good fracture data is the poor compliance with ERT (and for bisphosphonates as well), with discontinuation in most patients after 1 to 3 years possibly indicating that we are not really being very effective at all in this population in the protection of skeletal health. The major estrogen pharmaceutical producers are designing clinical trials to answer the fracture protection question in a prospective fashion.

BISPHOSPHONATES OR SELECTIVE ESTROGEN RECEPTOR MODULATORS FOR PREVENTION

The FDA has approved the bisphosphonates alendronate (5 mg/d) and risedronate (5 mg/d), as well as the SERM raloxifene (60 mg/d), for the prevention of postmenopausal osteoporosis. These agents will prevent early postmenopausal bone loss and should be considered as prevention strategies in women, especially those who cannot or will not take ERT. Although the BMD changes noted with 5 mg/d of alendronate or risedronate versus baseline values seem greater than those after 60 mg/d of raloxifene, the lack of fracture data (as anticipated in these early menopausal women who infrequently sustain fractures) makes women who decide to not use ERT for the protection of skeletal mass candidates for bisphosphonates or SERM, not based on fracture data, but on nonfracture considerations. For example, if women enter menopause with a low BMD (T scores lower than −1.5 SD) and have significant risk factors for osteoporosis, options for skeletal protection are the exception. Because BMD is normally distributed across all age ranges, determination of BMD is essential for deciding the timing of initiation of estrogens, bisphosphonates, or SERMs for prevention inasmuch as women with normal to increased T scores (+1 SD or higher) may not require these interventions for the prevention of bone loss for several years. The risk factors that should be used to decide on interventions in women with low T scores are maternal history of hip fracture, current smoking, fragility fracture after the age of 40 years, high bone turnover, and low body mass index.

For women who cannot or will not take ERT for prevention of skeletal loss, the decision between choosing a bisphosphonate or a SERM is not easily made on evidence: both prevent early postmenopausal bone loss. Because of the absence of fracture data in prevention trials, the choice between a bisphosphonate and a SERM is often based on physician preference and patient concerns. For example, if a patient cannot tolerate an oral bisphosphonate, a SERM is a clear choice. Alternatively, women with a history of deep vein thrombosis or those having hot flashes may not be candidates for the current SERMs. Even though raloxifene is not FDA approved for the prevention of breast cancer because the strong evidence of breast cancer prevention seen in the Multiple Outcome Raloxifene Evaluation (MORE) trial occurred in a group at low risk for breast cancer, many women still choose raloxifene for prevention of bone loss and physicians prescribe it for this indication off-label; clinically, this choice is quite acceptable. The trial of raloxifene for breast cancer protection in normal to high-risk patients is currently under way; until these data become available, it is suggested that raloxifene use be limited to 5 years' duration.

It is important that physicians understand that calcitonin (Calcimar)* is not approved for prevention and is registered specifically for women at least 5 years past menopause.

TREATMENT OF POSTMENOPAUSAL OSTEOPOROSIS

Treatment strategies for postmenopausal osteoporosis are shown in Table 4. As in prevention strategies, authorities recommend adequate calcium (1500 mg/d) and vitamin D (400 IU/d for postmenopausal women younger than 65 years and 800 IU/d for women older than 65 years and patients receiving long-term glucocorticoid therapy). In addition, interventions to reduce the risk of falls in the elderly have not been sufficiently applied and yet may offer the best opportunity to reduce fragility hip fractures because 90% of these fractures occur after a fall. Thus, improving eyesight, muscle tone, and balance, which may reduce the tendency of the elderly to fall, home safety checks for objects or cords that might contrib-

*Not FDA approved for this indication.

TABLE 4. **Treatment Strategies for Osteoporosis**

Calcium (1500 mg/d)
Vitamin D (400–800 IU/d)
Modification of risk factors that can be changed
Fall prevention strategies
Hip pads
Pharmacologic options: bisphosphonates, raloxifene, calcitonin

ute to falls, and restricted use of central nervous system–altering drugs may do more than pharmacologic therapy to reduce hip fracture rates. More recently, hip pad protectors have been shown to reduce the incidence of hip fractures.

The other interventions listed in Table 4 all have independent data showing positive effects on current (5-year) fracture rates in elderly postmenopausal women. Most of these agents affect bone mineral content, in part by inhibiting bone resorption (and are therefore classified as antiresorptive agents); one anabolic agent, parathyroid hormone (PTH), stimulates bone formation. Because these agents alter bone remodeling (bone turnover), a discussion of bone remodeling, the remodeling space, and the remodeling transient is in order.

It is important to also point out that even though all these agents (except PTH) have antiresorptive action, they inhibit bone resorption by dissimilar mechanisms; in that regard, even various bisphosphonates and SERMs may not inhibit bone resorption in the same way. We must keep an open mind about this issue—combinations of antiresorptive agents may have benefits beyond therapy with one agent alone, simply as a function of their different mechanism of action.

The Remodeling Space and the Remodeling Transient

Both cortical and cancellous bone has bone-remodeling units (BMUs) throughout their anatomic structure. Cancellous bone has more BMUs than cortical bone does because of its larger surface area, even though the most abundant bone type throughout the human skeleton is cortical bone (approximately 80% versus 20% for cancellous bone). It is estimated that the human skeleton has approximately 4 million BMUs. At any given point in time, approximately 30% of these BMUs are in some phase of bone metabolic activity, either bone resorption or bone formation, whereas the other 70% are in a quiescent phase of the bone-remodeling cycle. Because of the difference in BMU allocation between cancellous and cortical bone, it is logical to expect that drugs that alter the bone-remodeling cycle will have their measurable effect earliest on cancellous bone, which is exactly what we see in clinical practice when monitoring the response of bone to antiresorptive drugs: a greater change from baseline in bone sites that have predominately cancellous bone.

The remodeling space is therefore the amount of BMUs that is metabolically active at any point in time; because the pharmacologic agents presently at our disposal to alter the remodeling space are agents that inhibit bone resorption, that proportion of the remodeling space that is undergoing bone resorption is the proportion that our current therapies can affect.

In any individual BMU, bone resorption is intimately coupled with bone formation—and in the same direction; that is, whenever bone resorption increases, so does bone formation, and vice versa. This relationship is called "coupling."

However, the time frame of these BMU-coupling events is not exactly linked. Bone formation takes about 3 months longer than bone resorption, which on average takes less than 1 month. Thus agents that inhibit bone resorption without altering bone formation allow bone formation to continue for some time uncoupled to bone resorption; in the end, bone mineral content increases. It is believed that in time, bone formation will also decrease because bone resorption has decreased, and the natural biology of coupling mechanisms will prevail. Hence, the balance between bone resorption and bone formation will return, yet BMD will be higher as a consequence of the period when bone formation exceeded bone resorption, specifically the remodeling transient. The amount of bone mineral added during this transient period is a function of the following:

1. The amount of BMUs active at initiation of therapy with the antiresorptive agent.
2. The intrinsic osteoclastic inhibitory activity of any given antiresorptive agent (which is related to absorption, the intrinsic bone distribution of each antiresorptive agent, receptor binding, and other pharmacodynamics of the antiresorptive agent).
3. The biologic capacity of the osteoblast to respond (i.e., decrease) its activity in response to the decrease in osteoclast activity.

Thus for many known and unknown reasons, different antiresorptive agents might not be expected to behave the same for the reasons just stated, yet they are all classified as "antiresorptive agents."

This antiresorption action of bone metabolism often results in a "plateau" effect of these antiresorptive agents: a so-called leveling off of BMD after the first or second year of administration, which is believed to reflect "filling in" of the remodeling transient and return of the normal coupling of osteoclasts to osteoblasts. Nevertheless, for the bisphosphonates, the observations that BMD may continue to increase beyond 2 to 3 years of administration and that fracture rates may continue to decrease for a number of agents beyond the period that coupling should have returned to balance lend some theoretical insight into the possibility that certain antiresorptive agents may "stimulate" bone formation (directly or, more likely, indirectly).

Thus although the remodeling transient is a real biologic observation, the relationship between the intrinsic biology of the remodeling transient and alteration of the remodeling transient by pharmacologic agents that alter bone remodeling may not be direct (i.e., not coupled).

Finally, when we try to relate the seemingly small changes in BMD to the magnitude of fracture reduction seen in prospective trials of the various remodeling agents, we should keep in mind several issues that are, for the most part, unproven, yet actively discussed:

1. Small changes in BMD may be more important in improving bone strength if the baseline BMD is low than if the baseline BMD is not very low.
2. Bone antiresorptive agents may be unequally distributed within bone, so certain agents may have greater effect on some active resorptive sites than other agents, even in the same anatomic bone area.
3. Some antiresorptive agents may result in bone being deposited in areas where bone strength is disproportionately increased (i.e., more toward cortical surfaces than inner bone surfaces), thereby increasing the cross-sectional moment of inertia, which in turn will disproportionately increases bone strength.
4. Some antiresorptive agents improve bone strength (and quality) by mechanisms that may be independent of BMD (collagen architecture, mineral quality, and/or location, etc).

While the science of all these plausible hypotheses is being examined, the clinician is left with the knowledge that all antiresorptive agents reduce bone remodeling and that in turn, as BMD increases, fractures decrease. Hence, we have at our disposal a menu of choices for the treatment of postmenopausal osteoporosis to offer these patients.

Vitamin D and Calcium

Although not "officially" FDA approved for treatment, prospective data indicate that in certain subgroups, vitamin D and calcium reduce the risk of vertebral, nonvertebral, and hip fractures.

In one study by Recker and colleagues, calcium supplementation reduced vertebral fracture rates in elderly women with postmenopausal osteoporosis who had previously had vertebral fractures. In another study by Dawson-Hughes and associates, calcium (700 mg/d) and vitamin D (800 IU/d) reduced the rates of nonvertebral fractures in elderly women and men. Finally, in an elderly population of institutionalized frail nursing home patients who had low baseline plasma vitamin D levels, vitamin D and calcium replacement reduced the risk of hip fractures within 18 months. Hence, in the elderly population, vitamin D and calcium supplementation confers a fracture benefit.

Yet it is important to emphasize that even though calcium and vitamin D are important interventions, the addition of one of the FDA-approved agents for osteoporosis treatment bestows fracture benefit in addition to that of vitamin D and calcium. This finding has resulted from the FDA's requirement that osteoporosis clinical trials have no true "placebo" group; all patients must receive at least 500 mg/d of calcium supplementation, as well as 400 IU/d of vitamin D. Thus the fracture benefit seen with calcitonin, the bisphosphonates, or the SERMs is in addition to that observed with calcium and vitamin D alone.

Estrogen

Estrogens are FDA approved for the "management" of postmenopausal osteoporosis, even though the fracture reduction data are mostly retrospective or prospective and based on small numbers of patients or longitudinal cohort studies. The word "management" is a U.S. FDA stipulation that is now required for product labeling, as opposed to the word "treatment," which would indicate 3-year fracture reduction benefit. A well-powered prospective study of estrogen's fracture benefit has yet to be completed, although the Women's Health Initiative data may provide such information. Some pharmaceutical companies are planning such prospective fracture reduction trials with estrogen.

It seems that if estrogens are to have fracture benefit, they may need to be started early after menopause and continued indefinitely. Because estrogens probably act through the same receptor as raloxifene, they should show fracture benefit in older women as well, like raloxifene. The estrogen fracture trials simply have not been designed the same way as raloxifene. These trials are now in progress and are important.

A number of studies suggest that women who had previously been on ERT for 10 years but have not been taking it for 10 years have BMD and fracture rates similar to those of women who have never received ERT. In addition, data from large prospective fracture trials (SOF and EPIDOS) even suggest that elderly women receiving long-term ERT (average, 22 years) have a greater prevalence of osteoporosis or low bone mass and higher fracture rates than one would anticipate from such long-term ERT use. These results do not discount the possibility that ERT could reduce fractureates similar to raloxifene—the trials simply have not been designed in a similar fashion. Yet at the current time, the National Osteoporosis Foundation guidelines for BMD testing incorporate recommendations to perform BMD testing in elderly women (65 years or older), even those managed with long-term ERT, because of the lack of evidence of ERT fracture benefit in the older population and the higher than anticipated prevalence of low bone mass in these elderly women.

Age-related bone loss might not be mitigated by ERT because of the independent pathophysiology of age-related bone loss and estrogen-dependent bone loss. Thus, a recent iconoclastic viewpoint on the evidence (or lack of evidence) of estrogen's fracture benefit challenges us to be cautious in this regard in the elderly and indicates the need for a large prospective, randomized, placebo-controlled study to accurately define estrogen's fracture benefit.

Calcitonin

Injectable and nasal spray salmon calcitonin is also FDA approved for the treatment of postmenopausal osteoporosis. Until very recently, only a paucity of fracture data were available for this antiresorptive agent as well. The recently completed PROOF study of nasal calcitonin's significant vertebral fracture reduction benefit (200 IU/d) has furnished the best supportive data compiled to date, although the strength of these data is questioned for a variety of reasons.

Calcitonin, an inhibitor of osteoclastic activity and bone resorption, has been used for many years for osteoporosis treatment. Its duration of action is short, although once-daily administration is adequate for inhibition of bone turnover for 24 hours. It seems that, at least regarding surrogate markers for bone biologic effect (serial BMD and serial biomarkers of bone resorption), calcitonin is a less "potent" agent than bisphosphonates because the changes in BMD and resorption markers are less than for the bisphosphonates.

In fact, in the only head-to-head comparative study yet completed between 200 IU/d of nasal calcitonin and 10 mg/d of alendronate in women with postmenopausal osteoporosis, alendronate induced significantly greater increases in BMD and reductions in urinary biomarkers of bone resorption than calcitonin did. No fracture data exist in this 2-year head-to-head trial that was powered for BMD and biomarker changes and yet clearly documented the superior biologic effect of alendronate over calcitonin on these parameters of bone biology.

The data discussed later provide indirect evidence that the pharmacologically induced magnitude of changes in BMD does matter inasmuch as the improvement in BMD is related to the magnitude of fracture reduction. In this regard, it is likely that bisphosphonates or PTH (which increase BMD more) will reduce fracture rates to a greater extent than calcitonin or SERM will. In fact, such data are nonexistent in any head-to-head trial.

In contrast, when one compares the changes in BMD resulting from placebo with the reduction in the relative risk of vertebral and nonvertebral fractures resulting from any of the currently available antiresorptive agents (prospective vertebral fracture trials: non–head-to-head comparisons), no difference can be seen in the reduction in the relative risk (as well as 95% confidence intervals) of vertebral fractures produced by any of these agents, despite significant differences in changes in BMD mediated by the various agents. These data would suggest that antiresorptive agents produce equal vertebral and nonvertebral fracture reduction despite only minimal changes in BMD. These observations have led to the theory that changes in BMD mediated by these various antiresorptive agents are unimportant in explaining the fracture reduction. Yet a more compelling body of evidence would suggest that a strong relationship does exist between the amount of BMD added by antiresorptive agents and improvement in bone strength.

A linear relationship is found between the amount of bone mineral and bone strength. In both animal and human in situ models, 80% of the variance in bone strength is explained by BMC. Why adding bone mineral would be unimportant in increasing bone strength is illogical. One cannot have it both ways.

Alternatively, data suggest that the magnitude of change in BMD influences the magnitude of reduction in fracture risk.

In a post hoc analysis of Fracture Intervention Trial (FIT) data, Hochburg has shown that in patients who achieved an increase in BMD of greater than 3% with alendronate, the reduction in vertebral fractures was significantly greater than in patients whose BMD was either stable (no increase) or declined.

In addition, in three separate meta-analyses of prospective randomized controlled clinical trials assessing the relationship between the changes in BMD induced by various antiresorptive agents and fracture risk reduction (both vertebral and nonvertebral), a very statistically significant relationship was found between the magnitude of increase in BMD and the magnitude of reduction in fracture incidence. Meta-analyses of properly performed prospective randomized trials are the highest order of evidence-based medicine. It becomes irrational to discount the relationship between increased BMD and fracture reduction benefit. The latter evidence does not eliminate the fact that other non-BMD factors may contribute to bone strength—there is simply no evidence to date to support the non–BMD-related factors in clinical trial data.

Another analysis of BMD changes in the FIT and MORE trials suggests that patients who lost BMD in the first year often gained BMD in the second or those who gained BMD during the first year lost BMD during the second such that no differences in BMD (regression to the mean) were seen over the 2-year trial period (in these analysis). Fracture benefit was not assessed in this regression analysis. The observation of regression to the mean is not unique to serial BMD measurements—it is seen in all serial biologic measurements, including serial blood pressure and cholesterol testing. Furthermore, the article in the *Journal of the American Medical Association* did not show regression of BMD to the mean in the control group, a significant scientific design flaw because what is really a test of drug effect versus the intrinsic regression to the mean that is seen in all biologic (treated and control) measurements is the *difference* between the treated and control populations at the point of the regression. This BMD regression analysis cannot conclude that patients receiving alendronate or raloxifene do not differ over the 2 years at the regression average point in time because comparable points in the control group are not shown. In clinical medicine, regression to the mean occurs in every form of measurement performed over time, so *not* doing the measurement would reduce clinical practice in patients receiving treatment to simply guesswork. Finally, the phenomenon of regression to the mean was never intended to be applied to individuals, only groups of patients.

One also needs to keep one major point in perspective when making conclusions about even well-designed prospective, randomized clinical trials: clinical trial patients differ greatly from patients in clinical practice in that clinical trial patients are (1) highly motivated, (2) seen every 3 months by study coordinators, (3) have compliance pill counts, and (4) are excluded if they have concomitant medical diseases or are taking medications that alter bone metabolism. Therefore, the clinical, real-world response to any osteoporosis intervention cannot be expected to be exactly matched by clinical trial data, and extrapolating from one observation to another is neither realistic nor scientific.

Hence, possibly the most important reason for performing serial BMD measurements in patients receiving antiresorptive therapy is to ensure that BMD does not go *down*; although greater increases in BMD are, at least in part, reassuring that a greater fracture benefit should be seen, it is also true that a fracture benefit may be seen if the BMD remains stable and does not decline. A true decline in BMD should initiate queries about compliance, absorption, or factors that may blunt the bone biologic response. Such factors include asymptomatic celiac disease, mastocytosis, myeloma, hyperparathyroidism, and other not uncommon diseases often seen in clinical practice that may mitigate the otherwise good pharmacologic response usually seen with these medications.

In conclusion, regarding calcitonin's BMD effect, it should be emphasized that calcitonin has been around for a long time and has a trustworthy safety record. This observation, plus the facts that it is easy to administer, has FDA approval for treatment and very few side effects, and now has significant fracture reduction data, makes it an appealing therapy for postmenopausal osteoporosis. Many bone metabolism authorities reserve calcitonin for elderly patients who have low BMD, are not prone to fractures, and cannot tolerate oral bisphosphonates, a subgroup representing a large proportion of the elderly postmenopausal population.

Bisphosphonates

Bisphosphonates, biochemical analogues of naturally occurring pyrophosphates (adenosine triphosphate metabolic end products), have now been used clinically for more than 20 years. Their absorption by the oral route of administration is extremely specific and blunted by the ingestion of many substances such as milk, coffee, and other medications or "pills" and bisphosphonates have a long bone half-life.

The bisphosphonates are extremely safe, with no known toxicities. They may induce certain side effects such as upper gastrointestinal inflammation, myalgias, fever, headaches, or iritis, but they do not induce hepatic, renal, central nervous system, cardiac, or pulmonary abnormalities because their pharmacologic binding is specific to active bone-remodeling sites. These extraosseous symptoms may be mediated by transient release of cytokines from osteoclast precursors and may not recur on re-administration after temporarily being discontinued in patients in whom these extraosseous symptoms have previously developed.

Even though bisphosphonates are extremely safe compounds as a class, caution is advised in several circumstances, one being the use of intravenous bisphosphonates (pamidronate* [Aredia], zoledronate,† or ibandronate*) in dialysis patients or those with severe chronic renal failure (creatinine clearance <30 mL/min). In these patients, administration that is too rapid may be followed by prolonged and severe hypocalcemia or potentiation of the renal failure. It is believed that in patients in whom an intravenous bisphosphonate is necessary (severe hypercalcemia, patients with fractures who cannot tolerate oral bisphosphonates), a much slower rate of infusion will obviate these unfavorable consequences. A second caution regarding bisphosphonate use is in a healthy, premenopausal woman who could become pregnant. Bisphosphonates cross the placenta and the effect on human fetal development is unknown. Bisphosphonates should not be given to healthy, estrogen-replete premenopausal women who are discovered to have low bone mass because their low BMD more likely represents low peak adult bone mass and no data have shown that bisphosphonates affect BMD or unknown fracture risk in this healthy population. This latter population is different from the nonhealthy premenopausal population who may be having fractures because of amenorrhea or eating disorders—in this group who cannot or will not take higher dose ERT, bisphosphonates may have a role.

The upper gastrointestinal side effects noted with use of the aminobisphosphonates are real but have also been overstated. If clinicians recognize patients with clear-cut evidence of persistent severe upper gastrointestinal esophageal or gastric disease and instruct them to carefully dilute the bisphosphonate with adequate amounts of water (>8 ounces) and to not lie down for 30 minutes after consumption, true severe esophageal complications may occur at a lower rate than 1 in 10,000 doses. The newer aminobisphosphonate risedronate may or may not be better tolerated; until postmarketing experience with this bisphosphonate becomes available, equal caution in its application should be provided to patients as with alendronate. Both alendronate and risedronate have newer formulations that may improve the tolerability of both compounds. In either case, patients should be instructed that if upper gastrointestinal symptoms develop, use of the bisphosphonate should be promptly stopped and the next step discussed with their physician. In many cases, rechallenging the

*Not FDA approved for this indication.
†Investigational drug in the United States.

patient with a lower alendronate (5 mg/d) dose or trying an every-other-day dose schedule will be tolerated. Once-weekly alendronate (70 mg/wk) is now FDA approved, and risedronate trials with this formulation are being completed. Both may offer some help with regard to compliance and tolerability. Patients who have busy schedules often find the daily schedule of oral bisphosphonates very inconvenient, and the once-weekly dosage, if as effective, may solve many of the issues stated earlier.

Oral bisphosphonates are poorly absorbed, with less than 1% of any single daily dose being absorbed under the strictest conditions (i.e., no other food, pills, or beverages other than plain water for 30 to 45 minutes after consumption). If this amount of bisphosphonate is absorbed, it has a powerful bone biologic effect, even though half of the absorbed dose is excreted in the urine in 24 hours. One of the great limitation that the clinician faces is knowing whether the bisphosphonate is being absorbed, even in patients who take it correctly. Even though the BMD response in clinical trials is greater than 95%, this figure may not be the case in real practice for multiple reasons previously stated, and we often see patients who have had gastrectomies, gastrojejunal bypass, gastric stapling, and the like in whom we have no knowledge of whether the bisphosphonates are being absorbed. Bisphosphonates are absorbed in the upper part of the jejunum; hence diseases that alter function or surface area of the small bowel could preclude bisphosphonate absorption. It would be to our clinical benefit if clinical assays were available to measure bisphosphonate blood levels, but there are none. Therefore, we must use surrogate markers, such as serial BMD and serial biomarkers, to assess adequate compliance, absorption, and bone biologic effect.

In patients who need bisphosphonates for more compelling indications beyond early prevention strategies (such as patients prone to fractures, patients with high bone turnover markers and low bone mass, elderly patients with previous hip fractures, patients who require high-dose glucocorticoids) and in whom the physician is uncertain whether the oral bisphosphonate is being absorbed for reasons previously stated, the currently available intravenous bisphosphonate pamidronate offers an alternative.

The use of intravenous pamidronate ensures that the bisphosphonate is at least being delivered to bone. Registered in many countries for osteoporosis, pamidronate* is used off-label in the United States for this indication but is FDA registered for many nonosteoporotic indications. Pamidronate 30 mg, is administered over a 2-hour period every 3 months. It is important to ensure adequate calcium and vitamin D intake before pamidronate use and to warn patients of the potential for a "first-phase reaction," fever and myalgias, which occur infrequently, last 24 to 48 hours with no sequelae, and rarely happen again.

The newer aminobisphosphonates are taken up intracellularly by both osteoclasts and osteocytes after they adhere to the calcium phosphate surface of active bone resorption sites. Intracellularly, they alter the mevalonic acid pathway and lead to the loss of geranylgeranylated proteins, which are needed for essential osteoclastic function. Not only does this biochemical alteration mitigate many osteoclast cytoplasmic functions, such as cytoskeletal rearrangement, membrane ruffling, and vesicular trafficking, but osteoclast life span is also reduced (apoptosis). Thus, the aminobisphosphonates alter bone resorption by two mechanisms: first, a physiochemical one in which binding to the calcium phosphate resorption surface stabilizes the resorption induced by osteoclast enzymes and lowers surface pH and, second, a cellular one in which osteoclast function and life span are altered. How much of the inhibition of the bone resorption effects brought about by bisphosphonates is due to their physicochemical function versus their cellular function is not clear. However, because of the fact that over 70% of the distribution of all bisphosphonates is on the resorption surfaces, it is possible that most of the antiresorptive effect of bisphosphonates is predominately a physicochemical rather than a cellular one.

The bisphosphonates that adhere to the calcium phosphorate surface and are not taken up by osteoclasts or osteocytes become buried deeper in the bone as that particular remodeling unit ultimately becomes remineralized. This process results in the long bone "half-life" of bisphosphonates, which may have far different implications than the half-lives of other compounds in the classic pharmacodynamic sense. These deeply buried bisphosphonates, as far as we know, have no biologic activity. Yet they may be reintroduced to the circulation again when that resorption site is once again activated and resorption resumes. In this hypothetic model, the previously buried bisphosphonate may become recycled. It is unknown whether a recycled bisphosphonate has any more biologic activity or is inert. Even if active, it is believed that the amount re-released is so small (and half of this amount will be excreted) that it would probably have insignificant systemic bone effects. This latter statement is purely conjectural but may have two important clinical implications: the first is related to how long bisphosphonates need to be administered, and the second concerns the implication of treating fracturing amenorrheic or anorectic women who refuse oral contraceptives but could later become pregnant if their amenorrhea stops and fertility returns.

It is unknown whether bisphosphonate administration needs to be continued indefinitely or whether "honeymoon" periods may occur in which they might be temporarily discontinued and then restarted at a later time. Data have documented that etidronate use for 3 years with subsequent discontinuation is accompanied by a decline in BMD the following year but that etidronate use for 5 years with subsequent discontinuation maintains BMD for 2 years. Alendro-

*Not FDA approved for this indication.

nate data also suggest that the longer the administration and/or the higher the dose, the more likely that discontinuation is less likely to be followed by either a fall in BMD or a rise in biomarkers of bone resorption the following 1 to 2 years. The recent 8-year alendronate data showing that the downturn in activation frequency (~80%) was maintained with no continual decline are reassuring that "oversuppression" of bone turnover may not occur. In addition, from the long-term etidronate data, it is encouraging that in patients whose BMD declined after discontinuation, re-administration of etidronate was associated with another increase in BMD. This finding suggests that previous exposure to a bisphosphonate does not mitigate another favorable response on re-exposure. Hence, it may be that protocols will develop that entail the use of oral bisphosphonates in an "on-off-on" fashion. We may never have direct long-term data to support such a suggestion, but both from a cost and from a patient concern point of view, such an approach may be inevitable. Fortunately, patients in whom bisphosphonate use is discontinued, we can monitor both BMD and biomarkers of bone resorption as objective guides regarding when to restart therapy.

The issue of treating premenopausal women who have diseases that affect bone or are receiving chronic glucocorticoid therapy, either of which may be associated with fragility fractures, is a complicated one. Many of these women may become (or are) fertile and yet are sustaining fractures and need help. Obviously, maximizing the elimination of other risk factors (smoking, etc.) and ensuring adequate vitamin D and calcium intake are very important as adjuvant therapy. In those women who are estrogen deficient, adding adequate estrogen back is very important if it is possible. Nevertheless, many of these women may not be able or may refuse estrogen replacement, and no data have found calcitonin to be effective in this group. Likewise, no data are available on the use of SERMs in these younger women who may be having fractures because of their estrogen-deficient status. On the other hand, the increasing data that younger women receiving chronic glucocorticoid therapy (most of whom may be estrogen deficient) increase their BMD and may show a trend toward fracture reduction with bisphosphonate use are often compelling reasons to begin treatment with these agents, especially patients sustaining fractures or premenopausal women who have low BMD and need to be subjected to long-term steroid use. However, these women need to be completely informed that bisphosphonates cross the placenta and that even if use is stopped before any anticipated pregnancy, they may still be re-released into the circulation from previous bone stores.

Fracture Reduction With the Bisphosphonates: Alendronate and Risedronate

The strength of the bisphosphonate prospective fracture trails is the consistency of the data: in multiple studies of vertebral, nonvertebral, and hip fracture analysis, both alendronate and risedronate data show a significant fracture reduction benefit in all three of these fracture outcomes. In fact, the only prospective hip fracture data available (other than the Chapuy vitamin D data) have been acquired with alendronate and risedronate, with the latter bisphosphonate hip fracture reduction data being the only hip fracture data in which the primary efficacy end-point for planned analysis was the reduction in hip fractures. Both of these bisphosphonates significantly reduce vertebral and nonvertebral fractures within 12 months of initiation of therapy, and for both it appears that the fracture benefit is best observed in higher risk patients: those with baseline T scores lower than 2.5 SD and/or current vertebral compression fractures. In fact, the risedronate hip fracture trial did not show any significant fracture reduction in the group that was randomized on the basis of frailty and clinical risk factors for falling (>80 years of age and significant risk factors for falling). BMD was determined in only 31% of the 80-year-old and older age group in the risedronate trial, and "osteoporosis" as determined by *World Health Organization (WHO) criteria was seen in only 7% of this subgroup*. The risedronate data would suggest that in frail people who may fall more frequently, this bisphosphonate (and probably other ones) may not protect against hip fracture reduction, but in those who are less frail and have osteoporosis by WHO criteria at the femoral neck in accordance with the NHANES III reference population database, the drug has hip fracture reduction benefit.

It is important to emphasize that although the risedronate hip fracture data did not show a significant hip fracture reduction benefit in women 80 years of age and older who were randomized on the basis of only one risk factor for frailty, the conclusion that risedronate has no benefit in women older than 80 years must be confined to the strict context of the randomization criteria, which were designed in 1992 when known risk factors for hip fracture were limited. It is entirely plausible that in 2001, when many more hip fracture risk factors are known, and that in the context of patients having more than one risk factor (only one risk factor was required for risedronate randomization), elderly patients with more than one risk factor may have different outcomes than seen in the 80-year-old and older group of the risedronate trial. This hypothesis would be even more appealing in the group whose femoral neck T scores were below −2.5 SD.

Selective Estrogen Receptor Modulators

To date, only raloxifene has been shown to be of value not only in the prevention of early postmenopausal bone loss but recently also in the reduction of vertebral fracture risk in elderly postmenopausal women. In the MORE trial, raloxifene (60 or 120 mg/d) significantly reduced the incidence of new vertebral compression fractures. This antifracture benefit was seen in women who entered the trial both with and without current vertebral compression fractures. Because on average women in the MORE trial had T scores below 2.5 SD, the raloxifene data suggest (as did the risedronate hip fracture data and the alendronate data in women without current fractures) that women who have osteoporosis by WHO BMD criteria may benefit the most from intervention.

Neither nonvertebral fracture reduction (preplanned) nor hip fracture reduction was observed in the MORE trial despite the fact that the women randomized were similar in age and BMD status as those in the alendronate FIT trial. It is known that the BMD changes at the hip were less with raloxifene than with the bisphosphonates (~2% versus 4 to 5%), yet both BMD increases were significant within groups in comparison to placebo. However, the raloxifene trial was not powered for hip analysis, and the number of hip fractures was small and similar in the raloxifene and placebo groups. Equally as important is the possibility that in any of these large fracture trials the rate of falling might differ (even in the placebo and treated groups).

Although it is probable that the placebo and treatment groups should have fallen equally in the alendronate, risedronate, and raloxifene trials, these data were never captured, except in the raloxifene trials, where the frequency of falling was similar. Nevertheless, it is still possible that the placebo groups fell more frequently than the treatment groups, that the frequency was different in one study versus the next, or that the nature of the falls was different. It is known that a distinct fall on the hip is required in this population to cause a hip fracture. Fall "quality" may differ from one study to another—we do not know. Because more than 90% of hip fractures occur after falls, this uncaptured data element could influence comparative outcome analysis between any of the very large and important fracture studies.

A very important and underemphasized aspect of hip fracture reduction is the development of strategies by both physicians and other health care providers to reduce the incidence of falls. Most hip fractures in osteoporotic patients result from falls, specifically, falls on the hip. Certain strategies may reduce this fall risk, including eyesight improvement, improvement in depth perception (a well-recognized complication of macular degeneration), balance improvement with balance-enhancing exercises, avoidance of loose rugs, and well-placed hand rails in bathrooms and showers. Hip pads also reduce hip fracture rates in patients who are frail and may fall easily, but compliance with the use of hip pads may be less than ideal in the "real world." Nonetheless, we should try.

Making a Choice Between Antifracture Antiresorptive Agents

The selection of a bisphosphonate, calcitonin, or a SERM for the treatment of postmenopausal osteoporosis has become more difficult by the nature of the fracture data pertaining to each compound. The choices are often based on physician specialty (i.e., gynecologists tend to more comfortable with estrogen and estrogen-like compounds, geriatricians may prescribe more calcitonin because of its safety, and bone metabolism specialists may use more bisphosphonates in actively fracturing patients or the other agents in those who cannot tolerate oral bisphosphonates). Since publication of the MORE positive vertebral fracture data, raloxifene has become another strong choice for treatment of postmenopausal osteoporosis, but without a hip fracture benefit, its place may best be in postmenopausal women younger than 75 years, a group whose hip fracture incidence is low, and in postmenopausal women whose femoral neck T scores are not below −2.5 SD but have low spine BMD.

The availability of different agents should be viewed as a positive change; only a very few years ago, choices for osteoporosis treatment were limited, with little fracture data. Now, data are abundant. The final decision may often be based on cost, tolerability, secondary benefits (i.e., breast), advanced disease, or hip fracture risk at various BMD levels (oral or intravenous bisphosphonates). The biggest challenge is the problem of poor compliance in that most patients discontinue all the forementioned therapies within 1 year of prescription. If we could double the compliance, we would improve outcomes. If we could simply get patients who have already had a hip fracture to take any form of osteoporosis therapy (currently, <8%), we would have a greater impact.

Choices between the two currently available oral bisphosphonates in the United States are based on non–head-to-head trials and both physician- and patient-driven decisions. The fracture data pertaining to these two bisphosphonates in terms of their reduction in relative risk and the confidence intervals regarding the reduction in reductive risk all overlap, thus suggesting that outcome data may not be the best method of choosing. The same may be true of gastrointestinal tolerability, where competition between these two bisphosphonates is intense, yet the issue should really be the low level of market penetration, where there is more than ample opportunity for either bisphosphonate.

An even larger issue is that most patients (~90%) who have already suffered a hip fracture are not receiving *any* osteoporosis therapy! Why? There can be only speculations but a few are as follows:

1. Currently approximately 300,000 hip fracture events occur each year in the United States.
2. There are 100,000 primary care physicians.
3. Hip fracture patients are not seen (until months later) by their primary care physician because they are admitted to hospital orthopedic services.

We must develop policies where orthopedic services care or direct the care of a hip fracture patient to physicians who will assess and treat their metabolic bone disease.

Combination Antiresorptive Regimens

Combinations of alendronate and estrogen or raloxifene and estrogen have been shown to increase BMD of the spine and hip more than either one alone in prospective trials. When to add a bisphosphonate to estrogen or raloxifene is not clear, but the author has the following opinions about such approaches:

1. Bisphosphonates should be added to the treatment of elderly women who are having fractures, are losing BMD, or continue to have high biomarkers of bone turnover with estrogens.
2. Bisphosphonates should be added to estrogen or raloxifene in elderly women who have femoral neck T scores lower than 3 SD despite long-term ERT. These women, assuming that they have no other secondary causes of this degree of low BMD, may be estrogen nonresponders or have age-related bone loss that has dominated their bone metabolism beyond the capacity of estrogen (or possibly even SERMs) to protect the aged skeleton.

Although no fracture data are available with combination therapies, it seems reasonable in high-risk patients who appear to not be responding to ERT and/or are elderly and have an exceptionally high hip fracture risk to add another antiresorptive agent that may be additive, if not synergistic to, the BMD effect.

MONITORING CLINICAL RESPONSE TO ANTIRESORPTIVE THERAPIES

Fracture reduction is the most important outcome. However, waiting for the occurrence of fractures to declare effectiveness is not very appealing. Hence, surrogate markers have become the clinical means of defining pharmacologic response. These surrogate markers are:

1. Measured change in height
2. Changes in BMD
3. Changes in biomarkers of bone resorption or formation

Measuring a patient's height by accurate means (a stadiometer) is very beneficial because height changes may reflect current or future vertebral deformities. Patients who have lost more than 1.5 inches from their peak height should have lateral thoracic and lumbar spine radiograph, which at these levels of memory-measured height discrepancies has a great probability of detecting a current vertebral deformity (most of which are asymptomatic). Lateral dual energy x-ray absorptiometry (DXA) vertebral morphometry is an even more accurrate means of measuring for vertebral deformities and can now be done as a point-of-care procedure at the same time that DXA is performed. Patients who continue to lose height because of progressive vertebral deformities (incipient fractures) while receiving antiresorptive therapy need special consideration. It could be that the antiresorptive agent is totally effective in as much as antiresorptive agents will *reduce* fracture risk but not *abolish* this risk. Nevertheless, these patients should be queried regarding their compliance, potential malabsorption (i.e., celiac disease), secondary conditions that might mitigate the bone response, or true drug ineffectiveness.

If the physician has reason to believe that the bisphosphonate is not being absorbed despite correct use, patients losing bone or sustaining fractures may benefit from intravenous bisphosphonate administration. Because no serum assays are clinically available for ensuring bisphosphonate absorption, the intravenous route of administration at least removes any doubt about inadequate absorption of these fastidiously absorbed compounds. Currently, the only intravenous bisphosphonate available is pamidronate. Pamidronate* is FDA approved for several indications but not for osteoporosis, although data have been published on its efficacy in postmenopausal osteoporosis and it is widely used for this indication in many other countries. If used "off-label," the dose is 30 mg infused over a 2-hour period every 3 months. Before using intravenous bisphosphonates it is important that patients have adequate vitamin D and calcium intake and levels because intravenous administration and the subsequent inhibition of bone resorption may result in transient hypocalcemia symptoms in patients without adequate vitamin D or calcium levels or result in a blunted PTH response. Intravenous pamidronate may be monitored in a small percentage of patients by the "first-phase" reaction, a 24- to 48-hour "flulike" illness consisting of fever and myalgias that abate and usually never occur with the second infusion. Finally, intravenous pamidronate should be used very cautiously in dialysis patients because the bisphosphonates are not dialyzable; if they are used (as in hypercalcemic myeloma patients with end-stage renal disease), they should be given more slowly. If given at the usual rates of infusion, severe and prolonged hypocalcemia and hypophosphatemia may result, in which case the bisphosphonate can be removed by plasmapheresis.

BMD and/or biomarker changes as surrogate markers can be extremely valuable in measuring the pharmacologic response. Proper quality control of DXA instruments and interpretation of serial BMD changes are paramount to competent clinical analysis. For example, if the precision error of in vivo serial BMD change in a particular densitometry facility is 3%, often seen in patients with low BMD, rather than the manufacturer's stated 1% precision error, a 9% change (increase or decrease) must be observed for it to be real rather than a measurement error. How many patients have been told to discontinue an otherwise effective antiresorptive agent because the densitometry facility reported BMD changes that seem large but are unknowingly within the measurement error? Likewise, careful consideration of biomarker changes is important when deciding whether changes are real or within the reproduc-

*Not FDA approved for this indication.

ibility errors of the measurements and whether the changes represent a true bone biologic effect.

GLUCOCORTICOID-ASSOCIATED OSTEOPOROSIS

Glucocorticoids (steroids) induce bone loss, and both the rate and amount of loss are dependent on the dose and/or duration of the dose. High doses (>30 mg/d of prednisone or a prednisone equivalent) induce rapid loss, whereas low doses (5 mg/d) induce loss over a slower period, but cumulative doses are detrimental as well. Although the data are not strong, it may be that no dose of steroids or route of administration (oral, inhaled, or nasal) is truly safe as long as their use is prolonged. This latter negative effect of low-dose steroids may also depend on the disease that it is being used to treat: diseases that may be associated with bone loss in and of themselves (such as rheumatoid arthritis) may be more susceptible to the negative effects of steroids.

Glucocorticoids affect bone through several mechanisms:

1. They reduce gastrointestinal calcium absorption.
2. They increase urinary calcium excretion.
3. They induce both osteoblast and osteocyte apoptosis.
4. They reduce osteoblast function.

Hence, steroids are particularly detrimental to bone through multiple mechanisms. Several studies have now documented the ability of bisphosphonates to both prevent bone loss at initiation of steroid therapy and increase BMD and reduce fractures in patients with established steroid-induced osteoporosis.

Etidronate (Didronel)*, alendronate (Fosamax), and risedronate (Actonel) have been shown in prospective studies to have the beneficial effects listed earlier, with the fracture data being strongest for alendronate and risedronate, but all are associated with positive fracture reduction trends. In addition, although etidronate is registered as an indication for steroid-induced osteoporosis in Canada and the United Kingdom, alendronate and risedronate are FDA approved for this indication in the United States.

Some BMD data also suggest efficacy for both injectable and nasal calcitonin in the management of steroid-induced osteoporosis, but no fracture data are available for calcitonin use. Hence the bisphosphonates are the first line of therapy for steroid-induced osteoporosis.

Various guidelines can provide physicians some direction regarding when to begin bisphosphonates for the prevention of steroid-induced osteoporosis. Essentially, patients who may need long-term steroid therapy of 7.5 mg/d of prednisone or greater or a dose equivalent for 3 months or longer should have BMD testing. If their T scores are normal or high, it is reasonable to initiate more conservative therapy (vitamin D, calcium, gonadal steroids if deficient, and thiazides if the patient is hypercalciuric), with BMD measurement repeated 6 months later and annually thereafter. If BMD significantly declines in the 6-month period (or thereafter), the addition of a bisphosphonate is indicated. Alternatively, if the T score at the start of steroids therapy is low (T score lower than −1 SD), beginning bisphosphonates at the outset is indicated.

Patients requiring high doses of steroids (>30 mg/d) for potentially prolonged periods (>6 months), such as might be used in certain renal or rheumatologic diseases or after heart/liver/lung transplantation, should receive bisphosphonates from the beginning, regardless of their BMD levels. Baseline BMD determinations are important for the purpose of serially monitoring the efficacy of the bisphosphonate effect.

MALE OSTEOPOROSIS

Osteoporosis does develop in men, and fracture rates are increasing in men as well, in part because of the increased longevity in the male population. Men do not usually go to their physicians for BMD testing because they are not concerned about menopause. Men generally seek treatment for fractures or are referred after androgen ablation in the context of prostate cancer therapy or steroid use.

Yet in groups of men, BMD begins to decline around the average age of 65 years as a result of the same process of age-related bone loss that affects women, and in prospective studies, hip BMD declines in men after the age of 65 years at an average rate approximately of 1% per year, independent of their gonadal hormone status. For these reasons, it might be appropriate to do BMD testing on asymptomatic men at the age of 65 years to initiate both prevention and treatment strategies.

Possible etiologies of male osteoporosis are manifold but include:

1. Hypogonadism (hypothalamic-pituitary, post-orchiectomy, androgen-receptor blockade—the highest number now being the population of men with prostate cancer)
2. Estrogen eficiency (seen in men with aromatase deficiency or estrogen-receptor deficiency)
3. Low insulin-like growth factor type 1 levels
4. Alcoholism
5. Heavy smoking
6. Hypercalciuria (with or without renal stone formation)
7. Chronic liver disease
8. Vitamin D deficiency (malabsorption, hemigastrectomies, inadequate intake)
9. Chronic medication use that affects bone (phenytoin [Dilantin], heparin, etc.)
10. Mastocytosis
11. Hyperprolactinemia
12. Renal tubular acidosis

*Not FDA approved for this indication.

13. Hyperparathyroidism
14. Hyperthyroidism (or excess thyroid hormone replacement)

For all males 65 years or older regardless of their BMD, prevention strategies to mitigate age-related bone loss include 800 IU/d of vitamin D and 1500 mg/d. For males who have sustained fractures, fulfill the steroid guidelines previously mentioned, or are losing BMD for unknown reasons and have T scores lower than −2 SD, bisphosphonate use will benefit these patients.

Absolute BMD in males at the femoral neck has been shown in prospective studies to be as predictive of hip fracture risk as the absolute BMD of elderly white females. In addition, recent 10-year prospective hip fracture data from Sweden have shown that the absolute risk is also identical at the same age in white men and women at the same T scores as developed from the young white female NHANES III database. Hence it is possible that as pertaining to risk, elderly men and women should be assessed the same way—even using female young normal databases.

Alendronate has recently gained FDA approval for male osteoporosis. Entry criteria for this prospective, randomized, placebo-controlled study were 65 years of age or older, current vertebral fractures, or T scores lower than −2 SD. Whereas the "placebo group" received vitamin D and calcium, the alendronate group received 10 mg/d of this oral bisphosphonate in addition. Two years later, the BMD at the spine and hip significantly increased in the alendronate-treated group whereas the BMD declined in the control group. Although the study was not powered for fracture analysis, a trend was seen in vertebral fracture reduction in the alendronate-treated group, as well as significantly less height loss in this group. Hence, for the first time males have available a registered therapy for osteoporosis prevention and treatment.

In androgen-deficient osteoporotic males, androgen replacement might be considered. Although androgen replacement in hypogonadal men may increase BMD, fracture reduction data are limited, and androgen replacement has not been capable of augmenting BMD in eugonadal men. Furthermore, androgen administration is associated with substantial risks in elderly men: prostate issues, undesirable lipid changes, polycythemia, and for some androgens, hepatic enzyme changes. Therefore, the bisphosphonates offer a far safer option and established efficacy for male osteoporosis, even in eugonadal men. Cautious androgen use may have separate benefits.

Osteoporosis is very treatable, and patients can have substantial risk reduction with proper diagnosis and treatment. The challenges are to use these diagnostic and treatment tools responsibly and with correct patient selection.

PAGET'S DISEASE

method of
PAUL D. MILLER, M.D.
University of Colorado Health Sciences Center
Denver, Colorado

1. Paget's disease has no known cause.
2. Paget's disease is diagnosed by radiography, not by bone scan or magnetic resonance imaging.
3. Paget's disease is often asymptomatic.
4. Paget's disease may be active with normal biochemical markers of bone turnover: collagen cross-links or bone-specific alkaline phosphatase.
5. Bisphosphonates are the treatment of choice for Paget's disease.
6. Bisphosphonates should be used in asymptomatic patients with Paget's disease who have elevated bone turnover markers.
7. Paget's disease of bone may be *mono-osteitic* (single-bone involvement) or *polyostotic* (more than one bone). Once a patient is diagnosed with either type of Paget's disease (mono-osteitic or polyostotic), whatever bone or bones are involved will be the *only* bones ever involved by the pagetic process.

Paget's disease is most common in whites of Northern European extraction. Although the incidence seems to be decreasing in Northern England, the incidence in other nations may not be.

Paget's disease is a disease of bone turnover that may present with pain, or it may be detected when a routine biochemical panel reveals an elevated alkaline phosphatase. In the latter circumstance, once the physician determines that the elevated alkaline phosphatase is originating from bone, not liver, the cause of the elevated bone-specific alkaline phosphatase needs to be determined. Most of these other etiologies can excluded clinically using blood tests and radiographs. If metastatic disease and hyperparathyroidism are excluded, asymptomatic Paget's disease may be present. A complete radiographic skeletal survey is then used to look for Paget's disease. If total skeletal survey radiographs are normal, Paget's disease does not exist. Paget's disease is a radiographic based diagnosis. The only disease that may mimic Paget's disease on radiograph is metastatic prostate carcinoma. However, metastatic prostate carcinoma is usually associated with an elevated prostate-specific antigen; if not, then bone biopsy can clarify the distinction.

Painful Paget's disease needs treatment. The treatment of choice is the use of bisphosphonates. These agents may be capable of "curing" Paget's disease or, at least, putting the disease into an extended period of normal bone turnover (i.e., normal biochemical markers of bone remodeling, resorption as well as formation markers).

Asymptomatic Paget's disease also needs to be treated, especially because the consequences of long-term nontreatment may be unacceptable: fractures, high-output congestive heart failure, hearing loss, and skeletal disfigurement. The randomized prospective longitudinal data are insufficient to indicate which asymptomatic untreated patients will progress to clinical consequences. Because the bisphosphonates are exceptionally safe and because these drugs can be administered either orally or intravenously, there is no reason to withhold treatment in asymptomatic pagetic patients.

Patients with Paget's disease may also have normal bone-specific alkaline phosphatase (BSAP) and yet high bone resorption, which is indicated by elevated serum or urine collagen cross-links, both biochemical markers of bone resorption. I believe this combination is seen in two circumstances: early Paget's disease of a form that I describe as type 2 and type 1, Paget's disease. Paget's disease is a disease of the osteoclasts, the cells that induce bone resorption. These cells are larger and have multiple nuclei in these patients, and these cells induce excessive bone resorption. Thus, the first radiographic defect that is seen is an osteolytic lesion. Hence, early in the pagetic process one may see an increase in bone resorption markers before the bone formation increases in response to the coupling process between these bone-to-cell lines. During this early osteolytic process, the BSAP is normal. Ultimately, the bone formation increases and an osteoblastic effect is seen on radiograph as well as in the elevation of BSAP. This is the classic type 1 Paget's disease.

Type 2 Paget's disease looks similar on radiograph to type 1 in that the osteolytic lesion prevails and the bone resorption markers are elevated; however, the BSAP never becomes elevated and the lesion, by radiograph, does *not* resemble fibrous dysplasia. There is something different about this form of Paget's disease that I and my colleagues who see many pagetic patients have seen. The coupling between the two cell lines is not present or is inadequate. In some of these patients, it is possible that their BSAP was low to begin with and increased in response to the increase in bone resorption but to a level that remains within the normal range. It may also be that type 2 Paget's disease is different at the cellular level than type 1.

Do these two forms of Paget's disease respond differently to treatment? The answer is "no," although the proportion of patients with active Paget's disease who have high bone resorption without an increase in bone formation (that is, a normal BSAP) are few, and no well-performed studies have been done comparing the potential differences in response of types 1 and 2 Paget's disease.

TREATMENT

The treatment for Paget's disease may involve either bisphosphonates or calcitonin (Calcimar) as first lines of therapy and, in rare circumstances, gallium nitrate and/or plicamycin. Because the bisphosphonates are effective in treating this disease and can be administered orally rather than using a parenteral approach (subcutaneous injection for calcitonin or intravenous with pamidronate), the oral bisphosphonates should in most cases be the first treatment of choice for Paget's disease.

Daily etidronate was the first Food and Drug Administration (FDA)–approved bisphosphonate for Paget's disease nearly 20 years ago. However, in comparative head-to-head trials, etidronate (Didronel), is not as effective as the aminobisphosphonate, risedronate, at least on the biochemical markers of bone turnover. Both alendronate (Fosamax) and risedronate (Actonel), the biologically active aminobisphosphonates, are the first-line therapies for Paget's disease. Alendronate dosage is 40 mg/d for 6 months; risedronate dosage is 30 mg/d for 2 months. There are no head-to-head comparative studies examining efficacy between these two aminobisphosphonates. Selection is probably physician preference, tolerability, and costs. With either bisphosphonate, the biochemical markers of bone turnover should be measured at the end of the treatment regimen. If they have not normalized, either a second course of the bisphosphonate can be tried or intravenous bisphosphonate, pamidronate, is considered. Pamidronate (Aredia) is also FDA-approved for the treatment of Paget's disease and I often used it as first-line therapy in patients with very painful Paget's to induce rapid pain reduction, in patients who "fail" oral bisphosphonates, or just before surgery to reduce the chance of bleeding in patients having surgery in a pagetic bone involvement. I use 90 mg administered over 4 hours in two doses 1 week apart (total 180 mg). Often, either of these oral aminobisphosphonates or the intravenous pamidronate will induce prolonged clinical and biochemical remission for months or years before re-treatment is necessary. Patients can periodically (every 6 months) be monitored and re-treated whenever the BSAP and/or collagen cross-link rises above the normal range.

Normalization of the biochemical markers of bone turnover is achievable in most patients with the aminobisphosphonates or intravenous pamidronate, a feature that was not nearly as possible with etidronate.

Resistance to one or more bisphosphonates may be seen after repeated exposure. For example, patients who previously "responded" to one (clinically with pain reduction or biochemically) may not be as responsive to repeated dosing, if required. The exact nature of this resistance is unknown but seems to be specific to the particular bisphosphonate because use of alternate bisphosphonates often leads to rapid induction of remission. This suggests that resistance may not be similar among bisphosphonates. The good news is that physicians have several highly effective bisphosphonates available to use.

Injectable calcitonin has been used for more than 25 years as a therapy for Paget's disease and may be effective in patients whose ability to use bisphosphonates is limited by intolerance. Subcutaneous administration of 100 IU/d often leads to an average 50% reduction in markers of bone turnover 3 to 6 months after therapy. The nasal spray formulation of calcitonin (Miacalcin),* is not FDA registered for Paget's disease, and experience with its use is limited to anecdotal observations.

Finally, there are a few instances in which the clinician must use extra diligence in treating the pagetic patient. One is the patient with a painful osteolytic lesion in the proximal femur. Bisphosphonate administration will relieve the pain promptly, which may encourage the patient to increase activity and weightbearing on that hip a very short time after treatment is started, resulting in a hip fracture. In these circumstances, the patient should be cautioned about this possibility and provided a cane until a few weeks of therapy can allow additional mineralization of the osteolytic lesion. Another area of caution is in the patient who does not respond to any treatment

*Not FDA approved for this indication.

or relapses quickly and has a rapidly progressive radiograph of pagetic bone. Although rare, osteogenic sarcoma could be present in such a lesion, and it should be biopsed. Finally, a third area of caution is the patient in whom neurologic impairment may be related to the pagetic bone encroachment, spinal cord compression with long-tract signs, spinal stenosis, or basilar invagination with neural compromise. Close consultation with the neurosurgeon is needed to help select a surgical intervention through a vascular pagetic bone.

Paget's disease is manageable and may be put into very long-term remission by normalization of biochemical markers through the use of the newer bisphosphonates. Asymptomatic patients with high bone turnover should be treated to prevent potential long-term consequences. Treatment in these patients is very reasonable given the evidence that the newer aminobisphosphonates are highly effective and very safe.

PARENTERAL NUTRITION IN ADULTS

method of
BRUCE W. ROBB, M.D., and
ROBERT H. BOWER, M.D.
University of Cincinnati College of Medicine
Cincinnati, Ohio

Maintenance of nutritional status is recognized today as an essential component of patient care. However, scarcely more than 30 years ago, parenteral nutrition support was not used to treat patients. In 1969, Dudrick and Wilmore reported the successful use of parenteral nutrition to support an infant with intestinal atresia and initiated the modern era of nutritional support. In its early years, total parenteral nutrition (TPN) was complex therapy that was associated with considerable morbidity and even mortality. Through the use of multidisciplinary teams and the establishment of strict protocols for administration, TPN therapy has become a safe and standard form of therapy for patients in whom the enteral route is unavailable or nonfunctional. TPN is now an established part of the therapy for many disease states and allows the nutritional and metabolic support of patients who, without such support, would be unable to recover or survive.

NUTRITIONAL REQUIREMENTS

The primary goal of nutritional support is maintenance or replacement of lean body mass or protein mass. To accomplish this goal, there must be provision of both protein substrate and energy. There are three sources of energy for bodily processes: protein, carbohydrate, and fat. Under normal conditions, 85% of the daily energy requirements are provided from carbohydrate and fat, and the remaining 15% is from protein.

Ingested carbohydrates are converted to glucose and subsequently yield 4 kcal/g through glycolysis. Glucose may be stored as glycogen in the liver or skeletal muscle. Glycogen breakdown yields 1 to 2 kcal/g. Glycogen stores are exhausted within approximately 24 hours of initiation of a fast. The predominant source of carbohydrate in TPN is dextrose. Metabolism of dextrose yields 3.4 kcal/g.

Fat is an energy-dense substance that yields 9 kcal/g. Fat provides the greatest source of stored energy in the body. Most tissues of the body are able to use fat as an energy source, with the exception of red and white blood cells, brain tissue, and the renal medulla, which are dependent upon glucose in the early stages of fasting. After adaptation, the brain and renal medulla may use ketone bodies derived from fat breakdown.

Of the approximately 15% of energy requirements derived from protein, roughly half is from gluconeogenesis. The remaining half is from the direct oxidation of the branched-chain amino acids (valine, leucine, and isoleucine) to high-energy phosphate. Breakdown of protein yields 4 kcal/g. Use of protein for energy is detrimental both through its diminution of the lean body mass and because it is inefficient. More than four times as much energy is required to synthesize protein than is reclaimed in metabolism through gluconeogenesis.

ESTIMATION OF ENERGY REQUIREMENTS

Caloric needs in adults are approximately 25 kcal/kg/d in the healthy state and 30 to 35 kcal/kg/d during illness. Basal energy expenditure (BEE) in healthy adults at rest can be calculated on the basis of body weight, height, sex, and age using the Harris-Benedict equation:

$$\begin{aligned}\text{BEE (men)} = {} & 66.47 + (13.75 \times \text{weight in kg}) \\ & + (5 \times \text{height in cm}) \\ & - (6.76 \times \text{age in years})\end{aligned}$$

$$\begin{aligned}\text{BEE (women)} = {} & 655.1 + (9.56 \times \text{weight in kg}) \\ & + (1.85 \times \text{height in cm}) \\ & - (4.58 \times \text{age in years})\end{aligned}$$

Adjustment based on physical activity is made by multiplying the BEE by an activity factor of 1.2 for bedridden patients and 1.3 for other hospitalized patients.

The BEE may also be adjusted to account for additional caloric needs during times of stress by multiplying by an injury factor, as described by Long:

Minor operation = 1.2
Skeletal trauma = 1.35
Sepsis = 1.6
Severe thermal injury = 2.1

When all these factors are taken into account, total caloric needs are estimated by the following equation:

$$\text{BEE} \times \text{Activity Factor} \times \text{Injury Factor}$$

Studies have suggested that the Harris-Benedict equation is less accurate in patients who are ill. Under such circumstances, this equation underestimates caloric requirements. However, the multiplication by the activity factors generally results in overestimation of requirements. As an example, measurements of caloric needs after uncomplicated hernia repair by Kinney and coworkers revealed no increase over baseline.

As a general rule, most patients who are ill or are under metabolic stress require approximately 30 to 35 kcal/kg/d. However, in critically ill patients, these estimates are accurate in only approximately one third of cases. A more accurate clinical determination of caloric needs may be obtained through indirect calorimetry. Indirect calorimetry calculates Resting Energy Expenditure (REE) from measurements of oxygen consumption ($\dot{V}O_2$):

$$\text{Resting Energy Expenditure (kcal/h)} = \dot{V}O_2\,(\text{mL/min}) \times 60\ \text{min/h} \times 1\ \text{L}/1000\ \text{mL} \times 4.83\ \text{kcal/L}$$

Indirect calorimetry also calculates a respiratory quotient (RQ). RQ is determined by measuring the patient's carbon dioxide production ($\dot{V}CO_2$) and $\dot{V}O_2$:

$$RQ = \dot{V}CO_2 / \dot{V}O_2$$

The RQ of fat metabolism is 0.7 and the RQ of carbohydrate metabolism is 1.0. Administration of carbohydrate calories in excess of requirements results in lipogenesis and an RQ greater than 1. As a consequence, a measured RQ of 0.8 to 0.9 indicates utilization of mixed fuel substrates (carbohydrate, fat, and protein) and is desirable. An RQ less than 0.7 indicates ketogenesis and underfeeding or provision of fewer calories than required. An RQ greater than 1.0 indicates carbohydrate overfeeding or administration in excess of requirements.

Automated metabolic analyzers that measure gas exchange and calculate REE and RQ are increasingly available in larger intensive care units. Measurements are most accurate when performed in patients who are intubated. The measurements are accurate for the period of measurement but do not take into account changes in activity or stress during other times of the day.

It should be emphasized that although total energy needs are increased 20% to 40% during illness or stress, total protein needs are increased by an even greater amount. The disparity between the increases in energy requirements and protein requirements in critically ill patients requires the modification of TPN formulas in such patients to meet their metabolic needs and avoid the problems of overfeeding.

Protein

The recommended daily allowance (RDA) of protein for healthy adults is 0.8 to 1.0 g/kg ideal body weight per day. In states of metabolic stress, such as sepsis, thermal injury, or major surgical procedures, protein requirements may more than double. In these situations, both protein breakdown and synthesis may be increased, but there is greater breakdown than synthesis, resulting in net protein catabolism. The amino acids released from this protein catabolism are used for gluconeogenesis, wound healing, and in other components of the acute inflammatory response. Although this release of amino acids is essential in the short run, the continued breakdown of protein results in a loss of function since there is no nonspecific storage form of protein. The resulting functional losses include immune suppression, poor wound healing, and loss of skeletal muscle mass and strength.

Increasing protein intake can increase the rate of protein synthesis to match more closely the elevated rates of protein breakdown seen in stress states. Protein intake may need to be increased to 1.5 to 2.0 g/kg body weight/d in sepsis or stress and 2.0 to 3.0 g/kg body weight/d in major thermal injury.

Carbohydrate

Most of the calories in TPN are provided as carbohydrate in the form of dextrose. As previously noted, administered dextrose is converted into glucose. The maximum rate at which glucose can be metabolized via either the enteral or parenteral route is 5 mg/kg/min, or approximately 500 g/d in a 70-kg man.

Fat

Fat is an energy-dense substrate that is required for normal growth, development, and immune function. Fat is administered parenterally as emulsions of either safflower or soybean oil. These emulsions can be administered as separate infusions, but are more commonly admixed with other components of TPN in a total nutrient admixture or 3-in-1 infusion. Linoleic and α-linolenic acid cannot be synthesized endogenously and must be supplied in the diet or administered parenterally. Symptoms of essential fatty acid deficiency include dry skin, dermatitis, and alopecia. Administration of 4% to 6% of calories in the form of parenteral lipid emulsion is sufficient to prevent essential fatty acid deficiency. Although fat may supply as much as 45% of calories in the American diet, most nutritional formulations limit calories from fat to 30% or less of total calories.

Calorie-to-Nitrogen Ratio

An adequate number of calories must be provided to permit protein synthesis and to minimize catabolism of administered protein or amino acids for gluconeogenesis. In general, a ratio of 150 kcal for each gram of administered nitrogen (6.25 g of protein = 1.0 g of nitrogen) is recommended. As previously noted, the protein requirements increase more than the caloric requirements in states of metabolic stress, sepsis, and injury. Consequently, a calorie-to-nitrogen ratio (Cal:N) of 80:1 is recommended in stress states.

Micronutrients

In general, vitamins and trace elements should be administered according to the RDA. Multivitamin infusions are generally administered in TPN daily. Vitamin K is not administered as part of the multivitamin infusion and may be withheld in patients who require anticoagulation with warfarin. There have been manufacturing shortages of multivitamin infusions several times in the recent past. Under such circumstances, individual vitamins need to be administered in TPN. Deficiency states of the water-soluble vitamins are generally the first to occur. Thiamine deficiency can occur in as little as 1 week and is often precipitated by the high carbohydrate content of administered TPN. Acutely, thiamine deficiency can manifest as peripheral neuropathies, cranial nerve weakness, congestive heart failure, and encephalopathy.

Trace elements are also administered daily as combination injections containing zinc, copper, chromium, manganese, and selenium. Of the deficiency states related to trace elements, zinc deficiency is generally the first to become apparent. Zinc deficiency most often occurs in patients with large stool losses, such as from small-bowel stomas, diarrhea, or gastrointestinal (GI)-cutaneous fistulas. As much as 20 mg of zinc per day may be lost in the stool. Signs of zinc deficiency include skin rashes, especially in flexion creases; pustular perioral rashes; hair loss; and changes in sense of smell and taste. Deficiencies of copper may result in megaloblastic anemia. Chromium deficiency may become apparent due to glucose intolerance. Deficiencies of copper and chromium are rarely seen today owing to the routine daily administration of multiple trace elements.

INDICATIONS FOR NUTRITIONAL SUPPORT

Techniques of parenteral nutritional support are more effective in preventing loss of lean body mass than in its replacement. The decision to initiate nutritional support depends upon the patient's age, the severity of the illness, whether there is preexisting malnutrition and the estimated length of interruption of nutrition. Nutritional support is indicated in the following circumstances:

1. A normally nourished individual who has had no nutrient intake for 5 to 7 days is a candidate for nutritional support. Peripheral intravenous solutions containing 5% dextrose provide small amounts of energy and help to spare protein loss. However, significant deficits in body stores may occur within 7 days in severely ill individuals. Nutritional support should be initiated before physiologic functions become compromised.
2. An individual who is already malnourished should have nutritional support started immediately. In general, patients who have lost 10% to 15% of their usual body weight in the previous 6 months have an increased risk of complications.
3. An individual, even if normally nourished, who has an illness or type of therapy that is expected to render him unable to eat for 10 days or more should have nutritional support started immediately. Patients with multiple injuries, sepsis, pancreatitis, or other major disturbances of GI function are likely to require the prompt initiation of nutritional support.

In addition to the initial nutritional assessment, the changing conditions of patients, especially those who are critically ill, require re-assessment every 3 to 5 days to determine if adjustments in the formula are needed or whether there is continued need for nutritional support.

ENTERAL NUTRITION

Once it has been determined that nutritional support is indicated, the route of administration must be selected. The enteral route should be used whenever possible. Several studies of critically ill patients have demonstrated decreased rates of mortality and morbidity in those patients who received their nutrition enterally when compared with those who received TPN. There are numerous theoretical advantages of enteral nutrition over parenteral nutrition. Enteral feedings maintain the integrity of the GI mucosa and gut-associated lymphoid tissue, theoretically decreasing the translocation of bacteria from the GI tract to the systemic circulation. Delivery of nutrients into the GI tract maintains the normal metabolic pathways in the liver. When administered properly, there is minimal infectious risk associated with enteral feeding. Enteral nutrition is less expensive than parenteral nutrition.

Many of the previous benefits are realized even when only a small portion of a patient's nutritional needs are met enterally. Therefore, even when it is not possible to meet the patient's total nutritional needs via the GI tract, it is advantageous to provide a portion of the patients needs enterally.

Multiple enteral delivery systems are available depending on the condition of the GI tract and the duration of feeding anticipated. Those who will need only short-term nutritional support will benefit from a transnasal tube whose tip lies either in the stomach or beyond the pylorus in the duodenum or proximal jejunum. These tubes should be flexible, small-bore catheters (<10 French) designed as enteral feeding tubes, not those designed to aspirate the stomach. The decision to deliver nutrition into the stomach or as jejunal feedings is based on the patient's mental status, primary pathology, presence of gastroparesis, and risk of aspiration. Advantages of gastric feeding include ease of feeding tube placement, the ability to give bolus feedings, and the ability to use hypertonic formulations. Disadvantages include a higher risk of aspiration. Postpyloric or jejunal feeding tubes decrease the risk of aspiration but are somewhat more difficult to place and generally work better with continuous feeding of isosmolar feeding formulas.

All small-bore feeding tubes should have their position confirmed radiographically before the initiation of enteral feedings. As previously mentioned, enteral feedings may be administered for their salutary effects on the GI tract, even when the majority of nutritional requirements are provided as TPN. In such patients, enteral nutrition can be used safely, but caution must be observed. Enteral nutrition should be administered with caution to patients with hemodynamic instability. Initiation of enteral feeding should wait until patients are fully resuscitated and no longer require pressors to maintain hemodynamic stability. Modest advancement of rate should be the rule. It is important to monitor for signs and symptoms of intolerance such as diarrhea, increasing abdominal girth, and cramping. Feedings should be stopped immediately in the presence of intolerance and resumed only when symptoms have completely resolved.

Patients who require long-term support will benefit from more permanent options that include surgically placed gastric or jejunal feeding tubes, as well as percutaneous endoscopically placed gastrostomy tubes. Consideration of gastric versus jejunal feeding tubes is made on a similar basis as previously noted with nasal tubes.

Formulations

There are multiple commercially available tube feeding preparations. In most instances, a polymeric formula containing fiber will suffice. Although numerous specialty formulas are available commercially, specialty formulations are rarely required. Occasionally, patients with chronic renal insufficiency may benefit from formulations with higher caloric density and altered electrolytes. Patients with hepatic insufficiency in whom hepatic encephalopathy develops when standard formulas are administered may benefit from special hepatic formulations. Patients with compromised pulmonary function rarely require any special formula if care is exercised not to administer excessive carbohydrates. There also exist immunomodulatory formulations that have been shown to reduce infectious complications and length of hospital stay in severely stressed patients.

PARENTERAL NUTRITION

Indications

Parenteral nutrition is utilized when the GI tract is unavailable or has functional derangements that preclude its use for nutrition. TPN may be used as either primary or supportive therapy. Those instances where TPN has been shown to be an effective primary therapy include short-bowel syndrome (the condition for which TPN was developed), GI-cutaneous fistula, acute renal failure, and hepatic insufficiency. TPN has been shown to be an effective supportive therapy for numerous conditions that render patients unable to ingest nutrients for varying periods such as in radiation enteritis, chemotherapy toxicity, hyperemesis gravidarum, and prolonged ileus. There is controversy regarding the role of TPN in the preoperative support of patients and in the treatment of patients with cancer.

SHORT-BOWEL SYNDROME

The short-bowel syndrome results from the massive loss of small bowel due to mesenteric vascular thrombosis or embolism, resection for volvulus, or multiple resections for conditions such as Crohn's disease. The use of TPN has enabled the survival of patients who would otherwise have died from nutritional insufficiency. Patients with short-bowel syndrome undergo adaptation of their remaining bowel over time. This adaptation will allow many of them to maintain their nutrition enterally. Those patients who can tolerate some enteral intake should be allowed to eat even as they receive most of their nutritional needs from TPN. Those patients who have less than 60 cm of functioning small bowel (45 cm if a competent ileocecal valve is present) are likely to require lifelong TPN support.

GASTROINTESTINAL-CUTANEOUS FISTULA

Parenteral nutrition allows for the provision of nutrients while facilitating decreased fistula output through bowel rest. TPN may increase the rate of spontaneous fistula closure in comparison with enteral nutrition, thereby avoiding the need for operative repair. Most patients will benefit from a trial of TPN and bowel rest to facilitate spontaneous closure. If such closure does not occur, and operative therapy is required, the patient should have decreased morbidity from the operative procedure as a result of the treatment of his or her malnutrition along with an overall improved nutritional state.

ACUTE RENAL FAILURE

In transient acute tubular necrosis (ATN), the use of TPN may result in earlier recovery of renal function and delay, or even avoid, the need for dialysis. This may be of critical importance in patients too unstable to tolerate hemodialysis. The goal in such circumstances is to provide the nutritional requirements in a reduced volume and with a formula designed to minimize azotemia and electrolyte disturbances. TPN formulas containing essential amino acids and high concentrations of dextrose (70%) are given in low volume to decrease the proteolysis that accompanies renal failure and decrease circulating urea nitrogen. Once it has been determined that the patient requires hemodialysis, a balanced TPN formulation should be administered to meet the patient's nutritional needs while volume and electrolyte problems are managed by dialysis.

HEPATIC INSUFFICIENCY

Patients with liver disease are hypermetabolic and have energy requirements as great as 55 kcal/kg/d. Decreased mortality rates are seen in patients with hepatic failure who receive aggressive nutritional support. Unfortunately, administration of adequate protein to meet nutritional needs often results in hepatic encephalopathy. Patients who develop hepatic encephalopathy when receiving conventional TPN formulations, or whose encephalopathy does not respond to oral antibiotics or lactulose, may benefit from the use of specialized TPN or enteral nutritional support. Patients with encephalopathy often have an abnormal pattern of amino acids in their plasma. The abnormality is characterized by high concentrations of aromatic and sulfur-containing amino acids and low concentrations of the branched-chain amino acids. In general, patients whose encephalopathy is associated with such an abnormal plasma amino acid pattern will benefit from special parenteral amino acid formulas enriched with branched-chain amino acids and containing reduced amounts of the aromatic amino acids and methionine. Such a formula is designed both to meet the patient's protein needs and to do so in a way that normalizes the abnormal plasma amino acid pattern. Such formulas have been shown to be as effective as lactulose or neomycin in the treatment of hepatic encephalopathy.

PREOPERATIVE SUPPORT

Several studies have investigated the use of TPN in the preoperative preparation of malnourished patients who require major surgical procedures. Although biochemical markers of nutrition can be improved with such therapy, there is a paucity of evidence that complications and mortality are reduced significantly. Patients who receive TPN preoperatively have been shown to have higher rates of infectious complications. Of the groups studied, patients with the most severe malnutrition demonstrate the greatest net benefit. In general, patients who have malnutrition as demonstrated by loss of 10% to 15% of usual body weight and whose serum albumin concentration is less than 3 g/dL are likely to have the greatest benefit. The optimal duration of preoperative TPN is unknown; however, it is probably between 5 and 7 days.

CANCER

There is an abundance of research regarding the use of nutritional support in patients with cancer. It is often confusing and difficult to decide how this information should be applied to the therapy of individual patients. In general, TPN is indicated in patients with malignancy who are unable to tolerate enteral nutrition and who are receiving antineoplastic therapy. Patients with malignancy should have their nutritional needs met, but administration of nutrients in quantities greater than their requirements (overfeeding) should be avoided since this may contribute to tumor growth. The use of antioxidants should be reduced in those receiving chemotherapy.

ADMINISTRATION OF TOTAL PARENTERAL NUTRITION

Peripheral Versus Central Route

Peripheral parenteral nutrition is rarely used today. It may have limited value in situations where patients have no practical central venous access and nutritional support may be required for only a brief period. The peripheral route is limited by the inability of peripheral veins to tolerate the increased osmolarity of the nutrient solutions. The incidence of thrombophlebitis may be reduced by meticulous care of cannulation sites by members of an intravenous team.

In institutions where the rates of complications related to catheter insertion and subsequent septic complications are acceptable, a central venous catheter should be the first choice for delivery of TPN. Percutaneous subclavian or internal jugular vein catheters may be placed at the bedside. In general, a subclavian central venous catheter is the most comfortable option for patients and the easiest site for maintenance of a sterile occlusive dressing. Peripherally inserted centrally located catheters may be used when subclavian or jugular vein catheters are not feasible.

Initiation of Total Parenteral Nutrition

Before the initiation of TPN therapy, baseline laboratory studies are usually obtained, including serum electrolyte, blood urea nitrogen, creatinine, calcium, magnesium, phosphorus, liver enzyme, and triglyceride levels; prothrombin time; complete blood cell count; and nutritional proteins including albumin, transferrin, pre-albumin, and retinol-binding protein. In addition, the patient's vital signs and body weight should be recorded.

The protein and energy requirements of the patient are estimated using the techniques previously described. An appropriate formula is then ordered (usually from a set of standard formulas designed by the nutrition support team), which delivers the protein and energy requirements of the patient in approximately 2 L of infusate. Amino acid concentrations of standard formulas are usually 5% (4.25% to 6%). Dextrose concentrations for standard formulas range from 15% to 25%. Electrolytes, multivitamin infusions, and trace elements are added to the formula daily. Lipid emulsions may be added to the infusion within certain limits of solubility to provide all components of nutrition in a single infusion or total nutrient admixture. Insulin may be added as needed to keep blood glucose concentrations below 200 mg/dL. In addition, certain drugs, such as histamine receptor antagonists, may be added to the TPN formulation. In general, formulas deliver approximately 1 kcal/mL of infusion. The composition of the standard and specialty TPN formulas used at The University Hospital in Cincinnati are shown in Table 1.

Infusion is typically begun at 40 mL/h and increased by 20 to 25 mL/h daily to the target rate of administration. If TPN infusion is interrupted, a peripheral infusion of 5% dextrose with appropriate electrolytes should be initiated at the same rate as the TPN to avoid hypoglycemia.

Monitoring

Vital signs should be monitored at least every 8 hours. Intake and output should be measured and recorded daily. Body weight should be measured before the initiation of TPN and twice weekly thereafter during the period of TPN infusion. A complete laboratory panel as previously described should be obtained before the initiation of therapy and repeated at least weekly thereafter. Serum electrolyte, calcium, magnesium, and phosphorus levels and a liver profile may need to be monitored more frequently in patients at the initiation of therapy or who are clinically unstable. After these values have stabilized, twice-weekly measurements may suffice.

Blood glucose should be measured by fingerstick studies twice daily during the initiation of TPN and during periods of rate increase. In patients who have diabetes mellitus, or in whom glucose concentrations have been elevated, monitoring should occur every 6 hours. Hyperglycemia is treated with subcutaneous injections of regular insulin. The rate of TPN infusion should not be advanced until blood glucose is consistently below 200 mg/dL throughout the day. The amount of regular insulin required to control blood sugar for a 24-hour period may be added. Two thirds of the total amount may subsequently be added to the next day's TPN infusion with continued monitoring to determine if still more insulin will be required. Hyperglycemia that occurs without a change in TPN rate in a patient who was heretofore normoglycemic may be an early sign of sepsis.

COMPLICATIONS OF TOTAL PARENTERAL NUTRITION

The complications of TPN include those related to the access device and those complications of the

TABLE 1. **Composition of Parenteral Nutrition Solutions Available at the University Hospital, Cincinnati, Ohio**

Component*	Range	Standard	High Dextrose	Hepatic	Renal	Peripheral†
Dextrose (%)	10–47	15	20	25	46.7	5
Amino acids (%)	1.7–6.4	5	5	4‡	1.7§	3.5
Fat (grams as TNA)	0–40	40	40	40	0	40
Sodium (mEq/L)	0–154	30	30	5	2	40
Potassium (mEq/L)	0–80	18	18	12	0	10
Calcium (mEq/L)	0–9.4	4.5	4.5	4.7	0	4.7
Magnesium (mEq/L)	0–12	5	5	8	0	8
Phosphorous (mmol/L)	5–15	10	10	5	1.7	5
Chloride (mEq/L)	0–150	37	37	13.5	1	40
Acetate (mEq/L)	14–80	55	55	31	14	52
Insulin (U/L)	0–120	0	0	0	0	0
kcal/mL	—	1.1	1.3	1.3	1.65	0.71

*Trace elements (Zn, 3.0 mg; Cu, 1.2 mg; Mn, 0.3 mg; Se, 60 µg; and Cr, 12 µg) and a multivitamin solution (10 mL) are provided daily. Vitamin K, 5 mg, is given weekly to patients who are not anticoagulated.

†Peripheral solutions are not formulated as TNA (total nutrient admixture); lipids are given separately.

‡Enriched in branched-chain amino acids.

§Provides essential amino acids.

infusate. In general, those related to the access device are early and late technical complications as well as septic complications.

Technical Complications

Technical complications may be minimized by appropriate preparation of the patient before the procedure and meticulous attention to details of technique during catheter insertion. Insertion of a central venous catheter for TPN is never an emergency. Adequate time should be taken to prepare the patient. Preparation of the patient includes assurance of hydration (2–3 L of fluid overnight are often required); correction of clotting abnormalities, if any; an appropriate explanation of the procedure with the patient's informed consent; and conscious sedation to minimize anxiety and to allow the patient to be positioned properly. For subclavian vein cannulation, the patient should be positioned with the arms at the sides, the shoulders abducted by means of a rolled towel placed axially beneath the thoracic spine, and in Trendelenburg position. Positioning the patient in this way allows horizontal access to the subclavian vein, thereby minimizing the possibility of injury to structures deep to the vein. It also facilitates positive pressure in the vein to make it larger and easier to find, as well as minimizing the probability of air embolism.

The most common technical complication includes pneumothorax, which occurs in 3% to 6% of catheter insertions. It is more common in elderly, cachectic, and dehydrated patients. Its occurrence may be minimized by adequate hydration, proper positioning of the patient, sedation before catheter insertion, and the use of the Seldinger (or guidewire) technique. Lacerations of the subclavian artery (or carotid artery in the case of internal jugular vein cannulation) are rare. They can be minimized by proper positioning of the patient and through use of a small-bore "finder" needle to locate the jugular or subclavian vein before attempts to cannulate with the larger needle. Care should also be taken to avoid redirecting the needle when its tip is near the vein. Even rarer are lacerations of the brachial plexus and thoracic duct. Air embolism is prevented by adequate hydration, Trendelenburg positioning, and care to avoid opening the hub of the needle to atmospheric pressure without ensuring that the patient has positive thoracic pressure. Embolization of the catheter guidewire is a technical complication that results from withdrawal of the J-tipped wire through the insertion needle. As the curved J tip of the guidewire is forced against the bevel of the needle, it may be sheared off with subsequent embolization to the heart or pulmonary circulation. Should attempts to advance the guidewire be unsuccessful, the needle and wire should be removed together as a unit to prevent embolism. Care should be taken in patients with inferior vena cava filters not to pass the wire so deeply that it becomes engaged with the filter.

Thrombosis of the subclavian vein, internal jugular vein, or vena cava is a late complication and may occur in up to 5% to 10% of patients with central venous catheters. Of these, greater than one third may be clinically silent. Symptoms may include swelling of the ipsilateral arm or tenderness in the supraclavicular fossa or along the sternocleidomastoid muscle. The diagnosis may be confirmed with noninvasive vascular imaging, although venography represents the gold standard. Treatment consists of catheter removal and anticoagulation, at least until the symptoms resolve. Long-term anticoagulation therapy may be necessary.

Infectious Complications

Catheter-related sepsis is the greatest source of morbidity and mortality for patients receiving TPN. Catheter care directly affects sepsis rates. The occurrence of catheter sepsis can be minimized through the use of single-lumen catheters dedicated solely to TPN infusion. The establishment of nutrition support teams and the use of strict protocols for the infusion of TPN and care of catheters can result in catheter sepsis rates of 1% to 3%. Catheter sepsis can occur from contamination of the insertion site with subsequent descending infection of the fibrin sheath that surrounds the catheter. Meticulous attention to sterility of the skin surrounding the catheter site before insertion and maintenance of sterility through the use of occlusive dressings changed three times weekly minimizes catheter infection from this cause. Catheter-related infection may also occur by hematogenous seeding of the catheter from distant sites of infection. Such infection occurs more commonly with gram-positive bacteria than with gram-negative organisms. This may be due to the limited susceptibility of gram-positive organisms to complement lysis. The most common pathogen in many hospitals is *Staphylococcus epidermidis*. Detection of this organism may be difficult because of intermittent bacteremia. Three sets of blood cultures within a 24-hour period, drawn at least 30 minutes apart, have a very low probability of missing an occult bacteremia.

Fungal infections can be devastating in patients receiving TPN. The most common pathogens are *Candida* species that probably enter the bloodstream via the GI tract. When there is evidence of invasive fungal infection, TPN should cease, all catheters should be removed, and antifungal therapy should be initiated.

A suggested algorithm for the diagnosis and management of catheter-related infection is shown in Figure 1.

Metabolic Complications

Metabolic complications of TPN are most commonly due to disorders of glucose metabolism and deficiency states. Hyperglycemia can be caused by inappropriately rapid advancement of the TPN infusion rate. Increased serum glucose levels can be treated initially with intermittent peripheral administration of insulin with subsequent addition of insulin to the TPN as previously described (see Monitor-

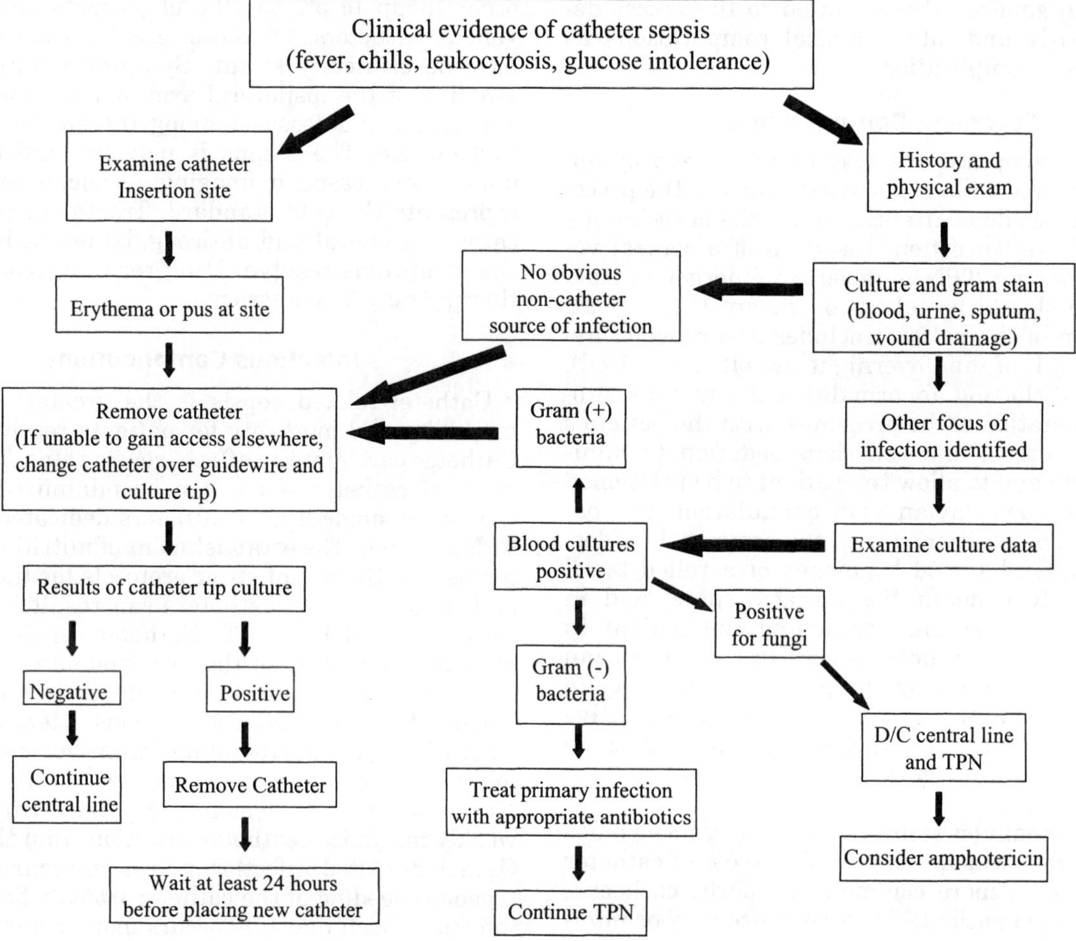

Figure 1. Suggested algorithm for the diagnosis and management of catheter-related infection.

ing). Hypoglycemia may result from excessive insulin administration or disruption of the TPN infusion. If the TPN infusion must be interrupted, infusion of 5% dextrose with appropriate electrolytes is generally sufficient to prevent symptoms.

Electrolyte abnormalities are common in patients receiving TPN, especially at initiation. These disturbances can be minimized by supplementation of electrolytes and frequent monitoring. In severely malnourished patients, the initiation of TPN may be associated with refeeding syndrome. Infusion of glucose and insulin may result in intracellular shifts of cations, resulting in hypokalemia, hypophosphatemia, or hypomagnesemia. Such decreases in serum concentrations may cause respiratory arrest, arrhythmias, or other sequelae. Potassium, phosphate, and magnesium should be supplemented routinely when TPN is initiated.

Mild disturbances of hepatic function may accompany the administration of TPN in adults. The cause of this dysfunction is not well understood. Biochemical abnormalities include elevated liver enzyme and alkaline phosphatase levels. The bilirubin level is almost never elevated as a consequence of TPN. Elevated serum concentrations of bilirubin should prompt a search for occult sepsis. Cholestasis and hepatic steatosis may be present. These abnormalities may be minimized by avoiding administration of carbohydrates in excess of calculated needs. Administration of even small amounts of enteral nutrition in combination with TPN may minimize these abnormalities.

Deficiencies of vitamins, trace elements, and essential fatty acids are prevented and treated by routine supplementation.

PARENTERAL FLUID AND ELECTROLYTE THERAPY IN PEDIATRICS

method of
BERNARD GAUTHIER, M.B., B.S.
Schneider Children's Hospital
New Hyde Park, New York

In planning parenteral fluid therapy it is convenient, conceptually and practically, to think in terms of maintenance therapy, designed to supply enough water and electrolytes to replace physiologic and continuing pathologic losses, and deficit therapy, designed to correct deficits already present at the time parenteral therapy is instituted.

MAINTENANCE THERAPY

Physiologic requirements of water and electrolytes are dependent on metabolic activity. Maintenance therapy therefore is most appropriately based on estimation of metabolic rate.

Estimation of Metabolic Activity

On the basis of metabolic studies published in the 1950s, the daily metabolic expenditure of a sick child in hospital may be calculated as follows for children weighing more than 3 kg (see later section on Parenteral Fluid Therapy in the Neonate for infants weighing less than 3 kg):

From the first 10 kg of body weight (BW), the metabolic expenditure is 100 calories/kg BW/d.

From the next 10 kg BW, the metabolic expenditure is 50 calories/kg BW/d.

For any weight above 20 kg BW, the metabolic expenditure is 20 calories/kg BW/d.

The calculation of maintenance is sometimes based on an estimation of "metabolic weight" in "metabolic kilograms" (metabolic kg) which may be defined as the body weight of a sick hospitalized child who generates a daily metabolic expenditure of 100 calories. For children weighing more than 3 kg this is done as follows:

For the first 10 kg BW, the metabolic weight is 1 metabolic kg/kg BW.

For the next 10 kg BW, the metabolic weight is 0.5 metabolic kg/kg BW.

For any weight above 20 kg BW, the metabolic weight is 0.2 metabolic kg/kg BW.

Whichever method is used, the resulting calculated maintenance therapy is the same.

Examples

The metabolic expenditure of a sick, hospitalized child weighing 8 kg, at 100 calories/kg BW/d, is

$$100 \times 8 = 800 \text{ calories per day}$$

and the metabolic weight, at 1 metabolic kg/kg BW, is

$$1 \times 8 = 8 \text{ metabolic kg}$$

With a body weight of 14 kg, metabolic expenditure at 100 calories/kg BW for the first 10 kg BW and 50 calories/kg BW for the next 4 kg BW, is

$$(100 \times 10) + (50 \times 4) = 1200 \text{ calories per day}$$

and the metabolic weight at 1 metabolic kg/kg BW for the first 10 kg BW and 0.5 metabolic kg/kg BW for the next 4 kg BW is

$$(1 \times 10) + (0.5 \times 4) = 12 \text{ metabolic kg}$$

With a body weight of 25 kg, metabolic expenditure at 100 calories/kg BW for the first 10 kg BW, 50 calories/kg BW for the next 10 kg BW, and 20 calories/kg BW for the next 5 kg BW is

$$(100 \times 10) + (50 \times 10) + (20 \times 5) = 1600 \text{ calories per day}$$

and the metabolic weight at 1 metabolic kg/kg BW for the first 10 kg BW, 0.5 metabolic kg/kg BW for the next 10 kg BW, and 0.2 metabolic kg/kg BW for the next 5 kg BW is

$$(1 \times 10) + (0.5 \times 10) + (0.2 \times 5) = 16 \text{ metabolic kg}$$

Relationship Between Metabolic Activity and Maintenance Water and Electrolyte Requirements

Water Requirements

With normal renal function, excess water may be excreted by excreting the solute load in dilute urine, or, if necessary, water may be conserved by excreting the solute load in concentrated urine. For this reason, with normal renal function, the choice of an amount of water designed to correct physiologic water losses is somewhat arbitrary. The long and well-established practice of supplying 100 mL of water per day per 100 calories of estimated metabolism or per metabolic kilogram has been based on the following considerations:

- Insensible water loss, through lungs and skin, amounts to about 45 mL/100 calories or metabolic kg/d
- In the absence of diarrhea, stool losses are no more than 5 to 10 mL/100 calories or metabolic kg/d
- In the absence of visible sweating, sweat losses are 0 to 25 mL/100 calories or metabolic kg/d
- Oxidation of carbohydrates and fats to carbon dioxide and water generates 12 to 17 mL/100 calories or metabolic kg/d
- Tissue catabolism during illness and undernutrition releases about 3 mL/100 calories or metabolic kg/d
- An allowance of 55 mL of water/100 calories or metabolic kg/d for replacement of urinary water losses allows a well-hydrated patient to excrete the daily solute load in a urine with a specific gravity of about 1010, or an osmolality approximately equal to that of plasma, when the solute load is the usual 17 to 20 mOsm/100 calories or metabolic kg/d in a child on parenteral fluid therapy. An allowance for urinary water losses of 55 mL/100 calories or metabolic kg/d would allow a high solute load (40 mOsm/100 calories or metabolic kg/d) to be excreted in a urine with an osmolality of 730 mOsm/L and would allow a low solute load (10 mOsm/100 calories or metabolic kg/day) to be excreted in a urine with an osmolality of 180

TABLE 1. **Summary of Maintenance Water and Electrolyte Requirements in Relation to Metabolic Expenditure or Metabolic Weight**

Insensible water loss	45 mL/100 calories or metabolic kg/d
Stool losses	5–10 mL/100 calories or metabolic kg/d
Sweat losses	0–25 mL/100 calories or metabolic kg/d
Urinary losses	55 mL/100 calories or metabolic kg/d
Water supplied by oxidation of carbohydrates and fats and by catabolism	12–20 mL/100 calories or metabolic kg/d
Usual water requirement added and rounded off from above	100 mL/100 calories or metabolic kg/d
Electrolyte requirements	Approximately 2 to 2.5 mEq each of sodium and potassium/100 calories or metabolic kg/d

mOsm/L. Therefore, 55 mL of water/100 calories or metabolic kg/d for replacement of urinary water losses provides extra free water in cases where the fluid requirements might have been underestimated and would not overtax the kidneys' diluting ability in cases where they might have been overestimated. The relationship between metabolic activity and maintenance fluid and electrolyte requirements is summarized in Table 1.

Electrolyte Requirements

Electrolyte requirements are approximately 2.5 mEq each of sodium and potassium/100 calories or metabolic kg/d. This figure is somewhat arbitrary. It is based on a consideration of the intake of sodium and potassium of a healthy infant on breast milk (about 1 to 1.5 mEq of each per 100 calories or metabolic kg/d) and on cow's milk (about 2 to 4.5 mEq of each per 100 calories or metabolic kg/d) and the recognition that intake of either electrolyte is compatible with good health. An intake of 2 to 2.5 mEq of sodium and potassium per 100 calories or metabolic kg/d therefore constitutes an adequate maintenance electrolyte intake.

Nutritional Requirements

It is impractical and it is not essential to provide full parenteral nutrition to every child who requires parenteral therapy for a short time. Nevertheless, the administration of maintenance fluids as a 5% glucose solution (dextrose 5% in water [D5W]) has the effect of providing 20% of caloric requirement when it is given in a amount equal to 100 mL/100 calories or metabolic kg/d, since it provides 5 g of glucose (i.e., 20 calories)/100 calories/d. This energy allowance minimizes tissue catabolism and ketosis and is adequate when parenteral therapy is required for a short time. Total parenteral nutrition should be considered when parenteral therapy in the absence of oral intake is needed, or when it is anticipated that it will be needed, for more than 5 to 7 days in a well-nourished child, or more than 2 to 3 days in a poorly nourished child.

Thus, maintenance fluid and electrolyte requirements and 20% of energy requirements as outlined earlier may be met by giving 100 mL/100 calories or metabolic kg/d of an appropriate electrolyte solution in 5% dextrose solution. The solution most commonly used at our hospital is 5% dextrose with 0.33% sodium chloride (i.e., 56 mEq sodium/L) solution (D5W ⅓ NS) and 20 mEq potassium chloride/L. Giving 100 mL/100 calories or metabolic kg/day of this solution provides 20 calories/100 calories or metabolic kg/d, 2 mEq potassium/100 calories or metabolic kg/d, and 5.6 mEq sodium/100 calories or metabolic kg/d. This sodium allowance exceeds the amount estimated from a consideration of the oral sodium intake of a healthy infant. Nevertheless, empirically, the use of this solution has worked well. Five percent dextrose with 0.45% sodium chloride (D5W ½ NS) is the maintenance fluid commonly used in older children. I do not know, and I have not been able to find in the literature, a physiologic basis for that practice.

A discussion of metabolic expenditure has been given to illustrate the basis for the plan of maintenance therapy in common use. However, it is not necessary to calculate metabolic expenditure and then calculate maintenance. Because maintenance fluid is given at 100 mL/100 calories/d, and because metabolic expenditure is calculated as 100 calories/kg BW/d for the first 10 kg BW, 50 calories/kg BW/d for the next 10 kg BW, and 20 calories/kg BW/d for any weight above 20 kg, it is simpler to calculate maintenance more directly as 100 mL/kg BW/d for the first 10 kg BW, 50 mL/kg BW/d for the next 10 kg BW, and 20 mL/kg BW/d for any weight above 20 kg.

Examples of Maintenance Fluid Regimens

For a child weighing 8 kg, at 100 mL/kg BW/d:

$$100 \times 8 = 800 \text{ mL/d of D5W } ^1/_3 \text{ NS with 20 mEq potassium/L}$$

For a child weighing 14 kg, at 100 mL/kg BW for the first 10 kg BW and 50 mL/kg BW for the next 4 kg BW:

$$(100 \times 10) + (50 \times 4) = 1200 \text{ mL/d of D5W } ^1/_3 \text{ NS with 20 mEq potassium/L}$$

For a child weighing 25 kg, at 100 mL/kg BW for the first 10 kg BW, 50 mL/kg BW for the next 10 kg BW, and 20 mL/kg BW for the next 5 kg BW:

$$(100 \times 10) + (50 \times 10) + (20 \times 5) = 1600 \text{ mL/d of D5W } ^1/_3 \text{ NS with 20 mEq potassium/L}$$

Because parenteral fluid administration needs to be ordered in milliliters per hour, the amount may be calculated more simply as 4 mL/100 calories or metabolic kg/h, or more directly as 4 mL/kg/h for the first 10 kg of body weight, 2 mL/kg/h for the next 10 kg of body weight, and 1 mL/kg/h for each additional kilogram. This calculation gives results that are essentially the same as the calculations based on 100 mL/100 calories or metabolic kg/d.

The different methods of calculation of maintenance fluid therapy are outlined in Table 2.

When metabolic activity may be expected to be higher or lower than normal, estimates of metabolic expenditures, calculation of metabolic weight, and hence calculation of fluid allowance may need to be modified. Fever greatly increases metabolic activity. Estimated fluid allowance should be increased by 12% for every degree Celsius (7% for every degree Fahrenheit) above normal if there are reasons to believe that fever will persist for longer than a few hours. Conversely, if hypothermia is expected to be prolonged, an unlikely possibility, estimated fluid allowance should be decreased by 12% for every degree Celsius (7% for every degree Fahrenheit) below normal. It should be increased by 25% to 75% in cases of salicylism or of hyperthyroidism and decreased by 10% to 25% in hypometabolic states.

Abnormal Maintenance Requirements

In estimating maintenance fluid requirements, allowance must be made, when appropriate, for visible sweating, continuing gastrointestinal losses (persistent diarrhea, vomiting, aspiration of gastrointestinal fluid), and the oliguria usually present in acute renal failure.

Sweating. Losses through sweating should be taken into account when environmental temperature exceeds 30.5°C (87°F). For persistently higher ambient temperatures, 30% extra maintenance fluid should be given for every degree Celsius above 30.5 (17% for every degree Fahrenheit above 87).

Gastrointestinal Losses. Gastrointestinal losses need to be taken into account if they continue to be significant for more than a few hours after the institution of intravenous therapy. This is only rarely a problem because vomiting and diarrhea most commonly cease or become minimal when oral intake is suspended. With significant and continuing vomiting, diarrhea, or aspiration of gastrointestinal fluid, maintenance therapy should be modified to correct those continuing losses. It is possible in some cases (e.g., nasogastric aspirate) to measure the composition of the fluid lost and replace it accordingly. When that is not possible, the composition of the fluid given to correct continuing losses should be chosen by taking account of the most common composition of gastrointestinal fluids. Ready-made solutions for this may not be available and may need to be prepared as needed.

VOMITING OR GASTRIC ASPIRATE. This loss should be corrected, volume for volume, with a solution containing 140 mEq sodium, 15 mEq potassium, and 155 mEq chloride/L.

SMALL INTESTINAL FLUID. This loss should be corrected, volume for volume, with a solution containing 140 mEq sodium, 15 mEq potassium, 40 mEq bicarbonate, and 115 mEq chloride/L.

DIARRHEA. This loss should be corrected, volume for volume, with a solution containing 40 mEq each of sodium, potassium, bicarbonate, and chloride/L. It is often possible in hospital to estimate the amount of diarrheal losses by weighing diapers. When it is impractical to quantify the amount of diarrhea, the allowance of this solution should be 10 to 25 mL/kg/d for mild diarrhea, 25 to 50 mL/kg/d for moderate diarrhea, and 50 to 75 mL/kg/d for severe diarrhea.

OLIGURIA DUE TO ACUTE RENAL FAILURE. Parenteral fluid therapy in states of acute renal failure is a specialized subject and its discussion is outside the scope of this article.

TABLE 2. **Different Methods of Calculation of Maintenance Requirements**

Preferred Method, Based Directly on Weight	
Daily fluid allowance	100 mL/kg BW for first 10 kg BW 50 mL/kg BW for next 10 kg BW 20 mL/kg BW above 20 kg BW
Other Methods	
Method Based on Estimation of Metabolic Expenditure	
Estimation of daily metabolic expenditure	100 calories/kg BW for first 10 kg BW 50 calories/kg BW for next 10 kg BW 20 calories/kg BW above 20 kg BW
Daily fluid allowance	100 mL/100 calories
Method Based on Estimation of Metabolic Weight	
Estimation of metabolic weight	1 metabolic kg/kg BW for first 10 kg BW 0.5 metabolic kg/kg BW for next 10 kg BW 0.2 metabolic kg/kg BW above 20 kg BW
Daily fluid allowance	100 mL/metabolic kg
Calculation of Fluid Allowance in mL/h	4 mL/100 calories or metabolic kg/h or 4 mL/kg BW for first 10 kg BW/h 0.5 mL/kg BW for next 10 kg BW/h 0.2 mL/kg BW above 20 kg BW/h

See text for examples of calculations. Note that these different methods all yield the same results and are applicable only to children of weight greater than 3 kg.
Abbreviation: BW = body weight.

DEFICIT FLUID THERAPY

Deficit parenteral fluid therapy is intended to replace deficits already present when parenteral fluid therapy is started. It is most effectively based on an estimate of the degree of dehydration from which may be calculated the amount of fluid that has to be given to correct the deficit (i.e., to rehydrate the patient). In its strictest meaning, the term *dehydration* refers only to a water deficit. This may indeed be present with diabetes insipidus or prolonged water deprivation. However, in most clinical situations, water deficits are accompanied by concomitant and usually proportional electrolyte deficits. By common usage, "dehydration" refers to a water and electrolyte deficit and is usually associated with fairly mild or no abnormalities of serum electrolytes, except in the rare cases of hyponatremic dehydration (serum sodium below 130 mEq/L) or hypernatremic dehydration (serum sodium above 150 mEq/L).

Estimating the Degree of Dehydration

This is done by applying the rule of 5-10-15 for children younger than the age of 2 years and the rule of 3-6-9 for older children. For children younger than the age of 2 years, mild (i.e., barely detectable) dehydration may be considered associated with a fluid and electrolyte deficit resulting in a 5% fall in body weight. This is said to be 5% dehydration. Dehydration may be considered to be 10% when it is obvious but is associated with good circulatory status (capillary refill <3 seconds, normal or slightly low blood pressure, no obtundation). It may be considered to be 15% when it is associated with hypotension or shock (capillary refill >3 seconds, low blood pressure, apathy). In children older than the age of 2 years, clinically similar degrees of dehydration correspond to 3%, 6%, and 9% dehydration, respectively.

For any particular fluid deficit, the signs of dehydration are less conspicuous in hypernatremic dehydration, because the hypertonicity of the extracellular compartment causes an extracellular shift of water, resulting in better preservation of the extracellular compartment at the expense of the intracellular compartment. The management of hypernatremic dehydration will be discussed separately. In hyponatremic dehydration the opposite is true: the extracellular compartment is further depleted by an intracellular shift of water. This tends to increase the signs of dehydration in relation to the true deficit and leads to an overestimation of the degree of dehydration. However, the error in the estimation of the deficit in hyponatremic dehydration is not important in practice.

Having estimated the percent dehydration, the deficit may be calculated as follows:

$$\%\ \text{dehydration} \times 10 \times \text{body weight in kg} = \text{deficit (in mL)}$$

(This calculation is based on the fact that x% dehydration means that for every 100 g of body weight, there is a fluid and electrolyte deficit equal to x g. Therefore, for every kilogram of body weight, there is a deficit equal to $10x$.)

A study in which weight on admission and weight after rehydration were used to determine the severity of dehydration retrospectively showed that the most reliable signs of mild to moderate dehydration were the following:

- Decreased peripheral perfusion, determined by examining capillary refill in the nail beds. This is done by compressing a fingernail bed, thus squeezing blood out of it and looking at the time it takes for the nail bed to become pink again. This normally takes less than 2 seconds. More than 3 seconds is indicative of severe dehydration.
- Deep breathing
- Decreased skin elasticity. This is judged by pinching the skin and subcutaneous tissue of the abdominal wall or the chest. In a well-hydrated child, the skin fold should disappear instantly when it is released.
- High blood urea nitrogen
- Low blood pH
- Large base deficit

That study also showed that dehydration tended to be overestimated: mild dehydration, classically considered to be 5%, was found to be associated with a deficit only of 3% to 4%; moderate dehydration (10%) was found to be only of 5% to 6%; and severe dehydration (15%) was only of 8% to 10%. Nevertheless, calculation of deficit therapy based on the preceding considerations and the rule of 5-10-15 and 3-6-9 outlined earlier has worked well in practice and does not seem to result in volume overload.

Rehydration

Treatment of Uncomplicated Dehydration

The dehydration of a child requiring parenteral therapy may be considered uncomplicated when circulatory status is well maintained and the condition of the child suggests that it will continue to be well maintained. In those cases, the degree of dehydration is usually 5% (3% in children older than 2 years). Rehydration may be accomplished by giving the same fluid as is given for maintenance (i.e., D5W ⅓ NS). Potassium should be added, to a concentration of 20 mEq/L, once the patient has passed urine and laboratory values confirm that the patient is not in renal failure. This should be given at a rate calculated to replace the deficit over 24 hours and provide maintenance therapy simultaneously.

Example

A child weighing 14 kg on admission is considered 5% dehydrated (for explanations of calculations, see earlier discussion of calculation of maintenance fluid and of deficit therapy):

Maintenance therapy: $(10 \times 100) + (4 \times 50) = 1200$ mL
Deficit therapy: $5 \times 10 \times 14 = 700$ mL
Total: 1900 mL over 24 hours (i.e., ~80 mL/h)

For a child with mild dehydration, a common practice that saves time and calculations is to provide parenteral fluids for the first 24 hours at a rate equal to 1.5 times maintenance. In children with a body weight below 10 kg, providing fluid at 1.5 times maintenance has the effect of providing an extra 50 mL of fluid per kg/24 h. This happens to be the amount required to correct 5% dehydration. Because maintenance fluid per kilogram of body weight decreases with body weights above 10 kg, this method of treatment in bigger children provides smaller deficit replacement. For example, in a child weighing 14 kg on admission and considered 5% dehydrated, maintenance requirement is 1200 mL and 1.5 times maintenance is 1800 mL in 24 hours. In such a child the deficit, calculated separately, is 700 mL (see earlier), and maintenance plus deficit then would come to 1900 mL in the first 24 hours. A difference of this magnitude is not clinically important. In any case, dehydration is uncommon in bigger children and the question is less likely to arise. In practice, giving 1.5 times maintenance in the first 24 hours for mild dehydration has worked well.

Treatment of Severe Dehydration (10% to 15%)

Children with 10% to 15% dehydration are hemodynamically compromised, or on the verge of being hemodynamically compromised, and the rapid administration of fluid is appropriate and urgent. The fluid of choice for this is lactated Ringer's solution (sodium 130 mEq/L, potassium 4 mEq/L, chloride 109 mEq/L, lactate 28 mEq/L, and calcium 3 mEq/L). This may be given initially as a bolus of 20 mL/kg over 30 minutes and may be repeated if necessary. Lactated Ringer's is a more physiologic fluid than 0.9% saline (NS) for this purpose. The recommendation to withhold intravenous potassium until urine has been passed does not apply to the bolus administration of lactated Ringer's solution because of its low physiologic concentration of potassium. However, emergency department staff more commonly use normal saline and this has worked well. It should be noted that a 20-mL/kg bolus corrects a 2% deficit. Thus, one bolus corrects 2% dehydration and two boluses correct 4% dehydration. Fluid boluses given in an emergency department should be subtracted from the total deficit therapy.

Example

A child weighing 8 kg is considered 10% dehydrated. The total deficit is

$$10 \times 10 \times 8 = 800 \text{ mL}$$

The patient is given a 20-mL/kg (i.e., 160 mL) bolus of lactated Ringer's or normal saline in 30 minutes. At the end of the first 30 minutes the patient looks better, capillary refill has improved, and pulse rate has decreased.

The balance of the deficit is

$$800 - 160 = 640 \text{ mL}$$

From this point on the patient may be given intravenous fluids as discussed earlier under "Uncomplicated Dehydration." That is, the child may be given D5W ⅓ NS with 20 mEq potassium/L (once urine has been passed) at a rate calculated to give maintenance and the balance of the deficit in the 24 hours after admission.

More commonly, house officers simply give the same fluid at 2 times maintenance. This provides 100 mL/kg/24 h for deficit replacement therapy in the case of children weighing 10 kg or less, thus correcting 10% dehydration. The amount of fluid given in the emergency department is usually not subtracted from subsequent deficit replacement therapy, but the method works well. In children who require more than one bolus, the total deficit may have been greater than 10% and providing 2 times maintenance might be considered inadequate. However, two 20-mL/kg boluses correct 4% dehydration and 2 times maintenance corrects 10% dehydration. Thus, the total amount of deficit therapy, by this method, still proves to be adequate, even for 15% dehydration.

Because recent data have shown that the rule 5-10-15 overestimates dehydration, which is in fact 3% to 4% for mild dehydration, 5% to 6% for moderate dehydration, and 8% to 10% for severe dehydration, it would be appropriate to give 1.3 and 1.7 times maintenance (after NS boluses if necessary) instead of 1.5 or 2 times maintenance.

Treatment of Hypernatremic Dehydration

Rapid restoration of an elevated serum sodium concentration to normal is frequently associated with cerebral edema, cerebral hemorrhages, and convulsions, thought to be due to swelling of brain cells due to lag between cerebral intracellular and extracellular osmolality.

The rehydration of a child with hypernatremic dehydration should aim at reducing the serum sodium by no more than 10 mEq/d (i.e., 0.4–0.5 mEq/h) and correcting dehydration and electrolyte abnormalities over 48 hours. This may be achieved as follows.

Half of the calculated deficit, and maintenance, is given at the same rate throughout the first 24 hours. The other half of the deficit, and maintenance, should be given in the same way in the next 24 hours. Hypernatremic dehydration is associated with a disproportionate water deficit, when compared with isonatremic or hyponatremic dehydration, and with a smaller sodium deficit. Therefore, the fluid of choice for hypernatremic dehydration is 0.25% sodium chloride solution (25 mEq sodium and chloride/L, i.e., ⅙ isotonic saline, ⅙ NS). Once urine has been passed and acute renal failure has been excluded, potassium should be added in a concentration of 40 mEq/L. The higher potassium concentration has the effect of minimizing cerebral swelling and the potassium influx into muscle cells takes water with it, thus minimizing the dilution of the extracellular fluid compartment. Optimally, this should be given with a glucose concentration of only 2.5% (D2.5W) to minimize the risk of hyperglycemia often seen with hypernatremic dehydration and calcium gluconate to a concentration of 9.6 mEq/L (10 mL of 10% calcium gluconate/500 mL of parenteral solution) to minimize the risk of hypocalcemia.

Example

A child weighing 8 kg is considered 10% dehydrated. He or she is initially given a bolus of 160 mL

NS (20 mL/kg). Shortly afterward, results of electrolyte determination on blood drawn at the time of admission become available, showing a serum sodium concentration of 165 mEq/L.

Balance of deficit after 160-mL fluid bolus: $(10 \times 10 \times 8) - 160 = 640$ mL, which should be given over 48 hours (i.e., at 13.3 mL/h).

Maintenance: 800 mL/24 h (i.e., 33.3 mL/h).

Fluid regimen: D2.5W ⅙ NS with 40 mEq potassium/L and 9.6 mEq calcium/L at $13.3 + 33.3 = 46.6 \sim 47$ mL/h for 48 hours.

Treatment of Hyponatremic Dehydration

Hyponatremic dehydration may be treated in the same way as uncomplicated dehydration. Neurologic complications of hyponatremia are unlikely with a serum sodium concentration above 120 mEq/L or when hyponatremia has been present for longer than 48 hours. In the rare patient with a serum sodium level below 120 mEq/L, if the history indicates that the illness is of less than 48 hours' duration, enough hypertonic saline (3% saline [i.e., 513 mEq/L]) should be given, as a bolus, to raise the serum sodium value by 3 to 5 mEq/L. The amount of sodium that will accomplish this may be calculated as follows:

Body weight × 0.6 × desired change in serum sodium = amount of sodium to be given (mEq)

where 0.6 is the volume of distribution of sodium.

Example

A dehydrated child is found to have a serum sodium concentration of 116 mEq/L. Enough hypertonic saline should be given to raise the serum sodium value by, say, 5 mEq/L. The child weighs 8 kg, and the amount of sodium needed therefore is $8 \times 0.6 \times 5 = 24$ mEq. This requires $1000 \div 513 \times 24 = 46.8 \sim 47$ mL of 3% saline. The same result may be reached more quickly by making use of the fact that to raise the serum sodium value by 1 mEq/L requires 1.2 mL/kg of 3% saline (by this calculation the same patient would have been given $5 \times 1.2 = 6$ mL/kg [i.e., 48 mL] to increase the serum sodium by 5 mEq).

Treatment of Acidosis

Acidosis is always present to some extent in dehydrated children but corrects itself with standard rehydration therapy. However, the partial correction of the more severe degrees of acidosis (blood bicarbonate value below 10 mEq/L, blood pH below 7.2) found with severe dehydration may improve patients' clinical status and is worthwhile. In this context, it should be noted that the measurement of "CO_2" on blood chemistry panels frequently yields misleading values, often considerably below the bicarbonate value obtained by measurement of blood gases. Therefore, correction of acidosis, if any, should preferably be done after measurement of blood gases. If the serum bicarbonate value is below 10 mEq/L, and especially if the blood pH is below 7.2, a small, rapid correction of acidosis is indicated and may be accomplished by giving a bolus of sodium bicarbonate calculated to increase the serum bicarbonate value to about 15 mEq/L. This may be calculated as follows:

Amount of bicarbonate to be given mEq/L = body weight × 0.5 × desired change in serum bicarbonate value

where 0.5 is the volume of distribution of bicarbonate.

Example

A child weighing 8 kg has severe dehydration and is found to have a blood pH of 7.15 and a bicarbonate concentration of 7 mEq/L. To raise the serum bicarbonate level to 15 mEq/L requires $8 \times 0.5 \times (15 - 7) = 32$ mEq/L bicarbonate.

Duration of Parenteral Therapy

Parenteral therapy is needed until rehydration has been accomplished to an extent sufficient to ensure a good circulatory status and until oral intake of fluids is tolerated. This is often accomplished in a few hours. Indeed, many children who come to an emergency department for dehydration because of an acute gastrointestinal illness are discharged after a few hours without having required hospitalization. In those children who do require hospitalization, usually because they do not tolerate oral intake, parenteral therapy is seldom needed for longer than 24 hours. In situations in which parenteral therapy is required for reasons other than an acute gastrointestinal illness, the duration of parenteral therapy depends on its original indication; after abdominal surgery for example, parenteral fluid and electrolyte therapy may be needed for several days.

Monitoring of Patient on Parenteral Fluid and Electrolyte Therapy

Weight and vital signs should be measured and recorded on arrival, and blood should be drawn for measurement of serum electrolytes, blood urea nitrogen, serum creatinine, and blood cell count. Subsequently, urinary output should be recorded and vital signs should be checked periodically, the frequency depending on the patient's initial status. Serum electrolytes should then be checked every 6 to 8 hours in the case of hypernatremic dehydration and every 12 to 24 hours in other cases. If a bolus of hypertonic saline is given, the serum sodium value should be checked as soon as possible after the bolus has been given. The same is true for blood bicarbonate; blood gases should be checked after a bolus of bicarbonate. Blood urea nitrogen and creatinine need not be measured again if they were normal on admission and if urinary output remains good.

PARENTERAL FLUID THERAPY OF THE NEONATE

This is a specialized subject outside the scope of this article and the discussions given earlier are not

TABLE 3. **Summary of Parenteral Fluid and Electrolyte Therapy**

Maintenance Fluid and Electrolyte Therapy

Fluid to be given: D5W ⅓ NS with 20 mEq potassium/L
Daily amount to be given:
100 mL/kg BW for the first 10 kg
50 mL/kg BW for the next 10 kg
20 mL/kg BW for any weight above 20 kg

Treatment of Uncomplicated Dehydration

D5W ⅓ NS with 20 mEq potassium/L at 1.3. to 1.5 × maintenance for the first 24 hours

Treatment of Severe Dehydration

One or two boluses of lactated Ringer's or NS rapidly, then D5W ⅓ NS with 20 mEq potassium/L at 1.7 to 2 × maintenance for the first 24 hours

Treatment of Hypernatremic Dehydration

D2.5 W ⅙ NS with 40 mEq potassium/L and calcium gluconate to a concentration of 9.6 mEq/L at maintenance + half of deficit in first 24 hours and the same again in second 24 hours

See text for example of calculations. Note plan of maintenance fluid therapy is applicable only to children weighing more than 3 kg.

applicable to infants in the neonatal period. Fluid requirements for the neonate depend on the age and on the size of the infant. For a full-term infant on day 1 of life, a maintenance allowance of 70 to 80 mL/kg/d is appropriate. This is gradually increased to 140 to 160 mL/kg/d by day 5 of life. The fluid of choice is D5W or D10W ⅙ NS with 10 mEq potassium/L and calcium as indicated. In infants of low birth weight, fluid requirements are much higher and depend on the infant's gestational age, skin texture, temperature control, and environment. In general, the smaller the infant is, the higher the fluid allowance per kilogram of body weight needs to be. In addition, because infants of very low birth weight cannot tolerate enteral feeding, parenteral nutrition is usually started immediately.

CONCLUSION

A summary of parenteral fluid and electrolyte therapy is presented in Table 3.

ACKNOWLEDGMENTS

The material in this article is largely derived from the work of R. W. Winters, M. A. Holliday, and W. E. Segar, L. Finberg, and A. Mackenzie, to whom I am indebted. I am indebted also to my colleagues and to members of our house staff for their help in preparing this article.

Section 8

The Endocrine System

ACROMEGALY

method of
SHEREEN EZZAT, M.D.
University of Toronto
Toronto, Ontario, Canada

Regardless of etiology, sustained growth hormone (GH) excess results in physical disfigurement associated with debilitating arthritis, cardiac dysfunction, colonic neoplasia, and reduced survival. Current understanding of the pathophysiology of GH hypersecretion as it relates to the diagnosis, complications, and treatment of patients with acromegaly is discussed here.

DIAGNOSIS

The diagnosis of acromegaly rests on the demonstration of excessive, autonomous secretion of GH. Isolated, random sampling of serum GH is usually insufficient to establish the diagnosis because GH secretion is rhythmic and under dual regulation by the hypothalamus. GH-releasing hormone (GHRH) stimulates GH synthesis and release, whereas somatostatin (SS) suppresses its release. SS secretion is also episodic and is increased during fasting, during sleep, and in obese individuals. In normal individuals sampled during a 12-hour period, at least 75% of serum GH values are below the limits of assay detection (<0.2 ng/mL) and circulating serum GH levels may spontaneously reach several times the normal range in healthy individuals. Patients with active acromegaly may have GH levels within the normal range. Therefore, based on currently available GH assays, the diagnosis of acromegaly requires demonstration of lack of GH suppression to less than 1 ng/mL after the oral ingestion of 75 g of glucose.

Although somatic growth in adults is primarily under the influence of GH, its effects are largely mediated through insulin-like growth factor I (IGF-I), previously known as somatomedin-C (Sm-C). This growth factor is produced in most tissues and acts locally to regulate cell growth and differentiation. Circulating IGF-I is mainly of hepatic and possibly adipose tissue origin and is GH dependent. Serum IGF-I levels are usually elevated in most patients with active acromegaly. Poorly controlled diabetes mellitus results in impaired hepatic production of IGF-I. Similarly, IGF-I levels decline with normal aging and during periods of starvation. IGF-I levels also rise during normal pregnancy, reaching two to three times nonpregnant values. With these exceptions, an elevated IGF-I level confirms the diagnosis of acromegaly. Moreover, circulating levels of total IGF-I do not fluctuate as rapidly as levels of GH. Indeed, serial IGF-I levels have proven to be a practical alternative for measuring disease activity in most acromegalic patients.

MONITORING OF DISEASE ACTIVITY

Traditional polyclonal radioimmunoassays were considered to result in suppression of GH to less than 2 ng/mL after an oral glucose challenge in normal subjects. This was also accepted as evidence for acromegaly disease remission. Most laboratories now use the more sensitive immunoradiometric assays, with a normal cutoff of less than 1.0 ng/mL after glucose ingestion. With the development of more sensitive IGF-I and IGF-binding protein-3 (IGFBP-3) assays, additional tools are now available to assess the GH/IGF-I axis. Studies have demonstrated that sensitive GH measurements by immunoradiometric assay are superior to the radioimmunoassay method in that overlap between patients with and without active disease is eliminated. Furthermore, whereas serum IGFBP-3 levels correlate overall with IGF-I levels, total IGFBP-3 levels are not always predictive of disease status. Up to a third of patients with active disease have normal total IGFBP-3 levels. Correlating patients' symptoms with these measurements is essential, especially in the unusual cases in which GH and IGF-I measurements are discordant.

TREATMENT OBJECTIVES

The aims of treatment in acromegaly include restoration of normal GH secretion and responsiveness to stimulation as well as attainment of a normal age-adjusted IGF-I level. The presence of any mass effect should be relieved. Most importantly, however, is the arrest or prevention of long-term complications and excess mortality associated with this condition.

The general consensus is that acromegaly is associated with double the risk of mortality, usually from cardiovascular and neoplastic diseases. Multivariate analysis revealed that survival was significantly influenced by the last known GH, presence of hypertension or cardiac disease at diagnosis, and duration of symptoms before diagnosis. Survival among acromegalic patients was reduced by an average of 10 years.

A more recent multicenter retrospective cohort study of 1362 patients from the United Kingdom also revealed that the mortality rate due to colon cancer was higher than expected. This and another U.S.-based study confirmed that overall mortality rate in patients with post-treatment GH levels less than 2.5 ng/mL was comparable with that of the general population. These data provide the framework for more rational objective measures to validate treatment outcomes.

THERAPEUTIC OPTIONS

Therapeutic options for management of acromegaly and/or gigantism include pharmacotherapy, surgery, and/or radiation. Regardless of the approach, it is important to recognize that the criteria that represent biochemical cure may be difficult to achieve. For each type of pituitary adenoma associated with a distinct clinical syndrome, over the years specialists have gravitated in attitude from one end of the spectrum to the other.

Surgery

Trans-sphenoidal adenomectomy by an experienced neurosurgeon has traditionally been viewed as the primary form of treatment. A subfrontal approach is sometimes necessary for patients with tumors demonstrating extensive suprasellar or parasellar extension. Rapid reduction in GH levels with concomitant improvement in clinical symptomatology can be achieved. GH levels are reduced to less than 5 ng/mL in up to 80% of patients with microadenomas and in 50% to 60% of those harboring macroadenomas. The frequency of surgical success, however, is closely correlated to the size and degree of invasiveness of the tumor, as well as to the surgical expertise.

Pharmacologic Approaches

The development of SS analogues has resulted in a more aggressive attitude toward the management of patients with persistently active disease. Although SS analogues reduce GH and IGF-I levels and alleviate symptoms in 50% to 70% of patients, tumor size reduction is limited to, at most, 30% of patients. These findings have supported the use of these agents as secondary therapy in patients who have had surgery and who continue to have elevated GH and IGF-I levels.

In addition, medical therapy has been advocated for acromegalic patients who refuse surgery or who are poor surgical candidates. The controversial issue revolves around whether medical therapy should be considered as *primary* therapy for patients with acromegaly. Limited data from nonrandomized studies demonstrate that SS analogues are effective as long-term agents in normalizing GH and IGF-I levels in approximately two thirds of patients who have not been operated on. The general consensus is that patients with GH-secreting microadenomas should undergo surgery to obtain definitive adenomectomy. For those with macroadenomas, medical debulking might be considered with the view that the two treatments may work synergistically. Medical therapy is better justified as initial management. Depending on the response, subsequent surgery may improve the benefits.

Octreotide (Sandostatin) was the first synthetic modified octapeptide analogue of SS that resists enzymatic degradation and had an extended half-life of nearly 2 hours, lending itself to clinical application for suppression of GH hypersecretion. This agent has now been in use for more than a decade. Its clinical effects, the rapid and significant improvement of most features of the disease, are well described. Mean GH levels decline by more than 25% in 70% of subjects, usually within an hour of administration of 100 μg of octreotide subcutaneously. Maximal suppression is reached within 2 hours and usually lasts for 6 hours. Because the GH response is rapid, this assessment can be done at the outset to identify responsive patients.

In subjects whose GH levels return to baseline before the end of the dosing interval, the frequency of administration can be increased. To address some of these shortcomings, newer formulations of SS analogues (octreotide, lanreotide) with even longer actions have been developed. Administered as a single intramuscular injection (10–30 mg every 10–28 days), they result in similar clinical benefits to those achieved with the subcutaneous form. Nevertheless, direct comparison between the subcutaneous and long-acting preparations of the SS analogues in controlling acromegaly-related complications remains to be demonstrated.

The impact of SS analogues on acromegaly-related complications is best studied in terms of impaired cardiovascular function. Glucose-suppressed GH levels to less than 1 ng/mL together with normalization of plasma IGF-I levels for 1 year have been shown to be associated with significant improvement, but not complete normalization, of left ventricular ejection fraction. In contrast, persistence of elevated GH was associated with increased systolic blood pressure and impaired cardiac performance.

SS analogues represent the current agents of choice in the medical treatment of acromegaly. Where they fall within the scheme of management of different patients, however, requires individual assessment. The use of SS analogues is of obvious potential benefit to those patients with persistently nonsuppressible GH and elevated IGF-I levels after pituitary surgery. It may also constitute primary therapy for those who cannot tolerate surgery. Less clear is the potential role of these agents as primary therapy for those with aggressive lesions in whom surgically induced remissions are difficult, if not impossible, to achieve.

GH-receptor antagonists represent a new class of therapy. The agent developed competes with natural GH for binding with the GH receptor. Unlike normal GH, this antagonist prevents GH receptor dimerization and signaling, thus blocking GH action and IGF-I generation. Daily subcutaneous administration (10–20 mg) of the first antagonist (Pegvisomant) resulted in normalization of IGF-I levels in nearly 80% of acromegalic patients. This investigational drug is under review by the Food and Drug Administration. Its long-term effects on pituitary tumor growth as well as other acromegaly-associated conditions are unknown.

Radiotherapy

This adjunctive therapeutic option is usually reserved for patients who have failed pituitary surgery and/or medical therapy. It has lost momentum in the past few years as more studies emerge reporting lack of efficacy in achieving normalization of IGF-I levels.

Multiple techniques for irradiation of pituitary tumors have been examined. Conventional external-beam irradiation results in GH reduction in most subjects. GH levels decline by approximately 15% per year such that values less than 5 ng/mL are reached by 40% and 70% of subjects after 5 and 10 years, respectively. Tumor growth is arrested, followed by size regression. Adverse effects include transient hair loss and irreversible hypopituitarism. However, IGF-I normalization rates are disappointing. More significant is the finding that a random GH concentration less than 1.5 ng/mL was associated with a pathologically high IGF-I in nearly half of patients. Recently, gamma knife stereotactic radiotherapy has been investigated. Mean time to normalization of GH and IGF-I levels was 1.5 years in the group treated with the gamma knife compared with 7.1 years in those treated with fractionated radiotherapy. These early results suggest that the use of stereotactic radiosurgery may become the preferred treatment of choice for patients with surgical and medically refractory disease.

CONCLUSION

Acromegaly is often a chronic debilitating condition that, if left uncontrolled, is associated with increased morbidity and mortality. The diagnosis is established by documenting autonomous GH hypersecretion and by imaging of the pituitary. Surgical

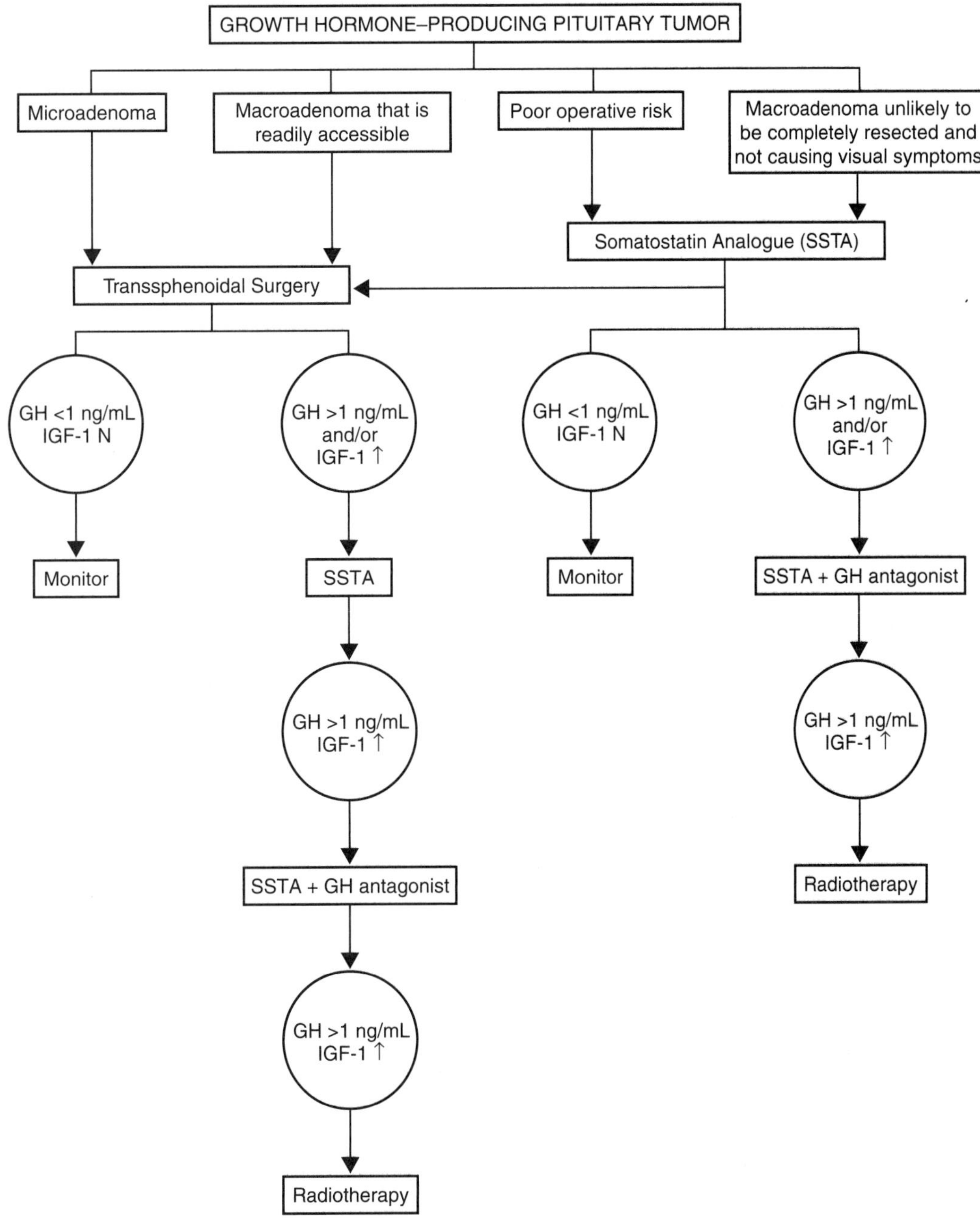

Figure 1. Therapeutic algorithm of growth hormone–producing pituitary tumor.

resection of the responsible pituitary adenoma represents the cornerstone of management. This has been challenged, however, because a strict target of normalization of IGF-I and a glucose suppressed GH to less than 1 ng/mL is difficult to achieve by surgery alone.

Adjunctive therapy is frequently necessary, because complete resection is often not possible. This has prompted the view that primary medical therapy may be a suitable option to consider for some patients. Persistent disease is now well documented to be associated with increased morbidity and mortality. A suggested therapeutic algorithm is shown in Figure 1. SS analogues are of particular benefit to those patients with persistently nonsuppressible GH and/or elevated IGF-I levels after pituitary surgery or during the interim period after radiation therapy. SS analogues may also constitute primary therapy for those who decline, are not likely to achieve a remission, or cannot tolerate surgery or irradiation. The use of GH antagonists alone or in combination with SS analogues, although pharmacologically rational, remains to be proven.

ACKNOWLEDGMENT

The author wishes to acknowledge the invaluable technical assistance of Ms. W. Maharaj.

ADRENOCORTICAL INSUFFICIENCY

method of
TREVOR A. HOWLETT, M.D.
University of Leicester Medical School and Leicester Royal Infirmary
Leicester, England

Adrenocortical insufficiency is a life-threatening hormonal deficiency that is readily treatable but that commonly presents with long-standing, vague symptomatology. It may be the presenting symptom of serious pituitary disease, may be associated with other endocrine deficiencies and autoimmune diseases, or may result from long-term corticosteroid therapy for other diseases. It is therefore essential that all physicians can recognize the condition and initiate appropriate investigations and emergency therapy.

ETIOLOGY

Adrenocortical insufficiency may result from disease of the adrenal itself—primary adrenal failure, or Addison disease—or from decreased adrenocorticotropic hormone (ACTH) secretion due to disease of the pituitary and/or hypothalamus—secondary adrenocortical insufficiency, or ACTH deficiency.

Primary Adrenal Failure

Primary adrenal failure is caused by autoimmune adrenalitis in more than 90% of patients. This is often associated with a personal, or family, history of other autoimmune conditions, most commonly hypothyroidism and vitiligo but also primary hypoparathyroidism, premature ovarian failure, diabetes mellitus type 1, and thyrotoxicosis, as well as pernicious anemia and ulcerative colitis.

Tuberculosis of the adrenal was historically the most common cause, as described by Thomas Addison; this had become a rarity in developed countries but is now increasing again in certain communities with the increasing incidence of AIDS. Other causes are relatively rare (Table 1).

Secondary Adrenocortical Insufficiency—ACTH Deficiency

ACTH deficiency usually occurs in the context of other pituitary disease but is often the presenting symptom of the pituitary disorder and may occasionally occur as an isolated deficiency. Other than iatrogenic suppression by corticosteroid therapy, the most common cause is an expanding benign pituitary macroadenoma, which either interrupts the passage of corticotropin-releasing hormone (CRH) from the hypothalamus to the pituitary in the portal vessels of the pituitary stalk or destroys the corticotrophs themselves. Other causes are listed in Table 2. Many of these affect the hypothalamus and CRH secretion rather than the pituitary itself.

CLINICAL PRESENTATION

Primary and secondary adrenocortical insufficiency usually present as long-standing, vague symptomatology of ill health, but both may present as a life-threatening emergency, or "adrenal (addisonian) crisis," when severe intercurrent illness occurs in the absence of a normal corticosteroid stress response.

Chronic symptoms include general malaise, tiredness, weakness, anorexia, weight loss, dizziness (often associated with postural hypotension), headache, and vague abdominal pain or discomfort. This may be superimposed on symptoms of hypothyroidism, due to associated autoimmune thyroid failure or thyroid-stimulating hormone (TSH) deficiency. Gonadal symptoms may occur, with loss of libido, menstrual irregularity, and sometimes loss of secondary sexual hair in women (due to loss of adrenal androgens), and these symptoms may be profound if associated with gonadotropin deficiency. In primary adrenal failure, pigmentation is common and caused by high circulating ACTH levels that are raised from loss of negative feedback from cortisol. Pigmentation classically involves

TABLE 1. **Causes of Primary Adrenal Failure**

Common
Autoimmune adrenalitis
Uncommon
Tuberculosis
Metastasis to adrenals
Hemorrhage or infarction of adrenals (e.g., meningococcal septicemia or antiphospholipid syndrome)
Iatrogenic: bilateral adrenalectomy or associated with nephrectomy
Rare
Other granulomatous disease
Adrenoleukodystrophy
Congenital adrenal hypoplasia
AIDS

TABLE 2. **Causes of ACTH Deficiency**

Pituitary Adenoma
Nonfunctioning, prolactinoma, acromegaly, TSH-oma
Other Pituitary and Parapituitary Tumors
Craniopharyngioma, Rathke pouch and other cysts, chordoma, meningioma, suprasellar germinoma, etc.
Metastasis to Pituitary
Hypophysitis
Lymphocytic, granulomatous, autoimmune
Granulomatous Disease of Pituitary/Hypothalamus
Sarcoid, tuberculosis, Wegener, histiocytosis X
Isolated ACTH Deficiency
Congenital or idiopathic
Pituitary Infarction or Hemorrhage
Iatrogenic
Hypothalamic and pituitary irradiation
Pituitary and parapituitary surgery
Medium to long-term corticosteroid therapy for other medical conditions (>7.5 mg prednisolone or >0.5 mg dexamethasone daily)

Abbreviations: ACTH = adrenocorticotropic hormone; TSH = thyroid-stimulating hormone.

palmar creases, buccal mucosa, recent scars, and pressure areas but may simply be apparent as an increased general "tan." Symptoms of hypotension and hypovolemia are more marked in primary adrenal disease, owing to associated mineralocorticoid deficiency (in ACTH deficiency the renin-angiotensin-aldosterone axis is intact).

In the general population, such chronic symptoms are common and usually due to other underlying disease, depression, chronic fatigue syndrome, or often no identifiable disease. The diagnosis of adrenocortical insufficiency is therefore primarily by biochemical investigation, but the challenge is to identify the rare case of adrenocortical deficiency among the many patients with nonspecific symptoms.

Adrenal crisis, in contrast, is dramatic and life-threatening. The patient presents as an emergency with hypotension, semiconscious or unconscious, and seriously ill—usually precipitated by another acute illness, commonly prolonged diarrhea or vomiting, infection at any site (e.g., pneumonia), infarction (e.g., myocardial), and emergency or elective surgery. Hypoglycemia or hyponatremia are frequently associated. Crisis may occur in the undiagnosed patient as the presenting feature or in an established case when corticosteroid replacement has been omitted or not appropriately increased for stressful illness. Biochemical features (see later) are characteristic.

INVESTIGATION

In suspected adrenal crisis, treatment should not be delayed while awaiting the results of biochemical investigations, but cortisol (and, if possible, ACTH) assay should be requested on the sample taken before immediate treatment is begun. Under other circumstances, the diagnosis should be confirmed biochemically before treatment.

Basal cortisol taken at 8:00 to 9:00 AM gives valuable guidance and may be diagnostic. In severe deficiency, cortisol is often undetectable (<25 nmol/L [<1 μg/dL]), and any level less than 100 nmol/L (3.6 μg/dL) is highly correlated with deficiency and demands further investigation but is occasionally seen in normal individuals. A cortisol level greater than 550 nmol/L (20 μg/dL) is usually taken to indicate normality, and more than 400 nmol/L (14.5 μg/dL) is highly correlated with a normal stress response. Levels lower than this during acute illness are highly suspicious. However, in severe intercurrent illness (when levels are often in the thousands of nanomoles per liter), even such levels may sometimes represent deficiency. Levels between 100 and 400 nmol/L represent a progressively decreasing likelihood of deficiency, but confirmation requires a dynamic test.

Short ACTH Stimulation Test (Synacthen Test)

Tetracosactrin (Cortrosyn/Synacthen*), 250 μg, is administered intravenously or intramuscularly, and cortisol is measured basally and after 30 minutes. Normal 30-minute responses vary slightly between genders and between different cortisol assays, so that an appropriate reference range must be used. In our laboratory, a peak cortisol value greater than 600 nmol/L (21.8 μg/dL) is normal and makes adrenal insufficiency very unlikely; however, occasionally normal individuals show slightly lower responses than this and patients with mild deficiency may "pass" the test (especially if the cause is ACTH deficiency and/or the patient is stressed). I therefore regard a peak response of 400 to 600 nmol/L as "equivocal," requiring further investigation, and also advise that additional investigations are required if a patient, especially with pituitary disease, remains typically symptomatic after a normal Synacthen test (SST).

Further Investigations and Differential Diagnosis

If an SST is abnormal, then an 8:00 to 9:00 AM ACTH level (before replacement) can confirm the differential diagnosis. The ACTH level is markedly elevated in primary adrenal failure and low or (inappropriately) normal in ACTH deficiency. If this test is not available, or not obtained until after some time on corticosteroid replacement, then other tests may be required to confirm the diagnosis.

Adrenal antibodies are frequently, but not always, positive in patients with autoimmune primary adrenal failure.

Basal tests of other pituitary hormone axes (free thyroxine + TSH, luteinizing hormone/follicle-stimulating hormone + testosterone or estradiol, prolactin) may demonstrate other pituitary deficiencies and hence clinch a diagnosis of ACTH deficiency. These tests may also be useful in a patient with symptoms suggestive of hypoadrenalism but a normal SST. If evidence of pituitary deficiency is established, then pituitary magnetic resonance imaging is mandatory to exclude a pituitary or hypothalamic mass (see Table 2).

Using depot tetracosactrin (Synacthen),* 1 mg and monitoring cortisol response over 24 hours can distinguish secondary adrenal insufficiency (cortisol slowly rises to normal between 30 minutes and 24 hours) from primary adrenal failure (no further response).

In a nonstressed individual the SST is usually sufficient to diagnose or exclude deficiency. However, in the presence of known pituitary disease, ACTH deficiency may occasionally be present when the SST is "normal" and further investigations are indicated if the patient is symptomatic (some endocrinologists would insist on an additional test even if the patient was asymptomatic). In this case, the gold standard is to assess the cortisol response to hypoglycemia using an insulin tolerance test, a complex test that

*Not available in the United States.

is potentially hazardous and should be performed only in experienced hands and in appropriate facilities. Alternatives include glucagon and metyrapone tests, but all require specialist interpretation.

Other Biochemical Abnormalities

Hyponatremia is a common biochemical marker of adrenocortical insufficiency, particularly under conditions of stress, and hypoadrenalism should always be excluded in a patient with persistent or recurrent hyponatremia. With the coexistent mineralocorticoid deficiency of primary adrenal failure, hyperkalemia and elevation of urea/blood urea nitrogen and creatinine also typically occur. This characteristic combination of low sodium, high potassium, and high urea/blood urea nitrogen in a sick patient should always lead to investigation for possible adrenocortical insufficiency, but note that electrolyte levels may remain normal in the absence of stressful illness.

Hypoglycemia may occur as part of an adrenal crisis but is rare otherwise.

Thyroid function tests in newly diagnosed severe primary adrenal failure commonly show the pattern of primary hypothyroidism; this may be due to coexistent autoimmune primary hypothyroidism but may also be a temporary finding that resolves with adequate glucocorticoid replacement.

Hypercalcemia is an occasional biochemical marker of adrenal insufficiency, particularly primary adrenal disease, which resolves with glucocorticoid replacement. Hypercalcemia may rarely be the presenting feature and can mask coexistent severe primary hypoparathyroidism until after glucocorticoid replacement.

Eosinophilia is typically present and may be the presenting abnormality.

TREATMENT

Acute

Adrenal crisis is a medical emergency, and treatment must begin as soon as the diagnosis is suspected (after drawing blood for cortisol). Hydrocortisone, 100 mg intravenously or intramuscularly, should be given immediately, with intravenous normal saline to correct fluid and salt depletion, and 5% dextrose if hypoglycemia is present. An underlying cause of stressful illness precipitating the crisis should be sought and treated.

Hydrocortisone can be continued at 100 mg intramuscularly or intravenously every 6 hours until the condition is stabilized and/or the patient is able to take oral medication. Thereafter, two to three times the usual oral replacement dose will usually be required for several days depending on the underlying stressful illness.

Long Term

After acute treatment or after diagnosis in a nonacute presentation, glucocorticoid replacement is usually given in the form of hydrocortisone (the generic drug name for cortisol). The plasma half-life of cortisol is fewer than 2 hours and, if very high peak levels are to be avoided, then adequate circulating levels of hydrocortisone can usually only be maintained throughout the day by thrice-daily dosing.

My usual starting dose is hydrocortisone, 10 mg immediately after rising, 5 mg at lunchtime, and 5 mg early evening—a dose that most commonly achieves optimal levels. Thereafter, dosage may be monitored and adjusted using a "hydrocortisone day curve." Patients collect a 24-hour urine sample for free cortisol on the day before the test, beginning and finishing the collection immediately before the morning dose of hydrocortisone, taken at the normal time, at home, on awakening. Plasma cortisol is measured at 9:00 AM, 12:30 PM (before any lunchtime dose), and 5:30 PM (before the evening dose) during a day-case attendance. I advise adjustment of doses to achieve a 9:00 AM cortisol and urine sample for free cortisol within the reference range for the normal population (to avoid overreplacement), with 12:30 PM and 5:30 PM levels above 50 nmol/L (2 μg/dL) to avoid underreplacement at these times. Such levels are most commonly achieved using 10-mg/5- to 10-mg/5-mg regimens, which correlate with recent estimates of normal cortisol production rates.

Patients with primary adrenal failure also require mineralocorticoid replacement in the form of fludrocortisone (Florinef), initially, 100 μg once daily, with dosage monitored clinically by means of blood pressure and biochemically by plasma renin levels (high if replacement is inadequate and suppressed on excessive treatment).

Intercurrent Illness

Patient education is an essential part of the management of adrenocortical insufficiency, in particular, knowledge about appropriate increases in replacement during intercurrent illness when adrenal crisis might otherwise occur.

No change in dose is usually required for minor illness such as a "cold," sore throat, or minor psychological stress, but doses should be doubled during more serious pyrexial or other stressful illness or major psychological stress (e.g., bereavement). During vomiting or diarrheal illness, doses need to be further increased and parenteral hydrocortisone therapy begun if the patient is unable to keep down the tablets or if hypotension occurs. This usually requires admission to a hospital, but if practical the patient should have an ampule of hydrocortisone and syringe available at home, which the patient or family members may be taught to inject.

For planned surgical procedures, hydrocortisone, 100 mg intramuscularly, will provide full cover for 6 hours, which may be sufficient for minor operations. For longer, more stressful procedures, hydrocortisone, 100 mg intramuscularly every 6 hours, is appropriate, followed by two to three times the normal oral dose when able to take oral medication. Alternatively, a continuous intravenous infusion of hydrocortisone, 5 mg/h (preceded by a 25-mg intravenous bolus), will maintain adequate high circulating levels, where an infusion can be reliably maintained and monitored.

Withdrawing Long-Term Corticosteroid Therapy

Numerically, ACTH deficiency most commonly results from supraphysiologic doses of glucocorticoid for other medical conditions (e.g., asthma). The degree of suppression depends on a combination of dose and duration but may be profound after months or years on high doses. A frequent clinical problem is to know when adrenal suppression has recovered and corticosteroids can be safely stopped. This is complex because if adrenals are suppressed then full replacement is indicated; yet this very replacement will tend to maintain the suppression. My approach in established suppression is as follows:

1. Reduce corticosteroids as underlying disease dictates and perform no adrenal test until reaching a dose of prednisolone, 5 mg daily (or equivalent).
2. After several weeks or months on this dose, measure cortisol at 8:00 to 9:00 AM one morning before the dose of corticosteroid (prednisolone cross reacts in most cortisol assays). Management depends on the result.
3. If more than 400 nmol/L (14.5 μg/dL), stop corticosteroids if underlying disease permits. Reassess further with SST some weeks after stopping to ensure a normal response.
4. If less than 100 nmol/L (3.6 μg/dL), continue corticosteroids in replacement dose. Consider a change to hydrocortisone in physiologic doses and subsequent slow withdrawal, starting with an evening dose and monitoring 8:00 to 9:00 AM cortisol levels.
5. If 100 to 400 nmol/L, slowly reduce corticosteroid replacement unless the patient is symptomatic, perhaps changing to hydrocortisone, but do not reduce below prednisolone 2.5 mg/hydrocortisone 10 mg daily unless the morning cortisol level is above 250 nmol/L. At this stage a normal SST may allow corticosteroids to be stopped.

Confounding factors include recurrence of the original corticosteroid responsive disease and ongoing ACTH and cortisol suppression by high-dose inhaled corticosteroids.

All patients on steroid therapy and within 1 year of stopping prolonged therapy are likely to require corticosteroid cover for serious intercurrent illness.

CUSHING'S SYNDROME

method of
WILLIAM F. YOUNG, Jr., M.D.
Mayo Clinic and Mayo Foundation
Rochester, Minnesota

Cushing's syndrome is a symptom complex that results from prolonged exposure to supraphysiologic concentrations of glucocorticoids. It is associated with an unmistakable phenotypic picture and is curable when correctly diagnosed and properly treated. When undiagnosed or improperly treated, it can be fatal. The source of excess glucocorticoids may be exogenous (iatrogenic) or endogenous. Endogenous Cushing's syndrome is caused by hypersecretion of adrenocorticotropic hormone (ACTH; ACTH-dependent Cushing's syndrome) or by primary adrenal hypersecretion of glucocorticoids (ACTH-independent Cushing's syndrome) (Table 1). The overall treatment program for patients with Cushing's syndrome includes the resolution of hypercortisolism; the concomitant treatment of the complications of Cushing's syndrome (e.g., hypertension, osteoporosis, and diabetes mellitus); and, following definitive treatment, the management of glucocorticoid withdrawal and hypothalamic-pituitary-adrenal (HPA) axis recovery.

PRESENTATION

Typical signs and symptoms of Cushing's syndrome include weight gain with central obesity, facial rounding and plethora, supraclavicular and dorsocervical fat pads, easy bruising, fine cigarette-paper skin, poor wound healing, purple striae, proximal muscle weakness, emotional and cognitive changes (e.g., irritability, spontaneous tearfulness, depression, restlessness), hypertension, osteoporosis, opportunistic and fungal infections (e.g., mucocutaneous candidiasis, tinea versicolor, pityriasis), altered reproductive function, and hirsutism. These clinical features may occur slowly; thus, comparison of the patient's current appearance with old photographs is invaluable. Standard laboratory studies may reveal fasting hyperglycemia, hypokalemia, hyperlipidemia, and leukocytosis with relative lymphopenia.

DIAGNOSIS

An accurate diagnosis of Cushing's syndrome and its subtype is essential to direct the appropriate treatment. The diagnostic evaluation of Cushing's syndrome typically proceeds as outlined in Table 2. Hypercortisolism must be suspected and then confirmed with measurements of serum and 24-hour urine cortisol concentrations. Autonomous hypercortisolism may be confirmed with the low-dose dexamethasone suppression test (dexamethasone 0.5 mg orally every 6 hours for 48 hours); a 24-hour urinary cortisol excretion greater than or equal to 20 μg confirms the

TABLE 1. **Causes of Cushing's Syndrome**

Exogenous glucocorticoid administration: most common cause
Endogenous
ACTH-dependent (85%)
Pituitary
Corticotrophic adenoma (70%)
Corticotrophic multinodular hyperplasia (rare)
Ectopic
Ectopic ACTH-secreting tumor (15%)
Ectopic CRH-secreting tumor (rare)
Ectopic ACTH- and CRH-secreting tumor (rare)
ACTH-independent (15%)
Unilateral adrenal disease
Adenoma (8%)
Carcinoma (7%)
Bilateral adrenal disease
Massive macronodular hyperplasia (rare)
Primary pigmented nodular adrenal disease (rare)

Abbreviations: ACTH = adrenocorticotropic hormone; CRH = corticotropin-releasing hormone.

TABLE 2. **Diagnostic Evaluation of Cushing's Syndrome**

Confirmation of hypercortisolism
Clinical assessment
Baseline glucocorticoids (serum cortisol levels, urinary free cortisol excretion), and low-dose dexamethasone suppression test
Subtype diagnosis
Plasma ACTH
Subtype and localization studies
Directed computerized imaging
Inferior petrosal sinus sampling for ACTH with oCRH stimulation

Abbreviations: ACTH = adrenocorticotropic hormone; oCRH = ovine corticotropin-releasing hormone.

diagnosis. However, the low-dose dexamethasone suppression test may produce false-negative results in patients with mild pituitary-dependent Cushing's syndrome. The plasma ACTH concentration classifies the subtype of hypercortisolism as ACTH-dependent ("normal" to high levels of ACTH) or ACTH-independent (undetectable ACTH).

Unfortunately, the diagnosis of Cushing's syndrome is not always straightforward. Baseline 24-hour urinary cortisol measurements may be elevated by alcoholism, depression, high urine volume (>5 L/24 h), carbamazepine (Tegretol), and severe illness. In addition, all forms of endogenous Cushing's syndrome can produce cortisol in a cyclical fashion that confounds the biochemical documentation and interpretation of suppression testing.

Because of their lack of precision, high-dose dexamethasone suppression, metyrapone (Metopirone) stimulation, and ovine corticotropin-releasing hormone stimulation tests are rarely performed to differentiate ectopic from pituitary-dependent Cushing's syndrome. If a well-defined pituitary tumor is not found on computed tomography, further evaluation with inferior petrosal sinus sampling for ACTH with ovine corticotropin-releasing hormone is indicated (Figure 1).

However, in patients with ACTH-independent hypercortisolism, the high-dose dexamethasone suppression test shows no suppression in urinary cortisol excretion (see Figure 1). In these patients, computed tomography of the adrenal glands usually indicates the type of adrenal disease (see Table 1).

The diagnosis and subtype evaluation are usually complicated. A delay in diagnosis of severe Cushing's syndrome may be fatal. Tertiary care centers are best equipped to provide prompt diagnosis and treatment.

PRINCIPLES OF TREATMENT

Selective pituitary adenectomy by transsphenoidal surgery (TSS) is the treatment of choice for patients with pituitary-dependent disease. The long-term surgical cure rate for ACTH-secreting microadenomas is approximately 90%. If pituitary surgery is not curative, bilateral laparoscopic adrenalectomy and/or pituitary irradiation are adjunctive treatment options. Surgical extirpation of an adrenal adenoma or carcinoma or the source of ectopic ACTH production is the treatment of choice for patients with primary adrenocortical disease or ectopic ACTH production. Bilateral laparoscopic adrenalectomy is the preferred treatment for patients with ACTH-independent bilateral macronodular or micronodular hyperplasia. Pharmacologic therapy is reserved for patients not cured with these surgical approaches.

Iatrogenic Cushing's Syndrome

Usually, iatrogenic Cushing's syndrome is the unfortunate accompaniment of the appropriate treatment of a life-threatening or debilitating inflammatory disorder (e.g., vasculitis, severe asthma) with supraphysiologic doses of glucocorticoids. The most frequently used preparation is prednisone (Deltasone). It has been suggested, but not proven, that alternate-day steroid therapy results in fewer side effects and less suppression of the HPA axis. HPA suppression can occur with high-dose (>25 mg prednisone or equivalent per day) glucocorticoid therapy for more than 1 week or lower doses (>12.5 mg prednisone or equivalent per day) for more than 4 weeks. If glucocorticoid therapy must be continued, the lowest possible dose that effectively treats the underlying disorder should be sought.

Pituitary-Dependent Cushing's Syndrome

The treatment of choice for pituitary-dependent Cushing's syndrome is transsphenoidal selective adenectomy by an experienced neurosurgeon. Inferior petrosal sinus sampling for ACTH should be considered in patients without an obvious pituitary tumor on sellar magnetic resonance imaging. In cases where an obvious tumor is not found intraopera-

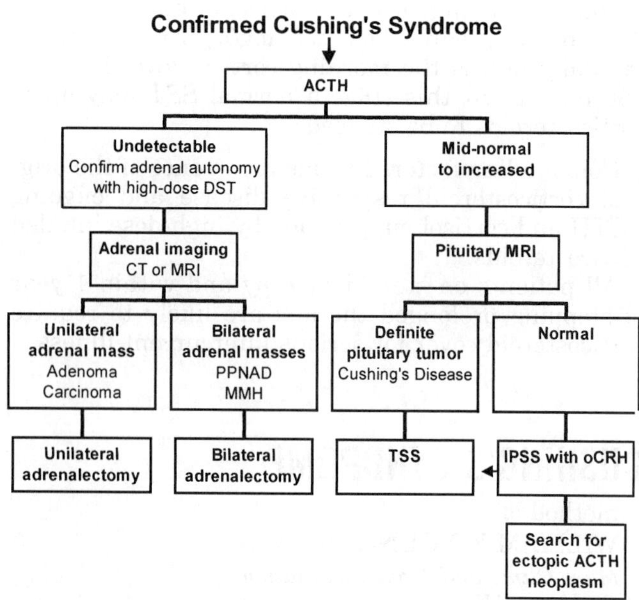

Figure 1. Diagnostic strategy for the evaluation of Cushing's syndrome. The details are discussed in the text. *Abbreviations:* ACTH = adrenocorticotropin; CT = computed tomography; DST = dexamethasone suppression test; MMH = massive macronodular hyperplasia; MRI = magnetic resonance imaging; oCRH = ovine corticotropin hormone; PPNAD = primary pigmented nodular adrenal disease; TSS = transsphenoidal surgery.

tively, lateralization of ACTH secretion from the preoperative inferior petrosal sinus sampling study guides the surgeon for a hemihypophysectomy. The goal of surgery is to remove the adenoma selectively and preserve normal pituitary tissue. At pituitary surgery centers, the mortality rate of TSS is less than or equal to 1%. The incidence of perioperative morbidity is approximately 10% and includes transient diabetes insipidus, hyponatremia (due to inappropriate secretion of antidiuretic hormone), cerebrospinal fluid leak, and meningitis. Potential permanent complications are infrequent (<5%) and include diabetes insipidus; partial or complete anterior pituitary failure; and injury to the carotid arteries, optic nerve, or cavernous sinus cranial nerves.

Postoperative Management

Sudden secondary adrenal insufficiency develops in patients who are cured with TSS. For this reason all of our patients receive a standard preoperative glucocorticoid preparation of 20 mg of methylprednisolone sodium succinate (Solu-Medrol) administered intramuscularly the morning of the operation and again the evening of the operation; the dosage is tapered to 10 mg every 12 hours on the first postoperative day and to 10 mg on the morning of the second postoperative day. Plasma cortisol concentrations are measured at 8 AM and 4 PM on the third postoperative day. Symptoms of adrenal insufficiency will develop 24 to 36 hours after the last dose of methylprednisolone in most patients who are cured. Patients are cautioned about these symptoms and advised to report them promptly—a blood sample is then obtained for cortisol measurement and 10 mg of methylprednisolone is promptly administered intramuscularly. If the plasma cortisol concentrations are less than 3 μg/dL, then a short-term cure is assured. We have observed some patients with long-term cures that had postoperative plasma cortisol concentrations between 3 and 20 μg/dL. Observation and reevaluation several weeks later with baseline 24-hour urinary cortisol excretion is indicated in these cases.

Most patients have been exposed to endogenous hypercortisolism for many years and abrupt postoperative institution of replacement doses of glucocorticoid results in significant withdrawal symptoms. Typically, patients leave the hospital taking prednisone 5 mg orally in the morning and 5 mg orally before the evening meal; 1 to 2 weeks later, the dosage is decreased to 5 mg in the morning and 2.5 mg in the afternoon. Even with this cautious tapering program, all patients have withdrawal (recovery) symptoms of myalgias, depression, and fatigue. Perioperative counseling about the anticipated recovery phase is necessary.

Full HPA axis recovery may require 6 to 24 months. The recovery of hypothalamic corticotropin-releasing hormone secretion is the primary and limiting determinant for recovery. Some degree of adrenal insufficiency must occur during recovery from HPA axis suppression. Two to 3 months postoperatively, it is important to change the dosage to a single morning dose of a short-acting glucocorticoid (e.g., 20 mg hydrocortisone). This lower dose of hydrocortisone facilitates HPA recovery by causing relative cortisol deficiency in the afternoon and evening. If the symptoms of adrenal insufficiency cannot be tolerated, then 5 to 10 mg of hydrocortisone may be added at 4 PM daily for 2 to 3 weeks. Morning plasma cortisol concentrations are measured every 1 to 2 months to assess HPA axis recovery. When the daily dosage of hydrocortisone is at 20 mg, it is rarely necessary to taper this dose further. When the basal level of plasma cortisol is greater than or equal to 10 μg/dL, therapy may be discontinued. Depending on the degree of HPA suppression, it may take up to 2 years before the plasma cortisol concentration normalizes. Cosyntropin (Cortrosyn) stimulation testing is superfluous in this setting. Also, alternate-day glucocorticoid administration is usually not necessary or helpful in the withdrawal process. Patients should receive stress glucocorticoid coverage and wear a Medic-Alert identification for 1 year after the use of exogenous glucocorticoids has been discontinued.

Finally, it is important to assess the status of the pituitary-thyroid and pituitary-gonadal axes 6 to 12 weeks postoperatively.

Failed Transsphenoidal Surgery

From 1974 to 1997, 349 patients underwent TSS at Mayo Clinic for pituitary-dependent Cushing's syndrome. Long-term clinical cure was achieved in 80%. A second TSS surgery was performed in 55 patients, with a reoperation success rate of 40%. If TSS fails to cure Cushing's syndrome, a second operation should be considered. The role of total hypophysectomy in this situation is controversial and many factors, such as hypopituitarism and the desire for future reproductive function, should be considered. In patients with severe Cushing's syndrome who have failed TSS (and certain patients with mild-to-moderate persistent disease), I favor a quick and definitive cure of the hypercortisolism with bilateral laparoscopic adrenalectomy, which can be lifesaving. Nelson's syndrome (an aggressive ACTH-secreting tumor) developed in 11% of our patients who required bilateral adrenalectomy for the treatment of Cushing's syndrome. In our experience, the development of severe Nelson's syndrome correlated with preoperative invasive features of the pituitary tumor and was not caused by adrenalectomy.

In patients with mild Cushing's syndrome who have persistent disease following TSS, combined sellar radiation and pharmacotherapy may be considered. If the residual adenoma can be identified on magnetic resonance imaging, gamma knife radiation surgery is preferred because it is more rapidly effective and associated with less hypopituitarism than conventional radiation therapy.

Until radiation therapy is effective, some form of pharmacotherapy must be continued. Drugs targeted at decreasing pituitary tumor ACTH secretion (e.g., cyproheptadine [Periactin],* bromocriptine [Parlodel],* valproic acid [Depakene],* octreotide) are rarely effective. The two most commonly used agents that inhibit steroidogenesis are ketoconazole (Nizoral)* and mitotane (1,1-dichloro-2[*o*-chlorophenyl]-2-[*P*-chlorophenyl]ethane; *o,p'*-DDD; Lysodren*). Ketoconazole is an imidazole-derivative antimycotic agent that inhibits 17,20-desmolase, 11-hydroxylase, and other enzymes in the adrenal cortex. Dosages range from 300 to 600 mg administered twice daily on an empty stomach. Because drug absorption requires an acidic environment, antacids and agents that decrease stomach acidity should be avoided. Side effects include hepatic dysfunction, renal dysfunction, gynecomastia, and gastrointestinal upset. Liver function tests, serum creatinine level, and urinary cortisol excretion should be followed up every 6 to 8 weeks. The use of mitotane is discussed below in the section on adrenocortical malignancy.

ECTOPIC ACTH SYNDROME

The optimal treatment in patients with ectopic ACTH production (ectopic ACTH syndrome) is resection of the ACTH- or corticotropin-releasing hormone–secreting tumor. However, this may not be possible for two reasons: (1) inability to localize the source of ectopic ACTH production (in 20% of cases at time of presentation), and (2) inability to completely resect the ectopic ACTH-secreting tumor (unresectable or metastatic disease). Ectopic ACTH syndrome was diagnosed in 106 patients at the Mayo Clinic between 1956 and 1998. Bronchial carcinoid was the most frequent cause (25%), followed by islet cell cancer (16%), small cell lung carcinoma (11%), medullary thyroid cancer (8%), disseminated neuroendocrine tumor of unknown primary source (7%), thymic carcinoid (5%), pheochromocytoma (3%), disseminated gastrointestinal carcinoid (1%), and other tumors (8%). No tumor was found in 16% of patients. Twenty-eight patients were treated medically, and the others had either curative tumor resection (13 patients) or bilateral adrenalectomy (65 patients). The diagnoses of Cushing's syndrome and ACTH-secreting neoplasm were usually made concurrently; however, there were remarkable cases in which the two conditions were diagnosed several years apart.

In the patient with an occult ectopic source of ACTH, I favor a quick definitive cure with bilateral adrenalectomy. Pharmacotherapy in these patients rarely completely controls the hypercortisolism, and the associated morbidity and risk of mortality persist.

In the patient with an occult ectopic source of ACTH and mild disease, it is reasonable to treat the hypercortisolism with ketoconazole and mitotane and evaluate the patient every 6 months (for up to 2 years) with magnetic resonance imaging of the chest and upper abdomen and octreotide scintigraphy. If the ectopic source of ACTH is found, then surgery is usually curative. The dosages of ketoconazole or mitotane are adjusted to maintain the 24-hour urinary cortisol level at the low end of the reference range. To prevent symptomatic adrenal insufficiency, I treat these patients with low dosages of dexamethasone (e.g., 0.25–0.5 mg daily). As previously discussed, liver function tests and serum creatinine level should be checked every 6 to 8 weeks in patients treated with ketoconazole, and the drug should be discontinued in the event of hepatic or renal toxicity.

Metastatic or Unresectable ACTH-Secreting Tumor

In the patient with unresectable or metastatic ACTH-secreting tumor, bilateral laparoscopic adrenalectomy offers a quick definitive cure and is the treatment of choice. Pharmacotherapy is rarely effective in controlling hypercortisolism due to the markedly elevated levels of plasma ACTH. In some cases, such as small cell lung carcinoma, tumor-specific chemotherapy may result in a hormonal cure.

The perioperative glucocorticoid therapy for bilateral adrenalectomy is the same as discussed previously for patients treated with TSS. However, prednisone at a dosage of 5 to 7.5 mg daily (or an equivalent of hydrocortisone) is required for the remainder of the patient's life. In many cases, the full replacement dosage is not needed because of a small amount of residual functioning adrenocortical tissue. We instruct patients on stress steroid coverage to wear medical identification. In addition, orally administered mineralocorticoid replacement in the form of fludrocortisone (Florinef Acetate) at a dosage of 0.05 to 0.1 mg/d is started before dismissal from the hospital. The proper dosage is determined by serum electrolytes and supine and standing blood pressures.

ADRENOCORTICAL CARCINOMA

The treatment of choice for adrenocortical carcinoma is complete surgical resection by the anterior abdominal approach. This malignant tumor should be suspected in patients with marked hypercortisolism (24-hour urinary cortisol >1000 μg) and adrenal tumors greater than 6 cm in largest lesional diameter on computerized imaging. Even when the resection is apparently complete, the recurrence rate is high and the 5-year survival rate is approximately 20%. Treatment with mitotane should be used in patients with incomplete tumor resection. This drug is an adrenal cytolytic agent that inhibits adrenal steroid synthesis and destroys normal and neoplastic adrenocortical cells. Treatment is started 3 to 6 weeks following adrenalectomy. The initial dosage is one 500-mg tablet with food twice daily. The total dosage is increased by 500 mg weekly until the maximum tolerated dosage or a maximum dose of 10 g daily is attained. In most patients, the dose is limited by nausea, anorexia, diarrhea, somnolence, skin rash, and pruritus. Mitotane is lipophilic and has a long

*Not FDA approved for this indication.

half-life (0.5–6 months). Therefore, mitotane is contraindicated in women desiring fertility within 2 to 5 years of treatment. This drug may also destroy the normal contralateral adrenal gland and concomitant therapy with dexamethasone (0.5 mg daily) or prednisone (5 mg daily) should be administered. In addition, low-dose mineralocorticoid replacement may be needed, and this is determined by periodic measurement of serum potassium concentration. If hyperkalemia develops, then treatment with fludrocortisone 0.05 mg daily is started and adjusted to maintain the serum potassium level in the normal range.

Because of the high recurrence rate of adrenocortical carcinoma, I favor adjuvant treatment with mitotane in patients who are apparent surgical cures. Reevaluation with computerized abdominal imaging is done at 1, 3, 6, 9, and 12 months following surgery. If recurrent disease is not evident at 12 months postoperatively, then the mitotane treatment is discontinued. Continued close follow-up is indicated in these patients.

ADRENAL ADENOMA

Patients with Cushing's syndrome caused by an adrenal adenoma are cured with unilateral adrenalectomy. This surgery is usually performed by the laparoscopic approach. The patient should be cautioned that it may take 4 to 18 months before the HPA axis recovers. The rate-limiting step in axis recovery is in the hypothalamic corticotropin-releasing hormone neuron and/or higher regulatory inputs. At approximately 6 weeks following surgery, patients are switched to a shorter acting glucocorticoid (e.g., hydrocortisone 20 mg in the morning and 10 mg in the afternoon). The afternoon dose is tapered and discontinued over 2 to 8 weeks. The single morning dose allows for relative nocturnal glucocorticoid insufficiency and stimulation of the hypothalamic neurons. The concentration of plasma cortisol at 8 AM (before hydrocortisone administration) is measured every 6 to 8 weeks. Hydrocortisone treatment may be discontinued when the plasma cortisol concentration is greater than or equal to 10 μg/dL. Patients are cautioned on the need for stress steroid coverage for approximately 1 year after exogenous treatment is discontinued. Mineralocorticoid replacement is usually not required in patients following unilateral adrenalectomy.

COMPLICATIONS OF CUSHING'S SYNDROME

Hypertension

Hypertension is present in approximately 75% to 80% of patients with Cushing's syndrome. The mechanisms of hypertension include increased production of deoxycorticosterone, increased vascular reactivity to catecholamines, and overload of cortisol inactivation with stimulation of the mineralocorticoid receptor. Deficient cortisol ring A reduction due to overload of metabolizing enzymes results in a type II variant of "apparent mineralocorticoid excess" in patients with severe hypercortisolism. The hypertension associated with Cushing's syndrome should be treated until a surgical cure is obtained. Spironolactone (Aldactone), at dosages used to treat primary aldosteronism, is effective in reversing the hypokalemia (see article on primary aldosteronism). Second-step agents include thiazide diuretics, β-adrenergic receptor blockers, angiotensin-converting enzyme inhibitors, and calcium channel antagonists. The hypertension associated with the hypercortisolism usually resolves several weeks after the surgical cure, and antihypertensive agents can be tapered and withdrawn. Approximately 26% of patients have persistent hypertension despite cure of the hypercortisolism.

Osteoporosis

In patients with iatrogenic Cushing's syndrome, it is important to quantitate and follow bone mineral density at the hip and spine. If long-term glucocorticoid treatment is planned, it is important to optimize several factors in an attempt to preserve bone density:

1. Increase daily elemental calcium ingestion to 1500 to 2000 mg daily.
2. Follow 24-hour urinary calcium excretion and, if it exceeds 300 mg, consider thiazide diuretic therapy to prevent renal lithiasis.
3. Ensure adequate vitamin D intake with one or two multiple vitamin tablets daily.
4. Initiate estrogen replacement therapy in postmenopausal women.
5. Decrease the glucocorticoid dosage to lowest effective single daily dose.
6. Consider preventive therapy with a biphosphonate (see article on osteoporosis).

A quick complete cure of hypercortisolism is the best therapy for osteoporosis in patients with endogenous Cushing's syndrome.

Hyperglycemia

Diabetes mellitus secondary to hypercortisolism is common in Cushing's syndrome. Insulin therapy is frequently indicated and may need to be continued indefinitely in patients who have iatrogenic Cushing's syndrome because of planned long-term glucocorticoid administration. A quick, complete cure of hypercortisolism is the best therapy for diabetes mellitus in patients with endogenous Cushing's syndrome, and frequently, insulin treatment can be tapered and discontinued over several weeks following surgery.

DIABETES INSIPIDUS

method of
TARIQ MUBIN, M.D., and
BARBARA A. CLARK, M.D.
Allegheny General Hospital
Pittsburgh, Pennsylvania

Diabetes insipidus (DI) is a disorder characterized by excessive urine output (>30 mL/kg body weight/d) due to inability of the kidneys to concentrate urine. It can be due to complete or partial resistance of the kidneys to the effects of antidiuretic hormone (ADH), intrinsic renal disease, or deficient ADH (decreased production or increased breakdown).

ETIOLOGY

For ease of discussion DI is divided into two main categories: central DI and nephrogenic DI.

Central Diabetes Insipidus

The most common cause of central DI is disruption of the pituitary-hypothalamic axis, which can be caused by surgery, trauma, infiltrative diseases, or tumors (e.g., histiocytosis, craniopharyngioma, astrocytoma, leukemia, lymphoma, or metastases from breast or lung cancer). The cause is idiopathic in up to 25% of the cases. Other rare causes include sarcoidosis, Wegener's granulomatosis, thrombotic thrombocytopenic purpura, anorexia nervosa, and heredity. Any form of central DI may be exacerbated during pregnancy due to increased production of vasopressinases, enzymes that degrade ADH.

Nephrogenic Diabetes Insipidus

Nephrogenic DI also can be inherited (autosomal recessive or X-linked) or acquired, which is much more common than the inherited form. Causes of acquired nephrogenic DI include drugs such as lithium (Lithobid), phenytoin (Dilantin), alcohol, colchicine, and furosemide (Lasix), with lithium being the most common. Other causes include chronic renal disease (polycystic kidney disease, medullary cystic disease, pyelonephritis) and systemic disorders including hypokalemia, hypercalcemia, sickle cell disease, multiple myeloma, and amyloidosis.

DIAGNOSIS

Differential diagnosis includes polyuric states; that is, osmotic diuresis of any cause and primary polydipsia. The main challenge is to differentiate between central DI, nephrogenic DI, and primary polydipsia. Plasma sodium level and osmolality can still be maintained within reference limits if the thirst mechanism is intact at the expense of polydipsia and polyuria.

Correct diagnosis can be achieved by a detailed history (i.e., central nervous system trauma/surgery, drugs, and the rate of onset of polyuria: abrupt in central DI but gradual in nephrogenic DI and primary polydipsia), laboratory values, and a water restriction test.

Water Restriction Test

The diagnosis of polyuria should be confirmed by water restriction test results. Patients should be monitored closely during the test. Baseline values of plasma osmolality and sodium should be obtained. If plasma osmolality is above 295 mmol/kg and sodium is more than 143 mmol/L, the diagnosis of primary polydipsia is excluded. Otherwise, one should proceed with the test. Urine volume and osmolality and plasma sodium concentration and osmolality should be measured every 1 to 2 hours. The test is continued until urine osmolality is greater than 600 mmol/kg (which indicates both ADH release and site of action are intact), the urine osmolality remains stable on two or three successive measurements despite a rising plasma osmolality, or the plasma osmolality exceeds 300 mOsm/kg. Once urine osmolality stabilizes or plasma osmolality reaches 300 mOsm/kg, 5 U of aqueous vasopressin (Pitressin Synthetic) subcutaneously or 10 μg of desmopressin (DDAVP) by intranasal route should be administered. If urine osmolality increases further at this point, then the diagnosis of central DI is established. The urine osmolality increases from 100% to 800% in complete central DI and from 15% to 50% in partial central DI, with an accompanying decrease in urine output.

Administration of ADH in partial nephrogenic DI may also result in an increase in urinary osmolality (up to 45%). It can be differentiated from partial central DI because patients with partial central DI usually achieve a urinary osmolality of 300 mOsm/kg or higher after water restriction. Subjects with nephrogenic DI have persistently dilute urine, the osmolality of which rises with ADH but remains well below 300 mOsm/kg.

In primary polydipsia, the maximum urinary concentrating ability is impaired due to partial washout of the medullary interstitial gradient. With water restriction, urinary osmolality may increase to 500 mOsm/kg, and there is no additional response to exogenous ADH because the endogenous response is intact.

TREATMENT

Hypernatremia is usually not the major presentation of DI because the thirst mechanism is intact in most cases. However, if the thirst mechanism is impaired or the patient does not have access to water, life-threatening hypernatremia can occur, which requires administration of electrolyte-free water. Because hypernatremia is frequently chronic in nature in DI, the rate of correction of sodium should not exceed 0.5 mEq/L/h or 12 mEq/L/d, to prevent cerebral edema and risk of herniation. The only exception is that if the patient has convulsions or some other central nervous system signs and symptoms, the serum sodium level should be rapidly corrected by 4 to 5 mEq/L. This usually relieves the seizures or other symptoms. Further correction should proceed slowly, as mentioned previously.

Central Diabetes Insipidus

Because the main defect in central DI is deficiency of ADH, the mainstay of treatment is administration of ADH. It is available as arginine vasopressin (AVP) or its analog 1-desamino-8-D-arginine vasopressin (desmopressin or DDAVP). DDAVP has virtually replaced AVP, given its ease of administration and lack of vasopressor activity. AVP can be administered only intramuscularly or intravenously, whereas DDAVP is available as an oral, a nasal, and a parenteral formulation. It is also available in intravenous and subcutaneous forms. The nasal form can be delivered via a dose-calibrated plastic tube or a nasal spray. In a cooperative patient, treatment is usually initiated at a dose of 5 μg of intranasal DDAVP at bedtime and gradually titrated upward in increments of 5 μg, based on the response of the nocturia, to a usual maximum dose of about 20 μg. It can also be administered in twice-daily divided doses.

The oral tablet form of DDAVP is also available in the United States in 0.1-mg and 0.2-mg doses. Only about 5% of the oral form is absorbed from the gut, and absorption may be erratic even in healthy people. Administration of the tablet with meals further decreases the absorption by 40% to 50%. Hence, the potency of the oral form is only one-tenth to one-twentieth of that of the nasal form, and a change from the nasal to oral form will require retitration of the dose. The usual starting dosage of the oral form is 0.05 mg at bedtime with gradual titration upward to a usual dose of about 0.1 mg to 1.0 mg in divided doses in most people. Doses greater than 0.2 mg have a longer duration of action but no greater antidiuretic effect.

The main use of the parenteral form of DDAVP or AVP is after head trauma or neurosurgery and in unconscious or uncooperative patients. It can also be used for the treatment of a brain-dead organ donor. Because DI can be transient or triphasic after head trauma, patients should be observed closely. Inputs, outputs, weight, blood pressure, and blood sodium level should be obtained frequently to avoid hyponatremia while pituitary function recovers. Therapy may need to be withheld periodically.

The main risk of treatment is the development of hyponatremia, because these patients now have insuppressible ADH activity and may not be able to excrete ingested water normally. The thirst mechanism is still intact but may be modified by other exogenous factors, such as drugs, diet, smoking, mouth breathing, and so on, that could lead to excess water ingestion. This problem can be avoided by patient education and the use of a minimum dose of vasopressin or DDAVP to control the polyuria.

Other Drugs

With the widespread use of desmopressin or DDAVP, the role of other drugs has decreased, but these drugs may still be useful in certain circumstances. In some patients with partial central DI, supplemental drugs can enhance the response to ADH or serve to increase ADH release. The most widely used drug for this purpose is chlorpropamide (Diabinese*; an oral hypoglycemic agent) in doses of 125 to 250 mg once or twice a day. Higher doses increase the risk of hypoglycemia. This drug may work by enhancing the effect of ADH on kidney (possibly by increasing the sodium chloride reabsorption in the thick ascending limb and thereby enhancing medullary hypertonicity). The other drug that enhances the response to ADH is carbamazepine (Tegretol*; antiseizure medication) in doses of 100 mg to 300 mg twice daily. Clofibrate (Atromid-S*; drug to treat hyperlipidemia) may increase ADH release at a dosage of 500 mg every 6 hours.

Other modalities include the use of diuretics* and nonsteroidal anti-inflammatory drugs* and sodium and protein restriction. These modalities also form the cornerstone of therapy for nephrogenic DI. Indapamide (Lozol*; a thiazide diuretic) has been shown to be effective at doses of 2.5 mg/d in patients with central DI. Each of these measures may lower the urine output by more than 50%.

Nephrogenic Diabetes Insipidus

In nephrogenic DI, the mainstay of treatment is correction of the underlying disorder (e.g., hypokalemia, hypercalcemia) or discontinuation of the offending agent (e.g., lithium). However, sometimes patients may have irreversible tubular injury and alternative strategies are needed to reduce polyuria.

One alternate strategy is to increase proximal sodium and water absorption (ADH independent) and thereby diminish distal delivery of water to ADH-sensitive sites in the collecting tubules. This can be achieved by inducing mild volume depletion with the use of a thiazide diuretic such as hydrochlorothiazide* at doses of 25 mg once or twice daily. Their effect can be enhanced by the concomitant use of potassium-sparing diuretics such as amiloride (Midamor),* which have the additional beneficial effect of diminishing the hypokalemia caused by thiazide diuretics. Amiloride is also the drug of choice for the treatment of lithium-induced reversible nephrogenic DI. It blocks the entrance of lithium by blocking luminal sodium channels of the collecting duct (through which lithium usually enters these cells) and may allow the lithium to be continued. Lithium levels still need to be closely monitored to avoid toxicity from increased proximal tubular reabsorption associated with volume depletion.

Loop diuretics (e.g., Lasix*) can also induce volume depletion but interfere with the generation of medullary hypertonicity, thus inducing relative ADH resistance, which is counterproductive in DI.

Nonsteroidal anti-inflammatory drugs inhibit renal prostaglandin synthesis. Prostaglandins antagonize ADH action by inhibiting the formation of cyclic adenosine monophosphate (AMP). In addition, the vasodilator action of prostaglandin increases medullary flow, which lowers medullary hyperosmolality. Therefore, prostaglandin inhibition may serve to potentiate ADH action and, by increasing medullary tonicity, contribute to more concentrated urine. Not all nonsteroidal anti-inflammatory drugs work equally well in a given patient. Some patients may respond better to one agent than to another. Indomethacin (Indocin,* 100–150 mg/d in two or three

*Not FDA approved for this indication.

*Not FDA approved for this indication.

divided doses) is the most frequently used agent. Nonsteroidal anti-inflammatory drugs may work more effectively when combined with a thiazide diuretic. In this circumstance, renal function must be monitored carefully to avoid adverse effects.

Polyuria can also be improved by a low salt and protein diet (reduction in urea generation and hence excretion) by decreasing net solute excretion.

Finally, some patients with nephrogenic DI may have persistent polyuria despite the previous measures. These patients might benefit by attaining supraphysiologic hormone levels from administration of exogenous ADH or DDAVP because the resistance to ADH may be incomplete. Occasionally, the combination of DDAVP plus nonsteroidal anti-inflammatory agents to enhance the action may be useful.

Diabetes Insipidus in Pregnancy

Some patients with subclinical or partial nephrogenic or central DI might present with overt DI (or worsening of a previously well-controlled DI) when they are pregnant. This condition is due to vasopressinases secreted by the placenta. These patients are resistant to vasopressin, due to increased catabolism, but remain sensitive to DDAVP (probably due to a different N-terminus that confers resistance to vasopressinases). Nephrogenic DI resistant to DDAVP and vasopressin may also occur in pregnant patients, which resolves after delivery of the infant. Central DI can also develop in women postpartum due to Sheehan's syndrome (infarction of the pituitary gland due to massive hemorrhage during childbirth).

HYPERPARATHYROIDISM AND HYPOPARATHYROIDISM

method of
JOHN D. WARK, M.B., B.S., PH.D., and
MARK S. STEIN, M.B., B.S., PH.D.
The Royal Melbourne Hospital
Victoria, Australia

HYPERPARATHYROIDISM

Primary Hyperparathyroidism

Primary hyperparathyroidism (PHPT) refers to excessive secretion of parathyroid hormone (PTH) due to intrinsic parathyroid disease. It is usually associated with a high circulating PTH level and with a high serum calcium concentration.

PHPT is the most common cause of hypercalcemia in nonhospitalized patients. The reported incidence appears to have fluctuated in the United States in recent decades and is currently around 8 in 100,000 per year. Seventy-five percent of patients are female, and they typically are postmenopausal.

ETIOLOGY AND PATHOGENESIS

The PTH excess arises from a single, benign parathyroid adenoma in 80% to 85% of cases. Most of these tumors are monoclonal or oligoclonal. Multigland benign disease—hyperplasia, multiple adenomas—explains most of the remaining cases. Multigland disease can be sporadic or hereditary (multiple endocrine neoplasia syndromes, hereditary PHPT). Etiologic factors in sporadic PHPT include external irradiation and long-term lithium therapy. Parathyroid carcinoma is found in less than 1% of patients with PHPT.

The ultimate cause underlying most cases of PHPT is not known but evidence suggests either overexpression of a growth promoter or inactivation of a tumor-suppressor gene.

It is believed that hypercalcemia occurs with parathyroid adenomas because the cells of the adenoma have reduced sensitivity to extracellular calcium. In contrast, in parathyroid hyperplasia, the excessive PTH secretion comes about because of the increased number of secretory cells.

CLINICAL MANIFESTATIONS AND PRESENTATION

Most commonly, PHPT is first suspected when mild-to-moderate hypercalcemia is found on biochemical screening. These patients may have nonspecific complaints such as lethargy or weakness. Patients with additional, classic features of hypercalcemia or of PHPT are less common (Table 1). A minority of these patients develop nephrolithiasis (~20%), and a smaller proportion develop diffuse nephrocalcinosis and/or renal impairment. Overt parathyroid bone disease, now very uncommon, causes bone pain and deformities associated with radiologic features of subperiosteal resorption, abnormalities in the skull, bone cysts, and brown tumors.

In some patients, PHPT causes osteoporosis or osteopenia on bone densitometry. Thus, some cases of PHPT are diagnosed after the serum calcium level is measured as part of an investigation of osteoporosis. The effect of PHPT on fracture risk is uncertain.

INVESTIGATION AND DIAGNOSIS

Almost all patients with PHPT will have hypercalcemia (may be mild and intermittent in mild cases). If PHPT is suspected, for example, because of the presence of kidney stones or osteoporosis, several measurements of the serum calcium level should be made to obtain good evidence against the diagnosis. Measurement of the serum PTH concentration is pivotal in diagnosing the cause of hypercalcemia. Measurement of PTH using current immunoradiometric and immunochemiluminometric assays for the intact molecule is generally very reliable. Using these techniques, the PTH level is increased in approximately 90% of cases of PHPT. In the remainder, the PTH level is within the reference range, in contrast to the suppressed PTH levels found in the great majority of patients with hypercalcemia due to nonparathyroid causes. If the PTH level is suppressed, nonparathyroid causes of hypercalcemia should be considered further (Table 2), with the most likely diagnosis being hypercalcemia of malignancy.

In addition to hypercalcemia and elevation of the PTH concentration, other typical laboratory findings include a low or low-normal serum inorganic phosphate level, mild

TABLE 1. **Classic Features of Primary Hyperparathyroidism**

Lethargy, depression, poor concentration
Myopathy, myalgia, arthralgia
Constipation, abdominal pain
Nephrolithiasis
Low bone mass, bone pain

TABLE 2. **Nonparathyroid Causes of Hypercalcemia**

Malignant Disease

Parathyroid hormone-related protein (PTHrP) production (carcinomas of lung, head and neck, esophagus, ovary, bladder, kidney)
Multiple myeloma
Breast cancer*
Ectopic production of 1,25-dihydroxyvitamin D (lymphoma)

Endocrine/Metabolic Disorders

Hyperthyroidism
Familial hypocalciuric hypercalcemia
Other endocrinopathies rarely (e.g., pheochromocytoma, adrenal insufficiency)
Milk-alkali syndrome
Hypophosphatasia

Granulomatous Diseases

Sarcoidosis
Various infective causes

Drug-Induced

Vitamin D
Thiazides
Lithium†
Gonadal steroids
Vitamin A intoxication
Aminophylline
Aluminum intoxication

Other

Immobilization with high bone turnover
Acute and chronic renal failure

*Bone lysis due to local PTHrP production.
†PTH-mediated.
Abbreviation: PTH = parathyroid hormone.

hyperchloremic metabolic acidosis, elevation of the serum total alkaline phosphatase (and of more specific bone turnover markers), and inconsistent elevation of the serum 1,25-dihydroxyvitamin D level. Urinary calcium excretion is elevated in approximately 25% of patients with PHPT, whereas urinary calcium excretion and the calcium–creatinine clearance ratio are low in the rare familial hypocalciuric hypercalcemia.

In many cases of confirmed PHPT, it is useful to measure bone density of the lumbar spine and proximal femur by dual-energy x-ray absorptiometry, a sensitive and precise indicator of bone loss. Because cortical bone is lost preferentially in PHPT, a deficit is more likely to be found at the hip (or the distal radius) than the lumbar spine. If evidence of renal involvement will influence management, ultrasonography (US) or radiography seeking stones or renal calcification is helpful. Parathyroid imaging is rarely indicated in the evaluation of patients with PHPT unless they have undergone previous neck surgery.

TREATMENT OF HYPERPARATHYROIDISM

The only definitive treatment for PHPT is surgical removal of the abnormal parathyroid tissue. The majority of patients have asymptomatic or mild disease; therefore, it is necessary to consider potential benefits and risks carefully when making treatment decisions. Although solid evidence that allows prediction of outcomes is generally lacking, recommendations from a National Institutes of Health consensus conference in 1990 remain useful. Thus, surgery can be advised in the following situations:

1. The serum calcium level is greater than 1 mg/dL (0.25 mmol/L) above the upper limit of the reference range.
2. There is a history of life-threatening hypercalcemia.
3. There is marked hypercalciuria (>400 mg/24 h [10 mmol/24 h]).
4. There are complications of PHPT, particularly overt bone disease, nephrolithiasis, or impaired renal function.
5. There is a moderate or severe reduction in bone mineral density, for example, a deficit of 2 or more SD below the age- and gender-matched mean value at any site.
6. The patient is younger than 50 years of age.
7. The patient has typical symptoms, for example, fatigue, weakness, myalgia, arthralgia, and abdominal pain.

These recommendations are for guidance only; many individual patient and physician factors also come into play.

If the decision is made in favor of surgery, the next step is to find a highly skilled parathyroid surgeon. The cure rate at first operation should be approximately 95% in the hands of an experienced surgeon. This cure rate generally exceeds the confirmed localization rate with parathyroid imaging modalities; therefore, these investigations usually are not needed before a first surgical exploration of the neck. Although surgical exploration of the neck with the patient under general anesthesia remains the standard surgical approach, minimally invasive endoscopic surgery with the patient under local anesthesia is being used increasingly. Although cure rates do not seem to match the standard surgical approach, minimally invasive surgery has potential advantages for patients at high operative risk. Of even greater importance than the cure rate is the complication rate. In the hands of experienced surgeons, recurrent laryngeal nerve palsy occurs in less than 1% of cases.

The surgical approach to patients who have had neck surgery is more difficult; preoperative localization studies usually are performed as an aid to the surgeon. Technetium-99m sestamibi scanning is widely regarded as the best, most convenient noninvasive localization technique; it can be combined with single-photon emission computed tomography to provide tomographic images. Standard computed tomography, magnetic resonance imaging, and US also can be used. When these noninvasive tests are unsatisfactory, arteriography and/or selective venous sampling for PTH in neck and mediastinal veins should be considered. These techniques can be very powerful when performed by a radiologist with special expertise, but they are very skill- and time-demanding procedures and should be undertaken only in centers where appropriate expertise and resources are available. The embryologic development and migration of the parathyroid glands explain why "failed" cases are often cured by removal of an additional parathyroid gland from the mediastinum.

The overwhelming majority of cases can be cured surgically. Most will have a single adenoma. Nevertheless, all glands should be identified at surgery to avoid missing multigland disease. There is some variation in operative approach when multigland disease is present. Many now favor total parathyroidectomy with implantation of parathyroid fragments into forearm muscle. These autografts have a high rate of function by 2 to 3 months after surgery. Parathyroid tissue should also be cryopreserved in case the fresh implant fails. The alternative to total parathyroidectomy with autografting is removal of 3.5 glands, marking the residual tissue with a surgical clip. This simpler procedure has an appreciable rate of recurrence of PHPT.

The perioperative course is relatively uneventful in most cases, and the serum calcium level is within the reference range within approximately 24 hours. Transient mild hypocalcemia is not uncommon. If symptomatic, it can be managed effectively using an intravenous calcium infusion. The serum magnesium level should also be checked and normalized through oral supplements.

When significant parathyroid bone disease is present (high alkaline phosphatase, radiologic changes of hyperparathyroidism), there is an appreciable risk of prolonged postoperative hypocalcemia that may be severe. This state is due to the marked influx of mineral into the healing skeleton (so-called hungry bone syndrome). Patients at risk for this complication seem to be best treated by starting a calcium infusion early postoperatively and using frequent monitoring of the serum calcium level to adjust the infusion rate. Several days of preoperative treatment with an active vitamin D metabolite is sometimes also recommended. Postoperative treatment with calcium and sometimes an active vitamin D metabolite may be required for weeks or several months. Other potential complications include postoperative permanent hypoparathyroidism and recurrent laryngeal nerve damage. Both are more likely when the surgery is complicated.

Medical Management

Patients who do not meet any of the above criteria for surgical intervention may be observed rather than undergoing surgery. These patients should be advised to maintain a generous fluid intake (at least 2 L/d) to avoid dehydration. Medical attendants should be aware that hypercalcemia may be worsened by periods of immobility and dehydration occasioned by intercurrent illness; therefore, attention to fluid balance and monitoring of the serum calcium level are required. Thiazide diuretics should be avoided because their hypocalciuric effect may exacerbate hypercalcemia. Caution is required in the use of loop diuretics such as furosemide (Lasix),* which can reduce the glomerular filtration rate, and thus renal calcium excretion, because of extracellular volume contraction. Dietary calcium intake should be moderate only (800–1000 mg/d), and calcium and vitamin D supplements avoided.

*Not FDA approved for this indication.

Clinical and laboratory evaluation should be undertaken at regular intervals to monitor for the onset of symptoms or other evidence of progression, under which circumstances surgery should be reconsidered. In most cases, a follow-up interval of 6 months is reasonable. Serum calcium, albumin, creatinine, and alkaline phosphatase levels should be measured at each monitoring visit. Bone densitometry should be obtained every 1 to 2 years and renal US approximately every 2 years. Patients who do not undergo surgery because of their unwillingness or because they present an unacceptable operative risk should be monitored clinically and with the investigations listed earlier; the follow-up intervals are determined by the degree of clinical concern. The same applies to the small proportion of patients in whom surgical cure is not achieved.

Unfortunately, there is no safe, effective medical therapy for PHPT. Oral phosphate therapy can achieve a mild-to-moderate reduction in the serum calcium level (0.5–1.0 mg/dL) but is not well tolerated, particularly because of diarrhea. There are concerns that oral phosphate therapy can lead to soft tissue calcification and a further increase in PTH levels.

Hormone replacement therapy may have a minor role in the medical treatment of postmenopausal women with PHPT by helping to prevent bone loss. Therapy with potent bisphosphonates is often moderately effective in the short term (days to weeks), reducing the serum calcium level through inhibition of bone resorption. This treatment is useful when surgical exploration of the neck must be delayed because of intercurrent illness. Potential options are intravenous pamidronate infusion and oral treatment with alendronate (Fosamax),* risedronate (Actonel),* or clodronate.† Etidronate is not effective. A new class of drugs under investigation are calcimimetic agents, which are agonists at the extracellular calcium-sensing receptor. These have the potential to depress PTH secretion and serum calcium levels.

Hypercalcemic crisis is present when patients are severely symptomatic and usually have metabolic derangements, including fluid and electrolyte depletion. Intravenous infusion of 0.9% saline is the cornerstone of treatment, often supplemented with calcitonin (Calcimar)* and/or intravenous pamidronate.* Salmon calcitonin (100–200 IU/6–12 h) usually has an onset of action within 12 hours. Pamidronate infusion (30–90 mg over 2 to 4 hours in 500-mL 0.9% saline) is effective but the benefit is often delayed by approximately 24 hours. Calcitonin* and pamidronate* can be used in combination for life-threatening

*Not FDA approved for this indication.
†Not available in the United States.

hypercalcemia. Dialysis also should be considered in the most serious cases.

A common error in this situation is the early administration of furosemide.* The rationale for giving furosemide is that it acts on the loop of Henle to reduce renal calcium reabsorption. However, the administration of furosemide to a dehydrated patient only worsens pre-renal renal failure. It further reduces the glomerular filtration rate and thus markedly reduces renal calcium excretion.

SECONDARY HYPERPARATHYROIDISM

In secondary hyperparathyroidism, PTH is elevated because of a lesion originally extrinsic to the parathyroid glands, most commonly vitamin D deficiency, reduced renal reserve, and medications (e.g., furosemide, glucocorticoids, and bisphosphonates).

Vitamin D and Vitamin D Deficiency

Etiology and Pathogenesis

Vitamin D is a fat-soluble vitamin that functions in the body as a steroid hormone.

Vitamin D acts on cells of the intestine, kidneys, and skeleton to promote intestinal calcium and phosphate absorption and renal calcium conservation.

Vitamin D_3 (also called *cholecalciferol*) is synthesized in the skin under the influence of ultraviolet light and is subsequently metabolized to a large number of metabolites. An important metabolic pathway includes hepatic hydroxylation to 25-hydroxyvitamin D_3 (25-OHD_3). This is the vitamin D metabolite present in serum in the greatest amount, and measurement of total serum 25-OHD_3 is performed to assess vitamin D nutritional status. The serum half-life of 25-OHD_3 is approximately 3 weeks. Vitamin D circulates bound to an α-globulin called *vitamin D–binding protein.* Age does not affect the serum levels of this binding protein.

When 25-OHD_3 undergoes 1α-hydroxylation in the kidney, the very potent metabolite 1,25-dihydroxyvitamin D_3 (also called *calcitriol*) is formed. The half-life of 1,25-dihydroxyvitamin D is approximately 2 days. The activity of the renal hydroxylase enzyme is very tightly regulated. It is increased by PTH and low plasma phosphate and inhibited by high plasma phosphate and by 1,25-dihydroxyvitamin D_3 itself.

The few dietary sources of vitamin D_3 include liver and fatty fish. Most vitamin D nutrition derives from exposure to sunshine. Some countries, including the United States, fortify their milk with vitamin D as a public health measure. Window glass filters ultraviolet rays and prevents vitamin D synthesis.

Vitamin D_2, or *ergocalciferol,* is a synthetic sterol produced by irradiation of the yeast or plant provitamin ergosterol. It is thought to follow the same metabolic pathways in humans as vitamin D_3 but may also have its own additional pathways. The relative potencies of vitamin D_3 and D_2 in human beings were thought to be equal, but this is currently undergoing reappraisal with investigations of the possibility that vitamin D_2 is less toxic. An international unit of vitamin D is equivalent to 0.025 μg of pure cholecalciferol (40,000 U = 1 mg of calciferol).

Those at increased risk for vitamin D deficiency largely are individuals who infrequently spend time outdoors. This includes institutionalized elderly people in nursing homes and hostels (up to 50% of whom may be vitamin D deficient), frail elderly people living at home, intellectually impaired people living in residential care, and people with a range of medical problems. Healthy individuals who wear clothes that limit skin exposure may also have a high prevalence of vitamin D deficiency. Long-term therapy with multiple anticonvulsant drugs may be associated with osteomalacia, but the mechanism of the association is uncertain. Phenytoin therapy is not associated with lower serum 25-OHD_3 levels, although it may cause bone disease.

Vitamin D deficiency leads to reduced intestinal calcium absorption and thus plasma calcium concentration falls. The reduction in plasma calcium level stimulates the parathyroid glands to increase PTH secretion. This secondary hyperparathyroidism returns the plasma calcium concentration to normal. This is mediated partly by PTH increasing the activity of the renal 1α-hydroxylase, with a consequent increase in the serum calcitriol level. This hormone in turn increases intestinal calcium absorption. Secondary hyperparathyroidism is associated with bone loss. This adverse outcome occurs because at mild elevations of PTH in subjects already in negative bone-remodeling balance, bone turnover is accelerated, although at even higher levels of PTH, negative bone-remodeling balance is engendered directly.

Treatment of Vitamin D Deficiency

Treatment of vitamin D deficiency is most appropriately done by provision of vitamin D itself, for example, ergocalciferol capsules (together with a calcium supplement if dietary calcium is also deficient). The body then synthesizes all the vitamin D metabolites from this replenished basic substrate. A common error is to provide calcitriol rather than vitamin D. Although calcitriol is a potent metabolite of the parent vitamin, provision of calcitriol does not enable synthesis of many other vitamin D metabolites and also bypasses the tightly regulated renal hydroxylase step, risking hypercalcemia, hyperphosphatemia, hypercalciuria, and hyperphosphaturia consequent upon unregulated intestinal calcium and phosphate hyperabsorption.

In older people who live in the community, vitamin D and calcium supplements may reduce both bone loss and nonvertebral fractures. In nursing home residents, treatment of secondary hyperparathyroidism by correcting vitamin D deficiency and supplementing with calcium has been associated with a 43% reduction in hip fracture incidence. This may be

*Not FDA approved for this indication.

due to improvement in bone mass. However, because vitamin D deficiency and secondary hyperparathyroidism may also impair neuromuscular function and thus affect falling, their rectification through treatment could also affect hip fracture incidence through a reduction in falls.

Prevention of vitamin D deficiency requires a high index of suspicion for diminished sunlight exposure. A daily oral supplement of 400 IU of vitamin D is commonly prescribed but this may not prove sufficient, and daily oral doses of 1000 IU may be more appropriate. This should be considered routinely for those subjects in the high-risk groups (see previous discussion). These subjects should also be considered for prescription of a daily oral calcium supplement of approximately 600 mg elemental calcium if dietary intake is poor. This is often given just before bed to maximize calcium absorption and minimize the nocturnal rise in PTH associated with the negative calcium balance of overnight fasting. A history of renal calculi is, of course, a relative contraindication to calcium prescription.

Subjects who suffer frank malabsorption may benefit from intramuscular vitamin D therapy where such preparations are available. In the absence of these preparations, high doses of oral vitamin D could be prescribed and the efficacy determined through measurement of serum 25-OHD_3. In the setting of hypocalcemia and malabsorption, use of the potent vitamin D metabolite calcitriol may be required to improve intestinal calcium absorption.

Reduced Renal Reserve

Renal tissue mass falls with age. The associated fall in the mass of the 1α-hydroxylase enzyme engenders an age-related secondary hyperparathyroidism that increases residual hydroxylase activity and thus leads to adequate calcitriol production. An additional stimulus for an age-related elevation in PTH may be co-incident age-related intestinal resistance to calcitriol. This is all distinct from the hyperparathyroidism of end-stage renal disease (see later section on this subject).

Medications

Furosemide (Lasix) therapy is associated with secondary hyperparathyroidism. This is most likely mediated through a furosemide-induced acute fall in plasma ionized calcium consequent upon calciuresis and a change in blood pH. The compensation for this is chronic secondary hyperparathyroidism. In contrast, thiazide diuretics are associated with reduced serum PTH levels due at least in part to a reduction in urine calcium excretion.

Glucocorticoids are associated with secondary hyperparathyroidism, although this effect may be mediated at least in part through the underlying disease processes. Potential mechanisms for this glucocorticoid effect include an increase in urine calcium loss, a possible reduction in intestinal calcium absorption, and a direct effect on the parathyroid glands to increase PTH secretion.

Bisphosphonates are associated with secondary hyperparathyroidism. This effect may be due to a fall in plasma ionized calcium consequent upon a perturbation in bone remodeling.

END-STAGE RENAL DISEASE AND TERTIARY HYPERPARATHYROIDISM

Etiology and Pathogenesis

With a more marked reduction in renal function than that described previously, phosphate excretion decreases and the plasma phosphate concentration thus increases. This metabolic disturbance has a positive direct post-transcriptional effect on PTH synthesis (through increased stability of the PTH messenger RNA) and also leads to parathyroid cell hyperplasia. The consequent secondary hyperparathyroidism promotes phosphate excretion through the remaining nephrons, but renal mass is so diminished that hyperphosphatemia often persists. With a general reduction in renal mass, there is a reduction in hydroxylase enzyme mass and thus total renal hydroxylase activity. Hyperphosphatemia reduces this activity even further. This exacerbates the impairment in calcitriol production previously noted that commenced with mild age-related renal impairment. With lower serum calcitriol concentrations, intestinal calcium absorption is reduced and plasma calcium concentration decreases. Hyperphosphatemia may also directly induce a decrease in the plasma ionized calcium concentration. Decreased plasma calcium is sensed by membrane calcium receptors of the parathyroid cell and causes an increase in PTH secretion. Low plasma calcium might also cause increased PTH synthesis through an increase in the stability of PTH mRNA. In addition, the inhibitory effect of calcitriol on PTH production (through an effect on gene transcription) is removed, and this further increases serum PTH levels.

Secondary hyperparathyroidism of end-stage renal disease differs from other forms of secondary hyperparathyroidism, being characterized by serum PTH levels that are typically an order of magnitude higher, calcitriol deficiency and calcium malabsorption, hyperphosphatemia, lack of renal function, and intercurrent systemic illness.

TERTIARY HYPERPARATHYROIDISM

This condition is present when secondary hyperparathyroidism evolves to a state of apparently autonomous parathyroid function, which is reflected by hypercalcemia and an unsuppressed serum PTH level. Often, this indicates the development of an adenoma, but it can be associated with a monoclonal or oligoclonal nodular expansion of parathyroid cells.

TREATMENT OF SECONDARY HYPERPARATHYROIDISM IN END-STAGE RENAL DISEASE

Treatment for this condition comprises dietary phosphate restriction, phosphate binders, oral calcium, calcitriol, manipulation of dialysate calcium concentration, and parathyroid surgery.

Because phosphate cannot be excreted in the absence of renal function, and given its critical role in the pathogenesis of hyperparathyroidism, reduced dietary phosphate input is critical. A low-phosphate diet can potentially prevent the development of secondary hyperparathyroidism. However, the coincidence of dietary phosphate and protein sources limits restriction of the former.

Agents are then prescribed that bind dietary phosphate in the gastrointestinal tract and thus reduce its absorption. These phosphate binders are taken with meals and include calcium acetate and calcium carbonate. Some calcium absorption may occur, however, which is a problem if there is hypercalcemia. Aluminum-based binders are no longer in common use because there is associated aluminum absorption and accumulation in renal failure with attendant risks for anemia, bone disease, and dementia. A relatively new phosphate binder that does not contain calcium or aluminum is composed of cross-linked poly(allylamine hydrochloride). It may also lower serum lipids but there is a theoretical concern about its long-term effect on acid-base balance. Iron-based binders are under investigation but pose the risk of iron accumulation.

Attempts are made to restore calcitriol action (and hence intestinal calcium absorption and suppression of parathyroid gene transcription) by pharmacologically bypassing the hydroxylase enzyme. The drug 1α-hydroxyvitamin D_3 is converted by the liver to calcitriol and, if given relatively early in renal disease, may prevent progression of secondary hyperparathyroidism. Oral calcitriol is effective in reducing serum PTH in dialysis patients. There is a narrow therapeutic range, however, between doses that usefully reduce serum PTH and those that cause hypercalcemia and hyperphosphatemia. The latter conditions place patients at risk for mineral deposition in cardiovascular structures and other soft tissues. In an effort to maximize its direct action on the parathyroid gland while minimizing its action on the intestine, the drug has been given in large intermittent oral doses (*oral pulses*) or via the intravenous or intraperitoneal routes. Less calcemic analogues of calcitriol have been investigated in the hope that they will have higher parathyroid gland:intestine therapeutic ratios, as has 1α-hydroxyvitamin D_2.

When given between meals, the same calcium preparations that act as phosphate binders when taken with food also serve as calcium supplements. This is relevant for patients whose secondary hyperparathyroidism is characterized by low-normal plasma calcium levels. Manipulation of dialysate calcium concentration is also sometimes adopted as a strategy to alter plasma calcium concentration.

The indications for parathyroidectomy in the setting of dialysis include the following:

- Tertiary hyperparathyroidism
- Radiographic changes of parathyroid bone disease
- Severe pruritus
- Large vessel and/or soft tissue calcification

Surgery is generally offered only after failure of medical therapy, which is reflected by high plasma calcium and phosphate concentrations in the setting of a PTH more than three times above the upper reference limit, despite full medical measures. Aluminum bone disease as a possible cause of the hypercalcemia should be considered because surgery in this setting may not be associated with improvement in the plasma calcium level and may be associated with worse bone lesions. *Calciphylaxis* is a term used to describe a rare syndrome in which there is small-vessel (medial) calcification. The intima may demonstrate proliferation. Infarction of skin and subcutaneous (adipose) tissue occurs, leading to ulceration, often with sepsis, and there is a high risk of mortality. Muscle lesions may also be present and muscle pain may precede the skin signs. Calciphylaxis is another indication for parathyroidectomy because it is hoped that through a reduction in the plasma calcium and phosphate concentrations, the chances for survival may improve.

The surgical procedure is usually total parathyroidectomy with reimplantation of a remnant (often in the forearm). In this manner, it is hoped that there will be appropriate residual parathyroid function. Should excess function develop at a later date, repeat surgery is then possible on the forearm. This avoids the morbidity associated with repeat neck surgery. Some surgeons consider subtotal parathyroidectomy as preferable, which may avoid postoperative hypocalcemia (see following section). It is critical that any parathyroid surgery is performed by surgeons experienced with these procedures to minimize morbidity.

The drop in PTH levels that occurs postoperatively may be associated with a precipitous fall in plasma calcium level. Intravenous calcium is usually required perioperatively. Patients not already taking calcitriol should begin this drug approximately 1 week before surgery (receiving at least 0.25 μg of calcitriol orally twice each day) to prime the intestine to permit maximum absorption of oral calcium supplements postoperatively to assist in maintaining plasma calcium level. Postoperatively, gross radiologic lucencies have been noted to heal, and this coupled with the profound demand for a positive calcium balance led to the name hungry bone syndrome. Patients now rarely present with such severe radiologic lesions preoperatively. Nevertheless, bone density increases rapidly after parathyroidectomy. Whether this conveys benefit for fracture risk in these patients is not clear. Surgery is also associated with a reduction in bone pain, irritability, and pruritus. The latter benefit may relate to reduced PTH induction of mast cell degranulation. Data on resolution of left ventricular hypertrophy are conflicting.

It may be possible to prevent hyperparathyroidism in renal failure. This could involve aggressive attempts to maintain the plasma phosphate level within the normal reference range, including early institution of dietary phosphate restriction and early prescription of phosphate binders. In practice, these measures are only instituted once renal disease is advanced and hyperparathyroidism already established. The clinical institution of these measures years earlier, at the stage of early renal impairment, however, is worthy of further clinical consideration and investigation because it may retard or prevent hyperparathyroidism. Similarly, calcitriol deficiency (as opposed to vitamin D deficiency) could be addressed long before end-stage renal failure by the early prescription of oral calcitriol, although careful monitoring of plasma and urine calcium levels to avoid renal calculi/nephrocalcinosis would then be required.

HYPOPARATHYROIDISM

Hypoparathyroidism is an uncommon disorder in which hypocalcemia occurs because either PTH secretion is inadequate for the maintenance of a normal extracellular fluid calcium concentration or there is impaired PTH action in target tissues.

Etiology and Pathogenesis

Most cases occur as a complication of neck surgery. The risk of transient hypoparathyroidism associated with parathyroid and thyroid surgery is in the range of 1% to 10%. Permanent hypoparathyroidism is less common after these operations but occurs in most patients having radical surgery for malignancies of the head and neck. Other causes are rare (Table 3). Autoimmune destruction, either isolated to the parathyroid glands or as part of a polyglandular syndrome, is found in a small proportion of cases. Hypomagnesemia is an important, reversible cause of impaired PTH secretion and may also result in target organ resistance to PTH.

TABLE 3. **Causes of Hypoparathyroidism**

Destruction of Parathyroid Tissue
Surgery
Autoimmunity
Radiation, including high dose radioiodine
Infiltration (iron or copper overload, malignancy, granulomatous disease)
Abnormal Regulation of PTH Secretion
Genetic
Hypomagnesemia
Maternal hyperparathyroidism
Impaired PTH Action
Hypomagnesemia
Pseudohypoparathyroidism
PTH receptor defects
Developmental Failure
Isolated hypoparathyroidism
Complex genetic syndromes

Abbreviation: PTH = parathyroid hormone.

Clinical Manifestations and Presentation

Most cases are diagnosed when hypocalcemia occurs in the first few days after neck surgery. Symptoms depend to some extent on the severity of hypocalcemia (and probably also on its rapidity of onset and duration). The less severe symptoms are circumoral and acral paresthesias and muscle cramping. More severe manifestations are spontaneous tetany (carpopedal spasm, laryngospasm), muscle weakness, impaired consciousness, and generalized seizures. Cardiac arrhythmias, hypotension, cardiac failure, and characteristic electrocardiographic abnormalities also may occur. Electrocardiographic changes may include prolonged ST segments with late T waves, giving prolonged QT intervals.

In long-standing hypoparathyroidism, symptoms typically are mild and less specific, including lethargy and depressed mood. Cataracts are common. Signs of latent tetany (Trousseau sign, Chvostek sign) are often positive in both acute and chronic hypocalcemia.

Investigation and Diagnosis

Hypocalcemia with an undetectable or low PTH level is diagnostic of hypoparathyroidism. A PTH level within the reference range (i.e., not appropriately elevated) suggests partial hypoparathyroidism. If serum protein concentrations are abnormal (hypoalbuminemia in particular), correction formulas can be applied to assess whether there is true hypocalcemia, but measurement of the ionized calcium concentration is generally more reliable for this purpose. The venipuncture should be performed without a tourniquet because of the decrease in ionized calcium induced by venous stasis. The serum magnesium should be measured to exclude hypomagnesemia as a reversible cause of hypocalcemia. The serum inorganic phosphate level rises with any cause of hypoparathyroidism. In contrast, when hungry bone syndrome occurs following parathyroid surgery, the phosphorus level decreases.

Treatment

The general aim of treatment is to prevent symptoms and complications of hypocalcemia in the safest way possible. In the absence of the hypocalciuric action of PTH on the kidney, during therapy urinary calcium excretion tends to become excessive with serum calcium concentrations within the reference range, which thus risks promoting renal calculi/nephrocalcinosis. As a compromise, the achievement of serum calcium levels in the low-normal range will usually control symptoms without hypercalciuria being a problem. The basis of long-term treatment is combination therapy with calcium supplements and a vitamin D compound. One to 2 g of elemental calcium should be taken daily in several divided doses. Higher doses tend to cause constipation. Suitable calcium salts include calcium carbonate and calcium citrate. Calcium phosphate should not be used and a high intake of dairy products should be avoided because of their high phosphate content.

Therapy with vitamin D compounds is required in addition to calcium in most patients. Calcitriol (1,25-dihydroxyvitamin D_3) is the agent of choice. It is the major active form of vitamin D and is deficient in hypoparathyroidism. Its main therapeutic action is to enhance intestinal calcium absorption. It has a relatively fast onset and offset of effect on the serum calcium level over 1 to 2 days, making it optimal for dose adjustment and avoidance of a major complication of therapy, which is hypercalcemia. Most patients require a maintenance dose of calcitriol (Rocaltrol) in the range 0.25 to 2.0 μg daily. Vitamin D_2 (*ergocalciferol*) and vitamin D_3 (*cholecalciferol*) had major roles historically in the treatment of hypoparathyroidism, but these fat-soluble sterols can accumulate and cause prolonged vitamin D intoxication. Thus, although they are inexpensive compared with shorter acting forms of vitamin D, they are considerably more hazardous at the doses required to treat hypoparathyroidism and should be avoided for this indication if possible. Typical dosages are in the range of 25,000 to 100,000 U daily. This use is quite distinct from the setting of vitamin D deficiency where low doses of ergocalciferol or cholecalciferol are the agents of first choice.

Patients should be seen every 1 to 2 weeks until therapy is stabilized. Symptoms, tolerability, and compliance with medications and the serum calcium and inorganic phosphate levels should be monitored on each occasion. When the treatment regimen is stable, 24-hour urinary calcium excretion should be measured to check for hypercalciuria. In the event of hypercalciuria, a gentle reduction in therapy might be attempted. If this maneuver precipitates symptomatic hypocalcemia, an alternate strategy is to introduce a small dose of thiazide diuretic to enhance renal calcium conservation. In the long term, clinical and biochemical monitoring at 3- to 6-month intervals is usually satisfactory. Ophthalmologic studies should be performed every 1 to 2 years to screen for cataracts.

The acute management of hypocalcemia due to hypoparathyroidism depends on the severity of the condition. If features of the hypocalcemia are mild, it is generally sufficient to commence treatment with oral calcium and calcitriol, starting at the lower dose ranges given previously. When hypocalcemia and its manifestations are more severe (as is often the case with postoperative hypoparathyroidism), treatment is urgent, and careful observation and monitoring are required. Intravenous 10% calcium gluconate (10–20 mL infused over 10–20 minutes) will usually relieve symptoms. This should be followed by a continuous intravenous calcium infusion. This may be maintained over the ensuing day or two until oral calcium and vitamin D compound therapy can be established. The goal is to maintain the serum calcium level within the reference range to control symptoms. During infusion, the serum calcium level should be monitored at 3- to 4-hour intervals. A convenient infusion can be made up by adding 100 mL of 10% calcium gluconate (8.9 mg calcium/mL) to 500 or 1000 mL of 5% dextrose in water. Typical infusion rates that are required are in the range of 1 to 2 mg calcium/kg body weight/hr. Patients require careful observation during calcium infusion.

Hypoparathyroidism following parathyroid surgery is often transient. Therefore, therapy should be aimed to control symptoms of hypocalcemia and to avoid moderate or severe reductions in the serum calcium level, in anticipation of recovery of parathyroid function. Recovery often ensues within days to weeks of surgery. Regular attempts should be made to decrease the level of treatment over this time, seeking evidence of recovery.

PRIMARY ALDOSTERONISM

method of
RICK SCHIEBINGER, M.D.
Susquehanna Health System
Williamsport, Pennsylvania

Recent estimates indicate that the incidence of primary aldosteronism (PA) is as high as 12% of the hypertensive population. The incidence has clearly increased, possibly owing to improved screening techniques. PA is now recognized to be the most common form of secondary hypertension.

PATHOPHYSIOLOGY

PA is characterized by an inappropriately high circulating plasma aldosterone concentration (PAC) for the level of plasma renin activity (PRA). The most common subtypes of PA are the adrenocorticotropic hormone (ACTH)-responsive aldosterone-producing adenoma (APA) and angiotensin II (AT II)-responsive bilateral hyperplasia, also known as *idiopathic hyperaldosteronism (IHA)*. Less commonly seen is AT II–unresponsive primary adrenal hyperplasia, which may be unilateral.

Two forms of familial hyperaldosteronism (FH) have been described: FH type I and FH type II. *FH type I* or *glucocorticoid-remediable aldosteronism* is autosomal dominant in inheritance. It is caused by a chimeric gene in which the ACTH-responsive 5′-promoter of the 11β-hydroxylase gene is fused to coding sequences of the aldosterone synthase gene. This results in ectopic expression of aldosterone synthase activity in zona fasciculata cells of the adrenal cortex under the regulation of ACTH, with resultant hyperaldosteronism and suppression of AT II–stimulated aldosterone production in the zona glomerulosa. The chimeric gene product generates hybrid steroids such as 18-hydroxycortisol and 18-oxocortisol in addition to aldosterone. FH type II is also autosomal dominant in inheritance. Aldosterone secretion is not dexamethasone suppressible, and patients present with APA, IHA, or both. The genetic cause of FH type II remains unknown. Thus far, it does not appear to be a mutation in aldosterone synthase (CYP11B2) or the AT II receptor.

The morbidity/mortality from PA is primarily due to its vascular effects. Hyperaldosteronism raises blood pressure (BP) by increasing sodium reabsorption and peripheral vascular resistance in addition to causing central nervous system effects that raise BP through alterations in renal nerve stimulation and baroreceptor function. Aldosterone induces vascular smooth muscle hyperplasia and hypertrophy that increase vascular tone. Its effects are both acute (nongenomic) and chronic (genomic). Aldosterone may also adversely effect the heart. It has been shown to cause cardiac fibrosis and hypertrophy. This effect appears to be influenced by salt intake. Aldosterone has recently been shown to increase plasminogen activator inhibitor-1 that appears to play a role in the development of glomerulosclerosis.

In addition, patients with PA have been shown to have insulin resistance that improves after surgical cure but not when treated with spironolactone alone. Finally, there is an increased incidence of hemorrhagic stroke in patients with FH type I: mean age 32 years, incidence 18%, mortality 61%. The underlying mechanism in most cases is intracranial aneurysm.

PRESENTATION

Most patients with PA present with hypertension. Exceptions have been noted, especially in patients with FH type I. Most patients with PA present with hypokalemia except those with the familial forms that rarely have unprovoked hypokalemia. Patients with the nonfamilial forms of PA almost never have a serum potassium above 4 mmol/L. The hypertension may be severe. Some patients may have headaches, muscular weakness, flaccid paralysis, muscle cramps, palpitations, or polyuria as symptoms of PA.

DIAGNOSTIC TESTING

The diagnostic approach consists of two phases: establishing the diagnosis and distinguishing between surgically remediable forms of PA and those that respond to medical management. Unprovoked hypokalemia in a hypertensive patient is a helpful clue to screen for PA; however, patients with FH are usually normokalemic.

In the normokalemic patient, age and family history of hypertension may prompt one to screen for PA. However, if the incidence of PA is truly around 10% as suggested by recent estimates, consideration should be given to screening most hypertensive patients younger than age 50.

It is best but not always necessary to screen patients off any antihypertensive drugs that influence the renin-angiotensin-aldosterone axis for 2 to 4 weeks. The simplest screening test is the ratio of PAC (in ng/dL) to PRA (in ng/mL/h). Patients with a ratio greater than 20 and a PAC greater than 15 ng/dL should be further evaluated to confirm the diagnosis of PA unless the ratio is greater than 70, which is considered diagnostic. The higher the ratio and PAC the greater the probability of PA. The specificity of the screening ratio is improved if patients are ambulatory at the time of blood sampling and if they are free of hypertensive nephropathy. A urinary potassium excretion rate of greater than 30 mmol/24 h lends further support to the diagnosis of PA.

Confirmation of the diagnosis of PA can be made several ways. Volume expansion by administration of fludrocortisone (Florinef Acetate) 0.4 mg/d for 3 days on a greater than 100 mmol sodium diet is considered one of the better tests to establish the diagnosis. At the end of day 3, a PAC greater than 5 ng/dL confirms the diagnosis of PA. Vigorous potassium replacement will likely be required during this test. Alternative tests include the infusion of 2 L normal saline over 4 hours. At the end of the infusion, a PAC greater than 8.5 ng/dL confirms the diagnosis. Volume expansion may also be achieved by the administration of a high salt diet followed 3 days later with a 24-hour measurement of urinary aldosterone. An excretion rate greater than 14 μg again confirms the diagnosis in the presence of high sodium excretion (>200 mmol/d).

DIFFERENTIAL DIAGNOSIS

Once the diagnosis of PA is established, one must make the distinction between APA and IHA. The hypertension caused by adenomas can be cured by surgical therapy, whereas the hypertension associated with bilateral hyperplasia is often not cured even by total bilateral adrenalectomy and is therefore treated medically. Adenomas tend to produce more severe hyperaldosteronism and consequently more severe hypertension, more profound hypokalemia, and more complete renin suppression, but these findings do not reliably differentiate them from hyperplasia.

The simplest way to distinguish between these two causes of PA is to demonstrate the presence of an adrenal tumor by high resolution computed tomography (CT). Unfortunately, a negative CT does not exclude the presence of a small APA. Conversely, a positive CT does not indicate the functionality of a tumor; however, it is reasonable to proceed with surgical removal of the tumor unless it does not have the appearance of a benign adrenal adenoma on CT. A negative CT requires further testing before concluding that the patient has IHA. The most definitive test is bilateral adrenal venous sampling with ACTH stimulation. In most cases, if an APA is present, the PAC-cortisol ratio will be greater than 5:1 when comparing the two sides and the PAC-cortisol ratio of the unaffected adrenal will be less than the ratio for the peripheral vein. Scintigraphy with NP-59 (iodomethylnorcholesterol) is frequently not sensitive enough to detect tumors not visualized by CT.

One widely used noninvasive test to distinguish hyperplasia from adenoma is based on incomplete suppression of renin activity in bilateral hyperplasia. PRA rises slightly and PAC increases significantly after stimulation of 2 to 4 hours of upright posture in these patients because the hyperplastic glands are AT II–sensitive whereas adenomas typically are not. In addition, PRA remains suppressed and PAC does not rise in patients with adenomas. PAC usually falls during the posture test in patients with adenomas, which are sensitive to the circadian fall in ACTH over the time of testing. Consequently, cortisol measurements should be taken during the posture test to reflect a fall in ACTH. The posture test has a diagnostic accuracy of 85% or less.

Another test that may be helpful is the measurement of plasma 18-hydroxycorticosterone. This steroid is produced in cells in which aldosterone synthase and 11β-hydroxylase are co-expressed, which occurs in APA. Normal glomerulosa cells do not express 11β-hydroxylase. Consequently, 18-hydroxycorticosterone is elevated in patients with an adenoma with plasma concentrations greater than 50 ng/dL and usually in excess of 100 ng/dL. In contrast, plasma concentrations in patients with hyperplasia are less than 100 ng/dL with most less than 50 ng/dL.

Finally, patients with a negative CT should be screened for FH type I. A 24-hour urine 18-hydroxycortisol excretion in excess of 1100 μg or direct genetic blood testing to detect the chimeric gene are diagnostic. Alternative, a PAC of less than 4 ng/dL after administration of dexamethasone (Decadron) 0.5 mg every 6 hours for 2 days is a useful screening test.

TREATMENT

Patients with an APA should have it laparoscopically removed. Patients with adenomas approaching 3 cm should undergo a dexamethasone suppression test before surgery. These tumors express 17-hydroxylase activity and are capable of making cortisol. The amount of cortisol produced is a function of tumor size.

If normal suppression is not demonstrated, the patient should be treated for adrenal insufficiency after surgery. Surgery is also recommended in patients with suspected primary adrenal hyperplasia. It is not common practice to perform bilateral adrenalectomy for IHA because hypertension is rarely normalized by surgery. Medical treatment is recommended especially with spironolactone (Aldactone) 200 to 400 mg/d because it is the most effective drug offering cardiac protection from aldosterone-induced cardiac fibrosis and hypertrophy. Unfortunately, spironolactone (Aldactone) is often not well tolerated, especially in men, due to its antiandrogenic effects. Alternative treatment with amiloride (Midamor),* 5 to 20 mg/d will diminish potassium wasting but will have no direct protective effect on the heart like spironolactone.

Unless new antimineralocorticoids come to market soon for those intolerant to spironolactone, one wonders if bilateral adrenalectomy may not be the best current treatment for these patients. Medical treatment usually includes a diuretic with the addition of a calcium channel blocker, β-blocker, or angiotensin-converting enzyme inhibitor as needed. The goal of treatment for patients with FH type I is ACTH suppression. It has recently been found that total suppression is not necessary to normalize BP. Dexamethasone (Decadron), 0.125 to 0.25 mg/d or prednisone, 2.5 to 5 mg/d is adequate in most patients. Higher doses of steroids are not recommended. BP not controlled on these lower steroid doses should be treated like that in patients with bilateral hyperplasia. Patients with FH type I should also be screened for intracranial aneurysms by magnetic resonance angiography. Patients with FH type II should be treated like any other patient with an APA or IHA. Hypertensive family members should be screened for PA.

*Not FDA approved for this indication.

HYPOPITUITARISM IN ADULTS

method of
DESMOND JOHNSTON, M.B.CH.B., PH.D.,
MA'EN A. AL-MRAYAT, M.B.B.S., and
TARA KEARNEY, M.B.B.S.
St. Mary's Hospital
London, England

Hypopituitarism is uncommon, affecting 10 to 15 in 1 million people per year. In view of the multiplicity of causes, patients may present through several medical disciplines but most frequently via endocrine and neurology clinics. Here, we focus on disease in adulthood and its biochemical evaluation and therapy.

ETIOLOGY

Hypopituitarism results from inadequate secretion of one or more pituitary hormones. It occurs most commonly in association with pituitary tumors, after pituitary surgery and/or irradiation, or secondary to hypothalamic disease. Deficiency of the hypothalamic-pituitary-adrenal (HPA) axis, as an isolated problem, occurs most commonly in patients who have received prolonged therapy with glucocorticoids in the recent past.

CLINICAL PRESENTATION

The presentation may be acute or chronic. Acute hypopituitarism, due to pituitary infarction or hemorrhage, causes sudden headache, collapse, and hypotension; it may be life-threatening. In chronic hypopituitarism, the onset of symptoms is often insidious. Clinical manifestations depend on the degree, the duration, and the specific hormones that are deficient. Symptoms include lack of well-being and fatigue. In children, growth hormone (GH) deficiency is a cause of growth failure. Decreased gonadotropin secretion causes the clinical features of hypogonadism in both sexes. Rare instances of prolactin deficiency result in failure of lactation. Vasopressin deficiency presents with thirst and polyuria.

FUNCTIONAL TESTING AND TREATMENT

Guidelines for the investigation of hypopituitarism have been published recently by national and international organizations; certain areas (assessment of adrenocorticotropic hormone [ACTH] reserve and of GH reserve; GH replacement therapy in adults) are contentious, and more emphasis is placed on them in this review (see the following sections).

Adrenocorticotropic Hormone

Assessment of Adrenocorticotropic Hormone Secretion

ACTH deficiency is classically associated with structural disease of the hypothalamus or pituitary gland. Hypopituitarism, including ACTH deficiency, may also follow more generalized central nervous system insults such as cranial irradiation or severe head injury. The assessment of ACTH reserve is also important in several clinical situations where there is not a strong suspicion of structural hypothalamic or pituitary disease (e.g., patients receiving systemic or topical glucocorticoids for prolonged periods, patients with unexplained hypoglycemia or hyponatremia).

BASAL CORTISOL LEVELS

Measurements of random circulating ACTH and 24-hour urinary-free cortisol are of limited value. Fasting plasma cortisol levels at 8 AM to 9 AM are considered by some to be of use. In one series of 232 tests, the response to hypoglycemia was consistently normal if the fasting cortisol concentration was greater than 400 nmol/L, and the authors suggested that subsequent dynamic testing was unnecessary if cortisol concentrations exceeded 400 mmol/L. Caution is required, however, in that there are instances in which a basal cortisol level greater than 400 nmol/L is associated with an unequivocally subnormal response to hypoglycemia (in up to one third of patients). Some of the differences in the literature undoubtedly reflect the variations in cortisol assays and reference ranges. If the basal cortisol concentration is greater than the threshold for a normal response to provocation with any particular assay, then dynamic testing is probably unnecessary.

A variety of dynamic tests have been devised and there has been much discussion of their relative merits.

INSULIN STRESS TEST

The insulin stress test (IST, also referred to as *insulin tolerance test;* Table 1) is generally regarded as robust. In suspected panhypopituitarism, a low dose of insulin (0.05–0.15 U/kg) is given to produce hypoglycemia (laboratory blood glucose level <2.2 mmol/L, with hypoglycemic symptoms). If hypoglycemia is not achieved, higher insulin doses are necessary on a separate occasion, and up to 0.3 U/kg may be necessary in particularly insulin-resistant patients, such as those who are obese or those with acromegaly. In patients with diabetes mellitus, the test has been performed following restoration of the fasting glucose level to normal with a continuous insulin infusion, although the test performed in this way has not been fully validated.

The IST has been used for many years. With this test, an adequate response to hypoglycemia indicates that the response to major illness or surgery will be sufficient without therapeutic glucocorticoid coverage. In early studies in which this was established, an 11-hydroxycorticosteroid response of greater than 20 μg/100 mL (measured using the fluorimetric Mattingly method, equivalent to 580 nmol/L) in an IST was defined as the *adequate response.* This was associated with normal clinical outcome and normal circulating 11-hydroxycorticosteroid levels during major surgery in patients who were receiving, or had received, treatment with systemic glucocorticoids and

TABLE 1. **Common Dynamic Tests for the Diagnosis of ACTH and GH Deficiency**

Test	Hormone(s) Tested	Threshold for Replacement Treatment	Contraindications	Comments
Insulin hypoglycemia test: 1. Insulin (0.05–0.1 U/kg) IV after overnight fast. Blood glucose must reach ≤2.2 mmol/L. 2. Measure serum GH, cortisol, and glucose at 0, 15, 30, 45, 60, 90, and 120 min.	GH and ACTH	GH increases to >20 mU/L (children), GH increases to >6–10 mU/L (adults). Cortisol increases to >500–580 nmol/L.	Ischemic heart disease, abnormal ECG, epilepsy, previous dysrhythmia, cerebrovascular disease, altered mental status, and generalized debility. Frequently restricted to patients <65 y.	Careful monitoring with bedside glucose 50% and hydrocortisone. Higher insulin doses (up to 0.3 U/kg) in insulin-resistant cases. Patients should receive a meal before leaving.
Glucagon test: 1. Glucagon 1 mg (children 0.5 mg) SC or IM after overnight fast. 2. Measure blood glucose, GH, and cortisol every 30 min for 4 h.	GH and ACTH	GH increases as for insulin hypoglycemia. Cortisol increases to >500–580 nmol/L.		May be used in patients with ischemic heart disease or epilepsy. Nausea and vomiting may occur. Some healthy subjects do not respond.
Short Synacthen test: 1. Tetracosatrin (250 μg) IM or IV 2. Collect blood for cortisol at 0, 30, and 60 min.	ACTH	Cortisol increases to >550–580 nmol/L at 30 min.		Patients need not fast.
Arginine test: 1. L-Arginine (0.5 g/kg to a maximum of 30 g) IV over 30 min after overnight fast. 2. Collect blood for GH level every 30 min for 2 h.	GH	Same as insulin hypoglycemia.		Women and children respond consistently better than men. 30% to 35% of healthy subjects do not respond.

Abbreviations: ACTH = adrenocorticotropic hormone; GH = growth hormone; IM = intramuscular; IV = intravenous; SC = subcutaneous.

The criteria for normal cortisol responses have varied in different studies and in different centers. Each center should establish its own criteria based on clinical experience and assay method. The dose of insulin required to produce hypoglycemia may need to be increased in insulin-resistant subjects.

were therefore at risk of adrenal insufficiency. A lower limit for the adequate IST response could not be devised for ethical reasons in these early studies because those with a lower IST response were given glucocorticoid coverage for anesthesia. There is, however, no better way to establish a threshold. An additional benefit with IST is that it provides an estimate of GH reserve.

Patients with ischemic heart disease, an abnormal resting electrocardiogram, previous dysrhythmias, or epilepsy are excluded. It should not be performed if the 9 AM serum cortisol is less than 100 nmol/L or in patients who are at risk of adrenal suppression through long-term glucocorticoid therapy, without first confirming that the adrenal cortex can respond normally (e.g., with a tetracosactrin [Synacthen] test). Intravenous hydrocortisone (100 mg) and glucose (50 mL of 50% weight/volume) must be available immediately for the patient undergoing an IST. With these exclusions and precautions, the IST in experienced hands is a safe diagnostic procedure in adults. It is recommended that only endocrine teams that routinely perform the IST should use this test.

THE SHORT SYNACTHEN TEST

The short Synacthen test in standard dosage (SST; 250 μg tetracosactrin given intramuscularly [or intravenously] with blood drawn for serum cortisol measurement at 0, 30, and 60 minutes after injection) was devised primarily as a test of adrenal reserve. Tetracosactrin is a synthetic peptide (ACTH 1-24) that has equimolar activity to natural human ACTH (1-39) in the stimulation of adrenal cortisol secretion. The SST also gives an estimate of ACTH secretion because the adrenal gland needs prior exposure to circulating ACTH to respond normally to tetracosactrin. The 30-minute cortisol response to tetracosactrin is better than the 60-minute value in discriminating secondary pituitary failure from reference levels, and the 30-minute values correlate with the peak cortisol level in an IST.

Discrepancies among the tests (typically an adequate SST but inadequate IST response) have been reported for individual patients with adverse clinical consequences in some instances. These discrepancies may be minimized by choosing a higher cortisol threshold for normality in the SST than in the IST. The advantage of the SST is that it is rapid and safe, and patients do not have to fast overnight. It is unsuitable in the period immediately following pituitary surgery (probably for a minimum of 2–3 weeks) because ACTH deficiency does not immediately result in an impaired adrenal cortical response. Some concerns remain regarding the discrepancies with the IST and the fact that a normal SST has not been demonstrated to indicate sufficient HPA activity for major illness or surgery. The SST is not recommended as a test of ACTH reserve following withdrawal of exogenous glucocorticoid therapy because the response may be normal when the IST response is clearly deficient (although it is useful to exclude primary adrenal suppression; to be discussed).

Variations in cortisol immunoassays influence the interpretation of provocation tests. In one study of 100 healthy volunteers and 44 newly diagnosed, untreated patients with pituitary disease, basal and 30-minute post-tetracosactrin cortisol levels were determined using four immunoassays. The *normal response,* defined as the fifth percentile, ranged from 510 to 626 nmol/L with the different methods. This emphasizes the need to establish reference ranges for each immunoassay method and to re-establish a reference range if the laboratory method is changed. A further observation from this study was a marked difference between genders, which was also variable between assays. Women had a higher 30-minute response to tetracosactrin than men, but the difference ranged from 6% to 17% depending on the assay used.

THE GLUCAGON TEST

The glucagon test (using 1 mg subcutaneously) may be substituted for those unable to tolerate the IST. This test is safe, although nausea and vomiting are common. It is probably less reliable than the IST in that some healthy subjects do not respond. It has the advantage over the Synacthen test of permitting GH reserve to be tested in the same procedure.

THE METYRAPONE TEST

The metyrapone test is used more frequently in North America than elsewhere. Metyrapone is an inhibitor of 11β-hydroxylase and inhibits cortisol synthesis. It assesses the adequacy of cortisol feedback and results are comparable to those of the IST in patients with pituitary tumors. It has, however, not been proven to indicate the ability to respond adequately to stress. In its traditional form, the test is cumbersome. Even in a form modified for overnight investigation, it requires measurement of 11-deoxycortisol, which is not generally available.

THE LONG SYNACTHEN TEST

The long (or depot) Synacthen test has been used to confirm ACTH deficiency. Depot tetracosactrin (1 mg intramuscularly) is given with blood drawn for serum cortisol level at 0, 24, 48, and 96 hours. Patients with ACTH deficiency have a poor 24-hour response but achieve a normal serum cortisol level at 48 to 96 hours. This long test has probably few advantages over the SST, while still suffering from most of the same drawbacks. It is very rarely used.

THE LOW-DOSE SYNACTHEN TEST

The low-dose Synacthen test (1 μg or 0.5 μg/1.73 m^2) attempts to refine the traditional (250 μg) SST. Because the aim is to demonstrate adrenal cortical atrophy, lower doses might be more sensitive than the standard 250-μg dose (which is a grossly supraphysiologic stimulus). Excellent concordance has been reported between cortisol responses to 1-μg tetracosactrin and the IST. In other studies, however, the low-dose (1 μg) test was no more sensitive than the standard 250-μg test in distinguishing patients with mild-to-moderate ACTH deficiency. A 10-μg

Synacthen test has also been reported but no low-dose test has yet gained acceptance. Some anxiety has been expressed about the adsorption of tetracosactrin to plastic tubing and cannulae with such low doses, in view of reports of variable results being obtained using different injection techniques. The low-dose Synacthen test cannot be recommended for general use at present.

SPECIAL SITUATIONS

Assessment of the Hypothalamic-Pituitary-Adrenal Axis Following Pituitary Surgery. During pituitary surgery, patients receive glucocorticoid coverage irrespective of their preoperative ACTH secretory status. Early postoperative (third or seventh day) plasma cortisol levels predict the subsequent requirement for cortisol replacement; levels less than 100 nmol/L indicate the need for lifelong glucocorticoid replacement, whereas values greater than 450 nmol/L suggest that this will be unnecessary. Nonetheless, exceptions occur and formal testing of ACTH reserve at a later stage is generally performed. As previously discussed, the SST alone is inappropriate in assessing ACTH reserve in the first 1 to 3 weeks postoperatively.

It is customary to re-evaluate ACTH reserve 4 to 12 weeks postoperatively using one of the tests previously outlined. An SST is traditionally performed first to ensure that some degree of adrenal suppression has not developed over this period of hydrocortisone replacement. Both the SST and the subsequent IST or equivalent (if an additional provocation test is desired) are performed in the morning, with the patients having taken no hydrocortisone replacement therapy since the previous day. Recent evidence suggests that there may be an advantage to delaying assessment of the HPA axis until this later postoperative stage, in that dysfunction observed in postoperative days 4 to 11 (observed using both low- and high-dose tetracosactrin, and during an IST) may normalize by 1 to 3 months.

Assessment of the Hypothalamic-Pituitary-Adrenal Axis Following Prolonged Glucocorticoid Administration. Transient suppression of the HPA axis occurs after short periods (up to 4 weeks) of glucocorticoid treatment administered orally or systemically at pharmacologic levels. This usually resolves within a few days and is of no clinical importance. In patients on glucocorticoid therapy for longer periods, ACTH deficiency (or adrenal suppression) may persist when treatment is stopped and may be permanent if treatment has been given over several years (although some may recover their HPA reserve despite many years of glucocorticoid treatment). It is often necessary to assess ACTH and cortisol reserve as the exogenous glucocorticoid dosage is reduced. Conventionally dosage reduction is gradual, for example, reducing the daily dose of prednisone (or equivalent) by 1 mg at 1- to 2-month intervals. There is no point assessing ACTH or adrenal secretion while patients are taking more than 5 mg of prednisone daily. Once below this dosage, adrenal suppression can be excluded with an SST. If the response to tetracosactrin is normal, then the HPA axis may be assessed with a central stimulant such as the insulin stress test or glucagon test. While some would not accept a normal response to either the SST or the IST alone as indicating adequate HPA reserve, most would accept that the axis is intact if both responses are normal. In view of the cross-reaction of prednisone in many cortisol immunoassay tests, the prednisone dose should be omitted on the mornings of the tests. Although the formulary advice is that tetracosactrin should not be given to patients with a known allergic history, many patients being weaned off glucocorticoid replacement are in this category (e.g., those with asthma or eczema) and the authors have never observed an adverse event when tetracosactrin was administered in this situation.

Although topical glucocorticoids (inhaled or preparations applied to the skin) were designed to target glucocorticoid therapy to the relevant tissues, systemic absorption occurs when high doses are used (e.g., inhaled beclomethasone 2000 μg/d or equivalent) and may lead to suppression of the HPA axis.

Assessment of the Hypothalamic-Pituitary-Adrenal Axis in Patients With Unexplained Hypoglycemia or Hyponatremia. ACTH deficiency in these circumstances may be isolated and may not be associated with structural disease of the hypothalamus or pituitary, for example, where there is chronic alcohol excess as the primary pathology. In severely ill patients, treatment must be commenced immediately but it is helpful for diagnosis to obtain blood samples for measurement of cortisol and ACTH before the first administration of glucocorticoid. Low levels of both cortisol and ACTH in an ill patient are suggestive of ACTH deficiency. The diagnosis may be confirmed at a later stage if necessary, as previously outlined.

Treatment of ACTH Deficiency

Hydrocortisone is the preferred glucocorticoid replacement therapy for ACTH deficiency, often taken orally on rising (10–20 mg) and mid-afternoon (5–10 mg), or as a thrice-daily regimen (e.g., 10 mg on rising, 5 mg at midday, 5 mg late afternoon). Prednisolone (3–6 mg) given in the morning, or in two divided doses, is an alternative. Fludrocortisone (Florinef Acetate; mineralocorticoid) is rarely required. Glucocorticoid therapy is monitored clinically; although it is not possible to reproduce with tablets the normal 24-hour circulating cortisol levels, a daily serum cortisol profile will help to indicate adequate or excessive concentrations throughout the day in patients taking hydrocortisone.

Patients must be educated to increase oral glucocorticoids (twofold to fourfold) with serious illness, and to receive systemic therapy if they are vomiting. Medic Alert or SOS bracelets/pendants are recommended in addition to carrying a steroid card.

Gonadotropins, Luteinizing Hormone, and Follicle-Stimulating Hormone

Assessment of Luteinizing Hormone and Follicle-Stimulating Hormone Secretion

Measurement of serum luteinizing hormone (LH) level with appropriate target organ hormone level (testosterone or estradiol) is usually adequate. A low target hormone value combined with a low or even normal LH level establishes LH deficiency. In women, measurements of target organ response (e.g., endometrial thickness, progestogen withdrawal test) are often more useful than measuring estradiol. Similarly a low serum follicle-stimulating hormone (FSH) level with low sperm count or evidence of anovulation suggests FSH deficiency.

The gonadotropin-releasing hormone test is rarely necessary to confirm LH and FSH deficiency.

Treatment of Luteinizing Hormone and Follicle-Stimulating Hormone Deficiency

In women, cyclical estrogen and progesterone should be given until 50 years of age or older, assuming there is no contraindication, for example, breast carcinoma. The duration of therapy will be influenced by factors such as bone mineral density. In certain patients (e.g., those with chronic estrogen deficiency) lower dosage regimens in the first instance may be advisable. Patients should have regular withdrawal bleeding. In those with a previous hysterectomy, unopposed estrogen is adequate. Treatment of infertility will require a specialist.

Replacement therapy in men with testosterone can be given orally (e.g., testosterone undecanoate 80–160 mg/d in divided doses), although the oral route is usually inadequate for satisfactory replacement. Transdermal testosterone via patches may provide a satisfactory regimen, although many patients find the patches unacceptable. Intramuscular injection of testosterone esters (100–250 mg every one to four weeks) is satisfactory, if inconvenient, for most patients. Subcutaneous testosterone implants are rarely required. Treatment should be monitored by measuring blood testosterone levels, which should be kept in the reference range while avoiding wide fluctuations in blood concentration. In patients receiving intramuscular replacement, adequate circulating testosterone levels should be ensured throughout the 1- to 4-week period. Some concerns exist about long-term therapy causing prostatic carcinoma, although there is no evidence for this using the standard therapeutic dosages for replacement. Stimulation of spermatogenesis, for example, with FSH and human chorionic gonadotropin, will require input from a specialist.

Thyroid-Stimulating Hormone

Assessment of Thyroid-Stimulating Hormone Secretion

Measurement of both serum thyroid-stimulating hormone (TSH) and thyroxine (T4) (free or total) is usually sufficient to determine TSH deficiency, which is defined by a low value of T4 in the presence of a low or normal TSH. Doubts may arise, for example, in the rare instances of thyroxine-binding globulin deficiency where subjects are clinically euthyroid, TSH is normal, but total T4 levels are low. Where doubt remains even with estimations of free hormone levels, the thyrotropin-releasing hormone (TRH) test may be of value.

Treatment of Thyroid-Stimulating Hormone Deficiency

Administration of L-thyroxine in a dose of approximately 125 μg daily (range, 75–200 μg) is usually adequate. Triiodothyronine as sole therapy offers no advantage. The benefits or otherwise of triiodothyronine in addition to thyroxine replacement are an area of current investigation. Therapy is monitored clinically and by measurement of serum thyroid hormone levels, keeping serum values in the reference range. Replacement is probably less precise than when patients with primary hypothyroidism are treated, in that the TSH level is of less value in assessing the adequacy of the dosage that is used.

Prolactin

Prolactin deficiency in women postpartum may be confirmed by a low serum prolactin value and confirmed by failure of response to a secretagogue such as TRH. Prolactin deficiency is not treated.

Growth Hormone

Assessment of Growth Hormone Secretion in Adults

GH deficiency in adults has assumed importance because recent studies have identified significant morbidity and mortality and since then, GH replacement therapy became an option. Because treatment is considered only for severe GH deficiency in adults, a stimulated level of less than 6 to 10 mU/L (<2.0–3.3 ng/mL) has been proposed. The IST is the conventional GH provocative test (with restrictions as previously outlined) and is a more effective stimulus than glucagon, arginine, L-dopa, and clonidine. GH responses are lower in obesity and with aging, and the diagnosis of GH deficiency in the obese and the elderly may be difficult. A low age-related IGF-1 concentration is of value in young adults with GH deficiency of childhood onset but less so in adult-onset disease, and many patients with unequivocal GH deficiency have IGF-1 levels in the low normal range. IGFBP3 levels are a poor discriminator in GH deficiency of adult onset.

Adults with multiple pituitary hormone deficiency are likely to be GH deficient. Indeed when two or more hormone deficiencies are present, there may be little need to test for GH deficiency. Newer tests of GH reserve are undergoing evaluation, for example, combined hexarelin–GHRH, and combined arginine–

GHRH, but they have not yet been validated for general use.

Treatment of Growth Hormone Deficiency in Adults

In children, biosynthetic GH is given as a subcutaneous injection 5 to 7 days each week. Growth and development are monitored in pediatric endocrine centers.

In adults, the decision to start GH replacement therapy is difficult. Morbidity associated with hypopituitarism, which may be caused by GH deficiency, includes altered body composition (reduced lean body mass and increased adipose tissue mass in a central distribution), together with decreased muscle strength and exercise capacity. There is also a reduction in bone density and an increased prevalence of osteoporosis. Patients have dry skin as a consequence of reduced sweating. Risk factors for vascular disease are present; increased low-density lipoprotein cholesterol and triglyceride levels; insulin resistance and impairment of glucose tolerance; increased fibrinogen and plasminogen activator inhibitor levels; and increased intima media thickening in the carotid arteries. In some patients, there is evidence of cardiac dysfunction. Life expectancy is reduced and mortality from cardiovascular disease is increased twofold. The quality of life in many patients is reduced in comparison with the general population.

The rationale for GH replacement in adults is based on the adverse cardiovascular risk factor profile, an increased risk of fracture, and the decrease in quality of life. GH replacement improves some of the conventional cardiovascular risk factors, increases lean body mass, and reduces body fat. Two years of GH replacement increases bone density in patients in whom it is reduced initially. Treatment has, however, not been available for a sufficiently long time to know if it will improve mortality and reduce fractures. Some patients do seem to have an improvement in quality of life when assessed in interviews and by questionnaire.

The decision to treat is therefore made on an individual basis and is guided by the initial assessment and patient wishes. Once a decision to start therapy has been made, patients are started on a low dose, typically 0.6 to 0.9 U/d (0.2–0.3 mg/d), increasing monthly until IGF-1 levels are in the middle of the age-related normal range. Clinical assessment, including anthropometry, measurement of vascular risk factors, and evaluation of quality of life, should be performed during GH replacement. The most common side effects are fluid retention and arthralgia, although these are minimized with the low-dose regimen. Fasting glucose level (or HbA1c) should be checked initially within 3 to 6 months of treatment, then every 6 months. It is reasonable to withdraw therapy after 6 months if there is no perceived benefit.

Vasopressin

Assessment of Vasopressin Secretion

A water deprivation test is usually necessary to determine vasopressin deficiency (24-hour urine volume >3 L in the presence of normal plasma sodium concentration). The test comprises a period of 8 hours of total fluid deprivation with measurement of plasma and urinary osmolality every 2 hours, followed by administration of desmopressin (2 μg intramuscularly) with subsequent urinary osmolality measurement at 5, 12, and 16 hours after injection. Rapid weight loss (>5% initial body weight) in the first part of the test requires cessation of fluid deprivation, but continuation of desmopressin injection. Vasopressin deficiency is recognized by poor urinary concentration (<300 mOsm/kg) after fluid deprivation but normal osmolality (>750 mOsm/kg) after administration of desmopressin. It is not unusual to have equivocal results. In ACTH deficiency, the water deprivation test will give spurious results. Patients should be tested once glucocorticoid replacement has been instituted.

Confirmation of vasopressin deficiency can be made by osmotic stimulation with 5% hypertonic saline infusion for 2 hours with blood measurements of osmolality and vasopressin. This is available in specialized centers only.

Treatment of Vasopressin Deficiency

Desmopressin is given orally (50–1000 μg/d) or intranasally (5–60 μg/d) in divided doses to reduce urine volume to 2.0 to 3.0 L/24 hours. Intermittent measurements of serum sodium level are advised to avoid the slow development of hyponatremia due to overdosage.

LONG-TERM CARE AND FOLLOW-UP STUDIES

Once stabilized on replacement therapy, patients should receive specialist follow-up care as outpatients every 6 to 12 months.

Anterior pituitary hormone deficiency may develop many years later in patients who have received radiation therapy. Formal testing for additional pituitary hormone deficiency should be performed every 1 to 3 years. Lifelong follow-up care by a specialist is required to monitor pituitary function and replacement treatment.

PERIOPERATIVE MANAGEMENT

Over the period of pituitary surgery, patients generally receive systemic glucocorticoid replacement therapy (hydrocortisone 100 mg preoperatively intravenously followed by a further 200–300 mg in the subsequent 24 hours). The dose is typically reduced over the following 7 to 10 days to the maintenance regimen. At 4 to 12 weeks postoperatively, patients should undergo full pituitary function testing (as previously outlined). Postoperative diabetes insipidus is common and may require desmopressin therapy. The diabetes insipidus is often transient (lasting 24 hours–1 week), however, and desmopressin should be withdrawn at intervals to assess posterior pituitary function. Perioperative antibiotic therapy for transsphenoidal surgery is conventional as prophylaxis against meningitis.

HYPERPROLACTINEMIA

method of
ERVIN E. JONES, PH.D., M.D.
Yale University School of Medicine
New Haven, Connecticut

Prolactin is a polypeptide hormone secreted by the lactotroph cells located in the anterior pituitary gland. Human prolactin is composed of 198 amino acids and has a molecular weight of 22,500 d. Like other anterior pituitary hormones, prolactin is secreted episodically. The physiologic secretion of prolactin is primarily under inhibitory control imposed by dopamine released from the hypothalamus. The primary physiologic function of prolactin in human beings is its effects on lactation. Pathologic secretion of prolactin leads to several endocrine disorders. The majority of such disorders are related to reproductive processes. Effects of hyperprolactinemia include galactorrhea, anovulation, hyperandrogenism, and decreased libido. Very high levels of prolactin can alter testicular function, androgen production, and spermatogenesis.

INCIDENCE

The reported incidence of supranormal prolactin levels may be as high as 38% in women with amenorrhea alone, whereas as much as 28% of galactorrheic women with normal menses may have prolactin levels above the normal range. When amenorrhea and galactorrhea occur concurrently, the incidence of hyperprolactinemia increases to 70% to 84%.

CAUSES

The etiology of hyperprolactinemia may be divided into five broad categories.

Tumors

The most common cause of hyperprolactinemia is prolactin-secreting adenomas. Prolactin-secreting adenomas of the anterior pituitary have been classified as microadenomas (≤10 mm) and macroadenomas (>10 mm). Other tumors of the pituitary gland and sella may also cause hypersecretion of prolactin. These tumors may be nonfunctioning, or they may secrete other protein and polypeptide hormones. Such tumors include chromophobe adenomas. These tumors may cause increased prolactin secretion by causing anatomic distortion of pituitary gland tissue or alterations in hypothalamic dopamine secretion.

Pharmacologic Causes

Drugs that interfere with the synthesis, metabolism, re-uptake, or receptor binding of dopamine can cause hyperprolactinemia. Drugs such as phenothiazines, thioxanthenes, and butyrophenones, which are used to treat certain psychiatric illnesses, are common causes of drug-induced hyperprolactinemia. Other drugs that cause hyperprolactinemia include antihistamines, antidepressants, antihypertensives, and antiemetics. Opiates increase prolactin secretion by acting through central endorphin systems to inhibit dopamine secretion. As dopamine secretion decreases, the lactotrophs are released from inhibition and pathologic prolactin secretion increases.

Metabolic Diseases

Metabolic disturbances caused by chronic diseases, such as renal failure and cirrhosis of the liver, are associated with increased prolactin secretion. Hypothyroidism may cause increased prolactin secretion via compensatory increases in thyroid-releasing hormone (TRH). As much as 40% of patients with acromegaly are found to have hyperprolactinemia.

Dopamine Deficiency

Lesions in or about the pituitary cause dopamine deficiency. Such lesions can occur from transection of the pituitary stalk, surgical trauma, and compression of the pituitary stalk secondary to extrinsic masses. Craniopharyngiomas, meningiomas, and pineal tumors can also cause increased prolactin secretion, although these are generally located in the suprasellar region. Infiltrative diseases such as the Hand-Schüller-Christian complex, sarcoidosis, and hemochromatosis may be associated with elevated prolactin levels.

Other Causes

Other causes of hyperprolactinemia include pregnancy, nipple stimulation, and increased estrogen secretion. Although exceedingly rare, prolactin may be produced in ectopic sites, such as breast carcinoma, bronchogenic carcinomas, and hypernephromas. Other nonspecific stimuli, such as anaerobic exercise, nipple stimulation, coitus, emotional stress, hypoglycemia, eating, venipuncture, surgical stress, and anesthesia may cause transient increases in prolactin secretion. Although no specific prolactin-releasing hormone has been identified, a number of hormones are known to induce prolactin release. These include TRH, which is a potent stimulator of prolactin secretion. Other stimulators are serotonin, estrogens, vasointestinal peptide, angiotensin II, endogenous opioids, histamine, neurotensin, and substance P.

EFFECTS OF HYPERPROLACTINEMIA ON FERTILITY AND SEXUAL FUNCTION

Women with hyperprolactinemia usually seek medical attention because of amenorrhea, infertility, menstrual abnormality, or galactorrhea, whereas men usually seek medical attention for headaches, visual loss, neurologic defects, decreased libido, or spermatogenesis. Prolactin-secreting tumors in women are usually microadenomas, and hypopituitarism is extremely rare. In contrast, prolactinomas in men are usually macroadenomas. Up to one third of men with a prolactinoma tumor may have galactorrhea, and nearly one half will have visual impairment.

Galactorrhea is a common presenting sign of hyperprolactinemia. Approximately two thirds of women with galactorrhea have menstrual dysfunction. Approximately one third of galactorrheic women with normal menses have hyperprolactinemia. Inappropriate lactation may be an important clue to the existence of hypothalamic-pituitary disease when accompanied by amenorrhea. Amenorrhea, oligomenorrhea, and polymenorrhea generally indicate ovulatory dysfunction. Hyperprolactinemia may be responsible for as much as 38% of patients with chronic anovulation. Menstrual dysfunction associated with hyperprolactinemia probably is not a function of prolactin itself but rather a disturbance of the hypothalamic dopamine system, with resultant acyclic gonadotropin secretion. Thus, the pulsatile secretion of gonadotropin-releasing hormone (GnRH) is abnormal, causing aberrant gonadotropin secretion. The amplitude and frequency of episodic secretion of luteinizing hormone (LH) is disturbed in individuals with hyperprolactinemia. This results in anovulation and infertility.

Defects of Ovarian Function

Although the significance of luteal phase abnormality remains controversial in female infertility, it has been speculated that luteal abnormality may be the first manifestation of hyperprolactinemia in infertility. Prolactin also has direct effects on ovarian function. High levels of prolactin impair folliculogenesis and decrease luteal function. Both estrogen and progesterone secretion from the ovary decrease in patients with hyperprolactinemia.

Clinical evidence of androgen excess is present in approximately 30% of women with hyperprolactinemia. Folliculogenesis, ovulation, and luteal function may be abnormal in hyperprolactinemic-androgenized women. Approximately 33% of women with hirsutism have associated polycystic ovarian disease. The exact mechanisms underlying elevated prolactin secretion in patients with polycystic ovarian disease are not clear. However, increased estrogen production is found in patients with polycystic ovarian disease.

DIAGNOSIS OF HYPERPROLACTINEMIA

Evaluation of the patient with suspected hyperprolactinemia should focus on relevant signs and symptoms. Patients with galactorrhea, menstrual dysfunction, hirsutism, diminished libido, or unexplained infertility should have a serum prolactin level determined. A proper history should exclude the ingestion of pharmacologic agents that may increase prolactin levels. Prolactin secretion follows a nyctohemeral rhythm with maximum concentration between 12 PM and 9 AM. Prolactin secretion is also entrained to food intake as well as the sleep-wake cycle. Therefore, serum prolactin should be drawn in the fasting state around 10 AM. Prolactin levels greater than 20 ng/mL should be repeated. It is particularly important to repeat marginally elevated levels of prolactin because slight elevations in circulating prolactin levels may affect fertility. Marginal elevations of prolactin may also be due to other, more serious lesions of the pituitary gland and/or sella. Clearly, lesions other than prolactinomas can cause increased prolactin secretion and must not be missed during the diagnostic evaluation. Primary hypothyroidism should also be ruled out and, thus, a thyroid-stimulating hormone (TSH) level should be drawn. When other disorders such as renal disease are suspected as the cause of hyperprolactinemia, appropriate laboratory tests should be ordered at the time of the initial workup.

Baseline prolactin levels coupled with imaging studies of the sella are the best means of diagnosing a pituitary tumor. When the cause of hyperprolactinemia is not readily apparent, nuclear magnetic resonance imaging with contrast should be employed to evaluate the pituitary and sella region. Location and size of the lesion must be determined. If the tumor extends to the supra sella region or laterally into the adjacent sinuses, the margins of the lesion must be delineated.

TREATMENT OF HYPERPROLACTINEMIA

Knowledge of the etiology of the patient's hyperprolactinemia is critical. Certainly, a patient with mildly elevated prolactin levels who wishes to conceive will be treated differently than a patient with a large, symptomatic macroadenoma. The crucial matter is to determine which form of therapy is correct for a given patient. It is important for all clinicians to realize that dopamine receptor agonists frequently cause significant side effects. Because of the side effects associated with bromocriptine (Parlodel), lack of compliance may be a problem. Gastrointestinal symptoms, such as nausea and vomiting, and cardiovascular effects, such as dizziness and syncope, are the most common. Nasal stuffiness during the first hour following administration of bromocriptine is also common. To ameliorate such "early dose" side effects, a graduated regimen is recommended. Gradually increasing small, divided doses taken daily with meals or at bedtime will usually result in the patient's ability to take the intended therapeutic dose. For example, treatment with bromocriptine should begin with a dose of 1.25 mg administered at bedtime with a snack. After 1 week, 1.25 mg can be added in the morning. At weekly intervals, the dose should be increased by 1.25 mg until the intended therapeutic dose is reached. Usually, 2.5 to 7.5 mg/d is required to normalize PRL levels up to 200 ng/mL. Larger doses may be required to treat macroadenomas, particularly when tumor shrinkage is the object of therapy.

The primary goals of treatment of hyperprolactinemia are to restore gonadal function by normalizing prolactin levels and to decrease the size of prolactin-secreting tumors. Oral administration of bromocriptine decreases both synthesis and secretion of prolactin (PRL). LH pulses increase in both frequency and amplitude following initiation of therapy, and restoration of normal LH and follicle-stimulating hormone (FSH) secretion results in recovery of normal ovarian function. Return of menstrual function occurs in approximately 80% of patients, usually within the first 6 weeks of therapy. Add clomiphene citrate (Clomid)* to the bromocriptine regimen for patients who fail to ovulate and for those who ovulate but fail to conceive. Document ovulation and establish a normal luteal phase with basal body temperature charts and endometrial biopsies. Insensitivity to clomiphene has been demonstrated in patients with hyperprolactinemia. Therefore, prolactin levels should be normalized before initiating clomiphene therapy. Hyperprolactinemic women who are anovulatory or oligo-ovulatory usually have good responses to appropriate doses of FSH. FSH therapy should be reserved for patients with insensitivity to clomiphene. Bromo-

*Not FDA approved for this indication.

criptine remains the drug of choice for ovulation induction in these women. FSH is the treatment of choice when hypogonadotropic hypogonadism occurs following surgery or radiotherapy.

Bromocriptine has also been used as specific therapy for PRL-secreting pituitary adenomas, regardless of fertility interests. Bromocriptine causes tumors to shrink in the majority of patients, and macroadenomas appear to respond particularly well. Bromocriptine-induced tumor shrinkage has particular relevance for patients whose neurologic signs and symptoms could be relieved by medical shrinkage of the tumor in lieu of surgery or radiotherapy. Unfortunately, the effect of bromocriptine on tumor size is transient and appears to be a function of its continuous use because once the drug is withdrawn, the tumor will usually return to its original size. Reduction in tumor size usually occurs within 4 to 6 weeks, and about 60% of women with macroadenomas will have more than a 50% reduction in tumor size. Bromocriptine must be given continuously to be effective, and discontinuation of the drug leads to a rapid return to pretreatment PRL levels and tumor reexpansion.

Pergolide (Permax)* has a longer duration of action, and dosages of 50 to 150 μg once daily are as effective as bromocriptine in normalizing PRL. Currently, pergolide is approved by the Food and Drug Administration (FDA) only for treatment of Parkinson's disease. Cabergoline (Dostinex) is a more potent dopamine agonist with a very high specificity for the dopamine (D_2) receptor and a long half-life. Dosages of 0.5 to 2 mg weekly are as efficacious as daily administration of bromocriptine and may be associated with fewer side effects.

Although dopamine receptor agonists should be first-line treatment for prolactinomas today, a surgical approach will often be necessary for patients with macroadenomas. A transsphenoidal approach is particularly useful in the removal of microadenomas or macroadenomas with superior midline extension. *Cure rates*—defined as restoration of serum PRL levels to normal, resolution of galactorrhea and/or amenorrhea, and preservation of pituitary function—as high as 90% have been reported. The major problem with the surgical approach to treat prolactinomas is that the recurrence rate is high and often requires adjunctive therapy to control the patient's hyperprolactinemia. Radiotherapy is probably best used in conjunction with the surgical or medical treatment of a macroadenoma or in areas in which those forms of treatment are contraindicated or have failed.

Partial or complete pituitary insufficiency occurs in approximately 5% to 10% of patients undergoing surgery or radiotherapy for a pituitary tumor. Therefore, all patients must be evaluated for pituitary reserve preoperatively and postoperatively with GnRH and TRH stimulation and insulin tolerance testing. If thyroid or adrenal insufficiency exists, replacement therapy must be instituted because such deficiencies are serious and potentially life-threatening. Conventional radiotherapy is a viable mode of adjunctive therapy for prolactinomas. Megavoltage techniques are used to deliver approximately 5000 rads to the tumor over approximately 1 month. Heavy particle beam radiotherapy may be somewhat more effective than conventional radiotherapy if the tumor is confined to the sella. Five thousand to 14,000 rads may be delivered to the pituitary in a single session without wide area spread.

MANAGEMENT OF HYPERPROLACTINEMIA DURING PREGNANCY

At present, it is impossible to predict which patients with pituitary tumors will experience enlargement sufficient to produce symptoms. Bromocriptine should be discontinued when pregnancy is diagnosed. All patients with prolactinomas who conceive should have a baseline neurologic examination and ophthalmologic consultation to assess visual field acuity. Most often, the pregnancy can be carried to term uneventfully, with delivery of a normal, healthy infant. However, complications may arise that are directly attributable to the pituitary lesion in 4% to 5% of patients. Headaches and visual disturbances are the most common tumor-related symptoms. Once symptoms develop, radiologic reevaluation of the sella is mandatory. Induction of labor and vaginal delivery of the infant may prove beneficial in the absence of obstetric indications for cesarean section. If the fetus is not mature, conservative medical management should be attempted. Bromocriptine in doses of 5 to 20 mg/d is now the treatment of choice for pregnant women with symptomatic pituitary adenomas. The presence of a pituitary tumor does not appear to markedly affect the outcome of pregnancy. Finally, the risk of teratogenicity resulting from the use of bromocriptine in pregnancy appears to be minimal.

Visual field testing is indicated in patients with macroadenomas and in those with documented suprasellar extension of a pituitary tumor. If ophthalmologic signs or symptoms are encountered, visual field examinations should be obtained. Similarly, visual field testing should be performed on all patients with either microadenomas or macroadenomas who become pregnant and on those who are attempting to conceive because close follow-up of potential tumor progression is necessary.

*Not FDA approved for this indication.

HYPOTHYROIDISM

method of
JEROME M. HERSHMAN, M.D., and
NALINI SINGH, M.D.
Veterans Affairs Greater Los Angeles Healthcare System and UCLA School of Medicine
Los Angeles, California

Hypothyroidism can be described as a state of thyroid hormone deficiency that results in a generalized slowing of the body's metabolism. It occurs in about 5% of adults of all ages, with a prevalence of 10% to 15% of the elderly, and a female-to-male ratio of about 3 or 4 to 1. Overt hypothyroidism can be classified as primary or central. In the primary form, the thyroid gland itself fails to synthesize and secrete thyroid hormone. The free thyroxine (T_4) is low, resulting in reduced negative feedback on the pituitary gland and an elevated thyroid-stimulating hormone (TSH) level. Thyroid gland failure can result from Hashimoto's thyroiditis, surgery (i.e., thyroidectomy for thyroid cancer), radioactive iodine therapy for Graves' disease, radiation therapy for Hodgkin's disease or laryngeal cancer, drugs (amiodarone, lithium, iodine, antithyroid drugs), severe iodine deficiency, and defects in hormone synthesis (Table 1).

In the much rarer central form, either the hypothalamus does not secrete enough thyrotropin-releasing hormone or the pituitary gland does not secrete enough functional TSH to stimulate the thyroid gland to synthesize a normal amount of thyroid hormone. As a result, the T_4 level is low, and the TSH level is usually low (in some cases the TSH is normal or slightly elevated but biologically inactive). Central hypothyroidism results from pituitary tumors or their surgical resection, radiation therapy, infiltrative disease (hemochromatosis), mass lesions (tumors, metastases), pituitary apoplexy, and autoimmune destruction (lymphocytic hypophysitis). It is usually accompanied by other evidence of pituitary or hypothalamic disease.

Subclinical (or minimal) hypothyroidism is characterized by a normal free T_4 level and an elevated TSH level. In population-based studies, it affected 5% to 10% of men and 5% to 17% of women over age 60. Overt hypothyroidism develops in about 5% of this subgroup per year, with further elevation of the TSH and a subnormal free T_4 concentration.

TABLE 1. **Etiology of Hypothyroidism**

- Hashimoto's thyroiditis
- Thyroid ablation
  - Surgical thyroidectomy
  - Following ^{131}I treatment of hyperthyroidism
  - Radiation of neoplasms (laryngeal cancer, Hodgkin's lymphoma)
- Drugs
  - Iodine, inorganic or organic (amiodarone)
  - Lithium
  - Interferon alfa
  - Bexarotene (Targretin)
- Hypopituitarism or hypothalamic disease
- Congenital
  - Dysgenesis
  - Biosynthetic defects

CLINICAL MANIFESTATIONS

Many clinical manifestations in hypothyroidism stem from the accumulation of glycosaminoglycans and the increased capillary permeability in interstitial tissues, which produce interstitial edema, especially in the skin, heart, and muscle.

Classic symptoms of hypothyroidism include fatigue, weight gain, muscle cramps, dry skin, cold intolerance, mental slowing, and depression. Patients also may complain of constipation, hair loss, hoarse voice, and paresthesias. Women may notice menorrhagia. Children may present with precocious puberty and short stature. Patients often have a family history of autoimmune thyroid disease. Some patients, especially the elderly, may present with few vague symptoms, such as fatigue, or no symptoms at all.

Physical findings include hair loss (especially thinning of the lateral eyebrows), dry skin, macroglossia, periorbital edema, peripheral edema, bradycardia, and diastolic hypertension. The physician should examine deep tendon reflexes for a delayed relaxation phase. The presence of a goiter may be suggestive of Hashimoto's thyroiditis. More advanced hypothyroidism may lead to pleural or pericardial effusions, joint effusions, carpal tunnel syndrome, hydroceles, ileus, decreased cardiac output, sleep apnea, and diminished mentation. Myxedema coma is a state of severe hypothyroidism characterized by hypercapnic ventilatory failure, stupor, and hypothermia. There is often a precipitating event, such as infection, congestive heart failure, myocardial infarction, pneumonia, fluid overload, or sedation of a hypothyroid patient.

LABORATORY EVALUATION

The patient with hypothyroidism has a low free T_4 level. The total T_4 level may not be reliable in states of thyroid-binding globulin deficiency, such as glucocorticoid use, androgen use, nephrotic syndrome, and cirrhosis. Thus, the diagnosis of hypothyroidism should be based on the free T_4 level. The physician should also be aware of concomitant medications that reduce serum free T_4 concentration by accelerating the metabolism of levothyroxine, such as phenytoin (Dilantin), carbamazepine (Tegretol), rifampin (Rimactane), and phenobarbital. The anti-arrhythmic agent, amiodarone (Cordarone), which contains 37% iodine, can precipitate hypothyroidism via the inhibitory effect of iodine on thyroid hormone synthesis and secretion. Lithium (Eskalith, Lithane, Lithonate), the mood-stabilizing agent, reduces T_4 levels by interfering with various steps in the synthesis and secretion of thyroid hormone.

If the free T_4 level is low and the TSH level is elevated, the patient has primary hypothyroidism. Antithyroid peroxidase antibodies may be ordered to diagnose Hashimoto's thyroiditis. A low free T_4 level and a low or normal TSH level are suggestive of central hypothyroidism. In patients with central hypothyroidism, it is important to detect and treat adrenal insufficiency before initiating treatment with thyroxine. When a patient exhibits serious comorbidities and similar aberrations in thyroid function tests, the differential diagnosis also includes nonthyroidal illness. In nonthyroidal illness, thyroid function tests usually normalize when the patient regains his or her baseline state of health. Nonetheless, it is advisable to evaluate overall pituitary function, especially the pituitary-adrenal axis, to detect and treat adrenal insufficiency in a patient facing critical illness. If the patient does show evidence of hypopituitarism, a magnetic resonance image of the brain is required to rule out a mass affecting the hypothalamus or pituitary gland.

The patient with hypothyroidism may display other abnormal laboratory findings, such as macrocytic anemia with spur cells, an elevated creatine kinase level, an elevated lactic dehydrogenase level, hyperprolactinemia, and an elevated cholesterol level (secondary to decreased hepatic low-density lipoprotein receptors and lipoprotein lipase activity). Some patients with subclinical hypothyroidism may also have hypercholesterolemia. Patients with myxedema coma may have hyponatremia and hypoglycemia. An electrocardiogram reveals a lengthened PR interval and low voltage.

THERAPY

Patients with primary or secondary hypothyroidism should be treated with synthetic T_4 or levothyroxine (Synthroid, Levoxyl). In primary hypothyroidism, the therapeutic goal is to achieve a TSH level in the midnormal range (1–3 mU/L). The average adult dosage of T_4 required to achieve these goals is 1.7 μg/kg/d (1.3 in the elderly). Adolescents (aged 11–20 years) require an average dose of 2 to 3 μg/kg/d.

Patients who have undergone thyroidectomies for thyroid cancer require a higher dose to suppress the TSH-mediated growth of residual thyroid tissue. The desirable level of TSH is less than 0.1 mU/L in a low-risk thyroid cancer patient and less than 0.02 mU/L in a high-risk patient.

The young patient without cardiac disease can be started on near full replacement, that is, 1 to 1.5 μg/kg/d of levothyroxine. Levothyroxine has a half-life of 7 days and about 70% of the oral dose is absorbed. The TSH and free T_4 levels should be checked after 6 weeks. For consistency, the blood should be drawn before taking levothyroxine. The dosage can be increased by 25 μg every 6 to 8 weeks until the TSH level is within the reference range.

In the therapy of central hypothyroidism, the free T_4 level should be in the reference range and the serum TSH level cannot be used to assess the adequacy of replacement therapy. The guidelines for the starting dose of levothyroxine in primary hypothyroidism also apply to central hypothyroidism. The dose should be increased by 25 μg every 6 weeks until the free T_4 level is normal.

Physicians should exercise greater caution in elderly patients, especially those with coronary artery disease. The effect of thyroid hormone on ischemic heart disease is manifold. Some studies have suggested that thyroid hormone replacement may exacerbate angina. Other studies have refuted this contention, and still others demonstrate that thyroid hormone improves cardiac contractility and reduces afterload. In any case, it is recommended that elderly patients begin therapy with 12.5 to 25 μg of levothyroxine per day. At 6- to 8-week intervals, the dosage should be titrated gradually upward (by increments of 25 μg) to achieve a TSH level (or free T_4 level if central hypothyroidism) in the reference range.

At the initiation of therapy, the physician should explain the possible side effects of levothyroxine to the patient. Side effects, usually at higher T_4 levels, include nervousness, tachycardia, diarrhea, tremulousness, and insomnia. Supranormal T_4 levels and a suppressed TSH level can also predispose patients to osteoporosis and atrial fibrillation. Levothyroxine increases the catabolism of vitamin K–dependent clotting factors and may potentiate the effect of oral anticoagulant agents. Thus, hypothyroid patients taking anticoagulant therapy should be observed closely when they start levothyroxine by checking the prothrombin time and adjusting the anticoagulant dose.

At subsequent visits every 2 months, the physician should follow thyroid function tests and monitor the patient for side effects. Overtreatment can be corrected by stopping levothyroxine for 3 days and then resuming therapy with a reduced dosage. When the patient appears euthyroid clinically and thyroid function tests have normalized, she or he can return for follow-up visits every 6 months.

Special Dosage Considerations

Patients on the same dose of levothyroxine for a long time may have an unexpected elevation in TSH level. Possible causes include noncompliance, an ineffective generic preparation, or worsening of thyroid failure (Table 2). Physicians should be aware of medications that decrease the absorption of levothyroxine from the gastrointestinal tract: calcium carbonate (Os-Cal, Tums), ferrous sulfate (iron), aluminum-containing antacids (Maalox, Mylanta), cholestyramine (Questran), colestipol (Colestid), and sucralfate (Carafate). They should counsel patients to take these medications 3 to 4 hours apart from levothyroxine. In addition, phenytoin, carbamazepine, rifampin, phenobarbital, and sertraline (Zoloft) accelerate the metabolism of levothyroxine. Patients on these medications may need a higher dose of levothyroxine to achieve or maintain euthyroidism. If the hypothyroidism is secondary to amiodarone or lithium, stopping the medication may result in normal thyroid function. If amiodarone or lithium is necessary for the patient's medical treatment, then the drug can be continued and thyroid replacement can be initiated.

TABLE 2. **Explanations for Increase in Thyroid-Stimulating Hormone in Patient on Same Dose of T_4**

Noncompliance or drug holiday
Ineffective generic preparation
Drug-induced malabsorption
Calcium carbonate (Os-Cal, Tums)
Ferrous sulfate (iron)
Sucralfate (Carafate)
Aluminum hydroxide (Maalox, Mylanta)
Cholestyramine (Questran), Colestipol (Colestid)
Accelerated metabolism
Phenytoin (Dilantin)
Carbamazepine (Tegretol)
Sertraline (Zoloft)
Rifampin (Rimactane)
Worsening of thyroid failure
Pregnancy

Pregnancy increases the dosage requirement of levothyroxine by 25 to 50 μg or more beginning in the first trimester, possibly because of increased demand for thyroxine synthesis and increased degradation of thyroxine. Thus, pregnant women on levothyroxine therapy should be observed with a TSH level early in pregnancy and every trimester thereafter for dosage titration of levothyroxine. Women with thyroid ablation require larger dose increments than those with Hashimoto's disease.

The importance of diagnosing hypothyroidism in pregnant women was elucidated in a recent study in which children of hypothyroid mothers who were not treated during pregnancy had lower IQ scores than the offspring of euthyroid mothers. To avoid this, pregnant women should be screened for hypothyroidism by TSH measurement at the end of the first trimester; if hypothyroid, they should be started on levothyroxine.

Subclinical Hypothyroidism

Not all patients with a slight elevation of serum TSH level require treatment. Those with a TSH level less than twice the upper limit of normal (8–10 mU/L) and no other clinical manifestations often do not benefit from therapy. However, patients with a TSH level greater than 10 mU/L, goiter, positive antithyroid peroxidase antibodies, or symptoms of hypothyroidism (i.e., fatigue, depression, weight gain, cognitive dysfunction) should receive levothyroxine. Patients with subclinical hypothyroidism who require chronic amiodarone or lithium treatment should also receive levothyroxine. In patients who have a slightly elevated TSH level and a free T_4 level in the lower 25% of the reference range, a trial of therapy is warranted. Studies have shown that, in patients with a TSH level greater than 12 mU/L and hypercholesterolemia, levothyroxine improves the lipid profile. Therapy should be initiated with 50 μg T_4 in younger people and 12.5 to 25 μg in older people. Because overt disease develops in 5% of patients with subclinical hypothyroidism each year, they should be monitored with thyroid function tests every 6 to 12 months.

Other Thyroid Hormone Preparations

Liothyronine (Cytomel, T_3) alone is not appropriate for chronic hormone replacement because of its 1-day half-life and transient effects. It has been used synergistically with antidepressant therapy in euthyroid patients.

The T_4-T_3 combination has been prescribed as desiccated thyroid (Thyroid USP), with 1 grain (60 mg) containing about 40 μg of levothyroxine and 10 μg of liothyronine. Another combination preparation is liotrix (Thyrolar), which is a 4:1 T_4-T_3 ratio. Some physicians believe that the T_4-T_3 combination seems more physiologic and that patients experience a heightened state of well-being while taking it. In a recent study, one group of patients took their standard dose of T_4, and another group took a T_4-T_3 combination that was formulated by adding T_4 (their usual dose minus 50 μg) to 12.5 μg of T_3 (in place of 50 μg of T_4). The patients on the T_4-T_3 combination reported an improvement in neurocognitive assessment when compared with those on T_4 alone. At this time, most physicians choose to prescribe levothyroxine alone because it is easier to titrate and normalizes serum TSH levels consistently, although it results in slightly higher levels of T_4 and lower levels of T_3 than those in the euthyroid population. It is likely that combination T_4-T_3 preparations will become available that are more likely to normalize both T_4 and T_3 levels in a high proportion of patients.

TREATMENT OF MYXEDEMA COMA

Patients with myxedema coma have a high mortality and require close monitoring in the intensive care unit. Patients in respiratory failure should be intubated and mechanically ventilated. Excessive fluid and sedation should be avoided. If known, the precipitating illness, such as infection, should be treated vigorously.

There are different opinions about the choice of thyroid hormone therapy. Some endocrinologists advocate an initial dose of 300 μg of levothyroxine delivered intravenously, followed by 50 μg of levothyroxine intravenously daily. Alternatively, because severely ill patients have decreased T_4 to T_3 conversion, some experts prefer intravenous liothyronine (Triostat, 10–25 μg two to three times daily). Yet another group favors initial treatment with T_4 and T_3 and continuation with T_4 only.

Because some patients with myxedema coma may also suffer from adrenal insufficiency, a cortisol level or a cosyntropin stimulation test should be done. Stress-dose hydrocortisone (100 mg intravenously, then 50 mg intravenously every 6 hours) should be administered initially and continued unless the cortisol value is found to be greater than 20 μg/dL or the cosyntropin test is within reference limits.

HYPERTHYROIDISM

method of
DOUGLAS S. ROSS, M.D.
Harvard Medical School and
Massachusetts General Hospital
Boston, Massachusetts

The symptoms of overt hyperthyroidism include weight loss, increased appetite, palpitations, tremulousness, heat intolerance, fatigue, dyspnea on exertion, frequent bowel movements, oligomenorrhea, muscle weakness, insomnia, and irritability. Mild hyperthyroidism may paradoxically be associated with weight gain due to appetite stimulation. Elderly patients may have weight loss and cachexia without tachycardia or tremulousness. Exacerbation of angina or congestive heart failure is common. Physical examination reveals tachycardia, a widened pulse pressure, tremor, stare, hyperreflexia, and onycholysis. Goiter may be absent, especially in the elderly. Exophthalmos, orbital inflammation, and pretibial myxedema are specific for Graves disease.

LABORATORY DIAGNOSIS

Overt hyperthyroidism is diagnosed in patients with a subnormal (usually undetectable) serum thyroid-stimulating hormone (TSH) concentration and an elevated serum free thyroxine (T_4) and/or serum triiodothyronine (T_3) concentration. *Subclinical hyperthyroidism* is diagnosed in asymptomatic patients with subnormal serum TSH and normal free T_4 and T_3 concentrations. Patients with subclinical hyperthyroidism have a threefold increased risk of atrial fibrillation, and postmenopausal women who are not taking estrogen replacement develop reduced bone mineral density. I therefore recommend treatment of subclinical hyperthyroidism when serum TSH concentrations remain under 0.1 μU/mL, especially in older patients and those with cardiac disease and risk factors for osteoporosis.

Low serum TSH concentrations do not always indicate hyperthyroidism. When associated with low or low-normal serum T_4 concentrations they may indicate central hypothyroidism, severe nonthyroidal illness, corticosteroid excess, depression, or concurrent dopamine therapy. Hyperthyroidism is rarely associated with normal or elevated serum TSH levels in patients with TSH-producing pituitary adenomas or partial pituitary resistance to thyroid hormone.

ETIOLOGY OF HYPERTHYROIDISM

Conceptually, there are two groups of thyroid disorders (Table 1). Hyperthyroidism associated with a high radioiodine uptake indicates de novo synthesis of hormone, and primary treatment modalities are antithyroid drugs, radioiodine, or surgery. Hyperthyroidism associated with low radioiodine uptake occurs when there is inflammation of thyroid tissue with release of preformed thyroid hormone (subacute thyroiditis) or when the source of thyroid hormone is exogenous. These entities are not treated with antithyroid drugs, radioiodine, or surgery.

TABLE 1. **Types of Hyperthyroidism**

Hyperthyroidism With a High Thyroidal Radioiodine Uptake
Graves disease
Toxic adenoma or toxic nodular goiter*
Trophoblastic disease
Thyroid-stimulating hormone–mediated hyperthyroidism
Hyperthyroidism With Extrathyroidal Radioiodine Uptake
Struma ovarii
Metastatic follicular thyroid cancer
Hyperthyroidism With a Low Radioiodine Uptake
Subacute thyroiditis
Subacute granulomatous thyroiditis (de Quervain)
Subacute lymphocytic thyroiditis (painless or silent)
Postpartum lymphocytic thyroiditis
Factitious ingestion of thyroid hormone

*The uptake may be subnormal in iodine-induced hyperthyroidism.

THERAPY

Hyperthyroidism With a High Radioiodine Uptake

Graves disease, the most common form of hyperthyroidism, is an autoimmune disorder characterized by immunoglobulins that stimulate the TSH receptor. Treatment options include a course of antithyroid drugs with the hope of attaining a remission, ablation of the gland with radioiodine, or surgery. *Toxic adenoma* and *toxic nodular goiter* result from autonomous function of thyroid tissue and are treated similarly to Graves disease, except that remission is not anticipated after a course of antithyroid drugs. Treatment of trophoblastic disease, TSH-producing adenomas, struma ovarii, and metastatic follicular cancer is directed primarily against the neoplastic process, but antithyroid drugs may provide useful adjunctive therapy, octreotide (Sandostatin) may be useful in patients with TSH-producing adenomas who have failed surgery, and radioiodine is useful in patients with metastatic struma ovarii and hyperthyroidism from metastatic thyroid cancer. Treatment of patients with resistance to thyroid hormone is controversial; some patients improve with liothyronine (Cytomel) or 3,4,3′-triiodothyroacetic acid (TRIAC). The following discussion addresses treatment of Graves disease and toxic adenoma and nodular goiter.

β-Adrenergic Blocking Agents

Because hyperthyroidism increases β-adrenergic receptors in many tissues, β-adrenergic blocking agents ameliorate the tachycardia, palpitations, heat intolerance, and anxiety associated with hyperthyroidism and are therefore useful adjunctive therapy for all patients who do not have contraindications to β-adrenergic blockade. Propranolol (Inderal)* in very high doses inhibits conversion of T_4 to T_3, but it must be given every 6 hours to be effective. I therefore prefer the use of long-acting β_1-selective agents such as atenolol (Tenormin),* 25 to 50 mg or more daily as a single or divided dose depending on the severity of the hyperthyroidism.

Thionamides (Antithyroid Drugs)

Methimazole (Tapazole) and propylthiouracil (PTU) are the two thionamides available in the United States; carbimazole,† which is metabolized to methimazole, is available in Europe and elsewhere. Thionamides block the synthesis of thyroid hormone by preventing the organification of iodine. They are used initially to control the hyperthyroidism before definitive therapy with radioiodine or surgery, or they may be used in Graves disease for prolonged periods in an attempt to achieve a remission. Controversy exists as to whether thionamides have immunomodulatory effects that make remission more likely or whether they simply control the hyperthyroidism until spontaneous remission occurs. Remis-

*Not FDA approved for this indication.
†Not available in the United States.

sion rates after 1 to 2 years of treatment vary from 20% to 40%. The lower rates are seen in men and patients with large glands and more severe hyperthyroidism; the higher rates occur in women with small glands and mild hyperthyroidism. In Japan, patients may be treated with thionamides for 10 years or longer and up to 75% of patients may achieve remission.

There are significant differences in the pharmacology of methimazole and PTU. The serum half-life of PTU is 75 minutes, versus 4 to 6 hours for methimazole. More importantly, intrathyroidal methimazole concentrations remain high for over 20 hours after a single dose, resulting in a more prolonged organification blockade compared with PTU. As a result, in most patients, methimazole is effective as a single daily dose, whereas PTU usually requires divided dosing. PTU, but not methimazole, inhibits conversion of T_4 to T_3. This theoretical advantage is realized only during the first 1 or 2 weeks of therapy and requires frequent dosing. Because methimazole is overall more effective than PTU, patients given methimazole normalize their serum T_3 concentrations weeks earlier than those given PTU. I therefore prefer methimazole for initial therapy (Table 2).

Initial Therapy. Thionamides only prevent new hormone synthesis. It therefore takes 3 to 12 weeks for patients to become euthyroid, because existing thyroid hormone stores must first be exhausted. Traditionally, high doses of thionamides are given initially: 30 to 40 mg of methimazole in a single or divided dose, or 100 mg of PTU three times a day. Once euthyroidism is restored, lower maintenance doses are substituted, such as 5 to 15 mg of methimazole daily. The time required to achieve euthyroidism is similar for most patients when these lower doses of methimazole are used for initial therapy. Because occasional patients do require maintenance doses in excess of 20 mg of methimazole, higher initial doses are appropriate in patients with severe hyperthyroidism and patients with large goiters. Most patients with mild hyperthyroidism and modest goiters can be started on a single dose of methimazole, 10 to 20 mg/d. Compliance is improved when a single dose of methimazole is combined with a single dose of a long-acting β-adrenergic blocking agent. For patients who have minor side effects from methimazole, PTU may be substituted.

TABLE 2. **Comparison of Antithyroid Drugs**

Advantages of Methimazole
Inhibits organification longer than PTU
May be given as a single daily dose
Euthyroidism is achieved more rapidly
Unlike PTU, pretreatment with methimazole is not associated with radioiodine failure
May be associated with a lower incidence of agranulocytosis when low doses used
Hepatic toxicity less severe: obstructive jaundice for methimazole versus hepatocellular necrosis for PTU
Unlike PTU, rarely associated with antineutrophilic cytoplasmic antibodies
Advantages of Propylthiouracil
Acutely lowers T_4 to T_3 conversion
Crosses placenta and is concentrated in breast milk less well than methimazole
Not associated with neonatal scalp defect (aplasia cutis)

Abbreviation: PTU = propylthiouracil.

Maintenance Therapy and Remission. With the control of chemical hyperthyroidism, the thionamide dose may need to be tapered to lower levels, especially if the initial dose of methimazole was greater than 10 to 15 mg. TSH measurements may be misleading during acute therapy for hyperthyroidism, because subnormal serum TSH concentrations may persist for weeks after euthyroidism has been attained. Therefore, it is essential to monitor both free T_4 and T_3 concentrations during titration of the thionamide dose. Patients should be seen initially at 4- to 6-week intervals but may be seen at 3- to 6-month intervals once stability has been achieved. Patients with Graves disease who opt for long-term therapy are traditionally treated for 1 to 2 years in the United States, but there is no compelling reason not to treat longer.

There is no reliable way to determine if the patient has achieved a remission other than cautiously tapering the thionamide dose to determine if hyperthyroidism is still present. Many patients will become chemically hyperthyroid within 1 to 4 weeks, whereas others may relapse weeks to months after stopping thionamides, and late relapses can occur even years after a remission. Patients who experience relapse may take another course of antithyroid drugs, or go on to radioiodine therapy or surgery.

Side Effects and Toxicity. Both thionamides have significant side effects. Up to 13% of patients cannot tolerate thionamides because of rashes, hives, nausea, vomiting, joint pains, or fevers. Patients allergic to one thionamide may tolerate the other, but cross-reactivity may occur in up to 50%. Agranulocytosis occurs in 0.2% to 0.5% of patients; it may be slightly less common with doses of methimazole under 30 mg and occurs most commonly during the first 3 months of therapy. One study detected agranulocytosis early when white blood cell counts were obtained every 2 weeks, but most endocrinologists check white blood cell counts only at follow-up visits and instruct patients to obtain a white blood cell count immediately if they develop a fever or sore throat. Leukopenia (3000–4000 cells/mm^3) is common in Graves disease due to antineutrophil antibodies and should not be confused with agranulocytosis. Cholestatic jaundice (methimazole) and hepatocellular necrosis (PTU) are uncommon toxicities of thionamides. In one study, it was found that a third of patients taking PTU, but not methimazole, developed antineutrophilic cytoplasmic antibodies. Many of these patients have arthralgias, but glomerulonephritis is rare. The significance of this finding is uncertain.

Use During Pregnancy and Lactation. Because PTU is less soluble than methimazole and bound to serum proteins, it crosses the placenta only one fourth as well as methimazole and is concentrated in breast milk only one tenth as well. Methimazole may also be associated with a rare scalp defect, aplasia cutis. PTU is therefore preferred over methimazole during pregnancy. Fetal goiter and hypothyroidism can be minimized by using the smallest dose possible to control maternal hyperthyroidism. Mild maternal hyperthyroidism may be tolerated to avoid fetal hypothyroidism. When monitoring thyroid function during pregnancy, it is important to note the effects of estrogen-induced thyroxine-binding globulin (TBG) excess on total serum T_4 and T_3 concentrations and rely on free hormone levels to titrate the dose. There are no case reports of adverse effects on the neonate due to nursing during maternal thionamide therapy.

Iodinated Radiocontrast Agents and Iodine

Iopanoic acid (Telepaque), a radiocontrast agent used for oral cholecystograms, is the most potent inhibitor of T_4 to T_3 conversion available and can normalize serum T_3 concentrations within 5 days. It has been used effectively in patients with thyroid storm or severe hyperthyroidism, preoperatively in patients allergic to thionamides, and in patients with excessive hyperthyroid symptoms from subacute thyroiditis. The usual dose is 500 to 1000 g/d.

Iopanoic acid should not be used routinely because it also provides pharmacologic amounts of iodine. Iodine will ameliorate Graves hyperthyroidism by blocking its own organification and blocking thyroid hormone release, but it may exacerbate hyperthyroidism due to toxic adenoma or nodular goiter by providing substrate for de novo synthesis of hormone. Iodine-containing medication should not be administered to patients with toxic adenoma or nodular goiter unless the patient has started to receive thionamides at least 2 hours previously. The use of iodine-containing medication may delay the subsequent use of radioiodine for up to 6 weeks.

Iodine itself may be given for adjunctive therapy of severe Graves hyperthyroidism as potassium iodide (SSKI), 5 drops two to four times daily. Iodine (SSKI 10 drops daily) has been used as adjunctive therapy beginning 1 week after radioiodine treatment in patients with Graves hyperthyroidism to normalize thyroid hormone concentrations more rapidly and is routinely used preoperatively in Graves disease to reduce gland vascularity.

Radioiodine

Radioiodine is used as definitive therapy for hyperthyroidism and is recommended as the therapy of choice by two thirds of thyroid specialists in the United States. It is administered as an oral solution or capsule and has no immediate side effects. Patients are advised to avoid close contact with children and pregnant women for approximately a week after treatment. The biologic half-life is 2 to 3 days, but destruction of thyroid tissue occurs after 6 to 18 weeks or longer. One percent of patients develops transient painful radiation thyroiditis and 10% require a second dose. There is no increased risk of cancer, leukemia, or birth defects. Controversy exists as to whether ophthalmopathy may worsen after radioiodine therapy, and many patients with severe ophthalmopathy now choose thyroidectomy, although concurrent corticosteroid administration has been reported to prevent exacerbation of ophthalmopathy after radioiodine therapy.

Because patients do not become euthyroid for several months after radioiodine, and because radioiodine may initially exacerbate hyperthyroidism due to the release of hormone from radiation-induced inflammation, elderly patients, patients with heart disease, patients with severe hyperthyroidism, and patients who are not tolerating hyperthyroid symptoms well are first pretreated with a thionamide to control hyperthyroidism and to deplete thyroid hormone stores. However, a recent study suggests that treatment failure occurs more commonly when PTU, but not methimazole, is given before radioiodine. Younger patients with mild to moderate hyperthyroidism do not need to be treated with thionamides before radioiodine.

Most centers recognize hypothyroidism as the goal of radioiodine. Patients with functioning thyroid remnants after radioiodine may develop recurrent hyperthyroidism or develop late hypothyroidism at a rate of 2% to 3% annually.

Surgery

Surgery is uncommonly chosen as therapy for hyperthyroidism. Indications include large obstructive goiters, patients whose glands are so large that they will require multiple doses of radioiodine, patients with coexistent nodules with suspicious or indeterminate biopsy results, pregnant hyperthyroid patients who are allergic to thionamides, patients with severe ophthalmopathy, and patients who fear radioiodine. It is critical that the surgeon be skilled at a near-total thyroidectomy. Complications include permanent hypoparathyroidism and recurrent laryngeal nerve injury. If a significant surgical remnant is left, the patient may be euthyroid, but persistent and recurrent hyperthyroidism may also occur, so many surgeons consider the goal of surgery to be permanent hypothyroidism.

Ideally, patients are given thionamides preoperatively and are euthyroid at the time of surgery. Iodine is given for 10 days preoperatively in Graves disease to reduce gland vascularity. Patients allergic to thionamides are given iopanoic acid and β-adrenergic blocking agents preoperatively for Graves hyperthyroidism or β-adrenergic blocking agents alone for toxic adenoma or nodular goiter. Long-acting agents such as atenolol given preoperatively maintain β-adrenergic blockade in the immediate postoperative period when the patient is not taking medication orally. Intravenous propranolol can be used intraoperatively.

Thyroid Storm

True thyroid storm with fever and altered mental status is rare, but severe hyperthyroidism is not uncommon and treated similarly. For Graves hyperthyroidism, high doses of methimazole (e.g., 10 to 15 mg every 6 hours) and iopanoic acid (500 mg twice daily) to block T_4 to T_3 conversion is most effective. Methimazole is absorbed equally well through the rectal mucosa and can be prepared by the hospital pharmacy for administration as a rectal suppository if the patient cannot take oral medication. Iodine (SSKI) may also be administered. Severe hyperthyroidism is less common from toxic nodular goiter, but when it occurs, iodine-containing drugs should be used cautiously because they may provide substrate for hormone synthesis, and PTU, 200 mg every 4 hours, may be preferred over iopanoic acid for inhibiting T_4 to T_3 conversion, even though it is less effective. Corticosteroids have traditionally been used for thyroid storm, although there is little evidence for their efficacy. Cholestyramine (Questran) may be used to reduce the enterohepatic circulation of thyroid hormone.

Hyperthyroidism With a Low Radioiodine Uptake

It is critical to recognize that patients with Graves hyperthyroidism and subacute lymphocytic thyroiditis may be distinguished only by the radioiodine uptake (see Table 1). Thionamides and radioiodine have no role in the treatment of subacute thyroiditis, because there is no ongoing synthesis of thyroid hormone. Hyperthyroidism occurs due to destruction of thyroid tissue and release of preformed hormone. β-Adrenergic blocking agents* are primary therapy for the hyperthyroidism, which is usually mild. Iopanoic acid may be given when the hyperthyroidism is more severe. The treatment of thyroiditis is discussed elsewhere in this book.

THYROID CANCER†

method of
KENNETH B. AIN, M.D.
University of Kentucky and Veterans Affairs Medical Center
Lexington, Kentucky

Thyroid malignancies include a broad range of tumors with unique properties and clinical behaviors that are different from most other cancers. The severity of these malignancies can range from the innocuous unifocal papillary microcarcinoma, with virtually no clinical significance, to the lethal anaplastic carcinoma, with rare survival past several months despite any therapeutic efforts. Unlike the situation for many other cancers, clinical follow-up for thyroid cancer is typically lifelong in most cases. Distinct therapeutic approaches to different types and presentations of thyroid cancer necessitate careful attention to details of histology, tumor stage, and functional features.

More than 18,000 new cases of thyroid cancer are identified each year. This number represents only a tiny portion of prevalent disease because most patients survive for many years or suffer no disease-specific mortality. The majority of patients are women, although male gender appears to confer some prognostic risk. Sparse, microscopic, intrathyroidal foci of typical papillary thyroid cancer are present in a large portion of the general population (occult papillary microcarcinomas) constituting a high incidence of nonclinical cancer. This is distinct from clinically relevant disease, which can be characterized as having one or more of the following: typical papillary cancers that are multifocal, larger than 1 cm, locally metastatic, and composed of an aggressive histologic subtype or of any-sized nonpapillary thyroid cancer.

Thyroid cancer is more common with increasing age, although this malignancy can be seen in children and is particularly evident in populations previously exposed to therapeutic radiation or radioactive fallout as children. Medullary thyroid cancers are noteworthy in that many are expressions of autosomal dominant, highly penetrant, gene mutations (*RET* proto-oncogene on chromosome 10), which places affected families at particular risk for this cancer, greatly in excess of the general population incidence. Clusters of cases of papillary carcinomas have been described in some families, prompting several active investigations to determine possible genetic predispositions. On the other hand, the vast majority of patients with thyroid cancer have no known inherited or environmental predilection for this malignancy.

TYPES OF THYROID CANCER

The thyroid gland is composed of a variety of cells, including thyroid follicular cells, parafollicular cells, vascular smooth muscle and endothelium, lymphocytes, and connective tissues. Each of these types of cells may produce malignant neoplasms with characteristic features (Table 1). Most thyroid carcinomas are derived from thyroid epithelial cells, producing general categories of papillary carcinomas, follicular carcinomas, and anaplastic carcinomas. The majority are papillary carcinomas, consisting of several different subtypes or variants: usual papillary, follicular variants and less common variants with particularly aggressive clinical courses (tall cell, columnar cell, diffuse sclerosing, and oxyphilic [Hürthle cell]). Typically, characteristic nuclear features have made the recognition of papillary cancers possible despite varied histologic growth patterns.

Although usual papillary thyroid cancers tend to disseminate regionally along lymphatic channels and respond to radioactive iodine therapy, because they constitute the majority of thyroid cancers, they are also highly represented among those patients with disease-specific mortality. On the other hand, the aggressive papillary variants tend to recur and spread distantly, often losing the expression of the sodium-iodide symporter (NIS), the membrane protein iodide pump responsible for the susceptibility of thyroid cancer to radioiodine therapy.

Follicular thyroid carcinomas also tend to concentrate radioiodine; however, they are likely to spread hematogenously to distant organs and bones, resulting in greater mortality than typical papillary carcinomas. In addition, because the discrimination between a follicular adenoma and follicular carcinoma requires extensive histologic examination for any tumor capsule or vessel invasion to define a carcinoma, it is not too uncommon for patients with previous surgery for "follicular adenoma" to be found with distant metastases of follicular carcinoma many years

*Not FDA approved for this indication.

†All material in this chapter is in the public domain, with the exception of any borrowed figures or tables.

TABLE 1. **Classification and Features of Clinically Relevant Thyroid Cancers**

Histologic Categories	Incidence % (Subset)	Functional Features	Tumor Markers	Systemic Therapy
Differentiated epithelial cancers				
Papillary carcinomas	75	NIS, TSH-R	TG	I-131
Usual papillary	(75)	NIS, TSH-R	TG	I-131
Follicular variant	(15)	NIS, TSH-R	TG	I-131
Tall cell variant	(4)	±NIS, TSH-R	TG	I-131
Columnar cell variant	(<1)	±NIS, TSH-R	TG	I-131
Diffuse sclerosing variant	(3)	NIS, TSH-R	TG	I-131
Oxyphilic (Hürthle cell) variant	(2)	±NIS, TSH-R	TG	I-131
Follicular carcinomas	10	NIS, TSH-R	TG	I-131
Oxyphilic (Hürthle cell) variant	(20)	±NIS, TSH-R	TG	I-131
Insular carcinoma	2	±NIS, TSH-R	TG	±I-131
Anaplastic carcinomas	2	None	None	Paclitaxel
Medullary (parafollicular cell) cancer	<8	None	Calcitonin, CEA	None
Other cell types (most are very rare)				
Lymphoma	<5	None	None	CHOP
Angiomatoid neoplasms, mucoepidermoid carcinoma, malignant adult thyroid teratoma, carcinomas with thymic features, paragangliomas	Very rare	None	None	None

Abbreviations: CEA = carcinoembryonic antigen; CHOP = cyclophosphamide, doxorubicin, vincristine, and prednisolone; I-131 = radioiodine therapy; NIS = sodium-iodide symporter; TG = thyroglobulin; TSH-R = thyrotropin (TSH) receptor.

later. Because this histologic distinction is so critical, it is wise to insist on careful review of all "benign follicular adenomas" to avoid such scenarios.

The cytologic indistinguishability of follicular adenomas from carcinomas requires any fine needle biopsy result of "follicular neoplasm" to be dealt with by a surgical thyroid lobectomy to permit histologic analysis. Inasmuch as the only effective systemic therapy is radioiodine, the tendency of oxyphilic thyroid carcinomas to lose iodine-131 (^{131}I) uptake may result in dire consequences from distantly metastatic and unresectable tumor. Outdated classifications of mixed papillary and follicular tumors are more correctly designated papillary carcinomas and, likewise, follicular variants of papillary carcinoma were often misclassified as follicular carcinomas, accounting for the higher incidence of follicular cancers described in older texts. Insular thyroid cancers were previously classified as anaplastic carcinomas until some were found to respond to radioiodine. Nonetheless, with nearly one third of patients having disease-specific mortality, insular cancers show clinically aggressive behavior midway between follicular and anaplastic carcinomas.

Anaplastic carcinomas are the ultimate malignant dedifferentiation of the thyroid follicular cell, constituting the most lethal solid tumor of humans. They occur in less than 2% of incident thyroid cancer patients but are uniformly fatal, with median survival from 4 to 12 months. These tumors do not concentrate radioiodine and have thyroid-stimulating hormone (TSH)–independent growth. Anaplastic cancer patients require aggressive measures to attempt local disease control but inevitably succumb to local progression or distant metastases.

Parafollicular cells secrete calcitonin and can undergo malignant transformation to medullary thyroid carcinomas. Because these malignancies intrinsically lack features of thyroid follicular cells, they do not concentrate radioiodine or produce thyroglobulin but are identified by secretion of calcitonin and carcinoembryonic antigen. Although most of these cancers develop sporadically, particularly in older patients, a sizable portion of them are consequent to germline autosomal dominant mutations of the *RET* proto-oncogene. They can be prevented by prophylactic thyroidectomy of affected family members when identified by genetic testing. Inherited medullary thyroid cancer presents as either isolated medullary carcinoma or an essential component of multiple endocrine neoplasia type 2a (MEN2a; including parathyroid adenomas and pheochromocytomas) or type 2b (MEN2b; marfanoid habitus, gastrointestinal ganglioneuromatosis, mucosal neuromas, and pheochromocytomas). Identification of a medullary carcinoma in the context of a potential MEN2a or MEN2b family should prompt evaluation for a pheochromocytoma before initiating surgical management of the thyroid cancer.

Thyroid lymphomas are uncommon malignancies; however, they show excellent clinical responses to a combination of local external radiation therapy (XRT) and systemic chemotherapy. On the other hand, the other rare thyroid malignancies, listed in Table 1, are nearly all clinically aggressive with no proven effective systemic therapies. Histologic confirmation of these cancers is important, using expert reviewers, owing to the scarcity of these cases and corresponding inexperience with these diagnoses.

CLINICAL PRESENTATION AND DIAGNOSIS

The majority of thyroid cancers are found as palpable thyroid nodules or enlarged cervical lymph nodes. There is no role for using thyroid ultrasonography to screen for thyroid nodules because nearly half of the population will have tiny thyroid nodules less than 1 cm in diameter (usually benign nodules or occult papillary microcarcinomas). Incidental thyroid nodules exceeding 1 cm may be discovered fortuitously during ultrasound evaluation of the carotid vessels or during unrelated radiologic procedures. Radiologic procedures that incorporate administration of iodinated intravenous contrast agents should almost never be used diagnostically because the stable iodine from these agents may impair radioiodine scanning and therapy of potential malignancies for 6 to 12 months. Less commonly, a distant metastasis may be the first evidence of a primary thyroid malignancy after histologic or cytologic evaluation (using immunohistochemistry for thyroglobulin or calcitonin to define the primary site).

Evaluation of thyroid nodules requires assessment for thyrotoxicosis, with iodine-123 (^{123}I) thyroid scanning reserved exclusively for thyrotoxic patients (with suppressed TSH levels). This will discern autonomously functioning ("hot") thyroid nodules, which are nearly never malignant, from the unusual hypofunctioning ("cold") nodule in the context of Graves' disease (which should be sampled). In nonthyrotoxic patients, thyroid nuclear scans should not be performed because they cannot distinguish benign from malignant nodules. Likewise, suppression of thyroid nodules with thyroid hormone provides no diagnostic benefit to discern thyroid cancer from benign nodules. Proper assessment of dominant thyroid nodules requires fine-needle aspiration biopsy with evaluation by appropriately trained cytopathologists, documenting sufficient thyroid follicular epithelial cells to render a diagnosis. The absence of sufficient thyroid follicular cells to demonstrate a benign or malignant process characterizes an "inadequate" biopsy that has no diagnostic value and should be repeated. Around 90% of dominant thyroid nodules are benign, and benign cytologic findings should be confirmed by follow-up clinical assessments to document lack of nodule growth over time. Biopsy results confirming cancer or demonstrating a suspicion for cancer or follicular neoplasia should result in surgical consultation for thyroid resection and final histologic confirmation. Fine-needle biopsy of cervical lymphadenopathy that reveals thyroid follicular cells is diagnostic of thyroid carcinoma, even in the absence of detectable thyroid nodules. Rapid enlargement of a thyroid mass is suggestive of lymphoma or anaplastic carcinoma, which requires equally rapid diagnostic evaluation with fine-needle or surgical biopsy.

THERAPY FOR DIFFERENTIATED PAPILLARY AND FOLLICULAR CANCERS

Surgical Management

Thyroid surgeons must demonstrate specialized skills and judgment because the complication rates of hypoparathyroidism and recurrent laryngeal nerve damage are inversely proportional to their experience and thyroid cancer caseload. The minimal acceptable surgery for a malignant or suspicious thyroid nodule is a total ipsilateral thyroid lobectomy and isthmusectomy, because this obviates any need for ipsilateral reoperation. This is appropriate final surgery for lesions shown to be benign neoplasms or unifocal, intrathyroidal, papillary microcarcinomas ($\leq$1.0 cm diameter). For all other thyroid cancers (except lymphomas, which do not require resection), the optimal procedure is a total thyroidectomy, either as a primary resection (if possible) or after a previous lobectomy (after cancer is histologically confirmed). Lesser resections are avoidable compromises in care and partial lobectomies or "nodulectomies" are unacceptably beneath any modern standard of care. Careful intraoperative assessment showing lymphadenopathy should result in resection of these nodes and modified neck dissections (ipsilateral and central) are appropriate for bulky nodal disease and invasive tumors. It is important to resect all macroscopic cancer because follow-up therapy is most effective with minimal residual disease. For medullary carcinomas, more extensive formal node dissection may be beneficial because there are no effective systemic postoperative therapies.

After thyroid surgery, prognostic variables may be assessed to provide the clinician with some guidance as to the future biologic behavior of this malignancy. Increased primary tumor size, vascular invasion, extrathyroidal penetration, local metastases, older age at diagnosis (>45 years), distant metastases, male sex, and aggressive histologic subtypes all presage worsening prognosis and permit appropriate therapeutic and diagnostic intensification. A variety of prognostic staging systems have been developed for evaluating differentiated thyroid carcinomas, with appropriate application in epidemiologic studies for statistical analyses of large patient populations and as stratification tools for designing clinical trials. None of them are sufficiently predictive of outcome to permit their use for determining therapy in individual patients.

Radioiodine Therapy

Preparation for Radioiodine Therapy

Radioiodine (^{131}I) as a treatment agent has specific application in differentiated thyroid epithelial carcinomas (papillary and follicular carcinomas) but is of no value in other thyroid malignancies. Effective ^{131}I therapy requires optimal patient preparation. After complete surgical thyroidectomy (or after stopping levothyroxine in previously thyroidectomized patients), patients are placed on liothyronine (Cytomel, 25 μg twice daily) for 4 weeks, which is then discontinued for 2 weeks along with implementation of a strict low-iodine diet. This results in sufficient elevation of thyrotropin (TSH >30 mU/L) to stimulate radioiodine uptake in both thyroid remnants and residual or metastatic thyroid carcinoma. Exogenous recombinant human thyrotropin has been used for preparation for diagnostic radioiodine scanning in low-risk patients but currently has no role in typical ^{131}I therapy owing to reduced radiation dose delivery to target tissues as compared with classic hypothyroid preparation (except in patients with pituitary insufficiency who are unable to generate endogenous TSH). Metastases in critical sites, such as in the brain, spinal cord, or bone, are best treated with assertive surgical resection before high-dose ^{131}I therapy. Alternatively, stereotactic XRT (gamma knife) may be used for intracranial metastases. Unfortunate use of iodinated contrast media in diagnostic radiographic studies can be a cause of ^{131}I treatment failure, persisting for up to 12 months. A low-iodine diet for 1 week terminating with a 24-hour urine iodine assessment will define when this stable iodine contamination has passed (when 24-hour urine iodine is <100 μg). Fertile female patients must have a negative pregnancy test before ^{131}I is administered and are advised to initiate birth control measures before withdrawing thyroid hormone therapy.

Radioiodine Ablation

Unifocal, nonmetastatic papillary microcarcinomas are not usually treated with ^{131}I; however, all other patients with more advanced papillary cancers or follicular cancers require definitive postoperative ^{131}I ablation. Radioiodine is appropriate in both child and adult thyroid cancer patients, as long as the ^{131}I dose can deliver tumoricidal radiation at a dose rate sufficiently high to avoid tumor cell recovery from sublethal radiation damage. For this reason, therapeutic efficacy is related to the adequacy of each administered dose, rather than to the total cumulative effect of small, insufficient doses. Consequently, our lowest therapy doses are 100 mCi for low-risk intrathyroidal cancers without evidence of metastatic disease (based on surgery and diagnostic ^{131}I scans). Regional metastases warrant doses of 150 mCi, whereas invasive or residual bulky disease may be treated with doses up to 200 mCi.

We administer activities under 120 mCi as outpatient therapy and hospitalize patients given higher doses for 24 to 48 hours. Patients should not be advised to force fluids during treatment because this may compromise tumor ^{131}I uptake and aggravates potential hyponatremia when hypothyroid. Radiation sialadenitis is common, self-limited, and unavoidable, often resulting in permanently decreased salivary function. Putative radioprotectants are not advised because the potential risk of compromising the therapeutic effects of ^{131}I has not been evaluated.

Distantly metastatic tumors require appropriately aggressive therapy with the maximal ^{131}I doses each patient can safely tolerate. Quantitative ^{131}I total-body dosimetry has been successfully applied for more than 35 years to individually delineate dose limits based on gamma probe counts of patients and their blood samples at multiple time intervals over 5 days ($<$200 REM red marrow exposure, $<$120 mCi retained in the body at 48 hours, and $<$80 mCi in the lung at 48 hours). This has permitted safe administration of single ^{131}I doses exceeding 600 mCi in some patients with aggressive tumors. Likewise, this method may also limit administered doses to less than typical empirical amounts, particularly with unresectable bulky tumor or compromised renal function. Few nuclear medicine facilities currently have sufficient experience in this method; thus, patients requiring aggressive therapy may warrant appropriate referral unless local consultants acquire such expertise. Serial peripheral blood cell counts, obtained weekly after maximal dose therapy, reveal a nadir of platelets, white blood cells, and reticulocytes approximately 1 month later, with recovery by 6 to 8 weeks. Radioiodine therapies are typically spaced at least 5 to 6 months apart to permit time for marrow recovery and sufficient opportunity for full therapeutic response.

There are several remediable causes of radioiodine treatment failure besides stable iodine contamination from iodinated contrast dyes or dietary noncompliance. Some tumors fail to retain ^{131}I long enough to deliver effective radiation. Lithium carbonate, administered before the radioiodine dose and maintained at standard therapeutic serum levels for 5 days after ^{131}I administration, can significantly prolong tumor radioiodine retention. Rarely, the radioiodine tracer dose used for diagnostic scanning "stuns" tumor deposits sufficient to impair uptake of a closely following ^{131}I therapy dose. This can be deduced from comparison of diagnostic scans with post-therapy scans performed at similar time intervals from ^{131}I administration and can be corrected by giving therapeutic ^{131}I, at least 6 months later, without a preceding diagnostic study.

As long as recurrent or metastatic tumors concentrate iodine, further ^{131}I therapy may be considered because there is no evidence of an intrinsic cumulative limit on therapy provided that clinical headway is evident and toxicity is monitored. Elevated thyroglobulin levels may reveal ^{131}I-treatable disease (with $\geq$200-mCi doses) in the absence of positive diagnostic ^{131}I scans or radiographic sites; however, there is no role for empirical ^{131}I therapy when radiographically evident macroscopic disease fails to concentrate diagnostic ^{131}I doses. Unfortunately, in such circumstances there are no known effective treatments aside from suppression of TSH with sufficient levothyroxine and XRT of localized tumor.

Levothyroxine Suppression of Thyroid-Stimulating Hormone

All thyroidectomized patients require lifelong therapy with levothyroxine sodium, but, unlike typical hypothyroid patients, differentiated thyroid cancer patients should be given sufficiently high levothyroxine dosages to maintain suppression of serum TSH. The average suppression dose of 2.0 μg/kg/d should be titrated to the minimal dosage sufficient to maintain TSH less than 0.10 mU/L, while avoiding thyrotoxic symptoms. This provides a valuable therapeutic benefit in improved survival and decreased tumor recurrence. A minority of patients note palpitations or tachycardia that is easily avoided by treatment with extended-release β-adrenergic blockers.* Concerns regarding possible accelerated bone loss with suppressive levothyroxine have shown to be of little significance, except in postmenopausal women, in whom they must be balanced against the potentially increased aggressiveness of thyroid cancer in this age group. The most vexing aspects of levothyroxine therapy are to maintain adequate compliance, avoid concomitant interfering medications (e.g., ferrous sulfate, sucralfate [Carafate], cholestyramine [Questran]), and prevent degradation of levothyroxine tablets by exposure to heat.

Additional Therapies

Chemotherapy is ineffective in differentiated thyroid carcinoma and has no place in the treatment of

*Not FDA approved for this indication.

patients whose tumors retain radioiodine uptake. In patients with thyroid carcinomas that have lost or never had ^{131}I uptake, such as dedifferentiated papillary or follicular carcinomas, medullary carcinomas, and rare thyroid cancers derived from other cellular lineages, surgical resection should be performed for bulky or critically located tumor masses. Distantly metastatic disease should be monitored for rate of progression because the risk of immediate morbidity from usually ineffective chemotherapy must be balanced against the delayed morbidity consequent to these metastases, which often grow remarkably slowly. Anaplastic thyroid carcinoma grows so rapidly that antineoplastic chemotherapy is usually warranted for treatment of distant disease. Paclitaxel (Taxol)* has provided the best response rate for these patients, although this agent merely delays inevitable mortality. On the other hand, systemic chemotherapy (CHOP—cyclophosphamide, doxorubicin [Adriamycin], vincristine [Oncovin}, and prednisolone), combined with XRT, can be curative of thyroid lymphomas. Newer agents with antiangiogenic activity may be useful as adjunctive or tumoristatic therapy.

The use of XRT is limited to tumors without radioiodine uptake and is usually directed toward the neck and superior mediastinum. Sometimes, XRT is used to treat metastases to bone; however, better results are seen if these metastases are resected before ^{131}I therapy or XRT, if dedifferentiated. There is no evidence that chemoradiosensitization provides better results than hyperfractionated XRT alone, but it causes significantly greater morbidity. Stereotactic XRT or gamma-knife treatment has proven particularly useful for intracranial metastases.

FOLLOW-UP MODALITIES AND STRATEGIES

Tumor Markers

Thyroglobulin is a unique protein product of thyroid follicular cells and serves as a specific tumor marker for papillary and follicular carcinomas. TSH stimulation of residual thyroid cancer (either by hypothyroidism or by recombinant human TSH administration) enhances thyroglobulin release, whereas levothyroxine suppression of TSH results in suppression of thyroglobulin. Tumor dedifferentiation is often discordant in regard to ^{131}I uptake and thyroglobulin production, so that measurable thyroglobulin denotes persistent disease, even with negative ^{131}I diagnostic scans. Unfortunately, in around one fourth of thyroid cancer patients, antithyroglobulin autoantibodies make thyroglobulin assessments unreliable. New techniques that assess for circulating thyroid cancer cells (using reverse transcriptase polymerase-chain reaction detection for thyroglobulin messenger RNA) may prove useful in such circumstances to denote the presence of residual disease.

Calcitonin and carcinoembryonic antigen levels provide tumor markers applicable to medullary thyroid carcinoma. Whereas these tests have been used to screen kindreds of inherited medullary thyroid cancer in the past, such use has been superseded by genetic testing. They still provide information regarding residual tumor burden after primary thyroid surgery in known medullary cancer patients. Previous use of pentagastrin to stimulate calcitonin release, increasing the sensitivity of this assay, is no longer possible because this agent is no longer manufactured.

Nuclear Medicine Scanning

Radioiodine scanning with ^{131}I is the hallmark of evaluation for differentiated papillary or follicular thyroid cancer in thyroidectomized patients. Preparation, with levothyroxine withdrawal and low iodine diet, is identical, as described earlier for ^{131}I therapy. We typically use ^{131}I scanning doses of 5 mCi, preceded by measurement of TSH and thyroglobulin, and obtain 24-hour and 48-hour whole-body scans, enabling assessment for residual tumor or remnant uptake as well as turnover rate. Positive scans result in therapeutic ^{131}I administration with reassessment by scanning after appropriate preparation 6 months later. Negative evaluations are followed by repeat studies at longer intervals of 1 year, then 2 years, then 3 to 5 years indefinitely, as long as the patient remains free of detectable disease. For patients with favorable prognostic tumor features and several years of negative follow-up studies, or in hypopituitary patients unable to produce TSH, recombinant human TSH (rhTSH) injections have been used in place of hypothyroid preparations. Although avoidance of debilitating hypothyroid symptoms and loss of employment productivity are significant advantages, they must be balanced against the high cost of rhTSH, the need to prolong scanning time threefold (to acquire at least 140,000 counts per whole-body image), the decreased sensitivity compared with hypothyroid preparation, and the need to initiate a full hypothyroid preparation should scans indicate the need for ^{131}I therapy. We do not use ^{123}I for whole-body imaging because its short half-life precludes accurate 48-hour imaging, turnover assessment, or radioiodine dosimetry analysis for high-dose therapy. It is important to perform post-therapy whole-body scanning after each administration of ^{131}I therapy. We perform this at 48 hours from the treatment dose to permit direct comparison with the 48-hour diagnostic scan and assess for tumor "stunning."

Alternative scanning techniques and isotopes provide further clinical information, particularly for tumors without radioiodine uptake. Whole-body scans with thallium-201 or technetium-99m-sestamibi may provide evidence of metastatic sites. Likewise, positron emission tomographic imaging with ^{18}F-fluorodeoxyglucose is useful to delineate dedifferentiated tumor, particularly in the lung or mediastinum.

*Not FDA approved for this indication.

Additional Radiologic Procedures

It is important that anatomic radiologic studies complement functional nuclear scans because loss of tumor function would result in false-negative clinical assumptions. We perform baseline computed axial tomography of the lung (without contrast medium enhancement), repeating it at intervals of 1 to 4 years based on prognostic features and known extent of disease and substituting conventional chest radiographs for very low risk disease. For anatomic regions requiring contrast agents, we use gadolinium enhancement of magnetic resonance imaging. Dedifferentiated tumors or tumors that are not treated or scanned with ^{131}I may be evaluated using computed tomography with standard iodinated contrast medium. Extensive ultrasound evaluation of the neck, in conjunction with fine-needle biopsies of all suspicious structures, has proven quite useful for locating local tumor recurrences despite loss of iodide uptake.

New Directions

Because the most effective systemic therapy has utilized radioiodine, loss of radioiodine uptake is a critical cause of treatment failure. Although retinoic acid has been proposed to restore ^{131}I uptake, our clinical trials with this approach have been uniformly negative. Research findings regarding epigenetic regulation of NIS expression have prompted additional trials with potentially useful agents. Likewise, ongoing preclinical studies of new antineoplastic and antiangiogenic agents may additionally delineate new therapeutic directions.

PHEOCHROMOCYTOMA

method of
McCLELLAN M. WALTHER, M.D.
National Institutes of Health
Bethesda, Maryland

Pheochromocytomas are catecholamine-producing tumors, notorious for an unpredictable and catastrophic clinical course of malignant hypertension. Pheochromocytomas occur in the sympathetic nervous system—from the glomus jugulare at the base of the skull to the urinary bladder. The majority, however, occur in the adrenal glands. Certain extra-adrenal pheochromocytomas, called *paraganglia*, have been given unique names, such as glomus tumor derived from the glomus jugulare, chemodectoma from the carotid body, and organ of Zuckerkandl tumor named for those paraganglia.

Clinical signs and symptoms of pheochromocytoma result from excessive tumor catecholamine production, with over 50% of patients developing marked hypertension. Fifteen percent to 20% of the adult population of western countries have sustained essential hypertension, and 0.05% to 0.3% of these patients are estimated to have chromocytomas. The diagnosis of pheochromocytoma in the general population is further complicated by paroxysmal hypertension in those patients with a baseline normotensive state. A pheochromocytoma is usually a benign tumor, curable if properly identified and removed, but it can be fatal if undiagnosed or not treated appropriately.

CLINICAL FEATURES

Sporadic pheochromocytomas are usually diagnosed in the fourth through sixth decades of life, with equal gender distribution. Solitary adrenal pheochromocytomas occur in 72% to 82%, bilateral adrenal pheochromocytomas occur in 3% to 11%, and extra-adrenal tumors occur in 9% to 19% of affected patients.

Patients with sporadic pheochromocytomas most often present with hypertensive crises. Other presentations include pallor, sweating, essential hypertension that responds poorly to conventional treatment, paroxysmal symptoms suggesting seizure disorder, or anxiety attacks. Hypertension can be paroxysmal or sustained, with similar occurrence of each. Marked blood pressure lability is characteristically present, with distinct crises occurring in patients with sustained hypertension. Hypertensive crises are often severe and can be resistant to standard medications used in the management of essential hypertension. Hypertensive crisis can occur on a daily basis or at intervals of weeks or months. The crises tend to increase in frequency, duration, and severity over time.

Other commonly found symptoms include profuse sweating, palpitations, tachycardia, and headache. Chest or abdominal pain, nausea and vomiting, and a feeling of apprehension or impending doom can also occur. Crises associated with marked vasoconstriction produce pallor or flushing. Myocardial infarction, congestive heart failure, cardiac arrhythmias, hypertensive retinopathy, cerebrovascular accident, dissecting aortic aneurysms, renal failure, or tumor hemorrhage can occur during a crisis. Long-term exposure to elevated levels of catecholamines has been associated with catecholamine cardiomyopathy, arteriosclerosis, and ischemic enterocolitis.

Pheochromocytoma catecholamine release is not mediated by neuronal activity but can occur with physical stimuli, tumor necrosis, or changes in blood flow. Classic presentations are an acute hypertensive crisis during surgery, physical activity, abdominal trauma, or, in patients with bladder pheochromocytoma, voiding. A number of drugs have a provocative effect on pheochromocytomas, including imaging agents, glucagon, histamine, guanethidine (Ismelin), metoclopramide (Reglan), and phenothiazines. Lower elevations of plasma catecholamines are present outside the times of crisis and are associated with increased metabolic rate and weight loss. Elevated catecholamine levels can also suppress insulin production and increase hepatic glucose output, leading to hyperglycemia, as well as cause vascular constriction with diminished plasma volume and elevated hematocrit.

DIFFERENTIAL DIAGNOSIS

Patients with signs and symptoms of pheochromocytoma can have a presentation similar to essential or secondary hypertension, hypertension of pregnancy, renovascular hypertension, hypertensive crises associated with withdrawal of some antihypertensive agents (clonidine) or drugs (cocaine), anxiety and panic attacks, intracranial tumors, or self-administration of sympathomimetic amines. Patients who should be considered for evaluation of pheochromocytoma have hypertension resistant to conventional therapy, hypertension of new onset, or a familial syndrome associated with pheochromocytoma. Patients with hereditary pheochromocytomas should be evaluated before contemplating pregnancy because a high incidence of fetal or maternal death is found in undiagnosed patients with pheochromocytoma.

ASSOCIATED DISEASES

Cholelithiasis has been found in 3% to 23% of patients with pheochromocytoma. Pheochromocytoma-associated paraneoplastic syndromes including Cushing syndrome, erythrocytosis, and hypercalcemia are cured after removal of isolated tumors. Renal artery stenosis with elevated peripheral plasma renins has been infrequently observed. Removal of the pheochromocytoma is often curative, but nephrectomy or renal artery reconstruction is occasionally required.

SPECIAL CLINICAL SITUATIONS

Pregnancy

Undiagnosed pheochromocytoma in pregnancy is associated with a high rate of fetal loss and maternal death. The effect of medical blockade is not well known but is necessary for patient survival. α-Blockade appears to be safe to the fetus. Delivery is preferably performed electively by cesarean section. Laparoscopic and open surgery have been performed in pregnancy, although the risk of spontaneous abortion increases as gestation increases using both techniques.

Epinephrine-Producing Tumors

Most pheochromocytomas are primarily norepinephrine-producing tumors, which causes their typical signs and symptoms. Epinephrine-producing tumors are more associated with headaches, panic attacks, chest pain and palpitations, leg and abdominal cramps, sweating, fever, and vomiting. Impaired glucose tolerance can also be seen in association with these types of tumors. The vasodilatory β-adrenergic action of epinephrine can produce hypotension and even shock, particularly after α-adrenergic blockade.

Malignant Pheochromocytoma

Malignant pheochromocytomas are diagnosed by the presence of metastases, as histologic findings are not informative. *Metastases* are defined as pheochromocytomas located outside normal sympathetic tissue and occur in 7% to 15% of patients. Pheochromocytoma metastases can be found in bone, liver, lung, regional lymph nodes, and the brain. Metastases are usually slow growing, and a median survival is more than 10 years. Use of α- and β-blockers is often necessary to minimize symptoms or prevent hypertensive crisis. A catecholamine synthesis inhibitor (metyrosine [Demser]) can be added if additional therapy is needed.

Treatment of metastatic pheochromocytoma is usually reserved until symptoms are present because no effective therapy currently exists. Treatment with meta-iodobenzylguanidine-^{131}I, cyclophosphamide, vincristine, and dacarbazine chemotherapy or with radiation has mixed results that are usually not durable. Isolated or slow-growing tumors have uncommonly been resected with long-term response.

HEREDITARY FORMS OF PHEOCHROMOCYTOMA

Familial tumors are thought to comprise about 10% of pheochromocytoma; described forms include von Hippel-Lindau disease (VHL), multiple endocrine neoplasia type 2 (MEN2), von Recklinghausen neurofibromatosis, hereditary paraganglioma syndrome (PGL), and hereditary pheochromocytoma. All are inherited in an autosomal dominant fashion, and the gene has been identified in several types.

Screening families with hereditary pheochromocytoma can identify patients with small nonfunctional tumors. Some of these patients have been followed every 6 months and surgery recommended in patients with localized tumors when catecholamine secretion becomes elevated, when associated signs or symptoms occur, or when tumor size approaches 4 cm in diameter. Partial adrenalectomy may be performed in patients with smaller localized tumors because larger tumors can be destructive to the gland and make adrenocortical preservation more difficult. Patients with hereditary pheochromocytomas should be evaluated and treated before any surgery or pregnancy is contemplated.

Von Hippel-Lindau Disease

VHL disease (VHL tumor suppressor gene, chromosome 3p25) is a multitumor syndrome characterized by central nervous system hemangioblastoma, endolymphatic sac tumors, retinal angiomas, renal cysts and carcinomas, neuroendocrine tumors and cysts of the pancreas, epididymal cystadenomas, and/or pheochromocytoma. VHL has been estimated to affect 1 in 45,500.

VHL pheochromocytomas identified by screening family members seldom (16%) have related signs or symptoms. Patients with VHL pheochromocytoma identified by screening affected families present at an earlier age (30 years), have fewer symptoms, have less hypertension, are less functional, have fewer diagnostic tests, and have smaller tumors than patients with sporadic pheochromocytoma. VHL pheochromocytomas are mainly norepinephrine-secreting tumors. Twelve percent of VHL tumors are extra-adrenal, and metastases occur in 1.6% of patients. Compared with other VHL gene germline mutations, missense mutations are most frequently associated with the development of pheochromocytoma, younger age at presentation, extra-adrenal tumors, and metastatic disease.

Multiple Endocrine Neoplasia Type 2

Multiple endocrine neoplasia type 2A (MEN2A) is a multitumor syndrome characterized by medullary thyroid cancer, parathyroid hyperplasia, and pheochromocytoma. Patients with MEN2B, a less common phenotype, also develop mucosal ganglioneuromas. The incidence of MEN2 (*RET* proto-oncogene, chromosome 10q11) has been estimated at 1 in 30,000.

Patients with MEN2 tumors usually have demonstrable elevations of catecholamines, although as many as 52% of affected patients are asymptomatic and only 35% hypertensive at initial diagnosis. The mean patient age at diagnosis is 37 years. MEN2 tumors usually secrete both norepinephrine and epinephrine. Seventy percent of MEN2 patients have bilateral adrenal tumors, and extra-adrenal tumors are rare. A *RET* germline mutation in codon 634 is found in as many as 85% of MEN2A families.

Von Recklinghausen Neurofibromatosis

Von Recklinghausen neurofibromatosis is characterized clinically by neurofibromas and café-au-lait spots, osseous lesions with a low penetrance of pheochromocytoma (0.1 to 5.7%), and carcinoid tumors. It is estimated to affect 1 in 3000 individuals (neurofibromatosis type 1 gene, *NF1*, chromosome 17q11). Patients with other types of neurofibromatosis are not thought to develop pheochromocytomas. About 40% of patients have no related symptoms or hypertension. Mean patient age at diagnosis is 42 years. Of affected patients, 9.6% had bilateral adrenal tumors and 6.1% had extra-adrenal tumors; metastases have been reported in 12% of patients. Both epinephrine and norepinephrine secretion are found in these tumors. About 9% of patients also develop gastrointestinal carcinoid tumors.

Hereditary Paraganglioma Syndrome

Hereditary paraganglioma (hereditary paraganglioma syndrome, *PGL1*, chromosome 11q23) is characterized by paragangliomas of the head and neck region (glomus tumors or chemodectomas, carotid body tumors). Multiple tumors occur in about two thirds of patients. Genomic imprinting occurs in PGL; children of affected men inherit the disorder in an autosomal dominant pattern, whereas children of affected women rarely develop the disease. It is estimated that 1 in 100,000 are affected with PGL. PGL paraganglia are usually not functional, and long-term cure has been associated with radiation treatment in a number of patients.

Hereditary Pheochromocytoma

Hereditary forms of pheochromocytoma that do not fit the previous syndromes have been described. Missense mutations of the VHL gene are often found in patients with only subtle retinal angiomas or central nervous system hemangioblastomas associated with their pheochromocytoma. MEN2 families with only pheochromocytoma have not been described. A small number of poorly characterized families with neither VHL nor *RET* mutations have been reported.

DIAGNOSTIC EVALUATION

Functional Studies

Standard testing for pheochromocytoma starts with 24-hour urinary determination of catecholamines and their metabolites. Biochemical metabolites are preserved by addition of acid to the container and by chilling the specimen until analysis is performed. Urine creatinine excretion and volume measurement can be used to determine if an adequate collection was obtained. Norepinephrine is converted to epinephrine by the action of phenylethanolamine-*N*-methyl transferase (PNMT). Expression of PNMT is regulated by corticosteroid release in the adrenal gland. Adrenal pheochromocytomas thus often secrete epinephrine in addition to norepinephrine. Tumors in extra-adrenal locations secrete mainly norepinephrine.

Plasma catecholamine evaluation has been infrequently used because of its greater expense and lower sensitivity and specificity than urine studies. Elevated plasma catecholamines are sometimes found associated with essential hypertension or an active sympathetic nervous system. Testing for plasma catecholamine 3 hours after an oral dose of clonidine (0.3 mg/70 kg), which will suppress sympathetic nervous activity in patients without pheochromocytoma, increases specificity (clonidine suppression test). Provocative testing, such as glucagon stimulation, has been used in patients with clinical suspicion of pheochromocytoma who have nondiagnostic catecholamine secretion studies. Glucagon stimulates pheochromocytoma release of catecholamines but has no effect in patients with an active sympathetic nervous system or essential hypertension. The evaluation of plasma catecholamines and provocative testing are complementary and used as clinically indicated when the diagnosis of pheochromocytoma is not clear. Measurement of plasma free metanephrines is a new test that is very sensitive and may be more cost effective.

Localization Studies

Computed tomography and magnetic resonance imaging are excellent for identification of pheochromocytoma. T2-weighted magnetic resonance imaging is associated with high signal intensity in pheochromocytoma that is characteristically very bright. Arteriography is not recommended because of the risk of inducing a hypertensive crisis. Adrenal vein or random venous sampling for catecholamines is sometimes used if standard imaging is not informative.

MIBG, an analogue of norepinephrine, is taken up by adrenal medullary tissue and pheochromocytoma, where it is stored in neural secretory granules. MIBG-123 (^{123}I) scintigraphy has been used for imaging the adrenal medulla and pheochromocytoma (extra-adrenal, metastatic, or recurrent tumors) and yields better images than MIBG-^{131}I. Metyrosine and catecholamine uptake inhibitors can interfere with MIBG imaging. Positron emission tomography is developing into a more sensitive test for pheochromocytoma.

CURRENT MANAGEMENT

Preoperative Blockade

Induction of anesthesia or tumor manipulation can cause massive catecholamine release, resulting in hypertensive crisis, arrhythmias, or stroke. Surgery without catecholamine blockade has been associated with a 24% to 50% mortality. The use of adrenergic blockade has resulted in a significant decrease in mortality.

Phenoxybenzamine (10 mg every 12 hours for 2 weeks before surgery) provides α-adrenergic blockade, contributing to vascular dilation with expansion of constricted fluid volume. The dosage can be increased 0.5 mg/kg/d in two divided doses to control blood pressure or symptoms. A common side effect is nasal congestion. An additional dose (1 mg/kg) is given at midnight the night before surgery. Because of associated orthostatic hypotension, patients are placed at bed rest with the siderails up. A β-blocker is added as necessary to blunt the reflex tachycardia (pulse >100 beats per minute) sometimes associated with α-blockade. Administration of a β-blocker before α-blockade can worsen hypertension secondary to unopposed vasoconstriction.

An important addition to preoperative medical blockade has been the addition of metyrosine (Demser), a competitive inhibitor of the enzyme tyrosine hydroxylase. Metyrosine blocks the conversion of tyrosine to DOPA, the rate-limiting step in catecholamine production. Use of metyrosine (250 mg every 6 hours for 2 weeks) can decrease tumor catecholamine content by 50% to 80%. After 1 week, 250 to 500 mg may be added every 2 to 3 days as needed for additional blockade. One gram of metyrosine is administered at midnight the night before surgery. The use of metyrosine has been associated with decreased doses of vasoactive medication to control blood pressure, lower intraoperative fluid requirements, and less blood loss. Excessive sedation, depression, hallucinations, sleep disturbances, extrapyramidal signs, and tremor occur in less than 10% of patients. A limited experience suggests carbidopa/levodopa (Sinemet) may control these symptoms. Urinary crystal formation may occur with doses greater than 4 g/d. Intravenous hydration overnight may help restore intravascular volume. Combined medical blockade with a liberal salt diet allows restoration of contracted plasma volume and blunts tumor catecholamine stores, making surgery and anesthesia safer.

Intraoperative Management

In addition to standard anesthetic monitoring, patients with pheochromocytoma are managed with arterial blood pressure monitoring. Large-bore intravenous cannulas are inserted to facilitate volume replacement during the procedure. Patients are sedated for the placement of an arterial catheter, or occasionally it can be placed after induction but before intubation. Anesthetic induction is accomplished with a potent sedative-hypnotic in combination with opioids and nondepolarizing neuromuscular blockade. Agents that cause histamine release are routinely avoided. Anesthesia is usually maintained with a potent inhalational agent, avoiding halothane because of its sensitization of the myocardium to catecholamines. Nitrous oxide may or may not be used for open procedures and is often avoided for laparoscopic procedures. A central line is placed after intubation for central venous pressure monitoring and the administration of certain medications. In patients with a cardiomyopathy or other indication, a pulmonary artery catheter is placed instead of a central line. Surgical manipulation of the tumor is minimized before controlling the venous drainage to limit the release of catecholamines into the circulation. Paroxysmal elevations of blood pressure are controlled with phentolamine or nitroprusside, and tachycardia and tachydysrhythmias are controlled with intravenous β-blockers (e.g., esmolol [Brevibloc], labetalol [Normodyne, Trandate], metoprolol [Lopressor], propranolol [Inderal]). After the venous drainage of the tumor is ligated, severe hypotension can develop. This hypotension is usually controlled with intravascular volume replacement with crystalloid, but it may also require intermittent doses of phenylephrine or infusions of phenylephrine or norepinephrine (Levophed) for a short period of time. Preoperative blockade can blunt the responsiveness to pharmacologic blood pressure support.

Surgery

Laparoscopic surgical removal of adrenal and extra-adrenal pheochromocytomas is rapidly becoming the standard of care. Modern imaging techniques have generally replaced full abdominal exploration and palpation to identify multifocal or extra-adrenal tumors. Compared with open surgery, laparoscopic surgery has been associated with lower narcotic requirements, shorter hospital stays, and more rapid return to normal activity. No difference was found between hemodynamic changes or need for intraoperative antihypertensive treatment during surgery, and patients have similar operative times, blood losses, and transfusion rates. Laparoscopic partial adrenalectomy has been used to preserve adrenal cortical function and maintain quality of life in patients with hereditary forms of pheochromocytoma.

Postoperative Care

After removal of the tumor, patients are predisposed to orthostatic or resting hypotension, which is treated with continued restoration of intravascular volume. The actions of pressor drugs are blunted for about 24 hours while the preoperative blockade wears off (phenoxybenzamine, half-life of 24 hours; metyrosine, half-life of 4 hours). Hypertension can occur with overcorrection of fluid volume or inadequately treated postoperative pain. Elevated levels of plasma catecholamines resulting from surgery can increase insulin production and lead to hypoglycemia, requiring monitoring of glucose levels until normal physiologic responses return.

Follow-Up

Patients are evaluated about 6 weeks after surgery to confirm return to baseline normal levels of circulating catecholamines. Persistently elevated levels may be associated with multifocal or metastatic disease. From 27% to 38% of patients have nonparoxysmal hypertension after removal of pheochromocytoma, attributed to essential hypertension. Overall 5-year patient survival after surgery has been 84% to 96%. Sporadic pheochromocytoma recurrence has been reported in 2% of patients at 10 years, 7% at 15 years, and 9% at greater than 20 years after surgery, necessitating yearly follow-up for recurrence of symptoms or hypertension. Patients with hereditary forms of pheochromocytoma are at high risk of developing new pheochromocytomas over the course of their life.

THYROIDITIS

method of
SARAH E. CAPES, M.D., and
HERTZEL C. GERSTEIN, M.D., M.Sc.
McMaster University
Hamilton, Ontario, Canada

Thyroiditis is an inflammation of the thyroid gland characterized clinically by thyrotoxicosis and/or hypothyroidism. It is occasionally associated with pain and tenderness over the thyroid gland and may manifest systemic symptoms such as fever and malaise.

Acute, subacute, and chronic forms of thyroiditis have been described (Table 1). Thyroiditis associated with medications may have an acute, subacute, or chronic presentation and is therefore considered separately.

ACUTE SUPPURATIVE THYROIDITIS

Bacterial infection of the thyroid gland, presenting as fever and a tender thyroid mass, is rare in developed nations but occurs more commonly in areas of the world with a high prevalence of endemic goiter. The most common infective organism is *Staphylococcus aureus*, with fewer cases due to *Streptococcus pyogenes* and *Pseudomonas*. Other agents reported to cause acute suppurative thyroiditis include *Salmonella typhi*, *Escherichia coli*, *Candida*, and *Pneumocystis carinii* (in patients with HIV). Acute thyroiditis may also occur in military tuberculosis. Among children, acute suppurative thyroiditis may indicate the presence of a fistula between the piriform sinus and the perithyroidal space that may be demonstrated by barium swallow or endoscopy. Treatment of acute suppurative thyroiditis consists of drainage and appropriate antimicrobial therapy. Pyriform sinus fistulas should be surgically resected to prevent recurrence of thyroiditis.

SUBACUTE THYROIDITIS

All forms of subacute thyroiditis are characterized by release of stored hormone from the thyroid gland and transient thyroid dysfunction. Thyroid dysfunction may consist of thyrotoxicosis alone, transient thyrotoxicosis followed by hypothyroidism, or hypothyroidism alone. Management of thyroid dysfunction is similar for all forms of subacute thyroiditis. β-Blockers (such as propranolol [Inderal],* 40–120 mg/d) may be needed to control symptoms of hyperthyroidism. Thionamide medications are not effective. Treatment with levothyroxine can be used for patients during the hypothyroid phase; in such cases, a low dose of levothyroxine (Synthroid) (e.g., 50 μg/d) should be used, with a trial of withdrawal after 6 to 12 weeks. Permanent hypothyroidism is common after subacute lymphocytic thyroiditis and postpartum thyroiditis, but it rarely occurs after subacute granulomatous thyroiditis. Specific considerations for each subtype of subacute thyroiditis are considered below.

TABLE 1. **Types of Thyroiditis**

Type of Thyroiditis	Clinical Presentation and Diagnosis
Acute suppurative	Painful thyroid mass; fever; pus and/or bacterial or fungal organism on aspiration biopsy
Subacute granulomatous	Pain and tenderness over thyroid; transient hyperthyroid and hypothyroid phases; high erythrocyte sedimentation rate and low radioiodine uptake
Subacute lymphocytic	Painless, transient hyperthyroid and hypothyroid phases; often associated with goiter and antimicrosomal antibodies; low radioiodine uptake
Postpartum	Painless hyperthyroid and/or hypothyroid phases occurring in the first year postpartum; low radioiodine uptake
Chronic	Painless hypothyroidism usually associated with goiter and antimicrosomal antibodies
Drug-induced	Thyrotoxicosis and/or hypothyroidism associated with drugs such as lithium, interferon alfa, amiodarone, or radioiodine

Subacute Granulomatous Thyroiditis (DeQuervain Thyroiditis)

The distinguishing characteristic of subacute granulomatous thyroiditis is pain and tenderness over the thyroid gland. The pain may start unilaterally but usually spreads to both lobes and may be aggravated by swallowing or turning the head. The thyroid gland is often enlarged. Systemic symptoms such as fatigue and low-grade fever may occur and may precede the pain by a few days. In most patients, the illness lasts 2 to 4 months. About half of patients develop transient hyperthyroidism, which may be followed by a transient hypothyroid phase beginning 2 to 4 months after the onset and lasting an additional 2 to 7 months. Subacute granulomatous thyroiditis is thought to be due to viral infection and often follows an upper respiratory tract infection. The finding of suppressed radioiodine uptake and an elevated erythrocyte sedimentation rate confirm the diagnosis. Symptoms can be ameliorated by anti-inflammatory agents (such as aspirin, 2.4–3.6 g/d, or naproxen [Naprosyn], 1–1.5 g in divided doses) (Table 2). In more severe cases, prednisone (40 mg/d) may be initiated and will usually relieve pain and tenderness within 24 to 48 hours. The dose of prednisone should then be tapered over several weeks.

Subacute Lymphocytic Thyroiditis

Silent (Sporadic) Thyroiditis

This is a painless form of subacute thyroiditis that is often associated with goiter, thyroid antibodies, and lymphocytic cell infiltration on biopsy. These findings support the conclusion that silent thyroiditis is an autoimmune disease; it is often considered a variant of chronic autoimmune (Hashimoto) thyroiditis. However, a subset of cases is not associated with goiter or thyroid antibodies and seems to have a seasonal and geographic variation in incidence; the etiology of these cases is less clear.

Postpartum Thyroiditis

Postpartum thyroiditis is characterized by either painless thyrotoxicosis or hypothyroidism in the first

*Not FDA approved for this indication.

TABLE 2. **Drugs Used to Treat Thyroiditis**

Drug	Indication	Example
β-Blockers	Symptomatic hyperthyroidism	Propranolol, 10–40 mg every 6 hours
Nonsteroidal anti-inflammatory drugs	Painful subacute thyroiditis; radiation-induced thyroiditis	Aspirin, 650 mg every 4–6 hours
Prednisone	Painful subacute thyroiditis; radiation thyroiditis; amiodarone-induced thyroiditis (type 2)	Prednisone, 40 mg/d
Thionamides	Amiodarone-induced thyroiditis (type 1)	Methimazole, 30 mg/d
Levothyroxine	Chronic thyroiditis; hypothyroid phase of subacute thyroiditis; drug-induced hypothyroidism	Levothyroxine, 100–150 μg/d

year postpartum. Associations with DR antigens and thyroid antibodies and the finding of lymphocytic infiltration of the thyroid suggest that postpartum thyroiditis is also an autoimmune disease, precipitated by postpartum changes in the immune system. The incidence of postpartum thyroiditis in the first postpartum year is about 5%; among women with type 1 diabetes, the incidence may be as high as 25%. Hypothyroidism alone is the most common finding, but transient hyperthyroidism followed by hypothyroidism or thyrotoxicosis alone also occurs. Postpartum thyroiditis usually resolves spontaneously, without treatment. If β-blockers are prescribed to treat thyrotoxicosis, breast-feeding should be discouraged. Postpartum thyroiditis recurs in subsequent pregnancies in as many as 70% of women, and permanent hypothyroidism develops in up to 25%.

CHRONIC THYROIDITIS

Most cases of chronic thyroiditis are due to Hashimoto's thyroiditis, a painless lymphocytic infiltration of the thyroid gland. Less often, Reidel's thyroiditis (fibrous infiltration of the thyroid) or atrophic thyroiditis (hypothyroidism without goiter) may occur. Treatment of hypothyroidism consists of levothyroxine in a dose adequate to normalize the thyroid-stimulating hormone (TSH). In most young patients or in patients who have undergone thyroidectomy, levothyroxine can be started at 100 μg/d. A TSH level should be drawn 2 to 3 months later; the dosage of levothyroxine can then be adjusted as necessary. In older patients or in those with coronary artery disease, levothyroxine should be initiated at a dose of 25 to 50 μg/d, and the dose should be titrated upward by 50 μg/d every 3 to 4 weeks to normalize the TSH. The average daily requirement of levothyroxine is about 1.7 μg/kg. Although recent research has suggested some benefit to the combination of triiodothyronine with levothyroxine, there is currently insufficient evidence to recommend use of triiodothyronine either alone or in combination with levothyroxine.

Once a stable dose of levothyroxine has been achieved, TSH should be monitored once per year. Fluctuations in TSH often indicate reduced compliance with medication but may reflect reduced absorption due to small bowel disease or drug interactions. The requirement for levothyroxine also increases in pregnancy in most patients. Women of reproductive age who are receiving levothyroxine should be informed of the need to increase the dose in pregnancy. TSH should be checked soon after conception and monitored in each trimester, and the dosage of levothyroxine should be adjusted accordingly. Children born to mothers who were hypothyroid during pregnancy have been shown to perform worse on neuropsychological tests compared with children of euthyroid women; this highlights the need to maintain euthyroidism in pregnancy.

Subclinical Hypothyroidism

Whether subclinical hypothyroidism (i.e., elevated TSH with normal thyroxine concentration) should be treated is controversial. One argument for treating subclinical hypothyroidism is to prevent the development of overt hypothyroidism (elevated TSH with low thyroxine concentration and symptoms of hypothyroidism). The incidence of overt hypothyroidism in people with raised TSH (>6 mU/L) and/or positive antithyroid antibodies is up to 4.3% per year. Whereas some researchers have proposed that subclinical hypothyroidism may be a risk factor for cardiovascular disease, epidemiologic research has not clearly demonstrated an association between elevated TSH or positive antithyroid antibodies and either mortality or ischemic heart disease. Nevertheless, treatment of subclinical hypothyroidism with levothyroxine may improve an individual's cardiovascular risk profile by lowering cholesterol levels.

The effect of levothyroxine therapy on total and low-density lipoprotein cholesterol is modest (reductions of ≤10 mg/dL [0.26 mmol/L]), and no significant effect on high-density lipoprotein cholesterol or triglycerides is seen. Some studies have also shown that treatment of subclinical hypothyroidism with levothyroxine improves nonspecific symptoms such as fatigue and weight gain. In summary, the available evidence suggests that treatment with levothyroxine may lower cholesterol levels and may improve subtle symptoms of hypothyroidism in patients with subclinical hypothyroidism. A 2- to 3-month trial of levothyroxine in patients with subclinical hypothyroidism (particularly those with symptoms or with elevated cholesterol levels) therefore can be considered.

DRUG-INDUCED THYROIDITIS AND THYROID DYSFUNCTION

Several medications have been associated with thyroiditis and/or thyroid dysfunction (Table 3).

TABLE 3. **Drugs Reported to Cause Thyroiditis or Thyroid Dysfunction**

Amiodarone
Lithium
Interferon alfa
Interleukin-2
Radioiodine

Lithium

Transient abnormalities in thyroid function tests are common in patients started on lithium; these changes often revert to normal within 1 to 2 years. Subclinical and overt hypothyroidism also are significantly more common in patients on lithium than in the general population, affecting 8% to 19% and up to 23% of patients on lithium, respectively. Patients with overt hypothyroidism should be treated with levothyroxine supplementation. Patients with subclinical hypothyroidism who require continued use of lithium may also be treated if they have symptoms or a TSH level greater than 10 mU/L. If lithium is discontinued, a trial off levothyroxine could be considered in patients with subclinical hypothyroidism.

Amiodarone

Amiodarone (Cordarone) is commonly associated with changes in thyroid hormone levels, which may lead to either thyrotoxicosis or hypothyroidism in up to 24% of patients. Two patterns of amiodarone-induced thyrotoxicosis have been described. Type 1 thyrotoxicosis occurs in patients with an underlying abnormal thyroid gland (multinodular goiter or latent Graves' disease) and is a result of iodine-induced synthesis of excessive thyroid hormone. It is associated with inappropriately normal or elevated radioiodine uptake. In contrast, type 2 thyrotoxicosis occurs in patients with normal thyroid glands and is thought to result from amiodarone-induced cytotoxicity with release of thyroid hormone from damaged cells; it is associated with raised serum interleukin-6 levels and low or undetectable radioiodine uptake.

Type 1 thyrotoxicosis may be treated with thionamide drugs (e.g., methimazole [Tapazole], 30 mg/d). Potassium perchlorate, 1 g/d, has also been used but may be associated with significant toxicity, particularly at higher doses. Type 2 thyrotoxicosis can be treated with prednisone, 40 mg/d. Refractory hyperthyroidism may require thyroidectomy. Because amiodarone is usually prescribed for serious atrial or ventricular arrhythmias, it is usually not feasible to discontinue amiodarone; even if amiodarone can be safely discontinued, hyperthyroidism may persist for as long as 6 months.

Amiodarone-induced hypothyroidism is most common in women with pre-existing antithyroid antibodies and may represent unmasking of subclinical thyroid dysfunction by exposure to excess iodine. Treatment with levothyroxine should start with 25 to 50 μg/d and increase by 25 μg/d at 4- to 6-week intervals. In one case series, a mean dose of 136 μg/d was required to normalize serum thyroxine levels.

Other Drugs

Patients receiving interferon alfa for chronic hepatitis C may develop transient thyrotoxicosis or hypothyroidism, which usually resolves after discontinuation of treatment. Hypothyroidism and hyperthyroidism may also occur in patients receiving interleukin-2 for cancer.

Radioiodine Therapy

Exacerbation of thyrotoxicosis and pain may also follow radioiodine treatment of Graves' disease and usually resolves within 1 week. Pain may be treated with a short course of anti-inflammatory drugs or prednisone.

Section 9

The Urogenital Tract

BACTERIAL INFECTIONS OF THE URINARY TRACT IN MEN

method of
STEPHEN R. JONES, M.D.
Legacy Health System and
Oregon Health Sciences University
Portland, Oregon

Bacterial urinary tract infection (UTI) in adult men is uncommon. When compared with women in similar age groups, the lower prevalence remains striking until middle age, when UTIs become associated with urethral obstruction. The low prevalence in men is thought to be secondary to the greater length of the male urethra and to the antibacterial activity of prostatic fluid.

UTIs and urethritis in men both present as dysuria, and they must be distinguished from each other because of public health and treatment requirements. Urethritis is usually a sexually transmitted disease caused by either *Neisseria gonorrhoeae* or *Chlamydia trachomatis*. UTIs are usually caused by Enterobacteriaceae, predominantly *Escherichia coli*, but occasionally by enterococcal species and *Staphylococcus saprophyticus*.

It is clinically useful to classify the urinary tract infections of adult men in one of three major clinical groups: (1) asymptomatic bacteriuria; (2) lower urinary tract infection with or without clinical evidence for prostatitis; and (3) upper urinary tract infection. Further classification may be made by the clinical tempo and/or the temporal occurrence, that is, acute versus chronic and isolated infections versus recurrent infection.

ASYMPTOMATIC INFECTIONS

In healthy adult men, bacteriuria without symptoms is uncommon, although it becomes more common in the frail elderly. Screening for bacteriuria in asymptomatic healthy men is not recommended. If bacteriuria is found by chance, it should lead to an investigation to exclude predisposing structural or functional abnormalities of the urinary tract. Routine antibiotic treatment in asymptomatic men is not supported by available data; however, such patients should be treated with the intent of eradicating the bacteriuria before genitourinary instrumentation. Alternatively, preventive treatment may be given in the perioperative period.

LOWER URINARY TRACT INFECTION

It is important to recognize the relationship between lower UTIs and prostatitis. Prostatitis may cause symptomatic infection with or without bladder infection. Bladder infection in men with mechanically normal urinary tract systems often is associated with bacterial prostatitis; however, uncomplicated lone cystitis does occur

Uncomplicated Cystitis

Cystitis without underlying prostatitis is most likely to occur in young men with acute symptoms. Risk factors include homosexuality with anal-rectal intercourse, a lack of circumcision, and AIDS. Instrumentation is the most common identifiable cause of these infections in older men.

The most common clinical symptoms at presentation are dysuria, increased frequency of urination, and urgency. These may be accompanied by perineal discomfort if prostatitis is present. If the gland is enlarged and exquisitely tender, acute prostatitis is likely; however, the results of the examination in chronic prostatitis are not usually abnormal. Sexually active men who present with dysuria without urgency and increased frequency usually have a sexually transmitted urethritis rather than a traditional UTI. Both UTIs and urethritis may be complicated by epididymitis

Diagnosis

If a urethral discharge is present it should be examined grossly, Gram stained, and cultured. This will usually allow the distinction between *Chlamydia* and gonococcal urethritis. For those patients without urethral discharge urinalysis and quantitative urine culture are essential. A prostate examination should be performed. The urinalysis will show pyuria (i.e., ≥ eight white cells per high-power field). The urine culture will usually show greater than or equal to 100,000 colonies/mL of urine, but any level of bacteriuria in a clean-catch specimen from a man should be considered significant.

Treatment

Initial therapy for the adult man with his first UTI is usually empirical because clinical urgency requires treatment before results of culture and sensitivity testing are available. A fluoroquinolone should be chosen because of its broad activity against the Enterobacteriaceae and because of the high therapeutic-to-toxic ratio. Examples include ciprofloxacin (Cipro), 250 mg twice daily, ofloxacin (Floxin), 200 mg twice daily, and levofloxacin (Levaquin), 250 mg once a day. A 7-day course is suggested if a prostatic focus seems unlikely.

Acute Bacterial Prostatitis

For those individuals with acute bacterial prostatitis it is important to exclude *Staphylococcus aureus*, and this can be done with acceptable accuracy by the Gram stain of the urine. If gram-positive cocci in clusters are present, it is important for the clinician to review the possibility of systemic staphylococcal infection, including bacteremia and endocarditis. Consideration should be given to intravenous therapy in patients with staphylococcal prostatitis.

Treatment

For other patients with acute bacterial prostatitis a fluoroquinolone is recommended because members of this antimicrobial class achieve high prostatic fluid tissue levels. The fluoroquinolone chosen by the physician's hospital, medical group, or the patients' health plan is likely to be preferred because there is little to suggest that one over another offers substantial benefit. The same doses of fluoroquinolones can be given as for uncomplicated cystitis. If prostatitis is accompanied by bacteremia, then the doses should be doubled. Although the optimum duration of therapy is not well defined, a minimum of 14 days is suggested, and, if there is a reasonable probability of chronic prostatitis, at least 6 weeks of treatment is recommended.

Chronic Bacterial Prostatitis

Chronic prostatitis is a more subtle condition than acute prostatitis. Bacteria in the mildly inflamed prostate are difficult to eradicate, and the prostate can remain a persistent source of UTI. The prostatic focus can repeatedly infect the bladder. The infection is usually due to gram-negative aerobic bacilli. Occasionally, enterococcal species may play a role either alone or in co-infection with other uropathogens.

Diagnosis

In that subset of patients who have prostatitis without cystitis, the bladder urine may contain ambiguously low numbers of bacteria or may be, in fact, sterile. Prostatic fluid expressed by prostatic massage should be cultured from these individuals. Prostatic localization studies have been suggested. These procedures are time consuming, expensive, and uncomfortable for patients and are therefore infrequently performed by clinicians. A critical review of the evidence of the utility of these studies suggests that they are not justified except for clinical research.

Treatment

A utilitarian alternative is to presume that the prostate is infected and to prescribe a course of antibiotics to which the bacterium is susceptible on the basis of in vitro testing and which are also known to penetrate the prostate, such as a fluoroquinolone (see earlier for doses of selected drugs) or trimethoprim-sulfamethoxazole (Septra), one double-strength tablet twice daily.

Recurrent Urinary Tract Infections

In men, the occurrence of two or more UTIs in a 3-year period is used to define the clinical problem of recurrent UTIs, instead of 6 months that is usually used for infections in women. The association of chronic prostatitis as a source of recurrent UTIs is strong for both upper and lower urinary tract infections. If a man with recurrent UTIs is not found to have structural defects of the urinary tract, chronic bacterial prostatitis is almost always found.

Treatment

Treatment of recurrent UTI requires the use of a prostate-penetrating antimicrobial agent. Fluoroquinolones are ideal, and if the bacterium is susceptible by in vitro testing, trimethoprim-sulfamethoxazole may be substituted because the cost is a fraction of that for a fluoroquinolone. The best chance of cure is with 6 weeks of therapy.

If treatment for 6 weeks fails and if recurrences are frequent and severe, it may be appropriate to prescribe chronic suppressive therapy with low doses of daily antibiotics for which the bacterium is susceptible. In this case, it is not necessary to prescribe antibiotics that penetrate the prostate because the goal of therapy is simply to prevent the bladder urine from becoming symptomatically infected. For example, if the bacterium is susceptible to ampicillin, 250 mg once a day of this drug will usually be effective.

Abacterial Prostatitis

Abacterial prostatitis is far more common than chronic bacterial prostatitis. This has been referred to as prostatosis because an infectious etiology in most patients has defied definition.

Diagnosis

Patients have similar complaints to patients with chronic bacterial prostatitis; their physical examination is indistinguishable and they have pyuria. However, bacteria are not cultured from urine or prostatic fluid.

Treatment

There is no accepted approach to therapy. Most clinicians would give at least one course of therapy directed toward chlamydiae using either a tetracycline such as doxycycline or a fluoroquinolone for 2 weeks.

Prostatodynia

A group of patients who do not have bacteriuria or evidence of pyuria and no increased number of leukocytes in their prostatic secretions nevertheless present with increased frequency of urination and urgency. Results of the physical examination for the most part are normal. Antimicrobial therapy should not be instituted.

UPPER URINARY TRACT INFECTION

The approach to pyelonephritis in the healthy adult man does not differ from that in the adult woman.

BACTERIAL INFECTIONS OF THE URINARY TRACT IN WOMEN

method of
KALPANA GUPTA, M.D., M.P.H.
University of Washington
Seattle, Washington

EPIDEMIOLOGY

Urinary tract infections (UTIs) are among the most common bacterial infections in women and account for over 7 million outpatient visits and 1 billion health care dollars annually in the United States alone. At least 50% of women will experience a UTI some time during their lifetime, and up to 30% will have recurrent episodes of UTI. Most UTIs in women are uncomplicated and occur in the absence of an anatomic or predisposing reason for infection. Factors associated with an increased risk of UTI in otherwise healthy women include sexual activity, use of a diaphragm and spermicide or spermicide alone, pregnancy, history of UTI, advancing age, and estrogen deficiency.

PATHOPHYSIOLOGY

More than 95% of UTIs in women occur via the ascending route. Colonization of the vaginal introitus with bacteria from the fecal flora, usually *Escherichia coli*, is the critical initial step in the pathogenesis of UTI. Sexual intercourse and the use of a diaphragm with spermicide or a spermicide alone are strongly associated with an increased risk of *E. coli* vaginal colonization and bacteriuria, probably because of alterations in the normal vaginal microbial flora. With advancing age, estrogen deficiency (leading to changes in the vaginal microbial flora and a rise in pH), instrumentation, and incomplete bladder emptying are some of the factors associated with a higher incidence of UTI.

Increasing evidence indicates that genetic determinants such as secretor status and ABO blood group may influence the susceptibility to recurrent UTI, particularly in older women who do not have other UTI-related factors such as diaphragm-spermicide use or frequent sexual intercourse. Uroepithelial cells from women who are nonsecretors of blood group antigens demonstrate enhanced adherence of uropathogenic *E. coli* as compared with uroepithelial cells from secretors, and nonsecretor status has been epidemiologically associated with recurrent UTI in several studies. In addition, women with recurrent UTI are more likely to have had their first UTI before age 15 and to have a maternal history of UTI. Finally, many bacterial virulence determinants have been demonstrated to be important in the pathogenesis of UTI. P-fimbriated *E. coli*, in particular, has been associated with more severe forms of UTI such as bacteremic pyelonephritis in otherwise healthy hosts.

MICROBIOLOGY

A narrow and predictable spectrum of agents cause uncomplicated UTI in women: 80% to 90% of infections are due to *E. coli*, 5% to 15% are due to *Staphylococcus saprophyticus* (particularly in younger women), and a small percentage are caused by enterococci and non–*E. coli* aerobic gram-negative rods such as *Klebsiella* species and *Proteus mirabilis*. In complicated UTIs, *E. coli* is still the predominant pathogen, but other gram-negative bacilli, enterococci, and candidal species are also frequently found. Although the spectrum of etiologic agents has remained stable, the susceptibility patterns of these organisms have changed considerably in the past several years and need to be considered when choosing a therapeutic regimen.

MANAGEMENT OF URINARY TRACT INFECTION

Several clinical syndromes of UTI can be differentiated on the basis of the site of infection (bladder versus kidney) and the presence or absence of complicating conditions. Uncomplicated UTI is an infection of the bladder or kidney in an otherwise healthy person without any predisposing reason for infection. The vast majority of these infections occur in women, but it is now becoming increasingly apparent that young adult men can also have uncomplicated cystitis. If factors such as pregnancy, diabetes, other comorbid conditions, or anatomic or functional abnormalities of the genitourinary system are present, the UTI is considered complicated. Defining the UTI syndrome is an important first step in management because the choice of antimicrobial agent, dosage, and duration of therapy will depend on this assessment (Figure 1).

Acute Uncomplicated Cystitis

The typical symptoms of cystitis include a sudden onset of dysuria and urinary frequency and urgency. Occasionally, patients will complain of suprapubic discomfort or hematuria. A history of new or multiple sexual partners, vaginal discomfort or discharge, or indolent onset of symptoms warrants evaluation for alternative diagnoses such as urethritis from *Chlamydia trachomatis*, *Neisseria gonorrhoeae*, or herpes simplex virus or vaginitis from *Trichomonas vaginalis* or *Candida* species. In addition, if the patient has a history of back pain, fever, nausea, or vomiting in association with cystitis symptoms, a diagnosis of pyelonephritis should be considered.

Laboratory assessment of patients with acute cystitis includes evaluation for pyuria and bacteriuria. Pyuria can be measured with microscopy or a leukocyte esterase dipstick. The latter method is less sensitive for pyuria but more readily available in the office setting. In otherwise healthy women with pyuria and cystitis symptoms, it is safe and cost-effec-

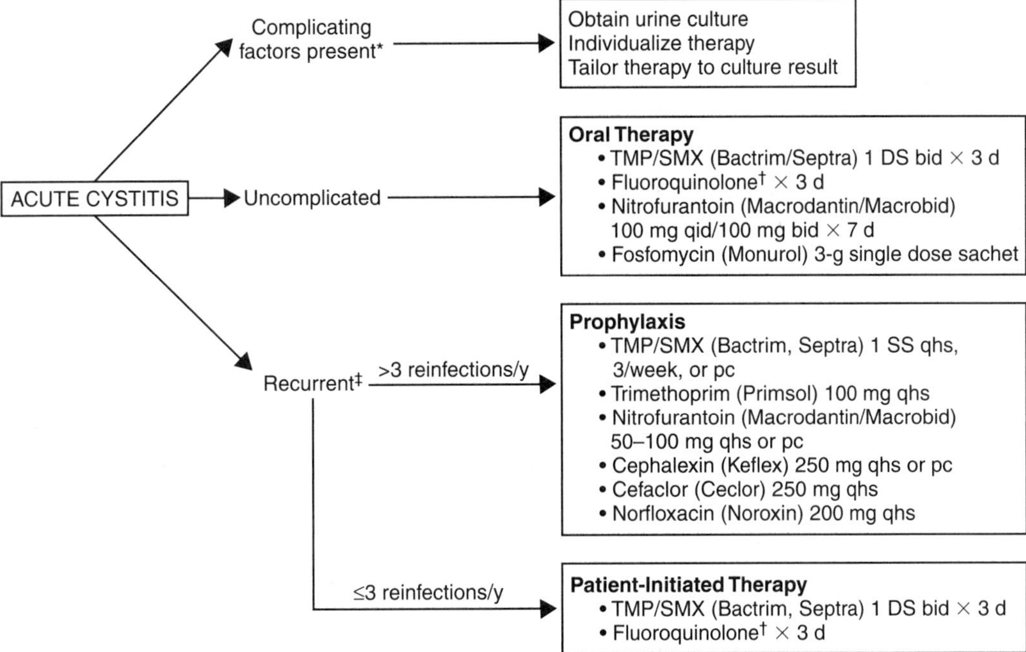

Figure 1. Management of women with acute cystitis. *See text for definitions and for management of pregnant patients. †Ofloxacin (Floxin) 200 mg twice a day, ciprofloxacin (Cipro) 250 mg twice a day, levofloxacin (Levaquin) 250 mg once a day, norfloxacin (Noroxin) 400 mg twice a day. ‡Assess modifiable risk factors first. *Abbreviations*: pc = postcoital; DS = double strength (160/800 mg); SS = single strength (80/400 mg); TMP/SMX = trimethoprim-sulfamethoxazole.

tive to omit the urine culture and initiate therapy empirically. However, if the diagnosis is in doubt or the patient has received multiple antibiotics in the past, urine culture and susceptibility testing are indicated to help confirm the diagnosis and optimize therapy. Traditionally, a urine culture was considered positive when 10^5 or more colony-forming units (cfu) per milliliter of a uropathogen were present. However, approximately one third of women with acute uncomplicated cystitis will have colony counts between 10^2 and 10^4 cfu/mL. Hence, a more sensitive threshold for significant bacteriuria in women with symptoms of cystitis is 10^2 cfu/mL or more of a uropathogen in a midstream urine specimen.

Several antimicrobial regimens are available for treatment of UTI (see Figure 1). Traditionally, trimethoprim-sulfamethoxazole (Bactrim) or trimethoprim (Primsol) alone has been recommended as the first-line agent for the treatment of acute uncomplicated cystitis in women. However, in communities in which resistance of uropathogens to trimethoprim-sulfamethoxazole approaches 20%, alternative agents should be considered. The fluoroquinolones are highly effective in this setting and have been shown to be cost-effective when used in a 3-day regimen. Nitrofurantoin is also effective against most uropathogens when used in a 7-day regimen. Fosfomycin (Monurol) is approved for use as a single-dose agent and should be considered when patient compliance is an issue. Avoid β-lactams due to lower efficacy rates and more side effects.

The duration of therapy depends on the antimicrobial used and associated factors. Single-dose therapy is effective in most women with uncomplicated cystitis but is associated with higher relapse rates, probably because of failure to eradicate the uropathogen from the vaginal reservoir. Three days is the optimal duration of therapy when trimethoprim-sulfamethoxazole or fluoroquinolones are used because efficacy is maximized while side effects and cost are minimized. Seven days of therapy should be considered when nitrofurantoin is used or in women with a history of recent UTI, symptoms of more than 7 days' duration, or diabetes. Follow-up urine cultures are not indicated unless the patient has persistent symptoms. If the patient is still symptomatic after completion of therapy and has a susceptible uropathogen identified on urine culture, a 14-day course of therapy should be given for the possibility of occult pyelonephritis.

Recurrent Cystitis

Recurrent episodes of cystitis in otherwise healthy women are common and can be classified as re-infections or relapses. In re-infection, a patient clinically improves after therapy and then has another UTI caused either by the same organism or by a different organism several weeks or months later. A relapse is clinically defined as recurrence of a UTI within 2 weeks with an organism of the same species and susceptibility pattern as the original causative organism and is suggestive of a nidus of persistent infection. Relapses require a longer duration of therapy and consideration of urologic evaluation. Most recurrent UTIs are uncomplicated re-infections and are generally caused by the same spectrum of organisms that cause sporadic UTIs. Thus, the antimicrobial regimens that are used for treatment of sporadic infections can generally be used to treat recurrent episodes.

Strategies for management of recurrent UTI include antimicrobial prophylaxis or patient-initiated therapy (see Figure 1). Before the initiation of any of these strategies, modifiable risk factors such as diaphragm-spermicide use or estrogen deficiency should be addressed. Antimicrobial prophylaxis can be given postcoitally, three times weekly, or daily, depending on whether the patient can temporally relate UTI occurrences to sexual intercourse. Typically, prophylaxis is used for a 6-month period. If the frequency of recurrences returns to the preprophylaxis pattern, a longer duration of prophylaxis can be given. Low-dose prophylaxis has been shown to be highly effective and safe, even over 5 years of use. In women with infrequent recurrences, patient-initiated therapy should be considered. The patient is provided with a 3-day course of an effective antibiotic by her physician and instructed to initiate therapy if symptoms of a UTI develop. She needs to see her provider only if her symptoms do not resolve with therapy or if the diagnosis is in doubt. This approach has many potential advantages for women who have few UTI recurrences, such as decreased antimicrobial use, improved patient convenience, and reduced overall cost.

Acute Uncomplicated Pyelonephritis

Patients with pyelonephritis most often have fever and flank pain. Symptoms of cystitis, nausea, vomiting, or sepsis may also be present. Urinalysis and urine culture almost always reveal pyuria and 10^4 cfu/mL or more of a uropathogen. The infecting pathogens are still usually *E. coli*, but other gram-negative rods and enterococci are also often isolated. Blood cultures should be performed if the patient is sick enough to be hospitalized because they are positive in 20% to 30% of these cases.

Pyelonephritis can be initially managed with oral outpatient therapy or with parenteral inpatient therapy, depending on the severity of the illness and comorbid conditions of the patient (Figure 2). Outpatient therapy for pyelonephritis should be used for patients with mild disease who are otherwise healthy and do not have significant nausea or vomiting. In this setting, oral trimethoprim-sulfamethoxazole or a fluoroquinolone has been shown to be highly effective for susceptible uropathogens. In areas with a high rate of trimethoprim-sulfamethoxazole resistance, fluoroquinolones are preferred. Amoxicillin-clavulanate (Augmentin) should be considered if the Gram stain suggests enterococci. The traditional length of therapy with most antimicrobials has been 14 days. However, based on the findings of a recent randomized trial, a 7-day course can be considered when using a fluoroquinolone. In patients who need additional observation before deciding about the best route of therapy, an initial intravenous dose of a fluoroquinolone or an extended-spectrum β-lactam can be given before initiating the oral regimen. Patients who are very ill or unable to take oral medications or in whom complicating conditions are suspected should be hospitalized for parenteral therapy. Various regimens can be used, including a fluoroquinolone, an aminoglycoside with ampicillin, or an extended-spectrum cephalosporin with or without an aminoglycoside (see Figure 2). Ampicillin-sulbactam with or without an aminoglycoside should be considered if enterococci are suspected. Therapy should be modified once the infecting organism and its susceptibility pattern are known. Oral therapy can be used

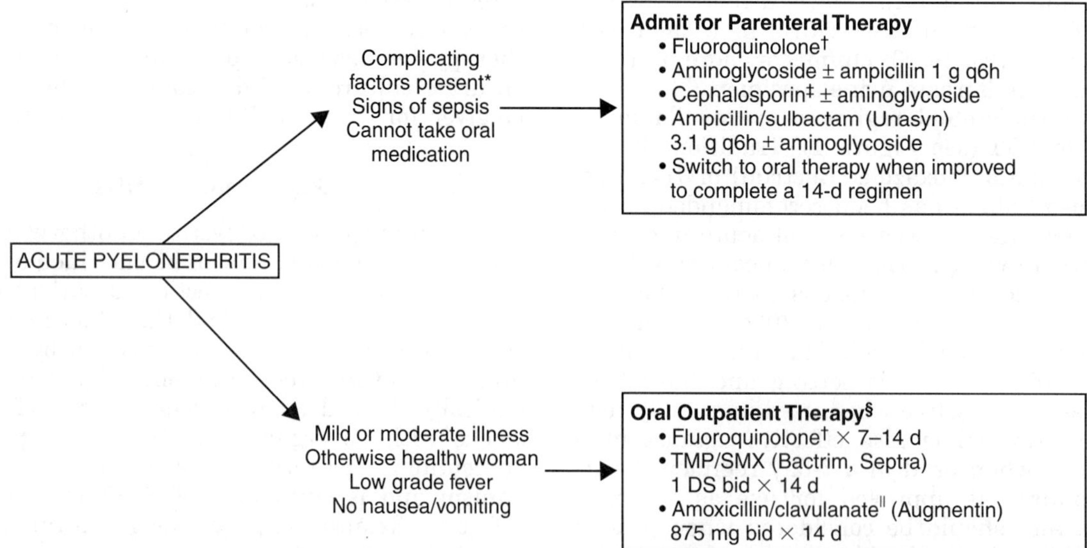

Figure 2. Management of women with acute pyelonephritis. *See text for definitions and for management of pregnant patients. †Ofloxacin (Floxin) 200 mg twice a day, ciprofloxacin (Cipro) 250 mg twice a day, levofloxacin (Levaquin) 250 mg once a day, norfloxacin (Noroxin) 400 mg twice a day. ‡Ceftriaxone (Rocephin) 1–2 g every 12 hours or ceftazidime (Fortaz) 1–2 g every 8 hours. §Consider an initial parenteral dose of antibiotic in more ill patients. ‖If enterococci are suspected. *Abbreviation*: TMP/SMX = trimethoprim-sulfamethoxazole.

to complete the 14-day course when the patient has improved.

Urinary Tract Infection in Pregnancy

UTI in pregnancy merits special consideration because even asymptomatic cases need to be identified and treated, therapeutic regimens are limited, and close follow-up is warranted. The incidence of asymptomatic bacteriuria in pregnant women is 4% to 10%. If left untreated, asymptomatic bacteriuria is associated with symptomatic UTI in 20% to 40% of cases. Conversely, women who do not have asymptomatic bacteriuria in early pregnancy have only a 1% to 2% chance of symptomatic UTI later in pregnancy. Symptomatic UTIs in pregnancy are associated with an increased risk of premature birth and other perinatal complications in the mother and fetus. Thus, screening for asymptomatic bacteriuria in the 16th week of gestation is routinely performed. If detected, a 3- to 7-day course of an antimicrobial is prescribed. Importantly, a follow-up urine culture should be performed approximately 1 week after completion of therapy because persistence of asymptomatic bacteriuria is associated with an increased risk of symptomatic UTI. If asymptomatic bacteriuria is still present, a 7- to 10-day course of antimicrobial therapy is indicated. Continued persistence of asymptomatic bacteriuria should be managed with suppressive antibiotics until delivery.

Nitrofurantoin (Macrobid), ampicillin (Omnipen), and cephalexin (Keflex) are safe and effective for treatment of UTI in pregnancy. Sulfonamides can also be used but should be avoided near term because of a risk of hyperbilirubinemia. Symptomatic cystitis should be treated for 7 to 10 days because shorter courses are associated with high failure rates. Pregnant women with pyelonephritis should be admitted to the hospital for parenteral therapy. The antimicrobial regimen should be tailored once susceptibility data are available.

Complicated Urinary Tract Infection

Complicated urinary tract infections encompass a heterogeneous group of patients with a wide variety of structural and functional abnormalities of the urinary tract or with co-morbid conditions. The microbiology of complicated infections is variable and depends on the specific host and complicating factors. Thus, although *E. coli* is still a common uropathogen, other aerobic gram-negative rods such as *Klebsiella*, *Proteus*, *Pseudomonas*, and *Serratia* species are not uncommon. Additionally, enterococci, *Staphylococcus aureus*, and even *Candida* species can be isolated. Therefore, all patients with complicated UTI need culture and susceptibility testing. Therapy is usually begun empirically with a broad-spectrum agent and then tailored appropriately once susceptibility data are available.

Catheter-Associated Urinary Tract Infection

Catheter-associated UTIs are among the most common of nosocomial infections. Placement of a bladder catheter is associated with a daily incidence of bacteriuria of 3% to 10%, and approximately 15% of nosocomial bacteremias are related to nosocomial UTI. Risk factors for catheter-associated UTI include the duration of catheterization, female sex, and the type of catheter being used (intermittent catheterization and condom catheters may result in a lower incidence of UTI). Thus, the best preventive strategy is to remove the catheter as soon as possible. Other maneuvers important for prevention of UTI include aseptic insertion and maintenance of a closed urinary system. Systemic antimicrobials or coating of the catheter with antibacterial substances such as silver alloy or nitrofurantoin may prevent or delay the onset of bacteriuria, but they also result in an increased rate of resistant organisms and increased cost and are therefore not routinely recommended as prevention strategies. Most patients with catheter-associated bacteriuria are asymptomatic and do not need treatment except in special settings. If a catheterized patient has symptoms of infection, pyuria, and a positive urine culture, removal of the catheter and administration of antibiotic therapy should be instituted. Colony counts of 10^2 cfu/mL or greater are considered indications for treatment because studies have shown that colony counts will increase within a few days if the catheter is left in place.

Asymptomatic Bacteriuria

Isolation of 10^5 cfu/mL or more of a uropathogen in two consecutive urine cultures in the absence of pyuria or symptoms referable to the urinary tract is the criterion traditionally used to define asymptomatic bacteriuria. It is commonly found in the elderly, as well as catheterized patients. In general, asymptomatic bacteriuria does not require therapy. However, if it is detected in pregnant women or in patients with neutropenia, or preceding urogynecologic surgery or renal transplantation, therapy is warranted. Asymptomatic bacteriuria in a patient who is scheduled for instrumentation of the urinary tract should also be treated.

Prevention of Urinary Tract Infection

The development of prevention strategies, specifically non–antibiotic-based ones, is an important area of current research. First, patients should be educated about modifiable behaviors that may decrease the risk of UTI, such as voiding immediately after sexual intercourse and using a non–spermicide-based method of contraception. Ingestion of cranberry juice has been shown to be effective in decreasing both bacteriuria and pyuria in an elderly population, but its efficacy in younger women and in preventing symptomatic UTI remains to be demonstrated. The use of a lactobacillus probiotic to restore normal vaginal flora and the use of antiadhesin vaccines to prevent UTI are newer strategies currently under investigation.

BACTERIAL INFECTIONS OF THE URINARY TRACT IN GIRLS

method of
PATRICK H. McKENNA, M.D.,
Southern Illinois University School of Medicine
Springfield, Illinois

and

MARVALYN DeCAMBRE, M.D.
Connecticut Children's Medical Center
Hartford, Connecticut

Urinary tract infections (UTIs) in girls occur with different frequency at different ages, and management and evaluation of their infections are dependent on the severity of infection and their age. Repeated pyelonephritis may result in renal scarring and the early development of hypertension. Pyelonephritis is more common when associated urinary anatomic abnormalities are present. Recurrent cystitis without pyelonephritis is seldom associated with renal injury, although the recurring symptoms are bothersome. Some girls have asymptomatic infections, but they should still be evaluated. Evaluation should occur after one documented UTI, and management should be directed at preventing further infections.

EPIDEMIOLOGY

During the first year of life, the incidence of UTIs in girls is considerably less than in their male counterparts. Many authors have attributed this difference to fecal contamination of the preputial skin in uncircumcised males and differences in bladder neck development that may predispose males to poor bladder emptying in the neonatal period. After 1 year of age, the incidence of UTIs in females exceeds that of their male counterparts. After age 5 the incidence of UTIs in females versus males is 9:1. No clear-cut rationale can be found for the increased incidence in females as compared with males after age 1; however, we believe that pelvic floor dysfunction and a shorter urethra in females account for these differences.

ETIOLOGY

Periurethral contamination by fecal flora with urethral retrograde migration of bacteria appears to be the major mechanism of UTI (Table 1). Stasis of fecal material in the rectal vault or sigmoid and stasis of urine in the bladder, ureter, or renal pelvis secondary to anatomic or functional obstruction provide a prime environment for bacterial overgrowth. Virulent strains of bacteria can multiply. Additionally, in the first several months of life, the bladder mucosa is not yet mature and IgA appears less prominent, which may help explain why the uroepithelium is more susceptible to adherence of virulent organisms. Gram-negative organisms such as *Klebsiella*, *Enterobacter*, and *Proteus* and gram-positive organisms such as *Enterococcus* and *Staphylococcus saprophyticus* are common bowel flora responsible for UTIs. However, *Escherichia coli* is the primary bacterial organism responsible for the pathology associated with most UTIs in girls. Pili fimbriae (p-fimbriae) that attach to bladder uroepithelium in cystitis and to the renal parenchyma in pyelonephritis have been identified in virulent *E. coli* strains. In girls, periurethral adherence of a class III p-fimbriae *E. coli* has been identified as the major mechanism of UTIs. *E. coli* comes from fecal flora and is more likely to translocate to the introitus when constipation and encopresis are present in a female child.

TABLE 1. **Factors That Predispose to Urinary Tract Infections**

Bacterial Factors	Host Factors
P-fimbriae (pili) for adherence	Constipation
Rigid cell wall resistance to urine osmolality	Voiding dysfunction
Rapid doubling time	Urinary anatomic abnormalities
Ability to colonize the lower intestinal tract	P1 blood group
Adherence to urothelium	Receptor density on urothelium
Cell wall porins to prevent lysis	Defective bladder mucosal immune protection
Capsular antigen to prevent phagocytosis	Insufficient urinary IgA
Elaboration of hemolysin injuries to urothelium	Lack of breast-feeding
Aerobactin to accumulate Fe for growth	Uropathogen receptors in colonic mucosa
	Eradication of vaginal flora by medications
	Blood group type (Lewis, ABH)

DIAGNOSIS

Accurate diagnosis of UTIs often requires a high level of suspicion, especially in neonatal and asymptomatic patients.

Signs and Symptoms

In neonates and infants, a fever may be the first sign of a UTI; however, nonspecific signs and symptoms should be identified and may lead one to suspect a UTI. Nonspecific signs and symptoms may include poor feeding, emesis, irritability, or lethargy. Toddlers and school-aged children may be able to verbally identify specific symptoms such as dysuria or point to the suprapubic area as the source of discomfort during voiding.

History and Physical Examination

Management of children with recurrent UTIs should begin with a thorough history including assessment of bladder and bowel history, and then proceed to physical examination. The caregiver may identify specific abnormalities, such as "holding" maneuvers consisting of squatting, curtsying, and sitting on their heels. They may notice urge incontinence (leaking of urine or stool before the child makes it to the bathroom). They may also identify foul-smelling, cloudy urine or gross hematuria. These patients often have diurnal incontinence. Such examples are clues to the diagnosis of a possible UTI. In the office, the physician can identify irritation of the external genitalia and/or perirectal area. They may identify labial adhesions or even palpate stool in the rectal vault or lower part of the abdomen. Close inspection of the base of the spine is important in children with UTIs and incontinence because a rare sacral abnormality may be identified.

Urine Dipstick, Urinalysis, and Culture

A urine dipstick is not a reliable test for the diagnosis of UTI when used in isolation. It is most sensitive when evaluating for leukocyte esterase (a measure of the presence of leukocytes) or positive nitrites (a measure of the presence of bacteria). A urine dipstick can be falsely positive; therefore, pyuria and/or bacteriuria should be confirmed by urinalysis and then by culture if infection is suspected. A positive culture with a single organism and more than 100,000 colonies is greater than 80% accurate in the diagnosis of UTI. Accurate urine samples in children should be obtained by suprapubic aspiration or transurethral catheterization in young patients who are not potty trained because the likelihood of contamination is greatest with a clean-catch specimen. Urine cultures should never be obtained from a Foley catheter bag or ostomy bagged specimen, for these specimens are normally contaminated. In older children, presumably toilet trained, a properly collected midstream specimen is also accurate.

Radiologic Imaging

In girls younger than 6 years who have a documented UTI, we begin our evaluation with a renal/bladder ultrasound and a voiding cystourethrogram (VCUG) (Figure 1). These studies are indicated because: (1) 35% to 40% of children younger than 4 years with a UTI have vesicoureteral reflux, including those who have asymptomatic bacteriuria; (2) a renal scar will develop in 10% of children after their first episode of a febrile UTI; (3) 90% will have a second UTI within the following 3 years after the first infection, so waiting for a second infection does not make sense; (4) ultrasound alone will miss most of the girls with reflux because the majority have low-grade reflux. In older girls who have infections and incontinence, we do the same initial screening studies. If the patient is older than 6 years and does not have incontinence, a VCUG is obtained only if the girl has evidence of pyelonephritis.

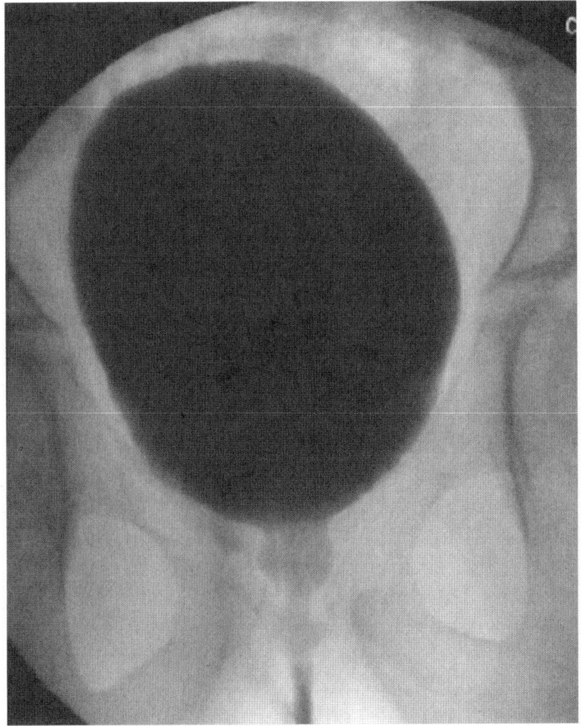

Figure 1. Voiding cystourethrogram. Spinning top deformity seen with dysfunctional voiding.

In girls, the combination of dysfunctional voiding, constipation, and vesicoureteral reflux are commonly associated with UTI. A kidney-ureter-bladder radiograph (KUB) obtained with a VCUG may often identify constipation. Girls younger than 10 years have a higher incidence of complicated UTIs in the form of pyelonephritis than the adult female population does. By age 10, however, most children with vesicoureteral reflux have been treated or have outgrown the reflux. Therefore, it is not always necessary to obtain a VCUG in this population.

The history, physical examination, and findings from the initial screening studies determine other radiologic imaging that may be required. Spinal magnetic resonance imaging is recommended if the history, physical examination, or KUB suggests a high likelihood of a spinal abnormality. If the patient has had multiple febrile UTIs or the ultrasound suggests renal scarring, a dimercaptosuccinic acid (DMSA) renal scan may be indicated. If the screening ultrasound reveals hydronephrosis or hydroureteronephrosis, a ^{99m}Tc-diethylenetriamine pentaacetic acid (DTPA) furosemide (Lasix) washout renal scan, an intravenous pyelogram, or a ^{99m}Tc-mercaptoacetyl triglycine (MAG-3) Lasix washout renal scan may be indicated.

MANAGEMENT

Management of UTIs in girls should concentrate on excluding anatomic abnormalities, followed by individual management based on age and the underlying pathology (Figure 2). In all cases, concentrating on preventing further infection should be the strategy. We use an escalating or stepwise treatment plan. Most organisms involved in UTIs are from the fecal flora. Many girls with recurrent infections have constipation, stasis of urine, and voiding dysfunction. The first step at our initial encounter is to initiate a four-point medical program: (1) correcting constipation, (2) improving voiding, (3) increasing fluid intake, and (4) improving hygiene. *Correcting constipation* is also a stepwise procedure. Initially, we recommend a high-fiber diet with maintenance of a diary to confirm daily bowel movements (twice daily in infants), followed by fiber supplements and bowel stimulants, if necessary (Table 2). Normal transit time from mouth to rectum increases from 8 hours in the first month of life to 16 hours by age 2 and 26 hours by age 10. Effective management of constipation has been demonstrated to significantly reduce the incidence of UTIs and improve voiding patterns in patients with dysfunctional voiding. *Improving voiding* initially includes frequent bladder emptying. We recommend timed voiding every 2 to 3 hours in a toilet-trained child. We also work on improving the flow of urine. Patients are trained to void with a continuous rather than a staccato voiding pattern. We encourage motivated families to engage the affected child in voiding tricks as a treatment addendum. One example in our practice entails placing Cheerios in the toilet bowl and having the girl void

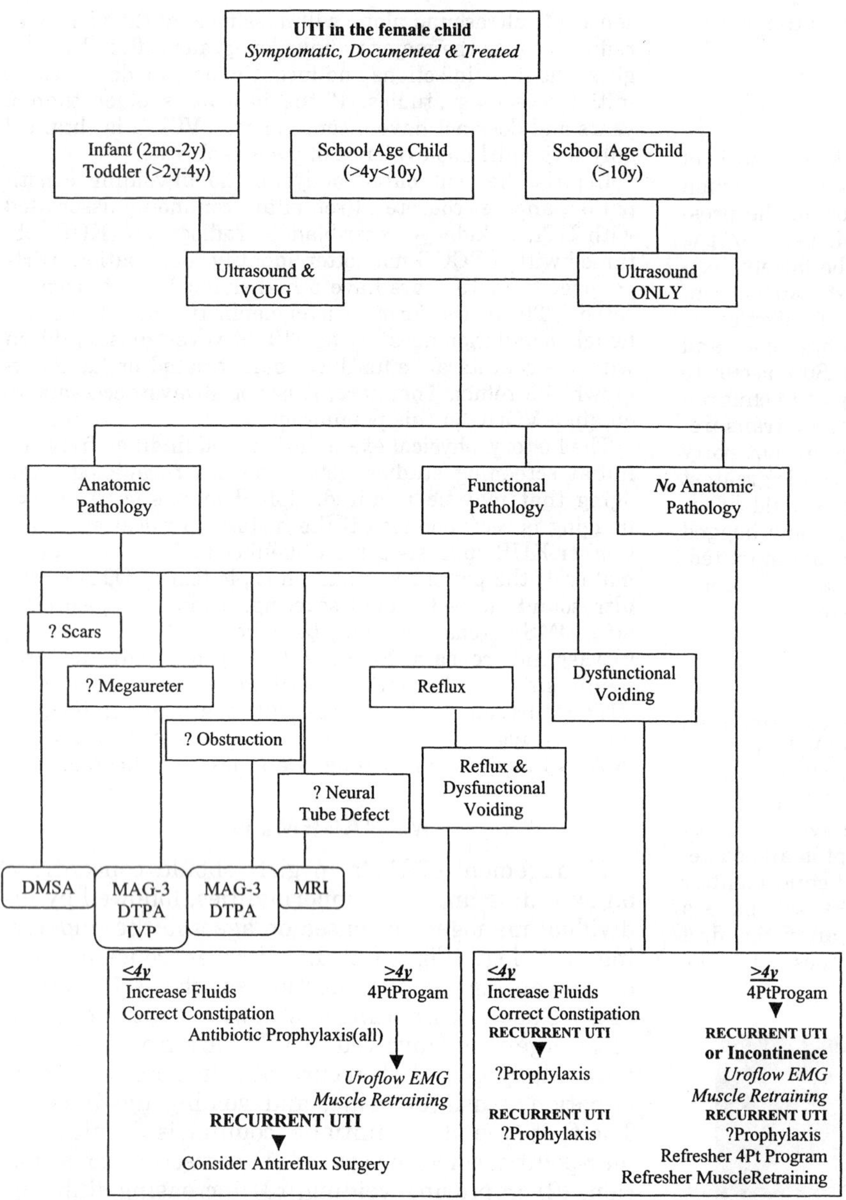

Figure 2. Evaluation of urinary tract infections in girls. *Abbreviations:* DMSA = dimercaptosuccinic acid (succimer); DTPA = diethylenetriamine pentaacetic acid; EMG = electromyography; IVP = intravenous pyelography; MAG-3 = ^{99m}Tc-mercaptoacetyl triglycine; MRI = magnetic resonance imaging; UTI = urinary tract infection; VCUG = voiding cystourethrography.

while sitting backward facing the toilet bowl cover and aiming to sink the Cheerios during voiding. *Increasing fluid intake* during the day not only improves gastrointestinal motility and softens the stool but also flushes the urinary tract, theoretically eliminating virulent bacteria and their endotoxins. We encourage *hygiene awareness and improvement*, where necessary, to ensure that the child wipes from front to back after stooling. Children should also avoid bubble baths because prolonged bathing may change the bacterial flora of the introitus. In infants, improving hygiene includes frequent changes of soiled diapers/underwear and wiping stool *away from* rather than toward the urethra, or the "front-to-back" method.

Antibiotic Prophylaxis and Treatment

In the belief that the underlying pathogenesis of recurrent infections is periurethral colonization with uropathogens, children have traditionally been thought to be biologically prone to the development of infection and subsequently managed primarily with prophylactic antibiotics (Table 3). The antimicrobial drug of choice for treatment or prophylaxis should be effective against *E. coli* because it is the most common organism associated with UTIs. Nitrofurantoin (Macrodantin) or trimethoprim-sulfamethoxazole (Bactrim) are good first-line antibiotics. Macrodantin and Bactrim/Septra are equally effective and do not adversely alter bowel flora. Bactrim has a unique advantage in that it decreases vaginal colonization. The better the bowel management, the less likely that resistant bacteria will develop because bacterial colony counts increase when stool is retained. Prophylaxis in children younger than 1 month is different because of delayed liver development, and in this case, amoxicillin is the drug of choice. If a UTI develops while the patient is receiving prophylaxis

TABLE 2. **Management of Constipation**

Method	Product
Oral/nasogastric	
Diet	Barley cereal/oatmeal/prunes (softeners)
Fiber	Cellulose (Citrocel), psyllium (Metamucil/Fiberall), polycarbophil (FiberCon/Konsyl Fiber)
Hyperosmolar	Fructose (prunes)/sorbitol/lactulose
Lubricant	Mineral oil
Stimulants	Salts (milk of magnesia/magnesium citrate)
	Senna (Senokot)
	Diphenylmethane (bisacodyl/Dulcolax)
	Prokinetic (cisapride [Propulsid], metoclopramide [Reglan])
Per rectum	
Lubricant	Mineral oil (Agoral/Kondremul)
	Surfactant (docusate [Colace])
	Hypertonic phosphate (Fleet Soap Suds Enema)
Stimulant	Bisacodyl (Dulcolax)
Surgical: antegrade continence enema	Reserved for severe refractory constipation
	Note: Phenolphthalein should not be used in children
Summary of Management of Constipation in Children	
Infant	Fiber + softeners (barley cereal/prune juice/lactulose)
Toddlers	Fiber + softeners +/− moderate- to high-dose stimulant
Children (school age; >4 y)	Fiber + softeners + moderate stimulant + muscle retraining

and the bacteria are sensitive to the prophylaxis, after the treatment has been completed, the prophylactic dosage should be increased. If the bacteria are resistant to prophylaxis, after the infection has been treated, the prophylactic dosage should be lowered. Hospital treatment of febrile UTIs is primarily with third-generation cephalosporin unless a complicated UTI is suspected, in which case a combination of ampicillin and gentamicin is initially indicated. The ultimate choice of antibiotic should be determined by culture sensitivities.

Children with a history of isolated UTI and no demonstrable anatomic abnormality after upper and lower urinary tract imaging studies may not require further treatment. Children with recurrent symptomatic UTIs and no anatomic abnormality should follow the four-point program and consider pelvic floor muscle retraining if associated voiding dysfunction or constipation is noted. If recurrent infections (more than four per year) occur despite this approach, patients may benefit from long-term antimicrobial prophylaxis. In a child in whom vesicoureteral reflux is not detected by standard VCUG but who continues to have symptoms of pyelonephritis, use of a nuclear VCUG may be contemplated because evidence suggests that this study is more sensitive than fluoroscopic VCUG in detecting vesicoureteral reflux.

Uroflow Electromyogram and Postvoid Residuals

Many female patients with UTIs have voiding dysfunction with or without vesicoureteral reflux. These females are almost always neurologically normal. Urodynamics has been recommended in the past for these patients, but this invasive study is probably only seldom necessary. We approach these patients conservatively and perform a noninvasive uroflow with simultaneous surface electromyography and check their postvoid residual with ultrasound (Figure 3). This approach can identify children with pelvic floor dysfunction. The most common pattern is increased pelvic floor muscle activity during voiding, with or without a small bladder capacity. Often, a large postvoid residual is present. By using this information and combining the four-point medical program with muscle retraining via computer games that are controlled by the pelvic floor, we have successfully cured pelvic floor dysfunction, incontinence, and constipation. Recurrent infections after this approach are rare.

Vesicoureteral Reflux and Urinary Tract Infections

The most common indication for surgical correction of vesicoureteral reflux in girls is a breakthrough UTI. The majority of girls with reflux and break-

TABLE 3. **Summary of Recommendations for Antimicrobial Therapy**

Drug*	Treatment Dosage	Daily Prophylaxis Dosage†
Nitrofurantoin (Macrodantin) (>1 mo)	5–7 mg/kg/d q6h	1–2 mg/kg/d (not with G6PD deficiency/toxic/febrile)
Trimethoprim-sulfamethoxazole (Septra)	8–10 mg/kg/d q12h	2–3 mg/kg/d (trimethoprim) (>2 mo)
Amoxicillin (Amoxil) (<1 mo)	20–40 mg/kg/d q8h	25 mg/kg/d q12h
Cephalexin (Keflex) (<2 mo)	25–100 mg/kg/d q6h	
Ceftriaxone (Rocephin) (IV)	75 mg/kg/d q24h	
Ampicillin (IV)	100 mg/kg/d q6h	
Gentamicin (Garamycin) (IV)	7.5 mg/kg/d q8h	
Tobramycin (Nebcin) (IV) instead of gentamicin	5 mg/kg/d q8h	

*Seven- to 10-day course for treatment and then consider long-term prophylaxis.
†*Note:* Follow-up culture should be performed 1 to 2 weeks after cessation of antibiotics.
Abbreviation: G6PD = glucose-6-phosphate dehydrogenase.

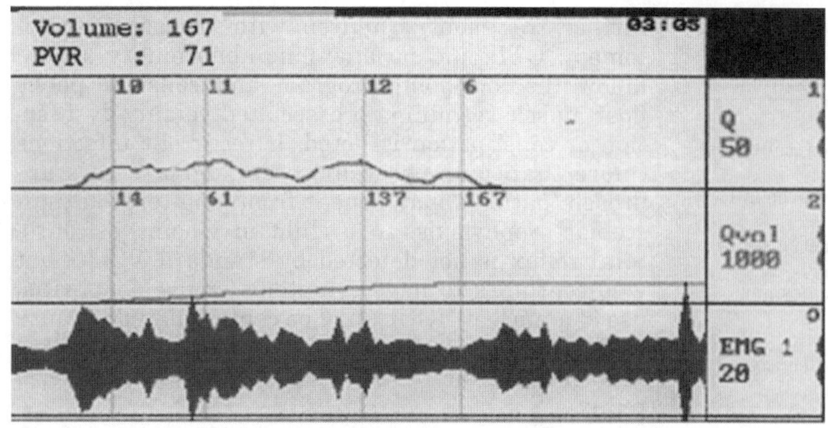

Figure 3. Uroflow electromyogram. Staccato-pattern high postvoid residual.

through infection have voiding dysfunction. Most girls who have surgery for reflux have voiding dysfunction, and girls with reflux and subsequent renal scars have often had breakthrough infection and voiding dysfunction. The best approach with these children is to prevent a breakthrough UTI. We have accomplished this goal by treating the voiding dysfunction with our four-point medical program and muscle retraining. In a small number of patients with limited bladder capacity and low postvoid residuals, the addition of an anticholinergic is occasionally helpful. Anticholinergic medication, however, predisposes to constipation, which is a risk factor for recurrent UTIs. Therefore, it should not be the first line of treatment in girls with UTIs and voiding dysfunction. We believe that dysfunctional voiding can be unlearned through pelvic floor muscle retraining, which can also improve constipation. The computer video games that we have developed have been effective in keeping children interested in the standard muscle-retraining techniques that the program provides. Our program has resulted in a significant decrease in breakthrough infections and a dramatic decrease in the need for antireflux surgery in our patient population.

The objective in the treatment of children with UTIs is to identify those with treatable anatomic abnormalities that may predispose to renal injury and the early development of hypertension, which is why screening studies should be obtained after the first documented UTI. The next objective is to prevent recurrent infections and concentrate on the underlying cause of the infection in girls. We believe that the main cause of infection is a combination of constipation, voiding dysfunction, and poor hygiene techniques. Attention to UTIs in girls, including prompt diagnosis, antibiotic therapy, radiologic evaluation, and implementation of a conservative medical program, including the four-point medical program and pelvic floor muscle retraining, prevents and decreases the associated risks of upper tract injury. This methodology decreases the need for long-term prophylactic antibiotics, anticholinergic medication, and surgical intervention for vesicoureteral reflux.

CHILDHOOD ENURESIS

method of
STEVEN J. SKOOG, M.D.
Doernbecher Children's Hospital, Oregon Health Sciences University
Portland, Oregon

Children with inappropriate wetting and voiding habits are common, constituting 20% to 25% of new patients seen in the pediatric urology office setting. A myriad of structural, neurogenic, and functional disorders can result in enuresis. However, the majority of these children will have functional abnormalities without overt neuropathic or anatomic disease. A thorough history and physical examination and an understanding of the normal development of urinary control direct the evaluation of these children. In the absence of associated urinary infection, invasive or complex procedures or radiologic imaging are rarely necessary. The focus of this discussion is on the healthy child who presents with enuresis after an age by which toilet training should have been accomplished.

ACQUISITION OF BLADDER CONTROL

The neurophysiologic mechanisms resulting in continence are complex. These processes result in various observed developmental stages of urinary control. In newborns, micturition is a reflex occurring 20 or more times per day. Bladder filling to an appropriate degree stimulates the efferent response of emptying with detrusor contraction preceded by relaxation of the sphincteric mechanism with complete bladder emptying. By 6 months of age, a noticeable increase in voided volume and decrease of urinary frequency is seen. This is attributed to unconscious inhibition of the voiding reflex. Between 1 and 2 years of age, the child develops a conscious sensation of bladder fullness, which sets the stage for voluntary control of voiding. Volitional voiding and inhibition of voiding at any degree of bladder fullness develops in the second and third years of life. By the age of 4 or 5 years, most children have developed an adult pattern of urinary control. The usual sequence of attainment of bowel and bladder control is as follows:

1. Nocturnal bowel control
2. Daytime bowel control
3. Daytime urinary control
4. Nocturnal urinary control

Children between 3 and 12 years of age void five to six times per day and have a bowel movement each day. Normal voided volume is more difficult to define, but bladder capacity can be approximated by the following formula:

$$\text{Age (years)} + 2 = \text{Volume (ounces)}$$

Comparisons of expected bladder capacity to measured bladder volumes provide insight into voiding dysfunction patterns and treatment.

Involuntary voiding beyond the age of anticipated control is the definition of enuresis. Diurnal enuresis is daytime wetting and nocturnal enuresis is nighttime wetting. Primary enuresis implies no interval of dryness, whereas secondary enuresis implies a 3- to 6-month dry interval. Twenty percent of wet children have diurnal enuresis and secondary enuresis comprises 25% of all wet children, but their evaluation, treatment, and response to therapy are no different from those of primary enuresis.

EVALUATION

The patient's history and the voiding log are the mainstays in separating patients with functional enuresis from those with anatomic and neurogenic incontinence. Most parents have poor knowledge of the specifics of their child's bowel and voiding habits. Sending a voiding log to keep for a few days before an appointment will clarify the frequency of voids and bowel accidents and the degree of wetness.

Continuous wetness between normal voiding episodes is a classic history in the girl patient with an ectopic ureter. Continuous wetness without voiding is seen in patients with neurogenic bladders and in patients with epispadias.

Children with episodic wetness are questioned regarding frequency of voiding, urgency, and posturing. Leg crossing, squirming, and heel sitting (Vincent's curtsy) are used to suppress the urgency associated with uninhibited bladder contractions. A small spot on the underwear immediately after voiding in girls may signal pseudoincontinence due to vaginal voiding. Boys also experience pseudoincontinence with urine trapped in the bulbar urethra and prepuce. Infrequent voiders will not usually empty their bladders upon awakening. The quality of the voiding effort should be reviewed. A dribbling urination may signify obstruction, a staccato character implies intermittent contraction of the external sphincter, and the use of Valsalva may suggest overflow incontinence or detrusor decompensation.

Other historical features important to note are the birth history, other conditions such as imperforate anus, vesicoureteral reflux, neurologic disease, and duplication anomalies. A history of a normal prenatal ultrasound suggests structural integrity of the urinary tract. A history of urinary tract infection and of constipation are important considerations in the treatment program.

How the family has dealt with their child's wetting and their immediate and future concerns will help guide subsequent treatment. A family history of nocturnal enuresis in the parent and knowledge of when the parent stopped wetting the bed assist in predicting the child's outcome with nocturnal enuresis.

PHYSICAL EXAMINATION

The physical examination is usually normal. However, abdominal examination and assessment of a palpable bladder, flank masses, or stool will help typify the elimination dysfunction. Careful examination of the spine for signs of occult spinal dysraphism includes inspecting for cutaneous lesions, dimples, lipomas, hairy tufts, and asymmetry of the gluteal cleft. Anal sphincter tone and anal wink are assessed. The gait is observed with testing of lower extremity reflexes. A high arched foot or slight leg length discrepancy is a significant sign of a tethered spinal cord. The external genitalia are inspected for epispadias, bifid clitoris, ectopic ureters, labial adhesions, and interlabial masses such as a ureterocele.

A urinalysis and urine culture are performed. If infection is present, it is treated with appropriate antibiotics. If no infection is present and the child is more than 5 years old with daytime wetting, a screening renal bladder ultrasound with prevoid and postvoid bladder assessment is performed. This will assess volitional voiding efficiency, residual urine, and the integrity of the upper urinary tract. A voiding cystourethrogram (VCUG) is performed on those children with a history of urinary tract infection and daytime incontinence. A kidneys-ureters-bladder (KUB) radiograph as part of the VCUG detects vertebral abnormalities and constipation. The VCUG rules out vesicoureteral reflux and urethral abnormalities.

If a spinal abnormality is detected, a neurologic origin is suspected, or the VCUG depicts an abnormal bladder, then formal urodynamics are performed. The results of urodynamics may confirm a neurologic origin and assist with management. These patients are usually studied with magnetic resonance imaging of the spine and referred to the pediatric neurosurgeon.

MANAGEMENT

The intent, interests, and cooperation of the child and family must be determined as treatment is planned. The length of treatment and commitment to various programs, such as behavior modification with an alarm system, need to be explained.

Diurnal Enuresis

Patients with urge incontinence are wet day and night. They may posture and when urine volume is assessed have a low functional bladder capacity. They may have a staccato type of urination due to contraction of the external sphincter during voiding. Many have concomitant urinary tract infections. Initial treatment consists of a timed voiding schedule, emptying the bladder every 2 to 3 hours. If this is not successful, then anticholinergic medication to treat the unstable bladder is helpful. Parents are instructed to listen to the child's voided stream and alert the child to intermittency and staccato urination. Overall, 87% of children with isolated overactive bladders will improve over a mean of 2.7 years. It is important that the child and parents understand this time commitment. Biofeedback training with reflex inhibition of detrusor contractions has also shown success in this group of patients.

Infrequent Voiding

Children with wetting and infrequent voiding are placed on a timed voiding schedule. These children frequently do not void on awakening and have associated urinary tract infections and constipation, which require ongoing treatment. A voiding log documenting time, wetting episodes, and volume of urine is kept by the child under parental supervision. The ultrasonic bladder scan to assess emptying has been used in the office and at home, providing immediate feedback on bladder emptying to the patient.

Hinman's Syndrome

The extreme form of dysfunctional voiding is the non-neurogenic neurogenic bladder or Hinman's syndrome. These patients have upper and lower urinary tract involvement due to detrusor instability and marked learned detrusor sphincter dyssynergia. The lack of coordination results in high-pressure inefficient voiding. High-pressure voiding leads to bladder decompensation, vesicoureteral reflux, residual urine, urinary tract infection, and, in worst-case scenarios, renal failure. The majority also have constipation and encopresis. They frequently come from families with abusive or overbearing parents. Treatment ranges from that previously discussed to adjunctive medications such as α-blockers to relax the bladder neck, clean intermittent catheterization, behavior modification, and psychological assistance. Help from the pediatric gastroenterologists to develop a good bowel program is sought. Behavior modification to teach relaxation of the external sphincter with voiding is also successful.

Giggle Incontinence

Complete loss of urinary control during the daytime precipitated by laughter is the hallmark of this voiding dysfunction. It is not usually associated with urinary tract infections or anatomic abnormalities. Giggle incontinence is not stress-related because there is no urinary loss with coughing, sneezing, or straining. It is often seen in adolescent girls and is a source of great embarrassment. Its cause is unknown. Giggle incontinence is very difficult to treat with behavior modification, and expedient bladder emptying is the most effective therapy. Anticholinergic agents are usually not efficacious. Methylphenidate (Ritalin,* 0.3–0.5 mg/kg every 4–6 hours while awake) has been successful in some patients with this disorder. Fortunately, in some girls the incontinence abates spontaneously.

Nocturnal Enuresis

Control of urination at night is the last step in the development of social continence. Our society standard for acquisition of nocturnal continence is 5 years of age. Fifteen percent to 20% of 5-year-old children wet the bed. Of these, 75% have always done so and 25% have secondary nocturnal enuresis. Fifteen percent of these children become dry at night each year, attesting to its developmental nature. It is important to remember nocturnal enuresis is a symptom and not a disease. The family history is one key because if one parent wet the bed, 44% of their children will do so and if both parents wet the bed, 77% of their children will do so. The age of attainment of nocturnal control will be similar to that of the parent.

*Not FDA approved for this indication.

The etiology of nocturnal enuresis is likely multifactorial. Conceptually, the triangle of bladder capacity, sleep arousal, and urine volume are the determinants of wetness at night. The bladder capacity is exceeded, the child is not aroused in response to the full bladder, and the bladder empties while the child continues to sleep. The pattern of sleep as measured by electroencephalography is normal; however, all the parents of these children will say how difficult it is to awaken the child. The daytime functional bladder capacity is decreased in some of these children. Also, a group of these children have increased nocturnal urine production due to a deficiency in the amount of antidiuretic hormone secreted at night. This loss of a normal diurnal increase in nocturnal antidiuretic hormone secretion combined with poor arousal results in a wet bed.

The evaluation of children with bedwetting is as previously outlined. The majority require a good history, physical examination, and urinalysis. No further imaging or studies are necessary if these results are normal. The decision to treat these children is based on the family and child's perception of the social and personal consequences of the bedwetting. If it prevents normal socialization or affects the child's self-esteem, then treatment is warranted. Many of the families just want to know that the condition will improve and reassurance is all that is necessary.

The mainstay of treatment of primary nocturnal enuresis is behavior modification because it provides the best long-term success. Motivational therapy, consisting of positive reinforcement and active patient involvement, is combined with conditioning therapy with an alarm. The alarm positioned on the pajamas is triggered by urine contact with a sensor in the underwear. When wetting occurs, the alarm sounds and the patient must awaken, which initially requires the assistance of his or her parents. The patient will stop urination upon awakening and is instructed to empty the remainder of urine into the toilet. This process ultimately results in awakening in response to a full bladder and a dry bed. The conditioning may take up to 15 weeks to occur. We require 25 consecutive dry nights prior to removal of the device. Numerous studies have reported a 65% to 100% cure rate after 4 to 6 months of treatment. Relapse may occur in up to 30% of children, but retreatment is successful if relapse occurs. Unfortunately, many families and patients are not willing to put in the time and effort to ensure success with conditioning therapy.

The primary pharmacologic agents utilized in treating nocturnal enuresis are anticholinergic agents,* tricyclic antidepressants, and desmopressin

*Not FDA approved for this indication.

acetate. Anticholinergic agents, specifically oxybutynin, decrease or abolish uninhibited bladder contractions and increase functional bladder capacity. Oxybutynin (Ditropan)* is of particular help in the child with both daytime and nighttime wetting. However, its use in children with only nocturnal enuresis is only rarely beneficial. In children with small functional bladder capacity, anticholinergic agents* with an alarm system have proven successful. In children 6 years of age or older, the dosage is 5 mg taken two to three times daily (0.2 mg/kg twice daily or three times daily). Parents need to be alerted to the facial flushing, dry mouth, and heat intolerance associated with the use of anticholinergic agents.

Imipramine (Tofranil), a tricyclic antidepressant, has success in the treatment of nocturnal enuresis. Its pharmacologic actions appear to be multiple because it acts centrally to cause arousal from sleep; it has weak anticholinergic effects on the bladder and mild α-adrenergic effects to close the bladder neck. It may also stimulate the secretion of antidiuretic hormone from the posterior pituitary gland. The dose of imipramine given 1 to 2 hours before bedtime should not exceed 50 mg in children 6 to 12 years old or exceed 75 mg in children 12 to 14 years old. On a weight basis, the usual recommended dosage is 0.9 to 1.5 mg/kg/day. Initial success with imipramine is as high as 50%; however, only 25% of patients have a long-term cure. It works best in older children who have minimal daytime wetness. Its effects are immediate, and it can be used on an as-needed basis for a dry night. Side effects include anxiety, insomnia, dry mouth, and personality changes. The medicine must be safely guarded and administered by the parents because fatal overdoses have occurred, with death due to cardiac arrhythmia, conduction blocks, and hypotension.

Desmopressin acetate (DDAVP), a synthetic analogue of arginine vasopressin, is the only other medication with FDA approval to treat nocturnal enuresis. In some patients with decreased nocturnal secretion of antidiuretic hormone, it is replacement therapy. In theory, the use of DDAVP combined with fluid restriction will result in a reduction in nocturnal urine output to a volume less than bladder capacity, resulting in a dry bed. It does not explain the sleep arousal–related problem in enuretic children. DDAVP is available as a spray or tablet. The spray delivers 10 μg per spray. The initial dose is 20 μg (one spray in each nostril). This dose can be titrated to a total of 40 μg (two sprays in each nostril). The tablet contains 200 μg of DDAVP. Treatment begins with one tablet and can be titrated to a total of three tablets per night (600 μg). In a number of blind controlled studies a *significant improvement,* defined as greater than 50% reduction in wet nights, is attained in greater than 50% of patients. Improved response to DDAVP is noted in older patients with fewer wet nights per week and patients with greater than 70% of predicted bladder capacity for age. This medication, like imipramine, has a high relapse rate when discontinued. It acts swiftly and can be used on an as-needed basis. The side effects of taking DDAVP have been negligible when strict fluid restriction is performed. Rare cases of hyponatremia and seizures have been seen. Fluid restriction beginning at least 2 hours prior to bedtime and voiding prior to going to bed are an important aspect of treatment with DDAVP. Patients with refractory nocturnal enuresis persisting into adulthood have been treated with various combinations of alarm system and pharmacotherapy. A recent study using hyoscyamine (Cystospaz)* and DDAVP reported success in 78% of patients. Combining the alarm system with oral DDAVP is particularly effective in children with the *most severe bed wetting,* defined as *more than 6* wet nights per week.

*Not FDA approved for this indication.

*Not FDA approved for this indication.

URINARY INCONTINENCE

method of
RODNEY A. APPELL, M.D.
Baylor College of Medicine
Houston, Texas

Urinary incontinence in an individual must be identified as a problem at the level of the bladder, at the level of the outlet, or both, to direct the most appropriate treatment. Urinary incontinence may be a symptom of which patients complain, a sign demonstrated on examination, or a condition (diagnosis) confirmed by definitive studies. Diagnostic accuracy is important to ensure appropriate choice of therapy. For example, therapies designed for outlet causes of incontinence will not improve and may worsen incontinence due to a bladder problem. Therefore, diagnostic accuracy is paramount and requires a complete history and physical examination.

The history should include the duration and frequency of the incontinence, as well as a clear description of how much of a problem the incontinence is for the patient. This may be objectified by the use of a 3-day voiding diary kept by the patient between the first and second appointment that details the patient's voiding habits and includes the voiding times and volumes of each voiding as well as incontinent episodes. This extension of the history then becomes a method of monitoring the progress of any therapeutic intervention and is extremely important in patient counseling with regard to behavioral modifications.

With regard to the physical examination, it is important to evaluate the prostate gland in males and whether any genitourinary prolapse is present in females. The extension of the physical examination to evaluate lower urinary tract function is called *urodynamic investigation* and provides graphic demonstration of pressure/volume relationships for urinary storage and voiding. Although this modality of testing is invasive requiring the use of urinary tract catheterization, it is imperative to allow observation of bladder and outlet (sphincteric) activity during the cycle of bladder filling and emptying (Tables 1 and 2) because incontinence and voiding dysfunction depend on intact bladder and urethral function. This implies low-pressure urine storage

TABLE 1. **Requirements of Bladder Filling**

Accommodation of increasing volume at low intravesical pressure and normal sensation
Absence of involuntary contractions
Bladder outlet closed at rest and with increases in intraabdominal pressure

during the filling phase of bladder function enhanced by intact outlet sphincteric function. As bladder capacity is reached, emptying is successfully completed by coordinated bladder and outlet activity initiated by outlet relaxation and immediately followed by a bladder contraction of adequate magnitude and duration to completely empty the bladder.

OVERACTIVE BLADDER AND DETRUSOR HYPERREFLEXIA

The term *overactive bladder* has recently been coined to describe frequency of urination and urgency of urination with or without urinary urge incontinence. This is a very large group of patients (17 million people in the United States); in fact, it is more prevalent than asthma, osteoporosis, and diabetes mellitus. In addition, it is a heterogeneous group including patients with bladder muscle overactivity either due to neurogenic causes such as spinal cord injury; multiple sclerosis; parkinsonism; and stroke; or non-neurogenic or idiopathic causes, which may include obstruction and even certain patients with outlet incompetence and stress urinary incontinence symptoms. When the motor overactivity can be directly related to a neurogenic cause it is referred to as *detrusor hyperreflexia*; otherwise, terms such as *overactive bladder, detrusor instability,* and *unstable bladder* are interchangeable. A third group of sensory/urge patients may have the symptoms of the overactive bladder but lack the urodynamic findings of abnormal motor contractions of the bladder. Nevertheless, these patients are part of the overactive bladder group.

Treatment goals for disorders affecting the lower urinary tract are obvious but are worth repeating before any discussion of a specific treatment modality. First and foremost, as in all of urology, maintenance of renal function is prioritized. Optimally, one would like to afford the patient a normal voiding pattern and to provide continence of urine. Realistically, if a cure is not feasible, then a significant improvement in symptoms is the aim to help the individual improve his or her quality of life.

Behavioral modification is the starting point for the treatment of the overactive bladder. Using the voiding diary, the patient can be instructed to modify fluid intake, adjust toileting frequency; additionally, dietary changes are recommended such as the elimination of caffeine, a bladder stimulant. Kegel pelvic floor exercises are recommended because contractions of the pelvic floor send impulses via pudendal and pelvic nerve afferent fibers to the sacral spinal cord, which results in inhibiting the pelvic nerve efferent fibers and allows for bladder relaxation and the slowing of the impending urge to void. More intensive pelvic muscle therapy involves biofeedback, electrical stimulation, or extracorporeal magnetic stimulation therapy to aid in pelvic muscle rehabilitation by allowing the individual to recognize the correct muscles to exercise by visual, auditory, or tactile sensation. The newest entry into this field is extracorporeal magnetic stimulation therapy, where the magnetic therapy induces electric current to flow and contract the muscles. There is no direct contact, thus no impedance and no probes in the vagina or rectum are necessary and the patient need not disrobe. Early clinical results of extracorporeal magnetic stimulation therapy are encouraging in the treatment of the overactive bladder.

Pharmacologic therapy is additive to behavioral and pelvic floor therapies. Oral antimuscarinic therapy with immediate-release oxybutynin chloride has been the mainstay of pharmacologic therapy for almost 30 years. Although efficacy has been satisfactory, high discontinuation rates due to anticholinergic side effects, such as dry mouth, constipation, blurred vision, and heat intolerance have reduced patient compliance. Recently two medications intended to improve tolerability and patient acceptance of antimuscarinic therapy for overactive bladder have become available. Tolterodine tartrate (Detrol) demonstrated efficacy in the reduction of urinary frequency as the primary clinical endpoint, and extended-release oxybutynin chloride (Ditropan-XL) has shown efficacy in the reduction of urge incontinence as the primary clinical endpoint. Tolterodine is normally prescribed as a fixed 4-mg dose (2 mg twice daily), whereas extended-release oxybutynin chloride doses are normally titrated (5–30 mg daily) to levels that achieve an optimal balance of tolerability and efficacy. Most recently, a study was completed comparing the effects of 12 weeks of treatment with these drugs on episodes of urge incontinence and micturition frequency in participants with overactive bladder symptoms. The findings demonstrated that a 10-mg dose of extended-release oxybutynin chloride was significantly more effective than the 4-mg (2 mg twice daily) dose of tolterodine as measured by end-of-study urge incontinence and micturition frequency episodes. Overall tolerability was excellent, with similar low rates of dry mouth and other adverse events in both groups.

Direct sacral nerve stimulation as a neuromodulation technique has provided an option to surgical augmentation cystoplasty using intestinal segments in patients refractory to the combined behavioral and

TABLE 2. **Requirements of Bladder Emptying**

Lack of outlet obstruction
Decrease in urethral and sphincteric resistance
Concomitant coordinated bladder contraction of adequate magnitude and duration to complete the emptying process

pharmacologic treatments. Satisfactory results in this difficult group of nonresponders is 50% for neuromodulation and 80% for augmentation cystoplasty.

INCONTINENCE ASSOCIATED WITH URETHRAL DYSFUNCTION

Stress urinary incontinence in men occurs clinically as a result of surgery on the prostate gland due to outlet damage, which may be direct or indirect with effects on the vascular or neurologic input to the smooth or striated component of the outlet. Of course, this can be the result of neurologic disease with injury to the sympathetic innervation of the bladder neck as seen in myelodysplasia or pelvic fractures.

Women are the primary group with urethral dysfunction resulting in urinary incontinence. When evaluating women with a history of stress urinary incontinence, the diagnosis cannot be established by history alone. Based on history alone the physician can expect to be incorrect at least 20% of the time about the cause of the incontinence. The physical examination is performed to determine if any associated prolapse is present. A postvoid residual urine assessment is recommended in every patient as an indication of emptying function. An elevated postvoid residual urine measurement may be the result of a poorly contractile bladder or outlet obstruction. This is not present in cases of pure stress urinary incontinence, and an elevated residual urine measurement warrants further search for another cause of the urinary incontinence.

In patients with symptoms suggesting stress urinary incontinence alone, documented urethral hypermobility, no significant prolapse, and minimal postvoid residual urine measurement, a filling cystometrogram is all that is required to confirm a stable, compliant reservoir. However, in patients with a suspected or established neurologic lesion, a history of pelvic surgery, or symptoms of mixed (urge/stress) incontinence, a more complex urodynamic investigation is indicated before selection of treatment. Prolapse should be reduced by pessary or packing to determine the Valsalva or abdominal leak point pressure during straining and the voiding pressures obtained to note the likelihood of the patient to void if urethral resistance is increased in any way. This is of significant importance based upon the fact that current management of stress incontinence in women is almost universally surgical.

All women with stress incontinence have at least some degree of intrinsic sphincteric deficiency. There may or may not be hypermobility of the outlet mechanism associated with the intrinsic sphincteric deficiency. Surgery for women with stress incontinence has changed substantially over the past few years. Following the evaluation of the literature by the American Urological Association, it is clear that many standard procedures (anterior repairs and transvaginal suspensions) did not provide the long-term success expected and that suburethral support to allow coaptation of the urethral mucosa is needed to attain successful treatment. This implied the need for sling surgery or the use of injectables to obtain the coaptation. The debates now center around the length of the sling, the exact position of the sling (bladder neck or mid-urethra), attachment of the sling, and the composition of the sling (autologous, homologous, heterologous tissue, synthetic material, and so on) and the clear answers in that regard are not yet known.

With respect to injectable therapy, the primary problem is that the materials currently approved by the FDA are not durable and reinjections are required to sustain the results. Currently there is one biomaterial and one synthetic material. The biomaterial is glutaraldehyde cross-linked bovine collagen (Contigen) and the synthetic material is carbon-coated zirconium beads (Durasphere) and the results 1 year after injection are almost identical. Many other materials are currently under study. It will literally take years to determine the remaining information needed to answer the questions on slings and injectables.

OVERFLOW INCONTINENCE

This type of incontinence is usually continuous and the diagnosis is made on physical examination and postvoid residual urine determination. This finding represents urinary dysfunction due to either detrusor hypocontractility or bladder outlet obstruction. Urodynamic investigation will determine the cause. The treatment for obstruction is to relieve the obstruction and the treatment for poor detrusor function is to teach the patient self-catheterization.

EPIDIDYMITIS

method of
L. KEITH LLOYD, M.D.
University of Alabama at Birmingham
Birmingham, Alabama

The *epididymis* is a coiled tubular structure that transports spermatozoa from the testicle to the vas deferens. It is located along the posterior border of the testicle with the head or caput at the upper pole of the testicle and the tail, which leads into the vas deferens, at the lower pole of the testicle. Epididymitis is an inflammation of the epididymis that causes pain and swelling of the epididymis and often of the adjacent testicle. It may be accompanied by abdominal pain and fever. It is usually seen in young men but may occur at any age. It is a significant cause of lost work and may at times be attributed to work-related injury.

ETIOLOGY AND PATHOGENESIS

It was thought at one time that most cases of epididymitis were idiopathic, but more recent evidence suggests that most cases result from retrograde spread of infection from the bladder or urethra. In heterosexual men younger than 35 years, genital infection with either *Chlamydia trachomatis* or *Neisseria gonorrhoeae* is the most common cause of epididymitis. The pathogens initially become established in the urethra and may not cause symptoms. The organisms then spread in a retrograde manner to the epididymis and result in the clinical syndrome of acute epididymitis. In older men, in some young boys, and in homosexual men who practice anal intercourse, the common pathogens are the coliform bacteria that usually cause urinary infection. In this case, the route of infection is initial bacteriuria with retrograde flow into the genital tract. Men who have neurologic disease and abnormal voiding or who require an indwelling catheter are especially at risk for urethritis and epididymitis and may have particularly severe infections. Young boys who have no pyuria or urethritis may have nonbacterial or sterile inflammations of the epididymis and hence not require antibiotic therapy. Viral infection may be the cause, but this has not been proved. Unusual systemic infections such as tuberculosis or systemic fungal infections occasionally result in bloodborne infection of the epididymis. The antiarrhythmic drug amiodarone (Cordarone) can cause epididymitis that is usually confined to the head of the epididymis. Lastly, a chronic epididymitis can occur many years after vasectomy. It is thought to be related to the surgical obstruction and development of sperm granulomas in the epididymis and has been called the *postvasectomy syndrome*.

CLINICAL PRESENTATION

Pain and swelling of the epididymis are the prominent features of the condition. Swelling usually begins in the tail of the epididymis and spreads to involve the entire epididymis and the testicle; it may involve the spermatic cord. Fever is usually present, and there may be associated abdominal pain. Patients may have noticed an antecedent urethral discharge or symptoms of frequency of urination and dysuria. If patients are examined early, there may be swelling of the epididymis only or even just a portion of the epididymis. It is usually exquisitely tender, and the pain can be relieved somewhat by gentle elevation of the involved side. Redness of the overlying scrotal skin and, in later stages, induration of the scrotal skin are frequently seen. If examined later, the epididymis and testicle may be swollen and matted together as one large mass with swelling extending up the spermatic cord.

LABORATORY EVALUATION

If a urethral discharge is present, a Gram stain should be performed. The presence of gram-negative intracellular diplococci indicates the presence of *N. gonorrhoeae*. If only white blood cells are seen, this suggests chlamydial infection as the likely cause. Urinalysis should be done to determine if there is any evidence of urinary tract infection, and a urine culture and sensitivity testing should be done when the urinalysis result is positive. A white blood cell count may be obtained in severely ill patients, but it is usually normal in most cases of epididymitis.

Imaging studies are helpful when the diagnosis is in doubt. Radionuclide scanning can differentiate among epididymo-orchitis, tumor, and testicular torsion but is often not readily available. Ultrasound (US) examination of the scrotum is more often used and with Doppler flow studies can usually reliably establish the diagnosis. Increased blood flow to the involved testicle should be seen along with a stronger arterial signal than that in the contralateral testicle.

DIFFERENTIAL DIAGNOSIS

The major concern is in distinguishing between epididymitis and testicular torsion. The presence of urethritis and a palpable swollen epididymis usually confirms epididymitis, but in young patients in whom torsion is a concern, Doppler US may be used to establish a diagnosis. Increased blood flow is compatible with epididymitis when poor flow to the affected testicle indicates torsion. If doubt remains, surgical exploration is indicated and should be done early. Testicular tumors usually present as painless swelling but occasionally present with acute swelling and pain. Persistent swelling after a course of antibiotics indicates a need for further evaluation to rule out tumor. US examination is usually helpful in this regard. If the swelling has not resolved or the US shows tumor, surgical exploration is indicated.

TREATMENT

Treatment is directed at the likely underlying cause. Antibiotic therapy is usually indicated, and supportive treatment consists of bed rest, elevation of the scrotum, and analgesics. In young men in whom chlamydial or *N. gonorrhoeae* infection is most likely, treatment with one of the tetracyclines is usually indicated. Doxycycline (Vibramycin) may be given in a dose of 200 mg initially and then 100 mg twice a day for 10 to 14 days. Tetracycline (Achromycin), 500 mg orally four times a day, may be used but will produce a greater incidence of gastrointestinal side effects. If Gram stain suggests *N. gonorrhoeae* infection, ceftriaxone (Rocephin), 250 mg, is administered intramuscularly. Alternatively, ciprofloxacin (Cipro), 500 mg twice a day for 3 days, can be administered. In older men and young boys with concomitant urinary tract infection, an agent directed toward the coliform bacteria is usually indicated. Initial treatment can be with trimethoprim-sulfamethoxazole (Bactrim, Septra), 1 double-strength tablet twice a day for 10 days or, particularly in patients with complex urinary problems, one of the fluoroquinolones such as levofloxacin (Levaquin), 500 mg a day, or ciprofloxacin, 500 mg twice a day for 10 days.

Prepubertal boys without pyuria or urethral discharge may be treated with scrotal support and analgesics and may not require antibiotic therapy. The major concern is to rule out testicular torsion. Patients with amiodarone-related epididymitis can be treated by reducing the dosage of the drug or changing to another agent if possible.

Postvasectomy epididymitis can occasionally be bothersome many years later. It is usually treated with nonsteroidal analgesics such as ibuprofen (Motrin) 400 mg four times a day for 10 to 14 days. Persistent pain and swelling with this or any other form of epididymitis may require surgical removal of the epididymis.

PRIMARY GLOMERULAR DISEASES

method of
WILLIAM A. WILMER, M.D.
The Ohio State University
Columbus, Ohio

Primary glomerulopathies are diseases of the kidney glomerulus that do not have identifiable causes. Secondary glomerulopathies are glomerular diseases that have identifiable, often systemic, causes. Examples of secondary glomerulopathies include diabetic nephropathy and glomerular injuries associated with systemic lupus erythematosus (SLE) or other connective tissue diseases. The primary glomerulopathies frequently occur in patients who have few symptoms and unremarkable medical histories. Their presentations can therefore be subtle, and commonly their diagnoses are made months or years after onset.

Glomerular diseases occur when any of the several cell types in the glomerulus undergo anatomic and/or functional changes that affect the ability of glomerular capillaries to selectively filter blood. The abnormal filtration that occurs in glomerular diseases allows abnormal urinary excretion of compounds that cause secondary changes in the kidney tubules, interstitium, and/or vasculature. Therefore, treatment of glomerular diseases can prevent more generalized kidney damage. The excretion of plasma proteins into the urine is an example of an inability to selectively filter blood and is a hallmark of most glomerular disorders. In general, the worse the glomerular pathology, the more severe the proteinuria, although obsolescence of diseased glomeruli may result in improvement of proteinuria despite advancing disease. Glomerular capillary injury can also cause red blood cell and white blood cell excretion into the urine. Excretion of these cells can be in the form of free-floating cells or in the form of cellular casts. Such cellular urine sediment is typically suggestive of an inflammatory glomerular process.

With time, the primary glomerulopathies can induce severe glomerular injury that prevents the filtration of metabolic solutes by the glomerular capillaries. This fall in glomerular filtration rate (GFR), indicated by elevated serum creatinine values, may progress until a patient requires renal replacement therapy in the form of dialysis or transplantation.

DIAGNOSIS

Many of the primary glomerulopathies are indolent. Even in inflammatory forms of glomerular disease, fever and other systemic manifestations of inflammation may be absent. This is in part due to the typically low-grade but chronic inflammation that causes many glomerular injuries. As a result, many glomerulopathies are first identified by abnormal screening urinalyses or routine blood chemistry profiles. With extensive glomerular injury that results in severe proteinuria and filtration loss, complications such as edema or hypertension are heralding signs. Nondescript symptoms such as fatigue, weight loss due to diminished appetite, or weight gain due to edema formation are often associated with glomerulopathies.

Urinalyses of patients with glomerular disease typically show proteinuria of more than 500 mg/24 h, the majority of which is albumin. Transient, mild proteinuria (less than 1 g/24 h) that is not due to glomerular disease occurs during fevers, after immunizations, or after exercise. Therefore, proteinuria of the glomerulopathies must be persistent. Up to 1 g/24 h of nonalbumin proteinuria can occur in tubule and interstitial kidney diseases. Kidney tubules, especially the proximal tubules, remove from the urine several proteins with molecular weights lower than albumin. With tubulointerstitial disease, these low-molecular-weight proteins are poorly reabsorbed by the tubules and are excreted in abundance into the urine. A urine protein electrophoresis is helpful in identifying the urine protein composition when proteinuria is about 1 g/24 h. An excessive excretion of low molecular weight proteins without significant albuminuria should alert the clinician to nonglomerular forms of kidney injury.

Most urine test strips measure the concentration of albumin in a random urine sample. The level of proteinuria on test strips may depend on the urine concentration—polyuria can underemphasize the amount of proteinuria, and oliguria will overemphasize it. A 24-hour urine collection is a standard way to quantitate proteinuria once a urine test strip identifies abnormal excretion. Proteinuria can also be quantified from a random urine sample, which is more easily obtained than a 24-hour urine collection. The protein concentration in a random urine sample is normalized to the concentration of urine creatinine. This urine protein:creatinine ratio estimates the number of grams of protein excreted if a 24-hour urine collection were obtained. The correlation of protein:creatinine ratios using a first morning urine void to a 24-hour urine collection is very good.

Most primary glomerulopathies cause proteinuria of more than 2 g/24 h. In the past, considerable emphasis was placed on determining if a patient had the "nephrotic syndrome," which is classically defined as proteinuria greater than or equal to 3.5 g/24 h/1.73 M^2, hypoalbuminemia, hyperlipidemia with lipiduria, and edema. When criteria for the "nephrotic syndrome" were met, it was implied that severe glomerular injury was present. Failure of a patient to meet the definition of the "nephrotic syndrome" does not necessarily portend a better prognosis because patients with severe glomerular disease can manifest extensive proteinuria but not lipid abnormalities or edema. A better term to indicate the presence of extensive glomerular disease is *nephrotic range proteinuria,* a term that indicates proteinuria greater than or equal to 3.5 g/24 h.

Even this term is misleading because the level of proteinuria is reflective of serum protein stores. If serum albumin stores are very low (less than 3 g/dL), patients with extensive glomerular disease may excrete only a few grams of albumin. In such patients, calculating an albumin clearance is helpful in identifying severe proteinuria. The albumin clearance is the amount of albumin excreted into urine in 24 hours divided by the serum albumin level. An albumin clearance greater than 150 mL/24 h is analogous to "nephrotic range proteinuria."

The excretion into urine of other components of the blood compartment (red cells, white cells) is helpful in determining if a glomerular lesion is inflammatory. The sediment of centrifuged urine allows the morphology of red cells to be determined, identifies the presence of casts, and, in general, provides a rapid and inexpensive way of identifying an inflammatory state. When inflammation is present, urine is called "nephritic." Glomerulopathies are commonly referred to as "nephritic" or "nephrotic" based on urinalyses and protein measurements. These definitions are helpful in the differential of glomerulopathies, but it should be remembered that every glomerulopathy can present with nonclassic urinalysis features. That is, variability of disease causes even those glomerulopathies that commonly have "nephritic" urine to present with unimpressive urine sediment, especially between injury exacerbations.

Identifying systemic illnesses that can cause glomerulopathy is important. Many of the glomerular diseases discussed in this article were first described as idiopathic. Over time, many have been linked to systemic inflammatory processes or malignancies. The reason to search for a secondary cause of a glomerulopathy is threefold. First, identifying a secondary cause may lessen the need for a native kidney biopsy. Second, identifying a secondary cause may provide an opportunity to improve or cure the glomerulopathy by treating the systemic illness. Third, glomerulopathy may lead to the diagnosis of a covert illness because renal involvement is often the first presentation of severe systemic illnesses or malignancy. The caveat of identifying a secondary, systemic illness in patients with obvious glomerular injury is incorrectly linking the two diseases. For example, diabetic nephropathy is classically a noninflammatory glomerular lesion. A patient with diabetes and proteinuria in whom the most likely diagnosis is diabetic nephropathy may actually have a different glomerular injury if the urine sediment is inflammatory or if a rapid loss of kidney function occurs. When such a diagnostic dilemma occurs, a kidney biopsy is often indicated.

A kidney biopsy is required for the proper diagnosis of the primary glomerulopathies. Although a urinalysis may focus a differential diagnosis, it is often insufficient for determining the true diagnosis. In addition to providing the histology of the glomerular process, a biopsy can help determine the chronicity of disease by determining the amount of fibrosis present in the biopsy sample. The amount of fibrosis present is often prognostic and, interestingly, may not be reflected by elevated serum creatinine values. The amount of fibrosis present may also direct the aggressiveness of immunosuppressive therapy. Patients with extensive fibrosis may not warrant the risks of aggressive immunosuppression.

With advancements in radiologic localization of the kidneys and mechanical devices that obtain the biopsy material, kidney biopsies can be safely performed. Indications for a biopsy include persistent albuminuria of more than 1 g/24 h, an inflammatory urine sediment, or loss of glomerular filtration (an abnormal serum creatinine or creatinine clearance). A rapid loss of kidney filtration is an indication for urgent kidney biopsy. Patients with low-grade proteinuria (less than 1 g albumin excretion/24 h) with preserved GFR and a benign (noninflammatory) urine sediment often do not require a kidney biopsy. This recommendation is based on the lower likelihood of needing immunosuppressive therapies in diseases with minimal and stable proteinuria. As outlined earlier, a urine protein electrophoresis is helpful in patients with such low-grade proteinuria. A kidney biopsy may also be required even if a secondary cause is suspected or known. For example, in patients with systemic lupus who have proteinuria, a kidney biopsy can help determine the presence of one of several histologic classifications of lupus glomerulonephritis that require different immunotherapies or even anticoagulation therapy.

OVERVIEW OF TREATMENT STRATEGIES

General Approach to Therapy

Two types of therapy are appropriate for most of the glomerulopathies. First, many primary glomerular lesions are treatable with corticosteroids and immunosuppressive therapies. Although the exact immunologic cause of the primary lesions may not be known, it is apparent that the immune system participates in many of these persistent glomerular injuries. Second, patients with glomerular injuries should also be treated with "renoprotective" interventions—therapies that control mechanical stress of glomerular cells and prevent secondary glomerular injury. Most of the primary glomerulopathies can cause permanent loss of kidney function, and therapies that protect remaining kidney function from mechanical injury of hypertension and hyperfiltration are extremely important in long-term preservation of kidney health. Therefore, it is wise to initiate "renoprotective" therapies at the onset of immunotherapy for a primary glomerulopathy.

Before discussing specific treatment strategies of the glomerulopathies, the general approach to using immunosuppressive therapies is discussed.

Corticosteroids

Interest in corticosteroid treatment of primary glomerulopathies has existed for decades, and their use is the foundation of most treatment strategies. Corticosteroids possess direct anti-inflammatory properties owing to suppression of leukocyte function, including inhibition of leukocyte trafficking, inhibition of granulocyte degranulation, and direct lymphocytotoxic effects. Corticosteroids also improve capillary permeability that occurs in inflammation. They also offer immunosuppressive effects by inhibiting inflammatory interleukins, altering lymphocyte responses to antigen, and, to a lesser extent, inhibiting antibody production. These latter effects generally require longer treatment periods to attain. The immunosuppressive effects of corticosteroids occur at a prednisone dose of 1 mg/kg/d. Doses of corticosteroid above that equivalent prednisone dose may not confer added immunosuppression, although higher doses do impart more anti-inflammatory effects. Anti-inflammatory doses of corticosteroids are often used in patients with severe forms of glomerular damage that require urgent treatment, such as kidney failure due to rapidly progressive glomerulonephritides. In these cases, a 3-day treatment with an intravenous corticosteroid (800 mg methylprednisolone [Solu-Medrol] or 1000 mg of prednisolone) may attenuate inflammation and even control glomerular cell proliferation (e.g., crescent growth). Use of high-dose corticosteroids beyond a few days should be done with caution because such use may limit a patient's ability to mount a response to infections.

The lupus plasmapheresis trial sponsored by the National Institutes of Health (NIH)[1] devised a rational treatment strategy for high-dose oral prednisone use. This approach confers adequate immunosuppression without overly risking the development of infection. This protocol is intended for the most severe forms of glomerular injury. Patients weighing less than 80 kg are started on prednisone, 60 mg/d in divided doses for 4 weeks, and the dose is decreased to 50 mg/d for 4 weeks (as a single dose), and then to

40 mg/d as a single dose for 4 weeks. The dose is then decreased to 30 mg/d as a single dose for 2 weeks. Thereafter the dose is tapered on alternate days by 5 mg, and a new tapered dose is begun each week (e.g., 30 mg/d alternate with 25 mg/d for 1 week, then 30 mg/d alternate with 20 mg/d for 1 week, then 30 mg/d alternate with 15 mg/d, and so on until 30 mg alternates with no prednisone every other day). The every-other-day prednisone dosage is thereafter tapered by 5 mg/wk. Patients weighing more than 80 kg are started at 80 mg/d in divided doses for 4 weeks then tapered by 10 mg/d every 2 weeks until the dose reaches 40 mg. Then alternate-day dosing with the same tapering protocol for patients weighing 60 kg should be followed.

The same dosing regimen can be adjusted to create a medium-dose protocol for less severe forms of glomerular injury. The medium-dose protocol simply tapers the prednisone dose twice as rapidly as the high-dose protocol.

Immunosuppressive Agents

Alkylating Agents

Alkylating agents such as chlorambucil (Leukeran)* and cyclophosphamide (Cytoxan)* have been useful therapies for a variety of primary glomerulopathies. Similar to corticosteroids, oral and intravenous preparations of alkylating agents have been used. These agents work by suppressing B-cell production of antibodies that contribute to immune-complex formation. Intermittent use of these agents, often in conjunction with oral or intravenous corticosteroids, is preferred over chronic therapy. An intermittent use is preferred due to the cumulative effects of these agents in causing malignancies and pancytopenia. I prefer to use oral preparations of the alkylating agents due to their ease of administration and the flexibility of titrating the medication dose depending on peripheral leukocyte counts.

Given slightly better gastrointestinal tolerance than chlorambucil, I use oral cyclophosphamide (Cytoxan) at doses starting at 1.5 to 2 mg/kg/d, not to exceed 150 mg/d. This dose can be taken for 8 to 12 weeks, but it is often used for 4-week intervals in conjunction with oral corticosteroids. The risks of oral cyclophosphamide include hemorrhagic cystitis and/or bladder carcinomas. My group's experience with many patients on oral cyclophosphamide is favorable if the patients maintain appropriate fluid intake and diuresis to ensure minimal contact of the excreted medication with the urinary bladder. Chlorambucil is less likely to cause bladder toxicity. Both agents can induce gonadal failure. Although gonadal failure typically occurs after several courses of these agents, patient variability exists and some patients may develop gonadal failure during the first course. Intravenous administration of these agents is certainly preferable in patients in whom compliance with oral medications is questionable or in those who develop gastrointestinal intolerance of the oral preparation. The usual dose of intravenous cyclophosphamide is 750 mg/M^2 every 4 weeks, often used for 6 months of total therapy. Peripheral leukocyte counts should be measured at least every 2 weeks. If leukopenia develops, subsequent intravenous cyclophosphamide dosing should be tapered and oral cyclophosphamide should be discontinued until improvement occurs. The oral dose should then be restarted at 50% of the previous dose.

*Not FDA approved for this indication.

Antagonists of Purine Biosynthesis

The agents azathioprine (Imuran)* and mycophenolate mofetil (CellCept)* can also be used in conjunction with corticosteroids for the treatment of glomerulopathies. In severe glomerulopathies requiring longer immunosuppression, these agents are also useful after a course of alkylating agent therapy. My opinion is that the alkylating agents are much more successful than azathioprine at initially controlling many of the immune-mediated renal diseases. However, once improvement in disease is established with corticosteroids and an alkylating agent, azathioprine use can help maintain the remission. The standard dose of azathioprine for use with most glomerulopathies is 2 mg/kg, adjusted downward if leukopenia is observed. Allopurinol can significantly prolong the biologic effects of azathioprine and even the alkylating agents. A dose reduction by 50% is appropriate in patients using daily allopurinol (Zyloprim). Mycophenolate appears to be more successful than azathioprine in suppressing the immune system, as has been shown by its superior ability to prevent renal transplant rejection. It also appears to be potent in the control of glomerular diseases that are refractory to corticosteroids and even alkylating agent therapy. In patients who are reluctant to use alkylating agents due to their risk of malignancy or gonadal failure, mycophenolate is often an appropriate choice. The dose of mycophenolate I use to treat glomerular diseases (500–2000 mg/d in divided doses) is less than that used for preventing transplant rejection. It is noteworthy that mycophenolate is a relatively new drug with limited published reports on efficacy and long-term safety in treatment of glomerular diseases. The few published reports on its use in glomerulopathies and my group's experience is that it is more potent than azathioprine, and, consequently, it does have therapeutic potential for some patients. Similar to azathioprine, a risk of transient leukopenia and/or thrombocytopenia exists with mycophenolate. Gastrointestinal side effects of mycophenolate include nausea and diarrhea, but the doses usually needed to treat the primary glomerulopathies are generally well tolerated.

*Cyclosporine (Sandimmune)**

The success of cyclosporine in transplantation has supported its use in the control of the glomerulopa-

*Not FDA approved for this indication.

thies. Much of the use of this medication has been in corticosteroid-resistant forms of disease. The usual dose for adults is 5 mg/kg/d in two divided doses. Although cyclosporine can induce improvements or remissions of proteinuria, withdrawal of the medication often causes relapse of proteinuria. A major concern of the chronic use of cyclosporine for treatment of the glomerulopathies is its association with interstitial fibrosis.

Renoprotective Therapies

Renoprotective interventions are therapies designed to preserve kidney function other than the immunosuppressive treatments outlined earlier. Renoprotective interventions should be initiated early in the treatment of glomerular diseases because their effects may be additive to standard immunosuppressive therapy. In some of the glomerulopathies, immunosuppressive therapies are often ineffective and renoprotective therapies may be the only interventions that prolong kidney health.

Renoprotective interventions are founded on an expanding body of literature that demonstrates how a progressive loss of kidney function occurs in many chronic renal diseases after the primary insult is controlled. When glomeruli are diseased and unable to efficiently filter, hyperfiltration of healthy glomeruli can lead to secondary glomerular injury. Renoprotective interventions attempt to temporize this secondary injury while the primary glomerular lesion is allowed to heal.

Many therapies considered as "renoprotective" were historically used to control the complications of glomerulopathies, such as edema formation or hypertension. It is more appropriate to consider these treatments as therapies that improve kidney integrity as well as controlling these complications. These renoprotective interventions are basically focused on improving proteinuria by means of alterations of glomerular hemodynamics. Excessive protein excretion, as well as the excretion of lipids and other immunoreactive compounds present in severe proteinuria, can induce tubule and interstitial damage. Therefore, excessive and prolonged proteinuria is considered not only a marker of kidney disease but a mediator of disease as well. Renoprotective treatment strategies include the following.

Control Systemic Hypertension

Systemic hypertension develops or worsens in glomerular diseases in part due to a diminished ability to excrete sodium and water. Long-term systemic hypertension is associated with progressive loss of kidney function, if renal impairment exists. An aggressive control of blood pressure (<130/85 mm Hg) should be the goal of therapy, as has been suggested in several large clinical trials. For example, in the NIH-sponsored Modification of Diet in Renal Diseases (MDRD) study, loss of kidney function was slower in patients with extremely aggressive systolic blood pressure control (systolic blood pressures <125 mm Hg).

Diuretics and dietary salt restriction are almost always necessary to achieve adequate blood pressure control when glomerulopathies exist. Furthermore, several medication types may be able to lower glomerular hypertension as well as systemic hypertension.

Control Glomerular Hypertension

Lowering glomerular hypertension can lessen proteinuria and theoretically protect against an additional mechanical stress within the hyperfiltering glomerulus. The renin-angiotensin axis is typically activated in renal injury, and this contributes to the increased intraglomerular pressure. Agents that antagonize the renin-angiotensin axis, such as angiotensin converting enzyme (ACE) inhibitors and angiotensin II, type 1, receptor blockers (ARBs), are therefore useful renoprotective therapies. These drugs not only lower glomerular blood pressure, but they also antagonize the profibrotic effects of the growth factor–promoting peptide angiotensin. A benefit of using low doses of these medications may exist in patients without systemic hypertension. Other antihypertensive medications that lower proteinuria include β-blockers and nondihydropyridine calcium channel blockers. Some dihydropyridine calcium channel agents have been shown to deleteriously affect renal afferent arteriole function and increase proteinuria.

The renoprotective benefits of these therapies will largely be negated if systemic hypertension is not controlled. Using an ACE inhibitor, for example, when systemic hypertension remains is not as helpful. Furthermore, the benefits of these medications on glomerular function and improvement of proteinuria may take months to achieve. For example, improvement of nephrotic-range proteinuria of diabetic patients in The Captopril Study, which followed patients with established diabetic nephropathy, took several months to be fully achieved.

Limit Salt Intake

Diets excessive in salt will exacerbate hypertension and edema formation in most of the glomerular diseases. Furthermore, a high-salt diet will increase glomerular hyperfiltration, which can induce secondary mechanical stress to glomerular structures. The antihypertensive and proteinuria-lowering effects of ACE inhibitors and ARBs can be attenuated by high-salt diets. Diuretic use in patients with excessive salt intake can also cause or worsen hypokalemia by presenting abundant cations at the distal tubule, the site of aldosterone effects. Chronic hypokalemia can thereafter stimulate interstitial fibrosis.

Dietary recall is generally ineffective at determining a patient's salt intake. Measuring sodium excretion in a 24-hour urine collection can provide a good indication of salt intake during the 24 hours of collection. Although some sodium is excreted in stool, the amount is minimal and of little clinical importance compared with urine excretion. When evaluating creatinine clearance or proteinuria in a 24-hour urine collection, I typically measure sodium excretion. I do not tell patients we are looking at sodium excretion until after the 24-hour urine is obtained, to prevent the patients from temporarily adjusting their diet. Some laboratories report urine sodium excretion as millimoles per 24 hours. Multiplication of the number of millimoles by 23 equals the number of milligrams of sodium excreted, which reflects the amount of sodium chloride eaten. Sodium not in the form of sodium chloride (such as sodium citrate present in vegetables) contributes minimally to the total sodium excretion in the urine.

Limit Dietary Protein Intake

Diets high in protein are deleterious to kidney function if filtration is impaired. Amino acids from high-protein diets induce glomerular hyperfiltration, which induces mechanical stress and increases proteinuria. The MDRD study demonstrated in patients with chronic renal impairment that benefits in long-term kidney survival are experienced when protein-restricted diets were followed. Protein intake ranging between 0.6 and 0.8 g/kg/d is suggested to confer renoprotection without risking protein malnutrition. The amount of protein a patient eats can be determined with a 24-hour urine measurement of urea. The amount of urea multiplied by 6.25 represents the number of grams of protein metabolized during the 24 hours of collection. This value can be divided by body weight to determine dietary protein intake.

Other Interventions

Other interventions include the control of hyperlipidemia, which is a risk factor for progression of renal and cardiovascular disease. Patients who use nonsteroidal anti-inflammatory drugs (NSAIDs) should also be cautioned about the deleterious renal effects of their excessive, chronic use.

COMPLICATIONS OF PRIMARY GLOMERULOPATHIES AND THEIR TREATMENT

Edema

Lower extremity edema often prompts the initial visit to a physician's office, although the presence of edema is largely a cosmetic concern. Abdominal striae can form when abdominal edema occurs in the setting of a negative nitrogen balance due to extensive proteinuria. Lower extremity edema may be severe enough to compromise normal tissue control of infection and aggressive forms of cellulitis may develop in patients with extensive edema. The tendency to develop edema is in part related to low serum protein levels, which generally reflect elevated urine protein excretion. Edema formation is also dependent on salt intake and compromised salt filtration by the diseased kidney. Many patients may develop edema with modest decreases in serum albumin levels if their dietary salt intake is high, whereas other patients with very low serum albumin levels may be edema free by eating a salt-restricted diet. The foundation of edema control therefore is restriction of dietary salt intake to less than 4 g/d, preferably to 2 g/d. Edema control also frequently requires diuretic use and mechanical compression of lower extremity edema with pressure stockings.

The diuretic regimen that works in the majority of patients is use of adequate doses of a loop diuretic such as furosemide (Lasix, 40–160 mg/d) or bumetanide (Bumex, 2–4 mg/d). Sulfa-allergic patients can be treated with ethacrynic acid. Dosing of furosemide can be twice daily, but to offset the inconvenience of nocturia the second dose can be taken 6 hours after the morning dose. Failure of a loop diuretic to improve and control edema may be due to inadequate dosing. Oral furosemide doses of greater than 80 mg twice daily are commonly needed. Because furosemide works at the luminal side of tubule cells, it has been argued that severe albuminuria may interfere with furosemide effects by intraluminal binding of the drug. Therefore, in patients with extremely high urine protein values, higher doses of furosemide may be needed to induce a natriuresis/diuresis and provide relief of edema. The addition of a thiazide diuretic (HCTZ, 12.5–25 mg/d, or metolazone [Zaroxolyn], 2.5–20 mg/d) may potentiate the effects of a loop diuretic.

Hyperlipidemia

Enhanced liver generation of albumin to offset serum albumin losses is frequently associated with elevations in serum lipid levels. Because the hyperlipidemia of severe proteinuria represents liver production of lipids, dietary interventions and even resin binding agents do not routinely work; however, the use of HMG-CoA reducing agents can control this form of hyperlipidemia. I generally initiate lipid control treatments early in the care of the glomerulopathies because the resolution of proteinuria to normal levels and the reversal of hyperlipidemia is frequently slow. Another reason to control serum lipid levels is the control of lipiduria, which is considered to be a mediator of interstitial fibrosis during severe proteinuria.

Hypercoagulopathy

Naturally occurring serum anticoagulants can be lost in the urine of patients with severe proteinuria, resulting in hypercoagulopathy. Patients at risk include those with membranous glomerulopathy, although other types of glomerulopathy can also give rise to a hypercoagulable state. Generally, patients have severe serum protein losses and serum albumin levels are in the range of 2 g/dL or below when a hypercoagulable predisposition exists. Renal vein thrombosis is a classic form of hypercoagulability, and its occurrence is indicated by an unexpected increase in proteinuria, a marked drop in serum albumin levels, and the development/worsening of lower extremity edema or development of scrotal edema. Magnetic resonance angiography is useful to detect renal vein thrombosis. Heparin therapy followed by warfarin (Coumadin) therapy is indicated until the nephrotic syndrome improves to restore serum protein levels.

Protein Malnutrition

Excessive loss of proteins into the urine can over time result in protein malnutrition. If wasting of serum albumin stores occurs, a tendency to want to feed patients high-protein diets may follow. A paradoxical increase in proteinuria will occur when high-protein diets are prescribed, however. Even when restricting oral protein intake as a renoprotective intervention, one must adjust for the number of grams of protein excreted into the urine. I typically increase daily dietary protein intake gram-for-gram of excreted urine protein. This usually helps prevent the development of protein malnutrition.

Infections

With severe proteinuria, immunoglobulins are lost and circulating immunoglobulin levels are depleted. This may place a patient at risk of developing infections, and often the infections are due to uncommon bacterial or fungal organisms. The extent of hypogammaglobulinemia must be considered when using immunosuppressive agents in patients who are severely proteinuric. Quantitative measurement of serum immunoglobulins, especially IgG, before and during immunosuppressive therapy in patients with extensive nephrotic syndrome is warranted.

SPECIFIC GLOMERULAR DISEASES

Minimal Change Disease

This classification of glomerular disease is based on the apparent absence of anatomic changes within the glomerulus, as assessed by light microscopy. In reality, electron microscopy shows foot process fusion, which occurs in other forms of glomerular injury as well. Other electron microscopic evidence of glomerular injury, such as the presence of fibrils suggestive of amyloidosis or fibrillary glomerulopathy, must be absent in this disease.

Due to alterations in the normal barrier to protein excretion, very large quantities of protein can be excreted in minimal change disease (MCD, nil disease, lupoid nephrosis). This disease has a bimodal distribution, with pediatric and older patients being common patient groups that develop MCD. In general, the urinalysis in MCD is not inflammatory, although hematuria may be present in severe, resistant forms of the disease.

The association of MCD with lymphomas and use of some drugs suggests that a circulating immune-mediated compound(s) may be responsible for at least some forms of the disease. Furthermore, the fascinating corticosteroid responsiveness and corticosteroid dependence of many patients with MCD confirms this as an immune-mediated disorder, likely a T-cell–mediated disorder. MCD can occur in patients taking NSAID medications. Therefore, patients with proteinuria who report daily NSAID use should be evaluated after a 2- to 3-week cessation of NSAIDs.

Most patients with MCD are responsive to corticosteroid therapy. I usually treat patients with prednisone at 1 mg/kg/d, not to exceed 80 mg/d in two divided doses. A prolonged course of prednisone is usually required, and it is recommended to keep doses stable for 6 or more weeks after remission of proteinuria. The prednisone dose can be titrated downward by 20 mg every 2 weeks and very slowly tapered when the daily dose reaches 20 mg/d. A very cautious lowering of prednisone dose is needed below 20 mg/d to prevent relapse of nephrotic-range proteinuria. It is impressive how some MCD patients can be controlled to normal protein excretion, only to rapidly relapse into nephrotic-range proteinuria when the prednisone dose is minimally tapered. Approximately 20% of patients will relapse more than once despite a slow prednisone taper. Frequent relapsers can be given oral cyclophosphamide for 8 to 12 weeks.

MCD has been argued to be a minor form of focal segmental glomerulosclerosis (FSGS). That is, a spectrum of disease may exist represented by MCD on one extreme and FSGS on the other. FSGS lesions may be seen in patients with MCD who have a second biopsy due to recurrence of proteinuria or refractoriness to corticosteroids and immunosuppression. It is therefore appropriate to consider those patients with an aggressive, refractory form of MCD as "at risk" for developing FSGS lesions.

Focal Segmental Glomerulosclerosis

FSGS represents a group of diseases in which some but not all glomeruli of a biopsy specimen are sclerotic and where only a focal area of each glomerulus is sclerotic. FSGS is a histologic lesion of a variety of renal and systemic diseases, and it should often be considered a secondary glomerular lesion. For example, FSGS lesions can occur as a consequence of hypertension in African Americans or of hyperfiltration that occurs in chronic renal failure or obesity. Heroin abuse can also cause FSGS. A unique form of FSGS termed *collapsing glomerulonephritis* (GN) develops in patients with chronic viremia, especially HIV viremia. The podocyte of the glomerulus is the site of initial injury in collapsing GN. Podocyte damage results in the involution of the glomerular capillary tuft and an apparent "collapse" of glomerular structures into a nonfunctioning mass of capillaries. Screening patients with collapsing GN for hepatitis and HIV is appropriate. Prednisone therapy has been advocated in HIV-associated collapsing GN.

FSGS may also be idiopathic and recur in renal transplants. This form of FSGS is similar to MCD and can be responsive to immunosuppressive therapies, although less so than MCD. The treatment of FSGS includes prednisone therapy dosed according to the severity of disease. Moderate-dose prednisone results in improvements in 25% to 30% of patients with normal kidney function. Responses to this prednisone approach suggest a favorable long-term prognosis. When GFR is impaired, proteinuria is severe, or when histologic evidence of kidney scarring exists, high-dose prednisone should be attempted. The long-term use of high-dose prednisone in corticosteroid-resistant FSGS has been reported to improve proteinuria in over half of patients enrolled into therapy. It is noteworthy that one protocol used by Nagai and colleagues is very high-dose prednisone (≥100 mg) on alternate days for 3 to 5 months.[2] This may benefit older patients with FSGS.

Some of the trials using cytotoxic agents such as cyclophosphamide* in FSGS have shown an advantage of this therapy. In some trials, as many as 50% of patients treated with cyclophosphamide showed some improvement in proteinuria. Therefore, I suggest that oral cyclophosphamide for 8 to 12 weeks may benefit some patients with corticosteroid-resistant forms of FSGS. Cyclosporine* has also been used in FSGS. It is suggested that a 6-month cyclosporine treatment, 3.5 mg/kg/d in divided doses, followed by a careful wean of the dose can help control proteinuria in corticosteroid-resistant FSGS. Chronic cyclosporine use does accelerate interstitial fibrosis, which may lessen the long-term renal survival. Therefore, the use of cyclosporine should be considered as a last alternative of FSGS treatment.

The use of renoprotective interventions is extremely important in FSGS because hypertension is common with this disorder and improvement in proteinuria by medications that lower intraglomerular hypertension occurs frequently.

Membranous Glomerulopathy

Membranous glomerulopathy is an immune-mediated disorder in which glomerular capillary membranes, as visualized by light microscopy, are thickened. Electron microscopy of these capillary membranes shows immune complexes at the membrane margins with varying stages of new membrane growth around the immune complexes. Despite the presence of immune complexes, this disorder rarely is associated with inflammation, and urine sediment is generally free of white blood cells or hematuria. The degree of proteinuria is variable, but nephrotic-range proteinuria is common. Only 20% or fewer of membranous glomerulopathy cases will demonstrate less than 2 g proteinuria in 24 hours. This disorder can occur as a complication of SLE, and measuring antinuclear antibodies and complement levels is advisable if membranous glomerulopathy with appropriate immunofluorescent staining is confirmed on kidney biopsy. Several medications and endogenous proteins have been identified as antigens in membranous immune complexes. Therapies for rheumatic diseases that can cause membranous glomerulopathy include pencillamine and gold salts. Nonsteroidal anti-inflammatory drugs (NSAIDs) also can induce membranous lesions. Membranous glomerulopathy that develops in patients with diabetes mellitus is thought to be due to antigenic forms of insulin. Although this is an uncommon development in diabetic patients, an unexpected worsening of proteinuria and/or fall in GFR in a tightly controlled patient with diabetic nephropathy should prompt a search for a separate glomerular lesion, such as a membranous lesion.

Perhaps the most important association with membranous glomerulopathy is malignancy. Tumor proteins are often antigens in the immune complexes of membranous lesions. Importantly, many malignancies are not clinically evident when membranous glomerulopathy is diagnosed on biopsy. A variety of malignancies are more commonly associated with membranous glomerulopathy, including colon, thyroid, pancreas, breast, and lung cancers. A thorough screening for malignancy is indicated in every patient diagnosed with idiopathic membranous GN. The literature reports, and I have seen, patients who successfully undergo chemotherapy for a malignancy resolve their proteinuria and membranous lesions.

Membranous glomerulopathy has a fairly high spontaneous remission rate, and some patients undergo cycles of spontaneous remissions and exacerbations of proteinuria. This has made clinical trials for the treatment of membranous glomerulopathy difficult to interpret. Patients whose disease likely will not spontaneously remit and in whom progression may occur include males, patients with very elevated proteinuria, patients with refractory hypertension, and patients with abnormal GFR. Membranous glomerulopathy that occurs in patients with diabetes may also be unlikely to spontaneously remit given experimental evidence that capillary membrane protein turnover is slowed in the diabetic milieu.

Membranous glomerulopathy responds better to alkylating agents and corticosteroids than corticosteroids alone. It is noteworthy that very high doses of prednisone (100 to 150 mg on alternate days) have been used as monotherapy with some success. However, the protocol constructed by Ponticelli and associates that uses alkylating agents has shown the best long-term outcome and is my preferred method of treating membranous glomerulopathy.[3] The original Ponticelli protocol includes intravenous methylprednisolone for 3 days followed by oral prednisone taper for 4 weeks and then by intravenous or oral chlorambucil* for 4 weeks. The cycle of corticosteroids and alkylating agents can be repeated until remission occurs. Ponticelli and associates have published that cyclophosphamide works as well as chlorambucil. Although patients receive the alkylating agents, they are generally maintained on oral prednisone (0.5 mg/

*Not FDA approved for this indication.

*Not FDA approved for this indication.

kg/d). Treatment of membranous glomerulopathy requires patience. Resolution of the immune complexes at the glomerular capillaries takes several weeks or months. Therefore, improvement in proteinuria is also often slow. Renoprotective interventions that lessen proteinuria are also important treatments.

Membranoproliferative Glomerulonephritis

Lesions of membranoproliferative glomerulonephritis (MPGN, mesangiocapillary glomerulonephritis, or lobular glomerulonephritis [GN]) demonstrate expansion of the number of mesangial cells within the glomerulus and classic capillary basement membrane changes. The deposition of matrix proteins within the glomerulus creates a nodule-like appearance of the glomerular capillary tufts, hence the term *lobular GN.* There are two classic forms of MPGN, classified as type I and type II MPGN based on differences in the location of immune complex deposition seen by electron microscopy. Some pathologists have described a third form of MPGN (type III MPGN). Type III MPGN is the diagnosis given when the histology closely resembles membranous glomerulopathy with increased mesangial cell proliferation, which is atypical of membranous glomerulopathy. Ultrastructurally, this type of MPGN has irregularly thickened glomerular basement membranes with numerous intramembranous deposits. Type III MPGN is otherwise very similar to type I MPGN.

Patients with MPGN lesions present at any age but are often younger than 30 years old when abnormal urinalyses are noted. Often the courses of these diseases are insidious, and most patients who present with MPGN have mild hematuria, proteinuria, and elevated serum creatinine values. In approximately half of patients, nephrotic-range proteinuria occurs. Hypertension is very common. An acute nephritic attack with gross hematuria can be the reason for referral to a physician. Many cases follow an upper respiratory tract infection, and sometimes an elevated antistreptolysin-O (ASO) titer is seen. The MPGN lesions are associated with depressed serum complement levels, particularly C3. C4 is usually depressed in type I MPGN but may be normal in type II MPGN. A rise in ASO titer and low C3 value often leads to the suspicion that a patient's proteinuria and loss of GFR is due to poststreptococcal glomerulonephritis (PSGN). However, MPGN has chronically depressed C3 values and recovery does not occur as in PSGN.

MPGN type I is associated with hepatitis C infections with and without cryoglobulinemia. The cryoglobulinemia associated with hepatitis C infections includes an IgM rheumatoid factor. Patients with nephritis, proteinuria, and low C3 values should have a full hepatitis C panel and rheumatoid factor and cryoglobulins measured. Interferon alfa (Intron A) therapy is reported to control MPGN associated with hepatitis C, and it may be worthwhile offering this therapy to affected patients even if histologic evidence of liver damage is absent.

Except for hepatitis-associated MPGN, the ability to control and reverse MPGN lesions is very difficult. Spontaneous remissions are reported, but many patients progress to end-stage renal disease. The majority of patients with nephrotic-range proteinuria progress to end-stage renal disease within 10 years. Controlled trials using prednisone and cyclophosphamide have not shown clear-cut benefits of immunosuppressive therapy in MPGN. It is reasonable to attempt to attenuate MPGN with moderate dosing of prednisone, administered every other day, and to offer renoprotective therapies to slow the progression to end-stage renal disease.

IgA Nephritis

IgA nephritis (IgAN) is the most common glomerulopathy in the world, although it is less common in North America. Patients with IgAN present with nephritic urine sediment and, at times, severe proteinuria. The disease is a spectrum that ranges from minimal hematuria in some patients to severe hematuria, nephrotic-range proteinuria, and rapid declines in GFR in others. Variability in clinical course range within the same patients, and many who are clinically silent for years can develop severe renal compromise in a short period of time. The cause of IgAN remains unknown, although flares of hematuria, proteinuria, and GFR decline typically follow within days of mucosal inflammation/infection, especially upper respiratory tract infections. On kidney biopsy, IgA staining within the mesangium of the glomerulus is typical, although not exclusive, of IgAN. Mesangial cell proliferation is also increased, as is glomerulosclerosis, although the mechanisms connecting the IgA deposition to these glomerular changes remain undetermined. Two interesting infections are associated with IgAN. First, reports of an association with *Haemophilus parainfluenzae* infection and IgAN flares have been made. It is argued that this bacterial infection may be one antigenic stimulus of IgAN flares. Second, patients with prolonged methicillin-resistant *Staphylococcus aureus* (MRSA) infections can develop IgAN and eradication of the MRSA infection may prevent renal impairment.

Immunosuppression may not be successful in many patients with IgAN. Immunosuppressive therapy should be reserved for those with risk factors of progression (male sex, hypertension, and nephrotic-range proteinuria). Severe histologic lesions on renal biopsy are another indication to attempt immunosuppression. IgAN is one glomerular disease in which glomerular crescents can be seen and, for this reason, kidney biopsies should be performed when IgAN is suggested, or even repeat biopsy if IgAN is known, if renal function deteriorates and/or proteinuria is in the nephrotic range. Alternate-day, moderate-dose prednisone can be attempted for short periods (months). Alkylating agents do not appear to be helpful in IgAN. Trials with omega fatty acids have shown promise in controlling IgAN flares. The control of mucosal infections, which are recognized as inducers of IgAN flares, is important. Early treatment of pharyngitis with oral antibiotics, including those that treat *H. parainfluenzae* (amoxicillin) is appropriate. Recurrent diarrheas should alert for a workup of celiac sprue, which occurs in a higher percentage of patients with IgAN. A gluten-free diet may improve the sprue and limit IgAN flares. Patients with recurrent cystitis may also experience IgAN flares, and suppressive antibiotics to limit cystitis may also he helpful.

Rapidly Progressive Glomerulonephritis

Rapidly progressive GN (RPGN) is an older classification of those glomerular diseases that cause a rapid fall in kidney function, usually associated with glomerular crescent formation. Usually, these diseases cause a 50% fall of kidney function in less than 3 months, although in many patients the loss of function occurs within days or weeks. The term *RPGN* is often mistaken as "crescentic GN," but several glomerular diseases can cause crescent formation with slower rates of GFR loss. Alternatively, rapid loss of glomerular function can occur without crescent formation, as in patients with collapsing FSGS and thrombotic thrombocytopenic purpura. Rarely, glomerular diseases without much immune-mediated damage (e.g., diabetic nephropathy) have been shown to develop crescents.

Crescents develop by two mechanisms. When capillary integrity is lost, serum components stimulate epithelial cells of the Bowman capsule to proliferate. Second, if the Bowman capsule loses its integrity, interstitial macrophages can migrate into the urinary space and contribute to crescent formation. Treatment of cellular crescents before they are replaced by fibrosis is a goal in the crescentic glomerulopathies.

Three important forms of RPGN exist: anti–glomerular basement membrane–associated RPGN (type I crescentic GN); crescent formation due to immune-complex deposition, as occurs in SLE and other connective tissue diseases (type II); and pauci-immune crescent formation, which may or may not be associated with positive antineutrophil cytoplasmic antibody (ANCA) (type III). To discriminate among these three forms of RPGN, immunofluorescent staining and electron microscopy of kidney biopsy specimens are needed.

Given that all three forms of RPGN are mediated by some component of the immune system, patients often present with symptoms of systemic inflammation: low-grade fevers, fatigue, arthralgias, loss of appetite, and weight loss. In patients with anti–glomerular basement membrane–associated RPGN, lung hemorrhage may occur (Goodpasture syndrome). The lung hemorrhage of Goodpasture syndrome can be severe and require ventilator support to ensure adequate oxygenation. An association of smoking and Goodpasture syndrome is noteworthy and a reason to advise patients with this form of RPGN to stop smoking. In pauci-immune GN, sinopulmonary complaints and cavitary lung lesions may develop, even in patients with end-stage kidney disease.

The urinalyses of patients with RPGNs can vary from severe proteinuria, pyuria, and hematuria with white and red blood cell casts to minimal proteinuria and minimal hematuria. Complement levels are low in immune-complex–associated forms of RPGN but are generally normal in other forms. Sedimentation rates and C-reactive protein levels, however, are often quite elevated. Measurement of serum anti–glomerular basement antibody levels to pursue a diagnosis of type I RPGN is sometimes helpful, but often the elevated levels return after a diagnosis is made on histologic findings of a kidney biopsy.

Treatment strategies of these three forms of RPGN differ enough to warrant a timely kidney biopsy to ensure a proper diagnosis. Cellular crescents may respond to high-dose corticosteroids but, if the crescents have become fibrotic, aggressive corticosteroid use may not be warranted. After an extensive search for infections, patients may be given 3 days of intravenous methylprednisolone (800 mg/d) and then oral prednisone at a starting dose of 1 mg/kg ideal body weight. Patients with linear IgG of capillary membranes that suggests the presence of anti–glomerular basement membrane antibody should be treated with plasma exchange to remove circulating antibody. Immune-complex–associated RPGN may also respond to immunosuppressive therapy with cyclophosphamide* or chlorambucil.* Similarly, patients with pauci-immune RPGN often respond to several-week courses of moderate-dose prednisone and low-dose daily oral cyclophosphamide. Unlike in membranous glomerulopathy, ANCA vasculitis often requires longer courses of alkylating agent treatment (e.g., several months of low-dose daily oral cyclophosphamide*). Recent reports suggest mycophenolate* may be able to control glomerular injury of some patients with ANCA vasculitis. Given the cumulative effects of alkylating agents, it is reasonable to attempt to convert patients with pauci-immune RPGN to mycophenolate for chronic treatment after control of the glomerulopathy is achieved by an alkylating agent. In those patients who are ANCA positive, following ANCA titers can offer a general idea of the efficacy of immunosuppressive therapy, but changes of ANCA titers often lag behind remission and recurrence of disease. A role of neutrophil priming by infections in ANCA vasculitides suggests that investigating for and treating bacterial infections is appropriate. Sinopulmonary forms of ANCA vasculitis can respond to prophylactic antibiotic therapies, but renal manifestations of ANCA vasculitis do not usually respond well to prophylactic antibiotics.

---

*Not FDA approved for this indication.

REFERENCES

1. Lewis EJ, Hunsicker LG, Lau SP, et al: For the lupus collaboration study group: A controlled trial of plasmapheresis in severe lupus nephritis. N Engl J Med 326:1373–1379, 1992.
2. Nagai R, Cattran DC, Pei Y: Steroid therapy and prognosis of focal segmental glomerulosclerosis in the elderly. Clin Nephrol 42:18–21, 1994.
3. Ponticelli C, Zucchelli P, Passerini P, et al: A randomized trial of methylprednisolone and chlorambucil in idiopathic membranous nephropathy. N Engl J Med 320:8–13, 1989.

ACUTE PYELONEPHRITIS

method of
KURT A. McCAMMON, M.D., and
CAROL F. McCAMMON, M.D.
Eastern Virginia Medical School
Norfolk, Virginia

Infection of the renal parenchyma and pelvis with associated inflammation is characteristic of acute pyelonephritis. Most patients presenting will complain of fever, chills, and flank pain (most commonly unilateral). Some experience gastrointestinal distress, such as nausea, vomiting, and diarrhea, and up to 75% report current or recent dysuria, frequency, or urgency. Physical findings include fever and generally ill appearance. Costovertebral angle (CVA) tenderness can be elicited, and mild abdominal tenderness is often present. Although the majority of patients may successfully be treated as outpatients, it is important to remember that inadequate or delayed eradication of infection can result in serious sequelae.

ETIOLOGY

The most common pathogens causing acute pyelonephritis are aerobic gram-negative bacteria. Most cases result from ascending lower urinary tract infections (UTIs); therefore, the etiologic agents parallel. Nearly 85% of community-acquired cases of acute pyelonephritis result from *Escherichia coli.* Other less common pathogens include *Proteus, Klebsiella, Enterococcus,* and *Staphylococcus saprophyticus.* Nosocomial infections are predominantly caused by *E. coli* as well (only ~50%) and other pathogens include (in order of frequency) *Enterococcus, Klebsiella, Enterobacter, Citrobacter, Serratia, Pseudomonas aeruginosa,* and *Staphylococcus epidermidis.*

PATHOGENS

The susceptible host frequently develops acute pyelonephritis from the lower urinary tract. Colonization of the perineum by the intruding organism may be the initial event. If untreated at the lower urinary tract level, the organism may further ascend the urinary tract via the ureters to the renal pelvis and renal parenchyma, resulting in the clinical manifestations of acute pyelonephritis. This retrograde progression may result from the presence of fimbriae on the surface of many bacteria that invade the urinary tract. Eighty percent of cases of acute pyelonephritis have culture-proven fimbriated organisms.

Hematogenous seeding of the renal parenchyma from a remote site of infection causes pyelonephritis in only about 5% of cases. These patients will more frequently exhibit bilateral flank pain and CVA tenderness, and sources other than the urinary tract must be sought and appropriately treated. Individuals at risk include those immunocompromised from chronic illness, those undergoing immunosuppressive therapy, and those with a history of intravenous drug use. A gram-positive bacterial urine culture is nearly always a result of a blood-borne, distant infection.

EPIDEMIOLOGY

Women are most frequently affected by acute pyelonephritis because the average woman has a 50% chance of developing a lower UTI in her lifetime. Only 2% of these lower UTIs are found to ascend. Pregnancy adds a significant risk, particularly in the second and third trimesters, when ureteral compression and urinary stasis from the enlarging uterus play anatomic roles in establishing urinary infection. For this reason, treatment of asymptomatic bacteriuria is recommended in pregnant women.

In children, vesicoureteral reflux and anatomic anomalies are most often associated with the development of pyelonephritis.

ANCILLARY TESTING

Urinalysis and urine culture are indicated before institution of antibiotic therapy because pyelonephritis, by definition, is a complicated UTI. Urinalysis and urine culture require adequate clean urine; in females, a catheterized specimen is recommended. The urinalysis frequently shows pyuria, bacteria, esterase, and nitrates. It should not contain epithelial cells, which indicate contamination and are not adequate for culture.

White blood cell casts are often seen in the setting of acute pyelonephritis. Taking blood for complete blood cell count and culture should also be considered because the

TABLE 1. **Oral Antibiotic Regimens for Outpatient Treatment**

Primary	Alternative
Ciprofloxacin (Cipro)* 500 mg bid	Amoxicillin/clavulanate (Augmentin)* 875 mg bid
Norfloxacin (Noroxin)* 400 mg bid	Cephalexin (Keflex)* 500 mg tid-qid
Ofloxacin (Floxin)* 400 mg bid	Cefadroxil (Duricef)* 1–2 g divided bid
Levofloxacin (Levaquin) 250 mg qd	Cefaclor (Ceclor) 250–500 mg tid
Lomefloxacin (Maxaquin)* 400 mg qd	Cefprozil (Cefzil)* 250–500 mg qd
Enoxacin (Penetrex)* 400 mg bid	Cefdinir (Omnicef)* 600 mg qd
	Cefixime (Suprax)* 400 mg qd
	Cefpodoxime (Vantin)* 100–400 mg bid
	Ceftibuten (Cedax)* 400 mg qd

*Not FDA approved for this indication.

No Criteria for Complicated Acute Pyelonephritis

Collect adequate urine specimen for culture
↓
Initiate oral antibiotic/oral antipyretic/analgesic therapy
↓
Re-evaluate at 72 h; check urine culture
↓
If successful progress, continue therapy 14–21 d
↓
Repeat urine culture after completion of course for test of cure

Figure 1. Treatment algorithm for uncomplicated acute pyelonephritis

white blood cell count can be followed for signs of response to treatment along with clinical progress. The blood culture is useful in the treatment of particularly ill-appearing patients, and 20% to 30% of patients will have a positive blood culture. Renal function should also be ascertained because acute pyelonephritis may cause renal dysfunction in severely affected patients, those with co-morbid conditions, or those with a single kidney. Antibiotic choice and further radiographic evaluation may be altered in the patient with a disturbance in renal function. Empirical treatment should promptly begin while awaiting culture results.

Patients with significant co-morbid conditions and those who do not respond well to initial antimicrobial therapy should be considered for radiographic evaluation. Indications include pyelonephritis in pregnancy, history of urolithiasis, prior genitourinary surgery, recurrent pyelonephritis, prepubescent age, fever for more than 5 to 7 days without appropriate medical evaluation, and elderly patients. Intravenous pyelogram (IVP) is the initial study of choice in the nonpregnant patient with adequate renal function. IVP will demonstrate segmental or global renal enlargement, delay in nephrogram, anatomic anomalies, and/or urinary tract obstruction. However, 75% of studies prove normal.

The advantage of ultrasound (US) is that it is less invasive, safe in pregnancy, and will not disturb renal function; however, it may not provide as much information as IVP. It is very sensitive in identifying the presence of perinephric or intrarenal abscess, segmental renal abnormalities, and hydronephrosis and may detect larger renal calculi.

TABLE 2. **Criteria for Complicated Pyelonephritis (Consider Admission)**

Anatomic or functional urinary tract abnormalities
Immunocompromised host
Prepubertal age
Pregnancy
Male gender
Sepsis
Nausea and vomiting
Significant co-morbid conditions

Computed tomography is recommended for patients who do not respond to adequate therapy after 3 days of treatment or who have had IVP and US evaluations that did not provide adequate information.

MANAGEMENT

First, it must be determined whether the patient has a complicated or uncomplicated case of acute pyelonephritis. Patients with uncomplicated cases of acute pyelonephritis are treated as outpatients (Figure 1). After an adequate urinalysis and culture are sent, the patient can be started on oral antibiotics, most often a fluoroquinolone or other antibiotic with similar coverage (Table 1). Antipyretics, analgesia, and fluids are recommended. The patient should be re-evaluated in 72 hours and, if the patient is appropriately improving, may continue outpatient treatment for 14 to 21 days. At the end of treatment, the patient should return for repeat urinalysis and culture to prove complete adequate treatment. If this culture is positive, re-treatment with an appropriately targeted antibiotic should be started and radiographic evaluation of the urinary tract considered. Nonsteroidal anti-inflammatory drugs and corticosteroids may potentially decrease renal scarring, and

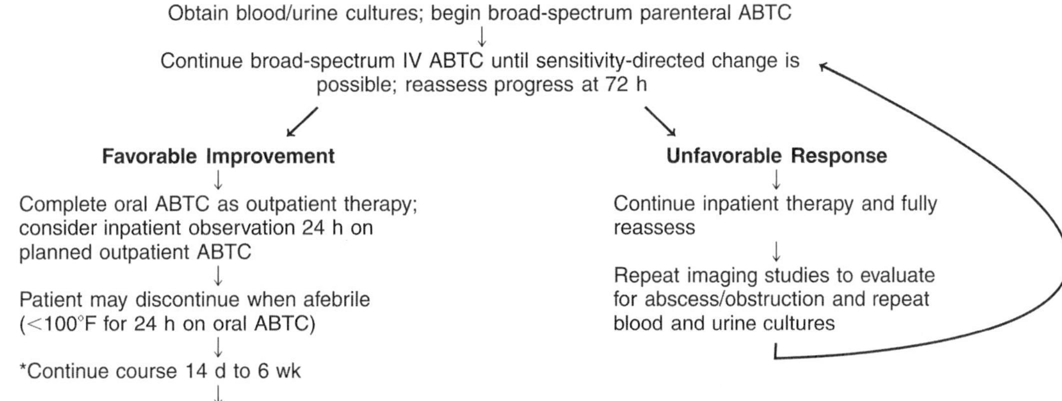

Figure 2. Treatment algorithm for complicated acute pyelonephritis. *Prolonged courses are typical for patients with underlying prostatitis, with indwelling foreign body, and after genitourinary surgical procedure. *Abbreviation:* ABTC = antibiotic.

TABLE 3. **Intravenous Antibiotic Regimens for Inpatient Treatment**

Primary	Alternative
Ciprofloxacin* 400 mg q12 h	Ticarcillin/clavulanate (Timentin)* 3.1 g q4–6 h
Levofloxacin 250–500 mg q24 h	Ampicillin/sulbactam (Unasyn)* 1.5–3 g q6 h
Ofloxacin* 200–400 mg q12 h	Piperacillin/tazobactam (Zosyn) 3.375 g q6 h
Ampicillin 1–2 g q4–6 h plus gentamicin 1 mg/kg q8 h	
Ceftriaxone (Rocephin)* 1 g q24 h	
Ceftizoxime (Cefizox)* 1–2 g q8–12 h	
Ceftazidime (Fortaz)* 1–2 g q8–12 h	
Cefotaxime (Claforan)* 1–2 g q6–8 h	

*For gram-positive organisms, consider adding vancomycin 1 g q12 h.

investigation of their use in this setting is currently underway.

Patients with complicated cases of acute pyelonephritis should be strongly considered for inpatient treatment with at least 3 days of intravenous antibiotics (Table 2 and Figure 2). These patients are at risk for serious sequelae in the face of treatment failure and should be monitored closely. After adequate urinalysis and culture, the patient should promptly be started on an intravenous broad-spectrum antibiotic regimen (Table 3). The patient should have a complete blood cell count, blood culture, and creatinine level drawn. Supportive measures of intravenous fluids, antipyretics, analgesia, and antiemetics should be administered. Radiographic evaluation in the hemodynamically stable patient should be considered early in the course of treatment. If the patient's fever abates and he or she clinically improves within 72 hours, the patient may be switched to a tailored oral regimen. A further day of observation is recommended to make certain the patient remains afebrile. If the patient does not improve within 72 hours, review cultures and sensitivity and perform studies to rule out renal abscess, perinephric abscess, urinary tract obstruction, or other abnormality. If any are present, appropriate management by a urologist is indicated.

MANAGEMENT IN PREGNANCY

Obstetric/gynecologic consultation in these patients is appropriate in management of acute pyelonephritis. Antibiotic regimens that are category B or C are acceptable under most circumstances, provided the patient has no allergies.

SPECIAL PEDIATRIC CONSIDERATIONS

Pediatric patients with acute pyelonephritis are highly likely to have urinary tract anomalies. These patients must have radiographic evaluation to include renal US and voiding cystourethrography to further evaluate the anatomy of the urinary tract. Once initial infection is eradicated, the patient should be maintained on daily antibiotic suppressive therapy until it is deemed unnecessary by the urologist or until the abnormality is appropriately corrected.

COMPLICATIONS

Aggressive early treatment of acute pyelonephritis prevents most complications of the disease. However, patients who are inadequately treated or who present late in a fulminant process can suffer significant complications, including sepsis and death. Emphysematous pyelonephritis is a rare form and occurs primarily in diabetics. It is a fulminant, necrotizing infection, commonly caused by *E. coli.* An examination of the kidney, ureter, and bladder may show air in the nephric shadow. The involved kidney functions poorly; therefore, an IVP is not helpful in confirming the diagnosis. Emphysematous pyelonephritis is an indication for emergency nephrectomy. Percutaneous drainage may be helpful in the appropriate clinical setting.

Renal and perinephric abscess should be evaluated by a urologist and may respond to antibiotics alone. Some may require percutaneous or surgical drainage or possibly nephrectomy.

Chronic renal scarring may lead to hypertension. Recurrent episodes can cause enough scar formation to contribute to chronic renal failure.

GENITOURINARY TRAUMA

method of
KEY H. STAGE, M.D., and
ARTHUR I. SAGALOWSKY, M.D.
University of Texas Southwestern Medical Center at Dallas
Dallas, Texas

In the United States, trauma is the leading cause of death among individuals under the age of 45. The most common cause of trauma is motor vehicle collision, and twice as many males as females are involved. Vehicle collision is also the most common cause of blunt trauma to the bladder and a significant cause of genitourinary (GU) trauma overall.

GU trauma is divided into either blunt or penetrating injury. Blunt trauma accounts for more than 90% of all renal injuries, and renal injury occurs in approximately

10% of patients who sustain abdominal trauma. Assessment of GU trauma may require clinical staging, radiologic evaluation, and surgical exploration. Clinical staging necessitates careful history, physical examination, urinalysis, and appropriate radiologic evaluation to determine the extent of injury. Radiologic assessment is obtained for any trauma patient who demonstrates gross hematuria, blunt trauma with microscopic hematuria and documented hypotension (systolic blood pressure <90 mm Hg), or penetrating trauma in proximity to GU structures. We also use it with all patients under age 16 who display any degree of microscopic hematuria associated with blunt or penetrating trauma.

Initial physical examination is crucial. A flank hematoma in a patient with blunt trauma suggests parenchymal renal injury and perirenal hematoma. A perineal butterfly hematoma in the presence of pelvic fracture implies posterior urethral injury. Speculum examination of female patients may reveal urethral injury or vaginal laceration. Rectal examination is important to check for rectal injury as well as assessment of the prostate gland. A high riding or nonpalpable prostate gland due to the presence of a large pelvic hematoma occurs following avulsion of the posterior urethra in patients with blunt trauma. Blood at the penile meatus requires a retrograde urethrogram to exclude urethral injury. The presence of gross hematuria in the Foley catheter mandates complete imaging of the urinary tract.

RENAL INJURY

Renal injuries occur in approximately 10% of patients sustaining abdominal trauma. Our standard radiologic evaluation of the GU tract consists of rapid infusion computed tomography (CT) using 2 mL/kg of intravenous contrast material, which is followed by CT cystography using a gravity fill technique of at least 300 mL of dilute contrast material via a Foley catheter. After the cystogram is obtained and the bladder is drained, the abdomen and pelvis should be rescanned to check for renal function and late extravasation of contrast material from the upper tracts. If emergency surgery precludes CT evaluation, a one-shot intravenous pyelogram can be obtained in the operating suite. CT is the gold standard for urinary tract imaging in trauma patients. A prompt nephrogram confirms renal blood flow and excludes complete renal artery occlusion. A delayed or absent nephrogram might be indicative of a renovascular injury or severe arterial spasm due to massive parenchymal injury.

CT allows detailed classification of the extent of renal injury and directs treatment. Pelvic hematoma and fractures on CT suggest a strong likelihood of bladder rupture or posterior urethral injury (see the following discussion).

Renal injuries are classified by severity (grade I–V) according to guidelines established by the 1989 American Association for the Surgery of Trauma (Figure 1). Grade I injuries represent simple renal contusions or small subcapsular hematomas. Grade II injuries involve a small cortical laceration with coexisting perirenal hematoma. Grade III injuries

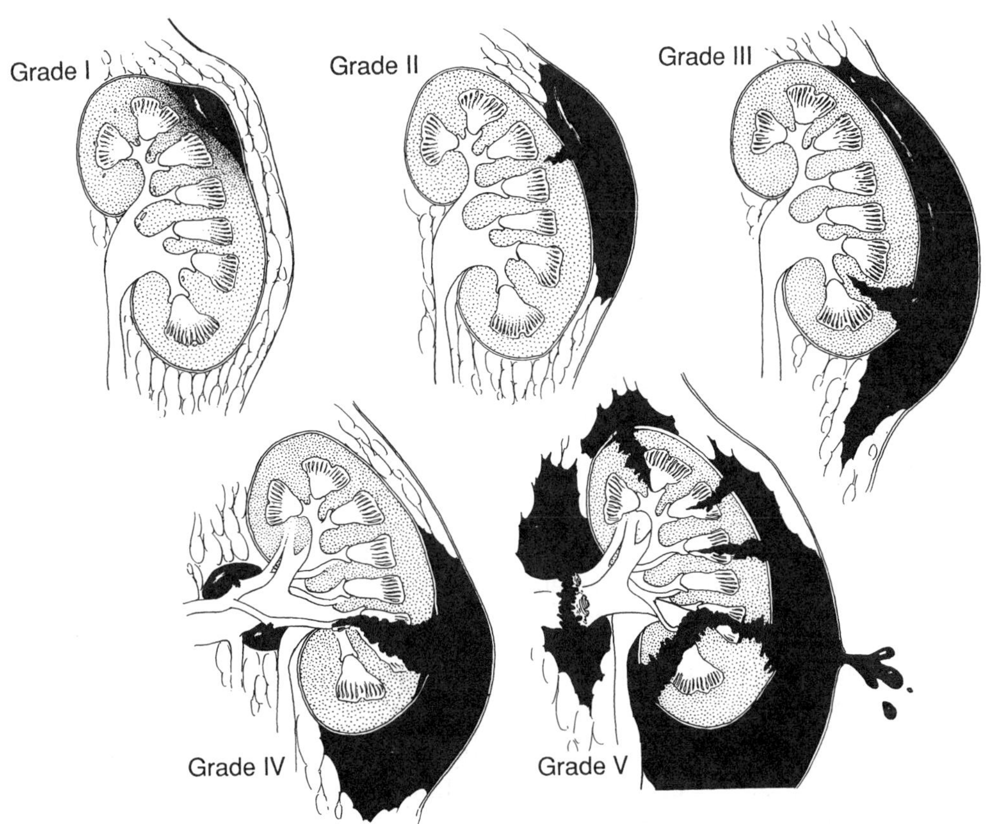

Figure 1. Classification of renal injury. (From Miller KS, McAninch JW: Indications for radiographic assessment in suspected renal trauma. In McAninch JW [ed]: Traumatic and Reconstructive Surgery. Philadelphia, WB Saunders, 1996, p 90.)

are cortical lacerations greater than 1 cm in depth, but without urinary extravasation of contrast material. Grade IV renal injuries are lacerations that extend into the collecting system with extravasation, or they may represent partial or segmental renal artery vein injuries with a contained perinephric hematoma. A grade V injury is a totally shattered kidney or complete avulsion of the renal pedicle. Fortunately, most renal injuries are secondary to blunt trauma. Less than 5% of these injuries require formal exploration, and only conservative management is required in most grade I, II, and III injuries.

Absolute indications for exploration of blunt renal trauma, especially in the hemodynamically unstable patient, include an expanding or pulsatile upper retroperitoneal hematoma. Nearly all penetrating injuries associated with hematuria should be surgically explored. Exploration may be avoided if adequate staging with CT scan suggests that there is a low-grade renal injury and a low risk for other nonrenal injuries, corroborated by findings such as a nontender abdomen, lack of bowel thickening on CT, negative peritoneal lavage, or normal abdominal sonography. This is especially true with stab wounds confined to the flank.

The relative indications for renal exploration are somewhat controversial and include incomplete preoperative staging, significant urinary extravasation due to a deep parenchymal laceration, presence of nonviable tissue from blunt or penetrating trauma, and arterial thrombosis (most commonly seen secondary to a deceleration injury with intimal tear to the renal artery). Warm ischemia time longer than 6 hours should mitigate against acute exploration because there is an extremely low salvage rate of kidneys with delayed operative exploration. However, exploration should be performed, regardless of warm ischemia time, in patients with renal artery injuries who either have a solitary kidney, bilateral renal artery thrombosis, or severely reduced overall renal function. The severity of accompanying nonrenal injuries often precludes prolonged and complex renovascular repair.

Renal exploration for trauma is performed through a midline vertical incision both for speed and because of the need for formal exploratory laparotomy. Nephrectomy is required most often for a fractured kidney with massive bleeding or little remaining viable parenchyma. Prior isolation of the renal pedicle allows for assessment and repair of lesser injuries without initial sudden hemorrhage, which might otherwise result in urgent nephrectomy. Débridement and/or partial amputation is performed for polar injuries. Débridement and wedge resection are common for mid-portion renal injury. Openings into the collecting system are carefully closed and may be identified by administration of intravenous indigo carmine. Defects in the renal parenchyma are addressed by a variety of techniques, including the use of absorbable gelatin sponges with bolsters, the argon beam coagulator, omental pedicle flap for defect coverage, and the occasional use of an absorbable mesh wrap, which is placed around the kidney to aid the renal repair and control hemorrhage. Main arterial injuries can be repaired with segmental resection and anastomosis or with the use of vein interposition grafts. Renal vein injuries are most commonly oversewn and controlled with 5-0 vascular sutures. Early complications of renal trauma can include hemorrhage, abscess, urinary extravasation, and sepsis. Late complications, such as hypertension, may be caused by external compression of the kidney by a surrounding hematoma. Arteriovenous fistulas may occur, especially after penetrating trauma, and can be treated with selective embolization by the interventional radiology team.

URETERAL INJURY

Ureteral injuries are uncommon and comprise less than 1% of all urologic trauma. Yet, they merit attention because they can cause significant morbidity if unrecognized. Eighty percent to 90% of ureteral injuries are associated with only microscopic hematuria, which means that unilateral ureteral injury may easily be missed even with appropriate preoperative staging radiographs. Consequences of a missed ureteral injury include urinoma, abscess, stricture, or fistula. Principles of ureteral repair include débridement of ischemic tissue and creation of a tension-free spatulated anastomosis with end-to-end approximation of mucosal and adventitial tissue. Generally, indwelling double-J ureteral stents are used in the repair, and a closed suction drain is placed.

Disruption of the ureteropelvic junction is a rare injury and is more common among children due to their greater musculoskeletal flexibility. High-speed injuries with hyperextension and rapid deceleration are the cause. Proximal ureteral injuries are most common secondary to penetrating trauma. A spatulated end-to-end ureteroureterostomy is completed over an indwelling double-J ureteral stent when possible. In other types of ureteral injury, the defect may be too long for primary repair, such as with a shotgun blast or other massive injury. If primary re-anastomosis is not possible, the ureter may simply be ligated, and a percutaneous nephrostomy tube placed postoperatively in the interventional radiology suite. A formal nephrostomy tube is almost never indicated at the time of the initial trauma exploration.

Injuries to the mid-ureter can be challenging. Some injuries may allow direct ureteroureterostomy, occasionally incorporating caudal mobilization of the kidney to gain proximal ureteral length. If the defect is too long to allow a tension-free direct anastomosis of the mid-ureter, reimplantation can almost always be accomplished either by mobilizing the bladder alone (psoas muscle bladder hitch) or by combining this maneuver with the creation of an elongated flap of the bladder wall (Boari-Ockerblad flap).

Injuries to the distal ureter require ureteral reimplantation; end-to-end ureteroureterostomy should be discouraged in this area. In a ureteral reimplantation, the distal end of the ureter is débrided, spatulated, and reimplanted in an antireflux fashion into the bladder. Once again, the repair is accomplished over a double-J ureteral stent.

When a patient suffers from massive trauma and is extremely unstable, there may not be time to address formal ureteral repair. The ureter may simply be catheterized with a 5-French to 8-French pediatric feeding tube after débridement of the traumatized distal end. The stent is secured by a ligature around the distal ureter and simply brought out in the lateral quadrant of the skin as a temporary intubated urostomy.

BLADDER TRAUMA

Blunt trauma to the bladder most commonly results from motor vehicle collision, motor-pedestrian collision, or crush injury that is associated with pelvic fracture. Penetrating trauma is caused by stab or gunshot wound, or direct perforation of the bladder from a bony spicule associated with a pelvic fracture and crush injury. Although nearly all bladder injuries from blunt trauma are associated with a pelvic fracture, the reverse is not true; the vast majority of pelvic fractures are not associated with a bladder injury.

CT cystography is invaluable in the diagnosis of intraperitoneal or extraperitoneal bladder injury. An intraperitoneal bladder rupture is diagnosed when contrast material is seen outlining loops of bowel. This should be treated with formal exploration, cystorrhaphy, and drainage with either a suprapubic cystostomy or Foley catheter. Extraperitoneal extravasation most often is associated with blunt trauma and pelvic fracture. These injuries may be treated conservatively with Foley catheter drainage alone.

POSTERIOR URETHRAL INJURY

Posterior urethral injuries are most commonly seen with pelvic fractures and should be suspected when blood is seen at the urethral meatus. In the presence of this finding, retrograde urethrography should be done before attempts at inserting a Foley catheter. Posterior urethral injuries may involve either partial or complete disruption of the posterior urethra at the level of the pelvic diaphragm. Management consists of formal placement of a suprapubic tube for urinary diversion alone, or placement of a suprapubic tube in combination with an attempt at primary urethral alignment at surgery.

Direct open formal re-anastomosis and acute repair of posterior urethral injury in the presence of significant pelvic hematoma and pelvic fracture should be discouraged. There is significant risk of bleeding and a low rate of success. Postoperative stricture rates are somewhat lower if primary realignment can be accomplished. During open surgical repair of the bladder, catheters may be passed gently via retrograde urethral and antegrade passage across the bladder neck, joined to establish an intact bladder catheter through the urethra. Four to 6 months should elapse before performing posterior urethroplasty for repair of residual urethral stricture. Complications of posterior urethral injury associated with pelvic fracture include incontinence, erectile dysfunction, and stricture. These complications are usually caused by the injury itself and not as a result of gentle intraoperative attempts at primary urethral alignment.

ANTERIOR URETHRAL INJURY

Anterior urethral injuries can occur from blunt trauma, penetrating trauma, or factitiously placed foreign bodies. A retrograde urethrogram may be used to assess the anterior urethra for trauma. Small crush injuries with or without partial tears may be treated by simple urinary diversion with a percutaneous suprapubic cystostomy or a urethral catheter. Blast effect from gunshot injury must be taken into account. Débridement of nonviable urethral margins should be performed, and a spatulated end-to-end repair done over a urethral catheter using interrupted absorbable sutures.

EXTERNAL GENITALIA TRAUMA

The etiology of penile injury varies. Strangulation, or even necrosis, may occur from factitious application of various devices such as tools, rings, or even condom catheters. Blunt injuries may result from falls, motor vehicle collisions, or power take-off injuries, and penetrating trauma frequently includes gunshot or stab wounds.

Diagnosis of penile trauma mainly rests with the physical examination. The integrity of Buck's fascia will determine a particular pattern to the hematoma. If Buck's fascia remains intact, the hematoma will be limited to the shaft of the penis (Figure 2); if Buck's fascia is violated by the injury, extravasation may extend proximally into Colles' fascia, resulting in the characteristic butterfly hematoma (Figure 3).

Management of penile injury most commonly involves surgical exploration. If a corporal injury is suspected, a circumferential incision is made around the coronal sulcus, and the penis is degloved to expose both corporal bodies. Anterior urethral injuries secondary to penetrating trauma also may be exposed ventrally on the penis by extending the incision into the perineum if necessary. End-to-end spatulated urethral anastomosis or repair of lacerations is accomplished using an absorbable suture.

Injury that degloves the penis is often a result of an accident involving power machinery. Part or all of the penile skin may be avulsed, and there may be violation of the scrotum that exposes the testicles. Wound repair includes débridement of ischemic and nonviable tissue and an attempt to cover the defect using the scrotal flaps. If lack of adequate skin precludes wound coverage, the testicles may be temporarily placed in bilateral subcutaneous thigh pouches for later reconstruction.

Partial or complete amputation of the penis may

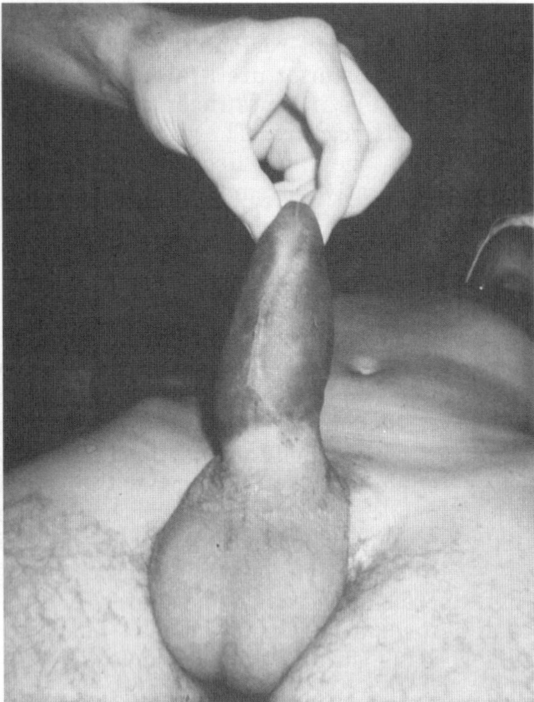

Figure 2. Penile hematoma confined to Buck's fascia. (From Sagalowsky AI, Peters PC: Genitourinary trauma. In Walsh PC, Retik AB, Vaughan ED Jr [eds]: Campbell's Urology, 7th ed. Philadelphia, WB Saunders, 1998, p 3113.)

result either from trauma or self-inflicted injury. If possible, the severed distal portion of the penis should be retrieved and placed in ice for possible microvascular reconstruction. Although erectile function may not return, the cosmetic appearance of the penis may be maintained in most circumstances and makes efforts to accomplish re-anastomosis worthwhile. Success of penile reimplantation is highest when the length of warm ischemia time is less than 12 hours.

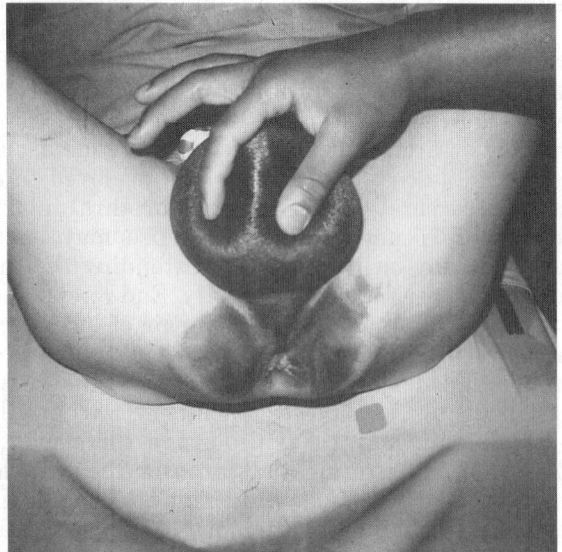

Figure 3. Pelvic hematoma extending through Colles' fascia, giving the classic butterfly appearance. (From Sagalowsky AI, Peters PC: Genitourinary trauma. In Walsh PC, Retik AB, Vaughan ED Jr [eds]: Campbell's Urology, 7th ed. Philadelphia, WB Saunders, 1998, p 3113.)

Testicular injuries are uncommon, due to their mobility and relatively protected position. Blunt or penetrating trauma can lead to serious testicular injury. Blunt trauma of significant force may rupture the very strong tunica albuginea that surrounds the seminiferous tubules. Scrotal exploration should be undertaken when there is significant blunt trauma with hematoma to the testicle or with gunshot or stab wounds. Testicular repair includes débridement of extruded seminiferous tubules, meticulous wound irrigation, and repair of the very dense tunica albuginea using absorbable suture to cover and contain the underlying seminiferous tubules. If the injury is severe or there is obvious lack of blood supply to the testicle, orchiectomy should be performed. With salvage, the affected testicle's ability to produce testosterone and spermatozoa can be maintained.

The external genitalia can also suffer burns and electrical injuries. Typical thermal injury involves the skin as well as the subcutaneous tissue and can produce deep necrosis. Standard management of the burned area includes débridement, topical therapy, and skin grafting with subsequent reconstruction. The mechanism of electrical burn is very different from that of thermal burn. Electrical wounds often involve an entry and exit site, and apparently minor wounds may have significant areas of tissue necrosis and soft-tissue injury in between.

Special mention should be made of injuries to the external genitalia in the female. Often, these are not considered and are missed in the diagnostic assessment of the female trauma patient. These injuries may result from physical or sexual abuse, straddle injury, or pelvic crush injury. Vulvar hematoma causes a swollen and tender ecchymotic mass to the labia. Vaginal lacerations may be associated with severe hemorrhage. They can be caused by perforation of the vaginal mucosa secondary to a bony spicule from a pelvic fracture or a stab or gunshot wound. Bladder and rectal injuries may be associated with vaginal injuries. Formal repair of the vaginal laceration is accomplished with interrupted or running absorbable sutures.

Four percent to 6% of female patients with associated pelvic fractures have an anterior urethral injury. Anterior urethral injuries may be easily missed and are being recognized more frequently. Diagnosis is made due to a high index of suspicion, and is confirmed with cystoscopy. Flexible cystoscopy may be performed in the emergency or operating room.

Anterior urethral injuries in females may involve the bladder neck or extend to the proximal urethra. Complete urethral disruption or traumatic urethrovaginal fistula may result. Injuries extending to the bladder neck should be repaired with absorbable sutures. Complex disruptions in the female patient should be treated with both a urethral catheter as a stent and a formal suprapubic cystostomy tube.

PROSTATITIS

method of
J. CURTIS NICKEL, M.D.
Kingston General Hospital
Kingston, Ontario, Canada

EPIDEMIOLOGY

Prostatitis is the most common urologic diagnosis in men younger than 50 years of age and the third most common diagnosis in men older than 50, representing almost 8% of visits to North American urologists and 1% of visits to family physicians. Four percent to 11% of men (depending on the type of survey) have a history of prostatitis, which affects men of all ages almost equally, and the overall prevalence of prostatitis-like symptoms is approximately 10%.

ETIOLOGY

Acute bacterial prostatitis is rare and is associated with a generalized infection of the prostate gland with typical uropathogens (*Escherichia coli, Klebsiella pneumoniae, Pseudomonas aeruginosa,* and *Enterococcus faecalis*). Chronic prostatitis is associated with similar uropathogenic bacteria in less than 5% of the cases. The ramifications of presumed nonuropathogenic bacteria, such as *Staphylococcus saprophyticus*, anaerobic bacteria, and *Corynebacterium species* and organisms such as chlamydia, mycoplasma, fungi, and viruses are unknown.

Anatomic (bladder neck hyperplasia, urethral strictures, refluxing prostatic ducts), and/or physiologic (vesical-sphincter dyssynergia) abnormalities may result in chemically or immunologically mediated inflammation of the prostatic ducts/acini or neurogenic damage within or around the prostate gland. The end result is pain (and to a lesser extent voiding and sexual disturbances).

CLASSIFICATION

The traditional classification system of acute bacterial prostatitis, chronic bacterial prostatitis, nonbacterial prostatitis, and prostatodynia attributes the symptoms of "prostatitis" to a specific prostate problem, which is not necessarily the case in many of these men.

The National Institutes of Health (NIH) classification system of prostatitis (Table 1) is similar to the traditional system in that categories I and II are identical to the traditional system of acute and chronic bacterial prostatitis. Category III (the majority of patients with prostatitis syndrome) would be categorized as chronic pelvic pain syndrome (CPPS). This category is further divided into category IIIA (or inflammatory CPPS) and category IIIB (or non-inflammatory CPPS), based on the presence or absence of excessive leukocytes in prostate-specific specimens (including semen). Category IV refers to patients with asymptomatic prostatic inflammation (being worked up for an elevated prostate-specific antigen, benign prostatic hyperplasia, or infertility). The NIH classification system for the prostatitis syndromes has now become accepted by the international urological community for use in research studies and clinical practice.

CLINICAL EVALUATION

Category I patients present with an acute febrile illness associated with obstructive and irritative voiding symptoms, varying degrees of urinary obstruction, and a soft prostate gland that is exquisitely painful on palpation.

TABLE 1. **The Prostatitis Syndromes**

Classification	Description	Presentation	Treatment
Category I (acute bacterial prostatitis)	Acute infection of the prostate gland	Acute febrile illness associated with perineal and suprapubic pain, dysuria, and obstructive voiding	Antibiotics Urinary drainage
Category II (chronic bacterial prostatitis)	Chronic infection of the prostate	Recurrent UTIs with variable pain and voiding disturbances	Antibiotics Prostate massage
Category III (CPPS)	Chronic genitourinary pain in the absence of uropathogenic bacteria localized to the prostate gland employing standard methodology	Chronic perineal, suprapubic, groin, testicular, penile, or ejaculatory pain associated with variable dysuria and obstructive and irritative voiding	See below (Category IIIA and Category IIIB)
Category IIIA (inflammatory CPPS)	Significant WBCs in EPS, postprostatic massage urine sediment (VB3), or semen	See above (Category III)	Trial of antibiotics Anti-inflammatories Phytotherapy Pentosan polysulfate Finasteride Prostate massage
Category IIIB (inflammatory CPPS)	Insignificant WBCs in expressed prostatic secretions, post-M urine sediment (VB3), or semen	See above (Category III)	α-Blockers Anti-inflammatories Muscle relaxants Phytotherapy Physical therapy Biofeedback
Category IV (asymptomatic inflammatory prostatitis)	WBCs (and/or bacteria) in EPS, post-M urine sediment (VB3), semen, or prostate pathology	No symptoms (assessed for infertility, elevated PSA, prostate cancer, or BPH)	No treatment necessary (unless infertile, elevated PSA, planned urologic endoscopy)

Abbreviations: BPH = benign prostatic hyperplasia; CPPS = chronic pelvic pain syndrome; EPS = expressed prostatic secretion; post-M = urine specimen after prostatic massage; PSA = prostate-specific antigen; UTIs = urinary tract infections; WBCs = white blood cells/inflammatory cells.

Before initiating therapy, patients require a midstream urine and blood culture.

The symptom complex of patients presenting with categories II and III chronic prostatitis/CPPS are really indistinguishable, except that patients with category II typically have a history of recurrent urinary tract infections (UTIs). The primary complaint is pain: perineal, suprapubic, testicular, and penile associated with ejaculation or voiding. The pain is associated with variable irritative and obstructive voiding symptoms. These chronic symptoms have a significant impact on the patient's quality of life. A history that includes recurrent UTIs, genitourinary problems, sexually transmitted diseases, stones, or urologic surgery may be extremely relevant. Physical examination is usually unremarkable. The prostate can be soft or normal and may be asymptomatic, tender, or painful on palpation.

The recently validated and published NIH Chronic Prostatitis Symptom Index (NIH-CPSI)[1] consists of nine questions that address the three most important domains of the chronic prostatitis experience: perception of pain, level of urinary function, and impact on quality of life. The NIH-CPSI has now been accepted by the international prostatitis research community as an accepted outcome measure and has proved useful in evaluation and follow-up of patients in general clinical practice.

The Meares-Stamey four-glass lower urinary tract localization test, which employs an initial stream urine (voided bladder 1 [VB1]), a midstream urine (VB2), an expressed prostatic secretion (EPS), and a postprostatic massage urine (VB3), remains the gold standard evaluation test. Most physicians find this test time-consuming, cumbersome, and expensive, and it rarely leads to significant change in management.

Physicians have abandoned this rigorous technique, and unfortunately, many have abandoned any standardized evaluation of the lower urinary tract at all. The pre- and postmassage (two-glass) test is a simple, cost-effective screen for patients presenting with chronic prostatitis syndrome (see Table 1). Other specialty tests, which include cystoscopy, simple urodynamics (urinary flow rate combined with bladder ultrasound), videourodynamics, transrectal ultrasound, and even biopsies may be warranted for specific urologic indications.

TREATMENT

Category I

Initial intravenous wide spectrum antibiotics (for example, combination gentamicin 80 mg every 8 hours and ampicillin 1 g every 12 hours or a third generation cephalosporin such as ceftriaxone [Rocephin] 1 g every 24 hours) followed by either a fluoroquinolone (such as ciprofloxacin [Cipro] 500 mg every 12 hours) or trimethoprim-sulfamethoxazole ([TMP-SMZ, Septra, Bactrim] 160/800 mg every 12 hours) is almost always successful in curing the patient unless there are significant structural abnormalities of the lower urinary tract or the patient develops a prostate abscess. Many patients require short bladder drainage with a urethral or suprapubic catheter. Antibiotics should be continued for 2 to 4 weeks.

Category II

Antibiotic therapy, employing either a fluoroquinolone or TMP-SMZ (similar dose as indicated for category I) should be initiated and continued for 4 to 12 weeks in patients with definite uropathogenic bacteria localized to prostate-specific specimens or to patients with a history of recurrent UTIs. For patients who are refractory to treatment, the addition of repetitive prostatic massage (performed once or twice a week for 4 weeks) may help a further one to two thirds of patients. Some patients with recurrent symptoms (and/or infection) will require long-term (many months) antibiotic suppression or prophylaxis (one fourth the daily dose of oral antibiotics indicated above).

Category III

There are few well designed randomized placebo-controlled trials evaluating various treatment options in CPPS, but there is sufficient evidence available in the literature to practice a "best evidence-based" approach to therapy that does take into account differentiation of the leukocyte status of prostate-specific specimens (see Table 1).

Approximately 40% of patients with chronic prostatitis (or CPPS) have some symptomatic improvement with antimicrobial therapy, and antibiotics should be considered as empiric therapy in at least category IIIA CPPS, but the benefits should be appraised after a minimum of 2 to 4 weeks of therapy. α-Blockers (terazosin [Hytrin]* 5 mg/d, doxazosin [Cardura]* 4 mg/d, tamsulosin [Flomax]* 0.4 mg/d) appear to reduce symptoms, particularly in men with obstructive voiding symptoms. Nonsteroidal anti-inflammatory agents (NSAIDs) (ibuprofen [Motrin]* 300 mg thrice daily or COX-2 inhibitors such as rofecoxib [Vioxx]* 25–50 mg/d) reduce inflammatory-type symptoms such as dysuria, stranguria, and painful ejaculation. Pentosan polysulfate ([Elmiron]* 100 mg thrice daily for 6 months), an anti-inflammatory glycosaminoglycan that has been used for the treatment of interstitial cystitis may be considered in men in whom irritative voiding and suprapubic pain are the predominant symptoms. Finasteride ([Proscar]* 5 mg/d for a least 6 months), a 5-α reductase inhibitor used in benign prostatic hyperplasia, reduces symptoms in some patients with category IIIA CPPS, particularly those who are older than 40 years and have a large "boggy" prostate on examination. Skeletal muscle relaxants such as diazepam ([Valium],* 5–10 mg) and baclofen ([Apo-Baclofen]* 10 mg thrice daily) combined with adjuvant medical and physical therapies can be helpful in some patients with category IIIB CPPS. Phytotherapeutic agents, including bee pollen extract ([Cernilton]* 1 tablet thrice daily) and bioflavonoids ([Quercetin]* 500 mg twice daily) have helped patients with CPPS and the effect of these plant extracts appears to be more than just a placebo effect.

Repetitive prostate massage was the main therapy for chronic prostatitis syndromes for most of the 20th century. Although it fell into disrepute over the past

*Not FDA approved for this indication.

30 years, it has recently made a comeback. About one to two thirds of patients do obtain some benefit when subjected to repetitive prostate massage for 4 to 6 weeks. Frequent ejaculation has been recommended by many urologists, and there is some evidence that it may be beneficial. Treatment of pelvic/perineal myofascial trigger points with heat therapy, physiotherapeutic massage, ischemic compression, stretching, anesthetic injections, acupuncture, and electroneuromodulation has been suggested for these patients. I have found that biofeedback ameliorates some specific prostatitis-like symptoms, particularly in category IIIB CPPS.

Minimally invasive therapies such as balloon dilation, balloon dilation with prostatic hyperthermia, transurethral needle ablation of the prostate and Nd:YAG laser therapy have all been advocated, but only microwave thermotherapy has been convincingly shown to be superior to placebo therapy in clinical trials. Surgery does not have an important role in the treatment of most patients with CPPS unless a specific indication is discovered during evaluation of the patient. Patients with urethral strictures or urodynamic evidence of bladder neck obstruction may benefit from endoscopic incision. Radical transurethral resection of the prostate and radical prostatectomy have been advocated and although the potential complications of radical prostate surgery are well known, the long-term potential benefits have never been adequately demonstrated.

REFERENCE

1. Litwin MS, McNaughton-Collins M, Fowler FJ Jr, et al: The National Institutes of Health chronic prostatitis symptom index: Development and validation of a new outcome measure. Chronic Prostatitis Collaborative Research Network. J Urol 162:369–375, 1999.

BENIGN PROSTATIC HYPERPLASIA

method of
DEBRA L. FROMER, M.D., and
STEVEN A. KAPLAN, M.D.
New York-Presbyterian Hospital
New York, New York

EPIDEMIOLOGY

Benign prostatic hyperplasia (BPH) is highly prevalent in men older than 50 years. Epidemiologic studies show that 38% of American men between 40 and 79 years of age experience moderate to severe symptoms of prostatism and that one in four U.S. men in their eighth decade will require treatment of BPH. Its prevalence is higher in Asian men, with 56% of Japanese men aged 40 to 79 years experiencing moderate to severe symptoms of BPH and 56% of Asian men between 70 and 79 years having enlarged prostates by transrectal ultrasound. The relative risk for the development of symptoms of urinary tract obstruction from prostatic enlargement doubles for each decade of life between the ages of 40 and 90 years. Age has not been shown to be a direct causal agent of BPH; however, the development of BPH has been associated with exposure to androgenic and estrogenic stimulation over time. Furthermore, substantial evidence supports a genetic component in the development of BPH. Other factors, such as race, sexual activity, smoking, socioeconomic status, vasectomy, alcohol, and diet, have not been proved to be etiologic agents in the development of BPH.

PATHOPHYSIOLOGY

The discovery of large numbers of α-adrenergic receptors in the smooth muscle of the prostate adenoma, prostatic capsule, and bladder neck in the early 1970s led to the conclusion that the outlet obstruction associated with BPH has both a static and dynamic component. The static component of urinary obstruction is largely a function of cellular overgrowth that results in encroachment of the hyperplastic prostate on the lumen of the urethra. Ultimately, this hyperplasia leads to sufficient urethral narrowing to cause symptoms of urethral obstruction. Superimposed on this structural problem is the variable degree of smooth muscle contraction controlled by the sympathetic nervous system by way of α receptors on the prostate capsule, the prostate adenoma, and the bladder neck.

BPH first develops in the transitional zone of the prostate. The transitional zone lies immediately external to the preprostatic sphincter. The prostatic stromal and epithelial cells maintain a paracrine type of communication whereby the growth of prostatic epithelium can be regulated by cellular interaction with the basement membrane and stromal cells. There is strong evidence that stromal cell production of an excretory protein regulates epithelial cell differentiation. BPH may therefore be due to a defect in a stromal component that normally inhibits epithelial proliferation, thereby allowing overgrowth of prostatic epithelial cells. It is evident that androgenic stimulation is required for normal development of the prostate. Testosterone is converted to dihydrotestosterone by two forms of the enzyme 5α-reductase. Type 1 isoenzyme is present in liver, skin, and other tissues and contributes to circulating levels of dihydrotestosterone. Type 2 isoenzyme predominates in urogenital tissue. In individuals with a deficiency in type 2 isoenzyme, normal external genitalia or prostates do not develop. Immunohistochemical studies with type 2 5α-reductase–specific antibodies show primarily stromal cell localization, thus emphasizing the importance of stromal cells in the development of epithelial cell proliferation.

Prostatic smooth muscle plays a significant role in the pathogenesis of BPH. It is well known that prostatic smooth muscle represents a significant volume of the gland. Stimulation of the α_1-adrenergic receptors in prostatic smooth muscle results in a dynamic increase in prostatic urethral resistance. Pharmacologic blockade of this stimulation results in a diminished response.

SYMPTOMS

Lower urinary tract symptoms relate to problems in bladder filling, storage, and voiding of urine. The traditional classification as either "obstructive" or "irritative" correlates poorly with urodynamic diagnoses and may therefore be both inaccurate and misleading. Symptoms should be carefully assessed to determine their cause, the diagnosis of BPH should be confirmed, and other bladder and prostate pathology should be excluded as appropriate.

Although BPH can lead to obstructive uropathy and renal failure, urinary retention, urinary tract infections, and bladder calculi, the vast majority of procedures performed for BPH are for symptomatic relief. It is therefore critical to determine whether and how much the patient's symptoms interfere with his quality of life, which can be reliably accomplished by using the American Urologic Association Symptom Score, also called the International Prostate Symptom Score (IPSS) (Figure 1). Symptoms can be classified as mild (0 to 7), moderate (8 to 19), or severe (20 to 35). Symptom scores alone, however, do not capture the impact of prostatism as perceived by the individual patient. Intervention may be more appropriate for a moderately symptomatic patient who is very bothered by his symptoms than for a severely symptomatic patient who finds his symptoms tolerable.

DIAGNOSIS

In addition to eliciting specific voiding complaints and a detailed medical history and obtaining an IPSS, it is important to search for other causes of symptoms, such as neurogenic bladder, urinary tract infection, urolithiasis, diabetes, urethral stricture, prostate carcinoma, or bladder carcinoma.

Physical examination should include a digital rectal examination to determine the size, consistency, symmetry, and tenderness of the gland, as well as rectal tone. It is important to understand that only the posterior lobe of the prostate can be palpated, not the lobes characteristically involved. In a patient in retention or with high postvoid residuals, a suprapubic or lower abdominal mass may be appreciated on abdominal examination.

Laboratory data should include urinalysis, a serum creatinine determination, and urine cytologic studies if irritative voiding symptoms are severe. It is recommended by the American Urologic Association that all men not at risk for prostate cancer receive an annual prostate-specific antigen determination beginning at age 50. Determination of the urinary flow rate and abdominal ultrasound to measure the postvoid residual are often performed before the initiation of therapy as baseline and then after treatment initiation to determine the response to therapy. More sophisticated urodynamic measurements, such as pressure-flow studies, are reserved for patients who fail medical therapy and who may require operative intervention.

TREATMENT

Watchful Waiting

Some men with symptomatic BPH choose not to undergo treatment for various reasons. On most occasions, the symptoms are not severe enough or are not enough of a bother to warrant long-term treatment with medication or surgical intervention. The patient can be urged to limit fluids in the evening, decrease caffeine intake, and avoid medications that impair voiding, such as decongestants and anticholinergics. A recent study of 556 men with moderate symptoms of BPH compared the outcome of patients treated with transurethral resection of the prostate (TURP) versus watchful waiting. During 3 years of follow-up, 8% and 17% subjects randomized to TURP and watchful waiting, respectively, failed treatment. Treatment failure in the watchful waiting group was mostly due to high postvoid residuals and significant increases in the IPSS.

Phytotherapy

Plant extracts are widely used in Europe, and numerous preparations claiming to benefit "the health of the prostate and bladder" are available in the United States. In Europe, phytotherapeutic preparations represent one third of the total sales of all therapeutic agents sold for the treatment of BPH. The mechanism of these herbal treatments has not been well established, however. The most common of these preparations is *Serenoa repens* (saw palmetto), which appears to offer a modest improvement in symptom scores and flow rates in comparison with placebo, with minimal side effects. A recent random-

American Urological Association Symptom Index

Question	Not at All	Less Than 1 Time in 5	Less Than Half the Time	About Half the Time	More Than Half the Time	Almost Always
1. During the last month or so, how often have you had a sensation of not emptying your bladder completely after you finished urinating?	0	1	2	3	4	5
2. During the last month or so, how often have you had to urinate again less than 2 hours after you finished urinating?	0	1	2	3	4	5
3. During the last month or so, how often have you found you started again several times when you urinated?	0	1	2	3	4	5
4. During the last month or so, how often have you found it difficult to postpone urination?	0	1	2	3	4	5
5. During the last month or so, how often have you had a weak urinary stream?	0	1	2	3	4	5
6. During the last month or so, how often have you had to push or strain to begin urination?	0	1	2	3	4	5
7. During the last month or so, how many times did you most typically get up to urinate from the time you went to bed at night until the time you got up in the morning?	None	1 Time	2 Times	3 Times	4 Times	5 or More Times
	0	1	2	3	4	5

Figure 1. International Prostate Symptom Score.

ized, placebo-controlled study showed that saw palmetto was associated with epithelial cell contraction, especially in the tranzition zone. However, no significant improvement in symptom score or flow rate was observed.

α-Adrenergic Blocking Agents

α-Adrenergic antagonists have been shown in numerous randomized, placebo-controlled trials to be both safe and effective in the treatment of BPH. All of the classic α-adrenergic-blocking agents (Table 1) in clinical use at present appear to be very similar in terms of clinical efficacy and safety; they produce an approximately 20% to 30% increase in urinary flow rate with a significant 20% to 50% improvement in symptom scores. Terazosin (Hytrin) and doxazosin (Cardura) were the first α-antagonists introduced for the treatment of BPH. However, because of postural hypotension with these agents, the doses had to be titrated. The introduction of tamsulosin (Flomax), a selective α-antagonist, eliminated the need for titration. The most common side effects include headache, dizziness, asthenia, and drowsiness. Sexual side effects, with the exception of retrograde ejaculation, are unrelated to treatment with α-antagonists.

5α-Reductase Inhibition

Finasteride (Proscar) inhibits the conversion of testosterone to dihydrotestosterone in the prostate. It has been shown to have its greatest effect in men with larger (>40 g) prostates, and at least 6 months of therapy is required for maximal effect to be observed. A recent placebo-controlled study compared finasteride with placebo and showed significant increases in maximal flow rates and decreases in prostate volume and bladder pressure on urodynamics. However, a 1-year placebo-controlled study of 1229 men with BPH demonstrated no improvement in IPSS and flow rate over placebo and only a small improvement with larger prostate volumes. In a 4-year randomized trial, finasteride reduced the risk of acute urinary retention and the probablity of surgical intervention.

Finasteride has likewise proved effective in suppressing the significant hematuria associated with BPH. It can also be used as a neoadjuvant therapy for minimally invasive techniques and as adjuvant therapy if symptoms return after other treatments.

The most common side effects include decreased ejaculatory volume and sexual dysfunction, which occurs in 6% to 8% of patients. Breast tenderness and gynecomastia have also been associated with the use of finasteride. In addition, finasteride causes a 50% reduction in prostate-specific antigen after 6 months of therapy.

Minimally Invasive Therapies

TURP has been the most effective treatment of BPH and has been regarded as the gold standard. During the last decade, a number of new minimally invasive therapies have been developed as alternatives to reduce the known complications of TURP, such as bleeding, TURP syndrome, incontinence, impotence, and retrograde ejaculation, and they are particularly useful in a patient who is a poor surgical risk. Most minimally invasive types of therapies use various kinds of energy, such as microwave, radio frequency, laser, ultrasound, and new applications of electrosurgical current (Table 2).

Transurethral microwave thermotherapy (TUMT) is designed to produce coagulative necrosis of the transitional zone by microwave radiative heating while water-conductive cooling of the urethral mucosa preserves the periurethral tissue. A prospective randomized study comparing low-energy TUMT and TURP showed significant improvements in symptom score, flow rate, and postvoid residual after both methods, although the observed improvements were more pronounced after TURP. Most clinical trials demonstrate a 75% reduction in symptom score and a 35% increase in peak flow rate. Higher energy TUMT provides enhanced efficacy but is associated with increased postoperative morbidity. Retrograde ejaculation, rarely seen after low-energy TUMT, developed in 33% of patients. Catheterization is needed for a mean of 2 weeks because of prolonged urinary retention.

Laser treatment of BPH has recently become popular among urologists. Visual laser ablation of the prostate (VLAP) is performed by using a side-firing Nd:YAG laser fiber. The results of several prospective randomized trials comparing VLAP and TURP were similar and showed equivalent improvement in symptom score and increases in flow rates in both groups, but higher in the TURP group. The major drawback of VLAP is the prolonged postoperative catheterization because of urinary retention. Furthermore, most patients have irritative voiding symptoms lasting 2 to 6 weeks on average, and retro-

TABLE 1. **α_1-Receptor Antagonists Approved for the Treatment of Benign Prostatic Hyperplasia**

Terazosin (Hytrin)
Doxazosin (Cardura)
Tamsulosin (Flomax)

TABLE 2. **Minimally Invasive Treatment of Benign Prostatic Hyperplasia**

Transurethral microwave therapy (TUMT)
Low-energy thermotherapy
High-energy thermotherapy
Laser prostatectomy
Visual laser ablation of the prostate (VLAP)
Interstitial laser coagulation (ILC)
Holmium laser resection of the prostate (HoLRP)
High-intensity focused ultrasound (HIFU)
Transurethral needle ablation of the prostate (TUNA)
Transurethral vaporization of the prostate (TUVP)

grade ejaculation occurs in 36% to 47% of patients. In contrast to VLAP, interstitial laser coagulation uses a laser fiber that is inserted into the prostate under cystoscopic control and induces coagulation necrosis well inside the prostate rather than at its urethral surface. Clinical results after 1 year showed marked improvement in symptom score and peak flow rate. Drawbacks include prolonged catheterization (18.3 days on average) and retrograde ejaculation in 0% to 12%. Holmium laser resection of the prostate uses an Ho:YAG laser to resect pieces of prostate tissue, which are then eliminated through the operating channel of the resectoscope. Prospective randomized studies show equivalent improvement in symptom score and flow rate when compared with TURP, a shortened length of hospital stay, and fewer side effects. However, operating time with holmium laser resection is significantly longer and performance requires considerable endoscopic skill.

High-intensity focused ultrasound uses focused ultrasound pulses delivered transrectally to a small area of tissue to cause a temperature rise to 80°C to 100°C. Long-term clinical results are still limited, and data from a randomized clinical trial are not yet available. Urodynamic results demonstrate relief of bladder outlet obstruction comparable with that of TUMT.

Transurethral needle ablation of the prostate (TUNA) applies low–radio frequency waves and thermal energy to the prostate via needles inserted transurethrally into the prostate. Tissue necrosis occurs at 80°C to 100°C in 3 to 5 minutes. A prospective study comparing TUNA with TURP showed comparable improvement in symptom score at 12 months. However, TURP was superior in improving flow rates and in pressure-flow studies. Currently, data on the durability of the clinical response extend to 3 years. Postoperative catherization for a mean of 1 to 3 days is required in 13% to 42% of patients. Although irritative voiding symptoms develop in 40% of patients, erectile dysfunction and retrograde ejaculation are rare.

Transurethral electrovaporization of the prostate (TUVP) is one of the most effective minimally invasive treatment options. In this technique, both electrosurgical vaporization and desiccation are combined into one effective simultaneous action. Current prospective randomized studies comparing TUVP and TURP show an equivalent clinical outcome. The risk of TURP syndrome and transfusion is minimal. Intermittent hematuria was noted in 57% of patients immediately postoperatively, and retrograde ejaculation was reported by 84% of patients.

Prostate Surgery

TURP remains the mainstay of surgical treatment of BPH. The procedure uses electrosurgical energy to remove prostatic tissue cystoscopically under anesthesia. With the advent of effective pharmacologic treatment of BPH, indications for surgical management have evolved (Table 3). Although patients with absolute indications are at risk for lower urinary tract decompensation and, subsequently, upper urinary tract damage, the most common indication for TURP remains bothersome symptoms. Men with moderate to high symptom scores have the greatest likelihood of a successful outcome after TURP. Objective outcomes such as those at cystoscopy are less prognostic of outcome. Overall satisfaction after TURP ranges from 75% to 87% with up to 17 years of follow-up. Short-term complications include transfusion (3%–7%), the TURP syndrome, and failure to void (10%–44%). Long-term complications include retrograde ejaculation (75%), impotence (4%), incontinence (1%), and urethral stricture or bladder neck contracture (3%). Approximately 15% of patients have persistent symptoms that may require further treatment, with a 5% risk of having a second TURP procedure within 7 years after the initial surgery.

TABLE 3. **Transurethral Resection of the Prostate**

Absolute indications
Recurrent acute urinary retention
Bladder stone formation
Renal deterioration secondary to bladder outlet obstruction
Recurrent gross hematuria from the prostate
Recurrent urinary tract infection
Relative indications
Bothersome lower urinary tract symptoms
High postvoid residual volume

Open prostatectomy remains the surgery of choice for patients with a prostate too large to be safely removed by TURP. This procedure is reserved for the minority (<5%) of patients with prostates in excess of 80 to 100 g.

CONCLUSIONS

BPH is an extremely common disease in aging men. Options for treatment include medical therapy with phytotherapy, α-blockers, TURP, and a wide variety of minimally invasive procedures. Watchful waiting is an acceptable option for men with low symptom scores who are not severely bothered by their symptoms. The efficacy of medical therapy has reduced the frequency of TURP. However, patients who fail medical therapy or opt against it have many newly available options for the minimally invasive treatment of BPH. Nevertheless, TURP remains the gold standard for surgical treatment of BPH.

ERECTILE DYSFUNCTION

method of
LAURENCE A. LEVINE, M.D.
Rush-Presbyterian-St. Luke's Medical Center
Chicago, Illinois

It has been estimated that more than 100 million men in the world suffer from erectile dysfunction (ED). A recent survey in the United States determined that 52% of men between the ages of 40 and 70 suffered from ED ranging from mild to complete. Yet, fewer than 1 in 10 sought evaluation or treatment by a medical professional. Demographic studies executed in Asia, Turkey, and the northern countries of South America have demonstrated a similar prevalence of ED to that shown in the U.S. study.

Although ED has been demonstrated to become more prevalent with aging, it is certainly not an inevitable result of aging. Rather, it appears to be the cumulative result of repetitive neurovascular insults resulting in a greater likelihood of injury to the vascular supply to and within the corpora cavernosa.

Much has changed in our understanding of ED. Advances in the field of neurovascular physiology and improved diagnostic techniques have given us a better understanding of the underlying causes and pathophysiology of ED. Twenty to 30 years ago, most ED was believed to be psychogenic in origin. We now know that in up to 80% of men with ED, there is a primary organic cause, although the psychogenic component will always remain an important factor owing to the emotional nature of sexual behavior. The most commonly recognized risk factors for ED are listed in Table 1 and include those disorders that might result in an accelerated atherosclerotic process, including hypertension, dyslipidemia, and diabetes.

Briefly, a normal erection is a hemodynamic event governed by the integrity of the smooth muscles in the arterial wall and cavernosal tissue as well as the network of veins of the corpora cavernosa—the two rods of spongy tissue housed in the penile shaft. When sexual stimulation occurs, a central erectile integration center—now thought to be in the vicinity of the medial preoptic area of the brain—causes a nerve impulse to be transmitted via the central nervous system and pelvic plexus to the corpora cavernosa, causing the local release of the neurotransmitter nitric oxide (NO) by noradrenergic, norcholinergic nerves. NO is a potent but short-acting vasodilator that acts by diffusing into the smooth muscle cell. There it activates the cytosolic enzyme, guanylate cyclase, to stimulate the production of cyclic guanosine monophosphate (cGMP) from guanosine triphosphate (GTP).

cGMP, via a series of processes that have not been completely elucidated, causes the sequestration of intracellular calcium. This precipitates a hyperpolarization event that results in smooth muscle relaxation. This process is transmitted quickly throughout the smooth muscle of the corpora cavernosa via gap junctions. As intracorporeal pressure increases, there is progressive occlusion of the small veins that traverse the tunica albuginea, preventing drainage of blood from the corpora. The result of these actions is an erection, which is maintained until a sympathetic neural impulse produces ejaculation and detumescence. Therefore, normal erectile function depends on healthy blood vessels, nerves, and connective tissue. Disease or disturbances in any of these systems, alone or together, may lead to erectile problems.

TABLE 1. **Risk Factors for Erectile Dysfunction**

Alcohol abuse	Hypogonadism
Anemia	Peyronie disease
Coronary artery or peripheral vascular disease	Smoking
Depression	Trauma to perineum (i.e., straddle-type injuries)
Diabetes mellitus	Trauma or surgery to the pelvis or spine
Hyperlipidemia	Vascular surgery
Hypertension	

TABLE 2. **Drugs Associated With Erectile Dysfunction**

Antihypertensives	Narcotics
Antidepressants	β-Blockers
Alcohol	Psychotropics
Cigarettes	Cocaine
Estrogens	Spironolactone
Antiandrogens	Lipid-lowering agents
H_2 receptor blockers	Nonsteroidal anti-inflammatory drugs
Ketoconazole	Cytotoxic drugs
Marijuana	Diuretics

Local mechanisms of control of the smooth muscle are currently under investigation. These include neurotransmitters responsible for smooth muscle relaxation, such as NO, cGMP, cAMP, vasoactive intestinal polypeptide (VIP), and prostaglandins. Neurotransmitters responsible for vasoconstriction may also, in the future, be manipulated to reduce cavernosal vascular tone. Endothelin is a potent vasoconstrictor released from the endothelium of the cavernosal vascular tissue that may be responsible for some forms of ED. Research on modulators of endothelin release and/or production may lead to future therapies for ED. Clearly, the most common factors that affect penile blood flow are those processes that result in injury to the smooth muscle, vascular endothelium, and connective tissue of the penis.

Hypogonadism has been associated with diminished sexual function. It appears that a below normal serum testosterone is rarely the sole cause of erectile insufficiency, but it may have significant bearing on libido. In the young man with primary ED (i.e., never experienced a satisfactory erection) and hypogonadism, testosterone replacement will typically result in recovery of normal erectile capacity. A proper circulating testosterone threshold (which as yet has not been established) may be important because the action of NO synthase, responsible for the production of NO, is an androgen-dependent enzyme.

It will also become increasingly important to recognize the contributions to nonsexual function that circulating androgens make to our male patients, including bone and lipid metabolism, muscle mass, and cognitive function. Suffice it to say, if a man presents with hypogonadism and erectile insufficiency, it is sensible to offer testosterone replacement therapy. Response to therapy should be checked periodically because many men will have a satisfactory blood level of testosterone without improvement in erectile/sexual function. Therefore, androgen replacement may not be needed. Also, there are potential adverse side effects associated with unnecessary androgen replacement, including exacerbation of lower urinary tract symptoms associated with benign prostatic hyperplasia, stimulation of an occult prostate cancer, worsening of sleep apnea, and polycythemia.

Many prescription drugs, including most of the antihypertensive medications and antidepressants, may exacerbate ED by interfering with blood flow or response to neurotransmitters. For other medications associated with ED, see Table 2.

Another important yet relatively uncommon form of erectile failure is that following pelvic or perineal trauma. These injuries may result in acute disruption of the common penile arteries and/or the cavernosal nerves in the perineum as they emerge from the deep pelvis. It has also been demonstrated that remote "relatively minor" perineal/penile trauma may also cause discrete vascular injury that, over time, causes accelerated atherosclerotic changes and subsequent ED. Similar injuries may also result from repeated trauma to the perineum from any saddle sport.

EVALUATION OF ERECTILE DYSFUNCTION

It has been suggested that owing to the absence of specific medical therapies for particular etiologies of ED, there is little value to performing an extensive and potentially expensive and invasive evaluation to determine the precise etiology of a man's ED. Therefore, in 1990, a goal-directed approach to the evaluation of ED was proposed and has been adopted worldwide by most experts. This includes a detailed medical and sexual history in which the nature, frequency, onset, and duration of ED is assessed. This detailed history includes questions about the presence of spontaneous morning and nocturnal erections and whether the patient experiences situational ED with different partners and is capable of having erections with self-stimulation.

In addition, a focused physical examination should be performed. Laboratory studies can be kept to a minimum, with a morning serum testosterone level that, if abnormal, can be evaluated further. Baseline complete blood cell count, chemical testing, glucose tolerance, and lipid surveys are indicated if not performed recently.

Therapy can then be initiated depending on the results of this limited evaluation or further testing may be initiated by specialists. More specialized evaluation may include penile brachial blood pressure index studies, which have little value and are not recommended. Pharmacologic penile duplex ultrasound is recognized as the most valuable test to assess penile vascular integrity, and it offers an opportunity to study erectile and emotional response to an intracorporal injection of vasoactive drugs. Nocturnal penile tumescence and rigidity monitoring is recognized as the best discriminator between organic and psychogenic ED and may aid in the referral to a sex therapist when the problem is primarily of psychogenic etiology. Other testing is rarely indicated unless the patient is a candidate for vascular reconstruction; candidates are primarily men younger than 40 to 50 years of age who have a traumatic etiology for their ED. In these patients, cavernosometry to evaluate venous drainage and phalloarteriography to evaluate arterial supply are indicated.

Following workup, it is important to have a discussion with the patient regarding assessment of the etiology of the ED as well the treatment options. This is certainly an opportunity for the physician to recommend lifestyle modifications to enhance not only sexual health but long-term general health. This discussion could include recommendations for changing diet, changing or increasing physical activity, reducing stress, decreasing alcohol consumption, and quitting smoking, although it is not clear that any of these changes will improve ED.

Treatment Options for Erectile Dysfunction

A panel of experts developed the "process of care" approach for the evaluation and treatment of men with ED, directed toward the primary care physician (Table 3). In this well conceived algorithm, therapy is offered in a step-wise fashion:

1. First-line therapy includes oral medications, external vacuum constriction devices, or psychosexual counseling, when indicated.

TABLE 3. **Treatment Options for Erectile Dysfunction**

First Line
Psychosexual counseling
Hormone replacement
Oral agents
Vacuum pumps and constriction devices
Second Line
Intracavernosal injection
Intraurethral instillation
Third Line
Penile prosthesis
Vascular reconstructive surgery

2. Second-line therapy includes penile injection therapy or intraurethral instillation therapy.
3. Third-line therapy includes penile implants and vascular reconstructive surgery.

Multiple oral therapies have been used over the past 20 years, including yohimbine (Yocon), trazodone (Desyrel),* and more recently L-arginine.* Controlled studies have failed to show any clear treatment advantage with these agents. In March 1998, sildenafil (Viagra), the first safe and effective oral agent for the treatment of ED, was approved. New oral agents under investigation and Food and Drug Administration (FDA) review include apomorphine (Uprima),† which is a central dopamine agonist that enhances central neural output to induce erection. Phentolamine (Vasomax)* is an α-adrenoceptor antagonist. It works by inhibiting the action of penile catecholamines, which may enhance arterial inflow.

Sildenafil works as a result of sexual stimulation causing the release of NO, as previously noted, with a subsequent increase in cGMP within the smooth muscle of the corpora cavernosa. Sildenafil acts to prevent the degradation of cGMP by phosphodiesterase type 5, which is the predominant type of this enzyme in the corpus cavernosum for which sildenafil is a selective and potent inhibitor. More than 11,000 patient-years of exposure have been monitored by the manufacturer, allowing extensive evaluation of patients receiving this agent. Men with virtually all co-morbidities associated with ED have been successfully treated, although men with more advanced neurovascular disease, particularly associated with diabetes, advanced hypertension, and pelvic surgery, may not respond as well as those with milder forms of vascular insufficiency. The side effect profile of sildenafil has also been clearly established with headache, flushing, and dyspepsia being the primary side effects due to peripheral inhibition of phosphodiesterase activity. Rarely do these cause patients to drop out from treatment.

There has been a good deal of concern, particularly fostered by the media, regarding the association of

*Not FDA approved for this indication.
†Not available in the United States.

sildenafil with life-threatening cardiac events. It is clearly recognized that coronary heart disease and ED share many of the same risk factors. In the man who has significant coronary disease, the cardiac work expended during sexual relations could tax the heart, which is not capable of responding, potentially causing a serious cardiovascular event. But multiple studies have demonstrated the overall safety of sildenafil, even in patients with severe coronary disease and angina. In addition, in a large survey, no statistically significant increased risk of myocardial infarction or death was found in patients receiving sildenafil over those receiving a placebo. Therefore, sildenafil does appear to be a safe and effective therapy for men with ED and does not appear to substantially increase risk for myocardial events.

For the man who fails therapy with sildenafil, various well established treatments remain including vacuum constriction devices, the most noninvasive but the least physiologic and least expensive approach. Many models of this now over-the-counter therapy are available, with patient satisfaction rates in the 20% to 80% range.

The previous gold standard therapy for ED—before the introduction of sildenafil—was vasoactive intracavernosal pharmacotherapy, in which a vasodilating drug is injected directly into the shaft of the penis to activate smooth muscle relaxation. Alprostadil (Caverject) is available commercially. It is the only FDA-approved drug for this purpose, but various mixtures of alprostadil with papaverine* and phentolamine* have been used successfully since the mid-1980s. Potential side effects from this therapy include corporal fibrosis, penile deformity, and priapism. Therefore, patients must undergo proper instruction for auto-injection and dose titration in the office by a qualified health care provider before initiation of home therapy. Intraurethral instillation of alprostadil (MUSE—medicated urethral system for erection) was approved by the FDA in 1997 and has also been a useful approach, although it maintains a very low percentage of market share due to a relatively low rate of efficacy (30%–50%) and a reasonably high level of genital pain caused by the drug (10%–40%).

A penile prosthesis remains an effective therapy but in most cases should be considered a procedure of last resort. However, it may remain the best option for men with the most advanced forms of ED associated with neurovascular disorders or corporal fibrosis. There has been significant improvement in design of these devices since the early 1970s, and the overall mechanical failure rate is in the 3% to 15% range over a 5- to 10-year period. These devices are placed inside the body. Although most devices contain silicone, there have been no silicone-related disorders reported of the 350,000 devices implanted. It should be recognized that although penile prosthesis is the most invasive approach, patient and partner satisfaction rates remain the highest of all therapies at 90% to 98%.

ED is a highly prevalent medical disorder, potentially associated with significant underlying medical disease. Although many men suffer with it, the great majority still do not seek evaluation. Substantial advances have been made in the understanding of the pathophysiology of ED as well as our ability to evaluate its etiology. New treatment options have brought us to the modern era of oral therapy. Still, the future of this field may lie in the proper education of physicians and health care providers in general. ED continues to carry a significant stigma. Nevertheless, we should be encouraged to question our patients, especially those over 40 years old, about their sexual function—not only for the significance this could have on their own life but possibly on their relationship with their partner.

*Not FDA approved for this indication.

ACUTE RENAL FAILURE

method of
YOUSRI M. BARRI, M.D., and
SUDHIR V. SHAH, M.D.
University of Arkansas for Medical Sciences and Central Arkansas Veterans Healthcare
Little Rock, Arkansas

DEFINITION AND ETIOLOGY

Acute renal failure (ARF) is a syndrome that can be broadly defined as an abrupt decrease in renal function sufficient to result in retention of nitrogenous waste (e.g., blood urea nitrogen and creatinine) in the body. The frequency of ARF varies greatly depending on the clinical setting. The frequency among hospitalized patients is about 5% but can be as high as 15% after cardiopulmonary bypass. Despite major advances in dialysis and intensive care, the mortality rate among patients with severe ARF requiring dialysis has not decreased significantly over the past 50 years. This may be explained in part by the fact that the age of the patients continues to rise and coexisting serious illnesses are increasingly common among these patients. Therefore, our efforts should be targeted at the prevention of ARF.

ARF can result from a decrease of renal blood flow (*prerenal azotemia*), intrinsic renal parenchymal diseases (*renal azotemia*), or obstruction of urine flow (*postrenal azotemia*). The most common intrinsic renal disease that leads to ARF is an entity referred to as *acute tubular necrosis* (*ATN*), which designates a clinical syndrome of abrupt and sustained decline in glomerular filtration rate occurring within minutes to days in response to an acute ischemic or nephrotoxic event. Its clinical recognition is largely predicated upon exclusion of prerenal and postrenal causes of sudden azotemia, followed by exclusion of other causes of intrinsic ARF (i.e., glomerulonephritis, acute interstitial nephritis, vasculitis). It is necessary to carefully exclude the other defined renal syndromes before concluding that ATN is present. Interstitial nephritis is the cause in 10% of the cases and acute glomerulonephritis is the cause in 5%. Although the name *ATN* is not an entirely valid histologic description of this syndrome, the term is ingrained in clinical medicine and is, therefore, used in this article. In this article, we detail the prevention of ARF and then describe management of ARF.

PREVENTION OF ACUTE RENAL FAILURE

The steps in the prevention of ARF include identifying the patients at risk; avoiding potentially nephrotoxic agents; and using strategies to prevent renal injury (Table 1). Patients at risk are the elderly, those with pre-existing renal disease, and those who are volume depleted. There is compelling evidence that aggressive restoration of intravascular volume dramatically reduces the incidence of ATN after major surgery, trauma, and burns. In patients at risk, specific measures should be taken to reduce the occurrence of ARF when surgery or intravenous contrast administration is planned. Avoidance of nephrotoxic agents is an important aspect of prevention. In case it is necessary to use potentially nephrotoxic agents, steps should be taken to reduce the risk of ARF. Hydration and high urine flow rates are protective against the toxicity of sulfonamides and chemotherapeutic agents, including methotrexate and cisplatin (Platinol).

In prerenal states in which renal perfusion is reduced, intrarenal vasodilator prostaglandins act to buffer the vasoconstrictor effect of angiotensin. Therefore, nonsteroidal anti-inflammatory drugs (NSAIDs) that block prostaglandin synthesis can markedly reduce renal blood flow in prerenal patients, leading to ischemic tubular injury. The prevention of NSAID-induced acute ischemic injury depends on eliminating prerenal factors before administration, or to avoid their use in patients with a fixed reduction in renal perfusion. NSAIDs may cause interstitial nephritis as direct toxins or ATN via an ischemic mechanism.

The production of renal prostaglandins is regulated by the inducible form of the enzyme cyclooxygenase (COX-1), whereas the synthesis of the inflammatory prostaglandins are mediated by COX-2. ARF caused by COX-2 inhibitors has been reported and preliminary studies have suggested that the incidence of ARF is similar with use of NSAIDs. In general, NSAIDs should be avoided or used with extreme caution in patients with underlying renal insufficiency. Diuretics, angiotensin-converting enzyme inhibitors, and other vasodilators should be used with caution in patients with suspected true or effective hypovolemia or renovascular disease because they may convert prerenal azotemia to ischemic ATN and make these patients more susceptible to the adverse effect of nephrotoxins. Careful monitoring of circulating drug level appears to reduce the risk of cyclosporine (Sandimmune) nephrotoxicity.

TABLE 1. **Prevention of Acute Renal Failure**

Identify Patient at Risk
Elderly patients
Patients with abnormal renal function and/or diabetics
Patients who are volume depleted
Following vascular surgery
Following trauma
Avoid Nephrotoxic Agents
NSAIDs
Aminoglycosides
Amphotericin B
Chemotherapeutic agents, e.g., Cisplatin
ACE inhibitors in volume-depleted patients
Specific Prevention Strategies
Contrast media
Rhabdomyolysis
Tumor lysis syndrome
Surgical procedures
Avoid multiple insults

Abbreviations: ACE = angiotensin-converting enzyme; NSAIDs = nonsteroidal anti-inflammatory drugs.

Aminoglycoside antibiotics constitute a frequent cause of hospital-acquired ARF. Dose adjustment for renal function and a single daily dose is less nephrotoxic and as effective as multiple daily doses. The risk of renal failure with aminoglycosides is increased with prolonged use and nephrotoxicity may occur even when plasma levels are in the therapeutic range. Amphotericin B is a relatively frequent cause of ARF in the setting of sepsis and hypotension. Recent studies suggested that amphotericin B in lipid emulsion is less nephrotoxic than the usual preparation of amphotericin B. Hydration with normal saline before amphotericin B infusion ameliorates nephrotoxicity. We usually infuse 500 mL of normal saline before amphotericin B infusion. In patients at high risk for nephrotoxicity, we recommend using liposomal amphotericin B.

As previously mentioned, prevention of postoperative ARF must start before surgery. Recognition of high-risk patients, such as those with pre-existing renal disease, chronic liver disease, cardiac failure, and elderly patients, is the first step. The preservation of renal function in these high-risk patients should start at the preoperative assessment of risk and volume status optimized. Thereafter, avoiding additional insults such as volume depletion, hypotension during surgery, and nephrotoxic agents are important preventive measures.

PREVENTION OF CONTRAST MATERIAL–INDUCED ACUTE RENAL FAILURE

It is important to identify patients at increased risk for contrast material–induced nephropathy. The most important risk factor is the presence of prior renal insufficiency. Several studies have shown that maintenance of high urinary flow rates during and after contrast material administration protects against renal failure. Extracellular fluid volume expansion with sodium chloride has been shown to prevent contrast material–induced ARF. Our protocol is to give at least 1 L of D5W in half-normal saline over 8 hours before the procedure and to continue to replace urinary losses after the procedure.

We do not recommend routine use of diuretics or mannitol because recent studies have shown that diuretics and/or mannitol do not benefit volume expansion and may be harmful. However, diuretics may be useful for fluid management in patients with volume overload or low cardiac output. Although nonionic contrast agents have been shown to attenuate contrast material–induced ARF in animal studies, their clinical superiority in reducing the incidence of ARF has not been established. We believe that further studies are necessary before recommending the use of acetylcysteine (Mucomyst) to prevent contrast material–induced ARF.

PREVENTION OF ACUTE RENAL FAILURE IN RHABDOMYOLYSIS

As soon as diagnosis is suspected, aggressive optimization of intravascular and extravascular fluid volume by using isotonic normal saline is the most important initial step in preventing ARF (Table 2).

PREVENTION OF ACUTE RENAL FAILURE IN TUMOR LYSIS SYNDROME

ARF may occur in patients with high turnover malignancies (acute lymphoblastic leukemia and poorly differenti-

TABLE 2. **Prevention of Acute Renal Failure in Rhabdomyolysis**

Correct Intravascular Volume Depletion
Infuse normal saline as determined by the severity of volume depletion. Infuse 200–300 mL/h; follow hemodynamics with invasive monitoring when indicated.

Alkalinization of Urine and Use of Mannitol
Add 2 ampules of mannitol (25 g in 100 mL) and 2 ampules of sodium bicarbonate (100 mEq in 100 mL) to 800 mL of 5% D5W and infuse at a rate of 250 mL/h.
If urine output is good, continue infusion until myoglobinuria resolves. If the patient continues to be oliguric, stop fluids and treat as established renal failure.

ated lymphomas) who either spontaneously, or more frequently, after cytotoxic therapy, release massive amounts of purine uric acid precursors, leading to uric acid precipitation in the renal tubules. During massive cell lysis, phosphate and potassium are also released in large amounts, resulting in hyperphosphatemia and hyperkalemia. The peak uric acid level is often greater than 20 mg/dL and a ratio of urinary uric acid to creatinine concentration greater than 1:1 suggests the diagnosis of acute uric acid nephropathy. Steps must be initiated before starting chemotherapy in patients with lymphoproliferative and myeloproliferative disorders.

Treatment With Allopurinol

Allopurinol (Zyloprim), a xanthine oxidase inhibitor that blocks the synthesis of uric acid, should be administered in dosages of 300 to 600 mg/d in patients with normal renal function starting 3 days before chemotherapy to prevent acute hyperuricemia. In patients with initial hyperuricemia, it is prudent to administer allopurinol and achieve a normal serum uric acid concentration before initiating chemotherapy.

Forced Diuresis

Intravenous normal saline should be used to supplement oral intake to maintain a urine output of more than 5 L/d provided the clinical condition of the patient permits. Forced diuresis maintains a lower intratubular concentration of uric acid and presumably helps to reduce intratubular obstruction.

Urinary Alkalinization

Urinary alkalinization increases the solubility of xanthine and uric acid and enhances excretion. This can be achieved by the infusion of sodium bicarbonate in amounts to keep urinary pH above 7 with or without the administration of acetazolamide (Diamox). This agent inhibits the reabsorption of sodium bicarbonate in the proximal tubule, thereby making the tubular fluid and the urine alkaline. An advocated regimen is to infuse 1 g/m^2 of acetazolamide/d accompanied by sodium bicarbonate 100 mEq/m^2 daily to balance urinary losses, and 40 to 80 mEq of potassium to avoid hypokalemia due to increased renal excretion.

CONSERVATIVE MANAGEMENT OF ACUTE RENAL FAILURE

The loss of the excretory function of the kidney makes the patient very vulnerable to derangements in the internal milieu unless special care is taken to monitor the fluid and electrolyte and nutritional intake of the patient. Daily assessment of patients with particular attention to daily weight, intake/output, and other laboratory parameters are described in Table 3.

MANAGEMENT OF VOLUME HOMEOSTASIS

The goal of management is to keep the patient euvolemic and daily assessment of volume status is an important part of the management. Daily measurement of supine and standing blood pressure and pulse, examination of the mucous membranes, skin turgor, examination of the lungs for pulmonary congestion, examination for edema, daily weight and daily intake and output records are important to assess volume status. In the intensive care unit, clinical assessment of volume status may be affected by

TABLE 3. **Daily Assessment of Patients With Acute Renal Failure**

Variable	Comments
Weight	Aim for a daily weight loss of 0.5–1.0 lb in patients with ATN to prevent fluid retention
JVD, basal crackles	Indicate volume overload or congestive heart failure: restrict volume and consider diuretics or dialysis when indicated
CVP and PCWP	May be indicated in the differential diagnosis of volume overload versus noncardiogenic pulmonary infiltrates; low PCWP (<10) suggests noncardiogenic pulmonary edema (e.g., ARDS)
Intake/output	In euvolemic patients, give the previous day's urine output volume plus 400 mL for insensible loss in stable patients
BUN	When disproportionately high, look for GI bleeding, medications such as steroids, or catabolic states such as sepsis
Serum sodium	Reflects body water status; hyponatremia suggests excess water intake in the face of impaired free water clearance by the kidney
Serum potassium	Hyperkalemia out of proportion to the renal failure suggests tumor lysis or catabolic states such as sepsis; in severe hyperkalemia, electrocardiogram is a better guide for therapy
Total CO_2	Decreases by 1–2 mEq/day and stabilizes at 16–18 mEq/L; generally no treatment is required; in case of more severe acidosis, look for other causes such as lactic acidosis, ketoacidosis, or toxin ingestion
Serum calcium	Hypocalcemia is usually asymptomatic and requires no treatment; in hypercalcemia look for hyperparathyroidism or underlying malignancy

Abbreviations: ARDS = acute respiratory distress syndrome; BUN = blood urea nitrogen; CO_2 = carbon dioxide; CVP = central venous pressure; JVD = jugular vein distention; GI = gastrointestinal; PCWP = pulmonary capillary wedge pressure.

surgical wounds, severe pneumonia, or edema due to capillary leak. Therefore, invasive monitoring such as central venous pressure or pulmonary capillary wedge pressure may be necessary to precisely evaluate volume status.

In addition to urine losses, water losses occur from diffusion and evaporation through the skin and expired water vapor. These losses normally amount to 0.5 to 0.6 mL/kg/h or approximately 850 to 1000 mL/d in a 70-kg afebrile resting adult. With fever, insensible water loss increases by about 13% for each 1°C (7% for each 1°F). Because insensible loss cannot be accurately determined, daily assessment and modification of fluid therapy are essential. Water is also continuously generated from endogenous sources by the oxidation of protein (41 mL/100 g), fat (107 mL/100 g), and carbohydrate (55 mL/100 g). Without carbohydrate supplementation, a 70-kg man burns 1 g of protein and 2 g of fat/kg of body weight with the generation of 0.25 to 0.35 mL/kg/h or approximately 450 mL of water. The addition of 100 g of carbohydrate reduces protein metabolism by 50% with a small but significant decrease in water generation.

Additional carbohydrate will not further reduce protein catabolism. Thus, to balance the difference between insensible water loss and endogenous water production in an afebrile 70-kg man, daily water intake must be limited to 400 mL plus an amount equal to that passed in urine. In hypercatabolic states, such as may occur with severe infections, trauma, or surgery, more water may be generated by enhanced protein and fat catabolism. In the patient maintained with intravenous fluids without protein or fat administration, the physician should target small daily weight losses of 0.2 to 0.3 kg to prevent fluid retention. Patients with evidence of volume depletion should be provided with additional fluid to maintain euvolemia because sustained hypovolemia may delay recovery.

Hypernatremia and Hyponatremia

Abnormal serum sodium concentrations are caused by disorders of water metabolism. Hyponatremia resulting from an excess water intake in the presence of impairment of free water clearance is very common in ARF. Sources for excess water intake that lead to hyponatremia include hypotonic solutions given as 5% dextrose, parenteral medication administered in 5% dextrose, or excess intake of free water with enteral or parenteral feeding. Hypernatremia is uncommon and is usually due to inappropriate administration of intravenous fluids.

Potassium Balance

Hyperkalemia is one of the most serious consequences of ARF and steps should be taken to prevent hyperkalemia in patients with ARF by dietary potassium intake restriction to less than 50 mEq/d (Table 4). Cardiac toxicity is the most threatening problem and the electromechanical effects of hyperkalemia on the heart are potentiated by hypokalemia, acidosis, and hyponatremia. Thus, the electrocardiogram, which measures the summation of these effects, is a better guide to therapy than a single potassium determination. The earliest change is the appearance of a peaked T wave followed by shortening of the QT interval. Later, the P wave may become flat and disappear. The QRS complex becomes wide followed by ventricular arrhythmia, fibrillation, or arrest.

TABLE 4. **Prevention of Hyperkalemia in Patients with Acute Renal Failure**

Restriction of potassium intake
Omit potassium from parenteral fluids and TPN
Discontinue drugs containing potassium, e.g., penicillin G
Avoid salt substitutes that contain potassium
Avoid drugs that impair potassium
Discontinue medications that inhibit potassium excretion
Potassium-sparing diuretics
NSAIDs
ACE inhibitors

Abbreviations: ACE = angiotensin-converting enzyme; NSAIDs = nonsteroidal anti-inflammatory drugs; TPN = total parenteral nutrition.

The treatment of hyperkalemia depends on the urgency and severity of the problem. In patients with hyperkalemia associated with electrocardiographic changes, intravenous calcium infusion in the form of calcium chloride or calcium gluconate immediately antagonizes the effect of the potassium on the heart. Potassium can be redistributed from the extracellular to the intracellular space by the administration of insulin and glucose, inhaled or intravenous β-adrenergic receptor agonists, or intravenous sodium bicarbonate. These measures require 30 to 60 minutes before they affect serum potassium and the duration of action is short-lived. Removal of potassium from the body is achieved by the use of the cation exchange resin sodium polystyrene sulfonate (Kayexalate), which may be administered orally or rectally. Oral polystyrene sulfonate is administered as 30 g in a solution of 20% sorbitol every 2 to 4 hours, whereas rectal polystyrene sulfonate is administered as a retention enema, 60 g mixed with 200 mL of water every 1 to 2 hours. The administration of sorbitol by rectum is contraindicated because of its association with colonic epithelial necrosis. Hyperkalemia that cannot be easily controlled by conservative means is an indication for dialysis.

ACID-BASE HOMEOSTASIS

An individual weighing 70 kg on a normal American diet will produce about 60 to 80 mEq of acid daily that is normally excreted by the kidney to maintain acid-base homeostasis. In patients with ARF, the serum bicarbonate level decreases by 1 to 2 mEq/d and stabilizes at about 16 to 18 mEq/L and does not require treatment except as an adjuvant treatment for hyperkalemia. A more rapid or a severe drop is either due to a very catabolic state related to the underlying disease leading to ARF, infection, or inadequate nutrition. In such patients, it is also important to exclude other causes of acidosis such as lactic acidosis, ketoacidosis, or drug overdose before it is attributed to ARF. Metabolic acidosis not related to ARF should be treated by removing the source of acid generation or bicarbonate loss. In patients with ARF, dietary protein restriction will slow the development of acidosis because acid is generated from protein metabolism. Adequate nonprotein calories must be provided to avoid a catabolic state and should be assessed carefully with the assistance of a dietitian. In the few patients requiring the correction of acidosis, sodium bicarbonate can be administered orally or parenterally depending on the urgency for replacement and the degree of acidosis. Parenteral sodium bicarbonate should be administered in isotonic solution by adding three ampules of sodium bicarbonate (50 mEq/50 mL) to 1 L of 5% dextrose in water. Acetate can be added to parenteral nutrition and adjusted to maintain acid-base homeostasis. The disadvantage of sodium bicarbonate or acetate is worsening of volume overload.

Calcium and Phosphate Balance

A reduction in the serum calcium concentration is commonly found in patients with ARF and may be particularly severe with rhabdomyolysis and hyperphosphatemia. Hypocalcemia may worsen the cardiac toxicity of hyperkalemia, as previously mentioned. Hypomagnesemia inhibits synthesis and release of parathyroid hormone and functional hypoparathyroidism may contribute to hypocalcemia. In most patients, hypocalcemia is asymptomatic and does not require specific treatment. Hypercalcemia may occur in the recovery phase of ARF in patients with rhabdomyolysis and generally requires no treatment.

Hyperphosphatemia occurs commonly in ARF but is most severe in tumor lysis syndrome and rhabdomyolysis. Hyperphosphatemia may contribute to secondary hyperparathyroidism and may cause metastatic calcification; therefore, treatment should be given with phosphate binders. Treatment should be given with calcium carbonate (Tums) 0.5 to 1 g with meals or aluminum hydroxide (Amphojel) 15 to 30 mL with meals. If calcium phosphate product is high (>70), it is preferable to use aluminum hydroxide. The risk of aluminum intoxication is low because of the short duration of use. Hypophosphatemia is unusual in ARF and is encountered most commonly in patients with burns, in patients with history of alcohol abuse, and in some patients on hyperalimentation. Severe hypophosphatemia may affect several organ systems and should be corrected either orally or parenterally.

Hypermagnesemia is common in patients with ARF. High levels occur in patients given magnesium-containing antacids or laxatives. Magnesium can be removed by dialysis. Hyperuricemia is usually modest, with no clinical consequences, and no treatment is usually required. The only exceptions are conditions associated with uric acid nephropathy such as tumor lysis syndrome, in which case the uric acid levels should be decreased by using hemodialysis.

NUTRITIONAL THERAPY

Although previous studies suggested that treatment with glucose and essential and nonessential amino acids as compared with glucose alone or no nutrition may improve the nutritional status and possibly survival, these reports are not conclusive. Nonetheless, a minimum goal of nutritional support is to minimize the catabolic state, and it appears prudent to administer sufficient oral or parenteral nutrition to attain the most optimal nutritional status. The need for nutritional therapy may be particularly important for patients who are wasted or very catabolic.

Urea Nitrogen Appearance

Calculation of the urea nitrogen appearance is a simple, inexpensive, and accurate measurement of net protein breakdown. The usefulness of the urea nitrogen appearance is that it usually correlates with total nitrogen output. Table 5 describes the formula to calculate urea nitrogen appearance and estimation of dietary nitrogen intake.

In patients with a low rate of urea nitrogen appearance (<4 to 5 g/d) who are not wasted and not on dialysis, a dietary intake low in nitrogen (0.6 g/kg/d) is recommended. This regimen will maintain neutral nitrogen balance and minimize the rate of accumulation of nitrogenous metabolites. For patients with a urea nitrogen appearance greater than 4 to 5 g/d or who are malnourished or on dialysis, it is necessary to provide 1 to 1.2 g/kg/d as both essential and nonessential amino acids. The larger nitrogen intake may reduce the patient's negative nitrogen balance. With appropriate dialysis, the high nitrogen intakes are well tolerated by most patients.

ORAL OR ENTERAL THERAPY

For patients able to receive nutrition by eating, enteral tubes, or gastrostomy, administration of nutrition by these routes is preferred to intravenous

TABLE 5. **Calculation of Urinary Nitrogen Appearance and Estimation of Dietary Nitrogen Intake**

UNA (g/d) = urinary urea nitrogen (g/d) + dialysate urea nitrogen (g/d) + change in body urea nitrogen (g/d)
Change in body urea nitrogen (g/d) = $(SUN_f - SUN_i) \times BW_i \times$ (0.6 L/kg) − $(BW_f - BW_i) \times SUN_f \times$ (1.0 L/kg)
Total nitrogen output (g/d) = 0.97 UNA (g/d) + 1.93
Dietary nitrogen intake = 0.69 UNA (g/d) + 3.3

Abbreviations: 0.60 = estimation of total body water; 1.0 = the volume of distribution of urea; BW = body weight in kilograms; i and f = initial and final values; SUN = serum urea nitrogen in g/L; UNA = urea nitrogen appearance.

administration. Parenteral nutrition is more hazardous, provides greater fluid loads, and is more costly. The diet should supply at least 30 kcal/kg/d. The diet should also contain no less than 0.65 g/kg/d of high biologic value protein. Patients on hemodialysis should ingest a higher amount of protein, that is, 1.0 to 1.2 g/kg/d with approximately 50% of high biological value. Urea nitrogen appearance should be monitored in these patients to ensure that there are no negative nitrogen values. For patients who must be fed by an enteric tube or a gastrostomy, many liquid proteins or defined formula diets are available. The electrolyte composition of the various preparations often differ. Thus, the potassium, protein, and phosphorus content should be evaluated and the preparation chosen should provide adequate protein intake in the lowest possible volume and potassium content.

Parenteral Feeding

If oral feeding is not possible, it is reasonable to limit treatment to intravenous fluids for 3 to 5 days. During this time, the goal is to supply about 100 g of glucose/d to achieve optimal fluid and electrolyte balance. If hypertonic glucose solutions are required, insulin must be administered to avoid hyperglycemia. Adequate supplementation of water-soluble vitamins, trace metals, and folic acid must be provided with all dietary regimens.

Total Parenteral Nutrition

Nitrogen imbalance can be improved by infusion of amino acids with additional calories in the form of 70% solution of hypertonic glucose. In noncatabolic patients (urea nitrogen appearance <4–5 g/d) who are not on dialysis, 20 to 30 g/d of essential amino acids may be infused. In catabolic patients (urea nitrogen appearance >4–5 g/d) who are undergoing dialysis or malnourished, infusion with 1.0 to 1.2 g/kg/d of essential and nonessential amino acids may be necessary.

CONSERVATIVE MANAGEMENT OF ORGAN SYSTEM COMPLICATIONS

Extrarenal manifestations of ARF are generally similar to those found in chronic renal failure. Many of the manifestations are due to volume and electrolyte abnormalities. However, some of these complications are secondary to uremia and may require replacement therapy. Table 6 summarizes the major complications associated with ARF.

TABLE 6. **Major Complications of Acute Renal Failure**

Cause	Complications
Impairment of Fluid and Electrolyte Excretion	
Water	Hyponatremia
Sodium chloride	Volume expansion Congestive heart failure
Potassium	Hyperkalemia Arrhythmias Muscle weakness
Hydrogen ion	Metabolic acidosis
Phosphate	Hyperphosphatemia Hypocalcemia Metabolic calcification
Magnesium	Hypermagnesemia
Uric acid	Hyperuricemia
Retention of Urea and Other Solutes	Cardiac: uremic pericarditis Neurologic: asterixis, confusion, somnolence, coma, seizures Hematologic: anemia, coagulopathy, bleeding diathesis Infection Gastrointestinal: nausea, vomiting, gastritis, bleeding Skin, pruritus Glucose intolerance
Synthetic Impairment	
1,25-Dihydroxyvitamin D_3	Hypocalcemia
Erythropoietin	Anemia
Impaired Drug Metabolism and Excretion	Drug toxicity, decreased diuretic effectiveness

INFECTIOUS COMPLICATIONS

Infection is frequently associated with ARF and is a major cause of increased morbidity and mortality. The most common sites for infections include pulmonary, urinary tract, surgical wounds, and peritoneum. Infections related to indwelling venous and arterial catheters can also occur. Meticulous attention to prevention of infection is crucial. Therefore, the urinary catheter should be removed as soon as possible and should not be kept in patients who are able to void. Similarly, parenteral sites and surgical wounds require extraordinary care in patients with ARF. Early recognition and appropriate antibiotic therapy for infections is important in improving the outcome of these patients. The dosage of antibiotics should be adjusted to the degree of renal function, and nephrotoxic agents avoided when possible.

GASTROINTESTINAL COMPLICATIONS

The primary gastrointestinal complications of ARF include symptoms of anorexia and vomiting and upper gastrointestinal bleeding. Gastrointestinal bleeding may be particularly serious in a postoperative or posttraumatic setting. Stress ulcers and gastritis are common and can be prevented by the use of antacids such as aluminum hydroxide or sucralfate (Carafate) 1 g three to four times per day. Magnesium-containing antacids should be avoided to prevent hypermagnesemia. The use of H2-receptor antagonists such as ranitidine (Zantac) 150 mg orally once a day, or 50 mg intravenously every 6 to 8 hours may be helpful as prophylaxis in high-risk patients. If cimetidine is used, dose adjustment is necessary because it is excreted by the kidney. Some centers have reported that gastrointestinal bleeding is associated with a high mortality rate. Prophylactic dialysis may reduce the incidence of this complication and associated mortality in patients with advanced ARF. An increase in serum amylase level may be observed in these patients because amylase is cleared by the kidney. Thus, lipase determination and clinical assessment are often necessary to diagnose acute pancreatitis in the setting of ARF.

CARDIOVASCULAR AND PULMONARY COMPLICATIONS

Cardiovascular problems such as arrhythmia, pulmonary edema, and hypertension are attributable to fluid overload and electrolyte abnormalities. In elderly patients (age >70 years), there is increased death from myocardial infarction. Uremic pericarditis may rarely complicate the course of ARF. The pericarditis usually resolves with intensive dialysis. If pericardial effusion is present and hemodynamically significant, pericardiocentesis may be required. Pericardial tamponade may not present with the classic clinical findings; therefore, it should be suspected in patients with unexplained hypotension. Pulmonary complications include infection, infiltrates, or hemorrhage associated with rapidly progressive glomerulonephritis. The presence of pulmonary complications adversely affects the prognosis of ARF.

BLEEDING ABNORMALITIES

The most common cause of bleeding abnormalities in ARF is due to platelet dysfunction associated with prolonged bleeding time. Dialysis usually corrects the disorder. If the bleeding tendency is not corrected or the patient is actively bleeding, the infusion of 10 U of cryoprecipitate, or 1-deamino-8-D-arginine vasopressin (Pitressin Synthetic) 0.3 units intravenously will correct the bleeding time abnormality. Conjugated estrogen was also found to be helpful but takes several days to be effective.

ANEMIA

Anemia may occur early in ARF secondary to blood loss, increased hemolysis, or decreased erythropoietin level that occurs rapidly after the onset of ARF. In most patients, anemia does not need treatment. However, patients with congestive heart failure, symptomatic coronary artery disease, or hypoxia may require treatment with blood transfusion. The role of parenteral erythropoietin is not clear but may be useful in prolonged ARF.

NEUROMUSCULAR COMPLICATIONS

Neuromuscular symptoms such as asterixis, irritability, somnolence, stupor, and coma are found early in the course of ARF and are caused by electrolyte abnormalities such as hypernatremia and hyponatremia, hypocalcemia and hypercalcemia, and hypophosphatemia. Late in the course of the disease, the symptoms are usually due to uremia. The aim of management is to correct electrolyte abnormalities and uremia by conservative management or dialysis when indicated.

PHARMACOLOGIC THERAPY IN ACUTE RENAL FAILURE

Diuretics

Furosemide (Lasix) is the most commonly used loop diuretic in patients with ARF. Whether use of diuretics in ARF favorably affects the outcome is controversial. We do not routinely use diuretics in patients with ARF because there is no evidence that this approach affects the outcome. However, patients with evidence of volume overload may warrant a therapeutic trial with furosemide. A higher dose in the range of 2 to 10 mg/kg/d intravenously may be required and should be given over 20 to 30 minutes to avoid ototoxicity. Continuous infusion of bumetanide (Bumex) produced more sodium excretion and less toxicity than bolus bumetanide. Therefore, continuous infusion should be considered when the response to bolus administration is not adequate. Diuretics may convert oliguric to nonoliguric ARF, which makes management easier with less volume overload and electrolyte imbalance. However, there is no evidence that it is effective in reducing mortality or the need for dialysis.

Mannitol

Mannitol is an osmotic diuretic and has been used in prophylaxis and treatment of ARF with the rationale of preventing cell swelling and decrease intratubular obstruction. We use mannitol in conjunction with volume replacement and sodium bicarbonate to prevent myoglobinuric ARF. We do not recommend the use of mannitol to prevent contrast-induced ARF because hydration is the most important single factor. We do not use mannitol to prevent ischemic ARF or during its course. In the absence of clinical evidence, mannitol cannot be recommended to prevent perioperative ATN.

DOPAMINE

Dopamine (Dopastat) dilates renal arterioles and increases renal blood flood and the glomerular filtration rate. Dopamine has been used for both the prevention and treatment of ARF in critically ill patients. However, in our opinion, the role of dopamine in the management of ARF is controversial. We do not recommend the routine use of dopamine in patients with ARF because clinical studies have not demonstrated the efficacy of this approach for the treatment or prevention of ATN. Proponents of dopamine recommend a trial of low-dose dopamine, 1 to 3 μg/kg/min, in a subset of euvolemic patients with oliguric ARF and believe that dopamine may help to convert oliguric to nonoliguric ARF. Main side effects of dopamine are tachyarrhythmia, pulmonary shunting, and gut and digital necrosis.

TABLE 7. **Advantages and Disadvantages of Renal Replacement Therapy**

Intermittent Hemodialysis
Advantages
More efficient for solute removal
Short duration
May be performed without heparin
Less complex and rapidly available
No need to train ICU staff
Disadvantages
Large shift in fluid and electrolytes
Risk of cardiac arrhythmias
High incidence of hypotension
Disequilibrium syndrome may occur

Continuous Renal Replacement Therapy
Advantages
Removal of large volumes of fluid
Hemodynamic stability
Permit unlimited nutrition
Removal of more large molecular weight solutes
Disadvantages
Need for heparin
Need training for ICU staff
Prolonged use and may be interrupted by tests
Needs careful follow-up of replacement fluid

Peritoneal Dialysis
Advantages
Hemodynamic stability
No anticoagulation needed
Ability to remove volume easily
Disadvantages
Need surgical insertion of Tenckhoff or acute catheter
Risk of bowel perforation
Technical drainage problems
Risk for peritonitis and exit site infection

Abbreviation: ICU = intensive care unit.

DIALYSIS THERAPY IN ACUTE RENAL FAILURE

Indications for the commencement of renal replacement therapy include diuretic-unresponsive volume overload, severe hyperkalemia, and metabolic acidosis unresponsive to conservative measures, uremic pericarditis, and uremic encephalopathy. In addition, most nephrologists initiate dialysis when the blood urea nitrogen level reaches approximately 100 mg/dL. Early dialysis makes the overall nutritional and fluid electrolyte management easier and may help to prevent some complications of uremia.

The choice of renal replacement therapy in ARF depends on the patient's circumstances. The main aim of dialysis in patients with ARF is to restore normal electrolyte levels and acid-base balance and to remove excess fluid. Intermittent hemodialysis can achieve these goals in hemodynamically stable patients in the absence of significant volume overload. Most patients typically undergo acute intermittent hemodialysis for 3 to 4 hours daily or on alternate days, depending on their catabolic state, volume status, and laboratory results. Intermittent hemodialysis is convenient, efficient in solute removal, and can be performed with or without anticoagulation if necessary.

There are different methods for continuous renal replacement therapy. Because the process is gradual, hemodynamic stability can be maintained even if the patient has low blood pressure. Continuous renal replacement therapy is also superior to intermittent hemodialysis in allowing more nutritional support. Despite the theoretical advantages of continuous renal replacement therapy in patients with ARF, there are no controlled studies that show superiority of this technique compared with intermittent hemodialysis or peritoneal dialysis. Furthermore, there are no studies to indicate the optimal dose of dialysis and whether early dialysis influences the outcome in ARF. Until such studies are available, the choice of dialysis modality and dose depend on individual patient circumstances and local preferences (Table 7).

CHRONIC RENAL FAILURE

method of
JEFFREY S. BERNS, M.D.
University of Pennsylvania School of Medicine
Philadelphia, Pennsylvania

There are more than 300,000 patients with end-stage renal disease (ESRD) in the United States. Among patients starting dialysis for ESRD, about 30% have type II diabetes mellitus and about 25% have hypertension identified as the primary cause of ESRD. Glomerulonephritis accounts for 10% to 15% of new cases and polycystic kidney disease accounts for about 3% of new cases of ESRD. Renovascular or ischemic renal disease is increasing in prevalence and may account for as many as 10% to 20% of new cases of ESRD in patients over the age of 65 years.

There is estimated to be more than 10 million people in this country with mild renal insufficiency who have serum creatinine levels of 1.5 mg/dL or greater and nearly 1 million with serum creatinine levels of 2.0 mg/dL or greater. With more than 80,000 new patients starting dialysis each year and Medicare expenditures for the care of patients with ESRD exceeding $12 billion annually, efforts to prevent or slow the progression of renal insufficiency can have great clinical and economic impact.

This article presents a brief review of the diagnosis and assessment of renal insufficiency then focuses on factors that are associated with progressive renal failure and ways to slow this progression. Management of some of the complications of renal failure are described. Finally, preparation of the patient for dialysis or transplantation and end-stage renal failure will be reviewed. The terms *chronic renal insufficiency (CRI)* and *chronic renal failure (CRF)* are used interchangeably, describing patients with any degree of impaired age-specific renal function who do not yet require dialysis or transplantation for survival.

DIAGNOSIS OF CHRONIC RENAL FAILURE

An important component of the early diagnosis and management of CRF is the identification of patients who are at increased risk for development of progressive renal failure and ESRD. This includes patients with type I or type II diabetes mellitus, hypertension, or family history of kidney disease; elderly patients; and patients with atherosclerotic vascular disease. Patients with hypertension or diabetes mellitus and microalbuminuria (urinary protein excretion below the limits of detection of urine dipsticks, ~300 mg/d, but with urinary albumin excretion of 30–300 mg/d or 20–200 μg/min), or overt proteinuria detected by urine dipsticks have an increased risk of ESRD and should be monitored closely.

Most patients with CRF will experience progressive loss of kidney function, eventually leading to ESRD. The normal glomerular filtration rate (GFR) is 100 to 130 mL/min. Symptoms associated with renal failure, such as anorexia, nausea, fatigue, malaise, and weight loss do not typically develop until the GFR falls below about 15 to 20 mL/min, and dialysis is often recommended when the GFR approaches 10 to 15 mL/min. Identification of patients with CRF only after they have symptoms and already have substantially reduced GFR leaves little opportunity for slowing progression of the renal failure. In addition, many of the manifestations of CRF (Table 1) that add substantially to overall morbidity will already have developed.

The presence of renal insufficiency is typically established by the presence of elevations of the blood urea nitrogen (BUN) and serum creatinine. Although readily available, these tests are both only very crude estimates of renal function. Because of the nature of the relationship between serum creatinine level and GFR (Figure 1), there may be little if any increase in serum creatinine level until 50% or more of renal function has been lost. Small increases in the serum creatinine level when renal function is relatively well preserved reflect much more substantial losses of GFR than similar changes in serum creatinine when GFR is more severely impaired. This notion cannot be overemphasized. By the time a patient's serum creatinine level has increased from 1.0 mg/dL to 1.5 mg/dL, the GFR may have fallen already from 100 mL/min to less than 50 mL/min, even though the serum creatinine level is still within the reference range.

TABLE 1. **Clinical and Laboratory Manifestations of Chronic Renal Failure**

Cardiac	**Endocrine**
Hypertension	Insulin resistance
Left ventricular hypertrophy	Hyperlipidemia
Dilated cardiomyopathy	Impotence
Pericarditis	Decreased libido
Hematologic	Amenorrhea
Anemia	Hypogonadism
Platelet dysfunction	**Pulmonary**
Metabolic bone disease	Pleuritis
Osteitis fibrosa	Pulmonary edema
Osteomalacia	Pneumonitis—uremic lung
Neurologic	**Miscellaneous**
Asterixis	Edema
Encephalopathy	Fatigue
Peripheral neuropathy	Muscle cramps
Restless legs	Hypothermia
Gastrointestinal tract	Sleep disorders
Nausea, vomiting	Weight loss
Anorexia	**Laboratory**
Hiccups	Elevated BUN and creatinine
Metallic or fishy taste	Hyperkalemia
Uremic fetor	Metabolic acidosis
Gastritis	Hyperphosphatemia
GI tract AV malformations	Hypocalcemia
Dermatologic	
Pruritus	

Abbreviations: AV = arteriovenous, BUN = blood urea nitrogen, GI = gastrointestinal.

The clinical assessment of renal function is most often based on the serum creatinine level and calculation of the creatinine clearance as an approximation of GFR. Creatinine is a byproduct of muscle metabolism and is excreted primarily by the kidneys. The relationship between creatinine clearance and muscle mass is reflected in the effects of age, weight, and gender on calculated estimates of creatinine clearance derived from the serum creatinine level, such as the Cockcroft-Gault formula:

$$\text{Creatinine Clearance} = \frac{(140 - \text{age}) \times (\text{weight in kilograms})\ (\text{in women} \times 0.85)}{72 \times \text{Serum Creatinine (in mg/dL)}}$$

and as seen in Figure 2.

Creatinine clearance is calculated based on a 24-hour urine collection as (UV/P) ÷ by 1440, where U is urinary concentration of creatinine in milligrams per deciliter, V is 24-hour urine volume in milliliters, and P is plasma creatinine concentration in milligrams per deciliter. Division by 1440, the number of minutes in a day, generates creatinine clearance in milliliters per minute. The completeness of a 24-hour urine collection, and hence the accuracy of the creatinine clearance calculation, can be assessed by measuring the total daily creatinine excretion; adult men typically excrete 1.5 to 2.0 g and women 1.0 to 1.5 g of creatinine per day.

In addition to being freely filtered across the glomerulus, creatinine is secreted into the urine by the renal tubules. Urinary creatinine excretion, and therefore creatinine clearance, is thus a function not only of glomerular filtration but also of tubular secretion of creatinine. Tubular secretion of creatinine typically contributes no more than 5 to 10 mL/min to creatinine clearance when renal function is relatively normal. However, as renal function declines, creatinine secretion increases both in absolute and relative terms and may account for as much as 40% to 50% of total creatinine clearance at low levels of renal function. This results in a substantial overestimation of actual GFR.

Urea clearance [(urinary urea nitrogen concentration in mg/dL × 24-hour urine volume in milliliters) divided by (BUN divided by 1440)] tends to underestimate GFR because of tubular reabsorption of urea. The average of these creatinine and urea clearances more closely approximates true GFR than either clearance alone or creatinine clearance calculated with the Cockcroft-Gault equation. The mean of the urea and creatinine clearance may be useful to measure in patients with advanced renal insufficiency, especially when there is a question as to the degree of renal dysfunction. This situation may arise, for instance, when a patient who presents with clinical features consistent with uremia but perhaps due to advanced age or small muscle mass has a relatively low serum creatinine level. In usual clinical circumstances, more precise measurement of GFR with inulin clearance or use of radioisotopes is unnecessary.

SLOWING THE PROGRESSION OF CHRONIC RENAL FAILURE TO END-STAGE RENAL DISEASE

Reversible Causes of Renal Failure

Reversible causes of renal dysfunction should be considered when evaluating patients with CRF, par-

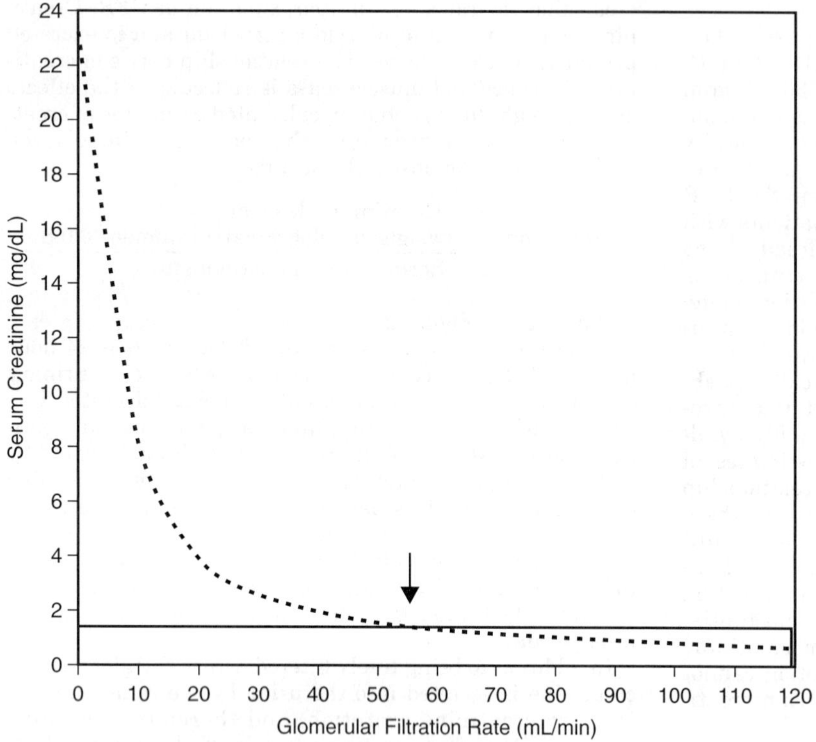

Figure 1. Relationship between glomerular filtration rate (GFR) and serum creatinine concentration. The serum creatinine concentration does not increase above 1.5 mg/dL until there has already been a substantial loss of renal function (*arrow*). At low levels of renal function, a further decline in the GFR results in a much greater increase in serum creatinine concentration than a similar decline in GFR starting from higher levels of renal function.

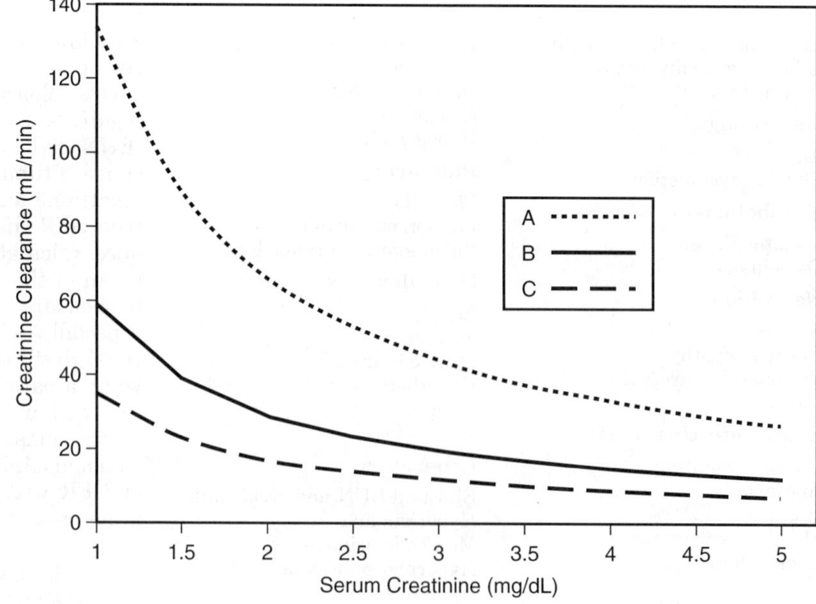

Figure 2. Relationship between serum creatinine and estimated creatinine clearance using the Cockcroft-Gault formula. Depending on the gender, age, and weight of the patient, a given serum creatinine concentration may be indicative of very different levels of renal function (creatinine clearance), as shown here for a 20-year-old man weighing 80 kg (A), a 40-year-old woman (B) and an 80-year-old woman (C), each weighing 50 kg.

ticularly when renal function has recently declined. These include renal hypoperfusion due to hypovolemia (i.e., diarrhea, vomiting, poor oral intake, diuretic use) or reduced cardiac output or blood pressure (BP) (i.e., heart failure, antihypertensive drugs) and drugs that can impair GFR, such as nonsteroidal anti-inflammatory drugs (NSAIDs) (including the newer cyclooxygenase-2 (COX-2) selective agents), angiotensin converting enzyme (ACE) inhibitors, and the newer angiotensin receptor blockers (ARBs). Use of nephrotoxic drugs, such as NSAIDs, aminoglycoside antibiotics, and iodinated radiographic contrast material should be avoided whenever possible in patients with preexisting renal insufficiency. Urinary tract obstruction should always be considered, especially in men who may have prostate gland enlargement and in patients with diabetes mellitus or other disorders that may result in neurogenic bladder dysfunction.

Systemic and Glomerular Hypertension

Experimental data, as well as clinical studies, indicate that both systemic hypertension and elevated intraglomerular pressure accelerate the rate of progression of renal disease. Intraglomerular hypertension results from compensatory responses to nephron loss and altered glomerular hemodynamics that attempt to maintain GFR but lead to altered glomerular permeability, cellular hypertrophy, endothelial and epithethial cell damage, release of cytokines and growth factors, and increase in glomerular mesangial matrix synthesis.

Arterial hypertension is common in patients with renal disease and either directly or through effects on intraglomerular pressure contributes to progression of renal insufficiency. BP reduction in hypertensive patients with calcium channel blockers, β-blockers, vasodilators, ACE inhibitors, diuretics, and other agents can reduce progression of renal insufficiency. Recent evidence indicates that BP targets for patients with renal insufficiency, particularly in patients with diabetes mellitus or other proteinuric renal diseases, should be lower than traditionally recommended. Systolic BP should be maintained below 130 to 135 mm Hg and diastolic BP should be maintained below 80 to 85 mm Hg in patients with hypertension and low-grade proteinuria (<1–2 g/d). Lower BP goals, with systolic BP below 125 mm Hg and diastolic BP below 75 to 80 mm Hg, are desired in patients with diabetes mellitus or more significant proteinuria.

Evidence indicates that ACE inhibitors are more effective than other antihypertensive therapies in reducing proteinuria and slowing progression of renal insufficiency in patients with type I diabetes mellitus and in those with type II diabetes mellitus and other forms of chronic renal disease associated with proteinuria. ACE inhibitors and to a somewhat lesser extent the nondihydropyridine calcium channel blockers diltiazem (Cardizem) and verapamil (Calan) seem to reduce proteinuria more consistently and to a greater degree than other antihypertensive agents. ARBs may have an effect similar to that of the ACE inhibitors, although data are limited and a long-term renoprotective effect of these newer agents has yet to be demonstrated. Although some of the benefit of ACE inhibitors compared with other drugs may be due in part to somewhat better BP control with the ACE inhibitors, an additional specific renoprotective effect seems likely. This effect seems to correlate with the degree of reduction in proteinuria, even in patients without hypertension. Thus, ACE inhibitors are the preferred drugs for treatment in most patients with diabetes mellitus or other nephropathies associated with proteinuria, even in the absence of significant hypertension. There is no definite evidence that one ACE inhibitor is better than any other as far as a renoprotective or antiproteinuric effect is concerned. Acute, self-limited declines in renal function often occur within the first few months after starting ACE inhibitors and should therefore not necessarily lead to discontinuation of the ACE inhibitor.

Diltiazem, verapamil, or one of the ARBs may be the best alternative for control of hypertension and for reduction of proteinuria in patients who experience cough with ACE inhibitors. Hyperkalemia, worsening azotemia that is not self-limited (and that might prompt closer evaluation for renovascular disease), and angioneurotic edema with ACE inhibitors may also occur with ARBs. Diltiazem or verapamil are preferred in patients with any of these reactions to ACE inhibitors. Use of one of these calcium channel blockers or an ARB in combination with an ACE inhibitor may reduce proteinuria more than either drug alone. Because fluid overload is common in patients with renal insufficiency and contributes to the development of hypertension, loop diuretics are often necessary as well. Treatment with loop diuretics also often enhances the antihypertensive and antiproteinuric effect of ACE inhibitors.

Hyperglycemia

Rigorous control of blood sugar in patients with type I diabetes mellitus using oral hypoglycemics or insulin slows the progression of diabetic nephropathy, as well as neuropathy and retinopathy. A less extensive body of literature suggests that the same is also probably true for type II or non–insulin-dependent diabetes mellitus. The glycosylated hemoglobin concentration should be maintained below 6.5% while avoiding hypoglycemia. Although insulin resistance occurs as part of the uremic syndrome, insulin and oral hypoglycemic requirements often fall as renal failure progresses due to altered insulin and drug metabolism and excretion, reduced muscle mass (and hence extrarenal metabolism of insulin), and reduced caloric intake.

Dietary Protein Intake

A beneficial effect of restricting dietary protein on the progression of diabetic nephropathy and certain other renal diseases has been suggested by both experimental and clinical studies. Dietary protein restriction may also ameliorate some of the clinical manifestations of uremia by reducing the generation of urea and other nitrogenous waste products. As such, it may be possible to delay initiation of dialysis by postponing the onset of symptomatic uremia even in the absence of any effect on the rate of decline of GFR. Dietary protein restriction also tends to reduce dietary phosphate intake and metabolic acid generation. Hormonal responses to dietary protein intake and effects of amino acids on intrarenal sodium handling and intraglomerular hemodynamics have been postulated to account for the beneficial response to low-protein diets.

Enthusiasm for dietary protein restriction has been tempered by concern about adverse nutritional effects of protein-restricted diets and by results of recent large clinical trials, which have suggested only a small clinical benefit. This area of therapy remains controversial, and the relative merits of dietary protein restriction compared to aggressive control of BP and use of ACE inhibitors is uncertain. In highly motivated and compliant patients who can tolerate the somewhat impalatable nature of this dietary restriction and who can have periodic review of their diets and overall nutritional status with an experienced dietitian, dietary protein restriction to 0.6 to 0.8 g/kg/d while maintaining total energy intake of at least 30 to 35 kcal/kg/d may be of some benefit in terms of slowing the progression of renal disease and delaying the onset of uremic symptoms.

Other Factors That May Accelerate Progression of Chronic Renal Failure

Although both hyperlipidemia and hyperphosphatemia have been implicated in the progression of renal insufficiency, there is no convincing clinical evidence that treatment of these conditions significantly ameliorates the progression of renal insufficiency. Despite this, control of hyperlipidemia and hyperphosphatemia are important in the overall management of the metabolic complications of CRF.

In addition to contributing to atherosclerotic renovascular disease and ischemic renal disease, cigarette smoking appears to be associated with an increased risk of microalbuminuria in diabetics, more rapid progression to overt diabetic nephropathy, and more rapid loss of GFR in established diabetic nephropathy. Similar findings have been noted in patients with other renal diseases and in patients with essential hypertension. Although smoking cessation has not yet been shown to slow the progression of renal disease, this still should be part of the recommended treatment of patients with renal insufficiency.

MANAGING COMPLICATIONS OF CHRONIC RENAL FAILURE

Hypervolemia

Excessive sodium and water retention frequently occur as GFR falls, particularly in patients with relatively high dietary salt intake, and result in hypertension, edema formation, and pulmonary vascular congestion. Therapy should be directed first at reducing dietary sodium intake to no more than 2 to 3 g/day. Fluid restriction is generally not needed unless hyponatremia is also present. Loop diuretics such as furosemide (Lasix, starting dose 20–80 mg once or twice daily), bumetanide (Bumex, starting dose 0.5–2 mg once or twice daily), ethacrynic acid (Edecrin, starting dose 50 mg once or twice daily) or torsemide (Demadex, starting dose 10–20 mg daily) are usually effective in controlling volume overload. The dosage should be slowly adjusted to achieve the desired response. Thiazide diuretics are not effective when used alone in patients with renal insufficiency but are useful in potentiating the effects of loop diuretics when patients do not respond adequately to loop diuretics alone. Metolazone (Zaroxolyn) is often used in this setting in a dose of 2.5 to 10 mg/d along with a loop diuretic. Combination diuretic therapy can be quite potent, so care must be taken to avoid potentially serious electrolyte imbalances such as hypokalemia, intravascular volume depletion, and exacerbation of renal insufficiency.

Hyperkalemia

Even with relatively advanced CRI, patients are often able to maintain normal serum potassium concentrations in the absence of excessive potassium intake, either dietary or from prescribed potassium supplements, or use of drugs that impair potassium excretion and/or aldosterone synthesis, such as potassium-sparing diuretics, ACE inhibitors, ARBs, and NSAIDs. Increases in the serum potassium concentration may be slightly less with ARBs compared to ACE inhibitors. Patients with renal insufficiency due to tubulointerstitial renal disease or hyporeninemic hypoaldosteronism (type IV renal tubular acidosis) are particularly likely to become hyperkalemic, even without additional exacerbating circumstances.

Dietary potassium restriction to less than 1 mEq/kg/d, use of diuretics in patients with evidence of volume overload, and avoidance of drugs that may exacerbate hyperkalemia are usually effective. Medications and nutritional supplements should be reviewed periodically to be sure that there are no additional exogenous sources of potassium or causes of impaired potassium excretion. Occasionally, the potassium-binding resin sodium polystyrene sulfonate (Kayexalate), usually administered in a solution with 70% sorbitol to avoid constipation, is needed. This can be given as a dose of 15 to 30 g a few times per week or as much as once to twice daily, although such frequent dosing is not likely to be tolerated by most patients.

Metabolic Acidosis

A metabolic acidosis often develops as kidney function declines, with the plasma bicarbonate concentration usually stabilizing in the range of 15 to

20 mEq/L. Metabolic acidosis may worsen bone disease associated with renal failure due to buffering of the retained hydrogen ions resulting in release of calcium and phosphorus from bone. Acidosis also increases skeletal muscle catabolism and reduces albumin synthesis. Alkali therapy is recommended to maintain the plasma bicarbonate concentration above 20 to 22 mEq/L, which typically requires about 0.5 to 1.0 mEq/kg/d. Sodium bicarbonate may be administered as tablets (650 mg tablets with 11.9 mEq of sodium and bicarbonate per gram, one to two tablets two to three times per day) or even baking soda (26.8 mEq/½ teaspoon), although the latter is not well tolerated by most patients. Sodium citrate solution (Bicitra, containing 1 mEq sodium citrate/mL, at a dose of 15–30 mL two to three times daily) is better tolerated but must not be given in patients who are also taking aluminum-containing phosphate binders because citrate enhances intestinal aluminum absorption. Citrate in this solution is rapidly metabolized to generate an equivalent amount of bicarbonate.

Hyperphosphatemia and Metabolic Bone Disease

Dietary phosphate intake typically exceeds urinary excretory capacity and hyperphosphatemia develops once GFR falls below about 25 to 30 mL/min. Phosphate retention without significant hyperphosphatemia may still be associated with development of hyperparathyroidism and early renal osteodystrophy with even milder degrees of renal insufficiency. Dietary phosphate restriction of 600 to 800 mg/d may ameliorate the hyperphosphatemia to some degree, but at the expense of what may be undesirable restriction of protein intake. Oral phosphate binders are often necessary to maintain the serum phosphorus concentration below 4.5 to 5 mg/dL.

The most commonly used phosphate binders are calcium carbonate (Os-Cal 500 and various others) or calcium acetate (PhosLo, 667 mg), from one to as many as five to six tablets (or more) with each meal. The dose must be adjusted to correct hyperphosphatemia while avoiding hypophosphatemia or hypercalcemia, which can occur as a result of absorption of calcium from these phosphate binders. Aluminum hydroxide and magnesium-containing antacids, although effective, are not usually used unless hypercalcemia develops with calcium-containing phosphate binders because of potential aluminum toxicity and hypermagnesemia, respectively. A new compound, sevelamer (Renagel, 400-mg and 800-mg tablets) is a cationic polymer that binds phosphate but does not contain calcium, aluminum, or magnesium. A similar number of pills, also to be taken with meals, is usually required as with calcium-containing phosphate binders.

Calcitriol (1,25-dihydroxyvitamin D_3) is produced by the kidneys, so as GFR falls, calcitriol synthesis declines. Calcitriol synthesis is also inhibited by hyperphosphatemia. Secondary hyperparathyroidism and osteitis fibrosa develop as a result of phosphate retention, low levels of calcitriol, and hypocalcemia. Calcitriol (Rocaltrol; 0.25–0.5 μg daily, or sometimes even less often) may be given to patients with hyperparathyroidism and/or hypocalcemia but should not be given unless hyperphosphatemia has been controlled. Calcitriol increases intestinal calcium and phosphate absorption, so patients need to be monitored for hypercalcemia as well as hyperphosphatemia.

Anemia

A normocytic, normochromic hypoproliferative anemia develops in most patients as GFR falls below about 30 to 40 mL/min, due primarily to reduced synthesis of erythropoietin by the kidneys. The hemoglobin usually remains above about 7 to 8 g/dL. Hemoglobin levels tend to be higher in patients with polycystic kidney disease compared to patients with other causes of CRF and ESRD. Iron deficiency may be an important contributing factor in some patients, and if present, should be corrected (and its etiology determined). Likewise, folate and vitamin B_{12} deficiency, although less common, should be excluded. It is neither necessary nor clinically useful to measure a plasma erythropoietin level in most patients once the serum creatinine concentration exceeds 2 mg/dL.

Recombinant human erythropoietin (epoetin alfa: Epogen, Procrit) is often used to treat anemia in patients with CRF, as well as most with ESRD. Many of the clinical manifestations attributed to "uremia" in patients with CRF, such as anorexia, fatigue, exercise intolerance, sexual dysfunction, and somnolence, may in fact be due to anemia or at least are improved with partial correction of anemia. Quality-of-life measurements, physiologic functions such as exercise capacity, sexual function, hospitalization rates, cardiovascular morbidity, and mortality rates improve in patients with CRF and ESRD when anemia is corrected to hemoglobin levels of at least 11 to 12 g/dL. Current recommendations support the use of epoetin alfa to maintain hemoglobin levels within this range in most patients with CRF and ESRD. Maintenance of normal hemoglobin levels (>13 g/dL) is not currently recommended because of concern about potential adverse effects as well as economic considerations, although there does appear to be some additional benefit compared to lower levels. Administration of epoetin alfa in patients not on dialysis does not affect the rate of progression of renal insufficiency.

In patients with CRF who are not yet on dialysis, epoetin alfa should be started at a dose of 4000 to 10,000 units subcutaneously once or twice weekly, then titrated to achieve and maintain the desired hemoglobin concentration. Use of benzyl alcohol–containing formulations of epoetin alfa reduces patient discomfort associated with injection of formulations without this preservative. Oral iron (i.e., ferrous sulfate 325 mg two to three times daily) will be needed in most patients to provide adequate iron for the stimulated erythropoiesis. Intravenous iron therapy is only rarely needed in patients with CRF, compared to patients on hemodialysis, most of whom receive parenteral iron.

ANTICIPATING AND PLANNING FOR DIALYSIS

Most patients with CRF will progress to ESRD and, unless inappropriate because of other co-morbid conditions such as malignancy, dementia or end-stage heart failure, will require dialysis or renal transplantation. Ample evidence documents that early referral of patients with renal disease to a nephrologist, well before the need for dialysis is imminent, reduces morbidity, frequency and length of hospitalization, and costs of care, and increases use of appropriate arteriovenous access while reducing dependence on vascular catheters for hemodialysis. A consensus panel of the National Institutes of Health in fact has recommended that patients should be referred to a nephrologist when the serum creatinine level is greater than 1.5 mg/dL in women and greater than 2.0 mg/dL in men. The nephrologist will include in a team approach, when the time is right, a renal dietitian, social worker, and nurses to best prepare the patient and family for dialysis. In addition to providing recommendations to primary care physicians concerning many of the issues previously addressed (such as delaying the progression of renal disease, BP management, and treatment of anemia and other complications), early involvement by a nephrologist increases the opportunity to have proper dialysis access in place before dialysis is necessary. Patients with ESRD respond less well to hepatitis B vaccine than patients without kidney disease or those who have milder CRF; vaccination should therefore be offered when patients are seen with mild renal insufficiency.

The initial step in preparing for ESRD is education and counseling of the patient and appropriate family members about renal failure and its symptoms, and the advantages and disadvantages of hemodialysis, peritoneal dialysis, and renal transplantation. This process should begin as soon as it is known that the patient has CRF. Ideally, all patients with CRF who are candidates for transplantation would receive a transplant just prior to needing renal replacement therapy; this unfortunately rarely happens. Patients can be placed on a cadaver-transplant waiting list once the creatinine clearance is 20 mL/min or less. Referral to a transplant center should occur prior to this to provide ample time for any necessary pretransplant evaluation, then wait-listing as early as possible. This evaluation will also include assessment of the options for living-related, living-unrelated, and cadaver kidney donation.

Hemodialysis requires access to the bloodstream. A primary arteriovenous fistula constructed in the nondominant arm from an anastomosis of the radial artery and cephalic vein, or alternatively the brachial artery and cephalic vein, is the preferred form of hemodialysis access. Patients should be advised to avoid needlesticks for blood drawing or intravenous access in the nondominant arm as soon as renal insufficiency is identified. Since it may take 3 to 4 months for a primary arteriovenous fistula to mature and be usable for dialysis, patients should be referred to a surgeon with an interest and expertise in this type of surgery when the GFR is about 25 mL/min or when dialysis is anticipated within 1 year. In addition to a careful history and physical examination, in selected patients venography, arteriography, and Doppler ultrasound studies may be needed for access planning. Iodinated contrast should be avoided if possible to avoid loss of residual renal function; CO_2 or gadolinium may be used instead.

If a primary arteriovenous fistula cannot be created or fails to mature, a synthetic arteriovenous graft using polytetrafluorethylene should be created. This type of access can be used within 2 to 3 weeks of placement, although it is preferable to wait 3 to 6 weeks if possible. Compared to primary arteriovenous fistulae, synthetic bridge grafts have a greater risk of infection and thrombosis, and need radiologic or surgical intervention to maintain long-term patency more often. Hemodialysis access can also be achieved with central venous double-lumen cuffed catheters. These catheters, although relatively easy to place and usable immediately after placement, are often uncomfortable and have a greater risk of infection, malfunction, and inability to achieve adequate dialysis blood flows than other forms of hemodialysis access. Although useful while waiting for other access sites to mature, their use as permanent hemodialysis access should be avoided unless all other potential arteriovenous access options have been exhausted.

Placement of a peritoneal dialysis catheter into the abdominal cavity should ideally be performed at least 10 to 14 days before the anticipated start of peritoneal dialysis. This allows adequate healing and minimizes the risk of fluid leaks once dialysis is started.

Starting Dialysis

The decision to start dialysis involves consideration of medical circumstances, nutritional status, the severity and tolerability of any uremic symptoms, and ultimately the willingness of the patient to begin dialysis treatments. Absolute indications for beginning dialysis are shown in Table 2. More subtle manifestations of uremia such as anorexia, occasional nausea (nausea and vomiting first thing in the morning seems to be very characteristic of uremia), declining edema-free weight, or pruritus should prompt serious consideration of starting dialysis. There is a spontaneous decline in dietary protein intake in most patients as renal function declines, often despite reports by the patient of well-preserved appetite and intake. The past several years have brought increasing awareness of the deleterious consequences, in terms of both morbidity and mortality, of declining nutritional status at the start of dialysis. As such,

TABLE 2. **Absolute Indications for Initiation of Dialysis**

Uremic manifestations
Persistent nausea and vomiting, encephalopathy, confusion, seizures, myoclonus, neuropathy
Fluid overload or pulmonay edema*
Hypertension*
Hyperkalemia*
Metabolic acidosis*
Uremic coagulopathy
Pericarditis

*When refractory to medical therapy.

even in the absence of other overt uremic symptoms, initiation of dialysis should be recommended for patients with advanced renal insufficiency in whom even minimal decrements in the serum albumin or prealbumin concentration develop. Most patients should start dialysis before the GFR falls below 10 mL/min. The BUN and creatinine concentrations that accompany this level of renal dysfunction vary tremendously, so it is not practical to establish firm levels for a BUN or creatinine above which dialysis should be started.

Dialysis can be a life-saving medical intervention, but it also unavoidably alters the lifestyle of the patient and close family members. Easing this transition requires education, planning, involvement of family members, nurses, dietitians, social workers and other health care providers, and cooperation between the primary care physician, access surgeon, and nephrologist.

MALIGNANT TUMORS OF THE UROGENITAL TRACT

method of
VIVEK NARAIN, M.D., and
DAVID P. WOOD, M.D.
Wayne State University
Detroit, Michigan

PROSTATE CANCER

Prostate cancer is the most commonly diagnosed cancer among men in the United States and is estimated to have affected approximately 180,400 men in the year 2000. At some point in the disease process, metastatic disease will develop, and approximately 31,900 patients with prostate cancer will die this year. The clinical course of metastatic disease is characteristically progressive and fatal with a median overall survival time between 24 and 36 months.

Owing to the complex cellular makeup of the prostate gland, it is difficult to discern which cells in the prostate are the origin of cancer. Adenocarcinoma of the prostate gland rarely causes symptoms early in the disease course because the major tumor mass is peripheral. The presence of symptoms suggests locally advanced or metastatic disease.

Age and race remain the strongest risk factors yet identified for prostate cancer from epidemiologic studies. In the United States, black men have a substantially higher incidence of prostate cancer than do age-matched white men. They tend to present with a tumor of a higher grade and stage and ultimately have a higher mortality rate. Geographic location seems to affect mortality rates; the highest rates are seen in Switzerland, Sweden, and Norway, and the lowest rates are seen in Asian areas, such as Singapore, Japan, and Hong Kong. The role of diet as a risk factor remains undetermined. A positive family history of prostate cancer is also a significant risk factor for the development of the disease. A form of hereditary prostate cancer has been linked to a locus on chromosome 1q24.24.

The American Cancer Society recommends that prostate cancer screening begin at age 45 for black men and age 50 for white men without a family history of prostate cancer; any male older than the age of 45 with a family history of prostate cancer should be screened as well. The use of prostate-specific antigen (PSA) testing in conjunction with digital rectal examination in early detection programs for prostate cancer has been linked to a marked increase in the detection of localized disease and a simultaneous decline in both regional and metastatic prostate cancer. Today, nearly 70% to 80% of men are diagnosed with prostate cancer while it is pathologically confined to one organ. Digital rectal examination is not suitable for early detection because about 70% of the palpable tumors have already spread beyond the prostate capsule. It has become routine to perform 4 to 18 systematic random biopsies of the prostate gland under transrectal ultrasound guidance in patients with a PSA greater than 4 ng/mL.

Although PSA has clearly revolutionized early detection, PSA alone is not the perfect screening tool. For example, 12% to 37% of patients with a normal PSA value of less than 4 ng/mL have clinically significant cancers. Four measures—PSA density, PSA velocity, age-specific PSA cutoff values, and PSA forms—have been proposed to improve the specificity.

The treatment options for clinically localized prostate cancer include radical prostatectomy, radiation therapy, cryosurgery, and watchful waiting.

TREATMENT

Watchful Waiting

Prostate cancer is relatively slow growing, with doubling times for local tumors estimated to be 2 to 4 years. The decision to adopt a strategy of watchful waiting for patients with newly diagnosed prostate cancer is advocated by many experts when certain conditions pertain: (1) life expectancy of fewer than 10 years, (2) presence of significant co-morbid disease, and (3) presence of a low-grade, low-stage tumor.

Radical Prostatectomy

With contemporary radical prostatectomy, about 70% of men with clinically localized disease will have long-term disease-free survival, depending on tumor grade, stage, and serum PSA level. The results of definitive treatment, whether radiation therapy or radical prostatectomy, for locally advanced cancer (clinical stage T3) are poor. Neoadjuvant total androgen deprivation in this setting has not been proven to be superior to radical prostatectomy alone. Postoperative adjuvant radiation therapy may be beneficial in patients with adverse pathologic findings. Salvage radical prostatectomy after radiation failure is associated with a significantly higher complication rate and limited prospects for cure.

Radiation Therapy

Although most external beam radiation therapy (EBRT) in the United States is performed without three-dimensional planning, several large centers have reported on the benefit of managing prostate cancer with three-dimensional planar or nonplanar beams. Radiation Therapy Oncology Group trials have suggested that survival rates are comparable to those expected following radical prostatectomy. Neoadjuvant hormone treatment has been shown to improve local control and disease-free survival in patients with locally advanced prostate cancer. Particle beams such as protons and neutrons used as monotherapy or in combination with photon therapy have also been used in select institutions to manage prostate cancer with good results.

Contemporary prostate brachytherapy involves the transperineal placement of radioactive seeds directly into the prostate under ultrasonographic or fluoroscopic guidance in an outpatient setting. For clinically localized prostate cancer with a low risk of extraprostatic disease, brachytherapy appears to be as effective as EBRT or radical prostatectomy. Because of the potential drawbacks of monotherapy in patients with intermediate and high risk of extraprostatic disease, EBRT has been added to brachytherapy. This combination approach allows the periprostatic tissues to be treated more effectively than brachytherapy alone and permits the administration of a higher intraprostatic dose of radiation than does EBRT alone.

Cryosurgery

Despite several recent technical improvements in cryoablation of prostate cancer, there is no evidence that it is superior to other forms of treatment, such as radiation or radical prostatectomy, for low-stage prostate cancer.

METASTATIC PROSTATE CANCER

Metastatic adenocarcinoma of the prostate has an overwhelming predilection to involve the bone. Expansion of tumor from the bone may cause bone pain, epidural cord compression, pathologic fractures, and major impairment in hematologic function by means of extensive bone marrow replacement.

Prostate cancer growth is largely dependent on the presence of androgens. Androgen ablation through surgical or medical castration successfully decreases or stabilizes both cancer symptoms and PSA in approximately 90% of patients. The major palliative effects of endocrine therapy include a decrease in pain and urinary symptoms and improved performance status. Despite its effectiveness as palliative treatment, a survival benefit has never been properly demonstrated in randomized trials of androgen deprivation therapy.

Gonadal androgen ablation by surgical castration (bilateral orchiectomy) or medical intervention is the mainstay of therapy for patients with evidence of metastatic disease. Surgical castration is still considered the gold standard for managing metastatic prostate cancer. The ultra–long-acting gonadotropin-releasing hormone analogues, such as leuprolide (Lupron) or goserelin (Zoladex), last for 3 months and have been found to be equally effective. The use of estrogens such as diethylstilbestrol (DES) has been largely abandoned owing to a relatively high incidence of cardiac and vascular toxicity.

Antiandrogens, pure and steroidal, counteract the effect of hormones at their target level. Steroidal antiandrogens (cyproterone acetate [Androcur],* megestrol acetate [Megace]†), owing to their progestational properties, act by suppressing gonadotropins and thereby lower plasma testosterone levels. Pure antiandrogens are nonsteroidal in structure and do not have any antigonadotropic effects. They act by directly binding to the peripheral androgen receptor. Currently available pure antiandrogens include flutamide (Eulexin), bicalutamide (Casodex), and nilutamide (Nilandron). Studies are under way to evaluate the impact of antiandrogen monotherapy in metastatic prostate cancer.

The concept of total androgen blockade continues to be controversial even after a decade of randomized controlled trials. To eliminate the effects of residual circulating androgens produced by the adrenal glands, investigators have combined surgical or medical castration with antiandrogens. The cell death process induced by androgen ablation fails to eliminate the entire malignant cell population, and after a variable period of time averaging 24 months, the tumor inevitably recurs, characterized by androgen-independent growth. The concept of intermittent androgen suppression was devised in an attempt to delay progression to the androgen-independent state by restoring apoptotic potential to cells surviving androgen ablation. This is still considered an experimental approach undergoing further evaluation.

More than half of the newly hormone-refractory patients will die within a year of disease progression. There are several second-line hormonal agents that have been used with varying degrees of success—the most common are high-dose bicalutamide, diethylstilbestrol, and ketoconazole.† Chemotherapeutic agents currently used as salvage therapy include doxorubicin (Adriamycin),† vinblastine (Velban),† estramustine (Emcyt), etoposide (Toposar),† mitoxantrone (Novantrone), prednisone,† and paclitaxel (Taxol).†

BLADDER CANCER

Among urologic cancers, bladder cancer remains second only to prostate cancer in prevalence and is

*Not available in the United States.
†Not FDA approved for this indication.

the fourth most common solid tumor in adults. This disease is more common in whites than in blacks, with an average age at diagnosis of 65 years. It is also more predominant in males than in females. Cigarette smoking, chronic bilharzial infection (schistosomiasis), chronic cystitis in the presence of indwelling catheters or calculi, phenacetin, cyclophosphamide (Cytoxan), ifosfamide (Ifex), perchloroethylene (used in dry cleaning), ochratoxin A, and exposure to arylamines used in chemical, rubber, dye, and textile industries have been linked to the development of bladder cancer. More than 90% of bladder cancers are transitional cell carcinomas.

A majority of the patients with bladder cancer present with painless gross or microscopic hematuria. A few will present with irritative symptoms such as urgency and frequency, which is associated with diffuse carcinoma in situ (CIS). Patients with symptoms suggestive of bladder cancer should initially undergo a complete urologic examination, including imaging (either ultrasonography or intravenous pyelography), cystoscopy, and urinary cytologic study. Upper urinary tract evaluation is also performed to rule out coexisting upper tract tumors. Urine cytologic studies are most useful in detecting CIS and high-grade tumors.

Bladder cancer is broadly classified into superficial and muscle-invasive disease. The superficial disease consists of tumors confined to the bladder mucosa (stage Ta) and those that penetrate the lamina propria (stage T1). CIS is a superficial disease that extends along the plane of the urothelium but does not penetrate the basement membrane. Approximately 75% of all newly diagnosed bladder cancers are considered superficial. Because the bladder mucosa is devoid of vessels and lymphatics, the incidence of metastatic disease with superficial disease is very low. Transurethral resection is the standard initial therapy for superficial bladder cancer; however, this is associated with a recurrence rate of 60% to 90% if used without adjuvant therapy. In patients at risk of disease progression or recurrence, intravesical therapy, usually intravesical bacillus Calmette-Guérin immunotherapy, is instituted to improve outcome. Indications for its use include CIS, high-grade stage Ta tumors, stage T1 tumors, and prophylaxis in patients with tumors refractory to intravesical chemotherapy. Bacillus Calmette-Guérin immunotherapy has been shown to reduce recurrences of superficial transitional cell carcinomas and to decrease stage progression, cystectomy rates, and disease-specific mortality. Bacillus Calmette-Guérin is also considered superior to treatment with intravesical chemotherapeutic agents, namely thiotepa (Thioplex), doxorubicin, and mitomycin (Mutamycin),* particularly for patients with CIS.

Of the patients with bladder cancer, approximately 25% will have muscle-invasive disease at initial presentation. Additionally, 15% of patients with superficial disease will experience progression to invasive disease. Clinical parameters associated with relapse and tumor progression in superficial bladder cancer are as follows: (1) failure after intravesical therapy, (2) the presence of multifocal CIS, and (3) endoscopically uncontrollable disease. The presence of a recurrent high-grade Ta lesion, any T1 lesion, or CIS refractory to optimal intravesical therapy portends an especially poor prognosis, with stage progression to muscle-invasive disease. Individuals with these conditions are considered appropriate candidates for cystectomy. The standard treatment for muscle-invasive disease is radical cystectomy with bilateral lymph node dissection and urinary diversion. This provides excellent local control, with pelvic recurrence rates of approximately 10%. The addition of preoperative radiation therapy does not appear to provide any additional benefit in terms of survival or local control. Almost 50% of all cystectomy candidates with high-grade tumors have unrecognized distant metastasis at the time of surgery and die of disseminated disease within 2 years of presentation. The role of systemic chemotherapy applied in either an adjuvant or a neoadjuvant setting is still evolving and is considered investigational.

*Not FDA approved for this indication.

RENAL CELL CARCINOMA

Renal cell carcinoma (RCC) is the third most common genitourinary tumor, accounting for more than 2% of cancers in the United States. It is more common among males and urban dwellers. RCC seem to arise from the proximal convoluted tubules, the same cell of origin as renal adenoma. Epidemiologic studies have incriminated tobacco. Other risk factors include a history of von Hippel-Lindau disease and acquired renal cystic disease of chronic renal failure. The most consistent chromosomal changes observed in RCC are deletions and a translocation involving the short arm of chromosome 3.

Traditionally, the diagnosis of RCC has been made after the investigation of any or all of the classic triad of symptoms (flank pain, flank mass, and hematuria). RCC is characterized by a lack of early warning signs, resulting in a high proportion (one third) of patients with metastases at diagnosis. For these patients, the prognosis is dismal, with a 5-year survival rate of less than 10% and an average survival time of only 6 to 12 months. For patients with apparently localized disease, metastasis will develop in almost 50%. With the advent and mainstream use of abdominal computed tomography and ultrasonography in recent years, the incidental detection of RCC in asymptomatic patients has increased. Incidentally discovered RCC tends to be smaller and of a lower stage and is associated with a better survival time and lower recurrence and metastasis rates than is disease detected in symptomatic patients. Symptomatic RCC presents at a significantly higher stage and grade and is substantially more aggressive than incidental lesions, particularly at later stages.

Radical nephrectomy remains the procedure of choice for surgically resectable lesions. Relapse occurs in 20% to 30% of patients with completely resected RCC after radical nephrectomy. Predictors of relapse include renal vein involvement and nodal metastasis. In these patients, administration of postnephrectomy radiation therapy or adjuvant interferon alfa does not delay time to relapse or overall survival compared with observation. Therefore, the standard of care remains observation following nephrectomy.

Nephron-sparing surgery has also become a successful form of treatment for this disease when there is a need to preserve functioning renal parenchyma. This need is present in patients with bilateral RCC, RCC involving a solitary functioning kidney, chronic renal failure, or unilateral RCC and a functioning opposite kidney that is at risk of future impairment from an intercurrent disorder such as calculus disease, renal artery stenosis, diabetes mellitus, or nephrosclerosis. Several studies have confirmed that nephron-sparing surgery provides curative treatment that is equally effective as radical nephrectomy for patients who have a single, small (<4 cm), unilateral, localized focus of RCC. It is also increasingly becoming recognized as being effective for small select, incidentally discovered tumors, even when the contralateral kidney is normal. The major disadvantage of nephron-sparing surgery is the small risk (4% to 6%) of local tumor recurrence in the operated kidney due to undetected microscopic multifocal RCC in the remnant kidney.

Historically, 4% to 10% of patients with RCC have tumor thrombus extending into the inferior vena cava, and 1% have tumor involving the right atrium. The prognosis for patients with resectable inferior vena caval extension or lymph node involvement approaches the prognosis for stage I disease. In the absence of metastases, an aggressive surgical approach provides the only hope for potential cure.

Lymph node involvement and metastasis are adverse predictors of survival. The outlook for patients with distant metastasis is poor, with a 5-year survival rate of less than 10% for those presenting with stage IV disease. If metastasis is discovered preoperatively, surgery is considered only for palliation, for entry into adjuvant treatment protocols, or possibly for a solitary metastasis. Metastases recognized at surgery, particularly hepatic metastases, are associated with poor outcome; further surgery should probably be abandoned in most of these patients. Unfortunately, the development of metastases is not uncommon after complete surgical resection, and the most common cause of death for these patients after surgery is metastatic RCC. Paraneoplastic syndromes, hemorrhaging, and tumor pain can be ameliorated by nephrectomy as well.

RCC is resistant to chemotherapy. Immunotherapy with aldesleukin (Proleukin) or interferon alfa-2a or -2b* for metastatic disease achieves responses in 10% to 20% of patients, some of which are durable.

*Not FDA approved for this indication.

TESTICULAR CANCER

Testicular cancer represents the most common malignancy in males in the 15- to 35-year-old age group. It is one of the most curable of all solid neoplasms. An undescended testis is more likely to undergo malignant degeneration than the normal testis. Additionally, about 20% of testicular tumors occurring in patients with cryptorchidism develop in the contralateral, supposedly normal, scrotal testis. The usual presentation for testicular cancer is a nodule or painless swelling of one gonad.

Germ cell tumors, which arise from germ cell elements from within the seminiferous tubules, account for 90% to 95% of all testicular tumors. Seminoma is the most common histologic type in adults and accounts for approximately 65% of all germ cell tumors. Nonseminomatous germ cell tumors arise mostly from gonadal stroma and mesenchymal structures. These tumors are histologically composed of embryonal carcinoma, teratoma, choriocarcinoma, and yolk sac elements.

Current staging of testicular cancer is based on primary histologic findings as well as serum markers (α-fetoprotein and β-human chorionic gonadotropin) and computed tomography of the abdomen/pelvis and chest. α-Fetoprotein may be produced by pure embryonal carcinoma, teratocarcinoma, and yolk sac tumor but not pure choriocarcinoma or pure seminoma. β-human chorionic gonadotropin, produced from syncytiotrophoblastic cells, is noted in choriocarcinoma, in embryonal carcinoma, and in up to 10% of patients with pure seminoma. Clinical stage I testicular cancer is defined by no evidence of metastasis after radical inguinal orchiectomy. Stage II disease implies spread to the retroperitoneal lymph nodes.

SEMINOMA

Approximately 75% of patients with seminoma present with stage I disease; however, 20% of those with clinical stage I disease harbor disease in retroperitoneal nodes despite normal imaging and negative serum markers. Postorchiectomy EBRT to the retroperitoneal nodes achieves a 90% to 95% cure rate. The optimal treatment for patients who present with distant metastasis or bulky retroperitoneal disease is chemotherapy initially. Treatment for persistent radiographic masses despite chemotherapy remains controversial. Some centers recommend resecting the residual mass (>3 cm) and administering subsequent radiation therapy or chemotherapy in patients in whom viable malignant disease is demonstrated.

NONSEMINOMA

In contrast to seminomas, 50% to 70% of patients with nonseminomas present with metastatic disease at diagnosis. Inguinal radical orchiectomy remains the initial therapeutic procedure for all nonseminomas. Approximately 30% of stage I cases will have clinically undetectable metastatic disease to the retroperitoneum. Treatment alternatives include retroperitoneal lymph node dissection (RPLND) and surveillance. RPLND is considered both diagnostic and therapeutic and achieves an overall survival rate of 99%. Surveillance with intense close follow-up with computed tomography, chest radiography, physical examination, and marker determinations has also achieved excellent long-term chance of cure in compliant patients. Salvage chemotherapy is administered to those patients who experience relapse. Surveillance is not recommended, however, in patients with disease with poor prognostic features, which carries a 50% relapse rate. Poor prognostic factors from the orchiectomy specimen include (1) vascular or lymphatic invasion, (2) a volume of embryonal carcinoma of greater than 40%, and (3) tumor invading the tunica vaginalis and beyond.

Primary RPLND and chemotherapy are treatment options in patients with clinical stage II disease. Immediate adjuvant chemotherapy or expectant management with salvage chemotherapy will also achieve similar overall disease-free survival. With primary chemotherapy, 75% of patients will achieve complete response. Partial responders will need to undergo RPLND to rule out the presence of viable tumor or teratoma. If cancer is found in the retroperitoneum, then additional courses of chemotherapy need to be administered. The presence of elevated serum α-fetoprotein and β-human chorionic gonadotropin levels is an accepted exclusionary criterion for adjunctive surgery following primary chemotherapy. Combination chemotherapy with three cycles of BEP (bleomycin [Blenoxane], etoposide [VP-16], and cisplatin [Platinol]) chemotherapy has become the standard treatment for patients with disseminated germ cell tumor. Cure rates of 70% to 80% can be achieved in patients with advanced germ cell tumor.

PENILE CANCER

Squamous cell carcinoma accounts for roughly 95% of all cases of penile cancer. It is a relatively uncommon malignancy in the United States, with an estimated incidence of 0.2 per 100,000. It is typically found in men between 50 and 70 years of age.

Circumcision seems to exert a protective effect by preventing the accumulation of smegma, which forms from desquamated epithelial cells. When circumcision is delayed until puberty, its protective effect is diminished. Smoking, phimosis, balanitis, and human papillomavirus have independently been associated with squamous cell carcinoma of the penis.

Erythroplasia of Queyrat and Bowen's disease are synonymous with squamous cell carcinoma in situ and are considered preinvasive malignancy. When diagnosed, in situ carcinomas of the penis respond well to local treatments such as excisional biopsy, 5% 5-fluorouracil cream, circumcision, Mohs' micrographic surgery, and laser ablation. Careful monitoring of signs of local recurrence is required in these cases.

In tumors that involve only the prepuce, circumcision can be both diagnostic and therapeutic. If the lesion involves the glans, the coronal sulcus, or the shaft, excisional biopsy is performed to determine the depth of invasion. When excisional biopsy reveals invasive disease, the primary tumor must be resected along with a 2-cm-wide margin. Depending on the location of the primary tumor, this may require partial or total penectomy. Laser therapy and Mohs' surgery have limited widespread application; however, they are effective only in select patients.

Radiation therapy yields local control approaching that of surgical resection in carefully selected patients. It is not recommended for patients with bulky tumor because the relapse rate is unacceptably high. All patients undergoing radiation therapy need local circumcision beforehand to reduce local morbidity.

Metastatic spread from penile cancer is by way of the lymphatic system to the regional nodes—the superficial and the deep inguinal nodes, then to the pelvic and the retroperitoneal nodes. This is followed by lung and bone metastasis. Adenopathy is noted in roughly half the patients who present with disease at diagnosis. Of these patients, metastatic carcinoma will be diagnosed in 45%. The remainder will have inflammatory lymphadenopathy, which will resolve following resection of the primary tumor and a 4- to 6-week course of oral antibiotics. Persistent lymph node enlargement indicates the need for therapeutic inguinal lymphadenectomy. Bilateral inguinal lymphadenopathy is recommended in patients with unilateral inguinal lymphadenopathy owing to the high incidence of bilateral disease. In patients who have surgically resected metastatic inguinal lymph nodes, the 5-year survival rate is 57% to 66%. Some 20% of patients with a clinically negative groin examination and invasive penile cancer at diagnosis will have occult metastases. Prophylactic inguinal lymphadenectomy in these patients has a significant survival advantage over the same procedure performed in patients after the emergence of adenopathy.

Chemotherapy for locally advanced and metastatic disease rarely achieves complete remission.

URETHRAL STRICTURES

method of
MICHAEL T. GAMBLA, M.D., and
ROBERT R. BAHNSON, M.D.
The Ohio State University
Columbus, Ohio

The male urethra has two anatomic divisions: the anterior and the posterior urethra. The anterior urethra comprises three regions: the glanular, the pendulous (penile), and the bulbous. The posterior urethra has two subdivisions: the membranous and, proximally, the prostatic urethra. Anteriorly, the urethra is centrally located within a thin smooth muscle layer known as the corpus spongiosum. At the level of the pubis this tissue becomes more developed and the bulbospongiosis muscles surround the urethra. Proximally, the bulbous urethra is positioned more anteriorly within the corpus spongiosum. Urethral location is important because incision by internal urethrotomy into the thick bulbar urethra is more successful than incision into the thin penile spongy tissue.

Urethral strictures are a consequence of the development of anterior urethral scar tissue. Scar tissue results from urethral epithelial tissue injury and is often progressive, resulting in concentric scar formation. Furthermore, contraction then leads to narrowing of the urethral lumen. The time from injury to symptomatology varies greatly, as does the degree of scarring (spongiofibrosis). Knowledge of the position and length of the spongiofibrosis is an important factor in determining surgical options.

The etiology of anterior urethral strictures is varied, and a detailed medical and sexual history can often provide clues to the cause. In the past, inflammatory strictures were most often due to gonococcal urethritis, which accounted for a majority of stricture disease. This has changed, however, owing to prompt use of effective antibiotics. The role of chlamydial infections in inflammatory stricture development is still unclear. At this time, the most common cause of anterior urethral strictures is iatrogenic injury from urethral catheterization or instrumentation. External penile and pelvic trauma accounts for a significant portion of strictures, whereas ischemic, idiopathic, and congenital causes occur rarely.

The phlegmatic process of urethral cicatrization may result in delayed symptoms years from the time of original injury. Acute trauma, however, such as a motor vehicle accident with associated pelvic trauma can cause severe injury or complete transection of the posterior urethra, leading to an early obliterative urethral stricture.

The normal caliber of the male urethra is 28 to 30 French (10 mm). Patients usually note urinary obstructive voiding symptoms when the lumen narrows to approximately 15 French (5 mm). Recurrent urinary tract infections such as epididymitis or prostatitis may also signal presence of a urethral stricture. Patients may describe a variety of symptoms from a slow stream to an inability to void. Post-void dribbling may also be present secondary to urine remaining in the dilated portion of the urethra proximal to the stricture. Uncommonly, hematuria can be present due to high urethral flow pressures causing small mucosal lacerations. Perhaps the most common complaint from patients with urethral strictures is spraying of the urinary stream. Because of the myriad of symptoms, this problem can be difficult to diagnose in an older man with concurrent benign prostatic hypertrophy.

Once patients are suspected of having a urethral stricture, they should be referred for a urologic consultation. Evaluation includes the history and physical examination, urinalysis, voiding flow rate, and possibly cystoscopy. Cystourethroscopy is done under local anesthesia with 2% viscous lidocaine as an office procedure. Patient discomfort is minimal and flexible cystoscopy provides detailed images of the urethra. Some patients may have a retrograde urethrogram (RUG) as an outpatient radiologic evaluation. This test identifies the stricture and also defines the urethra proximal and distal to it. In addition it can delineate the length, caliber, multiplicity, and proximity of the stricture to the urethral sphincter. Retrograde urethrography is the primary investigative radiologic test for evaluation of stricture disease. However, it can often underestimate bulbar stricture length. Therefore, if contrast medium passes into the bladder, then a voiding cystourethrogram can be performed to view the proximal extent of the stricture. Identifying the length and extent of spongiofibrosis preoperatively is an important criterion for determining therapy. Ultrasonography has found an expanding role in the diagnosis and evaluation of urethral stricture disease. It allows for a noninvasive, dynamic, precise assessment of anterior strictures, measures bulbar length more accurately than conventional retrograde urethrography, and can detail the extent of periurethral fibrosis and spongiofibrosis. It is performed in an outpatient office setting with minimal discomfort.

TREATMENT

The treatment regimen for patients with urethral strictures follows a three-step algorithim. The primary treatment is dilation. This is performed either by sequential dilation with filiforms and followers or cystoscopic balloon dilation. Both are office-based treatments done with local anesthetic and have become an optimal choice for patients with severe medical problems prohibiting aggressive surgical intervention. Rigid dilation is less frequently used because of associated complications, including significant discomfort, urethral bleeding, and mucosal tearing and trauma with resultant spongiofibrosis. Balloon dilation avoids traumatic shearing and is the best alternative primary treatment. Inflation of the device allows for a minimum 20 French diameter. The lasting success of balloon dilation has been variable, but it is clear that repeat treatments are often necessary. A resolution of symptoms usually follows the procedure; however, over time patients typically report a noticeable decline in urine flow rate and increased pressure needed to complete voiding. Occasionally, the patient with a small, short stricture can be cured with balloon dilation alone. Balloon dilating catheters have improved, and most recent data with use of the UrethraMax and coudé-tip balloon catheters by MacDiarmid supports this as an atraumatic, safe, effective office procedure. This treatment is usually not successful for long, narrow strictures nor appropriate in patients with associated false passages, urethral inflammation, or urethral fistula. After multiple dilations most patients advance to more aggressive therapy.

The second step in the algorithm for the treatment of urethral strictures is the direct visual internal urethrotomy (DVIU). This technique began with development of the cold knife in 1961 by Cervantes and its further adoption for use in the urethra by Sachse in 1972. It has gained increasing use over the decades and is the mainstay of treatment. An endoscopic urethrotome is inserted transurethrally and the stricture visualized. A cold knife placed at the 12 o'clock position is then passed beyond the stricture and incision is performed. Healthy corpus spongiosum must be identified for effective treatment. A Foley catheter is then placed and left indwelling for 3 to 7 days.

Identifying the appropriate patient for DVIU has led to many studies. In 1983, Holm-Nielsen treated 225 men with urethral strictures. Iatrogenic causes accounted for 59% of strictures. Cure rates were 54% with initial treatment and increased to 77% with subsequent repeat intervention. Minimal increase in cure was met after three urethrotomies. Success was also much better in shorter strictures (<5 mm). In 1996, Pansadoro and colleagues studied 224 men with urethral strictures in whom the primary etiology was iatrogenic (40%). Their long-term success rate was 42%. Subdivision by stricture etiology revealed congenital strictures to be much more effectively treated than traumatic ones by DVIU.

Later that year, Albers and coworkers reviewed 937 patients and reported a 65.7% long-term success rate for bulbous strictures. They concluded that DVIU is a safe, effective treatment; however, patients with more than one recurrence or stricture length greater than 1 cm are at a high risk for failure. In summary, DVIU is effective for short strictures with mild scarring. Success rates diminish significantly with each subsequent repeat procedure.

For patients who fail DVIU initially, endoscopic reevaluation should be performed. Depending on the amount of scar tissue seen one may choose a repeat DVIU or open surgical treatment. Whether one has balloon dilation or DVIU, there is supporting evidence that postprocedure clean intermittent catheterization (CIC) on a daily basis helps maintain urethral caliber for a longer period of time. We currently recommend patients perform CIC for 4 weeks to allow scar stabilization.

In the early 1990s a new alternative for the treatment of recurrent anterior urethral strictures was developed. The Urolume intraurethral stent (American Medical Systems) is a woven mesh of self-expanding superalloy wire. A single stent can be used for strictures up to 3 cm in length and offers an unconstrained diameter of 14 mm (42 French). Insertion is usually after balloon dilation or DVIU and should be at least 1 cm from the external sphincter. The wire mesh slowly becomes epithelialized over a 1-year period and cannot be removed except by excision. Success rates of preventing restenosis approach 75% to 80% in properly selected patients. Major risk factors for failure are prior failed urethroplasty and post-traumatic strictures. At this time Urolume is a promising alternative for recurrent strictures. Durability has been shown up to the 2-year mark, but long-term follow-up will fully characterize its natural history and ultimate role for recurrent urethral strictures.

After multiple failures with balloon dilation or DVIU, patients should be treated by open surgical repair. Urethral reconstruction is best suited for patients with long, narrow scar tissue or dense spongiofibrosis from prior procedures. A wide array of surgical techniques are available; however, procedure selection should be dictated by location, etiology, length, multiplicity, and local adverse conditions such as periurethral inflammation or urethrocutaneous fistula. Most repairs can be done in a one-stage procedure, especially with improved graft techniques. The optimal choice for most patients is excision with primary anastomosis. This requires mobilization of the bulbous urethra and limits this procedure to strictures up to 2 cm in length. The surgical technique involves placing the patient in a lithotomy position with elevation of the scrotum. A perineal incision is performed, and the urethra is then identified. Mobilization of the corpus spongiosum allows for identification of the stricture by a sound or bougie. Finally, the scar tissue is excised and the mobilized urethral ends are reanastomosed after spatulation. It is critical that the anastomosis be tension free. A Foley catheter is then left indwelling for 3 to 4 weeks. Long-term success rates approach 95% with this technique, and undoubtedly this provides the best results of all surgical repairs.

Patients with long, complex strictures in the bulbous or pendulous urethra often require a substitution urethroplasty. This form of surgical technique involves incising the stricture longitudinally until healthy tissue is identified. The urethral wall is then reconstructed with a flap or graft. A penile or preputial skin flap is developed by mobilizing and transferring an island of tissue maintaining its blood supply on a vascular pedicle. This ensures a proper blood supply to the healing tissue. Free grafts, such as buccal mucosa, are excised and transferred to the urethra without a pedicle. The host bed must be well vascularized for success with this technique. The results for substitution urethroplasty range from 85% to 93% with 2-year follow-up. After 4 years there is a steady attrition rate of about 5% per annum.

CONCLUSION

The etiology and management of urethral strictures has changed over the past 10 years. Our understanding of disease prevention and progression has improved as well. By integrating this knowledge we have effectively developed successful treatments for the majority of patients presenting with anterior urethral strictures. Long-term patient follow-up and clinical investigation will continue to guide our efforts.

UROLITHIASIS

method of
SCOTT TROXEL, M.D., and
ROGER K. LOW, M.D.
University of California, Davis
Sacramento, California

Urolithiasis is a common disorder affecting 20% of males and 10% of females, primarily during the second through fourth decades of life. The cost for treating these patients is estimated at $1 billion annually. Because of the high prevalence, it is imperative that all health care providers be familiar with the evaluation and treatment of patients with urinary stones. In this discussion the current initial evaluation, treatment, and subsequent metabolic evaluation of patients with urinary stones are reviewed.

PRESENTING SYMPTOMS AND SIGNS

Acute renal colic occurs primarily only in those patients with ureteral calculi. The classic presentation for ureterolithiasis is colicky flank pain that may radiate to the lower abdominal quadrant or groin. Pain is usually severe and incapacitating and may be accompanied with nausea and vomiting. Patients are often most symptomatic just before passage of stones from the distal ureter into the bladder. Stones near the ureterovesicle junction commonly cause irritative voiding symptoms, which may be confused as a lower urinary tract infection. Gross hematuria is uncommon, and other urologic causes should be suspected in those patients with painless hematuria. Stones contained within peripheral renal calyces may cause pain, but typically it is mild and chronic.

The appearance of a patient experiencing renal colic is typical and nearly unmistakable for any other condition. Typically, patients are in severe distress, writhing unsuccessfully to find a comfortable position. Tachycardia and a low-grade fever are common; however, a temperature greater than 100°F (37.8°C) should raise the suspicion for pyelonephritis or pyonephrosis. Patients usually have palpation tenderness overlying the ipsilateral flank at the costovertebral angle. Some may have deep palpation tenderness on abdominal examination but should not demonstrate signs of peritoneal irritation.

LABORATORY INVESTIGATION

The initial laboratory survey aids in the diagnosis and management of patients with urinary stones. This survey should include urinalysis, complete blood cell count, and basic chemistry panel. Some degree of hematuria on urinalysis occurs in 85% to 90% of patients with urinary stones. Finding a few white blood cells on microscopy is not uncommon; however, urine that is nitrite positive or exhibits severe pyuria suggests infection. The presence of urinary crystals does not always correlate with active stone disease. Calcium oxalate, calcium phosphate, and urate crystals may normally be present in persons without stone disease. Finding certain urinary crystals on microscopy, however, is pathognomonic for urolithiasis. Hexagonal crystals are pathognomonic for patients with cystinuria and finding coffin-lid–shaped crystals is indicative of patients with struvite stones. Urinary pH may be helpful in patients found to have urinary stones. An acidic urinary pH less than 5.5 in a patient with radiolucent stones is indicative of uric acid stones, whereas an alkaline urine (pH $>$ 8) in a patient with a history of urinary tract infection suggests struvite stones.

A mild leukocytosis is common in patients presenting with an acutely obstructing stone. Pyelonephritis or pyonephrosis should be considered in any patient with a significantly elevated white blood cell count. Serum creatinine concentration is usually normal or slightly elevated, often more related to dehydration than to renal impairment. Finding a significantly elevated serum creatinine value usually indicates underlying chronic renal disease, bilateral obstruction, or obstruction of a solitary kidney.

RADIOGRAPHIC EVALUATION

Noncontrast helical computed tomography (CT) has now replaced intravenous pyelography (IVP) as the diagnostic modality of choice to evaluate patients with acute renal colic. Advantages of CT over IVP are the lack of need for intravenous contrast, the rapidity of acquiring diagnostic images, and the high accuracy rate. Most series report an accuracy rate of 95% or better for CT in diagnosing patients with obstructing ureteral calculi. There are four radiographic findings of an obstructing ureteral stone: hydronephrosis/hydroureter, nephromegaly, perinephric/periureteral stranding, and visualization of the stone itself. Unilateral perinephric stranding as indicated by an irregular renal border is a sensitive indicator of acute obstruction (Figure 1). Severe stranding may represent urinary extravasation from a ruptured calyceal fornix. Even the smallest of stones brightly enhance on CT. Confusion of phleboliths for stones may be problematic in the pelvis. Diagnosis may rely on noting associated upper tract changes of obstruction or noting the "bull's-eye" sign, corresponding to the pattern of a stone outlined by the wall of the ureter. An abdominal radiograph should accompany the CT to better determine size and radiopacity of stones.

IVP still has a role in the diagnostic evaluation of stone formers. Patients with medullary nephrocalcinosis benefit from intravenous pyelography to determine whether they have medullary sponge kidney, an anatomic defect predisposing to kidney stones. In some instances, visualization of collecting system anatomy may also alter patient management.

TREATMENT

There are several therapeutic options to manage patients with urolithiasis. These include observation, medical dissolution, extracorporeal shock wave lithotripsy (ESWL), endoscopic stone manipulation, and open surgery. The use of minimally invasive techniques such as ESWL and endoscopy has made open stone surgery nearly obsolete except for the largest and most complex stones.

Observation is an option for those patients with asymptomatic renal calculi and minimally symptomatic small ureteral calculi. Typically, small calyceal stones are asymptomatic and warrant therapy only if a source of infection or symptoms. Patients with a history of urolithiasis often choose to electively treat asymptomatic stones to minimize their risk of future colic. Observation in hopes of spontaneous passage is recommended for most patients with small ureteral

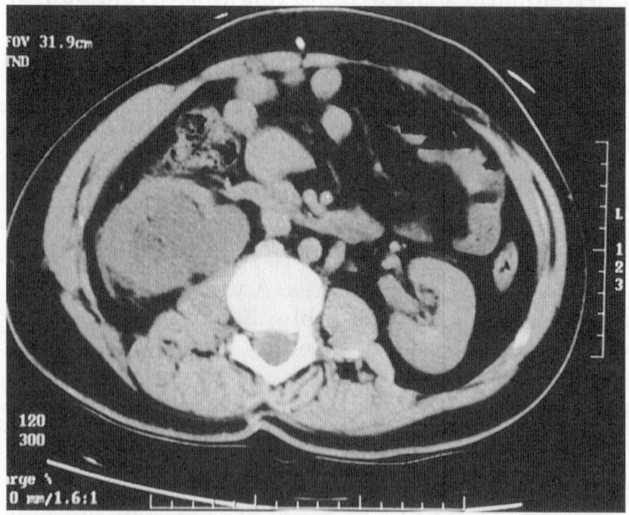

Figure 1. Nonenhanced abdominal computed tomogram demonstrating right hydronephrosis and perinephric stranding.

calculi. Stones less than 5 mm in diameter are capable of passing uneventfully without the need for intervention. Stones greater than 5 mm rarely pass, and patients should be counseled on the probable need for intervention. Most stones that eventually pass do so within 6 to 8 weeks of first becoming symptomatic. Stones failing to pass within this time period usually require intervention. Patients managed with observation are given analgesics and counseled to return if they experience fever, intractable pain, or nausea/vomiting. These symptoms suggest the presence of either infection or high-grade urinary obstruction requiring either hospitalization or intervention. The forcing of oral fluids is commonly recommended, although there is no scientific evidence to support this recommendation. Radiographic demonstration of renal obstruction, even urinary extravasation, alone is not an indication for intervention or the need for immediate evaluation by a urologist. Patients with potentially passable stones can safely be observed as long as they do not exhibit fevers, intractable symptoms, or renal insufficiency.

Dissolution of stones by either ingestion of oral agents or direct irrigation of the urinary tract is possible with some urinary stone types. Stone dissolution by oral agents is only an option for those patients with uric acid stones. Patients with radiolucent calculi and a history and urinalysis consistent for uric acid stones may consider treatment with oral urinary alkalinizing agents. Variability in patient compliance and stone composition greatly affect efficacy of alkalinizing regimens. Chemodissolution by direct irrigation of the urinary tract is an option for a variety of stones, but it is impractical in this day and age. Chemodissolution is best reserved as an adjunct to remove stones inaccessible to removal by other treatment modalities.

ESWL is the most common form of therapy for patients with upper urinary tract stones. ESWL involves the generation of focused acoustic waves capable of fragmenting stones into small particles. Fragments resulting from ESWL typically are 1 to 3 mm depending on the type of stone treated and the type of lithotriptor utilized. In most cases, ESWL is the treatment of choice for renal stones less than 2 cm and stones along the entire course of the ureter. Although ESWL revolutionized the treatment of kidney stones, we now recognize certain limitations to this technology. Both stone composition and location affect lithotripsy efficacy. Cystine stones and calcium oxalate monohydrate stones are particularly hard and refractory to ESWL energy. In addition, stones located in the lower pole calyces of the kidney are more commonly associated with retained fragments after ESWL than stones treated in other regions of the kidney and ureter.

Most of the recent technologic advances are in flexible endoscopy and intracorporeal lithotripsy. Flexible ureteroscopes in use today are 7 to 10 French in diameter and allow endoscopic access to the entire upper urinary tract (Figure 2). Smaller-diameter endoscopes result in less tissue trauma and less need for postoperative ureteral stenting. There are a variety of intracorporeal lithotrites, but the holmium laser has emerged as the lithotrite of choice for treating ureteral stones. Desirable characteristics of the holmium laser include a universal ability to destroy all urinary stone types while producing minimal urothelial trauma. The holmium laser differs from other intracorporeal lithotrites in its mechanism of stone degradation, which is photothermal rather than acoustic. The combination of latest-generation flexible ureteroscopes and the holmium laser make nearly every stone patient a candidate for transurethral endoscopic therapy. Patients with uncorrected bleeding diatheses, who are morbidly obese, or who possess severe skeletal abnormalities precluding treatment with other modalities have all been successfully treated with this combination.

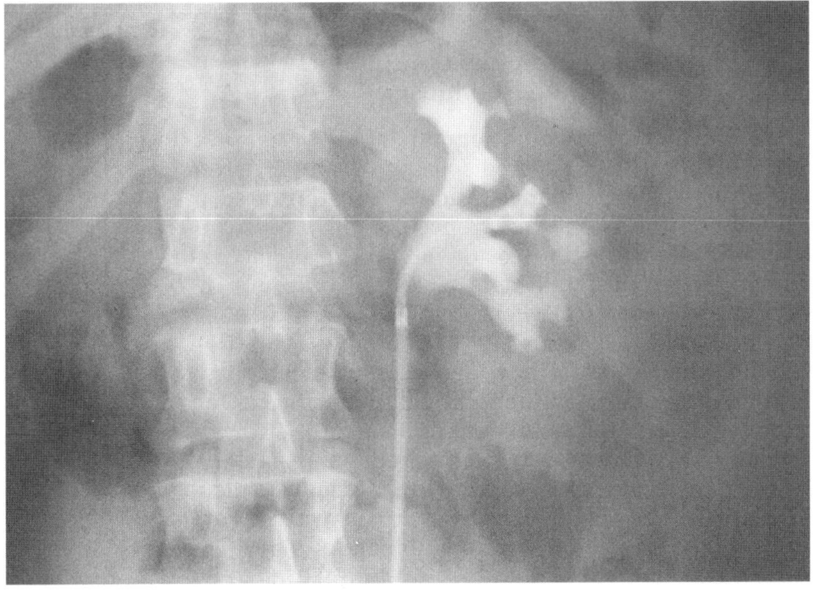

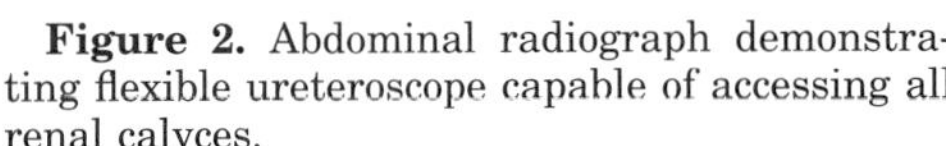

Figure 2. Abdominal radiograph demonstrating flexible ureteroscope capable of accessing all renal calyces.

Ureteral Stones

Patients with small ureteral calculi are best managed initially with a trial of observation. Intervention is suggested for those failing to pass their stone within 6 to 8 weeks of becoming symptomatic and for those developing fever or intractable symptoms. Patients with larger stones are best treated with ESWL or ureteroscopy. It is widely accepted that ESWL is the treatment of choice for stones located between the ureteropelvic junction and the pelvic ureter. It is controversial which therapy is best for stones located in the distal ureter. Proponents of ESWL cite the noninvasiveness and reasonable success rates afforded by ESWL. Those favoring an endoscopic approach cite higher stone-free rates associated with endoscopic intervention. Large, hard, or impacted stones are best treated endoscopically through either a retrograde or a percutaneous antegrade approach.

Renal Stones

Small renal stones less than 2 cm are typically best treated with ESWL. Larger stones benefit from percutaneous nephrostolithotripsy (PCNL), a technique in which an endoscope is placed in the kidney after creation of a retroperitoneal tract. This technique is favored for very large renal stones because of the ability to evacuate generated stone fragments. Large stones treated with ESWL are associated with a high risk of requiring ancillary or additional procedures to treat residual stones or complications. Recently, we have come to the realization that the anatomy of the renal collecting system also influences stone passage. Stones located in inferior calyces, which are long, narrow, or acutely angled relative to the ureteropelvic junction, are associated with a higher risk of retained stones after ESWL. Only the largest most complex stones require open surgery. Open surgery is also required for those with anatomic defects requiring reconstruction.

Medical Evaluation of Patients With Urolithiasis

We recommend evaluating all stone patients to determine risk factors predisposing to urinary stone formation. This recommendation is substantiated by the high risk of stone recurrences, even in first-time stone formers and the cost/benefit ratio of medical evaluation versus treatment of recurrences. An underlying risk factor predisposing to stone recurrences is found in 97% of patients undergoing evaluation. Studies demonstrate lower stone formation rates, fewer symptomatic episodes, and decreased intervention rates for patients given prophylactic therapy.

Medical evaluation is postponed until patients have fully recovered from therapy to remove calculi and are free of upper urinary tract obstruction and infection. The initial evaluation consists of stone analysis, serum chemistries, and quantitative 24-hour urine chemistries. The composition of the removed or passed stone directs evaluation and treatment. Urine should be tested for the presence of urease-producing organisms in patients having struvite or apatite (calcium phosphate) stones and patients with stones of unknown composition and a history of urinary tract infection.

All patients should have an SMA-7 to document baseline serum creatinine level and to evaluate patients for renal tubular acidosis. Serum calcium, phosphorus, and uric acid levels are useful in patients with calcium and uric acid stones. Patients with calcium stones require a 24-hour urine collection for the following chemistries: calcium, oxalate, citrate, magnesium, uric acid, volume, pH, sodium, and phosphorus. Laboratories specializing in the evaluation of stone formers' urine provide comprehensive testing, which is convenient for patients and easily understandable to treating physicians (Figure 3). Explaining to patients the importance of accurately collecting urine specimens is paramount, given reference values being based on a 24-hour collection. Table 1 lists the normal 24-hour urine excretory values. Validity of patient samples can be determined by urinary creatinine and body weight. Men excrete an average urinary creatinine concentration of 22 mg/kg/d compared with an average of 17 mg/kg/d for women.

Table 2 lists the most common stone types along with their frequencies. Recently, a new urinary stone type has been described, attributable to the use of medications for the treatment of human immunodeficiency virus (HIV). Protease inhibitors prevent the maturation of HIV, producing immature noninfectious viral particles. The most widely used protease inhibitor, indinavir sulfate (Crixivan), is associated with the highest risk of forming stones; however, all protease inhibitors are capable of forming stones. At normal urine pH, filtered, unaltered drug is capable of either precipitation or complexation with known

TABLE 1. **Normal 24-Hour Urinary Excretory Values**

Calcium	<250 mg/d
Oxalate	<44 mg/d
Citrate	>320 mg/d
Magnesium	>50 mg/d
Uric acid	<600 mg/d
Volume	>2 L/d
Sodium	<200 mEq/d
Phosphorus	<1300 mg/d
Cystine	<250 mg/d

TABLE 2. **Stone Types**

Calcium stones	
Calcium oxalate	70–80%
Calcium phosphate	5–10%
Uric acid	5–10%
Struvite	5–10%
Cystine	1–2%

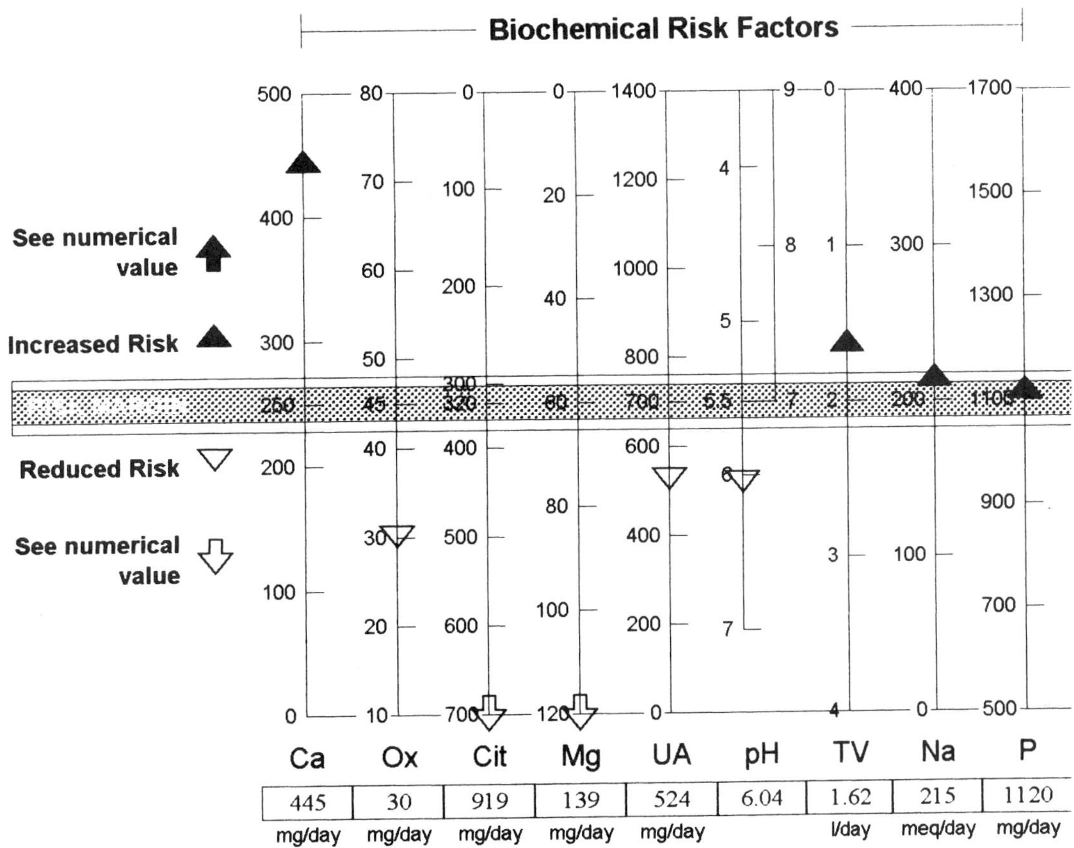

Figure 3. Comprehensive report of 24-hour urine chemistries indicating hypercalciuria, high urinary sodium, and low urinary volumes.

stone-forming salts. Up to 30% of patients using urease inhibitors may experience renal colic while on therapy. Stones associated with protease inhibitors are known for two unique properties, their radiolucency and their amenability to conservative therapy. Protease inhibitor calculi are radiolucent both on standard radiographs (IVP) and CT. Diagnosis often relies on clinical suspicion and finding indirect signs of upper tract obstruction on diagnostic radiography. Initial treatment consists of temporary cessation of the drug and forced hydration, which is successful in 70% of cases. Intervention is reserved for those not responding to conservative measures.

Calcium Stones

Most patients have calcium-based stones composed predominantly of calcium oxalate. Often, stones may contain a mixture of either calcium oxalate and calcium phosphate or uric acid. It is important to recognize that factors other than hypercalciuria and low urinary volume contribute to calcium oxalate stone formation. Counseling all patients with calcium oxalate stones to merely reduce their dietary calcium consumption and increase their oral fluid intake is inadequate. Elevations in urinary oxalate, sodium, uric acid, and deficiencies in urinary stone inhibitors also contribute to calcium oxalate stone formation.

Hypercalciuria for an adult is broadly defined as urinary calcium excretion greater than 250 mg/d. Utilizing calcium excretion more than 4 mg/kg/d is applicable to both sexes, children, and people of different body habitus. There are three main categories of hypercalciuria: resorptive (hyperparathyroidism), absorptive, and renal. All patients with hypercalcemia should be evaluated for primary hyperparathyroidism with a serum parathyroid level. Stone disease is now an uncommon presentation for primary hyperparathyroidism, given widespread routine screening. Parathyroidectomy is indicated in those found to have primary hyperparathyroidism and is successful in over 90% of cases.

Absorptive hypercalciuria refers to elevated urinary calcium level due to an increase in calcium absorption from the small intestine. Patients with absorptive hypercalciuria can be further subdivided into types I (severe) and II (mild). Patients with the milder type II can be managed with dietary restriction of calcium (400 mg/d). Patients with type I are most often managed with a combination of thiazide diuretics and potassium citrate. Thiazides reduce urinary calcium levels directly by increasing calcium resorption in the distal renal convoluted tubule and indirectly by increasing proximal tubular reabsorption resulting from natriuresis and volume contraction. Potassium citrate is recommended to avoid hypocitraturia and hypokalemia from thiazide usage. Renal hypercalciuria results from the inability of kidneys to resorb calcium. The cause of renal hypercalciuria is not entirely understood; however, infection, tubular dysfunction, and anatomical defects have all been postulated. The treatment of patients with renal hypercalciuria also is with thiazide diuretics in combination with potassium citrate.

Hyperoxaluria contributing to urinary stone disease is most often due to a condition called enteric hyperoxaluria. Any condition resulting in the absence/nonfunction of small bowel or defective intestinal absorption of fat or bile acids predisposes to this condition. Historically, patients having jejunoileal bypass for morbid obesity primarily were affected; however, patients with regional enteritis, previous small bowel resection, or chronic pancreatitis may also be affected. Ironically, patients with enteric hyperoxaluria are treated with supplemental oral calcium to bind and reduce free intestinal oxalate. Patients with enteric hyperoxaluria represent some of the most challenging stone patients due to the severity of hyperoxaluria and other urinary risk factors associated with this condition. Dietary contribution to urinary oxalate is minimal and comes in the form of green leafy vegetables, chocolate, tea, and nuts. Vitamin C is another potential external source of oxalate. Patients with calcium oxalate stones should be advised to limit their vitamin C supplementation to 500 mg/d. A recent report also warns that cranberry extract tablets taken as supplements may promote calcium oxalate stone formation due to their high oxalate content.

Dietary sodium influences the risk of calcium oxalate stone disease. High urinary sodium promotes calcium oxalate stone formation by increasing urinary calcium and by forming monosodium urate, a nucleator of calcium oxalate. Each incremental increase of 100 mEq of urinary sodium increases urinary calcium excretion by 50 mg/d. As a result, dietary sodium restriction to 100 mEq/d (one teaspoon) is generally recommended to all patients with calcium stones.

Urinary citrate is a potent inhibitor of calcium oxalate stone formation. Citrate inhibits calcium oxalate stone formation by forming soluble complexes with calcium and directly inhibiting calcium oxalate nucleation and growth. Any condition resulting in a metabolic acidosis produces hypocitraturia. Common clinical conditions associated with hypocitraturia are renal tubular acidosis, chronic strenuous exercise, and chronic diarrheal states. Dietary citrus fruits and juices increase urinary citrate, but they are more an adjunct than replacement therapy.

Uric Acid Stones

Two factors influence urinary uric acid solubility: uric acid concentration, and urine pH. Of these, urinary pH is the most influential factor governing uric acid stone formation. An acidic urinary pH less than 5.5 promotes supersaturation of undissociated uric acid and stone formation. Chronic acidic urinary states include gout, strenuous exercise, and certain gastrointestinal disorders. Hyperuricosuria also contributes to uric acid stones and may be a factor in 15% to 20% of patients with calcium oxalate stones. At normal urine pH greater than 5.5, hyperuricosuria promotes calcium oxalate stone formation by promoting heterogeneous nucleation of calcium oxalate. Under normal circumstances, endogenous uric acid production accounts for the majority of urinary uric acid. Hyperuricosuria can result from any condition producing high cellular turnover such as myeloproliferative states and tumor lysis. Purines in the form of animal meats represent the primary dietary source of urinary uric acid. Patients with uric acid stones are instructed to reduce their intake of animal meats and maintain a high fluid intake. Those with refractory stone formation are best treated with potassium citrate to alkalinize their urine pH between 6.5 and 7.0. Allopurinol (Zyloprim) is a less effective therapy than urinary alkalinization, but it represents an alternative for those intolerant of alkali therapy, those with hyperuricemia, or patients with renal insufficiency.

Struvite Stones

Struvite stones or magnesium ammonium phosphate stones are found predominantly in women with a history of recurrent urinary tract infections and people with urologic disorders predisposing to urinary stasis. Struvite stones are caused by urease-producing organisms capable of catalyzing urea into

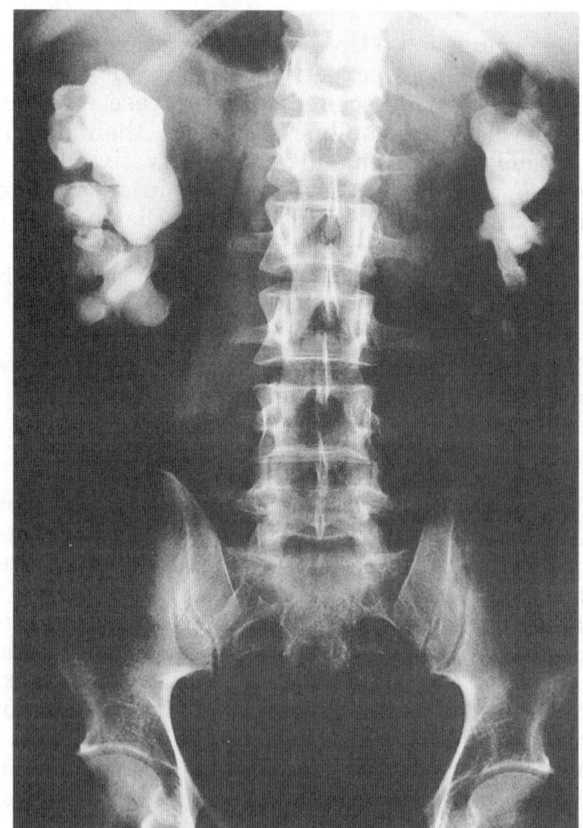

Figure 4. Abdominal radiograph showing bilateral staghorn renal calculi.

carbon dioxide and ammonia. Ammonia further dissociates into ammonium and hydroxide ions. The combination of urinary saturation with ammonium ion and an alkaline (urine pH > 7.2) environment promotes the development of struvite and calcium phosphate (apatite) stones. The most common urease-producing organisms associated with stones are *Proteus, Pseudomonas, Klebsiella,* and *Staphylococcus* species. *Escherichia coli* is not a urease-producing organism or organism associated with infection-related stones. Classically, infection-related stones are known for having a "staghorn" appearance, completely filling the renal collecting system (Figure 4). Complete removal of all stones utilizing a combination of percutaneous endoscopic and ESWL techniques is the mainstay of therapy. Culture-specific chronic suppressive antibiotic therapy, maintenance of hydration, and optimal urinary drainage are recommended. Urease-inhibiting agents such as acetohydroxamic acid have a limited therapeutic role owing to their high frequency of intolerable side effects.

Cystine Stones

Cystinuria is an autosomal recessive inherited disorder resulting in elevated levels of urinary cystine and recurrent cystine stones. Patients typically present in the second and third decades of life with stone formation the only clinical manifestation of the disease. Although cystinuric patients represent a small percentage of patients with stones, the severity of their stone disease often leads to renal loss.

Stone formation results from the poor solubility of cystine at normal urinary pH. Dietary restriction of foods rich in methionine, the main source of cysteine, is impractical. The mainstay of therapy consists of minimizing the number of stone insults to the kidneys and maintaining patients on a regimen of high oral fluid intake and urinary alkalinizing agents. Most cystinuric patients require the addition of agents such as tiopronin (Thiola) or D-penicillamine (Cuprimine), which reduce stone formation by forming soluble complexes with cystine.

Section 10

The Sexually Transmitted Diseases

CHANCROID

method of
GEORGE SCHMID, M.D., M.Sc.
National Center for HIV, STD, and TB Prevention, Centers for Disease Control and Prevention
Atlanta, Georgia

Chancroid, one of the three sexually transmitted diseases (STD) characterized by genital ulceration (genital herpes and syphilis being the other two) is caused by *Haemophilus ducreyi*, a small gram-negative bacillus. A common STD in the United States before World War II, chancroid cases decreased markedly with the introduction of penicillin. In the latter 1980s, however, chancroid resurged with the introduction of crack cocaine and an attendant high-risk sex-for-drugs trade. Since a peak of 4986 cases in 1989, case numbers have diminished for unclear reasons, and in 1999, only 143 cases were reported. In sub-Saharan Africa and parts of Asia, chancroid remains common and is responsible for facilitating transmission of the HIV epidemic.

Chancroid should be suspected if a patient has one or a few very painful genital ulcers; in about one half of patients, painful inguinal adenopathy occurs. The ulcers are raw and often deep with bleeding. Definitive diagnosis is difficult because special culture media required to grow *H. ducreyi* are not often available; PCR testing may be available from referral laboratories.

TREATMENT

Several therapies are equally effective: azithromycin (Zithromax) 1 g orally once; ceftriaxone (Rocephin) 250 mg intramuscularly once; ciprofloxacin (Cipro)* 500 mg orally twice a day for 3 days; and erythromycin base* 500 mg orally three to four times a day for 7 days. Antimicrobial resistance to these drugs has rarely, if ever, occurred.

Successfully treated patients report subjective improvement within 48 to 72 hours, and objective improvement is apparent within 3 to 7 days. If there is no clinical improvement by 7 days, the clinician should consider whether patients took their medication, antimicrobial resistance exists, there is coinfection with *Treponema pallidum* or herpes simplex virus (~10% of patients), or the diagnosis is wrong. Patients should be followed until there is complete healing of the ulcer.

Patients with fluctuant buboes benefit from drainage to prevent spontaneous rupture and fistula formation. This may be done by either needle aspiration or by incision and drainage with packing of the node. The former approach may require subsequent reaspiration; the latter approach is more invasive. Despite successful therapy, nodes not fluctuant enough for drainage when patients are initially seen may later become fluctuant and require drainage.

Patients who are uncircumcised or who have HIV infection do not respond as well as circumcised patients or those without HIV infection; some experts prefer multiple dose regimens for uncircumcised patients. All patients with suspected chancroid should have an HIV test initially and, if negative, have the test again 3 months later because HIV seroconversion rates are high among those who are initially HIV negative. It is prudent to schedule a follow-up visit several days after initial diagnosis to check for evidence of healing and for counseling about the results of the initial HIV test.

Sex partners within the 10 days before the appearance of the ulcer should be notified, examined, and treated. Asymptomatic ulcers occasionally occur in the vagina or on the cervix. Asymptomatic carriage of *H. ducreyi* in cervical secretions has been described, but is uncommon.

Suspected cases should be reported to the local health department.

*Not FDA approved for this indication.

GONORRHEA

method of
DANA WASSON DUNNE, M.D.
Yale University School of Medicine
New Haven, Connecticut

Gonorrhea has a long and colorful history, with references to the disease dating back to the time of Leviticus. With the advent of potent antibacterial therapy in the mid-1900s, control of this prevalent sexually transmitted disease seemed at hand; however, evolving antimicrobial resistance, complex demographic patterns, and social transmission networks have allowed gonorrhea to remain a major public health problem in the 21st century.

EPIDEMIOLOGY

The peak incidence of gonorrhea in the United States occurred in 1975, with 468 cases per 100,000 individuals. Over the following 22 years (1975 to 1997), there was a 72% decline in the reported rate of gonorrhea, largely owing to the introduction of a national control program. This trend, however, has been reversing in the past 2 years; the Centers for Disease Control and Prevention (CDC) reported 360,076 cases of gonorrhea in 1999. This calculated rate of 133.2 cases per 100,000 represents a 9.2% increase over the 1997 rate of 122 cases per 100,000 and remains well above the Healthy People 2000 goal of fewer than 100 cases per 100,000. Although some of this disturbing trend may be explained by the introduction of more sensitive assays for the detection of *Neisseria gonorrhoeae* infections, true increases in disease frequency in certain geographic areas and populations appear to have occurred. Demographically, higher rates of gonorrhea continue to be observed in urban areas (especially in the southeastern United States) and among adolescents (15 to 19 years old) and minorities.

Because humans are the only natural host for the gonococci, transmission is achieved by direct physical contact with the mucosal surfaces of an infected individual. There is no evidence that fomites can serve as a meaningful reservoir capable of transmitting the disease. The one-time risk of transmission of *N. gonorrhoeae* from an infected woman to the urethra of her male partner is 20%. This risk increases to 60% to 80% after four or more encounters. The approximate risk for male-to-female transmission is 50% to 70% per contact.

MICROBIOLOGY

N. gonorrhoeae are gram-negative organisms that occur in pairs. The organisms have adjacent sides that are flattened, giving them a "kissing kidney bean" appearance. They are nonmotile and do not form spores. *N. gonorrhoeae* divides by binary fission every 20 to 30 minutes. The organism does not tolerate drying and is best plated immediately on Thayer-Martin medium and incubated at 36°C in a 3% to 5% CO_2 environment. Other members of the genus include *N. meningitidis* and *N. cinerea* among others.

CLINICAL MANIFESTATIONS

The primary site of infection in men is the anterior urethra. More than 90% of men are symptomatic and will complain of dysuria and a purulent urethral discharge beginning 2 to 5 days after contact with an infected sexual partner. Rare complications include penile edema and lymphangitis, urethral strictures, prostatitis, epididymitis, and dissemination. Rectal involvement is usually seen in men who have sex with men and can be asymptomatic. Severe proctitis can occur, however, with tenesmus, rectal bleeding, discharge, and painful defecation.

The primary site of infection in women is the endocervix. In contrast to men, fewer than 50% of women are symptomatic with gonorrhea. When women are symptomatic, they will complain of vaginal discharge, menometorrhagia, and bleeding after intercourse. On examination, mucopurulent cervicitis, edema, and friability can be observed. Complications include rectal involvement, Skene's or Bartholin's glands abscesses, urethral involvement (in women who have undergone hysterectomy), pelvic inflammatory disease (PID), perihepatitis (Fitz-Hugh–Curtis syndrome), and dissemination.

Pharyngeal infection occurs after orogenital contact and often results in asymptomatic disease. When patients do have symptoms, clinical findings are often indistinguishable from those observed with acute streptococcal pharyngitis. A history of orogenital contact in sexually active persons should always be obtained when evaluating patients with exudative pharyngitis. Autoinoculation of infected genital secretions into the eye results in monocular purulent conjunctivitis.

Pelvic inflammatory disease is caused by ascending infection from the endocervix into the uterus, the fallopian tubes, or the ovaries. Organisms implicated in PID include *N. gonorrhoeae*, *Chlamydia trachomatis*, or anaerobes and are often polymicrobial in nature. An estimated 1 million cases occur among U.S. women annually. These women are typically young, between 15 and 24 years of age. In addition to the short-term morbidity, long-term sequelae include infertility, ectopic pregnancy, and chronic pain. Gonococcal PID is more often associated with a fever and a shorter duration of illness (3 to 5 days). The CDC, who developed minimum criteria for the diagnosis of PID, recommend empirical treatment of PID when the following are present in the absence of an alternate diagnosis: lower abdominal pain, cervical motion tenderness, and adnexal tenderness.

Disseminated gonococcal infection complicates 0.5% to 3% of cases. Disseminated gonococcal infection is more common in women than in men and frequently occurs within 7 days of menses. In both sexes, disseminated gonococcal infection results from bacteremia and presents with a characteristic rash and tenosynovitis with or without frank arthritis (arthritis-dermatitis syndrome). The typical rash is an acrally distributed sparse eruption (10 to 25 lesions) consisting of a pustular lesion on an erythematous base. When septic arthritis is present, synovial culture results are positive in 50% of cases. The diagnosis rests on the isolation of *N. gonorrhoeae* from a sterile site (blood, joint) or can be made by isolating the organism from a mucosal site in the correct clinical setting.

DIAGNOSIS

The methods used to diagnose gonorrhea include Gram stain and culture, antigen detection tests, and nucleic acid techniques with or without amplification. The Gram stain is the most rapid and inexpensive method. The sensitivity of the Gram stain depends on the presence or absence of symptoms and the site cultured. Sensitivity can be as high as 85% to 95% in men presenting with urethral discharge but drops to 70% in asymptomatic men and to 50% in those with symptomatic endocervical and rectal infections. Culture remains the gold standard for diagnosis and requires direct inoculation onto selective media for optimal results, as previously discussed. Under these conditions, sensitivity will reach 95% to 100% in symptomatic men with urethritis, but sensitivity decreases in those with manifestations in other anatomic sites (Table 1). Culture has the following advantages: (1) It is approved for diagnostic use for any anatomic site; (2) it remains the test of choice in medicolegal situations, and (3) it can be used for antibiotic susceptibility testing.

Antigen detection tests include direct fluorescent antibody and enzyme immunoassays. These relatively older techniques do not offer much of a benefit in regard to sensitivity over a Gram stain in symptomatic men and are largely being replaced by nucleic acid tests.

Nucleic acid tests (nonamplified) use a chemiluminescent DNA probe that binds to a complementary portion of 16S RNA of the target organism. The resulting DNA:RNA luminescent hybrid is read by a luminometer. This technique

TABLE 1. **Performance of Gram Stain Compared With Culture for Diagnosis of Gonorrhea**

Site	Sensitivity, %	Specificity, %
Symptomatic male urethritis	95–99	97–100
Asymptomatic male urethritis	50–70	86–95
Cervical infection	50	95
Pharyngeal infection	Not recommended	Not recommended
Symptomatic rectal infection	57	87–100

offers sensitivity ranging from 70% to 90% and is highly specific. It is used widely because it does not require viable organisms and can concomitantly test for the presence of *C. trachomatis*. It is approved for use only on genital and conjunctival specimens and cannot be used for antibiotic susceptibility testing.

Amplified DNA tests such as the ligase chain reaction or polymerase chain reaction represent the latest technology being applied to the diagnosis of gonococcal infections. A probe targets specific known *N. gonorrhoeae* nucleic acid sequences, binds, and creates copies of the target. This amplification process greatly enhances the sensitivity of the test, offering 94% to 100% sensitivity in both males and females, while retaining excellent specificity (Table 2). In addition, this technique can be used on first-voided urine and vaginal swabs, obviating the need for invasive specimen collection. Similar to other nonculture tests, amplified tests are not approved for use in all anatomic sites and cannot be used for antibiotic susceptibility testing.

TREATMENT

The use of sentinel antibiotic susceptibility centers has provided guidance for the recommended treatment of gonorrhea for many years. Data from the Gonococcal Isolate Surveillance Project reveal that fully 29% of all gonorrhea isolates reviewed in 1996 were resistant to penicillin, tetracycline, or both. Although there is now significant resistance to penicillin (penicillinase-producing *N. gonorrhoeae*) and tetracycline, there remain many effective antibiotic choices for the treatment of gonorrhea. In addition to receiving treatment for gonorrhea, the patient should always receive therapy for concomitant infection with *C. trachomatis* (which coexists in 15% to 50% of patients infected with gonorrhea). The patient should also be tested serologically for syphilis and counseled about and tested for HIV infection. Any sexual partners in the 60 days before onset of symptoms should be referred for evaluation and treatment.

TABLE 2. **Performance of Nonculture Tests for Diagnosis of Gonorrhea**

Method	Sensitivity, %	Specificity, %
Antigen detection (DFA, EIA)	70–85*	94–99
Nucleic acid (e.g., Gen-Probe)	85–100	96–100
Amplified nucleic acid test (LCR/PCR)	94–100	≥99.7

*Lower range in asymptomatic patients, females.
Abbreviations: DFA = direct fluorescent antibody; EIA = enzyme immunoassay; LCR/PCR = ligase chain/polymerase chain reaction.

Uncomplicated Gonorrhea in Adults

The recommended treatment regimens listed in Table 3 are based on the CDC's 1998 sexually transmitted disease treatment guidelines. The Food and Drug Administration has approved regimens other than those listed, including single-dose therapy of other licensed fluoroquinolones and a 2-g dose of oral azithromycin (Zithromax). All approved regimens for uncomplicated gonorrhea are single-dose therapies and are safe and effective for the treatment of genital, rectal, and pharyngeal infection. Ceftriaxone

TABLE 3. **Treatment of Gonorrhea in Adults**

Cervix, Urethra, Rectum	**Plus Treatment for Chlamydia**
Ceftriaxone (Rocephin) 125 mg IM × 1 day *or* Cefixime (Suprax) 400 mg po × 1 day *or* Ciprofloxacin (Cipro) 500 mg po × 1 day *or* Ofloxacin (Floxin) 400 po × 1 day	Azithromycin (Zithromax) 1 g po × 1 day *or* doxycycline (Vibramycin) 100 mg po bid × 7 days
Pharynx	
Ceftriaxone 125 mg IM × 1 day *or* Ciprofloxacin 500 mg po × 1 day *or* Ofloxacin 400 mg po × 1 day	
Conjunctiva	
Ceftriaxone 1 g IM × 1 day	
Pregnancy*	
Ceftriaxone 125 mg IM × 1 day	In pregnancy use erythromycin base 500 mg qid × 7 days
Pelvic Inflammatory Disease†	**Plus Treatment for Chlamydia**
Inpatient (regimen A or B) A. Cefotetan (Cefotan) 2.0 g IV q12h *or* cefoxitin (Mefoxin) 2.0 g IV q6h B. Clindamycin (Cleocin) 900 mg IV q8h *plus* gentamicin (Garamycin) 2.0 mg/kg IV once then 1.5 mg/kg q8h (or single daily dosing) Outpatient (regimen A or B) A. Ofloxacin 400 mg po bid × 14 days *plus* metronidazole (Flagyl) 500 mg po bid × 14 days B. Single-dose cefoxitin 2 g IM *plus* probenecid (Benemid)1 g po × 1 day *or* ceftriaxone 250 mg IM × 1 day	Doxycycline 100 mg IV *or* po q12h × 14 days

*If allergic to cephalosporins, use spectinomycin, 2 g IM × 1 day.
†See text for indications for hospitalization.

(Rocephin) and cefixime (Suprax) are both safe in pregnancy and have the added benefit of activity against incubating syphilis. At this time, all strains of gonorrhea remain sensitive to these drugs. Fluoroquinolones, although inexpensive and very effective, cannot be used in pregnancy and have no activity against *Treponema pallidum*. In addition, fluoroquinolone-resistant *N. gonorrhoeae*, already recognized in Asia, Japan, and Australia, has been recently reported in Hawaii. In Hawaii, the percentage of isolates resistant to ciprofloxacin (Cipro) increased from 1.4% in 1997 to 9.5% in 1999. Additionally, a small outbreak of gonorrhea with decreased sensitivity to azithromycin was recently described in Kansas City, Missouri. These events highlight the continued importance of the Gonococcal Isolate Surveillance Project and serve as a reminder to practitioners to remain aware of gonorrhea resistance profiles in their area. Pregnant women who are highly allergic to cephalosporins should be treated with spectinomycin (Trobicin), 2.0 g intramuscularly. Test of cure need not be done if patients are symptomatically improved unless suboptimal therapy was used (e.g., spectinomycin for pharyngeal infection).

Pelvic Inflammatory Disease

The recommended treatment for PID, based on knowledge of the polymicrobial nature of the disease, is listed in Table 3. Hospitalization should be considered for women with the following conditions: indefinite diagnosis, pregnancy, vomiting, severe pain, suspected abscess, adolescence, or HIV infection; it should also be considered in women for whom follow-up cannot be guaranteed. Regimens are given for inpatient or outpatient therapy. For inpatients, the parenteral regimen should be given until the patient is substantially improved; after 24 hours, doxycycline should be continued orally to complete 14 days of therapy.

Disseminated Gonococcal Infection

Accepted therapies include ceftriaxone, 1 g intravenously or intramuscularly every 24 hours until the patient is improved. Then the patient can be switched to either oral cefixime (400 mg/day) or a fluoroquinolone (ciprofloxacin 500 mg/day or ofloxacin [Floxin] 400 mg/day) to complete 1 week of therapy. Septic joints rarely require repeated arthrocentesis because the response to parenteral therapy is brisk.

Gonorrhea in Infants and Children

Neonatal infection may result from the vaginal delivery of an infant from an infected mother. Prophylaxis by instillation of 1% silver nitrate into the conjunctivae is an effective method of preventing neonatal conjunctivitis (ophthalmia neonatorum). Vaginal infection in prepubertal girls is almost always the result of sexual abuse and should set in motion support and legal services to investigate this possibility. Uncomplicated infections in children and neonates can be treated with ceftriaxone, 25 to 50 mg/kg, not to exceed 125 mg. Treatment for chlamydia infection is generally withheld unless infection is diagnosed because therapies used in adults have not been well studied in children.

Gonorrhea remains a significant public health problem as a cause of PID, infertility, and ectopic pregnancy, and it is associated with an increased risk of HIV infection. Practitioners need to be aware of the typical presentation of genital gonorrhea as well as the less common manifestations of conjunctival and disseminated disease. Culture and Gram stain remain the mainstays of diagnosis, but the superlative performance of nucleic acid amplification tests may result in their more widespread use as our experience with these technologies grows. There are many very effective single-dose treatment regimens available, but knowledge of changing antibiotic resistance patterns is essential if gonorrhea is to be controlled. Co-treatment with antibiotics effective against *Chlamydia* is essential and is already proving to be an effective strategy in decreasing the incidence of this disease in certain settings. The lack of an animal model has been a barrier in the development of an effective vaccine for gonorrhea, but the use of human experimental infection may soon pave the way for the introduction of novel protection strategies.

NONGONOCOCCAL URETHRITIS

method of
MICHAEL F. REIN, M.D.
The University of Virginia Health System
Charlottesville, Virginia

Nongonococcal urethritis (NGU) is usually manifested by some combination of dysuria (50%–75%) and urethral discharge. Symptoms may be subtle. The condition is diagnosed when urethral inflammation is detected, and gonococcal infection has been ruled out. In men, the diagnosis is initially based on a Gram-stained smear of urethral discharge that shows the presence of polymorphonuclear neutrophils (PMNs) but no gram-negative diplococci consistent with *Neisseria gonorrhoeae*. A calcium alginate swab is inserted into the urethra far enough to pass through the fossa navicularis and into the area of cuboidal epithelium. The swab is rotated during removal and is then rolled onto a microscope slide, Gram stained, and examined microscopically at 1000×. Although some texts use 5 PMNs per oil-immersion field as the criterion for urethritis, a smaller number of PMNs are seen in 16% to 50% of cases and should be regarded as indicating disease, especially if the patient has recently urinated.

Diagnosis in women is more difficult, because the symptoms of NGU mimic those of bacterial cystitis. NGU should be suspected in women whose dysuria and pyuria are associated with negative routine bacterial cultures of urine or in whom symptoms frequently recur after sexual contact. NGU in men and women may be asymptomatic.

Patients with gonorrhea are frequently co-infected with an agent of NGU, and treatment of gonorrhea should include a regimen effective for NGU as well.

Chlamydia trachomatis causes 16% to 50% of the cases of NGU. *Ureaplasma urealyticum,* formerly known as the T-strain *Mycoplasma,* has been isolated from about 80% of men with *Chlamydia*-negative NGU. The causes of the remaining 20% of cases are less well defined and appear to include *Trichomonas vaginalis* (1%–4%), herpes simplex virus, the recently identified *Mycoplasma genitalium,* and a variety of other bacteria and viruses. Clinical etiologic differentiation is impossible, and NGU is therefore initially treated as a syndrome.

TREATMENT

Treatments for NGU are listed in Table 1. Those regimens recommended for syndromic treatment are usually active against the common causes, whereas those recommended for known chlamydial infection will not treat ureaplasmal disease. None of the regimens listed in Table 1 is effective in herpetic or trichomonal urethritis. There is no apparent advantage to extending any initial regimen beyond 7 to 10 days. Tetracyclines are somewhat less active than other regimens against ureaplasmas. The addition of trimethoprim to a sulfonamide provides no benefit in this setting. Sexual partners of index cases should be treated with equivalent regimens on the basis of their high risk of infection (epidemiologic treatment). It is inappropriate merely to test a female sexual contact for chlamydial infection and deny treatment on the basis of a negative test. NGU may well be nonchlamydial, some 25% of women with chlamydial infection are positive only at the urethra, and many of the currently available tests for chlamydia lack sensitivity.

Management of Recurrences

The pattern of recurrence can serve as a guide to subsequent management. Patients noting complete resolution of symptoms only to have them return days to weeks after re-exposure to a sexual partner are likely suffering from re-infection and may be re-treated with the initial regimen. Efforts to ensure that sexual partners are treated should then be redoubled.

Patients whose symptoms persist after initial treatment must be re-evaluated. The disappearance of PMNs from the urethra suggests an adequate response to initial therapy, and such patients should be followed to ensure that symptoms indeed eventually resolve. Patients with objective evidence of persistent urethral inflammation must be regarded as being infected with a resistant etiologic agent. Two well-characterized organisms are *T. vaginalis* and tetracycline-resistant *U. urealyticum.* Patients with persistent urethritis may thus be empirically treated with metronidazole (Flagyl, Protostat, Metric 21), 2 g orally as a single dose. Patients initially treated with a tetracycline should also receive erythromycin, azithromycin (Zithromax), or ofloxacin (Floxin), to which these ureaplasmas remain sensitive. Patients whose urethritis still fails to resolve should be given thorough microbiologic and urologic evaluations.

Least well understood are those patients whose urethritis initially responds to treatment but then recurs in the absence of re-exposure. Such patients are not likely to be infected either with *C. trachomatis, U. urealyticum,* or *T. vaginalis.* Treatment of these patients remains somewhat controversial, but some are cured by extending regimens of doxycycline or erythromycin to 3 to 6 weeks. Some patients who repeatedly experience relapse and in whom urologic workup is unrevealing (e.g., of stricture or prostatitis) may need chronic suppressive therapy with a low dose of tetracycline (e.g., 500 mg/d PO). Patients should abstain from coitus until all partners have completed therapy.

Patients being treated for NGU should be carefully examined for other sexually transmitted diseases. Because any sexually transmitted disease is a behavioral marker for increased risk of infection with HIV, and, indeed, the lesions of other sexually transmitted diseases may increase the risk of spread of HIV, patients with NGU should be encouraged to undergo HIV testing.

TABLE 1. **Treatment of Nongonococcal Urethritis**

Syndromic Treatment of Nongonococcal Urethritis
Doxycycline (Doryx, Vibramycin, Vibra-Tabs, Monodox), 100 mg PO bid × 7 d
Tetracycline, 500 mg PO qid × 7 d
Azithromycin (Zithromax), 1 g PO as a single dose*
Minocycline (Minocin, Vectrin, Dynacin), 100 mg PO qhs × 7 d
Erythromycin base (E-Mycin, Ery-Tab, ERYC, E-Base), 500 mg PO qid × 7 d*
Ofloxacin (Floxin), 300 mg PO bid × 7 d
Treatment If Urethritis Is Known to Be Chlamydial
Sulfisoxazole (Gantrisin), 500 mg PO qid × 10 d
Amoxicillin (Amoxil, Polymox, Trimox, Amoxi, Wymox), 500 mg PO tid × 10 d*
Clindamycin (Cleocin), 450 mg PO tid for 10 d*

*May be used in pregnancy.

GRANULOMA INGUINALE

(Donovanosis)

method of
TED ROSEN, M.D.
Baylor College of Medicine and VA Medical Center
Houston, Texas

Granuloma inguinale, or donovanosis, is a disorder caused by the obligate intracellular, pleomorphic gram-negative bacillus *Calymmatobacterium granulomatis.* A study of genes coding for ribosomal RNA place this organism in a close phylogenetic relationship with the *Klebsiella* genus, and it has been proposed that the organism's name be modified accordingly. This disease is rare in the United States; only 19 cases were reported to the Centers for Disease Control and Prevention in 1999. The disease primarily occurs in endemic foci in tropical and subtropical areas of the world, most prominently in southeast India, Papua New Guinea, China, Vietnam, South Africa, Zambia, Brazil, and Australia. Both sexual and nonsexual modes of transmission have been documented; children and sexually inactive persons probably acquire the disease from contact with infectious exudates.

Though often cited as 1 to 12 weeks (average of 2–3 weeks), the incubation period is quite variable. Ultimately, one or more nontender papules or nodules appear. The latter rapidly erode to form painless ulcers with sharp, raised and rolled borders and clean, friable and "beefy-red" bases. Multiple lesions may coalesce, and lesions are prone to inexorable extension that may lead to mutilating tissue destruction. Rare clinical manifestations include soft, erythematous papules with velvety granulation tissue–like surfaces (nodular variant) and large vegetating masses that resemble condyloma acuminatum (hypertrophic variant). Lesions tend to occur on the prepuce, frenulum, and coronal sulcus in men and the labia in women. Perianal lesions may occur in either sex, and the vagina and cervix are rarely involved in women. Cervical disease may spread deeply into pelvic tissues and hematogenously disseminate to other sites. True inguinal adenopathy does not accompany genital ulcers, but subcutaneous lesions in this region may produce inguinal swelling (pseudobuboes). Complications include phimosis, urethral stenosis, genital elephantiasis, and the development of squamous cell carcinoma in untreated lesions of long duration. Extragenital donovanosis occurs in 5% of patients and may involve the mouth, extragenital skin, the lungs, the liver, the spleen, and the bones. Unlike cutaneous disease, visceral involvement is associated with constitutional symptoms such as fever, night sweats, anorexia, and weight loss.

The diagnosis is based on a compatible clinical manifestation in conjunction with direct demonstration of the etiologic intracellular organisms (Donovan bodies). Tissue crush smears or tissue biopsy specimens are stained with Giemsa, Wright, or Warthin-Starry silver stains to visualize the bipolar bacilli within macrophages. Laboratory culture on artificial media, complement-fixation and other serologic tests, and skin test antigens are not commercially available. Polymerase chain reaction has been used successfully to identify the organism, but this technique is not readily accessible to practitioners.

TREATMENT

Recommended first-line treatments include: doxycycline (Vibramycin, Monodox), 100 mg twice daily, and trimethoprim-sulfamethoxazole (Bactrim DS, Septra DS),* 160/800 mg twice daily. Therapy is administered for a minimum of 3 weeks and should be continued until all lesions are totally healed. An acceptable alternative to the two recommended drugs is ciprofloxacin (Cipro),* 750 mg twice daily. The latter has even proved effective in the treatment of patients co-infected with HIV. Pregnant and lactating women should be treated with erythromycin (PCE),* 500 mg four times daily; however, response is notably slower with this regimen. Recent work in Australia suggests that azithromycin (Zithromax),* 1.0 g weekly for 4 weeks or 500 mg daily for 1 week, may be efficacious. Intravenous gentamicin (Garamycin),* 1 mg/kg every 8 hours, is reserved for recalcitrant cases. Radical surgical resection may be necessary to correct long-standing fistulas, abscesses, and massive tissue destruction

Patients with granuloma inguinale should be screened for other sexually transmitted diseases. They should also receive appropriate counseling and serologic testing for HIV infection. Sexual partners should be examined, although strictly prophylactic treatment is optional.

*Not FDA approved for this indication.

*Not FDA approved for this indication.

LYMPHOGRANULOMA VENEREUM

method of
TED ROSEN, M.D.
Baylor College of Medicine and VA Medical Center
Houston, Texas

Lymphogranuloma venereum (LGV) is a sexually transmitted disease caused by virulent and invasive serotypes (L1, L2, and L3) of the obligate intracellular organism *Chlamydia trachomatis*. This disease is endemic in India, Southeast Asia, South America, and portions of Africa. LGV is rare in the United States, with only 62 cases reported to the Centers for Disease Control and Prevention in 1999. Acute disease is more commonly seen in men, whereas late complications are more commonly encountered in women.

LGV is classically divided into three stages. The incubation period is quite variable and ranges from 3 days to as many as 40 days. Subsequently, a small, painless eroded papule appears on the glans penis or on the mucous membranes of the vulva, vagina, cervix, or rectum. This transient lesion heals in 1 week or less and goes unnoticed in most patients. The second stage, which appears 2 to 6 weeks later, demonstrates painful regional lymphadenitis, low-grade fever, and constitutional symptoms (malaise, anorexia, myalgia, and arthralgia). Adenopathy is unilateral in two thirds of patients. In men, enlarged lymph nodes above and below the inguinal ligament (Poupart's ligament) creates a highly characteristic indentation known as the "groove sign." Left untreated, enlarged nodes progress to spontaneous rupture in about one third of cases. In women, primary lesions may occur at anatomic sites that drain into deep iliac or perirectal nodes; hence, lower abdominal, pelvic, or low back pain may be the initial symptom. The late stage of untreated LGV consists of various combinations of perirectal abscesses, anogenital fistulas, rectal strictures, perineal lymphedema, and genital elephantiasis.

The diagnosis is based on a compatible clinical picture and a positive LGV complement-fixation test titer of 1:64 or greater. Although serologic testing is only genus specific, complement-fixation titers from other forms of chlamydial infection are rarely over 1:16. Alternative serologic tests, such as microimmunofluorescence titer and enzyme-linked immunosorbent assay, are not readily available. Recovery of chlamydiae from cutaneous lesions and lymph node aspirates is technically difficult, expensive, and rarely attempted. Histologic examination of affected lymph nodes demonstrates a very suggestive pattern of stellate microabscess formation; however, lymph node biopsy is not practical in most ambulatory care settings.

TREATMENT

The treatment of choice is doxycycline (Vibramycin, Monodox), 100 mg twice daily for at least 21 days (or until lesions clear). An alternative regimen consists of erythromycin (PCE), 500 mg four times daily for the same duration of therapy. Pregnant and lactating women should receive erythromycin. Although a few cases have been successfully treated with ciprofloxacin (Cipro)* and azithromycin (Zithromax),* the optimum dosing regimens have not been determined. Fluctuant lymph nodes may be aspirated or surgically incised to prevent rupture and relieve symptoms.

As is true of all genital ulcer disease, patients infected with LGV should be screened for other sexually transmitted diseases and should receive counseling and serologic testing for HIV.

*Not FDA approved for this indication.

SYPHILIS

method of
JEFFREY T. KIRCHNER, D.O.
Temple University School of Medicine
Philadelphia, Pennsylvania

Syphilis has been discussed in the archives of medicine for more than 500 years. The first recorded mention of this infectious disease was in 1495 when French soldiers acquired the illness while occupying Naples. A new epidemic known as the "great pox" began. It presumably made its way from Europe to the United States via Christopher Columbus; however, recent data published by Rothschild strongly suggest that the Dominican Republic was the initial site of contact with syphilis, and that it subsequently spread from the New World to the Old.

Despite the decline in the incidence of syphilis over the past 10 years, it remains a disease with significant health consequences and substantial social and economic costs. The goal of U.S. health officials is to eliminate this sexually transmitted disease by the middle of the current decade. Syphilis will likely remain a condition that physicians will encounter in their clinical practices, however, albeit with decreasing frequency. Like other genital ulcerative diseases, syphilis has been associated with an increased risk of acquiring and transmitting human immunodeficiency virus (HIV), which causes AIDS. The latter is a disease that continues to be widespread throughout the world; this fact makes the elimination of syphilis doubtful.

BIOLOGY

The causative organism of syphilis is *Treponema pallidum*, which is one of a small group of treponemes from the order Spirochaetales that are virulent in human beings. Two other genera in this order include *Borrelia* and *Leptospira*. *T. pallidum* cannot be distinguished immunologically, morphologically, or on the basis of DNA homology from treponemes such as *T. pallidum* subsp. *pertenue* (which causes yaws) or *T. carateum* (which causes pinta). Other treponemes may have human hosts but are either nonpathogenic or cause disease only in animals.

T. pallidum is quite small, with a length of only 6 to 20 μm and a width of 0.15 μm, thus making it too minute for viewing with light microscopy. It can be viewed only with darkfield microscopy or, in investigational situations, with electron microscopy. Darkfield examination of a specimen reveals a white appearance of the treponeme along with flexion and back-and-forth motions typical of virulent treponemes. In vitro growth of the organism is very difficult but has been accomplished on a limited basis. The inability to sustain the spirochete in vitro has limited the investigation of the antigenic composition, the toxin production capabilities, and the metabolism of *T. pallidum*.

TRANSMISSION AND EPIDEMIOLOGY

The primary mode of contracting syphilis is through sexual contact. A second mode is transplacental transmission from an infected mother to her developing fetus. Infection via blood transfusion or direct inoculation is theoretically possible but quite rare. Transmission by sexual contact requires a break in the squamous or columnar epithelium to allow the spirochete to enter the body. The organism disseminates via the bloodstream or the lymphatic circulation.

The overall incidence of syphilis in the United States has declined over the past decade, with fewer than 7000 cases of primary and secondary syphilis (rate: 2.6 cases per 100,000) reported to the Centers for Disease Control and Prevention (CDC) in 1998. This represents a 19% decline from 1997, when the case rate was 3.2 per 100,000. The most recent syphilis epidemic peaked in 1990, when 50,578 cases were reported. The incidence remains highest in the South and lowest in the Northeast sections of the United States. African Americans are affected the most frequently, followed by American Indians and Alaskan natives (2.8). The incidence of primary and secondary disease is highest among men 30 to 39 years of age and among women 20 to 24 years of age. Public health officials in the United States have a national plan to eliminate syphilis (defined as the absence of sustained transmission) by the year 2005. This would translate to fewer than 100 cases per year, or a rate of 0.4 per 100,000. It remains to be seen whether this goal can be accomplished.

CLINICAL MANIFESTATIONS

Primary syphilis is manifested by one or more painless ulcers (chancres), which represent the site of inoculation. The ulcer is round with a clear base and reaches 1 to 2 cm in diameter. The chancre is typically on the genitalia but may occur on the cervix, the rectal and perianal area, or the oral mucosa. The incubation period ranges from 10 to 90 days but is generally 14 to 21 days after exposure. The chancre may be accompanied by regional lymphadenopathy with node enlargement. Most patients are asymptomatic at this stage, and the chancre may go unnoticed. It heals in 4 to 6 weeks whether or not treatment is instituted.

The secondary or disseminated stage of syphilis develops 6 to 8 weeks after the chancre has healed, although there may be some overlap with primary disease. Secondary syphilis is characterized by a macular or papular rash that begins on the trunk and spreads to the palms or the soles. The rash affects 75% to 100% of patients. This stage of the illness is also associated with systemic symptoms such as fever, malaise, myalgias, arthralgias, and generalized lymphadenopathy. Epitrochlear lymph nodes may be found, which are thought to be unique to syphilis. There is ongoing spirochetemia, which allows for multiorgan involvement. Other clinical manifestations seen with secondary syphilis include meningitis, glomerulonephritis, and hepatitis. The differential diagnosis of secondary syphilis is extensive; for this reason, secondary syphilis has been called "the great imitator."

The natural history of secondary syphilis is such that even in the absence of treatment, there will be spontaneous resolution of all symptoms after 3 to 12 weeks. During the first year, about 25% of untreated patients may experience a relapse to active secondary syphilis. This stage is known as early latent syphilis. Generally, by 2 years there are no further relapses, and the patient is in the stage of late latent syphilis. By definition, these patients are asymptomatic but will have positive serologic test results for syphilis. The CDC uses a somewhat arbitrary period of 1 year to differentiate early latent from late latent syphilis. This distinction is important for treatment purposes.

Tertiary (or late) syphilis develops in 10% to 40% of untreated persons. Patients in this stage of the disease may exhibit a variety of neurologic, cardiovascular, and systemic infections. Essentially, any organ of the body can be affected, and symptoms can develop years after the primary infection. An extensive body of literature has been published on late-stage syphilis, including natural history data from the Tuskegee and Oslo studies. With effective screening and antibiotic therapy, tertiary syphilis is uncommon.

DIAGNOSIS

Microscopic Examination

In patients with primary or secondary syphilis, darkfield examination or immunofluorescence staining of material from active lesions is the most rapid method of establishing a diagnosis. For darkfield examination, the suspected lesion should be first cleansed with saline solution, then mildly abraded with dry gauze. Any serous exudate can then be collected on a dry slide and examined with darkfield or phase-contrast microscopy. Technically, three examinations should be done to determine that a lesion is nonsyphilitic. Oral lesions cannot be used owing to contamination with nonvenereal treponemes. If a lesion is inadvertently cleansed with povidone-iodine solution or another bactericidal solution, immunofluorescence staining can be used to detect dead or nonmotile spirochetes.

Serologic Tests

Syphilis can be diagnosed based on physical findings but must be confirmed with laboratory testing. The current tests for screening or initial diagnosis are the rapid plasma reagin and the Venereal Disease Research Laboratory test. Two additional tests include the automated reagin test and the toluidine red unheated test. These tests are referred to as nontreponemal tests and detect IgM and IgG antibody against a lipoidal antigen. They are nonspecific and thus can produce false-positive results (Table 1). They can be carried out as either qualitative or quantitative measurements but are usually performed and reported quantitatively. The serum of a patient suspected of having syphilis is diluted serially, and the test is repeated until it is no longer reactive. The inverse of the last dilution that is positive is the patient's titer. Higher titers (1:16 to 1:128) are found in secondary and early latent syphilis. False-positive titers will usually be 1:4 dilutions or less.

TABLE 1. **Causes of False-Positive Test Results for Syphilis**

Viral infections (early HIV; varicella; Epstein-Barr virus)
Bacterial infections (mycoplasmal, pneumococcal)
Lyme disease
Intravenous drug use
Connective tissue diseases
Pregnancy
Advanced age
Multiple myeloma

The rapid plasma reagin or Venereal Disease Research Laboratory test titers are used to monitor response to treatment, with a progressive decline noted in the weeks to months following antibiotic therapy. Most patients with primary disease should have a nonreactive titer by 1 year after treatment. Patients with secondary syphilis should have no detectable antibody by 2 years. Persons treated with late infection often have a persistently lower titer (<1:8) for many years, a condition known as a *serofast state*. Other conditions associated with persistently positive low antibody titers include a biologically false-positive result, treatment failure, or re-infection.

A positive nontreponemal antibody test should be confirmed by a specific antibody test for *T. pallidum*. These tests include the fluorescent treponemal antibody absorption test, *T. pallidum* hemagglutination, and the microhemagglutination assay for antibodies to *T. pallidum*. Their expense and the number of false-positive test reactions make these tests unsuitable for screening purposes. In general, these test results remain positive for life, but about 10% of patients will revert to nonreactive status, especially if treated early in the course of infection.

The nontreponemal tests can also be used to diagnose neurosyphilis. Abnormalities of the central nervous system can occur at any stage of syphilis without the presence of true neurosyphilis. Moreover, many patients with abnormal cerebrospinal fluid findings will be asymptomatic. The decision to perform a lumbar puncture in a patient with syphilis should be based on disease stage and clinical findings (Table 2). A definitive diagnosis of neurosyphilis is dependent on the presence of cerebrospinal fluid pleocytosis (8 to 100 lymphocytes per milliliter), an increased cerebrospinal fluid protein level, a decreased plasma glu-

TABLE 2. **Indications for Cerebrospinal Fluid Examination in Patients With Syphilis***

Neurologic or ophthalmic symptoms
Evidence of active tertiary syphilis (e.g., aortitis, gumma, or iritis)
Treatment failure
HIV-infection with latent syphilis of syphilis of unknown duration

*Cerebrospinal fluid examination should also be considered if warranted by other clinical circumstances not defined previously. If the findings are consistent with neurosyphilis, patients should be treated accordingly.

cose level, and a positive cerebrospinal fluid Venereal Disease Research Laboratory test result.

TREATMENT

The primary goals of treatment are to prevent further progression of syphilis and disease transmission. Historically, mercury was used for many years in a variety of formulations to treat syphilis. Another therapy used during the preantibiotic era was Ehrlich's arsenic derivative, salvarsan. It was developed in 1909 and was hoped to be the magic bullet for curing syphilis. The use of induced-fever therapy was promoted by Julius Wagner von Jauregg, who actually won the Nobel Prize in 1927 for his use of malarial injections to treat paralytic dementia (neurosyphilis).

The modern treatment of syphilis in its various stages has remained fairly constant since the introduction of penicillin therapy in late 1943. This antibiotic remains the drug of choice for most patients (Table 3). Despite its extensive use for more than 50 years, there is no evidence of the development of *T. pallidum* resistance to penicillin. Standard therapy for primary, secondary, and early latent disease is benzathine penicillin (Bicillin L-A), 2.4 million U intramuscularly as a single dose. For patients with late latent syphilis, syphilis of unknown duration, or tertiary syphilis, the CDC's recommendation is 2.4 million U weekly for 3 weeks. Neurosyphilis and congenital syphilis require intravenous penicillin. There are some studies supporting parenterally administered ceftriaxone sodium for treating syphilis. Although not studied extensively in the United States, there are also data to support the efficacy of oral azithromycin (Zithromax) for incubating and primary syphilis.

Jarisch-Herxheimer Reaction

After receiving penicillin therapy, some patients will experience a systemic reaction manifested by fever, chills, myalgias, and headache. It usually begins within 2 hours after treatment and subsides within 24 hours. It is most common in primary and secondary syphilis, affecting about 50% and 75% of

TABLE 3. **Recommended Treatment for Syphilis**

Stage	Primary Treatment	Alternative Treatment	Recommended Follow-up
Primary	Penicillin G benzathine 2.4 million U IM	Doxycycline (Vibramycin) 100 mg bid for 14 d; Tetracycline 500 mg qid for 14 d; Erythromycin 500 mg qid for 14 d; Ceftriaxone sodium (Rocephin) 1 g IM for 8–10 d	HIV testing Repeat serology at 6 and 12 mo along with clinical examination*
Secondary	Penicillin G benzathine 2.4 million U IM	Same as above	Same as above
Early latent	Penicillin G benzathine 2.4 million U IM	Same as above	Same as above
Late latent or of unknown duration	Penicillin G 2.4 million U IM weekly for 3 wk	Doxycycline 100 mg bid for 28 d; Tetracycline 500 mg qid for 28 d	HIV testing Clinical examination for tertiary disease Consider CSF examination Repeat serology at 6, 12, and 24 mo†
Tertiary	Penicillin G 2.4 million U IM weekly for 3 wk	None acceptable	HIV testing Repeat serology at 6, 12, and 24 mo
Neurosyphilis	Aqueous penicillin G 18–24 million U in divided doses q4h for 10–14 d	Procaine penicillin G 2.4 million U IM daily for 10–14 d *Plus*, probenecid 500 mg PO qid for 10–14 d	HIV testing Repeat serology at 6, 12, and 24 mo Repeat CSF examination q6 mo until normal
Pregnancy (primary, secondary, or early latent)	Penicillin G benzathine 2.4 million U IM	None acceptable	Same as disease stages noted above

*Some experts recommended obtaining the first serology 3 months after treatment.
†There are limited data regarding the decline of titers in patients with latent or tertiary syphilis.
Abbreviation: CSF = cerebrospinal fluid.
From CDC Guidelines for the Treatment of Sexually Transmitted Diseases 47(RR-1): 1–118, 1998.

patients, respectively. Patients may be pretreated with aspirin or ibuprofen. Although of unproven efficacy, some experts advise the administration of prednisone for patients with late syphilis before giving penicillin.

FOLLOW-UP OF TREATED PATIENTS

All patients diagnosed with syphilis at any stage should be tested for HIV. If the patient is considered high risk, or in areas where the seroprevalence of HIV is high, repeat HIV testing at 3 months is recommended. Following antibiotic treatment, patients should be examined clinically and should also undergo repeat serologic testing at 6 and 12 months. For patients initially found to have latent disease, titers should be checked again at 24 months. If there is not at least a fourfold decline in the nontreponemal titer by 6 months, or if there is a fourfold or greater increase in the titer, treatment failure is likely. A lumbar puncture should be performed in this case to rule out neurosyphilis, and retreatment with three weekly injections of 2.4 million U of benzathine penicillin is recommended.

In some cases, the nontreponemal titer remains serofast, often at dilutions of 1:2 or 1:4. The clinician must be aware that a twofold difference between tests is not uncommon and does not necessarily represent treatment failure. It may require obtaining further follow-up serologic testing. Some studies have found that a fourfold difference in the titer is possible on the basis of laboratory variability. If the patient's clinical history is not reliable, repeat titers should be obtained every 3 months (along with clinical observation) to ensure cure.

SPECIAL CONSIDERATIONS

Pregnancy

Syphilis can cause significant complications in pregnancy, including spontaneous abortion, intrauterine growth retardation, and stillbirth. All women should be screened for syphilis in the first trimester with a rapid plasma reagin or Venereal Disease Research Laboratory test. High-risk patients should be screened again in the third trimester. Treatment in pregnancy is essentially the same as in the nonpregnancy state, except that nonpenicillin therapy is not recommended. Women with a true penicillin allergy should undergo desensitization.

Acquired Immunodeficiency Syndrome

As noted, syphilis and other genital ulcerative diseases increase the likelihood of HIV transmission. There have been some observations and data suggesting that syphilis in patients with HIV may follow a more protracted and complicated clinical course. The CDC's treatment guidelines are the same as those for persons with HIV infection, although many experts advocate a more extended course of penicillin. Serologic responses have also been aberrant in HIV-infected persons compared with those in normal hosts. Consequently, it is recommended that titers be checked every 3 months for a minimum of 24 months after completion of antibiotic therapy.

Sexual Partners

The sexual partners of all patients diagnosed with syphilis should be notified. For patients with primary disease, all partners within the previous 3 months should be identified owing to the 90-day incubation period. Forty percent to 60% of sexual partners will become infected. This period should be extended to 2 years for contacts of patients diagnosed with secondary syphilis or early latent disease. Empirical treatment is recommended unless the contact patient is agreeable to regular laboratory follow-up and clinical surveillance.

Section 11

Diseases of Allergy

ANAPHYLAXIS AND SERUM SICKNESS

method of
H. JAMES WEDNER, M.D.
Washington University School of Medicine
St. Louis, Missouri

ANAPHYLAXIS

The term "anaphylaxis," *against protection,* was coined by Porter and Richet in 1902 after their observation that in dogs immunized to a fish toxin, a rapid and fatal reaction occasionally developed when the toxin was reintroduced. In 1912 Richet wrote, "Anaphylaxis is the opposite condition to protection (phylaxis). I coined the word in 1902 to describe the peculiar attribute which certain poisons possess of increasing instead of diminishing the sensitivity of an organism to their action."

Anaphylaxis is a severe systemic allergic reaction that occurs after the massive release of mediators of anaphylaxis from tissue mast cells and circulating basophils. The release of mediators may be the result of contact of the individual with an allergen to which an IgE response has been made, or it may be the result of the release of mediators by a non-IgE–mediated mechanism. The former is often referred to as "true anaphylaxis" or just "anaphylaxis," whereas the latter is called an "anaphylactoid" or "pseudoallergic" reaction. Although subtle differences may be seen in the features of these two types of systemic reaction, in practice, they can be considered the same, and the therapeutic approach to either is identical. Anaphylactic reactions should always be considered life threatening; in actuality, however, most published cases of death from anaphylaxis are the result of failure of the clinician to recognize and promptly treat the reaction.

Anaphylactic reactions are type I, or *immediate hypersensitivity,* reactions. As such, they generally occur very rapidly after exposure of the individual. The reaction may be seen within seconds of contact with the allergen, and virtually all of the reactions occur within 60 minutes. For example, retrospective studies of allergic reactions to penicillin have demonstrated that over 96% of the reactions occur 30 minutes or less after a penicillin injection or the ingestion of an oral penicillin preparation. Although certain anaphylactic reactions, such as those to nonsteroidal anti-inflammatory agents (NSAIDs) such as acetylsalicylic acid, some foods and/or food additives, and insect stings, may occur at times greater than 1 hour after exposure, in general, evaluation of delayed reactions should concentrate on alternative mechanisms.

Because mast cells are found in every tissue in the body with the exception of the brain, symptoms of anaphylaxis can be seen in every organ system. As shown in Table 1, the most commonly affected organs include the skin, the upper and lower respiratory tract, the cardiovascular system, the gastrointestinal system, and the genitourinary tract (particularly prominent in women because of the heavy concentration of mast cells in the uterus). It must be remembered, however, that not every patient who experiences anaphylaxis will have all the symptoms described in Table 1. Indeed, even symptoms that are generally associated with an anaphylactic reaction may be missing, but this absence of symptoms does not invalidate the diagnosis.

Anaphylactic reactions are classified according to the severity of the reaction. As shown in Table 2, systemic allergic reactions range from mild reactions limited only to the skin (type I) to cardiopulmonary arrest (type IV). Whereas the term *anaphylaxis* covers each of the four types, the term *anaphylactic shock* is generally reserved for patients who have type III or type IV reactions.

Mediators of Anaphylaxis. As noted earlier, the symptoms of anaphylaxis are a result of the rapid release of potent mediators from mast cells and basophils. The mediators can be divided into three basic groups: mediators that are preformed and stored within the mast cell granules, newly formed mediators, and cytokines secreted by stimulated mast cells and basophils. Preformed mediators stored within mast cell granules include histamine, proteolytic enzymes and matrix proteoglycans, and heparin and chondroitin sulfate. The enzymes present in mast cells differ according to the tissue location of the cells. Mucosal mast cells have a trypsin-like enzyme called tryptase and are often called "T" mast cells; cells located in serosal areas contain both a trypsin-like enzyme and a chymotrypsin-like enzyme called a chymase. These cells are called "TC" mast cells.

The tryptase enzyme has been used as a specific marker of mast cell mediator release and can thus be used to determine whether a patient has had an anaphylactic reac-

TABLE 1. **Symptomatology of Anaphylaxis**

Organ	Reaction	Approximate Incidence (%)
Skin	Irritation/erythema	3
	Urticaria/angioedema	61
	Fever	6
Upper respiratory tract	Profuse rhinorrhea, itchy, scratchy, watery eyes	60
	Laryngeal edema	15
Lower respiratory tract	Wheeze/dyspnea	38
	Respiratory arrest	10
Gastrointestinal tract	Nausea	29
	Vomiting	15
	Defecation	3
Cardiovascular system	Tachycardia	57
	Hypotension	48
	Hypertension	2
	Cardiac arrest	10
Genitourinary tract	Uterine cramping	30 (female)

TABLE 2. **Classification of Anaphylaxis**

Reaction Type	Skin	Gastrointestinal	Respiratory	Cardiovascular
I	Pruritus Urticaria Flush	None	None	None
II	Pruritus Urticaria Flush	Nausea	Dyspnea	Tachycardia Hypotension
III	Pruritus Urticaria Flush	Vomiting Defecation	Bronchospasm Wheezing	Shock
IV	Pruritus Urticaria Flush	Vomiting Defecation	Respiratory arrest	Cardiac arrest

tion. Two forms of tryptase are identified: α and β. The β form is constitutively released, and high levels of this enzyme are associated with elevated mast cell numbers such as seen in systemic mastocytosis. By contrast, the α form is released only when the mast cell releases all of its mediators, and high levels of this form are presumptive evidence of anaphylaxis. Unlike histamine, which is rapidly destroyed after release and is thus not a particularly good marker for anaphylaxis, tryptase remains in the circulation for a number of hours, well after the acute episode has been treated. We recommend that any patient with possible anaphylaxis have a single-clot tube of serum drawn and stored in case the diagnosis is questioned and needs to be confirmed.

The second class of mediators released on stimulation of mast cells consists of those that are newly formed. These mediators include prostaglandin D_2, leukotriene B_4 (LTB_4) and C_4 (LTC_4) (current evidence suggests that LTC_4 is exported from mast cells via the multidrug-resistance protein and is converted to LTD_4 and then LTE_4 outside the cell), and platelet-activating factor (acetyl glyceryl ether phosphoryl choline). The native molecules of these lipid-derived mediators are rapidly destroyed and cannot be used to define anaphylaxis; however, LTE_4 is quite stable and can be measured in the urine. Likewise, the metabolic byproduct of PGD_2 (6-keto-$PGF_{1\alpha}$) is relatively stable and can be assayed in the urine. Nevertheless, neither of these metabolites is as stable or easy to measure as tryptase, and evaluation of this enzyme is the preferred method for determination of mast cell mediator release.

A third class of mediators consists of cytokines that are secreted by stimulated mast cells and basophils. Secretion of these mediators takes a significant amount of time to become manifested (2 to 6 hours), and thus it is dubious that these mediators, including interleukin-3, interleukin-5, and granulocyte-macrophage colony–stimulating factor, contribute to the symptoms of anaphylaxis.

Pathophysiology of Anaphylaxis. The rapid and profound release of mediators from mast cells and basophils leads to a number of profound changes in the pulmonary and cardiovascular systems. In the lung, histamine, leukotrienes, and to a lessor extent the enzymes and platelet-activating factor are all potent spasmogenics that can lead to profound bronchoconstriction. Such bronchoconstriction leads to marked wheezing and, if persistent, to decreased oxygenation. These changes in the lung are confounded by similar changes in the upper airway, the most important of which is edema of the vocal cords with stridor and, if untreated, a marked decrease in airflow and marked hypoxemia. Indeed, the airway obstruction resulting from laryngeal edema may be life threatening without any other changes in the pulmonary or cardiovascular systems.

The effect of these same mediators on the vasculature is to decrease vascular tone and increase capillary leakage. Loss of vascular tone leads to pooling of the blood in the area of least resistance, most notably the splanchnic bed. The splanchnic bed has an immense capacity, and up to half of the intravascular volume may pool in the abdomen. The increase in capillary permeability leads to the rapid movement of fluid out of the vasculature and into the perivascular space (often referred to as third spacing). These two complementary changes, decreased vascular tone and increased capillary leakage, permit fluid to move out of the vasculature (third spacing) and into an area where the blood is unavailable to support the blood pressure. Thus, within minutes of the onset of anaphylaxis, a profound decrease in blood pressure can occur and lead to ineffective perfusion of the organs (shock).

Early changes in the vasculature lead to a decrease in systemic vascular resistance, and capillary leak leads to a decrease in blood pressure. The heart rate increases, as does stroke volume, and cardiac output during these very early stages is actually increased. As a result, central venous pressure is normal. Unless it is rapidly corrected, the profound fall in both blood pressure and effective intravascular volume rapidly decreases venous return to the heart, and despite the increase in heart rate, stroke volume and cardiac output will decrease. At this stage, central venous pressure will be decreased and result in poor perfusion of vital organs. If severe anaphylaxis remains untreated, systemic vascular resistance may actually increase in an attempt to increase perfusion pressure, but this adaptation is ineffective.

The upper and lower respiratory tract and the cardiovascular abnormalities seen in anaphylaxis are the most profound and have the potential to lead to a fatal outcome. Involvement of other organs, including the skin and digestive and genitourinary tracts, does not carry the same dire consequences. For this reason, as discussed later, primary therapy is directed at reversing the cardiovascular and respiratory abnormalities.

Two other syndromes associated with anaphylaxis are worthy of mention, although both are rare. In some instances, the profound capillary leak in the pulmonary vasculature can lead to pulmonary edema. It is important to recognize that the pulmonary edema is the result of an anaphylactic reaction because treatment should be directed toward the allergic reaction and not the pulmonary edema. Cardiac anaphylaxis results in ineffective beating of the heart and a profound decrease in cardiac output, over and above what would be seen with anaphylaxis. This condition may be confused with myocardial infarction or congestive heart failure. Several reports have suggested that balloon counterpulsation is an effective treatment for this rare anaphylaxis variant.

Incidence of Anaphylaxis. The true incidence of anaphylaxis is not known. Most series include a number of estimates to account for under-reporting of reactions because of failure to recognize the condition or fear of having caused the reaction—particularly in cases of drug-related anaphylaxis. The author is aware of a number of instances in which true anaphylaxis was not reported for this very reason. Nonetheless, Table 3 gives some indication of the major causes of anaphylaxis and their incidence.

Types of Anaphylaxis. Like all allergic reactions, anaphylaxis may be monophasic or biphasic. Patients may have a systemic allergic reaction that is successfully treated, and 6 to 24 hours later, a second reaction may occur without the introduction of additional allergen. In some cases, the second or "late phase" reaction may be more profound than the initial reaction. In addition, several reactions may follow the initial phase. Finally, a rare form of anaphylaxis may occur that has been termed "prolonged" anaphylaxis. This group of reactions seems to represent a combination of the initial and late phase reaction. They tend to be quite severe and relatively resistant to therapy. In contrast to other milder forms of this disease, prolonged anaphylaxis carries a high mortality rate.

The recognition that a significant percentage of patients who experience anaphylaxis will have a biphasic reaction is an important part of the therapy for anaphylaxis. The use of corticosteroids, which as will be noted later are of little use in the acute phase of therapy, can blunt or largely prevent the late phase reaction.

Causes of Anaphylaxis. As noted earlier, severe systemic allergic reactions can be classified as either anaphylactic (IgE dependent) or anaphylactoid (non–IgE dependent). The latter group includes agents that are capable of inducing mediator release from mast cells directly or by the generation of endogenous compounds that directly affect the mast cell. For example, opiate narcotics directly induce mediator release from the mast cell; by contrast, radiocontrast media (particularly the high–ionic strength material) most likely act by cleaving complement with the resultant generation of C3a and C5a (the anaphylatoxins), which then induce mediator release.

TABLE 3. **Incidence or Prevalence of Anaphylaxis**

Reaction	Incidence
General	1 in 2700 hospitalizations
Insect stings	0.4% to 0.8% of the population—250 fatalities per year
Radiocontrast media	1 in 1000 to 1 in 14,000 procedures—intravenous injection has a higher frequency than intra-arterial injection
β-Lactam antibiotics	0.1% to >5% of the population—250–300 fatal outcomes per year
General anesthesia	1 in 300 inductions—usually hypotension; a fatal outcome is rare, 1 in 10,000 to <1 in 100,000
Hemodialysis	1 in 1000 to 1 in 5000 treatments
Allergy immunotherapy	1 in 15,000 to 1 in 10,000,000 injections; in the United States, approximately 1 death per year

In general, anything capable of inducing the generation of IgE is a potential cause of anaphylaxis, including proteins that are directly immunogenic, such as aeroallergens and food allergens, and lower molecular weight compounds that must bind to a tissue protein and serve as a hapten. The most common members of this latter group are pharmacologic agents. Thus, the list of potential causes of anaphylaxis is quite extensive, Table 4 gives a brief classification of the causes of anaphylaxis.

Diagnosis of Anaphylaxis. The most important consideration in the diagnosis of anaphylaxis is maintaining a very high index of suspicion. Indeed, an old saying in allergy is that "if you think that a patient has anaphylaxis and needs to be treated, the treatment should have already been started." Nonetheless, the detection of classic signs and symptoms of anaphylaxis coupled with a history con-

TABLE 4. **Classification of the Causes of Anaphylaxis**

Type of Reaction	Mechanism	Type	Examples
Anaphylactic—IgE	Proteins	Foods	Peanut, tree nut, shellfish, soy, milk, fish
		Protein drugs	Insulin (largely beef and/or pork), chymopapain, ACTH, animal sera, monoclonal antibodies
		Allergens	Insect stings, mold, pollen, animal dander, latex
	Haptens	Drugs	β-Lactam antibiotics (penicillins, cephalosporins, penems), sulfonamides
		Preservatives	Parabens, metabisulfite, benzoates
Anaphylactoid—non-IgE	Direct mast cell	Drugs	Opiates, colloids, tricyclic antidepressant
		Immune complex	Immunoglobulins, blood products, polysaccharides
	Indirect mast cell	Generation of anaphylatoxins	Radiocontrast materials, immune complexes
Unknown mechanism	? Mast cell related	Physical urticarias	Dermatographism, cold, pressure, solar, cholinergic
		Exercise-augmented anaphylaxis	Celery
		Inhibition of arachidonic acid metabolism	ASA, other NSAIDs
	Unknown	Idiopathic anaphylaxis	

Note: This table is not designed to be a complete list of the causes of anaphylaxis; rather it contains some well-known examples.
Abbreviations: ACTH = adrenocorticotropic hormone; ASA = acetylsalicylic acid; NSAIDs = nonsteroidal anti-inflammatory drugs.

sistent with exposure to an agent to which the patient is known to be allergic or may be allergic is often all that is necessary to make an accurate diagnosis. Thus, the presence of laryngeal edema, bronchospasm, and/or hypotension, coupled with other upper respiratory, ocular, gastrointestinal, genitourinary, and skin symptoms, is prima facie evidence that a reaction is in process. Although other historical factors such as recent exposure or in vitro or in vivo evidence of IgE are helpful, physicians do not have time for this type of confirmation except as an afterthought.

Differential Diagnosis. Few conditions can mimic the rapid onset and profound symptom complex of anaphylaxis. Vasovagal syncope is the single most common condition confused with anaphylaxis. In vasovagal syncope, the pulse is generally slow rather than rapid, blood pressure is generally within the normal range (for that patient), and the skin is cool and clammy. Although bradycardia can rarely be seen during an anaphylactic reaction, the combination of bradycardia and normal blood pressure is sufficient to rule out anaphylaxis. Hereditary angioedema may be confused with anaphylaxis; however, the swelling in this condition is not associated with concomitant urticaria and does not itch (it may be described as tingling). This distinction is also true for the angioedema associated with the use of angiotensin-converting enzyme inhibitors. Mastocytosis, particularly systemic mastocytosis, can result in flushing and hypotension. However, the history is one of frequent episodes of flushing, and urticaria is not generally present unless the patient has urticaria pigmentosa and the skin has been stroked or traumatized. Carcinoid syndrome is generally limited to flushing and hypotension, and the other signs and symptoms of anaphylaxis are missing. Other conditions that might be confused with anaphylaxis include globus hystericus and fictitious anaphylaxis (often caused by drug abuse). Myocardial infarction and pulmonary embolism may be confused in patients with no antecedent history of cardiac or pulmonary disease, but the lack of a true anaphylactic symptom complex is often sufficient to make the diagnosis.

TREATMENT OF ANAPHYLAXIS

Four basic steps should be followed in the management of anaphylaxis: (1) prevention, (2) recognition, (3) prompt therapy, and (4) early transport to an emergency care facility.

Prevention. Prevention of anaphylaxis involves the recognition of individuals who may be at risk for an anaphylactic reaction. When possible, the potential offending agent should be avoided. For example, in a patient with a drug allergy, avoidance of that drug or other drugs with similar chemical characteristics is mandatory. This group includes β-lactam antibiotics (penicillin, first-generations cephalosporins, the penems, and to a much less extent, second- and third-generations cephalosporins and the monobactams), as well as sulfonamide-containing drugs. When avoidance is not possible, use of a drug desensitization procedure can be attempted under appropriate conditions. Patients who are at risk for an anaphylactic reaction should always carry injectable epinephrine. I prefer the use of an EpiPen because of its ease of use and the fact that the patient does not see the needle until the injection has been given, but other kits containing epinephrine are also available. The EpiPen is available for both adults and children, and I generally prescribe two so that patients can carry one and have the other at home or at work. When a person comes to an emergency care facility with anaphylaxis, it is important that the final step in treatment be prescription of an injectable epinephrine. Unfortunately, several studies have shown that such prescription is done less than 50% of the time.

Patients with food allergy should be advised to avoid the food to which they are allergic and read labels for hidden ingredients. For example, peanut and soy protein are ubiquitous in prepared foods. Patients should be advised that food allergy, particularly to the more potent allergens such as peanut and shellfish, rarely goes away. Attempting to “see if I'm still allergic” is not a good idea.

Oral rather than parenteral medications are much less likely to cause an anaphylactic reaction and are preferred when possible. When parenteral medication must be given in the outpatient setting, patients should be advised to remain in the clinic setting for at least 30 minutes (for penicillin, 60 minutes is preferable). The same considerations also hold true for allergy immunotherapy; a 20- to 30-minute wait is mandatory.

Patients should also be closely questioned regarding other drugs that may have been added to their regimen since the last injection. β-Adrenergic agents are particularly important because these drugs can turn a mild reaction into a severe reaction and thus make the reaction harder to treat. When questioning a patient, physicians or their staff members should remember to ask about eyedrops. The use of timolol (Timoptic) for glaucoma has been associated with peripheral β-blockade and an increase in the frequency and severity of anaphylaxis. Similar considerations are important for other β-blockers used for hypertension. In patients prone to angioedema, the use of angiotensin-converting enzyme inhibitors is to be avoided.

Individuals who have had a reaction to radiocontrast media can be managed in several ways. First is avoidance of the use of these reagents, which can be achieved by using an alternative procedure, for example, a magnetic resonance angiogram as opposed to an angiogram. When contrast is necessary, the use of a low-osmolality reagent such as iopamidol is associated with a significantly lower frequency and severity of reactions. Unfortunately, in the United States the cost of the newer contrast agents is significantly higher than the cost of the older drugs. It should also be mentioned that the major risk for death from a reaction to radiocontrast media is cardiac disease, so these patients should be monitored closely.

Individuals who have a history of an adverse reaction to Hymenoptera stings should be advised about the most effective avoidance methods, including not wearing brightly colored clothes and not using perfumes. They should work in the garden in the early morning or late afternoon when the insects are less active. When riding in the car, the windows should be kept closed and the air conditioner on. Finally, if a wasp or hornet nest is spotted, a professional entomologist should take care of the problem rather than the patient or family.

Recognition. As noted earlier, a diagnosis of anaphylaxis should be entertained whenever the sign and symptoms point to this diagnosis and the patient is at risk. In many instances, a bad outcome of an anaphylactic reaction has been associated with failure to recognize and treat the reaction. In our clinics, we always err on the side of diagnosing and treating anaphylaxis aggressively.

Prompt Treatment. The primary therapy for anaphylaxis is the use of epinephrine and fluids. These two agents should always be started at the onset of the reaction. Other pharmacologic reagents, though important, are not a substitute for epinephrine and fluids. Of course, simultaneously with the administration of epinephrine and fluids, checking for an adequate airway and respiration is mandatory.

Of the two agents, administration of epinephrine is easier than infusion of fluids and is more rapidly acting, and this medication should be administered first. In all but the most severe reactions, subcutaneous or intramuscular epinephrine is the preferred route. Doses of epinephrine are shown in Table 5.

Other adrenergic agents that may be used include dopamine (Intropin), 10 to 30 μg/kg/min, and norepinephrine (Levophed), 0.1 to 0.5 μg/kg/min. With either agent, the blood pressure or, if necessary, pulmonary artery pressure should be titrated and adequate tissue perfusion maintained.

Fluids may be given in the form of colloid or crystalloid solutions. In either case, however, it is important to administer an adequate amount. Infusion of 5 to 7 L of fluid is not unusual for patients with profound vascular collapse. Colloid solutions have the advantage that they restore intravascular colloid oncotic pressure, which tends to draw fluid from the extravascular to the intravascular space. Many colloid solutions have been used, including blood-derived products such as plasma proteins, fresh frozen plasma, blood, red cell concentrates, and albumin. Blood-derived products carry with them the possibility of transmission of virus and should be avoided. Starches and dextrans have also been administered. We prefer the use of hydroxyethyl starch (hetastarch), which is available as a 6% solution. An initial infusion of 500 mL followed by the use of crystalloid solution has been very effective.

The choice of a crystalloid solution is of much less consequence. In our clinics, we generally use 5% glucose in 0.5-N saline, although normal saline and Ringer's lactated solution are equally effective. Rapid infusion of fluids should be continued until the blood pressure is greater than 90 systolic and stable.

Additional pharmacologic agents useful in the treatment of anaphylaxis include H_1 antihistamines and corticosteroids. Neither of these agents is useful for the immediate treatment period, but they are very effective later. The choice of H_1 antihistamine is based on the route of administration. For intravenous administration, only the first-generation, sedating agents may be used (a little sedation may not be bad). Both diphenhydramine (Benadryl) and chlorpheniramine (Chlor-Trimeton) are available for intravenous administration. Oral preparations of the newer nonsedating H_1 antihistamines can also be used. Liquid preparations of loratadine (Claritin) and cetirizine (Zyrtec), as well as a rapidly desolving form of loratadine (Claritin RediTab) can be effective. If itching is profound, doxepin (Sinequan)* may be the drug of choice.

Corticosteroids are very important because they are the most effective agents for blocking the late phase of any allergic reaction. Hydrocortisone, 4 to 6 mg/kg every 4 to 6 hours, hydrocortisone hemisuccinate (Solu-Cortef), 100 mg every 2 to 4 hours, methylprednisolone (Solu-Medrol), 1 to 2 mg/kg every 6 hours, and dexamethasone (Decadron), 3 mg every 2 to 4 hours, are equally effective. I prefer to continue steroids for 24 hours after the onset of the reaction to ensure that a delayed reaction will not occur.

Other therapy should be based on the patient's condition. Patients who have any respiratory compromise should be treated with oxygen, usually by nasal prongs. The use of continuous oxygen saturation monitoring is helpful in determining the need for O_2 and the correct amount.

β-ADRENERGIC BLOCKADE. The increasing use of β-blockers for patients with hypertension and after myocardial infarction, as well as their topical use in glaucoma, means that many patients with anaphylaxis may respond suboptimally or not at all to epinephrine. Three strategies are available for these patients. The use of glucagon has been advocated. Glucagon is believed to activate adenylate cyclase in a non–β-adrenergic fashion and thus bypass the β-blockade. Administration of 1.0 mg of glucagon should be considered in patients who are responding poorly to epinephrine. Patients who are obtunded should be monitored closely to avoid aspiration from

TABLE 5. **Doses of Epinephrine for the Treatment of Anaphylaxis**

Minor to moderate manifestation
0.3–0.5 mg (1:1000) IM or SC—adults
0.01 mg/kg (1:1000) IM or SC—children (up to 0.3 mL)
Repeat every 12 to 20 min × 4
Severe reaction
0.1–1.0 mg (1:1000) IM or SC—adults
0.01–0.02 mg/kg (1:1000) IM or SC—children
Repeat every 3 min × 4
Cardiopulmonary arrest
0.1–1.0 mg (1:10,000) IV—adults
0.01–0.02 mg/kg (1:10,000)—children
Continuous IV therapy (use if intermittent therapy fails)
0.1–1.0 μg/kg/min—titrate to maintain blood pressure
Upper respiratory compromise
1.0–4.0 mg racemic epinephrine by multidose inhaler or nebulizer

*Not FDA approved for this indication.

glucagon-induced vomiting. A combination of intravenous H_1 and H_2 blocking agents has been advocated on theoretical grounds in β-blockade. Although insufficient clinical data are available to confirm the efficacy of this drug combination, these drugs have few side effects and should be tried in a poorly responding patient. Finally, the use of anticholinergic agents is effective for patients with bronchospasm. Ipratropium bromide (Atrovent) or glycopyrrolate* (Robinul) by nebulizer is valuable in this situation.

LARYNGEAL EDEMA. Laryngeal edema is a life-threatening complication of anaphylaxis. In severe situations, rapid establishment of a patent airway is necessary. The use of an oral airway may be effective, but more aggressive measures may be required. If the practitioner is comfortable with the procedure, insertion of an endotracheal tube may be attempted. A large-bore needle inserted into the cricothyroid membrane, cricothyroidotomy, or tracheostomy may also be necessary. In each case, however, performance of any of these procedures should depend on the capabilities of the practitioner.

RAPID TRANSPORT TO AN EMERGENCY CARE FACILITY. Although most patients recover rapidly from a mild to moderate anaphylactic reaction, the possibility of a severe and/or prolonged reaction is always present. The necessary monitoring equipment is not generally available in the physician's office. Thus, it is a good idea to have the patient transported to the closest emergency care facility even if improvement in symptoms is noted.

SERUM SICKNESS

Serum sickness is a type III reaction (in contrast to anaphylaxis, which is a type I reaction). When the concentration of circulating immune complexes, either generated within the body or from the infusion of materials that contain antigen-antibody complexes, exceeds the normal capacity of the reticuloendothelial portion of the innate immune system to clear these complexes, they are deposited in the vascular endothelium of multiple organ systems. In the endothelium the complexes begin to fix complement. The classic complement pathway produces terminal complement components that are toxic to the endothelium, as well as complement fragments, which are capable of attracting phagocytic cells into the area of immune complex deposition. The anaphylatoxins C5a and C3a are also generated and interact with tissue mast cells in the area of the affected vasculature. Recent evidence has demonstrated that activation of mast cells is critical to generation of the serum sickness reaction because mast cell–deficient mice are not capable of contracting the murine equivalent of serum sickness.

Serum sickness can be divided into illnesses that result from the introduction of exogenous antigen, such as drugs or animal sera (Table 6), and those that are associated with autoimmunity, such as lupus erythematosus. In general, the onset of serum sickness from exogenous antigen depends on the ability of the organism to generate antibodies. If the antigen is new, it will take between 7 and 21 days for the generation of sufficient concentrations of antibody to result in a serum sickness reaction. If the individual has been previously sensitized, a reaction may be seen in as little as 2 to 3 days. The course of the serum sickness reaction will depend on the nature and quantity of the antigen. The disease is usually self-limited and not generally fatal.

TABLE 6. **Exogenous Antigens Associated With Serum Sickness**

Type of Antigen	Class	Examples
Protein	Heterologous sera	Antivenom—usually horse
		Antilymphocyte globulin—horse, goat, or rabbit
		Murine monoclonal antibodies ("humanized" antibodies are much less likely to induce serum sickness)
	Homologous sera	Antitetanus globulin, RhoGAM
		Intravenous immune globulin
Haptens	Antibiotics	Penicillin and other β-lactams, sulfonamides, fluoroquinolones, and metronidazole
	Anticonvulsants	Phenytoin (Dilantin), carbamazepine (Tegretol)

The severity of the serum sickness reaction depends on the amount of antigen introduced and the size of the immune complexes generated. In general, the reaction is characterized by the rapid onset of fever and malaise, accompanied by a morbilliform rash and arthralgias of the large (and occasionally smaller) joints. Frank arthritis is also seen but is less common. The rash may be urticarial, consistent with the activation of mast cell as noted earlier. In addition, the rash may include petechiae or purpura, which may be palpable. These lesions, which generally begin in dependent areas such as the legs and travel upward, are the hallmark of a true vasculitis (leukocytoclastic vasculitis, hypersensitivity vasculitis), defined as destruction of the vascular basement membrane with extravasation of red blood cell into the perivascular space. Microscopic examination also demonstrates dead or dying leukocytes (leukocytolysis) and "nuclear dust." Similar reactions may occur in virtually any organ, depending on the concentration of the immune complexes and their size. The most serious of these reactions are serum sickness nephritis, hepatitis, and neuropathy.

The diagnosis of serum sickness is based on the classic picture and the known exposure of the patient to exogenous antigen. Physical examination may be helpful, particularly if vasculitis or arthritis is present. Laboratory evaluation may also be of use. The sedimentation rate is generally elevated, with depression of the early complement components and total complement, measured as CH_{50} or total hemolytic complement. The white count may be slightly depressed or normal, and no significant alteration is generally noted in the differential count. Other changes are largely organ specific. Urinalysis may demonstrate hyaline or red blood cell casts, and a slight increase in urinary protein may be detected. Serum creatinine may be normal or elevated, depending on the severity of the reaction. In severe cases, microscopic hematuria may be present. Patients with hepatitis may have a mild elevation in liver enzymes, but jaundice is very rare.

*Not FDA approved for this indication.

TREATMENT OF SERUM SICKNESS

Treatment of serum sickness is based on removal of the offending antigen, if possible, and waiting for the body to clear the immune complexes. From studies in rabbits, the time necessary to clear a foreign protein is 2 to 3 weeks. This period is the usual time course for recovery from serum sickness caused by exogenous antigen—some series suggest that it may take as long as a month, but such extended recovery is rare. The use of antihistamines of the H_1 type has been advocated, and studies in children have clearly demonstrated that these antihistamines are protective against serum sickness nephritis. Thus, the use of either a sedating or nonsedating antihistamine is clearly indicated. These drugs may also help with the skin reactions, especially if urticaria is present.

The use of systemic corticosteroids is controversial, and only limited data suggest that they are effective. Nonetheless, most clinicians use a modest dose of prednisone (20 to 60 mg/d) for the first 48 to 72 hours, with gradual tapering of the dosage over the next 2 to 3 weeks. Whether the steroid actually alters the course of the clearance of immune complexes is not known; however, most patients report that they feel better after prednisone. Other drugs such as NSAIDs have also proved to be useful, particularly when arthralgias are present. In very severe cases, exchange transfusion or plasmapheresis has been used in an attempt to remove the immune complexes. This measure has been reported to have been successful.

A number of syndromes can mimic serum sickness, but it has not been possible to demonstrate that antigen-antibody complexes are present. These syndromes include the serum sickness–like reaction that is seen with the use of cefuroxime (Ceftin) and the reaction seen after the administration of the broad class of anticonvulsants (often referred to as the anticonvulsant hypersensitivity syndrome). In both cases, intensive investigation has been conducted to determine the cause of the syndrome, with little success. These syndromes are treated with removal of the drug and administration of NSAIDs and antihistamines (when itching is a problem). Prednisone is rarely necessary.

ASTHMA IN ADOLESCENTS AND ADULTS

method of
MARK E. BUBAK, M.D.
Dakota Allergy and Asthma
Sioux Falls, South Dakota

and

JAMES T. C. LI, M.D., PH.D.
Mayo Medical School
Rochester, Minnesota

Asthma is a chronic inflammatory disease with reversible airway obstruction. It clinically manifests with cough, wheeze, dyspnea, or tightness of the chest that comes and goes. Most asthmatics are atopic. It affects all ages, races, and socioeconomic groups and both genders. Asthma is an important cause of clinic visits, medication costs, hospitalizations, and deaths. Fifteen million Americans have asthma. The costs are significant. In 1994 asthma in the United States cost $11.9 billion. More than 9 million office visits occurred in 1996 for asthma and 1.9 million emergency department visits. Although the overall hospitalization rate may be steady or declining, it is increasing in children, especially from lower socioeconomic groups. These statistics point out the need for continuing to improve diagnostic and therapeutic options for asthmatic patients.

DIAGNOSIS

The diagnosis of asthma is based on the medical history, physical examination, and pulmonary function tests. The patient with asthma may have a history of recurrent cough, wheeze, shortness of breath, or tightness of the chest. These symptoms are often triggered by allergen, irritant, or cold air exposure; exercise; or viral infections. Nocturnal symptoms are typical. Asthma can begin at any age. It may remit spontaneously in some young patients, only to return later in life in approximately a third. Changes in severity are common and must be followed closely with appropriate therapy adjustments.

During the initial diagnostic evaluation (Table 1), objective air flow measurement should be obtained using spirometry. This measurement serves as a diagnostic tool for assessing degrees of obstruction and reversibility and as a baseline for future comparisons. An acute improvement after β-agonist therapy of 15% forced expiratory volume in 1 second (FEV_1) or 20% peak expiratory flow (PEF) is generally believed to show objective reversibility of airway obstruction. The asthmatic patient should have regular reassessment of FEV_1 or PEF to follow disease severity and responses to treatment and to detect early asthma exacerbations. This reassessment is especially critical in nearly half of asthmatic patients who do not accurately perceive the severity of their asthma.

An allergy evaluation including a detailed history and appropriate tests (allergy skin testing or specific IgE in vitro testing) should be performed. Of asthmatics, 80% have allergic triggers. Appropriate avoidance of the offending allergens improves symptoms significantly, decreases bronchial hyperreactivity and medication use, and identifies patients who may benefit from allergen-specific immunotherapy. Perennial allergens, such as dust mites, pets, cockroaches, and molds, as well as seasonal allergens, such as grass pollens, weed pollens, tree pollens, and certain molds, are important allergic triggers of asthma. Foods rarely cause only asthma symptoms.

Viral infections, respiratory irritants (e.g., tobacco smoke), exercise, occupational exposures, medications (i.e., aspirin and β-blockers), and cold air are other important

TABLE 1. **Initial Asthma Evaluation**

History and physical examination
Spirometry
Peak flow measurement
Trigger identification (allergy testing if indicated)
Action plan development
Asthma education (includes inhaler technique, peak flow meter)
Establishment of follow-up plans

TABLE 2. **Asthma Triggers**

Allergens	Drugs (aspirin, β-blockers)
Respiratory infections	Occupational exposures
Irritants	Meteorologic (cold air, dry air)
Exercise	

triggers of asthma (Table 2). The initial diagnostic evaluation should also search for common concurrent diseases, such as allergic rhinitis, atopic dermatitis, sinusitis, and gastroesophageal reflux.

Severity classifications proposed by the National Heart, Lung, and Blood Institute guideline publications assist the clinician in selection of appropriate long-term controllers (Table 3). The criteria used to assess asthma severity include frequency of symptoms, nighttime symptoms, frequency of exacerbations, and objective measures of lung function (FEV_1 or PEF). Patients commonly change their severity classification over time, and not all patients with asthma can be categorized neatly. At each clinic visit, a reassessment of severity is needed so that appropriate changes in therapy can be made.

The differential diagnosis of asthma includes disorders of the lungs, heart, and upper and lower airways as well as hematologic, endocrine, and psychiatric disease (Table 4). The clinician must use the history, physical examination, and selective diagnostic testing to clarify the diagnosis of asthma. Referral to an asthma specialist is recommended if the diagnosis of asthma is in question as well as for allergy testing or immunotherapy, asthma education, or asthma co-management.

It is essential for the physician and the patient to work as partners (including regularly scheduled clinic visits). This partnership involves re-evaluating asthma severity,

TABLE 3. **Asthma Severity and Treatment**

	Mild Episodic	**Mild Persistent**	**Moderate Persistent**	**Severe Persistent**
*Classification by**				
Symptom	≤2 times a week	>2 times a week and <1 time a day Flares may limit activity	Daily Flares limit activity	Continuous Limited physical activity
Nighttime symptoms	≤2 times a month	>2 times a month	>1 time a week	Frequent
Lung function				
FEV_1 or PEF	≥80% predicted	≥80% predicted	>60%–<80% predicted	≤60% predicted
PEF variability	<20%	20%–30%	>30%	>30%
Treatment				
Asthma education	Yes	Yes	Yes	Yes
Trigger avoidance	Yes	Yes	Yes	Yes
Relievers				
Inhaled β-agonist (i.e., albuterol, pirbuterol)†	1–2 puffs as needed	1–2 puffs as needed	2 puffs as needed	2 puffs as needed
Controllers				
Anti-inflammatory				
Inhaled corticosteroids	Not indicated	Low dose	Medium dose‡	High dose with long-acting bronchodilator‡
Cromolyn	Not indicated	Optional	Optional	Optional
Nedocromil	Not indicated	Optional	Optional	Optional
Systemic corticosteroid	Not indicated	Not indicated	Not indicated	If not controlled by topical
Immunotherapy	Optional in allergics	Optional in allergics	Optional in allergics	Optional in allergics
Long-acting bronchodilators				
Sustained-release theophylline	Not indicated	Optional	Optional	Often with ICS
Salmeterol (Serevent)	Not indicated	Optional	Optional with anti-inflammatory	Often with ICS
Formoterol (Foradil)	Not indicated	Optional	Optional with anti-inflammatory	Often with ICS
Long-acting $β_2$-agonist tablets	Not indicated	Optional	Optional with anti-inflammatory	Often with ICS
Leukotriene antagonists				
Zafirlukast (Accolate)	Not indicated	Optional	Optional with ICS	Optional with ICS
Montelukast (Singulair)	Not indicated	Optional	Optional with ICS	Optional with ICS
Leukotriene formation inhibitor	Not indicated	Optional	Optional with ICS	Optional with ICS
Zileuton (Zyflo)	Not indicated	Optional	Optional with ICS	Optional with ICS
Combination products				
Fluticasone/Salmeterol (Advair)	Not indicated	Not indicated	Optional	Often

*The most severe criteria select severity rating.
†With exacerbation, 4 puffs or 2.5–5 mg albuterol by nebulizer each 20 minutes × 3 doses, then each 1–4 as needed; strongly consider short burst of oral steroid (i.e., prednisone, 40 mg daily for 5 days).
‡Preferred.
Abbreviations: FEV_1 = forced expiratory volume in 1 second; ICS = inhaled corticosteroids; PEF = peak expiratory flow.

TABLE 4. **Differential Diagnosis**

Cardiovascular
- Congestive heart failure

Drugs
- Angiotensin-converting enzyme inhibitor cough

Pulmonary
- Chronic obstructive pulmonary disease
- Pulmonary embolism
- Interstitial lung disease
- Cystic fibrosis
- Obliterative bronchiolitis
- Bronchiectasis
- Tumor
- Enlarged lymph nodes
- α_1-Antitrypsin deficiency
- Eosinophilic lung diseases
- Carcinoid tumor
- Mechanical obstruction of the airways

Hematologic
- Anemia

Psychological
- Hyperventilation syndrome
- Vocal cord dysfunction
- Panic attacks

appropriateness of therapy, and compliance with management recommendations. Asthma education, including proficiency with inhaler devices and home peak flow meters, should take place at regularly scheduled follow-up visits. The frequency of follow-up visits must be individualized but should be about once a year for mild asthma, two to four times a year for moderate asthma, and more often for severe asthma.

TREATMENT

The goals of asthma treatment are prevention of attacks, relief of symptoms, maintenance of (nearly) normal lung function, maintenance of normal quality of life, and existence of minimal or no side effects. To accomplish these goals effectively, the treatment program must be tailored to the individual patient based on his or her triggers and lifestyle in partnership between patient (and family) and physician. From this interaction, a written action plan is developed and enacted.

The action plan clearly outlines the asthma treatment strategy. It includes trigger avoidance, monitoring instructions (symptoms and/or home PEF), baseline medications, medications for asthma exacerbations, symptoms (and PEF readings) to watch for exacerbation, and how to respond to these changes. The treatment plan states clearly how to obtain further help.

All asthmatic patients must receive education about their disease, the medications used, and how to follow their individual asthma action plan. They must also clearly understand how to access medical care further for uncontrolled symptoms and (preferably) for regular preventive asthma care. Allergic asthmatic patients receive avoidance information. All asthmatic patients learn irritant avoidance. Regular peak flow measurement may be helpful in select patients. Yearly influenza vaccination is recommended.

Allergen avoidance is important whenever possible for allergic asthmatic patients because this is a controller therapy. For dust mite allergy, encasements for mattresses and pillows combined with weekly washing of the bedding decrease allergen exposure. Pet-allergic asthmatic patients should not have animals in the home and need to minimize other exposures. This situation is difficult because cat exposure is a daily occurrence in the dust, air, and furnishings of most buildings and on pet owners' clothing. To decrease exposure to outdoor allergens, the house is closed up and central air conditioning and heating is used. For patients with occupational asthma, changes in workplace exposure are required. Medications for asthma can be categorized into (1) those that give fairly rapid relief of symptoms (*symptom relievers*) and (2) those that control the asthma on a more long-term or preventive basis (*symptom controllers*).

Symptom Relievers

Regardless of disease severity, use of symptom relievers is important for all asthmatic patients. These drugs are used *as needed* to relieve asthma symptoms such as cough, wheeze, dyspnea, and chest tightness. Relievers are inhaled short-acting β-agonist agents such as albuterol (Proventil, Ventolin), pirbuterol (Maxair), terbutaline (Brethine), and epinephrine. Inhaled administration is preferred, with a metered-dose inhaler working as well as a nebulizer if correct technique is maintained. β-Agonists are also helpful if used 10 to 15 minutes before exercise to prevent exercise-induced bronchospasm. In some patients with asthma, ipratropium (Atrovent) can also be used as a reliever.

Systemic corticosteroids are recommended for the treatment of asthma exacerbations. For many patients, prednisone (Deltasone), 40 mg daily for 5 to 7 days, is effective, but some patients need an alteration of this schedule. The routine use of antibiotics should be discouraged. Severe asthma exacerbations can require hospitalization and higher corticosteroid dosages in conjunction with bronchodilator therapy, supplemental oxygen, and close monitoring. Oral prednisone works as well as intravenous steroids when it can be used. Moderate doses of intravenous corticosteroids (e.g., methylprednisolone [Solu-Medrol], 40 mg every 6 hours) have been generally as effective as larger doses, with significantly fewer side effects.

Symptom Controllers

Patients with persistent asthma should use a controller medication every day (see Table 3). The most effective controllers are inhaled corticosteroids. These agents should be taken regularly to control airway inflammation and can be titrated based on asthma severity. Although any of the controllers can

TABLE 5. **Inhaled Corticosteroid Dosing**

	Daily Medication		
Type	*Low Dose*	*Medium Dose*	*High Dose*
Beclomethasone (Vanceril)			
42 μg	4–12 puffs	12–20 puffs	>20 puffs
84 μg, 40 μg HFA	2–6 puffs	6–10 puffs	>10 puffs
Budesonide (Pulmicort)	1–2 puffs	2–3 puffs	≥4 puffs
Flunisolide (AeroBid)	2–4 puffs	4–8 puffs	>8 puffs
Fluticasone (Flovent)			
44 or 50 μg/puff	2–6 puffs		
110 or 100 μg/puff		2–6 puffs	>6 puffs
220 or 250 μg/puff			>3 puffs
Triamcinolone (Azmacort)	4–10 puffs	10–20 puffs	>20 puffs

be chosen for mild persistent asthma, inhaled corticosteroids are the treatment of choice for moderate and severe persistent asthma (Table 5; also see Table 3). Inhaled corticosteroids can be used with a second controller, such as an inhaled long-acting bronchodilator. Some patients with severe asthma may require three controller agents.

Other controllers can be prescribed in mild persistent asthma as single agents or as adjunctive agents in moderate and severe persistent asthma. These controllers include cromolyn (Intal); nedocromil (Tilade); salmeterol (Serevent); theophylline; leukotriene receptor antagonists such as zafirlukast (Accolate) and montelukast (Singulair); leukotriene formation inhibitors such as zileuton (Zyflo); and allergen-specific immunotherapy. Some patients with severe asthma require the continuous (daily or alternate day) use of oral corticosteroids. The dose of corticosteroids must be individualized, balancing the need for asthma control with the risk of corticosteroid-induced adverse effects.

Controller choice is influenced heavily by patient variables. For example, allergic asthmatics may benefit from specific allergen immunotherapy, whereas patients with nonallergic asthma would not. The leukotriene-modifying drugs are convenient for patients who prefer pills to inhaler devices but may be ineffective in approximately 30% of cases. Similarly, nedocromil and cromolyn are alternatives to inhaled corticosteroids, particularly in children. Inhaled long-acting bronchodilators can be used in combination with inhaled corticosteroids. Theophylline, once or twice daily, can also be used in combination with inhaled corticosteroids or as a single agent in patients who prefer taking pills. Serum theophylline levels of 5 to 15 μg/mL are recommended, but adverse effects are common even at low drug levels. A major factor in successful controller therapy is convincing the patient to take the controller consistently, and great effort needs to be directed at this. Selecting a controller with therapeutic goals and patient preferences in mind aids success.

ASTHMA IN CHILDREN

method of
MITCHELL R. LESTER, M.D.
Fairfield County Allergy, Asthma, and Immunology Associates
Norwalk, Connecticut

Asthma is the most common chronic disease of childhood and is a major reason for hospitalizations, school absence, and decreased quality of life. The annual direct and indirect cost of asthma care in the United States is approximately $6 billion. Asthma prevalence and mortality have been gradually increasing for at least 20 years, particularly in teens, inner city residents, and African Americans. Thankfully, evidence that these trends may be leveling off has recently surfaced. In 1991, the first Expert Panel was convened to recommend guidelines for the diagnosis and management of asthma. Emphasizing that inflammation is pivotal in the pathogenesis of chronic asthma, the Expert Panel stressed the importance of treating asthma as a chronic disease with regular use of preventive anti-inflammatory medications in addition to as-needed use of bronchodilator symptom relievers. The use of inhaled anti-inflammatory medications in the United States has thus increased in recent years. The most recent revision of asthma guidelines, *Expert Panel Report II: Guidelines for the Diagnosis and Management of Asthma* (EPR II) (available online at www.nhlbi.nih.gov/guidelines/asthma/asthgdln.pdf), is an important reassessment and reaffirmation of previous guidelines, with a thorough review of the supporting data. Initial stepwise management is based on asthma symptom severity, with stress on the importance of gradually stepping therapy down to the lowest controlling dose. In addition to in-depth discussion regarding appropriate medication use, every set of consensus guidelines published also stresses nonmedical aspects of asthma care and self-management skills necessary for optimal control. In this article, I shall review the four components of asthma care addressed in the EPR II and concentrate on key areas that (in my experience) are most commonly misinterpreted or neglected by primary care providers.

COMPONENT 1: MEASURES OF ASSESSMENT AND MONITORING

Definition and Diagnosis

Asthma is a chronic disease characterized by eosinophilic airway inflammation, airway hyperreactivity, and episodic reversible bronchoconstriction and airflow obstruction. Patients with asthma usually have a cough and/or wheeze and a history suggesting reactivity of airways. A detailed medical history and physical examination are usually sufficient for making the diagnosis of asthma. Nonetheless, the diagnosis can be elusive because of the disease's variable expression and its lack of specific signs and symptoms. Delaying the diagnosis based on incorrect perceptions of what asthma is (or is not) may delay appropriate treatment, lead to persistent and bothersome symptoms, increase morbidity, and frustrate parents. Physicians vary widely in their individual diagnostic criteria and frequently rely on signs or symptoms not generally considered important by asthma experts. In distinct contrast to the EPR II definition, many pediatricians still identify a child being older than 2 years and afebrile as necessary or important to the diagnosis. Clinicians who pay close attention to historical aspects of the patient's symptoms can identify when asthma is likely to be present and, just as important, be able to identify when it not present.

Airway inflammation is the underlying pathophysiologic problem in asthma. The airway response after allergen exposure is well characterized. The early airway response occurs in 15 minutes to 2 hours after exposure and spontaneously resolves. This phase is associated with release of preformed mediators of inflammation (histamine and leukotrienes, among others) primarily from mast cells and macrophages and the direct action of these mediators on the airway and its smooth muscle. The most obvious effect is bronchoconstriction. A patient's clinical response to inhaled β_2-adrenergic medications is circumstantial evidence of reversible air flow obstruction.

Some preformed mediators are also chemotactic for other inflammatory cells and contribute to the late phase. The late airway response occurs 6 to 12 hours after allergen exposure, after inflammatory cells (and their mediators) have been recruited to the site. The late response is associated with inflammation and damage to the epithelium, edema, mucus formation, and cellular infiltration (primarily lymphocytes and eosinophils). Inflammatory mediators increase bronchial hyperreactivity (BHR), bronchospasm, and mucus production. The clinician can infer the presence of airway inflammation by a patient's response to oral or inhaled steroids. In contrast, if no clinical response occurs after an adequate dose of oral corticosteroids, the treating physician should question whether asthma is solely responsible for the patient's symptoms or whether a masquerader or complicator of asthma is present (Table 1).

The late airway response is followed by BHR, or the tendency of airways to constrict in response to nonsensitizing chemical or physical agents to a degree greater than seen normally. BHR is quantified by methacholine or histamine challenge, after which bronchoconstriction is present without inflammation. Incremental doses of the challenge substance are inhaled until the concentration required (provocative concentration, PC_{20}) to reduce the forced expiratory volume in 1 second (FEV_1) by 20% is reached. Increased BHR (lower PC_{20}) is only roughly correlated with the severity of asthma and medication requirement. The use of anti-inflammatory medications will diminish BHR, decrease symptoms, and reduce the medication requirement in most patients. Without their use, a cycle of increasing inflammation followed by BHR, increased need for symptom relief, and continued inflammation and BHR may be created. Therefore, it is necessary to address BHR by treating the inflammation. Patients who give a history of asthma symptoms after exposure to nonallergenic triggers are demonstrating the presence of BHR. The common phrases "twitchy airways" and "reactive airways" imply BHR. Bronchoconstriction is the hallmark of the early airway response, but it also occurs during periods of airway inflammation, throughout the airway response to allergen, and during periods of BHR.

TABLE 1. **Masqueraders and Complicators of Asthma**

α_1-Antitrypsin deficiency	Hypersensitivity pneumonitis
Allergic bronchopulmonary mycosis	Interstitial lung disease
Allergic rhinitis	Laryngeal cleft
Bronchiolitis obliterans	Laryngeal web
Bronchiolitis obliterans organizing pneumonia	Laryngo/tracheo/bronchomalacia
Bronchopulmonary dysplasia	Postnasal drip syndromes
Cardiac disease	Postviral bronchiolitis
Chronic aspiration	Primary ciliary dyskinesia
Chronic obstructive pulmonary disease	Psychogenic/habit cough
Chronic sinusitis	Pulmonary hemosiderosis
Cystic fibrosis	Pulmonary infiltrates with eosinophilia
Foreign body aspiration	Tracheal stenosis
Gastroesophageal reflux	Tracheobronchitis
Humoral immune deficiency	Tracheosophageal fistula
	Tumor
	Vascular ring
	Vocal cord dysfunction
	Vocal cord paresis

Asthma symptoms typically worsen with cold air exposure, during exercise, and in the middle of the night (3–4 AM), particularly in patients with poorly controlled disease. In fact, exercise or cold air challenge is often performed in lieu of methacholine or histamine challenge when the diagnosis of asthma is in doubt. The frequency of nocturnal symptoms is such a good marker of disease control that it is used in the classification of asthma severity (Table 2). I regularly question patients about nighttime and exercise-induced symptoms when establishing the diagnosis and when monitoring asthma control.

In summary, patients with asthma usually worsen at night or with exercise. They typically respond to oral or inhaled steroids and to inhaled bronchodilators. Particular historical attention is paid to identifying specific precipitants of symptoms (allergic or nonallergic). The severity as well as the frequency of asthma exacerbations should also be addressed. Finally, children with asthma usually have a personal or family history of atopy. Although these criteria are not diagnostic of asthma, greater consideration should be given to the presence of a complicator or masquerader thereof when they are not met.

The physical examination often provides evidence of other atopic disease, so a thorough examination of the nose and skin is essential. Examination of the chest might be entirely normal, particularly in patients with less severe disease who are not in the midst of flaring symptoms. In contrast, some patients have a prolonged expiratory phase of respiration or expiratory wheezing even when at their baseline. Wheezing can sometimes only be heard with forced expiration, a maneuver that can trigger cough in patients with BHR. Particularly in patients with more severe disease, air trapping is manifested by hyperexpansion of the thorax and the classic hunched-shouldered appearance of the asthmatic child.

Spirometry is a sensitive adjunct to the objective assessment of asthma and is one parameter used in classifying asthma severity. Spirometry is more sensitive than peak expiratory flow rate (PEFR) measurement, but it is highly effort dependent and can only be performed by older, more cooperative children. Changes in expiratory air flow rates and volumes can be monitored over time to evaluate response to therapy. Performing spirometry before and after administration of an inhaled β_2-agonist is useful for identifying reversible air flow obstruction. An improvement in FEV_1 of 12% or more is clinically and statistically significant.

Monitoring Asthma Control

The ultimate goal of asthma therapy is to control airway inflammation and decrease the risk of airway remodeling, thereby decreasing the risk of long-term morbidity. Without easily obtainable clinical markers of airway inflammation, short-term goals are monitored with the assumption that achieving them will increase the likelihood of long-term control. With adequate therapy, chronic and fre-

TABLE 2. **Asthma Severity Classification**

Severity	Daytime Symptoms	Nocturnal Symptoms	Pulmonary Function
Mild intermittent	Less often than 3 times per week Asymptomatic between flares Brief exacerbations (of any intensity)	Less often than 3 times per month	Normal (FEV_1 and PEFR $\geq$80% of predicted and PEFR diurnal variability <20%)
Mild persistent	3 or more times per week, but less often than daily Exacerbations may affect activity	3 or more times per month, but less than weekly	FEV_1 and PEFR $\geq$80% of predicted PEFR diurnal variability, 20% to 30%
Moderate persistent	Daily Exacerbations affect activity Exacerbations more often than twice per week	More often than once per week	FEV_1 and PEFR 60% to 80% of predicted PEFR diurnal variability >30%
Severe persistent	Continual Limited activity Frequent exacerbations	Frequently	FEV_1 and PEFR $\leq$60% of predicted PEFR diurnal variability >30%

Abbreviations: FEV_1 = forced expiratory volume in 1 second; PEFR = peak expiratory flow rate.

quently recurring symptoms and asthma exacerbations are prevented. As a result, children maintain normal activity levels and sleep patterns, so the asthma symptoms have little or no impact on quality of life. Normal pulmonary function is maintained in nearly all patients (although it cannot be measured in the very young in an office setting). Before asthma education, parents often have erroneous ideas of how well asthma can be controlled. Therefore, their initial expectations should at least be met and often exceeded. Optimal control of symptoms should be achieved with as little medication as necessary (see Component 3) and without adverse effects of medication.

Because asthma is a chronic, not an episodic, disease, patients should have regularly scheduled follow-up visits to assess symptom control, adjust medications as indicated, and review other related issues. The historical and physical parameters described earlier should be re-addressed at each follow-up visit. The frequency of required follow-up visits varies from one patient to another, depending on the severity of disease and the ease with which it has been controlled, the medication requirement for control, and the seasonal variation in symptoms. Asthma education (see Component 4) is an ongoing process and is therefore addressed at each follow-up visit. Parents are less likely to absorb the necessary information regarding long-term care of asthma when visiting the physician for an acute illness.

PEFR is a useful tool for monitoring, not diagnosis of asthma. It is an insensitive measure for many patients, however. Most primary care providers are familiar with its usefulness in the assessment and management of acute asthma flares ("red," "yellow," and "green" zones), but many physicians have patients check their PEFR only with the onset of asthma symptoms. PEFR is even more useful when measured regularly. The PEFR often begins to drop before recognition of significant symptoms and is therefore an early warning sign for patients in whom it is a sensitive measure. Regular monitoring of PEFR also provides an objective measure of disease control after adjustments in medications. Diurnal variation in PEFR is used in the classification of asthma severity, and early loss of asthma control is sometimes identified by an increase in diurnal variation. PEFR is effort dependent, so low values should be observed and confirmed by the parent or guardian. Peak flow meters are not well calibrated, and values obtained on one are not comparable with those on another. In fact, peak flow rates obtained on two meters of the same brand may vary by 20%.

Although primary care physicians are highly skilled in the care of asthma, many patients require consultation by an asthma specialist. In general, patients with life-threatening exacerbations, those not meeting other goals of therapy, and those unresponsive to medications and in whom the diagnosis is in doubt should be referred. Similarly, patients with moderate or severe persistent asthma (see Table 2) and those who require oral corticosteroids more than twice per year or high-dose inhaled steroids should see a specialist. Patients requiring intense education regarding asthma and its prevention and control should also be referred. Because most children with asthma have atopic disease, many pediatricians prefer referral to an allergist. In contrast, if another underlying pulmonary disease is present, a pediatric pulmonologist is the preferred choice. Patients with significant nasal disease, those suspected of having allergies, and those being considered for allergen immunotherapy should see a board-certified allergist. Whenever a masquerader of asthma is identified, referral to the appropriate subspecialist is indicated. Finally, even in this era of managed care, it is my belief that patients who request a second opinion by a specialist should be given that opportunity.

COMPONENT 2: CONTROL OF FACTORS CONTRIBUTING TO ASTHMA SEVERITY

Identification plus avoidance of triggers of asthma symptoms are pivotal for their optimal control. A thorough history directed at identifying exposure to specific (IgE-mediated) and nonspecific (non–IgE-mediated) triggers and whether symptoms worsen after these exposures is essential. Nonspecific triggers can precipitate symptoms in anyone, independent of atopic status. Exercise, cold air, strong odors (paint, perfume, cleaning fluid, etc.), viral infection, passive smoke, and air pollution are common examples. Although complete avoidance of all these factors is impossible and impractical, exposure can often be decreased and early measures taken when exposure is unavoidable (for example, treatment before exercise with an inhaled β_2-agonist).

The vast majority of children with asthma have inhalant allergies. Therefore, a complete environmental history is useful to identify potential allergenic triggers to asthma. Clinicians should attempt to correlate exposure with symptom pattern whenever possible. In so doing, the most relevant potential allergens are often identified by the history alone. Perennial problems with r without seasonal variation suggest indoor allergen sensitivity (dust mite, mold, animal dander, cockroach, rodent). Seasonal variation in symptoms can suggest pollen sensitivity. Of course, each clinician must consider the aerobiology of the particular geographic region. It is beyond the scope of this article to discuss environmental controls and allergen avoidance, but the reader is referred to the article "Allergic Rhinitis Caused by Inhalant Factors."

As discussed earlier, the symptom pattern and response to therapy may suggest a masquerader or complicator of asthma (see Table 1). If present, appropriate treatment is necessary. An important but often overlooked relationship between the upper and lower airways is seen in children with asthma. It is quite clear that control of nasal and/or sinus disease affects BHR and control of the lower airway disease. In fact, many children have significantly fewer asthma symptoms and require significantly less medication for asthma when their allergic rhinitis is well controlled with the regular use of intranasal corticosteroids.

COMPONENT 3: PHARMACOLOGIC THERAPY

Determining Asthma Severity

Asthma severity is a continuum ranging from mild and rare symptoms that resolve spontaneously to continuous symptoms that affect the quality of life and are life-threatening. Initial medical therapy for asthma is dependent on asthma severity. For simplicity in choosing initial therapy, the EPR II views the continuum of severity as four distinct steps: mild intermittent, mild persistent, moderate persistent, and severe persistent (see Table 2). It is overall control of symptoms even more than the frequency and severity of exacerbations that determines asthma severity. Even patients with mild intermittent asthma can have severe, life-threatening exacerbations. The clinician's history should identify the frequency of both daytime and nocturnal symptoms. Pulmonary function testing and peak flow monitoring are also considered when establishing asthma severity.

Clinical features and pulmonary function before initiation of therapy define asthma severity. It is essential to recognize that control of asthma symptoms with adequate therapy is not synonymous with resolution of the disease; that is, a patient with poor pulmonary function and frequent severe asthma symptoms who achieves control with high-dose inhaled steroid therapy should not be considered a mild asthmatic. Strictly speaking, the patient's asthma severity should be categorized as the most severe step into which any one of the features falls. Asthma experts (myself included) recognize that such rigorous adherence may fail to adequately characterize the patient's disease. For instance, some patients with frequent symptoms have otherwise mild clinical markers of disease and might not require the same amount of medication initially as other patients with severe persistent asthma. Complicators of asthma (e.g., allergic rhinitis or sinusitis) might be contributing in such cases and should be treated as well. In contrast, some patients categorized with mild intermittent asthma have severe exacerbations requiring hospitalization at least once a year. I sometimes describe these patients as having "severe intermittent" or "severe bronchospastic asthma," a category not recognized by the EPR II. They require aggressive therapy at the earliest sign of asthma exacerbation.

Medications for the Chronic Care of Asthma

Initial pharmacologic therapy for asthma is based on severity. I find it most efficient to treat aggressively enough at first to gain rapid control of the disease. Allergic inflammation begets more allergic inflammation, so therapy can usually be "stepped down" after asthma control is achieved. Because the clinical effects with each step-down in dose may not be immediately evident, small steps should be taken over months, rather than weeks. A step-down in therapy that is followed by increasing symptoms should prompt a "step-up" to the previous controlling dose. The lowest medication requirement that adequately controls disease is the optimal therapy. Patient compliance improves, the cost of therapy decreases, and the risk of adverse effects from medications is diminished. Some practitioners start with less aggressive therapy and increase doses until control is finally achieved. In some cases, this practice delays the time until adequate control of the symptoms. In either case, clinicians should remember that asthma therapy should not be rigid; that is, with continual and regular review of the patient's symptom pattern, appropriate adjustments in the medical regimen allow optimal (usually complete) control of symptoms with the least amount of medication necessary.

Mild Intermittent Asthma

Mild intermittent asthma is characterized by symptoms occurring twice or less per week. Patients may have exercise-induced bronchospasm as well. These patients rarely, if ever, awaken at night from asthma. Pulmonary function is normal, with normal diurnal variability between episodes, and reverts to normal after β_2-agonist inhalation during an episode. Patients with mild intermittent asthma are treated with as-needed β_2-agonists only.

Short-acting β_2-agonists (Table 3) are rescue medications and should therefore be used only for the relief of symptoms. They have no anti-inflammatory activity and no role in the prevention of chronic

TABLE 3. **Available Formulations of Short-Acting β-Agonists**

Drug	Parenteral	Oral	Inhaled
Albuterol (Proventil)	O	X	X
Levalbuterol (Xopenex)	O	O	X
Epinephrine (Adrenalin)	X	O	X
Isoproterenol (Isuprel)	X	O	X
Metaproterenol (Alupent)	O	X	X
Pirbuterol (Maxair)	O	O	X
Terbutaline (Brethine)	X	X	X

Abbreviations: O = not available; X = available.

asthma symptoms. However, as inhibitors of the early airway reaction, they may be useful for prevention when taken before known triggers such as exercise. They may be taken before anticipated allergen exposure, but patients should still be prepared for late airway reaction in these circumstances.

β_2-Agonists can be delivered via inhalation, orally, or parenterally. Inhaled forms have an onset of action and peak response at least as quickly as when delivered subcutaneously and faster than when taken orally. The peak response is greater with the inhaled and subcutaneous forms than with the oral. Finally, subcutaneous and oral delivery is associated with more α-adrenergic side effects than inhaled delivery. For these reasons, whenever possible, inhalation (either nebulized or metered-dose inhaler [MDI]) is the preferred route of delivery for β-agonists. MDI use requires meticulous attention to technique, which should be taught when the MDI is first prescribed and reviewed at subsequent visits. Young children should always be taught to use an MDI with a holding chamber (e.g., InspirEase, AeroChamber, AeroChamber/Mask). Use of the chamber eliminates the difficulty of coordinating actuation of the MDI and inhalation. For younger children or those who cannot coordinate the use of an MDI, nebulization is the preferred method for inhalation. The use of a mask or mouthpiece with the nebulizer will improve delivery of the nebulized medication to the airway in comparison with the "blow-by" method. Untoward effects from albuterol are diminished in many patients with nebulized levalbuterol (Xopenex). Subcutaneous delivery of adrenergic agents is used when the patient is unconscious or cannot generate significant inspiratory effort or in the setting of systemic anaphylaxis.

Short-acting β_2-agonists are only "rescue" medications for breakthrough symptoms. Their frequent need may be considered a treatment failure. As medications that provide symptomatic relief, β_2-agonists may mask the effects of increasing inflammation when used regularly and perpetuate the cycle of inflammation and BHR described earlier. It can therefore be useful to ask patients how often they require β_2-agonist rescue and how long one MDI dose lasts.

It has become apparent that regular use of short-acting β_2-agonists results in down-regulation of β_2-adrenergic receptor expression and is associated with heightened BHR to methacholine or allergen. The mechanisms underlying these findings are still not well defined but are undoubtedly the effect of β_2-agonists' influence on multiple airway and inflammatory cell types. What was once a controversy over the safety of prolonged and regular use of short-acting β_2-agonists is now resolved. When they are required frequently, regular use of a controller anti-inflammatory medication is indicated.

Mild Persistent Asthma

Patients who have asthma symptoms more often than once a week but less frequently than daily or who awaken more often than two to four times per month are classified as mild intermittent asthmatics. Patients with persistent asthma of any severity should receive regular treatment with anti-inflammatory medication in addition to as-needed rescue bronchodilators. Because asthma is a chronic rather than an episodic disease, anti-inflammatory medications are prescribed for long-term use rather than sporadically. It is essential for clinicians to recognize persistent asthma because poorly controlled airway inflammation results in a less than expected increase in pulmonary function during childhood, airway remodeling, and a faster than expected loss of pulmonary function in adulthood.

Low-dose inhaled corticosteroids (ICSs) (Table 4) are useful in the treatment of mild persistent asthma and are still considered the gold standard for anti-inflammatory medication in asthma. ICSs improve every clinical and physiologic marker of asthma severity and are the most effective long-term controller medication for asthma. Furthermore, ICS use decreases asthma morbidity and the cost of medical care. Nonetheless, unfamiliarity with different ICS preparations and concern regarding their safety limits their use by some practitioners. The long-term risks of regular oral steroids are well known. For some time after ICSs were introduced, they were assumed to be free of systemic side effects. Many studies of the adverse effects of ICSs are difficult to

TABLE 4. **Inhaled Corticosteroid Dosage Ranges (μg/d)**

		BDP	BUD	FLU	FP	TAA
Low	Adults	168–504	200–400	500–1000	88–264	400–1000
	Children	84–336	100–200	500–750	88–176	400–800
Medium	Adults	504–840	400–600	1000–2000	264–660	1000–2000
	Children	336–672	200–400	1000–1250	176–440	800–1200
High	Adults	>840	>600	>2000	>660	>2000
	Children	>672	>400	>1250	>440	>1200

Abbreviations:

BDP = beclomethasone dipropionate (Vanceril, Beclovent, 42 and 84 μg per puff). No comparative data are available for QVar, 40 and 80 μg per puff.

BUD = budesonide (Pulmicort Turbuhaler, 200 μg per inhalation). No comparative data are available for Pulmicort Respules by nebulizer.

FLU = flunisolide (AeroBid, 250 μg per puff).

FP = fluticasone propionate (Flovent, 44, 110, and 220 μg per puff from a metered-dose inhaler, or 50, 100, or 200 μg per inhalation from a dry powder inhaler).

TAA = triamcinolone acetonide (Azmacort, 100 μg per puff).

compare because of differences in the steroid preparation, delivery system, duration of use, outcomes measured, age and atopic status of the study population, and asthma severity. Despite the great controversy in the literature, the preponderance of data now suggests that long-term use of ICSs (particularly the newer ones) is safe, particularly when used in low to moderate doses. Of particular note, a recent study demonstrated that children who used budesonide for an extended period achieved predicted adult height. Because the risk of poorly controlled asthma far outweighs the risk of ICS side effects, the risk of adverse effects should not preclude their use in eligible patients. Even so, practitioners should not ignore the risk of ICSs and should monitor growth in children, be aware of the risk of hypothalamic-pituitary-adrenal axis suppression, and (particularly in those taking high doses) ensure adequate calcium intake and regular ophthalmologic examinations. The use of a holding chamber with ICSs decreases oropharyngeal deposition and subsequent systemic absorption of drug, thereby further decreasing the risk of an adverse effect. Nebulized budesonide (Pulmicort Respules) should be delivered via mask or mouthpiece rather than "blow-by" to direct the medication toward the airway and away from the eyes. Because normal lungs allow more systemic absorption of deposited ICSs than in lungs with increased inflammation, the importance of stepping the ICS dose down to the lowest controlling dose cannot be overstated. Alternative therapies such as nonsteroidal anti-inflammatory medications, allergen avoidance, and allergen immunotherapy should be considered in appropriate patients with persistent asthma.

Some patients with mild persistent asthma are successfully treated with nonsteroidal anti-inflammatory medications. Mast cell stabilizers (cromolyn sodium [Intal] and nedocromil sodium [Tilade]) are effective in mild disease, particularly when concomitant allergic rhinitis is treated. To achieve the same degree of control as with low-dose ICSs, mast cell stabilizers may require more puffs per day and more frequent dosing.

Leukotrienes are inflammatory mediators that contribute to allergic inflammation. A newer class of anti-inflammatory medications, the leukotriene receptor antagonists (LTRAs), also have a role in the treatment of mild persistent asthma. Because EPR II was published just as LTRAs were being released to the U.S. market, they receive only brief discussion therein. Montelukast (Singulair) and zafirlukast (Accolate) are highly effective for controlling asthma in some patients. Their oral dosing is an attractive alternative to MDIs or nebulizers for many patients, perhaps increasing compliance with their recommended use. Patients who do not respond to an LTRA as initial therapy should be given an ICS. Conversely, those controlled with an ICS can often successfully step therapy down to an LTRA.

Moderate Persistent Asthma

Moderate persistent asthma is characterized by daily symptoms, disturbance in daily activities, including exercise and sleep, and interference with quality of life. Pulmonary function tests show evidence of moderate air flow obstruction. Patients with moderate persistent asthma require daily moderate dose or high-dose ICSs.

ICS use is associated with a dose-response curve, that is, with a higher daily dose, patients have a greater clinical response. However, the dose-response curve reaches a plateau, frequently in the moderate dose ICS range (500 to 1000 μg/d of beclomethasone [Vanceril] or equivalent). Some patients reach their dose-response plateau at a lower dose and some at a higher dose. Increasing the dose of ICS without further clinical response only serves to increase the risk of ICS-related adverse effects. For these patients, combination therapy with other classes of medication is necessary. Excellent data indicate that the addition of montelukast, theophylline (Theo-Dur), or salmeterol xinafoate (Serevent) to ICS therapy improves asthma control in comparison with doubling the dose of the ICS.

By antagonizing the actions of the proinflammatory leukotrienes, LTRAs can provide a layer of protection beyond that of the ICS. Some patients who have reached the plateau of their ICS dose-response curve achieve improved asthma control with the addition of an LTRA. Furthermore, because LTRAs are anti-inflammatory medications, some patients can step their ICS dose down without clinical evidence of increased airway inflammation (i.e., increased BHR and need for β_2-agonist rescue).

The intent of long-acting bronchodilator therapy with theophylline, salmeterol, or oral sustained-release albuterol (Proventil Repetab, Volmax) is to provide a background of bronchodilation at all times to protect against nocturnal symptoms and to decrease the need for frequent β_2-agonist rescue. Although the EPR II classifies all these medications as "long-term controllers," it is important that they not be considered anti-inflammatory medications. For that reason, they may best be considered "long-acting symptom relievers" that are intended for use in an ongoing, continual manner. They should not be used as rescue medication alone or in the absence of adequate anti-inflammatory medication.

It is not yet clear how long-acting inhaled β_2-agonists fit into the β-agonist controversy. Some studies have shown tolerance to their protective effects over just 2 months of treatment, but others have not. Although these medications have a role in the management of moderate and severe asthma, they should be used with caution. Even when they are used, the frequency of β_2-agonist rescue is a measure of asthma control and an indicator of the need for improved symptom control.

Theophylline is an old standby in asthma therapy. It has fallen in and out of favor over the last 3 decades, but clearly has a role in therapy, especially for those with nocturnal asthma or frequent need for rescue medication. It does not have proven efficacy in therapy for acute exacerbations. One of the great concerns about theophylline use is its narrow therapeutic window. Mild side effects include the caffeine-like effects of jitteriness, insomnia, and gastrointestinal upset. Transient caffeine-like side effects may occur when initial dosing is too aggressive. They resolve over time or may be avoided by gradually increasing the initial dose. Potentially serious effects include tachycardia, central nervous system irritability, and electrocardiographic changes. Theophylline's serious side effects include seizures and arrhythmias. For these reasons, a serum theophylline concentration of 5 to 15 μg/mL is now accepted as therapeutic. Most children will achieve a therapeutic level with a dose of 15 to 20 mg/kg lean body mass per day. It is essential that theophylline levels be monitored with changes in dose, changes in preparation, growth, suspicion of toxicity, or suspicion of subtherapeutic levels, or when a second factor that alters theophylline clearance is present (Table 5).

Although combination therapy is necessary for patients who are poorly controlled at the plateau of their ICS dose-response curve, data are inadequate to make that conclusion for those who are not. Combination therapy in the latter group is therefore more controversial. Nonetheless, combination with an LTRA may allow for a lower daily dose of ICS in patients at risk of or concerned about adverse effects. Unfortunately, compliance with two daily medications is likely to be less than with one. The use of long-acting bronchodilators may mask the signs of increasing airway inflammation, thereby increasing the risk of airway remodeling over time or delaying the introduction of prednisone in an asthma flare. Therefore, I generally try to delay their introduction until the patient has reached the maximal achievable response to anti-inflammatory medications.

TABLE 5. **Factors Affecting Theophylline Elimination**

Decrease Elimination (Increase Serum Theophylline Concentration)	Increase Elimination (Decrease Serum Theophylline Concentration)
Diet* (high CHO, low protein, dietary xanthines)	Diet* (low CHO, high protein, charbroiled meat)
Bronchopulmonary dysplasia	Hyperthyroidism
Fever (sustained >24 h)	Medications:
Heart failure	Carbamazepine (Tegretol)
Hypothyroidism	Isoproterenol (IV) (Isuprel)
Liver disease	Phenobarbital
Medications:	Phenytoin (Dilantin)
Alcohol	Rifampin (Rifadin)
Allopurinol (Zyloprim)	Smoking (tobacco or marijuana)
Cimetidine (Tagamet)	
Ciprofloxacin (Cipro)	
Disulfiram	
Estrogen (oral contraceptives)	
Interferon	
Macrolide antibiotics	
Methotrexate	
Propranolol (Inderal)	
Verapamil (Calan)	
Zileuton (Zyflo)	

*Only if the change in diet is sustained and extreme.
Abbreviation: CHO = carbohydrate.

Severe Persistent Asthma

Patients with severe persistent asthma have nearly continuous symptoms with frequent exacerbations. They regularly have activity limitation and interrupted sleep. Pulmonary function testing shows severe air flow obstruction (FEV_1 <60% of predicted) with a large diurnal variation in PEFR (>30%). Pulmonary function will not usually normalize after β_2-agonist therapy.

Patients with severe persistent asthma are often treated with multiple medications in high doses and in combination. They may require daily or alternate-day oral corticosteroids when all else fails. These patients represent a relatively small proportion of asthmatics, but they require close attention and monitoring. Because of their risk of adverse effects from medications, identification and control of complicators of asthma should be aggressively addressed and medications stepped down to the lowest controlling dose.

COMPONENT 4: EDUCATION FOR A PARTNERSHIP IN ASTHMA CARE

The old adage "knowledge is power" applies to asthma. Patient education is a major component of complete asthma care. A full educational program is comprehensive, complex, and difficult to coordinate and relies heavily on the patient's behavior for success. Patient education is an ongoing process and must be fully integrated into routine asthma care. The time that a clinician spends educating patients sends an important message regarding that clinician's commitment to working with the family and the family's empowerment and self-management abilities.

Complete asthma education need not and cannot be accomplished in a single visit. Over time, patients will learn about basic asthma pathology and be able to distinguish the difference between airway inflammation and bronchospasm. In so doing, they will recognize and understand the difference between and the rationale for the use of regular controller anti-inflammatory medications and as-needed symptom reliever bronchodilators. They must learn numerous new skills, including the proper use of MDIs and holding chambers, trigger identification and avoidance, peak flow and symptom monitoring, early recognition of asthma symptoms, and what to do in case of symptoms (self-management and action plans).

For any program to be successful, basic educational principles must be applied. Participants must reach an agreement on goals. A big difference is often seen in the level of control that the physician and the patient or parent believe is possible and acceptable, particularly because of the public's perception of asthma as an episodic, not a chronic disease. Demonstration and hands-on rehearsal of the necessary skills described earlier are required. Repetition contributes to learning. By having patients recite their asthma medications and demonstrate an understanding of them, demonstrate the use of MDIs and peak flow meters, and so on at routine asthma follow-up visits, the clinician will be able to identify knowledge gaps requiring review. At the same time, patients will have a forum to ask their own questions. Each visit is therefore an opportunity for re-assessment. It is essential that patients be given only as much information as they are able to apply at a time. Finally, reinforcement from the positive results that patients achieve and in the form of praise from medical providers will encourage patients to continue in their pursuit of the best possible asthma control.

ALLERGIC RHINITIS CAUSED BY INHALANT FACTORS

method of
HUGH H. WINDOM, M.D.
University of South Florida
Tampa, Florida

Allergic rhinitis is the most common manifestation of allergic disease, affecting 20% of the U.S. population. The mucous membranes of the nose, eyes, and lower respiratory tract are repositories for airborne allergens, and in sensitized individuals these membranes serve as the target organs for allergic reactions. Although sensitivity to inhalant allergens is the most common reason for patients to experience rhinitic symptoms, there are a number of nonallergic causes of rhinitis (Table 1). About 50% of patients presenting to a general practitioner with complaints of rhinitis will have allergies as a cause of their symptoms. Differentiating allergic from nonallergic rhinitis can be accomplished through a careful history, physical examination, and limited diagnostic testing. Optimal treatment can depend on accurate identification of the patient's specific type of rhinitis.

Allergic reactions occur through the binding of allergen peptide fragments to specific IgE on mast cells, leading to the release of preformed and formed mediators capable of producing allergic symptoms. Mast cell substances include histamine, leukotrienes, prostaglandins, cytokines, and tryptase. Histamine acts on sensory nerves to produce sneezing and itching symptoms characteristic of the acute allergic reaction. Neural and humoral agents affect the nasal vasculature, resulting in rhinorrhea, congestion, or both. Other important cells include T lymphocytes and eosinophils. These cells are recruited to submucosal sites within 24 hours and in turn release their mediators and cytokines that amplify and prolong the allergic reaction.

Despite the advances in the understanding of the immunobiology of allergic rhinitis, measuring the severity of allergic rhinitis is not possible in the laboratory. Clinicians must rely on quality of life measures and the presence or absence of disease complications. Rhinitis has been shown to adversely affect quality of life (physical, emotional, social, and occupational) more than other chronic and more serious diseases such as asthma. The complications of rhinitis all relate to the anatomic connection between the upper airway and the ears, sinuses, and lower airway. Proper management of allergic rhinitis will minimize the occurrence of otitis media, sinusitis, cough, and asthma. The price tag for allergic rhinitis, often misconstrued as being of trivial importance, exceeds $2 billion in annual health care spending in the United States.

DIAGNOSING ALLERGIC RHINITIS

Establishing the proper diagnosis for a patient with nasal symptoms is important before considering treatment options. Patients usually perceive rhinitis as an allergic disease. Physicians contribute to this misconception by labeling many of their rhinitis patients with allergic rhinitis before diagnostic testing has established the true etiology. This leaves the allergist with the task of reviewing the long list of other causes seen in Table 1 to a patient shocked to find he or she has nonallergic rhinitis. The patient history and physical examination offer early clues to the type of rhinitis that will eventually be determined by diagnostic allergy tests.

Patient History

The following historical elements are useful in distinguishing between allergic and nonallergic rhinitis: age at onset of symptoms (the younger the age, the more likely the patient is atopic), type of rhinitic symptoms (sneezing, watering, and itching suggest atopy), timing of symptoms (seasonal suggests atopy; after exposure to irritants such as fragrances and chemicals suggests nonallergic rhinitis), past medical history (concomitant asthma or atopic dermatitis suggest atopy), and family history (atopic siblings or parents with asthma, rhinitis, or eczema suggest atopy). None of these are pathognomonic for the type of rhinitis, but collectively they are helpful in guiding the patient workup. Exceptions to the standard character types exist (e.g., the patient with chronic nasal obstruction who is allergic to the perennial dust mite). Specific forms of nonallergic rhinitis may be identified through the patient history, such as gustatory rhinitis in the patient describing profuse rhinorrhea occurring while or soon after eating.

The environmental history of patients with rhinitis can identify potential allergic triggers and is necessary to confirm clinical relevance of specific allergy test results. In addition to the obvious question of pets in the home, other

TABLE 1. **Etiology of Nonallergic Rhinitis***

Infectious	Other		Structural
Viral Bacterial	Vasomotor Atrophic rhinitis Pregnancy Occupational Granulomatous	Nonallergic rhinitis with eosinophils syndrome Gustatory Hypothyroidism Ciliary dyskinesia Rhinitis medicamentosa	Nasal polyps Septal deviation Adenoid hypertrophy Tumors Choanal atresia/stenosis

*These conditions are responsible for up to 50% of rhinitis cases. Once inhalant allergy is ruled out, this differential diagnosis should be considered

features of the home should be explored, such as type of air conditioning/heating, recent leaks or damp areas, type of flooring especially in the bedrooms, family members who smoke, and use of potpourri or air fresheners. A lot of attention in the press is given to sick buildings, and possibly because of this and the resulting high standards for air quality in the workplace, the home is a much more likely source of airborne triggers of rhinitis.

Physical Examination

The classic description of the allergic nose is pale with boggy, or edematous, membranes. Although this is very suggestive of atopy when seen, the fact is that only about one third of patients with allergic rhinitis will have such an examination; another one third of patients will have erythematous nasal membranes, and the final one third have normal pink membranes. Percussion may elicit sinus tenderness over the paranasal sinus cavities, and in cases of bacterial sinusitis purulent secretions can be seen in the nasal cavity or nasopharynx. "Cobblestoning" or lymphoid hypertrophy of the posterior pharyngeal wall is a result of ongoing postnasal drainage. Examination of the ear is rarely enlightening, with the exception of finding otitis media with effusion in younger patients.

In children, the examination takes on added importance because it compensates for their inability to recognize and verbalize a good symptom history. Children may have a darkening of the skin over their lower orbit, so-called allergic shiners, that develop as a result of nasal obstruction and suborbital edema. Years of performing the "allergic salute," upward rubbing of the nose with the palm of the hand, may lead to a transverse line above the tip of the nose (nasal crease). Finally, persistent nasal obstruction will lead to mouth breathing and a V-shaped upper palate often requiring dental manipulation.

Diagnostic Testing

Appropriate testing must be performed to add certainty to a diagnosis of allergic rhinitis. The definition of inhalant allergic sensitivity is based on the presence of specific IgE antibody to an airborne allergen. The patient must then have exposure to the particular allergen, which in turn induces nasal symptoms to establish the diagnosis of allergic rhinitis. These definitions highlight the importance of tying together the results of diagnostic testing and clinical history.

The standard measure of allergic sensitivity to inhalant allergens is the allergy skin test. This is a safe, quick, and relatively inexpensive means of documenting atopy. The allergy skin test involves introducing a small quantity of allergen into the skin and observing whether an allergic reaction takes place by measuring local erythema and wheal formation. The basis for the skin test is that mast cell–bound specific IgE will recognize the allergen being tested and this linkage leads to histamine release from the mast cell. Histamine produces the flare reaction, or erythema, and induration, or wheal. Commercial histamine is applied as a positive test control to ensure the test subject is capable of mounting a measurable wheal and flare reaction (some medications will suppress histamine, such as antihistamines, tricyclic antidepressants, and chronic corticosteroids). Diluent used in packaging of the test allergens is applied as a negative test control. Allergy testing cannot be interpreted without appropriately responding control tests.

Initially, the administration of control materials or allergen extract is by an epicutaneous route into the dermis using such techniques as the scratch, prick, or puncture test. After waiting 15 to 20 minutes the size of the reaction is read in millimeters and recorded as such or graded according to a defined 1 to 4+ scale. In clinical situations in which atopy is more strongly suspected, a negative epicutaneous test will be followed by a more sensitive test using an intradermal injection of 0.02 mL of diluted allergen. The reaction is recorded in a similar fashion after 15 to 20 minutes. Allergen concentrations used in both types of testing should be documented as well as the extract manufacturer. Systemic reactions, although exceedingly rare, are possible with allergy skin tests.

The alternative to skin testing is the in vitro measurement of specific IgE, a radioallergosorbent test (RAST). Unlike the skin test, patients do not need to avoid taking drugs affecting histamine or have normal skin available for multiple tests. Blood is drawn from the patient without regard to fasting and then exposed to a solid phase containing the test allergen. Specific IgE will bind to the allergen, and then radiolabeled anti-IgE is used to mark and measure the amount of IgE present in the patient's serum. This quantitative result is reported in absolute units and assigned to a class ranking from 0 to 5. This IgE RAST should not be confused with a similar methodology using radiolabeled IgG, an unproven measure of allergic sensitivity. Studies comparing allergy skin tests with IgE RAST have shown good correlation between them, with a small advantage going to the skin tests. The quality of both tests is highly dependent on technique, the person performing the skin test, and the commercial laboratory selected for the RAST.

CURRENT THERAPY

The management scheme for a patient with allergic rhinitis can be summated in three, often sequential, options: (1) avoidance of exposure to inhalant allergens, (2) pharmacologic treatment using both over-the-counter and prescription agents, and (3) allergen immunotherapy. There is no single best treatment option for all patients. The goal is to minimize symptoms and reduce disease complications such as sinusitis and asthma without undesired drug side effects that affect mental or physical function.

Allergen Avoidance

Allergen avoidance is only worth pursuing if diagnostic testing has clearly established the specific inhalant allergens to which the patient is sensitive. Empirical dust or mold avoidance efforts are often more costly than the testing to determine allergic sensitivity. The success of allergen avoidance can vary from absolute resolution of symptoms, in cases of animal removal from the home, to absolutely no benefit, typically in cases of panallergic individuals in whom altering exposure to a few indoor allergens does not offset the effects of ongoing exposure to other allergens. Patients should be educated about where and when the allergens are in their environment and by what means they can reduce exposure levels. The extent to which these suggestions are followed is left to patient discretion; continuing to golf during tree pollen season may be worth the discomfort and dismissing a beloved furry pet may not be up for discussion.

The allergen control measures most likely to succeed are directed at the indoor environment. Removing pets from the home is helpful, but not immediately, because it has been demonstrated that cat protein allergens remain in homes for up to and beyond 1 year. Washing cats once weekly will over time diminish cat allergen levels. Dust mites are best dealt with first from the bedding where a patient spends 7 to 10 hours a day and then working outward throughout the house as long as such efforts remain feasible. Simple plastic encasings of the mattress, bedsprings, and pillows for under $100 can reduce mite exposure in an area where patients spend 7 to 10 hours a day. Washing all bedding placed over the plastic encasings in hot water (>130°F) will eliminate mites in these areas. General household recommendations include reducing humidity below 50%, removing carpets in favor of solid surfaces, and removing dust-collecting upholstered furniture and curtains. Mold growth indoors is limited by humidity control, repairing water leaks, and eliminating moisture-prone areas. Air filtration systems, particularly with a high-efficiency particulate air (HEPA) filter, may be useful for some patients.

Antihistamines and Decongestants

First-generation antihistamines have been used in the treatment of inhalant allergies since the early 1940s (Table 2). The major drawback to these agents is their sedative properties and often subtle impairment of psychomotor function. A study has shown automotive driving ability to be more impaired by the use of diphenhydramine (Benadryl) than illegal levels of alcohol. Antihistamines reduce nasal secretions, sneezing, itching, and watery eyes. Because there is minimal improvement in nasal congestion, these agents are often marketed in combination with decongestants. Adding a decongestant to a first-generation antihistamine often can have the advantage of offsetting the sedative effects. The most commonly used oral decongestant is pseudoephedrine (Sudafed). Phenylpropanolamine (previously used in such over-the-counter combination products as Contac, Dimetapp, and Triaminic) was taken off the market in late 2000 by the FDA because of an association with cerebral hemorrhage in women.

Second-generation agents produce fewer central nervous system effects and unlike the classic antihistamines are administered only once or twice a day. School performance as measured by simulated class-

TABLE 2. **Histamine H_1-Receptor Antagonists**

Generic Name	Trade Name	Formulation	Sedating	Usual Dosage
Classic Antihistamines				
Azatadine	Optimine	Tabs: 1 mg	Yes	>11 y: 1 mg bid
Brompheniramine	Dimetane	Elixir: 2 mg/5 mL	Yes	0.35 mg/kg/24 h in 3–4 doses
		Tabs: 4, 8, 12 mg		4 mg q4–6h, 8–12 mg bid
Chlorpheniramine	Chlor-Trimeton	Tabs: 4, 8, 12 mg	Yes	4 mg q4h, 8 mg q8h, 12 mg bid
Clemastine	Tavist	Syrup: 0.67 mg/5 mL	Yes	0.67–1.34 mg bid
		Tabs: 1.34, 2.68 mg		1.34 mg q4–6h, 2.68 mg bid
Cyproheptadine	Periactin	Syrup: 2 mg/5 mL	Yes	0.25 mg/kg/24 h, in 3–4 doses
		Tabs: 4 mg		4 mg q4–6h
Diphenhydramine	Benadryl	Syrup: 12.5 mg/5 mL	Yes	5 mg/kg/24 h, in 3–4 doses
		Chewable: 12.5 mg		
		Caps: 12.5, 25 mg		25–50 mg q6h
Hydroxyzine	Atarax, Vistaril	Syrup: 10, 25 mg/5 mL	Yes	2 mg/kg/24h, in 3–4 doses
		Tabs: 10, 25, 50, 100 mg		25–50 mg q4–6h
Promethazine	Phenergan	Syrup: 6.25, 25/5 mL	Yes	1 mg/kg/24 h ½ qhs ½ in 2 day doses
		Supp: 12.5, 25, 50 mg		
		Tabs: 12.5, 25, 50 mg		12.5–50 mg tid
Newer Antihistamines				
Azelastine	Astelin	Nasal solution 0.1%, 137 μg/spray	+/− (12%)	5–11 y: 1 spray/nostril bid
				>11 y: 2 sprays/nostril bid
Cetirizine	Zyrtec	Syrup: 5 mg/5 mL	+/− (14%)	2–5 y: ½–1 tsp qd
		Tabs: 5, 10 mg		6–11 y: 1–2 tsp qd
				>11 y: 10 mg qd
Fexofenadine	Allegra	Caps: 60 mg	No	6–11 y: 30 mg bid
		Tabs: 30, 60, 180 mg		>11 y: 60 mg bid, 180 mg qd
	Allegra-D	Tabs: 60 mg fexofenadine, 120 mg pseudoephedrine		>11 y 1 tab bid
Loratadine	Claritin	Syrup: 5 mg/5 mL	No	2–5 y: 1 tsp qd
		Tabs: 10 mg		>5 y: 2 tsp or 10 mg qd
		Reditabs: 10 mg		
	Claritin-D 12 h	Tabs: 10 mg loratadine, pseudoephedrine 120 mg/12 h, 240 mg/24 h		>11 y: 1 tab bid
	Claritin-D 24 h			>11 y: 1 tab qd

room learning was improved in children taking loratadine (Claritin), whereas subjects on diphenhydramine (Benadryl) learned less than placebo controls. The first two second-generation drugs introduced in the United States, terfenadine (Seldane) and astemizole (Hismanal), have been removed from the market because of their potential to prolong the QTc interval and lead to fatal dysrhythmias. Cetirizine (Zyrtec) inhibits eosinophil migration in the skin, making it the slight favorite in the management of urticaria and pruritic skin conditions. Azelastine (Astelin), the only intranasal antihistamine preparation, has equivalent histamine antagonist properties of the oral agents, with some studies showing a significant decongestant effect. On the negative side, azelastine can be sedating and has a notable bitter taste after use. Among the second-generation products only loratadine (Claritin) and fexofenadine (Allegra) are marketed with a combined decongestant (pseudoephedrine), but cetirizine (Zyrtec) is expected to be available in combination with pseudoephedrine in 2001. Desloratadine and norastemizole are active metabolites of loratadine (Claritin) and astemizole (Hismanal), respectively, now undergoing final clinical trials. These agents according to abstract presentations should be slightly more efficacious with fewer side effects.

Intranasal Corticosteroids

Nasal corticosteroids are the most effective class of medications to treat the myriad of symptoms associated with allergic rhinitis (Table 3). They inhibit the acute and late-phase reaction after allergen challenge and reduce levels of inflammatory mediators found in nasal secretions. When administered appropriately all of the nasal corticosteroid preparations appear equally efficacious. Onset of action has been demonstrated as early as 5 hours after use, but more commonly within 1 to 3 days. Safety issues surrounding the use of corticosteroid products, decreased growth rate, osteoporosis, behavioral disturbances, and cataracts are rarely of concern in the case of topical nasal sprays. Nasal biopsies after 1 year of nasal corticosteroid administration show improved epithelial structures without evidence of tissue atrophy. Exquisitely sensitive biochemical measures of hypothalamus-pituitary-adrenal axis have enabled investigators to show axis suppression with chronic nasal corticosteroid use, but the clinical consequences of these findings are unknown. More relevant adverse effects are epistaxis, nasal irritation, and a very rare septal perforation.

Nasal corticosteroid sprays can be initiated in children as young as 4 years old (fluticasone or Flonase approved down to age 4). Physicians have a choice of dry (aerosols) or wet (aqueous) preparations to offer patients. Dosing is typically once daily and can be reduced after clinical benefit has been obtained. Patients should be instructed to direct the nasal applicator straight upward in the nostril or a little outward. Continuous spraying medially toward the nasal septum can lead to septal perforation. If epistaxis occurs, pretreatment with nasal saline and a brief respite from the nasal corticosteroid in the affected nostril may allow the patient to tolerate ongoing treatment. In difficult cases in which symptomatic relief is not achieved with a corticosteroid spray alone, adding an antihistamine/decongestant is appropriate.

Anticholinergic Agents

Ipratropium bromide (Atrovent)* is the treatment of choice of gustatory rhinitis. Other forms of rhinitis with the major feature of rhinorrhea will also respond to the antagonism of acetylcholine at the cholinergic receptor. As can be imagined, the side effects of inhibiting nasal serous and seromucous gland secretion are excessive drying and nasal irritation. This can usually be overcome by downward adjustment of the dose. Atrovent nasal spray is available in two strengths, 0.03% and 0.06%, the higher dose having the indication of treatment of the common cold. These agents do not relieve symptoms of postnasal drip, sneezing, or nasal congestion.

Cromolyn Sodium

Classified as a mast cell stabilizer, cromolyn sodium (NasalCrom) prevents the early- and late-phase mast cell–mediated reactions after allergen challenge. This over-the-counter product available in a 4% solution relieves the symptoms of rhinorrhea, sneezing, and nasal pruritus. Like antihistamines, to which its efficacy can be compared, there is often little effect on nasal congestion. The safety features of NasalCrom (no reports of significant adverse events) make it popular for pediatric patients fearful of corticosteroid preparations. Local side effects occur in less than 10% of patients, and they include sneezing, burning, and stinging. The drug can be used prophylactically, for example, before visiting a home with a cat, but chronic use is limited by its demanding four-times-a-day dosing schedule.

Leukotriene Modifiers

Sulfidopeptide leukotrienes are released in nasal and bronchial mucosa in response to allergen exposure. Drugs that interfere with leukotriene production and those that antagonize the leukotriene D_4 receptor were initially approved for the treatment of asthma but have since shown promise in reducing nasal congestion. These drugs are not yet indicated for allergic rhinitis. Montelukast (Singulair)* has been studied in combination with loratadine (Claritin) in subjects with allergic rhinitis. The combined product significantly improved daytime nasal symptom scores (congestion, rhinorrhea, itching, and sneezing) compared with placebo and the individual agents. Singulair is a once-a-day product available

*Not FDA approved for this indication.

TABLE 3. **Intranasal Corticosteroid Agents**

Generic Name/ Trade Name	Formulation	Dose/ Actuation (μg)	Doses/Unit	Age	Usual Starting Dosage
Beclomethasone					
Beconase or Vancenase pockethaler	Aerosol	42	200	6–11 y ≥12 y	1 spray/nostril bid 2 sprays/nostril bid
Beconase AQ or Vancenase AQ	Aqueous	42	200	6–11 y ≥12 y	1 spray/nostril bid 2 sprays/nostril bid
Vancenase AQ 84 μg	Aqueous	84	120	6–11 y ≥12 y	1 spray/nostril qd 2 sprays/nostril qd
Budesonide					
Rhinocort	Aerosol	32	200	≥6 y	4 sprays/nostril qd
Rhinocort Aqua	Aqueous	32	120	≥6 y	1 spray/nostril qd–bid
Flunisolide					
Nasalide or Nasarel	Aqueous	25	200	6–13 y ≥14 y	1 spray/nostril tid 2 spray/nostril bid
Fluticasone					
Flonase	Aqueous	50	120	4–11 y ≥12 y	1 spray/nostril qd 2 sprays/nostril qd
Mometasone					
Nasonex	Aqueous	50	120	3–11 y ≥12 y	1 spray/nostril qd 2 sprays/nostril qd
Triamcinolone					
Nasacort	Aerosol	55	100	≥6 y	2 sprays/nostril qd
Nasacort AQ	Aqueous	55	120	6–11 y ≥12 y	1 spray/nostril qd 2 sprays/nostril qd

in 10-mg tablets for patients 15 and older, 5-mg chewable tablets for 6- to 14-year-olds, and a 4-mg chewable tablet for 2- to 5-year-olds. Zafirlukast (Accolate)* is dosed twice daily and available in 20-mg tablets for 12 years old and older and 10-mg tablets for 6- to 11-year-olds. These agents are well tolerated and have a pregnancy category B.

Allergen Immunotherapy

Allergen immunotherapy is a treatment option to allergen avoidance and pharmacotherapy in patients with allergic rhinitis. Specific-allergen vaccines are prepared individually for each patient. Vaccines administered over many months produce a T-lymphocyte tolerance to the specific allergens contained in the vaccines, with a resulting reduction in tissue sensitivity, mediator release, and inflammation. Immunotherapy is indicated in the following situations: (1) patients who prefer this modality of treatment to pharmacotherapy for long-term management of their allergic symptoms, (2) patients who fail to respond to pharmacotherapy or suffer side effects from them, and (3) patients with more severe rhinitis and concomitant atopic conditions such as asthma that can also benefit from allergy shots. Allergen vaccines are administered subcutaneously in an office or clinic initially on a weekly basis as the allergen concentration is gradually increased. Once the maintenance dose is reached, injections are spread out to every 2 to 4 weeks. Injections can produce local reactions or more severe systemic allergic reactions, so it is important to administer shots in a medical facility with appropriate resuscitative equipment and personnel available. Immunotherapy is effective in the large majority of patients undergoing treatment. Recent work has suggested that early immunotherapy in children monosensitized to dust mites can prevent the development of additional sensitivities to pollens, molds, and animals. Furthermore, these children with allergic rhinitis are less likely to continue the "allergic march" toward asthma. Efforts are underway to use different routes of administration (particularly oral) and modified vaccines with less allergenic properties to reduce risks of treatment.

Managing Patients With Allergic Rhinitis

Physicians need to appreciate the significance of allergic rhinitis as a disease that seriously affects the well-being, quality of life, and capacity to work and learn, whereas increasing the risk for co-morbid conditions such as sinusitis, otitis media, cough, and asthma. Treatment should be individualized as to specific therapies but generally should follow a stepped approach that includes environmental con-

*Not FDA approved for this indication.

trol measures to limit allergen exposure, pharmacotherapy, and possibly allergen immunotherapy. Special subgroups such as pregnant women, elderly patients, and athletes demand individual considerations while still fitting within the stepped approach. Seasonal disease with the more dramatic itchy/watery naso-ocular symptoms can often be treated with antihistamines with or without a decongestant. Perennial disease with its more prominent chronic nasal congestion is often best treated with once-daily administration of nasal corticosteroids. Patients responding incompletely to initial treatment should receive additional medications to cover breakthrough symptoms (e.g., eye drops or antihistamines for ocular symptoms, ipratropium bromide [Atrovent] for rhinorrhea, or a nasal corticosteroid or oral decongestant for nasal stuffiness [intranasal decongestants used for longer than 1 week can cause rhinitis medicamentosa]). Allergen immunotherapy "turns off" allergic sensitivity rather than treats symptoms, making this an appealing option for patients with more severe symptoms. Early evidence suggests immunotherapy modulates disease progression in the form of preventing new specific allergies and halting transition from allergic rhinitis to other atopic conditions. Confirmation of these findings may lead to more widespread use of immunotherapy, particularly at a very young age. In whatever form, management of allergic rhinitis aims to improve quality of life, decrease prevalence of costly complications, decrease time loss from work/school, and cut related expenditures for antibiotics, emergency department services, surgery, and hospitalizations.

ALLERGIC REACTIONS TO DRUGS

method of
MUNIR PIRMOHAMED, PH.D.
The University of Liverpool
Liverpool, England

Adverse reactions to drugs (ADRs) are common; a recent meta-analysis suggested that ADRs were responsible for more than 100,000 deaths in the United States in 1994, making them the fourth most common cause of death after ischemic heart disease, cancer, and cerebrovascular disease. ADRs can also prolong a hospital stay by a mean of 2 days and can increase the cost of hospitalization by approximately $2500 per patient.

ADRs can be divided into two basic types: A (augmented) and B (bizarre, also termed idiosyncratic) (Table 1). Even within these two general types, however, the clinical manifestations of ADRs are protean, and indeed ADRs can mimic almost any disease process. Type A reactions account for 80% of all ADRs; these are not allergic drug reactions, although they are often mistakenly labeled as being allergic. These reactions are usually dose dependent and can be predicted from the known pharmacology of the drug.

The type B or idiosyncratic ADRs are unpredictable and do not show a simple dose-response relationship. All allergic drug reactions fall into the category of type B ADRs, but not all type B ADRs are allergic in origin. Clinical and laboratory features can be used to distinguish between allergic and nonallergic idiosyncratic ADRs (Table 2). Allergic reactions are so named because they are thought to be immune mediated and account for approximately 20% of all ADRs. In general, the mechanisms of allergic drug reactions are poorly understood; hence, it is not surprising that there are no specific therapies.

TABLE 1. **Characteristics of Type A and Type B Adverse Drug Reactions**

Characteristics	Type A	Type B
Dose dependency	Usually shows a good relationship	No simple relationship
Predictable from known pharmacology	Yes	Not usually
Host factors	Genetic factors may be important	Dependent on (usually uncharacterized) host factors
Frequency	Common	Uncommon
Severity	Variable, but usually mild	Variable, proportionately more severe
Clinical burden	High morbidity and low mortality	High morbidity and mortality
Animal models	Usually reproducible in animals	No known animal models

TABLE 2. **Distinction Between Allergic and Nonallergic Idiosyncratic Adverse Drug Reactions**

Feature	Nonallergic	Allergic
Time to adverse reaction	Variable but often rapid	Hours (anaphylaxis) 2–6 wk (hypersensitivity) 7–14 d (serum sickness) >2 y (systemic lupus erythematosus)
Time to toxicity on rechallenge	Similar to primary exposure	Sooner than on primary exposure
Associated symptoms	Symptoms of organ affected	Symptoms of organ affected plus rash, fever, adenopathy (hypersensitivity manifestations); fever, urticaria, and arthralgia (serum sickness manifestations)
Laboratory features		
Eosinophilia	No	Yes, in many reactions
Antibodies	No	Yes, but only demonstrated for a few reactions
Specific T cells	No	Yes, but only demonstrated for a few reactions

In this article, general aspects of the diagnosis and the clinical management of allergic ADRs are covered first, followed by a discussion of the two specific types of allergic drug reactions chosen to highlight important issues relating to either clinical management or recent therapeutic advances.

DIAGNOSIS OF DRUG ALLERGY

The diagnosis of an allergic drug reaction is essentially a clinical diagnosis (Table 3). A good accurate history is essential. Many patients claim to be allergic to a drug, but close questioning reveals that they are merely intolerant. For example, many patients who claim to be penicillin allergic have actually had vomiting or diarrhea, which are due to gastrointestinal irritation and not due to an allergic reaction. The timing between the start of drug therapy and the start of the reaction is important. Some allergic reactions such as anaphylaxis occur almost immediately (within 1 hour) after drug intake, whereas others are delayed. The majority of so-called hypersensitivity reactions occur within the first 6 weeks of drug intake. Rarely, as in the case of drug-induced systemic lupus erythematosus, prolonged drug intake (more than 2 years) is needed for the reaction to become clinically manifest. It is important to obtain a history of use of not only prescribed drugs but also over-the-counter medications or remedies from health food shops.

Allergic drug reactions usually improve with drug discontinuation. Rechallenge is often followed by recurrence, which occurs much more quickly than with primary exposure. This indicates the presence of specific drug-reactive memory T cells. With some drugs, the reaction is much more severe on rechallenge than on primary exposure. This is certainly true for abacavir (Ziagen), a nucleoside reverse transcriptase inhibitor used in human immunodeficiency viral disease, which leads to hypersensitivity reactions in 4% of patients. Rechallenge is strictly contraindicated because the reaction is more severe, and several deaths have been reported. In many situations, therefore, deliberate rechallenge to confirm a diagnosis is not ethical. There are circumstances, however, in which it may be deemed necessary to desensitize a patient, particularly when the drug in question is the best treatment available for that particular condition. The rationale behind desensitization is that by exposing the allergic individual to increasing doses of the allergen, it may be possible to inhibit the allergic reaction. The mechanism by which such a strategy is able to induce desensitization is not known. There is a great deal of experience with desensitization strategies in penicillin-allergic patients, and recently with trimethoprim-sulfamethoxazole (Septra) in patients infected with HIV. Successful desensitization has also been reported for nonsteroidal anti-inflammatory drugs, allopurinol (Zyloprim), paclitaxel (Taxol), and iron. Desensitization is not without risk and can result in death. Therefore, it should be performed only by specialists in settings where there are adequate resuscitation facilities. Furthermore, desensitization should be attempted only in patients who have had mild allergic ADRs. Stevens-Johnson syndrome, other blistering skin conditions, exfoliative dermatitis, and hepatitis should be considered contraindications to desensitization.

TABLE 3. Steps to Determine Whether a Drug Is Responsible for an Allergic Reaction

What Is the Timing Between the Start of Drug Therapy and the Reaction?

Most reactions occur soon after commencing drug therapy; anaphylactic reactions can occur within hours, whereas hypersensitivity reactions typically take 2–6 weeks. Other reactions such as drug-induced lupus may be delayed for years.

Does the Reaction Improve When the Drug Is Withdrawn or Dose Reduced?

Most reactions improve on drug withdrawal, although the recovery phase can be prolonged. In rare instances, an autoimmune phenomenon may be set up, and thus the reaction will not improve on drug withdrawal.

What Happens When the Patient Is Rechallenged With the Drug?

Recurrence on rechallenge provides good evidence that the drug is responsible for the adverse effect. This is, however, rarely possible, particularly for serious reactions, because of the danger to the patient.

Have Concomitant Drugs and Other Nondrug Causes Been Excluded?

An adverse drug reaction is a diagnosis of exclusion because there are no specific laboratory tests available. It is important to exclude nondrug causes clinically as well as by performing relevant investigations.

Has the Reaction Been Reported Before?

If the reaction is well recognized, it may be mentioned in the literature from the manufacturer or may have been reported in the medical literature. An opportunity should always be taken to search reference databases such as MEDLINE, which can provide valuable insight into the appropriate treatment of patients with what may be a relatively rare reaction.

The history should also elicit whether the patient has an underlying disease process that may increase the risk of developing an allergic ADR. For example, atopic patients are at increased risk of developing anaphylaxis with use of compounds such as penicillin and latex. Patients with autoimmune diseases may also be predisposed to developing allergic ADRs. It is important to determine whether the patient had an underlying viral infection, because this can increase the risk of certain types of ADRs. For example, almost all patients with infectious mononucleosis will develop an exanthematous eruption if they are given ampicillin; however, this reaction does not recur when the patient has recovered from infectious mononucleosis. Similarly, patients infected with HIV are at higher risk of developing hypersensitivity reactions with trimethoprim/sulfamethoxazole, which is used for the treatment and prophylaxis of *Pneumocystis carinii* pneumonia. This also seems to be dose dependent in that almost 50% develop the hypersensitivity reaction (most commonly manifested by a skin eruption) when the drug is used at high doses (up to 8 g/d) for treatment, whereas the frequency is 30% when the drug is used for prophylaxis (960 mg/d). Gradual initiation of trimethoprim-sulfamethoxazole over 2 weeks can reduce the frequency of rash and fever by more than 40% when compared with routine initiation of a 960-mg tablet.

Early diagnosis of an allergic ADR is essential to management, because delay in drug withdrawal can sometimes be deleterious. Early diagnosis is not helped by the fact that allergic drug reactions can have widely varied manifestations, can affect any bodily system (Table 4), and can be of variable severity. The skin is probably the most commonly affected organ. It is important that the clinician be aware of the potential of drugs to cause such widely varied manifestations and that he or she includes drug-induced disease in the differential diagnosis.

TABLE 4. **Examples of Organs Affected by Immune-Mediated Allergic Drug Reactions***

Organ System	Type of Reaction	Drug Examples
Generalized reaction	Anaphylaxis	Penicillins
Generalized reaction	Hypersentivity	Phenytoin (Dilantin)
Skin	Toxic epidermal necrolysis	Nonsteroidal anti-inflammatory drugs
Liver	Hepatitis	Halothane (Fluothane)
Hematologic system	Aplastic anemia	Felbamate (Felbatol)
	Agranulocytosis	Propylthiouracil (PTU)
	Hemolysis	Nomifensine†
	Thrombocytopenia	Quinidine (Quinaglute)
Central nervous system	Guillain-Barré syndrome	Zimeldine*
Kidney	Interstitial nephritis	Penicillins
Lung	Pneumonitis	Dapsone
Heart	Myocarditis	Clozapine (Clozaril)

*Although these reactions have been labeled as being allergic, in many instances, this is based on clinical symptoms, and there may be insufficient laboratory data to support an immune pathogenesis.
†Not available in the United States.

Diagnosis of a drug as the cause of a patient's symptoms usually includes the exclusion of nondrug-induced diseases, which can have very similar clinical features. For example, in children, drug-induced erythema multiforme and Stevens-Johnson syndrome can be mistaken for Kawasaki disease, whereas toxic epidermal necrolysis can be difficult to distinguish from staphylococcal scalded skin syndrome. In patients with mild allergic reactions, it may be sufficient to distinguish these reactions from those of nondrug-induced disease using clinical criteria. For more severe reactions, however, such as hypersensitivity syndrome, even though the diagnosis is largely clinical, it is important to perform laboratory tests to exclude nondrug-induced disease and to determine whether other organ systems are involved. Thus, at a minimum, patients should undergo a full blood cell count (including an eosinophil count), determination of renal and liver function, and urinalysis. Other tests will depend on the manifestations of the adverse reaction and can include chest radiography, measurement of autoantibody levels, thyroid function tests, and skin biopsy.

In general, there are no reliable diagnostic tests for allergic ADRs. Various tests have been described (Table 5); however, these are still largely used as research tools because they are neither sensitive nor specific enough and are expensive. It is true that the lack of suitable diagnostic tests reflects our ignorance of the pathophysiology of these adverse reactions.

GENERAL ASPECTS OF THE MANAGEMENT OF DRUG ALLERGY

Immediate discontinuation of the culprit drug is essential in patients who develop an allergic drug reaction. In mild cases, this is often the only maneuver necessary. There may be a need for symptomatic therapy in other cases; for example, antihistamines and topical corticosteroids can be used to alleviate symptoms. Nonsteroidal anti-inflammatory drugs may be required for muscular or joint symptoms, which may be prominent in drug hypersensitivity, or in patients with drug-induced systemic lupus erythematosus. Systemic corticosteroids are often used for more severe allergic reactions; however, this is largely based on anecdotal evidence of their effectiveness, and there is certainly a need for more robust randomized controlled clinical trial data. Patients with blistering skin conditions also require supportive measures such as careful wound care, hydration, nutritional support, and treatment of sepsis. Anaphylaxis should be regarded as a medical emergency and should be treated with epinephrine, oxygen, antihistamines, bronchodilators, and steroids.

Once a reaction has occurred, the patient should be told to avoid the causative drug in the future. The details of the reaction should be carefully documented in the notes, and the family physician should also be informed (if the reaction occurred in the hospital). There may also be a risk of cross-sensitivity with other drugs that have a similar chemical structure. This risk is not absolute, however (i.e., not every patient with a drug allergy will react to another drug that is chemically similar). There is no

TABLE 5. **Investigations Used for the Diagnosis of Allergic Drug Reactions**

Test	Comments
Antibody detection	Various techniques used including ELISA, immunoblotting, and immunofluorescence. Hampered by the fact that we often do not know the structure of the antigen derived from the drug. For autoantibodies, only few drugs lead to autoantibody formation.
Lymphocyte transformation test	Used for detecting drug-reactive T cells. Limited because tend to be positive in only 30–60% of individuals, and sometimes it is difficult to reproduce results between different laboratories.
Lymphocyte cytotoxicity assay	Labor-intensive and expensive. It is also relatively insensitive and has been used for a limited number of drugs including anticonvulsants and sulfonamides.
Patch testing	Used for the detection of T-cell–mediated disease. Positive in only 30% of patients.
Skin testing	Used for detection of IgE-mediated allergic ADRs. Requires a knowledge of the antigen with drugs such as penicillin, and should only be carried out where there are facilities for resuscitation.

Abbreviations: ADR = allergic drug reaction, ELISA = enzyme-linked immunosorbent assay.

way of predicting cross-sensitivity; therefore, it is probably safer to avoid drugs with similar chemical structures. A typical example is hypersensitivity to one of the aromatic anticonvulsants (phenytoin [Dilantin], carbamazepine [Tegretol], phenobarbital), in which there is a substantial, although not yet accurately defined, risk of cross-sensitivity. Thus, patients who have had a serious reaction to one aromatic anticonvulsant should avoid the other aromatic drugs. These patients can be safely started on sodium valproate (Depakene), which does not exhibit cross-reactivity. There is also evidence suggesting that many of these allergic ADRs are genetically determined. Familial occurrence of hypersensitivity has been reported with phenytoin, carbamazepine, and allopurinol. This predisposition is not inherited in a simple mendelian fashion, however, and is probably multigenic. Therefore, although the risk of a similar reaction occurring in a family member is higher than in the general population, it is difficult to quantify that risk. Family members requiring similar drug therapy should be counseled regarding the risk of reaction, and, if alternative therapies that are equally efficacious are available, the culprit drug should be avoided.

The occurrence of a serious allergic drug reaction should be reported to the drug regulatory agency in the country in question as well as to the manufacturer. Spontaneous reporting of ADRs is an important form of postmarketing surveillance that is essential for maintaining the safety of a drug throughout its life cycle. It suffers from the major disadvantage of underreporting, but despite this has generated important drug safety signals in many countries, including the United Kingdom and the United States. The reporting of an ADR to the drug regulatory agency should be seen as part of the overall care of the patient and not merely as an afterthought.

SPECIFIC ALLERGIC ADVERSE DRUG REACTIONS

Given the large number and types of allergic ADRs, it is beyond the scope of this article to review the specific management of all ADRs. To illustrate some specific issues and recent advances, two areas (penicillin allergy and blistering skin conditions) are discussed in greater detail.

Penicillin Allergy

All clinicians encounter penicillin allergy. The incidence of all allergic reactions ranges from 1% to 10%, whereas the incidence of true anaphylactic reactions is in the range of 0.004% to 0.015%. Many patients claim to be allergic to penicillin, but closer examination often reveals that the patients do not have a true drug allergy. True allergy to penicillin has a variety of clinical manifestations, including anaphylaxis (type I hypersensitivity), hemolysis (type II hypersensitivity), serum sickness (type III hypersensitivity), and cutaneous eruptions (type IV hypersensitivity). The IgE-mediated anaphylactic reactions are most feared because of their dramatic presentation and their severity. Skin testing for the presence or absence of penicillin-specific IgE antibodies may be useful. The test has a high negative predictive value because more than 98% of patients who have a history of penicillin allergy but whose skin test results were negative can safely receive the antibiotic (with respect to the risk of anaphylaxis). If the patient has a positive skin test result, then penicillin antibiotics should be avoided, and alternative antibiotics should be prescribed. Even when a patient has a positive skin test result, it does not necessarily mean that he or she will experience an allergic reaction to that particular drug. For example, in patients with maculopapular reactions to penicillin, skin test results may be positive in up to one third of patients, despite the fact that these reactions are cell mediated. Given that not all penicillin-allergic reactions are IgE-mediated, to improve the predictability of penicillin allergy, there have been attempts to investigate cellular immunity by using patch testing and lymphocyte transformation testing, with variable results.

Once a patient is labeled as being penicillin allergic, there is a natural tendency to prescribe non–β-lactam antibiotics, such as macrolides and vancomycin (Vancocin). This may be inappropriate in many cases because the patient may have been labeled as penicillin allergic on the basis of the (often inadequate) history. Fears have been expressed that the inappropriate use of antibiotics may lead to the emergence of resistant bacterial strains, as well as increased costs of treatment.

Penicillin allergy has been the subject of more research than any other allergic ADR. This has led to some interesting insights into the mechanisms of the immune reaction to a small molecule, and it has demonstrated that there are different antigenic determinants in different individuals. Clearly, further research is required. In patients claiming to be penicillin allergic, it is essential to obtain an accurate history. Skin testing and immunoassays using minor and major antigenic determinants of the β-lactam ring, as well as antigens derived from the penicillin side chains, will provide useful confirmation of an IgE-mediated reaction. It is important for clinicians to note that although skin testing is said to have a high negative predictive value, this was determined in a clinical trial situation. Whether this is also true in an everyday clinical setting where patients are unselected and have disparate histories is unclear. The problem is compounded by the fact that a precise diagnosis cannot be made, because not all penicillin determinants are currently available and there is no standardization of testing among different clinics. Therefore, if a patient has had a skin test, it should always be interpreted in conjunction with a carefully taken history.

Drug-Induced Blistering Skin Conditions

The skin is the most commonly affected organ in allergic ADRs. The most severe reactions are characterized by epidermal detachment, which ranges from an incidence of less than 10% in Stevens-Johnson syndrome to greater than 30% in toxic epidermal necrolysis. The latter has been reported to have a mortality rate of 30%. There is good evidence to show that these reactions are immune mediated, and the drugs most commonly implicated include nonsteroidal anti-inflammatory drugs, antibiotics (sulfonamides and penicillins), and anticonvulsants.

Early recognition is important. Prompt withdrawal of the causative drug reduces the risk of death by 30% per day. This is also consistent with the fact that the longer the half-life of the causative drug, the greater the risk of dying. If a patient is on more than one drug when a blistering skin condition develops and it is impossible to determine which drug is responsible, all drugs should be withdrawn. In the early stages, it may not be possible to distinguish between self-limited and serious skin reactions. Even then, however, it may be possible to discontinue all medications temporarily (if the culprit cannot be identified) and reintroduce the medications once it is clear whether the skin reaction is self-limiting or severe.

The mainstay of treatment for patients with toxic epidermal necrolysis is supportive and includes skin care, nutritional support, fluid management, and aggressive treatment of infections. Eye care is also important. Systemic steroids are often used in these patients; however, there are no good controlled trial data showing that these are beneficial. Indeed, some studies have suggested that steroids may increase morbidity and mortality by increasing the risk of sepsis. Data supporting the use of plasmapheresis and immunosuppressants are also relatively weak. More recently, it has been shown that human intravenous immunoglobulin, which contains antibodies that block *Fas*-mediated keratinocyte apoptosis, stopped the progression of disease in 10 patients with toxic epidermal necrolysis. This now needs to be tested in a randomized controlled trial.

The virtue of randomized controlled trials is highlighted by the fact that drugs may have unforeseen effects. For example, a study using thalidomide as an inhibitor of tumor necrosis factor-α in patients with toxic epidermal necrolysis was terminated prematurely because the mortality rate in the treatment arm was significantly higher than in the placebo arm.

ALLERGIC REACTIONS TO INSECT STINGS

method of
DAVID B. K. GOLDEN, M.D.
Johns Hopkins University
Baltimore, Maryland

Insect bites and stings normally cause localized swelling, redness, pain, and itching that are confined to the site of the sting and subside within hours. Allergic swelling can also result from the bites or stings of many kinds of insects, but it is the stinging insects of the order Hymenoptera that can cause anaphylaxis. Allergic reactions to stings from honeybees, vespids (yellow jackets, hornets, wasps), and fire ants are due to the presence in the blood and tissues of IgE antibodies directed against the protein allergens that are in the venoms (but not in the bodies or saliva) of these insects. Yellow jacket and hornet venoms are almost identical and are partially cross-reactive with wasp venoms, but honeybee venom and fire ant venom are each unique. Commercial venom vaccines are available for honeybee, yellow jacket, yellow hornet, white-faced hornet, and *Polistes* wasps (ALK Laboratories, Wallingford, CT; Hollister-Stier Laboratories, Spokane, WA).

Allergic reactions may be localized or systemic. Large local reactions have a late-phase inflammatory mechanism that develops 12 to 24 hours after the sting, causing painful induration often larger than 8 inches in diameter and lasting for 5 to 7 days. A large local reaction to a sting can mimic laryngeal edema (from a sting in the mouth or throat) or cellulitis (lymphangitic drainage from the reaction on an extremity). Systemic reactions are immediate hypersensitivity reactions with manifestations distant from the site of the sting, which can include any one or more of the signs or symptoms of anaphylaxis, including urticaria, angioedema, throat tightness, dyspnea, dizziness, or hypotensive shock. The reported frequency of 50 to 100 fatal reactions per year in the United States is certainly an underestimate. Elevated serum tryptase and venom-specific IgE antibodies have been reported in postmortem blood samples in cases of unexpected death in young individuals. Half of fatal reactions occurred in persons with no prior history of reactions to stings. The population at risk is greater than generally appreciated: 3% of adults in the United States have a history of a systemic allergic reaction to insect stings, and more than 20% have detectable IgE antibodies to venom allergens.

DIAGNOSIS

The most important diagnostic information is obtained from the patient by exploring the details of the history. It is important to determine the exact features and time course of the reaction to distinguish large local, systemic, and nonallergic reactions. Objective signs and documented clinical observations can be more reliable than subjective descriptions by the patient. The presence of venom-specific IgE antibodies can be demonstrated by skin testing or serologic methods (RAST) but must be interpreted in the context of the clinical history. Skin testing with the five Hymenoptera venoms (or fire ant whole-body extract) is recommended for patients who have had systemic allergic reactions to an insect sting, but it is not required for large local reactors. Skin tests are generally performed with a modified intradermal technique of very superficial injection

TABLE 1. **Clinical Recommendations Based on History of Sting Reactions, Age, and Results of Venom Skin Test (or RAST)**

Reaction to Previous Sting	Skin Test (or RAST)	Risk of Systemic Reaction	Clinical Recommendation
No reaction	Positive	10–20%	Avoidance
Large local	Positive	5–10%	Avoidance
Cutaneous systemic	Positive—child	1–10%	Avoidance
	Positive—adult	10–20%	Venom immunotherapy
Anaphylaxis	Positive	30–60%	Venom immunotherapy
	Negative	5–10%	Repeat skin test/RAST

Abbreviation: RAST = radioallergosorbent assay

of only 0.02 mL of the venom at concentrations starting at 0.001 μg/mL and increasing incrementally up to 1.0 μg/mL, if needed, until a positive wheal and flare reaction is elicited. Diagnostic laboratory measurement of venom-specific IgE antibodies (RAST) may be useful when skin testing is inconclusive. As with other allergen systems, the venom RAST is positive in 15% of affected patients with negative skin tests; and, conversely, the RAST is negative in 20% of patients with positive skin tests. A positive venom skin test in an individual with no history of sting reaction is associated with a 17% frequency of systemic reaction to a subsequent sting. The level of sensitivity on skin test or RAST has not been consistently correlated with the severity of the sting reaction.

The assessment of the risk of a systemic reaction to a future sting is based on the detailed history of the reaction, the presence of venom-specific IgE antibodies, and the known natural history of the condition (Table 1). In adults with positive venom skin tests and a prior history of systemic reactions, the risk of systemic reaction is 30% to 60%, with the higher risk being in patients with the most severe reactions (airway obstruction, unconsciousness) and the lower frequency in patients who had cutaneous systemic signs (urticaria, angioedema) and/or mild-moderate dizziness or throat tightness. With the passage of time, the risk declines by half over a 10-year period, but remains 15% to 20% even after 20 to 30 years. The risk of systemic reaction is known to be low in the general population and in some subgroups of affected patients (Table 2). The majority of affected children (age 16 and younger) have had systemic reactions limited to skin manifestations, including angioedema of the face or lips, but with no tongue or throat swelling or hypotension. In these children, subsequent stings cause no systemic reaction in 90%, cause mild cutaneous systemic reaction in 10%, and cause more severe reaction in less than 1%. Persons who have large local reactions generally have positive venom skin tests but have a less than 10% risk of systemic reaction to future stings.

TABLE 2. **Considerations in Starting or Stopping Venom Immunotherapy**

Severity/pattern of systemic reaction
Age (child/teen, adult, senior)
Skin tests (or RAST)
Exposure/activities
Time/duration
Reactions during venom immunotherapy

Abbreviation: RAST = radioallergosorbent assay

TREATMENT AND AVOIDANCE OF STING REACTIONS

Local allergic reactions can be treated symptomatically with ice and antihistamines. Large local reactions may require a burst of oral prednisone (e.g., 40 to 60 mg the first day, tapering over 4 to 7 days) but almost never require antibiotic treatment. Systemic reactions generally require the administration of epinephrine, 0.3 mg, in an adult (0.01 mg/kg in children), with the availability of oxygen, intravenous fluids, or airway support if needed. The recommended route of administration for epinephrine is now intramuscular (rather than subcutaneous) in both adults and children. Corticosteroids have no benefit in the acute stage but are often administered when the patient's condition stabilizes to prevent late-phase manifestations. The patient should be monitored for 3 to 6 hours because over 20% of cases develop recurrent or prolonged reactions. Any patient at risk for anaphylaxis should have a prescription for an epinephrine injection kit and detailed instructions on when to use or not use it. Commercial kits include the Epi-Pen and Epi-Pen Jr (Dey Laboratories, Napa, CA) and the Ana-Kit and Ana-Pen (Hollister-Stier Laboratories, Spokane, WA). Patients who have had allergic reactions to stings and have not been immunized should be counseled to take special avoidance precautions. Nesting areas should be avoided or eliminated and patients should avoid trash receptacles, eating outdoors, lawn mowing, or going barefoot. Insect repellants do not seem to prevent stings.

PREVENTION OF STING REACTIONS (VENOM IMMUNOTHERAPY)

Systemic reactions to insect stings can be prevented with 98% efficacy with venom immunotherapy. The indications for therapy are simply a positive history (of systemic reaction to stings) and positive venom skin tests (or RAST), although the severity of previous reactions and age are also important variables (Table 3). Venom immunotherapy, and therefore skin testing, is not considered necessary for low-risk patients because over 90% will never have a systemic reaction, such as in persons with large local reactions and in children with cutaneous systemic reactions.

Venom immunotherapy should begin with all of the venoms giving a positive skin test and follows a dose schedule described in the product package insert (ALK Laboratories; Hollister-Stier Laboratories). Injections are generally administered weekly for 8 to 26 weeks, to achieve the full maintenance dose of 100 μg of each venom. This dose is then maintained every 4 weeks for at least 1 year, then every 6 weeks for 1 to 2 years and every 6 to 8 weeks thereafter. During immunotherapy, systemic reactions occur in 5% to 15% of cases, with variable degrees of urticaria, airway obstruction, or hypotension. The majority of such reactions are mild, but some require aggressive treatment for anaphylaxis. Venom injections also cause large local reactions in many patients during the first few months of therapy. All reactions are much less common during maintenance treatment. The frequency of systemic reactions to venom immunotherapy is no different from that observed during immunotherapy with inhalant allergens, and there are no known nonallergic or long-term side effects. Periodic monitoring of venom skin test or RAST sensitivity is recommended every 2 to 5 years to determine possible early discontinuation of therapy. The level of venom-specific IgG antibodies has been correlated with clinical protection and may be measured during the first 1 to 4 years of venom immunotherapy, especially to determine whether protection is maintained when maintenance intervals are prolonged.

The duration of venom immunotherapy remains a matter of judgment. The product package insert advises that venom immunotherapy should be continued indefinitely. Venom skin tests become negative in only 20% to 25% of patients treated for 5 years but in 50% to 60% treated for 7 to 10 years. When venom immunotherapy is stopped after at least 5 years of maintenance treatment, the chance of reaction to a sting returns to 10% for each sting that occurs, even 10 to 15 years after stopping, even if there are uneventful intervening stings and even if skin tests become negative. The cumulative risk of reaction after discontinuing treatment returns to almost 20% after 10 years off therapy, but the risk of a very severe reaction exists primarily in the patients who had such a reaction before treatment. Patients with a very severe history should therefore consider remaining on therapy indefinitely. Another high-risk subgroup of patients who should consider remaining on treatment even after 5 years are those who had a systemic reaction during treatment, whether to an injection or a sting. Both the relapse rate, and level of venom-specific IgE (or skin test), are higher in patients who stop therapy after only 3 years compared with 5 years. Some investigators have suggested that lower-risk patients (e.g., children and mild reactors) might be able to safely stop after 3 years of treatment, but published data are limited.

TABLE 3. **Patients With Low Risk for Anaphylaxis**

Minimal (<5%)	General adult population
	Patients on venom immunotherapy
	Children with cutaneous systemic reactions
Low (5%–10%)	Patients with large local reactions
	Discontinued venom immunotherapy after 5 years

ACKNOWLEDGMENT

This work was supported by National Institutes of Health grant AI08270.

Section 12

Diseases of the Skin

ACNE VULGARIS AND ROSACEA

method of
GUY WEBSTER, M.D., PH.D.
*Jefferson Medical College
Philadelphia, Pennsylvania*

ACNE VULGARIS

Acne vulgaris is a common and variable disease that afflicts nearly all adolescents and adults at some time in their lives. Although not medically dangerous, the cutaneous scars, as well as the emotional ones, can last a lifetime. Studies exist documenting numerous psychological problems stemming from acne, even to the point of causing decreased employability in adulthood. Fortunately, acne is eminently treatable.

Pathogenesis

A sensible approach to therapy cannot exist without some understanding of the disease's pathogenesis. Acne is truly multifactorial, involving abnormal keratinization, hormonal function, and immune hypersensitivity, and each defect provides a potential target for therapy.

Acne is limited to the pilosebaceous follicles of the head and upper trunk. The primary lesion is the *comedo,* an impaction and distention of the follicle with improperly desquamated keratinocytes and sebum. The stimulus for comedogenesis is unknown. At puberty, when androgens stimulate sebum production, comedones become engorged and enlarge to the point of visibility. Subsequently, some individuals begin to show signs of inflammation as well. Inflammatory acne is the result of the host response to the follicular inhabitant *Propionibacterium acnes*, which is a member of the normal flora and is a harmless commensal, largely incapable of tissue invasion. The level of anti–*P. acnes* immunity is proportional to the severity of acne inflammation and appears to be causal. The response has many characteristics of hypersensitivity, rather than a necessary immune defense against a pathogen.

Treatment

The first step in the treatment of any disease is to determine the severity of the problem. In diseases such as diabetes and hypertension, severity can be measured and response to treatment followed with quantifiable markers. This is only partially the case in acne. Severity is often overestimated by the patient and minimized by the doctor. Teenagers in particular are stigmatized by fairly trivial acne: in their eyes, severe acne can mean ruination. Thus, simple pimple counts are only partially useful; it is of little benefit to clear 95 of 100 lesions if the patient is left with several large nodules. Grading schemes that rely solely on lesion counts are of greater use in clinical studies than in clinical practice. I prefer to focus on the most severe lesions because adequate treatment for them covers all lesser pimples. For the purposes of clinical practice, acne classification can be condensed to just a few categories: purely comedonal (i.e., noninflammatory acne); mild, pustular, scarring papular; and nodular.

Patients (and their parents) usually need to have a few common misconceptions addressed before treatment begins. The misconceptions share the feature of blaming the patient for the disease and are to be avoided. Above all, patients (and parents) need to realize that cleanliness has nothing to do with acne. The black tip of a comedo is oxidized sebum, not dirt, and cannot be removed by scrubbing. Vigorous washing may actually make things worse. Second, parental admonitions notwithstanding, diet has never been shown to affect acne. Finally, stress reduction does not play a big role in controlling the disease.

Comedonal Acne

Noninflammatory acne is the mildest form of disease but can be the hardest to treat. Comedones are usually firmly ensconced in the follicle and, untreated, cannot be expressed without some risk of scarring. Topical tretinoin (Retin-A) (retinoic acid) cream is the standard against which all other anticomedonal agents are compared. Applied once or twice daily, it inhibits comedo formation and clears even severe comedonal acne in a few months. The only significant drawback is that irritation is greatest after a few weeks, and it usually does not require intervention. If desired, a moisturizing lotion may be prescribed. Because their skin is inherently irritable, patients with atopic diseases may not tolerate topical tretinoin even with moisturization. Other drugs are also useful for noninflammatory acne. Adapalene (Differin) is a naphthoic acid derivative that binds to nuclear retinoid receptors. It is effective for comedonal acne and also has a measure of anti-inflammatory activity. It appears to be equivalent to topical tretinoin but with somewhat less irritation.

Tazarotene (Tazorac) is a potent anticomedonal cream that is only slightly more irritating than tretinoin. Azelaic acid (Azelex) is a dicarboxylic acid that has both antibacterial and comedolytic effects. Topical application is effective in reducing comedones, and it is the least irritating of the preparations. The side effect of hypopigmentation may be desirable in some patients.

Inflammatory Acne

TOPICAL THERAPY

Mild papulopustular acne rarely results in scarring and typically is responsive to aggressive twice-daily topical therapy. Usually, two drugs are prescribed, an antibacterial and a comedolytic (discussed in the preceding paragraph). Benzoyl peroxide from 2.5% to 10% is an extraordinarily effective anti–*P. acnes* drug. Its major disadvantage is irritation, which can be minimized by using lower concentrations in a cream. Topical erythromycin and clindamycin (Cleocin T) are available as alcoholic solutions, lotions, creams, and gels, all of which are about equally effective. Acne that does not respond to erythromycin is usually also resistant to clindamycin. A combination of erythromycin and benzoyl peroxide in gel form is often found to be superior to topical antibiotic alone. Azelaic acid 20% cream is also an effective alternative to topical macrolide preparations.

During the past 2 decades, several reports have documented the acquisition of antibiotic resistance by *P. acnes* during acne therapy, most commonly with topical clindamycin and erythromycin. Extracutaneous infections with resistant organisms resulting from acne therapy have not been reported. Relatively resistant *P. acnes* strains are more commonly seen in acne that is refractory to therapy, but not always. When resistance is suspected, culture and susceptibility testing is not needed because therapeutic failure in acne should automatically prompt a change in medication. The addition of benzoyl peroxide to the topical regimen is the easiest way to eliminate resistant organisms.

ORAL THERAPY

Acne that is resistant to topical treatment or that manifests as scarring or nodular lesions typically requires oral antibiotics to improve. Many of the antibiotics useful in treating acne also have an anti-inflammatory activity in the disease, which is nearly as important as the anti–*P. acnes* effect. Many physicians prefer to begin using tetracycline or erythromycin at 1 g/d in divided dosage. I find this drug to be often insufficient and usually begin with doxycycline (Doryx) or minocycline (Dynacin) at 100 to 200 mg/d. Most patients are significantly improved after 4 to 6 weeks. Patients are instructed to take the medication with food, a maneuver that minimizes stomach complaints and maximizes compliance at the cost of a slight decrease in absorption. Patients should be warned that they may sunburn more easily. Oral antibiotic therapy may be continued for months or years with little concern, given the decades-long track record of these drugs in treating acne.

If, for some reason, minocycline or doxycycline cannot be used, reasonable alternatives include trimethoprim-sulfamethoxazole (Bactrim, Septra),* clarithromycin (Biaxin),* azithromycin (Zithromax),* and ciprofloxacin (Cipro).* Long-term acquisition of resistance to these drugs has not been studied. In general, cephalosporins and penicillins are not very effective in acne therapy. The increased cost of some of these newer drugs may make using tretinoin an attractive option if long-term treatment is needed.

Because all acne begins with follicular impaction, it is appropriate to add a topical comedolytic such as tretinoin, azelaic acid, or adapalene to oral antibiotics, and most patients greatly benefit from it. Even with combination therapy, the physician should expect at least 4 to 6 weeks to pass before seeing maximal improvement.

Isotretinoin. Isotretinoin (Accutane) revolutionized the therapy of severe acne about 20 years ago. For the first time, a short course of medication was able to control severe acne and change the course of disease even after the drug was discontinued. Isotretinoin is a synthetic retinoid that inhibits sebaceous gland differentiation, corrects the keratinization defect in the follicle, and also has a measure of anti-inflammatory activity. Its major indication is severe nodular acne, but it is commonly used for significant acne that is resistant to oral antibiotics as well.

Side effects of isotretinoin are mostly dose related and are not always trivial. Most patients complain of dry skin, lips, and eyes. In dry seasons, it is common to see epistaxis and flares of atopic dermatitis due to the drug. About one third of patients show an elevation in triglyceride levels during the first month of therapy. Usually, dietary modification or dosage reduction keeps the triglyceride level from rising too high. Thinning of hair occurs infrequently but can be particularly distressing. Hair usually regrows after the drug is discontinued.

Patients with severely inflamed lesions may have a severe flare of disease accompanied by systemic complaints similar to those seen in serum sickness. Administration of prednisone, 20 to 40 mg/d, at the initiation of isotretinoin therapy is sensible in selected severe cases. Rarely, patients complain of myalgias while taking isotretinoin and show significant elevations of creatinine kinase and transaminase levels. Because creatinine kinase measurement is rarely ordered, hepatitis is often incorrectly diagnosed. Restriction of exercise and reduction of dosage usually correct the problem. Depression is another rare, but reported, adverse effect of isotretinoin. A convincing linkage to the drug has not been documented. Dosage reduction or discontinuation usually is required.

Isotretinoin is listed as a drug capable of causing pseudotumor cerebri, although tenuously, because most patients with pseudotumor related to isotretinoin use were also treated concurrently with a tetracycline, a well-established cause of the problem. It is therefore contraindicated to co-administer the two medications. Patients with a history of pseudotumor from another medication have safely taken isotretinoin without recurrence of disease.

The most feared side effect of isotretinoin is its teratogenicity. A majority of fetuses developing during isotretinoin therapy are severely malformed. Two means of birth control, hormonal or surgical and

*Not FDA approved for this indication.

barrier, are required for all fertile women taking the drug and should be continued for one menstrual period after therapy is stopped. It is now clear that after a course of isotretinoin, fertility and development are normal. There are no known deleterious effects on the fertility of male patients.

Some laboratory monitoring is required during treatment. A lipid panel, sequential multiple analyzer 12/60, complete blood cell count, and pregnancy test are sufficient pretreatment tests. At 1 month, tests are repeated, and if the results are normal, only the pregnancy test need be repeated each month unless the dosage is increased. The correct dosage of isotretinoin is a matter of some controversy, and clearly, there is a point at which greater efficacy is outweighed by increased side effects. I prefer to use 0.75 to 1 mg/kg/d. Lower dosages often require longer than the standard 4 or 5 months of treatment and have a higher long-term failure rate.

Hormonal Therapy. It is clear that virilized women have a higher incidence of acne, but it is mistaken to assume that any woman with acne has a hormonal derangement. In fact, the majority of hyperandrogenic women do not have significant acne. Treatment-resistant acne, especially in a woman with irregular menses, should be investigated with at least measurements of total and free testosterone as well as dehydroepiandrosterone sulfate. If these substances are elevated, two approaches may be taken: suppression with either low-dose oral corticosteroid or oral contraceptives. Currently, levonorgestrel–ethinyl estradiol (Triphasil) is the only contraceptive approved for acne therapy.

Acne and Pregnancy

No drugs can be unequivocally guaranteed to be safe in pregnancy, but several have come into general use in this situation. Erythromycin, topical or oral, is usually thought to be safe, although it is often poorly tolerated in patients whose lower esophageal sphincter is already relaxed. Benzoyl peroxide rapidly decomposes into benzoic acid and hydrogen peroxide and is certainly safe for use during pregnancy. Topical tretinoin use in pregnancy is theoretically safe because vitamin A blood levels do not change with topical therapy, but many doctors recommend it be avoided until after childbirth.

ROSACEA

Rosacea is largely limited to the fair-skinned, easily blushing patient. Early disease may simply be a more persistent blush on the cheeks or a fixed telangiectasia. Inflammatory papules that resemble acne, but lack a comedo, arise in some and often become granulomatous. Sebaceous hyperplasia is common and reaches its zenith on the nose, where a knobby, swollen overgrowth known as *rhinophyma* may develop. (The actor W.C. Fields is a great example.) About 50% of rosacea patients have significant ocular involvement, which may range from mild conjunctivitis to styes, hordeola, and even corneal damage.

Diet clearly plays a role in rosacea, but food never gave anyone the disease. Anything that increases blood flow to the face makes rosacea worse. Spicy food, hot food, and alcohol are most commonly identified as triggers, but it is hard to document that abstinence will ultimately make a difference for the patient.

Rosacea may be treated topically using metronidazole (MetroGel, Noritate) or azelaic acid. Available as a cream or gel, this preparation helps in mild to moderate inflammatory disease. The physician should allow about 6 weeks of therapy before switching to a stronger drug.

Topical steroids are often used to treat rosacea, a practice that should be discouraged. Although initially responsive to weak compounds, the rosacea quickly exhibits tachyphylaxis, requiring stronger and stronger preparations that both damage facial skin and eventually potentiate the rosacea.

Oral antibiotics are often the best therapy for severe rosacea and are most effective in ocular rosacea. Tetracyclines work best, but erythromycin may occasionally be useful. I generally prescribe doxycycline or minocycline (Minocin)* 100 mg twice daily for 1 or 2 months and then taper the dosage to daily or alternate-day dosing. Because the drug probably acts more as an anti-inflammatory than as an antibiotic, these low dosages are not as homeopathic as they might seem.

*Not FDA approved for this indication.

HAIR DISORDERS

method of
ELISE A. OLSEN, M.D.
Duke University Medical Center
Durham, North Carolina

The effective treatment of hair loss is totally dependent on the diagnostic acumen of the observing physician. Just as in cutaneous medicine in general, there are genetic, inflammatory, hormonally related, autoimmune-driven, infectious, and self-induced types of alopecia. Diagnosis can largely be made through history and physical examination, with the additional aids of a microscope and a few blood tests. Only occasionally is a scalp biopsy necessary to make a diagnosis of hair loss, and usually this is merely confirmatory.

The most important parts of the evaluation of the scalp are listed:

1. Determination of a patchy (or patterned) loss versus diffuse (evenly distributed or global) loss
2. Scarring versus nonscarring hair loss
3. Abnormal hair shedding versus breakage
4. Inflammatory versus noninflammatory changes of the scalp.

Mere observation of the scalp can determine the pattern of loss and whether scale, erythema, or induration exists. In nonscarring loss, the follicular openings are obvious on the scalp, even without hairs physically in the follicles. In scarring loss, this finding is absent, leaving slick areas where viable follicles once resided.

To help establish whether an abnormal amount of shedding is occurring, a hair pull is performed. This is done by grasping clumps of 25 to 50 hairs close to the scalp and gently pulling to the distal ends. Normally, six to eight such hair pulls should net no more than two to five telogen hairs. The proximal ends of the hair so collected should then be evaluated microscopically to confirm that they are indeed telogen and not distorted anagen hairs. *Anagen* (or actively growing) hairs have a malleable pigmented proximal end and are not normally removed with a hair pull. *Telogen* (resting) hairs have a nonpigmented proximal "club" end. Anagen shedding and telogen shedding stem from different etiologic factors and require different evaluations. The distal ends of the hairs obtained by a hair pull can also be evaluated to determine whether breakage is present and, if so, what type. This helps to further delineate the etiology of the hair loss.

Scalp biopsies are done primarily to confirm a scarring alopecia and to determine the subtype. Scalp biopsies may also be done to differentiate patchy alopecia areata from trichotillomania or to differentiate pattern hair loss in women from diffuse alopecia areata and telogen effluvium. There are a very few independently diagnostic scalp biopsies of alopecia. Because of this, scalp biopsies should be done only by those with a knowledge of the differential diagnosis involved and interpreted only by dermatopathologists experienced in the assessment of scalp pathology. To do less makes this an expensive and usually worthless exercise.

Most types of alopecia can be readily diagnosed and have effective therapeutic options for the control and/or reversal of the clinical abnormality (Table 1). The discussion that follows addresses only the most common forms of potentially reversible alopecia.

TABLE 1. **Differential Diagnosis of Nonscarring Hair Loss**

Diffuse
Breakage
Anagen effluvium
Hair shaft disorder
Physical or chemical processing
Telogen effluvium
Female pattern hair loss
Alopecia areata
Loose anagen syndrome
Failure of, or abnormal, hair production
Focal
Breakage
Infection
Trauma
Trichotillomania
Hair shaft disorder
Physical or chemical processing
Male pattern hair loss
Female pattern hair loss
Alopecia areata
Loose anagen syndrome
Developmental

TELOGEN EFFLUVIUM

Abnormal shedding of scalp hair can occur as a result of an increase in the percentage of telogen hairs. This is a very common problem, probably accounting for more than 40% of women with hair loss presenting to physicians. Normally constituting 10% of the scalp hair, telogen (or resting) hairs are shed with usual daily hair traction (brushing, shampooing) secondary to their relative lack of physical anchors in the scalp compared with anagen hairs. An increase in the percentage of telogen hairs, rarely beyond 50% of the total, may occur as a reaction to a variety of medical or psychological insults or with certain drugs (notably β-blockers, anticoagulants, and retinoids). The scalp is otherwise normal. The hair loss is diffuse or global on the scalp, an important differentiating point from female pattern hair loss.

Because the hair loss usually presents 3 to 4 months after the inciting event and many stresses are of brief duration, the patient typically presents at the time of worst loss and, unless the promoter of hair loss is still present, improvement generally follows over the next 6 to 12 months. All such patients should be screened for a potential underlying thyroid disorder, iron deficiency, and/or anemia, and all concomitant drugs should be considered potential offenders. In women, hormonal changes, such as going on or off an oral contraceptive pill, may trigger increased telogen shedding. Treatment is generally directed at the underlying offender, not the hair loss itself. However, in cases in which no obvious explanation is available and the problem is persistent, topical minoxidil (Rogaine) 2% or 5% applied twice daily may be of some benefit.

PATTERN HAIR LOSS

Male pattern hair loss (or male pattern baldness) is an androgen-dependent, hereditary type of alopecia that occurs in 50% of men or more. The onset is usually in the third and fourth decades but can begin as early as puberty. Affected men develop a recession and resculpturing of the frontotemporal hair line as well as loss of hair on the top and vertex of the scalp: this can proceed to frank baldness. The degree of hair loss is directly correlated to the shortening of anagen duration, increased percentage hairs in telogen, and the degree of miniaturization of the follicles in the involved area. Male pattern baldness appears to be dihydrotestosterone (DHT) related.

Patterned hair loss in women may also occur as early as puberty but generally presents either in the third to fourth decade or in the fifth decade. Women, unlike men, have a more generalized thinning of the hair over the top of the scalp often with accentuation toward the frontal scalp in a "Christmas tree" pattern. The process in women also involves progressive miniaturization of the involved hair follicles, but the miniaturization is not as extensive or uniform in a given area as in men: bald areas do not generally develop in women with this process. Abnormal telogen shedding, if present, is generally only a transient part of the clinical picture. In women with irregular periods, acne, or hirsutism, it is reasonable to screen with a serum dehydroepiandrosterone sulfate (DHEA-S) and free or total testosterone test: female pattern hair loss can be caused by androgen excess alone without a hereditary history of pattern hair loss. If androgens are elevated, further workup may be indicated. Most women with female pattern hair loss will, however, have none of these other signs of hyperandrogenism and results of an androgen screen will be normal.

Treatment of both men and women with pattern hair loss can be with either a hair growth promoter or hair transplants. The only hair growth promoter approved by the Food and Drug Administration (FDA) for both men and women is 2% topical minoxidil. This medication must be applied a minimum of twice a day to the scalp (less is subthreshold for response), with the earliest clinical response seen at about 6 months and a maximum response at 1 year. Only 20% to 25% of subjects will have notable regrowth, and generally these are the men and women whose involved hairs are finer than normal but not minuscule at treatment onset. Most patients will experience at least a stabilization of loss. Topical minoxidil 5% (Rogaine Extra-Strength) is currently approved for use in men with male pattern baldness and appears to have enhanced efficacy in men without additional safety concerns. In women who use 5% topical minoxidil there is a slight increased incidence (still <5%) of facial hypertrichosis over the 2% preparation, which may be related to either inadvertent facial exposure or to low blood levels of minoxidil in sensitive patients. Hypertrichosis is completely reversible when the drug is stopped.

Surgical treatment for androgenetic alopecia has dramatically improved in recent years. Donor dominance allows continued growth of hair transferred from the portions of the scalp genetically immune to hereditary thinning to those areas exhibiting baldness. Cosmetic coverage is limited by the amount and thickness of available donor hair and the expertise of the surgeon. Male candidates for this procedure should be those whose balding process is no longer active. A combination of standard 4-mm plugs of donor hair and/or minigrafts (1.5–2.5-mm grafts) and micrografts (1–2 hairs each graft) are used to fill in areas of baldness. The micrografts are particularly useful because they do not require removal of a plug of tissue to insert the graft into but rather a slit can be made to accommodate a single or a few donor hairs. Micrografts also make the transplantation process significantly less obvious than that seen with standard plugs. Micrografts are the surgical treatment of choice in women with female pattern hair loss who, unlike men, never develop complete baldness and for whom the use of standard hair transplants means a loss of recipient tissue that still has hair.

Drugs that block either the enzyme 5α-reductase type II alone or are joint 5α-reductase type I/II blockers have been shown to be effective in male pattern hair loss. Of 18- to 41-year-old men with Hamilton-Norwood patterns III_v, IV, or V of hair loss who were treated with 1 mg of finasteride (Propecia) daily, 50% showed a clinical increase in hair growth at 1 year and two thirds at 2 years of treatment. Side effects were minimal and limited to a slight increase in sexual adverse events, including decreased libido, erectile dysfunction, and ejaculation disorder in those on finasteride versus placebo (3.8% versus 2.1%, respectively). Five-year data show that use of finasteride long term has a stabilizing effect on hair loss.

Women of childbearing potential with female pattern hair loss have not been evaluated in a clinical trial of a systemic 5α-reductase inhibitor because of the risk of abnormal genital development in male fetuses exposed to this enzyme inhibitor. Postmenopausal women with female pattern hair loss who were treated for 1 year with finasteride did not show any improvement compared with placebo. Whether female pattern hair loss in postmenopausal women is different from that presenting in premenopausal women is unknown, but this clearly speaks to different etiologic factors in this age group of affected women compared with younger men with male pattern hair loss.

For women with female pattern hair loss who have evidence of androgen excess or hypersensitivity, the use of medications that either block the production or the cellular utilization of androgens may be helpful. Combination oral contraceptive pills that use a nonandrogenic progestin (such as norgestimate) decrease both ovarian and adrenal production of androgens. Systemic antiandrogens such as spironolactone (Aldactone),* in doses of 100 mg or more daily, and flutamide (Eulexin),* 250 to 500 mg daily, have shown effectiveness in small numbers of hirsute women with concomitant female pattern hair loss. Spironolactone is a potassium-sparing diuretic whose main side effects are hyperkalemia, irregular menses, and breast tenderness/bloating. Flutamide users must be monitored for potential hepatotoxicity. Because both drugs can cause feminization of a male fetus, they should be used only in women of nonchildbearing potential or in those women who are using effective contraception, preferably combination oral contraceptives.

ALOPECIA AREATA

Alopecia areata presents as patches of hair loss on the scalp with variable amounts of hair loss else-

*Not FDA approved for this indication.

where. The scalp is otherwise normal. Telogen hair shedding is increased in areas of hair loss with "exclamation point" hairs present in areas of active loss. The latter are short (<¼ inch) pigmented hairs that are broader at the tip than the base (the opposite of normal new hair growth) and are pathognomonic of alopecia areata. Some cases of alopecia areata are more diffuse (global) versus patchy on the scalp and can mimic a telogen or anagen effluvium. In these cases, a biopsy can be useful. A peribulbar chronic inflammatory infiltrate with sparing of the "bulge" area near the sebaceous gland is confirmatory evidence of alopecia areata.

Current effective treatments can be divided into three major categories: corticosteroids (or other immunosuppressive agents), topical irritants/allergens, and nonspecific hair growth promoters. Those patients with patchy scalp alopecia areata (the vast majority) are usually best served by an externally directed approach first. Intralesional (intradermal) corticosteroids are very effective in doses of 3 to 10 mg/mL of triamcinolone, usually showing subtle hair growth by 1 month after injection. Injections are painful, however, and should be repeated monthly until hair growth is complete. Intralesional corticosteroids can lead to depressions in the scalp surface secondary to inadvertent injection into the subcutaneous tissue or too high a concentration (this is generally reversible over time) as well as potential systemic effects when given repetitively over several months. Eyebrows can also be injected, but with utilization of the lower concentrations (3–5 mg/mL) of corticosteroid secondary to the greater risk of atrophy in these areas.

Topical corticosteroids are easy to use and to tolerate and are very effective for patients with patchy alopecia, whether limited or extensive in scope. The key to their effective use lies in consistent daily application of a mid- to high-potency corticosteroid through complete regrowth and beyond. I generally employ in adults a mid- to high-potency (class 1–3) corticosteroid in a solution or lotion vehicle, the latter to facilitate application to slick areas as well as areas with partial hair regrowth. Signs of regrowth are generally first apparent 3 to 4 months after topical treatment: a 25% regrowth is typical at this time point. With continued application, hair growth will gradually fill in. Treatment should be continued in a tapering fashion 3 to 6 months after clearing to prevent fallout of newly regrown hair. Children can also use midpotency corticosteroids topically on the scalp (this only represents approximately 3% body surface area) without development of systemic side effects: diprosone lotion is an ideal preparation, being a class 5 corticosteroid. Patients should avoid letting the topical agent drift down onto the face because this can lead to hair growth on the face and acne, both reversible conditions. Other classes of topical immunosuppressive agents are being developed, including FK506*: these may be effective alternative treatments for alopecia areata but have not been specifically tested.

*Investigational drug in the United States.

Systemic corticosteroids are always more effective in alopecia areata than intralesional or topical corticosteroids but have the risk of systemic side effects. Some cases of extensive or rapidly progressive alopecia areata, however, require systemic corticosteroids for either curtailment of hair loss or induction of hair growth. To minimize side effects, this is best served by a taper of prednisone* over a minimum of 6 to 8 weeks beginning at 40 mg/d or less in an adult. Patients *must* be on a concurrent topical regimen (not topical irritants or allergens) because the doses of prednisone fall below 10 to 20 mg/d and must be continued on this well beyond the end of the systemic taper: without this, approximately 50% of patients with systemic corticosteroid-initiated hair growth will experience fallout of the newly regrown hair. Cyclosporine (Sandimmune)* is another systemic immunosuppressive agent that has been effective in inducing hair growth in alopecia areata; however, its profile of side effects make it even less desirable to use in this setting than systemic corticosteroids.

The induction of contact dermatitis (irritant or allergic) in areas of alopecia will often induce hair growth in alopecia areata. Agents that can be used to this end include irritants such as anthralin or the allergens DNCB, diphencyprone (DPCP), squaric acid dibutylester, or *Rhus* antigen. Irritants require no prior induction of allergy and anthralin is more readily available in the United States than the other aforementioned chemicals. Anthralin (Anthra-Derm)* is FDA approved for the treatment of psoriasis, which notably, in a dose-dependent fashion, is irritating to nonpsoriatic skin. It can be used very effectively in alopecia areata in 0.5% to 1% concentrations applied daily to the involved areas of hair loss. Hair growth can be effectively induced by achieving a threshold minimal irritation (vs. blatant dermatitis), so that the length of application (15 minutes to overnight) is tailored to the time necessary to achieve this reaction, a time that is variable in each patient. The time course to signs of regrowth with anthralin is, as with topical corticosteroids, usually 3 to 4 months. Patients should be warned that a purple discoloration could occur in treated areas where the medicine is incompletely removed and can persistently discolor nails that come in contact with the medicine. The concomitant use of topical corticosteroids to ameliorate or modify irritation should be avoided because these two therapies presumably work through diametrically opposed mechanisms and co-treatment can be counterproductive.

PUVA may work in alopecia areata as an externally directed immunosuppressive agent. It is an arduous treatment and one best used in patients with very extensive alopecia areata. The initiation of hair growth may take 40 to 80 treatments and complete regrowth 1 to 2 years. However, PUVA is often effective when "all else" has failed. Potential risks include

*Not FDA approved for this indication.

acute erythema, PUVA lentigos, and skin cancer (including melanoma), the latter usually identified years later. Patients should be screened with an antinuclear antibody (phototoxicity is an issue here) and eye examination. Protective glasses must be worn for 24 hours after psoralen treatment to protect the eyes from the risk of cataracts or retinal damage.

A third possibility for treatment of alopecia areata is the category of drugs known as hair growth promoters, of which topical minoxidil is the prototype. Data suggest that 5% topical minoxidil can be an effective single agent in limited patchy alopecia areata or as an adjuvant to systemic corticosteroid or topical anthralin use in the treatment of more extensive alopecia areata.

TRICHOTILLOMANIA

Patients with trichotillomania are usually adolescents, primarily girls, who generally present with a history of inexplicable treatment-refractory hair loss. The hair loss is generally patchy, although it can be diffuse, and consists of a decrease in the density of hair as well as scattered short hairs generally 1 to 2 mm in length in the affected area. Examination of the remaining hairs, which generally must be removed by a forcible hair pluck versus hair pull, reveals anagen hairs with broken, tapered, or cut distal ends: the broken ends reflect the breakage associated with pulling anagen hairs, tapered tips reflect newly regrowing hairs, and the cut ends reflect the not uncommon habit of these children to cut, if not pull out, their hair.

Trichotillomania is not a diagnosis likely to be supported by history because usually the child is not prepared to be honest regarding the etiology and the distraught parents are generally clueless and actually defensive about the potential self-induced nature of this problem. Confirmatory evidence can be produced by a scalp biopsy in an affected area that will show an increase in catagen hairs, pigment casts in the isthmus or infundibular area of the follicle, and damaged or empty follicles. Treatment requires acceptance of the diagnosis by the child and parents, reassurance that this is not necessarily evidence of a life-long disabling psychiatric disorder, and referral for counseling.

TINEA CAPITIS

Tinea capitis is a common problem that can occur at any age but is most common in poor African-American children. There are three clinical presentations: (1) a seborrhea-like scale on the scalp with thinning of the hair in the involved areas, (2) areas of noninflammatory, nonscaly alopecia with hairs broken off flush or near flush to the scalp (so-called black-dot ringworm), and (3) inflammation and induration of the scalp with associated hair loss that can progress, in extreme cases, to a kerion. Potassium hydroxide (KOH) preparation is less likely, especially in cases of inflammatory tinea, to be positive than a culture: both should be done. A positive KOH generally demonstrates spores versus hyphae. The most common causative agent in the United States is *Trichophyton tonsurans.*

Treatment must be systemic, although 2.5% selenium sulfide shampoo* or 2% ketoconazole shampoo two to three times per week is an effective adjuvant that decreases shedding of viable spores. Griseofulvin (Fulvicin), in doses of 10 to 25 mg/kg given with a fatty meal (glass of milk) for at least 8 weeks is effective in most cases. Side effects are infrequent but include headaches, gastrointestinal disturbances, and photosensitivity. A fungal culture should be negative before discontinuation of treatment.

Ketoconazole (Nizoral)* is a much less effective drug for tinea capitis than griseofulvin. The triazoles, either fluconazole (Diflucan),* in doses of 5 to 6 mg/kg or itraconazole (Sporanox)* or terbinafine (Lamisil),* in a standard dosing regimen by weight (<20 kg = 62.5 mg/d, 20–40 kg = 125 mg/d, and >40 kg = 250 mg/d) are effective alternative treatments of tinea capitis when given daily for 4 weeks. Itraconazole can also be dosed at 3 to 5 mg/kg/d for 1 week, with repeat courses every 2 to 3 weeks for an additional 1 to 3 pulses. The triazoles have a greater potential for drug-drug interactions because they affect the cytochrome P-450 system. Household and other close contacts should be checked for simultaneous infection and treated: to not do so invites incomplete eradication or recurrence of infection in the proband.

*Not FDA approved for this indication.

CANCER OF THE SKIN

method of
LEONARD DZUBOW, M.D., and
EYAL K. LEVIT, M.D.
University of Pennsylvania
Philadelphia, Pennsylvania

Nonmelanoma skin cancers account for over a third of all cancers in the United States. They are the most common cancers among whites worldwide. Over 95% of these are basal cell carcinoma (BCC) and squamous cell carcinoma (SCC). Their incidence is estimated between 0.9 and 1.2 million new cases per year. BCC accounts for 80%, with the remaining 20% being SCC.

The pathogenic mechanism is most likely related to the malignant transformation of keratinocytes in a monoclonal fashion. Damage to DNA, due to mutated tumor suppressor gene (especially high frequency of ultraviolet [UV] light–induced mutations of the *p53* tumor suppressor gene and/or activation of oncogenes as *ras* proto-oncogenes), if uncorrected, leads to the initiation of a "weakened" cell. On further exposure to carcinogens, months or years later, a second "hit" to the "weak" cell promotes the progression into a malignantly transformed cell. This theory is known as the "two (or multiple)-hit theory."

Today, as more carcinogens involved in the pathogenesis of skin cancer are identified, it is imperative that physicians educate patients about their existence. A preventive approach through identifying premalignant skin cancers as actinic keratoses and informing patients about possible carcinogenic factors is important. A lag of about 20 years between the initial exposure to carcinogens and the appearance of clinically evident malignancy hinders such tasks. The use of a variety of products to halt the initiation or promotion of the "weakened cell" into a transformed malignant cell seems promising. Such products include antioxidants, corticosteroids, and free radical scavengers, such as vitamin C, vitamin E, selenium, and retinoids. These agents may help halt the initiation phase of tumor progression. The tumor promotion phase could be slowed by antiproliferative drugs or antioxidants such as protease inhibitors (e.g., leupepin*), as well as a diet high in retinoic acid, vitamin D, and green tea.

Once a skin cancer has appeared, definitive treatment is needed.

BCC is the most common skin cancer type, with incidence ranging from 1/100 in Australia and 146 to 317/100,000 in the United States. It usually affects middle-aged whites, although prepubertal lesions can appear in certain genodermatoses such as basal cell nevus syndrome, xeroderma pigmentosum, and albinism, among others. The most commonly involved sites are the head and neck. BCC is only locally aggressive, with rare metastases in less than 0.005% of patients (usually enlarged, ulcerated, and recurrent tumors). It is estimated that once a person has one BCC there is a 47% chance of developing a second unrelated BCC within 3.5 years.

Although UV radiation plays a major role in the formation of BCC, unlike SCC, it is not related to the cumulative UV dosage. This is evident by the fact that 20% of BCCs occur in non–sun-exposed areas. Celtic ancestry (red/blond hair and blue eyes) and family history of skin cancer independently confer an increased risk of skin cancer. Outdoor occupation appears to propagate skin cancer rather than be an independent risk factor. Although chemical carcinogens such as arsenic, ionizing radiation, immunization scars, chronic ulcers, and immunosuppression can lead to BCCs, they more often promote the formation of SCCs.

Recent keratin studies support the origin of BCC from the hair follicle (outer root sheath below the isthmus). This explains why BCC, unlike SCC, occurs only on hair-bearing skin. Clinically, BCC often resembles a "pimple" or a "pearly" telangiectatic cyst that lasts over a month. Other forms appear as red scaly plaques, scarlike patches, or even brown to black pigmented papules. They often bleed on trauma and may be associated with itching.

SCC of the skin is the second most common skin cancer. Its incidence has been increasing by 4% to 8% per year. It is directly related to the cumulative UV exposure, with UVB (290–320 nm) wavelength (mostly blocked by the ozone layer) more so than UVA (320–400 nm). This explains why over 70% of SCCs occur on the sun-exposed regions of the head and neck. The reported incidence is higher in men than in women. In the United States each year, 156 new cases are reported in men and 100 new cases are reported in women per 100,000 population. The rate in African Americans is much lower, being 3 per 100,000, and is associated with burn scars rather than UV exposure.

SCC commonly occurs in middle-aged whites. The incidence of metastasis from sun-induced SCC ranges from 0.5% to 25%. This is less than that from SCC arising in a chronic ulcer, scar, or radiation dermatitis, which is 18% to 38%.

*Not available in the United States.

Although only 6% to 10% of actinic keratoses progress into SCC, 60% of SCC arise from an actinic keratosis that had been present at least 1 year earlier.

SCC clinically appears as a red scaly patch or nodule, at times with central erosions or ulcerations. When located on mucosal surfaces such as the lips or genitalia, they may look like whitish or red nonscaly patches or plaques. When SCC is associated with HPV, it may appear as a fungating verrucous lesion.

TREATMENT OPTIONS

Factors that should be considered when choosing a treatment modality include skin cancer location, size and duration, histologic type, and previous treatment. Patients' concurrent medical conditions should also be considered.

The main disadvantage of the first four mentioned modalities is the lack of tissue for histologic conformation. The outcome is thus highly variable and correlates with the choice of cancer treated as well as the clinical skill and experience of the operator.

Cryotherapy

This is a method that uses heat removed from tissue by application of cold. The most common cryogen material used is liquid nitrogen with a boiling point of −195.8°C. The liquid nitrogen is typically delivered from either a spray bottle or by using a cotton-tipped applicator. A proper procedure includes a rapid freeze and slow thaw repeated twice with a minimum temperature of −50°C at the base of the tumor. Rapid cooling leads to intracellular ice formation with subsequent cell lysis during thawing.

Patients allergic to local anesthesia, with anticipated poor wound healing, or necessitating a bloodless method, are excellent candidates for cryotherapy.

If used as a treatment for skin cancers, it is advisable to use thermocoupling electrodes that ensure proper freeze at the base of the tumor. Although this method is indispensable for precancerous lesions as actinic keratosis and can be used with BCC in experienced hands, it is not advisable for use in SCC because it may hide residual cancer that has a metastatic potential.

Electrodesiccation and Curettage

This method uses a medium-sized curet (a looplike metal with a handle and sharp edge on one side of the loop) to debulk the skin cancer. It relies on the fact that most skin cancers produce a gelatinous-like matrix that can be differentiated from the normal, hard dermis. This is followed immediately by electrodesiccation using a high-frequency, high-voltage, low-amperage damped current, which results in approximately 1 mm of surrounding tissue distraction. This process is repeated two more times with a smaller curet used to explore the base and margins for possible pockets of tumor. The use of the electrodesiccation provides a 3-mm margin (1 mm per step) beyond the skin cancer. Because the method depends on the differentiation of the soft tumor from the hard dermis it cannot be used for skin cancers that extend into fat. It is also very difficult to perform reliably over cartilaginous surfaces as the ear and nose. Because of the use of a current this method is better off avoided in patients with pacemakers, although the modern pacemakers are very well shielded from standard electrosurgical current. It should not be used in the perianal and oxygen enriched (close to a nasal canula) areas to avoid fire. The plume from the cautery is carcinogenic and may also carry viral particles.

In experienced hands a recurrence rate of less than 6% can be achieved for primary skin cancers that do not fit the criteria for Mohs surgery.

A resultant white, depressed, or hypertrophic scar may appear.

Radiation Therapy

This method uses ionizing radiation between 4000 and 7000 cGy, fractionated over 4 to 6 weeks, three to five times per week. We do not recommend this modality for patients younger than age 50 who are able to undergo one of the other-mentioned treatments because ionizing radiation is itself a nonselective DNA-damaging modality that can lead to future skin cancers. Depending on the location and fractionation, this may be a well-tolerated treatment with good to fair cosmetic results, albeit being time consuming.

Laser Surgery

Ablative surgery with laser resurfacing such as CO_2 or erbium:YAG is a blind technique that results in superficial burn. Although it may be used to treat precancerous lesions, it is not advised for the treatment of skin cancer because it may lead to an insufficient and superficial treatment, allowing a residual tumor to grow hidden beneath a scar.

Photodynamic therapy (PDT) is a modality that has been gaining acceptance in the treatment for bladder, esophageal, and lung cancer and, more recently, for superficial skin cancers and precancers. It uses the combination of a photosensitizer, which preferentially accumulates in malignant cells, and photoactivation by visible light to kill the tumor cells. The only currently Food and Drug Administration–approved chemical is photophrin, which is administered intravenously, costing over $2000 and resulting in an undesirable, generalized photosensitivity for a period of 2 months. Stage three clinical trials are ongoing with the use of a topical photosensitizer (5-aminolevulinic acid). Whereas this topical medication will allow for fewer side effects, it will also result in decreased cure rate, owing to the physical limitation of the cream's penetration depth. In one study, 50% of skin cancer showed residual tumor, with the recurrence rate in another study over 16% within 2.5 years.

Surgical Excision

A 4- to 5-mm margin is recommended around a BCC or SCC. Using this method one usually removes the skin cancer in an elliptical fashion and sends the specimen for pathologic evaluation. Because of the method used by the laboratory to process the specimen, it is impossible to examine all edges of the specimen received. A "clear" margin, thus, does not necessarily ensure clear margins, resulting at best in a 95% cure rate offered by this method for primary skin cancers. The advantage of this method, aside from providing a specimen for pathologic evaluation, is the ability to reconstruct the surgical defect immediately.

Mohs Micrographic Surgery

This method allows a 99% cure rate of SCC and BCC. It involves removing the skin cancer initially with less than a 1-mm margin. The tissue is then processed keeping the orientation it had on the patient. The processing is done by frozen section to allow examination of all skin edges. The Mohs surgeon/pathologist examines the cut sections under the microscope and maps out the involved edges. This map is used as a guide to the edges needing further attention. The surgeon removes only the involved edges taking a millimeter of skin at a time in the direction of the involved edge. The process is repeated until negative margins are achieved. The advantage of this method is the ability to provide the highest cure while having the smallest surgical defect (corresponding as closely as possible to the size of the original skin cancer).

Mohs surgery is especially indicated for cancers of long duration, located on cosmetically sensitive regions of the body such as the face, with a history of recurrence, and located on the "H" region of the face (midface and ears, where other therapeutic modalities show a 9%–18% 5-year recurrence). A lesion of greater than 2 cm (has a 26% recurrence if removed by regular excision) or with aggressive histology (morpheaform, micronodular, infiltrative) (12%–30% recurrence with other treatment modalities) should also be referred for Mohs surgery. The previous use of radiation therapy as a treatment of the cancer also may increase the aggressive nature of the cancer and require a more precise tissue-sparing technique, as is offered by the Mohs surgery.

Emerging Alternative Therapies

Recently, a number of immune and differentiation modulating creams have been used for superficial skin cancers. Because no sufficient long-term follow-up is available, their efficacy is still to be proven. These creams are listed below:

1. Imiquimod (Aldara)* is a 5% cream invented for the treatment of anogenital warts. It works by

*Not available in the United States.

increasing interferon alfa locally, which in turn increases the TH1 (cell-mediated) immune response. It is currently in study for superficial BCC only. It is applied three times per week for a period of 8 to 10 hours (usually at night). Side effects are mainly irritation and/or ulceration. Although it shows promise, there is no long-term follow-up. Patients may also develop significant irritation and itching at the treatment site, with resultant poor compliance.

2. Tazarotene (Tazorac)* is supplied as a 0.1% or 0.05% gel. It selectively binds to the retinoid receptors involved in the promotion of epithelial differentiation. A recent study using 0.1% gel daily for 5 to 8 months showed 100% improvement (decrease in size); 80% clearance of superficial BCC, and less than 30% clearance of nodular BCC. The study was small and lacked a long-term follow-up. Similar side effects are seen as with imiquimode.

3. Isotretinoin (Accutane)*: As chemotherapy, an oral dose of 4.5 mg/kg/d for 8 months shows a 10% complete clinical and histologic remission of BCC. As chemo*prevention,* an oral dose of 0.5 to 1.5 mg/kg/d is used. No new tumors are seen during the treatment period. No remission of present BCCs is seen on a chemoprevention regimen. Once the chemotherapy or chemoprevention is stopped (usually due to side effects) there is a rapid appearance of BCCs or "rebound."

4. The use of interferon alfa-2b (Intron A)* can give a 50% to 80% cure rate.

5. A new cream investigated for lymphoma called Targretin† may show promise in skin cancer treatment.

6. Because BCC is thought to arise from hair, it would be interesting to see whether the incidence of BCC would decrease in patients getting laser treatment for unwanted hair.

*Not FDA approved for this indication.
†Investigational drug in the United States.

CUTANEOUS T-CELL LYMPHOMAS

method of
PETER W. HEALD, M.D.
Yale University School of Medicine
New Haven, Connecticut

BIOLOGY OF CUTANEOUS T-CELL LYMPHOMA

The immunologic protection of the skin has antigen-specific and nonspecific components. T cells regulate the specific arm of the skin's immune system. Cutaneous T-cell responses are the function of a subgroup of T cells (aptly named "cutaneous T cells") that express specific homing affinities for the skin. One of the molecular mediators of skin homing has been delineated. T cells that express the cutaneous lymphoid antigen (CLA) are found in cutaneous lymphoid infiltrates but not in lymphoid infiltrates of other tissues. In addition, the malignant cells of cutaneous T-cell lymphoma (CTCL) have been shown to express CLA. The skin homing protein CLA binds to E-selectin. The latter is upregulated on endothelial cells in inflamed skin. Thus, the circulation contains a readily recruitable reserve of immune cells for skin-based reactions. After tethering to the endothelial cells, CLA expressing T cells migrate to the cutaneous site of inflammation. Cells can then reenter the circulation by way of the thoracic duct or in local lymph nodes. This model of cutaneous T-cell–based immunity explains why patients with this disease often have multifocal skin infiltrates with no readily detectable peripheral blood involvement.

Patients with CTCL present with inflammatory skin lesions of varying sizes, from 4 cm up to total-body erythroderma. One histologic finding is that the T-cell infiltrates will frequently show epidermotropism. Investigations have shown that while in the epidermis the malignant cells of CTCL often express markers of activation and cell division, implying that there is a crucial step in the life cycle of the cell occurring in the epidermis. Presumably the malignant cells traffic the same pathways as normal T cells, freely moving about the skin and the blood. Sophisticated molecular studies have demonstrated circulating malignant cells where routine staging tests reveal normal peripheral blood parameters. As immunologically active cells, the CTCL cells can produce cytokines that probably mediate the clinical findings of erythema, pruritus, and tissue and peripheral blood eosinophilia. As the disease progresses there are several changes that may occur. One is transformation to high-grade large cell lymphoma. This histologic change of the disease signals a much more aggressive course. Another is that normal immune cells senesce in the presence of the expanding lymphoma population. This incurs a state of immunosuppression from the disease and manifests itself as increased susceptibility to infection and second malignancies. The various components of the biology of CTCL: skin homing, activation in the epidermis, recirculation, cytokine production, immunosuppression, and transformation, all come to bear on the therapy of the disease. Undoubtedly, the varying degrees of these components in different patients create the clinical variants of CTCL.

STAGING

The goals of therapy are remission, palliation, and improvement of survival. Given the chronic nature of the disease, surrogate markers for survival are used in clinical trials. Tumor burden measurements and measures of palliation are the markers most commonly used. Skin score systems and health assessment questionnaires are the tools used to assess both discrete and global manifestations of the disease. The primary goal of therapy is to prolong life while an equally important goal is to improve the quality of life. Clinical studies of CTCL patients began initially to measure the quantity more than the quality of life, with the first meaningful data being the survival curves for different stages. The first staging of CTCL was done on the basis of skin involvement in a multicenter project by the Mycosis Fungoides Cooperative Group. This working group established a T staging system as shown in Tables 1 and 2. Patients are segregated by the degree of skin involvement and the type of lesion. Three stages were defined by surface area: less than 10% (T1), greater than 10% (T2), and T4 as erythroderma (generally believed to be >80% body surface area but without sharp margins). The other stage defined was T3, signifying the presence of tumors but not quantifying the number or body surface area involved. The strength of this staging system was that it segregated the patients into groups that differ in-

TABLE 1. **TNM Classification of Mycosis Fungoides/Sézary Syndrome**

Skin-T

T0—Clinically and/or histopathologically suspicious lesions
T1—Patches and/or plaques; <10% body surface area
T2—Patches and/or plaques; ≥10% body surface area
T3—Tumors with/without other skin lesions
T4—Generalized erythroderma

Lymph Nodes—N

N0—Not clinically enlarged; histopathologically negative
N1—Clinically enlarged; histopathologically negative
N2—Not clinically enlarged; histopathologically positive
N3—Clinically enlarged; histopathologically positive

Peripheral Blood—B

B0—Atypical cells <5% of leukocytes
B1—Atypical cells ≥5% of leukocytes

Visceral Organs—M

M0—Absent
M1—Present

Based on Bunn PA, Lamberg SI: Report of the Committee on Staging and Classification of Cutaneous T-Cell Lymphomas. Cancer Treat Rep 63:725–728, 1979.

prognosis. Thus, with this system the physicians who deal with CTCL embraced the concept of grading skin involvement by the T system. The T staging provided the only underpinning for linking tumor burden with survival in that from limited patch to 100% involvement, the more the skin was involved, the worse was the prognosis. In addition to skin staging, there are other factors that contribute to the heterogeneity of CTCL. This heterogeneity has undermined the utility of the TNM staging system. One recent report looking at this noted that within the same T stage, patients with more than 20% suppressor T cells in their biopsy specimens fared better than those with less than 15%. Furthermore, it has not been shown that the reduction of a patient's disease from a stage T3 to a T1 is accompanied by any benefit in survival. However, the correlation of survival with extent and depth of skin involvement from CTCL has led to the use of various skin tumor burden indices as surrogate markers for survival in clinical trials. With a chronic disease such as CTCL, surrogate markers are a necessity.

THERAPY PRINCIPLES

The approach to initiating therapy in a given patient begins with identifying the goals of therapy and defining the parameters (skin score, palliation parameters) that will guide therapy. Palliation or remission is the first decision. Based on the time frame of a particular therapy, a schedule for when a therapy would be judged a success or failure should also be identified. There are a few principles that help design therapy strategies. Excellent long-term results have been reported with the localized therapy for localized disease. More widespread disease requires total skin or systemic therapy. However, it is not known at what percentage of skin surface involvement it becomes imperative to treat the entire skin. Another principle is that CTCL induces immunosuppression and, as a result, nonimmunosuppressing systemic therapies are preferred and helpful. A final principle of therapy is based on the chronic nature of the disease. Because many patients will have therapies that span decades, it is important to minimize exposure to therapies that have cumulative toxicities on keratinocytes (mutagens) or the bone marrow.

TABLE 2. **TNM Staging System for Mycosis Fungoides/Sézary Syndrome**

Stage	Skin	Lymph Nodes	Viscera
IA	T1	N0	M0
IB	T2	N0	M0
IIA	T1, T2	N1	M0
IIB	T3	N0, N1	M0
III	T4	N0, N1	M0
IVA	T1–T4	N2, N3	M0
IVB	T1–T4	N0–N3	M1

Based on Lamberg SI, Bunn PA: Cutaneous T-cell lymphomas: Summary of the Mycosis Fungoides Cooperative Group–National Cancer Institute Workshop. Arch Dermatol 115:1103–1105, 1979. Copyright 1979, American Medical Association.

The success of skin-directed therapies (SDTs) for CTCL implies that a significant portion of the life cycle of the skin-homing malignant cells is within reach of the therapeutic impact of SDTs. These treatments are typically palliative and often remittive. Long-lasting remissions of localized lesions can be induced by spot radiotherapy, topical carmustine,* and topical bexarotene. Frequently, high-potency topical corticosteroids are used, although primarily as palliative, not remittive, therapy. Total skin treatments include total skin electron-beam radiotherapy, topical nitrogen mustard, and phototherapy with photochemotherapy with 8-methoxypsoralen and ultraviolet A (PUVA) light or ultraviolet B (UVB) light. Each of the therapies mentioned will be discussed in terms of their usefulness based on patient-specific features.

THERAPY FOR CUTANEOUS T-CELL LYMPHOMA

Spot radiotherapy is the most reliable and rapid method of inducing a remission of localized CTCL. There is widespread availability of radiotherapy, and most lesions, no matter where they occur on the body (e.g., eyelid, buttock crease, ear), can be treated with this modality. There are no compliance problems because each session is recorded by professional radiotherapists. The toxicity is minimal acutely, but the chronic toxicity of radiation dermatitis and cutaneous malignancy is what encourages the conservative use of this modality.

The limitations of topical carmustine therapy are the systemic toxicity from absorption of this chemotherapeutic agent. As a result, topical carmustine is primarily used for limited (<15%) body surface area. The initial protocols for using carmustine involved an alcohol-based solution kept in the refrigerator; however, the ointment-based protocols are now more

*Not FDA approved for this indication.

common. Carmustine can be easily made up in 20-, 30-, or 40-mg/dL ointments in petrolatum. Patients typically apply carmustine at night and wash it off in the morning. Locally, there may be a dose-responsive irritation and/or hyperpigmentation that appears over the 8 to 20 weeks needed to clear lesions. Monitoring includes complete blood cell counts every 2 weeks looking for marrow suppression. The cumulative toxicity of carmustine is primarily structural damage with skin thinning and telangiectasia. Reliable and compliant patients are needed for this therapy to succeed.

Similarly, the limitations of topical bexarotene (Targretin [1%]) gel are primarily due to the dose-responsive irritant response. Hence, bexarotene gel is typically used for less than 15% body surface area (most of the patients in the pivotal trial). The gel is commercially available at 1% so that dose intensity is varied by the frequency of application. Patients will typically initiate therapy with nightly applications of bexarotene gel just to the lesions. After a week, the frequency is increased to twice daily and the patient cautioned about an irritant dermatitis at the site of the lesions. Complete clearance of lesions will usually occur after 12 to 16 weeks of therapy. Irritant responses can be managed by decreasing the frequency of application or by the use of topical corticosteroids. Successful topical bexarotene therapy also requires a compliant patient willing to put up with the irritating properties of this vitamin A derivative. As a retinoid, there should be no cumulative toxicity with regard to cutaneous carcinogenesis or structural damage. In fact, the retinoids typically have activities that counter these effects of the mutagens.

In considering total skin therapy options, there are several features that affect the choice of therapy. The first is availability of the modality and the second is the availability of the lesions. Nitrogen mustard (Mustargen) therapy is widely available. As an initial dose, a 10-mg vial is mixed with 2 oz (50 mL) of tap water. The entire volume is then applied to the whole body surface by the patient. A delayed hypersensitivity reaction may complicate treatment. Ointment-based mechlorethamine (10 mg/dL) may be less sensitizing and is stable on the shelf over a long period of time. Other side effects from mustard therapy, besides hypersensitivity reactions and primary irritant reactions, include the development of second cutaneous malignancies and hypopigmentation and hyperpigmentation.

The total skin treatment with radiation therapy is accomplished with electron-beam radiation. Electrons penetrate only to the upper dermis; electron beam therapy may be used without systemic effect. The total dose of irradiation is important, and a dose of 30 Gy or more gives better complete remission rates and disease-free survival than do lower doses. With a rotational six-field technique, it is possible to administer 1 to 2 Gy per treatment session. Those areas not exposed with the six-field approach need additional therapy: soles, scalp, perineum, and flexural areas in obese patients. These need supplemental therapy. Individual tumors can be spot treated in the midst of the total skin electron-beam therapy. Eyeshields and nailshields minimize toxicity in these areas. This therapy is only available at select centers, and patients undergo four treatments per week for 9 weeks. The major disadvantages are that this type of therapy requires a specialized center and takes up to 3 months for complete treatment. Local side effects include alopecia, atrophy of sweat glands and skin, radiodermatitis, and edema. As the total radiation dose increases, so does the risk of squamous cell carcinoma and radiodermatitis.

The phototherapies used for total skin therapy are PUVA and UVB. These are only available through dermatology offices, limiting their availability to those in remote rural areas. UVB is technically easier because patients need not ingest oral photoactivators nor use photoprotection on the eyes and skin after therapy. Patients having a successful response to UVB (and PUVA) will have lesions that are on easily exposed skin, whereas patients with lesions deep in the groin, buttock crease, and hairy scalp will not have as great a chance at remission. Another clinical finding in UVB-responsive patients is that thin lesions ("patches") clear better than thick plaques, but there are no histologic or easily reproducible guidelines for this distinction. PUVA therapy involves the ultraviolet A light activation of psoralen in the epidermis and dermis at doses that are cytotoxic to lymphocytes but not to the structural elements of the skin. The use of the oral photosensitizer 8-methoxypsoralen (Oxsoralen Ultra), dosed at 0.5 mg/kg, incurs several risks for patients: gastrointestinal intolerance may occur, patients may not reach therapeutic levels of psoralen (particularly in obese patients), and photosensitivity of the eyes and skin occurs for 24 hours after therapy. Treatment frequency is typically three times per week until the disease starts clearing. At that point, the therapy can be decreased to twice weekly for purposes of convenience. A major advantage of the phototherapies is that the recording of treatment frequency and light dosing of each therapy session provides for the analysis of treatment failures. In general, phototherapy doses are increased to the point of toxicity and then decreased to be certain that the patient is in the therapeutic range of the modality. Once clear from phototherapy the patient may continue on with a maintenance treatment schedule (discussed later). If there is partial responsiveness to phototherapy the patient can continue with the modality and clear with the addition of interferon or oral bexarotene systemic therapy.

The decision to use systemic therapy can be arrived at based on easy availability, on widespread disease not amenable to irradiation therapy, or on the need for therapy for erythrodermic disease when skin-directed therapies can often aggravate the erythroderma. As monotherapies, the systemic treatments are more palliative than remittive, necessitating their use in combination therapy regimens to achieve remission. The systemic therapies used for

CTCL include interferon injections, photopheresis, oral bexarotene therapy, low-dose methotrexate therapy, oral chlorambucil* therapy, and infusional cytotoxic therapy.

Interferon (Roferon, Intron)* injections are administered initially at doses of 1 MU three times a week and increased to 5 MU daily as tolerated by the patient's symptoms or bone marrow suppression. The major symptoms are depression, apathy, and fatigue, all aspects important to the quality of life. Interferon appears to synergize with PUVA therapy. Photopheresis therapy is administered at select referral centers, limiting its availability. Sessions are typically performed at 4-week intervals for 3 to 6 months to see a response. Photopheresis has been used in conjunction with total skin electron-beam radiotherapy. Oral therapy with bexarotene (Targretin capsules) can be performed by the patient at home, with little subjective toxicity at doses of 300 mg/M^2. The major toxicity of oral bexarotene is metabolic with hyperlipidemia and hypothyroidism. As a result, patients with pre-existing hyperlipidemia or pancreatitis should not be considered for therapy. Bexarotene oral therapy has been shown to improve signs and symptoms of CTCL gradually over a 12- to 16-week period. Patients can then be maintained on oral bexarotene if it is being used as a palliative agent or tapered off it if it was used as an adjunct to inducing a remission. To date, bexarotene has been used in combination with PUVA, UVB, and photopheresis without any adverse interaction. The low-dose chemotherapy agents methotrexate (Rheumatrex) and chlorambucil (Leukeran)* are useful palliative agents for managing CTCL. Methotrexate is dosed weekly and increased to the maximal tolerated dose (typically, 15–40 mg). The major toxicities are bone marrow suppression, mucositis, and chronic hepatotoxicity. Methotrexate can be used to help manage noncompliant patients because the weekly dose can be administered by injection in the office. Chlorambucil* is taken daily at doses of 2 to 6 mg/d and often combined with prednisone at 20 mg/d to control symptoms and signs of CTCL. Marrow toxicity and the potential for secondary hematopoietic malignancies limit the widespread use of chlorambucil.

Alongside all of the skin directed and systemic therapies for CTCL, topical corticosteroids can provide palliative relief. Class I topical corticosteroids such as clobetasol (Cormax) can be used twice daily for 2 months to help clear lesions. For widespread involvement, triamcinolone cream can be used with sauna suit occlusion to provide total-skin palliation of symptoms while a primary therapy is reducing the tumor burden of CTCL. Another common use of topical corticosteroids in the management of CTCL is in the first-line therapy for suspected relapse. Patients who have achieved remission may develop nondescript lesions that have similarly nondescript histopathology. These areas can frequently be cleared with aggressive use of topical corticosteroids that, if unsuccessful, should be stopped 2 weeks before repeating any biopsies.

The decision to use intravenous infusional cytotoxic therapy is arrived at when the physician and patient face unresponsive disease, widespread lymph node involvement, or rapidly progressing disease. There are several concerns about using infusional therapy in CTCL. Permanent indwelling catheters are difficult to manage in CTCL patients. Skin lesions of CTCL are compromises in the skin barrier function, and this undoubtedly contributes to the seeding of central lines and subsequent sepsis. In addition, as mentioned, the disease is immunosuppressing so that further immunosuppression is best avoided. For these reasons, the fusion toxin denileukin diftitox (Ontak, 9–18 mg/kg) is the first infusional therapy to be considered. This agent is a protein generated from genetic engineering that has fused the interleukin 2 protein with a portion of the diphtheria toxin protein. The drug is given through a peripheral intravenous line for a 30-minute infusion 5 days in a row, every 3 weeks. Patients who will improve with denileukin diftitox will show a response within the first two cycles of therapy. The major toxicities from the fusion toxin are a vascular leak syndrome and an extremely rare anaphylactic reaction to the protein. Most infusion therapy centers are equipped to premedicate patients to manage these events. For patients not responding to the fusion toxin or who might not tolerate the vascular leak syndrome, traditional chemotherapy can often be palliative for all phases of advanced CTCL. Combination chemotherapies can be administered with heightened awareness for the propensity of CTCL patients to develop infections and bone marrow toxicity. The roles of autologous and allogeneic transplantations are currently being explored.

MAINTENANCE THERAPY

Once a patient's disease has cleared with a total-skin therapy, it is common practice to continue intermittent total-skin therapies to maintain a remission. The biology that underlies this common practice is the normal recirculation of T cells. The clearing of a skin lesion does not imply clearing of the disease. Any CTCL cells recirculating have the ability to home to the skin and recapitulate lesion production. For practical purposes, patients are typically started at once-weekly maintenance therapy and over time tapered to one treatment a month of phototherapy or topical nitrogen mustard therapy. The decision to discontinue maintenance would be affected by any ongoing chronic toxicity from these therapies, which are normally well tolerated.

*Not FDA approved for this indication.

PAPULOSQUAMOUS DISEASES

method of
JOHN A. ZIC, M.D.
Vanderbilt University School of Medicine
Nashville, Tennessee

Papulosquamous skin diseases are defined as inflammatory skin disorders characterized by erythema and scale, usually with pruritus. There are many skin diseases that present as red, scaly, itchy rashes. In Table 1, the papulosquamous diseases are grouped by their common primary lesion at presentation. Note that some papulosquamous diseases can present with more than one type of primary lesion.

Diagnosis is important, obviously, in helping the patient. Early in the disease, enough clinical clues may be lacking to accurately diagnose the condition. A skin biopsy is usually helpful, but the early histopathology may be just as nonspecific as the early gross morphology. One challenge to the clinician is being able to sort out which eruptions can be cured and which can be controlled.

MORBILLIFORM DRUG ERUPTIONS

Morbilliform drug eruptions must be considered in the differential diagnosis of papulosquamous disorders. In terms of frequency, morbilliform drug eruptions are rivaled only by psoriasis and, possibly, eczema. A morbilliform drug eruption can mimic most other papulosquamous disorders; therefore, like secondary syphilis, it can be considered a great masquerader. This eruption is often described as a "maculopapular rash," a term that should be discarded and replaced with a more precise description of the morphology. "Papules coalescing into plaques" or "macules coalescing into patches" more precisely defines the morphology of morbilliform drug eruptions. This also distinguishes morbilliform drug eruptions, the most common type of drug eruption, from drug-induced skin reactions characterized by blisters, pustules, erythroderma, and so on. Consider a morbilliform drug eruption if a patient has started a new drug 7 to 14 days before the onset of the eruption. Some patients, however, may develop an allergy to a drug that has been taken for months to years. A skin biopsy can be most helpful if eosinophils are present in the dermis and the biopsy specimen lacks the classic features of other papulosquamous diseases.

Treatment is obvious; stop the offending drug. Because of the fact that hundreds of drugs can cause morbilliform drug eruptions, deciding which drug is the culprit may be a challenge. Statistically, antibiotics, allopurinol (Zyloprim), and thiazides are more likely to cause drug eruptions than others and a trial off the most likely drug is indicated. A 6-week trial off the suspected drug is recommended; it can occasionally take up to 6 weeks for a sustained remission to evolve. A drug stopped for only 1 or 2 weeks without improvement may still be the offender. Patients can usually be supported with triamcinolone (Kenalog), 0.1% cream or ointment topically, and oral antihistamines during the 6-week drug holiday.

PSORIASIS

Psoriasis vulgaris is, perhaps, the most common papulosquamous disorder, affecting 1% to 3% of the adult population. It is an immunogenetic disease characterized classically by the presence of well-defined plaques on the extensor surface of the extremities. Within the skin is a complex sequence of antigen presentation and T-cell activation, resulting in the release of cytokines and chemoattractants. These local chemical mediators induce a hyperproliferative state in the epidermis and increased vascularity in the dermis. An obvious inherited component is found in almost one third of affected patients. It appears that some inherit, or through a spontaneous mutations evolve, a T-cell defect leading to an activated state after exposure to a variety of antigens, including *Streptococcus*, neurochemicals induced by stress, alcohol, certain drugs (β-blockers, lithium, antimalarials), and others.

Patients with psoriasis can display a myriad of clinical presentations, ranging from nail-only involvement to generalized pustules or erythroderma. Pitting of the nails can be a subtle but important clue in making the diagnosis. Guttate psoria-

TABLE 1. **Papulosquamous Diseases: Primary Lesion at Presentation**

Plaque	Patch	Papule
Chronic and subacute cutaneous lupus erythematosus*	Atopic eczema	Guttate psoriasis
Morbilliform drug eruptions†	Morbilliform drug eruptions†	Lichen planus
Mycosis fungoides*	Mycosis fungoides*†	Lymphomatoid papulosis*
Pityriasis rubra pilaris	Nummular eczema	Morbilliform drug eruptions†
Psoriasis vulgaris	Parapsoriasis	Pityriasis lichenoides et varioliformis acute (PLEVA)
Secondary syphilis†	Pityriasis rosea	Pityriasis lichenoides chronica
	Seborrheic dermatitis	Secondary syphilis†
	Secondary syphilis†	
	Systemic lupus erythematosus*	
	Tinea corporis*†	

*Discussed elsewhere.
†Potentially curable skin conditions. The others can only be controlled. Note that patch stage mycosis fungoides has the potential for cure, but plaque stage does not.

sis is a less common variant that presents with scaly papules on the trunk more so than the extremities, usually in response to T-cell stimulus by streptococcal antigens. Therefore, a throat swab for culture and antistreptolysin-O antibody titers may be indicated with this variant.

Treatments for psoriasis are aimed at one or more of three cellular targets: the T cell, the hyperproliferative epidermal cells, or other inflammatory cells. Topical corticosteroids, the basis of therapy for limited disease, primarily act on inflammatory cells and T cells. Tar-containing products such as anthralin show anti-inflammatory effects. Topical and oral retinoids and topical vitamin D analogues (calcipotriene [Dovonex]) primarily affect epidermal cell differentiation. Oral methotrexate and cyclosporine (Sandimmune) are T-cell activation inhibitors and therefore target an early step in the pathogenesis of psoriasis. Ultraviolet light induces apoptosis in T cells and also has effects on other inflammatory cells. This explains why psoriasis usually flares during the winter. Several factors to be considered in the treatment of psoriasis include the age of the patient, co-morbid conditions, extent of disease, availability of treatments, and skin type.

The importance of good skin care in the treatment of psoriasis and other papulosquamous diseases cannot be stressed enough. Dry skin (xerosis) is the most common cause of itching and will contribute to patient discomfort no matter what the cause. Hot baths and showers can contribute to xerosis and should be avoided. Because fragrance-containing skin products tend to dry out the skin, recommending fragrance-free skin cleansers/soaps, moisturizers/skin lubricants, and laundry detergents will have a sustainable impact on a patient's skin disease. Psoriasis, like many other papulosquamous disorders, can be controlled, not cured, and good skin care can help patients achieve a higher level of comfort and satisfaction.

Localized Plaque Psoriasis

Localized plaque psoriasis on the trunk and extremities can be treated with a group 1 or 2 potent topical corticosteroid applied twice daily for 1 or 2 weeks to induce significant clearing. Overuse can lead to tachyphylaxis, skin atrophy, and striae, especially in the axillae and groin. At this point, a long-term maintenance program is begun, including good skin care, a group 3 or 4 midpotency topical corticosteroid for flares at bedtime, and, possibly, topical calcipotriene ointment or cream twice daily. Over half of patients with psoriasis will respond to the vitamin D analogue calcipotriene after 2 or 3 weeks of application. This agent avoids the complication of skin atrophy seen with topical corticosteroids. A rare complication of calcipotriene therapy is hypercalcemia, occurring primarily in children and the elderly when more than 100 g is applied weekly. Facial lesions should be treated with a group 5 to 7 low-potency topical corticosteroid up to twice daily on an intermittent basis.

Patients who have failed the just-described regimen may benefit from topical tazarotene (Tazorac) gel applied daily in addition to topical corticosteroids nightly. This topical retinoid will induce a retinoid dermatitis characterized by redness and irritation and, therefore, should be used on less than 20% of the body surface area. The addition of topical corticosteroids appears to reduce this adverse effect and make patients more adherent to the treatment plan.

For stubborn plaques on the trunk and extremities, short contact therapy with anthralin cream (Drithocreme) may be helpful. The cream is applied thinly just to the affected plaque(s), left in place for 15 to 45 minutes, and then washed off. Irritation is a common side effect and may result in modification of the regimen from once-daily to less frequent application. Discoloration of the skin, clothing, and furniture may occur.

Scalp psoriasis is usually responsive to tar-containing shampoos that should be lathered and left on the scalp skin for at least 5 minutes before rinsing. Topical corticosteroid solutions (e.g., fluocinolone [Synalar], 0.01% solution) can be applied twice daily for help with the pruritus, and group 3 topical corticosteroid creams on thicker plaques may be needed. Applying peanut oil or olive oil to the scalp at bedtime can help loosen thick scale before shampooing the next morning.

Extensive Plaque Psoriasis

Patients with more extensive plaque psoriasis (20% body surface area involvement) will usually require phototherapy and/or systemic therapy to achieve significant clearing. Natural and artificial (tanning bed) sunlight will improve psoriasis, but the risks of sunburn reactions, accelerated photoaging, and skin cancers must be strongly considered. Phototherapy delivered in the office of an experienced dermatologist and nursing staff can significantly improve psoriasis while exposing patients to the least amount of ultraviolet energy to induce and maintain clearing. Ultraviolet B (UVB) (290–320 nm) phototherapy is effective in thin extensive plaque psoriasis and guttate psoriasis. The minimal erythema dose (MED) is calculated before therapy, and treatment is begun at 50% MED three to five times weekly. Significant improvement is usually achieved by 4 to 6 weeks. To maintain response, UVB treatments may be continued at biweekly to once-monthly intervals.

PUVA (psoralen and UVA) phototherapy is more effective than UVB phototherapy for patients with widespread thick plaques. UVA (320–400 nm) energy penetrates deeper into the skin than UVB energy. The addition of oral psoralen (methoxsalen [Oxsoralen]) has a synergistic effect on inducing apoptosis of T cells. Methoxsalen is given at a dose of 0.6 mg/kg 60 to 90 minutes before UVA exposure. The UVA energy is slowly increased over time and is delivered at thrice-weekly intervals until significant clearing occurs, usually after 4 to 6 weeks. As with UVB phototherapy, twice- or once-monthly PUVA treatments can maintain remissions. Side effects of oral psoralen include nausea and photosensitivity lasting up to 18 hours. Because of the additional risk of cataracts with UVA combined with psoralen, protective eyeglasses must be worn for the rest of the day after a treatment. Recently, a variant of UVB phototherapy called narrow-band UVB has become available in the United States. The nonerythromogenic wavelength (314 nm) allows a 10-fold increase in energy delivered to the skin without the same increased risk of burning. Furthermore, patients can achieve the same level of clearing with narrow-band UVB phototherapy as PUVA without the side effects of psoralen. The long-term risks of narrow-band UVB phototherapy are not as well defined as those of the other phototherapies. The potential risks of basal and squamous cell skin cancers must be considered with any phototherapy. There also appears to be a slight increased risk of malignant melanoma in psoriasis patients receiving more than 10 years of chronic PUVA phototherapy.

The three FDA-approved oral agents used to treat extensive or recalcitrant psoriasis are methotrexate, acitretin (Soriatane), and cyclosporine (Neoral). These agents are used in patients who are poor candidates for phototherapy (unavailability, history of skin cancer) or those who have failed other therapies discussed earlier. Methotrexate and acitretin have the potential to cause liver toxicity, and cyclosporine may lead to nephrotoxicity. Both methotrexate and cyclosporine may lead to immunosuppression, which is expected to a certain extent in achieving therapeutic response. Because of these potential side effects, these drugs require careful monitoring by a physician with experience using them. Baseline laboratory evaluations for liver and kidney function and complete blood cell count are required. Pregnancy is contraindicated for patients on these agents.

Methotrexate has the advantage of decades of experience and the potential to help psoriatic arthritis that affects one in seven patients with psoriasis. The drug is begun with a test dose of 2.5 to 5.0 mg followed by laboratory evaluation of liver enzymes and complete blood cell count 6 days later. The drug is then continued once weekly with a gradual dose escalation of 2.5 mg weekly until significant clearing occurs or a maximum dose of 20 mg weekly has been given. Most patients require a 7.5- to 10.0-mg maintenance dose; much higher doses may indicate the need for another therapy. Laboratory evaluations should continue weekly (the day before dosing) until a steady-state dose is reached. Most patients will respond 4 weeks into therapy with significant clearing by 8 to 12 weeks. After 1.5 g of methotrexate is ingested, a liver biopsy should be performed to rule out occult fibrosis that may not be evident on laboratory evaluations. Side effects include nausea, anemia, anorexia, headaches, and fatigue.

Acitretin (Soriatane) is an oral retinoid especially helpful for pustular variants of psoriasis, hand and foot (palmoplantar) psoriasis, and severe plaque psoriasis. Initial doses range from 25 to 50 mg/d with dose escalation to achieve response as high as 100 mg/d. Responses can be expected in 4 to 6 weeks. Acitretin may be combined with PUVA phototherapy (Re-PUVA) to allow a lower daily dose of acitretin and a lower energy requirement of PUVA to achieve faster response and longer remissions. Side effects include moderate xerosis, dry mucous membranes, hyperlipidemia, photophobia, and joint and muscle aches. Women should avoid drinking alcohol because it can induce the metabolism of acitretin to etretinate, a retinoid with a clearance of over 3 years that is also a potent teratogen.

Cyclosporine (Neoral) can be used successfully to induce remissions in patients with severe plaque psoriasis or erythroderma, but its long-term use should be limited to avoid irreversible nephrotoxicity. A low dose of 2.5 to 3.0 mg/kg/d can induce remissions within several weeks while another oral agent or phototherapy is initiated for long-term maintenance. As with other oral agents, a flare of psoriasis will occur after stopping the drug.

PITYRIASIS RUBRA PILARIS

Well-defined plaques that may mimic psoriasis but show head-to-toe progression and unique follicular hyperkeratotic papules characterize *pityriasis rubra pilaris.* Smooth, thick, yellowish palmoplantar keratoderma and well-defined islands of sparing are also common findings. The acquired form seen in adults may resolve in several years, but the congenital form has a poorer prognosis for improvement.

Pityriasis rubra pilaris is usually responsive to oral retinoids, but not to the extent one sees in psoriasis. Doses of acitretin (Soriatane)* in the range of 25 to 100 mg/d or doses of isotretinoin (Accutane),* 1 to 2 mg/kg/d, may be required. See section on psoriasis for monitoring guidelines. Methotrexate* has been less helpful. Like psoriasis, topical corticosteroids and good skin care have a role in decreasing itching.

ECZEMA

Eczema is a general term referring to the finding of ill-defined red scaly patches, not due exclusively to external factors. In other words, eczema is a diagnosis made only after excluding dermatophyte fungus, allergens, heat, cold, food, and drugs as the sole cause of the eruption. These factors may exacerbate eczema, but they do not cause it. The cutaneous lymphoma mycosis fungoides should also be excluded, especially in adults with the progressive onset of "eczema" in sun-protected areas. There are many forms of eczema, including nummular eczema, which shows more well-defined scattered patches often with crusting. The diagnosis of hand eczema

*Not FDA approved for this indication.

should be made after excluding possible contact allergens.

Atopic eczema is the best-defined variant of eczema, emerging usually in the first several years of life as ill-defined red patches first on the cheeks and extensor limbs and then moving to primarily the flexural surfaces. Like psoriasis, atopic eczema is an immunogenetic disease, characterized, however, by a TH-2 dominant T-cell phenotype. There is an increased susceptibility to develop asthma and allergic rhinitis in the patient and family members. Luckily, over two thirds of affected infants will outgrow the disease by midchildhood.

Good skin care, as outlined in the section on psoriasis, is the hallmark of eczema treatment. Occasional bursts of topical corticosteroids (groups 2–4) for 7 to 10 days are usually necessary for flare-ups. Some patients may require low-potency topical corticosteroids (groups 4–7) for chronic maintenance therapy. Patients with extensive disease may gain control with UVB phototherapy using a psoriasis protocol. Rarely will patients need chronic intramuscular corticosteroids or oral low-dose weekly methotrexate* (5–10 mg) for control.

PARAPSORIASIS

Parapsoriasis is a chronic lymphoproliferative disorder of the skin with no relationship to psoriasis vulgaris. The etiology is unknown. A small percentage of patients with the large plaque (6 to >15 cm) variant will progress to develop mycosis fungoides. This variant can be indistinguishable, clinically, from early patch stage mycosis fungoides, and a skin biopsy is necessary to confirm the diagnosis. Scaly pink, often-atrophic patches (*plaques* in French) scattered predominantly on the trunk and sun-protected areas of the skin characterize both the small- and large-plaque variants. UVB and PUVA phototherapy twice to thrice weekly are quite effective in controlling the chronic eruption. Patients will often only require therapy during the winter months when casual sun exposure is less. Consider a repeat biopsy if the disease progresses or the patient develops thicker plaques.

PITYRIASIS LICHENOIDES

Pityriasis lichenoides is a benign inflammatory skin disorder of unknown etiology with an acute form seen primarily in children—pityriasis lichenoides et varioliformis acuta (PLEVA)—and a chronic form—pityriasis lichenoides chronica (PLC). An acute polymorphic eruption of pink papules evolving into vesicles and crusted shallow scars typifies PLEVA. Fever and constitutional symptoms may accompany the eruption that resolves over several months. In contrast, PLC is characterized by reddish brown papules covered with an adherent thin micacious scale and may wax and wane over many years. Both forms may show a lymphocytic vasculitis histologically and white patches (leukoderma) clinically.

*Not FDA approved for this indication.

PLEVA may respond to oral erythromycin,* albeit temporarily. UVB phototherapy is usually helpful in symptomatic patients, and tetracycline,* 1 to 2 g/d for 4 weeks, is an option for adults. Education about the natural history of the diseases is most important.

PITYRIASIS ROSEA

Pityriasis rosea is a benign self-limited skin disorder diagnosed in the spring through fall and thought to be of viral etiology. Recent studies have not identified a likely pathogen. A well-defined red patch, often the largest, precedes a generalized eruption of pink oval macules and small patches with a characteristic peripheral rim of fine scale. The herald patch may precede the truncal eruption by days to weeks. The eruption fades over 4 to 6 weeks and may be accompanied by intense itching. Topical corticosteroids (groups 3–6) and oral antihistamines are helpful in controlling the itching. Unusually intense or chronic cases will respond to UVB phototherapy thrice weekly in 2 to 3 weeks. Secondary syphilis should be ruled out with appropriate serologic studies.

SECONDARY SYPHILIS

Secondary syphilis, "the great imitator," may present as generalized patches, plaques, papules, and pustules but rarely vesicles. The palms and soles are characteristically involved. Onset of the asymptomatic eruption occurs 6 to 8 weeks after the primary chancre and is usually accompanied by peripheral adenopathy. A single intramuscular 2.4-million unit dose of benzathine penicillin G is administered for primary and secondary syphilis and for disease present for less than 1 year. Three weekly intramuscular doses of benzathine penicillin G are administered to patients with infection of undetermined length or greater than 1 year's duration. Tetracycline,* 2 g/d, may be given to penicillin-allergic patients for 15 or 30 days with infection of undetermined length or greater than 1 year's duration. The benefits and risks of erythromycin orally versus penicillin desensitization in penicillin-allergic pregnant patients should be weighed carefully and appropriate expert consultation obtained.

SEBORRHEIC DERMATITIS

Seborrheic dermatitis is a chronic inflammatory skin condition that presents as a greasy fine scale overlying ill-defined patches on the nasolabial folds, eyebrows, scalp, ears, chest, and, uncommonly, the groin. Infants may have localization to the scalp—"cradle cap." Children are usually spared until puberty when androgens stimulate sebaceous glands. The etiology is unknown, but the yeast *Pityrosporum ovale* has been implicated. Support for this

*Not FDA approved for this indication.

hypothesis comes from the fact that many patients are helped by the application of the antifungal ketoconazole (Nizoral)* cream twice daily. Daily application of hydrocortisone 1% cream is safe and effective in a majority of patients. Selenium sulfide, ketoconazole, and tar-containing shampoos are helpful for scalp involvement. Efficacy is increased if the lather sits on the scalp skin at least 5 minutes before rinsing. The condition will eventually relapse off therapy.

LICHEN PLANUS

Lichen planus (LP) is an inflammatory skin and mucous membrane disease associated with hepatitis C infection in a large minority (~20%) of patients. Drugs are another common trigger for the disease. LP is thought of as a reaction pattern of the skin characterized histologically by an intense bandlike infiltration of lymphocytes hugging the dermoepidermal junction. The primary skin lesion of classic LP is an intensely pruritic, flat-topped, violaceous, polygonal, 3- to 6-mm papule. Well-developed lesions may show white streaks on the surface called Wickham's striae. Similar white reticulated patches may be seen on the buccal mucosae. The disease may persist for 3 to 5 years. Several clinical variants exist: hypertrophic LP, erosive oral LP, atrophic LP, LP/lupus erythematosus overlap, and bullous LP.

Treatment of the skin lesions of classic LP includes high-potency (group 1 or 2) topical corticosteroids twice daily over 2 to 3 weeks followed by midpotency topical corticosteroids (group 3 or 4) daily for maintenance. Deep postinflammatory hyperpigmentation is expected. Early erosive oral lesions will usually respond to fluocinolone (Synalar) 0.05% topical gel up to three times daily for 7 days. Widespread mucocutaneous lesions require systemic treatment with prednisone, 20 to 40 mg/d, tapering off over 2 to 6 weeks. Intramuscular corticosteroids may also be tried. For recalcitrant cases, PUVA phototherapy has been used successfully. Isotretinoin (Accutane),* 0.5 to 1 mg/kg/d may also be helpful in recalcitrant cases.

*Not FDA approved for this indication.

CONNECTIVE TISSUE DISORDERS

method of
VIOLETA RUS, M.D., and
CHARLES S. VIA, M.D.
University of Maryland School of Medicine and Baltimore VA Medical Center
Baltimore, Maryland

SYSTEMIC LUPUS ERYTHEMATOSUS

Systemic lupus erythematosus (SLE) is a prototypical multisystemic, autoimmune disease, characterized by the presence of autoantibodies directed against components of the cell nucleus. SLE is highly variable in its presentation and clinical course. Typically, patients present with generalized or constitutional symptoms such as fever, fatigue, myalgias, anorexia, rashes, arthralgias, or arthritis, as well as any combination of organ involvement, including kidneys, lungs, heart, nervous system, or hematologic system. Antinuclear antibodies (ANAs) are positive in 95% to 98% of SLE patients. However, the presence of ANA positivity alone does not mandate a diagnosis of SLE. Suggestive clinical features must be present because 5% of the normal population may be ANA positive at a significant titer of 1:320. A negative test is strong evidence against SLE. Among ANA specificities, anti-dsDNA and anti-Sm antibodies are highly diagnostic of SLE.

Skin Manifestations

Over 90% of patients with SLE eventually will have cutaneous manifestations during the course of their disease. Skin lesions may be specific for SLE, such as discoid lupus, malar rash, and subacute cutaneous lupus, or nonspecific, such as photosensitivity reactions, urticaria, vasculitis, alopecia, ulcerations, papules, and nodules. Sun protection using broad-spectrum sunscreens with a sun-protective factor (SPF) of 15 or greater is an important measure. Antimalarial drugs are also effective in controlling not only most skin lesions but also arthritis, mild serositis, and fatigue. Once the disease has been brought under control, antimalarial therapy is typically continued, especially in patients who have more than just dermatologic manifestations.

Of the antimalarial agents, hydroxychloroquine (Plaquenil) is the most widely used in the United States. Although chloroquine has a similar efficacy and is cheaper, it may have a greater incidence of retinopathy. Antimalarial agents have long half-lives and a slow onset of action. We initiate therapy at 200 mg/d orally, with the dose taken at night for 1 to 2 weeks to reduce side effects, such as anorexia, nausea, abdominal cramps, or diarrhea. These complaints disappear usually with continued use, and the dose can be increased to 400 mg/d. Other toxicities of antimalarial agents include corneal deposition, which may be asymptomatic or result in complaints such as blurred vision, visual halos, and focusing difficulties. These complaints usually appear during the first several weeks of therapy and do not require discontinuation of the drug. The major ocular toxicity of antimalarial agents is retinal damage due to binding of the drugs to the melanin of the pigmented epithelial layer. Retinal toxicity is related to the daily, and not the cumulative, drug dose. At doses below 6.5 mg/kg/d for hydroxychloroquine and 4 mg/kg/d for chloroquine, retinal toxicity is exceedingly rare. An ophthalmologic examination to include visual acuity, slit-lamp, funduscopic, and visual field testing should be performed at or before drug initiation and biannually thereafter. Other side effects include rashes, pruritus, alopecia, hyperpigmentation, and, rarely, exfoliative dermatitis, neuromyopathy, and cardiomyopathy. Hematologic side effects are rare and can affect all three cell lines.

Topical corticosteroids applied directly to skin lesions are effective and frequently used when skin lesions are not extensive. The more potent fluorinated forms are avoided on the face because of the possibility of skin atrophy. Injection of corticosteroids in discoid lesions or into a joint or tendon sheath may be beneficial.

Dapsone* is used in the management of various cutaneous forms of SLE, including discoid, subacute cutaneous, vesiculobullous, and lupus profundus. Therapy is usually started at 25 to 50 mg/d and is gradually increased to 100 to 200 mg/d. The major side effects are hemolytic anemia, especially in patients with glucose-6-phosphate dehydrogenase (G6PD) deficiency and methemoglobinemia. Prescreening for G6PD deficiency before initiating therapy with either dapsone or antimalarial agents is recommended.

Musculoskeletal Manifestations

Arthralgias and arthritis are the most common presenting manifestations of SLE. Other manifestations such as avascular necrosis may occur either as a manifestation of lupus or as a complication of corticosteroid therapy. Nonsteroidal anti-inflammatory drugs (NSAIDs) are the first line of therapy for musculoskeletal manifestations such as arthralgias, arthritis, and myalgias. They are also used for mild pleuritis and/or pericarditis. Patients with SLE are prone to develop NSAID-induced hepatitis, particularly with salicylate compounds. NSAIDs should be avoided in patients with suspected lupus nephritis or impaired renal function. When musculoskeletal symptoms are not well controlled by NSAIDs, Plaquenil is useful in suppressing synovitis. Occasionally, low-dose prednisone (<10 mg/d) may be required. In patients with arthritis unresponsive to hydroxychloroquine or requiring higher doses of corticosteroids, methotrexate, a dihydrate folate reductase inhibitor, in low weekly doses of 10 to 15 mg, may be useful. Folic acid, 1 mg/d, should be added to diminish side effects. Periodic blood monitoring for hematologic and hepatic toxicity is required.

Renal Manifestations

Overall, two thirds of patients with SLE have some degree of kidney involvement during their course. It is one of the major prognostic factors with chronic morbidity related to end-stage renal disease and hemodialysis. Early lupus nephritis is often silent; therefore, urinalysis and renal function tests should be performed as screening tests. Although clinical manifestations may correlate with the pathologic features early in the course of lupus nephritis, renal biopsy is often necessary to determine the status of the renal parenchyma.

*Not FDA approved for this indication.

The World Health Organization (WHO) classification of lupus nephritis identifies six forms of glomerulonephritis that are not static and may progress or regress to another WHO class. No therapy is necessary for WHO class I, in which the biopsy shows normal glomeruli. WHO class II nephritis is characterized by mesangial disease. Although usually a mild form of lupus nephritis with minimal urinary abnormalities, it can be the initial stage of a more severe form. For patients with mesangial hypercellularity (type IIb pattern) and more than 1 g of proteinuria per day, high anti-dsDNA, and low C3 complement, low doses of corticosteroids (20 mg/d) are generally used for 6 weeks to 3 months and then tapered, depending on the degree of remaining activity. WHO classes III and IV include focal-segmental and diffuse proliferative nephritis, respectively. Both forms, except for the very mild forms of focal proliferative nephritis, require aggressive therapy with corticosteroids and cytotoxic drugs. Corticosteroids may be administered either as intravenous "pulse doses" of 1000 mg methylprednisolone (Solu-Medrol), given for 3 consecutive days, or as high-dose oral prednisone (1 mg/kg/d) usually given in twice- or thrice-daily dosing for 6 to 8 weeks, after which the dose can be gradually tapered over the next 2 to 3 months. An alternate-day regimen can be initiated when the single daily dose has reached 30 mg/d.

Cyclophosphamide (Cytoxan),* either orally (1–3 mg/kg/d) or as a monthly intravenous pulse therapy, is concomitantly started. Equally efficacious, intravenous pulse therapy has fewer side effects. The intravenous pulse is given monthly in a dose of 0.75 g/m^2 (0.5 g/m^2 if the glomerular filtration rate is less than one-third normal). The dose of the next pulse is adjusted by increments or decrements of 0.25 g/m^2 to maintain the white blood cell count above 1500/mm^3 (between days 10 and 14 after pulse). An extended course of intravenous cyclophosphamide (not to exceed maximum 3 years) is given monthly for 6 months and then quarterly for 1 year after remission. Cyclophosphamide has substantial toxicities. Nausea and vomiting can be particularly severe with the intravenous pulse regimen and require antiemetic therapy. The addition of dexamethasone and antiemetics (ondansetron [Zofran] or granisetron [Kytril]) has markedly improved tolerance. Alopecia may occasionally be severe but is reversible. Ovarian failure leading to amenorrhea and infertility occur with extended courses of intravenous cyclophosphamide. The risk of premature ovarian failure increases with the number of cyclophosphamide pulses and with patient age. Bladder complications include hemorrhagic cystitis and bladder cancer. Vigorous hydration with 2 to 3 L/d of fluids and the use of 2-mercaptoethane sulfonate sodium (mesna [Mesnex]) lowers the risk of bladder complications. An alternative maintenance therapy, especially for patients who wish to preserve fertility, uses azathioprine (Imuran),

*Not FDA approved for this indication.

2 mg/kg/d, along with alternate-day therapy with prednisone.

Class V biopsy specimens are characterized by membranous nephropathy. About one third of patients with membranous nephropathy develop renal failure at 10 to 15 years. Patients with nephrotic-range proteinuria are treated with high doses of prednisone for 2 to 3 months, which is then tapered to alternate-day therapy or discontinued depending on whether a response has been documented. Cyclophosphamide or cyclosporine (Sandimmune)* can be added to prednisone, especially when a proliferative component is detected. Additionally, hypertension should be aggressively controlled, preferably with angiotensin-converting enzyme inhibitors, which have an additional effect of lowering proteinuria. Patients with membranous nephropathy have an increased risk for cardiovascular disease due to the hypercholesterolemia that accompanies nephrotic syndrome; therefore, lipid-lowering agents should be started if hypercholesterolemia persists for more than 3 months.

Hematologic Abnormalities

These include anemia, leukopenia, lymphopenia, and thrombocytopenia. The most characteristic anemia in lupus is autoimmune hemolysis; however, anemia due to chronic disease, renal failure, blood loss, or medications may occur. Autoimmune hemolytic anemia typically develops gradually but may present as a rapidly progressive hemolytic crisis. Systemic high-dose corticosteroids are the mainstay of therapy, and approximately 75% of patients respond to treatment. In patients who fail corticosteroids, azathioprine,* 2 to 2.5 mg/kg, danazol (Danocrine),* high-dose intravenous human immunoglobulin (IVIG),* and, ultimately, splenectomy may be required.

White blood cell counts between 2500 and 4000/mm^3 are present in over 50% of patients with SLE. White blood cell counts below 1500/mm^3 are rare and often associated with active disease; however, this does not require therapy by itself. Other causes for leukopenia such as drug toxicities and infection must be ruled out. Lymphocytopenia (a lymphocyte count $<$1500/mm^3) is present at some point in the majority of patients and correlates with disease activity.

Thrombocytopenia is primarily immune mediated by antiplatelet or antiphospholipid antibodies; however, infection or drug-related causes may contribute. Most patients have a mild degree of thrombocytopenia that may parallel other manifestations of disease activity, whereas a minority of patients may have an isolated, chronic thrombocytopenia that can drop below 50,000/mm^3. Bleeding usually presents as petechiae, ecchymoses, and bleeding from the gastrointestinal tract, kidneys, bladder, and uterus. Severe bleeding manifestations such as spontaneous intracranial hemorrhage are rare, especially in younger patients, but can be fatal.

*Not FDA approved for this indication.

Patients with bleeding manifestations or with platelet counts of less than 20,000/mm^3 are treated with high-dose corticosteroids by either oral or intravenous pulse administration. In the presence of antiplatelet antibodies, platelet transfusions are ineffective because the transfused thrombocytes are rapidly destroyed. IVIG may be useful in inducing a rapid increase in platelet counts in emergency situations such as surgery. In patients unresponsive to corticosteroids, medications such as danazol,* azathioprine,* monthly intravenous cyclophosphamide,* and *Vinca* alkaloids (vincristine* and vinblastine*) can provide an alternative to splenectomy.

Among clotting abnormalities, the most common is the secondary antiphospholipid syndrome, which is clinically manifested as venous or arterial thrombosis, recurrent pregnancy loss, and/or thrombocytopenia. Laboratory diagnosis consists of an enzyme-linked immunosorbent assay for IgG, IgM, and IgA anticardiolipin antibodies and in vitro phospholipid-dependent coagulation assays such as activated partial thromboplastin time or dilute Russell viper venom test. Confirmation of the lupus anticoagulant in the latter assays is performed by phospholipid neutralization, resulting in normalization of the prolonged test. Treatment of arterial or venous thrombotic episodes relies on acute treatment with heparin followed by lifelong anticoagulation with warfarin or low molecular weight heparin.

Neuropsychiatric SLE (NP-SLE)

A variety of focal and diffuse manifestations can present in the context of active SLE or independent of disease activity. NP-SLE is a diagnosis of exclusion and other potentially correctable causes such as infections, uremia, hypoxia, electrolyte abnormalities, severe hypertension, and medication side effects should be ruled out. Supportive evidence for NP-SLE is provided by corticospinal fluid analysis showing pleocytosis, increased protein, increased IgG index, oligoclonal bands, and antineuronal antibodies. Imaging studies, computed tomography or preferably magnetic resonance imaging, may demonstrate white matter abnormalities. Diffuse manifestations include cognitive dysfunction, organic brain syndrome, psychosis, lupus headache, and coma. Despite short studies demonstrating improvement of cognitive dysfunction with corticosteroid or immunosuppressive medication, no therapeutic consensus currently exists. Treatment of acute lupus headache is commensurate with its severity. If empirical treatment fails, a short trial of low-dose prednisone may be beneficial. Lupus psychosis may respond to antipsychotic medication such as haloperidol, but when the functional impairment is severe and antipsychotic medication is ineffective, high-dose corticosteroids may be necessary. Corticosteroid-induced psychosis may also occur and typically presents as a manic state in a patient with a personal or family history of bipolar disorder.

*Not FDA approved for this indication.

Delirium (organic brain syndrome) is characterized by fluctuating attention and confusion. Correctable causes, if present, must be treated before using corticosteroids.

Focal neurologic manifestations are generally believed to result from a vascular process (e.g., vasculopathy, vasculitis, in situ thrombosis, or embolism). Seizures occur in 15% to 20% of patients with SLE. In addition to anticonvulsive therapy, high-dose corticosteroids should be used if signs of central nervous system inflammation can be demonstrated. Stroke may be a devastating event and results in significant disability. Treatment depends on whether hemorrhage, embolism, thrombosis, or vasculitis is present.

Transverse myelitis is rare but may be the presenting feature of SLE. High-dose corticosteroids plus intravenous pulse cyclophosphamide* are most beneficial if given early. Neuropathies in SLE patients can affect peripheral, cranial, or autonomic nerves. Both mononeuritis multiplex and a diffuse, symmetric polyneuropathy may be present. When an inflammatory or vasculitic mechanism is suspected, corticosteroids are indicated.

Pulmonary Manifestations

Approximately 60% of patients will at some point in their disease have symptomatic pulmonary involvement, involving the pleura, the lung parenchyma, the vasculature, and/or the diaphragm. Pleuritis is the most common manifestation and usually responds to NSAIDs or to a brief course of low-dose prednisone. Lupus pneumonitis is a dramatic manifestation with high mortality and is characterized by abrupt onset of dyspnea, cough, fever, hemoptysis, and hypoxia, with bilateral diffuse infiltrates in the absence of infection. Patients should be promptly treated with intravenous pulse corticosteroids and an immunosuppressive drug (azathioprine* or cyclophosphamide*). Pulmonary hemorrhage due to lupus pneumonitis may be fatal and requires aggressive therapy to include plasmapheresis. Chronic (fibrotic) pneumonitis is a more insidious process, slowly evolving from a potentially reversible alveolitis to irreversible interstitial fibrosis. High-resolution computed tomography and bronchoalveolar lavage may be helpful in determining the presence of active alveolitis, which calls for treatment with high-dose corticosteroids and oral cyclophosphamide.* Pulmonary hypertension is rare but inevitably progresses to right-sided congestive heart failure. Multiple pulmonary emboli must be excluded by pulmonary angiography. Shrinking lung syndrome is believed to be the result of diaphragmatic dysfunction. In patients whose pulmonary function declines, a trial of 40 to 60 mg of prednisone may be beneficial.

INFLAMMATORY MYOPATHIES

Dermatomyositis (DM) and polymyositis (PM) are inflammatory myopathies that share many clinical manifestations but have distinctive pathogenetic and clinical differences. Both DM and PM present clinically with symmetric, proximal muscle weakness, usually of insidious onset. Dysphagia or regurgitation of swallowed food with possible aspiration may occur secondary to involvement of striated esophageal muscle. Both myopathies may be associated with malignancy, but the incidence is higher in DM. Two classic skin manifestations are seen in DM: (1) the Gottron sign, an erythematous, symmetric, nonscaling rash over the extensor surfaces of the metacarpophalangeal/interphalangeal joints, elbows, and knees; and (2) heliotrope rash, a reddish-violaceous erythema of the upper eyelids. Pathogenetically, DM is associated with immune complex deposition in the vessels, whereas PM appears to result from T-cell–mediated cytotoxicity. A clinical diagnosis is supported by an increase in muscle enzymes (creatine phosphokinase, aldolase, lactate dehydrogenase, aspartate and alanine aminotransferases) and an electromyogram showing increased membrane irritability. A muscle biopsy specimen obtained usually from a clinically weak muscle demonstrates muscle fiber necrosis, degeneration, and regeneration and an inflammatory cell infiltrate that is perifascicular or perivascular in DM and intrafascicular in PM. Other typical histologic features for DM are perifascicular atrophy and fibrosis. More than 80% of the patients have autoantibodies to nuclear and/or cytoplasmic antibodies such as anti-RNP, anti-SSA, or anti-PM-Scl. Myositis-specific antibodies (anti-Jo-1, anti-Mi2, and anti-SRP) are present in approximately half of the patients, define clinically discrete subgroups of patients, and appear to have predictive value for the response to treatment.

Other possible causes that can cause muscle weakness—such as amyotrophic lateral sclerosis, myasthenia gravis, muscular dystrophies, endocrine diseases, drugs such as lipid-lowering agents, zidovudine (AZT, Retrovir), colchicine, and viral infections such as influenza, mononucleosis, rickettsia, HIV, and parasites—need to be excluded.

Corticosteroids are the mainstay of therapy in inflammatory myopathies. Treatment is initiated with 1 mg/kg/d and tapered gradually once a therapeutic response is obtained. The response to corticosteroids, assessed by the improvement in muscle strength and normalization of muscle enzymes, is evaluated at 3 months. Failure to improve or an incomplete response justifies the use of the immunosuppressive drugs such as azathioprine* and/or methotrexate*; however, a corticosteroid myopathy or an alternative diagnosis such as inclusion-body myositis, muscular dystrophies, or hypothyroidism should be considered and excluded before adding these drugs. Methotrexate has the advantage of a convenient once-a-week dosing but should be avoided in patients with a history of liver disease or in those who cannot abstain from alcohol. Monitoring for methotrexate liver toxicity is difficult in the presence of elevated aspartate

*Not FDA approved for this indication.

*Not FDA approved for this indication.

and alanine aminotransferases of muscle origin. In patients with myositis-associated interstitial lung disease, the possibility of methotrexate pulmonary toxicity may present diagnostic difficulties; therefore, azathioprine may be preferred in this setting. The rash from DM responds to topical corticosteroids and/or antimalarial agents.

SYSTEMIC SCLEROSIS

Systemic sclerosis is a multisystemic disease characterized by fibrosis of the skin and internal organs and an obliterative small vessel vasculopathy. Patients with limited cutaneous systemic sclerosis have skin thickening limited to extremities distal to the elbows or knees, whereas patients with diffuse cutaneous systemic sclerosis (diffuse scleroderma) have skin thickening involving the trunk and the extremities in areas both distal and proximal to knees and elbows. CREST syndrome (*c*alcinosis, *R*aynaud's phenomenon, *e*sophageal dysmotility, *s*clerodactyly, *t*elangiectasia) is a subgroup of limited scleroderma distinguished by skin thickening limited to the fingers and face and often association with anticentromere antibodies. In scleroderma overlap syndromes, features of limited or diffuse scleroderma coexist with features of polymyositis, rheumatoid arthritis, systemic lupus erythematosus, or Sjögren's syndrome. Raynaud's phenomenon is present in 95% of cases of limited or diffuse scleroderma. The absence of Raynaud's phenomenon and sparing of the fingers from skin thickening raises the possibility of diagnoses other than scleroderma.

Many patients with limited scleroderma have a more benign onset and course than patients with diffuse scleroderma, but interstitial lung disease or pulmonary artery hypertension may occur. Anticentromere antibodies are found in 20% to 30% of patients with limited scleroderma, especially in those with the CREST variant, and are associated with relative protection from interstitial lung disease but not from pulmonary artery hypertension. In contrast, patients with diffuse scleroderma often have a more abrupt onset, with constitutional symptoms, clear-cut skin thickening with proximal involvement, significant arthralgias, and onset of major internal organ involvement within the first few years of disease. Typically, skin involvement regresses spontaneously after 18 to 36 months of disease whereas organ involvement may remain fixed. Antibodies against DNA topoisomerase 1 (Scl-70) are found in 15% to 25% of patients with diffuse scleroderma. Their presence is often associated with interstitial lung disease.

Treatment of scleroderma is based on the extent and severity of organ involvement. No treatment has been shown to accelerate the spontaneous improvement in skin thickening. The mainstays of treatment for Raynaud's phenomenon are cold exposure avoidance, warm clothing, and calcium channel blockers. When digital ulcers occur, general measures such as local wound cleansing with soap and water and topical antibiotic creams may be useful. Antibiotic therapy and débridement of infarcted tissue is sometimes necessary. When severe ischemia or frank infarction occurs, Doppler examination of the palmar arch may identify a surgically approachable lesion or need for thrombolytic therapy.

Dysmotility of the gastrointestinal tract is responsible for multiple complaints such as heartburn, dysphagia, postprandial bloating, early satiety, abdominal cramps, and pseudo-obstruction. Proton pump inhibitors and prokinetic/motility agents are beneficial in relieving symptoms and prevent the development of esophageal erosions. Dysphagia may respond to metoclopramide (Reglan). Intestinal dysmotility symptoms may be improved by treatment with prokinetic agents such as low-dose erythromycin* and the somatostatin analogue octreotide (Sandostatin). Diarrhea due to bacterial overgrowth and malabsorption is treated with antibiotics. Pulmonary fibrosis is suggested by dyspnea on exertion, dry cough, bibasilar crackles, and restrictive pulmonary function test abnormalities. High-resolution computed tomography and bronchoalveolar lavage can be used to estimate the degree of lung inflammation. When alveolitis is present, treatment with 100 to 150 mg/d of cyclophosphamide (Cytoxan)* for 12 to 18 months has been reported to improve lung function outcome and survival. Pulmonary hypertension due to scleroderma may improve with calcium channel blockers in approximately 20% of patients. Continuous intravenous epoprostenol (Flolan) (prostaglandin I_2), has been used and approved for use in pulmonary hypertension in patients with scleroderma. Lung transplantation may be considered in patients with end-stage lung disease.

Scleroderma renal crisis presents as diastolic hypertension and rapid decline in renal function, which can be associated with microangiopathic hemolytic anemia, retinopathy, proteinuria, or hematuria. Antecedent high-dose corticosteroid therapy is associated with scleroderma renal crisis. Aggressive therapy with angiotensin-converting enzyme inhibitors is the first-line therapy for renal crisis. An inflammatory myositis indistinguishable from polymyositis occurs in a small number of patients and usually responds to corticosteroid treatment. Methotrexate* may be helpful as a corticosteroid-sparing agent.

*Not FDA approved for this indication.

CUTANEOUS VASCULITIS

method of
IRENA SPEKTOR, M.D., and
ROBERT A. SWERLICK, M.D.
Emory University School of Medicine
Atlanta, Georgia

The most common form of cutaneous vasculitis is *cutaneous necrotizing vasculitis* (CNV) (also known as small-vessel necrotizing vasculitis, leukocytoclastic vasculitis, allergic angiitis, or hypersensitivity vasculitis), which appears clinically as crops of palpable purpuric lesions, usually at the same stage. The initial lesions may be erythematous macules or urticarial plaques that rapidly become hemorrhagic and purpuric. A small but significant percentage of patients develop atypical lesions characterized by pustules, bullae, plaques, and ulcerations. Lesions occur most frequently on the skin below the knees and, less commonly, on other dependent areas. Facial and mucous membrane lesions may be seen, particularly in patients with severe nausea and vomiting.

HISTOPATHOLOGY

On histopathologic examination of CNV lesions, leukocytoclastic vasculitis (LCV) is most commonly demonstrated. Pathogenesis of this form of CNV is mediated by immune complexes that are formed after antigenic exposure (type III hypersensitivity reaction) and deposited in the vessel walls of small postcapillary venules, activating the complement cascade and inducing neutrophil influx and inflammatory mediator release. The inflammatory reaction results in segmental vessel wall destruction, endothelial cell swelling, fibrinoid necrosis of the vessel walls, and erythrocyte extravasation. A cellular infiltrate within and around the blood vessel walls consists mainly of neutrophils exhibiting nuclear fragmentation. Fibrin, complement, and immunoglobulin deposition may be seen on immunofluorescent examination, particularly of early lesions. In addition to the leukocytoclastic variant, a distinct lymphomonocytic form of CNV of presumed immune cell-mediated pathogenesis has been described.

DIFFERENTIAL DIAGNOSIS

Differential diagnoses of CNV include both inflammatory and noninflammatory purpuras. Palpable purpura may result from embolic phenomena such as left atrial myxoma, endocarditis, or cholesterol emboli. In patients with paraprotein disorders, such as essential mixed cryoglobulinemia or hyperglobulinemia, the pathologic lesions can be vasculitic or result from occlusive vasculopathy. Cutaneous infarctions in patients with disseminated intravascular coagulation or other hypercoagulable states, noninflammatory dependent purpura in patients with thrombocytopenia, as well as fragile blood vessels in disorders such as scurvy may also mimic cutaneous lesions of vasculitis. Other inflammatory skin conditions such as erythema multiforme may appear clinically similar to LCV.

EVALUATION

The critical elements of evaluation of a patient with CNV are confirmation of the diagnosis, identification of any treatable precipitating factors, and definition of whether the vasculitis is limited to the skin or involves extracutaneous sites. Although cutaneous vasculitis can be diagnosed clinically in many cases, it is prudent to obtain a biopsy specimen to confirm the diagnosis histologically. Additionally, fresh frozen tissue or tissue preserved in Michel media can be examined for deposition of immunoglobulins or complement in dermal blood vessels. This may be useful to identify individuals with Henoch-Schönlein purpura, who demonstrate deposits of IgA in dermal blood vessels, whereas IgG or IgM deposits are seen in most other types of LCV.

It is generally assumed that vasculitis results from an aberrant immune response to exogenous or endogenous antigens, although an inciting agent or underlying illness can only be identified in about half of cases of cutaneous vasculitis. In those individuals in whom an agent can be identified, up to 60% are presumed to have drug-induced vasculitis, although patients are almost never rechallenged. The most commonly implicated medications are penicillins, diuretics, sulfonamides, nonsteroidal anti-inflammatory agents (NSAIDs), antihypertensives, and anticonvulsants.

Infection may be associated with cutaneous vasculitis in approximately 10% of reported cases. Acute necrotizing vasculitis may be seen in cases of dental abscess, bacterial endocarditis, meningococcal meningitis, or Rocky Mountain spotted fever. Chronic infections, such as hepatitis B and/or C, or chronic streptococcal infections have also been associated with CNV. Other infections linked to cutaneous vasculitis are hemorrhagic fever, *Mycoplasma* infection, syphilis, gonorrhea, and fungal infection.

The clinical course of patients with collagen vascular diseases is not infrequently complicated by cutaneous vasculitis, with or without visceral involvement. The true incidence of systemic involvement in patients who present with CNV is not certain and is difficult to define. Arthritis and arthralgias may be seen in up to 40% of patients, although frank arthritis is often associated with pre-existing rheumatologic disease. The actual incidence of renal involvement in patients with cutaneous vasculitis is also uncertain. Renal disease is the leading cause of end-organ failure in those affected with cutaneous vasculitis.

A subset of patients with malignancy may present with cutaneous vasculitis in association with other constitutional symptoms. Concurrent expression of CNV is associated with a variety of bone marrow dyscrasias, leukemias, and solid tumors. These patients tend to have a very poor prognosis.

The history and careful physical examination are crucial in determining the extent of laboratory workup necessary for evaluation of cutaneous vasculitis. A minimal laboratory screening evaluation should include a complete blood cell count with differential, as well as measurement of the platelet count; serum creatinine, blood urea nitrogen, liver enzyme, and bilirubin levels; sedimentation rate; urinalysis; and stool sample test for occult blood. Evaluation for renal disease is particularly important because renal disease associated with CNV may be completely asymptomatic.

Further tests should be dictated by the findings of the history or the physical examination. Prominent pulmonary symptoms are not characteristic of CNV and should alert the examiner to the possibility of Wegener's granulomatosis or allergic granulomatosis. Neurologic findings or prominent gastrointestinal pain may suggest a diagnosis of polyarteritis nodosa. Additional studies may include serologic testing for rheumatoid factor, antinuclear antibodies, antineutrophil cytoplasmic antibodies, complement levels, cryoglobulins, cryofibrinogens, anticardiolipin antibodies, serum protein electrophoresis, and hepatitis B and C antigens. Further diagnostic examination may include chest radiography, arteriography, or biopsy of extracutaneous sites.

THERAPY

Most patients with CNV have a self-limited disease with no extracutaneous manifestations. One needs to be certain to identify any treatable causes, including any possible drug-induced etiology. It may be necessary to include a history of occult or illicit drug use. Most patients have minimal to moderate symptoms associated with multiple crops of cutaneous lesions that develop and resolve over a period of a few weeks to a few months. Therapy should be supportive and directed toward symptoms. Mild burning or itching may benefit from antihistamines, and pain or arthralgias may be relieved by NSAIDs or acetaminophen. Leg elevation, use of support hose, or both may improve swelling. A graded pressure stocking is preferable to antiembolism hose, and its usefulness alone or as an adjunct to any other therapy instituted should not be underestimated.

Certain patients have more severe cutaneous disease that, although limited to the skin, requires more aggressive therapy. After careful examination for extracutaneous disease or infection, a short course of oral corticosteroids may be extremely useful in controlling severe cutaneous disease. When treating patients with non–life-threatening vasculitic syndromes, a short-acting oral preparation (prednisone or methylprednisolone, 0.5–1 mg/kg/d) should be given in a single daily dose to minimize the chance of adrenal suppression.

Systemic corticosteroids are extremely effective agents for patients with severely debilitating disease, but long-term use is limited by predictable toxicity. Long-term management of patients with persistent disease should be directed toward using alternate-day corticosteroid therapy, a corticosteroid-sparing agent, or both.

Colchicine,* 0.6 mg given once to three times daily, may be a very effective agent either alone or in conjunction with alternate-day corticosteroid therapy. Gastrointestinal intolerance, most commonly diarrhea, may limit colchicine's usefulness, although most patents tolerate up to 0.6 mg twice daily with minimal difficulty. Bone marrow toxicity has been reported, and it is prudent to monitor complete blood cell and platelet counts during therapy. In addition, colchicine is teratogenic; thus, it should be avoided in potentially pregnant women.

Dapsone* has also been shown to be useful in the management of subsets of individuals with cutaneous vasculitis. All patients should be screened for glucose-6-phosphate dehydrogenase (G6PD) deficiency before use. Dapsone is generally used at doses of 100 to 200 mg/d, although higher doses can be used if tolerated. All patients develop some degree of hemolysis and methemoglobinemia, and patients with compromised cardiac or pulmonary function should be started on lower doses. Hemolysis may be alleviated to some degree by daily administration of vitamin E (800 U/d). Methemoglobinemia associated with high-dose dapsone therapy may be monitored with venous blood and can be controlled by the administration of methylene blue tablets* (Urolene Blue), 65 to 130 mg one to three times daily with meals. Dapsone may be associated with idiosyncratic reactions that tend to occur early in the treatment course. These reactions may include flulike illness associated with elevated liver enzymes and potentially life-threatening neutropenia. Blood cell counts with differential and liver function studies should be obtained on a biweekly basis for the first 2 to 3 months, and then every 3 to 4 months thereafter. High doses of dapsone may also be associated with a peripheral neuropathy.

*Not FDA approved for this indication.

The use of immunosuppressive agents for systemic vasculitis has been well described. Patients with life-threatening vasculitic syndromes such as Wegener's granulomatosis, polyarteritis nodosa, or allergic granulomatosis of Churg and Strauss are often treated with a combination of divided dose corticosteroids and immunosuppressive agents, including cyclophosphamide (Cytoxan)* or azathioprine (Imuran).* However, the use of these immunosuppressive agents in skin-limited vasculitis is of unproven benefit.

Additional therapeutic considerations include pentoxifylline (Trental),* mezoglycan,† mycophenolate mofetil (CellCept),* leflunomide (Arava),* chlorambucil (Leukeran),* thalidomide (Thalomid),* dapsone,* methotrexate,* cyclosporine (Sandimmune),* interferon alfa,* and intravenous immune globulin.*

*Not FDA approved for this indication.
†Not available in the United States.

DISEASES OF THE NAILS

method of
MARTIN ZAIAC, M.D., and
LISA BARBA, A.R.N.P.
Mt. Sinai, Miami Beach, Florida

The primary functions of the nail are to protect the fingertip, aid in tactile discrimination, assist in manipulating small objects, and be a convenient tool for many everyday purposes. Apart from compromising the manipulative function of the nail, nail disease can be disfiguring and a source of embarrassment to the affected individual. Numerous studies have shown that quality of life values are lower in patients affected by nail disorders. Rough, thickened, discolored, or disfigured nails are unsightly and often a source of embarrassment. Smooth and even-colored nails are considered an essential component in personal hygiene. Thus, the esthetic importance of nails should not be overlooked.

An overview of basic nail anatomy, general nail hygiene measures, and common nail disorders and their management is provided here. Common terms in nail disease are given in Table 1. Nail disorders vary in their cause and presentation and are generally divided into different categories: infectious, inflammatory, neoplastic, and miscellaneous causes.

NAIL ANATOMY

When treating nail disorders, the knowledge of nail anatomy is important. The nail unit is composed of four different parts and includes the proximal nail fold, nail bed, nail

TABLE 1. **Glossary of Common Terms for Nail Disease**

Anonychia	Absence of nail plate of nail unit
Hyponychium	Distal component of the nail unit, beneath the nail bed
Koilonychia	Spoon shaped nail plate
Leukonychia	Whitening of the nail plate
Lunula	Visible, half moon pattern of the distal matrix
Median nail dystrophy	Medical split in the nail plate
Onychalgia	Nail unit pain
Onychauxis	Hypertrophied nail plate
Onychogryphosis	Curved pattern nail plate grows in a ram's horn shape
Onycholysis	Distal separation of the nail from the nail bed
Onychomadesis	Proximal separation of the nail plate from the matrix
Onychomycosis	Fungal infection of the nail unit
Onychophagia	Nail biting
Onychorrhexis	Longitudinal striations of the nail plate
Onychoschizia	Distal splitting of the nail plate parallel to the nail bed
Onychotillomania	Compulsive pulling or picking of nails
Paronychia	Inflammation or infection of the nail unit
Trachyonychia	Rough nails
Unguis incarnatus	Ingrown nail

matrix, and hyponychium. The proximal nail fold is an extension of the overlying epidermis and produces the cuticle, which adheres to the nail plate. The cuticle acts as a barrier and seal to protect the growing nail unit from the environment. The nail bed lies under the nail plate and begins at the distal end of the matrix and reaches the hyponychium. The hyponychium is the most distal component of the nail unit and is the area under the free edge of the nail plate. The matrix is the most important component of the nail unit because it is responsible for the formation of the nail plate. The rate of nail plate growth varies from the fingernails to the toenails, with the fingernails growing faster than the toenails at a rate between 0.5 and 1.2 mm/wk. It takes 5 to 6 months to completely regrow a fingernail and 8 to 12 months to regrow a toenail.

GENERAL NAIL HYGIENE MEASURES

It is important to educate patients with and without nail disorders on proper nail hygiene measures to prevent damage to the nail unit. Patients should be taught not to clean the underside of the nail plate aggressively with any sharp tools. A soft toothbrush or nail brush can be used for this purpose. Patients should be instructed to keep nails short and filed smooth with a nail file. Manicures should be performed, ideally, with the patient's own tools to prevent possible cross contamination in nail salons. If a patient desires to have manicures, emphasis should be placed on avoiding manipulation and trauma to the nail unit to prevent compromise of the nail unit structures. Special attention should be placed on protecting the cuticle, which acts as a natural barrier to the environment. Aggressive cleaning may lead to infection.

To protect the nails from potential irritants, it is suggested that individuals wear gloves when working with water or chemicals. The regular use of a moisturizer for the nails is also recommended to prevent excessive drying of the nail plate and nail folds.

FUNGAL INFECTIONS

Onychomycosis

Onychomycosis is the term used for any fungal infection of the nail and accounts for more than 50% of nail conditions seen in office settings nationwide. Onychomycosis can be divided into fungal infections caused by dermatophytes, yeasts, and nondermatophyte molds. Dermatophytes are the most common cause of onychomycosis.

Dermatophyte infections can be classified into three subtypes: distal subungual onychomycosis (DSO), white superficial onychomycosis (WSO), and proximal subungual onychomycosis (PSO). DSO occurs when fungus from the palmar and plantar epidermis invades the hyponychium and lateral nail folds and advances to the underside of the distal free edge of the nail plate and into the nail bed. DSO does not invade the nail plate. Manifestations include hyperkeratosis, subungual debris, and discoloration of the nail. *Trichophyton rubrum* is the most common organism found in DSO.

WSO exists when fungus invades only the superficial surface of the nail plate. Manifestations include patchy white streaks on the nail plate. *Trichophyton mentagrophytes* is commonly identified as the cause of WSO, although other types of fungi have also been detected.

PSO is a rare form of onychomycosis seen most commonly in the immunocompromised host (e.g., a person with HIV infection, on chemotherapy, or with leukemia) caused by invasion of fungus through the proximal nail fold. A white-brown patch at the proximal subungual aspect of the nail plate is the most common presenting sign. PSO is considered a marker for HIV infection.

Management of onychomycosis has improved significantly over the years. Before treatment, it is essential to establish the diagnosis of onychomycosis because it can mimic other conditions, especially psoriasis. A potassium hydroxide 10% slide preparation, a fungal culture using subungual nail bed debris or scrapings from the superficial nail plate, and a biopsy of a nail clipping are appropriate diagnostic tests to confirm the diagnosis.

Systemic antifungal agents are the treatment of choice in the management of onychomycosis. Systemic medications diffuse into the nail bed and incorporate into the growing nail plate to act as a barrier to the fungus. The Food and Drug Administration (FDA) has approved terbinafine (Lamisil), 250 mg/d for 3 months, as a treatment option for onychomycosis. Itraconazole (Sporanox) pulse dosing at 200 mg twice a day for 7 days every month for a total of 3 months is another FDA-approved treatment option. Alternative methods have been shown to be effective and include pulse dosing with terbinafine at 250 mg every day for 7 days each month (unpublished study). Anecdotal evidence suggests that terbinafine pulse dosing at 250 mg every day for 7 days on alternating months may also be helpful in eradicating onychomycosis.

Topical preparations have limited value in the treatment of DSO. They do not penetrate through the nail plate into the nail bed and therefore are not as effective as systemic medications. However, WSO, a fungal infection of the nail plate, can be successfully treated with topical preparations because the fungal infection is on the surface of the nail plate. Ciclopirox (Penlac) is a new antifungal nail lacquer that may be useful for patients who refuse or cannot take systemic medications. Another approach is to remove or debulk the nail or smooth the nail plate with a nail file followed by twice-daily applications of an antifungal cream such as terbinafine.

Dr. Nardo Zaias, a leading nail specialist, has suggested a novel approach to monitoring and evaluating the treatment of onychomycosis with systemic medications. He suggests that a nail wedge be placed using a No. 15 scalpel blade to mark the most proximal point of clinical invasion by the fungus. The growth of healthy normal nail can be measured at subsequent visits to monitor progress and will assist in determining whether improvement is occurring with the use of systemic medications. It is also suggested that treatment with systemic antifungal agents continue until complete regrowth of the affected nail has occurred.

The most common form of onychomycosis caused by yeast and molds is caused by *Candida*. Candidal onychomycosis is found only in individuals who have *chronic mucocutaneous candidiasis,* a term used to describe a group of syndromes characterized by chronic, treatment-resistant, superficial candidal infections of the skin, nails and oropharynx. Candidal onychomycosis may also be found as a secondary infection in patients who have onycholysis, or separation of the nail plate from the nail bed.

Candida affects the nail plate of both the fingernails and toenails by invasion through the hyponychium. The nails become thickened, rough, and discolored. The appearance of the nails may mimic DSO. However, an inflammatory paronychia may accompany candidal onychomycosis.

Management of candidal onychomycosis requires identification of the pathogen with the use of a potassium hydroxide preparation or fungal culture. Onychomycosis caused by *Candida* can be treated by avoiding any contact with water by using gloves, limiting hand washing, and drying the hands carefully after washing. Treatment should also be focused on the treatment of onycholysis. Topical ketoconazole (Nizoral) may be applied twice a day to the affected nails in resistant cases.

VIRAL INFECTIONS

Verruca

Verrucae are caused by the human papillomavirus (HPV) and can often affect the periungal area. Verrucae present as firm, hyperkeratotic, skin-colored vegetative papules on the nail folds. Reddish-brown dots in the lesion represent thrombosed capillaries and are pathognomonic for verruca. Occasionally, very large warts may interfere with the normal growth pattern of the nail by applying pressure at the nail matrix.

Management of verruca in the periungal area is similar to treatment of verruca on other parts of the body. Spontaneous regression of verruca is reported, but patients will often request treatment. Liquid nitrogen applied on a regular schedule until completely resolved is an option. Other treatment options include surgical excision, carbon dioxide laser, cantharidin, imiquimod (Aldara),* and over-the-counter preparations that contain salicylic acid. Intralesional bleomycin (Blenoxane)* by an experienced practitioner has been reported to be successful in the treatment of recalcitrant warts. Treatment of warts by any means can be painful and can lead to scarring.

Refractory lesions require a biopsy because verruca can often mimic squamous cell carcinoma. A low threshold of suspicion for a squamous cell carcinoma should be held for any lesion that does not respond to treatment.

BACTERIAL INFECTIONS

Pseudomonas Infection

Pseudomonas is a gram-negative bacterium that commonly invades the nail unit and thrives in the moist, warm environment beneath the nail plate. Clinically, this infection produces a dark green pigment known as pyocyanin in an irregular-sized patch under the nail. *Pseudomonas* often occurs secondary to onycholysis.

Management of *Pseudomonas* infection includes treatment of onycholysis. Soaking the affected nail in a 1:4 concentration of water to bleach or vinegar solution four times a day is a simple and cost-effective treatment option. Clipping the affected nail may assist with a more rapid clearing of the infection. The use of a blow dryer on a warm setting after hand washing is a novel approach to thoroughly drying underneath the nail plate. General nail hygiene measures should also be employed.

INFLAMMATORY DISEASE

Psoriasis

Psoriasis is a chronic, relapsing, inflammatory disorder of the skin that can also affect the nails. Psoriasis in the skin presents as sharply demarcated pink-colored plaques with overlying silvery scales on various areas of the body. Psoriatic nail disease affects between 10% and 15% of patients seen with psoriasis. Psoriasis can manifest itself in the nail without evidence of cutaneous signs and can affect a single nail or all 20. The most common manifestations of nail psoriasis include nail pitting, furrows or transverse depressions, onycholysis, splinter hemorrhage, and subungual hyperkeratosis. The "oil drop

*Not FDA approved for this indication.

sign," a reddish-brown discoloration of the nail bed, as seen through the nail plate, is pathognomonic for nail psoriasis.

The nail abnormalities that occur with nail psoriasis can mimic other nail disorders, the most common being onychomycosis. In this case, it is helpful to examine a sample of subungual debris on a slide with potassium hydroxide 10% for the presence of hyphae or obtain subungual debris for culture evaluation. Histologic examination of a nail clipping, which reveals confluent parakeratosis with neutrophils, will also assist in making the final diagnosis.

Many topical preparations are available in the treatment of psoriasis of the skin but have limited value in the treatment of nail psoriasis, because they do not penetrate into the nail unit. Topical preparations that are available for treatment of nail psoriasis include daily applications of high-potency corticosteroids (e.g., clobetasol propionate [Temovate], ointment), retinoids (e.g., tazarotene [Tazorac] gel), and the vitamin D derivative calcipotriene (Dovonex).

Patients who receive systemic medications for skin disease often see an improvement in their nails. Methotrexate, acitretin (Soriatane), and cyclosporine (Neoral) are available to treat psoriasis and are very useful in controlling psoriasis. However, the use of systemic medications in psoriatic nail disease should be used only in individuals with extensive psoriatic skin disease because of potential side effects associated with long-term use. However, recurrence after treatment is common and patients should be made aware of this before instituting a regimen. Intralesional injections into the nail matrix with 2.5- to 3.0-mg/mL triamcinolone acetonide (Kenalog) every 4 to 6 weeks may have some benefit in controlling psoriasis limited to the nails. Intralesional injections are painful and should be limited to the treatment of individual nails or in patients who are motivated to undergo this procedure.

Lichen Planus

Lichen planus is a common inflammatory skin condition of unknown etiology that can affect both the skin and nails. Only 1% to 2% of all individuals affected by lichen planus have disease limited to the nails. Lichen planus of the skin appears as erythematous to violaceous, flat-topped, polygonal papules with fine, white lines on the surface, also known as Wickham's striae. The most common manifestations to occur with lichen planus of the nails include thinning, longitudinal ridging, and distal splitting of the nail plate, onycholysis, and subungual hyperkeratosis. Nail bed pterygium appears as adhesions between the epidermis of the proximal nail fold and nail bed and is pathognomonic for lichen planus. The presence of pterygium leads to the eventual destruction of the nail matrix and loss of the nail plate.

Management of the patient with lichen planus includes early detection and intervention to prevent irreversible destruction of the nail unit. If only one nail is affected, intralesional injections of 2.5 to 3.0 mg/mL triamcinolone acetonide using a 30-gauge needle into the nail matrix has been found to be effective in slowing the progression of lichen planus.

If all nails are affected, systemic corticosteroids at 20 to 40 mg/d may be indicated for several months. However, if systemic medications are to be considered, it is best to provide histologic evidence of lichen planus before beginning oral corticosteroids.

NEOPLASMS

Melanoma

Melanoma of the nail unit is rare but can be fatal if not treated early. Five-year survival figures for invasive melanoma are low. Melanoma of the nail unit is usually asymptomatic and often overlooked, resulting in a delayed diagnosis. Pain and discomfort is rare, as is nail dystrophy. Specific signs in any dark brown or black pigmented lesion in the nail unit should make the provider suspicious for melanoma and include single nail involvement, occurrence in middle age or older, widening or darkening of a lesion, and/or leaching of pigment into the proximal nail folds (Hutchinson's sign).

Threshold suspicion should be low for melanoma of the nail unit. It should be assumed that an acquired, longitudinal pigmented band in the nail of a white patient is a melanoma until proven otherwise. Heavily pigmented individuals often have benign longitudinal brown and black bands in the nails known as melanonychia striata. Melanonychia striata is a benign condition, especially in patients with darker skin.

Management of melanoma in the nail unit includes early detection of a pigmented lesion. A biopsy is essential in confirming the diagnosis of melanoma. Treatment options include surgical removal of the pigmented lesion with adequate surrounding margins. A radiograph of the site will assess possible bony involvement. If necessary, systemic chemotherapy and localized irradiation should be implemented.

Squamous Cell Carcinoma

Squamous cell carcinoma (SCC) is a slow-growing, uncommon lesion that can affect the nail unit. The signs and symptoms of SCC are nonspecific and include bleeding, swelling, and ulceration of a thickened, granulated papule on the nail folds. Pain and nail plate deformity may also occur as a result of the tumor impinging at the nail matrix. SCCs are commonly mistaken for verruca, resulting in delayed diagnosis; thus, recalcitrant verruca requires a biopsy. Any lesion that does not respond to treatment in an adequate time period should be evaluated for a malignant process.

Management of squamous cell carcinoma in the nail unit includes a low threshold of suspicion with early detection followed by a biopsy. Treatment consists of conservative surgical removal of the lesion with adequate margins. Mohs' surgery is the surgical method of choice for excision of SCC in the nail unit.

MISCELLANEOUS CONDITIONS

Paronychia

Paronychia is a common occurrence and is characterized by damage or loss of the cuticle due to trauma, followed by inflammation. Loss of the cuticle facilitates exposure of the nail to the environment and its irritants such as pathogens, chemicals, solvents, food products, and water. Redness, warmth, tenderness, and edema surrounding the nail folds are classic presenting signs.

Acute paronychia is a primary infection of the nail folds following trauma. Aggressive manicuring and self-induced traumatic manipulation of the nails are examples of trauma that can cause an acute paronychia. Bacterial infection by *Staphylococcus aureus* and *Streptococcus* are common. Paronychia can also be caused by yeast, the most common which is *C. albicans*. Unless trauma is avoided, acute paronychia will progress to the chronic state.

Management of acute paronychia includes patient education on proper nail hygiene and the avoidance of trauma and irritants to the cuticle. Culture and sensitivity studies should be performed to identify the infectious organism followed by administration of appropriate antibiotic therapy. Warm saline soaks for 10 to 15 minutes two to four times a day may help resolve the inflammation of acute paronychia.

Chronic paronychia is a more insidious process than acute paronychia. Chronic paronychia occurs most frequently in people whose jobs require their hands to be in a moist environment (e.g., bartenders, waiters, chefs, hair salon employees). Frequent immersion in water or other irritants results in a compromised cuticle. A good history is necessary to determine the offending irritant or cause. The primary cause must be avoided for healing to take place and prevent recurrence.

Management of chronic paronychia includes patient education. Patients are encouraged to use gloves whenever in contact with aqueous solutions. The use of a blow dryer on a warm setting will adequately dry the nails after immersion in water. Patients must understand that the cause of the paronychia is a compromised and damaged cuticle. Appropriate nail hygiene measures should be encouraged.

Onycholysis

Onycholysis is defined as separation on the nail plate from the underlying nail bed. A single or multiple nails may be affected. A white opaque patch of varying size and shape reflects the portion of the nail plate that is separated from the nail bed. Common causes of onycholysis include trauma (external or self-induced), contact with irritants, systemic and cutaneous disease (psoriasis, lichen planus, dermatitis), infection (fungal, bacterial, viral), systemic medications, neoplasms (verruca), and prosthetic acrylic nails.

Management of onycholysis is challenging. The longer the nail separation is present, the longer it takes the nail plate to reattach to the nail bed, owing to cornification and granulation of the nail bed. Management includes eliminating factors that cause the separation. General nail hygiene measures should be encouraged. Patients must be advised that the nail needs to grow out independently on its own. Manipulation of the separated nail edge will not assist the improvement but will only worsen the condition. Women should be encouraged to paint the nails in a color dark enough to prevent their paying constant attention to the affected nail.

Dry and Brittle Nails

Dry and brittle nails are extremely common. Dry and brittle nails appear as dull, splitting, fragile nails with distal layering. Excessive hydration-dehydration cycles, contact with occupational and recreational irritants, the frequent application and removal of nail polish, and age are the most common causes of dry and brittle nails.

Management of dry and brittle nails includes education of the patient and elimination of the primary cause, which is usually chemicals and water. The use of protective gloves is a good way to protect the nails. General nail hygiene methods should be emphasized. The nails should be kept short with mild buffing to induce a sheen. Moisturizers should be applied on a regular basis, and nail polish removal should be kept to a minimum because of the dehydrating chemicals found in nail polish remover. In recalcitrant cases, the use of nail prostheses or nail wrap applications might be warranted to protect the underlying nail plate.

CONCLUSION

Nail disorders can be disfiguring and can cause a significant amount of psychological stress owing to the pressures by society to maintain a neat appearance. As health care providers, we play a key role in educating patients on how to prevent further damage and destruction to the nail unit. We can also provide valuable information about the different treatment options that exist for different nail disorders. Most importantly, we can provide realistic expectations by educating and informing patients as to what they may expect in the course of their condition.

KELOIDS

method of
ERROL J. QUINTAL, Sr., M.D.
Xavier University of Louisiana
New Orleans, Louisiana

The word *keloid* comes from the term *cheloide,* originally coined by the French dermatologist Jean Louis Alibert in 1806. Actually, he first thought the disfiguring scars were malignant and initially described them as *cancoides.*

Keloids are tumors that develop as a response to dermal injury to the outer covering, and largest organ of the body, the skin. Characteristically, the lesion is protruberant and extends beyond the boundary of injury. Keloids may be asymptomatic, but in most cases, symptoms such as pruritus, stinging, pain, and, occasionally, superficial ulceration and punctate hemorrhaging may occur when the keloid enlarges rapidly.

African Americans appear to be more prone toward the development of keloids. Keloids also occur in people of other ethnic background and in whites. There appears to be no correlation between the degree of pigmentation of the skin and an increased tendency toward the formation of keloids.

With the growing popularity among young people of increasing the number of piercings for earrings from two to as many as possible and the return to the old trend of body piercing and tattooing, physicians will see more patients with preventable keloids. In regard to body piercing, allergy to the metal nickel in jewelry inserted or clamped onto the skin accompanied by a superimposed secondary infection can stimulate the development of a keloid tumor. Contrary to the popular belief that stainless steel jewelry should be worn when one is allergic to jewelry containing nickel, it has been found that stainless steel may contain as much as 37% nickel plus other sensitizing metals such as chromium and cobalt. Besides the ears, keloids can affect the eyebrows, tongue, umbilicus, and genitalia. Anatomic boundaries do not seem to exist. Frequently, keloid formation is a postsurgical complication. Children sometimes develop keloids in excoriated lesions of varicella.

Previously, it was thought that keloids in certain areas of the body, such as the shoulders, chest, back, and arms, were spontaneously induced and some were coined *safety-pin keloids* because of the unusual configuration of the lesion. Actually, these keloids are the result of either a subtle or pronounced folliculitis of the skin. Lesions of this variety also develop in the face and trunk in patients with papulonodular and cystic acne. Ingrown hairs in the scalp, face, neck, and pubic area similarly may eventuate into a keloid. Thermal and chemical burn victims have the most disfiguring and sometimes very extensive keloidal scars. Keloids have also been reported to form in the lesions of Kaposi sarcoma.

GENETICS

In this age of unraveling the human genome, we can probably look forward to a clearer understanding of the genes that program the predisposition to form keloids. Certainly, individuals of parents with keloids are more likely to express this genetic problem. In families in which a parent and a sibling are affected, this suggests inheritance of the dominant type. Unfortunately, ascertaining a relevant family history is not always feasible in this era of nonmarital procreation. Confusing this malady is another not well understood observance—those who form keloids secondary to piercing the ears may not necessarily form keloids elsewhere on the body after sustaining dermal trauma. Frequently, individuals with a past history of having major surgery without forming a keloid may develop a keloid on the ear after ear piercing. Genetics, metal contact allergy, and infection should all be considered as causative factors.

HISTOPATHOLOGY

During initial development, the immature keloid is proliferatively composed of fibroblasts in an unrestrained, highly vascularized, myxoid stroma. As the lesion matures, the number of fibroblasts decreases and the end result is a mature layer of eosinophilic, acellular collagen. Plasma cells and mast cells are seen in increased numbers; however, elastin is usually sparse or absent. The presence of fibroblasts and myofibroblasts and a disarrangement of collagen have been elucidated with the electron microscope.

PATHOGENESIS

Although it is not completely understood what biochemical and pathologic factors initiate the formation of a keloid, we have begun to elucidate a clearer insight of the mechanisms through which keloids tend to develop. It has been suggested that keloid formation is biochemically related to the growth factors or cytokines. Plasminogen activator inhibitor type 1 is secreted by fibroblasts. Elevated levels of this protein may result in the formation of keloids. Another protein that has been shown to affect keloid production is cytokine transforming growth factor-beta (TGF-β), which induces both the activation of fibroblasts and the extracellular matrix deposition and formation of collagens and proteoglycans. Platelet-derived growth factor (PDGF) and an insulin-like growth factor 1 that are known to regulate cell proliferation, differentiation, and growth are enhanced by plasminogen activator inhibitor type 1 in keloid fibroblasts but not in normal fibroblasts. High levels of connective growth factor are also stimulated by PDGF. Such biochemical abnormalities are compatible with a maverick healing process. Additionally, a gene called *Smad3* has been found to produce a protein that mediates TGF-β concentrations. Studies have determined that keloid tissue expresses proteins made by the *p53* and *bcl-2* genes that are not expressed by normal skin.

Electron microscopic findings suggest that the release of fibrin stimulates endothelial cell proliferation, which leads to the blood vessel occlusion, and, consequently, anoxia, which stimulates keloid formation.

SOCIOECONOMIC RAMIFICATIONS

The social and psychological impairment, compounded by severe physical disability in some cases, endured by these patients demands the utmost of the art and scientific skills within the scope of the physician's capabilities. Keloids on the face and other exposed areas of the body lead to significant social embarrassment and, at times, may lead one into social introversion. It is not uncommon for children to be harassed and adults discriminated against when applying for employment because of this affliction.

TREATMENT

Corticosteroids

Topical corticosteroids are not particularly effective but may have an adjuvant effect when used in conjunction with intralesional corticosteroids and surgery. The exact mechanism by which corticosteroids work is unknown.

Some problems associated with the use of topical and intralesional corticosteroids are suppression of the pituitary-hypothalamic axis, skin atrophy, hypopigmentation, striae, telangiectasia, folliculitis, exacerbation of pre-existing superficial fungal infections, and acne. Exacerbation of pre-existing medical problems such as diabetes mellitus, intestinal ulcers, depression, suicidal proclivity, and hypertension have also been reported.

Compression

Compression therapy is used by some physicians; however, it is difficult to explain therapeutic responses, realizing that, pathologically, compression in itself could also lead to anoxia, which is thought to promote the development of keloids.

Silicone

Silicone sheets alone or in combination with vitamin E have shown promise in the treatment of keloids. Problems associated with the use of this kind of treatment arise when keloids affect surfaces with grooves and crevices such as the ear where the sheets cannot be applied properly. The mechanism of action of silicone on keloids is not well understood. There is conjecture that silicone works by promoting hydration of the keloid. One study questioned the therapeutic effect of silicone on keloids and found that a non–silicone-containing cream alone was beneficial in improving the appearance of keloids. More in-depth, controlled research is needed to prove or disclaim the therapeutic effect of silicone.

Surgery

Surgical approaches to the treatment of keloids should always be used in conjunction with intralesional corticosteroids. Patients must be advised that the surgical excision of any keloid may be followed by a recurrence of the keloid to one of similar size or, unfortunately, to one even larger than the primary mass.

When removal of a keloid is surgically necessary the simplest approach is to perform an elliptical excision followed by biweekly to monthly intralesional injections of 10 to 40 mg/mL of triamcinolone acetonide or acetate for 1 to 2 months, then once monthly if indicated. At the same time the patient is monitored for any untoward effects. Postoperative intralesional therapy requires good patient compliance for the most successful therapeutic outcome.

Surgical removal of keloids on the ear presents unique therapeutic problems in that therapy is performed on a small external organ of the body with little resources for attaining adjacent tissue to cover the surgical defects when a simple elliptical excision does not suffice. Consequently, creation of an acceptable cosmetic outcome dictates considerable ingenuity. Although it has been reported that perhaps as much as one third of an ear can be resected and repaired to provide an acceptably configurated ear, conscientiously it is through the art of tissue manipulation that a superiorly reconstructed ear results. In performing an ear keloidectomy it is important to also remove the pierce that is surrounded by the keloid tissue to minimize the chance of recurrence. Some physicians choose to perform the simple shaving technique for the so-called dumbbell configurated keloids of the earlobe.

Surgery and Irradiation

A success rate implementing the use of surgical excision followed within 24 hours by irradiation in doses between 1000 to 3000 R was reported to be as high as 75%. Recurrences that did occur were seen more often among nonwhites and in the auricular and sternal regions.

Postexcisional kilovoltage irradiation to prevent regrowth was found to control recurrences when the sites were irradiated in the 600- to 900-cGy dosage range.

Irradiation

Irradiation is more effective for the treatment of extensive keloids. For small keloids, however, it is debatable whether irradiation is more effective than using the combination of excision and intralesional steroid therapy. Because of the discomfort that can be associated with intralesional treatment, patient compliance with irradiation is better.

Laser Surgery

Laser treatment of keloids with the carbon dioxide laser followed by healing with secondary intention has not controlled regrowth of keloids and necessitates postoperative intralesional therapy to suppress recurrences.

Electron-Beam Irradiation

Low-dose electron-beam irradiation has been found to be of clinical value. Superficial therapy of this type has not been associated with an increased incidence of radiation carcinogenesis after long-term follow-up.

Cryotherapy

Cryotherapy using liquid nitrogen weekly to biweekly appears to produce a response in about 30% of those treated for keloids; however, it appears to work better for hypertrophic scars. Liquid nitrogen has been shown to destroy melanocytes so this particular form of therapeutic approach may not be appropriate for treating keloids in people with darker skin.

Immunomodulators

Interferon

Interferon gamma (Actimmune),* known to be a potent inhibitor of collagen, has been used with limited success and may be considered as an alternative form of therapy. Successful treatment of keloids with

*Not FDA approved for this indication.

interferon alfa-2a (Roferon-A) in an intramuscular loading dose of 0.6 MU/cm^2 three times weekly for 2 weeks followed by 1 MU/cm^2 weekly for 6 weeks in extensive keloids that developed secondary to severe burns has been rewarding. In a small study, interferon alfa-2b (Intron A) given intralesionally was found to significantly reduce the rate of postoperative recurrences of keloid. Injection of interferon is, however, uncomfortable and costly.

Imiquimod

The use of topical 5% imiquimod (Aldara)* after keloid excision of the ear is under investigation. Initial results appear promising. Imiquimod, which is presently being prescribed for the treatment of human papillomavirus infections, works by stimulating the production of interferon that is thought to intensify collagenase activity while concomitantly reducing collagen and glycosaminoglycan formation.

PREVENTION AND COUNSELING

Nowadays, the importance of providing preventive therapy to patients who are susceptible to keloid formation cannot be overrated. Genetic counseling regarding the predisposition toward these tumors of both patient and family is invaluable. Obviously, the main method of preventing keloids due to body piercing would be to encourage our young people, those mainly affected, not to debase themselves.

African Americans and others of Mediterranean descent are more susceptible toward the formation of keloids after the onset of puberty. The risk of keloidal assailment is significantly greater in the younger age groups and decreases as one ages. Unusually, the elderly may develop keloids. Whether individuals with an atopic diathesis are more susceptible to nickel contact dermatitis and consequent keloid formation is a debatable matter. It is known that contact allergy to nickel is probably the main culprit that initiates the development of a keloid when adornment is involved. Inform your patients that nickel is the major component of costume jewelry. Stainless steel jewelry is less frequently associated with keloidal lesions. Keeping the site of the pierce clean prevents infection, which is another provocative element. Many patients complicate the problem with the use of polymyxin B/neomycin/bacitracin (Neosporin) and other medicaments, which cause further injury to the skin. The use of broom straws to maintain patency of the pierce remains a problem in some socioeconomic levels. In patients who form keloids and are candidates for major surgery, intralesional corticosteroid therapy around the surgical site postoperatively may help hinder keloid formation. Adequately controlling the pruritus associated with varicella and using intralesional steroid injections in patients with papulonodular and cystic acne are somewhat less than miraculous in preventing the development of keloids.

*Not FDA approved for this indication.

CONCLUSION

The treatment of keloids may be very formidable at times. As our therapeutic armamentarium and understanding of the genetic expressions of keloids expand in concert, modern medicine will have more to offer our patients to not only ameliorate their lives but maybe to end this malady.

WARTS AND THEIR MANAGEMENT

method of
ARTHUR D. JACKSON, B.Sc., M.Phil.
University of Wales College of Medicine,
Cardiff, United Kingdom

PREVALENCE

At least 10% of the population has warts at any one time, and few individuals escape them. Over the past 5 decades, the incidence of warts has increased considerably. Whereas previously they were more common in young children, the age range has increased, probably as an outcome of wider participation in recreational activities and changing social habits.

ETIOLOGY

Warts are caused by infection of the skin with a human papillomavirus (HPV). The virus gains entry through a breach in the epidermal surface. It replicates in the cells of the stratum spinosum, causing localized changes in epidermal behavior, giving rise to the clinical lesion. Infection is spread from direct contact from without, not through the tissues or the bloodstream.

Conditions that favor softening of the horny surface facilitate traumatic damage, providing both a portal of entry and an inoculum of infected keratin to be trodden, rubbed, or pressed into that breach. Thus, plantar warts are spread on floors, especially after the feet have been immersed in water. Facial warts are spread by shaving, nail biting, or finger sucking, which spreads warts between hands and lips. Occupations entailing damage to the hands, especially in association with wet work, spread hand warts. Genital warts are spread by sexual intercourse.

About 50% of warts will disappear spontaneously within 2 years. Some warts, however, can cause discomfort and can be a source of considerable incapacity, especially when on fingertips or the weight-bearing areas of the foot. In the United Kingdom, where practitioners are increasingly prepared to treat troublesome warts in primary care, viral warts account for 10% to 20% of new referrals to dermatology outpatient clinics.

IMMUNITY

Good evidence exists that those who develop warts have a lowered immunologic response. All types of warts are more persistent in those whose cell-mediated immunity is suppressed, such as renal transplant patients. In the normal individual, warts undergo spontaneous cure. This may occur within 3 months or take a number of years. In most cases, resolution takes place silently over 3 or 4 weeks. Although resolution may be preceded by itching, occasionally, especially in plantar warts, the lesions become suddenly and acutely painful due to hemorrhage into the surface of the wart. After spontaneous cure, the skin at the site of the warts is restored to normal, leaving no scars. Circulating protective antibodies appear at the time of the cure of the warts and persist for 3 to 4 years. It is not known whether the immunity conferred by one type of HPV confers immunity against others.

MANAGEMENT

Most warts resolve spontaneously, and unless they become painful or are a significant cosmetic problem, such as with someone handling food and serving customers, this can be explained to patients in a helpful information leaflet about warts. In spite of the increased prevalence among swimmers and active sports enthusiasts, I do not discourage these activities but simply advise the use of waterproof bandages during swimming and other physical activities and good skin hygiene.

Warts on Hands

If treatment is considered necessary by patient or parent, first-line treatment is the use of a simple keratolytic agent. This can be in the form of a salicylic acid gel such as salicylic acid 12% and lactic acid 4% gel (Salactic gel) or salicylic acid 11%, lactic acid 4%, copper acetate—equivalent to 1.1 mg copper per 100 g as a gel (Cuplex gel). The latter is less irritating to the surrounding skin and does not need to be covered with a bandage. Good instructions are most important and are provided on a simple advice sheet about warts and their management. Patients should be prepared to spend the time paring down their warts after soaking the skin and applying the wart gel daily for several weeks or even a few months.

Large or Isolated Verrucae

As explained earlier, verrucae on the sole of the foot can become very painful and require treatment. However, the clinician must avoid making the problem worse. Salicylic acid ointment such as Verrugon (salicylic 50%) supplied with self-adhesive corn ring plasters is available. The patient is advised to pumice the verrucae during or after a bath or foot soak. A self-adhesive ring is applied over the verruca, some salicylic acid ointment is squeezed into the space directly over the verruca, and the plaster disk is then applied to seal in the treatment. Patients are advised to repeat this treatment daily or on alternate days after gently using a pumice to wear away the dead part of the verruca. Care should be taken to avoid treatment of skin that is already infected or broken. If pain occurs, medical advice should be sought. An alternative salicylic acid treatment in the form of Cuplex gel is simpler to use, accompanied by thorough preparation of the skin.

Smaller, More Diffuse, and Shallow Verrucae or Mosaic Warts

Five percent formalin in an aqueous solution is a most suitable, painless, and effective way of treating this form of plantar wart. A good instruction sheet about the background of warts and the use of regular formalin soaks is given to the patient. The patient applies a protective layer of petrolatum (Vaseline) to the surrounding normal skin and then immerses the wart tissue for 10 to 20 minutes in a saucer containing the 5% formalin solution. This is repeated daily, and regular paring away of the dead hardened skin is required. After 2 to 3 weeks the warts become smaller and desiccated and can be pared away or curetted out with ease and little pain.

Liquid Nitrogen Cryosurgery

All the treatments discussed so far are readily available from pharmacists or can be prescribed by a primary care physician. Many primary care health centers run regular wart clinics or sessions using liquid nitrogen cryosurgery. As can be seen from Table 1, other refrigerants, such as carbon dioxide snow, have been used in the past for the same purpose. However, liquid nitrogen with its boiling point of −196°C is the most effective cryogen, especially if applied by means of a liquid nitrogen spray as opposed to the cotton pledget technique. Used in the right manner, liquid nitrogen cryosurgery can be of great benefit for the treatment of warts and some verrucae when previous treatments, used properly and adequately, have failed. Cryosurgery of warts does not work by damage to the virus (viruses are sometimes stored in the laboratory in liquid nitrogen) but by destruction of the wart tissue at a cellular level. However, the subzero temperatures used also stimulate the body's immune system and help to effect a more permanent cure. Liquid nitrogen is usually readily available at relative low cost from a hospital pharmacy department or an independent supplier. However, there are some basic rules and facts that need to be understood and adhered to before using cryosurgery for this benign skin condition:

- The majority of warts will eventually undergo spontaneous cure if left alone.
- Eighty percent of warts respond to the application of a keratolytic within 100 days.

TABLE 1. **Surface Tissue Temperatures Attainable With Various Cryogens**

Cryogen	Temperature (degrees Celsius)
Carbon dioxide snow	−79
Nitrous oxide	−75
Liquid nitrogen	−20 (cotton-wool bud) −180 (spray) 196 (probe)

- Cryosurgery is painful and badly tolerated in children.
- The operator must have had proper training and adequate experience in the use of cryosurgery.
- Whether undertaken by a physician or experienced, trained nurse, cryosurgery for a wart lesion should only be considered if there is no doubt about the diagnosis.
- Clear instructions (preferably backed up by an information sheet) about the nature of the treatment and its possible outcome are previously explained to the patient.
- The patient's (and parent in the case of a child) consent is obtained.
- Cryosurgery should not be used on tanned skin or other than white individuals if pigmentary cosmetic problems are to be avoided.

Cotton Pledget Technique

The simplest mode of delivery of liquid nitrogen is with a cotton pledget dipped in liquid nitrogen and firmly applied to the wart until a narrow halo of white ice forms. Because liquid nitrogen applied in this way cannot produce temperatures lower than −20°C, the method is only suitable for treating flat thin warts and can result in considerable surrounding tissue reaction with unnecessary pain.

Closed Delivery System of Cryosurgery

A much more efficient way of using a cryogen is by means of a closed delivery system in which the liquid nitrogen is sprayed directly on the wart lesion. Several designs of the hand-held cryosurgical units are now available. By using the spray spot-freeze technique and holding the spray-tip about 1 cm from the skin over the center of the lesion, a circular "icefield" is formed. The cryogun with its trigger action offers precise control, enabling the clinician to limit the size of the ice ball created to what is required. When the ice has developed within the desired field, spraying is continued to maintain the field size for the length of time considered adequate, from 5 to 20 seconds, depending on the size and thickness of the wart being treated. A record of the freeze-time used should always be entered in the patient's medical records; for example, a single 20-second liquid nitrogen spray freeze would be abbreviated to "Liq.N2 20s single FTC (freeze-thaw-cycle)." It is important to warn the patient about the likely degree of pain and outcome of the procedure beforehand. I always give a simple information sheet of explanation and advice (Table 2). Because patients react differently to liquid nitrogen cryofreeze, it is wise to limit the first freeze to 5 to 8 seconds. The patient is advised to return for review in 3 to 4 weeks to assess the response. If the first freeze has had little effect, then one can increase the length of freeze at the second or subsequent freeze until a cure has been achieved.

Warts Suitable for Cryosurgery

Warts on the Face. Plane warts, particularly on the face, are best left alone. Salicylic acid gel in the less irritating form of Cuplex gel may accelerate spontaneous clearance in persistent lesions. Liquid nitrogen therapy is best avoided on the face. Filiform warts that are not uncommon on the face and can look quite unsightly are best treated by using a very fine ring curet under local anesthetic and lightly cauterizing the base.

TABLE 2. **Information Sheet About Cryosurgery for Warts and Verrucae**

Your wart(s) or verruca(e) has been treated with liquid nitrogen. This destroys the wart tissue by freezing. Some stinging starts during treatment and may continue for a short time afterward but usually settles within a few minutes. If you get pain later, taking a simple analgesic such as acetaminophen can readily relieve it.
Redness and some swelling can be expected and in 1 or 2 days a blister may form over the treated area. This is normal and should be covered with a bandage. If you have any cause for concern, please contact the practice nurse for advice.
You should return to the wart/verruca clinic in 4 weeks to check that the wart has been adequately treated.

Localized, Thick Warts on Open Areas. If thicker warts on the back of the hand or knees fail to respond to adequate paring down and salicylic acid therapy, they can be very effectively treated using a liquid nitrogen spray gun and an appropriate-sized otoscope earpiece. The wart is first pared down using a new scalpel blade. An otoscope earpiece of the size to fit neatly over the wart is applied to the skin. A 10- to 20-second freeze using the appropriate spray is undertaken, spraying down the earpiece until an ice halo is achieved around the base of the lesion. By this method, a deep localized cryosurgical freeze is obtained, preventing unnecessary damage to the surrounding tissue. The procedure can be repeated as required.

Periungual Warts. Warts present quite commonly around the fingernails. They can be painful and unsightly. These can be suitably treated using a liquid nitrogen spray. Because cryosurgery of warts in this site is painful and to avoid damage to the nail matrix and subsequent abnormal nail growth, the spray freeze should be restricted to 6 to 12 seconds and repeated every 3 to 4 weeks until cure is achieved. Cryosurgery of warts over knuckle joints, nerves, and tendons also should be undertaken with care.

Plantar Warts. As already stated, mosaic plantar warts are best treated by the use of formalin solution soaks. However, the most resistant localized plantar wart can be treated by cryosurgery. Liquid nitrogen spray, with the use of an otoscope earpiece for deeper lesions, may be used after adequate paring away of overlying keratin, which is remarkably resistant to cryosurgery. Alternatively, liquid nitrogen spray using a closed probe and K-Y jelly applied to the probe as a means of contact between probe and wart tissue can also be used. Both methods ensure a good depth of freeze while limiting collateral tissue damage and pain both during and after the procedure. Some clinicians treat the more recalcitrant solitary plantar warts by curettage under local anesthetic, but the procedure and subsequent healing phase can be extremely painful, especially if secondary infection occurs.

Referral and Other Forms of Therapy

Genital Warts. These warts tend to develop in large clusters. They affect the penile and vulvar skin, mucous membrane, and also the perianal area. Genital warts can be persistent and difficult to treat. It is probably wiser to refer such patients and their partners for a full urogenital assessment. A full vaginal and/or rectal examination is required to establish the extent of the problem before starting treatment with alternate-day application of podophyllin 25% to 50% in soft paraffin, which needs regular supervision, or intermittent use of cryosurgery for as long as necessary. In the case of children presenting with genital warts, referral to a pediatrician to exclude sexual abuse may be appropriate.

Immunocompromised Patients. Transplant or AIDS patients are more prone to develop diffuse warts, which may even progress to form carcinomas. Inosine pranobex (Imunovir)* is sometimes used in conjunction with liquid nitrogen cryosurgery when three or four treatments with liquid nitrogen alone have failed to produce a cure. Some centers treat very resistant warts at any site with lasers and others with intralesional bleomycin (Blenoxane)† or systemic interferon.† The immune status of these patients must always be checked.

*Not available in the United States.
†Not FDA approved for this indication.

CONDYLOMA ACUMINATUM

method of
JOSEPH I. LEE, M.D., PH.D.
George Washington University Hospital
Washington, D.C.

Genital warts are a very common sexually transmitted disease. Approximately 1% of sexually active people have clinically visible genital warts. Although exact figures are not available, it is thought that as many as 14% of the population may have subclinical infections that can only be detected through DNA hybridization studies. These people may be infectious. Transmission of the virus occurs through exfoliated infected cells during sex. The role of condoms in preventing transmission is still an area of controversy, and studies are underway to resolve this question. The majority of patients with genital warts are in the 16- to 39-year age group. More than 90% of condylomata acuminata are caused by human papillomavirus (HPV) types 6 and 11. These HPV types that cause external genital warts are considered low-risk HPVs and are not associated with increased risk of developing cervical cancer.

MORPHOLOGY

Genital warts can appear as soft digitate papules on the mucosal surfaces, especially the vagina, the anus, the introitus, the urethral meatus, the labia minora, and the intertriginous areas of the groin, perineum, and anal area. The warts on keratinized epithelium tend to be more hyperkeratotic and can be pigmented. It is important to thoroughly inspect the genital area. Genital warts must be distinguished from seborrheic keratosis and skin tags.

TREATMENT

The goal of treatment is the removal of the visible genital warts (Table 1). This is not a cure of the HPV infection. No current available treatment method eradicates HPV infection or affects the natural history of HPV infection. It is reasonable for the patient to expect that treatment will bring about a wart-free period. Being wart-free may not decrease the infectivity of the patient. Latency periods of HPV infections may last years before visible warts appear. Some warts, if left alone, are known to clear spontaneously. It is believed in these cases that the immune system was able to mount a cellular immune response that led to wart regression.

The immune system plays a vital role in response to treatment. Vaccines for genital wart infections are under development. Immune-compromised patients are at higher risk for infection and recurrence of genital warts. In all patients, as a general rule, it is best to treat the warts early when they are smaller and fewer in number. Home and office therapy options are available to the patient. These treatments are not exclusive of each other. There is no reason why home therapy cannot be supplemented by office therapy. In fact, most patients benefit from this dual attack on the warts.

Home Therapy

Podophyllotoxin Topical Solution or Gel

Podophyllotoxin 0.5% (also called *podofilox* [Condylox]) is applied twice daily to external genital and anal warts for 3 consecutive days and then discontinued for 4 days. This cycle can be repeated up to four times. Podophyllotoxin is an extract of the podophyllum plant that binds to cellular microtubules and inhibits mitotic division in the condyloma cells. The wart becomes necrotic about 5 days after application, leaving a shallow erosion that heals within a few days. Over half the patients using podo-

TABLE 1. **Comparison of Therapies for Genital Warts**

Therapy	Cure Rate	Recurrence Rate (at 6 mo)
Scissor excision	100%	20%–30%
Cryosurgery	63%–89%	10%–30%
Trichloroacetic acid 80%	70%–81%	36%
Podophyllin		>50%
Imiquimod 5% (Aldara)	50%–80%	13%
Podophyllotoxin (Condylox)	11%–86%	17%–38%

phyllotoxin experience transient burning, tenderness, and erythema; scarring occurs in rare cases. The clearance rate is as high as 86% in the prepuce lesions in some studies and as low as 11% in other areas in other studies. The recurrence rate for podophyllotoxin ranges from 17% to 38% in various studies.

Imiquimod Cream

Imiquimod (Aldara) 5% cream is an immune response modulator that induces local production of interferon alfa and interferon gamma and the recruitment of immune cells such as CD4 T cells. It is thought that the stimulation of the cellular immune response results in the regression of the treated wart. The cream is applied three times a week at bedtime and washed off in the morning. Treatment continues until the wart is gone, or up to 16 weeks. The most common adverse affect with imiquimod use is erythema. In rare cases, ulcers can occur, as well as pigmentation changes in the treated skin. It is about 50% effective in males and 80% effective in females. The recurrence rate is about 13%.

Office Procedures

Surgical removal is an excellent option for small pedunculated warts on the keratinized genital skin. The area is infiltrated with a small amount of lidocaine, and iris or Gradle scissors are used to remove the wart. Hemostasis can be controlled with cautery or aluminum chloride solution. Genital skin tends to heal well, and infection is usually not a problem if patients are able to do careful wound care. A scalpel can be used to do tangential excisions of genital warts. These wounds should be allowed to heal by secondary intention, and suturing of the wound site is not recommended for most cases.

Surgical removal has the advantage over other modalities in that the patient is wart free in one visit. However, it is more time-consuming and still has a 20% to 30% recurrence rate. Surgical treatment of warts on the anal area should be approached with caution. Hemostasis can be a problem in the anal area, where access and visualization can be limited. Carbon dioxide lasers are useful for their ability to give good hemostasis while ablating the warts and for treatment of anal warts. A smoke evacuator is needed when using a laser. Circumcision is the treatment of choice when the foreskin has extensive warts. Treatment by other means may cause phimosis. Care must be taken when doing any surgical procedure near the urinary meatus. Scarring and stricture may lead to urinary retention.

Cryotherapy with liquid nitrogen is an excellent mode of therapy of genital warts of any size and location. It is simple, is efficient, and rarely causes scarring. Liquid nitrogen should be applied to the wart so that a halo of a white ice ball forms out to at least a few millimeters of the normal-appearing tissue surrounding the wart. Patients should be warned that swelling, blistering, and crusting will occur after treatment. The treatment usually needs to be repeated at weekly to biweekly intervals until the wart is gone. Cryotherapy has an efficacy range of 63% to 89%, with a recurrence rate of 10% to 30%.

Trichloroacetic acid (TCA) 80% solution can be applied to the wart to induce lysis of the wart cells. A white frosting will develop. Care should be taken that the acid does not wick to unaffected skin during application. TCA therapy requires multiple treatments and has a success rate of 70% to 81% but a recurrence rate of up to 36%. Podophyllin resin can be applied alone or in conjunction with TCA. The resin comes in 10% to 25% concentration compounded most commonly in tincture of benzoin. A thin layer of the resin should be applied to the wart. Sometimes TCA can be applied first to the wart to enhance the penetration of the podophyllin in thickly keratinized skin. The podophyllin resin should be allowed to dry before coming in contact with clothing. Podophyllin blocks the cellular mitotic machinery and is highly toxic. Only small amounts of the resin should be applied because systemic toxicity is possible with large doses. Podophyllin is an adequate alternative for the treatment of mucosal surfaces such as the urethral meatus, intertriginous areas of the vulva, and the anal area. It has a high recurrence rate.

NEVI

method of
PHILIP R. COHEN, M.D.
University of Texas—Houston Medical School
Houston, Texas

DEFINITION

The term *nevi* often refers to the plural form of a melanocytic nevus (mole). Typically, melanocytic nevi consist of groups (nests) of melanocytes located in the epidermis, the dermis, or both. Melanocytic nevi do not include other benign, often flat, pigmented lesions that show an epidermis in which the basal layer is hyperpigmented or contains an increased number of individual melanocytes or both (Table 1). The term *nevus* is also used to define a hamartoma of either epithelial or adnexal origin (Table 2); although some of these lesions (such as an epidermal nevus) may be pigmented, they are not melanocytic nevi.

CLINICAL PRESENTATIONS (Table 3)

An acronym for the clinical evaluation of pigmented lesions is ABCD: asymmetry, border, color, and diameter.

TABLE 1. **Benign Pigmented Lesions That Are Not Melanocytic Nevi**

Becker melanosis
Café-au-lait macule
Ephelides (freckles)
Lentigo simplex
Solar lentigo

TABLE 2. **Hamartomas: Nevi That Are Not Melanocytic**

Epithelial Hamartomas		Adnexal Hamartomas	
Name	*Tissue*	*Name*	*Tissue*
Connective tissue nevus	Collagen, elastic fibers	Apocrine nevus	Apocrine glands
Epidermal nevus	Epidermis	Eccrine nevus	Eccrine glands
Nevus lipomatosis	Adipose	Hair follicle nevus	Hair follicles
Smooth muscle nevus	Smooth muscle	Nevus sebaceus	Sebaceous glands

Benign nevi typically have (1) symmetry in their shape, (2) a border whose contour is smooth, (3) color that is uniform, and (4) a diameter of less than 6 mm. A pigmented lesion may appear unusual when one or more of the morphologic features frequently associated with a benign nevus is absent. Biopsy or excision of "unusual pigmented lesions" for histologic evaluation is commonly performed.

A pre-existing nevus that changes in appearance may warrant additional evaluation. *Nevus with cyst* refers to a benign melanocytic nevus that suddenly becomes larger and darker after either rupture or inflammation of a cyst or follicle that is surrounded by the nests of melanocytes; the rapid clinical changes in the previously stable pigmented lesion often prompt the patient to seek immediate medical attention fearing that the lesion is a melanoma. However, because melanoma can develop in a dysplastic nevus or a previously benign-appearing nevus, it may be prudent to microscopically examine all or part of a pre-existing nevus in which there has been a change in symmetry, border contour, color, and/or size.

Nevi usually appear in the first few decades of life. Pigmented lesions that initially appear in older people include solar lentigines (flat, sun-induced patches), seborrheic keratoses (raised epithelial plaques), and melanomas. Most melanomas develop de novo and not in a pre-existing melanocytic lesion. Therefore, although a new pigmented lesion in an older individual is often not a melanocytic nevus, microscopic examination may be warranted to exclude the possibility of melanoma.

Junctional nevi, compound nevi, and intradermal nevi are benign melanocytic lesions (Table 4). The latter two types are raised or pedunculated lesions that may be pigmented (compound nevi) or often flesh colored (intradermal nevi); they can be located anywhere on the body. Some individuals consider them to be unattractive and desire that they be removed for cosmetic reasons. Alternatively, when they are located beneath the bra strap or the pants waistline, they can become irritated by the clothing rubbing against them. Traumatized nevi may become tender and painful, prompting the person to request their removal.

The partial or complete removal of nevi is sometimes either unintentional or unsuspected. For example, some of the flesh-colored pedunculated papules from the thighs, axillae, and neck that are clinically thought to be skin tags (acrochordons) are actually intradermal nevi. Similarly, some of the verrucous and keratotic plaques that appear to be seborrheic keratoses are actually compound nevi; it is important to submit these lesions that are clinically suspected to be benign and nonmelanocytic for pathologic evaluation because verrucous malignant melanoma also morphologically mimics a seborrheic keratosis. In a child, the initial differential diagnosis of a red nodule—most commonly on the face—might not include a melanocytic lesion; however, microscopic examination can show a spindled and epithelioid cell (Spitz) nevus.

A *recurrent nevus* (which is really a persistent nevus that has become clinically apparent) often appears as pigmentation in the scar that resulted from the prior partial removal of a nevus at that location. The pigmentation may be asymmetric with irregular borders and varying colors, mimicking melanoma. Some of the microscopic changes can also be difficult to differentiate from melanoma.

Congenital nevi are present at birth or appear during early infancy. They range in size from small (<1.5 cm), to medium (1.5–20 cm) to large (>20 cm). Melanoma may develop in these lesions, and the risk is greatest for patients with large congenital nevi.

The definition and nomenclature of *dysplastic nevi* continues to evolve. It has been suggested that the clinical lesion be referred to as an *atypical mole* and that the corresponding pathologic diagnosis is a *nevus with architectural disorder with either mild, moderate, or severe cytologic atypia.* Morphologically, dysplastic nevi can have one or more of the following features: asymmetry, irregular borders, multiple colors, and size greater than 6 mm. Dysplastic nevi can be precursor lesions of melanoma, and their clinical characteristics are the same as those observed in melanoma.

TABLE 3. **Clinical Presentations for Melanocytic Nevi That Are Treated**

An unusual-appearing pigmented lesion
A change in a pre-existing nevus
A new nevus in an older person
An asymptomatic nevus electively "treated" for cosmetic reasons
A traumatized nevus
A microscopically diagnosed, clinically unsuspected nevus
A recurrent nevus
A congenital nevus
A "dysplastic" nevus

TABLE 4. **Clinical and Histologic Characteristics of Junctional, Compound, and Intradermal Nevi**

Characteristic	Junctional Nevus	Compound Nevus	Intradermal Nevus
Color	Brown	Brown	Flesh-colored
Morphology	Flat	Raised	Raised
Melanocyte location	Epidermis*	Epidermis* and dermis	Dermis

*Nests of melanocytes are present along the basal layer of the epidermis at the dermal-epidermal junction.

DIAGNOSIS AND TREATMENT OPTIONS FOR MELANOCYTIC NEVI
(Table 5)

Clinical Monitoring

Many nevi are asymptomatic and benign in appearance. Hence, they do not require additional investigation or treatment. For individuals with benign nevi, clinical monitoring of their melanocytic lesions—perhaps every 1 to 3 months by the patient and every 6 to 12 months by the clinician—may be appropriate.

Punch Biopsy/Excision

This procedure uses a circular cutting edge that ranges in diameter from 1 to 6 mm to remove either part (biopsy) or all (excision) of the lesion. The size of the instrument used determines the diameter of the specimen and the depth of the specimen depends on how firmly the clinician presses the instrument into the skin.

Advantages of the punch procedure include the ability to better evaluate (1) the dermal component of the lesion and (2) the depth of the lesion. However, this procedure requires more time to perform than the shave procedure. Another disadvantage of the punch procedure is the necessity for the patient to return to the office for suture removal.

Shave Biopsy/Excision

This procedure uses either a scalpel or a razor blade. The length, width, and depth of the specimen are determined by the clinician. This procedure can be rapidly performed in the office, and the patient does not need to return for the removal of sutures. However, the healing time is usually longer than that of either the punch or the ellipse procedures, and the site from which a deeper specimen has been removed may heal noncosmetically. Also, if nevus melanocytes (i.e., adjacent to a hair follicle) extend into the deeper dermis, the shave procedure may not be of sufficient depth to completely excise the nevus; hence, another surgical procedure would be required if complete removal of that lesion was necessary.

Elliptical Biopsy/Excision

This procedure usually uses a scalpel. The dimensions of the specimen are determined by the clinician, who, in most cases, attempts to completely remove the lesion. This procedure takes longer than the punch or the shave procedures to perform, and suture removal often requires that the patient return to the office. A prophylactic oral antibiotic is usually prescribed for a few to several days after the procedure, and an oral medication for local pain may be necessary during the first few postoperative days.

MANAGEMENT

The procedure used to evaluate or remove a nevus depends on the morphologic presentation of the patient's lesion and the clinical differential diagnosis entertained by the clinician. In many circumstances, more than one approach for the diagnosis and/or treatment of a nevus may be appropriate. When a suspected nevus is smaller than 6 mm and is either unusual in appearance, a new lesion in an older person, or a change in a pre-existing lesion, then it may be reasonable to attempt to excise the entire lesion using the punch procedure. For larger lesions, either a shave biopsy or a 3- to 4-mm punch biopsy can be performed to establish the diagnosis; if complete removal is required, an elliptical excision can subsequently be performed.

Either a punch, a shave, or an elliptical procedure can be used to remove all or part of an asymptomatic nevus for aesthetic purposes or a traumatized nevus. A recurrent nevus can potentially develop if residual nevus remains after a shave procedure in which the depth is too superficial; however, when the depth is deeper, healing may be prolonged and result in a noncosmetic depressed scar.

When the unexpected diagnosis of a nevus is estab-

TABLE 5. **Characteristics of Methods Used for Biopsy or Excision of Melanocytic Nevi**

Method	Diameter	Depth	Wound Management	Procedure Duration	Suture Removal
Punch	1–6 mm	Deeper dermis to subcutaneous fat	Cutaneous, or less commonly layered (dermal and cutaneous), suture placement or secondary spontaneous healing	Shorter than ellipse, yet longer than shave	Yes/No
Shave	1 to 15–20 mm (variable)	Mid to deeper dermis; occasionally subcutaneous fat	Secondary spontaneous healing	Shortest	No
Ellipse	Variable	Subcutaneous fat	Layered or cutaneous closure with either staples and/or sutures	Longest	Yes

lished microscopically, subsequent management depends (1) on whether the lesion has been entirely removed and (2) on the histologic type of nevus. Even if residual nevus remains, additional treatment is usually not necessary for an intradermal nevus (when acrochordon was suspected) or for a compound nevus (when seborrheic keratosis was suspected).

Conservative excision of residual Spitz nevi, recurrent nevi, and congenital nevi is often recommended. Even when a benign nevus is confirmed as the original diagnosis of a recurrent nevus, the new pigmented lesion is often completely excised. Because melanoma usually does not occur during childhood, the excision of a congenital nevus is often able to be postponed until late childhood or early adolescence when the procedure can be performed using local anesthesia.

There are several approaches for the management of dysplastic nevi. Some clinicians excise all of these lesions; their preoperative diagnosis is based on prior microscopic confirmation and/or clinical presentation. Other clinicians photograph and/or record (map) the clinically suspected dysplastic nevi every 3 to 6 months and only sample or excise those lesions that have changed.

MELANOMA

method of
PHILLIP M. WILLIFORD, M.D.
Wake Forest University
Winston-Salem, North Carolina

The incidence of melanoma is increasing faster than that of any other cancer. It now represents the leading cause of death in women between the ages of 25 and 29. It is estimated that 1 in 75 people born in the year 2000 will develop melanoma in their lifetime. Including in situ disease, there are approximately 80,000 patients diagnosed with melanoma in the United States each year and approximately 7700 deaths.

EPIDEMIOLOGY

The typical melanoma patient presents phenotypically as a blue-eyed, blond-haired individual who tends to burn rather than tan, freckles, has several dysplastic (clinically atypical) nevi, and more than 20 nevi overall. Blacks and Asians have one-twentieth the risk of whites. Children younger than 10 years are rarely affected. Those patients with a previous history of melanoma have a 3% to 6% risk of a second primary lesion. Recently, several melanoma susceptibility genes have been identified, and familial melanoma represents 8% to 12% of all cases.

SIGNS AND SYMPTOMS

Cardinal features of melanoma are change in size and color of a lesion over the course of 3 to 12 months. Fifteen percent to 25% of melanomas arise out of pre-existing nevi, with the remainder occurring de novo from melanocytes along the dermal-epidermal junction. Amelanotic lesions account for 1% to 2% of all lesions. Hypopigmentation (melanoma-associated leukoderma) is a feature of more advanced disease. Pruritus is a secondary feature noted in about 25% of patients. Bleeding is rarely a manifestation of early disease.

SUNSCREEN AND MELANOMA RISK

There is no evidence that sunscreen users suffer from hypovitaminosis D, nor is there evidence for a role of vitamin D in the development or spread of malignant melanoma. There are a number of epidemiologic studies investigating the relationship of sunscreen usage and melanoma with contradictory findings. Most of these studies suffer from recall bias, inclusion of patients using products of low-potency sun protective factor (SPF) with inadequate ultraviolet A (UVA) screens, undefined regularity of usage, small size, and retrospective design. It is not known whether sunlight is causative in the development of melanoma and if so what is the action spectrum associated with risk. However, until further information is available, recommendations to patients should include the sensible mantra popularized in Australia as *Slip Slap Slop Wrap* for slip on a shirt, slap on a hat, slop on some sunscreen, and wrap with sunglasses.

DIAGNOSIS

Consideration of the possibility is required before the ability to diagnose. Recognition of a suspicious lesion based on patient phenotype, history, and physical examination including the ABCDs (asymmetry, border, color, diameter) leads to the need for biopsy. The value of epiluminescent microscopy (skin surface microscopy) is gaining support among practitioners, increasing clinical acumen and reducing the need for unnecessary biopsy. When possible, it is most appropriate to excise a suspicious lesion with narrow margins. This approach allows the dermatopathologist to best evaluate the symmetry, breadth, and other histologic features that make diagnosis possible while excluding a variety of atypical pigmented lesions that may masquerade as true disease.

If the anatomic site or size of the pigmented lesion is not amenable to easy complete removal, consideration of an ellipse through the lesion with inclusion of clinically normal-appearing tissue on either side is reasonable. Finally, a shave of the lesion is only to be considered if it involves a scoop method that will provide adequate depth to achieve the important prognostic information garnered by measurement of the Breslow depth. The inclusion of photography as a means of documenting the morphology of pigmented lesions with use of software systems to manipulate images can be useful in patients with large numbers of atypical nevi and can direct the physician to those nevi that have demonstrated clear evolution of unusual features over time.

TREATMENT

The margin of excision recommended by pundits is based on dogma and a few small studies evaluating local recurrence and mortality. The original recommendations of 3- to 5-cm margins were based on an autopsy study of a patient with widespread metastases. Studies that do exist are not uniform in the manner in which deep subcutaneous tissue was removed in addition to dermal and epidermal tissues.

Despite these limitations, there are generally agreed-on recommendations governing margins for excision that should include, with the possible exception of in situ disease, subcutaneous tissue to fascia as part of the specimen (Table 1).

Prognostic Features

As is true with most solid malignancies, the single most salient feature predicting survival is status of lymph nodes and disease. Other features that are important regarding prognosis include tumor thickness (Breslow depth) and the presence of ulceration. Pregnancy seems not to worsen overall mortality.

Sentinel Lymph Node Biopsy, Lymphadenectomy, and Interferon Alfa-2b

The World Health Organization (WHO) has suggested that sentinel lymph node biopsy after lymphoscintigraphy is the standard of care for those patients with lesions larger than 1 mm in depth or Clark's level 4 to 5 lesions. This technique employs a vital blue dye such as isosulfan blue in conjunction with a radiocolloid tracer such as technetium sulfur to map lymphatic drainage and isolate the sentinel (first) node in the lymphatic basin. This node can then be examined for the presence of tumor, sparing true-negative patients extensive surgery. The false-negative rate is 1% based on data from a number of centers. There is far from uniform acceptance, however, of the WHO recommendation as standard of care.

First, there is no study that has shown survival benefit for elective lymphadenectomy without resorting to subgroup analysis that introduces the potential for bias. Those patients possibly benefiting based on the Intergroup Melanoma Trial data were those with lesions between 1 and 2 mm that were nonulcerated and who were younger than 60 years of age.

Second, it is not yet known whether the routine performance of sentinel node biopsies in newly diagnosed melanoma will alter survival. The Multicenter Selective Lymphadenectomy Trial may answer this question, but data will not be available until 2003.

Third, the role of interferon alfa-2b (Intron A) as adjuvant therapy for those with stage 3 disease is uncertain. The results of a recent Eastern Cooperative Oncology Group (ECOG) 1690 trial demonstrated no survival benefit, although disease-free survival improved. If there is no benefit, then there currently exists no adjuvant treatment regimen that is beneficial, making the prognostic information from sentinel node biopsy academic. It is possible that earlier lymph node dissection and the institution of adjuvant interferon alfa-2b before bulky disease may, in fact, benefit a subset of patients with limited disease burden. The Sunbelt Melanoma Trial may finally answer the question of efficacy in adjuvant therapies.

TABLE 1. **Suggested Margins of Excision for Melanoma**

Thickness (mm)	Excision Margin (cm)
In situ	0.5–1.0
0–1	1.0
1–2	1–2
2–4	2
>4	2

TABLE 2. **Simplified Staging System for Melanoma***

Stage	Breslow Depth	Lymph Nodes	Distant Metastases
1	<1.5 mm	Negative	None
2	>1.5 mm	Negative	None
3	Any	Positive	None
4	Any	Negative/positive	Positive

*In situ disease not included.

Staging and Evaluation

Initial evaluation of all patients should include a complete history and physical examination with attention to those organ systems likely to be impacted by metastatic disease, including lymphatics, brain, bone, and liver. The utility of diagnostic studies for stage 1 and 2 disease is not proven. (See simplified staging system, Table 2.)

Most authors argue against routine chest radiography and laboratory studies for stage 1 disease and suggest limited studies for stage 2 disease, depending on physician recommendations. Routine computed tomography is more likely to detect false positives than true positives related to melanoma. For those with stage 3, consider computed tomography of the head, abdomen, chest, and pelvis and/or positron emission tomography, although the yield is low. Those with stage 4 disease should have comprehensive studies.

Chemotherapy/Vaccine Therapy

At this time the role of vaccine therapy remains investigational. Many chemotherapeutic regimens have been studied, and none has demonstrated superiority to dacarbazine (DTIC) alone, with response rates of 10% to 20% and complete responses of 5%. Some reports of long-term responses with cisplatin and interleukin-2 in metastatic disease raise the possibility of cure, albeit with significant and severe toxicity.

SKIN CANCER PRECURSOR LESIONS

method of
ASHFAQ A. MARGHOOB, M.D.,
KLAUS J. BUSAM, M.D., and
DANA SACHS, M.D.
Memorial Sloan-Kettering Cancer Center
New York, New York

Skin cancer is the most common human malignancy, accounting for half of all cancers diagnosed in the United States. Most skin cancers develop de novo on normal-appearing skin. However, some cancers of the skin can arise in association with certain benign cutaneous neoplasms. These are the so-called skin cancer precursor lesions (Table 1).

The four most common types of skin cancer are basal cell carcinoma, squamous cell carcinoma, malignant melanoma, and cutaneous T-cell lymphoma. Inheritance of nonfunctional tumor suppressor genes or oncogenes, the phenotypic characteristics of an individual, environmental factors such as excessive sun exposure, and other host factors such as immunosuppression may all play a role in determining the magnitude of the risk for an individual for developing skin cancer. In addition to these risk factors, each one of the four common skin cancers may also develop in association with benign "precursor" lesions.

PRECURSORS TO BASAL CELL CARCINOMA

Basal cell carcinoma is the most common cancer of the skin and most frequently develops on the sun-exposed skin of the head and neck in middle-aged to elderly individuals. This malignancy is thought to develop from the basal cell keratinocytes located in the hair follicle, and mutations in the patched gene play an important role in the development of many basal cell carcinomas. Basal cell carcinomas almost always develop de novo; however, some have been reported to develop within seborrheic keratoses and in nevus sebaceus. The occurrence of a basal cell carcinoma in conjunction with a seborrheic keratosis is a rare event and is probably coincidental. On the other hand, the development of a basal cell carcinoma within a nevus sebaceus occurs at a frequency greater than can be explained by chance alone.

TABLE 1. **Skin Cancer Precursor Lesions**

Skin Cancer	Precursor
Basal cell carcinoma	Nevus sebaceus
Squamous cell carcinoma	Actinic keratosis and arsenical keratosis
	Porokeratosis
	Human papillomavirus
	Bowenoid papulosis
	Epidermodysplasia verruciformis
	Leukoplakia
	Lichen sclerosus (balanitis xerotica obliterans or kraurosis vulvae)
Melanoma	Congenital melanocytic nevus
	Dysplastic (atypical) nevus
Cutaneous T-cell lymphoma (mycosis fungoides)	Parapsoriasis en plaques

Nevus Sebaceus

Nevus sebaceus of Jadassohn is a hamartoma of the pilosebaceous unit and is composed primarily of sebaceous glands, hair follicles, and apocrine glands. Nevus sebaceus is present at birth or becomes apparent shortly after birth. It is a yellow to orange, mammillated, well-demarcated plaque, which frequently occurs on the scalp or face. During puberty, and under hormonal control, these lesions can become larger and develop a verrucous or nodular surface. Many textbooks state that approximately 20% of sebaceous nevi will develop a basal cell carcinoma within them. However, recent investigators have suggested that this is an overestimate because many tumors previously classified as basal cell carcinomas were, in fact, benign tumors that histologically resemble basal cell carcinomas. Two such benign tumors that can resemble basal cell carcinomas are trichoblastomas and basal cell hamartomas. Besides trichoblastomas, numerous other benign tumors can also develop within sebaceous nevi and include syringocystadenoma papilliferum, nodular hidradenoma, syringoma, sebaceous epithelioma, chondroid syringoma, and trichilemmoma. Recent reviews now estimate that 1% to 7% of sebaceous nevi will develop an associated basal cell carcinoma. Deletions in the patched gene have been identified in up to 40% of sebaceous nevi, lending credence to the theory that some of these sebaceous nevi may be true basal cell carcinoma precursor lesions. Rarely, large and extensive sebaceous nevi can be associated with skeletal and neurologic defects.

Decisions on how to manage patients with nevus sebaceus depend on weighing the risks of developing basal cell carcinoma versus the risks of prophylactic excisional surgery, anesthesia, and resulting scars or cosmetic defects. Removal of sebaceous nevi to improve cosmesis may be appropriate in some individuals, however; prophylactic excision of all sebaceous nevi in children is not warranted. Close clinical surveillance to help detect the development of malignant tumors is an appropriate alternative to prophylactic excision. Suspicious growths developing within nevus sebaceus need to be sampled. If malignancy is detected, complete surgical excision is advisable. Baseline clinical photographs can aid in the clinical surveillance of these lesions. Basal cell carcinomas can develop in sebaceous nevi of children, but the risk of malignancy is apparently highest after puberty, and therefore some physicians suggest close clinical follow-up of sebaceous nevi until puberty, followed by consideration for prophylactic excision.

PRECURSORS TO SQUAMOUS CELL CARCINOMA

Squamous cell carcinoma, a malignancy derived from the keratinocyte, is the second most common skin cancer. Many names have been given to squamous cell carcinomas depending on their stage of evolution, differentiation, and location. An in situ squamous cell carcinoma is called Bowen's disease; some well-differentiated squamous cell carcinomas are called keratoacanthomas; squamous cell carcinomas developing in chronic wounds are called Marjolin ulcers; and a squamous cell carcinoma on the penis is called *erythroplasia of Queyrat.* In addition, verrucous carcinoma, a low-grade squamous cell carcinoma, has three different names, depending on the location of the cancer. Verrucous carcinoma of the oral cavity is called *oral florid papillomatosis;* that of the genitoanal region is called *giant condylomata acuminata of Buschke and Lowenstein;* and that of the plantar surface is called *epithelioma cuniculatum.*

Clinically, squamous cell carcinoma can resemble warts, irritated seborrheic keratosis, or eczema and can sometimes be found at the base of a cutaneous horn. Some squamous cell carcinomas have developed in association with seborrheic keratosis and nevus sebaceus; however, this association is probably coincidental. As many as 90% of squamous cell carcinomas harbor mutations in the *p53* tumor suppressor gene, and some have been noted to harbor human papillomavirus DNA.

Potential precursors to invasive squamous cell carcinoma include actinic keratosis, arsenical keratosis, porokeratosis, leukoplakia, lichen sclerosus, and papillomas resulting from infection with specific human papillomavirus types.

Actinic Keratosis

Actinic keratoses are considered to be squamous cell carcinoma precursor lesions; however, this concept has recently come under considerable debate. Some researchers consider actinic keratoses to be premalignant lesions, whereas others believe them to be early forms of squamous cell carcinoma in situ. Both squamous cell carcinoma and actinic keratosis frequently harbor *p53* mutations.

Actinic keratoses, also known as *solar keratoses,* are linked to chronic and excessive ultraviolet light exposure. Ultraviolet light is considered to be both the initiator and the promotor of actinic keratosis/squamous cell carcinoma tumorgenesis. Clinically, actinic keratoses are rough, red, scaly macules or papules that develop on sun-exposed skin surfaces. Often it is difficult to visualize actinic keratoses; however, because most have a rough texture they can easily be located by lightly stroking the skin. There are five clinical variants of actinic keratoses: erythematous, hyperkeratotic, verrucous, pigmented, and cutaneous horn.

It is estimated that 10% of actinic keratoses will regress spontaneously; however, every year, approximately 1 per 1000 actinic keratoses will progress to invasive squamous cell carcinoma. The chance of an untreated actinic keratosis transforming into an invasive squamous cell carcinoma has been cited to be between 0.25% and 20%. Furthermore, nearly 60% of squamous cell carcinomas are found to arise from actinic keratoses.

Management of patients with actinic keratoses consists of efforts at preventing the development of new lesions and the destruction of existing lesions. Prevention starts with sun protection, which consists of trying to avoid unnecessary ultraviolet light exposure, using appropriate clothing, and regularly using sunscreens. It is recommended that patients frequently and liberally apply a broad spectrum (UVA and UVB) sunscreen with a sun protective factor of at least 15. Daily use of sunscreens can prevent the development of actinic keratoses and can also help in the remission of existing lesions. Daily use of topical retinoids such as tretinoin emollient cream 0.05% can also help in the prevention and treatment of some actinic keratoses.

Therapy for existing actinic keratoses consists of destructive procedures. Actinic keratosis can be treated by cryotherapy (liquid nitrogen), topical 5-fluorouracil, curettage, chemical peels, carbon dioxide laser, dermabrasion, shave excision, and/or photodynamic therapy. Photodynamic therapy utilizes 20% aminolevulinic acid, a topical photosensitizer, followed by exposure to blue light. However, the most commonly used methods of treating actinic keratoses are cryotherapy or use of topical 5-fluorouracil. Topical 5-fluorouracil 5% cream is usually applied to the affected skin twice a day for 2 weeks. The actinic keratoses tend to become red and crusted and, unless the patient develops an irritant or contact dermatitis, the uninvolved skin will not react and hence will remain normal in appearance. Once the therapy is complete the redness and irritation can be treated with a low- to mid-potency topical corticosteroid cream. If any lesions persist after attempted treatment they should be sampled to rule out invasive squamous cell carcinoma.

Brief mention of arsenical keratosis is warranted here. Arsenical keratoses are similar to actinic keratoses; however, they are due to exposure to arsenic and not to ultraviolet light. The management of patients with arsenical keratoses is to find and eliminate the exposure to arsenic and to treat existing lesions with one of the destructive modalities described earlier.

Porokeratosis

Porokeratosis is a disorder of keratinization that clinically presents as round, oval, or linear plaques. On close inspection the peripheral rim of the lesion frequently has a grooved, keratotic ridge. The center of the lesion is often atrophic. There are four main types of porokeratosis: disseminated superficial actinic porokeratosis, porokeratosis of Mibelli, porokeratosis palmaris et plantaris, and linear porokeratosis. Risk factors for developing porokeratosis include immunosuppression, sun exposure, and radiation exposure. Many lesions of porokeratosis have an overexpression of *p53* protein.

It is estimated that 7.5% of the lesions of porokeratosis eventually develop a squamous cell carcinoma. Lesions at greatest risk are those that are relatively large, of long duration, and have a linear configuration.

Besides close clinical follow-up the treatment options for porokeratosis include cryotherapy, topical 5-fluorouracil, carbon dioxide laser ablation, surgical excision, curettage, and electrodesiccation.

Human Papillomavirus (Bowenoid Papulosis and Epidermodysplasia Verruciformis)

Human papillomavirus (HPV), a double-stranded DNA virus, can elaborate oncoproteins that may result in cellular proliferation and immortalization. In addition, some of the viral proteins may be able to degrade the *p53* protein, thereby unblocking DNA synthesis, preventing cell death (apoptosis), and allowing cell division to occur. Current evidence suggests that infection with certain types of HPV may be involved in the pathogenesis of some squamous cell carcinomas. For example, HPV 6 and 11 have been detected in cases of giant condylomata acuminata of Buschke and Lowenstein and HPV 18, 31, 33, and 51 have been found in cases of oral florid papillomatosis.

Two potential squamous cell carcinoma precursor lesions, linked to HPV, are bowenoid papulosis and specific warts that occur in patients with epidermodysplasia verruciformis. Bowenoid papulosis consists of small brown to red papules that usually develop on the genitalia and can resemble condyloma. Histologically, they have features of squamous cell carcinoma in situ; however, most have a benign course and some lesions may regress spontaneously. Many of these lesions are found to harbor HPV 16 DNA. Bowenoid papulosis on the glans penis or vaginal area may, on rare occasions, progress to invasive squamous cell carcinoma, especially in older individuals. Individual lesions of bowenoid papulosis can be treated by shave excision, curettage, electrodesiccation, or carbon dioxide laser ablation. Topical therapy can be attempted by applying topical 5-fluorouracil 5% cream to individual lesions twice daily for 3 to 4 weeks.

Patients with epidermodysplasia verruciformis, an autosomal recessive trait, have a defective cell-mediated immune system. Hence, these patients have a tendency to acquire various HPV-related lesions. Most of these lesions are flat warts; however, they also develop flat macules that frequently coalesce to form larger red to brown plaques resembling tinea versicolor. The most common warts occurring in patients with epidermodysplasia verruciformis are flat warts due to HPV 3 and 10. However, the tinea versicolor–like lesions, seen almost exclusively in patients with epidermodysplasia verruciformis, are due to HPV 5 and 8, and they have oncogenic potential. It is estimated that 30% to 60% of patients with epidermodysplasia verruciformis will develop squamous cell carcinoma and that 90% of these squamous cell carcinomas are due to either HPV 5 or 8.

Treating patients with epidermodysplasia verruciformis is challenging because there are no specific treatments available for epidermodysplasia verruciformis. High doses of oral vitamin A, isotretinoin, or interferon may prevent the formation of squamous cell carcinoma. However, these medications have many unpleasant side effects and are effective only for as long as they are being taken. Once they are stopped the squamous cell carcinomas tend to develop once again. Avoiding exposure to ultraviolet and ionizing radiation plays an important role in preventing the formation of squamous cell carcinomas. The squamous cell carcinomas that develop in patients with epidermodysplasia verruciformis can be successfully treated by using any of the acceptable treatment modalities for squamous cell carcinoma, with the exception of radiation therapy. Radiation therapy is contraindicated in patients with epidermodysplasia verruciformis because of its potential to induce malignant transformation of warts.

Leukoplakia (Erythroplakia)

Leukoplakias are white, sharply demarcated, and irregular patches that can be found on the oral or vulvar mucosal surfaces. Erythroplakia are similar lesions that are erythematous instead of white. Unlike candidiasis, these plaques cannot be rubbed off. Leukoplakia may develop secondary to chronic irritation from tobacco, chemicals, or ill-fitting dentures. Those lesions of leukoplakia that are idiopathic or do not resolve within 4 weeks after stopping a presumed offending irritant may require a biopsy. It needs to be stressed that leukoplakia is a clinical diagnosis. Histologically, some lesions of leukoplakia may be benign, showing only parakeratosis; others may have atypia, whereas others may be malignant. Those plaques of leukoplakia that have atypia may be the precursor lesions. Many of these atypical lesions resemble actinic keratosis, and squamous cell carcinoma has been documented to develop in association with these lesions. HPV 11 and 16 have been found in some cases of leukoplakia.

Biopsy-proven benign leukoplakia does not need to be treated but should be monitored. The preferred methods of treating biopsy-proven leukoplakia with atypia include excision, cryotherapy, curettage and electrodesiccation, and laser ablation.

Lichen Sclerosus (Balanitis Xerotica Obliterans or Kraurosis Vulvae)

Lichen sclerosis et atrophicus can affect the skin and mucous membranes. It commonly presents as hypopigmented, flat-topped papules with surrounding erythema. These papules coalesce or enlarge to form larger atrophic patches of skin. The affected skin develops a wrinkled appearance, can develop erosions, and may be pruritic or have a burning sensation. Eventually the skin scars. Untreated lichen sclerosis et atrophicus of the male genitalia, known as *balanitis xerotica obliterans,* can result in phimosis or meatal stenosis. Lichen sclerosis et atrophicus of the female genitalia, known as *kraurosis vulvae*, can lead to vulvar and perianal sclerosis, resulting in labial stenosis. Some researchers have noted a loss of androgen receptors whereas others have found an association with HPV 16 in skin affected by lichen sclerosis et atrophicus. The significance of these findings is not clear.

Many lichen sclerosis et atrophicus lesions show epithelial dysplasia, and it is estimated that between 2% and 6% of genital lichen sclerosis et atrophicus will develop an associated squamous cell carcinoma. Treating lichen sclerosis et atrophicus may prevent the development of squamous cell carcinoma. First-line therapy for both men and women with genital lichen sclerosis et atrophicus is the topical application of clobetasol dipropionate (Temovate)* 0.05% cream applied twice daily for approximately 10 weeks. Testosterone therapy can also be used to treat lichen sclerosis et atrophicus; however, one needs to closely monitor women for signs of virilization. Topical testosterone (Androgel)* can be administered as 2% testosterone propionate ointment twice daily for 3 months. Oral stanozolol (Winstrol),* an anabolic steroid and synthetic derivative of testosterone, can be given at a dose of 2 mg twice daily for 3 months.

PRECURSORS TO MELANOMA

Melanoma is the deadliest form of skin cancer. The incidence and mortality rates of melanoma continue to rise at alarming rates. Despite advances in surgery, chemotherapy, and immunotherapy the prognosis for advanced disease remains poor. The key to survival lies in the early diagnosis of melanoma. Melanoma has been associated with two potential precursor lesions—the atypical mole and the congenital melanocytic nevus.

Some physicians categorize lentigo maligna of the face as a melanoma precursor lesion. However, most dermatopathologists agree that lentigo maligna is, in fact, an in situ melanoma. If left untreated, these lesions grow, invade the dermis, and can metastasize.

Lentigines are benign brown macules that occur on sun-exposed skin. These lesions are not normally considered to be melanoma precursor lesions. However, lentigines found in patients with xeroderma pigmentosum, a rare genetic syndrome, may be melanoma precursor lesions and should be monitored closely.

Congenital Melanocytic Nevi

A *congenital melanocytic nevus* is a melanocytic nevus that is present at birth or becomes apparent shortly after birth. They usually present as brown, multishaded pigmented lesions with sharply demarcated borders, often with a mammillated surface and hypertrichosis. Congenital melanocytic nevi generally grow in proportion to the growth of the child. They are usually classified according to the size they are predicted to attain in adulthood. Congenital melanocytic nevi that are less than 1.5 cm in greatest diameter are classified as small, medium congenital nevi measure between 1.5 and 19.9 cm, and large congenital melanocytic nevi measure at least 20 cm in greatest diameter.

Melanoma can develop within any congenital melanocytic nevus; however, the risk for developing melanoma is roughly proportional to the size of the nevus. Individuals at greatest risk are those with large congenital melanocytic nevi. The lifetime risk for developing melanoma in patients with large nevi is between 4.5% and 10%, and the relative risk is between 101 and 1046. Most of these melanomas develop before puberty and can occur within the skin or central nervous system. Patients with large congenital nevi that are at greatest risk for developing melanoma are those that have multiple satellite congenital nevi, and those in whom the large congenital nevus is located on the back, head, or neck area.

Congenital melanocytic nevi that are less than 20 cm in diameter have a reported lifetime risk for developing melanoma of between 0% and 6.3%. Two recent studies evaluating medium-sized congenital nevi did not reveal an increased risk for melanoma developing in nevi of this size. However, there are many case reports and series of cases that clearly show that melanomas can and do develop in congenital nevi that are less than 20 cm in diameter, and, therefore, these lesions do need monitoring. In contrast to large congenital melanocytic nevi, melanomas developing in smaller congenital nevi tend to develop at or after puberty.

Although the risk may be low, any congenital melanocytic nevus can potentially give rise to melanoma; therefore, prophylactic removal or lifelong observation of these nevi is warranted. Surgical removal of a congenital nevus may lower the risk for developing melanoma; however, it cannot eliminate the risk. If surgical excision is selected as the treatment of choice, it should ideally address the risk of malignant transformation, achieve satisfactory cosmetic results, and maintain adequate function. Because the risk for developing melanoma in patients with large congenital nevi is greatest in the first decade of life, many physicians believe it is preferable to excise these lesions during early childhood if possible. Because melanoma can develop even after surgical removal of the nevus, these patients require periodic and lifelong total cutaneous examinations and periodic neurologic examinations to aid in the detection of central nervous system melanomas. An alternative to prophylactic excision of large congenital nevi is close clinical surveillance. Any changes judged suspicious for melanoma should be sampled and appropriately treated. Baseline photographs of the nevus can be used for comparison during subsequent skin examinations to help detect subtle changes within these often heterogeneous-appearing large nevi.

*Not FDA approved for this indication.

The management of small and medium congenital nevi remains controversial. Because it is rare for smaller congenital nevi to undergo malignant transformation before puberty, many physicians agree that these lesions can be followed clinically and generally need not be considered for excision until later in childhood (8 to 10 years of age). Nevi that may warrant excision at an earlier age include relatively large medium-sized lesions and those that are difficult to follow clinically, such as those on the scalp. Some recommend the excision of congenital nevi that are clinically atypical or have unusual morphologic features. On the other hand, nevi that are uniform, light-colored, even textured, and without nodules can be photographed and followed periodically for change.

Atypical Nevi (Dysplastic Nevi)

Atypical nevi are acquired melanocytic nevi that are also referred to as atypical moles or dysplastic nevi. Unlike common acquired nevi, atypical nevi are frequently asymmetrical and have irregular borders, multiple colors, and diameters greater than 5 mm. Patients with many melanocytic nevi, some of which are atypical, may have an autosomal dominant genetic trait known as the atypical mole syndrome or dysplastic nevus syndrome. Individuals with the atypical mole syndrome have a markedly elevated risk for developing melanoma. Furthermore, the presence of atypical nevi, independent of the total number of nevi, is a powerful risk factor for developing melanoma even in the absence of the atypical mole syndrome. One study examining the number and type of nevi present on individuals revealed that patients with only one clinically atypical nevus had a twofold increased melanoma risk whereas those with greater than 10 atypical nevi had a 12-fold increased risk. Not all patients with dysplastic nevi are at equal risk for developing melanoma. The magnitude of the risk depends on factors such as number of nevi, personal history of melanoma, and family history of melanoma.

Atypical nevi are both markers that identify individuals at increased risk for developing melanoma and may also be precursors to melanoma. The precursor status of these nevi is supported by the fact that 24% to 50% of melanomas have an associated dysplastic nevus.

Management of patients with atypical moles consists of close clinical evaluation and follow-up. Any evidence of change in size, color, contour, symptoms, and/or consistency of a melanocytic neoplasm should prompt close inspection; and, if warranted, a biopsy should be performed. Any melanocytic neoplasm that looks like melanoma and cannot clinically be differentiated from a benign lesion should be sampled without delay. Although some physicians have advocated prophylactic excision of all atypical moles, this is impractical. Removal of every dysplastic nevus will not eliminate the risk for developing melanoma because up to 50% of melanomas develop in normal skin and not in association with a dysplastic nevus. Furthermore, individuals with the atypical mole syndrome tend to develop new atypical moles throughout life and therefore would require periodic excisions of these "new" melanocytic lesions. The alternative to prophylactic excision is close clinical follow-up with excisional biopsy performed only on those nevi that develop a suspicious change. Baseline clinical photographs of the entire cutaneous surface may greatly facilitate subsequent follow-up skin surveillance examinations and help detect new or changing lesions.

PRECURSORS TO MYCOSIS FUNGOIDES (CUTANEOUS T-CELL LYMPHOMA)

Cutaneous T-cell lymphoma (CTCL), a relatively uncommon skin cancer, is due to a clonal proliferation of skin homing T cells. The earliest lesions of CTCL are usually scaly patches or plaques, most commonly developing on the torso. CTCL may progress to form large plaques, nodules, or tumors. In advanced disease, the malignant T cells may be found in lymph nodes, other organs, or the peripheral circulation as seen in Sézary syndrome. The prognosis for patch stage CTCL is excellent, but Sézary syndrome is associated with a high mortality. The existence of a precursor lesion to CTCL remains controversial, although parapsoriasis en plaques may represent one such precursor lesion.

Parapsoriasis en Plaques

Parapsoriasis en plaques refers to a heterogeneous group of persistent, scaling, inflammatory, and psoriasiform dermatoses. Parapsoriasis usually presents as oval, erythematous to tan or yellow plaques with fine scale. In rare cases, some of the lesions of parapsoriasis may be atrophic. Parapsoriasis has a predilection for occurring on the buttocks, thighs, hips, and torso. Parapsoriasis has been divided into small and large plaque types. It is estimated that 10% to 30% of large plaque parapsoriasis will eventually develop into mycosis fungoides. The risk may be higher in individuals who have many lesions or pruritus or who develop thickening of the involved skin.

Generally, small plaque parapsoriasis does not require therapy. Emollients, phototherapy, and topical corticosteroids have been used with some effect. Large plaque parapsoriasis is usually treated more aggressively with high-potency topical corticosteroids, ultraviolet-B phototherapy, or psoralens plus ultraviolet A phototherapy (PUVA), in an attempt to prevent progression to mycosis fungoides. Patients with parapsoriasis should be clinically followed and skin biopsies performed, if indicated, to ensure that progression to overt mycosis fungoides has not occurred.

BACTERIAL DISEASES OF THE SKIN

method of
MICHAEL G. WILKERSON, M.D.
University of Oklahoma College of Medicine
Tulsa, Oklahoma

Bacterial diseases of the skin range from trivial annoyances to life-threatening emergencies that, if left unrecognized, result in severe morbidity with loss of limbs and systemic complications (Table 1). Death may occur in more severe cases, often to otherwise healthy individuals. The skin is the body's first line of defense against the onslaught of microorganisms from the environment, including bacteria, fungi, and viruses. Common normal skin flora include staphylococci, streptococci, diphtheroids, and propionibacteria.

Gram-negative bacteria may also be found, particularly "below the waist" and in immunocompromised patients. Yeasts such as *Candida, Pityrosporum ovale,* and other saprophytic fungi are commonly found on the skin. Knowledge of common bacterial flora and sensitivities to common antibiotics is essential for initial empirical treatment of patients and is usually sufficient without cultures. However, this is changing because of the emergence of bacterial resistance from overuse of antibiotics and incomplete treatment of infections. The most important resistant organism at this time is methicillin-resistant *Staphylococcus aureus* (MRSA), which is becoming more common in the community without obvious nosocomial exposure.

IMPETIGO AND ECTHYMA

Impetigo is a well-known disease. It is common in school-aged children and is easily transmitted. In past years, it was thought that much of impetigo was secondary to group A β-hemolytic streptococci; however, most cases now involve *Staphylococcus aureus.* Occasionally, one sees mixed infections of streptococci and *S. aureus.* Impetigo has a predilection for areas of traumatized skin, such as contact dermatitis or eczemas. Warm moist environments and poor and close living conditions aggravate impetigo.

Impetigo is classified as bullous or nonbullous. The nonbullous form is much more common (~70%) of cases. Bullous impetigo is often linked to *S. aureus* phage group II. The bullae usually appear on the trunk, buttocks, perineum, or face. A toxin produced by this particular type of *S. aureus* is thought to induce the bullae. Complications of impetigo include glomerulonephritis, septicemia, pneumonia, septic arthritis, osteomyelitis, and necrotizing fasciitis. Nephritogenic strains of *Streptococcus* may produce postinfectious glomerulonephritis after 18 to 21 days, particularly in young children 3 to 7 years of age. Unfortunately, antibiotic treatment does not appear to prevent this complication in susceptible individuals.

Ecthyma is a clinical variant of impetigo that affects mainly immunocompromised patients with diabetes, HIV infection, and neutropenic states from cancer chemotherapy and other immunosuppressants. The same causative organisms as impetigo are found. The lesions are more "punched out" and painful than impetigo and are not responsive to topical therapy.

Treatment

Limited superficial impetigo can be treated with topical therapy such as mupirocin (Bactroban) ointment or cream. This product must be applied two to three times a day for 2 to 3 weeks. Treatment of the anterior nares with Bactroban Nasal ointment is helpful because this is a harbor for chronic carriage. In limited disease, this treatment is helpful and avoids use of systemic antibiotics. All known isolates of group A β-hemolytic streptococci are sensitive to mupirocin; however, some isolates of *S. aureus* appear to be becoming resistant as use of mupirocin for long periods occurs. More extensive cases of impetigo and ecthyma should be treated with systemic antibiotics, which are β-lactamase resistant, such as dicloxacillin (Dynapen), cephalexin (Keflex), amoxicillin-

TABLE 1. **Bacterial Skin Infections**

Infection	Primary Organisms	Recommended Treatments
Impetigo, nonbullous	Group A *Streptococcus* or *Staphylococcus aureus*	If mild, topical mupirocin twice daily × 1 wk; dicloxacillin, cephalexin, erythromycin, or clarithromycin.
Impetigo, bullous	*Staphylococcus aureus* group II	Dicloxacillin, cephalexin, amoxicillin-clavulanate, clarithromycin.
Folliculitis	*Staphylococcus aureus* (most common); *Klebsiella, Enterobacter* (long-term acne antibiotics); *Pseudomonas* (hot tub exposure)	Superficial: topical mupirocin, erythromycin, clindamycin, and personal hygiene measures. For other than superficial: dicloxacillin, cephalexin, amoxicillin-clavulanate, clarithromycin. Cultures and sensitivities for non-*Staphylococcus* varieties. Hot tub folliculitis resolves spontaneously.
Cellulitis	Beta-hemolytic streptococci; *S. aureus*; *Haemophilus influenzae* (young children); Gram negatives "below the waist" especially in immunocompromised patients	Localized, nontoxic presentation: dicloxacillin, amoxicillin-clavulanate, cephalexin, and clarithromycin. Progressive, toxic, or immunocompromised: β-lactamase–resistant intravenous antibiotics.
Staphylococcal scalded skin syndrome	*S. aureus* phage group II	β-Lactamase–resistant antibiotics. Mupirocin for nares.
Necrotizing fasciitis	Polymicrobial infections with aerobic and anaerobic organisms	Surgical consultation, early débridement, broad-spectrum intravenous antibiotics for aerobic and anaerobic bacteria.

clavulanate potassium (Augmentin), erythromycin (E-Mycin), and clarithromycin (Biaxin). Use of macrolides such as erythromycin and clarithromycin should be reserved for penicillin and/or cephalosporin-sensitive individuals owing to potential for resistance, which appears to be increasing with time. Basic hygiene should be enforced, along with warm compresses to help remove crusts, followed by application of mupirocin ointment or cream. In cases of underlying dermatitis, control of the dermatitis is also helpful.

FOLLICULITIS

Folliculitis is a common infection involving the hair follicle or pilosebaceous unit. It usually presents as follicular-based yellow pustules. Sometimes these have been excoriated or shaved away, which may make the diagnosis less obvious. Spreading with scratching or shaving is a helpful clue. Patients who shave, work, or exercise in sweaty environments are particularly predisposed.

Treatment

Superficial folliculitis frequently responds to changes in local environment. Use of topical antibacterial soaps, changes in razors, less frequent shaving, and use of adequate shaving cream or lubricants are helpful. Most cases are due to *S. aureus* and can be treated with topical antibiotics such as mupirocin (Bactroban), erythromycin 2% (A/T/S), or clindamycin 1% (Cleocin T). More severe recalcitrant cases may require systemic β-lactamase–resistant antibiotics. Cultures are helpful in some cases if good initial response is not obtained. Less common causes include gram-negative bacteria such as *Klebsiella* or *Enterobacter*, which may be seen as a consequence of antibiotic therapy for acne vulgaris. *Pseudomonas aeruginosa* and *Pseudomonas cepacia* are associated with hot tub exposure ("hot tub folliculitis"). Low disinfectant levels in hot tubs need to be addressed before patients re-enter the hot tub. Hot tub folliculitis is usually self-limited and resolves in 7 to 10 days. *Proteus* infection is occasionally seen as a deeper, more nodular type of lesion.

FURUNCLES AND CARBUNCLES

Furuncles are more involved infections of the pilosebaceous unit resulting in indurated, red, painful nodules. *Carbuncles* are further extensions of this process to include multiple lesions that are interconnected to form multiloculated abscesses. The most common organism is *S. aureus*. Environmental factors include sweating, friction, oils and grease, poor hygiene, pre-existing dermatoses, nutritional factors, and immune status. The most common areas of involvement include the face, buttocks, thighs, perineum, breast, and axillae. Carbuncles involve the neck more commonly due to the thickness of the skin in this area.

Treatment

Good hygiene and warm compresses along with appropriate systemic antibiotic therapy will clear most cases. Large abscesses may require incision and drainage. Recalcitrant cases should be cultured if they do not respond to standard antistaphylococcal therapy. Hidradenitis suppurativa is a condition that at first may resemble chronic furunculosis. Primary involvement is seen in the axillae, nape of the neck, inframamillary area, and perineum. These patients form large abscesses, which are usually subcutaneous without evidence of follicular origin. Hidradenitis is treated with incision and drainage, antibiotics, and, in severe cases, extirpation with grafting of the involved skin.

CELLULITIS AND ERYSIPELAS

Cellulitis is a more invasive infection of the skin and associated soft tissues. *Erysipelas* is a more superficial form of cellulitis and occurs predominately on the face and legs. Due to the acute onset and fiery red appearance, it has been called *St. Anthony's fire.*

Cellulitis is frequently preceded by some type of superficial injury to the skin. Tinea pedis, dermatitis, varicella, or traumatic injuries are common precipitators. *S. aureus* and β-hemolytic streptococci are the most common causes. *Haemophilus influenzae* (less common since the HIB vaccine), group B streptococci in newborns, and pneumococcal cellulitis in immunocompromised patients also occur. Less common causes include atypical *Mycobacterium, Vibrio* species, and gram-negative bacteria such as *Pseudomonas* and *Klebsiella*.

Localized skin abscesses with necrosis, gangrene, septicemia, ascending lymphangitis, along with thrombophlebitis may occur. Anaerobic infections with *Clostridium* originating from soil and *Bacteroides* from fecal material are also seen. Many of these infections are polymicrobial and can be quite aggressive, dissecting along fascial planes.

Treatment

Treatment of cellulitis begins with a choice of systemic antibiotics on an empirical basis, bearing in mind the wound, immune status of the patient, and observed toxicity of the patient. Localized disease may be treated in an otherwise nontoxic healthy individual with oral antibiotics and outpatient follow-up. More aggressive infections in immunocompromised patients require intravenous antibiotic therapy along with incision and drainage and/or débridement if abscesses or necrotic tissue are present. Simpler infections require antibiotics that will cover *S. aureus* and streptococci. In children, *H. influenzae* must be considered, as it is best treated with amoxicillin/clavulanate (Augmentin) or other effective antibiotics. Needle aspiration and tissue cultures are helpful in some cases; however, yield from such procedures is typically less than 10% to 20% recovery of causative organisms. In infections that do not appear to respond or progress despite adequate therapy, the clinician should consider the possibility of necrotizing fasciitis.

STAPHYLOCOCCAL SCALDED SKIN SYNDROME

Staphylococcal scalded skin syndrome (SSSS) is a toxin-mediated manifestation of infection with staphylococci, usually phage group II. It occurs mainly in children and presents as acute fever, skin tenderness, and a scarlatiniform erythema. Flaccid bullae and erosions develop in 1 to 2 days, followed by desquamation.

Treatment

Treatment is directed at the *S. aureus* with β-lactamase resistant antibiotics. Sicker children and adults should be admitted for initial stabilization and then may be discharged on oral antibiotics once stable. Most cases heal without significant scarring although darker individuals may have variation of pigmentation, which may persist for some time.

NECROTIZING FASCIITIS

Necrotizing fasciitis is a deep infection of subcutaneous soft tissue including fascia caused principally by *S. pyogenes,* but often it is polymicrobial with other species including *Vibrio* species, *Zygomycetes,* Group C and G *Streptococcus, S. aureus,* Enterobacteriaceae, and other anaerobes. Immunocompromised individuals including diabetics, patients with peripheral vascular disease, young children, and the elderly are at increased risk. It may follow minor injuries, varicella, and trauma. Initial presentation is not always dramatic and may be localized swelling of an extremity, followed by a dusky, purple non-blanching skin, and localized tenderness to underlying muscle groups. Most cases progress rapidly to frank septicemia, hypotension, and necrosis. Despite adequate intervention with systemic antibiotics and surgical débridement mortality may approach 40% to 50%, particularly in patients with multiple underlying medical conditions. If necrotizing fasciitis is considered in the diagnosis, prompt surgical consultation with a surgeon experienced in management of these patients may be lifesaving.

VIRAL DISEASES OF THE SKIN

method of
JENNIFER C. ZAMPOGNA, M.D., and
FRANKLIN P. FLOWERS, M.D.
University of Florida College of Medicine
Gainesville, Florida

RUBELLA (GERMAN MEASLES)

Also known as *German measles, rubella* is a common communicable disease that afflicts school-aged children and young adults. Most infections occur in unvaccinated individuals during spring and summer after a 2-week incubation period.

The asymptomatic morbilliform exanthem of rubella is characterized by the development of 1- to 4-mm erythematous macules and papules on the face that spread to the trunk. Although lesions on the torso coalesce to cause a diffuse erythema, papules and macules on the extremities remain discrete. The presence of prominent cervical lymphadenopathy plus an enanthem of pinpoint erythematous macules known as Forschheimer spots offers additional support for the diagnosis of rubella. Transient arthralgias commonly occur in infected adults, but rare sequelae may include thrombotic thrombocytopenic purpura or encephalitis. The rash of rubella usually resolves within 3 days, in contrast to the exanthem of measles, which may persist for more than a week.

Roughly half of infants whose mothers are primarily infected with rubella during the first trimester will suffer an array of congenital abnormalities, including cardiac, visual, and sensorineural defects and bone marrow suppression. Rubella virus can be cultured from the urine, cerebrospinal fluid, and nasopharynx of infected neonates. Hemagglutination assays, acute and convalescent titers, and polymerase chain reaction can be used to diagnose current or prior infection.

Because there is no treatment for this self-limited infection, the primary goal is prevention of rubella via vaccine administration. The measles, mumps, and rubella vaccine (MMR) is recommended for infants 12 to 15 months of age and again at 4 to 6 years. It should not be given to pregnant women, and women should be advised to avoid pregnancy for 3 months after receiving the vaccination. Secretion of virus is negligible after vaccination, so it is safe to vaccinate family members in a home with a pregnant woman.

MEASLES (RUBEOLA VIRUS)

Measles has become an uncommon communicable disease in the United States since the implementation of aggressive vaccination programs. Caused by an RNA paramyxovirus, measles requires an incubation period of 1 week, followed by 2 to 4 days of high fever, upper respiratory tract symptoms, conjunctivitis, cough, and exanthem. The presence of 1- to 2-mm blue-gray macules on the buccal mucosa (Koplik spots) is pathognomonic. The rash of measles first appears behind the ears and then generalizes as a confluent morbilliform eruption of the trunk and extremities that resolves in 1 week. Common complications of measles include bacterial pneumonia (in up to half of patients) and otitis media.

Although serum diagnostic tests are not usually needed to confirm the diagnosis, a fourfold rise in titers of hemagglutination inhibition antibodies in acute and convalescent sera indicates rubeola infection. Appropriate supportive care is usually sufficient treatment. Childhood MMR vaccination confers lifelong immunity to this disease. Immune serum globulin, if administered within 5 to 6 days of exposure, may modify or prevent disease manifestations. This treatment is recommended for rubeola-exposed infants younger than the age of 5 months and in HIV-infected or other immunosuppressed patients who have not been vaccinated.

HAND-FOOT-AND-MOUTH DISEASE

Hand-foot-and-mouth disease is one of several manifestations of enterovirus infection in children. Enteroviruses, echoviruses, and coxsackieviruses are members of the same family of viruses that cause the vast majority of childhood exanthems in the summer and fall. These infections are spread by fecal-oral contamination and require an average incubation period of only 3 to 5 days. Nonspecific morbilliform, urticarial, vasculitic, or pustular skin lesions may develop secondary to these infectious agents, making specific diagnosis difficult.

In contrast, hand-foot-and-mouth disease is a very distinctive enterovirus infection that can be caused by coxsackievirus A16 or enterovirus 71. A brief prodrome of low-grade fever and malaise may occur 2 to 3 days before the onset of a characteristic exanthem of the hands, feet, and mouth. The most frequent symptoms of infection are sore throat and decreased feeding, owing to the presence of tender ulcerative oral lesions. Papules on the palatal or buccal mucosa form 2- to 6-mm dusky, blue-gray vesicles on an erythematous halo and progress to yellow-gray erosions. Similar vesicles on an erythematous background develop on the dorsa of the hands and feet and the sides of the toes and fingers. These skin lesions do not erode or ulcerate but can be very tender. Enzyme-linked immunosorbent assay detection of virus-specific IgM antibody is available but rarely indicated for the diagnosis. Anesthetic mouthwashes may be used for symptomatic relief, but this benign infection resolves within 7 to 10 days without sequelae.

HERPANGINA

Herpangina is a pharyngeal infection caused by group A coxsackievirus and other enteroviruses. It usually occurs in young children as an epidemic during the summer. An abrupt onset of fever and sore throat is followed by the appearance of 1-mm gray vesicles and erosions on a hyperemic base limited to the pharyngeal and tonsillar mucosa. The enanthem resolves within 1 week and requires no treatment. Anesthetic throat sprays can provide symptomatic relief, and the pharyngeal lesions have been noted to resolve more rapidly with the use of allopurinol mouthwashes.

ERYTHEMA INFECTIOSUM OR FIFTH DISEASE

Fifth disease is caused by parvovirus B19 infection and tends to occur in epidemics in school-aged children. By adulthood, up to 60% of individuals are seropositive for parvovirus B19. The virus is spread by means of respiratory droplets, blood products, and maternal-fetal transmission, with an incubation period of 6 to 16 days. Mild prodromal symptoms are followed by the development of remarkably erythematous patches on the cheeks that bestow a "slapped cheek" appearance. By day 4, a papular or reticulated macular exanthem develops on the extremities. The skin lesions may wax and wane or persist for several days to weeks. Although children are otherwise asymptomatic, adults infected with parvovirus B19 frequently have associated arthralgias that may persist for several weeks to months. Acral petechiae and purpura may develop during parvovirus B19 infection and is referred to as the papular purpuric *gloves and socks* syndrome.

Once the rash appears, the patient is no longer contagious. Maternal infection during the first or second trimester can result in hydrops and fetal demise in 19% of cases. Because parvovirus B19 specifically infects red blood cells, patients with chronic hemolytic anemias such as sickle cell disease are prone to the development of a parvovirus-induced transient aplastic crisis. Blood transfusion may be required until the aplastic crisis spontaneously resolves within 7 to 10 days. Rarely, a prolonged viral-induced anemia may occur in immunodeficient patients. This resolves promptly with intravenous immunoglobulin (IVIG)* therapy. Measurement of anti–parvovirus B19 IgG and IgM antibody is indicated to rule out infection in an exposed pregnant patient. Pregnant women who are acutely infected require close monitoring with frequent fetal ultrasound examinations. Several studies have revealed that a pregnant woman sustains a 1.0% to 2.5% risk of fetal compromise after household or occupational exposure, which is important to consider in teachers and other women of reproductive age who work with children. Therapy is largely supportive, and initial infection confers lifetime immunity.

ECTHYMA CONTAGIOSUM (HUMAN ORF)

Human orf typically presents as a single asymptomatic 1- to 2-cm nodule on the hand of an individual exposed to an infected animal. It is caused by a poxvirus that is endemic to sheep and goats. The incubation period of 3 days to 1 week is followed by the development of a blister or papule with an umbilicated crust that becomes nodular and heals spontaneously within 30 days. Regional lymphadenopathy is common. A similar disease known as *milker's nodules* occurs in patients exposed to cows infected with a similar poxvirus. These lesions are nonscarring and self-limited, therefore requiring no specific therapy. Excision, curettage and desiccation, and cryotherapy have been used successfully in some patients to facilitate healing. Glucocorticoids should be avoided.

MOLLUSCUM CONTAGIOSUM

Molluscum contagiosum is an extraordinarily common and highly infectious viral skin disease of childhood that is transmitted by skin-to-skin contact or autoinoculation by a human poxvirus. Although there are two serotypes of molluscum contagiosum, MCV-1 and MCV-2, the most common etiologic agent is MCV-1. An incubation period of 4 to 8 weeks is followed by the appearance of asymptomatic or mildly pruritic, umbilicated, translucent, or erythematous papules that may become irritated with manipulation. Healthy children manifest an average of 10 to 20 individual lesions of variable size on the thighs, pubis, face, arms, and legs. New lesions may appear as older ones heal without scarring. Molluscum contagiosum is a benign and self-limited skin disease that spontaneously clears within several months in most immunocompetent patients. In contrast, individuals with impaired cell-mediated responses can present with persistent cutaneous dissemination that is often refractory to treatment.

The diagnosis of molluscum contagiosum is often made clinically or in conjunction with manual expression and light microscopic examination of the central molluscum body (characterized by the appearance of Henderson-Patterson bodies) that is present in each skin lesion. Skin biopsy is particularly valuable in the evaluation of an HIV-infected patient with suspected molluscum contagiosum, because disseminated *Cryptococcus* or *Histoplasma* infections in this population can manifest as umbilicated cutaneous papules and nodules that mimic the appearance of molluscum contagiosum lesions.

Because molluscum contagiosum is a self-limited skin disease, patient and parent education and support is of utmost therapeutic benefit. Patients should be advised that

*Not FDA approved for this indication.

although this infection is easily transmissible to playmates and siblings, isolation or prevention methods are usually not warranted and may only exacerbate the psychosocial effects of this skin disease. Multiple methods of treatment for molluscum contagiosum are available and easy to use in an office setting, but patients should be counseled regarding the risk of scarring that exists with virtually any topical therapy.

Molluscum "evisceration" (i.e., removal of the umbilicated core) can be performed with a No. 11 surgical blade, toothpick, or hollow needle. Curettage and cryosurgery are other common modalities that can be repeated every 3 weeks as needed until cure is achieved. Podophyllin 25% may be applied on a weekly basis by a physician and rinsed off by the patient in 4 to 6 hours, but podophyllotoxin (Condylox)* (the active ingredient in podophyllin) is a safer alternative that can be applied by the patient twice daily for 3 days. Cantharidin (blistering beetle juice), salicylic acid plasters, and iodine solutions can also be used to treat molluscum contagiosum lesions.

Twice-daily application of topical tretinoin* (0.05% to 1.0%) to select lesions may achieve cure within 2 weeks, but mild to moderate local skin irritation should be anticipated. Oral cimetidine (Tagamet),* 40 mg/kg/d divided into two daily doses over a 2-month course, is another therapeutic alternative that may be used in conjunction with or in place of irritating topical treatments, although its efficacy rates remain questionable. Topical 10% potassium hydroxide solution, pulse dye laser (585 nm), and tape stripping methods are additional therapeutic options. Thrice-weekly application of the topical immune modulator imiquimod (Aldara 5% cream)* has cleared this infection in some patients.

Patients with advanced HIV disease may develop large or disseminated lesions of the skin that are frequently refractory to the aforementioned conventional therapies. Intravenous cidofovir (Vistide),* 2 mg/kg/wk for 2 weeks, or cidofovir 3% cream (Dermovan),* applied 5 days per week for 2 weeks, may improve or clear molluscum lesions in these patients. Further investigational studies of these drugs are currently underway.

HUMAN HERPESVIRUSES 1 AND 2 (HERPES SIMPLEX)

Herpes simplex virus (HSV) infection is increasingly prevalent in the U.S. population. More than 20% of individuals are seropositive for genital HSV, and over 90% of the population is seropositive for orolabial infection. The majority of orolabial herpes simplex infection is caused by HSV-1, whereas most genital disease is caused by HSV-2. The virus is transmitted through direct contact with active lesions or infected mucosal secretions and may even be spread during periods of asymptomatic shedding (particularly in genital infections). After primary inoculation, HSV migrates into the dorsal root ganglion of the spinal cord, where it remains latent indefinitely or until recurrence is precipitated.

Primary orolabial HSV infection of childhood may present with fever, malaise, and a painful erosive gingivostomatitis that resolves within 2 to 3 weeks. More commonly, children and adolescents experience subclinical primary oral HSV infection, thereby making the determination of seropositivity difficult based on clinical history alone. Most episodes of recurrent herpes labialis ("cold sores" and "fever blisters") develop in the same location on the lip or mucosal surface. Local itching, burning, and paresthesias often begin 24 to 48 hours before the development of tender erythematous papulovesicles. Physical and emotional stress and ultraviolet light exposure can precipitate orolabial recurrences, which usually heal within 7 to 10 days. It is uncertain why some individuals develop HSV seropositivity yet remain free of clinical infection, whereas others experience primary and/or recurrent episodes of oral or genital disease.

Genital herpes infection is an enormous public health concern. Prevention of infection through education and protective measures is essential. Abstinence or condom use must be recommended when active lesions are present, but the patient must understand that asymptomatic viral shedding is common (an estimated 5% to 50% of days per month) and can also spread disease. Nearly 70% of primary genital HSV infections are transmitted during these periods of subclinical shedding. Although HSV-2 causes most genital disease, HSV-1 has become an increasingly prevalent etiologic agent. Prodromal symptoms of low-grade fever, tender inguinal lymphadenopathy, malaise, genital burning, itching, and tingling may develop 7 to 10 days after initial exposure to HSV. Painful grouped papules, vesicles, and erosions that are highly infectious subsequently develop at the sight of inoculation. Crusting and healing of skin lesions usually occurs within 2 weeks of a primary genital infection.

Symptoms of recurrent genital HSV are variable and often far less severe than those of primary infection. Development of painful, erythematous anogenital papules, macules, or pustules plus-or-minus burning, dysuria, vulvodynia, discharge, and even urinary retention may herald primary or recurrent infection; therefore, a detailed clinical and HSV-exposure history is required to pinpoint the diagnosis and appropriately counsel each patient. The risk and frequency of mucocutaneous herpes simplex disease recurrences cannot yet be accurately predicted.

Other clinical variants of herpes simplex infections include *herpetic whitlow* (seen in HSV-1 infected children due to thumb-sucking) and *herpes gladiatorum* (which can occur on the torso of wrestlers or other athletes with frequent skin-to-skin contact and is also caused by HSV-1 inoculation). *Eczema herpeticum* is a diffuse cutaneous HSV infection seen in patients with chronic and often severe underlying inflammatory skin disorders (such as atopic dermatitis) that compromise skin integrity. Most cases of recurrent erythema multiforme are presumed to be caused by recurrent herpes simplex disease, and chronic suppressive antiviral therapy may improve morbidity. Herpes proctitis and lumbosacral herpes can present diagnostic challenges, yet need to be considered in immunosuppressed patients. Clinicians must educate patients that HSV-compromised skin is also at high risk for HIV transmission. HIV testing should be strongly considered once a patient is diagnosed with genital herpes.

Vertical transmission of genital herpes simplex virus to a neonate during vaginal delivery can have devastating and even fatal consequences. A previously seronegative mother who is infected during the third trimester is at highest risk for fetal compromise. Severe neurodevelopmental disabilities can afflict HSV-infected neonates, and the mortality rate approaches 40% despite aggressive therapeutic measures.

There are several diagnostic tools available to confirm the diagnosis of HSV infection and/or to determine its serotype. A Tzanck smear can be performed in the office by staining and microscopic evaluation of skin scrapings retrieved from the base of an intact vesicle. The presence

*Not FDA approved for this indication.

of multinucleated giant cells indicates a herpesvirus infection but cannot distinguish between HSV-1, HSV-2, and varicella-zoster virus. Viral skin culture is a helpful tool as well but must be obtained during early active infection for maximum sensitivity. It has virtually no yield if obtained more than 7 days after onset of symptoms. Fluorescent antibody testing is often used to rapidly diagnose HSV infection and distinguish between HSV serotypes. A new generation of enzyme-linked immunosorbent assays has been developed and can be performed in the office setting. The POCkit HSV-2 Rapid Test (Diagnology, Research Triangle Park, North Carolina) can be done in the office to detect type-specific HSV-2 antibodies with greater than 95% sensitivity and specificity any time after 2 weeks from inoculation. The Premier type-specific HSV-1 IgG test (Meridian Diagnostics, Research Triangle Park, North Carolina) is another rapid ELISA test available for the diagnosis of HSV-1 seropositivity.

Several oral antiviral drugs may be considered for the treatment and chronic suppression of HSV infections. Famciclovir (Famvir), valacyclovir (Valtrex), and acyclovir (Zovirax) have been proven to diminish shedding of herpesvirus and hasten healing of skin symptoms and lesions. No antiviral agent has been developed that can eliminate the latency of HSV infection. Primary and recurrent oral and genital herpes can be safely and effectively treated if diagnosis and initiation of appropriate therapy occurs within 48 to 72 hours of the onset of prodromal symptoms. Treatment after this window of opportunity may still diminish pain and time to healing, but it may not be as efficacious as early intervention (see Table 1 for complete guidelines for HSV therapy.)

Chronic suppressive antiviral therapy decreases asymptomatic shedding of HSV by 95% and should be strongly considered in discordant couples (i.e., a seropositive and a seronegative partner) to prevent transmission of disease. Chronic suppressive therapies decrease the frequency of recurrence of oral herpes by 50% to 78% and genital herpes by 80% to 90%. Unfortunately, once the antiviral agent is discontinued, recurrent episodes of clinical disease resume at the pretreatment rate. Chronic suppressive therapy has not been shown to increase the risk of resistant HSV strains in immunocompetent patients, even with long-term use for more than 6 years. Pre- and post-exposure HSV vaccines are under investigation for immunization of at-risk patients.

Topical acyclovir 5% cream can be used in lieu of oral antiviral agents for genital and oral herpes, although oral treatment is usually more efficacious. Topical penciclovir cream (Denavir) can also be used every 2 hours for 5 days to treat mild to moderate recurrent orolabial herpes infection. No topical therapy has proven effective in prevention of recurrent disease. Other investigative treatments for herpes infections include topical interferon,* undecylenic acid cream,* DIP-253 (Genivir)* 1% cream, foscarnet 0.3% cream,* and edoxudine (EDU) 3% cream.*

Immunocompromised patients are at especially high risk for severe or disseminated herpesvirus infections with life-threatening sequelae; therefore, aggressive therapy is indicated. Although oral acyclovir (Zovirax) offers effective treatment for localized disease recurrences, intravenous administration is indicated for moderate to severe HSV manifestations in this patient population. Chronic suppressive therapy in HIV patients with famciclovir (Famvir) has been demonstrated to decrease viral shedding and severity of recurrent disease (see Table 1). Up to 5% of immunosuppressed patients will experience at least one episode of acyclovir-resistant HSV infection that will require an alternative antiviral therapy. Intravenous foscarnet is the only drug that is FDA-approved for treatment of resistant HSV strains, but vidarabine and cidofovir (Vistide or Dermovan) are under investigation as potential therapeutic agents as well. Most acyclovir-resistant varicella-zoster virus and HSV strains become acyclovir-sensitive subsequent to foscarnet therapy.

HUMAN HERPESVIRUS 3 (VARICELLA-ZOSTER VIRUS)

Varicella-zoster virus (VZV) causes primary varicella infection (chickenpox) and zoster (shingles). Varicella afflicts more than 90% of young children and is less common in adults. It is transmitted to seronegative patients by direct contact with skin lesions or respiratory secretions and usually requires 14 days of incubation. A prodrome of fever and myalgia usually manifests before development of the characteristic exanthem. Pruritic macules, papules, and vesicles (2–6 mm) first arise on the scalp and face, followed by rapid spread to the trunk and extremities within 24 to 48 hours. Highly infectious VZV skin lesions appear to be in many different stages of evolution (papules, pustules, vesicles, and crusts) at any given time. Older patients who are primarily infected by VZV have a higher morbidity than children, and the risk of complications is predictably increased with larger numbers of lesions, persistence of fever, and severity of constitutional symptoms. Patients are considered contagious for at least 4 days before and 5 days after onset of the varicelliform eruption. Secondary bacterial impetiginization with subsequent scarring is the most frequent complication of varicella in children due to manipulation of pruritic lesions. Although varicella is usually benign and self-limited in the pediatric population, immunosuppressed patients may suffer from bacterial superinfection, encephalitis, hepatitis, neurologic complications, or pneumonitis. Varicella pneumonia is far more common in adults, and 1 in 400 may be hospitalized due to this complication, with a mortality rate ranging from 10% to 30%.

Diagnosis of varicella infection is based primarily on history of exposure and clinical examination. A Tzanck smear can be obtained to identify the presence of multinucleated giant cells by scraping the base of a vesicle for microscopic examination. However, this prep cannot distinguish between herpes simplex virus (HSV) and VZV infection. Viral culture can be obtained from an early vesicle, but viral lability results in a large number of false negatives. Even after 2 weeks of incubation, culture detects VZV infection in only 50% of patients known to have varicella or zoster. Currently, the most effective diagnostic tool for confirmation of the presence of VZV is the fluorescent antibody test for specific viral antigens. It is more rapid and sensitive than traditional culture techniques and can distinguish between VZV and HSV infection based on skin scrapings.

Treatment of primary varicella infection is warranted in adolescents, adults, pregnancy, and immunocompromised patients. Recent studies have suggested that it is cost-effective and therapeutic to treat all infected children with an oral antiviral agent. No risk of resistant strain selection or long-term immunologic compromise has been demonstrated in healthy children with the use of acyclovir (Zovirax); therefore, many clinicians begin oral antiviral therapy in patients with primary varicella infection. Treatment should be instituted within 24 to 48 hours of rash onset,

*Not FDA approved for this indication.

TABLE 1. **Treatment of Herpesvirus Infections**

Diagnosis	Therapeutic Options	Dosage Regimens
Primary and recurrent herpes orolabial infection	Penciclovir (Denavir) 1% cream	Apply q2h while awake for 5 days
	Acyclovir 5% cream	Apply 5 times a day for 5 days
	Acyclovir (Zovirax)*	400 mg PO 5 times a day for 5 days
	Famciclovir (Famvir)*	500 mg PO tid for 5 days
Chronic suppressive treatment of orolabial infection	Acyclovir*	400–1000 mg PO qd divided into bid or tid dosing
Primary genital herpes infection	Acyclovir cream or ointment	Apply q3h for 7 days
	Acyclovir	200 mg PO 5 times a day for 10 days or 400 mg PO tid for 10 days*
	Valacyclovir (Valtrex)*	1000 mg PO bid for 10 days
	Famciclovir*	250 mg PO tid for 5–10 days
Recurrent genital herpes infection (immunocompetent host)	Acyclovir cream or ointment*	Apply q3h
	Acyclovir	200 mg PO 5 times a day for 5 days or 400 mg PO tid for 5 days*
	Famciclovir	125 mg PO bid for 5 days
	Valacyclovir	500 mg PO bid for 5 days
Chronic suppressive therapy for genital infection	Acyclovir	400 mg PO bid
	Valacyclovir	1000 mg PO qd or 500 mg PO bid (if >10 recurrences annually) or 500 mg PO qd (if <10 recurrences annually)
	Famciclovir	250 mg PO bid or 125 mg PO bid*
Recurrent genital infection in the immunocompromised	Acyclovir	400 mg PO 5 times a day for 10–21 days or 5 mg/kg q8–12h for 7 days
	Acyclovir 5% ointment	Apply 6 times a day for 10 days
	Foscarnet (for resistant HSV strains)	IV 40 mg/kg q8–12h for 10 days
	Cidofovir ± probenecid*	IV 5 mg/kg/wk
	Cidofovir gel*	Apply qid
Neonatal infection	Acyclovir	500 mg/m²/d for 7 days

*Drug regimen or dosage has been shown to be successful in clinical trials but has not yet been approved by the FDA.

because viral replication and therefore drug efficacy diminishes after this time period.

Acyclovir (Zovirax) is the only FDA-approved drug indicated for treatment of primary varicella disease, although famciclovir (Famvir)* and valacyclovir (Valtrex)* are often used as well (see Table 2 for details of treatment regimens). The live attenuated Oka strain vaccine (Varivax) has proven effective in preventing and/or diminishing the severity of primary varicella in children older than 12 months old, patients with chronic disease, immunocompromised patients and their caregivers, and health care workers. The vaccine may also prove helpful in preventing zoster. It is well tolerated and currently recommended for universal immunization of children in the United States.

If maternal varicella infection occurs during the first trimester of pregnancy, fetal compromise is common, with

*Not FDA approved for this indication.

TABLE 2. **Treatment of Varicella-Zoster Virus Infections**

Diagnosis	Therapeutic Options	Dosage Regimens
Primary varicella in immunocompetent children	Acyclovir (Zovirax)	20 mg/kg (max 800 mg) PO qid for 5 days
Adult varicella	Acyclovir	800 mg PO 5 times a day for 7 days
	Famciclovir (Famvir)*	500 mg PO tid for 7 days
	Valacyclovir (Valtrex)*	1000 mg PO tid for 7 days
Adult zoster	Acyclovir	800 mg PO 5 times a day for 7 days
	Famciclovir	500 mg PO tid for 7 days
	Valacyclovir	1000 mg PO tid for 7 days
	The use of an antiviral plus oral corticosteroid may be helpful in adults > 50 year old*	
Immunocompromised adult with VZV	Acyclovir	10 mg/kg IV q8h for 7 days
Immunocompromised child with VZV	Acyclovir	500 mg/m² IV q8h for 7–10 days
Acyclovir-resistant VZV	Foscarnet	40–60 mg/kg IV q8h for 10 days

*Given drug regimen or dosage has been shown to be successful in clinical trials but has not yet been approved by the FDA.
Abbreviation: VZV = varicella-zoster virus.

abnormalities ranging from atrophy and scarring of the skin to central nervous system defects, optic damage, or fetal demise. VZV-specific immune globulin therapy (VZIG) (125 U/10 kg) is used for postexposure prophylaxis in pregnant women and the immunocompromised population without prior VZV infection. It is only effective in preventing or diminishing the incidence and/or severity of infection if administered within 4 days of known or presumed exposure to VZV.

Once a patient is infected with the varicella-zoster virus, he or she may develop zoster (shingles) any time in the future. Zoster is characterized by a prodrome of local tingling, burning, pain, and sometimes low-grade fever, followed by the appearance of erythematous vesicles, pustules, and papules in a unilateral dermatomal distribution. It is caused by the reactivation of VZV, which establishes latency in the dorsal root ganglion of patients after primary varicella infection. Up to 20% of the general population will experience one episode of zoster, which is more likely to occur in older age as T-cell–mediated immunity wanes. Only 5% of patients will experience more than one episode of shingles, and recurrences occur in the same dermatome 50% of the time. The cervical and thoracic dermatomes are most commonly affected, but involvement of the ophthalmic branch of the trigeminal nerve warrants most clinical concern.

Rarely, dermatomal pain can develop after VZV reactivation in the absence of any cutaneous lesions. This is referred to as *zoster sine herpete* and can mimic acute cardiac or abdominal pain. It is important to educate patients that zoster cannot beget zoster. In other words, a patient with shingles can only infect someone who is seronegative for VZV (i.e., someone who has not had chickenpox in the past). Viral skin culture suffers the same inherent problems in zoster as it does in varicella infection. The most rapid and sensitive confirmatory test for zoster is the fluorescent antibody assay, which is performed on scrapings from a vesicle floor. The Tzanck smear is often used in the clinical setting but is subject to misinterpretation and sampling error.

Most zoster eruptions heal within 1 month, but the persistence of neuropathic pain in the affected area is not uncommon. Treatment of zoster with oral antiviral agents is indicated to reduce viral shedding and reduce the duration of postherpetic neuralgia. There is a significant risk for severe and permanent visual compromise if the ophthalmic branch of the trigeminal nerve is involved. Up to 50% of these patients may develop conjunctivitis, iritis, retinal arteritis, or retinal necrosis; therefore, rapid diagnosis, ophthalmologic evaluation, and aggressive antiviral treatment is essential. If ocular involvement is suggested, topical acyclovir is indicated as an adjunct to systemic therapy.

Acyclovir (Zovirax) has been demonstrated to reduce shingles pain and hasten resolution of the associated exanthem. Like varicella, it is most effective if initiated within 48 hours of the development of prodromal symptoms. The recommended oral antiviral regimen is similar in the management of both varicella and zoster. Oral acyclovir (Zovirax), valacylovir (Valtrex),* or famciclovir (Famvir)* can be prescribed, and all three drugs may reduce the duration of postherpetic neuralgia as well (see Table 2 for complete treatment regimens). As with varicella infection, immunosuppressed patients may require intravenous acyclovir therapy. VZV immune globulin (VZIG) may also be used for postexposure prophylaxis if given to at-risk patients within 4 days of exposure to an individual with zoster. Although zoster is less contagious than varicella, VZV-seronegative patients who are immunocompromised or pregnant have a significant risk for acquiring infection on exposure to shingles and should be considered for VZIG therapy. Although the adjunctive use of oral corticosteroids in the treatment of zoster remains controversial, some dermatologists are now recommending their concurrent use in a select group of patients. Adults older than the age of 50 who have no contraindication for corticosteroid therapy may benefit from the combination of oral acyclovir and oral glucocorticoids for short-term reduction of pain.

No oral therapy has been shown to reduce the incidence or completely prevent the occurrence of postherpetic neuralgia. This debilitating neuritis affects nearly 50% of elderly patients after an episode of zoster. Early oral antiviral treatment of shingles lesions can potentially decrease the duration of postherpetic neuralgia. Several topical therapies may afford symptomatic relief. These include capsaicin (Zostrix-HP) and other local anesthetics such as EMLA cream,* ELA-Max,* and lidocaine patches (Lidoderm).* Although nonsteroidal anti-inflammatory drugs offer ineffective relief of postherpetic neuralgia, low doses (25–50 mg/d) of tricyclic antidepressants* are frequently beneficial. Carbamazepine (Tegretol),* gabapentin (Neurontin),* oral narcotics, and nerve blocks may be necessary in some patients for adequate pain relief. Patients should be advised to avoid manipulation of the affected area, wear loose-fitting clothes, and use Domeboro's soaks* or antihistamines for temporary relief of itching.

HUMAN HERPESVIRUS 4 (EPSTEIN-BARR VIRUS)

Epstein-Barr virus (EBV) is a member of the herpesvirus family that is primarily spread via oral secretions and infects epithelial cells as well as B lymphocytes. Once infected, the virus remains latent in B cells for the duration of a patient's lifetime, or until immunosuppression results in reactivation and viral replication. EBV has been associated with several diseases, including oral "hairy" leukoplakia in HIV patients, B-cell lymphoma, mononucleosis, nasopharyngeal carcinoma, Hodgkin disease, and some T-cell lymphomas.

Relevant to this discussion is the occurrence of a generalized rash in 5% to 15% of children with acute mononucleosis from EBV. The exanthem may be macular, papular, urticarial, or even erythema multiforme–like and occurs in association with fever, nasal congestion, lymphadenopathy, sore throat, and hepatosplenomegaly. If ampicillin or other penicillin-like antibiotics are inadvertently administered to a patient with acute EBV infection, a distinctive and diffuse morbilliform rash that may involve acral surfaces may erupt and persist for 7 to 10 days. This hypersensitivity reaction is not a true drug allergy; therefore, afflicted patients should not be labeled as penicillin-allergic.

EBV infection can be diagnosed by performing a heterophile (monospot) test in the office setting. Lymphocytosis and the presence of atypical lymphocytes in the peripheral blood are common supportive laboratory findings. The monospot test may not be sensitive until the third week of illness. It also loses sensitivity (by reverting back to a negative result) if obtained more than 12 weeks after onset of mononucleosis-associated symptoms. If clinical suspicion remains high after a negative monospot, IgM and IgG antiviral capsid antigens can be assayed.

*Not FDA approved for this indication.

*Not FDA approved for this indication.

Treatment of infectious mononucleosis is largely supportive. Acyclovir (Zovirax)* and oral corticosteroid therapy have not been shown to alter the clinical course of the disease in most patients. The use of ampicillin and amoxicillin should be avoided during the acute phase of EBV infection to avoid development of the aforementioned hypersensitivity exanthem.

Oral leukoplakia (also referred to as oral hairy leukoplakia) is a manifestation of reactivated EBV infection in HIV-positive and other immunosuppressed patients. Painless white plaques develop on the lateral margins of the tongue and can be distinguished from oral candidiasis by scraping the area. Hyperplastic EBV-infected cells of oral hairy leukoplakia do not scrape off, whereas yeast can be easily removed. Potassium hydroxide examination is recommended to confirm the absence of oral candidiasis. Treatment is usually unnecessary, but the condition does respond readily to oral acyclovir (Zovirax),* 400 to 800 mg five times daily, topical tretinoin,* trichloroacetic acid,* podophyllum resin,* or glycolic acid.* Unfortunately, the plaques of oral hairy leukoplakia will recur once any of these treatment modalities are discontinued.

HUMAN HERPESVIRUS 5 (CYTOMEGALOVIRUS)

Cytomegalovirus (CMV) is a herpesvirus that uncommonly presents as cutaneous disease. It is spread through body fluids such as saliva, semen, urine, and tears. Most people are seropositive for CMV by late adulthood, and many are asymptomatically infected as infants or young adults. Patients with HIV infection and other forms of immunosuppression or malignancy are at risk for skin manifestations secondary to disseminated disease. These lesions are extremely variable and nonspecific. Perianal ulcers in HIV-positive patients with CD4-positive cell counts less than 100/mm^3 can be caused by CMV, although recurrent HSV or VZV infections are far more common etiologic agents in this population. In an otherwise healthy patient, the only manifestation of CMV infection may be associated with a mononucleosis-type syndrome and a secondary morbilliform eruption.

Congenital CMV infection occurs in neonates whose mothers are primarily infected during the first or second trimesters. It is the most common congenital viral infection and the leading infectious cause of mental retardation and deafness. CMV is a component of the congenital TORCH syndrome, which includes toxoplasmosis, other (syphilis, bacterial causes), rubella, CMV, and HSV. Each of these congenital infections can present similarly with hepatosplenomegaly, central nervous system abnormalities, and purpuric cutaneous lesions. These "blueberry muffin" macules and nodules on the skin are a manifestation of a compensatory dermal hematopoiesis in infected neonates. They manifest in the first few days of life in approximately one third of infants afflicted by any of the TORCH agents.

Viral culture from the pharynx or urine is the best diagnostic test for confirmation of congenital CMV infection. Skin culture and biopsy for histology and polymerase chain reaction can be used reliably to diagnose cutaneous CMV infection in immunosuppressed patients. Enzyme-linked immunosorbent assays for IgM and IgG antibody are also commonly used to support the diagnosis and establish a timeline for the infection. The presence of IgM anti-CMV antibody indicates infection within the past 4 months. Despite the success of ganciclovir (Cytovene), foscarnet (Foscavir), and cidofivir (Vistide) drug therapies for treatment of many cutaneous and systemic manifestations of CMV, the development of CMV-associated skin lesions in immunosuppressed patients often portends a grave prognosis.

*Not FDA approved for this indication.

HUMAN HERPESVIRUSES 6 AND 7 (EXANTHEM SUBITUM, ROSEOLA INFANTUM, OR SIXTH DISEASE)

Human herpesviruses 6 and 7 (HHV-6 and -7) are ubiquitous in the general population, and most individuals are infected by the first year of age. They are believed to establish latent infections after oropharyngeal transmission. Although most primary infections are asymptomatic, many infants between the ages of 6 months and 2 years exhibit a nonspecific exanthem. The incubation period of 5 to 15 days is followed by the sudden onset of a high fever (102°–103°F [38.9°–39.4°C]) that remains elevated and then abruptly diminishes on the fourth day. Characteristically, the exanthem appears only after the prodromal fever has subsided. Rose-colored 2-mm macules and papules typically appear on the neck and back on the background of a white halo.

The temporal association of fever followed in several days by rash is essential for the diagnosis of roseola. Palpebral edema (the Berliner sign) commonly develops and can be a helpful diagnostic indicator. Despite the high fever, infected infants rarely appear toxic. The rash of exanthem subitum usually resolves without sequelae within several hours to days, but meningoencephalitis and seizures can occur as rare complications. Although HHV-6 and HHV-7 are susceptible to the same antiviral treatments as CMV, they are rarely indicated in this self-limited disease.

HUMAN HERPESVIRUS 8 (KAPOSI'S SARCOMA)

Kaposi's sarcoma (KS) is a malignancy of vascular origin caused by HHV-8 infection. Immunosuppressed patients (particularly HIV-infected homosexual men) are at significant risk for development of this disease. Although primary HHV-8 infection is common, it appears that this subset of the population is especially prone to viral reactivation and clinical manifestations due to insufficient cell-mediated immunity.

KS lesions may appear on cutaneous and mucosal surfaces as violaceous or brown patches, plaques, or nodules that can be susceptible to hemorrhage. Lesional skin biopsy confirms the diagnosis. Variants of KS include asymptomatic, indolent disease (classically found on the lower extremities of immunocompetent males of Mediterranean descent) to aggressive KS variants seen most often in immunosuppressed patients with associated gastrointestinal, pulmonary, bone marrow, or multiorgan involvement.

Cryotherapy, excision, and intralesional bleomycin can be used for treatment of localized disease. Limited cutaneous disease also responds to topical and systemic retinoids. Alitretinoin (Panretin) may be applied topically two to four times daily for treatment of Kaposi skin lesions and can achieve a 35% response rate in HIV-infected patients. Radiotherapy can achieve an 80% response rate, whereas systemic chemotherapeutics are reserved for treatment of severe, progressive disease. Vincristine,* bleomycin,* vinblastine, and interferon alfa are only a few among many agents under investigation for treatment of KS. Aggressive antiretroviral cocktails (HAART) prescribed for treatment of HIV-infection may also minimize the risk and progression of Kaposi's disease by improving cell-mediated immunity.

*Not FDA approved for this indication.

PARASITIC DISEASES OF THE SKIN

method of
PHILIP D. SHENEFELT, M.D.
University of South Florida
Tampa, Florida

Parasitic afflictions of the skin are caused by protozoa, helminths, and arthropods. Table 1 lists cutaneous parasites, the geographic distribution, parasitic diseases, and their treatment. Although a number of the cutaneous parasites occur primarily in the tropics, world travel exposes increasing numbers of individuals from temperate climates to these pathogens. Travel history and recreational/occupational history are important when cutaneous findings indicate that parasitic skin disease is in the differential diagnosis spectrum.

PROTOZOAL INFECTIONS

Amebiasis

Cutaneous amebiasis caused by *Entamoeba histolytica* is rare and occurs by direct inoculation from feces or an abscess. The lesion typically is an irregular painful ulcer on the perineum, buttock, or abdomen. Metronidazole (Flagyl), 750 mg orally every 8 hours for 5 to 10 days, is recommended, followed by iodoquinol (Yodoxin), 650 mg three times daily for 20 days, to eliminate the intestinal source.

Leishmaniasis

Cutaneous leishmaniasis is transmitted by the bite of an infected sandfly, with several *Leishmania* species involved. See the article Leishmaniasis for details on how to diagnose and treat cutaneous leishmaniasis.

Trypanosomiasis

Chagas disease, caused by *Trypanosoma cruzi,* often is clinically inapparent on the skin but may manifest as the *Romaña sign* (unilateral eyelid edema and conjunctivitis) or a *chagoma* (an erythematous indurated subcutaneous nodule). This occurs at the bite site from an infected reduviid bug. Early treatment is important to prevent late sequelae of cardiomyopathy or gastrointestinal involvement. Nifurtimox (Lampit) is available through the Centers for Disease Control and Prevention Drug Service and is given 8 to 10 mg/kg/d in four divided doses for 120 days.

African sleeping sickness is transmitted by the bite of the tsetse fly infected with *Trypanosoma brucei* var. *gambiense* or *rhodesiense.* About half of patients develop an initial 2- to 5-cm erythematous nodule surrounded by a white halo at the bite site 5 to 15 days after the bite. An evanescent macular eruption may occur weeks to months later. Early treatment is very important to prevent central nervous system involvement. For *Trypanosoma brucei* var. *gambiense,* eflornithine (Ornidyl), available from the World Health Organization, is given at 400 mg/kg intravenously in four divided doses for 2 weeks, followed by 300 mg/kg/d orally for 3 to 4 weeks. Suramin sodium (Antrypol), available from the Centers for Disease Control and Prevention Drug Service, can be used to treat *Trypanosoma brucei* var. *gambiense* or *rhodesiense.* The dosage is a 100-mg test dose followed by 1 g intravenously on days 1, 3, 7, 14, and 21.

HELMINTHS

Creeping Eruption (Cutaneous Larva Migrans)

Cutaneous larva migrans, or *creeping eruption,* occurs when the larvae of the cat and dog hookworm, *Ancylostoma braziliense,* penetrate skin in contact with the ground. The infestation usually occurs in warm, moist, sandy areas, such as at the beach, at playgrounds, in sandboxes, and under houses. Within a few hours of contact an erythematous papule appears at the site of skin penetration. In 1 or 2 days, pruritic erythematous serpiginous tracks develop. They usually progress at 1 to 2 cm per day. The larvae are accidental intruders and usually die within a few weeks, although some may persist for up to a year with cycles of remission and exacerbation.

Small numbers of lesions can be treated with ethyl chloride or liquid nitrogen freezing. Larger numbers can be treated topically with thiabendazole 10% (Mintezol) suspension applied three times a day until the lesions have resolved. Oral thiabendazole, 5 mg/kg/d in two divided doses up to a maximum of 1.5 g/d for patients weighing more than 70 kg may be given for 2 consecutive days after weighing the benefits with the potential adverse reactions. Oral ivermectin (Stromectol),* 200 μg/kg orally in a single dose, is a good alternative.

Patients should be instructed in preventive measures. Minimizing contact with the ground, covering sandboxes when not in use, and draping the ground with plastic before performing work in areas frequented by domestic animals help to prevent further exposure.

Dracunculiasis

Dracunculiasis occurs when the larvae are swallowed inside infected water fleas. *Dracunculus medinensis,* the Guinea worm, can be extracted by winding it around a small stick as it emerges from the subcutaneous tissues. Metronidazole (Flagyl),* 250 mg orally three times daily for 10 days, reduces inflammation and facilitates removal of the worm.

Loiasis

Migratory angioedema, called *Calabar swellings,* and worms visible in the scleral conjunctiva typify

*Not FDA approved for this indication.

TABLE 1. **Cutaneous Parasites, Parasitic Diseases, and Their Treatment**

Class	Causative Organism	Geographic Distribution	Cutaneous Manifestations	Recommended Treatment
Protozoa	*Entamoeba histolytica*	Worldwide	Amebiasis cutis	Metronidazole (Flagyl), 750 mg q8h PO for 5–10 d
	Leishmania species	Africa, Asia, Middle East, Central and South America	Cutaneous leishmaniasis	See article on leishmaniasis.
	Trypanosoma cruzi	Central and South America	Chagas disease	Nifurtimox (Lampit), 8–10 mg/kg/d in four doses for 120 d
	Trypanosoma brucei	Africa	Trypanosomal chancre or macular eruption	Eflornithine or suramin
Helminths	*Ancylostoma braziliense*	Worldwide	Cutaneous larva migrans	Topical 10% thiabendazole suspension (Mintezol), bid for 2 d; invermectin (Stromectol),* 200 μg/kg
	Ancylostoma duodenale/ *Necator americanus*	Africa, Asia, Mediterranean, Central and South America, Southeastern North America	Ground itch, Dew itch	Mebendazole (Vermox), 100 mg PO q12h for 3 d
	Dracunculus medinensis	Asia, Africa, Middle East	Guinea worm	Surgical removal
	Loa loa	Africa	Calabar swellings	Diethylcarbamazine (Hetrazan), 6 mg/kg/d PO for 21 d
	Onchocerca volvulus	Africa, Central and South America	Onchodermatitis River blindness	Ivermectin (Stromectol),* 50 μg/kg
	Schistosoma species	Africa, Asia, Middle East, Caribbean, South America	Schistosomiasis Cercarial dermatitis Swimmer's itch	Praziquantel (Biltricide), 20 mg/kg bid or tid for 1 d
	Strongyloides stercoralis	Worldwide	Larva currens, urticaria	Ivermectin (Stromectol),† 200 μg/kg PO
	Wuchereria bancrofti/ *Brugia* species	Asia, Africa, Caribbean, South America	Lymphatic filariasis, elephantiasis	Diethylcarbamazine (Hetrazan), 6 mg/kg/d PO for 6–12 d
Arthropoda	*Dermatobia hominis*/ botflies	Worldwide	Myiasis	Surgical removal
	Pediculus humanus *Phthirus pubis*	Worldwide	Head lice Body lice Pubic lice	1% permethrin (Nix Creme Rinse) for 10 min; repeat in 1 wk
	Sarcoptes scabiei	Worldwide	Scabies	5% permethrin cream or ivermectin (Stromectol),* 200 μg/kg PO
	Tunga penetrans	Central and South America, Africa	Tungiasis	Surgical removal

*Not FDA approved for this indication.
†Ivermectin (Stromectol) is officially indicated only for onchocerciasis and gastrointestinal strongyloidiasis.

the cutaneous manifestation of infection with *Loa loa.* Transmission is by infected tabanid fly bite. Treatment is with diethylcarbamazide (Hetrazan), 8 mg/kg/d orally in three divided doses for 21 days.

Lymphatic Filariasis

Elephantiasis occurs as a late sequelae of lymphatic channel obstruction by *Wuchereria bancrofti* or *Brugia* species, which are transmitted by infected mosquito bite. Microfilariae may be visible in blood samples viewed under the microscope. Treatment is with diethylcarbamazide (Hetrazan), 6 mg/kg/d orally in three divided doses for 6 to 12 days.

Onchodermatitis

Pruritic dermatitis and subcutaneous nodules are characteristic of *Onchocerca volvulus* infections. Transmission is by the blackfly. These infections tend to occur adjacent to the rivers where the blackfly larvae develop, hence the name *river blindness* for the ocular manifestations. Microfilariae may be visible in blood samples viewed under the microscope. Treatment with ivermectin (Stromectol), 150 μg/kg orally every 6 to 12 months, keeps the microfilariae under control. The adult worms are resistant to this treatment, hence the need for ongoing suppression of the microfilariae.

Schistosomiasis

Skin exposure to contaminated water is the cause of *schistosomiasis.* The duck/snail schistosome causes cercarial dermatitis or swimmer's itch with pruritic erythematous papules that last 5 to 7 days. Infection with the nonhuman species of *Schistosoma* is self-limited and does not require treatment. Human/snail schistosomaisis can be treated with praziquantel (Biltricide), 20 mg/kg two to three times in a single day.

Larva Currens

Strongyloides stercoralis often causes a serpiginous eruption similar to cutaneous larval migrans, but migration is much more rapid, up to 10 cm/d. It is often accompanied by diarrhea and proximal bowel infection. Ivermectin (Stromectol), 150 to 200 μg/kg orally as a single dose, is very effective for both the bowel and cutaneous involvement.

Uncinarial Dermatitis

The human hookworms *Ancylostoma duodenale* and *Necator americanus* cause dew itch or ground itch similar to cutaneous larval migrans, but the larvae penetrate venules, exit into the lungs, ascend the trachea, are swallowed, attach to the small intestine, and mature. Treatment is with mebendazole (Vermox), 100 mg orally every 12 hours for 3 days.

ARTHROPODS

Myiasis

Human myiasis may occur with *Dermatobia hominis* or one of several other species of botfly, screwworm fly, or flesh fly. These diptera deposit eggs on the skin and the larva burrow into the skin, creating an erythematous pruritic papule with a central punctum within which the tip of the larval abdomen periodically appears. Occlusion of the central punctum with petroleum jelly may force the larva to emerge to avoid suffocation. Otherwise, diagnosis and treatment is accomplished by surgical extirpation.

Pediculosis

Human lice are of three types. *Phthirus pubis,* the pubic louse or crab louse, prefers the pubic hair but can be found on body and axillary hair, eyebrows, eyelashes, and occasionally the occipital scalp. *Pediculus humanus* var. *capitis,* the head louse, and var. *corporis,* the body louse, are elongate and fast moving. The head louse prefers the scalp, whereas the body louse hides in seams in clothing. The eggs or nits of the pubic and head louse are cemented to the bases of hairs and those of the body louse are laid on clothing. Nits remain viable for up to a month. They hatch and evolve into adults within 2 or 3 weeks. Spread occurs from one person to another by close contact or sharing a bed or clothing. The louse bite results in a red pruritic macule with a central hemorrhagic center.

Pediculosis Pubis

Crab lice are identified by their characteristic shape and slow movement. They are difficult to see unless one looks closely. The nits also can be seen attached to the bases of hairs. In addition to the pubic hair, the body hair, axillary hair, eyebrows, eyelashes, and occipital scalp should also be examined. Pruritus and excoriations are common, and secondary impetiginization may supervene. Scattered bite sites may be seen on the skin near hairs.

Lindane (Kwell, Gamene) shampoo should be applied to the affected areas for 5 to 10 minutes and then showered off. A fine-toothed nit comb may be used to remove nits by combing the hairs. The treatment may be repeated once in 5 to 7 days. Eyelash infestations may be treated with careful mechanical removal of nits and lice using a fine forceps. Alternatively, petrolatum may be applied in a thick layer twice a day for a week. Clothing and bedding should be laundered in hot soapy water and mechanically dried for at least 20 minutes. Close contacts should be treated if infested.

Pediculosis Capitis

Head lice move quickly, so one must be alert for sudden movement when parting the hair. The nits are easier to find. The areas of heaviest nit involvement typically are at the occipital scalp. Nits are attached at the bases of hairs. Pruritus with excoriations is usually present. Secondary impetiginization may occur. Because head lice are highly contagious in children, all closely associated children should be treated.

Permethrin (Nix) is effective as a single dose treatment. It is applied after shampooing and toweling dry. After 10 minutes it is rinsed out with water. A nit comb is used to remove nits.

Pyrethrin piperonyl butoxide liquid (RID) is applied to dry hair and then shampooed out after 10 minutes. Because it is less effective as an ovicide, treatment should be repeated once in a week. Nits should be removed using a nit comb.

Lindane (Kwell, Gamene) shampoo has poor ovicidal activity. It is applied in contact with the scalp and hair for 4 minutes and then removed by shampooing. Nit combing must be thorough. Repeat treatments may be necessary.

Pediculosis Corporis

Body lice are most commonly found on homeless people or in wartime. Because the louse lives in the seams of clothing, it is not often observed on the skin. Typical feeding sites are on the trunk and buttocks. The resulting red papules are often extensively excoriated. Secondary impetiginization is common. Nits and lice should be sought in the seams of clothing for diagnosis.

Laundering or dry cleaning the clothes and bedding kills the lice and nits. After cleansing the skin with soap and water, pruritus may be treated with topical corticosteroid creams and oral antihistamines.

Scabies

Scabies is a skin infestation by the mite *Sarcoptes scabiei*. The mite lives and breeds in the stratum corneum. Usually the human host does not notice the initial exposure infestation until several weeks have passed. Sensitization to the mite or its scybellae (fecal droppings) then results in intense pruritus, accentuated at night. Reinfestation will result in pruritus usually within a day. Because of the asymptomatic initial phase of infestation, close contacts of a scabies patient should be treated even if not symptomatic. A successfully treated patient may continue to experience pruritus for a couple of weeks after treatment.

The distribution of scabies on the body typically involves the fingerwebs, wrists, ankles, elbows, axilla, waistline, area under the breasts and on the nipples in women, umbilicus, genitalia, and buttocks. Typically, lesions are small red papules that often are excoriated. Secondary impetiginization may supervene. Uncommonly, nodules may appear on the genitalia, groin, or axilla. Vesicles can occur, especially in children. A pathognomonic lesion, the burrow, can sometimes be identified as a tiny line on a fingerweb or lateral finger. Lesions do not ordinarily occur above the neck except in infants and toddlers. If the reaction to scabies has been partially suppressed by topical or systemic corticosteroids, scabies incognito may occur and be difficult to recognize. At the other extreme, a mentally retarded or debilitated or immunocompromised patient may have thick crusted areas and thousands of mites and even burrowing into the fingernails. This condition is known as Norwegian scabies.

A presumptive diagnosis of scabies can be made from the clinical presentation. To confirm the diagnosis, using a No. 15 scalpel blade dipped in mineral oil, one should scrape several lesions down almost to the point of pinpoint bleeding and transfer the scrapings to a drop of mineral oil on a clean glass slide. After placing a coverslip over the specimen, one then examines the slide under a microscope using the 10× or 40× objective. Finding the mite, its eggs, or its scybellae (droppings) clinches the diagnosis. Treatment of scabies is generally quite effective. To prevent reinfestation, asymptomatic close contacts should be treated simultaneously. Bedsheets and all clothing worn in the past 3 days should be laundered in hot soapy water or dry cleaned.

Permethrin 5% (Elimite) cream is applied from the neck down and left on overnight for 8 to 12 hours. Reapplication after 5 days is often advisable. If used on infants and toddlers, it should be applied to the head and scalp also.

Lindane 1% (Kwell, Gamene) lotion is applied from the neck down and left on overnight for 8 to 12 hours. Reapplication after 5 days is often advisable. Lindane should usually be avoided in infants, pregnant women, and epileptics because of its neurotoxicity. Up to 40% of scabies mites may be resistant to lindane.

Precipitated sulfur 6% in petrolatum is applied daily for 3 consecutive days without removal or bathing during the 3-day time interval. Treatment of infants and toddlers should include the face and scalp. This agent is preferred for infants, toddlers, and pregnant women because of its minimal toxicity.

Oral ivermectin,* 200 μg/kg orally in a single dose, may be useful for crusted scabies or scabies in an immunocompromised host.

Tungiasis

Infection with the burrowing female flea *Tunga penetrans* typically manifests as an erythematous papule with a central black spot. Location is usually on the foot. Diagnosis is confirmed, and treatment is accomplished by surgical removal of the embedded flea.

*Not FDA approved for this indication.

FUNGAL DISEASES OF THE SKIN

method of
JEFFREY M. WEINBERG, M.D.
St. Luke's–Roosevelt Hospital Center and Columbia College of Physicians and Surgeons
New York, New York

The predominant types of fungal infection of the skin include dermatophytosis, candidiasis, and tinea versicolor.

Proper diagnosis of these diseases, using methods including potassium hydroxide preparation, culture, and biopsy, is important because nonfungal diseases can often simulate these entities. Treatment of these diseases consists of topical or oral antifungal therapy, depending on the clinical setting.

DERMATOPHYTOSIS

The *dermatophytes* are fungi that infect keratinous tissue of people and animals and that have the ability to invade the hair, skin, and nails of the host and cause a host-mediated immune response. Dermatophyte infections, referred to as *tinea infections,* are named according to the body region infected. Infections of the scalp, glabrous skin, groin, feet, hands, beard, and nails are referred to, respectively, as *tinea capitis, corporis, cruris, pedis, manuum, barbae,* and *unguium* (also known as *onychomycosis*). Dermatophytes belong to three genera: *Trichophyton, Microsporum,* and *Epidermophyton.* Most infections in the United States are due to five species: *Trichophyton rubrum, Trichophyton tonsurans, Trichophyton mentagrophytes, Microsporum canis,* and *Epidermophyton floccosum.*

Tinea capitis, dermatophytosis of the scalp, most commonly occurs in African American children between the ages of 3 and 7, although 10% of culture-positive cases occur in adult women. The most common etiologic agent in the United States is *T. tonsurans.* Clinical presentations include a seborrheic type, black dot infection, and an inflammatory type, kerion. Many children and caretakers are asymptomatic carriers of infection. The most common methods for diagnosing tinea capitis are potassium hydroxide (KOH) preparation and fungal culture. Fungal culture can be performed using a soft toothbrush that is rubbed firmly over the involved scalp and then gently applied over the culture surface.

The gold standard of therapy for tinea capitis is oral griseofulvin. Topical therapy is most often unsuccessful because topical medications cannot penetrate the hair follicle. The dosage of microsized griseofulvin (Fulvicin)* is 20 to 25 mg/kg/d for 6 to 8 weeks. The medication is usually given to young children as a 125 mg/5 mL suspension, in conjunction with a fatty meal. In addition, the patient and family members should use selenium sulfide shampoo 2.5% three times per week to reduce the spread of infectious spores. For patients who fail therapy with griseofulvin or cannot tolerate the medication, treatment with itraconazole (Sporanox)* or terbinafine (Lamisil)* is an option. The dosing for itraconazole depends on the weight of the patient: 100 mg every other day for less than 20 kg, 100 mg/d for 20 to 40 kg, and 200 mg/kg for more than 40 kg. Similarly, terbinafine is dosed as follows: 62.5 mg/d for less than 20 kg, 125 mg/d for 20 to 40 kg, and 250 mg/d for more than 40 kg. The duration of treatment for the newer antifungal agents varies from 2 to 4 weeks according to different studies. All members of the patient's family should be evaluated for infection to prevent recurrences.

Tinea corporis refers to dermatophytosis of the glabrous skin. Types of clinical presentations include annular lesions, bullous lesions, granulomatous eruptions, pustular lesions, psoriasiform plaques, and verrucous lesions. The disease occurs worldwide and is generally more prevalent in tropical areas. *T. rubrum* is the most common cause of tinea corporis, and *T. mentagrophytes* is also a common pathogen. Tinea corporis caused by *M. canis* frequently presents as multiple lesions that tend to be more inflammatory and symptomatic than infections caused by anthropophilic dermatophytes. Tinea cruris refers to dermatophyte infection of the groin, including the suprapubic areas, proximal medial thighs, perineum, gluteal cleft, and buttocks. Infection is most commonly caused by *T. rubrum* and *E. floccosum* and most often occurs in men. Women less commonly develop tinea cruris, with candidiasis occurring more frequently.

First-line therapy for both tinea corporis and tinea cruris consists of topical antifungal agents. Topical antifungal agents used in the treatment of dermatophytosis include several classes of medications: imidazoles, allylamines, naphthiomates (tolnaftate), and the substituted pyridone ciclopiroxolamine. Commonly used imidazoles include clotrimazole (Lotrimin, Mycelex), miconazole (Micatin, Monistat), econazole (Spectazole), ketoconazole (Nizoral), oxiconazole (Oxistat), and sulconazole (Exelderm). The allylamines are fungicidal and include terbinafine (Lamisil AT), naftifine (Naftin), and butenafine (Mentax). Treatment with oral antifungal agents may be necessary in patients with extensive infection or with involvement of hair follicles. These individuals may be treated with itraconazole,* 200 mg twice daily for 1 to 2 weeks, or with terbinafine, 250 mg/d for 2 to 4 weeks.

Tinea pedis is a dermatophyte infection of the plantar surface and toe webs of the feet; it is the most common dermatophyte infection in human beings. Tinea manuum is a similar process involving the palm and interdigital spaces. Often, only one hand or foot is involved. Tinea pedis is most commonly caused by *T. rubrum,* followed by *T. mentagrophytes* and *E. floccosum.* There are four clinical patterns of infection: the moccasin type, with erythema, scale, and crusting of the plantar surfaces; the inflammatory type, with vesicles and bullous lesions involving the toes or the instep; the interdigital type, in which scale, crusting, and maceration develop in the interdigital spaces; and the ulcerative type, which is usually an extension of interdigital tinea pedis complicated by bacterial infection. Topical treatment with an imidazole or allylamine for 4 to 6 weeks will help to alleviate symptoms, but recurrences are common and require either intermittent therapy or chronic use of an antifungal powder such as miconazole (Zeasorb-AF). In patients with chronic or extensive infection, itraconazole or terbinafine may be used, with the same dosing schedules used for tinea corporis.

Onychomycosis, or *tinea unguium,* is caused by dermatophytes in the majority of cases but can also be caused by *Candida* and nondermatophyte molds. There are four types of onychomycosis: distal subungual onychomycosis, proximal subungual onychomycosis, white superficial onychomycosis, and *Candida* onychomycosis. The most common form is distal subungual onychomycosis, most often caused by *T. rubrum,* which is characterized by subungual debris, nail discoloration, and onycholysis (separation of the nail plate from the nail bed). Before initiation of therapy, it is important to document the presence of fungi using one or more diagnostic techniques, including KOH preparation, fungal culture, and nail plate biopsy with periodic acid–Schiff stain. Proper diagnosis is necessary because other disorders can mimic onychomycosis, including psoriasis, irritant dermatitis, and trauma.

In the past, patients with onychomycosis were treated with griseofulvin, with a cure rate of about 25% after 1 year of therapy for toenail disease. Over the past several years, the emergence of itraconazole and terbinafine has

*Exceeds dosage recommended by the manufacturer.

*Not FDA approved for this indication.

allowed much shorter and more effective courses of therapy. Itraconazole can be administered in a continuous or pulse fashion. In the continuous regimen, the dosage of itraconazole is 200 mg/d for 3 months for toenail disease and 2 months for fingernail disease. Pulse dosing of the medication involves a dosage of 200 mg twice daily for 1 week per month, with no therapy for the remaining 3 weeks. Toenails are treated with three pulses,* whereas fingernails are treated with two pulses. The dosage of terbinafine is 250 mg/d. Fingernail infection is treated for 6 weeks, and toenail infection for 12 weeks. Laboratory monitoring, including liver function tests, should be performed at baseline and at variable intervals (at 4 and 8 weeks for itraconazole, at 6 weeks for terbinafine, for 3-month courses) on patients taking either medication for over 1 month. It is important for clinicians to be aware of the drug interactions of itraconazole and avoid concomitant use of itraconazole and drugs metabolized by the cytochrome P-450 3A enzyme system. Terbinafine has fewer drug interactions than itraconazole, and there are no drugs that are contraindicated for simultaneous use.

CANDIDIASIS

Cutaneous infections caused by yeast of the *Candida* species occur in individuals of all ages but are seen most frequently in the newborn and elderly. Types of common infections include oropharyngeal thrush, balanitis, intertrigo, diaper dermatitis, onychomycosis, and congenital and neonatal candidiasis. In a minority of cases, individuals with defective cellular immunity can develop chronic mucocutaneous candidiasis.

Factors predisposing to *Candida* infections include the following: the presence of an impaired epithelial barrier, as in burns or wounds; systemic disorders, such as diabetes and hypothyroidism; neutrophil and macrophage disorders; immunosuppression (both primary and acquired); malignancy and hematologic disorders; and treatment with antibiotics or systemic corticosteroids. The most common form of infection is *Candida* intertrigo, which is characterized by erythema, superficial erosion, satellite pustules, and pruritus and pain in the skin folds and intertriginous areas of the body (the gluteal, perineal, and inguinal folds, the scrotum, the axillae, the inframammary and pannus folds). Cutaneous candidiasis can be effectively treated with topical imidazoles applied twice daily for 2 weeks.

TINEA VERSICOLOR

Pityriasis versicolor, also referred to as *tinea versicolor,* is a superficial mycotic infection of the skin. The causative agent is the lipophilic yeast *Malassezia furfur,* which is a normal colonizer on the skin. In certain individuals, overgrowth of the organism causes the typical clinical findings, most commonly consisting of asymptomatic, slightly scaly patches on the upper trunk and proximal upper extremities. The involved skin may be slightly hypopigmented, hyperpigmented, or erythematous. The most important predisposing factors in the pathogenesis of disease are high temperature and high relative humidity, which explains the high incidence of pityriasis versicolor in the tropics.

Pityriasis versicolor can be treated topically or orally. Effective topical medications include selenium sulfide shampoo 2.5%, topical imidazoles, and terbinafine spray or cream. For severe, extensive, or resistant cases, oral itraconazole,* 200 mg once or twice per day for 5 to 7 days, is effective. To avoid recurrence, prophylactic treatment regimens with either oral or topical therapies may be necessary.

*Not FDA approved for this indication.

*Not FDA approved for this indication.

DISEASES OF THE MOUTH

method of
CYNTHIA L. KLEINEGGER, D.D.S., M.S.
University of Iowa College of Dentistry
Iowa City, Iowa

This article is intended to aid the clinician in establishing a differential diagnosis for an unknown oral condition and to provide guidance in initial, if not definitive, management. A reasonable differential diagnosis relies on a complete medical and dental history, including detailed information about medications, dental home care products, and oral habits. Clinical examination of lesions should include observation of location, distribution, size, color, shape, borders, and surface contour and texture. In addition, lesions should be evaluated for consistency, fixation or mobility, drainage or bleeding, and association with obvious dental or periodontal disease. The diagnosis and management of several common and important oral conditions are addressed in the following discussion, separated on the basis of clinical appearance into surface lesions and soft tissue enlargements.

SURFACE LESIONS

Surface lesions involve the superficial mucosa and are flat, slightly raised, or slightly depressed. They may be separated into three categories based on clinical appearance: white, vesicular-ulcerated-erythematous, and pigmented.

White Surface Lesions

Leukoplakia. *Leukoplakia* is a clinical term used to describe an asymptomatic rough white surface lesion that will not rub off and has not been otherwise defined. Most white lesions of the oral cavity are the result of thickening of the epithelium (acanthosis) and/or of the superficial keratin layer (keratosis). These changes may be idiopathic or the result of mechanical, thermal, or chemical irritation. Biopsy is indicated if a source of irritation cannot be identified or if a lesion persists after removal of the suspected irritant.

Focal Keratosis (Hyperkeratosis), Epithelial Dysplasia, Carcinoma in Situ, and Squamous Cell Carcinoma. Focal keratosis is a benign asymptomatic form of leukoplakia that usually develops as a result of frictional irritation. Lesions may be translucent or opaque and smooth or rough, and borders are variably well defined. Focal keratosis may occur on any mucosal surface but more commonly involves the buccal and labial mucosa, edentulous alveolar ridge, and lateral tongue margins.

It is difficult or impossible to clinically differentiate focal keratosis from epithelial dysplasia, carcinoma in situ, or squamous cell carcinoma. Clinical features that should raise suspicion of precancerous changes or carcinoma include irregular thickening, areas of ulceration or erythema, induration, and fixation to underlying tissues. Lesions in high-risk areas (floor of mouth, ventrolateral tongue, soft palate, and retromolar trigone) should also be suspect. Microscopically diagnosed moderate to severe epithelial dysplasia, carcinoma in situ, or carcinoma should be excised or patients should be referred for oncologic management.

Smokeless Tobacco Keratosis (Snuff Dipper's Pouch). Smokeless tobacco keratosis presents in its early stage as a wrinkled white lesion in the area where the product is placed. This change is usually reversible if the habit is discontinued. More advanced lesions exhibit a thick furrowed appearance and may appear tan due to tobacco staining. Lesions with erythema at the base of the furrows, nodular thickening, ulceration, induration, or fixation are suggestive of epithelial dysplasia or carcinoma, and a biopsy is indicated. Lesions that persist after discontinuation of the habit should also undergo biopsy.

Nicotinic Stomatitis. Nicotinic stomatitis is most often seen in pipe or cigar smokers and is limited to the palatal mucosa. It presents as diffuse white mucosal thickening, often with scattered red puncta, which are inflamed ducts of minor salivary glands. Although the condition is not premalignant, the intensity of smoking required to produce these changes increases the risk of carcinoma in general. Management should be aimed at smoking cessation, which may result in resolution of nicotinic stomatitis.

Actinic Cheilosis. Actinic cheilosis is a form of hyperkeratosis resulting from long-term sun exposure of the lip vermilion. In its early form, the condition presents as a localized or diffuse, patchy white change and loss of distinction between the skin and the vermilion border. Early involvement may be reversed by diligent use of sun-blocking agents. As the condition advances, irregularly thickened plaques form. Areas of recurrent or persistent ulceration, induration, or fixation are suspicious for squamous cell carcinoma. Depending on the extent of involvement, these areas should be managed with excisional biopsy or vermilionectomy with mucosal advancement.

Lichen Planus. Lichen planus is a chronic, immunologically mediated mucocutaneous condition, most commonly occurring in middle-aged females. Oral lichen planus affects approximately 2% of the population. It is usually multifocal and may involve any mucosal surface. Oral lichen planus exhibits a variety of clinical presentations, all of which exhibit some degree of hyperkeratosis. The hyperkeratotic lesions associated with lichen planus may be reticular, papular, or plaquelike. The reticular form, which presents as lacy white striae, is often asymptomatic. In the absence of symptoms, ulceration or significant erythema, lichen planus does not require treatment. Management alternatives for lichen planus are presented in Table 1. Patients with symptomatic lichen planus should be evaluated for candidosis because approximately 25% of lichen planus patients present initially with concomitant candidal infection. The erosive form of oral lichen planus is discussed later

TABLE 1. **Management of Nonmicrobial Mucositis: Aphthous Stomatitis, Lichen Planus, Mucous Membrane Pemphigoid, Pemphigus Vulgaris, Erythema Multiforme**

Medication or Product	Dosage and Directions*
Triamcinolone acetonide (Kenalog) 0.1% or 0.2% aqueous suspension†	5 mL mouthrinse and expectorate qid (pc and hs). NPO 30 min after use.
Triamcinolone acetonide (Kenalog) 0.1% or 0.5% ointment‡	Apply thin film to inner surface of medication tray(s)§ and seat for 30 min bid–tid *or* apply to involved area qid (pc and hs). NPO 30 min after use.
Fluocinonide (Lidex) 0.05% ointment‡ or clobetasol (Temovate) 0.05% ointment‡	Apply thin film to inner surface of medication tray(s)§ and seat for 30 min bid *or* apply to involved area bid–qid (pc and hs). NPO 30 min after use.
Triamcinolone acetonide (Kenalog) 0.5% ointment 1:1 with Orabase	Apply thin film to dried mucosa bid–tid. *Do not rub in.* NPO 30 min after use.
Fluocinonide (Lidex) 0.05% or clobetasol (Temovate) 0.05% 1:1 with Orabase	Apply thin film to dried mucosa bid. *Do not rub in.* NPO 30 min after use.
Prednisone	30–60 mg PO qd (AM 90 min after arising) for 5 days, then 5–20 mg qod (AM 90 min after arising) for 10 days.
Triamcinolone acetonide (Kenalog) injectable 40 mg/mL diluted to 10–20 mg/mL with local anesthetic with vasoconstrictor‖	Anesthetize area and inject 10–40 mg into base of lesion.
Misoprostol (Cytotec)¶**	Available in various topical forms and dosages through a compounding pharmacist. May be mixed with corticosteroids and/or antifungals.
Biotene toothpaste††	Use in place of regular toothpaste.

*In most patients decreased frequency and dosages may be used if maintenance therapy is required.

†May be compounded in nystatin suspension.

‡May be mixed 1:1 with clotrimazole 1% or ketoconazole 2% cream or prepared by a compounding pharmacist in ointment form or mucoadhesive base to provide full strength of both medications.

§Custom tray(s) fabricated by a dentist.

‖For management of recalcitrant solitary lesions.

¶Contraindicated in women of childbearing age. Decreases pain and increases rate of healing of ulcerated mucosa.

**Not FDA approved for this indication.

††Does not contain sodium laurel sulfate, an anionic detergent found in most commercial toothpaste that tends to dry and irritate the mucosa. Patients who choose to use commercial mouthwash should select an alcohol-free product.

in the section on vesicular-ulcerated-erythematous lesions.

Candidosis. Candidosis is a common oral fungal infection usually caused by *Candida albicans*, an organism present as a commensal in approximately 50% of people. Local and systemic factors that predispose an individual to develop candidosis include xerostomia, intraoral prosthetic devices, other mucosal diseases, broad-spectrum antibiotic use, immunocompromising diseases and medical treatments, nutritional deficiencies, and metabolic disorders.

Oral candidosis has several clinical variants, two of which exhibit white mucosal plaques. Pseudomembranous candidosis, also known as thrush, presents as soft white plaques that can be rubbed off, revealing an erythematous base. Patients frequently complain of mucosal burning and dysgeusia. Chronic hyperplastic candidosis presents as focal white plaques that do not rub off. The hyperplastic variant is uncommon, is typically asymptomatic, and is most often found on the buccal mucosa. Based on clinical appearance alone, hyperplastic candidosis cannot be distinguished from other white lesions, such as focal keratosis or epithelial dysplasia, and biopsy may be required for diagnosis. Other clinical variants of oral candidosis, including angular cheilitis, are discussed in the section on vesicular-ulcerated-erythematous lesions.

Clinical diagnosis of candidosis may be confirmed with cytologic preparations. An important part of the management of candidal infection is identification and, if possible, removal or control of predisposing factors. A variety of topical and systemic medications are available for treatment of oral candidosis (Table 2).

TABLE 2. **Management of Oral Candidosis**

Medication	Dosage and Directions*
Chlorhexidine 0.12% oral rinse (Peridex, PerioGard)† or 0.2% alcohol-free aqueous‡	15 mL mouthrinse and expectorate tid. NPO 30 min after use.
Nystatin oral suspension (Mycostatin), 100,000 units/mL§	5 mL mouthrinse 1 min and expectorate‖ qid (pc and hs). NPO 30 min after use.
Clotrimazole, 10 mg/mL suspension¶	Swab 1–2 mL on affected area qid (pc and hs). NPO 30 min after use.
Ketoconazole 2% cream (Nizoral) or clotrimazole 1% cream (Lotrimin)	Apply thin film to inner surface of denture(s) and/or corners of mouth qid (pc and hs). NPO 30 min after use.
Clotrimazole 200 mg vaginal tablets (Gyne Lotrimin)**	Dissolve ½ tablet slowly in mouth bid. NPO 30 min after use.
Clotrimazole 10 mg oral troches (Mycelex)	Dissolve 1 troche slowly in mouth 5× daily. NPO 30 min after use.
Ketoconazole 200 mg tablets (Nizoral)	1 tablet PO qd for 7–10 days. Do not take antacids within 2 h of this medication.††
Fluconazole 100 mg tablets (Diflucan)	1 tablet PO bid for first day, then 1 tablet PO qd for 10–14 d.

*In most patients decreased frequency and dosages may be used if maintenance therapy is required.
†High alcohol content (11.6%) will irritate mucosa and enhance xerostomia. Should not be prescribed for recovering alcoholics.
‡Must be prepared by experienced compounding pharmacist. Many formulas include flavorings that decrease efficacy.
§High sucrose content. Not first-line choice.
‖May be swallowed for pharyngeal involvement.
¶Compounded in confectioner's glycerin.
**Not FDA approved for this indication.
††Acidic environment is required for absorption.

Hairy Leukoplakia. A condition thought to be caused by the Epstein-Barr virus, hairy leukoplakia occurs primarily in immunocompromised patients. In HIV-positive patients, the development of hairy leukoplakia is often associated with a decline in immune status. It typically involves the lateral tongue and may be unilateral or bilateral. The involved area appears white and may be vertically corrugated, shaggy, or smooth. Biopsy is required for diagnosis, and no treatment is indicated unless the condition is an aesthetic concern or interferes with eating or speech. Treatment with acyclovir, 800 mg four times a day, is often effective, but lesions usually recur when treatment is discontinued. Application of podophyllin resin 25% results in temporary remission but is not well tolerated by patients.

White Hairy Tongue. White hairy tongue is characterized by elongation of the filiform papillae on the dorsal tongue. In many cases, elongated papillae become stained with food, tobacco, or bacterial pigment. The condition has been associated with several predisposing factors, including cigarette smoking, poor oral hygiene, radiation therapy, and a variety of therapeutic agents such as antibiotics, corticosteroids, antacids, and oxygenating mouthrinses. Patients may complain of halitosis, dysgeusia, or, in severe cases, gagging. Management is geared toward regular mechanical débridement by the patient with a tongue scraper or the edge of a spoon, improvement of oral hygiene, and, if possible, elimination of predisposing factors. Severe cases may be treated with surgical excision of elongated papillae.

Vesicular-Ulcerated-Erythematous Surface Lesions

A wide variety of infectious, inflammatory, and neoplastic conditions result in erythema or ulceration of the oral mucosa. Several conditions result in formation of vesicles or bullae; however, in the oral cavity these rupture quickly, leaving ulcerated or desquamated mucosa.

Epithelial Dysplasia, Carcinoma in Situ, and Squamous Cell Carcinoma. These conditions commonly present clinically as red (erythroplakia) or mixed red and white (erythroleukoplakia) lesions. As discussed earlier under leukoplakia, any lesion that cannot be definitely diagnosed clinically and/or does not respond to treatment must undergo biopsy. Approximately 50% of erythroplakias demonstrate invasive squamous cell carcinoma on biopsy, compared with about 5% for leukoplakia. An additional 40% of erythroplakias demonstrate severe epithelial dysplasia or carcinoma in situ. Management of these conditions was addressed earlier.

Aphthous Stomatitis. Aphthous stomatitis, commonly referred to as "canker sores," is an immune-mediated mucosal disorder. It has been inconsistently associated with a wide variety of factors, including allergies, genetic predisposition, hormonal influence, trauma, stress, nutritional deficiencies, hematologic disorders, and infectious agents. There are three recognized clinical variations: aphthous minor, aphthous major, and herpetiform aphthae. Aphthous minor is the most common variant. It often presents initially in childhood or adolescence, manifesting as 3- to 10-mm diameter shallow but painful ulcerations, which typically heal in 7 to 14 days. Ulcers occur almost exclusively on nonkeratinized mucosa, with the buccal mucosa, labial mucosa, and ventral tongue being the most common locations. Patients experience recurrent episodes varying from 2 weeks to a year or more apart, with 1 to 5 ulcers per episode. Prodromal tingling or burning may precede ulcers. Deeper ulcers measuring 1 to 3 cm in diameter characterize aphthous major. Major aphthae require 2 to 6 weeks to heal and may scar. This variant may occur on any mucosal surface but most commonly involves the labial mucosa, soft palate, and tonsillar fauces. Frequency of recurrences is variable with 1 to 10 ulcers per episode. Herpetiform aphthae, the most frequently recurring variant, presents as multiple 1- to 3-mm diameter ulcers. Lesions typically occur on nonkeratinized surfaces, but any mucosal surface may be involved.

Diagnosis of aphthous stomatitis is usually based on clinical and historical features. Patients should be evaluated for systemic conditions that may present as aphthous-like lesions, including Behçet syndrome, inflammatory bowel disease, hematologic disorders, and HIV infection. Biopsy may be required for long-standing major aphthae to rule out malignant and infectious causes of chronic ulceration. Management options for aphthous stomatitis are presented in Table 1.

Erosive Lichen Planus. As discussed under white lesions earlier, lichen planus is a relatively common mucocutaneous condition with a variety of clinical presentations, all of which exhibit some degree of hyperkeratosis. Erosive lichen planus is a symptomatic form of the condition, which exhibits an erythematous or ulcerative component. In some cases, the presence of striated hyperkeratosis surrounding erythematous or ulcerated mucosa allows the diagnosis to be made clinically; however, a biopsy is often required. Depending on the patient's history, the differential diagnosis of lichen planus would include a mucosal reaction to a drug or chemical agent (see Mucosal Reactions to Drugs and Chemical Agents, later). Patients with lichen planus should be evaluated for candidosis because approximately 25% of lichen planus patients present initially with concomitant candidal infection. Treatment options for lichen planus are presented in Table 1. Most patients require maintenance therapy to prevent recurrent lesions.

Mucous Membrane Pemphigoid (Cicatricial Pemphigoid). This autoimmune condition is the result of antibodies directed against the epithelial basement membrane. It is seen more commonly in older adults. Mucous membrane pemphigoid may involve mucosa, skin, or both. Intraorally the condition manifests as painful ulcers, which are preceded by vesicles or bullae that rupture easily and may not be observed by patient or clinician. The condition may involve any intraoral location; however, it is commonly limited to gingiva. Although it may vary in severity over time, untreated mucous membrane pemphigoid typically persists without remission.

The diagnosis of mucous membrane pemphigoid requires biopsy of perilesional tissue with light microscopic examination and direct immune staining techniques. Standard therapy relies on topical or systemic corticosteroids (see Table 1). Because of its anticollagenase activity, doxycycline,* 100 mg once or twice daily, may be beneficial as alternative or adjunct therapy. Optimal oral hygiene, including dental prophylaxis at 3- to 4-month intervals, improves response to drug therapy. Oral lesions may require several weeks to demonstrate improvement, and most patients require maintenance therapy. Patients should be evaluated by an ophthalmologist because untreated ocular involvement may result in blindness secondary to conjunctival scarring.

Pemphigus Vulgaris. This chronic mucocutaneous blistering disease is caused by circulating antibodies to epithelial desmosomal complexes. The condition is most commonly diagnosed in the fourth to sixth decades of life. Oral lesions are common and often precede skin involvement. Intraepithelial vesicles and bullae form but rupture rapidly and are rarely observed by either patient or clinician. The remaining erosions and ulcerations may be observed on any oral mucosal surface. The differential diagnosis for pemphigus vulgaris includes pemphigus-like lesions secondary to certain medications or in association with malignant disease, such as lymphoma and chronic lymphocytic leukemia. Definitive diagnosis is made by biopsy of perilesional tissue with light microscopic examination and direct immunofluorescence. Indirect immunofluorescence for circulating antiepidermal antibodies is helpful in making the diagnosis and evaluating the response to treatment. Management of pemphigus vulgaris requires systemic corticosteroid therapy, often combined with another immunosuppressive agent, such as methotrexate,* azathioprine (Imuran),* or cyclophosphamide (Cytoxan).* Adjunctive topical therapy may be required for management of oral lesions (see Table 1).

Erythema Multiforme. Erythema multiforme is a mucocutaneous disorder that is most likely immune mediated. Most cases occur in young adults, and about half are triggered by drugs or infection. Patients may report prodromal fever, malaise, head-

*Not FDA approved for this indication.

ache, or sore throat 1 week before the outbreak of mucocutaneous lesions. Severity of outbreaks varies from limited oral mucosal or skin involvement to extensive oral, ocular, genital, and skin lesions (Stevens-Johnson syndrome). Oral lesions begin as areas of erythema or bullae, which progress rapidly to irregular painful ulcerations. The distribution of oral lesions is typically diffuse. Any intraoral location may be involved, although labial mucosa, buccal mucosa, soft palate, and tongue are more common sites and the gingiva is often spared. Hemorrhagic lip crusting is a common finding. In the absence of classic target-shaped skin lesions, it may be difficult to differentiate erythema multiforme from primary herpes simplex virus infection. Lymphadenopathy, a common finding in the latter, is not seen in erythema multiforme. In addition, the gingiva is commonly involved in primary herpes simplex virus infection.

The diagnosis of erythema multiforme is usually based on clinical and historical features. The condition is treated with topical or systemic corticosteroids, depending on the severity and extent of involvement (see Table 1). Recurrent episodes of erythema multiforme triggered by recurrent herpes simplex virus infection may be prevented with prophylactic antiviral drug therapy as described later.

Herpes Simplex. Primary oral infection with herpes simplex virus (primary herpetic gingivostomatitis) most commonly occurs in children but may occur in adulthood. Symptomatic patients present with multiple painful vesicles and ulcers, which may involve any mucosal surface, and painful edematous, erythematous gingiva. Fever, lymphadenopathy, and malaise accompany oral symptoms. In the immunocompetent patient, the infection usually resolves in 1 to 2 weeks. After primary infection, the virus remains dormant in the regional nerve ganglion. Reactivation, often due to exposure to ultraviolet radiation, trauma, or immune suppression, results in a localized recurrent infection. Prodromal tingling or burning may precede recurrent lesions. Lesions manifest as small clusters of microvesicles and ulcers on the lip (herpes labialis) or keratinized oral mucosa and typically heal within 7 to 10 days.

Supportive management, particularly for primary infection, may include a topical anesthetic mouthrinse for pain relief and assurance of adequate hydration. Systemic acyclovir (Zovirax), 200 mg five times per day for 10 days (longer for immunocompromised patients), will shorten the course of the primary infection. A 5- to 7-day regimen of acyclovir at the same dosage, initiated at prodrome or within 72 hours of onset of the infection, has been demonstrated to decrease the extent and duration of recurrent lesions. In some patients, use of sunblock before sun exposure may prevent recurrent herpes labialis. Patients who experience frequent recurrences may require prophylactic antiviral drug therapy such as acyclovir, 400 mg twice daily.

Varicella-Zoster. The skin lesions of primary varicella-zoster virus infection (chickenpox) may be accompanied, or even preceded, by oral lesions. Oral lesions, most common on the buccal and palatal mucosa, present as 3- to 4-mm opaque white vesicles that rupture, leaving ulcerations. These lesions are relatively painless, which helps to differentiate them from lesions of primary herpes simplex virus infection. After primary infection, the varicella-zoster virus remains latent in a regional nerve ganglion. It may be reactivated later in life to cause recurrent infection (herpes zoster or shingles) involving the distribution of the sensory nerve. Recurrent varicella-zoster infection is seen most often in older adults and immunocompromised patients. Recurrent lesions on the facial skin or oral mucosa reflect involvement of one or more divisions of the trigeminal nerve. Recurrent lesions are preceded by pain, which may be accompanied by fever, malaise, and headache. When the second or third division of the trigeminal nerve is involved, prodromal pain may masquerade as a toothache. Individually, recurrent oral lesions appear similar to those seen in the primary infection. However, recurrent lesions may involve any mucosal surface, exhibit a classic unilateral presentation, and may be quite painful. Recurrent oral lesions are often accompanied by involvement of the overlying skin. A potential sequela of herpes zoster is *postherpetic neuralgia,* which is defined as pain persisting for more than 1 month after the resolution of lesions.

Use of antiviral drugs may be helpful in the management of herpes zoster if begun within 48 to 72 hours of onset of symptoms. Decrease in the duration and severity of skin and mucosal lesions may be seen with acyclovir (Zovirax), 800 mg five times daily for 7 to 10 days, famciclovir (Famvir), 500 mg three times daily for 7 days, or valacyclovir (Valtrex), 1000 mg three times daily for 7 days. These drugs, particularly valacyclovir, also decrease pain during outbreaks and reduce the incidence of postherpetic neuralgia. Concurrent use of prednisone, 10 to 20 mg/d, may further decrease incidence of postherpetic neuralgia.

Other Viral Conditions. A variety of other viral infections may exhibit oral manifestations. *Herpangina,* one form of coxsackievirus infection, presents as small vesicles or ulcers that are few in numbers and are confined to the soft palate and tonsillar region. Another form of coxsackievirus infection, *hand-foot-and-mouth-disease,* presents as similar oral lesions, although they are typically more numerous and may occur on any mucosal surface. As the name implies, patients with hand-foot-and-mouth disease also develop vesicular lesions on the hands and feet. The rash of *rubeola* (measles) is usually preceded by small erythematous macules with white necrotic centers on the buccal mucosa (Koplik spots). Patients with *infectious mononucleosis* may exhibit palatal petechiae or acute necrotizing ulcerative gingivitis (see later). Chronic mucosal ulceration secondary to *cytomegalovirus infection* may occur in immunocompromised patients.

Erythematous Candidosis. Acute or chronic atrophic candidosis presents primarily or exclusively as erythematous mucosa. The acute form is associated with mucosal soreness or burning. Chronic atrophic candidosis, often observed on denture-bearing mucosa (denture stomatitis), is frequently asymptomatic. It is typically associated with 24-hour denture wear, ill-fitting dentures, or poor denture hygiene. When associated with a maxillary denture, the chronically inflamed palatal mucosa may exhibit papillary change (inflammatory papillary hyperplasia). Atrophic candidosis of the tongue manifests as localized or generalized loss of the filiform papillae (atrophic glossitis) and may be associated with dysgeusia. Another clinical entity associated with *Candida* is median rhomboid glossitis. This raised, red, depapillated area of the mid-dorsal tongue is usually asymptomatic, in which case it does not require treatment.

Angular cheilitis is most often the result of candidal infection of the labial commissures. It manifests as erythematous fissuring, is often sore, and may crack and bleed with wide mouth opening. Patients with *Candida*-related angular cheilitis usually exhibit intraoral candidosis.

Predisposing factors for candidosis are discussed previously in the section on white lesions, and pharmacotherapeutic management is presented in Table 2. Patients with denture-related candidosis should be educated regarding proper denture use and should have their prostheses evaluated by a dentist. Severe cases of inflammatory papillary hyperplasia require surgical excision.

Atrophic Glossitis. Atrophic glossitis is characterized by loss of filiform papillae, giving the dorsal tongue a patchy or diffuse, smooth red appearance. It is typically associated with burning symptoms. In addition to candidosis (discussed earlier), several other conditions must be included in the differential diagnosis of this condition. Iron deficiency anemia and pernicious anemia may result in atrophic glossitis, as well as atrophy of other mucosal surfaces and angular cheilitis. Anemia-related glossitis may be associated with candidosis; however, the condition does not resolve with antifungal therapy alone. Atrophic glossitis may also be a manifestation of erosive lichen planus (see earlier).

Patients with *xerostomia* frequently present with mucosal atrophy. Causes of xerostomia include medication side effects, head and neck radiation therapy, mouth breathing, Sjögren syndrome, and HIV infection. Several commercial products are available to relieve oral dryness. Among the more effective are buffered citric acid tablets (Salix SST), which can be dissolved slowly in the mouth to stimulate saliva flow, and a topical gel (Oral Balance), which provides longer lasting relief than rinses or sprays. Patients without medical contraindication may benefit from the use of pilocarpine 4% ophthalmic solution, 1 to 2 drops in 2 tablespoons of water; this solution can be swished and swallowed up to four times daily. Use of ophthalmic solution is economical and allows titration to the minimal effective dose. Patients with xerostomia should avoid alcohol and limit caffeine intake. They should use detergent-free toothpaste and, if desired, an alcohol-free mouthwash (see Table 1). Patients with xerostomia are at increased risk of dental caries, periodontal disease, and candidosis and should seek regular dental evaluation. The use of supplemental high-potency topical neutral sodium fluoride, such as PreviDent 5000-Plus brush-on or Karigel-N delivered in custom fluoride trays, will reduce the risk of dental caries.

Erythema Migrans (Benign Migratory Glossitis, Geographic Tongue). This common condition of unknown cause presents as patchy erythematous areas, often surrounded by a narrow hyperkeratotic border. Characteristic of the condition is the "migration" of involved areas from one location to another. Although patients with erythema migrans may be more sensitive to hot or spicy foods, the condition is otherwise asymptomatic and no treatment is required.

Acute Necrotizing Ulcerative Gingivitis. Fusiform bacteria and spirochetes are believed to cause this unique form of gingivitis. Predisposing factors include stress, smoking, poor nutrition, poor oral hygiene, and local trauma. The condition may be associated with HIV infection or mononucleosis. Acute necrotizing ulcerative gingivitis (ANUG) is characterized by inflamed, ulcerated, and necrotic gingiva that is painful and bleeds easily. The condition most severely affects the interdental gingiva. It is usually accompanied by fetid oral odor. Patients with ANUG may exhibit fever, malaise, and lymphadenopathy. Management centers on thorough débridement, improved oral hygiene, and close follow-up. Twice-daily rinsing with 15 mL chlorhexidine gluconate 0.12% (Peridex or PerioGard) followed by expectoration will improve response to therapy. Metronidazole (Flagyl), 250 mg four times daily for 7 days, is the antibiotic regimen of choice for severe cases or those with systemic symptoms.

Mucosal Reactions to Drugs and Chemical Agents. A wide variety of medications, dental products, and food additives have been associated with oral mucosal changes. Medication-induced changes often mimic other conditions, such as lichen planus or aphthous stomatitis. Ulcerative, erythematous, or lichenoid mucosal changes may be seen in response to cinnamon-flavored products and certain toothpaste formulas. Topical application of caustic agents, such as aspirin, results in mucosal necrosis, sloughing, and ulceration. The diagnosis of drug- or chemical-induced oral lesions relies on a complete and accurate patient history. A biopsy may be required to rule out other conditions. Elimination of the suspected agent is often sufficient management. Severe cases, or cases in which a medication cannot be eliminated for medical reasons, may be managed according to the recommendations for other nonmicrobial forms of mucositis (see Table 1).

Pigmented Surface Lesions

A wide variety of pathologic conditions and lesions associated with mucosal pigmentation have been identified. Pigmented lesions may be categorized into those deriving their color from melanin (melanocytic), from blood or blood cell breakdown products (vascular), or from other sources (miscellaneous). Brown, black, or gray discoloration is most often due to accumulation of melanin, hemosiderin, or foreign material, whereas red, blue, or purple color changes suggest a vascular process. Blanching upon pressure further supports a vascular process, although the failure to blanch does not rule out this possibility. Multifocal or diffuse mucosal hyperpigmentation may be a sign of an underlying systemic disorder or drug toxicity.

Localized Melanocytic Lesions

Melanotic Macule (Focal Melanosis). Melanotic macules develop as the result of focal increased melanin production. They are tan to dark brown, nonpalpable, well delineated, less than 1 cm in diameter, and usually solitary. They occur more often on the lower lip, buccal mucosa, gingiva, and palate. Although they are not premalignant, intraoral melanotic macules should be followed closely because early melanoma may have a similar appearance. Indications for biopsy include large or enlarging lesions, irregular pigmentation, recent onset, and unknown duration.

Acquired Melanocytic Nevus. The acquired melanocytic nevus is the result of melanocytic (nevus) cell proliferation, variably associated with increased melanin production. Clinically, the intraoral nevus is a solitary, well-demarcated, elevated lesion, typically less than 7 mm in diameter and most commonly observed on the palate or gingiva. Lesions may be nonpigmented. Those associated with increased melanin production appear tan, brown, or black. The intraoral nevus is considered premalignant and should be excised and examined microscopically to rule out melanoma.

Melanoma. Melanoma is a malignant neoplasm of melanocytic origin. Intraoral melanoma most often occurs on the palate, gingiva, or alveolar mucosa. The early lesion presents as an irregularly outlined brown to black macule. As the lesion progresses, it enlarges, thickens, and may ulcerate. Intraoral melanoma, although uncommon, is usually fatal. Any lesion suspected of being melanoma should be biopsied. Diagnosed intraoral melanoma requires aggressive oncologic management.

Localized Vascular Lesions

Submucosal Hemorrhage. Submucosal hemorrhage may present as petechiae, purpura, ecchymosis, and/or hematoma. It is usually secondary to trauma, but it may be a sign of coagulopathy or, in the case of petechiae, viral infection. Submucosal hemorrhage results in flat or elevated, nonblanching lesions, which are red, blue, purple, or, in later stages, brown. Traumatic submucosal hemorrhage occurs most commonly on the labial and buccal mucosa. On the soft palate it may be the result of fellatio, violent coughing, or vomiting. Unless it is secondary to a persistent habit or coagulopathy, submucosal hemorrhage will resolve without intervention.

Varix (Varicosity). The varix is an abnormally dilated vein, which manifests clinically as a blue or purple papule. Varices are soft and blanch with compression unless they are thrombosed. Multiple varices on the ventral tongue are a common finding in older adults. The solitary varix is more common on the lips and buccal mucosa. The solitary lesion may require excision for aesthetic concerns, if it is frequently traumatized, or to confirm the clinical diagnosis.

Hemangioma. This benign proliferation of blood vessels may be present at birth, develop early in life, or, less commonly, develop later in life. Hemangioma may involve any intraoral location. Superficial hemangiomas present as flat or slightly raised, smooth or multilobular lesions, which are red, blue, or purple and blanch with compression. Lesions vary greatly in size, and borders are often diffuse. Congenital and early childhood hemangioma may enlarge rapidly for several years and then gradually involute. Persistent lesions may require management for cosmetic reasons or if recurrent bleeding is a problem. Treatment alternatives include surgical excision, laser ablation, cryotherapy, and injection of a corticosteroid or other sclerosing agent. It is difficult to clinically differentiate later-onset hemangioma from other vascular lesions, such as Kaposi's sarcoma, and therapy should be instituted only after the diagnosis has been confirmed by biopsy. Difficulty in clinically differentiating hemangioma from a vascular malformation, which is associated with increased risk of intraoperative hemorrhage, should be considered when planning surgical management.

Kaposi's Sarcoma. This malignant vascular tumor is most commonly diagnosed in patients with AIDS. The oral cavity is frequently involved in AIDS-related cases, with the hard and soft palates and the gingiva being the most common locations. Early lesions present as red, blue, purple, or brown areas of discoloration. As the lesion progresses, plaques or nodules develop and the mucosal surface may become ulcerated. Lesions vary in size, and borders are typically diffuse. Blanching on compression is variable. The clinical differential diagnosis is broad, and biopsy is required for definitive diagnosis.

Treatment options for intraoral Kaposi's sarcoma include surgical excision, laser ablation, intralesional injection with a cytotoxin or sclerosing agent, and radiation therapy. The most common cytotoxin used for intralesional injection is vinblastine. Although this technique has produced complete resolution in a large percentage of patients, it is associated with significant postoperative pain. Intralesional injection with 3% sodium tetradecyl sulfate, a sclerosing agent, has also had a high rate of success and results in less postoperative pain. Radiation therapy is usually reserved for more extensive intraoral lesions, with total dosage in the range of 800 to 2000 cGy. Treatment of Kaposi's sarcoma is rarely curative, and recurrences are common.

Miscellaneous Localized Pigmented Lesions

Foreign Body Tattoo. Tattooing of the oral mucosa is caused by implantation of foreign material such as dental amalgam or pencil lead. Tattooing typically appears as single or multiple gray, black, or blue pigmented macules, which may be palpable if associated with soft tissue fibrosis. Unless foreign material is demonstrated radiographically or there is a clear history of traumatic implantation, excision and microscopic examination is indicated.

Black Hairy Tongue. Black hairy tongue is characterized by elongated filiform papillae, which have assumed a black or brown discoloration secondary to food, tobacco, or bacterial pigment. Predisposing factors and management of this condition are discussed in the previous section on white hairy tongue.

Generalized Hyperpigmentation

Oral mucosal pigmentation is a common finding, and it is most often due to normal melanin production. Recent onset and asymmetric or changing mucosal pigmentation suggest a systemic cause, such as a metabolic disorder or drug toxicity. Systemic causes to be considered include *adrenal insufficiency, Peutz-Jeghers syndrome, hemochromatosis, polyostotic fibrous dysplasia, hyperparathyroidism,* and *neurofibromatosis. Heavy metal poisoning* as a cause of abnormal pigmentation has become infrequent due to decreased industrial and domestic exposure to these elements. Although it is rare, abnormal oral pigmentation may be a sign of systemic malignancy such as *bronchogenic carcinoma. Acanthosis nigricans,* a condition that manifests as oral mucosal thickening and pigmentation, may be associated with gastrointestinal cancer. Mucosal hyperpigmentation is a relatively common finding in HIV-infected individuals, sometimes due to adrenal insufficiency or drug therapy. *Drug-related hyperpigmentation* has been associated with a broad variety of medications, including cancer chemotherapeutic agents, tranquilizers, hormones, carotenoids, phenolphthalein, heavy metal salts, and antimicrobial agents. Among the antimicrobial drugs more commonly implicated are ketoconazole, minocycline, zidovudine, clofazamine, and several antimalarial agents. *Tobacco-related mucosal melanosis* presents as diffuse or multifocal involvement; and, in some cultures, the habit of chewing certain seeds, bark, or leaves may result in unusual patterns of mucosal discoloration.

Diagnosis of diffuse or multifocal pigmentation suspected to be nonphysiologic involves a thorough patient history and physical evaluation and may require laboratory and radiographic studies. In some drug- or tobacco-related cases, pigmentation may gradually fade when the causative agent has been discontinued.

SOFT TISSUE ENLARGEMENTS

A wide variety of reactive, neoplastic, and cystic processes may result in localized oral soft tissue enlargement. An enlargement overlying bone may represent extension of an intraosseous process. In general, management of soft tissue enlargement involves complete excision and microscopic diagnosis; however, for large lesions or those suspected to be malignant, incisional biopsy should first be performed to guide definitive treatment.

Reactive Soft Tissue Enlargements

Reactive soft tissue enlargements frequently occur secondary to acute or chronic infection or chronic irritation. These lesions are typically asymptomatic unless they become ulcerated. In most cases, management includes excision, microscopic diagnosis, and, if possible, elimination of the suspected irritant. Many reactive lesions exhibit a tendency to recur, particularly when the source of irritation is not eliminated.

Reactive Mesenchymal Lesions

A variety of oral lesions represent reactive hyperplasia of fibrous tissue. The *fibroma* (irritation fibroma) presents as a variably sized, smooth nodular mass. It may occur on any mucosal surface, although it most commonly develops on the buccal mucosa as a result of cheek biting. It may appear pink or white due to surface keratinization or erythematous and ulcerated secondary to trauma. *Inflammatory fibrous hyperplasia* (epulis fissuratum) is characterized by folds of moderately firm, slightly erythematous soft tissue associated with the flange of an ill-fitting denture. Reactive fibroepithelial proliferation results in *inflammatory papillary hyperplasia,* a lesion typically seen on denture-bearing palatal and alveolar mucosa. The involved tissue appears erythematous and pebbly or papillary. This lesion is more common in patients with ill-fitting dentures or poor denture hygiene and those who wear their dentures 24 hours a day. The mucosa may be sore, particularly if it is concomitantly infected with *Candida* (see previous discussion of erythematous candidosis).

Reactive soft tissue enlargement frequently develops on the gingiva as a result of bacterial or mechanical irritation. Extension of a periapical dental abscess through the bone may produce a painful red pus-filled gingival swelling known as a *parulis.* The *pyogenic granuloma* is a smooth or lobulated mass of hyperplastic fibrovascular tissue. Although it is most common on the gingiva, pyogenic granuloma may occur in any location. The color of the lesion varies from red or purple to pink, depending on the relative proportion of the vascular and fibrous components. This lesion is more common in females, particularly during puberty and pregnancy. *Peripheral ossifying fibroma* and *peripheral giant cell granuloma* are unique reactive lesions that occur exclusively on gingiva. Both are composed of hyperplastic fibrous tissue containing mineralized material and osteoclast-type giant cells, respectively.

Reactive Epithelial Lesions

Reactive proliferation of oral epithelium most often occurs in association with human papillomavirus infection. The most common lesion in this group, *squamous papilloma,* presents as a solitary pink or white, pedunculated mass of finger-like projections. *Verruca vulgaris* (common wart) is less common in the oral cavity. Oral lesions exhibit a cauliflower-like appearance and may be pedunculated or sessile. Squamous papilloma and verruca vulgaris rarely measure more than 0.5 cm in diameter. *Condylomata acuminata* (venereal warts) in the oral cavity present as multiple sessile pink pebbly lesions, usually no larger than 1.5 cm in diameter. In general, reactive epithelial lesions are asymptomatic unless inflamed as a result of trauma. Verruca vulgaris and condyloma are both contagious and may spread to other areas by autoinoculation.

Neoplastic Soft Tissue Enlargements

A wide range of benign and malignant neoplasms is encountered in the oral cavity. Benign neoplasms commonly arise from mesenchymal or salivary gland tissue. Malignant lesions may arise from surface epithelium, salivary glands, mesenchymal tissue, or lymphoid tissue. Lesions that are slow growing, asymptomatic, well defined, mobile, and covered with normal mucosa are usually benign. However, there are several exceptions to this rule, and all soft tissue enlargements should be microscopically evaluated. Clinical features suspicious for malignancy are rapid growth, fixation, mucosal ulceration, and pain or paresthesia. Benign lesions are typically treated by surgical excision. Management of malignant lesions is determined based on microscopic diagnosis, location, and extent of disease.

Cystic Soft Tissue Enlargements

Soft tissue cysts typically present as compressible, mobile, subepithelial nodules. Cysts that contain keratin (e.g., epithelial inclusion cyst, lymphoepithelial cyst, and alveolar cyst of the newborn) usually appear white or yellow, whereas those containing mucin or serous fluid (e.g., salivary duct cyst and gingival cyst) may appear pale blue. A common lesion that may clinically resemble a cyst is *salivary extravasation reaction* (mucocele). This lesion results from traumatic damage to a salivary duct, which allows saliva to escape and pool within the adjacent connective tissue. Any benign or malignant salivary gland neoplasm with a significant cystic component may also clinically resemble a cyst. Cystic lesions should be excised and microscopically diagnosed. Salivary extravasation reactions have a tendency to recur, but recurrence is less likely if the associated minor salivary glands are removed with the lesion.

LEG ULCERS

method of
CLAUDE S. BURTON III, M.D.
Duke University
Durham, North Carolina

Lower extremity ulcers are the most common chronic wounds in our population and perhaps the *only* chronic wound that often develops in otherwise entirely healthy individuals during the most productive period in their lives. An estimated 1 million individuals harbor an active leg ulcer in the United States at any given time. The financial burden of lost work and productivity for affected individuals greatly exceeds the cost of treatment of these ulcers, although it is estimated that treatment costs alone exceed $1 billion a year in the United States. Unfortunately, specialists in chronic wound management suspect that more than half of these dollars are wasted on ineffective or potentially damaging therapies and unnecessary diagnostic tests and procedures. Most leg ulcers are easily diagnosed and respond to simple outpatient therapies.

DIFFERENTIAL DIAGNOSIS

Although the differential diagnosis of a patient with leg ulcers is lengthy, a single condition, venous insufficiency, dominates the list and accounts for 80% to 90% of ulcers in most reported series (Table 1). One can exclude the next two common etiologies, arterial insufficiency and neuropathy, simply by evaluating the peripheral pulses and sensation at the bedside. With intact sensation and normal arterial blood flow, the likelihood that an ulcer is due to venous disease is well above 90%. That being the case, an expensive diagnostic evaluation is not advisable for most patients. Rather, empirical treatment based on a clinical diagnosis is preferable. Improvement in a venous ulcer after application of appropriate dressing and a compression device is rapid. For any patient who does not respond to the treatment measures discussed later, additional studies are advisable, especially histopathology of the ulcer and adjacent tissue.

PATHOPHYSIOLOGY

A brief look at the anatomy and hemodynamics of the lower limb explains the leg's unique vulnerability to nonhealing wounds. Although the heart pumps blood to the foot, it is largely the calf muscle pump that moves blood back to the heart during upright posture. Effective calf muscle pumping requires full range of motion in the ankle, patent veins in both the superficial and deep systems with intact one-way valves that ensure forward flow and prevent reflux, and enough muscle to empty the deep system during muscular contraction. Although injury to any of these elements contributes to calf muscle pump dysfunction, the venous valves are most prone to early failure. These delicate valves direct blood from the superficial, relatively low-pressure veins of the saphenous system and its tributaries through perforating veins (because they "perforate" the fascia) that drain into the deep veins (Figure 1). During muscular activity, surprisingly high pressure develops in the deep veins. Varicosities do not develop in the deep veins because they are well supported by muscle and fascia. The superficial system is not so well supported. If the one-way valves in the perforators allow high-pressure regurgitation into the saphenous system, varicosi-

TABLE 1. **Differential Diagnosis of Leg Ulcers**

Vascular Diseases	**Hematologic Abnormalities**
Arterial (hypertensive atherosclerotic, vasospastic)	Hypercoagulable states (protein C, S, antithrombin III deficiency, antigen-presenting cell resistance, prothrombin gene polymorphism)
Venous (venous stasis ulcer)	Lupus anticoagulant syndrome
Lymphedema	Paroxysmal nocturnal hemoglobinuria
Metabolic Disorders	Sickle cell anemia
Diabetes mellitus	Thalassemia
Necrobiosis lipoidica diabeticorum	Polycythemia vera
Porphyria cutanea tarda	Leukemia
Gout	Dysproteinemia (cryoglobulinemia, macroglobulinemia)
Pancreatitic (pancreatitis, carcinoma)	**Tumors**
Infections	Cutaneous (basal cell cancer, squamous cell cancer, sarcoma, malignant melanoma, Merkel cell)
Bacterial (especially *Staphylococcus aureus, Streptococcus*)	Secondary (metastatic carcinoma, lymphoma)
Spirochetal (syphilis)	Kaposi's sarcoma
Fungal (deep fungal, mycetoma)	**Miscellaneous**
Opportunistic in immunocompromised hosts	Pyoderma gangrenosum
Viral	Trauma (including factitial)
Vasculitis	Burns
Hypersensitivity vasculitis	Pressure ulcers, neuropathic ulcers
Polyarteritis	Insect bites (brown recluse spider)
Systemic lupus erythematosus	Ulcerative lichen planus
Rheumatoid vasculitis	Bullous diseases (epidermolysis bullosa)
Wegener's granulomatosis	Sweet's syndrome
Lymphomatoid granulomatosis	Idiopathic
Lymphedema	
Congenital	
Postinfectious	
Postsurgical	
Postirradiation	
Drugs	
Halogens (bromide, iodide)	
Ergotism	
Drug-induced vasculitis	
Anticoagulant necrosis (warfarin [Coumadin], heparin)	
Hydroxyurea (Hydrea)	

ties and soft tissue injury will follow. Considerable debate continues regarding the molecular events that lead to tissue damage. Nevertheless, ambulatory venous hypertension initiates the cascade of events that lead to venous ulceration. Although ulceration may develop spontaneously, in many cases a minor episode of trauma leads to a wound that refuses to heal.

EVALUATION

Initial evaluation of a leg ulcer begins with evaluation of the arterial circulation in both extremities. Identification of a good, strong palpable pulse is often adequate to ensure good blood flow, but measurement of arterial pressure by Doppler is the gold standard. In normal individuals, systolic arterial pressure in the ankle is greater than or equal to systolic arterial pressure in the brachial artery (both pressure measurements should be obtained by Doppler). The product of these two measurements is the ankle brachial index (ABI). An ABI of less than 1 indicates the presence of arterial disease. The lower the ratio, the more severe the obstruction. As the ABI approaches 0.6 or thereabout, symptoms of ischemia develop and wound healing is impaired. Furthermore, atherosclerotic disease in the lower extremities is almost always accompanied by disease in the coronary and carotid circulations that may not have previously been diagnosed or treated. Having confirmed adequate blood flow, the prognosis for eventual healing is excellent. Patients with significant arterial disease may require arterial reconstruction for healing. If the ABI is abnormal, consultation with a vascular specialist is recommended, and the patient's primary care physician should consider the issue of clinically silent cardiovascular or cerebrovascular disease.

To exclude neuropathy, protective sensation should be confirmed by the use of a nylon quill that flexes when the applied force equals 10 g. When neuropathy is present, extra attention should be paid to protecting bony prominences when choosing compression techniques.

CLINICAL FINDINGS

The majority of venous ulcers are painful, and the open wounds frequently drain heavily. Most patients will report ankle edema and discomfort preceding the development of ulceration. A surprising number of patients will have received diuretics for the ankle edema with little improvement, thus suggesting a mechanical cause for the edema.

A number of physical findings support a clinical diagnosis of venous disease (Figure 2). Virtually all patients will have edema of the affected limb or limbs. Unlike the pitting edema of salt-retaining states such as heart failure, cirrhosis, and nephrotic syndrome, the edema fluid in patients with venous disease is often associated with exquisite soft tissue tenderness. As noted earlier, the edema fluid in venous disease accumulates under high pressure and is associated with soft tissue injury. The discovery of soft tissue tenderness while checking a patient for edema is often the earliest physical finding in venous disease. Fine petechial hemorrhage resembling the sprinkling of cayenne pepper on the skin may be noted and indicates leakage of red cells from damaged vessels. The hemoglobin deposited in the tissues will be digested, and the iron remains in the dermis as hemosiderin and produces brownish discoloration of the skin (Figure 3). Soft tissue injury occurs early in the delicate subcutaneous fat. This panniculitis, when acute, may be confused both clinically and histologically with idiopathic erythema nodosum or cellulitis if the presence of venous disease is overlooked. The acute panniculitis will in time lead to fibrosis of the subcutis and produce an indurated feel and appearance to the distal portion of the limb. Taken together, these changes are referred to as lipodermatosclerosis.

Varicosities are common in these patients and by definition indicate venous abnormalities. Patients should be examined while erect to distend large varicosities that might "disappear" when recumbent. More superficial varicosities are seen about the dorsum of the foot and ankle in patients with a venous ulcer. Dermatitis develops in many patients and may spread throughout the skin as an "id" reaction. The dermatitis is often pruritic, frequently excoriated, and prone to colonization with *Staphylococcus aureus*. The *S. aureus* carriage rate in venous disease with stasis has been reported to be 100%.

The term *atrophie blanche* describes the porcelain-white atrophic skin that develops before and after ulceration in most patients with long-standing venous disease (Figure

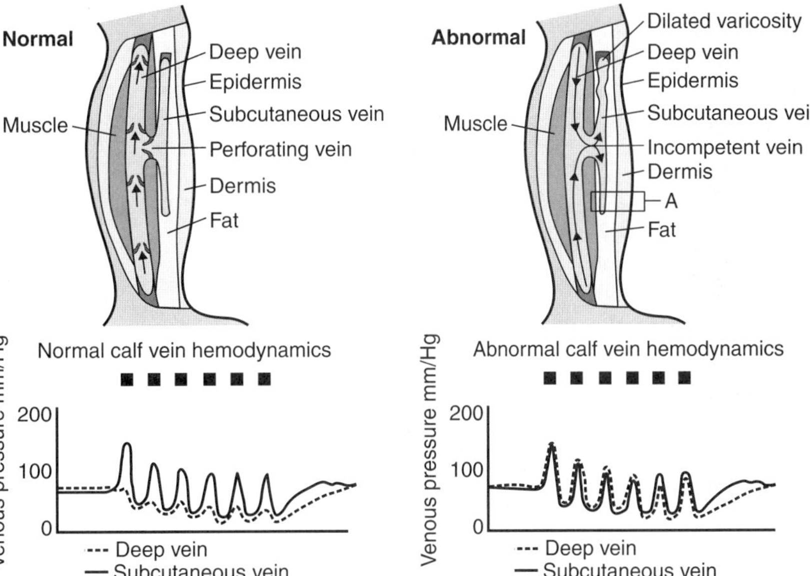

Figure 1. Anatomy and hemodynamics of the calf muscle pump.

4). Dilated capillary loops are often visible, and small thrombi may frequently be seen in these vessels. A variety of biochemical abnormalities predisposing to thrombosis have been noted in most patients with venous ulceration.

TREATMENT

Hippocrates, the father of medicine and a leg ulcer sufferer, emphasized the importance of gravity in the management of venous ulcers. He championed leg elevation, which though effective, has many drawbacks. Compression bandaging is a far more attractive alternative and allows most patients to continue full activity and employment. I tell patients that the bandage will "fool" the leg into thinking that they are in bed with the leg propped up while they go about their business.

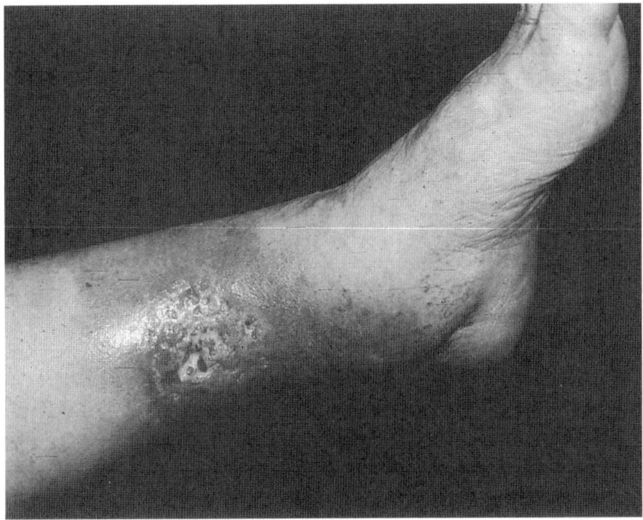

Figure 2. Venous ulceration. Note the superficial varicosities, hemosiderin staining, and inflammation of surrounding soft tissues with an exudative ulcer.

Not all forms of compression are alike. Ideally, application of a compression bandage will not allow additional fluid to accumulate. Such inelastic wraps provide a firm surface that directs the full force of calf muscle activity toward enhancing venous return. An elastic wrap or stocking will stretch with muscle activity and greatly reduce its effectiveness.

Unna, a prominent dermatologist of the 19th century, developed a zinc paste–impregnated inelastic gauze wrap for this purpose. Highly effective, the Unna boot enjoyed over a hundred years of unmodified success. Several manufacturers produce zinc paste wraps, but applying these wraps in such a way to achieve consistent graduated compression is difficult to learn and teach. When wrapped improperly, the Unna boot does more harm than good. Perhaps worse because once patients have a bad experience with any type of leg wrapping, they are reluctant to try another.

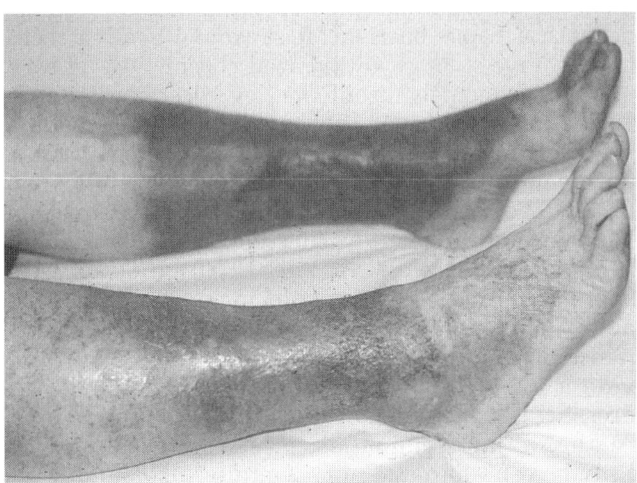

Figure 3. Venous dermatitis with marked hemosiderosis and excoriation.

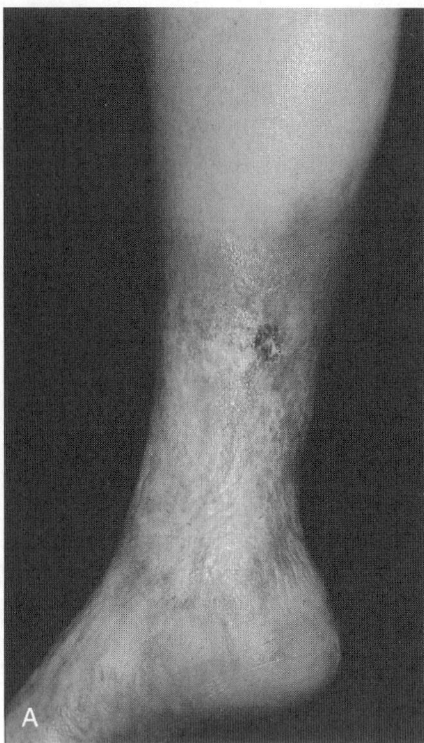

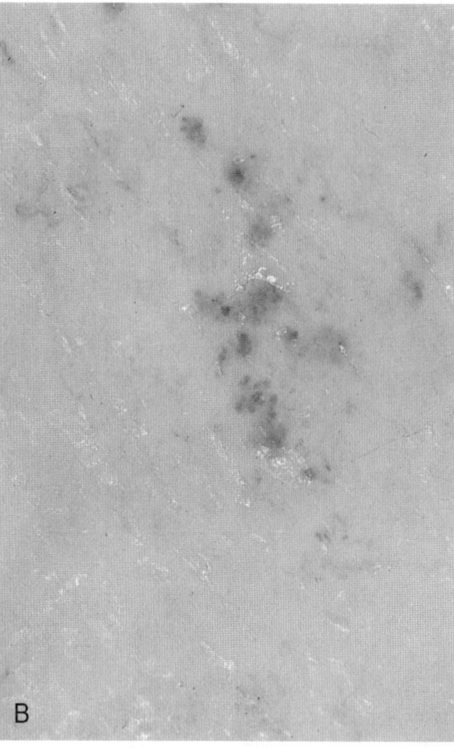

Figure 4. Leg ulcer with atrophie blanche, close-up of dilated vascular loops with thrombi.

We have championed a modified wrap widely known as a Duke boot that overcomes these limitations. A 4-inch-wide × 10-yard zinc oxide–impregnated wrap such as the Dome paste wrap is first applied *without tension*, beginning at the metatarsal heads and continuing in an overlapping (~50%) fashion up to the infrapatellar notch. Next, a self-adherent wrap such as Coban wrap is applied on top of the zinc wrap, again starting at the metatarsal heads and continuing in an overlapping fashion to the knee at *full stretch*. For both, a figure-of-eight wrap is used at the ankle. It is important that the ankle joint be held at about 90 degrees at the time of wrapping to prevent bunching of the materials when patients are walking (Figure 5).

In 1962, George Winter reported 100% improvement in the healing rates of experimental wounds beneath a vapor barrier. Moist wound-healing techniques have since revolutionized chronic wound care and are extremely useful for leg ulcer patients. A variety of dressings are now available that provide a moist environment for the ulcer and are compatible with compression bandages. These dressings also protect the ulcer from the fabric of the compression bandage and are highly effective in relieving pain. Innumerable choices in a variety of materials with subtle differences are available, including gas permeability, ability to absorb wound exudate, and maintenance of pH beneath the dressing, yet they all provide a moist healing environment. The choice of dressing is determined by the condition of the wound. At the initial examination, most chronic ulcers are heavily contaminated and contain considerable fibrinopurulent exudate. Anaerobic hydrocolloids such as Duoderm promote autolytic débridement of this exudate and encourage the wound bed to fill with granulation tissue (Figure 6). Once a wound has fully granulated, epithelialization in the moist environment beneath any of these dressings is fairly rapid.

Whenever the amount of wound drainage overwhelms the ability of the dressing to contain it, the dressing should be changed. Typically, patients are seen once or twice a week for dressing changes. Only tap water or saline should be used for wound cleaning during dressing changes. Antiseptics in particular are harmful to the delicate tissue in a healing wound and are to be avoided. Although these wounds are heavily contaminated with a variety of bacteria,

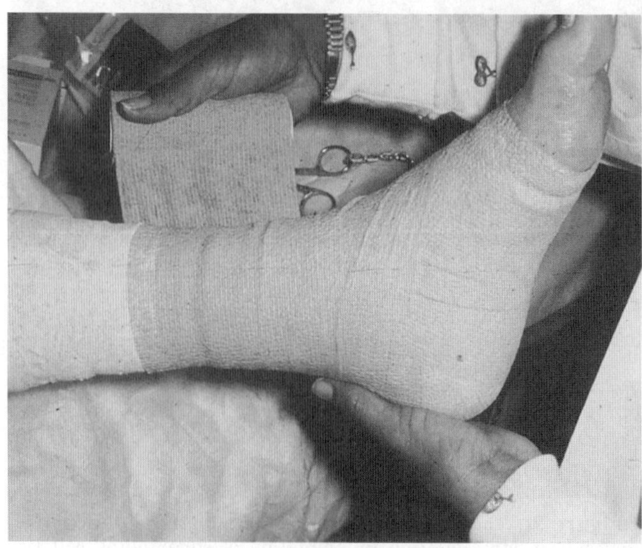

Figure 5. Application of the Duke boot.

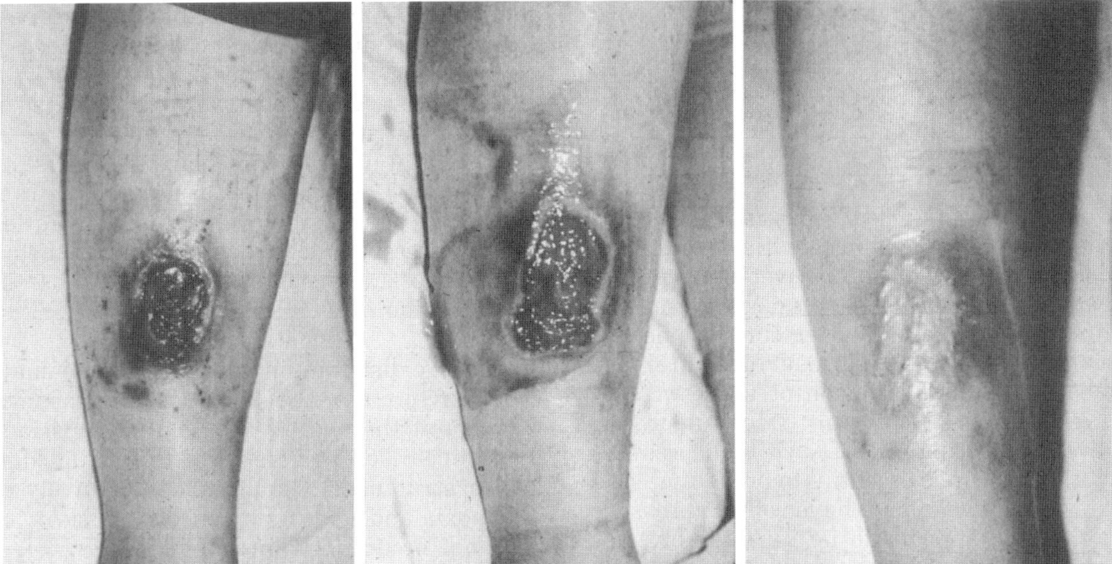

Figure 6. Autolytic débridement and healing over an 8-week period using Duoderm and a Duke boot.

antibiotics have been found ineffective at enhancing healing rates in patients with venous ulceration.

Adjunctive Measures

If dermatitis is present, it should be treated with topical corticosteroid ointment at the time of dressing changes or with a short course of systemic corticosteroid therapy (especially if the dermatitis is severe, if the panniculitis is highly inflammatory, or if the dermatitis is generalized). In patients with calf muscle pump dysfunction resulting from neuromuscular or skeletal abnormalities, it may be necessary to add sequential pneumatic pumping to the aforementioned regimen. The most useful approach is to initiate 30 to 60 minutes of compression immediately before a dressing change. Pain may be severe in ulcer patients and often requires narcotics (Figure 7). Many patients are not able to tolerate compression until the pain is controlled.

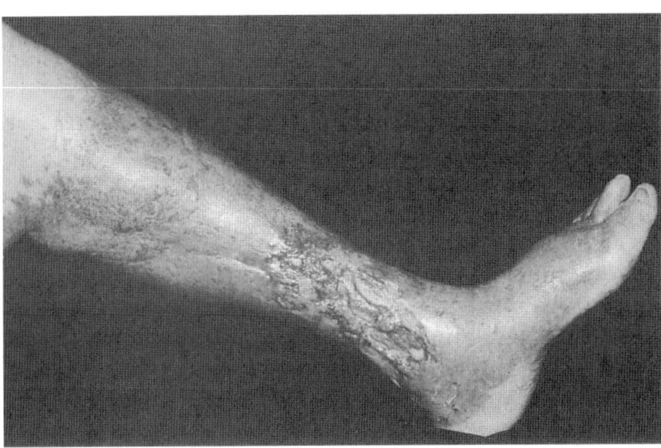

Figure 7. An example of painful venous ulceration.

Recent Approaches

Although the vast majority of patients heal without grafting, allogeneic and xenogeneic human skin substitutes are now marketed for ulcer patients. Several studies have produced promising results in carefully selected patients. Studies comparing these expensive bioengineered products with xenografts and autografts are pending.

One might suppose that adding growth factors to chronic wounds would hasten the healing process, but experience with these agents has been disappointing even though one product, a human recombinant platelet-derived growth factor, did win approval for use in neuropathic ulcers in diabetic patients.

PREVENTION

Ulceration is a late manifestation of venous disease and may be prevented if patients are treated early with compression bandages, followed by supportive stockings. It is not wise to suggest stockings until the leg is free of edema and tenderness.

Once ulcers have healed, supportive stockings are crucial to prevent relapse. The choice of stockings is important, and minimal compression of 30 to 40 mm Hg at the ankle is indicated. Knee-length stockings are adequate for most patients and are suitable for warm environments. A variety of assist devices (such as the stocking butler) are available to help patients step into their stockings. When stockings are not possible, compression devices that attach with Velcro (Circ-aid, Circ-plus) are a useful option.

PRESSURE ULCERS

method of
MARK J. ROSENTHAL, M.D.
Greater Los Angeles VA
North Hills, California

Pressure sores (once termed *decubitus ulcers*) develop on the hips, buttocks, and feet. Sustained high pressure localized to skin mainly over bony prominences becomes relevant when pressures exceed the tissue's threshold of pressure over time. Some hypothesize that a tissue-support surface interface pressure above capillary perfusion pressure will deprive tissues of nutriments and induce necrosis. Hence, preventing occurrence of such high pressure or limiting its duration is essential to prevention and treatment of such wounds. The absolute pressure needed for healing appears to be considerably less than that which causes formation of sores, but longitudinal studies have not yet been performed to verify this. This logic has been the genesis of most modalities for prevention and treatment of pressure sores.

Costs for care are high—more than $8 billion per year in the United States. Such care was previously provided at the acute hospital level but is now usually managed at a lower level of care, although some long-term care facilities may exclude patients with advanced pressure sores.

Pressures increase, "mature" over time because the skeleton settles into surrounding soft tissues and into the support surface as shown by radiologic study. Various systems have been developed, but flaws in design of such testing means that pressure measures were often too inaccurate to be clinically useful. Two interface pressure mapping systems were shown to have low creep (spurious increase due to compression of the pressure-measuring metal finger diode) and low hysteresis (sustained readings when actual pressure has been changed). Validated measures of pressure change over time are useful to gauge the timewise increased interface pressures causing tissue destruction. Such reliable systems are not yet in widespread clinical usage. Such testing should be routinely used to evaluate any support system to verify the best clinical approach for individual patients.

Although tissues can generally tolerate high pressure for short periods of time, if such pressure is maintained, blood supply and lymph drainage are impaired. The resulting tissue trauma is a multidimensional process with externally applied pressure identified as a primary contributing factor. Shear is produced when contiguous parts slide relative to each other in a direction parallel to the plane of contact. This angulates subcutaneous structures. Friction removes stratum corneum, causing superficial erosions by sliding, rolling, or flowing tissue. Injury from friction or shear shortens the period of ischemia necessary to produce necrosis.

Malnutrition and illness heighten the likelihood that any of these insults will lead to tissue breakdown. Some suggest serum albumin concentration as a marker of vulnerability to wounds. Sores develop early during the hospital stay, typically within the first 2 weeks. Commensurate with limited mobility and poor nutrition, 3% of patients entering an acute care hospital develop a pressure sore (most on orthopedic wards). This can be compared with the 30% rate for those in chronic care facilities. Patients who develop pressure ulcers have five times the mortality of non–pressure ulcer patients, and those in whom the ulcers do not heal have yet a greater risk of dying.

Pressure distribution results in a cone-shaped area over bony prominences, with the apex near the skin. Damage at the skin surface may be misleading and may appear less severe than the actual damage to deeper structures. The dermis is relatively resistant to hypoxia and ischemia. Hence, necrosis of this layer does not occur until late in the course of pressure injury. Muscle tissue is the most susceptible to high pressure, followed by subcutaneous fat.

Débridement of nonviable necrotic tissue decreases bacterial counts of wound tissue. To augment healing, infection should be treated, generally with topical application of disinfectants. Because agents such as benzalkonium chloride, povidone-iodine (Betadine), Dakin solution, or hydrogen peroxide are toxic to fibroblasts and epithelial tissues, their use is less advisable. These should be used very briefly to eliminate overt cutaneous infection, but silver sulfadiazine (Silvadene) can be used to the same effect with less toxicity.

Fever, elevated white blood cell count, purulent drainage, local tissue warmth, or tissue erythema indicate a need for systemic antibiotics, which are more effective in eliminating true infection than are topical antibiotics. Mortality runs as high as 60% for systemic dissemination of wound infections in older patients. Tissue biopsy or needle aspiration is recommended to determine the etiology of wound infection, particularly with osteomyelitis. A 1-cm^2 area of the wound can be swabbed for 5 seconds until slight fluid is extracted from the wound bed to provide adequate culture information.

Wounds are routinely graded by the Shea scale (I–IV) and can be scored by standard inventories using multiple descriptive criteria. Progression of stage I and II wounds can be managed by elimination of physical risk factors such as maceration from extended moisture (e.g., from urinary incontinence) or from unrelieved pressure. Early wounds can be successfully treated with hydrocolloid occlusive dressings. Occlusive dressings may be more cost-effective in terms of nursing time. Potential complications include wound infection and maceration. Adequate dietary intake is essential for healing of ulcers, and increased protein intake to 1.2 to 1.5 g/kg/d has been associated with faster healing. Zinc may augment wound healing, but delivery and utilization by tissues may be problematic. Deeper wounds may require aggressive and expensive therapies. Full-thickness skin grafts are often used in less functionally impaired patients, but transient bacteremia occurs.

Débridement of necrotic eschar accelerates wound healing. This should be performed surgically for infected eschar. Débridement removes healing as well as necrotic tissue. Topical application of gauze soaked with sterile saline is used for nonselective tissue removal. Such "wet-to-dry" therapy may be painful, and because this retards epithelialization, it should be discontinued when necrotic material is removed and only granulation tissue is visible. Desiccation impairs wound healing and epithelialization. Maintaining a moist environment leads to more rapid healing and is best applied with fine mesh gauze dressing moistened with normal saline. Moist dressings also lessen wound pain. The choice of a particular agent depends on clinical circumstances. Nonpermeable polymers can be macerating to normal skin. Most films have an adhesive backing that may remove epithelial cells when the dressing is changed. The herbal lotion aloe has been reported to improve wound healing of selected wounds, but trials in pressure sores are limited. Growth factors have shown promising results but are as yet poorly validated.

The primary means to prevent wounds is by frequent moving of vulnerable tissues and shifting weight off pressure-prone anatomic regions. Even with the best nursing care, sores may develop in patients who have inherently high pressures induced by contractures because these create extremely high pressure. Some advocate lysis of adhesions for such patients, but these drastic measures are not often employed because of the fear of additional functional impairment. However, once sores have developed, pressures are too high for routine bed therapy to allow healing. Static devices may lower pressure and improve healing; but lacking studies to verify benefit for stages III or IV wounds, most clinicians use dynamic bed therapy. A recently validated option is topical hyperbaric oxygen therapy. This was shown to accelerate healing of advanced wounds, in part by decreasing tumor necrosis factor and accelerating growth of granulation tissue.

In comparison to arterial or venous ulcers, the relationship of generally poor circulation is less overt. This is true even though tissue breakdown in pressure ulcers occurs largely as a result of impaired arterial flow into tissues and limited lymphatic drainage from tissues. The pathogenesis suggests best approaches to therapy. Generally, high pressure should be resolved to promote healing. The absolute threshold for healing varies dependent on location of wounds being lower over the sacrum than over the hip. Posterior thighs sustain more than 80 mm Hg without trauma, the subtrochanteric shelf less than 60 mm Hg, the ischia less than 40 mm Hg, and the coccyx less than 14 mm Hg. Normally innervated skin can withstand ischemia nearly 3 hours longer than skin of a spinal cord–injured individual without signs of breakdown and pressures nearly threefold as high as in older hospitalized patients.

A pressure reduction surface is indicated for advanced wounds or for patients at risk for progression from a stage II lesion. Because of cost, such treatment is generally reserved for advanced wounds, although some would use it to prevent wound progression. For advanced wounds, limited studies have shown that air-fluidized or low air loss beds may increase rate of healing more than routine hospital measures, but response of deep wounds has not been consistent and some patients developed new sores while on such beds. Air-fluidized support was previously the best treatment but is less widely used now due to cost and maintenance difficulties. Low air loss beds are currently in wide use, but some believe their benefits are "inadequately" studied. Hydrotherapy may also benefit severe wounds, but the conditions of many patients deteriorated while they were on such treatment.

Because no device has yet been shown to be effective to reduce heel pressure, bridging with pillows is often used. Unless overtly infected, heel ulcers are better left undébrided because of their poor vascularity. Consideration of pain reduction where indicated is often overlooked, and analgesics are indicated.

ATOPIC DERMATITIS

method of
HEIDI HWONG, M.D., and
MOISE L. LEVY, M.D.
Baylor College of Medicine
Houston, Texas

Atopic dermatitis (AD) is a chronic, relapsing inflammatory skin disease characterized by intense pruritus. This skin disorder is associated with an early age of onset and a familial predisposition for the atopic triad of allergic rhinitis, asthma, and AD.

Lesions are intensely pruritic, erythematous papules and vesicles. Other findings include scaling, lichenification, thickening, fissuring, and hyperpigmentation or hypopigmentation. The distribution of skin findings varies with age. In infants, the distribution is most commonly seen on the cheeks, forehead, scalp, and extensor surfaces of extremities. Areas affected in children are wrists, ankles, antecubital fossae, and popliteal fossae. Adolescents and adults typically present with lesions in flexural folds and on the face, neck, hands, and feet.

Simple criteria for diagnosis of AD are listed in Table 1. The differential diagnosis includes seborrheic dermatitis, psoriasis, fungal infection, contact dermatitis, drug eruption, scabies, and mycosis fungoides. Although the pathogenesis of AD is not completely understood, elevated IgE production, increased histamine release, and T-cell dysregulation demonstrate immunologic disturbance.

MANAGEMENT

The management of AD is often difficult. Patient and parent education is required, particularly about the chronic nature of AD and about compliance using dry skin and medicated therapies. These treatments

TABLE 1. **Simple Criteria for Diagnosis of Atopic Dermatitis**

Pruritic skin and at least three additional criteria
- History of flexural dermatitis
- History of asthma or hay fever in patient or in first-degree relative if <4 years old
- History of dry skin in the past year
- Skin rash occurring before the age of 2 years
- Visible flexural atopic dermatitis

From Williams HC, Burney PGJ, Pembroke AC, Hay RJ: The U.K. working party's diagnostic criteria for atopic dermatitis, III: Independent hospital validation. Br J Dermatol 131:406–416, 1994.

will not cure the disease but can help minimize acute flares (Table 2).

General Skin Care

Both sufficient lubrication of the skin and avoidance of irritants and other exacerbating factors are important long-term therapies in AD patients. Patients may take short daily baths using lukewarm water and gentle cleansers. Emollients should be applied to the skin within 3 minutes of bathing and reapplied at least once daily. Ointments are recommended for more effective moisturizing. The greasy feel of ointments may not be acceptable to patients. Creams are preferable to lotions except in very humid, warm environments. Products with hydroxy acids, alcohol, preservatives, and urea can irritate inflamed skin and should be used cautiously.

Triggers such as irritants, allergens, emotional stress, and infections can exacerbate AD. Patients should avoid irritants such as detergents, harsh chemicals, perfumed skin care products and soaps, bubble baths, and woolen and nylon clothing. Low humidity from cold winter temperatures and central heating dries skin, resulting in flares of AD. High temperatures with high humidity create sweat retention, which irritates skin and causes exacerbations of the dermatitis. We recommend that patients wear cotton clothing and thoroughly rinse them to remove the soap residue of detergents. Despite the controversial role of allergy in AD, allergens such as pollens, house dust, tobacco smoke, and animal dander from feathered or furry pets are best avoided.

Topical Medications

Topical steroids are the mainstay of treatment for reducing inflammation and pruritus in AD. The need to control acute exacerbations must be balanced with the potential side effects of chronic steroid therapy. In addition to generalized application of emollients, inflamed and pruritic skin should be treated two to three times daily until the flares are controlled, which often occurs within 2 weeks. Prolonged daily use of corticosteroids results in tachyphylaxis and side effects such as skin atrophy, telangiectasia, striae, and bruising. Sufficient quantities should be prescribed with refills monitored carefully. The exact choice of topical steroids is dependent on the medium, the patient's age, and the disease severity.

Ointment bases have more efficient absorption, contain fewer preservatives, and are more lubricating. They may, however, be poorly tolerated in hot, humid climates. Creams are more cosmetically acceptable and thereby increase compliance. Active areas can be treated with low- to mid-potency steroids except the face, groin, axillae, and under diapers. These areas and infants and young children with mild disease can be treated with 1% hydrocortisone. Moderate disease responds to 2.5% hydrocortisone or 0.05% desonide. Triamcinolone acetonide (Kenalog) 0.1% ointment, which comes in 1 lb jars, is a cost-effective, mid-potency steroid. In resistant lichenified areas on the limbs and trunk, more potent fluorinated steroids such as 0.01% to 0.025% fluocinolone acetonide (Synalar) cream, 0.1% mometasone furoate (Elocon) ointment, or 0.005% fluticasone propionate (Cutivate) ointment may be necessary for short, closely monitored periods. Topical steroids should be applied after bathing and before emollients for better skin penetration. Once exacerbations have subsided, topical steroids should be discontinued with the focus of therapy returning to proper skin hydration.

Mild shampoos are used for AD of the scalp. When

TABLE 2. **Management of Mild, Moderate, and Severe Atopic Dermatitis**

Mild	Moderate	Severe
Sufficient skin hydration Avoid triggers Short-term class 6 or 7 topical steroids, i.e., 1% hydrocortisone, 2.5% hydrocortisone, 0.05% desonide ointment +/− other tar preparations Tar shampoo Control of pruritus Treat any superinfection	Sufficient skin hydration Avoid triggers Short-term class 4 or 5 topical steroids, i.e., 0.2% hydrocortisone ointment (a short-term class 3 topical steroid may be necessary, i.e., 0.1% triamcinolone acetonide ointment) Tacrolimus ointment Consider advanced therapies Tar shampoos with short-term topical steroids, i.e., 1% hydrocortisone scalp lotion, 0.1% halcinonide solution, 0.05% fluocinonide acetonide solution Control of pruritus (oral medication) Treat any superinfection	Sufficient skin hydration Avoid triggers Topical steroids Tacrolimus ointment Advanced therapies Control of pruritus (oral medication) Treat any superinfection *Reconsider original diagnosis*

shampoos are inadequate, lotions and solutions containing corticosteroids such as 1% hydrocortisone scalp lotion, 0.1% halcinonide (Halog) solution, and 0.05% fluocinonide acetonide solution can be applied after shampooing for short-term use. A cosmetically acceptable but more expensive alternative is betamethasone valerate mousse.

Tar preparations have anti-inflammatory properties and can decrease use of topical corticosteroids. Tar therapy is often less cosmetically acceptable and can stain clothing and sheets as well as cause irritation.

Control of Pruritus

Topical medications help control pruritus, but patients may require additional modalities. Colloidal oatmeal (Aveeno Baths, Aveeno Anti-Itch cream or lotion) or camphor and menthol (Sarna Anti-Itch) lotion can lessen pruritic symptoms. The latter preparation should be used cautiously owing to the possibility of skin irritation from menthol and camphor. Hydroxyzine (Vistaril), 50 to 100 mg (2–4 mg/kg/d) divided into three to four doses a day and diphenhydramine (Benadryl) 5 mg/kg/d are sedating and help with nighttime itching. Doxepin (Sinequan),* 25 to 150 mg at bedtime, can be effective but is not approved for this indication; lower dosages have been used in very young children (1 mg/kg). Cetirizine 5 to 10 mg once or twice a day is nonsedating but may be less effective.

Treatment of Infection

If lesions have associated edema, serous discharge, and crusting, patients are often superinfected with *Staphylococcus aureus*. Patients with refractive lesions may also be secondarily infected and may benefit from antimicrobial therapy. Systemic antibiotics such as cephalexin or erythromycin are used for secondary infections. Appropriate cultures with sensitivity testing is important especially with increasing rates of antibiotic resistance. Aluminum acetate (Burow) soaks or wet compresses ameliorate crusted, infected patches. Localized disease may respond to topical mupirocin 2% ointment (Bactroban).* Superinfection with herpes simplex virus is treated with oral or intravenous acyclovir depending on the extent and severity of infection. Superficial fungal infections may result in generalized flares of AD and should be treated concurrently.

Advanced Therapy

Topical tacrolimus (FK506) (Protopic),* a potent macrolide immunosuppressant, is a newer therapy shown to be effective for lesions refractive to topical steroid treatment with minimal immediate side effects. Tacrolimus can be used on affected areas for short-term or extended intermittent therapy in

*Not FDA approved for this indication.

adults as a 0.1% or 0.03% ointment and in children older than 2 years of age as a 0.03% ointment. Studies of topical SDZ-ASM-981, a macrolactam ascomycini, have shown it also to be effective in the management of AD without local side effects. Cyclosporine (Sandimmune)* is an effective, well-tolerated treatment that is safe with carefully monitored, short-term use. Because rebound flaring can occur with cyclosporine, dosage should be tapered. Renal function also should be monitored. Phototherapy with ultraviolet B, ultraviolet A, psoralen with ultraviolet A, or combined ultraviolet A/ultraviolet B is effective in adolescents and adults with chronic refractive disease. Systemic corticosteroids are rarely indicated as a result of well-known side effects and rebound with discontinuation.

*Not FDA approved for this indication.

ERYTHEMA MULTIFORME, STEVENS-JOHNSON SYNDROME, AND TOXIC EPIDERMAL NECROLYSIS

method of
MARCIA G. TONNESEN, M.D.
State University of New York at Stony Brook
Stony Brook, New York

Historically, erythema multiforme (EM), Stevens-Johnson syndrome (SJS), and toxic epidermal necrolysis (TEN) are considered as a disease spectrum. Current evidence, however, supports a clear distinction between EM, with characteristic acrally distributed target lesions and an etiologic link to herpes simplex virus (HSV) infection, and SJS/TEN, with focal-to-widespread skin and mucous membrane involvement characterized by epidermal destruction and an etiologic link to adverse drug reactions.

Optimal therapeutic intervention is hindered by the fact that specific pathogenic mechanisms of tissue injury have not yet been completely defined. In addition, few controlled studies have been performed to evaluate the effectiveness of therapeutic interventions. Elimination of any identified or presumed precipitating factors is of prime importance. Successful therapy should combine symptomatic and supportive measures with observation for and treatment of associated complications, depending on the clinical characteristics and severity of the episode. Typically, EM is mild and self-limited and requires only symptomatic care. However, because of the degree and extent of epidermal and mucosal involvement that occurs in SJS and TEN, careful monitoring is critical, hospitalization is often required, and supportive care is usually necessary.

ERYTHEMA MULTIFORME

EM is an acute, self-limited, but frequently recurrent, inflammatory cutaneous disorder, characterized by the sudden onset of a symmetric erythematous eruption with primarily an acral distribution. Mucosal involvement, when present, is usually limited to the lips and oral cavity. Skin lesions begin as fixed erythematous macules, develop into edematous papules, and may become bullous. Some further evolve to form distinctive target lesions with at least three zones of color (dusky center, pale edematous halo, erythematous border). Individual lesions occasionally burn or itch, appear in successive crops, and spontaneously resolve within 1 to 4 weeks.

The majority of cases of recurrent EM are associated with HSV infection and typically occur up to 10 days after the appearance of a recurrent HSV lesion (oral, genital, or other location). Subclinical episodes of herpes can also induce EM. Viral HSV DNA, but not infective HSV, can be detected in EM lesions. Herpes-associated EM is currently believed to result from an HSV-specific host immune response to viral proteins in the skin.

THERAPEUTIC APPROACH

Elimination of Etiologic Factors

In recurrent HSV-associated EM, a course of acyclovir (Zovirax), 200 mg orally five times daily for 5 days, should be initiated at the first symptom of HSV infection. Acyclovir therapy is not effective if initiated after EM lesions have developed.

Symptomatic Measures

For pruritic or painful skin lesions, systemic antihistamines or analgesics may provide symptomatic relief. Topical acyclovir and topical corticosteroids have not been shown to be of benefit. Care for skin and mouth erosions is addressed in the following section.

Preventive Measures

Because of the common etiologic association between recurrent HSV infections and EM, measures that attempt to prevent recurrences of HSV may lessen the frequency of subsequent episodes of EM. Avoidance of sun exposure through the use of sunscreens (SPF 15 or higher), sunsticks (sunscreen-containing lip balm), and protective clothing, and by minimizing sun exposure from 10:00 AM to 3:00 PM (the peak period for ultraviolet B light) may reduce ultraviolet light–induced HSV recurrences. Attempts should be made to minimize stress, a well-known precipitating factor of HSV. Topical antiviral preparations have not been clearly shown to prevent or abort recurrent HSV infections.

Prophylactic administration of acyclovir has resulted in abolition of recurrent HSV infections and of ensuing episodes of EM. Therefore, in patients with frequently recurring, debilitating, herpes-associated EM, the treatment of choice is daily oral acyclovir for 6 months or longer. The recommended starting dose is 400 mg orally twice daily, with tapering of the dose after the disease is brought under control. Because asymptomatic subclinical HSV episodes can also trigger EM, patients with idiopathic recurrent EM often benefit from prophylactic antiviral therapy. If acyclovir fails to prevent recurrences of HSV, newer antiviral agents with enhanced bioavailability, such as valacyclovir (Valtrex) or famciclovir (Famvir), should be tried, although their efficacy in EM has not yet been determined. Because of the known occurrence of acyclovir resistance and the unknown long-term side effects of chronic acyclovir therapy, the drug should be stopped periodically and the need for its continuance reassessed.

Patient Education

Patients should be reassured regarding the usual benign, self-limited course of EM, educated regarding the frequent association with recurrent HSV infections, and advised regarding preventive measures.

STEVENS-JOHNSON SYNDROME AND TOXIC EPIDERMAL NECROLYSIS

SJS is a severe mucocutaneous illness characterized by an extensive blistering eruption with a primarily truncal distribution, and mucosal erosions, typically involving the mouth and conjunctivae. A prodrome with constitutional symptoms often heralds the onset of the eruption. Skin lesions begin as erythematous or purpuric macules, frequently develop central vesiculation, and may progress to bullae formation with epidermal necrosis. Epidermal detachment may involve up to 10% of the body surface area (BSA). Painful mucosal erosions result in characteristic hemorrhagic crusted lips, foul-smelling mouth, and decreased oral intake. Ocular involvement with photophobia and painful conjunctival erosions may lead to residual scarring and lacrimal abnormalities. Permanent visual impairment can occur. The disease duration is 4 to 6 weeks. Recurrences are infrequent. SJS is now recognized as strongly related to adverse drug reactions and linked to some infections, particularly *Mycoplasma pneumoniae*, but never to HSV infection.

TEN is characterized by widespread sheetlike necrosis and sloughing of the epidermis involving greater than 30% of the BSA. (Epidermal detachment between 10% and 30% of the BSA is now classified as SJS/TEN overlap.) Following a 1- to 3-day prodrome of fever and flulike symptoms, the cutaneous eruption characteristically begins with painful erythema, often distributed symmetrically on the face and upper body. It then rapidly extends to involve significant or total BSA within hours to 2 to 3 days. Involvement of multiple mucosal surfaces is present in nearly all patients. The order of frequency is oropharynx (which in severe cases may extend to involve the larynx and tracheobronchial tree), eyes, genitalia, and anus. TEN can be considered a manifestation of acute skin failure with abnormal barrier function resulting in fluid, electrolyte, and protein loss, increased susceptibility to infection, impaired thermoregulation, altered immune status, and increased energy expenditure. Morbidity is significant and the mortality rate is 25% to 40%. The leading cause of death is sepsis. Adverse drug reactions are now considered by many to be the only documented cause of TEN. Common offenders include sulfonamides, anticonvulsants (phenytoin [Dilantin], phenobarbital, carbamazepine [Tegretol], lamotrigine [Lamictal], valproic acid), and nonsteroidal anti-inflammatory agents (especially piroxicam-related agents), although many other drugs have been implicated. The pathogenic mechanisms resulting in epidermal necrosis have not been fully elucidated. Current evidence supports important roles for cytotoxic T cells, cytokines, fas-fas ligand-mediated apoptosis, and specific defects in detoxification of reactive drug metabolites in induction of keratinocyte death.

Therapeutic Approach

Strategies to Limit Disease Progression and Reduce Morbidity and Mortality

ELIMINATION OF ETIOLOGIC FACTORS

Immediate withdrawal of any suspected or potential causative drugs is critical because cessation of the offending agent no later than the stage of early blister formation may decrease mortality. *Mycoplasma pneumoniae* and other infections, if diagnosed, should be appropriately treated.

INTERVENTION WITH SYSTEMIC THERAPY TO STOP PROGRESSION

The use of systemic therapy in SJS/TEN is highly controversial because no randomized, controlled trials document efficacy of any systemic intervention. However, because widespread epidermal necrosis is associated with a high mortality rate, early administration of systemic therapy in the progressive phase of the disease process has been advocated by some to attempt to limit the extent of tissue damage. Use of systemic glucocorticosteroids has proven to be particularly controversial because some retrospective studies have indicated that patients treated with systemic steroids have an increased incidence of morbidity, prolonged hospitalization, and mortality. Therefore, other agents are currently being assessed.

Case studies or uncontrolled trials involving few patients have reported benefit from a variety of systemic agents. The most promising, but expensive, to date is the early administration of high-dose intravenous immunoglobulin to inhibit epidermal apoptosis mediated by the fas-fas ligand death receptor. Immunosuppressive therapy with oral cyclosporine (Sandimmune)* or high-dose intravenous cyclophosphamide (Cytoxan)* has been claimed to help several patients. Plasmapheresis has been found to be of great benefit, of some benefit, and of no benefit. Innovative treatment is not without risk, however. For example, a double-blind, placebo-controlled trial of thalidomide, which suppresses production of tumor necrosis factor-α, had to be aborted because of a dramatic increase in mortality, later determined to be related to thalidomide.

In the absence of documented efficacy, use of systemic therapy to limit disease progression in a specific patient remains at the discretion of the physician. However, it is now clear that if systemic intervention is administered, once disease progression ceases and the wound healing process begins, or if no response is noted within 2 to 4 days, treatment should be abruptly discontinued to minimize the risk of associated complications.

SUPPORTIVE CARE

Because of the extensive epidermal and mucosal necrosis and detachment that can occur in SJS and TEN, careful monitoring is critical and hospitalization is often required. Early referral of severe cases to a burn unit has been shown to decrease mortality.

SKIN CARE

For crusted erosive discrete skin lesions, mild drying, débridement, and cleansing as well as a soothing antipruritic effect can be achieved with open wet to damp compresses of tepid water applied for 20 minutes three or four times daily. Lesions should be observed for signs of secondary infection, cultured when indicated, and treatment initiated with the appropriate systemic antibiotic. Topical corticosteroids have not been shown to be of benefit. For pruritic or painful skin lesions, systemic antihistamines or analgesics provide symptomatic relief.

If extensive, advanced tissue necrosis occurs or is already evident (approaching 20% total BSA involvement), immediate transfer of the patient to a burn unit under the care of a surgical burn specialist is strongly advocated. Therapeutic burn unit protocols consist of the following:

1. Measures to guard against iatrogenic infection, including withdrawal from systemic steroids; limitation of antibiotic use to specific culture-proven infections; avoidance of indwelling lines and catheters whenever possible; daily cultures of skin, blood, and urine; and aggressive treatment of sepsis if it occurs
2. Supportive care consisting of use of an air-fluidized bed, respiratory and physical therapy, intravenous fluid therapy, tube feedings, adequate pain relief, and continuing care by an ophthalmologist
3. Avoidance of all unnecessary medications, particularly those that are known etiologic factors of SJS/TEN, such as sulfonamides (including sulfa-containing eye preparations and topical dressings)
4. Skin care with emphasis on early gentle débridement followed by application of dressings to protect the denuded dermis from desiccation and to facilitate rapid re-epithelialization. Reduced mortality and faster healing result from the use of synthetic dressings, biologic dressings, silver nitrate dressings, allografts, or porcine xenografts.

MOUTH CARE

When extensive painful mouth lesions are present, good oral hygiene is critical to minimize infection and discomfort. Hydrogen peroxide (1.5%) mouthwash every 2 hours provides cleansing and gentle débridement. Topical anesthetics, such as dyclonine

*Not FDA approved for this indication.

(Dyclone), viscous lidocaine, or a 1:1 mixture of attapulgite (Kaopectate Advanced Formula) and elixir of diphenhydramine (Benadryl), used as a mouthwash often provide pain relief. A liquid or soft diet, usually better tolerated, contributes to the maintenance of hydration and nutrition. More aggressive nutritional support is usually required for severe oral involvement.

EYE CARE

Because of the potential for long-term sequelae resulting in loss of vision, careful monitoring of eye involvement is mandatory and early consultation and daily continuing care by an ophthalmologist is strongly recommended. Suggested therapeutic measures include irrigation and compresses to cleanse the eye, lysis of adhesions, and instillation of topical antibiotics.

Preventive Measures

In drug-associated SJS or TEN, future avoidance of the causative drug or chemically related agents is mandatory.

Patient Education

For SJS and TEN, patients should be advised that the course is self-limited but potentially severe and life-threatening, educated regarding the association with adverse drug reactions, and warned to avoid future use of the implicated medication.

BULLOUS DISEASES

method of
LAWRENCE S. CHAN, M.D.
Northwestern University Medical School and Lakeside Medical Center
Chicago, Illinois

Skin blisters are defined as clear fluid-filled lesions, palpable by hand. A small skin blister (<1 cm in diameter) is called a *vesicle,* and a larger skin blister (>1 cm) is termed a *bulla.* Skin blisters can arise from both non-autoimmune or autoimmune causes. The etiology of skin blisters of the non-autoimmune nature includes genetic (epidermolysis bullosa group), infectious (herpes simplex, herpes zoster, impetigo), metabolic (bullosis diabeticorum, porphyria cutanea tarda), and allergic (poison ivy, toxic epidermal necrolysis) causes. Most of the non-autoimmune blisters, except the heritable epidermolysis bullosa group, are usually self-limited.

By contrast, most of the autoimmune blisters are chronic and inflammatory, therefore typically requiring long-term treatment and management by physicians. The following section is a discussion of the essential clinical and laboratory features and therapies for these autoimmune, chronic, inflammatory blistering skin diseases. A complete list of these diseases and their corresponding target antigens is presented in Table 1. Because these diseases are infrequently seen, large, well-controlled, clinical trials have not been performed. The following recommendations are generally not based on Food and Drug Administration–approved protocol but rather on the author's personal experience and current dermatology literature.

Autoimmune blistering diseases are best classified, by the location of lesion, into two major groups: the pemphigus group and the pemphigoid group. Pemphigus is derived from the Greek word *pemphix,* meaning "blister" or "bubble." *Pemphigoid* means "pemphigus-like." Although the pemphigus group includes a variety of intraepidermal blisters (i.e., blister occurs within the epidermis layer), the pemphigoid group also includes a variety of subepidermal blisters (i.e., blisters occur below the epidermis layer, with an intact epidermis layer). Two extremely rare variants of pemphigus (pemphigus herpetiformis and IgA pemphigus) and bullous systemic lupus erythematosus are not included in this discussion, owing to space limitation. Dermatitis herpetiformis is included because of its similarity to other autoimmune blistering diseases. However, strictly speaking, dermatitis herpetiformis is not an autoimmune disease because the skin target antigen for this disease has not yet been found.

TABLE 1. **Autoimmune Blistering Skin Diseases**

Disease Grouping	Skin Target Antigens
Pemphigus Group	
CLASSIC PEMPHIGUS	
Deep	
Pemphigus vulgaris (PV)	Desmoglein 3
Pemphigus vegetans (localized PV)	
Superficial	
Pemphigus foliaceus (PF)	Desmoglein 1
Pemphigus erythematosus (localized PF)	
NEW PEMPHIGUS VARIANTS	
Pemphigus herpetiformis	Desmogleins 1 and 3
Paraneoplastic pemphigus	Desmoplakins I and II, Envoplakin, Periplakin, Desmoglein 3, and BPAg1
IgA pemphigus	Desmocollin 1, Desmoglein 3
Pemphigoid Group	
Bullous pemphigoid	BPAg1, BPAg2
Gestational pemphigoid	BPAg2
Mucous membrane pemphigoid	BPAg2, laminin-5, laminin-6, type VII collagen, integrin β4 subunit
Linear IgA bullous dermatosis	BPAg2
Epidermolysis bullosa acquisita	Type VII collagen
Bullous systemic lupus erythematosus	Type VII collagen

PEMPHIGUS VULGARIS

Essential Clinical and Laboratory Features

Pemphigus vulgaris is the most severe form of autoimmune bullous diseases. It was invariably fatal before the availability of corticosteroids. In the majority of the patients affected with pemphigus vulgaris, oral mucosal blisters and erosions occur weeks to months before any skin lesions surface. When skin lesions develop, the most common lesion observed is erosion, with rare flaccid bulla arising from normal-appearing or erythematous (inflamed) skin in a generalized manner.

In its localized variant, pemphigus vegetans, lesions are formed primarily on intertriginous areas (neck, axillae, groin) and manifested as granulation and vegetative plaques. Histopathologic examination of an intact blister usually reveals an intraepidermal blister located just above the basal layer of epidermis and acantholysis (epidermal cells separated from each other). Direct immunofluorescence microscopy performed on the patient's perilesional skin detects IgG deposition at the surfaces of epidermal cells (a "chicken wire" pattern). Indirect immunofluorescence microscopy performed with the patient's serum on monkey esophagus epithelium (the recommended substrate) usually detects IgG circulating autoantibodies of the patients that bind to the surfaces of epithelial cells. The target antigen of the IgG autoantibodies of pemphigus vulgaris is a desmosomal protein termed *desmoglein-3,* a member of the cadherin superfamily.

Therapy

The mainstay of treatment for pemphigus vulgaris (and its localized vegetative variant) is systemic corticosteroids. For early localized disease, a moderate dose of prednisone (40–60 mg/d) should be initiated, along with an immunosuppressive agent, such as azathioprine (Imuran),* 100 mg/d. For generalized disease, a higher prednisone dose (60–150 mg/d) should be initiated, along with an immunosuppressive agent (azathioprine, 100 to 200 mg/d). Tapering of prednisone should be attempted when all or most of the existing active lesions are clear and no new lesions are observed in the 2 months before the initiation of taper. It would be helpful to examine the patients' pemphigus autoantibody titer (by indirect immunofluorescence microscopy) just before the attempt of tapering because pemphigus titer is somewhat correlated with the patients' disease activities.

When tapering prednisone, it is recommended that the dose reduction of 5 mg/d occur monthly. When the prednisone dose of 40 mg/d is reached, tapering of the dosage should be initiated to achieve alternative-day dosing (at the same reduction scheduling, 5 mg every other day, monthly) until a regimen of 40 mg of prednisone alternating with no prednisone is reached. At this time, reduction of 5 mg/d prednisone monthly should be attempted on the 40-mg/d alternative day schedule until all prednisone is eliminated. Thereafter, tapering of immunosuppressive agents could be attempted if no new lesions are observed for 3 consecutive months after all prednisone is eliminated.

*Not FDA approved for this indication.

Alternative immunosuppressive or adjuvant agents to Imuran include cyclophosphamide (Cytoxan),* 100 to 200 mg/d; cyclosporine, (Sandimmune),* intravenous IgG,* dapsone,* 100 to 200 mg/d, hydroxychloroquine (Plaquenil),* 200 mg/d, and mycophenolate mofetil (CellCept).* It is well known that prednisone and azathioprine (and other adjuvant) each carry significant side effects. For prednisone, monitoring developments of diabetes mellitus, cataracts, gastrointestinal bleeding, osteoporosis, infection, and central nervous system abnormalities is essential. For azathioprine, monitoring hepatotoxicity, malignancy, and bone marrow suppression (particularly lymphopenia) is necessary. For cyclophosphamide, monitoring for bone marrow suppression, hemorrhagic cystitis, and malignancy is important. For cyclosporine, monitoring renal toxicity is of utmost importance. For dapsone, monitoring neurologic and hematologic abnormalities is important. For hydroxychloroquine, monitoring retinal toxicity by ophthalmologists is required.

PEMPHIGUS FOLIACEUS

Essential Clinical and Laboratory Features

Pemphigus foliaceus usually presents as crusted, inflammatory, scaly plaques, with rarely observed flaccid small blisters, primarily on seborrheic areas (face, scalp, and upper chest and back). In its localized variant, pemphigus erythematosus, lesions are also observed in a malar distribution of the face, resembling that of lupus erythematosus. In Brazil, an endemic form of pemphigus equivalent to pemphigus foliaceus is identified and is named *fogo selvagem,* a Portuguese term meaning "wild fire." Histopathologic examination of an intact blister usually reveals an intraepidermal blister located just below the stratum corneum layer of epidermis and acantholysis. Direct immunofluorescence microscopy performed on the patient's perilesional skin detects IgG deposition at the surfaces of epidermal cells. Indirect immunofluorescence microscopy performed with the patient's serum on guinea pig esophageal epithelium (the recommended substrate) usually detects IgG circulating autoantibodies of the patients that bind to the surfaces of epithelial cells. The target antigen of the IgG autoantibodies of pemphigus foliaceus is the desmosomal protein *desmoglein-1,* a member of the cadherin superfamily.

Therapy

The therapeutic approach for pemphigus foliaceus is essentially the same as that for pemphigus vulgaris. For early localized disease, high-potency topical corticosteroids such as clobetasol (Temovate) oint-

*Not FDA approved for this indication.

ment applied twice a day, with or without an immunosuppressive agent, may be sufficient to control the disease. For generalized disease, the treatment approach should be the same as for pemphigus vulgaris, although a reduction of 15% medication dosage may be appropriate because pemphigus foliaceus is generally more receptive to treatment. The tapering strategy and side effect monitoring should follow that of pemphigus vulgaris.

PARANEOPLASTIC PEMPHIGUS

Essential Clinical and Laboratory Features

Paraneoplastic pemphigus is manifested clinically as a mucocutaneous blistering disease associated with underlying benign or malignant neoplasms, the most common of which are non-Hodgkin lymphoma, chronic lymphocytic leukemia, Castleman tumor, and thymoma. The most observed clinical feature of paraneoplastic pemphigus is an intractable stomatitis, consisting of painful erosions and ulcerations of the oropharynx and vermilion borders of the lips. The skin manifestations are variable, comprising blisters, erosions, and targetoid lesions that resemble erythema multiforme. In some patients, lichenoid papules and plaques predominate. Histopathologic findings in paraneoplastic pemphigus are variable, and the most characteristic observations include intraepidermal blister with acantholysis, necrosis of keratinocytes, vacuolar change of basilar epidermis, and mononuclear cell infiltration. Direct immunofluorescence microscopy performed on a perilesional skin biopsy specimen usually detects IgG deposits at the epithelial cell surfaces plus granular C3 deposition at the skin basement membrane zone. Indirect immunofluorescence usually detects IgG circulating autoantibodies that bind not only to epithelial cell surfaces of the squamous epithelium (monkey esophagus) but also to that of the transitional epithelium (rat bladder) in about 75% of the cases. The epidermal antigens recognized by the IgG autoantibodies from patients with paraneoplastic pemphigus include desmoplakins I and II, BPAg1, envoplakin, periplakin, desmoglein-3, and plectin.

Therapy

The therapy for paraneoplastic pemphigus should be first directed to elimination of the neoplasm. Every effort should be made to surgically remove those resectable tumors and to prescribe medical treatments for unresectable tumors. The therapeutic approach for the mucocutaneous disease should follow that of pemphigus vulgaris. Complete clinical resolution of paraneoplastic pemphigus can be observed in patients whose benign tumors were removed. However, patients with paraneoplastic pemphigus and unresectable malignant tumors are very resistant to medical treatments available to physicians and face very poor prognoses.

BULLOUS PEMPHIGOID

Essential Clinical and Laboratory Features

Bullous pemphigoid is manifested as localized or generalized tense bullae arising from normal-appearing or erythematous skin, particularly on the intertriginous areas. Bullous pemphigoid affects elderly individuals, with an average age at onset about 65 years. Histopathologic examination of an intact blister usually reveals a subepidermal blister located just below the epidermis and prominent eosinophil infiltration along the blistering areas. Direct immunofluorescence microscopy performed on the patient's perilesional skin detects linear IgG deposition at the epidermal basement membrane zone. Indirect immunofluorescence microscopy performed with the patient's serum on salt-split normal human skin (the recommended substrate in which the skin is artificially split at the middle lamina lucida) usually detects IgG circulating autoantibodies of the patients that bind to the upper surfaces of split (at the roof). The target antigens of the IgG autoantibodies of bullous pemphigoid are hemidesmosomal proteins BP antigen 1 (BPAg1) and BPAg2 (BP180); the latter protein is also named *type XVII collagen.*

Therapy

For the localized form of bullous pemphigoid, topical corticosteroids, with or without an adjuvant, may be sufficient to control the disease. Successful management with anti-inflammatory adjuvants (tetracycline,* 1 g twice a day, plus nicotinamide,* 2–2.5 g/d) along with high-potency topical corticosteroids (clobetasol ointment twice a day) can be achieved. Alternatively, low doses of prednisone (20–40 mg/d) along with topical corticosteroids may be used. For generalized disease, prednisone (40–80 mg/d) and azathiprine* (100 mg/d) should be initiated. The tapering strategy and side effect monitoring should follow that for pemphigus vulgaris. However, the examination of autoantibody titers (by indirect immunofluorescence microscopy) before tapering is not useful because the autoantibody titers by this method do not correlate with the patients' disease activities. Because even without treatment, the prognosis for patients with bullous pemphigoid is fairly good, every attempt should be made to use a minimally sufficient dose and duration of medication, to avoid severe side effects that may contribute to the morbidity and mortality of these elderly patients.

GESTATIONAL PEMPHIGOID (HERPES GESTATIONIS)

Essential Clinical and Laboratory Features

Gestational pemphigoid (originally named *herpes gestationis*) is a pregnancy-related disease mani-

*Not FDA approved for this indication.

fested as pruritic urticarial plaques and tense bullae on the trunk and abdomen, frequently observed at the periumbilical location. Gestational pemphigoid most frequently has its onset during the period between the fourth and seventh months of pregnancy, but it can occur in the first trimester and the immediate postpartum period or recur in subsequent pregnancies. Histopathologic examination of an intact blister usually reveals a subepidermal blister located just below the epidermis and prominent eosinophil infiltration along the blistering areas. Direct immunofluorescence microscopy performed on the patient's perilesional skin detects linear C3 deposition at the epidermal basement membrane zone. Indirect immunofluorescence performed with the patient's serum on salt-split normal human skin detects IgG circulating autoantibodies in about 25% of the patients that bind to the upper surfaces of split (at the roof). The target antigen of the IgG autoantibodies of gestational pemphigoid is BPAg2.

Therapy

A combination of antihistamine and topical clobetasol ointment (twice daily) may be sufficient for patients with localized disease. Alternatively, low doses of prednisone (20–40 mg/d) usually control the blister formation and relieve the pruritus. Exacerbation during the parturition may require a higher dose. An immunosuppressive adjuvant such as azathioprine* is rarely needed, and its use should be approved by the patient's obstetrician. Infants born of mothers receiving prednisone treatment should be monitored for adrenal suppression. Infants born of affected mothers may develop transient blistering disease but do not require treatment.

MUCOUS MEMBRANE PEMPHIGOID

Essential Clinical and Laboratory Features

Mucous membrane pemphigoid is defined as "a putative autoimmune, chronic inflammatory, subepithelial blistering disease predominantly affecting mucous membranes that is characterized by linear deposition of IgG, IgA, or C3 along the epithelial basement membrane zone" by a recently developed First International Consensus on Mucous Membrane Pemphigoid. Mucous membrane pemphigoid has previously been called *cicatricial pemphigoid* and *benign mucous membrane pemphigoid.* Oral mucosa is the most frequently affected, followed by ocular mucosa. The other affected mucosae include nasal, nasopharyngeal, anogenital, laryngeal, and esophageal. Minor skin involvement may be observed. The common manifestations are inflammatory patches, erosions, and blisters. Scarring is a hallmark of the disease except in the oral mucosa. Multiple target antigens have been identified by the autoantibodies from patients with mucous membrane pemphigoid, including BPAg2, laminin-5, laminin-6, integrin β4 subunit, and type VII collagen.

*Not FDA approved for this indication.

Therapy

According to the First International Consensus on Mucous Membrane Pemphigoid, the logical approach for therapy should be based on the relative risk of the type of disease. The Consensus defines *high-risk patients* as those with disease affecting ocular, genital, nasopharyngeal, esophageal, and laryngeal mucosae. The initial treatment of these high-risk patients should include prednisone (1–1.5 mg/kg/d) and cyclophosphamide* (1–2 mg/kg/d). Furthermore, these patients should be managed by a team of physicians experienced in the special care of these organ systems. Azathioprine* (1–2 mg/kg/d) may substitute for cyclophosphamide. For patients with less severe disease, dapsone,* 50 to 200 mg/d, can be used as an initial regimen. Other useful medication includes subconjunctival mitomycin C* injection by experienced ophthalmologists. For patients with low-risk disease affecting the oral cavity as the sole mucosal involvement, topical clobetasol gel may be sufficient to control the disease. Alternatively, tetracycline,* 1 to 2 g/d, and nicotinamide,* 2 to 2.5 g/d, can be used. If a satisfactory response is not achieved, dapsone,* 25 to 200 mg/d, can be initiated. In some patients, a low dose of prednisone, 0.5 mg/kg/d, with or without a low dose of azathioprine, 100 mg/d, may be needed to control the disease.

LINEAR IgA BULLOUS DERMATOSIS

Essential Clinical and Laboratory Features

Linear IgA bullous dermatosis is manifested most commonly as generalized pruritic papules and blisters. In children affected with this dermatosis, the disease is frequently called *chronic bullous dermatosis of childhood* and is characterized clinically by blisters forming along an annular ring, giving the appearance of a "cluster of jewels." Histopathologic examination of an intact blister usually reveals a subepidermal blister located just below the epidermis and prominent neutrophil infiltration along the blistering areas. Direct immunofluorescence microscopy performed on the patient's perilesional skin detects linear IgA deposition at the epidermal basement membrane zone. Indirect immunofluorescence microscopy performed with the patient's serum on salt-split normal human skin detects IgA circulating autoantibodies in about 30% of the patients that bind to the upper surfaces of split (at the roof). One of the target antigens of the IgA autoantibodies of linear IgA bullous dermatosis is BPAg2.

*Not FDA approved for this indication.

Therapy

The best medication for linear IgA bullous dermatosis is dapsone,* 1 to 1.5 mg/kg/d, or sulfapyridine,* 1 to 2 g/d. For most patients, this monotherapy is sufficient to control the disease, but for a minority of patients, additional low-dose therapy with prednisone (10–20 mg/d) is needed for complete control of the disease. Most children affected with linear IgA bullous dermatosis go into clinical remission within 2 years of onset of disease, whereas a minority of them persists into puberty.

EPIDERMOLYSIS BULLOSA ACQUISITA

Essential Clinical and Laboratory Features

Epidermolysis bullosa acquisita is manifested in two major clinical forms. The more common form is a mechanobullous form that is manifested as noninflammatory or minimally inflammatory blisters predominantly at the trauma-prone areas (knees, elbows, ankles, and dorsal hands) with scar and milia formation. The less common form is a generalized form that is manifested with generalized tense bullae that heal without significant scarring. A form of mucous membrane–predominated disease, previously categorized under epidermolysis bullosa acquisita, should now be included under mucous membrane pemphigoid, according to a recently developed First International Consensus on Mucous Membrane Pemphigoid. Epidermolysis bullosa acquisita affects mostly elderly patients. Histopathologic examination of an intact blister usually reveals a subepidermal blister located just below the epidermis with or without a mixed inflammatory infiltration along the blistering areas. Direct immunofluorescence microscopy performed on the patient's perilesional skin detects a thick band of IgG deposition at the epidermal basement membrane zone. Indirect immunofluorescence performed with the patient's serum on salt-split normal human skin (the recommended substrate) usually detects IgG circulating autoantibodies of the patients that bind to the lower surfaces of split (at the base). The target antigen of the IgG autoantibodies of epidermolysis bullosa acquisita is an anchoring fibril protein type VII collagen.

Therapy

Therapy for this epidermolysis bullosa acquisita is difficult because the disease, especially the mechanobullous form, is very resistant to conventional treatments useful for pemphigus vulgaris or bullous pemphigoid. A commonly used initial treatment regimen is systemic corticosteroids with either or both azathioprine* and dapsone* as corticosteroid-sparing agents. A combination of prednisone (1–1.5 mg/kg/d), azathioprine (1–2 mg/kg/d), and dapsone (100–200 mg/d) can be initiated. Alternative treatment can be considered should this regimen not offer much clinical improvement. These methods include colchicine* (1–2 mg/d), cyclosporine* (5–9 mg/kg/d), extracorporeal photochemotherapy, and intravenous IgG* (common initial dose: 400 mg/kg/d).

*Not FDA approved for this indication.

DERMATITIS HERPETIFORMIS

Essential Clinical and Laboratory Features

Dermatitis herpetiformis is manifested as a very pruritic blistering disease primarily affecting the extensor skin (elbows, knees, buttocks, scalp). It closely resembles linear IgA bullous dermatosis clinically and histopathologically. However, direct immunofluorescence microscopy detects granular (not linear) IgA deposits at the papillary dermis. Indirect immunofluorescence microscopy detects no IgA circulating autoantibodies to skin component. No skin target antigen has been found for dermatitis herpetiformis.

Therapy

Like linear IgA bullous dermatosis, dermatitis herpetiformis is very responsive to dapsone (1–1.5 mg/kg/d) or sulfapyridine (1–2 g/d). Alternatively, a strict gluten-free diet can achieve complete clinical remission.

*Not FDA approved for this indication.

CONTACT DERMATITIS

method of
MARK V. DAHL, M.D.
Mayo Clinic Scottsdale
Scottsdale, Arizona

Eczemas are poorly marginated, scaling inflammatory plaques or patches with epithelial disruption such as wetness, excoriations, fissures, crusts, and scale yellowed by plasma exudate. Contact dermatitis is an eczema produced either from cutaneous irritation or from allergy. These two diseases, irritant dermatitis and allergic contact dermatitis, are really quite different. The chemicals that elicit them are different, the amounts of chemicals necessary to elicit them are different, and their courses are different.

IRRITANT DERMATITIS

Irritant dermatitis results when the skin is injured by a chemical or solvent or by repeated desiccation. For example, if a strong acid is spilled on the skin or if a detergent is taped to the skin, the skin will rather quickly become red and tender or itchy, and if the irritation is severe enough, it may weep, crust, and scale. These are examples of strong irritants. After exposure, healing usually follows a straight line, although scarring may result.

Chronic, cumulative weak irritant dermatitis is less intuitively understood. Here, the skin is repeatedly irritated by exposures to chemicals that by themselves might likely not produce clinical eczema. For example, a dishwasher might develop a chronic, cumulative weak irritant dermatitis on the hands as a consequence of frequent dish washing, whereas he or she might not develop clinical contact dermatitis from intermittent dish washing in the home. In chronic, cumulative weak irritant dermatitis the insults are recurrent, small, and repetitive. The skin has no chance to heal before the next insult occurs. After a series of these weak irritant exposures, the skin becomes itchy and develops eczematous dermatitis. Because the stratum corneum protective barrier has been damaged, reverting to less frequent exposures does not necessarily allow the dermatitis to heal; the eczema often becomes chronic and less obviously related to known episodes of irritant damage.

ALLERGIC CONTACT DERMATITIS

The causes and mechanisms for allergic contact dermatitis are quite different. *Allergic contact dermatitis* is an immunologic reaction mediated by T lymphocytes. An example of allergic contact dermatitis is *Rhus* dermatitis (a dermatitis from poison ivy or poison oak). First exposure to an antigen does not elicit dermatitis. If an immune reaction is induced, however, then a secondary contact with it at some later time often produces an extremely itchy, often weeping or blistering eczematous dermatitis in the areas contacted by the allergen. Even small amounts of allergen can elicit dermatitis; the reaction is relatively dose independent.

EVALUATION

The appearance of chronic, cumulative weak irritant dermatitis, allergic contact dermatitis, and other eczemas, like atopic dermatitis, is quite similar. History and location of rash can awaken suspicions of irritations being causal. Patch testing can be used to discover occult antigens or to confirm a suspected diagnosis of allergic contact dermatitis to a particular one. The principle of patch testing is simple: a chemical is applied to skin and the site is observed for development of eczema 48 or 96 hours later. Chemicals for patch testing are usually incorporated into petrolatum in a concentration below that known to produce cutaneous irritation but at a concentration high enough to elicit an allergic reaction in allergic patients.

Although the principle of patch testing and the procedure of patch testing are simple, interpretation and determining relevance are difficult. A number of factors can create false-negative and false-positive reactions. A positive patch test may simply be a historical residual of a previous episode of allergic dermatitis, or it may be irrelevant. Once discovered, the patient must avoid contact by avoidance or allergen substitution, and this often requires special knowledge. Therefore, patch testing is usually done by dermatologists and often by a dermatologist with special interest in contact dermatitis or at tertiary medical centers.

TREATMENT

The treatment of choice for contact dermatitis, whether irritant or allergic, is to eliminate the cause. In most cases, contact with strong irritants is incidental and repeat contact is unexpected if appropriate protective measures are followed. Eliminating the cause of chronic, cumulative weak irritant dermatitis is much more difficult. Multiple environmental mild irritants can also play a role in making the dermatitis become an ongoing one. Protective measures, such as rubber gloves and protective clothing, are often useful. Substitutions sometimes also work, such as substituting a harsh soap for a mild one or discontinuing the use of soap entirely. Applications of medium-strength corticosteroids such as triamcinolone cream or ointment often aid the healing process but are unlikely to cure the process if chronic, cumulative irritations persist. Also, topical corticosteroids make the skin look better than it really is, often leading patients to prematurely cease precautionary maneuvers. After apparent healing, the barrier function of skin requires time to normalize. During this period, protective ointments such as petrolatum alba hasten the process and provide some degree of protection and skin hydration.

Similarly, allergic contact dermatitis ceases when contact with the allergen stops. Because allergic contact dermatitis is very dose independent, decreasing the frequency of exposure is no help. Once contacted, allergic contact dermatitis can continue for 2 to 3 weeks. However, because the allergy is usually specific for a specific chemical, it is often possible to substitute an alternative one. For example, a person allergic to a metal watchband could substitute a leather one. Although protective clothing and gloves theoretically should help, incidental contact or leaching of chemical through gloves often leads to ongoing dermatitis despite these maneuvers.

For acute allergic contact dermatitis such as acute *Rhus* dermatitis, systemic corticosteroids may be indicated. In this case, the diagnosis is rather well established and the systemic corticosteroids prevent much of the morbidity of itch and weeping eczema during the healing process. A usual regimen would be prednisone, 40 to 60 mg every morning for 1 week, and then reducing the daily dose in 20-mg increments over the next week or two. Systemic corticosteroids are generally not used to treat ongoing repetitive exposures to allergens, for example in the workplace. Topical corticosteroids can help, but the ferocity of chronic or acute allergic contact dermatitis usually makes them less than completely effective. If the eczema is weeping or if blisters are present, intermittent applications of compresses just less than dripping wet with saline, tap water, or Burow solution are often quite useful, especially when combined with topical or systemic corticosteroid therapy.

SKIN DISEASES OF PREGNANCY

method of
KIM B. YANCEY, M.D.
Medical College of Wisconsin
Milwaukee, Wisconsin

Skin changes during gestation include normal physiologic manifestations of pregnancy itself, exacerbations of existing skin disorders, coincidentally acquired skin diseases, and specific dermatoses of pregnancy. The last vary widely in their incidence and potential severity and often require specialized care to ensure their correct diagnosis and management.

PRURITIC URTICARIAL PAPULES AND PLAQUES OF PREGNANCY

Diagnosis

Pruritic urticarial papules and plaques of pregnancy (PUPPP, also called *polymorphic eruption of pregnancy*) is a distinctive pruritic eruption that typically presents during the third trimester of gestation in primigravidas. Although the exact incidence of PUPPP is unknown, it is generally regarded to be the most common specific dermatosis of pregnancy.

Lesions in patients with PUPPP almost always begin on the abdomen and typically present in periumbilical striae distensae. Other common sites of involvement include the buttocks and proximal extremities; facial involvement is rare. Lesions in PUPPP consist of small, erythematous, urticarial papules that usually coalesce into large urticarial plaques. Although uncommon, vesicles may be seen. In severe cases, large portions of the body are involved. Although pruritus in patients with PUPPP is characteristically severe, excoriations are uncommon. Biopsy specimens from skin lesions show a superficial or mid-dermal perivascular mononuclear cell infiltrate, dermal edema, and occasional eosinophils. Although not diagnostic, these findings are consistent. Anti–basement membrane autoantibodies are not present in these patients' circulation or skin. Because there is no specific laboratory test for PUPPP, its diagnosis is largely based on its characteristic clinical presentation.

PUPPP usually responds to treatment or resolves soon after delivery; it does not tend to flare post partum, recur in subsequent pregnancies, or develop in patients later exposed to oral contraceptives. PUPPP is not associated with an increased risk of fetal morbidity or fetal and maternal mortality. Lesions in infants born of affected mothers are uncommon. Several studies have demonstrated that patients with PUPPP have an increased average maternal weight gain, a newborn with increased birth weight, and an increased incidence of twinning—findings suggesting that abdominal distention (or a reaction to it) may play a role in the development of PUPPP.

Treatment

PUPPP is best treated by the application of potent topical corticosteroids (i.e., 0.05% fluocinonide [Lidex] or 0.1% triamcinolone acetonide [Kenalog]) four to six times daily. This treatment usually relieves pruritus and halts lesion formation. Less potent topical corticosteroids as well as less frequent treatment schedules should be employed once the eruption is controlled. In patients who are improving, therapy should be gradually tapered rather than abruptly stopped. Patients with severe disease may require treatment with 20 to 40 mg of daily prednisone each morning. This treatment usually promptly controls the eruption as well as the associated pruritus. Prednisone can be tapered fairly quickly (e.g., by 5 mg at 2- to 3-day intervals) in patients with PUPPP. Oral antihistamines are generally less effective in relieving pruritus than is aggressive use of potent topical corticosteroids; the former, however, may facilitate sleep.

HERPES GESTATIONIS

Diagnosis

Herpes gestationis (also called *pemphigoid gestationis*) is a rare, nonviral, vesiculobullous and/or urticarial skin disease of pregnancy and the puerperium. Herpes gestationis has no relationship to an existing or prior viral infection. Instead, its designation refers to the characteristically grouped (i.e., herpetiform) distribution of lesions in patients with this disorder. Herpes gestationis may present during any trimester of pregnancy or begin within 24 to 72 hours of delivery. Interestingly, severe exacerbations of herpes gestationis often occur immediately after delivery, and it is crucial to evaluate all patients carefully at that time (including women whose earlier disease was controlled by treatment or was relatively inactive). Herpes gestationis usually resolves within several weeks of delivery, although temporary flares of disease may develop when patients resume menses or are exposed to oral contraceptives. Herpes gestationis tends to recur in subsequent pregnancies and often presents earlier in such gestations.

Patients typically present with lesions on their abdomen and extremities; interestingly, the umbilicus is often involved. In severe cases, lesions may also affect the palms, soles, chest, and back; mucous membrane involvement is rare. Herpes gestationis is a polymorphic skin disease (i.e., lesions may demonstrate a variety of different morphologies). Classically, lesions consist of erythematous, urticarial papules and plaques that enlarge peripherally and are often rimmed by vesicles and blisters. Lesions are typically pruritic and often interfere with these patients' ability to sleep or perform routine activities comfortably. Infants born to affected mothers also occasionally demonstrate skin lesions of the same character. However, such lesions are usually limited in extent, transient, and require minimal supportive care.

Biopsy specimens of skin lesions demonstrate teardrop-shaped subepidermal blisters and an eosinophil-rich leukocytic infiltrate along the epidermal basement membrane and within the upper dermis. Although characteristic, these findings do not specifically distinguish herpes gestationis from other subepidermal blistering or inflammatory skin diseases. This distinction is typically provided by direct immunofluorescence microscopy studies revealing continuous deposits of C3, the third component of complement, in the epidermal basement membrane of these patients' normal-appearing perilesional skin. These C3 deposits, the immunopathologic hallmark of herpes gestationis, signify the existence of complement-fixing IgG autoantibodies directed against epidermal basement membrane. Current experimental evidence indicates that herpes gestationis is an autoantibody-mediated disease in which subepidermal blisters develop as a consequence of complement activation, mast cell degranulation, and granulocyte accumulation. Although the cause of autoantibody formation in these patients is unknown, the relationship of herpes gestationis to pregnancy and other endocrinologic stimuli (e.g., oral contraceptives) suggests that the pathophysiology of this disease is hormonally modulated.

Studies have shown that only 40% to 60% of patients with herpes gestationis have IgG anti–basement membrane autoantibodies in their circulation. Such findings illustrate the importance of studying these patients' skin for evidence of cutaneous deposits of C3 (rather than testing their sera for evidence of circulating autoantibodies that are demonstrable in a minority of patients). Because these patients' autoantibodies are of the IgG isotype, they are able to cross the placenta, enter the fetal circulation, deposit in fetal skin, and cause skin lesions. Although prior studies suggested that herpes gestationis is associated with an increased risk of fetal morbidity and mortality, this notion is now somewhat controversial. At present, there is general agreement that such pregnancies have an increased risk of prematurity and require specialized care.

Treatment

The goal of therapy in patients with herpes gestationis is to prevent new lesions, relieve intense pruritus, and care for sites of blisters and erosions. Decisions about treatment should be directly based on the character, extent, and severity of each patient's disease. In mild cases, vigorous use of potent topical corticosteroids such as 0.05% fluocinonide (Synalar) or 0.1% triamcinolone acetonide (Aristocort, Kenalog), four to six times each day may control the eruption and relieve symptoms. However, at some point in the course of their disease, most patients require treatment with moderate doses of systemic corticosteroids administered daily. Doses of 20 to 60 mg of prednisone each morning usually relieve pruritus and halt lesion formation within several days. Dividing doses of daily corticosteroids into morning and evening doses (i.e., given every 12 hours) has been used to hasten improvement in patients with severe disease.

Once the eruption and pruritus have been controlled, daily doses of prednisone should be tapered by approximately 5 mg every 1 to 2 weeks until lesions develop or symptoms recur. For postpartum flares of disease, daily prednisone should be restarted (or increased) at a dose of 20 to 40 mg each morning; postpartum patients unable to tolerate oral medications should be treated with an equivalent daily morning dose of hydrocortisone given intravenously. Severe postpartum flares of disease may require as much as 60 mg of prednisone given each morning (used in combination with other systemic immunosuppressive agents in rare cases). In managing this disease, the minimal effective dose of corticosteroids should be employed to control the eruption. Moreover, a modest amount of disease activity (e.g., several new vesicles or urticarial plaques developing every 2–3 days) is acceptable and should not warrant aggressive therapy. Patients using corticosteroids after delivery should be counseled about appropriate nursing practices. If systemic corticosteroids are used during pregnancy, physicians should be alert to possible reversible adrenal insufficiency in newborns. Studies have indicated that there is no significant difference in the incidence of uncomplicated live births in herpes gestationis patients treated with systemic corticosteroids versus those managed with more conservative forms of therapy.

For local care, open wet dressings of saline or tap water for 10 minutes three to four times each day should promote drying and débridement of weeping and/or eroded lesions. Individual blisters should be allowed to remain intact to promote wound protection and re-epithelialization; large blisters can be drained by aspiration. Lesions should be examined carefully for evidence of secondary bacterial infection; such sites should be cultured and treated appropriately. As noted earlier, lesions in newborns are usually transient, require only local care, and resolve as maternal autoantibodies are cleared from these infants' circulation.

PRURIGO GRAVIDARUM

Diagnosis

Prurigo gravidarum (also known as *recurrent cholestasis of pregnancy*) is a hepatic condition that usually occurs late in pregnancy and demonstrates cutaneous manifestations of pruritus and (in severe cases) jaundice. The initial manifestation of prurigo gravidarum is pruritus that may be either localized or generalized in distribution; secondary excoriations may be observed. In general, pruritus exceeds the onset of jaundice by 2 to 4 weeks. Prurigo gravidarum tends to remit soon after delivery but typically recurs in subsequent pregnancies. It may also recur in susceptible individuals after their exposure to oral contraceptives. Although the exact cause of this disorder is unknown, prurigo gravidarum is believed to be hormonally induced in susceptible individuals. Underlying hepatic impairment in these patients is often supported by elevated determinations of liver enzymes (e.g., transaminases, alkaline phosphatase). Some reports have suggested that there is an increased incidence of prematurity, stillbirth, and postpartum hemorrhage in patients with prurigo gravidarum. The incidence of such adverse events is highest in patients with both pruritus and jaundice. The diagnosis of this disorder is based on clinical and laboratory findings as well as on a personal and/or family history.

Treatment

Therapy in patients with prurigo gravidarum is entirely symptomatic. Emollients, topical antipruritics, topical corticosteroids, and, in selected cases, antihistamines with or without cholestyramine (Questran)* may be beneficial. Some have suggested that patients with prurigo gravidarum (because of potential fat malabsorption) receive supplemental vitamin K immediately before delivery to avert the potential of hemorrhage.

IMPETIGO HERPETIFORMIS

Diagnosis

Impetigo herpetiformis is the nosologic designation for a form of pustular psoriasis whose onset is triggered by pregnancy. Although extremely rare, this disease may be life threatening. It is often accompanied by significant constitutional symptoms (e.g., fever, chills, nausea, vomiting, diarrhea); in severe cases, it may be complicated by hypoalbuminemia, hypocalcemia, and tetany. Impetigo herpetiformis typically begins as a series of grouped erythematous plaques rimmed by small sterile pustules. Lesions predominate in flexural areas, expand peripherally, and show new pustules forming at the leading edge. Impetigo herpetiformis may progress to involve substantial portions of the body surface. In advanced cases, involvement of mucous membranes and nail beds also occurs. Biopsy specimens of skin lesions demonstrate alterations identical to those seen in pustular psoriasis.

Treatment

Systemic corticosteroids are the mainstay of treatment for impetigo herpetiformis. Prednisone in daily doses as high as 60 mg each morning is often required to control the eruption; this agent should be tapered slowly to avoid flares of disease. All patients should be closely monitored for evidence of hypoalbuminemia, hypocalcemia, fluid loss, or infection. Patients with impetigo herpetiformis require specialized care and careful monitoring by dermatologists, obstetricians, and pediatricians.

*Not FDA approved for this indication.

PRURITUS ANI AND VULVAE

method of
MARILYNNE McKAY, M.D.
Lovelace Medical Center
Albuquerque, New Mexico

Acute-onset perineal itching is most often due to one of the following: *Candida* infection, irritant and contact dermatitis, urinary tract infection, hemorrhoids, pinworms, and condylomata. Fecal contamination of the anus can be extremely irritating, as can overcleansing; contact dermatitis may develop after application of medications such as neomycin, benzocaine, or those containing preservatives such as ethylenediamine. Cleanliness, the use of bland emollients, and treatment of infection or infestation will generally resolve perineal itching that has been present for a few days to a few weeks.

Diagnostic tests for acute itching should specifically rule out infection, and examination of the female patient should include a vaginal smear for *Candida, Trichomonas,* and bacterial vaginosis (*Gardnerella*). Even though bacterial vaginosis is not typically itchy, the characteristic odor often induces patients to overcleanse or douche with irritating solutions. Recurrent candidiasis is common; culture specimens for *Candida* should be taken from the vagina, and anal culture should be considered in both sexes. Risk factors for *Candida* infection include antibiotics for sinusitis, urinary tract infections, or acne; corticosteroids or other immunosuppressants; HIV infection; and estrogen therapy (oral contraceptives, estrogen replacement). Itching resulting from estrogen deficiency may be important in perimenopausal women, because dry mucosal epithelium is easily irritated. Systemic disorders that may be associated with itching include diabetes, uremia, and hepatitis.

Chronic perineal itching is more difficult to evaluate than itching of recent onset, because the likelihood of discovering an underlying cause is significantly diminished when itching has persisted for months. With chronic pruritus, repeated episodes of itching and scratching cause local thickening of the skin called lichen simplex chronicus (LSC). LSC is identified by a leathery scaly texture with accentuation of normal skin lines. Irritable nerve endings in LSC lesions trigger an "itch-scratch-itch" cycle that typically continues long after the initial insult has resolved. LSC is secondary to rubbing and scratching, and this chronic skin change must be treated separately from the usual primary causes of acute perineal itching. Lichen sclerosus is an entirely different condition that may itch or burn; this dermatosis typically presents as thin, pale, friable skin around the anus and/or vulva.

If there are visible skin changes, a biopsy should be considered to differentiate LSC from other genital dermatoses such as psoriasis, lichen planus, or lichen sclerosus, as well as to rule out malignant neoplasms such as intraepithelial neoplasia (carcinoma in situ) or extramammary Paget disease. A 3- to 4-mm punch biopsy specimen should be taken from the thickest areas of any lesions (plaques, scarring, thickening). Acetowhitening (application of vinegar or 3% to 5% acetic acid for 1 to 2 minutes) can be used to highlight thickened areas if there is a history of genital warts (human papillomavirus [HPV]). If HPV infection is found on the vulva, colposcopy of the vagina and cervix is recommended; if it is found on the anus, proctoscopy should be done. Biopsy of multifocal lesions, typical of HPV-associated intraepithelial neoplasia, should be performed.

THERAPY

As mentioned earlier, the etiology of acute-onset perineal itching is most likely to be discovered by diagnostic testing. Therapy for infections should reduce itching within a few days, but *Candida* may be especially recalcitrant. Women with a tendency for recurrent candidiasis may need to use vaginal creams such as clotrimazole (Gyne-Lotrimin) or terconazole (Terazol) once a week for several months. An effective *Candida* suppression regimen is oral fluconazole (Diflucan), 150 to 200 mg weekly for 2 months, tapering to every 2 weeks for 2 months, then monthly. For relatively mild itching, 1% hydrocortisone cream is effective, especially when it is mixed with pramoxine, a mild anesthetic (Pramosone, Zone-A Forte).

Proper cleansing is the single most important factor in management of perineal itching. After each bowel movement or possible soiling, the patient should cleanse gently with Tucks pads, Balneol Perianal Cleansing or Cetaphil lotion, or a mild soap (Neutrogena, Purpose) followed by cool-water rinses. Plain white unscented toilet tissue is recommended, but Tucks cloth pads are probably better. The patient should be advised to pat the skin gently, because rubbing can be irritating. Tight or occlusive garments should be avoided; this includes plastic-backed panty shields, which can contribute to maceration. Perfumes in these products can be irritating as well. Wearing cotton underwear and avoiding the use of fabric softeners are often helpful.

There is debate over whether spicy or caffeine-containing foods contribute to pruritus ani; probably the best course is to advise the patient to adopt a bland diet at first and then add back one or two items a week to see whether symptoms are exacerbated. Some patients already realize that certain foods worsen their problem. Food allergens are another possible factor, and an elimination trial of milk, tomatoes, corn, and nuts should be considered.

Older patients who complain of burning or stinging rather than itching (and who usually have minimal skin change as a result) may actually suffer from a cutaneous dysesthesia. Low-dose tricylic antidepressants such as amitriptyline (Elavil)* or nortriptyline (Pamelor)* are especially effective. Begin with 10 to 20 mg at bedtime and increase by 10 mg weekly to a dose of 30 to 50 mg/d. It may take 4 to 6 weeks to reach an adequate therapeutic dose. Once improvement has been maintained for 1 or 2 months, the dosage can gradually be tapered.

For LSC, the mainstay is topical corticosteroid therapy. Caution is always advised in using fluorinated topical corticosteroid preparations in intertriginous areas; side effects include skin thinning, striae formation, and rebound erythema and burning. On the other hand, nonfluorinated class VII preparations such as hydrocortisone are unlikely to be effective in severe thickened LSC. Short-term application of a high-potency class I corticosteroid ointment such as betamethasone dipropionate 0.05% (Diprolene) or clobetasol propionate 0.05% (Temovate) can be extremely effective; I prescribe twice-daily applications for 3 to 4 weeks, then once daily for 3 to 4 weeks. Evaluation of the patient at 6 to 8 weeks almost always reveals significant improvement, sometimes for the first time in years. At this point, the potency and/or frequency of application should be decreased, using only the strength necessary to control symptoms. Triamcinolone acetonide 0.1% (Kenalog, Aristocort) may be used as a short-term step-down to maintenance therapy with 1% hydrocortisone. Fluorinated corticosteroids are recommended for use only on LSC or severe lichen sclerosus; they are contraindicated for erythema and burning, both of which can be worsened by their use. Overuse of potent topical corticosteroids on vulvar skin will cause rebound dermatitis with burning and erythema; perianal skin is more likely to develop thinning and telangiectasia.

It often takes 3 or 4 weeks for a topical corticosteroid to begin to affect well-established LSC, and itching typically flares from time to time during the healing process. The patient must be told that this does not mean that the medication is not working, especially if symptom-free intervals indicate that treatment is progressing satisfactorily. The patient's anxiety is often a significant factor in episodic itching, and reassurance is an important part of therapy.

*Not FDA approved for this indication.

URTICARIA

method of
JERE D. GUIN, M.D.
University of Arkansas
Little Rock, Arkansas

Urticaria represents a complex of conditions that are characterized by wheals. Angioedema is a deeper form of swelling that may or may not be associated with hives. The approach to treatment will be determined by the form of urticaria present. Classifications vary in complexity, but most patients will have some form of acute, chronic, physical, or contact urticaria or urticarial vasculitis.

EVALUATION

Acute and chronic urticarias may or may not be associated with dermographism or angioedema, and they are separated by lasting more or less than a certain duration, usually 6 to 8 weeks. Physical urticarias are easily recognized by their location, pattern, and history and, not infrequently, by a characteristic lesion, such as the linear wheals in dermographism or the 3- to 5-mm wheals with a large flare seen in cholinergic urticaria. Often, these conditions can be confirmed by relatively simple tests. Contact urticaria is common, but often it goes unrecognized because it is not presented for medical treatment.

Urticarial vasculitis is a special case. It represents an immune-complex vasculitis involving complement consumption. A diligent search for an underlying problem is indicated in patients with this condition, and its treatment is very different from that of most other conditions manifesting as urticaria. Lesions often persist for 1 to 3 days, leaving a discolored, scaly, or purpuric mark; frequently, the lesions burn or sting rather than itch. Other symptoms found include arthralgias, gastrointestinal complaints, fever, adenopathy, erythema multiforme–like lesions, and neuralgic disorders. Laboratory abnormalities include an elevated erythrocyte sedimentation rate, sometimes a depressed complement level, and a histologic appearance of vasculitis in a high percentage of patients. The latter may be the most reliable laboratory criterion, but no one finding is absolute.

The history in acute and chronic urticaria should concentrate especially on medications and, in cases of the chronic type, the physician should tactfully and empathetically look for emotional stress. One should also identify previous therapy and vasodilating influences. Treatment of chronic urticaria is both challenging and time-consuming, but it should not be considered hopeless. Searches for a specific cause are indicated, although as few as 10% may be positive if one eliminates emotional causes and physical urticarias, in which the cause is obvious and the eruption is identifiable. A more aggressive approach is probably indicated for persons who are unresponsive to treatment. A history of a prior urticarial reaction to penicillin indicates the need for a trial of avoidance of dairy products, which may be penicillin contaminated. Internal disease such as hepatitis, rheumatologic and other autoimmune disease, parasitic infestation, malignancy, hepatitis, or a focus of infection may rarely be found as an underlying cause in a specific patient, but workups for problems should be ordered on a case-by-case basis, because extensive testing for routine screening has been shown not to be cost-effective. In my experience when a cause for chronic urticaria is found, it is most commonly a drug and often after a totally negative history on a number of earlier occasions. In some cases, such as estrogens, progesterone, or a corticosteroid, the drug might not be suspected.

In chronic urticaria, certain dietary ingredients, although not obvious to the patient, may represent a source of aggravation. Use of a printed questionnaire in taking the history allows the patient to mark the various foods containing salicylates, benzoates, and azo dyes (especially FD&C Yellow No. 5 and Yellow No. 6). In patients who demonstrate an immediate skin test reaction to yeast, it may also help to look for foods containing yeast and perhaps tyramine; this can also be accomplished with the same printed form. Such dietary factors probably do not represent a source of allergy but are probably pharmacologically aggravating.

Identifying the presence (or absence) of emotional stress can also be helpful in chronic urticaria. This requires tact and empathy on the part of the physician, and it is best done personally in a quiet environment, where an unhurried and sympathetic attitude to the patient's plight demonstrates genuine care and concern for what is often an impressively stressful situation. Formal psychological testing may help prove that stress is present, but this is not usually necessary. Developing a relationship of trust and understanding is helpful in another way. Compliance with the routine required of patients with chronic urticaria is difficult at best, and the patient is much more likely to be compliant if the physician is perceived as being genuinely involved.

ACUTE URTICARIA

It is obvious that a known cause should be eliminated whenever possible. Although diet can be important as a source of allergy in acute urticaria, patients with acute urticaria due to food allergy are not often a problem because the patient generally identifies the offending food. Traditionally, treatment in adults with oral cyproheptadine (Periactin), 4 mg four times daily, or hydroxyzine (Atarax),* 10 to 25 mg three or four times daily, has been helpful in controlling symptoms, although most today start with nonsedating antihistamines, as in chronic urticaria. Intramuscular or intravenous diphenhydramine (Benadryl), 25 to 50 mg, can be helpful in severe reactions. When a known cause can be found and eliminated (as in an urticarial drug reaction), one might consider a course of oral corticosteroid therapy for those without contraindications. Initial dosage depends on severity, but a typical course might comprise an initial dose of 30 to 40 mg of prednisone by mouth daily after breakfast and tapered over a 10- to 14-day period.

Severe laryngeal edema or other life-threatening situations may require subcutaneous or intramuscular administration of 0.3 to 0.5 mL of 1:1000 epinephrine. Intravenous use, limited to severe anaphylaxis with signs of shock, requires dilution to 1:10,000 concentration, administering 1 mg at a time and repeating if no response is obtained. Maintenance of an airway may require intubation or even tracheostomy, and maintaining an intravenous saline drip has been recommended for patients with severe reactions.

CHRONIC URTICARIA

Adults have been traditionally treated with oral cyproheptadine (Periactin), 4 mg four times daily, or hydroxyzine (Atarax),* 10 to 25 mg three or four times daily, or both, with drowsiness being a limiting factor. For most people who are sensitive to the sedative effects or intolerant to the anticholinergic effects of antihistamines, fexofenadine (Allegra), 60 mg twice daily, cetirizine (Zyrtec), 10 mg daily, or loratadine (Claritin), 10 mg daily, by mouth are also preferred by the patient. Unresponsive patients sometimes improve with either oral doxepin (Sinequan)* or amitriptyline (Elavil).* This is started with a relatively low dose, perhaps 25 mg at bedtime or 10 mg three times daily, but an effective dose is usually somewhat higher. However, one must be wary of many doxepins colored with FD&C Yellow No. 6, which can be a problem. These agents are much better antihistamines than most other tricyclic antidepressants; for patients who already are taking another such medication, it may be helpful to substitute doxepin. Addition of an H_2 blocker should theoretically reduce the effect of histamine on blood vessels but adversely affect mast cells, which form histamine and other inflammatory mediators. This may explain the conflicting reports on the effectiveness of such treatment in chronic urticaria.

Leukotriene receptor antagonists are sometimes

*Not FDA approved for this indication.

helpful in anecdotal reports. Of these, montelukast (Singulair)* seems preferable at an adult dosage of 10 mg/d.

Elimination of vasodilating factors such as heat, exercise, and alcohol and the avoidance of nonspecific histamine-releasing agents such as opiates are indicated. A putative association with *Helicobacter pylori* has been difficult to establish and may be largely due to the associated flushing tendency.

Exposure to nonsteroidal anti-inflammatory drugs, aspirin and dietary salicylates, and certain azo dyes, especially FD&C Yellow No. 5 (tartrazine) and FD&C Yellow No. 6, tend to aggravate the problem, especially in more severe cases and at higher levels of challenge. Diet lists of foods high in salicylate content are available, and foods and over-the-counter medications containing FD&C Yellow No. 5 or FD&C Yellow No. 6 should have this on the label.

Ketotifen† looks promising but is not yet available. Other treatments that have been used in a few cases include stanazolol,* acupuncture, plasmapheresis, intravenous immunoglobulin,* and cyclosporin (Sandimmune).*

URTICARIAL VASCULITIS

Urticarial vasculitis is frequently associated with an underlying cause including medications, hepatitis C and B, mononucleosis, a variety of rheumatologic conditions, and immune dysregulation after therapy for Hodgkin disease. There are uncontrolled reports of benefit with oral colchicine, 0.6 mg twice daily; dapsone (Avlosulfon),* 100 mg daily after checking for G6PD deficiency; indomethacin (Indocin),* 75 to 200 mg daily in divided doses; or hydroxychloroquine (Plaquenil),* 200 mg twice daily. I have seen good results with colchicine. The minimal effective dose of prednisone is likely to be high, so another agent would seem preferable for initial treatment. Cyclophosphamide (Cytoxan)* has been used, although it is usually reserved for more severe forms of vasculitis.

PHYSICAL URTICARIAS

Dermographism can usually be adequately controlled with normal doses of loratadine, 10 mg daily, cetirizine, 10 mg daily, or fexofenadine, 60 mg twice daily, or low doses of cyproheptadine or hydroxyzine along with avoidance of unnecessary trauma and vasodilating factors, especially heat. For an adult, one might start with cyproheptadine, 2 to 4 mg four times daily, or hydroxyzine,* 10 mg three or four times daily by mouth, and adjust the dosage to the patient's response. In some cases, 2 to 4 mg daily of oral cyproheptadine is adequate for maintenance. Treatment is directed at preventing the response to injury. The duration of the eruption is short so one cannot wait until the eruption appears to treat it. Effectiveness of treatment can be measured by controlled stroking of skin of the upper back.

*Not FDA approved for this indication.
†Not available in the United States.

Some cases of cold urticaria may require a serologic test for syphilis and a test for cryoproteins to rule out symptomatic cold urticaria, but the most common cause is essential acquired cold urticaria, which can be treated in adults with avoidance of cold and the administration of oral cyproheptadine (Periactin), 4 mg four times daily, cetirizine, 10 mg daily, or ketotifen (Zaditor).* When an IgE-mediated allergy is known, elimination of exposure (in the case of penicillin allergy, avoidance of dairy products) is sometimes associated with clearing. Control here can be measured with change in response to a 5-minute application of an ice cube in a plastic bag.

Recommended treatment for cholinergic urticaria involves avoidance of sweating, avoidance of aspirin, and oral cetirizine, 10 mg daily, or hydroxyzine, 25 mg three times daily. Ultraviolet light can help, but this may not be appropriate for those who do not tolerate it. Danazol* and β-blockers* have also been used.

Aquagenic pruritus reportedly improves with antihistamines and erythema doses of ultraviolet B (UVB) light, and graduated exposure to ultraviolet A (UVA), UVB, and psoralen and UVA plus antihistamines raises the threshold in at least some cases of solar urticaria.

Acute treatment of hereditary angioedema sometimes requires maintenance of an airway and intravascular volume. Long-term treatment is with oral anabolic steroid therapy, especially danazol (Danocrine),* 200 mg twice or three times daily, tapered to 200 mg/d or alternate days according to the patient's response. An alternate drug is stanozolol (Winstrol),* 2 mg three times daily initially, reduced to 2 mg/d. The maintenance dose is individual, but there is a high incidence of flares on less than 2 mg/d. About 50% of women treated with 2 mg/d will have an androgenic effect; 20% will show this effect at 0.5 mg/d, a dose that is not adequate to prevent episodes in most patients. Both drugs require monitoring of blood pressure, and birth control is required in sexually active females.

Delayed pressure urticaria and nonhereditary angioedema associated with lymphoproliferative disease may also respond to this treatment approach, but acquired angioedema without lymphoproliferative disease (with antibodies to C1INH) may not, and corticosteroids have been recommended. For delayed pressure urticaria, montelukast and topical corticosteroid therapy have reportedly been helpful. Sulfasalazine (Azulfidine),* starting at 500 mg/d and increasing 500 mg weekly up to 4000 mg, has been used as a corticosteroid-sparing agent.

CONTACT URTICARIA

Contact urticaria may be immunologic or nonimmunologic, but treatment of the latter in most cases

*Not FDA approved for this indication.

is not a problem, because most patients do well by avoiding the offending substance. The mediators for contact urticaria vary, and antihistamines are helpful for some agents but not others. Nonsteroidal anti-inflammatory agents benefit nonimmunologic contact urticaria from several mediators but have less effect on nonimmunologic contact urticaria from cinnamic aldehyde. Antihistamines do not markedly reduce nonimmunologic contact urticaria from these three mediators but may reduce its severity from many other mediators.

Immunologic contact urticaria to latex gloves and other rubber objects has become a widespread problem in health care workers and their patients. Contact with many protein materials and certain medications can cause wheals, eczema, and even anaphylaxis requiring immediate treatment, as with acute urticaria. Glove powder may be an allergen itself and may carry the latex allergen. The most dangerous exposure is usually mucosal. One should be especially circumspect with atopic health care workers and persons with spina bifida, urogenital anomalies, or paraplegia. Latex-sensitive persons should also avoid certain foods, such as banana, kiwi, avocado, and chestnut. Even medications from rubber-stoppered bottles can be a problem. Use of non-latex gloves and supplies and latex-free resuscitation equipment is mandatory.

Contact urticaria comprises a diverse group of immediate "urticarial" reactions, and it includes reactions following exposure to certain plants and animals (e.g., nettles, jellyfish, and caterpillars). Pretreatment with topical corticosteroids also helps in prevention but does not totally eliminate the reaction. For most patients with contact urticaria, avoidance of the cause is the most important treatment.

PIGMENTARY DISORDERS

method of
KOWICHI JIMBOW, M.D., PH.D.
Sapporo Medical University School of Medicine
Sapporo, Japan

Red, yellow, brown, and blue are the four major colors of human skin. Of these colors, brown is the major determinant of the difference in skin color, primarily reflecting the presence of melanin. Melanin is produced within the melanosomal compartment of the melanocyte. Increased melanin pigmentation of the skin (hyperpigmentation, hypermelanosis) is primarily related to the increased synthesis; increased size; and altered shape, type, and color of melanosomes. It is also related to their distribution patterns in melanocytes and keratinocytes.

In contrast, hypopigmentation (hypomelanosis) of the skin is related to the absence of (amelanosis) or decreased function of the melanocyte, which may result in the decreased synthesis; decreased size; altered shape, type, and color of melanosomes and their distribution patterns in melanocytes and keratinocytes. The partnership of a melanocyte and a neighboring group of keratinocytes is called an *epidermal melanin unit*. Abnormal pigmentation (*hypermelanosis* [brown] or *hypomelanosis* [white]) reflects the alteration of the epidermal melanin unit. Hypermelanosis, however, also includes the blue or slate-gray color of the skin, which derives from abnormal accumulation of melanosomes within the dermis, which reflects the presence of abnormal melanocytes in the dermis (*dermal melanocytosis*) or incontinence (dropping off) of epidermal melanosomes to the dermis. The classification for hypermelanoses and hypomelanoses is presented in Table 1. Clinically, this approach may be relevant in that it is often possible to distinguish epidermal hypermelanosis from dermal hypermelanosis after clinical examination and inspection with a Wood lamp. Epidermal pigmentation is accentuated under Wood lamp examination, whereas dermal pigmentation becomes less prominent.

The two components of hypopigmentation—decreased or absent melanin pigmentation—can also be differentiated by a Wood lamp examination. The distinction of hyperpigmentation as well as hypopigmentation by a Wood lamp examination has therapeutic implications in that one can choose the most effective medical treatment based on the location of abnormal pigmentation in the skin. For example, most topical treatment modalities are best suited to treat epidermal causes of hyperpigmentation, whereas surgical options (e.g., laser surgery) are effective for both epidermal and dermal types of hyperpigmentation.

Not all the congenital pigmentary disorders, particularly hypomelanosis, are obvious initially. In a fair-skinned child who is not exposed to sunlight in the first year or early years of life, hypopigmented lesions that are, in fact, congenital, may be thought to be acquired. A white infant born in the late fall may not become tanned for at least a year; hence, the hypomelanosis may be invisible until the child goes outside to play and becomes tanned after sun exposure.

MELASMA

Melasma is a common, patchy, irregular, tanned brown pigmentation that is usually located on the face of women. It occurs exclusively in sun-exposed areas and is more apparent during and after sun exposure and less obvious in winter months when there is little sun exposure. Multiple factors have been reported to affect the degree of melasma pigmentation: pregnancy, oral contraceptives, endocrine dysfunction, genetic factors, medication, nutritional deficiency, and hepatic dysfunction.

Currently, hydroquinone (Melanex) is most commonly used for topical therapy of melasma. Treatment modalities include the topical application of hydroalcoholic lotion of hydroquinone at the concentrations of 2% to 5%. The decrease in skin color may be observed after 4 weeks of therapy, and the optimal depigmentation is achieved after 6 to 10 weeks of therapy. The effectiveness of hydroquinone is enhanced by concomitant daily use of an effective broad-spectrum sunscreen. However, the daily and prolonged use of hydroquinone at high concentrations (4%–5%) produces a high incidence of primary irritant reactions. Good results can be obtained with the combination of tretinoin (Retin-A)* 0.1%, hydro-

*Not FDA approved for this indication.

TABLE 1. **Major Pigmentary Disorders**

Hyperpigmentation	
Epidermal / Brown	
CONGENITAL	ACQUIRED
POEMS syndrome	Suntan
Albright syndrome	Melasma
Café au lait macules	Freckles
Becker's melanosis	Solar lentigo
Nevus spilus	Lentigo maligna
Lentigenes syndrome (e.g., Peutz-Jeghers syndrome, centrofacial neurodysraphic lentiginosis, Moynahan's syndrome, LAMB syndrome, Sotos' syndrome)	Postinflammatory (porphyria cutanea tarda, lichen planus, tinea versicolor, atopic dermatitis, arsenical ingestion, lupus erythematosus, pellagra, etc.)
Urticaria pigmentosa	Macular amyloidosis
Cronkhite-Canada syndrome	Drugs (e.g., phenytoin, contraceptives, estrogens, bleomycin, psorlaen, tar, cyclophosphamide)
Acanthosis nigricans (benign familial)	Systemic diseases (hyperthyroidism, renal insufficiency, biliary cirrhosis)
Dyschromatosis (universalis/symmetrica)	Addison's disease
Acropigmentatio reticularis	Hemochromatosis
	Acanthosis nigricans (malignant)
Dermal / Blue, Slate Gray	
CONGENITAL	ACQUIRED
Nevus of Ota	Riehl's melanosis
Extrasaccral Mongolian spots	Melasma
Incontinentia pigmenti	Fixed drug eruption
Franceschetti-Jadassohn syndrome	Ochronosis
	Erythema dyschromicum perstans
	Chronic nutritional insufficiency
	Metastatic melanoma with melanogenuria
	Tattoos
	Drugs (e.g., minocycline [Minocin], amiodarone [Cordarone], phenothiazine, antimelarials, chlorpromazine [Thorazine])
	Heavy metals (e.g. bismuth, chrysiasis, argyria)
	Hemosiderin
	Alkaptonuria
	Erythema abigne
Hypopigmentation	
Epidermal / White	
CONGENITAL	ACQUIRED
Piebaldism	Vitiligo
Tuberous sclerosis	Postinflammatory (e.g., lupus erythematosus, eczema, psoriasis)
Albinism	
Phenylketonuria	Chemicals (e.g., arsenicals, chloroquine, hydroquinone, glucocorticoids, retinoids)
Nevus depigmentosus	
Ataxia telangiectasia	Pityriasis alba
Nevus anemics	Leprosy
Nevus of Ito (incontinentia pigmenti achromians)	Sarcoidosis
Waardenburg's syndrome	Syphilis
Ziprowski-Margolis syndrome	Tinea versicolor
Woolf's syndrome	Burns
Idiopathis guttate hypomelanosis	Scleroderma
Menke's steely hair disease	Systemic diseases (e.g., Addison's disease, hypopituitarism, hypothyroidism)
Hemocystinuria	
Dermal / White	
CONGENITAL	ACQUIRED
None	None

quinone (4.0%), and triamcinolone acetonide* (0.025%). Formulations containing 2% hydroquinone and 0.05% or 0.1% tretinoin can also result in the best lightening effect in melasma. At high concentrations (>1.5%), tretinoin can be an irritant. Patients with macules of dermal melasma do not respond satisfactorily to hydroquinone therapy.

Azelaic acid (Azelex)* is a dicarboxylic acid originally isolated from *Pityrosporum ovale*, the organism responsible for pityriasis versicolor. It has been shown to be a competitive inhibitor of tyrosinase in vitro. It can be used successfully in the treatment of melasma. Azelaic acid is associated with fewer side effects, however, which suggest that its use might be beneficial if prolonged treatment is necessary. Kojic acid† is a fungal metabolite produced by *Aspergillus*

*Not FDA approved for this indication.

†Not available in the United States.

and *Penicillium* spp. It is structurally related to maltol. Like maltol, it is a good chelator of transition metal ions and has been shown to inhibit tyrosinase activity. Kojic acid was shown to inhibit tyrosinase isolated from black goldfish and standard goldfish and to suppress melanogenesis in cultured pigment cells. When kojic acid was ingested by the fish, the black goldfish became almost yellow-brown. Kojic acid, however, has a high sensitizing potential, and a comparatively high frequency of contact sensitivity has been observed. Phenolic thioethers such as 4S-cysteaminylphenol* (*N*-acetyl or *N*-propionyl) represent a new family of depigmenting compounds related to phenols. These agents derive from sulfur homologues of phenols, and are selectively melanocytotoxic. A preliminary clinical study using a 4% preparation of *N*-acetyl 4S-cysteaminylphenol was conducted on patients with melasma. Marked-to-moderate improvement was seen. The compound appeared less irritating to the skin than hydroquinone. Side effects were minimal. The depigmentation was associated with decreased numbers of functioning melanocytes and melanosomes transferred to keratinocytes. Both *N*-acetyl and *N*-propionyl 4S-cysteaminylphenols are the tyrosinase substrate. The in vivo study indicated that *N*-acetyl and *N*-propionyl 4S-cysteaminylphenols have both cytostatic and cytocidal effects on melanocytes.

Chemical peels, also referred to as *chemexfoliation,* have become an established technique for improving or treating hyperpigmentation disorders, including facial melasma. Superficial, medium, and deep chemical peels are often used to treat melasma. Topical application of glycoric acid* in the form of chemical peels is a safe and effective method for treating hyperpigmentation disorders. The effectiveness of peels can be enhanced by the use of 10% to 15% glycoric acid lotion plus hydroquinone (2%). Resorcinol,* an isomer of catechols, at 15% concentration results in medium-depth peels and has been useful in the treatment of patients suffering from not only melasma but also freckles and solar lentigenes. Kojic acid chemical peels at 2% concentration can be performed if hyperpigmentation of melasma persists after initial kojic acid gel treatment. Kojic acid peels may be less drying to the skin than glycoric acid chemical peels.

Salicylic acid chemical peels, at concentrations of 20% to 30%, can also be used for hyperpigmentation in melasma. Moderate to significant improvement was observed in patients suffering from postinflammatory hyperpigmentation. Trichloracetic acid can be used when treatment of hyperpigmentation by kojic acid peels is not satisfactory. Trichloracetic acid medium-depth peels can be used as an adjuvant to treat diffuse, persistent hyperpigmentation of melasma lesions.

FRECKLES (EPHELIDES)

Freckles are small, usually less than 0.5 cm in diameter, discrete brown macules that appear on the sun-exposed skin. In freckled skin, there is no increase in the number of functioning melanocytes, but these melanocytes are highly dendritic, strongly DOPA-positive, and have many stage IV mature melanosomes. In addition to topical depigmenting agents with or without chemical peels, freckles can be treated with other methods such as gentle freezing with liquid nitrogen. For dark-skinned patients, the lesions need to be carefully frozen because of the risk of permanent depigmentation.

Freckles respond to a variety of pulsed and continuous-wave lasers. The most commonly used pulsed lasers are the frequency-doubled Q-switched Nd:YAG laser at 532 nm, the Q-switched ruby laser (694 nm), the Alexandrite laser, and the pulsed dye green laser (510 nm).

SOLAR LENTIGENES

Solar or senile lentigenes are dark brown macules, usually 1 to 3 cm in diameter, that occur on the chronically sun-exposed surface of elderly individuals. They must be carefully distinguished histologically from lentigo maligna. The treatment of solar lentigenes is primarily the same as that of freckles. Laser treatment, previously listed, is effective. Liquid nitrogen treatment is also effective but often leaves some marginal pigmentation and may also cause depigmentation in dark-skinned patients.

CAFÉ AU LAIT MACULES

Café au lait macules are flat, pigmented lesions with a uniform pale brown color, serrated or irregular margins, and variable sizes. They are present in 10% of the normal population and can be seen in association with neurocutaneous syndromes such as neurofibromatosis (NF), Albright syndrome, tuberous sclerosis, Silver-Russell syndrome, Westerhof syndrome, Watson syndrome, and Bloom syndrome. Multiple lesions are especially common in NF of Recklinghausen disease (NF type 1). Café au lait macules can be good candidates for treatment with Q-switched lasers because submicrosecond laser pulses interact selectively with melanosomes in melanocytes and in keratinocytes of the epidermis. However, treatment with Q-switched lasers may not consistently yield successful results. Complete and partial clearance followed by recurrence may appear in some cases. Nonetheless, Q-switched ruby or Q-switched Nd:YAG lasers are the treatment of choice.

NEVUS SPILUS

Nevus spilus is a circumscribed tan-colored macule containing smaller darkly pigmented spots or papules. Nevus spilus can be treated as a combined disease of a café au lait macule with small junctional nevi. Q-switched lasers are the treatment of choice; however, careful follow-up is necessary because melanoma has been reported to occur in nevus spilus.

*Not available in the United States.

VITILIGO

Vitiligo is a common idiopathic or acquired disease with loss of normal melanin pigments and functioning melanocytes from otherwise healthy looking skin. When it is acquired, a genetic predisposition is considered. The leukoderma of vitiligo does not contain any functioning melanocytes. At present, there is no universally effective medical or surgical treatment for vitiligo. However, a number of active therapeutic approaches are known to be effective. Oral or topical application of psoralen plus ultraviolet A (PUVA) is the most popular therapy for vitiligo. Although the use of methoxsalen (Oxsoralen) is the treatment standard, the new ultramicronized methoxsalen (Oxsoralen-Ultra) has been introduced. It has a faster bioavailability and requires less time in waiting for the drug absorption before PUVA than that of traditional methoxsalen. Intradermal and topical corticosteroids have been used to treat vitiligo with mixed results. Recently, successful treatment for vitiligo has been reported with topical application of pseudocatalase and calcium followed by short-term, ultraviolet B-wave light exposure. This treatment appears to rely on the presence of tyrosinase activity in the depigmented epidermis. Furthermore, surgical grafting of an autologous epidermal sheet or cultured melanocytes (often combined with keratinocyte co-cultures) has been introduced to repigment the depigmented areas where PUVA is ineffective. PUVA therapy after autologous skin grafting can enhance repigmenting efficiency. Although PUVA with or without surgery is a useful tool in vitiligo treatment, one should also attempt to assess the degree of psychological impairment caused by vitiligo. In addition, normal skin of vitiligo can be totally depigmented by monobenzyl ether of hydroquinone to match the skin color in certain patients with generalized vitiligo.

ALBINISM

Albinism refers to genetic abnormalities of melanin synthesis associated with a normal number and structure of melanocytes. Reduced melanin synthesis in the melanocytes of the skin, hair, and eyes is termed *oculocutaneous albinism*, and hypopigmentation primarily involving the retinal pigment epithelium of the eye is termed *ocular albinism*. The precise definition of albinism includes specific changes in the development and function of the eye and optic nerves, and ocular changes are necessary to make the diagnosis. The ocular system changes in albinism include a reduction in iris and retinal pigments, foveal hypoplasia, misrouting of the optic fibers at the chiasm, nystagmus, and alternating strabismus.

Any child or adult with cutaneous hypopigmentation must have these ocular changes to make the diagnosis of albinism. Once it is established that the individual has albinism, then the determination of the specific type can be made with a family history and clinical examination. A family history of affected males related through unaffected females, indicative of X-linked inheritance, is consistent with ocular albinism. For oculocutaneous albinism, the family history is usually negative or there is an affected sibling of either gender, indicative of autosomal recessive inheritance (Table 2).

TABLE 2. **Classification of Albinism**

Type	Subtypes	Gene Locus	Includes	Mechanism
Related to Mutations of Tyrosinase Family Genes				
OCA1	OCA1A	Tyrosinase	Tyrosinase-negative OCA	Inactive/missing enzyme due to tyrosinase gene mutation
	OCA1B	Tyrosinase	Minimal pigment OCA	Partially active enzyme due to tyrosinase gene mutation
			Platinum OCA Yellow OCA Temperature-sensitive OCA Autosomal recessive OCA	
OCA2		P	Tyrosinase-positive OCA impaired tyrosine transport? Brown OCA Autosomal recessive OCA (some)	Partially active enzyme due to tyrosinase gene mutation
OCA3		TRP1	Rufous OCA Red OCA	Partially active enzyme due to TRP-1 gene mutation
OA1		OA1	X-linked OA	Partially active enzyme due to tyrosinase gene mutation
Unrelated to Mutations of Tyrosinase Family Genes				
HPS		HPS	Hermansky–Pudlak syndrome—mutation of AP-3, leading to impaired vesicular transport	Active enzyme
CHS		CHS	Chediak–Higashi syndrome—mutation of PI3-kinase, leading to impaired vesicular transport	Active enzyme

Abbreviations: AP = adaptor protein; OA = ocular albinism; OCA = oculocutaneous albinism; PI3-kinase, phosphatidyl inositol 3-kinase; TRP1 = tyrosine-related protein 1.

All individuals with albinism should be under the care of an ophthalmologist and should undergo annual examinations until they reach adulthood. Most are hyperopic or myopic and may have significant astigmatism. Protection from the ultraviolet radiation of the sun is necessary for individuals with oculocutaneous albinism, who have little or no skin and hair pigment. The care is the same as that for individuals without albinism who have type I or II skin and includes the use of sunblock, hats, and long sleeves and avoidance of the sun.

SUNBURN

method of
BARBARA A. GILCHREST, M.D.
Boston University School of Medicine
Boston, Massachusetts

and

HENRY W. LIM, M.D.
Henry Ford Hospital
Detroit, Michigan

Sunburn is the inflammatory reaction that follows sufficient sun exposure or irradiation from another ultraviolet (UV) light source. The most prominent component is erythema (rubor or redness), but, like all inflammatory reactions, sunburn also includes *tumor* (swelling), *dolor* (pain), and loss of function.

The sunburn action spectrum, or efficiency of different wavelengths of light in producing sunburn, was determined experimentally in human subjects nearly 20 years ago. Of light penetrating the Earth's ozone layer and thus present at the Earth's surface, the shortest and most energetic photons are most effective, with the erythemic efficiency of UV wavelengths decreasing by approximately four orders of magnitude (10,000-fold) between 300 and 400 nm. For convenience, the UV portion of the electromagnetic spectrum is divided into UVC (200–290 nm), so-called germicidal light, not present in terrestrial sunlight but emitted by germicidal lamps, welding arches, and other man-made sources; UVB (290–320 nm), so-called sunburn spectrum UV, wavelengths that penetrate the earth's ozone layer but are not transmitted through window glass; and UVA (320–400 nm), so-called black light or near UV, wavelengths transmissible through glass and responsible for drug-induced photosensitivity. Beyond the UV spectrum is the visible light spectrum (400–700 nm), whose biologic role is largely confined to vision, followed by infrared energy or heat. UVB constitutes on average approximately 0.5% of the sun's energy reaching the Earth's surface but is responsible for most of sun's effects on normal skin. Its intensity varies markedly over the course of the day and in temperate climates from winter to summer. UVA constitutes approximately 5% of the sun's energy at the Earth's surface, varies relatively little in intensity over the course of the day or year, and appears to have less impact on normal skin, although possible UVA contributions to chronic photodamage are an area of active investigation. UVA is, however, principally responsible for drug photosensitivity reactions that may include exaggerated sunburn.

Photons (packets of light energy) have biologic effect only when absorbed by a molecule in the tissue, termed a *chromophore*. In general, depth of penetration of photons into tissue is inversely related to their wavelength. UVC photons penetrate only into the superficial epidermis; UVB photons penetrate well into the epidermis, with approximately 10% entering the dermis in fair-skinned individuals; and UVA photons penetrate even deeper, with approximately half the incident energy reaching the dermis. Sunburn is thus a fairly superficial injury, concentrated in the epidermis and very superficial dermis within 100 to 200 μm of the skin surface.

CLINICAL AND HISTOLOGIC FEATURES

Erythema

The minimal exposure necessary to produce perceptible redness in skin is termed the *minimal erythema dose* (MED). Depending on the individual's complexion and sun intensity, at midday this sun exposure may be as little as 5 to 10 minutes or more than an hour. A 3-MED exposure usually produces bright red erythema that is painful to touch. An 8- to 10-MED exposure usually produces blistering and swelling in addition to painful erythema and may also be accompanied by fever, leukocytosis, and malaise. After a sufficient sun exposure, the sunburn reaction is delayed, with redness rarely perceptible before 3 and 4 hours. The erythema usually peaks at 12 to 24 hours and then gradually resolves over an additional 1 to 3 days (Table 1). In older individuals, the erythema tends to be less intense but may be more persistent. In all but extremely fair-skinned persons, the erythema is followed days later by tanning; and severe sunburn is usually also followed by *desquamation* (peeling) of the damaged epidermis.

UVA-induced erythema is rarely seen outside experimental laboratory settings, with the exception of tanning parlors, most of which use lamps greatly enriched in UVA compared with sunlight. This erythema is biphasic, with an immediate component that decreases over several hours after the irradiation and a delayed component that peaks between 6 and 24 hours. Similar to UVB-induced erythema, UVA-induced erythema in older individuals also tends to be more persistent. More severe reactions tend to peak later and persist longer. Sunburn-like phototoxicity reactions, for example, due to psoralen-UVA (PUVA), a treatment for psoriasis and other dermatoses, or to ingestion of a photosensitizing medication such as doxycycline or certain psychotropic medications, may peak as late as 48 hours and persist considerably longer.

Thus, a clinically severe sunburn evaluated less than 12 hours after the exposure usually warrants more aggressive therapy than an equally intense reaction evaluated 24 hours or longer after the causative exposure.

Loss of Function

Sunburned skin is strikingly deficient in two important functions: thermoregulation and immune surveillance. The fixed vasodilation that characterizes sunburn prevents the skin's extensive vascular network from expanding and contracting to dissipate or conserve core body heat appropriately. This peripheral vascular compromise is compounded by central temperature dysregulation due to interleukin-1 (IL-1) release from the inflamed skin.

In skin, Langerhans cells normally present antigens to lymphocytes and thus alert the immune system to the presence of microbes, foreign chemicals, or malignant cells. After UV irradiation, the number of Langerhans cells is

TABLE 1. **Acute Cutaneous Effect of Ultraviolet Radiation**

Cutaneous Effect	UVB (290–320 nm)	UVA (320–400 nm)
Erythema	Onset at 3–4 h; peaks at 12–24 h	Present immediately after exposure; second peak at 6–24 h
Immediate pigment darkening		Fades within minutes to hours
Persistent pigment darkening (tanning)	Peaks at 3–5 days; fades over days to weeks	Blends with immediate pigment darkening; plateaus at 2–24 h; lasts for days
Skin thickening	Moderate	Minimal

reduced markedly for several days, resulting in a temporary state of immunosuppression or even immune tolerance. The clinical consequences of these immune deficits are poorly understood. Some have suggested they prevent autosensitization to DNA during the period it is structurally altered by the presence of UV-induced photoproducts. Other evidence suggests they may prevent immune rejection of incipient skin cancers or predispose to chronic skin infections such as leishmaniasis, a disease prevalent in sunny climates.

Histologic Changes

UVB irradiation produces *apoptotic* ("suicide") cells with pyknotic nuclei and eosinophilic cytoplasm (known as *sunburn cells*) in the epidermis. Sunburn cells appear within 30 minutes and reach a maximum at 24 hours. In addition, epidermal spongiosis or edema is noted. There is also a significant decrease in epidermal Langerhans cells, most prominent at 24 hours. UVA irradiation does not usually induce sunburn cells nor reduce Langerhans cells, but spongiosis does occur.

Both UVB and UVA transiently degranulate dermal mast cells. Endothelial cell swelling and mixed perivascular infiltrate also occurs 24 to 48 hours after irradiation, an effect that is more prominent after UVA irradiation. Overall, histologic changes after UVB are observed more superficially in the skin than after UVA irradiation, presumably reflecting the deeper penetration of UVB versus UVA photons.

TREATMENT

Treatment of sunburn is primarily symptomatic. Because of the critical role of membrane-generated eicosanoids in the pathophysiology of sunburn, a nonsteroidal anti-inflammatory agent, if taken within 4 hours of excessive sun exposure, may reduce the subsequent erythema. For mild to moderate reactions, cool compresses are soothing; pruritus can be managed by oral antihistamines; and topical anesthetic sprays may be used judiciously, albeit at the risk of allergic sensitization. For severe reactions, a short course of oral corticosteroids (e.g., prednisone 40–60 mg tapered over 5 days) is sometimes used to reduce the pain and inflammation. Unfortunately, no after-the-fact treatment can undo UV-induced DNA damage that cumulatively leads to photoaging and skin cancer.

PHOTOPROTECTION

Prevention of sunburn and other forms of photodamage is achieved by a combination of sun avoidance, protective clothing, and sunscreens. Because UVB is responsible for at least 80% of sunburn incurred from sun exposure, blocking penetration of UVB photons into skin is paramount.

UVB is by far most abundant in sunlight at midday, in spring and early summer, near the equator, and at high altitudes. Thus, arranging outdoor activities to minimize ambient UVB exposure is very helpful. For example, engaging in outdoor summer activities before 10:00 AM or after 3:00 PM can reduce sunburn risk 10-fold or more. Broad-brimmed hats substantially reduce ambient sun exposure to the face, and tee shirts or other coverups over bathing suits similarly help prevent casual overexposure of large body areas. However, for most persons, sunscreen use is critical to optimal sun protection.

Sunscreens are classified as over-the-counter drugs and required by the Food and Drug Administration to display a sun protection factor (SPF) rating. The SPF is the exposure time (to sun or a commercial sun lamp) required to cause a 1-MED sunburn while wearing the product divided by that required for unprotected skin. If sunburn would normally result from a 10-minute exposure, after application of an SPF 15 sunscreen, a 150-minute or 2½-hour exposure would be required. Thus, use of an SPF 15 sunscreen should effectively prevent sunburn under all but extreme situations, such as an all-day trip to the beach. A major caveat is that sunscreens must be liberally applied to achieve the stated protection level. Most individuals spontaneously apply approximately half the recommended amount and are proportionately less protected. Sunscreens must also be reapplied after swimming or sweating, although products labeled "waterproof" continue to protect even after a 90-minute immersion in water. Sunscreens are available in cream, gel, and spray formulations and in a wide price range, facilitating user choice. Routine use of a product with an SPF of at least 15 is recommended by the American Academy of Dermatology.

Of note, the SPF rating applies specifically to sunburn and the degree of protection against UVA is usually far less. For example, a standard SPF 15 sunscreen blocks only 50% to 70% of UVA, as opposed to 93% of UVB, and may thus be only marginally helpful in preventing an "exaggerated sunburn" or photosensitivity reaction in patients using certain antibiotics or antihypertensive agents. Sunscreens labeled "broad spectrum" give relatively better UVA protection, but no quantitative rating system is available. Furthermore, the relative importance of UVA versus UVB in chronic sun damage is unknown. UVB is strongly implicated in causing most skin cancers, but some authorities question whether UVA may contribute disproportionately to melanoma and photoaging. As a result, the use of sunscreens to *prolong* sun exposure, and thus potentially increase total UVA exposure, is strongly discouraged.

Section 13

The Nervous System

ALZHEIMER'S DISEASE

method of
GREGG WARSHAW, M.D.
University of Cincinnati Medical Center
Cincinnati, Ohio

CLINICAL ASSESSMENT

Cognitive impairment is common in the older adult and often represents an underlying and undetected clinical condition. When accompanied by other medical or social problems, cognitive impairment can precipitate stressful problems for and require decisions from families, caregivers, and clinicians. Impaired memory, especially recent memory, typically indicates the onset of the clinical syndrome of chronic, progressive dementia. Other changes are impaired judgment, loss of insight, flattening of affect, and eventually a change in personality. As the illness progresses, these changes are commonly followed by trouble in swallowing, walking, controlling bladder and bowel functions, and maintaining mobility. Alzheimer's disease (AD), the most frequent cause of dementia in this age group, probably accounts for at least 50% of the progressive dementias in the elderly. The next most common causes of dementia are vascular disease, Lewy body disease, and alcohol-related dementia.

A thorough history is critical for successful diagnosis and treatment. Initially, the history should include a careful review, with both the patient and the family, of the chronologic course of the changes in mental status. The pace of the progression and the duration of the symptoms are assessed. It is important to determine if there has been a dramatic clinical course; a steady, slow, subtle change; or a wide fluctuation of changes of mental status. Sudden onset is not consistent with AD.

It is advised to administer an objective test for mental status and an assessment of functional capacity should also be obtained from family or friends. When office cognitive testing and family observations are discordant, more formal neuropsychological testing may be required. Focal neurologic findings, seizures, and gait disturbance are also features that are rare early in the course of AD. Although the clinical course of AD may consist of good and bad days, the general trend is slow deterioration. Periods of steady improvement are not consistent with the diagnosis.

LABORATORY EVALUATION

Depending on the circumstances and clinical information, some of the procedures listed in Table 1 should be performed. These tests are selected to carefully exclude other possible causes of confusion. Computed tomography (CT) of the brain is appropriate in the presence of a history suggestive of a mass, or focal neurologic signs, or in dementia of brief duration. Magnetic resonance imaging is more sensitive than CT for detection of small infarcts, mass lesions, and subcortical structures; however, CT is adequate for the assessment of most dementia patients. Attempts to identify a reliable diagnostic test for AD continue. Positron emission tomography, single-photon emission CT, and magnetic resonance spectroscopy have identified areas in brains of patients with AD that show reduced metabolic activity. The availability and costs of these procedures, however, limit their use in routine diagnostic work.

GENETICS

AD has a genetic component; the risk for an individual in a family with AD increases by a factor of three or four. The importance of the genetic risk in AD is complicated by the fact that the diagnosis is not always certain and that many individuals within families may not live to an old enough age to manifest symptoms. The two basic types of AD are familial (FAD) and sporadic AD.

FAD accounts for less than 10% of all AD cases. It is associated with gene mutations on chromosomes 1, 14, and 21. Most FAD cases are characterized by earlier onset (many before age 60).

The apolipoprotein E (apoE) gene on chromosome 19 has been linked to sporadic, late-onset AD. ApoE is a substance that helps transport cholesterol in the blood. The apoE gene has three different alleles: apoE2, apoE3, and apoE4. Having one copy (30% of U.S. population) or two copies (2% of U.S. population) of the apoE4 allele may increase a person's risk for AD. At age 70, 50% of those with apoE4/4 will have AD, as compared with 28% with apoE3/4 and 6% with apoE2/4 and 3/3. ApoE2, in particular, appears to be protective for AD. Individuals with mild cognitive impairments that progress to AD are more likely to carry the apoE4 allele. In summary, the apoE4 allele is neither nec-

TABLE 1. **Laboratory Assessment of Chronic Confusion**

Depending on the circumstances and clinical information, some or all of the following procedures should be performed. (Items 1–5 are obtained in most instances.)

1. Complete blood cell count
2. Measurement of serum electrolyte levels
3. Biochemical screening (calcium, glucose, blood urea nitrogen/creatinine, liver function studies)
4. Serum vitamin B_{12} level
5. Thyroid function tests
6. Urinalysis
7. Toxicology screening
8. Arterial blood gases
9. Serologic tests for syphilis
10. Human immunodeficiency antibodies
11. Chest radiography
12. Lumbar puncture (spinal fluid analysis)
13. Neuroimaging studies, computed tomography, or magnetic resonance imaging

essary nor sufficient for the development of AD, and some with apoE4 live into the ninth decade with no signs of dementia. At this time it is not recommended that apoE status be used in routine clinical practice for diagnosis or for predictive testing.

MANAGEMENT OF ALZHEIMER'S DISEASE

Organization of Medical and Health Services

Many family members report that obtaining medical care for relatives with AD is both difficult and frustrating. An adequate diagnostic assessment is the chief concern of families. After diagnosis, families also report difficulty communicating with physicians. For physicians, the addition of a third party to the clinical encounter is awkward, time-consuming, and poorly reimbursed. Many physicians and other health professionals view AD as incurable and therefore untreatable. This view can lead some professionals to place little emphasis on general health care for persons with AD. The AD patient's resistance to health care visits can complicate matters further. Also, access to medical care can be limited if these patients are homebound or living in long-term care institutions.

AD patients are at particular risk for adverse responses or injury from medical interventions (iatrogenic disease). This may result from unsupervised access to medications, relocation confusion (delirium) resulting in agitation, increased fall risk, inappropriate pharmacologic therapy for behavioral disturbances, overuse of indwelling catheters, and lack of adequate supervision while hospitalized.

To be effective, the primary care physician should be available, interested, and willing to talk with the family. Patients should see their doctor every 4 to 6 months. Even if all is going well, it is important for the doctor to be aware of the patient's current mental and physical condition. The mental status of AD can be further impaired by many other disorders, such as heart disease or infections. Recognition and aggressive treatment of a coexisting illness can result in a noticeable improvement in the patient's mental condition.

Many older people are taking several prescription medications, and even if they are being prescribed appropriately and being taken correctly, any medication poses a threat to the AD patient. A regular and careful review of the patient's medications is one of the most important aspects of good disease management. Sedative and psychotropic drugs and antihypertensive and cardiac medications are just a few examples of drug classes that can further impair the brain and worsen the functional mental status of patients.

Pharmacologic Treatment

There is consistent evidence that enzymes related to the cholinergic system are reduced in brains of patients with AD. Specific treatment of the memory loss associated with AD is currently limited to acetylcholine agonists: tacrine (Cognex), donepezil (Aricept), galantamine (Reminyl), and rivastigmine (Exelon). All four medications have a similar magnitude of cognitive effect. One third of patients who reach a therapeutic medication level obtain some benefit from acetylcholine agonists. Expected treatment responses may include improvement in short-term memory or functional capabilities or slowing of clinical decline. Dramatic responses are rare. These medications have been most effective in patients with mild to moderate symptoms.

With tacrine, the initial dosage is 10 mg orally four times daily. At 6-week intervals, if the medication is tolerated, the dose can be increased by 40 mg/d, not to exceed a total dosage of 160 mg/d. The most serious adverse event associated with tacrine is hepatotoxicity associated with elevations in alanine aminotransferase. Alanine aminotransferase levels should be measured every other week for at least the first 16 weeks of tacrine therapy. Elevations above three times normal require dose reduction or withdrawal of the medication. Other side effects include nausea, diarrhea, dizziness, headache, myalgia, and ataxia. Theophylline doses may need to be reduced if coadministered with tacrine.

Donepezil is not associated with hepatotoxicity and can be prescribed once daily. The initial dosage is 5 mg/d, and the dosage can be increased to 10 mg/d if side effects are tolerated (including nausea, diarrhea, dizziness, headache, myalgia, and ataxia).

Rivastigmine is also not associated with hepatotoxicity. It is prescribed on a twice-daily schedule. The occurrence of nausea, vomiting, and loss of appetite may be more frequent than that with donepezil, and a low starting dose of the medication is recommended (1.5 mg twice daily for 2 weeks, with subsequent increases of 3 mg/d, at 2–4 week intervals, as tolerated, up to a maximum dosage of 6 mg twice daily).

Ginkgo biloba* is a widely used, natural compound that may have some benefit in the treatment of AD. It has been studied extensively, with positive outcomes, but many of the clinical trials have been criticized for weak study design. A recent well-designed, 24-week trial with 214 subjects demonstrated no benefit. The recommended dose of ginkgo is 120 to 160 mg/d of the pure extract. Ginkgo can inhibit platelet aggregation, and increases in bleeding time can be seen, especially in association with other anticoagulant or antiplatelet therapy.

Interventions designed to slow or stop the neurodegenerative basis for AD have been tested with the objective of delaying the onset or slowing the progression of the disease. Trials of estrogen therapy in middle-aged and older women have been disappointing. High dosages (1000 IU twice daily) of vitamin E* may have some impact on the rate of progression of AD. It is not yet known if lower doses (400 IU twice daily) would have a similar effect. Also, regular

*Not FDA approved for this indication.

use of nonsteroidal anti-inflammatory medications* has been associated with a lower incidence of AD.

BEHAVIORAL PROBLEMS

Adjusting the Environment

Simple care in adjusting a demented person's environment can avoid unnecessary accidents and limit confusion. In general, the patient should be allowed as much freedom as possible. However, structure in the daily schedule and familiar positioning of objects in the environment are important. Meal routines, medication routines, and exercise should all occur at regular times. Bedtime should be set at the same time each evening. Avoid clutter and furniture that has sharp corners or is unstable. The environment needs to be checked for possible poisons or potential hazards for the patient. AD patients have difficulty evaluating the environment and in new situations, they are very prone to accidental falls.

Depression and Dementia

Depression is a common accompaniment of dementia, particularly in the early stages. It may be necessary to initiate treatment with antidepressant medications in patients with mild or moderate dementia who appear depressed. Sometimes the patient's mood will improve and their cognition will also improve. Nortriptyline (Pamelor) (10–25 mg/d), and serotonin uptake inhibitors (e.g., sertraline [Zoloft], 25–50 mg/d; citalopram [Celexa] 10–20 mg/d) are good choices. Depressed patients are also more likely to use alcohol or tranquilizers. This, of course, has a catastrophic effect on their mental functioning. Rather than being depressed, some demented patients, particularly late in the disease, are simply apathetic and listless. It can be helpful to encourage activities by trying to reinvolve the patient at a comfortable level in a familiar activity. Occasionally, the patient will become upset or agitated even with a small amount of stimulation.

Wandering

Wandering is a frequent, serious problem that deserves careful consideration. Patients should be evaluated for pain or other discomfort. When confused patients are taken to new places, they may feel lost or believe they are not where they are supposed to be. When wandering appears to be aimless, it is sometimes helpful to plan daily exercise for the patient to see if this will reduce wandering during other parts of the day. Physical restraints should be a last resort and should only be used in consultation with the patient's family. Reclining geriatric chairs are preferred rather than tying arms and bodies into chairs. Many people with AD are restless at night, and this sundowning can be very challenging. A sedating tranquilizer is just as likely to aggravate the problem as to help it.

*Not FDA approved for this indication.

TABLE 2. **Physical Problems Associated With Alzheimer's Disease**

Throughout the Course of the Illness
Iatrogenic illness
Delirium
Hearing and vision impairment
Infections
Falls and injury
Urinary incontinence
Constipation and fecal incontinence
Pain
Oral health issues
Later in the Disease Course
Fecal incontinence
Pressure sores
Malnutrition
Seizures

If medication is prescribed for wandering or nighttime agitation, the drugs should only be used after all nondrug interventions have been tried and a medical evaluation is completed to eliminate potential coexisting medical problems. If paranoid or violent behavior is a predominate symptom, then an antipsychotic medication can be used (e.g., haloperidol [Haldol], 0.25–2 mg/d, risperidone [Risperdal] 0.25–2 mg/d). For agitation without psychotic features, an antianxiety agent can be prescribed (e.g., lorazepam [Ativan] 0.5–2 mg/d or buspirone [BuSpar] 10–30 mg/d). Some anticonvulsant medications have also been helpful for the management of aggression associated with AD (carbamazepine [Tegretol]* 50–100 mg twice daily, valproate [Depakote] 125–250 mg twice daily). All psychotropic medications prescribed to patients with AD have the potential to adversely affect cognitive function or worsen agitation. Careful evaluation of target symptom–response and side effects is essential.

Reducing and Managing Co-Morbidity

AD is similar to other chronic illnesses (e.g., arthritis, heart disease) in that good medical management can slow functional decline and limit unnecessary complications. Some medical problems either occur more commonly in AD patients or result in excess disability. Correction of even minor physical problems may greatly help these patients. The types of coexisting medical conditions that commonly occur in association with AD are listed in Table 2 and are briefly discussed.

Delirium

Delirium occurs frequently in patients with AD. A number of prospective studies have documented that dementia is a significant risk factor for the develop-

*Not FDA approved for this indication.

ment of delirium during hospitalization for medical problems and after surgery. The occurrence of delirium in the hospitalized elderly has been associated with excess mortality. If possible, ill patients with AD should be treated outside the hospital. If hospitalization is required, the family should be encouraged to stay with the patient 24 hours a day, or, if affordable, sitters should be assigned to stay in the patient's room. Intravenous therapy and urinary catheter use should be brief. The use of physical restraints should be avoided, and sedative use should be kept to a minimum.

Hearing and Vision Impairment

It is important that patients with AD have optimal hearing and vision. Decreased sensory input secondary to poor vision or deafness may aggravate existing confusion and result in paranoia, delusions, or hallucinations. Careful hearing and vision evaluations should be part of the routine medical care of these patients.

Infections

Poor nutrition and inadequate diets can place patients with AD at greater risk for infection. Patients with AD frequently fail to recognize, understand, or verbalize early symptoms of infection. Fever may be absent or inapparent (frail adults may have lower baseline body temperatures) in older adults with infection. Pneumonia and urinary tract infections are common in patients with AD and result in considerable morbidity and use of health services. Infection is also a common cause of delirium associated with AD. The management of infections associated with AD, particularly with coexisting delirium, is a significant challenge to even the most experienced clinician. The treatment of serious infections in a familiar environment (home or nursing home) may result in better outcomes than hospitalization.

Falls and Injury

AD is a risk factor for falls and fractures among older adults. Among community-dwelling elderly persons with AD, the fracture rate is double that of cognitively intact controls. It is known that AD is a risk factor for poor functional recovery after hip fracture. Simple care in adjusting a demented person's environment can avoid unnecessary accidents and limit confusion. Hospitals and nursing homes report that falls are most common during the first several weeks of a patient's stay. It is also possible that medications or coexisting illnesses (e.g., Parkinson's disease or an unsuspected anemia) can be the cause of falling; therefore, any patient with AD who suddenly develops instability or falling should receive a thorough medical evaluation.

Urinary Incontinence

If the incontinence is the result of the AD, it usually represents the inability of the brain to inhibit bladder contractions (urge incontinence). This results in the bladder emptying without the patient being able to choose when and where this should occur. Supervised toileting programs that encourage voiding before the patient develops the urge to urinate can frequently lead to considerable improvement. It is important to emphasize that fluid restriction is not an acceptable treatment for urinary incontinence. These patients are at risk for dehydration (they may forget to drink enough liquids), which can lead to a worsening of their mental condition. Urinary incontinence remains one of the most difficult complications of AD for caregivers to manage in the home or institution.

Constipation

A forgetful person may not remember to go to the bathroom. Changes in diet that decrease the fiber content and less physical activity may both contribute to the development of constipation. Medications with anticholinergic effects and narcotics can also cause constipation. When a person with AD has the recent onset of constipation, the presence of a colonic obstructing disorder (e.g., cancer, volvulus) should be considered. Complications of constipation include fecal impaction, intestinal obstruction, megacolon, fecal incontinence, pain, increased confusion, and agitation. Hydration, dietary fiber, and the appropriate use of laxatives are required to avoid these complications.

Pain

AD is not known to cause physical pain, although people with AD can experience pain from the same conditions common to older adults: musculoskeletal problems, headache, malignancy, herpes zoster, pressure injury, lacerations, skin rashes from poor hygiene, and dental problems. In order to recognize pain in the patient with AD, the caregiver must carefully evaluate worsening behavior, facial expressions, moaning or shouting, and restlessness. Narcotic analgesics have the potential to worsen cognitive function.

Oral Health

In AD, salivary gland flow is decreased and tooth decay and gingival disease are more common. The decrease in saliva production appears to be independent of medication use and places patients with AD at increased risk for tooth decay. Preventive and treatment goals for these patients are similar to those in all adults: to preserve and maintain oral health and function.

Fecal Incontinence

Fecal incontinence is less common than urinary incontinence but occurs in the later stages of AD. A medical evaluation is essential. Reversible causes for this problem include stool impaction (constipation leading to fecal incontinence), laxative misuse, dietary habits, bowel infections, or other bowel disease. If a reversible explanation is not found for the incontinence, a neurogenic cause—spontaneous rectal contractions usually associated with the gastrocolic reflex—is likely. Bowel training programs can help to regulate stools and can be supervised by family, caregivers, or visiting nurses.

Pressure Ulcers

In the later stages of AD, patients may no longer be ambulatory and the risk of pressure damage to the skin and underlying tissues increases. Most pressure ulcers are preventable through recognition of risk and strategies to relieve pressure or shear. Daily inspection of the skin is essential for preventing skin damage. Regular repositioning is important, and, in advanced disease, pressure-relieving seat cushions and mattresses are needed.

Malnutrition

Patients with AD will often lose weight. This weight loss is not always an indication of poor nutritional intake; it may represent a hypermetabolic state. The patient's weight, hydration, and oral intake should be regularly evaluated. Malnutrition is not an inevitable consequence of advanced AD. In later stages of AD, nutrition is usually provided by soft or pureed diets. When choking or aspiration develops, semisolid foods will be safer than liquids. Vitamin and mineral supplements can be added to the diet. The use of chronic gastrostomy tube feeding should be instituted only after a careful review of the patient's advance directives and consultation with the family.

Seizures

Generalized seizures or myoclonus occur in 10% to 20% of patients with late-stage AD. If the patient examination does not reveal focal neurologic findings, brain scans seldom reveal new pathosis. Phenytoin (Dilantin) or carbamazepine are the anticonvulsant agents commonly used to control generalized seizures in this group of patients. There is no effective drug treatment for myoclonus or myoclonic jerking. Seizure activity may accelerate the course of AD.

ALZHEIMER'S DISEASE SPECIAL CARE UNITS

In an attempt to develop improved environments for patients with AD, many health facilities have developed special outpatient and inpatient programs for these patients. Adult daycare programs for individuals with dementia are sponsored by community health agencies, hospitals, and nursing homes. The goals of these programs are to allow patients to function in safe environments and participate in activities that are stimulating but not frustrating. Playing and listening to music, interacting with pets, and gardening are examples of frequently successful activities. An important achievement of daycare programs has been to relieve stress on home caregivers. This respite has enabled family caregivers to keep their relatives at home further into the course of the illness.

Inevitably, in many cases, patients with AD will eventually require assisted living or nursing home care. Some nursing facilities have developed units especially designed for the demented patient. These units encourage activity and exercise. The environment is free of hazards and disturbing stimulation. As with daycare programs, appropriate activities are encouraged. The use of physical restraints or sedatives is discouraged.

TABLE 3. **The Family and Alzheimer's Disease: A Framework for Professional Providers**

Early Stage

Family Issues
Denial, cure seeking, hiding the diagnosis
Asking the patient to try harder
Fear

Areas to Assess
Premorbid personalities and relationships
Previous and concurrent caregiving responsibilities
Informal supports (family and community)

Interventions
Conduct a medical evaluation and provide primary care and information
Discuss coping with ambiguities, embarrassing situations; how, when, and what to tell whom; coping with role changes; modifying expectations; enhancing support system; legal/financial precautions

Middle Stage

Family Issues
Protection versus allowing risks, role fatigue or overload
Behavior, mood, and sleep disorders management
Isolation, preliminary grief

Areas to Assess
Caregiver health status, tolerance for stress
Family conflicts regarding care
Cultural/religious proscriptions
Community resources (respite, daycare)

Interventions
Prescribe respite and ways to conserve energy
Discuss coping with crushed expectations; helplessness, anger, guilt; replacing lost confidant; accepting help: review old promises, how much, when, from whom?

Late Stage

Family Issues
Terminal care, guilt, limbo status

Areas to Assess
Family attitudes toward terminal care, nursing homes
Losses and gains with institutional care

Interventions
Encourage the locating and evaluation of long-term care facilities
Discuss coping with feelings and decisions regarding terminal care; planning for surviving family; coping with separation, new freedom; meeting altruistic needs

Modified from Gwyther LP: Care of Alzheimer's Patients: A Manual for Nursing Home Staff. Chicago: American Health Care Association and the Alzheimer's Disease and Related Disorders Association, 1985.

THE FAMILY AND ALZHEIMER'S DISEASE

The physician caring for a patient with AD can provide crucial support to the family and caregivers. Families of patients with AD have frequent questions and need advice and information. The issues on the minds of relatives change as the disease progresses. Table 3 reviews the common family issues that occur during the early, middle, and late stages of AD. Several excellent books on caring for relatives with AD are widely available (see Suggested Reading). Additional information for caregivers and professionals is available from local chapters of the Alzheimer's Association or from the Alzheimer's Association National Office: Alzheimer's Association, 919 North Michigan Avenue, Suite 1000, Chicago, IL 60611-1676; 800-272-3900; www.alz.org.

Suggested Reading

Mace NL, Rabins PV: The 36 Hour Day, 3d ed. Baltimore: Johns Hopkins University Press, 1999.

INTRACEREBRAL HEMORRHAGE

method of
MARC MALKOFF, M.D., and
ASHRAF EL-MITTALLI, M.D.
University of Texas Houston
Houston, Texas

Intracerebral hemorrhage (ICH) is a common cause of stroke and accounts for 5% to 10% of all strokes. In consecutive series of 938 stroke patients enrolled into the Stroke Data Bank of the National Institute of Neurological and Communicative Disorders and Stroke, primary ICH accounted for 10.7% of cases. Age-adjusted annual incidence rates for primary ICH range from 11 to 31 per 100,000 population in predominantly white population based-studies with a high rate of computed tomographic (CT) scanning. The risk of ICH in blacks is 1.4 times the risk in whites. The most common risk factors in the 403 black patients with ICH were pre-existing hypertension (77%), alcohol use (40%), and smoking (30%). Among the 91 nonhypertensive patients, hypertension was diagnosed in 21 (23%) after the onset of ICH. ICH remains a significant cause of morbidity and mortality in this population.

RISK FACTORS

Hypertension was the main causative factor of ICH in the autopsy study of McCormick and Rosenfield. The frequency of hypertension in series of patients with ICH varies widely and ranges from 40% to 89%, even in studies applying careful definitions of hypertension. Whereas chronic hypertension still appears to be the most important risk factor for ICH, studies suggest that its role in causing ICH is less dominant than previously thought.

Moderate drinking of alcohol increases the risk of both intracerebral and subarachnoid hemorrhage in diverse populations. Epidemiologic evidence is insufficient to conclude whether recent alcohol use affects the risk of either ischemic or hemorrhagic stroke.

CAUSES OF INTRACEREBRAL HEMORRHAGE

Chronic hypertension produces fibrinoid necrosis, lipohyalinosis, and medial degeneration, which make vessels susceptible to rupture. ICH that originates in the putamen, thalamus, pons, or cerebellum is most likely linked with hypertension; ICH at these sites is often referred to as *hypertensive ICH*, even in patients in whom the prestroke blood pressure level is unknown. However as mentioned earlier, recent studies suggest that the role of hypertension in causing ICH is less obvious than previously thought. Lobar hemorrhage is much less frequently associated with hypertension and often has other etiologies.

Cerebral amyloid angiopathy is characterized by the deposition of amyloid in small and medium-sized arteries of the cortex and leptomeninges, is confined to the cerebral vessels only, and increases steadily with age. Lobar ICH, often recurrent, is the main consequence of cerebral amyloid angiopathy and one of the most common causes of ICH in persons 70 years and older.

An abrupt, dramatic increase in blood pressure in normotensive patients has been documented to precipitate ICH. Their autoregulatory functions have not adjusted to high blood pressure, in contrast to chronically hypertensive patients. This state may be associated with *sympathomimetics* (amphetamines, pseudoephedrine, phenylpropanolamine [formerly contained in many over-the-counter nasal decongestants and appetite suppressors], and cocaine [especially in its precipitate form known as crack]).

Arteriovenous malformations are important causes of nonhypertensive ICH and tend to occur in relatively young patients. Intracranial aneurysms characteristically cause subarachnoid hemorrhage, but they may also bleed into the adjacent brain parenchyma and cause ICHs. Halpin and associates, however, found that among ICH patients thought to have underlying lesions, 13% of hypertensive patients, 31% of patients with hematoma involving the basal ganglia, and 18% of those with posterior fossa ICHs all had underlying aneurysms or angiomas.

Another common etiology is the presence of coagulopathy. ICH is the most common and least treatable neurologic complication of oral anticoagulants in the elderly. Unfortunately, risk factors for ischemic stroke and ICH overlap in many patients (e.g., advanced age, hypertension, previous stroke). Patients who are elderly (>70 years) with hypertension have an inherent risk for ICH that is multiplied by oral anticoagulants to absolute rates approaching 1% per year.

Transformation of stroke into hemorrhage is another cause of lobar hemorrhage. ICH during heparin treatment is less common. Risk factors for ICH during heparin therapy for acute cerebral infarction are large infarct size and uncontrolled hypertension. Thrombolysis in acute ischemic stroke increases the risk of severe, life-threatening hemorrhagic complications by up to 10 times versus controls (absolute rates of 3%–15%).

Bleeding into brain tumors is rare (5%–6% in autopsy-based studies), with the exception of pituitary adenomas, which may bleed in 16% of cases. Common etiologies include glioblastoma multiforma, metastatic melanoma, choriocarcinoma, and renal cell and bronchogenic carcinoma.

Trauma is a common cause of ICH. Trauma usually occurs in the occipital lobes, the temporal tips, and the orbital frontal cortex. Nontraumatic ICH is rarely seen in these locations.

CLINICAL FEATURES

ICH is generally manifested as stroke, a sudden, nonconclusive, focal neurologic deficit. Differentiation from ischemic stroke is difficult solely on clinical information.

General Clinical Manifestations

ICH characteristically occurs during activity (rarely during sleep). Headache, emesis, and decreased level of consciousness are more commonly seen in ICH than ischemic stroke, but they are not always present. Mohr reported headache in about 36% and vomiting in about 44% of patients alert enough to report the symptoms. Seizures are uncommon in the onset of ICH (7% of cases) but are found in 32% of lobar hemorrhages. Hypertension is frequent (91% of cases) and correlates with other physical signs indicative of hypertension such as left ventricular hypertrophy and hypertensive retinopathy. Classic neurologic findings are summarized in Table 1.

Investigations

CT remains the primary means of diagnosing ICH because it is easy to obtain quickly and can distinguish ICH from acute infarction. Magnetic resonance imaging (MRI) is less sensitive to hyperacute ICH, especially if only routine sequences are preformed. MRI and angiography have a role in diagnosing nonhypertensive etiologies or ICH in lobar or other atypical locations (or settings). MRI may also help in finding old (previous) hemorrhages in as much as differentiation of a posthemorrhagic pseudocyst from old contusions, ischemic lesions, or even astrocytomas may be difficult. Lumbar puncture is rarely necessary and may be contraindicated.

TABLE 1. **Classic Neurologic Signs and Symptoms by Intracerebral Hemorrhage Location**

Putamen

Hemiparesis/hemiplegia
Hemisensory syndrome (usually anesthesia)
Eye deviation (toward the lesion)
Dysarthria
Aphasia (left-sided lesion)
Hemineglect (right-sided lesion)

Caudate

Hemiparesis
Gaze deviation

Thalamic

Hemiparesis/hemiplegia
Hemisensory loss
- Less common
- Aphasia
- Anosagnosia
- Other neuropsychological deficits
- Skew deviation

Lobar

As per area involved

Cerebellar

Gait and truncal ataxia
Emesis
Nystagmus
Headache
- Less common
- Decreased level of consciousness (implies need for surgery)
- Gaze abnormalities

Brainstem

Crossed motor deficit (face-body)
Cranial nerve palsies
Decreased level of consciousness

Course and Prognosis

ICH often has a poor outcome. In one 6-month study, 34% of patients died, 36% were dependent on outside help for daily living, and 30% were capable of independent existence. Age greater than 60 years, Glasgow Coma Scale (GCS) score of 6 or less at the time of admission, ICH volume greater than 30 mL, a midline shift in the CT scan of more than 3 mm, and the presence of intraventricular hemorrhage and hydrocephalus all had an adverse impact on outcome. Young age, GCS score of more than 8, ICH volume of less than 20 mL, presence of lobar hemorrhage, and absence of intraventricular hemorrhage/hydrocephalus were associated with a relatively favorable outcome.

The most important predictor of 28-day survival is the level of consciousness on admission, followed by first-day mean arterial pressure (MAP). Hypertension is the most important predictor of first-day MAP, followed by age, which had an inverse effect on the MAP level. At all levels of consciousness, high first-day MAP (especially if >145 mm Hg) worsened the 28-day survival rate.

GUIDELINES FOR THE MANAGEMENT OF SPONTANEOUS INTRACEREBRAL HEMORRHAGE

Initial Management in the Emergency Department

Initial management should first be directed toward the basics of airway, breathing, circulation, and detection of focal neurologic deficits. In addition, particular attention should be given to detecting signs of external trauma. A complete examination should also include a search for complications such as pressure sores, compartment syndromes, and rhabdomyolysis in patients with a prolonged depressed level of consciousness (patients "found down").

Airway and Oxygenation

Although intubation is not required for all patients, airway protection and adequate ventilation are critical. Patients who exhibit a decreasing level of consciousness or signs of brainstem dysfunction are candidates for aggressive airway management. Imminent respiratory insufficiency should guide intubation.

Blood Pressure Management

The optimal level of a patient's blood pressure should be based on individual factors such as chronic hypertension, elevated intracranial pressure (ICP), age, presumed cause of hemorrhage, and interval since onset. High blood pressure treatment goals should be a MAP between 110 and 130 mm Hg in persons with a history of hypertension (level of evidence V, grade C recommendation). Recommended agents in order of preference are labetalol (Normodyne) (intermittent or drip), nicardipine (Cardene), and nitroprusside (Nitropress) (drips). Hypotension and wide swings in blood pressure should be avoided.

Management of Increased Intracranial Pressure

Elevated ICP is considered a major contributor to mortality after ICH; unfortunately, its management is difficult. A therapeutic goal for all treatment of elevated ICP is an ICP less than 20 mm Hg and cerebral perfusion pressure greater than 70 mm Hg. Optimal head position can be adjusted according to cerebral perfusion pressure values (default, 30 degrees).

Patients with suspected elevated ICP and deteriorating level of consciousness are candidates for invasive ICP monitoring. In general, ICP monitors should be placed in (but not limited to) patients with a GCS score of less than 9 and all patients whose condition is thought to be deteriorating because of elevated ICP (level of evidence V, grade C recommendation). Because secondary hydrocephalus may contribute to elevated ICP, ventricular drains should be used in patients with or at risk for hydrocephalus. Drainage can be initiated and terminated according to clinical performance and ICP values (level of evidence V, grade C recommendation).

Medical management consists of mild hyperventilation (P_{CO_2} of 32–35 mm Hg), osmotherapy, and sedation. For osmotherapy, mannitol at 0.25 to 1 g/kg every 6 hours is recommended. Urinary loss should replaced for 2 hours after the dose. Mannitol is unlikely to be effective if the serum osmolality is greater than 310, so osmolality should be measured just before each dose. Sedation and paralysis may be helpful.

Fluid Management

The goal of fluid management is euvolemia. Fluids should be isotonic and given according to need. Electrolytes (sodium, potassium, calcium, and magnesium) should be checked and substituted to attain normal values. Acidosis and alkalosis should be corrected according to blood gas analysis.

Prevention of Seizures

In patients with ICH, prophylactic antiepileptic therapy (preferably phenytoin with doses titrated according to drug levels [14–23 μg/mL]) may be considered for 1 month (especially in lobar ICH). This therapy should be tapered and discontinued if no seizure activity occurs during treatment, although data supporting such therapy are lacking (level of evidence V, grade C recommendation).

Management of Body Temperature

Body temperature should be maintained at normal levels unless deliberate hypothermia is attempted. Acetaminophen, 650 mg, or cooling blankets should be used to treat hyperthermia.

Other Medical Management Issues

Many patients who are delirious or stuporous are agitated. If psychological support is insufficient, prudent use of minor and major tranquilizers is recommended. Short-acting benzodiazepines or propofol are preferred. Other drugs such as analgesics and neuroleptics can be added if necessary. Doses and the regimen should be titrated to clinical need.

Pulmonary embolism is a common threat during the recovery period, particularly in bedridden patients. Pneumatic devices and heparin (and related compounds) can decrease the risk of pulmonary embolism. Ulcer prophylaxis is often recommended. Depending on the patient's clinical state, physical therapy, speech therapy, and occupational therapy should be initiated as soon as possible.

GUIDELINES FOR SURGICAL EVACUATION OF INTRACEREBRAL HEMORRHAGE

Patients with cerebellar hemorrhage greater than 3 cm in diameter who are neurologically deteriorating or who have brain stem compression and hydrocephalus from ventricular obstruction should have surgical evacuation of the hemorrhage as soon as possible (levels of evidence III through V, grade C recommendation).

Surgical treatment of other sources of ICH remains controversial. Young patients with large lobar hemorrhages (≥50 cm^3) who deteriorate during observation often undergo surgical evacuation of the hemorrhage. A structural lesion such as an aneurysm or a vascular malformation causing ICH may be removed if the patient has a chance for a good outcome and the structural vascular lesion is surgically accessible (levels of evidence III through V, grade C recommendation). Other surgical treatments remain promising, but unproven.

In conclusion, therapy for ICH is largely supportive. Surgery has a definite role in cerebellar ICH and may play an increasing role in supratentorial ICH. Medical management remains supportive and largely untested.

ISCHEMIC CEREBROVASCULAR DISEASE

method of
DAVID LEE GORDON, M.D.
University of Miami School of Medicine
Miami, Florida

Stroke is the third leading cause of death in the United States behind heart disease and cancer and the leading cause of long-term disability. Over 700,000 Americans suffer a new or recurrent stroke each year. The current cost of stroke in the United States is estimated to be over $50 billion per year. Post-hospitalization costs account for over half of the expense. A proactive, organized approach to the management of patients with acute stroke leads to successful performance improvement (quality of care) and utilization review (efficiency of care) efforts. This includes the implementation of an emergency stroke response team, a stroke multidisciplinary team, a stroke unit, prewritten stroke orders, and a stroke clinical pathway that addresses each aspect of stroke care (acute treatment, supportive medical care, rehabilitation, etiologic evaluation, secondary stroke prevention, and discharge planning) on each day of hospitalization.

Within the first few hours of onset, an ischemic stroke consists of a central zone of irreversible infarction surrounded by a zone of reversible ischemia called the ischemic penumbra. The patient's symptoms are due to both reversible ischemia and irreversible infarction. One cannot determine by neurologic examination or computed tomography (CT) how much brain tissue can still be saved. Preservation of the penumbra is the theoretical aim of any acute stroke therapy. Thrombolytic (or, more specifically, fibrinolytic) therapy with tissue plasminogen activator (t-PA, alteplase [Activase]) restores blood flow to the penumbra. Seizure, hypotension, hyperglycemia, and hyperthermia all damage the penumbra or hinder its recovery.

One should evaluate all patients with acute cerebral dysfunction urgently to discover what caused their symptoms, including those whose symptoms are transient. A transient ischemic attack (TIA) is, in essence, an ischemic stroke without permanent sequelae. By definition, a TIA lasts less than 24 hours, but this duration is arbitrary and outdated because we can now identify evidence of stroke on cerebral magnetic resonance imaging (MRI) in patients whose ischemic symptoms last just a few hours. In most cases, TIA symptoms last 2 to 20 minutes. Among patients who present to an emergency department with TIA, 25% have a stroke or other adverse event within the next 3 months and over 5% have a stroke within the next 2 days. Only by knowing the cause of the patient's first stroke or TIA can one determine the proper therapy to prevent a second, more disabling event.

TABLE 1. **Indications and Contraindications for Stroke Patients**

t-PA Indications

These statements must be true in order to consider t-PA administration:

1. Ischemic stroke onset ≤3 h of drug administration
2. Measurable deficit on NIHSS
3. Computed tomography without hemorrhage or nonstroke cause of deficit
4. Age ≥18 y

t-PA Contraindications

Do NOT administer t-PA if any of these statements are true:

1. Symptoms minor or rapidly improving
2. Seizure at onset of stroke
3. Suspected aortic dissection associated with stroke
4. Recent acute myocardial infarction
5. Suspected subacute bacterial endocarditis or vasculitis
6. Symptoms suggestive of subarachnoid hemorrhage
7. Another stroke, serious head trauma, or intracranial surgery within past 3 mo
8. Major surgery or serious trauma within 14 d
9. Known history of intracranial hemorrhage, AVM, or aneurysm
10. Gastrointestinal or urinary tract hemorrhage within 21 d
11. Arterial puncture at noncompressible site within 7 d
12. Lumbar puncture within 7 d
13. Received heparin within 48 h and has elevated PTT
14. PT >15 sec or INR >1.7
15. Platelet count <100,000/mm³
16. Serum glucose <50 or >400 mg/dL
17. Sustained systolic blood pressure >185 mm Hg
18. Sustained diastolic blood pressure >110 mm Hg
19. Aggressive treatment necessary to lower blood pressure

t-PA Warnings

If either statement is true, use t-PA with extreme caution owing to possible increased risk of intracranial hemorrhage:

1. Very large stroke with NIHSS score >22
2. Computed tomography shows evidence of large MCA-territory infarction (sulcal effacement or blurring of gray-white junction in more than one third of MCA territory)

Abbreviations: AVM = arteriovenous malformation; INR = international normalized ratio; MCA = middle cerebral artery; NIHSS = National Institutes of Health Stroke Scale; PT = prothrombin time; PTT = partial thromboplastin time; t-PA = tissue plasminogen activator.

EMERGENCY STROKE INFRASTRUCTURE

Intravenous t-PA (alteplase) decreases morbidity without increasing mortality and is cost effective if given within 3 hours of symptom onset per the National Institute of Neurological and Communicative Diseases and Stroke (NINCDS) protocol (Table 1). The short time window necessitates that medical centers proactively develop an approach to handling these patients on an emergency basis that includes developing stroke code teams and forming networks with other medical centers to enable rapid evaluation and treatment 24 hours a day, 7 days a week. The efficient stroke center takes approximately 1 hour to fully evaluate a patient and begin administration of t-PA (Table 2), typically by utilizing preprinted orders (Tables 3 and 4) and a unified paging system. In most centers, it is most practical to train emergency department (ED) personnel to administer t-PA. Centers wishing to give t-PA to stroke patients should have access to a neurosurgeon within 2 hours of t-PA administration in the event of a hemorrhagic complication of therapy.

Stroke centers should train personnel in the use of the National Institutes of Health Stroke Scale (NIHSS), a rapid and quantifiable neurologic examination designed for use by physicians and nurses in clinical trials of patients with ischemic stroke. It has good interrater and intrarater reliabilities and takes 5 to 7 minutes to perform. A low NIHSS score indicates a mild stroke, and a high score indicates a

TABLE 2. **Emergency Department Timeline for a "Stroke Alert"**

Stage I: ED Triage

Complete within 10 min of ED arrival:

1. Identify t-PA candidate (last known to be without symptoms ≤2 h).*
2. Notify Stroke Code Team via unified paging system.
3. Obtain fingerstick glucose and STAT labs: CBC with platelets, PT/PTT, chemistry 7.

Stage II: ED Medical Care

Complete within 25 min of ED arrival:

1. Elevate head of bed; give O_2 2 L if Sao_2 <92%; keep NPO.
2. Monitor BP.
3. Perform ECG 12-lead and rhythm strip.
4. Place intravenous catheter in each arm: administer NS 75 mL/h and saline lock.
5. Obtain patient weight.
6. Send for computed tomography.

Stage III: Computed Tomography and Laboratory Tests

Complete within 45 min of ED arrival:

1. Review STAT blood laboratory results.
2. Perform and interpret noncontrast brain computed tomography.
3. Transport patient to ED for t-PA if criteria met.

Stage IV: Acute Treatment

Begin t-PA within 60 min of ED arrival; must begin within 3 h of stroke onset:

1. Give intravenous t-PA per stroke protocol.
2. Monitor BP and neurologic examination every 15 min.
3. Treat BP elevations per stroke t-PA protocol.
4. Watch for signs of intracranial hemorrhage and follow protocol if necessary.
5. Do NOT give antiplatelet agent or anticoagulant.
6. If patient is stable, transfer to Acute Stroke Unit 30 to 60 min after t-PA completed.

*Because one must begin intravenous administration of t-PA within 3 h of stroke onset and because it takes approximately 1 h to complete the ED evaluation, the patient must actually enter the ED within 2 h of stroke onset.

Abbreviations: BP = blood pressure; CBC = complete blood cell count; ED = emergency department; ECG = electrocardiogram; NPO = nothing by mouth; NS = normal saline; PT = prothrombin time; PTT = partial thromboplastin time; t-PA = tissue plasminogen activator.

severe stroke. In the NINCDS t-PA trial, patients with a score of more than 22 who received t-PA had a higher incidence of intracranial hemorrhage than those with a lower score but still fared better than patients with a score of more than 22 who received placebo. Any center caring for stroke patients should have the ability to perform and interpret nonenhanced cerebral CT 24 hours a day, 7 days a week. Although CT may not demonstrate ischemic changes for several hours after stroke onset, its performance is necessary to eliminate intracranial hemorrhage or a nonstroke cause of the patient's symptoms.

MEDICAL CARE OF THE ACUTE STROKE PATIENT

The emergency management of acute ischemic stroke patients consists of measures to preserve the penumbra and prevent medical complications. It is especially important to avoid iatrogenic worsening of the patient's condition by avoiding excessive treatment of hypertension, not giving glucose-containing solutions, and not allowing aspiration. My specific emergency protocol is outlined in Tables 3 and 4. Table 3 consists of the initial emergency department orders for any stroke patient—ischemic or hemorrhagic—before obtaining a CT scan. Table 4 consists of orders specific to the ischemic stroke patient who qualifies for t-PA administration.

Acute hypertension at the time of stroke is most often a result of—and not a cause of—the stroke. This rise in blood pressure is necessary to supply the reversibly ischemic brain with enough blood to survive. In acute stroke, cerebral autoregulation, the normal mechanism by which the brain maintains a constant cerebral blood pressure despite sudden changes in systemic blood pressure, is damaged. Thus, the acutely damaged brain cannot protect itself from sudden decreases in blood pressure that may occur with antihypertensive therapy. Hypertension associated with acute stroke usually resolves spontaneously over the first few hours or days after stroke and, consequently, the response to antihypertensive agents in acute stroke patients may be exaggerated. In addition, many patients with acute stroke have a history of chronic hypertension and, thus, were accustomed to higher systemic pressures before the stroke. One should not treat hypertension in ischemic stroke patients unless the patient has evidence of another condition that necessitates lowering the blood pressure, such as acute myocardial infarction, acute congestive heart failure, aortic dissection, or acute renal failure. Although treatment of high blood pressure may benefit patients with hemorrhagic stroke (by decreasing intracranial pressure), because 85% of strokes are ischemic, it is best not to treat hypertension until after CT demonstrates intracranial hemorrhage. In patients with acute ischemic stroke who do not qualify for t-PA therapy, there is no good evidence that treating blood pressure elevation with fast-acting parenteral agents is beneficial, no matter how high the value. Based on cumulative data from many sources, I consider lowering the

TABLE 3. **Initial Emergency Department Orders for All Acute Stroke Patients**

1. Place cardiac, noninvasive blood pressure, and Sao_2 monitoring.
2. Perform glucose fingerstick and send for laboratory values STAT: CBC with platelets, PT/PTT, and chemistry 7.
3. Elevate head of bed ≥30 degrees.
4. Place or continue O_2 at 2-L nasal cannula if Sao_2 ≤92%.
5. Suction patient as needed.
6. Keep patient NPO (including no liquids or oral medications).
7. Monitor vital signs and neurologic checks every 15 min.
8. Obtain ECG 12-lead and rhythm strip.
9. Place an intravenous catheter in each arm: start NS 75 mL/h and saline lock.
10. Weigh patient using a scale.
11. Obtain STAT noncontrast computed tomographic scan of brain.

Abbreviations: CBC = complete blood cell count; ECG = electrocardiogram; NPO = nothing by mouth; NS = normal saline; PT = prothrombin time; PTT = partial thromboplastin time.

TABLE 4. **Emergency Department t-PA Orders for Stroke Patients**

1. Give t-PA total dose of ______mg (0.9 mg/kg up to maximum dose of 90 mg) as follows:
   a. Give 10% as IV bolus over 1 min.
   b. Give remaining 90% as constant IV infusion over 60 min.
2. Monitor BP and neurologic checks every 15 min during and for 1 h after t-PA administration.
3. If SBP >180 mm Hg or DBP >105 mm Hg for two or more readings 5–10 min apart, follow NINCDS Study Group protocol for blood pressure treatment in patients receiving t-PA.
   a. If SBP 180–230 mm Hg or DBP 105–120 mm Hg for two or more readings 5–10 min apart,
      i. Give IV labetalol, 10 mg over 1–2 min.
      ii. May repeat or double dose every 10–20 min to maximum dose of 150 mg.
      iii. Monitor BP every 15 min for hypotension.
   b. If SBP >230 mm Hg or DBP 121–140 mm Hg for two or more readings 5–10 min apart,
      i. Give IV labetalol, 10 mg over 1–2 min.
      ii. May repeat or double dose every 10–20 min to maximum dose of 150 mg.
      iii. Monitor BP every 15 min for hypotension.
      iv. If no satisfactory response, infuse sodium nitroprusside, 0.5–10 μg/kg/min.
         (1) Monitor BP with arterial line.
         (2) Watch every 15 min for hypotension.
         (3) Watch carefully for bleeding from arterial line site.
   c. If DBP >140 mm Hg for two or more readings 5–10 min apart,
      i. Infuse sodium nitroprusside 0.5–10 μg/kg/min.
      ii. Monitor BP with arterial line.
      iii. Watch every 15 min for hypotension.
      iv. Watch carefully for bleeding from arterial line site.
4. Do NOT give heparin, warfarin, aspirin, ticlopidine, clopidogrel, dipyridamole, or NSAIDs for 24 h after t-PA.
5. During or after t-PA administration, if patient has acute neurologic deterioration or new headache or acute hypertension or nausea and vomiting, then follow protocol for possible intracranial hemorrhage:
   a. Discontinue t-PA.
   b. Send blood for laboratory values STAT: PT/PTT, CBC with platelets, fibrinogen, type and cross 3 units.
   c. Prepare to administer 4–6 units of cryoprecipitate.
   d. Prepare to administer 6–8 units of platelets (or 1 unit of single-donor platelets).
   e. Obtain STAT noncontrast CT scan of brain.
   f. Consult neurosurgery if CT scan reveals intracranial hemorrhage.
6. If patient is stable, transport to Acute Stroke Unit 30–60 minutes after t-PA completed.

Abbreviations: BP = blood pressure; CBC = complete blood cell count; CT = computed tomography; DBP = diastolic blood pressure; IV = intravenous; NINCDS = National Institute of Neurological and Communicative Diseases and Stroke; NSAIDs = nonsteroidal anti-inflammatory drugs; PT = prothrombin time; PTT = partial thromboplastin time; SBP = systolic blood pressure; t-PA = tissue plasminogen activator.

blood pressure only if the mean arterial pressure is more than 135 mm Hg, aiming for a value between 125 and 135 mm Hg.

Hyperglycemia damages the ischemic penumbra by increasing local lactic acidosis and is associated with worse outcomes in patients with acute ischemic stroke. One should avoid administering glucose-containing solutions (and hypotonic solutions in general because they worsen cerebral edema) and attempt to maintain normoglycemia with insulin. Only if the patient is hypoglycemic on admission should one administer glucose; in this case, the hypoglycemia—not stroke—is the most likely cause of the focal neurologic deficit.

Most acute stroke patients have weak oropharyngeal musculature and are thus at high risk for aspiration pneumonia. Aspiration pneumonia is a major cause of morbidity and mortality in stroke patients. Aspiration prophylaxis consists of elevating the patient's head at 30 degrees, not allowing oral intake (including no oral liquids or medications) until the patient undergoes a swallowing evaluation, and placing the patient in the lateral decubitus position if emesis occurs. If necessary, one may place a nasogastric feeding tube 24 hours after t-PA administration or on admission if t-PA is not given.

There is no evidence that administration of supplemental oxygen is beneficial in acute stroke patients. High-flow oxygen may cause oxygen free-radical formation and damage the penumbra. One study of hospitalized patients suggested that 3 L of oxygen was not beneficial. I prefer that prehospital providers administer 2 to 4 L of oxygen, but in the hospital I continue low-flow oxygen only if the oxygen saturation is 92% or less. Hypothermia is neuroprotective, and preliminary evidence suggests that relative hyperthermia is associated with worse outcomes. At the very least, one should treat infections aggressively and lower any elevation in temperature with acetaminophen (Tylenol). Further study is necessary to determine if the use of cooled intravenous solutions and cooling blankets is of benefit in acute stroke patients.

Deep vein thrombosis (DVT) is common in stroke patients, and pulmonary embolism is unfortunately too common a cause of death in acute stroke patients. Optimal DVT prophylaxis includes combining pneumatic compression stockings, low-dose heparin (5000 units subcutaneously every 12 hours), and early mobility and rehabilitation. If the patient receives t-PA, delay the onset of subcutaneous heparin until 24 hours after t-PA administration. Early mobilization and rehabilitation are also effective in the prevention of aspiration, decubitus ulcers, constipation, urinary tract infection, and reflex sympathetic dystrophy. Post-stroke depression is common 1 to 2 weeks after the stroke and may interfere with recovery. I treat post-stroke depression with a selective serotonin reuptake inhibitor such as citalopram (Celexa) or sertraline (Zoloft).

EMERGENCY FIBRINOLYTIC AND ANTITHROMBOTIC THERAPY

In the NINCDS study, t-PA afforded a 30% decrease in risk of disability if given within 3 hours of stroke onset and did not increase mortality despite a 6.4% rate of intracranial hemorrhage. Multiple other community studies have confirmed the NINCDS study results—when administered within 3 hours of ischemic stroke onset in accordance with the NINCDS study protocol, t-PA is safe and effective. Based on other trials, however, if one does not adhere to the NINCDS protocol when administering t-PA, and especially if one gives t-PA beyond the 3-hour window, the drug is not effective and carries an increased risk of intracranial hemorrhage. For the purpose of t-PA administration, stroke onset is defined as the "last time the patient was seen without symptoms"; that is, if a patient goes to bed at 10 PM and awakens with a stroke at 4 AM, the time of stroke onset is 10 PM.

Although it is best not to treat hypertension in acute ischemic stroke, acute hypertension is believed to increase the risk of intracranial hemorrhage in patients receiving thrombolytic therapy. In the NINCDS t-PA study, patients with persistent systolic blood pressures greater than 185 mm Hg or diastolic blood pressures more than 110 mm Hg were excluded from participation in the study, as was any patient who received "aggressive" treatment to decrease the blood pressure below those parameters (see Table 1). In the NINCDS protocol, patients received one or two intravenous doses of labetalol (Normodyne) at 10 to 20 mg to lower blood pressure before t-PA administration; I prefer the lower dose of 10 mg. If a patient develops hypertension while receiving t-PA antihypertensive treatment, it is imperative to treat the blood pressure more aggressively, owing to the risk of intracranial hemorrhage and I follow the NINCDS protocol very closely (see Table 4). The dose of t-PA for stroke patients is less than the dose for patients with acute myocardial infarction. Administering even slightly too much t-PA increases the risk of intracranial hemorrhage. The intravenous dose of t-PA for stroke patients is 0.9 mg/kg, with a maximum dose of 90 mg (see Table 4).

Administering aspirin, 325 mg, within 48 hours of stroke onset decreases the risk of recurrent stroke and death. If the patient receives t-PA, one should give the aspirin 24 hours after t-PA is given. There is still no evidence that intravenous heparin is safe or effective in patients with acute ischemic stroke, and I do not routinely prescribe it. I primarily prescribe intravenous heparin (no bolus and maintaining an activated partial thromboplastin time of 50 to 70) when I believe patients require chronic warfarin for secondary prevention. I start oral warfarin concurrent with the intravenous heparin and discontinue the heparin when the international normalized ratio (INR) is 2 to 3.

SECONDARY STROKE PREVENTION

Whereas primary stroke prevention strategies are based on risk factor modification alone, secondary stroke prevention strategies are based on both risk factor modification and the cause of the patient's previous stroke or TIA. A *risk factor* is a condition that, when present, increases the likelihood of suffering a disease. A *cause* is the actual pathophysiologic mechanism by which a disease occurs. Many conditions are risk factors for more than one cause of stroke; for example, hypertension is a risk factor for intracerebral hemorrhage and at least three causes of ischemic stroke: atherosclerosis, small artery disease, and cardioembolism.

Clinical criteria alone are not sufficient to determine cause: one must have access to and utilize diagnostic testing. In the last several years, there have been many advances in secondary stroke prevention strategies and the diagnostic tools available to stroke clinicians, such as MRI. MRI is more sensitive than CT for detecting ischemic lesions, and preliminary evidence suggests that certain MRI modalities may be useful for detecting acute hemorrhage. In addition, new MRI technologies such as diffusion-weighted and perfusion imaging can delineate the ischemic penumbra, although their application in the emergency setting is not always feasible. Atherosclerosis is the most common cause of ischemic stroke, whereas small artery disease and cardioembolism are the next most common causes. In young adults (i.e., ages 18–55), hypercoagulable states, cardioembolism, and nonatherosclerotic vasculopathies occur more frequently. However, in any individual patient, any of the six pathophysiologic mechanisms may be responsible for causing the ischemic stroke or TIA. Proper utilization of diagnostic studies often results in the determination of the cause of stroke and, once the cause is determined, one can prescribe the proper secondary prevention measures (Table 5).

TABLE 5. **Determining Secondary Stroke Prevention Strategy***

Etiologic Evaluation	Cause of Ischemic Stroke	Secondary Prevention Strategy
Day 1		
Cardiac monitor and 12-lead electrocardiogram	Atherosclerosis (large-artery disease)	*Antiplatelet Agent*
Carotid duplex and transcranial Doppler	Lacunar stroke (small-artery disease)	Aspirin
Transthoracic echocardiography	Cardiogenic embolism	Ticlopidine (Ticlid)
Magnetic resonance imaging	Hypercoagulable state	Clopidogrel (Plavix)
Magnetic resonance angiography (intracranial)	Nonatherosclerotic vasculopathy	Aspirin + dipyridamole XR (Aggrenox)
Hypercoagulable evaluation (if patient ≤55 years old)	Hypoperfusion (watershed strokes)	*Anticoagulant*
Day 2		Warfarin (Coumadin)
If indicated by day 1 evaluation		*Surgery*
Transesophageal echocardiography		Carotid endarterectomy
Catheter angiography		*Risk Factor Modification*

*Based on results of etiologic evaluation, determine stroke cause and subsequent secondary prevention strategy. See text for details.

For patients with extracranial atherosclerosis, stroke prevention includes risk factor control, antiplatelet agents, carotid endarterectomy, and treatment of concurrent heart disease (atherosclerosis is a systemic disease, and the most common cause of death among stroke patients is actually heart disease). Among antiplatelet agents, aspirin, 325 mg/d, is my first choice in most cases and clopidogrel (Plavix), 75 mg/d, is my second choice. Carotid endarterectomy decreases risk of stroke and death in symptomatic patients with 50% or more stenosis through specific angiographic measurement criteria and has a complication rate of less than 6%. Endarterectomy does not preclude the need for antiplatelet therapy. If the cause of the patient's stroke is a high-grade intracranial stenosis due to atherosclerosis, surgery is not possible. In such patients, I prescribe warfarin (Coumadin), maintaining an INR of 2 to 3, and aim for a higher blood pressure (mean, 110–115 mm Hg or sytolic, 150–160 mm Hg). Cerebral angioplasty and stenting are currently experimental but may be considered in special circumstances. It is important to realize that not all occlusions of small arteries are due to primary small artery disease. If, after the diagnostic evaluation, one determines that the stroke is due to primary small artery disease, then stroke prevention measures include tight control of stroke risk factors, an antiplatelet agent, and treatment of concurrent heart disease.

Prevention of cardioembolism depends on the specific cardioembolic source. In most cases chronic anticoagulation is warranted (e.g., atrial fibrillation, akinetic left ventricular segment, dilated cardiomyopathy, or mechanical prosthetic heart valve). In patients with a patent foramen ovale and/or interatrial septal aneurysm as the cause of stroke, it would be wise to perform a hypercoagulable profile before determining if chronic anticoagulation is indicated. If the hypercoagulable profile is negative, one may treat temporarily with anticoagulation and then consider a surgical or interventional procedure to repair the septal abnormality. Certain cardioembolic sources are not treated with anticoagulation, such as infective endocarditis (antibiotics and possible valve replacement) and cardiac tumors (e.g., atrial myxoma, resected surgically).

Patients with stroke due to a hypercoagulable state are treated with chronic warfarin, in most cases maintaining an INR of 2 to 3. If a stroke is caused by hypotension, any systemic bleeding is treated and/or antihypertensive medications are decreased. The secondary prevention strategies for patients with stroke due to nonatherosclerotic vasculopathies (e.g., arterial dissection, vasculitis, or moyamoya disease) vary considerably depending on the specific condition.

Systolic and diastolic hypertension are independent risk factors for stroke. In patients who have already suffered a cerebral or cardiac ischemic event, it is best to maintain systolic blood pressure under 130 mm Hg and diastolic blood pressure under 85 mm Hg to decrease risk of a recurrent event, but one should achieve these levels gradually over weeks to months and not aim for ideal values by the time of discharge.

Lowering cholesterol levels with a statin medication such as pravastatin (Pravachol) or simvastatin (Zocor) decreases the risk of stroke. For patients who have suffered a stroke or myocardial infarction, a low-density lipoprotein level of less than 100 mg/dL is optimal. Although diabetes mellitus is "modifiable" in the sense that blood glucose values can be controlled with diet and medication, there is no current evidence that tight control of the blood glucose concentration decreases the risk of stroke. Likewise, although hyperhomocysteinemia is now an established risk factor for stroke and myocardial infarction, there is not yet proof that lowering homocysteine levels (e.g., by prescribing folate, vitamin B_6, or vitamin B_{12}) lowers the risk of a recurrent event. Stroke risk may decrease with increased dietary potassium* intake or daily vitamin E,* 400 to 800 IU.

Bupropion (Zyban) and nicotine patches, gum, or spray are helpful in efforts in smoking cessation. Drinking more than 2 ounces of alcohol per day results in hypertension and an increased risk for stroke. Drinking 2 or less ounces of alcohol per day, however, decreases stroke risk by decreasing blood pressure and raising high-density lipoprotein cholesterol. Binge drinking is just as harmful as excessive daily use of alcohol, so patients should be advised to drink in moderation on a consistent basis. Cocaine, amphetamines, and chronic use of phenylpropanolamine (in some diet pills and decongestants) and ephedrine increase blood pressure and stroke risk.

*Not FDA approved for this indication.

REHABILITATION OF THE STROKE PATIENT

method of
BARBARA J. BROWNE, M.D.
Jefferson Medical College and Magee Rehabilitation Hospital
Philadelphia, Pennsylvania

Stroke is the leading cause of adult disability in the United States. Approximately 600,000 Americans suffer a stroke each year, 200,000 of which are fatal. Hemiparesis is the most common manifestation. The initial level of stroke severity affects the level and course of recovery. Most survivors experience some degree of recovery in strength, including those with dense hemiplegia. Of those who survive, 10% experience full or nearly full spontaneous recovery. Another 10% fail to benefit from rehabilitative attempts. The remaining 80% have neurologic impairments that will benefit from rehabilitative intervention.

Most stroke recovery occurs in the first 90 days but a more protracted recovery may continue for 6 months or longer. Patients and families need to know the expected time course of recovery for rational planning of long-term care.

Survivors of ischemic stroke have a 35% to 65% prevalence of significant coronary artery disease (CAD). Heart disease is the third leading cause of death in the first month following stroke and the leading cause of death among long-term survivors. Uncontrolled hypertension, angina, cardiac arrhythmia, and congestive heart failure occur in 40% of stroke rehabilitation patients with CAD. These patients can safely participate in a rehabilitation program but need additional monitoring. Initially, blood pressure should be slowly decreased to 180/100 in patients with pre-existing hypertension or 160/95 in patients without pre-existing hypertension. Subsequently, blood pressure should be decreased gradually. Precautions for maximal heart rate should be determined individually based on the degree of CAD and age. Patients with congestive heart failure tolerate exercise best in an upright position and should be monitored for a hypotensive response to exercise, warning of further left ventricular failure.

Given the association between diabetes mellitus, hypertension, hyperlipidemia, and CAD, it is not surprising that many stroke survivors also have diabetes mellitus. Frequent adjustment of medications is required because of changes in feeding regimens and activity levels.

Self-administration of insulin is an important goal requiring an interdisciplinary approach. Specialized training to perform one-hand injection techniques can be successful.

TREATMENT OF COMPLICATIONS OF STROKE

Dysphagia

Dysphagia occurs in 50% of stroke patients. Aspiration pneumonia is the most common cause of nonneurologic death in the first month following a stroke. Videofluoroscopic swallowing studies have identified rates of aspiration as high as 70%. Early bedside evaluation can greatly reduce the incidence of aspiration pneumonia. Bedside predictors of aspiration include cough after swallow, wet vocal quality, dysphonia, dysarthria, abnormal gag reflex, lethargy, and inability to follow commands. Up to 60% of stroke patients aspirate silently and require videofluoroscopic study. Aspiration is most common in brainstem and large vessel strokes. A combination of bedside evaluation and videofluoroscopic study can identify 90% of patients with dysphagia and aspiration. Factors that increase the risk of pneumonia in the context of dysphagia and aspiration include nasogastric feeding, tracheostomy, lethargy, vomiting, and reflux. Stroke patients believed to be at high risk for aspiration should use enteral feedings. A gastrostomy or jejunostomy tube is placed if long-term enteral feeding is anticipated.

Compensatory strategies for dysphagia include chin-tuck with turning the head to the paretic side, an upright feeding position, and tactile thermal stimulation to stimulate the swallow reflex. Dietary modifications include thickened liquids and pureed or soft solids. Many patients benefit from a quiet, nondistracting dining location that allows quiet observation and assistance. Dehydration and malnutrition can result from use of unpalatable thickened liquids and lack of feeding assistance. Fortunately, most patients with dysphagia do eventually recover their ability to safely swallow. Even the majority of patients who require gastrostomy tubes are relieved of them on completion of an inpatient dysphagia program.

Thrombophlebitis

The risk of thrombophlebitis may be as high as 70% in unprotected stroke patients. At greatest risk are older patients with large strokes, severe immobility, infection, prolonged hospitalization, recent surgery, and a history of deep vein thrombosis. Patients who can walk 100 feet away from the parallel bars are at low risk for venous thromboembolism. All other patients should be considered for prophylaxis.

Unfractionated heparin at a dosage of 5000 U twice a day produces a 21% absolute risk reduction for thrombophlebitis. Low molecular weight heparin (LMWH) may be superior to unfractionated heparin because of superior bioavailability after subcutaneous injection. An added advantage of LMWH is once-daily dosing. Examples include enoxaparin (Lovenox) at 30 U twice daily or dalteparin (Fragmin) at 5000 U once daily. The use of antiembolic stockings may offer additional protection and limit lower limb–dependent edema. The safety of unfractionated heparin or LMWH following intracranial hemorrhage has not been well studied. Their use in hypertensive hemorrhage in which the blood pressure is stable and the cerebral hematoma has been unchanged for 1 week appears safe. Additionally, low-dose heparin can be used after cerebral aneurysm clipping if the neurologic examination has been stable for 48 hours. Alternatives for patients who cannot be given anticoagulant medications are intermittent pneumatic compression stockings. Intermittent pneumatic compression stockings are most effective when used around the clock but can be effective when used for 12 hours nightly. They are even more effective when paired with LMWH at prophylactic doses.

Urinary Dysfunction

Urinary dysfunction including retention, incontinence, and infection are commonly seen following stroke. Reports of retention vary from 47% in the first 72 hours to 21% at 3 weeks following stroke. The neurophysiologic explanation for poststroke detrusor areflexia is unknown, but there is a higher incidence in those with aphasia, cognitive impairment, and lower functional status. Diabetic stroke patients with neuropathy also have higher rates of retention, possibly due to diabetes-related detrusor paresis. Although poststroke urinary retention is generally a transient phenomenon, failure to recognize it can result in damage to the detrusor muscle from overdistention. Retention also predisposes the patient to urinary tract infection (UTI). UTI is the most common type of poststroke infection, although it may arise for other reasons including indwelling catheters. Postvoid residual urine should be checked in all stroke patients with urinary dysfunction.

Resolution of retention can be facilitated by avoidance of medications with anticholinergic side effects, voiding in the sitting or standing position, and treatment of UTI if present. α-Receptor antagonists such as tamsulosin (Flomax), terazosin (Hytrin), or doxazosin (Cardura) may help alleviate underlying outlet obstruction from prostate gland hypertrophy or in patients with suspected detrusor sphincter dyssynergia. Urodynamic studies with electromyographic recording from the urethral sphincter may provide diagnostic clarification.

Urinary incontinence is a frequent consequence of stroke and can be a burden to both the patient and caregiver. Uncontrolled incontinence can be a major factor in institutionalizing a patient for long-term care instead of providing care at home. The pattern of incontinence is that of an uninhibited neurogenic bladder in which the desire to void is closely coupled with a detrusor contraction resulting in incontinence. This can be treated in most cases with a schedule of time voiding in which the patient is asked to empty the bladder every 2 to 3 hours during the day and before bed. Additionally, judicious use of fluids, avoidance of caffeine and diuretics when possible can be very helpful. Anticholinergic medications such as oxybutynin (Ditropan) and tolterodine (Detrol) can increase bladder capacity and reduce the frequency of voiding. Their use can be limited by the side effects of dry mouth and sedation. Care must be used if there is a history of glaucoma. An effective combination is 5 mg of oxybutynin at bedtime and time voiding during the day.

Spasticity

Spasticity is an expected complication of stroke, given the upper motor location of the injury. *Spasticity* is defined as a velocity-dependent resistance to passive range of motion. Moderate spasticity can provide greater stability with standing secondary to extensor tone in the lower limb. However, spasticity can impair gait, dressing skills, and hygiene of the hand, axilla, and perineal areas. Additionally, spasticity may cause pain, result in limb contracture, and mask volitional motor recovery.

Several options have emerged as safe and effective treatments for poststroke spasticity. Tizanidine (Zanaflex) is an α_2-adrenergic receptor agonist that reduces spasticity by blocking the presynaptic release of excitatory neurotransmitters and facilitating inhibitory neurotransmitters. Its use is limited by its common side effects: sedation, dry mouth, and dizziness. Elevated liver enzyme levels have been reported and should be monitored periodically. Tolerance is best achieved by starting with low doses of 2 to 4 mg at night and slowly titrating by 2 mg every few days. Lower doses than the recommended 8 mg three times a day and nighttime doses alone are often effective.

Oral baclofen (Lioresal) and diazepam (Valium) are less effective with stroke related spasticity than with spinal cord spasticity and often cause unacceptable levels of sedation and confusion.

Dantrolene sodium (Dantrium) is an effective oral treatment that targets the sarcoplasmic reticulum of skeletal muscle. A touted advantage is preservation of cognitive function. Drowsiness and dizziness may occur, although the effect is usually transient. Unacceptable generalized weakness can limit its usefulness. Both fatal and nonfatal hepatitis have been reported at various doses, and the drug should not be given with active hepatic disease. Appropriate titration to the lowest effective dose and monitoring of liver function is needed. Dosing can be started at 25 mg per day and titrated by 25 mg thrice-daily up to 100 mg thrice-daily if needed.

Stroke patients with focal spasticity can be greatly helped by local muscle injections of botulinum toxin, type A (Botox).* Botulinum toxin type A blocks the release of acetylcholine from the nerve terminal, causing a chemical denervation. Botulinum toxin A injections are short-term therapy with reversible effects. Botulinum toxin type A requires 14 days to reach a peak effect with a duration of 2 to 4 months. Flulike symptoms are the most frequent side effect. Injections should be given no more frequently than every 12 weeks to avoid development of resistance. A more permanent effect can be achieved with the chemoneurolytic agent phenol. Care must be used because phenol-induced neurolysis of mixed nerves, containing both motor and sensory branches, may cause permanent dysesthesias. Phenol is best suited for large muscles such as the hip adductors and extensors, the pectorals, latissimus dorsi, and biceps brachii. Phenol has an immediate onset of action, low cost, and long duration. It should not be used in muscles where further motor recovery is expected to occur.

Before or in conjunction with medication, collaboration with a physical and occupational therapist is essential to achieve and maintain effective functional gains. A skilled therapist can provide stretching, serial casting for contractures, supportive splints, and electrical stimulation to facilitate antagonistic muscle activity. An ankle-foot orthosis set in neutral or 5 degrees of dorsiflexion can facilitate knee flexion, control foot drop, and correct minor equinovarus foot position.

Intrathecal baclofen delivers much lower doses of medication directly into cerebrospinal fluid thus avoiding lethargy while preserving therapeutic effects. Surgical implantation of the pump delivery system is required. Intrathecal baclofen is more effective with lower limb than upper limb spasticity.

Surgery to cut and transfer tendons can also reduce the negative effects of spasticity. Walking ability can be improved with a split anterior tibial tendon transfer. This procedure moves half of the anterior tibial tendon to the outside of the foot, limiting excessive inversion and facilitating proper foot position.

Up to 85% of stroke survivors experience some degree of shoulder pain in the paretic limb. Although many different causes have been proposed, the best

*Not FDA approved for this indication.

TABLE 1. **Poststroke Shoulder Pain**

Cause	Signs	Diagnosis	Treatment
CRPS I*	Pain with rest and activity Swelling of hand Temperature changes of skin	Painful compression of MCP joints and finger extension Triple phase bone scan	10–14 d of oral steroids Stellate ganglion block
Adhesive capsulitis	Limited external rotation Early scapular motion	Arthrography	PT/ROM Reduction of internal rotator spasticity Intraarticular steroids†
Impingement syndrome	Pain with abduction of 70°–90°		Subacromial steroid injection PT/ROM Scapular mobilization Reduction of internal rotator spasticity
Rotator cuff tear	Positive abduction and drop arm tests	Radiography MRI	PT/ROM Steroid injection Surgical repair Reduction of internal rotator spasticity
Inferior subluxation	Acromiohumeral separation	Radiography	Sling when upright Tray or table support when seated

*CRPS I is also known as reflex sympathetic dystrophy and shoulder-hand syndrome.
†The efficacy of intraarticular steroid injection in poststroke shoulder pain remains unproven.
Abbreviations: CRPS I = complex regional pain syndrome type I; MCP = metacarpophalangeal; MRI = magnetic resonance imaging; PT/ROM = physical therapy/range of motion.

treatment remains elusive. Poststroke shoulder pain interferes with the rehabilitative process and can prolong the hospital stay. Table 1 provides a summary of the most likely causes of poststroke shoulder pain and potential treatments. Additional use of analgesics is usually necessary. Gabapentin (Neurontin)* and tricyclic antidepressant drugs* can be especially useful with central or neuropathic pain. Topical capsaicin (Zostrix) and transcutaneous electrical nerve stimulation may be useful adjuncts. Routine use of slings has not been shown to be beneficial and may encourage disuse and contracture formation. However, limited use to support a flaccid arm during ambulation may increase comfort. Caregivers must be taught proper positioning and transfer techniques to avoid further injury.

Depression

Depression affects 30% of stroke survivors. Studies have failed to definitively show a correlation with the side or location of the lesion. Female patients with higher levels of education appear to be at greater risk for depression. Distinguishing between a major and minor depression can be difficult because some symptoms stressed by *Diagnostic and Statistical Manual of Mental Disorders,* fourth edition (DSM-IV) criteria can be a result of the brain lesion itself. Failure to treat poststroke depression can negatively affect rehabilitation outcome.

The serotonin-specific release inhibitors are safe and effective agents for treatment and have a superior side effect profile compared with the tricyclic antidepressants. Fluoxetine (Prozac) has been shown to alleviate depression and facilitate functional recovery. The psychostimulant methylphenidate (Ritalin)* has been shown to improve mood as well as enhance motor recovery and daily living skill ability. Methylphenidate provides a rapid onset of action, has a good safety profile, is well tolerated, and enables some patients to better participate in therapy during the critical period of inpatient rehabilitation. Use beyond 4 weeks is cautioned secondary to issues of dependency and unproven long-term benefit. Serotonin-specific release inhibitors are also effective treatment for poststroke emotional lability characterized by socially inappropriate outbursts of crying and sometimes laughter.

*Not FDA approved for this indication.

Seizures

Early seizures (<2 weeks) after stroke occur at rates of 2.5% to 15% with the highest rate occurring in lobar hemorrhages. The risk of recurring early seizures is unclear as is the need for long-term antiepileptic medication. Seizures occurring more than 2 weeks after stroke are related to scar formation, are likely to recur, and can usually be controlled with monotherapy.

Aphasia

Aphasia occurs in 24% of stroke patients. Broca's aphasia is common in infarctions involving the left

*Not FDA approved for this indication.

middle cerebral artery. Various speech therapy techniques have been shown to be helpful, although no single approach has proven superior. Case reports have suggested improvements in initiation, content, and fluency using the dopamine agonist bromocriptine (Parlodel)* in expressive aphasia.

Apraxia

Apraxia, a disorder of learned movement not caused by muscle weakness or sensory loss, is often seen in patients with left middle cerebral artery infarctions. Deficits include difficulty initiating speech, masticating, and using the paretic and nonparetic upper limbs.

Treatment of stroke patients on a dedicated stroke unit during both the acute and rehabilitative stages has been shown to improve outcome. Conventional methods of rehabilitation include range-of-motion exercises, mobilization activities, and compensatory techniques. More controversial are therapeutic exercise programs that incorporate neuromuscular reeducation. The Brunnstrom technique uses proprioceptive and cutaneous stimuli to enhance specific synergies. No rehabilitative technique has proven superior to the others. Most programs combine aspects of conventional and neuromuscular re-education techniques because specific techniques may be more beneficial in individual cases.

Only 5% of adults recover full use of the paretic upper limb and 20% fail to recover any functional use. Traditionally, compensatory strategies using the nonparetic limb are emphasized to maximize functional gains quickly. The emphasis on compensatory strategies and belief in the plateau of neural recovery after 3 months have recently been challenged.

Several small studies have demonstrated functional gains at more than 1 year after stroke. Monkey subjects with chronic stroke have demonstrated functional recovery following forced use of the paretic upper limb. Constraint-induced movement technique has demonstrated that additional recovery can occur greater than 6 months after stroke in certain cases. This technique is based on the theory that there is learned nonuse of the paretic limb that can be reversed with forced use by restraining the unimpaired side. Controlled trials of this technique in both subacute and chronic stroke patients are underway. Other promising techniques to enhance recovery include functional electrical stimulation to increase muscle strength. Although still largely experimental, implantable electrodes with neurocontrol systems have been used to enhance function after stroke and spinal cord injury.

REHABILITATION OF THE PATIENT

Stroke rehabilitation may be provided in several settings. Acute rehabilitation provides 3 hours of therapy a day, 5 to 7 days a week. Care is based on a multidisciplinary team approach usually led by a physiatrist or physician specializing in rehabilitation medicine. Patients receive daily physician visits and there is a strong emphasis on patient and family training. This level of care is most suitable for patients who require minimal to maximal assistance for mobility and self-care and have the physical and cognitive ability to participate and learn. Patients with language and swallowing impairments also benefit from this intensive level of care.

Subacute and skilled rehabilitation programs provide varying amounts of therapy. Patients may receive single or multiple therapies 1 to 2 hours a day, 3 to 5 days a week. Physician visits are one to three times per week at the subacute level and monthly at the skilled care level. This level of care is most appropriate for patients with physical or cognitive limitations that preclude participation at a more intensive level.

Outpatient and day programs are appropriate for patients with adequate functional mobility, medical stability, and social supports to manage safely in their homes. Home health programs have the added advantage of teaching patients in their home environment but lack professional equipment and personnel.

Discharge planning should begin during the acute care of the stroke patient. Typically, this involves the physician and social worker to assess anticipated need for 24-hour assistance and supervision, available caregiver support, and home accessibility. Further planning occurs throughout the inpatient stay with involvement of the patient and family in setting appropriate goals.

Outpatient follow-up visits with the rehabilitation physician are generally done at 1-month after discharge. Future visits are done at various intervals as warranted by progress and complications. Patients should retain their primary care physicians for general medical care and medication renewals. Good communication with the primary physician is essential.

Rehabilitation physician visits should address not only medical and neurologic status but also proper medication usage, daily activity levels, stroke prevention tactics, and compliance with the home exercise program. Direct inquiry about psychosocial issues and depression should be made. All orthotics and equipment should be inspected for fit and stability. The need for further therapy must be assessed. Unfortunately, many patients and families view the reduction or termination of therapy as the end of future progress. Gradually reducing therapy sessions while the patient resumes leisure activities and enrolls and participates in community exercise and socialization programs can ease the transition.

The successful return to work eludes most stroke patients, although it can be an important contributor to life satisfaction. Enrollment in a vocational rehabilitation program can provide training for the patient and employer. A gradual approach with initial part-time hours is most successful.

*Not FDA approved for this indication.

Some patients may be able to resume driving, but those with visual field deficit and right- or left-sided neglect should avoid it. When recovery is incomplete, participation in a driving program for stroke survivors is recommended. Patients with poststroke seizures must be seizure-free for 6 to 12 months according to state laws.

Stroke rehabilitation faces an exciting and challenging future. New information about recovery processes and neural plasticity may change the types and duration of rehabilitative services. Managed health care will continue to emphasize shorter lengths of stay. The physician caring for a stroke survivor has many responsibilities including preventing medical complications, assisting patients and families in choosing appropriate therapeutic options, and setting realistic goals. Knowledge of recovery patterns and coordination of care with therapists, consulting physicians, and social workers will greatly assist patients in achieving their maximal functional potential and improve their quality of life.

SEIZURES AND EPILEPSY IN ADOLESCENTS AND ADULTS

method of
NATHAN B. FOUNTAIN, M.D.
University of Virginia School of Medicine
Charlottesville, Virginia

Seizures and epilepsy have long been misunderstood by physicians, but a logical framework for the approach to seizures has emerged in recent years. Such an approach is especially important today because eight new antiepileptic drugs (AEDs) have been approved for use in the United States since 1993, and their proper use is contingent on a systematic approach.

This chapter follows the systematic analysis that should accompany the approach to treating patients with seizures and epilepsy by dividing the process into five steps. *Step 1* is to confirm that the paroxysmal symptom of concern is a seizure. *Step 2* is to determine the specific type of seizure present by classifying it as focal or generalized in onset. *Step 3* is to determine the neuroanatomic site of seizure onset to direct investigations toward identifying pathology at that site. *Step 4* is to identify the etiology or determine the epilepsy syndrome if the etiology is not identifiable. *Step 5* is to select the appropriate therapy.

Some terms used to describe seizures or epilepsy have definitions that are unique to the study of epilepsy. *Seizures* are behavioral changes that result from abnormal paroxysmal neuronal discharge and are a symptom of an underlying brain problem. A seizure may result from a transient perturbation of neuronal physiology such as occurs during acute head trauma, alcohol withdrawal, or hypocalcemia, or a seizure may result from an enduring tendency to seizures, commonly referred to as epilepsy. *Epilepsy*, therefore, is not a single "disease" but, instead, is any disease characterized by the spontaneous recurrence of seizures. Epilepsy syndromes are diseases that are characterized exclusively or primarily by the occurrence of seizures with few other systemic or neurologic symptoms. When the etiology of the seizures is definitely known, for example, when caused by a brain tumor or penetrating brain injury, then classification into an epilepsy syndrome is less important. However, when the etiology is not known because it is not identifiable or the evaluation is incomplete, then classification becomes useful. Patients grouped into a specific epilepsy syndrome are presumed to share a similar pathophysiology and therefore a similar natural history and response to therapy.

DIAGNOSIS

Differential Diagnosis of Paroxysmal Symptoms

Several entities cause symptoms similar to seizures. *Syncope* is commonly accompanied by motor movements, especially clonic or brief tonic arm movements, termed "convulsive syncope" or a "syncopal seizure," during which the electroencephalogram (EEG) shows profound suppression of brain activity because of cerebral anoxia; it does not show seizure discharges and is not an epileptic seizure. Syncope is distinguished from a true seizure by the presence of presyncopal symptoms (nausea, flushing, and lightheadedness), brief loss of consciousness, and return of normal cognition within a few seconds after arousal. *Migraine* headaches may occasionally be accompanied by complex visual phenomena or sensorimotor symptoms that could be confused with seizures. Postictal headaches may be confused with migraine. Complicated migraine with hemiparesis may be mistaken for postictal paralysis. A history of migraine headaches and preservation of normal consciousness help identify the spells as migraine. Transient ischemic attacks should almost never be mistaken for seizures because these attacks cause focal negative phenomena, such as weakness, aphasia, or ataxia, whereas seizures usually cause positive phenomena such as jerking, automatisms, or movements.

Psychiatric disease can cause symptoms nearly identical to seizures. Anxiety attacks can be characterized by anxiety, palpitation, facial flushing, and incoherence, and so can seizure auras. Seizure auras generally progress to complex partial seizures at some point in the evolution of the epilepsy, and auras are usually more stereotypical than anxiety attacks. Pseudoseizures, which have also been termed *psychogenic nonepileptic seizures*, may be identical to seizures in their characteristics. However, pseudoseizures are more likely to be long in duration, may involve bizarre or unusual symptoms and movements, can include pelvic thrusting or thrashing, and may be precipitated by psychologically stressful events, and they persist despite AED therapy. Unfortunately, epileptic seizures may also have these characteristics and video/EEG monitoring may be the only way to definitively distinguish seizures from pseudoseizures. Surprisingly, as many as 30% of patients admitted to inpatient epilepsy units for the diagnosis of spells are proved to have pseudoseizures.

Seizure Classification

The International League Against Epilepsy has developed a classification of seizures based on the site of seizure origin to facilitate communication (Figure 1). Seizures are divided into partial (or focal) and generalized classes. Consciousness is preserved in partial seizures because only a small region of the brain is affected, whereas it is lost in generalized seizures because the entire cortex is affected. Partial seizures may secondarily generalize. "Primary" generalized seizures involve the whole brain from the onset.

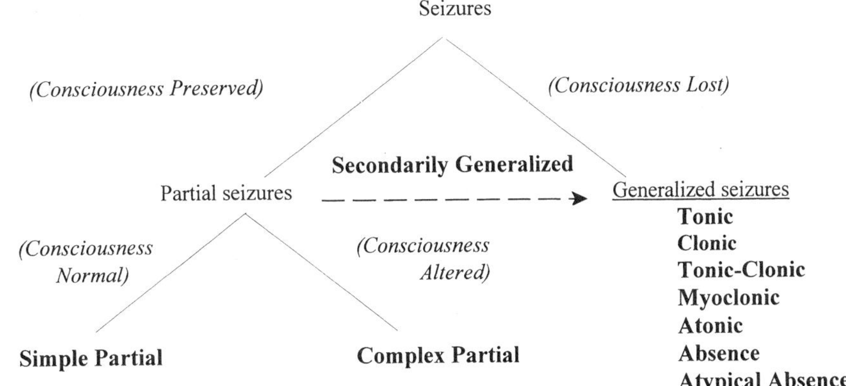

Figure 1. Algorithm for seizure classification.

Partial seizures are subdivided into simple partial and complex partial subtypes. *Simple partial seizures* arise in a small region of cortex and produce discrete symptoms without altering consciousness, depending on the area from which they arise. For example, seizures arising in the primary motor cortex in the frontal lobe cause clonic jerking of the contralateral limb, usually the hand. The most common simple partial seizures are indescribable auras arising in the temporal lobe and causing autonomic symptoms. *Complex partial seizures* are characterized by staring with a fixed gaze and lack of distractibility to examiners. Automatisms are common, especially picking or pulling at clothing, lip smacking, and swallowing.

Generalized seizures are classified according to the predominant motor activity. *Generalized tonic-clonic seizures* begin with sudden tonic extension of the extremities, often with an expiratory scream, followed by clonic rhythmic jerking of the extremities. Postictally, patients are always unresponsive for at least a brief period and usually sleep for minutes to hours. *Tonic seizures* contain only the tonic phase and *clonic seizures* contain only the clonic phase. *Myoclonic seizures* are a brief lightning-like jerk, most commonly of the arms. *Atonic seizures* consist of sudden unprotected falling with loss of muscle tone. *Absence seizures* are associated with nondistractible staring, similar to complex partial seizures, but they are very brief, frequent, found primarily in children, and associated with a generalized 3-Hz spike-and-wave pattern on EEG. *Atypical absence seizures* are similar but more prolonged and often accompanied by brief myoclonic jerks or loss of tone, and the EEG shows a slow or atypical generalized spike-and-wave pattern.

Etiology and Epilepsy Syndrome Classification

The underlying pathology or etiology of seizures ultimately determines the natural history and, to some degree, the response to therapy. Historically, the etiology was either unknown or not considered important, and the selection of an AED was based solely on the type of seizure present. In fact, all available AEDs were studied for their efficacy in treating specific seizure types without regard to etiology. This reasoning is rational for partial-onset seizures because partial seizures of all etiologies seem to respond to the same drugs. However, various types of generalized seizures selectively respond to certain AEDs. Overall, this logic is still widely applied, but when the etiology is known, it should be taken into account when selecting an AED.

Common etiologies of seizures are brain diseases that involve the cortex. The most frequent identifiable etiologies in adults are trauma, developmental malformations, stroke, and mass lesions. Mesial temporal sclerosis is the most commonly identified pathology in the temporal lobe, but its etiology is unknown. When the etiology cannot be identified or is not known, classification into an epilepsy syndrome is valuable. The epilepsy syndromes with the most value are those in which an etiology or underlying pathology is never found.

Epilepsy syndromes have been classified by the International League Against Epilepsy, similar to the classification of seizures (Table 1). The most important groupings of epilepsy syndromes are *localization-related epilepsies* (or focal), in which the pathology is localized to one region of the brain, and *generalized epilepsies*, in which the pathol-

TABLE 1. **Examples of Epilepsy Syndromes in Adolescents and Adults**

	Localization Related	Generalized
Idiopathic	Benign childhood epilepsy with centrotemporal spikes Benign occipital epilepsy Autosomal dominant nocturnal frontal lobe epilepsy	Childhood absence epilepsy Juvenile absence epilepsy Juvenile myoclonic epilepsy Epilepsy with generalized tonic-clonic seizures on awakening
Symptomatic	Temporal lobe Frontal lobe Parietal lobe Occipital lobe	Cortical malformations Cortical dysplasias Metabolic abnormalities West's syndrome Lennox-Gastaut syndrome
Cryptogenic	Any occurrence of partial seizures without obvious pathology	West's syndrome (unidentified pathology) Lennox-Gastaut syndrome (unidentified pathology)

ogy is expressed throughout the whole brain. The etiology can be further subdivided into three categories: (1) those that are "*symptomatic*" of underlying brain disease, (2) "*idiopathic*" causes in which an identifiable lesion is never identified, and (3) "*cryptogenic*" causes in which an anatomic lesion is suspected to be present but cannot be identified. Idiopathic and cryptogenic usually mean unknown in medical terminology, but in the epilepsy syndromes, the idiopathic syndromes are thought to be due to inherited abnormalities of neurotransmission without any anatomic lesion, whereas the cryptogenic syndromes are those that are actually symptomatic but the brain pathology cannot be identified with current technology. The importance of this distinction is that an aggressive search for underlying pathology is not necessary or indicated for idiopathic epilepsies but is necessary for cryptogenic cases.

Complex partial seizures are the most frequent type of seizure in adults. The etiology is most commonly not identifiable, and thus most patients have "cryptogenic focal epilepsy." The most common single identifiable syndrome is temporal lobe epilepsy, which is characterized by refractory complex partial seizures originating in the temporal lobe with occasional secondary generalization. Magnetic resonance imaging (MRI) most often demonstrates atrophy and gliosis of the hippocampus in the temporal lobe. Histopathologically, this condition is characterized by neuronal loss and gliosis of the hippocampus and several mesial temporal structures, which has given rise to the term "mesial temporal sclerosis." Mass lesions in the temporal lobe may be manifested in a similar manner and include malformations and tumors such as astrocytomas and dysembryoplastic neuroepithelial tumors. This syndrome is important to recognize because temporal lobectomy renders more than 70% of patients essentially seizure-free.

Generalized tonic-clonic seizures are the second most common type of seizure in adults. Partial-onset, rapidly secondary generalized seizures may appear identical to primary generalized seizures, so it is important to consider all of the information, especially EEG and imaging studies, before determining that a seizure is primary generalized. The syndrome causing primary generalized tonic-clonic seizures is most often not identifiable. However, the most common identifiable syndrome in adults is juvenile myoclonic epilepsy, which is named for the characteristic onset in adolescence of brief myoclonic arm jerks and generalized tonic-clonic seizures. Juvenile myoclonic epilepsy is associated with a characteristic generalized polyspike-and-wave EEG pattern in between seizures. Imaging studies are normal, as is the case for all idiopathic generalized epilepsies. The etiology is undoubtedly an abnormality in neurotransmission, and it has been localized to at least two separate chromosomal loci, but the pathophysiology is still unknown.

Many epilepsies commonly encountered in adults begin in childhood, and these epilepsies are addressed in a separate article. Childhood absence epilepsy is characterized by absence seizures and a typical generalized 3-Hz spike-and-wave EEG pattern. Absence seizures usually abate by 14 years of age, but about 30% persist into adulthood. Symptomatic focal epilepsies are due to underlying identifiable pathology and may thus arise at any age after head trauma or tumors.

Diagnostic Evaluation

Evaluation of *new-onset seizures* is aimed at finding acute transient causes such as metabolic abnormalities and excluding acute life-threatening etiologies such as infection or neoplasm. Most patients seek emergency care after the first seizure. At that time it is not usually possible to determine whether this seizure represents epilepsy or an acute medical illness. Consequently, simple screening laboratory tests may be indicated, including electrolytes, complete blood count, liver enzymes, and a urine drug screen. If central nervous system (CNS) infection is suspected, lumbar puncture should be performed. An EEG is always indicated because it may reveal interictal epileptiform discharges of the type present in patients with epilepsy, but it is not needed acutely. Neuroimaging is always indicated in the evaluation of a partial-onset seizure to exclude acute or serious focal pathology.

The evaluation of *established epilepsy* is aimed at defining the underlying cause of the epilepsy syndrome, which is usually more subtle. An EEG is always indicated because it may reveal focal epileptiform discharges and assist in classifying the seizure type and epilepsy syndrome. However, a normal EEG does not exclude epilepsy. The first EEG is abnormal in only about 40% of patients with clinically definite localization-related epilepsy. The EEG will remain normal in approximately 20% of these patients, even after as many as seven EEGs. The diagnostic evaluation of intractable epilepsy is intertwined with the presurgical evaluation and is discussed later.

ANTIEPILEPTIC DRUG THERAPY

Pharmacokinetic Principles

No logical system has been devised to classify AEDs. One convenient method is to divide them into conventional, new, unconventional, and experimental categories (Table 2). Conventional AEDs are those that were available before the onslaught of new AEDs that were approved starting in 1993. Although several conventional AEDs are available, only phenytoin, carbamazepine, valproate, phenobarbital, and primidone are widely used. New AEDs are those that have been approved since 1993. Unconventional AEDs are those that are either outdated, used only in specific circumstances, or primarily used for non–epilepsy-related purposes. This discussion focuses on the conventional and new AEDs.

The side effect profile of AEDs is important because conventional AEDs are frequently accompanied by side effects that often depend on the pharmacokinetics of the drug (Table 3). Half-life is important with AEDs because it determines the dosing interval and is often affected by concomitant AEDs. Infrequent dosing is important to improve compliance, and thus drugs with a long half-life are desirable. Some AEDs have a narrow therapeutic window, so patients may experience side effects at the peak of the serum level. More frequent dosing of smaller amounts may avoid peak-dose side effects.

Problematic AED interactions are common, especially among conventional AEDs. Pharmacokinetic interactions most often result from hepatic enzyme induction, which is reflected by changes in the blood level (Table 4). Overall, AED interactions are less common with the new AEDs than with the conventional ones because most new AEDs do not induce hepatic enzymes and are not heavily protein bound (see Table 3). All AEDs necessarily affect the brain, so pharmacodynamic interactions make the CNS side

TABLE 2. **Conventional, New, Unconventional, and Experimental Antiepileptic Drugs**

Conventional	New	Unconventional	Experimental
Carbamazepine	Felbamate	Acetazolamide	Clobazam (Frisium)†
Ethosuximide	Gabapentin	Adrenocorticotropic hormone*	Eterobarb‡
Phenobarbital	Lamotrigine	Amantadine*	Ganaxolone‡
Phenytoin	Levetiracetam	Bromides*	Harkoseride‡
Primidone	Oxcarbazepine	Clomiphene*	Losigamone‡
Valproic acid	Tiagabine	Ethotoin	Nitrazepam (Mogadon)†
	Topiramate	Mephenytoin	Piracetam (Nootropil)‡
	Zonisamide	Mephobarbital	Pregabalin‡
		Methsuximide	Progabide‡
		Trimethadione	Remacemide‡
			Retigabine‡
			Rufinamide‡
			Stiripentol‡
			Vigabatrin (Sabril)†

*Not FDA approved for this indication.
†Not available in the United States, but approved in other countries.
‡Investigational drug in the United States.

effects of lethargy, ataxia, and blurry vision more common when more than one AED is taken at a time. Even as monotherapy, all AEDs cause CNS side effects at high doses.

Several principles can be used to guide dosing and avoid problems. When initiating therapy, it is best to "start low and go slow." Most side effects are experienced at the initiation of therapy and can be avoided by starting with a low enough dose and increasing more slowly than recommended by the manufacturer. Table 5 provides general target doses that will usually be therapeutic. However, the "maintenance" doses given cover a wide range because none of the AEDs have a set final dose. The only method to verify that a given dose is "therapeutic" is to determine that the seizure frequency has decreased. Serum drug levels can provide a general guide, but many patients will be taking a "therapeutic dose" while their blood level is below the usual "normal" range. On the other hand, blood levels can help guide dose increases by warning that toxic side effects may occur with further increases when the blood level is at the upper limit of the established "therapeutic range." It is important to increase each drug to the maximal tolerated dose before labeling it ineffective. This process usually requires increasing the dose until

TABLE 3. **Pharmacokinetics of Conventional and New Antiepileptic Drugs**

Drug	Metabolized by Inducible Enzymes (Mechanisms)	Induces Hepatic Enzymes	Half-Life (h)	Protein Bound (%)
Carbamazepine	Yes (oxidized)	Yes	12–17	76
Ethosuximide	Yes (oxidized)	No	30–60 (30 in child)	0
Felbamate	Yes (multiple mechanisms)	No	20–23	25
Gabapentin	No	No	5–7	<3
Lamotrigine	Yes (glucuronidated)	No	25 alone or w/both 60 w/valproate 12 w/EI	55
Levetiracetam	No	No	6–8	<10
Oxcarbazepine	Yes (converted to MHD → glucuronidated)	Mixed	9–11 (for MHD)	67
Phenobarbital	Yes (hydroxylated, glucuronidated)	Yes	80–100	45
Phenytoin	Yes (hydroxylated, glucuronidated)	Yes	22	90
Primidone	Yes (similar to phenobarbital)	Yes	8–15 (shorter w/EI)	20
Tiagabine	Yes (glucuronidation, oxidation)	No	7–9 (alone) 4–7 (w/EI)	96
Topiramate	Yes (hydroxylated, hydrolyzed, glucuronidated)	No	20–24	13–17
Valproic acid	Yes (glucuronidated, oxidized)	No	9–16 (shorter w/EI)	70–90 (varies with level)
Zonisamide	Yes/no	No	63	40

Abbreviations: EI = enzyme inducer; MHD = monohydroxy derivative.

TABLE 4. **Antiepileptic Drug Interactions Influencing Serum Concentrations*†**

Drug Added	Serum Level Influenced												
	CBZ	*ESM*	*FBM*	*GBP*	*LMT*	*LEV*	*OXC*	*PB*	*PHT*	*TGB*	*TPM*	*VPA*	*ZNS*
CBZ	↓	↓	↓	–	↓↓	–	↓	–	↑↓	↓↓	↓↓	↓	↓
ESM	?–	– –	?–	?–	–	?–	?–	?–	?↑	?–	?–	?–	?–
FBM	↓ epox. ↑	?–	– –	?–	–	?–	?–	↑	↑↑	?–	?–	↑↑	?–
GBP	–	?–	?–	– –	?–	–	?–	–	–	?–	?–	–	?–
LMT	–	–	–	?–	– –	–	?–	–	–	?–	?–	↓	?–
LEV	–	?–	?–	–	–	– –	?–	–	–	?–	?–	–	?–
OXC	–	?	?–	?–	↓	?–	– –	–	–	?	?–	–	?–
PB	↓	↓	↓	–	↓↓	–	↓	– –	–	↓↓	↓	↓	↓
PHT	↓	↓	↓	–	↓↓	–	↓	–	– –	↓↓	↓↓	↓	↓
TGB	–	?–	?–	?–	?–	?–	?–	?–	–	– –	?–	↓	?–
TPM	–	?–	?–	?–	?–	?–	?–	–	↑	?–	– –	↓	?–
VPA	↓ epox. ↑	↑↓	–	–	↑↑	?↑	–	↑↑	–	–	↓	– –	–
ZNS	?–	–	?–	?–	?–	?–	?–	–	–	?–	?–	–	– –

*Effect of adding the drug listed in the first column on the blood concentration of the drugs listed in the other columns.

†Clinically significant effects are double arrows; other effects (single arrows) are not usually clinically relevant. Question marks indicate unknown interactions.

Abbreviations: CBZ = carbamazepine; ESM = ethosuximide; FBM = felbamate; GBP = gabapentin; LMT = lamotrigine; LEV = levetiracetam; OXC = oxcarbazepine; PB = phenobarbital; PHT = phenytoin; TGB = tiagabine; TPM = topiramate; VPA = valproic acid; ZNS = zonisamide.

side effects occur and then reducing the dose by one step. Patients must be informed of this strategy or they may refuse to take the drug, even at a lower dose. When substituting one AED for another, it is important to start the second drug and determine that it is effective before gradually withdrawing the first drug. This technique affords at least some protection from seizures at all times.

Conventional Antiepileptic Drugs

Phenytoin is probably the most widely used and familiar AED despite having the most problematic side effects. The metabolism of phenytoin (Dilantin) is saturable, which means that it shows zero-order kinetics at high blood levels. Very steep elevations in the blood level may occur with even small dose increases when the level is near 20 μg/mL, despite the occurrence of a linear increase in the blood level with dose increases when blood levels are below 20 μg/mL. For example, the blood level may be 10 μg/mL with 200 mg/d, increase to 15 μg/mL with 300 mg/d, and then increase to 20 μg/mL with 400 mg/d, but with an increase to 500 mg/d, the level may skyrocket to more than 30 μ/mL if metabolism is saturated.

TABLE 5. **Titration Guidelines for Conventional and New Antiepileptic Drugs**

Generic Name	Common Brand Name	Dosing Schedule	Adult			Child	
			Initial Dose (mg)	*Increment (mg)*	*Maintenance (mg/d)*	*Initial Dose (mg/kg/d)*	*Maintenance (mg/kg/d)*
Carbamazepine	Tegretol Tegretol-XR, Carbatrol	tid–qid bid	200 bid	200 qwk	600–1800	10	10–35 (for <6y.o.)
Ethosuximide	Zarontin	qd–bid	250 qd	250 q3–7d	750	15	15–40
Felbamate	Felbatol	tid	600–1200 qd	600–1200 q1–2wk	2400–3600	15	15–45
Gabapentin	Neurontin	tid	300 qd	300 q3–7d	1200–3600	10	25–50
Lamotrigine	Lamictal	bid	25 qd	25 q2wk	100 w/VPA 400 alone 600 w/EI	0.15–0.5	0.5–5 w/VPA 5 alone 5–15 w/EI
Levetiracetam	Keppra	bid	500 qd	500 qwk	2000–4000	20	40–60
Oxcarbazepine	Trileptal	bid	300 qd	300 qwk	900–2400	8–10	30–46
Phenobarbital	(Generic)	qd–bid	30–60 qd	30 q1–2wk	60–120	3	3–6
Phenytoin	Dilantin Kapseals Liquid, Infatabs	qd bid–tid	200 qd	100 qwk	200–300	4	4–8
Primidone	Mysoline	tid	125–250 qd	250 q1–2wk	500–750	10	10–25
Tiagabine	Gabitril	bid–qid	4 qd	4–8 qwk	16–32	0.1	0.4 w/o EI 0.7 w/EI
Topiramate	Topamax	bid	25 qd	25 q1–2wk	200–400	3	3–9
Valproic acid	Depakene, Depakote Depakote ER	tid–qid bid	250 qd	250 q3–7d	750–3000	15	15–45
Zonisamide	Zonegran	bid	100 qd	100 q2wk	200–400	4	4–12

Abbreviations: EI = enzyme inducer; ER = extended release; VPA = valproic acid.

Phenytoin's idiosyncratic side effects of hepatitis and blood dyscrasias are rare. One benefit of phenytoin is that Dilantin Kapseals and other slow-release preparations are available so that it can be taken once per day, unlike other phenytoin preparations, such as the suspension or the Infatabs, which must be taken at least twice daily. Cumulative side effects of phenytoin occur over many years and include gum hypertrophy, hirsutism, coarsening of features, ataxia from cerebellar atrophy, and peripheral neuropathy.

An intravenous phenytoin solution is very basic (pH 11) and frequently causes venous irritation, "purple glove syndrome," and severe acute necrosis leading to amputation. Intravenous phenytoin is mixed in polyethylene glycol, which causes bradycardia and hypotension, complications that limit the rate of infusion to less than 50 mg/min. This problem can be significant in the treatment of status epilepticus or frequent seizures. Fosphenytoin (Cerebyx) is a phenytoin prodrug in which the phosphate group is rapidly cleaved off when entering the bloodstream to yield phenytoin. It is mixed in an aqueous solution and has a more neutral pH; thus, it is much better tolerated and can be given as fast as 150 mg/min.

Carbamazepine (Tegretol), like phenytoin, is metabolized by and induces hepatic enzymes. It also undergoes autoinduction, or induces its own metabolism, for up to 3 weeks after initiation of treatment, so steady-state blood levels are not achieved for several weeks. Carbamazepine has a relatively narrow therapeutic window, with usual therapeutic blood levels of between only 7 and 12 μg/mL. It commonly causes acute toxicity (ataxia, diplopia, and lethargy) with only a small increase in dose. Carbamazepine does not have cumulative side effects, but it may rarely cause serious idiosyncratic side effects, including blood dyscrasias, hepatitis, and hyponatremia secondary to the syndrome of inappropriate antidiuretic hormone secretion. Mild leukopenia is common and does not require intervention unless the white blood cell count falls below 3000. Extended-release preparations that can be taken twice daily are now available.

Valproic acid (or valproate) is a very useful drug because it is effective for both partial and generalized seizures (see later). It is available as valproic acid (Depakene), sodium divalproex (Depakote), and an extended-release form (Depakote ER). Valproic acid (Depakene) frequently causes dyspepsia and other gastrointestinal side effects. Sodium divalproex (Depakote) is immediately cleaved to valproate in the stomach, but this preparation is tolerated much better. Valproate is usually taken three times daily because of its relatively short half-life. Delayed-release Depakote was recently approved for once-per-day administration for migraine headaches, but it is actually released over less than a 24-hour period, so twice-daily dosing will probably be more useful for the treatment of epilepsy. Valproate is now available as an intravenous preparation, with the frequency of dosing identical to that of the oral forms.

Valproate is usually well tolerated, but it occasionally causes weight gain, alopecia, tremor, and thrombocytopenia. It can cause potentially fatal hepatitis and pancreatitis. Hepatitis occurs in only 1 in 40,000 adult patients exposed, but it is much more common in children (as often as 1 in 500) taking multiple AEDs and those with mental retardation, possibly because they have an undiagnosed metabolic abnormality. It has been suggested that carnitine supplementation may reduce the risk of hepatitis. Although this benefit has not been demonstrated, it is prudent for children with unknown causes of mental retardation who are receiving valproate to take carnitine. The overall risk of birth defects associated with valproate is not substantially greater than the risk with other AEDs, but it is more often associated with neural tube defects, which are more serious. Folic acid supplementation at 5 mg/d can reduce this risk. Women of childbearing potential who are taking valproate should practice an effective method of birth control and take folic acid.

Phenobarbital has fallen out of favor as an AED because it occasionally induces lethargy, depression, and learning difficulties. However, it is usually well tolerated in adults, is effective for partial-onset and primary generalized tonic-clonic seizures, is inexpensive, and can be given intravenously. It can be taken once per day and has a very long half-life, which is an advantage in poorly compliant patients. Primidone (Mysoline) is a prodrug of phenobarbital that also has its own antiseizure effects but less often causes lethargy.

Ethosuximide (Zarontin) is unique because it is the only AED that is effective exclusively for absence seizures, with no efficacy for other types of seizures. It is usually well tolerated but occasionally causes nausea, anorexia, headache, and blood dyscrasias. It can be taken once per day because of its very long half-life, but it is generally better tolerated when taken twice daily.

New Antiepileptic Drugs

Felbamate (Felbatol) was approved in 1993 as the first "new" AED since valproate in 1978. It held great promise because it was highly effective for the most intractable epilepsies, such as the Lennox-Gastaut syndrome, as well as for partial-onset seizures, despite the frequent side effects of anorexia, insomnia, and agitation and the occurrence of frequent AED interactions. However, in 1994, after approximately 100,000 prescriptions had been dispensed, 35 cases of aplastic anemia and 18 cases of fulminant hepatitis were reported. These complications led to a sudden change in practice and labeling so that it is now indicated only for intractable epilepsy, in cases where the potential benefit outweighs the risk of potentially fatal side effects. Some obtain written consent from patients before prescribing felbamate, and its use should probably be limited to epilepsy centers.

Gabapentin (Neurontin) is very well tolerated and has no pharmacokinetic interactions because it is renally excreted unchanged. It has engendered an unwarranted poor reputation as an AED because some have thought that it is ineffective. Clinical studies examined doses that statistically reduced the frequency of seizures with minimal side effects, but the doses were not high enough to determine the maximal tolerated dose; thus, it was approved and initially used at relatively low doses of 900 to 1800 mg/d. However, clinical experience suggests that doses as high as 3600 mg/d may be required to be effective for most patients. On the other hand, high doses may not increase blood levels because drug absorption may be saturated at doses above 4000 mg/d.

Lamotrigine (Lamictal) is particularly useful because it is the only drug other than valproate that is effective for both partial and generalized seizures. It is severely affected by other AEDs, so its dosing is drastically different depending on concomitant AEDs (see Table 5). When taken alone or with a combination of an enzyme inducer and inhibitor, the half-life of lamotrigine is around 25 hours, but this time is reduced to 12 hours when taken with an enzyme inducer (such as phenytoin, phenobarbital, carbamazepine) and prolonged to as much as 60 hours when taken with valproate (an enzyme inhibitor). This interaction is important to recognize because the anticipated maintenance dose and dose escalation rate will be different depending on the concomitant AED. The only potentially serious side effect of lamotrigine is rash, whose occurrence is also dependent on concomitant AEDs. Mild rash is common and was present in as many as 1 in 50 children and 1 in 1000 adults during initial clinical studies. The rash can be life-threatening in the form of Stevens-Johnson syndrome or toxic epidermal necrolysis, but the incidence of serious rash is probably only about 1 in 40,000. The rash is most likely to occur after the first 3 weeks of therapy but can occur at any time, and it is more common with high initial doses and titration rates and when taken with valproate. The titration rates in Table 5 have been used with a very low incidence of rash, probably because the titration rate is so slow. As a matter of fact, the rate is so slow that patients are unlikely to see an effect for many weeks or months and may require encouragement from the physician. When a rash is reported, the patient must be examined immediately and serious consideration given to stopping use of the drug.

Levetiracetam (Keppra) is approved as add-on therapy for partial seizures in adults, and studies in children are ongoing. It is very well tolerated and has not been associated with serious side effects. It can be titrated relatively rapidly, so its effectiveness in a patient can be determined in a few months. It is primarily excreted unchanged, with only 24% hydrolyzed before excretion, and thus it is unlikely to have significant drug interactions.

Oxcarbazepine (Trileptal) was recently approved in the United States but has been used in Mexico and elsewhere for many years. It is a derivative of carbamazepine. The primary CNS side effects of carbamazepine are due to epoxide-10,11-carbamazepine, a metabolite produced by oxidation. Oxcarbazepine cannot undergo this conversion and thus does not produce this metabolite. Therefore, it is better tolerated than carbamazepine and is much less likely to cause diplopia and ataxia. The incidence of blood dyscrasias also appears to be lower than with carbamazepine. It may be associated with hyponatremia. Oxcarbazepine does not induce AED-metabolizing liver enzymes (although it does induce other liver enzymes) or undergo autoinduction. The daily dose cannot be directly converted from the carbamazepine dose. It is effective as monotherapy, so it is likely that in the future oxcarbazepine will entirely replace carbamazepine.

Tiagabine (Gabitril) is approved as add-on therapy for partial-onset seizures. The only AED that was designed for a specific mechanism of action, tiagabine inhibits the reuptake of γ-aminobutyric acid (GABA) in the synaptic cleft. It has a very short serum half-life, but it affects the GABA transporter for at least 12 hours, so it can be taken twice daily. Some patients may require more frequent dosing. Tiagabine is not associated with any end-organ toxicity, but it can precipitate nonconvulsive status epilepticus in those who are predisposed, usually patients with generalized epilepsy.

Topiramate (Topamax) is effective for partial seizures and the Lennox-Gastaut syndrome. It has acquired an unwarranted reputation for causing cognitive side effects. The source of this reputation is probably the design of clinical studies, which appropriately determined the maximal tolerated dose by finding the dose at which an unacceptable frequency of side effects occurs. If all topiramate clinical studies are considered together, the incidence of subject dropout in those treated with more than 400 mg/d was twice that of the group receiving less than 400 mg/d, which was approximately equal to placebo. This finding indicates that the average maximal tolerated dose is about 400 mg/d. Topiramate is a weak carbonic anhydrase inhibitor and can cause kidney stones, so the concomitant use of other carbonic anhydrase inhibitors is relatively contraindicated. End-organ toxicities have not been reported with topiramate.

Zonisamide (Zonegran) is the most recently released AED, although it has been available for several years in Japan. Its pharmacology is not well described, but it is metabolized by multiple mechanisms and has a very long half-life, which may allow it to be taken once per day. Zonisamide rarely causes kidney stones. It may also cause oligohidrosis (reduced sweating) and has rarely been associated with blood dyscrasias.

Choosing an Antiepileptic Drug

Drugs of Choice by Seizure Type and Epilepsy Syndrome

Selection of AEDs should be based on the epilepsy syndrome when it is known (see below), but because the etiology is often unknown, the choice of an AED must be based solely on the type of seizures present. This approach is consistent with clinical studies of AEDs that have investigated the efficacy of AEDs for specific seizure types without regard for the epilepsy syndrome. In adults, this method is probably reasonable because the most common situation in adults is the occurrence of complex partial seizures of unknown etiology.

All types of *partial-onset seizures* respond to the same medications, so they can be considered together. The most obvious question is which AED is most effective for partial seizures. Unfortunately, very few head-to-head comparisons of these drugs have been made. The available data suggest that they are equally effective, although most new AEDs are better tolerated than the conventional AEDs. The only AED that is not effective for partial seizures is ethosuximide. Therefore, to select among them, consideration must be given to the relative importance of the side effect profile, dosing interval, pharmacokinetics, and cost for each patient. In general, the new AEDs have less frequent side effects, daily or twice-daily dosing, and simple pharmacokinetics, which suggests that they are more desirable than conventional AEDs. On the other hand, conventional AEDs are familiar, have a proven track record, and are inexpensive. Most neurologists still prefer to start therapy with a conventional AED but move quickly to a new AED if necessary. It is likely that the new AEDs will replace the conventional AEDs in the next few years for the initial treatment of partial seizures.

Each type of generalized seizure must be considered individually. *Generalized tonic-clonic seizures, tonic seizures*, and *clonic seizures* seem to respond to the same AEDs as partial-onset seizures do, but this similarity may be due to the fact that historically, little distinction was made between primary generalized and secondary generalized seizures during drug development. All conventional AEDs, except ethosuximide, seem to be effective. Few studies on the efficacy of new AEDs for generalized seizures have been published, but lamotrigine, felbamate, and zonisamide seem to be effective; the efficacy of the others is unknown. *Absence seizures* respond to valproate, ethosuximide, and lamotrigine and not to carbamazepine, gabapentin, or tiagabine. The efficacy of other new AEDs has yet to be demonstrated. *Myoclonic seizures* respond to valproate and lamotrigine and occasionally to benzodiazepines.

A few epilepsy syndromes in adults and adolescents respond particularly well to specific AEDs. Myoclonic and generalized tonic-clonic seizures occurring in *juvenile myoclonic epilepsy* respond very well to valproate or lamotrigine. Atonic, tonic, and atypical absence seizures occurring as part of the *Lennox-Gastaut syndrome* respond very well to valproate, lamotrigine, and topiramate. This case is one in which the potential benefit of felbamate usually outweighs the risk. Approximately 30% of patients with *childhood absence epilepsy* have seizures that persist into adulthood, and valproate or lamotrigine is often a better alternative than ethosuximide when they have generalized tonic-clonic seizures in addition to absence seizures.

Special Considerations

Children represent a special population because the seizure types, epilepsy syndromes, etiologies, and pharmacokinetic responses of children are different from those of adults. This dissimilarity leads to important dosing differences such as doses based on body weight rather than absolute amounts (see Table 5). The long-term cosmetic cumulative side effects of phenytoin make it a poor choice for the chronic treatment of children, especially girls. Children are addressed elsewhere in this volume, but it is important to recognize that many childhood epilepsies persist into adulthood and may evolve.

The elderly deserve special consideration because they are more likely to have side effects, be taking multiple medications, and have hepatic and renal impairment. Seizures beginning in late adult life are always partial seizures from acquired etiologies, especially stroke. Phenytoin is particularly poorly tolerated in the elderly and, in addition, may have a prolonged half-life, so levels are unexpectedly high. Some new AEDs are better tolerated and less likely to cause drug interactions. Gabapentin is particularly desirable because it has no drug interactions.

Women pose several potential problems when selecting an AED. Women with epilepsy have increased rates of infertility because of intrinsic hormone changes, anovulatory cycles, irregular menstrual cycles, and altered sexuality. This increased infertility can be compounded by the effects of AEDs, especially valproate, which is associated with polycystic ovarian disease. Hysterectomy with bilateral oophorectomy may seem like reasonable therapy for seizures clustering around the menstrual period, but it is usually ineffective and deprives patients of the protective effects of estrogen. Osteopenia is common in postmenopausal women and is augmented by chronic phenytoin use.

Potential teratogenicity is an important consideration for women of childbearing potential, but data in humans are available only for the conventional AEDs. The incidence of birth defects in women taking an AED is approximately 5% to 6% as compared with 1% to 2% in the general population. The rate of birth defects appears to be the same for all conventional AEDs. Most birth defects associated with phenytoin, carbamazepine, and phenobarbital are considered mild or cosmetic, but valproate frequently causes neural tube defects. Folic acid reduces the rate of teratogenicity, especially neural tube defects, and is thus indicated for women taking valproate, in addition to being good practice for all women of childbearing potential. Some new AEDs are teratogenic in animal models, but the effects in humans are unknown.

Hepatic disease may impair the ability to clear hepatically metabolized drugs (see Table 4). Such impairment is particularly a problem for conventional AEDs, which are all hepatically metabolized. Among the new AEDs, gabapentin is not hepatically metabolized at all and is not affected even by severe liver disease. The new AEDs are not affected until liver disease is severe. The dose reduction of hepatically metabolized AEDs in hepatically impaired patients is determined by the prolongation in drug clearance, which is different in each patient. Therefore, no standard dosing recommendations can be made. Blood levels may guide therapy and are available for conventional AEDs, lamotrigine, gabapentin, and topiramate.

Renal disease may impair the clearance of AEDs eliminated unchanged by the kidneys. All conventional AEDs are primarily deactivated by hepatic metabolism before urinary elimination of inactive metabolites. Therefore, they are not significantly affected by renal disease until the onset of end-stage renal disease, in which case the small amount that is normally excreted unchanged may build up. Some new AEDs such as gabapentin, levetiracetam, oxcarbazepine, and topiramate have a significant portion excreted unchanged by the kidneys and will therefore require empirical or calculated dose reduction with renal impairment.

A more significant problem in the treatment of renally impaired patients is the removal of free drug during hemodialysis. The amount of drug removed depends on the free fraction, duration and volume of dialysis, and other factors, so a predictable change in blood levels cannot be determined. After each hemodialysis session, the blood level and effectiveness must be determined to decide how much drug must be given until a steady state of postdialysis dosing is reached. Phenytoin is not significantly affected by hemodialysis because only 10% exists in the free dialyzable form, but free levels should be monitored. A mild to moderate amount of phenobarbital is removed during dialysis, but if the level falls significantly after dialysis, a bolus can be given. Changes in valproate dosing are not usually necessary because although 20% is removed by dialysis, the half-life increases by 20%, which compensates. Among the new AEDs, gabapentin is the most severely affected; 60% is removed by hemodialysis, but the half-life becomes nearly infinite, so only very small doses are required once the patient becomes anuric, such as only 300 mg after each dialysis.

REFRACTORY EPILEPSY

Evaluation of Intractable Seizures

The definition of what constitutes refractory epilepsy has evolved in recent years. In statistical terms, patients who continue to have seizures after trying therapeutic doses of two AEDs are very unlikely to respond to additional AEDs, although some do. The definition is becoming increasingly important because refractory patients should be referred to an epilepsy center for diagnosis and consideration of the many therapeutic options now available, including epilepsy surgery to resect the seizure focus, palliative surgery to reduce the severity of some seizure types, unconventional AEDs, and experimental AEDs.

The evaluation of intractable seizures is dependent on a careful history and physical examination directed at elucidating the seizure type, neuroanatomic site of seizure origin, and the epilepsy syndrome or etiology. The most important diagnostic test is prolonged (24 h/d) simultaneous video and EEG monitoring to capture seizures. Video/EEG is vitally important to determine that the spells in question are indeed seizures, to define the seizure type, and to localize the site of origin. Video/EEG may need to continue for days or weeks to capture enough spells to make a correct diagnosis. MRI of the brain with special acquisition protocols to define fine brain anatomy often reveals abnormalities that are not obvious on routine MRI, especially in the temporal lobe, where seizures often arise. Positron emission tomography may reveal focal hypometabolism in the region of seizure onset. Interictal single-photon emitted computed tomography (SPECT) occasionally reveals focal hypoperfusion at the focus. To perform an ictal SPECT scan, the radiotracer is injected within 90 seconds of seizure onset and subsequent scanning often reveals focal hyperperfusion in the region of seizure onset. Magnetic resonance spectroscopy is primarily a research tool but can reveal focal changes in the region of the seizure focus. Neuropsychological testing may demonstrate dysfunction and lateralized or localized deficits.

Epilepsy Surgery

Surgery to resect the epileptic focus is the only method of curing epilepsy available today. Successful surgery is, of course, heavily dependent on correctly localizing the seizure focus. Presurgical evaluation is usually carried out in three phases. Phase 1 consists of extracranial monitoring and the noninvasive tests noted earlier. If the findings yield a general area from which the seizures arise but do not pinpoint the exact site of onset, the patient may proceed to phase 2, which is intracranial EEG monitoring through electrodes placed on or into the brain. Phase 3 is removal of the seizure focus. Fortunately, most patients do not require intracranial monitoring now because neuroimaging often identifies an anatomic abnormality to corroborate the EEG findings.

Any area of the brain is a candidate for resection, but in reality, the vast majority of patients have temporal lobe epilepsy and undergo anterior temporal lobectomy to remove the anterior 4 to 5 cm of the temporal lobe containing the hippocampus and amygdala. Approximately 70% of patients are essentially seizure-free after anterior temporal lobectomy, and the risk of stroke or other serious complications is less than 1%. Extratemporal resections are more complicated. The seizure focus must be more pre-

TABLE 6. **General Guidelines for Use of New Antiepileptic Drugs**

Select an antiepileptic drug by seizure type and epilepsy syndrome
Use a conventional drug first
Increase the dose to the maximal tolerated dose (toxicity) before changing
Substitute 1 drug at a time in attempt to achieve monotherapy
All new drugs are equally efficacious for partial seizures
Select by side effects, dosing, pharmacokinetics, cost
Refer to an epilepsy center for consideration of surgery if seizures are refractory to 2 antiepileptic drugs

cisely localized, and electrical brain mapping or other methods must be used to ensure that important brain functions will not be removed during surgery, which usually requires intracranial monitoring. Approximately 50% of patients are essentially seizure-free after surgery. The risk of complications, such as a motor deficit, is only slightly higher than with anterior temporal lobectomy. More drastic surgeries, such as hemispherectomy or corpus callostomy, are indicated in special circumstances.

Vagus nerve stimulation is a recently developed novel approach to seizure control. A small generator is placed subcutaneously in the left chest wall with wire electrodes leading to the left vagus nerve. The generator supplies a few seconds of current every several minutes at predetermined settings. Its efficacy in blinded controlled trials is about the same as that of a new AED; it reduces the frequency of seizures by 50% in about half of the subjects.

CONCLUSION

Treatment of epilepsy is rapidly changing and more complex than in previous years because 14 AEDs are now available to choose from, technologic advances have made diagnostic tests more useful, and epilepsy surgery is safer and more readily available. A systematic approach yields some basic guidelines for therapy (Table 6).

EPILEPSY IN INFANTS AND CHILDREN

method of
KATHERINE HOLLAND, M.D., PH.D., and
ELAINE WYLLIE, M.D.
The Cleveland Clinic Foundation
Cleveland, Ohio

Seizures are abnormal electrical discharges of nerve cells in the brain that cause changes in a person's level of consciousness, behavior, movement, or sensation. The form of a seizure depends on where in the brain it starts and where it spreads. Seizures are a symptom of abnormal brain function due to either medical or neurologic disturbances. Epilepsy is a chronic disorder characterized by recurrent unprovoked seizures. The clinical manifestations of seizures are varied and must be distinguished from nonepileptic disorders that can also produce recurrent paroxysmal changes in movement, consciousness, or behavior.

NONEPILEPTIC CONDITIONS THAT CAN BE MISTAKEN FOR EPILEPSY

The initial diagnostic consideration when evaluating a child with possible seizures is whether these paroxysmal events are seizures or nonepileptic events. The differential diagnosis is broad and includes a variety of physiologic or behavioral events and psychiatric disorders that are summarized in Table 1.

In infants, benign sleep myoclonus is the most commonly encountered nonepileptic paroxysmal event. These often occur in the first few months of life and are characterized by rapid, forceful movements of the extremities. The trunk may also been involved. These movements typically migrate from one muscle group to another and are not repetitive in the same muscle group. These movements occur in clusters and sporadically in all stages of sleep and stop when the infant is fully awakened. No treatment is necessary.

In toddlers, breathholding spells are common nonepileptic paroxysmal events, occurring in up to 5% of children. Crying precedes these spells. The child stops breathing in expiration, then becomes cyanotic, limp, and loses consciousness. Tonic posturing or generalized tonic-clonic seizures can rarely occur after the child loses consciousness.

TABLE 1. **Differential Diagnosis of Nonepileptic Paroxysmal Disorders in Infants and Children**

Unusual Motor Phenomena
Startle response
Shuddering
Hyperreflexia
Paroxysmal dystonia or chorea
Tics
Unusual eye movements
Opsoclonus-myoclonus
Spasmus nutans
Breathing or Circulatory Disturbances
Apnea
Cyanotic breathholding spells
Pallid infantile syncope
Hyperventilation
Syncope
Cardiac arrhythmias
Behavioral Disorders
Headbanging
Temper tantrums/rage attacks
Infantile masturbation
Self-stimulatory behaviors
Daydreaming
Attention deficits
Pseudoseizures
Migraine Variants
Benign paroxysmal torticollis
Benign paroxysmal vertigo
Basilar migraine
Sleep Phenomena
Benign sleep myoclonus
Sleep walking
Nightmares/night terrors
Narcolepsy/cataplexy

After a short spell, the child returns to normal. However, on occasion children will fall asleep after a spell. No treatment is necessary, although if iron deficiency anemia is present, it may decrease the frequency of the events.

Pallid infantile syncope occurs less frequently. These are usually evoked by pain or minor trauma. The child becomes pale and limp. Crying is absent or may be minimal. Tonic posturing may be seen. Electrocardiograms obtained during events show asystole for several seconds. These conditions are also benign and self-limited. Occasionally, atropine is used in cases when a child has frequent episodes.

Episodic staring is a common paroxysmal phenomenon that can be a manifestation of epilepsy (complex partial or absence seizures) or may represent daydreaming or inattention. Nonepileptic staring is characterized by no interruption of play, initial identification by a health care or teaching professional rather than by a parent, and responsiveness to touch during the staring.

In contrast, twitches in the arms or legs, loss of urine, or upward eye movement during staring suggest epileptic absence seizures. An initial warning or aura, longer duration (minutes versus seconds), and postictal lethargy or confusion suggest complex partial seizures as opposed to absence seizures. Semiautomatic hand movements, lip smacking, or chewing may be seen in either seizure type.

The distinction between nonepileptic paroxysmal events and epilepsy can be made largely from a detailed history. However, sometimes ancillary testing such as electroencephalography (EEG) or prolonged video-EEG monitoring is necessary to make the correct diagnosis.

EVALUATION

The most important issue in the evaluation of a clinical episode is a detailed, eyewitness description of the clinical event. The initial evaluation of a child with a new onset seizure in the acute care setting should include an evaluation of electrolyte levels (including calcium and magnesium), blood glucose level, and blood screening for toxic substances. A lumbar puncture should be considered when an infant or child presents with a seizure and altered mental status, fever, or meningismus. If there are focal findings on the neurologic examination, or a history of head trauma, then computed tomography of the head should be done prior to the lumbar puncture.

EEG should be done as part of an evaluation of suspected seizures. This is important because it can help define the seizure type (focal onset versus generalized onset). Results of a standard 30-minute awake EEG are abnormal in about 50% of patients with known epilepsy. This yield increases if sleep is attained during the recording. In contrast, epileptiform abnormalities can be recorded in some people who have never had a seizure. Therefore, it is important to interpret the results of the EEG in clinical context. Normal results on an EEG do not eliminate the possibility of epilepsy and abnormal EEG results alone do not confirm that diagnosis.

Neuroimaging studies, preferably magnetic resonance imaging, should be obtained if the seizure is partial or has focal features, if there are focal findings on the neurologic examination, or if the EEG has focal abnormalities. An exception to this is if seizures are a result of benign focal epilepsy with centrotemporal spikes.

TREATMENT

Anticonvulsant medications are the primary treatment for epilepsy. The goal of therapy is to prevent seizures without causing side effects with medication. This goal can be achieved in about 75% of children with epilepsy. Because medical treatment is not without risks (Table 2), it should not be initiated until there is a reasonable expectation that seizures will recur. The risk of recurrent seizures in a normal child after a single generalized tonic-clonic seizure is approximately 60%; this increases to 90% after the second seizure. Although the risk of seizure recurrence is higher if there is epileptiform activity on the EEG, an abnormal neurologic examination, or abnormal development, the increased risk generally does not outweigh the risks of treatment complications. Therefore, it is reasonable to defer treatment until after at least a second seizure.

With certain seizure types and in some age groups, the risk of injury from a seizure is low. For example, a 4-year-old child with infrequent nocturnal seizures is at a low risk of injury from seizures. Therefore, treatment may be deferred beyond a second seizure in select cases. Regardless of whether treatment is initiated, a review of safety measures is important to minimize the risks of physical injury from seizures. This includes restricting bathing or swimming without close supervision, emphasizing the importance of wearing a helmet when riding a bicycle, and limiting climbing.

The selection of medication is based on the seizure type, seizure frequency, and severity of medication side effects. Some medications are effective for seizures with a focal onset, others are effective for seizures with a generalized onset, and others are useful for a broad spectrum of seizure types (Table 3). Although there are no direct comparative studies in children, carbamazepine (Tegretol) and oxcarbazepine (Trileptal) are probably considered to be the most effective and well-tolerated medications for partial onset seizures. Selection of medications for generalized onset seizures is more difficult because of side effect profiles. Ethosuximide (Zarontin) is probably the best initial choice for absence seizures because of good efficacy for this seizure type and a favorable side effect profile, but this medication is not effective for generalized tonic-clonic seizures. For primary generalized tonic-clonic seizures, valproic acid (Depakene) is a standard treatment but should be used with caution in young children due to a high risk of potentially fatal hepatotoxicity in children younger than 2 years of age.

TABLE 2. **Risks and Benefits of Medical Treatment for Childhood Epilepsy**

Risks of Therapy	Risks of Seizures
Medication-related	Physical injury during seizure
Cognitive impairment	Status epilepticus
Adverse behavioral effect	Cognitive effects of frequent seizures
Systemic toxicity	Restriction of activity
Idiosyncratic reactions	Social stigmata
Teratogenicity	
Expense (of drug and monitoring)	

TABLE 3. **Medication Selection Based on Seizure Type**

Seizure Type	First Choice	Alternatives
Partial Onset Seizures		
Simple/complex	CBZ, OXC	LTG, TPM, VPA, LEV, GBP, PHT, TGB
Secondarily generalized	CBZ, OXC	LTG, TPM, VPA, GBP, PHT, TGB, PB
Generalized Onset		
Absence	ESM, VPA	LTG, TPM
Myoclonic	VPA, TPM, LTG	ZNS, BDZ
Tonic-clonic	VPA, LTG	TPM, BDZ, PB
Atonic	VPA, LTG	TPM, FBM, BDZ

Abbreviations: BDZ = benzodiazepines (clonazepam [Klonopin]); CBZ = carbamazepine (Carbatrol, Tegretol, Tegretol-XR); ESM = ethosuximide (Zarontin): FBM = felbamate (Felbatol); GBP = gabapentin (Neurontin): LEV = levetiracetam (Keppra); LTG = lamotrigine (Lamictal); PB = phenobarbital (Luminal); TGB = tiagabine (Gabitril); TPM = topiramate (Topamax); VPA = valproic acid (Depakene, Depakote); ZNS = zonisamide (Zonegran).

In general, the adverse effects of antiepileptic treatment fall into two broad categories: dose-related toxicity and idiosyncratic reactions. Toxic effects include sedation, cognitive changes, and behavioral disturbances. These are typically dose-related. In contrast, idiosyncratic reactions are not necessarily dose-related. These include hypersensitivity reactions (rash, fever, and lymphadenopathy), blood dyscrasias, and hepatotoxicity. Periodic monitoring of blood cell counts and hepatic enzyme levels is recommended with some medications (e.g., carbamazepine, valproic acid, and felbamate [Felbatol]). Additionally, long-term exposure to some medications is associated with changes in cosmetic appearance, changes in body weight, and teratogenicity. It is important to thoroughly review the side effects of the medication with the patient and family before beginning treatment.

Antiepileptic drugs should be started at a low dose. The dose should be increased slowly to the dose where seizures are prevented or intolerable side effects occur. Recommended dosing and titration of these medications are outlined in Table 4. Some mild side effects may be seen transiently when a medication is started or when the dose is changed but do not persist. Thus, a medication should not be abandoned prematurely, but slowing of the initiation schedule may be necessary. Medication levels can be a useful adjunct to clinical assessment of the patient; however, medication levels should not substitute for the clinical response. Therapeutic levels are indicators of average responses to medications. Some patients have adequate seizure control at levels that are lower than the therapeutic range, and other patients require levels higher than the therapeutic range for seizure control. Also, the level at which a patient experiences side effects may vary among individuals. Therefore, changes in the dose should not be made based solely on drug levels. Drug levels can be useful in the assessment of medication compliance. Noncompliance should be considered in a patient who has a low level despite taking a high daily dose of medication. In patients with infrequent seizures, the initial maintenance dose should be at the low end of the maintenance range, with a medication level at the lower end of the therapeutic range.

For the majority of antiepileptic medications, after a change in dose, it takes 1 to 2 weeks until the concentration of the drug reaches steady state.

TABLE 4. **Usual Pediatric Antiepileptic Drug Dosages (mg/kg/d)**

Drug	Starting	Escalation	Maintenance	Frequency
Carbamazepine, (Tegretol)	5–10	5–10 per wk	15–45	TID*
Clonazepam (Klonopin)	0.01–0.03	0.02 per wk	0.1–0.3	BID to TID
Ethosuximide (Zarontin)	10	5–10 per wk	15–40	BID or TID
Felbamate (Felbatol)	15	15 per wk	45–60	TID
Gabapentin (Neurontin)	10	10 per day	30–100	TID
Lamotrigine (Lamictal)†	0.6	1.2 every 1–2 wk	5–15	BID
Lamotrigine (Lamictal)† added to VPA	0.15	0.3 per 2 wks	1–5	QOD to BID‡
Levetiracetam (Keppra)§	10	10–20 per wk	20–60	BID
Oxcarbazepine (Trileptal)	8–10	10 per wk	20–45	BID
Phenobarbital‖	3–6		3–6	QD or BID
Phenytoin (Dilantin)‖	4		4–8	BID
Tiagabine (Gabitril)	0.1	0.1 every 1–2 wk	0.6–2	BID to QID
Topiramate (Topamax)	0.5–1	0.5–1 per wk	5–10	BID
Valproic acid (Depakene)	10–15	10–15	30–60	BID or TID
Zonisamide (Zonegran)	1–2	1–2	4–10	QD or BID

*BID dosing using extended-release carbamazepine formulations (Tegretol-XR and Carbatrol).

†When patient is taking other anticonvulsant medications that induce hepatic enzymes (e.g., carbamazepine, phenytoin, phenobarbital) and is not also taking valproic acid. When added to regimes that do not contain valproic acid or enzyme-inducing drugs then the dose should be about half of that listed for patients on enzyme-inducing medications.

‡When initiated every other day dosing may be needed for the first 2 weeks.

§Not FDA approved for use in children.

‖Can be initiated at a therapeutic dose.

Abbreviations: BID = twice daily; TID = thrice daily; QD = once daily.

Therefore, the full effect of a dose change will not be evident until then. As a result, it may take some time before treatment is effective.

If one antiepileptic medication is ineffective after maximally tolerated doses have been administered, then it should be replaced by a second medication. At that time, an evaluation to identify any factors that contributed to the treatment failure is indicated. In addition to the lack of efficacy of the medication, other common reasons for treatment failure include incorrect diagnosis of the seizure type (partial versus generalized), misdiagnosis of a paroxysmal event as epilepsy, and medication noncompliance. In the case of medical noncompliance, evaluation of the factors leading to compliance problems is important and the least complicated treatment regime should be used. If a second antiepileptic medication fails, referral to an epilepsy specialist should be considered.

Other treatments can be used for epilepsy that is refractory to conventional antiepileptic therapy. These include surgical resection of the epileptic focus in children with partial epilepsy, institution of the ketogenic diet, and use of the vagal nerve stimulator. These treatments should be coordinated through an epilepsy center with experience in pediatric epilepsy.

DISCONTINUATION OF THERAPY

Children on antiepileptic medications who have been seizure-free for at least 2 years have a good chance of remaining seizure-free off medication. Approximately 50% to 75% of such children will remain seizure-free off medication, and the majority of seizure recurrences occur within the first 6 to 12 months of discontinuation. The risk factors for seizure recurrence off medication include abnormal neurologic examination or development, epilepsy that is a result of a symptomatic brain lesion, and history of multiple different seizure types. An epileptiform pattern on the EEG combined with an area of focal slowing is also a poorer prognostic finding, but an epileptiform pattern alone does not increase the risk of recurrence unless certain patterns associated with idiopathic generalized epilepsy are present. However, even when risk factors are present, a trial off medications is usually indicated if there has been a prolonged seizure-free period.

Most medications can be discontinued over a 1- to 2-month period. However, slower tapering (over 3–6 months) of benzodiazepines and phenobarbital is indicated because of the risk of withdrawal seizures. The discontinuation process should be planned at a time that is convenient for the family and should not coincide with a time when the family plans to be away. If possible, tapering should be done at least 1 year before a child reaches driving age. The family should be instructed to seek emergency care in the event of a prolonged seizure, have instructions on how to resume treatment if a brief seizure occurs, and be reminded of seizure safety suggestions. They should also be instructed to contact the physician in the case of seizure recurrence so that follow-up visits can be arranged.

COMMON PEDIATRIC EPILEPSY SYNDROMES

Epilepsy syndromes are defined on the basis of a constellation of clinical and EEG characteristics. When a child's seizures result from a specific epilepsy syndrome, the most effective treatments and prognosis are better defined.

Febrile Seizures

Febrile seizures are the most common type of seizures and cause of status epilepticus in young children (the treatment of status epilepticus is outlined in Table 5). Typically, febrile seizures are brief generalized convulsions that occur in association with a fever. They occur in children between 6 months and

TABLE 5. **Treatment of Convulsive Status Epilepticus in Children**

1. Establish IV access, maintain airway, provide supplemental oxygen. Monitor ECG, BP, pulse oximetry	
2. Measure electrolyte levels (including Ca and Mg), CBC, glucose, toxic screen, drug levels	
3. If hypoglycemia cannot be ruled out give 2 mL/kg dextrose 25% IV	
4. Medications to be used:	
a. Lorazepam (Ativan)	0.1 mg/kg/dose IV (maximum dose 4 mg); repeat after 5 minutes if seizure continues. If no IV access established diazepam 0.3–0.5 mg/kg prn
b. Fosphenytoin (Cerebyx) *or*	20 PE/kg at rate of 3 PE/kg/min IV. If no IV access can be given IM
Phenytoin	20 mg/kg at rate of 1 mg/kg/min IV. *Cannot* be given IM or with dextrose containing IV
5. If seizure persists:	Additional 10 PE/kg of fosphenytoin
6. If seizure persists:	(Be prepared to intubate)
Phenobarbital	20 mg/kg IV at a rate of 2 mg/kg/min. Give additional 10 mg/kg if seizure continues
7. For refractory status epilepticus will need intubation (if not already done) and EEG monitoring to achieve cessation of seizure activity or burst suppression.	
Options:	
a. Pentobarbital	Loading dose 10–15 mg/kg; then continuous infusion of 1–3 mg/kg/h (associated with hypotension; may need pressor support)
b. Midazolam (Versed)*	Loading dose 0.2 mg/kg; then continuous infusion of 1–10 μg/kg/min

*Not FDA approved for this indication.

Abbreviations: BP = blood pressure; CBC = complete blood cell count; ECG = electrocardiography; EEG = electroencephalography; IM = intramuscularly; IV = intravenously; PE = phenytoin equivalent.

6 years of age and happen in approximately 5% of children. One third of these children will have recurrent febrile seizures, and the risk of recurrence increases if the child is younger than 18 months or if the seizure occurs at a temperature of less than 40°C. Epilepsy will develop in only a few (<2%) children with febrile seizures. *Complex febrile seizures,* defined as prolonged (>5 minutes), focal, or multiple seizures in one febrile illness, increase the chances of epilepsy. But a history of abnormal neurologic examination results or developmental delay is more strongly associated with epilepsy. The diagnosis of febrile seizures is a diagnosis of exclusion. If a central nervous system infection is suspected, a lumbar puncture is indicated because meningitis can also present with fever and a seizure.

Prophylactic therapy is usually not indicated for simple febrile seizures but may be considered in a child with a history of frequent or prolonged febrile seizures. Antipyretic therapy may also be helpful. Continuous treatment with phenobarbital is an alternative but this is not recommended due to side effects associated with its chronic use. Rectal diazepam (Diastat) 0.2 to 0.5 mg/kg given for prolonged (>5 minutes) or repeated seizures can be useful.

Absence Epilepsy Syndromes in Children

There are three common epilepsy syndromes with childhood onset that have absence seizures as a common feature. Because there is considerable overlap between the absence epilepsy syndromes, it may not be possible to differentiate them initially.

Childhood Absence Epilepsy

Childhood absence epilepsy begins between 4 and 8 years of age. Typically, these children have many absence seizures daily. Generalized tonic-clonic seizures may also occur, but these are infrequent. The EEG is abnormal due to 3-Hz generalized spike-and-wave activity. The seizures generally respond to ethosuximide; valproic acid can be used as an alternative, especially if generalized tonic-clonic seizures occur. This disorder typically resolves in adolescence.

Juvenile Absence Epilepsy

Juvenile absence epilepsy is a similar disorder, except the age of onset is later (6–10 years) and absence seizures are less frequent. However, generalized tonic-clonic seizures are more frequent. Therefore, valproic acid should be used as the treatment of first choice and lamotrigine considered as an alternative.

Juvenile Myoclonic Epilepsy

Finally, *juvenile myoclonic epilepsy* is characterized by myoclonic, absence, and generalized tonic-clonic seizures. The EEG may have generalized spike and polyspike-and-wave activity and epileptiform response to photic stimulation. In contrast to the other two absence epilepsy syndromes, this disorder does not resolve and lifelong treatment may be necessary. Valproic acid is considered the treatment of choice but owing to its teratogenicity, lamotrigine and topiramate should be considered as alternatives, especially in women, because treatment will likely continue into childbearing age.

Benign Rolandic Epilepsy or Benign Epilepsy With Centrotemporal Spikes

Children with benign rolandic epilepsy with centrotemporal spikes (BECTS) typically have seizures beginning with unilateral facial paresthesias then ipsilateral clonic activity of the face. Drooling and speech arrest are common. The seizures are infrequently generalized and are exclusively nocturnal in the majority of the children. There is often a family history of epilepsy and the EEG demonstrates unilateral or bilateral centrotemporal spikes with a characteristic morphology. Although there are exceptions, most children have rare nocturnal seizures and many do not need to be treated. When the seizures are frequent, occur during the day, or are generalized, often the medications used are those effective for partial seizures. The seizures remit spontaneously by adolescence regardless of treatment. There are other benign focal epilepsy syndromes in childhood that differ from BECTS because of the clinical manifestation of the seizures and location of the characteristic appearing spikes. However, the treatment and natural history of these is similar to that of BECTS.

Infantile Spasms and Lennox-Gastaut Syndrome

These are two severe pediatric epilepsy syndromes in childhood. *Infantile spasms* begin before 1 year of age and are characterized by clusters of extensor or flexor movement that often occur shortly after awakening. The EEG demonstrates a characteristic pattern called hypsarrhythmia. *Lennox-Gastaut syndrome* is characterized by atypical absence, myoclonic, and atonic seizures, slow spike-wave complexes on the EEG, and mental retardation. The onset of the seizures is typically between 2 to 5 years of age, although the child is often not neurologically normal before seizure onset. In both syndromes, the seizures are often difficult to treat and these syndromes are associated with a poor developmental outcome, especially if the seizures are not controlled. As a result, children with these syndromes should treated by a pediatric neurologist or epilepsy specialist.

Symptomatic Focal Epilepsy in Childhood

With improvements in neuroimaging, it is clear that childhood epilepsy may result from a variety of structural brain lesions such as malformations of cortical development, tumors, or mesial temporal sclerosis. Symptomatic epilepsy is often difficult to control medically. Because developmental and psychosocial outcomes are better with early seizure control, early surgical therapy for children with symptomatic focal epilepsy should be considered. If a child fails aggressive therapy with two medications, then referral to an epilepsy center is indicated, even if the duration of the symptoms has been relatively short.

ATTENTION DEFICIT HYPERACTIVITY DISORDER

method of
DAVID C. AGERTER, M.D.
Mayo Clinic
Rochester, Minnesota

Attention deficit hyperactivity disorder (ADHD) has been referred to by various names throughout the years, including minimal brain dysfunction, minimal cerebral dysfunction, the "all-boy" syndrome, dyslexia, and neurosis. It is a diagnosis given to children and adults who exhibit a cluster of maladaptive behavioral characteristics as specified in the *Diagnostic and Statistical Manual of Mental Disorders* (Table 1).

ADHD is a major clinical and public health problem and the most common pediatric psychiatric problem that physicians encounter. ADHD affects 30% to 50% of adults who had ADHD in childhood. Epidemiologic studies indicate that ADHD has a prevalence of at least 3% to 5% of all school-aged children. It is believed that up to 4% of adults have this disorder.

The central feature of ADHD is a persistent pattern of inattention and/or hyperactivity-impulsivity that is more frequent and severe than typically observed in other individuals at a comparable level of development.

Researchers generally agree that the disorder represents a disturbance in brain functioning. Imaging studies over the last decade have pointed to the prefrontal cortex, part of the cerebellum, and areas of the basal ganglion as regions that might malfunction in patients with ADHD.

ASSESSMENT

It is important to obtain a thorough personal history, as well as a family history. The history needs to be obtained from more than one source, including parents, teachers, and others who know the patient well. After a careful clinical history, a complete general medical examination should be undertaken to uncover any existing condition that warrants further investigation and appropriate treatment.

The use of various standardized instruments such as Conners' Rating Scale, including both the parent and teacher versions, is of great value to clinicians. In using Conners' Rating Scale, each item is rated with one of the following four responses: never, seldom; occasionally; often, quite a bit; and very often, very frequent. The responses are coded 0, 1, 2, or 3. Scores are obtained for the categories of oppositional, cognitive problems/inattention, hyperactivity, and the ADHD index. The scale has parent, teacher, and self-report forms. The parent and teacher forms are normed on children aged 3 to 17.

Additional assessments may be used for patients with ADHD or suspected of having this condition, including the Achenbach Checklist. These instruments are multiaxial, empirical-based assessment devices measuring a broad range of internalizing and externalizing behavior.

Interest has been expressed in the development of computerized assessment tools to include the Conners' Continuous Performance Task, which is a 14-minute computerized continuous-performance test. Respondents are required to press a bar when any letter except X appears. This test is presented in a gamelike format. The primary measures are omission, or an "index of inattention," and commission, or a "measure of impulsivity." This test is normed on community and clinical samples in the 14 to 18+ age range.

Another computerized test called the Test of Variables of Attention (TOVA) was developed by Dr. Lawrence Greenberg, Professor of Psychiatry. The TOVA is a 22.5-minute computerized continuous-performance test. It is non–language based, requires no right or left discrimination, and has negligible practice effects. The primary measures are omission errors, or an "index of sustained attention"; commission errors, or "a measure of impulse control";

TABLE 1. ***Diagnostic and Statistical Manual of Mental Disorders, Fourth Edition,*** **Criteria for Attention Deficit Hyperactivity Disorder**

A. Either 1 or 2:
  1. Six (or more) of the following symptoms of *inattention* have persisted for at least 6 mo to a degree that is maladaptive and inconsistent with the developmental level:
     Inattention
     a. Often fails to give close attention to details or makes careless mistakes in schoolwork, work, or other activities
     b. Often has difficulty sustaining attention in tasks or play activities
     c. Often does not seem to listen when spoken to directly
     d. Often does not follow through on instructions and fails to finish schoolwork, chores, or duties in the workplace (not because of oppositional behavior or failure to understand instructions)
     e. Often has difficulty organizing tasks and activities
     f. Often avoids, dislikes, or is reluctant to engage in tasks that require sustained mental effort (such as schoolwork or homework)
     g. Often loses things necessary for tasks or activities (e.g., toys, school assignments, pencils, books, or tools)
     h. Is often easily distracted by extraneous stimuli
     i. Is often forgetful in daily activities
  2. Six (or more) of the following symptoms of *hyperactivity-impulsivity* have persisted for at least 6 mo to a degree that is maladaptive and inconsistent with the developmental level:
     Hyperactivity
     a. Often fidgets with hands or feet or squirms in seat
     b. Often leaves seat in classroom or in other situations in which remaining seated is expected
     c. Often runs about or climbs excessively in situations in which it is inappropriate (in adolescents or adults, may be limited to subjective feelings of restlessness)
     d. Often has difficulty playing or engaging in leisure activities quietly
     e. Is often "on the go" or often acts as though "driven by a motor"
     f. Often talks excessively
     Impulsivity
     g. Often blurts out answers before questions have been completed
     h. Often has difficulty awaiting turn
     i. Often interrupts or intrudes on others (e.g., butts into conversations or games)

B. Some hyperactive-impulsive or inattentive symptoms that have caused impairment were present before the age of 7 y

Table reprinted with permission of Minnesota Medicine. From Agerten DC, Rasmussen NH: Diagnosing and treating ADHD in children. Minn Med 83(6):51–54, 2000.

response time (RT); and RT variability. Norms are published for ages 4 to 80+.

One may also use the Utah Adult Inventory Checklist, which may be beneficial for screening adults suspected of having ADHD. In assessing adults with ADHD, particular emphasis needs to be placed on two critical factors: documenting childhood onset and examining for other psychiatric disorders. Psychiatric disorders to consider in the differential diagnosis of adults with ADHD include major depression, bipolar disorder, generalized anxiety, substance abuse or dependence, and personality disorders, particularly borderline and antisocial personality.

In almost all patients with ADHD, the physical examination will be normal. Laboratory testing should be performed only when indicated by the history and physical examination. However, it needs to be kept in mind that co-morbidity is seen in as many as 30% to 40% of patients with ADHD. Therefore, it is often important to conduct psychometric testing to rule out coexisting conditions such as learning disability, anxiety disorder, depression, and the possibility of a bipolar affective disorder. Persons with ADHD and its associated co-morbid conditions have a significantly increased risk of cigarette smoking and alcohol and drug abuse.

It is believed that males are more commonly affected with ADHD than females; however, the ratio is not as great as once thought, probably a 3:2 ratio of males to females.

TREATMENT

Treatment of ADHD is often multifaceted and may include medications, behavioral modification, or alternative therapies. Behavioral modification is frequently effective therapy for ADHD because it incorporates direct contingency management, clinical behavior therapy, and cognitive behavioral procedures. It has not been well documented, however, whether these focus therapies are effective independent of the use of medications.

It is important to determine whether an individual has a coexisting learning disability. If so, specialized educational management will certainly be beneficial to the child. Such testing needs to be done and is supported through a federal law passed in 1973 that mandates that all suspected children have the necessary testing be made available.

Specific strategies for the student include a daily assignment notebook and an organizational flow chart with specific colors. It is important that they be allowed to work in a quiet space both at school and at home. In addition, it may be beneficial for the student to be given additional time to take examinations. It is now possible for students with ADHD to have additional time allotted to take college entrance examinations. It has been clearly shown that their scores will be improved. Many universities and colleges now have additional help available and programs to assist college students with ADHD to be more successful academically.

Special advice for teachers is that they should monitor the student's work on a daily basis and issue daily report cards that are straightforward and simple and provide the necessary information to the student and parents. Ideally, teachers will be flexible, patient, and consistent in their interaction with students and seek to provide positive feedback whenever possible. Their instructions and expectations must be clear and concise.

Children and adults with attention deficit disorders (CHADD) is a national organization with many regional and local chapters that are a great resource for parents, families, and others.

Pharmacotherapy remains the mainstay in the treatment of patients with ADHD, but there continues to be ongoing concern in the United States about the use of stimulant medications and their safety. However, it needs to be clearly understood that patients with ADHD will respond to the use of psychotropic medications greater than 80% of the time. Recent publications report that stimulant medications have shown efficacy and safety in studies conducted for at least 24 months.

Psychostimulants are considered first-line agents for ADHD. Stimulants are sympathomimetic drugs that increase intrasynaptic catecholamines (mainly dopamine) by inhibiting the presynaptic reuptake mechanism and releasing presynaptic catecholamines. The most commonly used stimulant medications in the United States are methylphenidate (Ritalin) and dextroamphetamine (Dexedrine).

Pemoline (Cylert) has been used in the past, but this drug should no longer be considered a first-line medication for the treatment of ADHD because of the potential risk of hepatic failure.

The most common side effects that patients and physicians will see with psychostimulant medications are appetite suppression and insomnia. Additional side effects that patients may experience include abdominal pain, irritability, weight loss, and headache, especially when they first start the medications. Before the patient starts taking a psychostimulant medication, it is important to ensure that the patient has no previous history of a movement disorder or a family history of such. On rare occasions, tics and Tourette's syndrome are seen as potential side effects.

Concern has been raised regarding the use of psychostimulant medications and whether such use may lead to potential abuse. It has now been shown that individuals with ADHD rarely abuse psychostimulant medications and that such abuse is primarily by non-ADHD individuals. Another key point is that children in whom ADHD is diagnosed and who are treated with the recommended doses of stimulant medications do not go on to abuse these drugs or other drugs. Key points to remember regarding stimulant medications are listed in Table 2.

Methylphenidate (Ritalin), the most commonly used stimulant medication in the United States, has been in use for the last 40 to 50 years and, overall, has been shown to be very effective, with limited side effects. Methylphenidate is now also being manufactured as Concerta, which can be given in a once-a-day dose. Concerta uses osmotic pressure to deliver methylphenidate at a controlled rate. The system resembles a conventional tablet in appearance, but

TABLE 2. **Stimulant Medications—Points to Remember**

For Physicians

- Know local regulations for the prescription of schedule II medications
- Carefully diagnose and document evaluations and different diagnoses
- Take and document evaluations and different diagnoses
- Inform the family of the diversion potential and instruct families on careful storage of all medications
- Be alert for early prescription renewals
- Be alert for "scams" in which individuals see multiple physicians
- Do not prescribe without seeing the patient

For Parents

- Do not leave stimulants in accessible places
- Monitor medication administration carefully if any suspicion of misuse exists for a child with attention deficit hyperactivity disorder
- Never send supplies of medication to school with any child. Medication should be hand-delivered to school personnel by parents
- Talk to children about the penalties for selling or giving medication to others

For Schools

- Need a clear-cut policy for administration and self-administration of medication by students in school
- Store medications in a locked place with limited access. Document and keep accurate records

Table reprinted with permission of Minnesota Medicine. From Agerten DC, Rasmussen NH: Diagnosing and treating ADHD in children. Minn Med 83(6):51–54, 2000.

it is composed of an osmotically active trilayer core surrounded by a semipermeable membrane with an immediate-release drug overcoat. This formulation allows the medication to be absorbed over a sustained period, and its duration of action is 8 to 12 hours. It is manufactured in 18- and 36-mg tablets and may be taken with or without food. The use of once-a-day medication increases compliance and avoids the potential embarrassment of the student needing to take the medication at school. Many students have found such dosing to be much more acceptable. The side effects with Concerta are the same as with methylphenidate (Ritalin) in its previous form.

Other medications used in the past have included antidepressants, primarily the tricyclics.* On occasion, tricyclics can be effective if patients are unable to tolerate stimulant medication. The side effects of tricyclics, however, are greater and include dry mouth, constipation, and the potential for electrocardiographic changes.

It is interesting that antihypertensive medications, including clonidine* (Catapres) and guanfacine* (Tenex), have been found to be a potential help. These medications have a central and a peripheral action. One of the advantages, especially with clonidine (Catapres), is that it can be given as a patch with once-a-week dosing.

*Not FDA approved for this indication.

On occasion, combined pharmacologic approaches can be used for the treatment of ADHD. Examples include the use of antidepressant along with stimulant medication. The selective serotonin reuptake inhibitors are often used in combination. Such regimens are likely to be effective in patients who have co-morbid conditions, possibly including bipolar affective disorder.

In summary, ADHD is a significant health problem. It is now understood that ADHD and its causes are multifactorial, including genetic predisposition and underlying neurobiologic factors. Although no specific laboratory test is available to make the diagnosis, physicians have several assessment tools at their disposal. It is very important that one obtain a thorough history, including a family history, and an appropriate examination. This approach should help screen for coexisting conditions. A team approach involving the patient, family members, teachers, coworkers, and physicians should be used to treat patients with ADHD. Such an approach should allow the patient to succeed at school or in the work environment. It is likely that a combined treatment approach that includes behavioral modifications and the use of psychostimulant medications may be of greatest benefit. It must be recognized, however, that a patient in whom ADHD is diagnosed will not outgrow the condition but will always have this disorder. Nevertheless, with effective treatment, symptoms related to the disorder can be greatly improved.

GILLES DE LA TOURETTE SYNDROME

method of
ROBERT A. KING, M.D.,
LAWRENCE SCAHILL, M.S.N., PH.D., and
JAMES F. LECKMAN, M.D.
Yale University School of Medicine
New Haven, Connecticut

Gilles de la Tourette Syndrome (TS) is a developmental neuropsychiatric disorder characterized by waxing and waning motor and phonic tics that have persisted for at least a year.

CLINICAL FEATURES AND COURSE

Simple motor tics include blinking, grimacing, head turning, shoulder shrugging, abdominal tensing, and so on. *Complex motor tics* include touching, tapping, hitting, and orchestrated sequences of simple tics or sustained dystonic tics. *Common simple phonic tics* include sniffing, snorting, throat clearing, or grunting. *Complex vocal tics* may include repeated syllables, words, phrases, obscenities (coprolalia), or changes in prosody. Complex tics are rare in the absence of simple tics.

The most common age of tic onset is about 6 years of age. Tics typically wax and wane in severity. Although the course of TS is difficult to predict in any individual case, on average, the severity of tics subsides markedly by later adolescence, and only a small minority of individuals continue to experience troublesome tics into adulthood.

CO-MORBID CONDITIONS

Individuals with TS often have a variety of other clinically significant psychiatric symptoms. Attention deficit hyperactivity disorder (ADHD) is seen in 25% to 50% of children with TS. Obsessive-compulsive disorder (OCD) is also common in TS and in many families appears to share a common genetic diathesis. TS-related forms of OCD often center on characteristic "just-right" phenomena (e.g., a need to arrange objects or touch things symmetrically, to repeat acts until they feel, look, or sound just right).

Individuals with TS also have an increased vulnerability to anxiety and depression. Although this may partially reflect the social burden and stigma that accompany prominent tics, there may also be an underlying neurologic vulnerability to these problems. Neuropsychological testing commonly reveals subtle visual-motor integrative difficulties in many individuals with TS and these may be functionally apparent in the form of graphomotor and learning difficulties.

For many individuals with TS, these various co-morbid difficulties are more burdensome than the tics. For example, the social and academic difficulties of children with TS are more closely correlated with the severity of ADHD symptoms than with tic severity.

Hence, beyond assessing the range and severity of tic symptoms, careful evaluation for the presence of ADHD; OCD; and anxiety, mood, or learning disorders is essential in determining the focus and choice of treatment in TS.

GENERAL CONSIDERATIONS REGARDING TIC-SUPPRESSANT MEDICATION

The decision of whether to initiate medication for tics is not automatic. Because pharmacologic treatment does not appear to influence the long-term course of the disorder, tics require treatment only if they are causing impairment or distress sufficient to outweigh the possible side effects of medication. Indications for treatment include pain or injury due to tics, disruption of the patient's concentration or the classroom or workplace environment, and teasing or social stigma.

Another consideration in deciding to initiate pharmacologic treatment for tics concerns their natural waxing and waning pattern. Tics are often exacerbated by stress and excitement (e.g., the start of school, impending holidays or birthdays, vacation trips). Furthermore, whether viewed over minutes, days, or months, tics occur in bouts, and these in turn occur in bouts of bouts. Hence, even without intervention, it is likely that many sharp escalations of tics will be followed by a period of spontaneous subsidence. Because tic-suppressant medication often requires a couple of weeks to have its full effect, it may be difficult to distinguish a therapeutic response to medication from a spontaneous regression. As a result, we try to avoid beginning or increasing medication as soon as an exacerbation begins, preferring to wait a couple of weeks unless the tics cause serious impairment. Because stopping or reducing the dose of tic-suppressant medications must be done gradually to minimize rebound exacerbations, it is important to avoid an immediate increase in the dosage with each exacerbation, which runs the hazard of ratcheting up to higher and higher doses that cannot be easily reduced. A final, related consideration is to adopt the goal of reducing tics to tolerable level, rather than suppressing them completely. Attempts to eliminate tics completely are usually not successful and result in excessive levels of medication with attendant side effects that may cause more impairment than the tics.

Choice of Tic-Suppressant Medication

Two general classes of medication are most widely used to control tics associated with TS.

α-Adrenergic Agents

Guanfacine (Tenex)* and clonidine (Catapres)* are two α-adrenergic agents originally developed as antihypertensive agents in adults. In low doses, clonidine reduces central noradrenergic activity by stimulating presynaptic α_2-adrenergic autoreceptors; guanfacine is believed to act more selectively on postsynaptic α_2-adrenergic receptors in the prefrontal cortex. Although they are not as potent as the neuroleptics in suppressing tics, guanfacine and clonidine are more benign than the neuroleptics in terms of potential short- and long-term side effects and are hence our first choice in previously untreated individuals, especially those with mild-to-moderate symptoms.

Treatment is usually initiated at a low dose and gradually titrated upward. For example, we usually begin with one quarter to one half of a 0.1 mg tablet of clonidine in the morning; if tolerated well for several days, an afternoon dose is added and then, after several days, a lunchtime dose. A fourth, evening dose may also be helpful if there are problems falling asleep or if tics awaken the patient during the night. The size of each dose may be gradually titrated upward to a total dose of 0.2 to 0.3 mg daily. Although the effect of each individual dose of clonidine appears to wear off after about 3 to 5 hours, the full tic-suppressant effects of the regimen may require 10 to 12 weeks to be apparent. An oral syrup formulation may help in titrating small fractional doses. Although some clinicians use clonidine as a transdermal patch, we have found it unreliable in children, prone to fall off or wear off in less than a week, and likely to produce a rash or irritation.

Guanfacine is longer acting than clonidine but is titrated in a similar fashion in a range of 0.25 to 1.0 mg two or three times a day.

The principal side effects of clonidine and guanfacine in the recommended dose range are sedation, sometimes accompanied by irritability. This effect often wears off after a few days but may require dose reduction or a change of medication. Reversible cardiac arrhythmias have been infrequently reported with clonidine; however, the need for electrocardiographic studies are advisable at baseline and once a stable dose level is reached remains controversial.

*Not FDA approved for this indication.

Hypotension has not been a common problem in children taking α-adrenergic agents except for those taking clonidine and guanfacine simultaneously, which is therefore not recommended. Rebound exacerbations may be seen with abrupt withdrawal of clonidine or guanfacine. Gradual tapering is advisable to avoid tic flare-up or rebound hypertension.

Neuroleptics

Several typical and atypical neuroleptics are commonly used for treating TS, especially those patients with more severe tics or those unresponsive to the α-adrenergic agents. The efficacy of these agents appears to be related to their potency as postsynaptic dopamine-2 (D_2) receptor blockers. Pimozide (Orap), haloperidol (Haldol), and fluphenazine (Prolixin)* are the most commonly used typical neuroleptics; risperidone (Risperdal)* and ziprasidone are two atypical neuroleptics with demonstrated tic-suppressant efficacy. Clozapine (Clozaril)* is not beneficial for tics and may even exacerbate them, whereas olanzapine (Zyprexa)* has not been systematically studied for TS. Direct comparisons suggest that pimozide may be less cognitively blunting than haloperidol and that fluphenazine was less likely than haloperidol to produce extrapyramidal symptoms. It is best to start out with a low daily dose, for example, 0.5 mg of haloperidol or fluphenazine or 1 mg of pimozide and gradually titrate upward. In our experience, increasing the neuroleptic dose above 3 to 5 mg/d rarely produces additional improvement and very often produces bothersome side effects. As with clonidine* or guanfacine,* abrupt withdrawal can produce a rebound tic exacerbation; hence, gradual tapering is necessary when reducing or discontinuing a neuroleptic.

Although neuroleptics are very widely prescribed for TS, many patients are noncompliant owing to frequent bothersome side effects. The most common, dose-related side effects of the neuroleptic are sedation or dysphoria. Weight gain is also a problem with most of these agents, especially risperidone. Some children taking neuroleptics develop de novo separation anxiety and school refusal. Although the atypical neuroleptics are believed to have a lower risk of tardive dyskinesia, acute extrapyramidal reactions (e.g., torticollis, oculogyric crisis, akathisia) do occur with the atypical neuroleptics and may require anticholinergic medication (e.g., diphenhydramine [Benadryl], 25 mg, as a first-aid measure, or a standing dose of benztropine [Cogentin]). Because of potential QT changes, baseline and follow-up electrocardiography is recommended for risperidone, ziprasidone, and pimozide. It is also essential for the prescribing clinician to be familiar with potential cytochrome P-450–related drug interactions because fatal interactions have occurred with pimozide and erythromycin-related antibiotics.

*Not FDA approved for this indication.

Other Tic-Suppressant Agents

Tiapride* and sulpiride* are two neuroleptics not available in the United States that have proved useful for tics in European clinical trials. Tetrabenazine, another antidopaminergic agent not available in the United States, has been mildly effective in open-label trials. Low doses of pergolide (Permax),† a mixed D_2-D_1 agonist, were effective in reducing tics in an open label trial and a recently reported double-blind clinical trial. Pergolide is usually started with a single daily oral dose of 0.025 mg and gradually titrated up to 0.075 mg thrice daily. The major side effect is nausea.

In open trials, brief administration of nicotine, either as chewing gum or transdermal patch, produced short-lived (i.e., 1–2 weeks) positive effects in potentiating the tic-reducing effectiveness of a concomitant neuroleptic. Mecamylamine (Inversine),† another agent acting at the nicotinic receptor, produced some apparently similar beneficial potentiating of neuroleptic effectiveness in two open but difficult to interpret trials. Clonazepam has also been used in open trials for tics and may be useful for patients with co-morbid OCD or anxiety disorder. However, the potential side effects of sedation, disinhibition, and dependence limit its usefulness, especially in children. All three of these agents await adequate controlled double-blind studies.

Locally injected dilute botulinum toxin may provide several weeks of improvement in tics in the area of injection, making it potentially useful for specific severe and refractory tics (e.g., head-snapping or loud vocal tics). Remarkably, some patients report a marked reduction in the premonitory sensory urges that often precede tics.

TREATMENT OF RELATED ADHD SYMPTOMS

The treatment of ADHD symptoms in patients with personal or family histories of tics is common, complex, and controversial. Stimulants, such as methylphenidate (Ritalin) and dextroamphetamine (Dexedrine), are the most effective agents for uncomplicated ADHD. However, although some experts claim that these drugs may be used with impunity in individuals with tics, in our experience, they can precipitate de novo tics or exacerbate pre-existing tics in many individuals. We prefer to begin with the various second-line treatments for ADHD, which, although not as potent as the stimulants, appear less prone to exacerbating tics. The α-adrenergic agents, clonidine† and guanfacine,† appear to be helpful for both ADHD symptoms and for tics (see previous section). The tricyclic antidepressants, such as nortryptyline,† also appear effective for ADHD but require electrocardiographic monitoring and careful dosing. Unfortunately, for many children with TS in whom ADHD is more disabling than the tics, alternative

*Not available in the United States.
†Not FDA approved for this indication.

medications are not sufficiently effective, and the addition of a low dose of a stimulant may be ultimately necessary despite some resultant increase in tic severity.

TREATMENT OF RELATED OBSESSIVE-COMPULSIVE DISORDER

The serotonin-reuptake inhibitors (clomipramine [Anafranil], fluoxetine [Prozac], sertraline [Zoloft], paroxetine [Paxil], citalopram [Celexa], and fluvoxamine [Luvox]) are useful in treating the OCD symptoms found in TS but may not produce as full a therapeutic response as in individuals with non–TS-related OCD. Augmentation with a low dose of a neuroleptic may increase these agents' antiobsessional efficacy. At higher dose levels, the serotonin-reuptake inhibitors may occasionally precipitate or exacerbate tics.

Antibiotic and Immunotherapies

Although it has been proposed that some cases of TS may be a sequela of group A β-hemolytic streptococcal infections, this connection remains controversial and is likely to be a contributing mechanism in only a minority of TS cases. Antibiotic prophylaxis and arduous investigational interventions such as plasma exchange or intravenous immunoglobulins have been successfully used in a small number of cases with well-documented exacerbations following streptococcal infection. Such measures should be considered only with expert child psychiatric and pediatric consultation. At present, the principal mandate for the clinician is to be vigilant in assessing children with pharyngitis or those exposed to streptococcus and vigorously treating and following up those with positive throat culture results.

PSYCHOSOCIAL MEASURES

The various manifestations of TS are best treated in the context of a long-term relationship with a clinician who can help the patient, family, and school deal with the changing manifestations of the disorder through the years. Because acute and chronic stress can exacerbate tics, psychotherapeutic attention to problems of self-esteem, social coping, family issues, and school adjustment may have nonspecific ameliorative effects on tic severity, as well as on attendant anxiety and depression. Parents should be encouraged to build on their child's strengths. Behavioral management training and parent guidance is important in dealing with the disruptive behavioral problems often associated with childhood TS. Specific cognitive behavioral techniques (such as habit reversal or exposure/response prevention training) may be useful for selected compulsions or tic behaviors.

HEADACHE

method of
DAVID E. TRACHTENBARG, M.D.
University of Illinois College of Medicine Peoria
Peoria, Illinois

Headache is a common medical problem. Ninety-three percent of patients report having a headache by age 29. One way of evaluating headaches is to divide them into primary and secondary headaches (Table 1). Primary headache disorders include migraine, tension-type headache, and cluster headache, diagnosis and treatment of which are emphasized in this article. Secondary causes of headache, including common problems such as sinusitis and serious causes such as meningitis, are important to rule out. Their treatment is discussed elsewhere in this book.

HISTORY AND PHYSICAL EXAMINATION

The history is the most important part of a headache evaluation. One example of questions specific to headaches is included in Table 2. The family history is ideally obtained by directly asking parents and siblings, who are about twice as likely to report the headaches as the patient. In addition to a neurologic examination, potentially helpful items from the physical examination include palpation of the muscles of the head and neck for tender areas, palpation of the temporomandibular joints (TMJs), percussion and transillumination of the sinuses, and palpation of the temporal artery area for tenderness. The time spent taking the history and performing the physical examination is ideal for reviewing misconceptions about headaches. Many patients call any severe headache a "migraine" even

TABLE 1. **A Clinical Classification of Headaches**

Primary Headache Disorders
Acute
Tension-type headache
Vascular headaches
Migraine
With aura
Without aura
Migraine with prolonged aura
Aura without headache
Basilar migraine
Menstrual
Cluster
Chronic
Transformed migraine
Chronic tension-type headaches
Secondary Headache Disorders
Common
Sinus
Temporomandibular joint
Visual
Medication
Potentially Serious Causes
Meningitis
Subarachnoid hemorrhage
Brain tumor
Pseudotumor cerebri
Temporal arteritis
Exertional

TABLE 2. **Headache History**

Date of onset
Frequency: How often do the headaches occur?
Duration
Time of day, night, week, month, year that headaches occur
Precipitating factors, including food and injuries
Type of onset: Do the headaches have premonitory symptoms or a preceding aura. Did the headache start suddenly?
Course: Are the headaches getting better, worse, or the same?
Severity of pain: Do the headaches interfere with activity?
Quality of pain: Constant or throbbing
Location of pain
Radiation of pain
Aggravating and alleviating factors
Tenderness at site
Effect of pressure
Effect of posture
Effect of head jolt
Associated factors
- Ear, nose, and throat: Congestion, rhinorrhea
- Gastrointestinal: Nausea, vomiting, constipation, diarrhea
- Genitourinary: Polyuria
- Visual: Scotoma, photophobia, homonymous hemianopia, rings round lights, ptosis
- Neurologic: Vertigo, dizziness
- Musculoskeletal: Soreness
- Family history of headache

though their headache may actually be a tension-type headache. Other patients report headache as a symptom of elevated blood pressure, although studies of patients with mild to moderate hypertension have found no correlation between headache and blood pressure.

DIAGNOSTIC TESTS

Laboratory testing is not routinely indicated for headache patients. Additional testing should be based on the patient evaluation, such as radiographs or computed tomography (CT) of the sinuses if sinusitis is suspected or a sedimentation rate if temporal arteritis is suspected (Table 3). The question of performing neuroimaging often arises, but headache severity does not predict intracranial pathology. Some indications for neuroimaging include the following:

1. Unexplained abnormal neurologic examination
2. Sudden onset of a severe headache (thunderclap headache)
3. Exertional headache
4. Progression of headache with time
5. Headaches that wake the patient up at night
6. Acute onset of a new type of headache, especially after middle age
7. Headaches that are consistently unilateral
8. Failure of the headache to fit a benign pattern
9. Risk factors such as immune deficiency or history of a malignancy that may metastasize to the brain

DIFFERENTIAL DIAGNOSIS

Table 4 contains information to help distinguish between the primary headache types. Frequently, patients have different types of headaches, and each must be evaluated and treated separately. Although no clear distinction can often be made between vascular and tension-type headaches, the symptoms that are significantly more common with migraine than tension-type headache are: nausea, photophobia, phonophobia, exacerbation during physical activity, and occurrence of an aura. Many more types of headache have been identified than can be discussed in the space of this article. The headache classification by the International Headache Society[1] is the most commonly recognized guideline used to classify and diagnose headaches.

MANAGEMENT

Whenever possible, the medications listed in this article are restricted to those with at least one study found in the literature. Care of patients is limited because many studies of headache treatment do not meet the highest standards of evidence-based medicine. In addition, many drugs related to well-studied medications may work as well but have even less evidence of headache efficacy.

General Measures

Headache triggers should be avoided whenever possible. For most patients, cold is more effective than heat for relieving headache pain.

Biofeedback and Other Behavioral Approaches

Relaxation therapy may be helpful for selected patients. Biofeedback is another behavioral modality that appears effective for selected patients. Temperature biofeedback and muscle relaxation biofeedback are helpful for migraine and tension-type headaches. Behavioral therapy may be combined with medication to obtain maximal clinical benefit.

Other Therapies

A review of manipulation for headache concluded that although the evidence indicates that manipulation may benefit some patients, more high-quality research needs to be done to make definitive recommendations. Acupuncture, hypnosis, occlusal adjustment, and hyperbaric oxygen are not established evidence-based treatment modalities.

TABLE 3. **Indications for Additional Testing**

Frontal pain, sinus tenderness, or other signs and symptoms of sinusitis	Radiograph of sinuses, CT scan of sinuses
Tender temporal artery, thickened temporal artery on palpation	Sedimentation rate, temporal artery biopsy
Temporomandibular joint tenderness, malocclusion of the teeth, decreased range of motion of the jaw	Dental consultation, single-contrast joint arthrography, panoramic dental radiographs, MRI of the joint, diagnostic arthroscopy
Suspected pseudotumor cerebri	Dilated eye examination by an ophthalmologist, visual fields, neuroimaging of the brain, lumbar puncture
Neck stiffness, sudden onset (thunderclap headache), mental confusion	CT, lumbar puncture
Blurred vision, pain behind the eyes, pain associated with reading, using a computer monitor, or watching TV	Dilated eye examination by an ophthalmologist, refraction testing

TABLE 4. **Typical Symptoms of Primary Headache Syndromes***

	Tension Type	Migraine	Cluster
Distribution	Bilateral	Unilateral	Unilateral orbital, supraorbital, or temporal
Pain	Constant pressure not aggravated by walking	Throbbing worse with physical activity	Throbbing
Untreated duration	30 min to 7 d	4 h to 3 d	15 min to 3 h
Typical time of onset	Later in day	Any time of day	At night
Associated symptoms	Less common than vascular headaches	Photophobia, phonophobia, nausea, vomiting, and scotoma are common	Conjunctival injection, lacrimation, nasal congestion, facial sweating, miosis, ptosis
Triggers	Stress	Stress, foods	Rarely identified
Gender	About 10% more common in females	Female-to-male ratio approximately 3:1	More common in males, approximately 2:1
Other		Family history is common. May have preceding aura	Occurs in periods lasting 7 d to 1 y separated by pain-free intervals of at least 2 wk

*Many patients will have the atypical pattern.

TREATMENT OF SPECIFIC TYPES OF HEADACHE

Primary Headache Disorders

Migraine

Migraine headaches are typically unilateral throbbing headaches that last 4 to 72 hours. In about 40% of patients the pain is bilateral. Other neurologic symptoms are usually present, including photophobia, phonophobia, osmophobia, visual changes, nausea, and vomiting. In about 15% of migraine patients the headache is preceded by an aura by 20 to 30 minutes. The most common type of aura is visual, and patterns include scintillating scotomas and flashing lights.

The International Headache Society classification includes many types of migraine, the main types of which include *migraine with an aura*, which has been called *classic migraine* in the past. What was previously called *common migraine* is now called *migraine without an aura*. Other types include *migraine with a prolonged aura*, which is defined as an aura that lasts 60 minutes or more. *Migraine aura without a headache* has been called *acephalic migraine* or *migraine equivalent*. *Basilar migraine* is migraine with basilar artery symptoms. The International Headache Society criteria for basilar migraine include two or more of the following symptoms: visual symptoms in the temporal and nasal fields of both eyes, dysarthria, vertigo, tinnitus, decreased hearing, double vision, ataxia, bilateral paresthesias or paresis, and decreased level of consciousness.

GENERAL TREATMENT MEASURES

A summary of medications used to treat migraine is presented in Table 5. Much of the management of migraine in this chapter is from a recent evidence-based review. Migraine-specific agents such as the triptans are advised for patients with moderate to severe headaches and those who do not respond to nonsteroidal anti-inflammatory drugs (NSAIDs). Patients with nausea and vomiting may be given intranasal, orally dissolving, or parenteral medications. Antiemetics such as metoclopramide can also be helpful in these patients.

ACUTE HEADACHE

Ergot Preparations and Triptans. The classic medications in this category are ergotamine (Ergostat) and dihydroergotamine (DHE) (Migranal). Ergotamine tartrate with caffeine is available in tablet and suppository form. DHE causes less vasoconstriction than ergotamine does and may be given intravenously, intramuscularly, or subcutaneously. An intranasal preparation is also available. Newer medications such as sumatriptan produce less nausea but are not significantly more effective.

The nasal and orally dissolving preparations work about as well as the oral ones. Patients who do not respond to the initial choice of medication may respond to a different triptan or a different route of administration. Longer-acting triptans such as zolmitriptan (Zomig) may have less rebound, although comparative data are limited. The parenteral forms of the ergot and triptan medications are significantly more effective and should be considered for patients who fail to respond to less effective routes of administration. Major contraindications to these medications include hypertension, coronary artery disease, cerebrovascular disease, peripheral vascular disease, and hemiplegic migraine. They should be used with caution in patients with basilar artery migraine. The ergot and triptan medications should not be combined. Caution is advised if taking them with serotonin reuptake inhibitors and other medications affecting serotonin metabolism.

NSAIDs. In randomized clinical trials, NSAIDs work as well as the triptans for migraine. Many patients have tried several NSAIDs without success before consulting a physician for their migraine headaches. For patients with mild to moderate migraine who have not tried an NSAID, these drugs are the most cost-effective to try initially.

TABLE 5. Migraine Treatment

Abortive

Ergot Preparations and Triptans

- Naratriptan (Amerge), 1–2.5 mg PO initially. May repeat in 4 h, up to 5 mg/d
- Rizatriptan (Maxalt), 5–10 mg PO initially. Available in orally disintegrating tablets. May repeat q2h up to 30 mg/d. If taking a β-blocker (e.g., propranolol), use 5 mg per maximal dose up to 15 mg/d
- Sumatriptan (Imitrex), 25–100 mg PO initially. May repeat q2h up to 200 mg/d.
  - 5–20 mg spray nasally. May repeat q2h up to 40 mg/d
  - 6 mg SC initially. May repeat in 1 h, up to 12 mg/d
- Zolmitriptan (Zomig), 1.25–2.5 mg initially. May repeat q2h up to 10 mg/d
- DHE SC, IM, IV, 1 mg initially. May repeat hourly up to 3 mg/attack and 6 mg/wk
- DHE nasal spray (Migranal), 1 spray in each nostril. May repeat in 15 min, up to 4 sprays per attack and 8/wk
- DHE IV plus an antiemetic: prochlorperazine* (Compazine) and metoclopramide* (Reglan) are the best studied
- Ergotamine, 1 mg/caffeine, 100 mg (Cafergot, Wigraine), 1–2 tablets PO q30min prn up to 6 mg/d and 10 mg/wk of ergotamine
- Ergotamine, 2 mg/caffeine, 200 mg (Cafergot, Wigraine) rectal suppositories, q30min prn up to 2 suppositories per attack and 10 mg of ergotamine per week
- Ergotamine tartrate sublingual (Ergomar), 2 mg. One tablet under tongue. May repeat at half-hour intervals, up to 3 per attack and 5 tablets/wk

NSAIDs

- Aspirin, 650 mg PO q4h prn
- Ibuprofen (Motrin), 400–800 mg/dose PO. Maximum, 3200 mg/d
- Naproxen (Naprosyn, Anaprox). Usual dose, 250–500 mg PO bid. Maximum, 1500 mg/d for 5 d
- Diclofenac (Cataflam, Voltaren). Usual dose, 50 mg PO tid. Maximum, 150 mg/d
- Flurbiprofen (Ansaid), 50–100 mg PO tid. Maximum, 300 mg/d
- Acetaminophen, 650–1000 mg per dose in 4–6 divided doses, up to 4000 mg/d (believed to be less effective, consider for pregnant migraineur)

NSAIDs (Continued)

- Ketorolac (Toradol), 60 mg IM/IV initially, 30 mg for repeat doses. Maximum, 120 mg/d. Use for no more than 5 d total

Narcotic Analgesics

- Butorphanol (Stadol), 1 mg IV or 1–4 mg IM q3h prn
- Butorphanol (Stadol) nasal spray in one or both nostrils q3h prn
- Meperidine (Demerol), 50–150 mg IM q3h prn or 25–50 mg IV q3h prn

Antiemetics

- Prochlorperazine* (Compazine), 10 mg IV or IM, maximal dose of 40 mg/day. 25-mg rectal suppository, maximum of 50 mg/d
- Metoclopramide* (Reglan), 10 mg IV or IM qid prn
- Chlorpromazine* (Thorazine), 25 mg IM, IV q4h prn

Combination

- Acetaminophen, 250 mg/aspirin, 250 mg/caffeine, 65 mg (Excedrin Extra Strength), 2 tablets PO at start of attack
- Acetaminophen, 300 mg/codeine, 30 mg (Tylenol No. 3), 1–2 tablets PO q4h prn, up to 12 tablets/d
- Aspirin, 325 mg/butalbital, 50 mg/caffeine, 40 mg (Fiorinal), 1–2 tablets q4h prn, up to 6 tablets/d
- Aspirin, 325 mg/butalbital, 50 mg/caffeine, 40 mg/codeine, 30 mg (Fiorinal with Codeine), 1–2 tablets q4h prn up to 6 tablets/d

Steroids

- Dexamethasone (Decadron), 16 mg IM or IV only once q3wk. May also be combined with an antiemetic
- Prednisone, 40–60 mg for 3–5 d

Miscellaneous

- Isometheptene mucate, 65 mg/dichloralphenazone, 100 mg/acetaminophen, 325 mg (Midrin), 2 capsules PO initially, followed by 1 capsule until headaches relieved every hour up to 5 capsules in 12 h and 8 capsules/d
- 0.4 mL of lidocaine 4% intranasally (Xylocaine)

Preventive

β-Blockers

- Propranolol (Inderal), start at 80 mg/d. Maximal dose, 240 mg/d in appropriately divided doses or a daily time release preparation
- Timolol (Blocadren), 10 mg PO bid or 20 mg PO qd. Maximal dose, 60 mg/d
- Atenolol* (Tenormin), 50–200 mg/d
- Metoprolol* (Lopressor, Toprol), 50–200 mg/d in 2 divided doses if not using a time release form
- Nadolol* (Corgard), start at 20–40 mg/d. Maximal dose, 120 mg/d

Anticonvulsants

- Divalproex sodium (Depakote), 500–1000 mg/d in 2 divided doses with food
- Gabapentin* (Neurontin), 300 mg PO tid, gradually titrating from 300 mg on day 1 over at least 3 days. Maximal dose, 3600 mg/d
- Tiagabine* (Gabitril), 4 mg/d to start. 56 mg/d maximum in 2–4 divided doses with food
- Topiramate* (Topamax), start at 50 mg PO qd up to 200 mg PO bid

Calcium Channel Blockers

- Verapamil* (Calan, Isoptin), 160–480 mg/d in appropriately divided doses if not using a time release form
- Diltiazem* (Cardizem), 120–360 mg/d in appropriately divided doses if not using a time release form
- Nimodipine* (Nimotop), 90–180 mg/d in 3–4 divided doses

NSAIDs

- Aspirin, 650 mg bid
- Ibuprofen (Motrin), 300–800 tid–qid. Maximum, 3200 mg/d
- Flurbiprofen (Ansaid), 50–100 mg PO tid. Maximum, 300 mg/d
- Ketoprofen (Orudis), 75 mg q8h or 50 mg q6h
- Naproxen (Naprosyn, Anaprox), 250–500 mg PO bid

Antidepressants

- Amitriptyline* (Elavil, Endep), start at 25–50 mg qhs. Maximum, 150 mg/d. May divide dose.
- Doxepin* (Sinequan), start at 25–75 mg qhs. Maximum, 300 mg/d. May divide dose.
- Imipramine* (Tofranil), 25–300 mg PO qhs. Start at 25–50 mg

Antidepressants (Continued)

- Mirtazapine* (Remeron), 15–45 mg PO qhs. Start at 15 mg qhs
- Nortriptyline* (Pamelor, Aventyl), start at 25–50 mg qhs. Maximum, 150 mg/d. May divide dose.
- Fluoxetine* (Prozac), 10–80 mg/d. Usual starting dose, 20 mg qAM
- Paroxetine* (Paxil), 10–50 mg/d. Usual starting dose, 20 mg PO qAM
- Protriptyline* (Vivactil), 5–10 mg PO tid–qid. Maximum, 60 mg/d
- Sertraline* (Zoloft), 50–200 mg/d. Start at 50 mg/d
- Trazodone* (Desyrel), 50–100 mg bid–tid. Maximum, 400 mg/d
- Venlafaxine* (Effexor), 37.5–225 mg/d in appropriately divided doses or as a daily long-acting dose. Start at 37.5–75 mg

Other

- Feverfew*
- Magnesium,* 600 mg trimagnesium dicitrate per day
- Vitamin B_2* (riboflavin), 400 mg/d PO
- Cyproheptadine* (Periactin), 4–8 mg PO tid–qid

Concerns About Possible Adverse Effects

- Methylergonovine, 0.2 mg qid for maximum of 1 week
- Phenelzine* (Nardil), 15 mg PO tid to start, up to 30 mg PO tid
- Methysergide (Sansert), 2–8 mg/d in divided doses

No More Effective Than Placebo

β-ADRENERGIC BLOCKERS

- Acebutolol* (Sectral)
- Pindolol* (Visken)

CALCIUM CHANNEL BLOCKERS

- Nicardipine* (Cardene)
- Nifedipine* (Procardia, Adalat)

ANTICONVULSANTS

- Carbamazepine* (Tegretol)

ANTIDEPRESSANTS/ANXIOLYTICS

- Clomipramine* (Anafranil)
- Clonazepam* (Klonopin)

NSAIDs

- Indomethacin* (Indocin)

MISCELLANEOUS

- Clonidine* (Catapres)

*Not FDA approved for this indication.

Abbreviations: DHE = dihydroergotamine; NSAIDs = nonsteroidal anti-inflammatory drugs; prn = as needed; qhs = at bedtime.

Adapted from Silberstein SD: Practice parameter: Evidence-based guidelines for migraine headache (an evidence-based review). Report of the Quality Standards Subcommittee of the American Academy of Neurology. Neurology 55:754–763, 2000.

Antiemetics. Antiemetics alone have been shown to help migraine. They can also be combined with other treatment to help nausea and vomiting.

Steroids. Many clinicians believe that a course of corticosteroids is helpful for terminating a prolonged attack. However, there is a lack of randomized controlled studies showing efficacy.

Narcotic Analgesics. Narcotic analgesics are generally limited to use as rescue medication for migraine patients who have failed to respond to specific treatment.

Miscellaneous. Intranasal lidocaine* relieved migraine headache pain in 55% of patients in one study.

Combination. Many combination drugs are available. Caffeine increases the efficacy of aspirin, acetaminophen, and other analgesics. Other medications such as butalbital and narcotic analgesics may likewise increase their efficacy, but their use increases the risk of dependence.

PREVENTION

Published criteria for prophylactic therapy include migraines that (1) occur more than twice a month, (2) last over 48 hours, (3) are severe, (4) are unable to be adequately treated acutely, (5) have a prolonged aura, and (6) make the patient unable to cope psychologically.

Diet. About one fifth of patients with migraine may benefit from avoiding triggering foods. Common trigger food components include cheese, chocolate, and citrus fruits. Other reported dietary triggering factors include nitrates, monosodium glutamate, and alcohol, especially red wine.

β-Blockers. Both selective β-blockers such as atenolol (Tenormin)* and nonselective β-blockers such as propranolol (Inderal) are effective prophylactic agents. β-Blockers with adrenergic activity such as pindolol (Visken)* are not effective.

Anticonvulsants. Divalproex (Depakote) is the best studied anticonvulsant agent. Gabapentin (Neurontin),* tiagabine (Gabitril),* and topiramate (Topamax)* also appear to be effective but have not been studied as well.

Calcium Channel Blockers. Verapamil (Calan)* and nimodipine (Nimotop)* both appear to be effective. Nimodipine's use is limited by cost. Diltiazem has less evidence of effectiveness. Other calcium channel blockers have not been as well studied or have not been found to be effective.

NSAIDs. Although NSAIDs are commonly used for the treatment of acute migraine, they can also be used for prophylaxis if given on a continuous basis. The newer cyclooxygenase-2 inhibitors* have not been well studied for effectiveness.

Antidepressant Medication. Many of the older tricyclic antidepressants,* as well as the newer antidepressants, including the serotonin reuptake inhibitors,* are effective prophylactic agents.

Drugs Limited by Adverse Effects. Methysergide and methylergonovine* are very effective in preventing attacks, but their use is limited by side effects. Use of the monoamine oxidase inhibitor phenelzine is also limited by potentially serious food and drug interactions.

Miscellaneous. Vitamin B_2 (riboflavin)* has been found to reduce the frequency of migraine headache, but it has to be given for several weeks to see an effect. Magnesium in the form of 600 mg of trimagnesium dicitrate* a day reduced the frequency of migraine attacks by 42%. The herbal preparation feverfew* also appears to be effective, but its use is limited by the lack of required standardization and quality control.

Menstrual Migraine

Menstrual migraine may be defined as migraine that always occurs within 2 days of the onset of menses. Menstrual-associated migraine is defined as migraine that additionally occurs at other times in the menstrual cycle. One key trigger for these headaches appears to be a drop in estrogen levels.

ACUTE TREATMENT

Medications for acute treatment of menstrual migraine are the same, but prophylaxis is different. NSAIDs are commonly used for first-line therapy. If one does not work, another from a different pharmacologic family may be tried. Ergotamine preparations and the triptans are also effective.

The NSAIDs have been successfully used for prophylaxis. Regimens vary from starting 3 to 7 days before the expected onset of menses and stopping 1 to 3 days after the start of menses. Ergotamine preparations such as Caffeine/ergotamine (Cafergot), one to two times a day, or ergonovine (Ergotrate), three to four times a day premenstrually, may also be successful. The dose of ergotamine should be restricted to less than 10 mg/wk to reduce the risk of ergot dependency. Ergotamine should also not be combined with the triptans. Two studies of sumatriptan from 1 day before to 4 days after menses and 3 days before to 5 days after menses showed that the drug was successful in aborting attacks. A typical dose of sumatriptan (Imitrex) for prophylactic use is 25 mg orally three times daily. β-Blockers and calcium channel blockers* can be tried for selected patients but clinically appear to be less effective for menstrual migraines.

Preventing drops in the estrogen level has also been tried. Using 100-μg estradiol (Estraderm) patches premenstrually may be effective. Lower dose patches do not appear to work as well. For women who are prescribed oral contraceptives, giving monophasic pills will reduce the variation in estrogen dose that may trigger headaches. Combining three packages of pills to give 9 weeks (63 days) of active pills followed by 7 days of reminder pills may also reduce the number of menstrually related migraines. This technique is called tricycling.

Medications that block estrogen effects are also

*Not FDA approved for this indication.

*Not FDA approved for this indication.

effective, but they should be considered only when other treatments have failed. Bromocriptine (Parlodel),* 7.5 mg/d, danazol (Danocrine)* 200 mg twice a day for the first 25 days of the menstrual cycle, and tamoxifen (Nolvadex),* 10 to 20 mg/d premenstrually and 5 to 20 mg/d for 3 days after the start of menses, have been reported to be effective.

Some patients taking prophylactic medication for their migraines who experience menstrual-associated migraine may respond by increasing the dose perimenstrually. Magnesium, 120 mg orally three times daily from the 15th day of the menstrual cycle until menstrual flow, has also been reported to reduce menstrual migraines.

Oral Contraceptives

Patients with migraine have about twice the chance of an ischemic stroke. This risk increases to about six times normal for migraine patients with aura. Use of the combined oral contraceptives appears to double the risk. Although the overall rate of stroke is still very low for women of childbearing age, patients with migraine should be informed about the risks versus benefits of oral contraceptives, and those with aura should consider alternative contraception. Migraine patients with other risk factors, including a prolonged aura, hypercoagulable blood, hypertension, smoking, diabetes, and a history of transient ischemic attack and stroke should be strongly discouraged from using oral contraceptives. Postmenopausal estrogen replacement therapy, which has the goal of replacing "normal" hormonal levels, is believed to be less risky.

Cluster Headache

Cluster headache occurs in about 0.4% of men and 0.08% of women. The headaches are typically unilateral throbbing headaches in the orbital temporal area that occur every day or every other day and last 15 minutes to 3 hours. They are associated with ipsilateral lacrimation, rhinorrhea, facial sweating and conjunctival redness. Horner's syndrome may also be present on the affected side. Cluster headaches tend to occur at the same time of day and take place at night in about 50% of patients. Unlike migraine and tension headache sufferers, cluster headache patients will frequently pace the floor. According to International Headache Society criteria, episodic cluster headache occurs in periods lasting 7 days to 1 year with pain-free intervals of at least 14 days. The rarer chronic forms will not be discussed in this article. Table 6 gives a summary of medications for the treatment of cluster headache. Abortive agents include 100% oxygen for 10 minutes, which provides relief in 82% of patients, but it may need to be repeated. Other proven agents are similar to those for migraine and include ergot and triptan preparations. Capsaicin (Zostrix) applied to the nostril on the affected side appears to be effective in aborting and preventing attacks. It commonly irritates the nostril and causes burning, sneezing, and a runny nose.

*Not FDA approved for this indication.

TABLE 6. **Episodic Cluster Headache Treatment**

Abortive
100% O_2 for 10–15 min, repeat as needed
Sumatriptan (Imitrex), 25–100 mg PO initially. May repeat q2h up to 200 mg/d
Sumatriptan (Imitrex), 6 mg SC initially. May repeat in 1 h, up to 12 mg/d
Sumatriptan (Imitrex), 20-mg spray nasally. May repeat q2h up to 40 mg/d
Zolmitriptan (Zomig), 5 mg initially. May repeat in 2 h. Maximal dose, 10 mg/d
Ergotamine, 1 mg/caffeine, 100 mg (Cafergot, Wigraine), 1–2 tablets PO q30 min prn up to 6 mg/d and 10 mg/wk of ergotamine
Ergotamine, 2 mg/caffeine, 200 mg (Cafergot, Wigraine), rectal suppositories, q30min prn up to 2 suppositories per attack and 10 mg of ergotamine per week
Ergotamine tartrate sublingual (Ergomar), 2 mg. One tablet under the tongue. May repeat at half-hour intervals, up to 3 per attack and 5 tablets/wk
DHE SC, IM, IV, 1 mg initially. May repeat hourly up to 3 mg/attack and 6 mg/wk
DHE nasal spray (Migranal), 1 spray in each nostril. May repeat in 15 min. Up to 4 sprays per attack and 8/wk
Capsaicin* 0.025% (Zostrix) applied to the nostril on the affected side
0.4 mL of 4% lidocaine* in the nostril on the affected side
Preventive
Lithium,* 600–900 mg/d to maintain levels 0.5–1.5 mEq/L
Methysergide (Sansert). Usual range, 2–8 mg/d in divided doses; start with 2 mg/d
Prednisone, 40–80 mg/d initially, followed by gradual taper
Verapamil* (Calan, Isoptin), 160–480 mg/d
Ergotamine, 1 mg/caffeine, 100 mg, 1–2 tablets PO qd–tid 1–2 h before usual time of attack
Capsaicin,* 0.025% (Zostrix), applied to the nostril on the affected side once or twice a day
Baclofen* (Lioresal), 15–30 mg in 3 divided doses

*Not FDA approved for this indication.
Abbreviation: DHE = dihydroergotamine.

Prednisone, 40 to 80 mg with a gradual taper, may break a bout of cluster headache. The headaches may recur, however, when the dose is reduced below 20 mg/d. If limited to short-term prophylaxis for episodic cluster headache, methysergide is safer to use than for migraine. Other preventive agents include lithium (Lithobid)* and verapamil (Calan).* Lithium* is highly effective but needs to be carefully monitored. Verapamil* is a less effective, but safer alternative. Anticonvulsant medications such as divalproex (Depakote)* are thought to be effective prophylactic agents clinically but are not well studied. In one study, 100 mg of sumatriptan orally three times daily for 7 days did not reduce the frequency of cluster headaches. Surgical procedures may be helpful when all else fails.

Tension Headache

About 40% of adults report at least one episodic tension-type headache a year. About 8% of patients

*Not FDA approved for this indication.

with episodic tension-type headaches reported lost workdays and about 40% reported decreased effectiveness at work. The term *tension-type headache* was chosen by the International Headache Society rather than the older term "muscle contraction headache" because with many of these headaches, patients do not have objective signs of muscle contraction. Although tension-type headaches are the most common type of headache seen in primary care, less evidence-based information is available for them than for migraine. The relationship between tension-type headaches and migraine is also controversial. Some authors believe that they are different manifestations of the same disease or that many people in whom tension-type headache is diagnosed actually have mild migraine headache. Others believe that they are distinct entities.

General measures include regular diet, sleep, and exercise. Stress management and relaxation therapy, including home relaxation training, may also be helpful for selected patients. Biofeedback may likewise be helpful. Cold is usually more helpful than heat, but both may be tried to see what works best for individual patients. Although commonly tried by patients, evidence that chiropractic manipulation improves tension-type headaches is limited.

A stepped treatment approach is helpful. Start with non-narcotic analgesics. If these agents do not work, combination medications may help. Muscle relaxer, barbiturate, anxiolytic, and narcotic use should be limited. Preventive treatment should be considered if headaches occur more than twice a week, if the headaches last over 4 hours, or if the headache causes significant medication overuse or disability. Although tricyclic antidepressants* are the best studied medications for tension headache prophylaxis, serotonin reuptake inhibitors* also appear to be effective. A summary of selected treatment options is presented in Table 7.

TABLE 7. **Selected Tension Headache Treatment Options**

Abortive

OTC Medications

Ibuprofen (Motrin), 400–800 mg initially, up to 2400 mg/d
Acetaminophen (Tylenol), 650 mg q4h or 1000 mg q6h prn
Aspirin, 650 mg q4h prn
Ketoprofen (Orudis), 25–50 mg PO q4h prn. Maximal dose, 300 mg/d
Naproxen (Aleve, Anaprox, Naprosyn), 200–500 mg. Maximal dose for regular administration, 1000 mg/d and 1500 mg/d for short periods

Prescription NSAIDs

Diflunisal* (Dolobid), 500–1000 mg followed by 500 mg bid as needed
Meclofenamate (Ponstel, Meclomen), 250–500 mg initially, followed by 250 mg q6h up to 8 per day

Combination Medications

Acetaminophen, 250 mg/aspirin, 250 mg/caffeine, 65 mg (Excedrin Extra Strength), 2 tablets PO at the start of the attack, up to 8 per day

Muscle Relaxers†

Carisoprodol* (Soma), 350 mg PO qid prn†
Cyclobenzaprine* (Flexeril), 10 mg PO tid prn†

Combination With Barbiturates or Narcotic Analgesics

Acetaminophen, 325 mg/butalbital, 50 mg/caffeine, 40 mg (Esgic, Fioricet), 1–2 tablets q4h prn, up to 6 tablets/d†
Acetaminophen, 500 mg/butalbital, 50 mg/caffeine, 40 mg (Esgic-Plus), 1 tablet q4h prn†
Aspirin, 325 mg/butalbital, 50 mg/caffeine, 40 mg (Fiorinal, Fiormor), 1–2 tablets q4h prn, up to 6 tablets/d†
Aspirin, 325 mg/butalbital, 50 mg/caffeine, 40 mg/codeine, 30 mg (Fiorinal with Codeine), 1–2 tablets q4h prn, up to 6 tablets/d†
Acetaminophen, 325 mg/butalbital, 50 mg/caffeine, 40 mg/codeine, 30 mg (Fioricet with Codeine), 1–2 tablets q4h prn, up to 6 tablets/d†
Isometheptene mucate, 65 mg/dichloralphenazone, 100 mg/acetaminophen, 325 mg (Midrin), 1–2 capsules q4h prn, maximum of 8/d†

Preventive

*Antidepressant Medications**

Amitriptyline (Elavil, Endep),* start at 25–50 mg qhs. Maximum, 150 mg/d. May give tid
Nortriptyline (Pamelor, Aventyl),* start at 25–50 mg qhs. Maximum, 150 mg/d. May give qid
Desipramine (Norpramin),* 25–75 mg qAM as a starting dose. Maximum, 300 mg/d. May divide dose
Doxepin (Sinequan),* 25–75 mg qhs as a starting dose. Maximum, 300 mg/d. May divide dose
Fluoxetine (Prozac),* 10–80 mg/d. Usual starting dose, 20 mg qAM
Paroxetine (Paxil),* 10–50 mg/d. Usual starting dose, 20 mg PO qAM

β-Adrenergic Blockers

Propranolol (Inderal), 80 mg/d as a starting dose. Maximal dose, 240 mg/d in appropriately divided doses or a daily time release preparation
Nadolol (Corgard),* 20–40 mg/d as a starting dose. Maximal dose, 120 mg/d

Antianxiety Agent

Buspirone (BuSpar),* 7.5 mg PO bid as a starting dose. May increase by 5 mg every 3 d. Typical dose, 30 mg/d. Maximal dose, 60 mg/d

*Not FDA approved for this indication.
†Use limited because medication can be habit forming.
Abbreviations: NSAIDs = nonsteroidal anti-inflammatory drugs; OTC = over the counter; prn = as needed; tin = three times a night.

Chronic Headache

Chronic daily headaches account for 35% to 40% of patients seen at headache clinics. About 2% of adults report that they have chronic tension-type headaches every year. Although less common in primary care, these patients are therapeutic challenges. According to International Headache Society criteria, these headaches occur an average of 15 days per month or more. Most of these patients have chronic tension-type headache or transformed migraine. Most patients with transformed migraine have a history of migraine headache or some migraine features to their headache. In addition, the majority of these patients have a history of analgesic misuse. Commonly, this type of chronic headache is characterized by transient relief of the headache with analgesics, followed by rebound pain when the analgesic wears off. Patients who take analgesics at least three times a day for 5 or more days a week are prone to rebound headaches. Ergotamine (Ergostat), acetaminophen,

*Not FDA approved for this indication.

aspirin, codeine, butalbital, caffeine, and propoxyphene (Darvon) are all reported to cause rebound headache. Many of these patients also have psychiatric diagnoses such as depression, anxiety, and panic disorder.

Gradual reduction of medication may be tried as an outpatient after starting prophylactic medication such as amitriptyline (Elavil)* for chronic tension headache or divalproex sodium (Depakote) for transformed migraine. Although many medications have been used for chronic headache prophylaxis, few randomized studies have been performed. Withdrawal symptoms, including nausea, vomiting, agitation, restlessness, and sleep problems, in addition to headache, may last for 2 weeks. Headaches may take up to 6 weeks to improve and 6 months to stop. Referral to a headache specialist should be considered for patients who do not respond to gradual withdrawal. Although hospitalization is common for these patients, a study comparing outpatient and inpatient withdrawal found no difference in outcome. The long-term success rate in patients referred to headache centers is about 70%. Patients with significant associated psychiatric problems have a poorer prognosis and may benefit from a multidisciplinary approach and psychiatric referral.

Secondary Headaches

Common Secondary Headache Disorders

SINUS

Sinus headache is typically associated with respiratory symptoms and tenderness over the sinus area. Its treatment is discussed elsewhere.

TEMPOROMANDIBULAR JOINT

Symptoms of TMJ dysfunction include clicking or catching of the jaw. Patients may have pain in the joint, facial pain, ear pain, headache, or neck pain. Tenderness to palpation of the TMJ joint or joints is usual. Obvious malocclusion of the teeth or decreased range of motion of the jaw may be present. Diagnostic options include single-contrast joint arthrography, panoramic dental radiographs, magnetic resonance imaging of the joint, and diagnostic arthroscopy. Dental consultation is often helpful for differential diagnosis and treatment.

VISUAL

Headaches from refractive errors are typically associated with pain behind the eyes after reading, watching television, or using a computer screen. There is little evidence that correcting refractive errors will prevent other types of headache such as migraine.

POST-TRAUMATIC HEADACHE

Post-traumatic headaches may be intermittent or constant. The headaches may be typical of tension-type headaches or migraine headaches, but they are often mixed. Pharmacologic treatment should be based on evaluating the type of headache and treating appropriately. Trigger point injections, spray and stretch, physical therapy measures such as heat, and therapeutic exercises may be used to alleviate musculoskeletal pain.

MEDICATION

In studies at headache centers, 4 to 5% of patients have drug-induced headache. As discussed earlier, overuse of analgesics may also produce an analgesic withdrawal headache. In addition, drugs may produce headaches as a side effect, from withdrawal, or by iatrogenically causing a condition that has headache as a symptom.

Nitroglycerin is an example of a drug that commonly causes headache as a side effect. Selected drug classes that cause headache as a side effect are listed in Table 8. Ironically, some medications used to treat headaches such as calcium channel blockers may also cause them as a side effect. To rule out medication-induced headache, both prescription and nonprescription drugs should be reviewed.

The most common drug withdrawal headache probably produced by stopping caffeine use. Caffeine withdrawal is often manifested as a weekend headache that occurs because the patient does not drink caffeine. Idiopathic intracranial hypertension is an example of a disease associated with headache that may be caused by medication.

Potentially Serious Causes

MENINGITIS

Meningitis is a life-threatening cause of headache. However, the symptoms of headache and nausea by themselves are too common to help with the diagnosis. If no fever, stiff neck, or altered mental status is present, meningitis is virtually ruled out. The Kernig and Brudzinski signs have a low sensitivity, but high specificity for meningitis. Jolt accentuation of head pain is another useful sign with a reported sensitivity of 100% and a specificity of 54%. Lumbar puncture is necessary to definitively rule out the disease.

TABLE 8. **Selected Drug Classes That May Cause Headache as a Side Effect**

ACE inhibitors and antagonists, e.g., captopril (Capoten), losartan (Cozaar)
α-Adrenergic blockers, e.g., prazosin (Minipress)
Antibiotics, e.g., trimethoprim (Trimpex), sulfamethoxazole (Gantanol), metronidazole (Flagyl)
Calcium channel blockers, e.g., nifedipine (Adalat)
Central antihypertensive agents, e.g., methyldopa (Aldomet)
H_2 blockers, e.g., ranitidine (Zantac)
Hormonal agents, e.g., combined oral contraceptives
Nitrates, e.g., isosorbide dinitrate (Isordil)
NSAIDs, including COX-2 inhibitors, e.g., naproxen (Naprosyn), celecoxib (Celebrex)

Abbreviations: ACE = angiotensin-converting enzyme; COX-2 = cyclooxygenase-2; NSAIDs = nonsteroidal anti-inflammatory drugs.

*Not FDA approved for this indication.

SUBARACHNOID HEMORRHAGE

About 80% of patients with subarachnoid hemorrhage have ruptured saccular aneurysms. A thunderclap headache is a clue to the diagnosis. This type of headache has a sudden onset within minutes and lasts hours to days. The headache may originate in any location. Associated nausea, vomiting, or a stiff neck may be encountered. The lack of exertion during onset of the headache does not rule out subarachnoid hemorrhage. Patients with suspected subarachnoid hemorrhage should have a CT scan for initial evaluation. CT scanning is about 98% sensitive within the first 12 hours and 93% sensitive during the next 12 hours, with sensitivity dropping to about 50% by 1 week. If the CT scan is negative, a lumbar puncture should be performed to look for bloody fluid. In selected cases, angiography may be necessary to make the diagnosis.

BRAIN TUMOR

Although a common concern of patients, brain tumors are infrequent in headache patients with no abnormal findings on neurologic examination. Only about half of patients with brain tumors have headaches. The pain is typically bilateral, similar to a tension-type headache that is worse on one side. In 32% of patients the pain is worse when bending over, and concomitant nausea and vomiting are seen in 40% of patients. The findings are similar in patients with primary brain tumors and metastatic disease.

PSEUDOTUMOR CEREBRI (IDIOPATHIC INTRACRANIAL HYPERTENSION)

This condition primarily occurs in obese women between the ages of 20 and 44. The headache is typically generalized. Clues to the diagnosis are transient visual loss that may occur many times a day and papilledema on opthalmoscopic examination. Medication, including tetracycline, minocycline, and isotretinoin, may contribute to or cause this condition. A high spinal fluid pressure is noted on lumbar puncture. Treatment with diuretics such as acetazolamide (Diamox)* is often used to lower cerebrospinal pressure. Surgery is indicated for severe cases.

TEMPORAL ARTERITIS

Temporal arteritis occurs at an average age of 70 years and is rare before the age of 50. The headache from temporal arteritis usually has a gradual onset in the temporal area. Clues to the diagnosis are tenderness over the temporal artery and palpable thickening of this artery. The sedimentation rate is nearly always high. The diagnosis requires temporal artery biopsy for confirmation. Steroids are the treatment of choice.

*Not FDA approved for this indication.

TABLE 9. **Acute Headache Treatment**

Migraine
Sumatriptan (Imitrex), 6 mg SC. May give a second dose in 1 h. Maximal dose, 12 mg/d. Do not combine with DHE
DHE, 1 mg initially SC, IM, or IV. May repeat hourly up to 3 mg/attack and 6 mg/wk. Do not combine with the triptan medication within 24 h
An antiemetic such as metoclopramide or prochlorperazine is usually given beforehand
Dexamethasone, 16 mg IM or IV only once every 3 wk. May also be combined with an antiemetic
Migraine or Tension-Type Headache
Ketorolac (Toradol), 60 mg IM or IV initially, 30 mg for repeat doses. Maximum, 120 mg/d. Use for no more than 5 d total
Prochlorperazine (Compazine),* 10 mg IV or IM with a maximal dose of 40 mg/d; 25-mg rectal suppository with a maximum of 50 mg/d
Metoclopramide (Reglan),* 10 mg IV or IM qid prn
Chlorpromazine (Thorazine),* 25 mg IM or IV q4h prn

*Not FDA approved for this indication.
Abbreviations: DHE = dihydroergotamine; prn = as needed.

EXERTIONAL HEADACHE

Coughing, exercise, or sexual activity may precipitate headache. Although many of these cases are benign, analysis of 72 patients found that 42% had intracranial lesions. Chiari type I malformation was the most common cause of cough headache, and subarachnoid hemorrhage was the most common cause of exertional headache.

ACUTE HEADACHE TREATMENT

Many patients will come to the physician's office, prompt care, or the emergency room with an acute headache. For patients with an acute headache, it is important to evaluate the patient to diagnose the type of headache and rule out serious causes of headache. Treatment of vascular and nonvascular headache is listed in Table 9.

Headache is a common and challenging diagnosis, with the history being the most important part of the evaluation. Serious causes need to be ruled out, and treatment should be specific to the patient's diagnosis.

REFERENCE

1. Headache Classification Committee of the International Headache Society: Classification and diagnostic criteria for headache disorders, cranial neuralgia, and facial pain. Cephalalgia 8(Suppl 7):1–96, 1988.

EPISODIC VERTIGO

method of
JOHN G. OAS, M.D.
Cleveland Clinic Foundation
Cleveland, Ohio

Treatment of patients with vestibular disorders causing episodic vertigo has greatly improved with recent advances in both diagnostic testing and treatment protocols. With highly effective treatments now available, it is critical for the clinician to gather specific clues regarding the cause of the disorder at its onset. It is now as unacceptable to render the diagnosis of "vertigo" as a specific medical condition as it is to prescribe symptomatic antivertigo medications for its treatment. Vertigo is a symptom too unreliable by itself to identify the source. For example, vertigo is often not reported by patients during vestibular testing (despite robust nystagmus) and in conditions expected to cause vertigo (benign paroxysmal positional vertigo [BPPV]). Examples of other symptoms reported in vestibular disorders are many (Table 1). These symptoms are also reported in other medical conditions ranging from the side effect of a newly added medication to the prodromal symptom of life-threatening cardiovascular or cerebrovascular disease. Although the differential diagnosis is challenging, correct identification and successful treatment outcome are rewarding.

Despite the diagnostic imprecision of descriptions of vertigo, the history still remains the most critical area of patient assessment. Details concerning episodes of vertigo are most critical, with careful scrutiny given to how random or provoked the episodes are, the precise duration of episodes, the exact episode frequency, and the temporal characteristics of the episodes with other symptoms. Recording these details early in the course of the illness, even when the importance is not immediately obvious, may be critical later when symptoms of concomitant conditions can obscure details of past symptoms. Episodic vertigo is commonly accompanied by the unpleasant vegetative symptoms of motion sickness. A history of childhood motion sickness is important because it often defines the severity of these symptoms in vestibular disorders. Episodic vertigo is nearly always accompanied by the disturbing psychological symptoms of anxiety. A predisposition to anxiety symptoms may well define the extent to which episodic vertigo is accompanied by these symptoms. The presence or absence of hearing symptoms helps identify an otogenic source of episodic vertigo. Meniere's original description of the syndrome, which bears his name today, required hearing loss to distinguish it from migraine. Any abrupt onset of unilateral, fluctuating, or rapidly progressive hearing loss or tinnitus should be noted as distinct from slowly progressive bilateral hearing loss or tinnitus. Specific historical details matching the clinical features of the vestibular disorders causing episodic vertigo are discussed here.

TABLE 1. **Symptoms Other Than Vertigo Reported in Vestibular Disorders**

Spinning	Dizzy
Lightheaded	Giddy
Whirling	Veering
Turning	Imbalanced
Head tilting	Tumbling
Rocking	Moving
Sinking	Floating

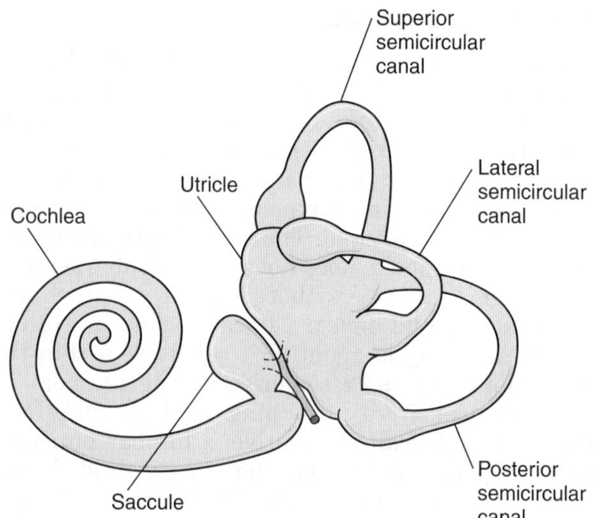

Figure 1. Endolymphatic anatomy of the inner ear. The vestibular labyrinth includes five structures: the saccule, utricle, superior semicircular canal, posterior semicircular canal, and lateral semicircular canal.

The vestibular system is a special sense distinct from the five classic senses. It functions as an autopilot to maintain upright balance against gravity, clear vision with head movement, and three-dimensional orientation. The vestibular system uses a pair of highly specialized sensory organs known as the vestibular labyrinth (Figure 1). The otolith organs, the saccule and utricle, sense head orientation in reference to the upright position (parallel to gravity), as well as tangential forces caused by head movement. They have a unique ultrastructural composition of thousands of microscopic stones (otoconia) that appear to form in a continuous process of mineralization and demineralization. A disturbance in this metabolism is an important step in the pathogenesis of BPPV. The semicircular canals sense head movement in three planes, yet by their anatomic design are incapable of sensing gravity. Upper cervical spine proprioceptive sensory input is used by the vestibular system to provide biomechanical information about head orientation relative to the body. Vision is used by the vestibular system to both enhance (optokinetic) and inhibit (pursuit) other vestibular sensory input. Central vestibular pathways link this otologic, proprioceptive, and visual sensory input via reflexes to control eye, head, and body stabilization. The vestibular system also connects directly to the autonomic nervous system, which controls both sympathetic and parasympathetic tone. Finally, the vestibular system combines this input with other sensory information to provide a cognitive sense of spatial orientation. Thus, pathologic processes affecting the vestibular system have considerable impact (Table 2). Perhaps because the vestibular sense is so critical for species survival, the vestibular system has an unusual neural plasticity. As long as these critical neural pathways are not disturbed, recovery from any acute vestibular disturbance will occur with time. Therefore, treatment of vestibular disorders causing episodic vertigo must be designed to limit the extent of damage to the system acutely while augmenting and facilitating adaptation in the long term.

Narrowing the differential diagnosis of vestibular disorders causing episodic vertigo often requires a careful proc-

TABLE 2. **The Effects of Vestibular System Dysfunction**

Vestibular Function	Consequence of Vestibular Disorder
Eye stabilization	Blurred vision, vertigo, oscillopsia, nystagmus, diplopia
Head stabilization	Head tilt, torticollis, cervicogenic headache
Body stabilization	Imbalance, veering, falls, ataxia, slowed gait
Parasympathetic tone	Diaphoresis, nausea, vomiting, diarrhea, vasovagal responses, motion sickness
Sympathetic tone	Tachycardia, anxiety
Spatial orientation	Disorientation, confusion distinguishing self from environmental movement

ess of inclusion or exclusion to differentiate the clinical features of an otogenic source from neurogenic, cervicogenic, cardiogenic, or psychogenic sources. Such differentiation is particularly important in chronic cases in which more than one source may be involved. What follows are the salient clinical features of the most common vestibular disorders encountered in a primary care setting, along with advanced treatment protocols used at the most specialized tertiary care clinics.

BENIGN PAROXYSMAL POSITIONAL VERTIGO

Clinical Features

BPPV is the most common single cause of recurrent otogenic vertigo, with an incidence of 6000 per million in those whose illness persists for more than 30 days. The majority of patients with recurrent episodes report that most of their previous bouts resolved within a couple of weeks, so this 30-day incidence greatly underestimates the true prevalence. Because the incidence and prevalence of this disorder increase with age, a near pandemic is anticipated as the mean age of the U.S. population increases. Curative treatment can be rendered in over 90% of cases with a simple 5-minute office procedure. Recurrence months to years later is the rule rather than the exception, yet no practical means of prevention exists. The differential diagnosis of episodic vertigo requires exclusion of this common, benign, and self-limited otogenic disorder *before* resorting to an expensive workup or costly hospitalization.

The pathogenesis of BPPV requires a disruption in otolith metabolism that allows for the accumulation of otoconia within the utricular sac, a pathologic condition termed *utriculolithiasis*. Because the utricle is also where the three semicircular canals originate, these freed otoconia under the influence of gravity move into the semicircular canals, usually while the patient sleeps. Anatomy again defines those places in the semicircular canals most vulnerable to this entrapment process. Once trapped, gravity causes their movement to stimulate the semicircular canal and induce positional vertigo in a pathologic state defined by the term *canalolithiasis*. Treatment is designed to reverse this process and place the otoconia back into the utricle. Utriculolithiasis resolves when the patient is kept in the upright position long enough (usually 48 hours) for the otoconia to be completely resorbed.

Diagnosis

A history of acute vertigo on awakening from bed is typical, followed by brief vestibular symptoms provoked by head position changes. The side involved can often be identified by the patient as the side most provocative of symptoms while recumbent. Concurrent otologic signs or symptoms indicate BPPV as a consequence of otologic disease. The most common cause is idiopathic, especially in those older than 65 years. Other causes include recent or remote head trauma, prolonged bed rest or extended periods of anesthesia, and pre-existing otogenic vestibular disorders (vestibular neuronitis, neurolabyrinthitis, Meniere disease). BPPV can occur without vertigo as a symptom, especially in the elderly, who figure that a few extra minutes spent dangling their feet at their bedside is just part of getting older. This observation is particularly haunting from a public health perspective inasmuch as vestibular disorders present clear risks for a hip fracture, a condition associated with 30% 1-year mortality in the elderly.

BPPV is confirmed when canalolithiasis can be demonstrated by a positive Dix-Hallpike positioning test (DHT) of the involved ear. Although the DHT can be performed safely and effectively at the bedside in most cases by clinicians with sufficient training, referral to a standardized vestibular test laboratory that uses videonystagmographic techniques is advised in all other situations. A positive DHT for BPPV requires provocation of the classic paroxysmal mixed vertical and torsional nystagmus in the head-hanging position of the involved side. A positive DHT made on the basis of the paroxysmal vertigo alone is discouraged because a host of other vestibular disorders can be expressed in this manner. Rarely, a malignant form of positional vertigo mistaken as BPPV results from a posterior fossa neoplasm, stroke, or multiple sclerosis. False-negative tests are also common in BPPV because a positive test documents only canalolithiasis and not utriculolithiasis, despite the role of the latter in BPPV described earlier.

Treatment

As with any acute vertigo, acute management of the accompanying unpleasant autonomic and disturbing anxiety symptoms with medications that provide antivertigo, antiemetic, and anxiolytic effects is often necessary to prevent the systemic complications that result from emesis and excessive sympathetic stimulation. The choice of agent and route administered should be carefully tailored to the patient's medical status (Table 3). Sublingual lorazepam* (Ativan) is helpful to reduce the intensity of vertigo in cases in which it causes vomiting. BPPV treatment protocols are collectively called particle-repositioning therapy (PRT). Techniques have evolved from evidence-based studies that have demonstrated their efficacy over the past two decades. All are useful but vary in their efficacy and complexity. Regardless of technique, PRT must be followed by a 48-hour period in which the patient remains upright without exception, including during sleep. Because body position cannot be regulated during sleep, the patient must sleep in a chair with provision made to support the neck and elevate the feet. Deviations from this strict requirement risk recurrence of BPPV

*Not FDA approved for this indication.

TABLE 3. **Medications Useful in the Management of Vertigo**

Medication	Indication	Duration of Use
Meclizine (Antivert), 12.5–50 mg PO q6h	Vertigo	>5 min but <72 h
Dimenhydrinate (Dramamine), 50 mg PO q4–6h, 100 mg pr q12h	Vertigo	>5 min but <72 h
Lorazepam* (Ativan), 0.5–1.0 mg sublingually q4h†	Vertigo*	>5 min but <8 h
Lorazepam (Ativan), 0.5–2 mg/IM/IV q4h	Anxiety	>24 h but <72 h
Diazepam (Valium), 2–10 mg PO/IV/IM q6–8h	Anxiety	>24 h but <72 h
Droperidol* (Inapsine), 2.5–5 mg IV/IM q3–4h	Nausea/vomiting	>24 h but <72 h
Promethazine (Phenergan), 12.5–25 mg PO/pr/IV/IM q4–6h	Nausea/vomiting	>24 h but <72 h
Prochlorperazine (Compazine), 5–10 mg PO/pr/IV/IM q6–8h	Nausea/vomiting	>24 h but <72 h
Prochlorperazine (Compazine Spansule), 10 mg PO q12h	Nausea/vomiting	>24 h but <10 d
Scopalamine patch (transderm Scōp), 0.5 mg/24 h q3d	Motion sickness	>24 h but <10 d

*Not FDA approved for this indication.
†Generic formulations are not tolerated for this use.
Abbreviation: pr = per rectum.

soon after PRT because of incomplete clearance of the original otoconia. The few cases that do require extended post-PRT upright periods (4 to 7 days) to resolve the utriculolithiasis demonstrate this point.

The Brandt-Daroff PRT technique (1980) requires the following positional exercise sequences repeated up to 10 times each session performed two or three times daily until the positional vertigo ceases. Starting from a sitting position with feet dangling at the edge of a bed, the patient first performs a controlled fall to a lateral decubitus position onto a pillow with the involved side down and holds the position for 2 minutes. This step is followed by a return to the sitting position without stopping, with another controlled fall to the lateral decubitus position onto another pillow with the opposite side down and holding that position for 2 minutes. The cycle is completed by a slow return to the sitting position with the chin tucked down on the chest. Although not a provision in the original studies, remaining in the upright position is now advised each day of treatment, with the patient instructed to remain upright for another 48 hours after the procedure no longer causes positional vertigo in the initial position of the first cycle.

The Sémont PRT technique (1988) requires a modification of the Brandt-Daroff technique and is done by the clinician at the time of the visit. The patient's head is held by the clinician and turned 45 degrees away from the involved ear, and this position is maintained throughout each cycle. This maneuver causes the initial position to be roughly the same head positioning as the DHT, with the second and final positions similar to those used in other PRT techniques. Cycles are repeated until paroxysmal nystagmus is no longer seen in the primary position. This technique ensures higher velocity than patients can achieve on their own but must be done very carefully in the frail elderly and anxious.

The Epley PRT technique (1992) requires both premedication and the use of continuous vibration from a vibrating massager applied to the mastoid bone of the involved ear. Like the Sémont technique, the initial stage is identical to that of the DHT. The next two stages are defined by head and body rotations away from this initial DHT position at 90- and 180-degree intervals opposite the involved ear. The last two stages are a return to a chin-tucked sitting and then the upright sitting position. The patient is held in each stage for a duration equal to twice the duration of the initial paroxysmal nystagmus. Cycles are repeated until the paroxysmal torsional nystagmus is no longer seen or until five to six cycles have been reached. After a 48-hour period of remaining upright, the patient returns to normal activities, including sleep. The patient is seen weekly until the positional vertigo resolves.

The PRT technique used in my tertiary center BPPV clinic requires direct observation of the positioning nystagmus with the same real-time digital videonystagmography used in the vestibular laboratory. A three-segment physiotherapy treatment table allows for comfortable positioning of the patient. Care is taken to avoid neck strain, motion sickness, and anxiety. Vibration is not used. One minute after a positive DHT (initial stage), the patient is rolled 90 degrees away from the initial DHT position with the head hanging down 45 degrees from supine (prepenultimate stage). One minute later, the patient is rolled another 90 degrees with the head hanging down 45 degrees from the prone position (penultimate stage). One additional minute later, the patient is moved from the lateral decubitus position to a sitting chin-tucked position (final stage). PRT success is demonstrated by a repeat DHT followed by another cycle of PRT before the patient leaves the procedure room. PRT failure is demonstrated by a persistent positive DHT and is often predicted by reversal of the paroxysmal nystagmus in the penultimate stage of PRT. Because these patients probably represent cases in which otoconia are trapped in the short arm of the semicircular canal, they are given specific instructions for a home-based treatment protocol designed to reposition these otoconia back in the utricle and told to return in 1 week for reassessment and additional PRT. Patients who report positional vertigo within a week before their visit and who have a negative DHT at the time of their visit are not treated with PRT but are still required to remain upright for a 48-hour period after their visit. This protocol has enjoyed a nearly 99% success rate since its implementation. Surgery to plug the posterior semicircular canal is offered to the remaining 1%

who still have a positive DHT when PRT attempts fail over a 1-year period. Outcome in these few cases is satisfactory, but not as favorable as the outcome after PRT, which leaves semicircular canal function undisturbed.

Interested clinicians are advised to complete graduate or postgraduate instruction in these techniques of testing and bedside treatment of BPPV. Such training will become increasingly more critical as the prevalence of this disorder in our elderly increases.

ACUTE VESTIBULAR LOSS

Clinical Features

The acute loss of vestibular function results in a biphasic illness characterized initially by an abrupt onset of vestibular symptoms most intense at onset or within several hours thereafter. Continuous vertigo that intensifies with any head movement and in all recumbent positions is accompanied by nausea and vomiting, even in those without pre-existing motion sickness. Nystagmus can be easily observed during the initial phase and usually has a mixture of torsional and horizontal components. The resulting gait ataxia spares the limbs and is generally accompanied by veering to the side opposite the loss (bilateral losses from aminoglycoside ototoxicity are an exception). Vestibular symptoms gradually improve over a period of several weeks but never completely resolve. This second phase of the illness is characterized by much milder vestibular symptoms that are never spontaneous, including oscillopsia in response to head movement and gait ataxia when visual cues are lacking. The intensity of symptoms in this phase of the illness depends on the severity of the loss and the extent to which the brain is able to adapt to these losses through alternative vestibular pathways.

The differential diagnosis of disorders causing acute peripheral vestibular loss is presented in Table 4. Vestibular neuronitis is differentiated from neurolabyrinthitis by the absence of ipsilateral hearing loss. Both are presumed to be viral in origin, although the latter generally results in more severe loss. Vestibular neuronitis can recur and usually results in progressively greater loss with each recurrence. Multiple sclerosis lesions can also result in acute vestibular loss as a result of demyelination at the vestibular root entry zone. Usually, the diagnosis of multiple sclerosis has already been made, but it is important to document the vestibular loss as a new exacerbation in cases in which doing so may change the course of its management. Although the vestibular loss after certain neuro-otologic procedures (vestibular nerve section, labyrinthectomy, or transtympanic aminoglycoside administration) is never in question, the treatment required to manage the results of these procedures is identical. Both aminoglycoside ototoxicity and autoimmune ear disease result in bilateral loss. Symptoms are milder in the initial phase and are more severe in the second phase than is the case with other causes. Aminoglycoside ototoxicity occurs idiosyncratically after weeks of treatment and is related to a total cumulative toxic dose effect rather than toxic serum levels. Usually it is too late by the time that the initial symptoms develop to rescue much vestibular function, although up to 10% of patients can recover some function within 6 months of onset. With more research it is hoped that those at risk can be identified prospectively. Autoimmune ear disease is caused by the effects of direct immunologic destruction of the inner ear organs. Its most common form is limited to the ear and results in subacute progressive bilateral hearing and vestibular loss Autoimmune ear disease can also be part of other immune disorders such as Cogan's syndrome, relapsing polychondritis, and polyarteritis nodosum. The diagnosis of acute bacterial labyrinthitis is often made after a careful search for the source of acute bacterial meningitis reveals otitis media or cholesteatoma and the patient regains consciousness with vestibular symptoms. Labyrinthine concussion is diagnosed when head trauma is closely followed by vestibular symptoms without accompanying hearing loss and confirmed by vestibular testing. This condition must be differentiated from post-traumatic BPPV and post-traumatic perilymphatic fistula, which is diagnosed by noting stepwise progressive hearing and vestibular loss and only confirmed by arrest of this progression with bed rest or fistula surgery. Thrombosis of the anterior inferior cerebellar artery results in a syndrome of acute unilateral vestibular and hearing loss coupled with ipsilateral brainstem dysfunction because the inner ear receives its sole blood supply from the vertebrobasilar system.

TABLE 4. **Causes of Acute Vestibular Loss**

Vestibular neuronitis
Neurolabyrinthitis
Multiple sclerosis
Neuro-otologic procedures
Aminoglycoside ototoxicity
Autoimmune ear disease
Acute bacterial labyrinthitis
Labyrinthine concussion
Perilymphatic fistula
Thrombosis of the anterior inferior cerebellar artery

Diagnosis

Although not required in all cases, clinical tests of hearing function (basic audiogram, otoacoustic emissions, electrocochleography, and auditory evoked responses) and vestibular function (basic electronystagmogram, rotational chair testing) are helpful to localize the site and extent of the loss when the differential diagnosis is not obvious, bilateral losses are suspected, or phase 2 of the illness is marked by persistent, bothersome vestibular symptoms. Serial audiograms are necessary to document the progressive hearing loss of autoimmune ear disease or stepwise hearing loss. Varicella zoster and herpes simplex titers are seldom helpful in vestibular neuritis and viral neurolabyrinthitis. The leukocyte transformation test to detect inner ear antigens can be helpful in cases of suspected autoimmune ear disease. Computed tomography of the temporal bones and cerebrospinal fluid studies are required tests in acute bacterial labyrinthitis. Magnetic resonance imaging (MRI) of the brain or magnetic resonance angiography (MRA) of the vertebrobasilar arteries can be helpful when multiple sclerosis or anterior inferior cerebellar artery thrombosis is suspected.

Treatment

As with any acute vertigo, management of the first phase of the illness requires aggressive treatment of the constitutional symptoms with medications that provide antivertigo, antiemetic, and anxiolytic effects and careful selection of the dosage and route of administration (see Table 3). Acute treatment should include recommendations to minimize head movement until the nausea subsides. Acute management of vestibular neuronitis and labyrinthitis should include the combination of an antiviral agent (valacyclovir [Valtrex],* 1000 mg orally three times daily or acyclovir [Zovirax],* 800 mg orally five times daily for 7 to 10 days) with a course of corticosteroids (prednisone [Deltasone], 60 mg/d orally, or methylprednisolone [Medrol] 48 mg/d orally as a starting dose tapered over 10 days). If multiple sclerosis is suspected, prompt neurologic referral regarding treatment of the exacerbation is advised. Autoimmune ear disease is managed acutely with prednisone (Deltasone), 60 mg/d orally, or methylprednisolone (Medrol), 48 mg/d orally for 30 days, with referral to a tertiary care otologist or rheumatologist for long-term management of this rare condition. Similarly, prompt referral to a tertiary care otologist is advised in cases of suspected post-traumatic perilymphatic fistula. Hospitalization and stroke protocols should be implemented in cases of suspected anterior inferior cerebellar artery infarction.

Management of the second phase of the illness involves gradual tapering of all antivertigo, antiemetic, and anxiolytic medications used in the first phase of the illness within 3 weeks of the onset of the illness. These medications can significantly impair central adaptation to vestibular loss. The patient should be advised to gradually and progressively increase physical activity to foster central vestibular adaptation. The development of neck pain during this period may indicate significant biomechanical compromise of the upper cervical spine as a result of activation of the vestibulocollic reflexes. Such pain should prompt referral for neck physiotherapy evaluation and treatment consisting of soft tissue and joint mobilization techniques to restore normal cervical spine function. Referral to a physical therapist with special training in vestibular rehabilitation should be made in cases in which the risk of falls and other safety issues are significant, when patients fail to advance their own level of physical activity beyond sedentary levels, and in all cases in which bilateral vestibular loss is documented. Physical therapy has proven efficacy in restoring agility and reducing the risk of falls in patients with vestibular loss.

*Not FDA approved for this indication.

MENIERE DISEASE

See the article "Meniere Disease."

VERTEBROBASILAR INSUFFICIENCY

Clinical Features

The inner ear receives all of its arterial supply from the vertebrobasilar system. A transient drop in mean basilar artery pressure can produce watershed ischemia in either labyrinth and thereby result in brief episodes of vertigo. Watershed ischemia can also occur in the lateral pontomedullary areas, affecting central vestibular structures as well. Vascular disease leading to stenosis in the proximal anterior inferior cerebellar artery or posterior inferior cerebellar artery can lead to ischemia affecting the vestibular labyrinth, vestibular nerve, vestibular nucleus, or vestibulocerebellum. Small-vessel disease can affect the arterial supply of the vestibular nerve, as well as the lateral pontomedullary areas critical for function of the vestibular system. Determining the source of the transient ischemia can be difficult because such ischemia provides few cues. The vestibular disturbance is varied in description but always starts abruptly and has a duration of less than 5 minutes. Most ominous is an escalating frequency or increasing duration of these episodes, which implies impending infarction.

Diagnosis

MRI/MRA of the brain and cerebrovascular arteries and their origins should be performed in cases in which vertebrobasilar ischemia is suspected. Selective vertebral angiography should be considered only in those in whom MRI/MRA fails to provide clear treatment guidance.

Treatment

Anticoagulant and antiplatelet medications are the mainstay of treatment in vertebrobasilar cerebrovascular disease. Low-dose buffered aspirin (82 to 325 mg/d orally) is sufficient in most cases when a crescendo pattern of event frequency is not a concern. Referral to a tertiary care stroke service is advised should low-dose aspirin therapy fail or MRA indicate a hemodynamically critical vertebral artery stenosis potentially amenable to endovascular therapy.

MIGRAINE

Clinical Features

Migraine is now recognized as an inherited neuronal calcium channelopathy. Transient visual disturbances have been recognized for centuries as migraine events even without close temporal association with migraine-type headaches. The pathogenesis of isolated vestibular events in migraine remains obscure but is probably similar to that of other transient neurologic events in migraine, including hemiplegia, visual aura, and hemicranial headache. Few features of the isolated episodic vestibular symptoms in migraine can differentiate it from other vestibular syndromes. Certainly, episodes punctuated by a typical migraine headache more than 50% of the time or an increase in the frequency of other migraine phenomena coincident with the development of episodic vestibular symptoms supports the diagnosis. It is the exception rather than the rule that the vestibular symptoms occur within a full-blown sequence of events described by the International Headache Society criteria for basilar migraine. The absence of fluctuating hearing loss or tinnitus distinguishes vertigo attacks in migraine from Meniere disease.

Diagnosis

The diagnosis of migraine as the source of episodic vertigo requires the exclusion of hearing loss typical of Meniere disease. Audiometric studies (basic audiogram, otoacoustic emissions, electrocochleography, and auditory evoked responses) are particularly helpful here. MRI/MRA of the brain is only helpful to exclude brain disorders or cerebrovascular disease. Vestibular tests that show mild central vestibular dysfunction are promising yet not proven as a technique to differentiate migraine from other vestibular disorders.

Treatment

Treatment of migraine includes lifestyle modifications consisting of improved diet, exercise, and sleep hygiene and the correction of endocrine or metabolic dysfunction. When these measures fail, migraine prophylaxis is advised. A 3-month trial of a medication with proven efficacy in migraine headache prevention (sodium valproate [Depakote delayed-release tablets], 1000 mg at bedtime; fluoxetine [Prozac],* 20 mg/d; propranolol [Inderal], 60 to 320 mg daily in divided doses; amitriptyline [Elavil],* 75 mg at bedtime; and verapamil [Calan],* 80 to 120 mg three times daily) should be tried along with an event diary to document efficacy.

CERVICOGENIC DIZZINESS

Clinical Features

Cervicogenic dizziness occurs because of altered upper cervical proprioception and not as a consequence of vertebrobasilar ischemia caused by vertebral artery occlusion. Proprioceptive afferents from joint and muscle spindles of the three uppermost cervical spine segments project directly to the vestibular nucleus. The upper two cervical vertebrae have no intervertebral disks and are held together by a complex set of muscles innervated by upper cervical motoneurons that receive dense vestibular projections from the vestibulospinal tract to form the vestibulocollic reflexes. This arrangement provides for considerable feedback to ensure head and neck stabilization during ambulation. Cervico-ocular reflexes dominate in very young children and disappear as the vestibulo-ocular time constant lengthens in early childhood, thus making it difficult to assess with vestibular testing. These vestigial reflexes become manifested when the vestibular system struggles to accommodate BPPV and compensate for otogenic losses.

Diagnosis

Cervicogenic dizziness is difficult to differentiate from the symptoms of uncompensated otogenic loss. A history of previous neck strain or relentless unilateral head pain provides important clues. Association with the clinical features of a cervicogenic headache is helpful. The diurnal pattern of the dizziness is also helpful in that it worsens as the day goes on, which is opposite the maturational onset of dizziness in uncompensated otogenic loss. Examination of the cervical spine often shows asymmetry in range of movement and isometric strength with unilateral myofascial trigger points. Nystagmus provoked at one extreme of neck torsion or provoked by vibration applied to one side of the neck can be the only abnormality noted on vestibular testing. This entity will remain controversial until more is known.

Treatment

Successful treatment of cervicogenic dizziness requires expert neck physiotherapy. Physical therapy techniques include manual therapy consisting of gentle segmental mobilization to restore normal upper cervical biomechanics. At the same time, exercises are needed to strengthen the neck and maintain normal posture. Close cooperation between the physical therapist and clinician is necessary throughout treatment.

MENIERE'S DISEASE

method of
BRUCE JAY GANTZ, M.D., and
RAVI N. SAMY, M.D.
University of Iowa
Iowa City, Iowa

Meniere's disease was initially described by Prosper Meniere in 1861. It is an inner ear disorder that involves both the cochlear and vestibular labyrinths and encompasses a

*Not FDA approved for this indication.

specific complex of symptoms. These symptoms are secondary to endolymphatic hydrops, which is manifested as excess fluid and pressure. The classic form of the disease consists of four symptoms in the affected ear:

1. Episodes of fluctuating hearing loss, particularly in the low frequencies
2. Recurrent, spontaneous episodes of vertigo
3. Roaring or buzzing tinnitus
4. Aural fullness

However, variations of the classic form may occur and are termed *cochlear* or *vestibular Meniere's disease.* These variants tend to evolve into a classic Meniere's pattern with time. Although some have stated that bilateral disease occurs in up to 50% of patients, in our series at the University of Iowa, only 2% of patients displayed bilateral symptoms while being followed up to 15 years. This suggests that in some studies, the patients may have incorrectly been diagnosed with Meniere's disease.

The incidence and prevalence of the disease varies among countries, with a prevalence in the United States of approximately 15:100,000. Over 100,000 Americans suffer from this disease each year. It is unknown to what extent geographic, genetic, environmental, and diagnostic factors play a role in the diagnosis and pathogenesis of the disease.

The symptoms are explained by fluctuating pressure and volume relationships in the endolymphatic system of the inner ear. Accumulation of endolymph causes distortion of the membranous labyrinth, breaking of the membrane, changes in pressure, and changes in the electrolyte composition of the fluid. Proposed etiologies include immune, allergic, vascular, infectious, and anatomic abnormalities. Yet in two thirds of patients, a cause is never discovered. However, the final common pathway is that of endolymphatic hydrops.

DIAGNOSIS

Although Meniere's disease was initially described in 1861, since then, temporal bone histopathologic examinations and clinical studies have helped to elucidate the pathophysiology of the process. In 1972, the American Academy of Ophthalmology and Otolaryngology provided official guidelines for diagnosis of the disease. The definition and diagnosis have since been refined.

As with all types of dizziness, a thorough history forms the most important part of the evaluation. Subjective historical information usually provides more information regarding the diagnosis of the disease than does objective laboratory testing or radiologic imaging. If the true diagnosis is not initially evident, serial observation and audiograms will eventually reveal the diagnosis. The diagnosis requires documentation of the symptoms over time with objective evidence that hearing is fluctuating.

The vertiginous spells, the most distressing feature of this disease, are not caused by motion or position changes but may be exacerbated by them. The dizziness is usually described as rotatory but may also include a sense of imbalance. The vertigo may be accompanied by nausea and vomiting. In severe episodes, vagal symptoms may occur, including pallor, sweating, and rarely, bradycardia. These may contribute to drop attacks, termed *crisis of Tumarkin.* These are spontaneous, unprovoked spells of falling to the ground without a loss of consciousness. These rare occurrences are also related to aberrant discharges down the spinal motor neural tracts.

Following resolution of the vertiginous spells, the patients have no long-term balance dysfunction. In addition, long remissions between episodes are common. The attacks of spontaneous, rotational vertigo last 20 minutes to 24 hours and are prostrating. However, the frequency and duration of episodes are variable. Episodes that last just a few seconds or minutes or days is not caused by Meniere's disease. Some patients are able to detect the onset of an attack by noticing that their tinnitus and aural fullness are increasing. The hearing loss and episodes of vertigo may or may not occur in tandem, but the hearing usually worsens as the tinnitus and aural fullness increase. Early in the disease process, after a spell of vertigo, it is common for hearing to improve, tinnitus to decrease, and aural fullness to resolve.

The physical examination is unremarkable in patients with Meniere's disease. However, a thorough head and neck examination is required to rule out other causes of dizziness. Horizontal or horizontal rotatory nystagmus is present on physical examination during acute attacks. Otologic testing reveals a normal outer and middle ear examination and normal Weber and Rinne tuning fork examination. Pneumatic otoscopy using both positive and negative pressure is useful to determine if dizziness or nystagmus is induced. If so, another cause for the dizziness is sought. The neurologic examination reveals no cranial nerve or cerebellar function abnormalities.

Laboratory tests are unrewarding, and most are used primarily for research purposes. However, the minimal baseline tests include an audiogram and an electronystagmogram. Caloric tests provide an excellent demonstration of a peripheral vestibular disorder and serve as a reference against which patients can compare their symptoms. Many patients with Meniere's disease have symmetric caloric responses and an otherwise normal electronystagmogram until late in the disease. Their positional tests are normal, and there is no evidence of spontaneous or latent nystagmus. Imaging studies, such as magnetic resonance imaging, are obtained only if symptoms warrant further evaluation.

Audiometric investigation includes an audiogram with pure-tone and speech discrimination tests and acoustic reflex decay. A low-frequency sensorineural hearing loss is present in early stages on the audiogram, but a flat pancochlear loss is present in the late stages of the disease. All types of hearing loss have been documented with Meniere's disease, including high-frequency loss. It is not unusual for hearing to be normal between episodes. Serial audiograms are needed to document the progression and the fluctuating nature of the disease. In addition, the late stages often involve a loss of speech discrimination. Immittance testing reveals a normal tympanogram, confirming normal external auditory canal and middle ear function.

The differential diagnosis of Meniere's disease is extensive and includes conditions that may also present with hearing loss and vertigo unrelated to position change: labyrinthitis, vestibular neuronitis, otosyphilis, sarcoidosis, Cogan's syndrome, autoimmune inner ear disease, perilymph fistula, vertiginous migraine, and retro-cochlear processes (including acoustic neuroma, multiple sclerosis, vascular compression, vertiginous epilepsy, and vertigo of brainstem origin). Meniere's should always be considered in the differential diagnosis of a patient with acute onset of severe vertigo with peripheral characteristics. The features that distinguish it from other causes of vertigo are spontaneous onset of recurrent attacks, limited duration of symptoms during each discrete attack, associated tinnitus, ear discomfort, and sensorineural hearing loss, recruitment on audiometry, and normal brainstem and cerebellar function.

TABLE 1. **Review of Treatment Modalities for Meniere's Disease**

Treatment Modality	Chance of Hearing Loss Due to Treatment
Low salt diet	No
Diuretic*	No
Transtympanic aminoglycoside*	Moderate
Endolymphatic sac procedures	Minimal
Transcanal/transmastoid labyrinthectomy	Yes
Middle cranial fossa vestibular nerve section	Minimal

*Not FDA approved for this indication.

TREATMENT

Failure to alter any of the symptoms of Meniere's disease with an adequate trial of medical management should bring the diagnosis into doubt. A vast number of therapies have been tried since the disease was first described. If the disease is suspected, patients are initially placed on a low sodium diet (1500–1800 mg/d for the average weight patient) and a diuretic. A combination thiazide* and triamterene* medication such as Dyazide* is prescribed either once or twice a day and is potassium-sparing. Control of acute episodes, when severe, can occur with the use of vestibular suppressants, such as benzodiazepines,* and antiemetics.* However, one should avoid their daily use to prevent addiction. In a few instances, high-dose steroids have been helpful in patients with repeated spells and significant drops in hearing. Long-term use of meclizine (Antivert)* is avoided because it may prevent vestibular compensation. Psychological and behavioral therapy may also play a role in reducing patient response to the disease process. After 1 year of treatment without recurrence, the conservative treatment may be tapered. This medical regimen controls the spells of vertigo in more than two thirds of patients with Meniere's disease (Table 1).

For those patients with severe, recurrent episodes and those patients refractory to medical treatment, several surgical procedures offer a chance to avoid the debilitating vertiginous attacks associated with the disorder. Treatment is individualized. Unfortunately, hearing can continue to deteriorate even when the attacks are controlled medically or surgically. A review of our experience at the University of Iowa reveals that 84% (n = 286) who experienced medical failure for treatment of Meniere's disease had their spells of vertigo controlled with an endolymphatic shunt procedure. Significant hearing loss occurred in 1% of patients. The advantage of these procedures is that hearing is preserved, which can be important because some patients may develop a bilateral form of the disease.

Surgical and chemical labyrinthectomies can be performed and work by ablating the vestibular organs. The surgical labyrinthectomies can either be done by a transcanal or transmastoid approach and have a 95% success rate. Chemical labyrinthectomies are reserved for patients with poor hearing and who cannot tolerate a surgical procedure owing to significant co-morbidities. The transtympanic application of gentamicin* is the most commonly used approach, but it may cause up to a 40% incidence of hearing loss. Long-term ataxia has also been reported with this procedure. Failures of the surgical treatments listed can be controlled with a posterior or middle fossa vestibular nerve section.

*Not FDA approved for this indication.

*Not FDA approved for this indication.

VIRAL MENINGITIS AND ENCEPHALITIS

method of
ALEX TSELIS, M.D., PH.D.
Wayne State University School of Medicine
Detroit, Michigan

Viral infections of the central nervous system fall into one of two categories: viral meningitis and viral encephalitis. The former is generally self-limited and usually requires no more than symptomatic therapy. The latter is a serious and frightening illness, is often difficult to diagnose, and requires intensive therapy.

The most important viral encephalitides in the United States are herpes simplex encephalitis, La Crosse encephalitis, St. Louis encephalitis, eastern and western equine encephalitis, and, more recently, West Nile virus encephalitis. Lymphocytic choriomeningitis is rarely seen. Rabies encephalitis and Powassan encephalitis are very rare (Table 1).

CLINICAL PRESENTATION

Viral meningitis presents as headache, fever, photophobia, and stiff neck. The fever may be moderate or high. There are usually no symptoms of brain involvement.

Viral encephalitis also presents as headache and fever, but symptoms of parenchymal involvement invariably ensue. Often, there is a prodrome of fever, malaise, muscle aches, headache, backache, nausea, and vomiting. Within a few hours to a few days, this evolves to unusual or

TABLE 1. **Viral Encephalitides Seen in North America**

Herpes simplex encephalitis
Enteroviral encephalitis
St. Louis encephalitis
La Crosse encephalitis
Eastern equine encephalitis
Western equine encephalitis
West Nile encephalitis
Lymphocytic choriomeningitis
Rabies encephalitis*
Powassan encephalitis*

*Very rare.

bizarre behavior, confusion, disorientation, focal weakness, abnormal reflexes, seizures, dysconjugate gaze, delirium, and drowsiness. This tempo of disease is unusual in other illnesses mimicking viral encephalitis. Rare cases evolving over 1 or 2 weeks have been described.

DIFFERENTIAL DIAGNOSIS OF FEBRILE HEADACHE AND ENCEPHALOPATHY

The differential diagnosis of febrile headaches includes toxic vascular headache, which can be seen in any systemic febrile illness, such as influenza, as well as viral meningitis, but the main item on the list is bacterial meningitis, which is important to detect quickly because early treatment is essential to prevent complications or death.

The differential diagnosis of a febrile encephalopathy is very broad and includes, besides viral encephalitis, illnesses that are listed in Table 2. As in meningitis, various historical and clinical features can narrow the differential diagnosis. Recent medication with neuroleptics suggests neuroleptic malignant syndrome. A history of heavy alcohol abuse suggests the possibility of delirium tremens. A symmetric rash suggests the possibility of enterovirus infection, Rocky Mountain spotted fever, or the HIV seroconversion syndrome (which can be accompanied by a febrile encephalopathy). Abnormal bleeding (e.g., hemoptysis or from venous puncture sites) suggests thrombotic thrombocytopenic purpura. Human monocytic ehrlichiosis is seen in the southeastern and south central part of the United States and is characterized by leukopenia, thrombocytopenia, abnormal results of liver function tests, and occasional encephalopathy.

In immunosuppressed patients, toxoplasmosis and cerebral aspergillosis, present in AIDS patients and transplant recipients, respectively, are high on the list of differential diagnoses, although their presentations can be atypical.

TABLE 2. **Diseases That Can Resemble Viral Encephalitis**

Infections
Sepsis
Pneumonia
Urosepsis
Bacterial meningitis
Neurosyphilis
Subdural empyema
Human monocytic ehrlichiosis
Toxic-Metabolic
Drug intoxication
Hypoxic encephalopathy
Hyponatremia
Hypoglycemia
Thyroid storm
Delirium tremens
Neuroleptic malignant syndrome
Vascular
Subarachnoid hemorrhage
Sagittal sinus thrombosis
Vasculitis
Other
Acute disseminated encephalomyelitis
Neoplasm
Acute multiple sclerosis
Neurosarcoidosis
Behçet syndrome
Acute psychosis

HISTORY AND CLINICAL SETTING

The history and clinical setting of the current illness is important to help delineate the diagnostic possibilities. Certain items in the history are crucial. These include time course, travel history, history of exposure to an epidemic, animal exposure, and history of immunosuppression.

Many virus infections display seasonality and geographic distribution, which are relevant to formulating the differential diagnosis. Thus, enterovirus disease is most common in the summer and early fall. Arboviral diseases are present only when the mosquito vectors are abundant, usually in the summer or fall, so that a patient with encephalitis occurring in midwinter cannot have any of these, in the absence of travel to an endemic region in the South. St. Louis encephalitis occurs in the late summer and early fall and is seen throughout the United States, with epidemics occurring along the Eastern seaboard, particularly in the south, in the midwest, and in the gulf states as well as in the Caribbean islands. La Crosse encephalitis usually occurs in the midwest and in West Virginia. Eastern equine encephalitis outbreaks occur along the eastern seaboard. Western equine encephalitis occurs in the western states. Lymphocytic choriomeningitis virus can cause either meningitis or encephalitis and is carried as a persistent infection in mice. The disease occurs in the winter, when mice come inside human habitations to escape the cold.

Where does the patient live? What viruses are circulating in the area of the patient's residence? Discussion with the local state public health authorities is important. St. Louis encephalitis, La Crosse encephalitis, eastern and western equine encephalitis, Rocky Mountain spotted fever, and human monocytic ehrlichiosis all have characteristic geographic distributions as discussed earlier.

Has the patient traveled recently? Travel to Central or Eastern Europe implies the possibility of Central European tick-borne encephalitis. Travel to the Far East and to Southeast Asia suggests Far Eastern tick-borne encephalitis (Russian spring-summer encephalitis) and Japanese encephalitis. Recently, Nipah virus encephalitis has been added to the differential diagnosis of encephalitis in parts of Southeast Asia, especially Singapore and Malaysia, and is seen in pig farm and abattoir workers. Rabies is enzootic in many parts of the tropics.

Has the patient been exposed to any sick animals? Rabies is present in the wildlife in Texas, along the east coast, and in Kentucky. Exposure to bats or coyotes should be ascertained. Exposure to mice is a risk factor for lymphocytic choriomeningitis, although the disease has become very rare in the past several decades. Has the patient had contact with monkeys? If so, herpes B encephalitis must be considered. Exposure to sick pigs in parts of Southeast Asia suggests the possibility of Nipah virus encephalitis.

Is the patient immunosuppressed? Does the patient have HIV disease? Has the patient had cancer chemotherapy or a transplant? Has the patient had a preceding dermatomal zosteriform rash? If so, relevant infectious considerations include varicella-zoster encephalitis and cytomegalovirus encephalitis, as well as cerebral toxoplasmosis. In advanced HIV disease, primary central nervous system lymphoma must also be considered.

DIAGNOSTIC STUDIES

A list of diagnostic studies is summarized in Table 3.

Laboratory Testing

Routine laboratory tests, such as determinations of levels of electrolytes, glucose, calcium, and magnesium; a

TABLE 3. **Workup of Suspected Viral Encephalitis**

Blood

Complete blood cell count with differential count and platelets, electrolytes, glucose, calcium, magnesium, blood urea nitrogen/creatinine, liver function tests, erythrocyte sedimentation rate, blood cultures, toxicology screen, thyroid function tests, antinuclear antibodies, HIV, rapid plasma reagin, Epstein-Barr virus panel

Urine

Urinalysis, with culture and sensitivity testing, if appropriate. Urine toxicology screen

Chest Radiograph

Magnetic resonance imaging of the brain with T1- and T2-weighted images

Cerebrospinal Analysis

Cell count with differential
Protein/glucose
Gram stain and bacterial culture
Acid-fast bacilli smear and culture
VDRL
Cytology
Viral culture
Cryptococcal antigen
Polymerase chain reaction for herpes simplex virus, cytomegalovirus, Epstein-Barr virus, varicella-zoster virus
IgM specific for La Crosse encephalitis, St. Louis encephalitis, eastern equine encephalitis, western equine encephalitis

Biopsy

complete blood cell count; and a urine toxicology screen should be obtained in all patients with suspected encephalitis. A chest radiograph can show the scarring of tuberculosis, the mediastinal adenopathy of sarcoidosis, or a mass suggesting lung cancer. In addition, laboratory tests to rule out the other possible causes discussed earlier should be done. These include antinuclear antibody, rapid plasma reagin, an Epstein-Barr virus (EBV) panel, angiotensin-converting enzyme, and antiphospholipid antibody titers. Blood cultures to rule out bacterial endocarditis should be done.

Lumbar puncture is mandatory in all cases of suspected viral encephalitis. Cerebrospinal fluid (CSF) examination can rule out other elements of the differential diagnosis, such as bacterial meningitis, neurotuberculosis, and subarachnoid hemorrhage, as well as positively diagnose viral encephalitis. Routine studies that should be done on the CSF include cell count and differential, Gram stain and culture, acid-fast bacterial stain and culture, and cytology. The cell count and differential can be useful in differentiating some viral encephalitides. For example, herpes simplex encephalitis and eastern equine encephalitis may show a polymorphonuclear pleocytosis.

Polymerase chain reaction (PCR) testing of the CSF is becoming the standard method for diagnosis of many viral infections of the central nervous system. A search for viral DNA by polymerase chain reaction can diagnose herpes simplex, cytomegalovirus, and Epstein-Barr virus encephalitis. In particular, CSF PCR testing for herpes simplex virus DNA is very sensitive and specific and can confirm the diagnosis from the CSF obtained on admission to the hospital. The RNA viruses, which commonly infect the nervous system, such as enterovirus, can be detected by reverse transcriptase PCR.

Serologic tests of the CSF, by an IgM antibody capture assay, can confirm eastern equine encephalitis, western equine encephalitis, La Crosse encephalitis, and St. Louis encephalitis and are available in kit form. These tests are often positive early in the illness and can confirm the diagnosis from specimens obtained from the admission lumbar puncture.

Imaging Studies

Magnetic resonance imaging of the brain is important in the diagnosis of viral encephalitis. Certain patterns of abnormality are characteristic of particular viruses. Thus, areas of abnormal signal (increased signal on T2-weighted images) and mass effect in the temporal lobe are especially suggestive of herpes simplex virus encephalitis, an important diagnosis to make because specific antiviral therapy is available. Multifocal white matter areas of hyperintensity on T2-weighted images suggest acute disseminated encephalomyelitis. The presence of areas of increased intensity in the basal ganglia and thalamus on T2-weighted images suggests eastern equine encephalitis. Ependymal enhancement in an AIDS patient suggests cytomegaloviral encephalitis. White matter lesions with a variegated appearance in an AIDS patient suggest varicella-zoster virus encephalitis. Furthermore, the diagnosis of illnesses that can resemble viral encephalitis, such as subdural empyema, sagittal sinus thrombosis, and brain abscess, can be readily ascertained by their characteristic imaging findings.

Electroencephalography

The electroencephalogram shows characteristic changes in herpes simplex encephalitis: there are periodic lateralized temporal lobe discharges on one or both sides. It is also useful in ruling out seizure activity in comatose patients in whom seizures can be very subtle.

Brain Biopsy

The role of brain biopsy in viral encephalitis is controversial and has in the past mainly been used to diagnose herpes encephalitis. Its role in this situation has been replaced by the detection of herpes simplex virus in the CSF by PCR. In a patient with a focal lesion with enhancement, without a clear diagnosis, whose condition is deteriorating steadily, biopsy should be considered. The biopsy should be directed to the affected tissue, rather than of normal-appearing tissue, which may be easier to access surgically. In one case seen at my institution, a patient with a prodrome of malaise and aching rapidly became delirious, and magnetic resonance imaging showed temporal lobe changes typical of herpes encephalitis. When the CSF by PCR was negative for herpes simplex virus and the patient did not respond to acyclovir, a biopsy of the affected area was done and revealed a T-cell lymphoma. Careful coordination between the neurologist, neurosurgeon, and neuropathologist is necessary for the optimal use of the brain biopsy.

MANAGEMENT

Viral meningitis is managed symptomatically because the disease is self-limited and recovery is spontaneous and complete. There are no data showing any advantage to using antiviral therapy in viral meningitis.

The management of viral encephalitis encompasses three dimensions: supportive care, specific antiviral therapy, and treatment of complications. In any case of viral encephalitis, it is imperative that the diagnosis of herpes simplex encephalitis be definitively ruled out because there is specific and effective antiviral therapy for this disease, which otherwise is frequently severely disabling or fatal.

Supportive care includes hydration (with care to avoid overhydration, which can exacerbate cerebral edema); nutrition; treatment of malignant fever; prevention of deep venous thrombosis; avoidance of decubiti; respiratory toilet, including intubation if necessary to protect the airway; bladder drainage; and prevention and treatment of urinary tract infection. Patients who require this care are probably best managed in an intensive care setting with the help of a skilled intensivist.

The only approved specific antiviral therapy currently available is acyclovir (Zovirax) for herpes simplex virus encephalitis. The drug is given intravenously at a dose of 10 mg/kg every 8 hours. It is important that an adequate course of therapy be given. In the past, cases of recurrent herpes encephalitis have followed 10 days of therapy, and it is considered that at least 2 to 3 weeks of acyclovir is necessary. The drug should be given at the first suspicion of herpes encephalitis, while the diagnostic workup is proceeding, because early treatment is imperative for a positive outcome. Renal function should be monitored when using acyclovir.

In the rare cases of cytomegaloviral encephalitis, it would be prudent to use ganciclovir or foscarnet because these drugs are active against the virus and the few cases described in the literature had poor outcomes. There have been no studies examining the role of these drugs in cytomegaloviral encephalitis, and they should be used with this in mind. A reasonable regimen would be to use ganciclovir (Cytovene), 5 mg/kg intravenously twice daily, or foscarnet (Foscavir), 90 mg/kg intravenously twice daily for 1 to 2 weeks, depending on clinical response. Serum calcium and magnesium levels, as well as renal function, must be monitored when using foscarnet. Similarly, for EBV encephalitis, there are no data to guide antiviral therapy. In cases of EBV infectious mononucleosis, acyclovir does not seem to affect the disease and its role in the treatment of EBV encephalitis is unclear, although it can be used because it is fairly nontoxic.

No specific antiviral therapy is available for other forms of encephalitis, although ribavirin has been used in La Crosse encephalitis and may be useful in West Nile virus encephalitis. However, the drug is available only in aerosol and oral forms and special arrangements must be made with the Centers for Disease Control and Prevention to obtain parenteral forms of the drug.

Complications of viral encephalitis include seizures and cerebral edema. Seizures can complicate the management of encephalitis and must be treated vigorously. If the patient has a clinical seizure, or if there is seizure activity on the electroencephalogram, antiseizure medication should be given. A reasonable regimen would be to infuse phenytoin (Dilantin) at a loading dose of 15 to 20 mg/kg intravenously, in saline, at a rate of no more than 50 mg/min with a target serum free phenytoin level of about 20 μg/mL. The patient's vital signs need to be monitored while the infusion is proceeding.

In patients who are very drowsy, cerebral edema is an important consideration and computed tomography of the brain can show the typical effacement of sulci and ventricles as well as mass effect. Mild degrees of cerebral edema can be monitored closely. If the edema is severe, with mass effect and if herniation is threatened, then more active measures need to be taken. An intracranial pressure monitor can be a useful guide to therapy, although it requires special skills to install, interpret, and maintain. Normal intracranial pressure is usually less than 10 mm Hg. Treatment of cerebral edema includes osmotic dehydration of the brain, hyperventilation, or intravenous dexamethasone. Hyperventilation constricts cerebral blood vessels and acts immediately, but the effect is not sustained for longer than a few hours to a day or so and must often be supplemented by osmotic dehydration. It is useful in cases with incipient central or uncal herniation, which are immediately life threatening. Osmotic dehydration of the brain acts within 15 minutes or so. Dexamethasone (Decadron)* acts within an hour. Osmotic dehydration is accomplished by the use of osmotic dehydrating agents such as mannitol (Osmitrol) 0.5 to 1.0 g intravenously every 3 to 4 hours, with a serum osmolality not to exceed 320 mOsm. Hyperventilation is achieved by intubating the patient and targeting for a P_{CO_2} of 25 to 35 mm Hg. Dexamethasone is given intravenously at a dose of 16 mg, followed by 4 mg intravenously every 4 to 6 hours. These doses should be tapered as the increased intracranial pressure and edema resolve.

It is important to be prepared for a long course with these patients because they can improve rapidly and dramatically many months after appearing to be making no progress at all. After the acute illness is over, rehabilitation becomes important.

*Not FDA approved for this indication.

MULTIPLE SCLEROSIS

method of
R. PHILIP KINKEL, M.D., and
RICHARD A. RUDICK, M.D.
Cleveland Clinic Foundation
Cleveland, Ohio

Multiple sclerosis (MS) is the most common cause of nontraumatic, neurologic disability afflicting young adults in the United States, with 250,000 to 350,000 estimated cases. In temperate zones of North America and Europe the prevalence may reach 0.1% to 0.3% of the population, making this disorder common enough to be seen regularly in most primary care and neurology practices. The chronic and protean nature of MS and its variability over time create many management challenges. To simplify our description of management strategies, we have divided this process into four separate areas:

1. Diagnosis
2. Education and counseling
3. Symptomatic treatment
4. Disease-specific therapies

The recent approval and marketing of disease-specific therapies has increased the complexity of patient management, leaving less time for clinicians to focus on important areas of management such as counseling, education, and symptomatic therapies. This occurs at a time of aggressive testing to establish a diagnosis of MS more quickly and to initiate preventative disease-specific therapies at the earliest stages of the disease. The availability of partially effective disease-modifying drugs does not eliminate the need for appropriate education, counseling, and symptom management.

DIAGNOSIS

Traditionally, the diagnosis of MS has been based on clinical features supplemented by diagnostic testing. The process of establishing a diagnosis is inherently complex, requiring, at a minimum, the consultative services of a neurologist. Clinical criteria require symptoms and signs reflecting multiple areas of central nervous system (CNS) demyelination spread over time in the absence of an alternative diagnosis capable of presenting in this fashion. Laboratory tests such as magnetic resonance imaging (MRI), cerebrospinal fluid (CSF) analysis, and sensory evoked potentials supplement clinical criteria and thereby play a major role in confirming the diagnosis and eliminating alternative diagnostic possibilities.

None of the existing clinical diagnostic criteria for MS allows a physician to render a definitive diagnosis after a single episode of symptomatic demyelination. Nevertheless, certain initial syndromes, such as monocular optic neuritis, partial transverse myelitis, or various brainstem syndromes, particularly internuclear ophthalmoplegia, are so commonly associated with MS that most neurologists strongly consider this diagnosis at the onset of symptoms. Before the era of MRI, it was impossible to determine which of these individuals would go on to develop typical MS and which individuals would be found to have another diagnosis or never experience further neurologic symptoms. Patients were considered "at risk to develop MS" after experiencing typical symptoms for the first time but were often not informed of this risk, because the probability of MS was uncertain and no therapies were available to reduce this risk or alter the future course of the disease. It took, on average, 5 years to establish a certain diagnosis of MS, a period of significant uncertainty and anxiety for many patients. MRI of the cranium and spinal cord revolutionized this diagnostic process. First, MRI allows clinicians to exclude many alternative mimic conditions that respond best to appropriate therapies initiated as early as possible. Second, MRI allows clinicians to finally establish a relative risk for the development of MS. For instance, 50% of patients have typical MS-appearing white matter changes at the time of their first symptoms. The number and location of these abnormalities are strongly associated with the short-term risk of developing a clinical diagnosis of MS. Specifically, those individuals in the correct demographic group with two or more typical white matter abnormalities have a greater than 50% risk of developing clinically definite MS within 3 years of symptom onset. These individuals are now considered at "high risk" to develop MS. Alternatively, those individuals without typical white matter abnormalities, especially those individuals with normal CSF studies, are considered at low risk to develop MS, with a 5-year diagnosis rate of less than 10%. Therefore, imaging abnormalities at the onset of MS symptoms can be used to educate and counsel patients appropriately and, as will be discussed later, make decisions regarding early initiation of disease-specific therapy.

Despite our current ability to establish a diagnosis of MS earlier and with greater certainty in many individuals, there are still cases in which the diagnosis remains uncertain even with extensive testing. In these cases, the diagnosis should not be made prematurely; rather, patients should be educated and counseled about diagnostic uncertainty from the onset. When uncertainty in the diagnosis of MS or the risk of developing MS exists, this should be discussed directly with the patient. Education and follow-up plans, including repeat MRI at 1- to 2-year intervals should be established. Repeat MRI will determine if characteristic white matter abnormalities have developed in the absence of new symptoms. Those patients unable to cope with an uncertain diagnosis, even after appropriate education, frequently give a history of maladaptive coping patterns to stresses and uncertainties in their lives. Such individuals may benefit from psychotherapy, either individually or in a group setting.

Although establishing a diagnosis is beyond the scope of this discussion, it is useful to mention two common diagnostic errors. The first is diagnosing MS in patients with no definable neurologic disease. It is quite common for us to see patients who have been diagnosed with MS because of nonspecific neurologic symptoms such as general weakness, fatigue, or tingling, at times supplemented by minimal changes on the MRI. By far the most common syndrome in this group of patients is recurrent paresthesias (usually described as pins and needles) in the extremities without any discernible abnormalities on neurologic examination or diagnostic testing. The condition is so frequent that we often characterize the syndrome as "benign paresthesias." Often the sensory symptoms are accompanied by a history of chronic fatigue and/or chronic diffuse pain suggesting an overlap with fibromyalgia and chronic fatigue syndrome. We have followed a number of patients with this condition for many years. Although a small minority eventually develops MS, most never develop a neurologic disease. In some cases, a somatization disorder becomes apparent over time.

The second type of diagnostic error is incorrectly diagnosing MS in a patient who has some other neurologic disease. As mentioned earlier, the widespread use of MRI has helped to eliminate many diagnostic errors but they still occur, often as a result of misinterpretation of MRI findings. We have listed a number of "red flags" that should alert the physician to the possibility of an alternative diagnosis (Table 1). When any of these red flags exist, an evaluation should be undertaken to exclude alternative causes.

EDUCATION AND COUNSELING

As with other chronic illnesses of uncertain etiology and prognosis, education and counseling may not only be therapeutic but may also be the main treatment required. During the early stages of MS, patients may be inappropriately

Table 1. **Red Flags Casting Doubt on the Diagnosis of MS**

Absence of eye findings—reflecting optic nerve or oculomotor dysfunction
Absence of remission—particularly in a patient younger than 30
Localized disease—particularly posterior fossa, craniocervical junction, or spinal cord
Atypical clinical features—particularly absence of sensory findings, reflexes, or bladder involvement
Normal results of magnetic resonance imaging
Normal cerebrospinal fluid examination

Adapted from Rudick RA, Schiffer RB, Schwetz K, Herndon RM: Multiple sclerosis: The problem of misdiagnosis. Arch Neurol 43:578, 1986. Copyright 1986, American Medical Association.

Table 2. **Essential Clinical Features of MS**

Peak age at onset is 18 to 35 (any age possible)
More common in females (approximately two thirds)
More common in temperate climates
Demyelination can cause motor, sensory, visual, bowel, bladder, cognitive, affective, and autonomic disturbances.
Relapsing-remitting course at onset in 85% of cases
Progressive course from onset more common in older onset cases (>40)
Ninety percent of relapsing cases eventually enter a secondary progressive phase

reassured by being told they have "benign MS" or given no significant information except to "call if new problems develop." Many health care resources are brought to bear on establishing a diagnosis, but little time remains to address the questions and concerns of patients and their families. This, in turn, leads to frustration and a breakdown in communication between the patient and health care provider.

What follows is a list of commonly encountered questions with suggested explanations. Neither the list nor the responses are meant to be an exhaustive compendium of information for the practitioner. Instead, these responses are offered as a starting point in the education process.

What Is Multiple Sclerosis?

Accumulating evidence suggests that MS (literally translated as multiple scars) is the result of organ-specific autoimmunity initiated and perpetuated by immune dysregulation in a genetically susceptible host. The inflammatory or autoimmune target in MS appears to be some component(s) of the myelin sheath that wraps around CNS axons. During the inflammatory process, myelin and the underlying axon are injured. The peripheral nervous system is *not* involved by the MS process, but peripheral nerve rootlets and cranial nerves are commonly affected where they exit from the CNS. Pathologically, acute MS lesions are characterized by perivascular cuffs of intense inflammation in the white matter of the CNS surrounded by a zone of macrophage infiltration and demyelination. A classic pathologic tenant held that there was "relative preservation of axons" in areas of inflammation. However, recent evidence suggests that axonal transection and wallerian degeneration occur often and early in the disease course. Furthermore, axonal damage may be responsible for most of the permanent injury occurring after an episode of inflammation. Much of the current research in MS focuses on the design of therapies to protect axons from injury.

During acute episodes of demyelination (i.e., when a new lesion is formed or an older lesion enlarges), breakdown of the blood-brain barrier occurs, which can be detected with gadolinium (Gd)-enhanced MRI. Because Gd enhancement persists for a few weeks, Gd-enhanced MRI helps to determine the activity of the disease at a given point in time. As the inflammatory process subsides, gliosis or scarring ensues. At unpredictable points in time, even during the recovery of recent inflammatory lesions, new inflammatory lesions occur in adjacent or totally different areas of the CNS.

The essential features of the disease are given in Table 2. The plethora of symptoms and signs observed is a testament to the importance of CNS myelin in the conduction of electrical impulses throughout the CNS. When stripped away from axons, electrical impulses are blocked, slowed, or produce aberrant signals. In the case of motor system involvement this can produce weakness, exertional fatigue, or paroxysmal muscle contractions. Of course, the same mechanisms can affect virtually any centrally mediated neural system, creating a variety of symptoms that are at times difficult to explain. Nevertheless, certain syndromes, listed in Table 3, are commonly associated with MS and should alert a physician to this diagnosis in the correct clinical setting.

Two additional points regarding the disease process should be emphasized. First, most new MS lesions do not produce symptoms or signs. This is particularly noticeable in the early relapsing-remitting (see later) phase of the disease. Most new lesions occur in areas of the CNS that are clinically silent. For instance, serial MRI has demonstrated that the majority of new lesions, even early in the course of the disease during clinical remissions when patients are asymptomatic, occur in these silent areas. Therefore, the absence of symptoms cannot be taken as evidence that the disease is in remission. Second, early in the disease process the CNS is capable of recovery after inflammatory demyelination. This contributes to the dramatic recovery often observed, even after severe attacks. However, with recurrent inflammatory demyelination, recovery becomes less complete, perhaps as a result of

Table 3. **Characteristic Clinical Syndromes in MS**

Optic neuritis: Acute, unilateral (rarely bilateral) loss of central vision with pain on eye movement and an afferent pupillary defect.
Partial transverse myelitis: Ascending numbness and/or paresthesias with hyperreflexia and, frequently, a "tight-band"–like sensation at the level of spinal cord involvement: variable motor, bowel, and bladder involvement.
Acute brainstem syndromes: Commonly a unilateral or bilateral internuclear ophthalmoplegia; variable additional presentations.
Trigeminal neuralgia: MS until proven otherwise in patients <40 years old.
Lhermitte phenomenon: Electric or shocklike sensations down the spine and/or into the limbs with forward neck flexion.
Useless hand syndrome: Clumsy unilateral hand and arm movements with relatively preserved strength and primary sensation (i.e., light touch and pinprick) but variable loss of joint position sensation and an inability to recognize objects placed in the hand.
Tonic spasms: Paroxysmal, painful, unilateral dystonic muscle contractions with a flexion posture of the upper extremity and an extension posture of the lower extremity, if the latter is involved.

mounting gliotic scarring, axonal injury, and neuronal loss. This permanent injury can be visualized on imaging studies as "black holes" in the white matter on T1-weighted imaging studies or as parenchymal atrophy with compensatory enlargement of ventricular spaces and cortical sulci.

What Can I Expect Will Happen to Me?

Unlike most debilitating diseases of young adults, life expectancy after MS onset is only a few years short of normal. Recent studies suggest that most of the variance is explained by suicides. Not unexpectedly, the majority of patients tend to develop considerable disability over time. Twenty percent of patients are unable to walk unassisted or conduct normal work activities 5 years after diagnosis, increasing to 50% at 15 years and to 80% at 30 years. Only 10% of patients with MS experience a truly benign course, defined as the absence of significant disability after decades of observation.

A hallmark of MS is the unpredictable course of the disease. It is not possible early in the disease to determine the rate at which an individual patient will develop disability, or the pattern of clinical features. Eighty-five percent of patients with MS experience a relapsing-remitting (RRMS) course during the early years of their disease. Each relapse (also called an exacerbation) is characterized by a rapid decline in neurologic function; each remission is characterized by spontaneous improvement that ranges from complete recovery to only slight improvement. When recovery is complete, there may be no persisting symptoms between exacerbations. The average patient experiences approximately two relapses every 3 years. After a variable period of time and after a variable number of relapses, MS patients tend to develop less clear attacks and a more or less steadily progressive course. Acute exacerbations may be superimposed on this steady worsening. This stage of the illness, termed *secondary progressive MS*, occurs in about 50% of patients within 10 to 15 years after onset. In 10% to 15% of patients a progressive course occurs from the onset (i.e., primary progressive MS) without exacerbations. In its most common form this consists of a progressive myelopathy. The *primary progressive* form of MS is age dependent, occurring more commonly in older patients. The risk of this form of the disease is over 50% in patients with MS onset when older than the age of 40. Clinical, genetic, imaging, and histopathologic differences between exacerbating remitting and primary progressive MS suggest that there may be etiologic differences between the two types.

Befitting a disease known for its unpredictable nature, MS patients can experience long intervals of stability after periods of progressive decline or may even go decades between relapses. In general, the course of MS during the first 5 to 10 years after symptom onset can be used to guide patients about their eventual course. Favorable prognostic signs after the first 5 years of MS include predominance of sensory involvement with relatively little motor impairment, long intervals between relapses (especially, the interval between the first and second attack), substantial or complete recovery between relapses, and minimal disease on brain MRI. Unfavorable prognostic signs include prominent motor and cerebellar involvement, frequent relapses, poor recovery between relapses or a progressive course, and a large T2 lesion burden on the brain MRI. Even with these guidelines, however, precise predictions cannot be made in an individual case with great accuracy; predictions should be made to reassure patients who appear to have more benign MS and to explain and justify more aggressive medical management for patients who appear to have a worse prognosis.

How Can I Make My Illness Better, and What Makes It Worse?

Most patients and their families harbor certain beliefs about the effects of certain behaviors on MS. These beliefs vary a great deal between patients and families, but generally they represent a need to gain some measure of control over the illness. Patients will not generally articulate these beliefs and rarely have insight into their need for more control over the disease. We encourage patients to verbalize what they think will improve or worsen their MS. If possible, active control measures should be directed toward healthy behaviors such as proper eating, exercise, and stress management. We discourage beliefs that could result in behavior with detrimental consequences, such as seeking dangerous or expensive alternative therapies without proven value. Many patients regain a sense of control by instituting a fitness program, improving their diet, reducing their weight, and eliminating negative behaviors such as smoking, alcohol, and drug abuse.

Most patients also believe certain events or activities precipitate MS disease activity. These beliefs are often held with surprising conviction. The most common of these is the belief that stress precipitates MS worsening or relapse. According to a survey in our center, over two thirds of our patients believe that stress makes MS worse. Although the evidence on this relationship is mixed and by no means conclusive, we often use the perceived relationship to recommend stress management to patients. Furthermore, patients selectively remember events just preceding relapses. For example, a patient experiencing a relapse shortly after a divorce or a minor car accident is likely to assign a causal relationship. Patients often believe that inoculations or vaccinations precipitate MS disease activity. Recent evidence suggests there is no increased risk with vaccination. We currently recommend that patients who are wheelchair restricted or residing in nursing homes and patients at high risk for influenza (e.g., day care or health care workers) receive yearly influenza vaccination. The precipitants that are recognized should be discussed with patients. Rigorous studies have established viral illnesses, usually of the upper respiratory tract, as known precipitants of relapses. Other febrile illnesses, particularly urinary tract infections (UTIs), commonly aggravate MS symptoms or precipitate significant new disease activity. Consequently, significant infection should be treated aggressively in MS patients, and UTI should be specifically ruled out in an MS patient experiencing a decline in function. Recurrent UTIs should be prevented by eliminating the cause, if possible (i.e., calculi, poor hygiene, poor catheter technique, chronic urinary retention). Similarly, chronically infected decubitus ulcers should be treated aggressively and the cause managed (i.e., poor nutrition, contracture, and excessive pressure from immobility).

Patients should be counseled that increased core body temperature, either with infection or hot weather, may result in the reappearance of many MS symptoms. Most patients are heat sensitive. Each individual patient should be advised about the relationship between body temperature and MS symptoms, but it is not necessary for MS patients generally to avoid heat exposure. Most MS patients can tolerate warm or hot showers, a day on the beach, or aerobic exercise. Few MS patients with moderate or severe disability, however, tolerate significant fever. Even in heat-sensitive patients, there is little evidence that heat worsens the course of MS or provokes new disease activity. Moderation and common sense are the only requirements.

Can I Have Children?

Most studies have found that women with MS have normal fertility, normal pregnancies, and normal infants. There seems to be little evidence to suggest that one or more pregnancies accelerate progression of disease, and women with MS who wish to become pregnant should be encouraged. However, numerous studies have suggested that pregnant women with MS experienced fewer exacerbations in the second and third trimesters of pregnancy and a higher risk of relapses in the first 4 to 6 months post partum. We advise women with mild to moderate disability to plan pregnancies on the basis of issues other than MS. The pregnancy should be planned to avoid the use of potentially teratogenic medications during any portion of the pregnancy. Disease-modifying therapies (see later) are discontinued before conception, if possible, and reinstituted after breast-feeding is complete or at any time post partum in women electing not to breast-feed. Pregnancy, labor, and delivery management should be routine. There is no reason to avoid epidural anesthesia. Breast-feeding should be supported if this is the wish of the patient. To avoid exhaustion, we advise breast-feeding mothers to pump their breasts at night and sleep while another family member feeds the infant by bottle.

Will Any of My Family Get MS?

We inform our MS patients that the lifetime risk of MS to a first-degree relative (e.g., child or sibling) is 3% to 5%. Although 30 to 50 times greater than the risk to the general population, this is still a small risk. Dizygotic twins have an identical MS concordance rate as nontwin siblings; monozygotic twins have a 40% concordance rate.

SYMPTOMATIC TREATMENT

Spasticity

Spasticity is defined as a velocity-dependent increase in muscle tone. This sign and associated symptoms are closely associated with other components of the upper motor neuron syndrome—loss of dexterity and weakness, hyperactive reflexes, clonus, spasms, and extensor plantar responses. Spasticity in MS is usually of spinal cord origin and predominantly affects lower extremities and trunk. Problems range from easy fatigue, loss of dexterity, and difficulty with stressed gait maneuvers such as running or hopping to stiffness, pain, severe weakness, involuntary spasms, and eventually contractures. The spastic gait appears stiff with short steps at times with scissoring of the legs. Stiffness is enhanced by more rapid ambulation, frequently causing a bouncing or jiggling appearance. Spasticity is more directly evaluated by passively stretching muscle groups with the patient seated or supine, which produces a "catch," or resistance to further movement after the limb is displaced. In mild cases this catch can only be demonstrated with rapid rates of passive movement across a joint (i.e., usually flexion and extension of the knee but any muscle group can be tested). In severe cases slow passive movements are difficult to perform against the extreme resistance in antagonist muscle groups.

The management of spasticity *must* involve a comprehensive approach. First, medication alone is often inadequate to prevent the complications of contractures, joint malalignment, and pain. Second, the functional consequences of spasticity vary from patient to patient. For example, spasticity may be beneficial in certain cases by allowing severely weak patients to ambulate. Therefore, treatment of spasticity must be tailored to the patient's impairment and disability. Most patients benefit by evaluation and treatment by a physical therapist experienced in this field. Patients with significant upper extremity spasticity or mobility problems (usually wheelchair dependent) should also be assessed by an occupational therapist. Physician and therapist should outline the goals of treatment and communicate this to the patient or caregivers. It is generally useful to reduce pain when possible and to treat infections, both of which exacerbate spasticity. Proper positioning also helps reduce spasticity. Simple measures such as flexion at hips and knees during sleep can reduce spasticity significantly. Examples of common therapeutic goals include alleviating knee pain from a spastic footdrop, improving perineal hygiene by eliminating hip adductor spasticity, decreasing nocturnal leg spasms, or reducing contractures in a bedridden patient.

Medications are considered adjuncts to physical measures. Antispastic drugs fall into four categories: γ-aminobutyric acid (GABA) agonists, benzodiazepines, skeletal muscle relaxants, and α_2-agonists. Baclofen (Lioresal), the only selective GABA-B agonist available, is usually the drug of first choice. The therapeutic window for this medication is wide, and the optimal dose must be individually determined. We usually begin treatment at 5 mg three times a day and instruct the patient to increase the dose by 5- to 10-mg increments every 3 days as needed. Mild cases may respond to doses ranging from 5 mg three times a day to 10 mg four times a day. Moderate spasticity usually requires 10 to 20 mg four times a day. More severe cases may require in excess of 120 mg/d, if tolerated. The principal limitations of baclofen are the unmasking of underlying weakness as spastic muscle tone is reduced and confusion, especially in cognitively impaired individuals. All patients should be instructed not to suddenly discontinue baclofen, because this may precipitate withdrawal seizures.

Noradrenergic α_2-agonists act within the spinal cord to enhance noradrenergic-mediated polysynaptic inhibition. In addition to demonstrated effects on spasticity and spasms, these drugs exert antinociceptive effects mediated by α_2 receptors in the dorsal horn of the spinal cord. Tizanidine (Zanaflex), the only drug of this class approved for the treatment of spasticity in the United States, is considered another first-line agent for the treatment of spasticity. Clinical trials of tizanidine monotherapy demonstrated clinical benefits on spasticity and spasm reduction similar to the benefits observed with oral baclofen. Although tizanidine therapy tends to create less weakness than baclofen, this benefit is offset by a relatively high incidence of sedation. Other side effects include dry mouth, dose-dependent hypotension, hepatic transaminase elevations, and, rarely, clinically evident hepatic dysfunction. The usual starting dose is 2 mg at bedtime with gradual escalation of the dose to a maximum of 36 mg/d in three to four divided doses. Combination therapy with oral baclofen has not been formally tested, but it offers many benefits and is used routinely in clinical practice. Hepatic transaminases must be monitored periodically throughout therapy.

Gabapentin (Neurontin),* an anticonvulsant approved as adjunctive therapy for partial seizures, has been very useful as a treatment of many paroxysmal motor and sensory phenomena in MS patients. Although structurally similar to the neurotransmitter GABA, gabapentin does not interact with the GABA receptor and its mechanism of action is unknown. We have found that gabapentin is a useful third-line adjunctive agent for the treatment of spasticity, especially nocturnal spasms. We often use gabapentin in combination with lower doses of baclofen or tizanidine in patients who tolerate these later medications poorly at higher doses. Gabapentin therapy is initiated at a dose of 100 mg three times a day and increased gradually to a maximum dose of 900 mg three times a day. Although tolerated at higher doses, it is rare to observe further benefit with dose escalation beyond 900 mg three times a day. For the treatment of nocturnal spasms, we prescribe gabapentin as a single bedtime dose. The only side effect associated with gabapentin for this indication has been sedation, usually only at the onset of therapy.

Benzodiazepines, principally diazepam (Valium), were previously used in conjunction with baclofen to control spasticity and spasms. However, with the availability of tizanidine and intrathecal baclofen, benzodiazepines are now principally used as third- or fourth-line agents. The only exception is the use of bedtime doses for the treatment of nocturnal spasms refractory to treatment with baclofen and tizanidine or gabapentin. For this indication we generally prescribe diazepam (5–15 mg qhs) or clonazepam* (Klonopin) (0.5–2 mg qhs). Single doses of diazepam at bedtime are frequently well tolerated, even in patients with severe forebrain disease.

Dantrolene (Dantrium) is usually reserved as a third-line agent in nonambulatory patients because of its potential hepatotoxicity and tendency to aggravate muscle weakness. Dantrolene acts at skeletal muscles by producing a dose-dependent reduction in myofibril contraction. Therapy is initiated at 25 mg given at bedtime and gradually increased to a maximum dose of 100 mg four times a day. As a single bedtime dose, dantrolene is well tolerated and effectively controls nocturnal cramps and spasms in patients unable to obtain relief with the previously mentioned agents. As the dose is increased and spread throughout the day, patients predictably develop diarrhea, anorexia, nausea, and sometimes vomiting. Some patients do not tolerate effective doses, because gastrointestinal side effects are dose dependent. Dantrolene may cause toxic hepatitis. The incidence of this potentially fatal complication increases with doses above 400 mg/d and is more common in women and patients older than age 35. Because of this complication, we monitor transaminase levels throughout the course of therapy and discontinue dantrolene in patients with aspartate amino transferase levels greater than two times the upper limit of normal.

Intrathecal administration of baclofen in the lumbar subarachnoid space (ITB therapy) through an implantable, externally programmable pump has revolutionized the treatment of severe spasticity in both ambulatory and nonambulatory patients. Management of spasticity is difficult in the case of wheelchair-restricted or bedridden MS patients because these patients either do not respond to oral therapies or tolerate high doses of baclofen or other oral antispasticity medications poorly. Without adequate spasticity management, caregiving, especially perineal hygiene and positioning of limbs, is difficult and contractures develop rapidly. This may result in skin breakdown and frequent UTIs that further aggravate spasticity and spasms. In these severely disabled patients, ITB therapy dramatically reduces spasticity and spasms in more than 90% of cases nonresponsive to conservative management and oral medications. Importantly, side effects from baclofen are minimal because it is concentrated in the thoracolumbar CSF, and many patients can discontinue centrally acting and sedating medications after the ITB pump is implanted and the dose titrated.

ITB therapy is also beneficial in a selected group of ambulatory patients with severe spasticity. Generally, in these patients the disease must be relatively stable and the patients able to transfer and walk after receiving a screening injection of ITB through a lumbar puncture. This patient population does not tolerate higher doses of ITB therapy, and screening injections should be administered at one half (25 μg) or one fourth (12.5 μg) the recommended screening dose. Implantation of a pump and use of intrathecal baclofen should be done at experienced centers to optimize outcome.

Bladder Dysfunction

Eighty percent of MS patients experience significant bladder dysfunction at some point in their illness. Fifty percent of mildly affected MS patients demonstrate abnormalities amenable to treatment early in their disease course. Bladder dysfunction results in restricted social, vocational, and leisure activities, disruption of sleep, UTI, kidney and bladder stone formation, and renal disease and interferes with normal sexual activities. There are three com-

*Not FDA approved for this indication.

mon categories of neurogenic bladder dysfunction observed in the MS patient: (1) failure to store urine (small capacity or irritable bladder); (2) failure to empty urine (large capacity, atonic bladder, or failure to relax the urinary sphincter); and (3) combined failure to store and failure to empty urine (usually due to an irritable bladder, and inability to relax the urinary sphincter, termed *detrusor-sphincter dyssynergia [DSD]*). An accurate diagnosis cannot be made by history alone. Bladder management strategies are most effective when the underlying bladder pathophysiology has been fully defined. All three categories of bladder dysfunction may produce urgency and frequency, nocturia, and urge incontinence. Similarly, hesitancy may imply an inability to relax the urinary sphincter or poor bladder contractions. Therefore, a history of bladder symptoms in an MS patient requires testing. The initial evaluation consists of a urinalysis. If the urinalysis shows evidence of infection, a culture should be obtained and appropriate antibiotics initiated. If symptoms do not clear after a course of antibiotics or no infection is found, a measurement of voided volume and post-void urinary residual volume should be obtained. Optimally, this measurement should be made when the bladder is full and when the patient experiences the usual urge to void. Table 4 outlines our management approach based on this testing. If the post-void residual volume is high, one cannot distinguish a hypotonic bladder from DSD or from mechanical outlet obstruction. However, one can empirically manage the patient with high residual volume. Management should be initially directed at DSD, because this is much more common in MS patients than bladder hypotonia. Second, both scenarios require intermittent catheterization (ISC) at least temporarily. If initial management strategies fail or the patient is reluctant to perform ISC, urodynamic studies will be necessary.

Patients with significant symptoms should cut down on caffeinated beverages. Fluid restriction should be discouraged. Patients should be encouraged to acidify their urine with cranberry juice daily to avoid UTIs. Patients with frequent UTIs despite good hygiene and catheterization technique require a complete urologic evaluation. Prophylactic antibiotics should be avoided unless all other measures fail. It has been our experience that suprapubic catheters, at least in women, do not prevent UTIs; our experience with catheterization in men is too limited to form an opinion.

Severe cases of nocturia unresponsive to evening fluid restriction, anticholinergic medications, and ISC at bedtime usually respond to desmopressin acetate nasal spray (DDAVP), 0.1 to 0.2 mL (10–20 μg) given at bedtime. Desmopressin is well tolerated and rarely results in a significant drop in serum sodium levels. Nevertheless, sodium levels should be monitored weekly for 2 weeks then every 3 months.

Bowel Dysfunction

Constipation is common in MS patients. The etiology is multifactorial with poor dietary habits, immobility, fluid restriction, and concurrent medications (e.g., anticholinergics) contributing significantly. Laxatives should be avoided, if possible. Bowel incontinence is relatively rare in patients with mild to moderate MS. Addition of an anticholinergic medication, particularly hyoscyamine (Levsin), may decrease excessive bowel motility. Patients should be counseled to defecate at regular intervals, preferably 30 to 60 minutes after eating when the gastrocolic reflex occurs.

Sexual Dysfunction

Sexual dysfunction is common in even mild cases and does not invariably co-exist with bladder or

TABLE 4. **Management of Bladder Dysfunction**

	Failure to Store	Failure to Empty	Combined*
Void Volume	200–300 mL	<200 mL	100–300 mL
Post-Void Residual Volume	<100 mL	>300 mL	100–300 mL
Treatment	1. Anticholinergics: oxybutynin (Ditropan), 2.5 mg bid to 5.0 mg tid *or* propantheline (Pro-Banthine),† 15 mg tid to 30 mg qid *or* hyoscyamine (Anaspaz)† (time release), 0.375 mg bid to tid *or* Tolterodine (Detrol), 2 mg bid 2. If ineffective, urodynamic testing	1. Intermittent catheterization 4 to 6 times per day 2. If ineffective add an anticholinergic 3. If ineffective urodynamic testing	1. α-Adrenergic blocker (also use ISC if post-void residual >200 mL) terazosin (Hytrin),† 1 mg qhs *or* clonidine (Catapres),† 0.05 mg bid to 0.1 mg bid‡ *or* imipramine (Tofranil), 10 to 25 mg tid 2. If ineffective add an anticholinergic 3. If ineffective urodynamic testing

*Combined failure to store and failure to empty is a complex management problem that benefits from early urodynamic testing to guide therapy.
†Not FDA approved for this indication.
‡May also use clonidine patches (TTS 0.1–0.3 mg) applied weekly.

bowel problems. Most MS patients do not spontaneously report sexual dysfunction, but many will readily report it with gentle direct questioning. Erectile dysfunction is the most common problem in men. Women commonly experience decreased libido, decreased perineal sensation, and decreased lubrication. The problem is often multifactorial. Involvement of the lower spinal cord may contribute to symptoms, but psychological factors such as depression and marital discord, as well as the effects of medications need to be considered. The treatment of erectile dysfunction in men with MS changed dramatically with the introduction of sildenafil (Viagra). Few of our patients have any of the known contraindications for therapy with this medication (i.e., cardiac disease), and most respond to doses of 50 to 100 mg taken 1 hour before intercourse. Unfortunately, there are still no medications of proven benefit for female sexual dysfunction in MS patients. Even with effective medical management available in our clinic, the treatment of sexual dysfunction in both men and women with MS often requires a comprehensive sexual dysfunction clinic to assess for secondary causes of sexual dysfunction and provide therapy and advice for sexual partners.

Tremor and Ataxia

Cerebellar tremor and ataxia are among the most disabling physical MS symptoms but are poorly responsive to drug therapy. Therefore, pharmacotherapy should always be buttressed by a rehabilitation approach. Occupational therapists can provide adaptive equipment to help maintain independence, and physical therapists can assist in gait training. Patients with a predominantly ataxic gait should be equipped with a rollator-type walker for safe ambulation.

Many drugs have been advocated as treatment for intention tremors in MS. In our experience, clonazepam (Klonopin) is the most effective and warrants a trial in most significantly affected patients. Before initiating treatment a simple trial of wrist weights should be tried. If weights are ineffective or only partially effective, we begin clonazepam at a dose of 0.5 mg given at bedtime. A morning and afternoon dose is gradually added over a period of 10 to 14 days. Thereafter, the daily dose is increased by 0.5 mg every 5 days, always beginning with the evening dose. The dose is gradually increased to an endpoint of effective control or unacceptable sedation. Rarely do patients tolerate doses in excess of 6 mg/d. Patients should be cautioned to discontinue clonazepam slowly.

Carefully selected patients may benefit from stereotactic ablation of the ventrolateral thalamic nucleus or implantation of a thalamic stimulator. The ablative procedure reduces the amplitude of tremor in the contralateral arm; complications include contralateral weakness and cortical deficits such as contralateral neglect or aphasia. Therefore, stereotactic thalamotomy should only be done in neurosurgical centers with demonstrated experience. We have performed this procedure in more than 20 MS patients in the past 10 years. In most cases tremor was dramatically decreased or eliminated. Most of the patients developed some degree of weakness in the contralateral limbs, and ambulatory patients found it more difficult to walk.

Thalamic stimulators are currently preferable to ablative procedures. The incidence of postoperative hemiparesis is extremely low when performed in experienced centers. The disadvantage of thalamic stimulators is the need for frequent visits to adjust the stimulator settings. Without these periodic adjustments, patients often re-develop tremor.

Ideal candidates for thalamic stimulators have relatively stable MS, have a moderate to severe proximal tremor of an upper extremity that limits activities of daily living, and have relatively preserved strength and sensation in the affected limb.

Fatigue

Classically, MS-related fatigue is described as a feeling of exhaustion that comes on with exertion, usually late in the day. The pathophysiology is unclear because patients can display significant fatigue in the absence of demonstrable motor dysfunction. Patients should first be evaluated for specific causes of fatigue that are amenable to specific treatments, including coexisting medical conditions such as thyroid disease or anemia, primary or secondary sleep disorders (the later includes frequent awakening due to nocturia), depression, and aggravating medications. If no alternative etiology can be found, the patient may benefit from amantadine (Symmetrel),* 100 mg in the morning and early afternoon. Recently, modafinil (Provigil),* a selective wakefulness agent approved for the treatment of narcolepsy, has been shown to benefit MS-related fatigue without significant side effects in doses of 400 mg or less every morning. The mechanism of action is unclear, but it appears to have far fewer side effects than typical CNS stimulants. We generally prescribe modafinal as a second-line agent in patients nonresponsive to amantadine. The dose is initiated at 100 mg orally every morning and increased to a maximum of 400 mg as needed. The most common side effect is headache.

Other CNS stimulants, such as pemoline (Cylert)* or methylphenidate (Ritalin),* have been prescribed for the treatment of MS-related fatigue for many years despite a lack of controlled trials demonstrating a significant degree of efficacy. We currently consider these medications as a third-line option in severe refractory cases of MS-related fatigue nonresponsive to comprehensive management or first- and second-line agents. All patients should be re-evaluated for alternative causes of fatigue, especially depression and the use of sedating medications. Medical management should be supplemented with a

*Not FDA approved for this indication.

regular exercise program to enhance aerobic capacity and endurance.

Heat Sensitivity

MS symptoms frequently worsen or recur in the heat, and increased ambient temperature may lead to exhaustion. This arises from conduction failure in partially demyelinated axons. Air conditioning may be required for almost all environments during the summer. If troublesome neurologic symptoms occur due to overheating, we advise cool showers or baths until the symptoms subside. Fevers from infections should be treated promptly with antipyretics and, if necessary, cooling blankets. Some individuals who are dramatically heat sensitive or have occupations that preclude air conditioning (e.g., factory or construction workers) benefit from custom-fitted cooling vests. The local chapter of the National MS Society should be able to provide information about available vendors in your area.

Pain Syndromes

Pain syndromes are very common in MS patients and can be separated into four broad categories: (1) neuralgia; (2) pain from meningeal irritation; (3) centrally mediated dysesthesias; and (4) secondary musculoskeletal pain. The dorsal root entry zone of virtually any peripheral or cranial sensory nerve may become irritated by an MS plaque, creating neuralgia. This sharp, lancinating pain occurs spontaneously or is triggered by certain movements or tactile stimulation within the distribution of the affected nerve. Trigeminal neuralgia is a classic example, but glossopharyngeal neuralgia and occipital neuralgia are quite common. MS plaques in the cervical spinal cord may produce a pseudoradicular pain, which can be difficult to differentiate from spondylitic radiculopathy. In addition to paroxysmal, neuralgic pain, MS patients may experience constant, severe, aching pain in the same sensory distribution as the neuralgia. At times this type of pain is more difficult to treat than the neuralgia. For neuralgia, we begin treatment with gabapentin (Neurontin) at a dose of 100 mg three times a day and increase the dosage as tolerated to a maximum of 3600 mg/d in three or four divided doses. For a second-line agent we usually use carbamazepine (Tegretal),* often in combination with gabapentin, beginning at a dose of 100 to 200 mg twice daily. The dose is titrated to pain relief or until unacceptable toxicity occurs. For patients who do not respond to or cannot tolerate carbamazepine,* an alternative is monotherapy with phenytoin,* (Dilantin),* amitriptyline (Elavil),* or baclofen (Lioresal).* Patients who do not respond to medications frequently respond to percutaneous rhizotomy.

Pain from meningeal irritation frequently occurs during episodes of optic neuritis or transverse myelitis in which the pain-sensitive dura is stretched or inflamed by involvement of adjacent optic nerve or spinal cord, respectively. Because this usually occurs during acute episodes of inflammation, we treat this pain with high doses of intravenous corticosteroids (see section on MS exacerbations).

Spontaneous dysesthesias, usually of a burning quality, are common and difficult to treat. At times, dysesthesia is accompanied by temperature and vasomotor changes in the limb, suggesting sympathetically mediated pain. Unfortunately, local blocks to sympathetic ganglia are not usually effective. Gabapentin,* tricyclic antidepressants,* and carbamazepine* are the most effective drugs for dysesthesias. The dosage should be increased gradually to allow patients time to develop tolerance to side effects. Doses of 150 to 200 mg/d of amitriptyline* are commonly required. We have had no success with mexilitine. Occasional patients with severe refractory pain may require perphenazine (Trilafon)* or fluphenazine (Prolixin)* in combination with amitriptyline,* although the risk of tardive dyskinesia should be considered.

Musculoskeletal pains, frequently in the lumbar spine, hip, knees, or shoulders, are common in patients with abnormal gait, poor sitting posture, or weakness in the upper extremities. Treatment must be directed at the underlying cause. Lumbar back pain in ambulatory patients should initially be treated with exercise to strengthen the paraspinal and abdominal muscles. Some patients too weak to benefit from exercises may benefit from an elastic lumbar corset. Gait training may improve posture and pain in selected patients. Nonsteroidal anti-inflammatory drugs, with or without a transcutaneous electrical nerve stimulation (TENS) unit, may relieve pain enough for patients to undergo physical therapy. Narcotics should be avoided except for short courses to control acute exacerbations of pain. Wheelchair-bound patients with lumbar pain may benefit from a lumbar roll or other types of lumbar support. In many cases, custom cushions for the wheelchair are effective in relieving pain.

Knee and hip pain are common in patients with a spastic gait, especially with a footdrop. Custom-fitted ankle-foot orthotic devices not only improve ambulation but also relieve pain in the majority of patients. If a well-fitted ankle-foot orthosis fails to relieve knee pain, the addition of a Swedish knee cage or Don Joy brace will further alleviate hyperextension at the knee joint. Unfortunately, patients who hyperextend the knee to compensate for weak knee extensor muscles may not be able to walk with a knee brace that prevents hyperextension.

Frozen shoulders from acute or chronic tendinitis are common in wheelchair-dependent or bedridden MS patients. This must be treated aggressively to preserve residual upper extremity function. Patients should receive intra-articular infiltration with a glucocorticoid combined with an anesthetic to allow aggressive physical therapy. Stretching exercises

*Not FDA approved for this indication.

*Not FDA approved for this indication.

should be continued indefinitely to prevent further recurrences. Hip pain is also common and may be a result of avascular necrosis of the femoral heads, particularly in patients receiving frequent pulses of corticosteroids. If the hip pain does not respond to conservative management, MRI of the femoral heads must be done to evaluate for this possibility.

Lastly, MS patients experience an accelerated rate of osteoporosis from a combination of immobility and corticosteroid treatments. Patients at risk (postmenopausal females, all patients with decreased ambulation ability, and patients receiving repetitive pulses of corticosteroids) should receive prophylactic treatment with calcium supplementation, vitamin D, and hormonal replacement, as appropriate. Yearly bone mineral density studies of the lumbar spine and femoral heads should be obtained to monitor bone density and determine the need for specific osteoporosis treatment. Patients with persistent poorly explained bone pain should be evaluated for fractures related to osteoporosis.

Paroxysmal Motor Symptoms

Paroxysmal motor phenomena are common in MS. The classic type has been variously described as *tonic spasms* or *tonic seizures*, the later term deriving from the superficial resemblance to focal motor seizures. During a spasm, one arm is forcibly contorted in a dystonic flexion posture while the ipsilateral leg is unaffected or forcibly extended. These spasms last seconds, occur repeatedly, and are frequently painful. Gabapentin* and carbamazepine* are both remarkably effective at controlling these spasms, even at subtherapeutic, anticonvulsant doses. We use the same dosing regimens described previously for these medications. For minor symptoms without pain, the dose can be increased more slowly. Patients unable to tolerate or poorly responsive to gabapentin or carbamazepine* may respond to phenytoin (Dilantin)* or, rarely, baclofen. We usually continue treatment for 6 months and then gradually taper the medication. The spasms do not usually require long-term treatment.

Other forms of paroxysmal motor phenomenon are less common in MS patients. Hemifacial spasm, a forceful, grimacing contortion of one side of the face, responds to the same treatments as tonic spasms. Rarely, patients describe "drop attacks" where their legs suddenly go out from underneath them with no warning. Because this complaint is so rare, it is unclear whether this phenomenon represents bilateral, tonic extensor spasms of the leg.

True seizures occur in 5% of MS patients, usually late in the course of the disease. A diagnostic evaluation to exclude alternative etiologies, including MRI with and without contrast medium and, sometimes, CSF analysis, should be performed after the first seizure. Seizures should be treated in the same manner as other symptomatic seizure disorders.

*Not FDA approved for this indication.

Vertigo, Nystagmus, Oscillopsia

Vertigo or dizziness may be disabling in MS. Acute vertigo is usually observed in the setting of a brainstem exacerbation. Treatment consists of intravenous corticosteroids combined with a 1- to 2-week course of a vestibular suppressant. We prefer diazepam (Valium) at a dose of 2 to 5 mg thrice daily. Residual vestibular symptoms may respond to vestibular rehabilitation exercises. Chronic ill-defined dizziness is much more difficult to treat. Vestibular testing may be helpful in clarifying the underlying pathophysiology. Alternate diagnoses, such as Meniere disease, benign positional vertigo, or cerebellopontine angle tumor are rarely found.

Abnormal eye movements, such as nystagmus, may degrade vision and create an illusory motion of the visual environment termed *oscillopsia*. Pharmacotherapy is generally ineffective, but one trial reported that gabapentin did help stabilize images. Some patients may benefit from optical stabilization devices, available at specialized neuro-ophthalmologic centers. Effective treatment can have a profoundly beneficial effect on the patient's quality of life.

Affective Disorders and Emotional Distress

Emotional distress is common in MS and tends to occur in response to a perceived loss or threat. Although this can occur at any time, it is most common at diagnosis, when symptoms become persistent rather than intermittent, and with the development of significant disability. It is often difficult to identify major depression in MS patients. Symptoms may overlap with certain MS-related symptoms such as fatigue, diminished attention and concentration, and pain. We have a very low threshold for exploring emotional issues, referring patients to a psychologist, and treating with antidepressants. We generally prefer the use of the selective serotonin reuptake inhibitor (SSRI) class of antidepressants. For patients with prominent sleep disruption we often add a small bedtime dose of trazodone (Desyrel)* 25 to 50 mg, for the first 4 to 8 weeks of therapy with any SSRI. For patients with pain syndromes or decreased libido with fluoxetine (Prozac), sertraline (Zoloft), paroxetine (Paxil), or citalopram (Celexa), we generally prefer the use of venlafaxine (Effexor). Lastly, for patients with prominent sleep disturbances and weight loss, we will often begin with mirtazapine (Remeron) or an older tricylic antidepressant, such as amitriptyline or nortriptyline (Pamelor). In fact, the tricylic antidepressants are often preferred if the anticholinergic effects are required to improve urgency and nocturia from a neurogenic bladder.

Bipolar disorders are 15 times more common in MS patients than in the general population. In rare cases an organic bipolar disorder is triggered by dis-

*Not FDA approved for this indication.

ease involving the mesial temporal lobes. Treatment is no different from that used to treat bipolar disorders in the general population. Emotional lability, so-called pathologic laughing and crying, is less common than depression but equally disabling. This tends to occur with extensive frontal lobe white matter disease. It is usually controllable with an SSRI or low doses of amitriptyline (i.e., 25 to 75 mg at bedtime).

Cognitive Impairment

MS-related cognitive impairment can be demonstrated in approximately 50% of patients. It is generally circumscribed rather than global; recent memory and information processing are most commonly affected. Cognitive impairment may have a devastating impact on everyday function, including activities at school, work, and home. It is important to consider the possibility of cognitive impairment in an MS patient who is having difficulty with any of his or her roles if the severity of motor or visual impairment is inadequate to explain the problems. Neuropsychological testing is required to determine the extent and type of cognitive impairment. Although there is no current specific drug treatment for cognitive impairment, it is important to accurately diagnose the problem for vocational and educational planning.

DISEASE-SPECIFIC TREATMENTS

Disease Classification and Relationship to Disease-Specific Therapies

Traditionally, MS is classified on the basis of clinical characteristics alone. Eighty-five percent of cases are initially classified as relapsing-remitting. All currently approved, disease-specific therapies are partially effective in the treatment of relapsing forms of MS. There is some recent evidence that those therapies are also effective in nonrelapsing forms of MS, but generally progressive disease is more difficult to control.

Patients with relapsing MS experience, on average, one relapse per year followed by some degree of spontaneous recovery. By definition, the presence of a relapse implies new or recurrent inflammation in the CNS. As pointed out previously, most new or recurrent episodes of inflammation do not result in a clinical relapse, however. Over time, patients tend to experience less frequent relapses, and many patients enter a more steadily progressive phase, termed *secondary progressive MS*. Even during the early secondary progressive phase of the disease, as currently defined, relapses may continue. At any stage in the illness it may be difficult even for an experienced clinician to determine if a patient is truly experiencing a relapse. Most patients experience periods of time when they are more symptomatic than other times and often consider these episodes as relapses. If patients are left to define relapses, they will often tell you that their relapses occur as frequently as once a month. If therapies are intended to treat new or recurrent inflammation, it is obviously a problem if the outcome patients use to monitor their treatment correlates poorly with the extent and severity of inflammation. Objective criteria for defining relapses help resolve this issue, but these criteria underestimate the true extent of disease activity. The best current definition of a relapse is the development of new or recurrent symptoms in the presence of neurologic stability for at least 1 month and the absence of an identifiable confounding condition that can lead to an increase in MS-related symptoms, such as a febrile illness or a UTI. In most cases the symptoms will develop steadily over a period of hours or days (80% of patients develop maximal symptoms and deficits within 2 weeks of onset and more than 90% do so within 1 month) with no significant resolution of symptoms for at least 48 hours. However, it is not unusual for patients to awaken with a fully developed relapse. When the symptoms are primarily sensory (especially the combination of paresthesia and fatigue) there may be little, if any, change on examination. To be certain that a relapse is occurring, there must be changes on examination that are consistent with the patient's symptoms or the symptoms must follow some recognizable pattern. The latter could include the report of ascending paresthesia to the waist with a "tight band" sensation around the trunk, even in the absence of changes on examination.

Regardless of the definition used for a relapse, it is important to remember three important pieces of the puzzle when selecting and monitoring patients on disease-specific therapies. First, the pathogenic mechanisms underlying the relapse may be different from one patient to next. In most patients cell-mediated immunity appears to be the predominant mechanism of inflammation, whereas tissue analysis from other patients reveals immunoglobulin-mediated tissue damage. It is reasonable to expect that patients with different mechanisms of inflammation require different treatment approaches. But until we can characterize the underlying mechanism in individual patients ex vivo, we must take an empirical approach to our treatment strategies based on clinical and MRI features.

Second, symptomatic relapses occur only when new or recurrent inflammation develops in a clinically eloquent area of the CNS, such as the optic nerve, brainstem, or spinal cord. Most new areas of inflammation occur in clinically silent areas of the brain such as the centrum semiovale or periventricular regions. When monthly MRI is done on relapsing MS patients, new or recurrent areas of inflammation by imaging criteria occur 7 to 10 times more frequently than clinically defined relapses. Therefore, it is important to supplement clinical monitoring of relapses and disease progression with serial MRI to assess a patient's response to therapy.

Third, the presence or absence of inflammatory activity is only partially responsible for clinical activity and severity of MS. Patients experience a variable degree of permanent tissue injury as a result of this inflammatory activity. Permanent tissue injury correlates better with physical disability and can now be monitored by MRI techniques. As the disease progresses and patients enter the secondary progressive phase, these areas of permanent tissue injury increase, whereas new areas of inflammation on MRI become less common or cease. Therefore, it is possible that the disease begins only as an inflammatory process with superimposed axonal injury and tissue loss related to the severity and extent of inflammation. Eventually, evidence of ongoing inflammation ceases, although patients experience worsening symptoms as a result of ongoing axonal and neuronal degeneration.

This new understanding of the varied pathogenic mechanisms underlying disease severity and progression is extremely important in selecting patients for treatment and in determining the response to treatment. First of all, relapses are a poor marker of disease activity and severity. Although it is true that patients with high rates of relapses (e.g., three or more per year) have a greater probability of experiencing more severe disease in a shorter period of time, the vast majority of patients experience only occasional relapses but still enter into a progressive phase of neurologic deterioration. Cerebral MRI helps to determine the true activity of the disease and the risk of disease progression. Those patients with enhancing lesions on random MRI have a greater probability of experiencing short-term disease activity. Furthermore, those patients accumulating new T2 lesions with a higher T2 lesion burden of disease have a greater probability of displaying evidence of cognitive dysfunction and eventually entering a progressive phase of the disease. Lastly, those patients with a greater degree or rate of parenchymal tissue destruction during the relapsing phase are more likely to enter into the secondary progressive phase of the disease in the shortest amount of time.

But how do we use this information to select patients for therapy and monitor their response to therapy? First, all current therapies are preventative not restorative. Therefore, disease-specific therapies must be initiated early, often before a patient has any outwardly obvious evidence of disease. To wait until the disease appears more severe or until the patient demonstrates a certain degree of symptomatic disease activity only limits the ability of the therapy to prevent an event that has already occurred. Second, clinical and MR characteristics in an individual patient must be used to set appropriate expectations for therapy. The ideal candidate for current disease-specific monotherapy has early relapsing disease, little if any disability, and a low T2 lesion burden. For these patients, it is reasonable to set a goal of completely preventing the development of any significant disability, although many will require proactive monitoring, and the use of combination therapies to reach this goal. On the other hand, patients with long-standing disease, large T2 lesion burdens on MRI, evidence of progressive disease, fulminant clinical features such as rapid progression from onset often accompanied by evidence of severe widespread inflammation on MRI, or significant cerebral atrophy are unlikely to demonstrate more than a partial response to monotherapy. These patients have features that are more difficult to manage and often benefit from consultation with an expert in MS-specific therapies.

Lastly, it is important to monitor the response to disease-specific therapy using both clinical observation and serial MRI. Yearly cranial MRI is often the only means of detecting subclinical disease activity signifying an inadequate response to monotherapy. Ideally, serial MRI should be done with and without Gd enhancement using repositioning protocols and identical imaging techniques to assist in the comparison of serial images.

Treatment of Exacerbations

Corticotropin and high-dose intravenous methylprednisolone (Solu-Medrol) have been documented in controlled trials to hasten recovery from acute exacerbations of MS. Evidence suggests that high-dose intravenous methylprednisolone may have a more rapid onset of action and may be more effective over time than other corticosteroid preparations. Furthermore, conventional doses of oral prednisone alone (1 mg/kg/d) in a study of optic neuritis were associated with an increased recurrence rate of optic neuritis in the same or opposite eye. The similarities between monosymptomatic optic neuritis and exacerbations in established MS should make physicians pause before prescribing conventional doses of oral prednisone alone in MS patients. Our current practice is to treat most patients with verifiable relapses regardless of the degree of functional impairment. However, physicians should resist the temptation to treat patients with corticosteroids for symptom fluctuations without functional consequences. A period of observation or additional testing is often necessary to determine if a relapse is indeed the cause of the patient's symptoms. All patients should be seen and evaluated for alternative causes of neurologic decline, particularly UTIs. We use a standard protocol of intravenous methylprednisolone 1000 mg/d for 3 to 5 days. This is followed by a short course of oral prednisone beginning at 60 mg every morning and tapering the dose by 20 mg every 4 days. If clear deterioration occurs during the prednisone taper, the dose is increased to 60 mg/d and tapered over 6 weeks. Prednisone tapers of longer duration should be avoided if possible. This protocol has been well tolerated and safely administered in the outpatient setting. Patients are hospitalized if they have concurrent medical conditions requiring close monitoring during intravenous treatment with methylprednisolone, such as diabetes, severe hypertension, or coronary artery disease.

Patients are also hospitalized for severe exacerbations resulting in the loss of independent function (i.e., ambulatory patients no longer able to walk).

Common side effects include a metallic taste during the infusion, gastrointestinal upset or rarely ulcers, insomnia, flushing, a temporary increase in blood pressure, fluid retention, weight gain, easy bruising, muscle pains (usually during the prednisone taper), and hiccups. We commonly prescribe ranitidine (Zantac) or another H2 blocker as a single bedtime dose during the entire 15 days of corticosteroid treatment. Patients with insomnia should be given appropriate sedation with a short-acting hypnotic. Diuretics should be avoided because of the risk of electrolyte imbalances. Edema is best managed with tight stockings, fluid restriction, and leg elevation. Rarely, patients experience significant depression, mania, or psychosis during or after treatment with corticosteroids. Premedication with trazadone (Desyrel), lithium, or an antipsychotic drug is usually effective at preventing recurrent episodes with repeated corticosteroid courses.

Preventative Therapy for Relapsing Forms of MS

Three drugs—recombinant interferon beta-1a (IFN-β1a, Avonex), recombinant IFN-β1b (Betaseron), and glatiramer acetate (Copaxone)—are approved for marketing in the United States based on efficacy and safety data from phase III clinical trials. An additional formulation of recombinant IFN-β1a (Rebif)* has been approved in Canada, Europe, and other parts of the world but is not currently approved in the United States. This discussion only applies to therapies currently approved by the U.S. Food and Drug Administration.

All phase III trials of disease-specific therapies involved somewhat different study populations and different primary outcome measures. Because of the differences in trial design, direct comparison of study outcomes is problematic. In the following section the primary outcome results from the major phase III trials are summarized. This is followed by editorial commentary by the authors regarding their thoughts on the use of these agents.

Beta Interferons

Interferon beta-1b (Betaseron) was tested in 372 patients given 8 million units (250 μg), 1.6 million units (50 μg), or placebo by subcutaneous injection every other day for up to 5 years. The primary outcome was a comparison of relapse rates between the three groups. Higher dose IFN-β1b reduced relapses by 33% and reduced the number of moderate or severe relapses by 50%. These effects were maintained in patients continuing under double-blind conditions for up to 5 years. Importantly, IFN-β1b therapy resulted in a significant reduction in new or enlarging T2 lesions and reduced the accumulation of T2 lesion burden on MRI. The results of this study led to the approval of the 8 million-unit dose of IFN-β1b to reduce the frequency of relapses in ambulatory RRMS patients. This was the first agent approved for the treatment of RRMS.

IFN-β1a (Avonex) was tested in 301 patients given weekly intramuscular injections of IFN-β1a (6 million units, 30 μg) or placebo for up to 2 years. The primary outcome for this study was a comparison of the rate of sustained disability progression as a result of incomplete recovery from relapses or progressive disease. Sustained disability progression was defined as worsening from baseline Expanded Disability Status Score (EDSS) by at least 1 point sustained for at least 6 months. IFN-β1a therapy resulted in a 37% reduction in the rate of sustained disability progression compared with placebo. IFN-β1a therapy also reduced the relapse rate, the number of new or enlarging T2 lesions at 1 and 2 years, and the number and volume of Gd-enhanced lesions at 1 and 2 years.

More recently, IFN-β1a was testing in patients at risk to develop MS after the first clinical demyelinating event involving optic nerve, brainstem/cerebellum, or spinal cord with at least two asymptomatic white matter abnormalities on cranial MRI. The study was designed to test effectiveness of therapy initiated at the first opportunity. The goal was to determine if IFN-β1a therapy could forestall development of clinically definite multiple sclerosis (CDMS) in this high-risk population and if treatment would be acceptable to patients who did not, as yet, carry a diagnosis of definite MS or have significant neurologic deficits. IFN-β1a therapy decreased the rate of CDMS by 44% and was well tolerated. Most importantly, patients on IFN therapy who did not develop CDMS experienced a significant reduction in disease activity measured by MRI. This was the first study to demonstrate the benefits of initiating therapy early, even before a definitive diagnosis can be rendered by traditional clinical diagnostic criteria.

Management of Side Effects of Interferon Therapy

The major side effect of IFN therapy is the "flulike syndrome." This usually begins 4 to 8 hours after subcutaneous or intramuscular injection and may persist until the next day. This syndrome consists of a variable combination of headache, fever, muscle aches, chills, anorexia, insomnia, weight loss, lassitude, or fatigue. When therapy is first initiated, flulike symptoms may persist up to 48 hours. Sixty percent of patients experience some degree of flulike symptoms at the onset of therapy, but only 10% experience persistent symptoms 3 months after starting treatment. In most cases symptoms are controlled with acetaminophen (Tylenol) or a nonsteroidal anti-inflammatory agent. In some cases, initiating therapy at one-half dose and increasing the dose over 4 to

*Not available in the United States.

12 weeks will minimize flulike symptoms commonly associated with therapy.

Injection site reactions occur frequently with subcutaneously administered IFN but are rare with intramuscular injections. Injection site reactions tend to be more persistent than flulike symptoms. In approximately 5% of cases, skin reactions to subcutaneous IFN-β results in skin necrosis. The more common skin reactions consist of swelling and redness, which is sometimes painful or pruritic but respond well to icing, antihistamines, or topical corticosteroids. Additional occasional side effects of IFN-β injections include elevated serum transaminase levels, neutropenia, leukopenia, anemia, palpitations, or menstrual irregularities. Hepatic transaminase elevations appear to be more common with IFN-β1b but rarely require discontinuation of therapy.

All interferons commonly increase spasticity transiently in patients with moderate to severe disability or significant spasticity before initiating therapy. This is best managed with gradual dose escalation and adjustment of antispasticity medications.

There are reports that IFN therapy may worsen psoriasis or result in hyperthyroidism. The latter is more common in patients with pre-existing thyroid disease.

Neurobehavioral side effects including irritability, anxiety, depression, suicidal ideation, paranoid ideation, or delirium are rare but usually result in drug discontinuation. Depression is best managed with SSRIs (i.e., fluoxetine) and temporary reduction in dosage. Patients should be closely monitored and treatment discontinued if a prompt response to treatment does not occur.

Glatiramer Acetate

Glatiramer acetate (Copaxone) is a mixture of synthetic polypeptides composed of four amino acids—L-alanine, L-glutamic acid, L-lysine, and L-tyrosine—in a molar ratio of 4.2, 1.4, 3.4, and 1.0, respectively. It was first synthesized at the Weizmann Institute of Science in Israel in 1967. The exact mechanism of action is unknown. Proposed mechanisms in MS include binding to Class II major histocompatibility complex with consequent inhibition of myelin-reactive T cells or generation of glatiramer-specific T cells that cross react with myelin antigens and inhibit the inflammatory response.

Glatiramer acetate was tested in 251 patients given daily subcutaneous injections of the active drug, 20 mg, or placebo for 2 years. The primary outcome was the effect of treatment on relapse rate. The original 2-year study reported a 29% reduction in relapse rates in glatiramer acetate–treated patients. The majority of patients continued in a 1-year blinded extension of the 2-year phase III trial. The reduction in relapse rates was maintained during this additional year of observation.

MRI was only performed on a small number of patients at one site participating in the U.S. phase III trial. No significant treatment effects were noted in this small population. Subsequently, a European trial was organized to determine the effect of glatiramer acetate on monthly, Gd-enhanced MRI. Eligibility for this study was restricted to patients with relapsing-remitting MS and at least one Gd-enhanced lesion on pre-study MRI obtained 1 month before study entry. Patients were randomized to receive glatiramer acetate (20 mg/d subcutaneously) or placebo for 9 months followed by an open-label phase where all patients received glatiramer acetate. MRI was obtained monthly during the 9-month placebo-controlled phase and then every 3 months for an additional 9 months. The primary outcome—a comparison of the total number of Gd-enhanced lesions during the 9-month placebo controlled phase—demonstrated a 30% to 35% reduction of total enhancing lesions. Similar reductions were reported for new enhancing lesions and new T2 lesions. This study demonstrated that the effect of glatiramer acetate on MRI measures of disease activity required 4 to 6 months to develop. Continued observation did not show any further increase in the MRI effect at 18 months. Similarly, a significant reduction in relapse rates did not occur until the last 3 months of the study (months 6–9). This study suggested that therapeutic effects from glatiramer acetate required months to develop.

Management of Glatiramer Acetate Side Effects

Glatiramer acetate is generally well tolerated. Mild skin reactions occur in the majority of patients and can include swelling or tenderness, both managed with ice and topical corticosteroid preparation. With prolonged administration patients may develop focal lipodystrophy at injection sites. The exact incidence of this reaction is unknown. Approximately 15% of patients experience a systemic reaction post injection that consists of flushing, shortness of breath, palpitations, diaphoresis, and anxiety. The exact cause of this reaction is unknown. It can occur early in therapy or much later. In some patients it recurs, and in others it is a one-time event. Fortunately, this reaction is self-limited, lasts only minutes, and has never been associated with any significant sequelae. However, patients should be educated about this potential reaction to avoid undue panic or concern, if it should occur. They should also be advised to seek medical attention if similar symptoms should occur and last more than a few minutes.

Commentary: Therapies for Relapsing-Remitting MS

There are now three disease-specific therapies approved in the United States for the prophylactic treatment of relapsing-remitting MS (RRMS): IFN-β1b (Betaseron), IFN-β1a (Avonex), and glatiramer acetate (Copaxone). All three therapies have demonstrated a reduction in relapse rates, a decrease in MRI measures of disease activity, and good long-term tolerability and safety. Nevertheless, there are differences between the three therapies that raise important questions when selecting the most appropriate therapy for any individual patient.

First, how should IFN-β therapy be selected, because two agents are currently available? It is our opinion that current evidence supports the use of IFN-β1a over IFN-β1b in IFN-naïve recipients. Most patients choose IFN-β1a over IFN-β1b because of the ease of once-a-week administration and the absence of skin reactions. But are there biologic reasons to select one interferon over the other? Unlike IFN-β1b, IFN-β1a is completely identical to human IFN-β and associated with low incidence (2% to 5%) of neutralizing antibody (NAB) formation. In contrast, IFN-β1b is a nonglycosylated, serine-substituted version of IFN-β that is prone to aggregate formation and associated with a high incidence (>30%) of NAB formation. Mounting evidence indicates that NAB to IFN-β that persist in the blood interfere with the biologic effects and clinical benefits of therapy. Additionally, many NABs are cross reactive and may neutralize the effect of other preparations of interferon. Therefore, it is most reasonable to initiate therapy with a less immunogenic preparation of IFN. Because NABs rarely develop after 18 months of therapy, patients who are doing well on IFN-β1b should continue on this therapy.

Second, how do you choose between interferon and glatiramer acetate treatment in naïve recipients? Both IFN-β and glatiramer acetate are appropriate first-line agents based on FDA approval for RRMS. Both therapies demonstrated a similar reduction in relapse rates. However, the effects on MRI parameters of disease activity appear to be different and may favor IFN therapy. Multiple studies of both IFN-β1a and IFN-β1b have shown a rapid, sustained 70% to 90% reduction in Gd-enhanced lesions and T2-weighted lesion activity. In contrast, a single study of glatiramer acetate demonstrated an MR effect of treatment that was delayed in onset and somewhat more modest in magnitude. Although it is difficult to compare the different study populations, these results raise the possibility that glatiramer acetate may be less effective than IFN therapy on MRI measures of disease activity. For these reasons, we usually initiate IFN-β1a in treatment of naïve-relapsing MS patients and use glatiramer acetate as an alternative therapy.

Disease-Specific Therapy for Early Secondary Progressive Multiple Sclerosis or Relapsing-Remitting MS Patients Worsening Despite Prophylactic Monotherapy

The clinical and pathologic distinction between late relapsing and early secondary progressive MS is ambiguous. Therefore, it is reasonable to assume that therapies effective in early relapsing MS may be effective in later stages of the disease, albeit with different expectations for a response to therapy. We have, therefore, combined this section to include treatment approaches for RRMS patients worsening despite monotherapy, as well as early secondary progressive MS patients worsening on monotherapy or naïve to monotherapy. There are no current therapies of demonstrated efficacy in the late secondary progressive phase of MS, defined as slow deterioration in the absence of relapses over many years with no evidence of inflammatory activity (Gd enhancement) on MRI.

The early secondary progressive phase of MS begins, on average, 10 years after onset of the relapsing-remitting phase, although there is wide variability in the time to disability progression. Ninety percent of relapsing patients eventually enter into this phase of the disease. The transition from relapsing-remitting to secondary progressive MS is often heralded by a period of instability with limited recovery from relapses with or without steady progression between relapses. Once the secondary progressive phase becomes readily identified, relapses tend to decrease in frequency or disappear altogether.

Treatment for this phase of MS is problematic. As mentioned previously, all currently approved therapies are preventative, but at this stage of the disease there is already considerable dissemination throughout the CNS and permanent tissue destruction. Whether administration of currently approved therapies as monotherapy in this patient population will result in clinically meaningful, long-term benefits is still unclear. Ideally, early administration of effective monotherapy may forestall the development of this phase. But it is unreasonable to expect all relapsing patients to remain stable on monotherapy with long-term observation even if therapy is initiated early.

So how do we approach therapy in this patient population? As always, we inform ourselves from the results of clinical trials. First, whenever possible therapy must begin early in the relapsing phase and patients must be monitored both clinically and by MRI. If a patient continues to deteriorate or show evidence of unacceptable disease activity on monotherapy, therapy with drug combinations must be considered. The selection and administration of combination therapies is currently an active area of clinical research. Therefore, patients should be referred to centers with active clinical research programs and expertise in monitoring and selecting appropriate regimens.

For patients naïve to treatment in the late relapsing or early secondary progressive phase, IFN therapy has demonstrated clinical benefits in phase III trials. This was demonstrated most clearly in the European phase III trial of IFN-β1b (Betaseron) for secondary progressive MS. Phase III trials of IFN-β1a (Rebif)* and IFN-β1a (Avonex) as well as a North American trial of IFN-β1b selected patients with disease characteristics more typical of the late secondary progressive phase. Not surprisingly, treatment

*Not available in the United States.

results appeared less robust at this stage of the disease.

Only one therapy, mitoxantrone (Novantrone), has been specifically approved for unstable relapsing MS despite monotherapy with IFNs or glatiramer acetate. The specific indication cited by the FDA in October 2000 approved mitoxantrone for "reducing neurologic disability and/or the frequency of clinical relapses in patients with secondary-progressive, progressive-relapsing or worsening relapsing-remitting MS." Mitoxantrone is a chemotherapeutic agent with potent effects on cellular and humoral immune mechanisms. In clinical trials, mitoxantrone treatment significantly reduced relapse rates, disability progression, and MRI measures of disease activity in active RRMS and secondary progressive MS. The major limitation of therapy is dose-dependent cardiac toxicity that limits the duration of therapy to approximately 2 years. Mitoxantrone therapy has also been associated with the development of leukemia in breast cancer patients receiving treatment in combination with radiation therapy and other chemotherapeutic agents. The risk of leukemia in MS patients receiving mitozantrone treatment is unclear at this time. Other common adverse effects include nausea, bone marrow suppression, amenorrhea, and infertility. Because of the potential toxicity, mitoxantrone should be prescribed by clinicians with expertise in MS treatments and administered by practitioners familiar with its use.

Smaller phase II studies suggest that bimonthly pulse therapy with intravenous methylprednisolone or low doses of oral methotrexate may slow disability progression in late relapsing or early secondary progressive MS. Also, several studies have reported benefits from pulse intravenous cyclophosphamide treatment in this phase of the disease. Generally, one of these options may be combined with IFN or glatiramer acetate therapy for patients showing evidence of continued disease activity despite monotherapy. However, until randomized controlled clinical trials are completed, it is not possible to provide evidence-based treatment recommendations for patients progressing despite approved monotherapy.

Treatment of Primary Progressive MS

This form of MS occurs in 15% of cases. Clinical, pathologic, MRI, and genetic differences between relapsing forms (relapsing-remitting and secondary progressive) and primary progressive MS (PPMS) suggest that this may be a different disease process. PPMS patients tend to be older at onset, more often male, to have few abnormalities on cranial MRI, and to not respond well to current disease-modifying therapies. Therapeutic approaches focus on rehabilitative strategies and experimental trials.

MYASTHENIA GRAVIS*

method of
DAVID S. SAPERSTEIN, M.D.
Wilford Hall U.S.A.F. Medical Center
San Antonio, Texas

and

RICHARD J. BAROHN, M.D.
University of Kansas Medical Center
Kansas City, Kansas

Myasthenia gravis (MG) is the best understood acquired autoimmune disorder of the nervous system. Antibodies directed against acetylcholine receptors (AChRs) on skeletal muscle produce weakness. Double vision and speech and swallowing difficulties are also common manifestations. Fluctuation and fatigue are clinical hallmarks of this disorder. Although, as with most diseases, the clinical history and physical examination are of paramount importance, specific serologic and electrophysiologic testing play an important role in facilitating the diagnosis. Pharmacologic manipulation of neuromuscular transmission and immune function is the cornerstone of management.

CLINICAL FEATURES AND NATURAL HISTORY

MG has a prevalence of approximately 125 cases/million population. Although this disease can occur at any age, MG peaks in the third and sixth decades. Overall, more females develop the disease (3:2 female to male ratio); however, males predominate among older patients.

MG is characterized by weakness and fatigability of ocular, bulbar, and extremity muscles. The ocular manifestations are ptosis and diplopia; respiratory manifestations consist of dysarthria, dysphagia, and dyspnea. In the extremities, proximal muscles are typically weaker than distal muscles. Although weakness occurring after repeated exercise or late in the day is regarded as a classic feature, such temporal symptoms are often not present.

MG usually begins with ocular symptoms (~80%), although the majority of patients will exhibit progression. One year after onset, the disease remains purely ocular in 40%, but over the course of follow-up, manifestations remain restricted to ocular muscles in only 15%. In other words, generalized weakness will develop in 85% of patients. If patients with ocular MG are going to experience progression, they usually do so relatively early. Among patients who present with purely ocular disease, generalized weakness develops in more than half by 6 months. If, after 3 years, a patient still has only ocular involvement, further progression is unlikely.

The initial onset of symptoms may be precipitated by systemic illness, such as thyroid disease or an upper respiratory infection. A number of medications may also invoke symptoms or worsen function in a patient with previously well-controlled MG (Table 1).

In recent years, mortality statistics for MG have improved significantly. Between 1940 and 1957, the mortality rate for MG was 31%, compared with only 7% from 1966 to 1985. The two primary reasons for this reduction in

*The views expressed herein are those of the authors and do not reflect the official policy of the United States Air Force or the Department of Defense.

TABLE 1. **Drugs That May Worsen Myasthenia Gravis**

Antibiotic agents
Aminoglycosides
Fluoroquinolones
Erythromycin and other macrolides
Tetracyclines
Sulfonamides
Clindamycin
Anesthetic agents
Neuromuscular blocking agents
Lidocaine
Procaine
Cardiovascular drugs
β-Blockers
Calcium channel blockers
Procainamide
Quinidine
Miscellaneous
Corticosteroids
Magnesium salts
Lithium
Neuroleptics
Iodinated radiographic contrast material

mortality are improvements in intensive respiratory care and the introduction of corticosteroids. In the 21st century, death from MG should be a rare event.

KEY POINTS IN BEDSIDE EVALUATION

On the cranial nerve examination, it is important to look for lid ptosis. We generally measure and record the maximum distance between the upper and lower eyelids (palpebral fissure) for each eye. Having the patient maintain upward gaze for several minutes can often bring about a decrease in the palpebral fissure (ptosis). Any restriction of ocular motility is noted, as is the development of diplopia. Testing for weakness in the orbicularis oculi muscle is often overlooked. Many patients with symptomatic MG have bilateral weakness of this muscle group. Strength should also be tested in the lower facial muscles (blowing out cheeks against resistance) and in the tongue. One should listen closely for dysarthria or nasal speech. Dysarthria may be provoked by having the patient read aloud.

Neck flexion and extension weakness are frequently present in MG. Some patients have dramatic neck extension weakness and present with head drop. These individuals may need to hold their head up by placing a hand under their chin. In other patients, neck weakness may be more subtle and should be tested in the supine (flexion) and prone (extension) positions against gravity and resistance.

DIAGNOSTIC TESTS FOR MYASTHENIA GRAVIS

In most instances, the clinician can be confident about the diagnosis of MG based on abnormalities brought out through the neurologic history and examination as previously noted. However, usually one or more tests are performed to support the clinical diagnosis of MG.

Edrophonium (Tensilon) Test

The intravenous (IV) administration of up to 10 mg of edrophonium is often the first diagnostic test performed in evaluating a potential MG patient. The edrophonium test, however, has a number of pitfalls. The most common mistake is that the physician performing the test does not have an objective parameter to follow. The most useful parameter is the degree of ptosis in each eye. The best indication of a positive test is a significant increase in the palpebral fissure distance, or if a completely closed eye opens up. Significant improvement in dysarthria is also a good yardstick for assessment.

If a patient simply reports a history of episodic ptosis or diplopia but the examination is normal or shows only mild proximal limb weakness, an edrophonium test will probably be of little use. Mild improvements in limb strength or subjective changes in diplopia or well-being are not sufficient to claim a positive test result. It is important to be aware that edrophonium can cause a transient improvement in other neurologic disorders such as motor neuron disease or peripheral neuropathy.

Even if there is a suitable parameter to follow, not all MG patients need to undergo an edrophonium test. If a patient has the appropriate clinical findings for MG and an elevated AChR antibody level (see following section), an edrophonium test is superfluous.

The edrophonium test can be kept quite simple. One milliliter (10 mg) of edrophonium is drawn up into a 1-mL tuberculin syringe. We often inject the edrophonium directly into a vein (usually antecubital), but alternatively, a small butterfly IV line can be used. Initially, we inject 0.2 mL (2 mg) and wait 30 to 60 seconds. If the patient experiences no side effects (fasciculations, sweating, nausea), we inject another 0.2 mL. More serious side effects such as bronchospasm or lightheadedness due to bradycardia are quite uncommon. Some patients will either experience side effects or will have a positive response, even at these low doses. If side effects or a positive response results, no further edrophonium needs be given. If neither side effects nor a positive response occur after 0.4 mL, we inject the remaining 0.6 mL (for a total dose of 10 mg). If an IV line is used, the line must be flushed with saline following each edrophonium injection. Nearly all patients experience some mild side effects, but these resolve—and the neuromuscular findings improve—in several minutes. Injectable atropine should be available in case severe bradycardia or hypotension develops. However, atropine is in reality seldom required. For most patients, the edrophonium test can be performed in an office setting.

Some practitioners use a placebo injection. However, if a patient has an objective parameter to follow, a placebo is probably not necessary. If a patient has no objective finding that can be easily measured, the test probably should not be performed. Therefore, we rarely use a placebo injection.

Before the use of immunosuppressive therapy, edrophonium tests were frequently performed in patients using oral acetylcholinesterase inhibitor therapy to determine if they were underdosed or overdosed. This is an old concept that is not useful in the modern management of MG.

Electrophysiologic Testing

Routine nerve conduction studies and electromyography results are typically normal in patients with MG. However, the technique of repetitive nerve stimulation can be used to diagnose MG. It is important to appreciate that an abnormal result is more likely to be observed in a clinically weak muscle. In a patient with generalized MG, the sensitivity of repetitive nerve stimulation in distal muscles is 66% and in proximal muscles, 83%. In patients with ocular MG, repetitive nerve stimulation is much less sensitive, demonstrating a positive result in only about 40% of cases. As with the edrophonium test, repetitive nerve stimulation does not need to be performed if one is already certain of the diagnosis based on the clinical findings and positive results on the AChR antibody test.

Single-fiber electromyography is a technique that is very sensitive for detecting disorders of neuromuscular transmission. It is abnormal in 94% of patients with generalized MG and in 80% of patients with ocular MG. This procedure is time-consuming and many neurologists in practice will either not have the training, equipment, or time to perform single-fiber electromyography. As with the other diagnostic tests discussed, single-fiber electromyography is seldom necessary for the diagnosis of MG in most patients.

Antibody Testing

Finding AChR antibodies in the serum of patient suspected of having MG is the most specific and reassuring test for supporting the diagnosis. The AChR antibody test that is most often obtained is the binding radioimmunoassay utilizing bungarotoxin. As previously noted, given the right clinical presentation, if the AChR antibody assay result is definitely positive, one can argue that no other diagnostic studies for MG are needed. AChR antibodies, however, are not elevated in all patients with MG. This test is most helpful in generalized MG in which results are positive in 85% of patients. AChR antibodies are elevated in only 50% of patients with ocular MG. Children make up an additional group of patients with MG who often have negative antibody titers.

AChR antibody titers correlate poorly with MG severity. Although a patient's AChR antibody titer may decrease as his or her clinical condition improves, as a general rule, we do not use antibody titers to guide our therapeutic decisions. AChR antibody levels may remain elevated in patients with MG in clinical remission, but this is not an indication to continue therapy. Borderline AChR antibody elevations can be a spurious laboratory finding and should be repeated in a different reference laboratory. Patients with antibody-negative MG are clinically indistinguishable from those with AChR antibodies, and our clinical approach is the same for both groups.

Radiographic Tests

Thymoma occurs in 10% to 15% of patients with MG. Although most thymomas are benign, these can be locally invasive and some are malignant. All newly diagnosed patients should undergo chest computed tomography. Routine chest radiographs may not detect up to 25% of thymic tumors. Patients who appear to have ocular MG but lack AChR antibodies and electrophysiologic confirmation should undergo brain magnetic resonance imaging to exclude an intracranial structural lesion.

Other Laboratory Tests

Other autoimmune disorders, such as diabetes mellitus, hyperthyroidism or hypothyroidism, pernicious anemia, and systemic lupus erythematosus may occur in association with MG. Appropriate screening laboratory studies are recommended.

TREATMENT

Anticholinesterase Medications

Anticholinesterase medications are the first line of therapy for MG. These drugs block the breakdown of acetylcholine at the neuromuscular junction. Pyridostigmine (Mestinon) is the anticholinesterase medication that is typically used. Other anticholinesterase drugs, such as neostigmine (Prostigmin), are rarely prescribed. Pyridostigmine is a symptomatic therapy and does not alter the underlying autoimmune pathosis. Nevertheless, many patients with mild MG can be successfully treated with pyridostigmine alone. Pyridostigmine comes in 60-mg crossed/scored tablets so that the drug can be given in 15-mg increments if necessary. Following an oral dose of pyridostigmine, improvement can be noticed in 15 to 30 minutes; the effect can last 3 to 4 hours. However, most patients require no more than 60 mg three or four times a day. Although pyridostigmine can be given in doses of 120 mg every 3 to 4 hours, our general rule is that if a patient requires more than 60 mg four times a day, then it is time to add immunosuppressive therapy.

Although very high doses of cholinesterase inhibitors can produce weakness from so-called cholinergic crisis, this should be a rare event in the modern management era because immunosuppressive therapy is usually initiated before excessive pyridostigmine doses are used. One of the common mistakes practitioners make in the treatment of patients with MG is to use increasingly higher doses of pyridostigmine in a patient who is steadily worsening instead of beginning immunosuppressive therapy.

Another frequent error is the improper use of slow-release pyridostigmine (Mestinon Timespan). These are 180-mg tablets that presumably have a delayed absorption and thus a longer duration of action. Slow-release pyridostigmine tablets have been suggested for bedtime use to prevent weakness on awakening. However, we find that patients are often placed on excessive pyridostigmine doses with these tablets, such as 180 mg every 3 to 4 hours. In addition, patients with MG usually do not have excessive weakness on awakening and taking a standard pyridostigmine tablet in the morning is usually sufficient. In addition, it is more difficult to regulate total pyridostigmine dosage with the slow-release tablets and, therefore, we generally discourage their use.

The use of pyridostigmine is not typically limited by weakness, which is a nicotinic receptor side effect, but by muscarinic side effects, such as gastrointestinal cramps and diarrhea. Many patients may also experience muscle fasciculations. Muscarinic side effects can limit the total dose of pyridostigmine that a patient can tolerate. Oral atropine (Sal-Tropine) in doses of 0.4 mg can be used to treat or prevent these side effects. Alternatively, the oral anticholinergic medication hyoscyamine sulfate (Levsin or Anaspaz),* available in 0.125-mg tablets, can be prescribed. These medications can be taken when symptoms develop or prophylactically with each pyridostigmine dose.

*Not FDA approved for this indication.

Corticosteroids

When a patient's symptoms are no longer adequately controlled by pyridostigmine alone, a decision must be made to use some form of immunosuppressive therapy. Prednisone is typically the first choice. Although the dose can be calculated at 1 or 1.5 mg/kg, we typically start prednisone at a high dose of 100 mg per day in most adults. After 2 to 4 weeks, we switch to alternate-day doses of 100 mg every other day to minimize side effects. If steroid therapy is initiated at moderate to high doses, improvement is ordinarily seen in 2 to 3 weeks. However, beginning prednisone at these doses can produce transient worsening in nearly 50% of patients. The mechanism may involve a direct effect of corticosteroids that worsens neuromuscular junction function. In one study, almost 10% of patients who became worse required intubation. Therefore, it is our practice to hospitalize patients with MG for 5 to 7 days when we initiate high-dose prednisone therapy. During this period, we monitor bulbar function and forced vital capacity daily. If patients are stable after 1 week, they can be safely discharged when they are still receiving oral prednisone.

An alternate approach that avoids transient worsening is to start with low prednisone doses and slowly build up to the target dose. One can begin at 10 to 20 mg/d and increase every 3 to 5 days by 5 mg/d. However, with this approach it takes much longer to achieve a beneficial response. If a patient has significant weakness, our preference is to begin the higher prednisone dose immediately in the hospital. If a patient has only mild generalized or ocular MG and a decision has been made to use prednisone, the outpatient go-low, go-slow approach is reasonable.

Following significant clinical improvement on prednisone, one should not rush to taper the drug. Premature tapering of prednisone is a common management error. We generally maintain patients on 100 mg every other day for 2 to 4 months before considering tapering the dose. We like to continue this dose until the patient's neurologic function returns to baseline or improvement plateaus. When we do begin to taper the dose, this is done very gradually by 5 mg every 2 weeks. Therefore, patients are on high-dose, alternate-day prednisone for 6 to 8 months. When the prednisone has been reduced to 20 mg every other day, we taper even more slowly. We attempt to get patients completely off of prednisone; however, it is not uncommon for patients to require low-dose therapy (5–10 mg every other day) for many years, or even indefinitely.

We use a number of measures in an attempt to minimize the side effects that may result from prednisone therapy. Alternate-day dosing will generate fewer complications than daily steroids. All patients are referred to a dietitian and placed on a calorie-restricted, low sodium, low carbohydrate diet. To prevent osteoporosis, patients are placed on supplemental calcium and vitamin D. Electrolyte levels, blood glucose levels, and blood pressure need to be monitored. We obtain bone density scans at baseline and then every 6 to 12 months. If osteoporosis is present we prescribe bisphosphonates. We do not prescribe H_2 blockers or proton pump inhibitors unless patients develop symptoms or clinical evidence of gastric irritation.

Azathioprine

Azathioprine (Imuran) is an antimetabolite that blocks cell proliferation. Presumably, inhibitory effects on T cells produce the benefit azathioprine has in the treatment of MG. Azathioprine is relatively easy to use, well tolerated, and typically used as a second-line immunosuppressive agent in patients already on prednisone. It is used most often in patients who relapse while on prednisone or who have been on prednisone for lengthy periods. In the latter circumstance, azathioprine is used as a steroid-sparing agent to permit the prednisone dose to be decreased or eliminated. The response to azathioprine is slow; it may take 6 to 18 months before improvement is seen.

Azathioprine is supplied as a 50-mg, dumbbell-shaped tablet that can be easily broken in half. The starting dose is 50 mg per day. If after 1 week there are no adverse effects, the dose can be immediately increased to the target dose of 2 to 3 mg/kg/d. Therefore, after the initial test dose, most patients with MG are placed on 150 mg/d. Although azathioprine is usually well tolerated, there are three important, limiting side effects. Approximately 10% of patients experience an idiosyncratic systemic reaction within the first several weeks of therapy, consisting of fever, abdominal pain, nausea, vomiting, and anorexia. If the medication is stopped, these symptoms resolve quickly. If the patient is rechallenged with azathioprine, these symptoms commonly recur. In addition, leukopenia and hepatotoxicity can develop. Blood cell counts and liver enzyme levels need to be monitored at least monthly. If the white blood cell count drops below 4000 cells/mm^3, the dose must be decreased; if it falls below 3000 cells/mm^3, the drug should be temporarily stopped. If liver enzyme levels become significantly elevated, the dose should also be held. Once laboratory values normalize, patients can sometimes be successfully rechallenged, although similar toxicity will often recur requiring discontinuation of the medication.

Cyclosporine

Cyclosporine (Sandimmune, Neoral) is increasingly being used as an immunosuppressive option in MG. This drug inhibits helper T cells and enhances expression of suppressor T cells. The onset of clinical benefit produced by cyclosporine is 1 to 3 months. Thus, although this is slower than the response seen with prednisone, it is appreciably faster than that seen with azathioprine. The dose of cyclosporine is 3 to 6 mg/kg/d given in two divided doses. Cyclosporine is available in 25- or 100-mg gelatin capsules or as an oral solution (100 mg/mL).

Side effects of cyclosporine include hirsutism, tremor, gum hyperplasia, headache, paresthesias, and hepatotoxicity. However, hypertension and nephrotoxicity represent the main limitations to therapy. Blood pressure, renal function, and trough plasma cyclosporine levels should be monitored monthly. Trough cyclosporine levels should be kept below 300 ng/mL.

Cyclophosphamide

Cyclophosphamide (Cytoxan) is a nitrogen mustard alkylating agent that blocks cell proliferation. There is little literature on the benefits of cyclophosphamide in MG and this drug is not typically used in patients with MG. In addition to bone marrow suppression and leukopenia, hemorrhagic cystitis and an increased risk of bladder cancer are serious limiting factors to the use of this medication, especially because other less toxic immunosuppressive agents are available.

Plasmapheresis

Plasmapheresis removes AChR antibodies from the circulation of patients with MG and can be a very effective therapy. The time to improvement following plasmapheresis is measured in days (usually 2–3 days), rather than weeks for corticosteroids and months for azathioprine and cyclosporine. The benefits of this procedure, however, usually last only a few weeks. In addition, the usefulness of this therapy is limited by the need for IV access (often a large double-lumen central line); complications such as pneumothorax, hypotension, and sepsis; as well as expense.

The are two clear indications for plasmapheresis: myasthenic crisis and weak patient before thymectomy (see following section). Not all patients require plasmapheresis before thymectomy if they are reasonably strong and have good pulmonary function. A more subjective indication for plasmapheresis is for severely weak patients hospitalized for initiation of prednisone therapy. Plasmapheresis can be administered as a temporary therapy until the prednisone starts to work. In rare instances, a patient with MG will require chronic intermittent plasmapheresis if all other therapies are unsuccessful.

Generally, a course of plasmapheresis consists of four to six exchanges in which 3 to 5 L of plasma are removed at each session. However, there is no exact science regarding the number of exchanges or the amount removed. To a large extent this depends on how the patient tolerates the procedure.

Intravenous Immunoglobulin

IV immunoglobulin (IVIG) is being used with increasing frequency by neurologists for the treatment of a number of immune-mediated neuromuscular diseases. However, although randomized, controlled studies have proven the benefit of IVIG in Guillain-Barré syndrome and dermatomyositis, the evidence is not as strong for MG. The precise mechanism of action of IVIG remains unknown. In a recent study, IVIG was compared to plasmapheresis in patients with exacerbations of MG. IVIG was as effective as plasmapheresis and had fewer side effects. However, we do not believe IVIG should be considered a substitute for plasmapheresis when a patient is in myasthenic crisis.

The initial dose of IVIG is 2 g/kg. This can be given over 5 days (0.4 g/kg/d), but more recently we have moved to administration over 2 days (1 g/kg/d). We usually admit the patient for 2 days (1 night) to give this large dose, which runs nearly continuously during the admission. IVIG is initially given as 5% or 6% solution. If it is well tolerated, subsequent infusions can be given at 10% or 12% concentrations. Patients are next given two or three subsequent infusions of 0.4 g/kg each, scheduled at 4- to 8-week intervals. These are usually administered on an outpatient basis. We then re-evaluate the patient to determine if further treatments are needed.

The advantages to IVIG are that side effects are minimal in most patients. Some lightheadedness or a mild headache can develop. Less often, patients can develop a severe headache due to aseptic meningitis. Nephrotoxicity can develop in patients with underlying renal impairment and hypertension, especially in those with diabetes mellitus.

A significant limitation to the use of IVIG is the great expense of this therapy. A number of insurance carriers are reluctant to approve this medication, especially because it has not been approved by the Food and Drug Administration (FDA) for the treatment of MG. In addition, IVIG is often difficult to obtain due to production shortages.

Thymectomy

There appears to be a general consensus that patients with generalized MG who are between puberty and 60 years of age can benefit from thymectomy. However, all evidence on the possible effectiveness of thymectomy is from retrospective or case-control studies. A critical review of the literature on thymectomy continues to raise questions about the effectiveness of the procedure for inducing remission or producing clinical improvement. A randomized study has yet to be performed despite calls for such a trial by some experts in the neuromuscular community.

Clinicians vary with respect to how they fit thymectomy into their therapeutic arsenal. Some advocate thymectomy for essentially all generalized MG after the diagnosis is made. Others wait and see if remission can be obtained with a trial of immunosuppressive treatment, usually prednisone. We tend to reserve thymectomy for patients not responding to initial medical therapies. Whether or not patients with ocular should have thymectomies is controversial. We generally do not send these patients for thymectomies. Thymectomies can be performed in children but this procedure should probably be avoided during the first few years of life. Thymectomy is probably less effective in the elderly due to atrophy of the tissue. However, whether to make any restriction based on age or at what point to set this cut-off is another unresolved issue. We generally do not recommend thymectomy to patients over 60 years old. The presence of a thymoma is the one absolute indication for thymectomy, regardless of age or disease severity.

Based on available data, what should a patient with MG be told regarding potential improvement from a thymectomy? A recent review of the available literature concluded that patients with MG undergoing thymectomy are 2.1 times more likely to achieve remission and are 1.7 times more likely to improve. Remissions attributed to thymectomy are often not immediate, and patients should be prepared for this. Some series have reported remissions occurring as long as 7 to 10 years after the thymectomy.

Yet another unresolved issue surrounding thymectomy regards the optimal surgical approach. A sternal-splitting technique is probably best for removing all thymus tissue and may be preferable to a transcervical approach. Thoracoscopic thymectomies have been introduced recently. More experience and data from this technique need to be published and, ideally, a randomized study comparing the transsternal and endoscopic procedures should be performed.

NEW THERAPIES

Mycophenolate mofetil (CellCept) is an immunosuppressive agent used to prevent rejection in patients with transplants. This medication inhibits aspects of protein synthesis that result in suppressing both T- and B-cell proliferation. The use of mycophenolate in patients with MG has been gaining increasing interest. The onset of action of mycophenolate may occur more quickly than with azathioprine. In this way it is similar to cyclosporine, but mycophenolate does not produce nephrotoxicity. Myelosuppression, however, can occur and blood counts need to be monitored. Typical doses used for MG are 1 to 3 g/d in two divided doses. This drug is expensive and the degree of benefit as well as the precise response time remain unknown. Future studies should help better define the role of mycophenolate in the management of MG.

TRIGEMINAL NEURALGIA

method of
RONALD BRISMAN, M.D.
College of Physicians and Surgeons of Columbia University
New York, New York

Trigeminal neuralgia is an extremely painful disorder characterized by sudden bursts of face pain that are often triggered by light touch around the mouth or face or by talking, eating, or brushing the teeth. The pain sometimes worsens or lessens for periods of weeks or months. The pain is in the area supplied by the trigeminal nerve (i.e., cheek, jaw, teeth, and gums or lips and less often around the eye or forehead). The pain is usually on one side of the face, but in 5% to 10% of patients, pain occurs on both sides of the face although not at the same time. The pain responds to carbamazepine (Tegretol), although sometimes the dose has to be increased and unpleasant side effects may occur.

When atypical features coexist with some of the previously described symptoms, the condition is called *atypical trigeminal neuralgia.* These atypical features may include a constant pain that is not always triggered by light touch. The treatments for trigeminal neuralgia are likely to relieve the sharp, electric-like pains that are triggered by light touch even in these patients but are less likely to relieve the constant, untriggered pains.

CAUSE

The cause of trigeminal neuralgia is not always certain. Approximately 5% of patients have a tumor pressing on the trigeminal nerve where it leaves the brain.

About 5% of patients with trigeminal neuralgia have multiple sclerosis. Patients with trigeminal neuralgia and multiple sclerosis are about 10 years younger (in their 40s) when they first develop face pain. They are more likely to have pain on both sides of the face and often have other neurologic abnormalities. Although these patients may have constant pain, it is the brief electric-like pains triggered by light touch that are most likely to respond to treatments for trigeminal neuralgia. However, most patients in their 40s or 50s who have trigeminal neuralgia do not have multiple sclerosis.

Some patients have a blood vessel that presses on the trigeminal nerve close to the brain. In other patients, the cause cannot be determined.

DIAGNOSIS

In addition to a thorough history and physical examination, magnetic resonance imaging (MRI) of the brain is recommended. This helps diagnose a brain tumor in the rare cases in which it is present. It may also help diagnose multiple sclerosis. Often, when the MRI is performed, some contrast material is injected into the vein so that the appearance of a small tumor or other structures in the brain can be enhanced and made easier to detect. High resolution MRI with 1-mm cuts often show a blood vessel in contact with or near the trigeminal nerve. The relationship of the blood vessel to the nerve as seen on MRI is not always diagnostic of a causal relationship. However, when there is no blood vessel near the nerve, it is very unlikely that the patient's trigeminal neuralgia symptoms are caused by blood vessel compression.

NONSURGICAL TREATMENT

There are some patients who have very mild face pain that may subside and even disappear without treatment. For pain that is bothersome, medication, especially carbamazepine, is often highly effective. Most patients will respond to 200 mg of carbamazepine three or four times a day. There are many possible side effects of carbamazepine. Some of the more common ones are sleepiness, forgetfulness, confusion, drowsiness, dizziness, and nausea. Elderly patients and those with multiple sclerosis are more likely to be bothered by carbamazepine. Carbamazepine can also cause more serious problems such as bone marrow suppression with anemia and leukopenia. Rarely, these are life-threatening. Blood counts have to be monitored. Carbamazepine also interacts with many medicines, and it may cause liver toxicity.

Another anticonvulsant, oxcarbazepine (Trileptal), has recently been approved and released for use in the United States. It works very well for trigeminal neuralgia, as does carbamazepine, but has fewer side effects. Unlike carbamazepine, oxcarbazepine does not cause bone marrow suppression or liver toxicity and has fewer interactions with other medicines. About 25% to 30% of patients who develop a rash from carbamazepine will also develop a rash from oxcarbazepine. Oxcarbazepine is more likely than carbamazepine to cause hyponatremia, especially when it is taken with other medicines, such as diuretics. Oxcarbazepine is taken twice a day and the dose is 50% more in milligrams than carbamazepine.

There are other medicines that can be used either alone or in combination. These are usually less effective than carbamazepine. They include gabapentin (Neurontin), baclofen (Lioresal), phenytoin (Dilantin), clonazepam (Klonopin), and lamotrigine (Lamictal). All of them, except baclofen, are also used to prevent seizures.

SURGICAL TREATMENT

A surgical procedure is recommended for patients who continue to be bothered either by pain or side effects of medicines.

There are peripheral nerve procedures, which damage the branches of the trigeminal nerve on the surface of the face. These procedures are less likely to be recommended because they are more likely to provide only temporary relief, cause much numbness that is often bothersome, are more difficult to repeat, and usually require general anesthesia.

Procedures that treat the trigeminal nerve near the brain are more desirable because pain and bothersome numbness are less likely to occur. Advances in technology have made some of the procedures (especially gamma knife radiosurgery) so safe and well tolerated that they should be considered before the pain becomes agonizing.

There are five important neurosurgical procedures:

1. Gamma knife radiosurgery (GKRS)
2. Radiofrequency electrocoagulation (RFE)
3. Glycerol injection (GLY)
4. Balloon microcompression (BMC)
5. Microvascular decompression (MVD)

RFE, GLY, and BMC are percutaneous procedures that are done with intravenous sedation. MVD is a more major procedure that requires a craniotomy and general anesthesia.

GKRS is a method for treating certain problems in the brain without making a surgical cut. In GKRS, 201 beams of radiation are focused precisely on the trigeminal nerve just where it leaves the brain. The intracranial structures are visualized on high resolution MRI scans. The treatment does not require general or intravenous anesthesia. The patient stays in the hospital for fewer than 4 hours. GKRS is as effective as the other neurosurgical procedures, but it is safer and has the fewest complications. Major complications have not been reported; thousands of cases have been done safely. Bothersome dysesthesias occur in less than 15% of patients and usually diminish within a few months. It works well whether or not there is a blood vessel compressing the trigeminal nerve. GKRS can be recommended for anyone with trigeminal neuralgia who is bothered either by pain or side effects of medicines.

OPTIC NEURITIS

method of
VALÉRIE BIOUSSE, M.D., and
NANCY J. NEWMAN, M.D.
Emory University School of Medicine
Atlanta, Georgia

Optic neuritis is an inflammatory disorder of the optic nerve that typically occurs in young adults. It is characterized by a subacute, painful loss of central vision. Visual loss is acute but may progress for 7 to 10 days. Visual acuity varies from a mild reduction to severe loss. Pain is usually exacerbated by eye movement and may precede or coincide with visual loss. Color vision is usually impaired out of proportion to visual acuity.

Examination reveals a relative afferent pupillary defect if the process is unilateral or asymmetric. The classic visual field defect has been said to be a central scotoma; however, almost any type of visual field defect is possible. The term *retrobulbar optic neuritis* is applied when the optic nerve appears normal in the acute phase; *anterior optic neuritis* or *papillitis* is used to refer to those cases with optic disk swelling. In both cases, temporal pallor of the disk develops 4 to 6 weeks after visual loss.

There are multiple causes of inflammatory optic neuritis, including infectious diseases such as syphilis, cat-scratch disease, and Lyme disease and noninfectious inflammation such as sarcoidosis. However, in most cases, optic neuritis remains idiopathic or is associated with multiple sclerosis. Idiopathic demyelinating optic neuritis is the most common acute optic neuropathy in people under age 45. At least two thirds of patients are women. In high-risk areas, such as northern Europe and the northern United States, the yearly incidence is about 3 in 100,000; in lower risk areas, the incidence is about 1 in 100,000. Patients typically improve over several weeks, regardless of treatment. The risk of subsequent development of multiple sclerosis after an isolated attack of idiopathic optic neuritis has been estimated to be as high as 75% at 15 years.

The Optic Neuritis Treatment Trial (ONTT), a large, multicenter trial designed to evaluate the effects of corticosteroid treatment on acute idiopathic optic neuritis, has provided important information regarding the natural history, prognosis, and treatment of this disorder. A total of 457 patients between the ages of 18 and 45 years with acute unilateral optic neuritis were examined within 8 days of onset of visual symptoms. All patients were followed 6 months or longer.

The study subsequently completed 5-year follow-up on a cohort of 388 patients with isolated optic neuritis. Seventy-five percent of the patients were women, and the mean age was 32 years. Pain, typically exacerbated by eye movement, was reported by 92% of patients. The optic disk was swollen in 35% of patients and normal in 65%. Visual field defects in the central 30 degrees were found frequently, and their configuration included arcuate and altitudinal defects as well as true central scotomas.

Initial diagnostic evaluation, including antinuclear antibodies (ANA) and free treponemal antibody (FTA) blood tests, chest radiograph, brain magnetic resonance imaging (MRI), and cerebrospinal fluid analysis, rarely revealed an alternative diagnosis, leading the study group to conclude that these tests are not diagnostically necessary for a patient with the typical features of optic neuritis. However, the ONTT found that brain MRI was a powerful predictor of the subsequent risk of multiple sclerosis. Indeed, patients with three or more T2 lesions on brain MRI had a 2-year risk of multiple sclerosis of about 32%, whereas patients with a normal MRI had a risk of about 5%. At 5-year follow-up, the risk of multiple sclerosis was 51% in patients with three or more lesions on MRI and 16% for patients with normal MRI. These findings are in accordance with a European study in which 82% of patients with abnormal MRIs versus 6% of those with normal MRIs at the time of optic neuritis had developed definite multiple sclerosis 5.5 years later.

Among those patients with abnormal MRI, other less powerful predicting factors for the development of multiple sclerosis among ONTT patients included prior nonspecific previous neurologic symptoms and a history of optic neuropathy in the fellow eye (previous optic neuropathy in the study eye was an exclusion criteria and therefore could not be evaluated). Among those patients with normal baseline MRI and no history of neurologic symptoms, positive predictive factors for the development of multiple sclerosis included white race, family history, female gender, retrobulbar location, pain, and a preceding viral illness. Lack of pain, the presence of optic disk swelling, and mild visual loss were features of the optic neuritis associated with a low risk of multiple sclerosis in patients with normal baseline MRI.

TREATMENT

Treatment of isolated idiopathic optic neuritis has included oral, retrobulbar, and intravenous steroids, and immunoglobulin. The ONTT has recently questioned the usefulness of oral prednisone, and a practice parameter was recently developed by the American Academy of Neurology to provide recommendations regarding the management of idiopathic optic neuritis. In this evidence review, 24 publications reflecting about 20 studies were analyzed (the largest and most important of which being the ONTT).

Patients in the ONTT were randomized to three treatment arms:

1. Oral prednisone (1 mg/kg/d) for 14 days
2. Intravenous methylprednisolone (250 mg, 4 times daily) for 3 days, followed by oral prednisone (1 mg/kg/d) for 11 days
3. Oral placebo for 14 days

Compared with the placebo and the oral prednisone regimens, intravenous therapy provided a more rapid recovery of vision but no long-term benefit. Most of the difference in rate of recovery among groups was seen within the first 2 weeks. Thereafter, differences in visual function among groups were small. After 1-year follow-up, there were no significant differences among the groups in visual acuity, contrast sensitivity, color vision, or visual field. The regimen of oral prednisone alone not only provided no benefit to vision but also was associated with an increased rate of new attacks of optic neuritis in both the initially affected eye and the fellow eye. Within the first 2 years of follow-up, new attacks of optic neuritis in either eye occurred in 30% of the patients in the oral prednisone group and 14% in the intravenous group. Side effects of the corticosteroid treatments generally were mild and no patients had lasting adverse effects, suggesting that administration of high-dose intravenous steroids in outpatients should be safe.

Visual recovery from optic neuritis, including visual acuity and visual fields, was rapid and occurred within the first month in nearly all patients. At 6 months, 94% of all patients had vision of 20/40 or better and 75% had improved to 20/20 or better. Therefore, the absence of visual improvement within the first month after the onset of treated and untreated optic neuritis or the worsening of visual symptoms after termination of a course of steroids should be considered atypical and warranting of further diagnostic investigations. The ONTT also found that the group receiving the intravenous regimen had a lower rate of development of multiple sclerosis within the first 2 years (7.5%) than did the placebo (16.5%) or oral prednisone (14.7%) groups. However, this protective effect was no longer appreciable after 3 years: 17.3% of patients treated with intravenous steroids and 20.7% of those treated with placebo had developed multiple sclerosis.

In the evidence review, seven other corticosteroid treatment trials relevant to this practice parameter were identified. All were prospective, randomized, and placebo-controlled studies, although sample sizes were considerably smaller than in the ONTT. These studies suggested that higher dose oral or parenteral methylprednisolone or adrenocorticotropic hormone may hasten the speed and degree of recovery of visual function, but there is no evidence of long-term visual benefit. The decision to use these medications to speed recovery but not to improve ultimate visual outcome should therefore be based on other non–evidence-based factors such as quality of life, risk to the patient, and visual function in the fellow eye, or other factors that the clinician deems appropriate.

The recently published CHAMPS trial (Controlled High Risk Subject Avonex Multiple Sclerosis Prevention Study) has suggested that interferon beta-1a should be initiated immediately following a first episode of idiopathic optic neuritis accompanied by abnormal brain MRI. A total of 383 patients with a first demyelinating event, including 100 patients with a

TABLE 1. **Recommendations for the Management of Patients With Idiopathic Optic Neuritis**

1. Consider brain MRI to assess the risk of future neurologic events of multiple sclerosis.
2. Do not use procedures such as chest radiograph, blood tests, and lumbar puncture to evaluate patients with the typical clinical features of optic neuritis (i.e., young adult with sudden visual loss with progression of symptoms of ≤1 week accompanied by pain on eye movements, with visual improvement beginning within 1 month, with either a swollen or normal optic disk but no more than a minimal vitreous cellular reaction, and with no history of systemic disease that might produce optic neuritis).
3. Avoid treatment with oral prednisone.
4. Consider treatment with intravenous methylprednisolone if the brain MRI demonstrates multiple signal abnormalities consistent with multiple sclerosis or if the patient wants to recover vision faster (severe visual loss, bilateral optic neuritis).
5. Consider treatment with interferon beta-1a in patients with at least two lesions suggestive of demyelinating disease on brain MRI, in order to reduce the rate of subsequent development of clinically definite multiple sclerosis.

Abbreviation: MRI = magnetic resonance imaging.

first isolated idiopathic optic neuritis and at least two clinically silent T2 lesions on the brain MRI were included. All patients received intravenous methylprednisolone, according to the ONTT protocol, within 8 days after the visual loss. Patients were randomized to either interferon beta-1a (30 μg intramuscularly once weekly) (49 patients) or placebo (51 patients). In this study, interferon beta-1a treatment of patients with acute idiopathic demyelinating events such as optic neuritis reduced the rate of developing definite multiple sclerosis by 43%. This effect was observed within 6 months and was sustained throughout the study (34 months).

Based on these results, several recommendations can be made for the clinician managing patients with acute optic neuritis (Table 1). It is important to remember that these recommendations are only strictly applicable to patients with typical acute optic neuritis seen early in the course of their disease.

GLAUCOMA

method of
TONY REALINI, M.D.
University of Arkansas for Medical Sciences
Little Rock, Arkansas

and

ROBERT D. FECHTNER, M.D.
New Jersey Medical School
Newark, New Jersey

RATIONALE FOR TREATMENT

Glaucoma is not, strictly speaking, a disease but rather a collection of diseases (more aptly referred to as *the glaucomas*) representing the final pathway of various idiopathic, ocular, and even systemic conditions. These diseases commonly share several characteristics, including progressive loss of optic nerve fibers that eventually leads to loss of the peripheral (and eventually central) visual field. Some are indolent and very slowly progressive, as in many cases of primary open angle glaucoma, whereas others are rapid and devastating to the eye and to vision, such as neovascular glaucoma commonly seen in the setting of posterior segment ischemia from diabetes or a retinal vascular occlusion.

Historically, elevated intraocular pressure (IOP) was considered the initial etiologic event in glaucomatous eyes, leading in a causal fashion to nerve damage and field loss. More recently, the role of IOP in the etiology of glaucoma is less clear. Although some forms of glaucoma appear to be very pressure dependent (pigmentary glaucoma and pseudoexfoliation glaucoma, for instance), others such as normal pressure glaucoma are less strongly linked to IOP. Early research suggests possible roles for IOP-independent mechanisms such as neurotoxins, vasospasm, and reduction of ocular perfusion in the pathogenesis of glaucoma. Our current understanding of the glaucoma-IOP relationship can be summarized as follows: although elevated IOP is not essential for the disease process or its diagnosis, there is an association between IOP and damage in glaucoma.

In the absence of any other potential treatable etiologic parameter of the glaucomatous process, we treat glaucoma by lowering IOP. In those glaucomatous eyes in which an underlying cause for elevated IOP is identified, therapy is aimed at the underlying cause. Although usually effective, these interventions are rarely curative, for once the trabecular meshwork (the drain of the eye) has been involved in any disease process, permanent damage usually results, with permanent outflow obstruction and persistent IOP elevations even if the causative process resolves completely. For this reason, most cases of secondary glaucoma, as well as virtually all cases of primary (idiopathic) glaucoma, require chronic therapy to lower IOP.

APPROACH TO IOP REDUCTION

Three treatment modalities exist to lower IOP, and these are generally applied in a stepped regimen. As a first line, medications are used to lower IOP. Typically, these are applied to the eye topically, although some systemic medications are occasionally used as well. In eyes judged to have an inadequate IOP-lowering response to medications, or for patients in whom medications are poorly tolerated or deemed unsafe owing to potential side effects, laser therapy is often the second step. If laser therapy to improve outflow is contraindicated or ineffective, incisional surgery to construct a new outflow pathway for the eye is performed. This stepped therapeutic approach is designed to maximize both efficacy and safety by saving more invasive—and potentially more complicated—procedures only for patients not well controlled by relatively safer means. This is our general approach to therapy, although there are numerous exceptions for individual patients. What follows, then, is a general outline for therapy.

Medications

Glaucoma medications generally lower IOP by one of two mechanisms: reduction of aqueous production or enhancement of aqueous outflow. Inflow suppressors work on the ciliary body, located behind and at the root of the iris, to block production of aqueous humor. Classes of these medications include the β-blockers, carbonic anhydrase inhibitors, and α_2-adrenergic agonists. Outflow enhancers can promote traditional outflow through the trabecular meshwork or may open nontraditional outflow channels through the so-called uveoscleral outflow tract. The parasympathomimetic agents are meshwork enhancers, and the prostaglandin analogues stimulate uveoscleral outflow.

With the myriad choices available to ophthalmologists, choosing an appropriate medication for a given patient is often as much art as science. Our decision process focuses on selecting the drug most likely to reduce IOP to a safer level (our target IOP) while avoiding any medication with a side effect profile that poorly matches the patient's systemic health.

Since the introduction of timolol in 1978, topical β-blockers have been the agent of choice for the long-term medical management of glaucoma. These agents are powerfully effective in reducing IOP in most patients and are generally well tolerated. Once- or twice-daily dosing makes them convenient, and the proliferation of generic choices renders them affordable. Side effects such as bronchospasm, cardiac arrhythmias, congestive heart failure, depression, impotence, and, rarely, death from cardiopulmonary collapse are very uncommon and were deemed worth the slight risk when these agents were the only powerful antiglaucoma agents available. But the rapid introduction of newer, equally powerful agents with significantly more favorable side effect profiles has led to a shift in the importance of β-blockers in glaucoma therapy.

Alternatives to ophthalmic β-blockers, long the mainstay of glaucoma therapy, are now commonly considered for initial therapy, in large part because of the unfavorable systemic effects associated with β-blockade. In general, we like the α_2-agonist brimonidine (Alphagan) and the prostaglandin analogue latanoprost (Xalatan). Brimonidine has come into widespread use recently for its powerful IOP-lowering effect and relatively favorable ocular and systemic side effect profile. This drug, widely used as initial monotherapy, is approved by the Food and Drug Administration for use three times daily, although common usage is twice daily. Brimonidine has efficacy similar to the ophthalmic β-blockers and less potential for systemic adverse effects, although ocular allergy is common and lethargy and sedation are also reported. There are some emerging data that this drug may have neuroprotective effects in certain experimental models (although this has not been confirmed in glaucoma). Latanoprost also provides excellent IOP reduction (at least as effective as β-blockers) and offers convenient once-daily dosing. This agent has a clinically significant nonresponse rate among glaucoma patients, however, and we avoid this drug in patients with active ocular inflammation or cystoid macular edema because there have been reports associating these pathologic problems with latanoprost. The topical carbonic anhydrase inhibitors dorzolamide (Trusopt) and brinzolamide (Azopt) are also indicated for use three times daily. With efficacy less than the nonselective β-blockers, they are not commonly used as first-line therapy. The ocular and systemic adverse effect profiles for these drugs are very favorable, with local irritation, blurring, and taste perversion as the common effects. A thorough discussion of the available glaucoma agents and their mechanisms of action, efficacy, and side effect profiles is beyond the scope of this article.

Once we have chosen a target IOP level and a drug to reach that target, we assess the results of a short, 3- to 6-week drug trial. If the medication is well tolerated and achieves our target IOP, we continue its use. If the chosen medication is not well tolerated, we immediately discontinue its use and try a different agent, selecting it in the same way we selected the first. If the medication was well tolerated but failed to achieve our target IOP, we are faced with the decision to switch to another agent or add an additional drug to the first drug. In general, if the IOP reduction we were seeking is within the drug's pharmacologic power but the drug failed to deliver as expected, we switch to monotherapy with an agent from a different class of drugs. If the drug delivered its expected pharmacologic power but we are still above our target IOP, we consider if our target IOP reduction is beyond the range of any single drug's reach, and, if so, we add an additional medication to the first drug, rather than switching. Once our target IOP is met, we monitor the patient regularly for evidence of progression by following the appearance of the optic nerve and the status of the visual field. If progression does not occur, we ask ourselves if the target IOP may safely be a bit higher and, if so, can we achieve this with less medication (fewer agents, lower concentrations, or less frequent dosing). The introduction of modern combination drops (two medications in one bottle) such as Cosopt (dorzolamide-timolol fixed combination) often allows us to reduce the total number of bottles and drops. If progression does occur, we set a lower target IOP and advance through the stepped therapeutic choices to reach our new goal. Again, there is no single algorithm we follow. As each new drug is added, we assess efficacy and monitor for adverse effects.

Laser

Because glaucoma medications are expensive, have side effects, and compromise our patients' quality of life in many ways, we try to achieve IOP control with no more than two medications. If two medications, both performing well, fail to achieve our target IOP, we consider the role of laser trabeculoplasty; and for patients already on three medications with inadequate IOP control, we routinely offer trabeculoplasty. Laser trabeculoplasty is a minimally invasive office procedure with few complications. In eyes with open angle glaucoma, the trabecular meshwork impedes outflow, and trabeculoplasty can effectively increase outflow in these eyes by counterintuitively selectively destroying some meshwork tissue. In laser trabeculoplasty, small laser burns are carefully placed throughout the circumference of the trabecular meshwork, focally shrinking tissue through photocoagulation. The tissue that is directly treated is destroyed, but the tissue between adjacent focal burns is put on stretch, opening more widely the outflow channels between treatment spots and perhaps actively stimulating neighboring tissue to improve functioning, thus enhancing outflow.

Trabeculoplasty's IOP-reducing power, generally on the order of 15% from baseline, is comparable to that from most single agents. When offered as primary therapy at the time of diagnosis (instead of medications), this procedure lowers IOP effectively in most patients, but its effects are transient—only 44% of eyes treated with trabeculoplasty were still controlled without additional medications 2 years later. In our experience, trabeculoplasty may be even less effective when used after medical therapy fails.

Given the chronic nature of glaucoma, the transient nature of IOP control associated with trabeculoplasty limits its clinical usefulness. There are circumstances, however, when trabeculoplasty is an appropriate therapeutic choice. Some forms of glaucoma, especially those seen in the pigment dispersion and pseudoexfoliation syndromes, often respond particularly well to trabeculoplasty. This may be due in part to the nature of these conditions: both can be viewed etiologically—from the standpoint of the associated glaucomas—as primarily trabecular diseases; treating the trabeculum may be especially beneficial in this setting. Also, trabeculoplasty is useful early in the stepped treatment paradigm for patients who cannot use drops for a variety of reasons: contraindications to all the medication choices, local intolerance to topical therapy (due to ubiquitous preservatives, for instance), physical or mental handicaps that preclude the ability to administer eyedrops, noncompliance with medical therapy, or the desire to live (at least temporarily) an eyedrop-free lifestyle. Trabeculoplasty can sometimes be repeated successfully in patients who had a good initial response.

Because laser trabeculoplasty is typically offered to patients only when reasonable medical therapy has failed, poor IOP control after trabeculoplasty often becomes a surgical disease. Patients reluctant to undergo incisional surgery may elect to add a third or fourth medicine to their daily regimen (if safe medication choices are still available), but the financial burden of this choice may be prohibitive—the most commonly used glaucoma medications cost $40 to $70 each for a month of therapy, and the inconvenience of such a medical regimen can be considerable. For most patients whose IOP is still poorly controlled after reasonable medical therapy and trabeculoplasty, we proceed with incisional trabeculectomy as the appropriate next step.

Incisional Surgery

In normal eyes, aqueous passes through the trabecular meshwork into a scleral duct called the *Schlemm canal,* from which it is shunted through the sclera in small collector channels that deliver aqueous to the external episcleral veins of the periocular tissue bed. In trabeculectomy, a new drain is fashioned in the sclera, creating an outflow tract that bypasses the nonfunctioning trabecular meshwork. Aqueous then drains into the subconjunctival space, where small vessels resorb the fluid. In a successful operation, the healing process partially scars the flap to its bed, providing some restriction to flow but not completely impeding flow. The surgeon's goal is to make the hole the right size, suture the flap under the right tension, and modulate the healing process pharmacologically so that the end result is a fistula with enough flow to keep IOP at a safe level. Antifibrosis agents such as mitomycin C and 5-fluorouracil inhibit scarring and increase the likelihood of good long-term filtration and IOP control postoperatively, but they increase the complication rate of surgery. Unlike ophthalmic surgery for cataract extraction, glaucoma surgery commonly has postoperative complications and can require fairly intensive postoperative care.

Complications of trabeculectomy include, in addition to failure due to excessive scarring, the following: overfiltration with too great a reduction in IOP and collapse of the eyeball due to the elastic contraction of the sclera; cataract formation; and late breakdown of the surgical site, leading to hypotony and intraocular infections. A reasonable estimate of surgical success for trabeculectomy may be about 50% still functioning after 5 years.

If trabeculectomy fails because of scarring, a repeat operation might include insertion of a small silicone tube through the eye wall to prevent the hole from scarring shut completely. One end of the tube is left in the anterior chamber, through which aqueous is shunted to its opposite end, at which a flat plate is secured to the posterior aspect of the eyeball externally. Fluid drained to this location is resorbed into the systemic circulation by orbital veins. These glaucoma drainage devices are associated with complications similar to those seen with trabeculectomy.

As a final resort, if these surgical procedures fail, the ciliary body can be focally destroyed using either laser energy or cryotherapy. Destruction of the ciliary body permanently reduces the production of aqueous fluid. Therefore, this procedure must be performed conservatively so as not to destroy too much of the ciliary body or the eye will collapse.

GOALS OF THERAPY

The glaucomas are a collection of diseases generally characterized by elevated IOP. We do not fully understand the pathogenesis of the glaucomatous process and cannot determine which of several proposed mechanisms may predominate in an individual patient. At this time, even in light of the questions surrounding its role in the disease process, all of our therapeutic efforts are directed at lowering IOP. We accomplish this with a minimum-necessary combination of medications, laser therapy, and incisional surgery.

Our target IOP becomes our easily measurable goal, but, of course, we do not treat pressure—we treat people who have glaucoma. Our true goals are to preserve visual function and to preserve quality of life for our patients. Although it is easy to measure IOP in the office, we recognize that this instantaneous sampling does not tell us very much about IOP at other times. It is well known that IOP is subject to diurnal fluctuations and at best we measure only "office pressure." Furthermore, our current techniques for testing visual function (visual field) and for detecting progressive optic nerve loss are limited; we can only detect substantial changes with certainty. The nature of glaucoma—its insidiousness, its lack of patient-detected symptomatology (no pain, no red eye, visual field loss so gradual as to be imperceptible over time)—and the limitations of diagnostic technology render those two goals almost impossible to reach. Glaucoma has no symptoms, but the therapies we employ to save our patients' vision often cause discomfort, systemic illness, and, on rare occasions, perhaps even death.

Simply stated, our approach to glaucoma therapy is to preserve sufficient visual function to allow a satisfactory quality of life while balancing the benefits with the burdens of therapy. We do so with an appalling lack of prospective data regarding outcomes. And the value of such data, even if they did exist, would be limited because each patient is an individual and deserves an individually tailored therapeutic approach. Thus, the notion of quality of life becomes a series of tradeoffs: chronically red eyes that see are better than quiet blind eyes. We try to make sure our patients know this. Most of them understand.

ACUTE FACIAL PARALYSIS
(Bell's Palsy)

method of
PAUL R. LAMBERT, M.D.
Medical University of South Carolina
Charleston, South Carolina

Paresis or paralysis of the face can have severe implications for the afflicted individual. The language of facial expression is fundamental to our interactions with others and conveys much about our personality. Damage to the facial nerve imparts an unnatural grimace to our countenance, which normal animation even exaggerates. It follows that facial nerve dysfunction not only produces a physiologic impairment, but also a psychological one.

This chapter will focus on one cause of facial paralysis, Bell's palsy. Current concepts on etiology, natural history, evaluation, and treatment will be presented.

ETIOLOGY

Over the past decade, a number of experimental studies have strongly supported the hypothesis that Bell's palsy is a viral neuropathy caused by herpes simplex virus type 1. For example, injection of this virus into the tongue or ear of mice will produce a facial paralysis, and herpes simplex virus-1 antigens can be detected in the geniculate ganglion of the mouse's facial nerve. Herpes simplex virus-1 DNA also has been detected in the endoneurial fluid of patients undergoing facial nerve decompression for Bell's palsy. In a recent human temporal bone study, herpes simplex virus-1 DNA was identified in the geniculate ganglion of a patient who died soon after the onset of facial paralysis.

It appears probable that herpes virus spreads from the oral cavity, where it frequently does cause infection, along the chorda tympani nerve to the geniculate ganglion. It is known that viruses can remain dormant in sensory ganglia for long periods, then reactivated by various physiologic stresses.

NATURAL HISTORY

A thorough understanding of the natural history of Bell's palsy is fundamental to formulating optimal diagnostic and therapeutic strategies. An excellent Danish study has been published on 1011 patients with untreated Bell's palsy collected during a 15-year period in Copenhagen. Several notable observations were made:

1. Every patient recovered at least some facial function by 4 to 6 months.
2. Greater than 90% of patients with only a paresis recovered completely.
3. Approximately 75% to 80% of patients with a full paralysis recovered completely or had only minor sequelae.
4. There was a good correlation between recovery and age, with each succeeding decade beyond age 40 showing a greater incidence of sequelae (residual weakness and/or synkinesis).
5. Three months after the onset of Bell's palsy was an important point. Nearly all patients in whom the first signs of recovery were delayed beyond this interval experienced significant sequelae.

EVALUATION

Differential Diagnosis

The facial nerve takes a complex path from the brainstem to the facial muscles. After traversing the cerebellopontine angle in approximation to the auditory-vestibular cranial nerve, it takes a winding course through the temporal bone to the stylomastoid foramen. Its extracranial segments then pass through the parotid gland on their way to the motor end plates of the muscles of facial expression. Both benign and malignant (primary and metastatic) tumors involving structures along this route can cause a facial paralysis. Inflammatory processes of the middle ear and mastoid process represent another common cause of facial nerve dysfunction. Primary tumors of the facial nerve (schwannoma or neurofibroma) can also cause a facial paralysis. Table 1 presents a number of entities that must be considered in the evaluation process of a patient who presents with a paralyzed or weak face.

History and Physical Examination

The history and physical examination are extremely important in ruling out other causes of facial paralysis. Strongly suggestive of Bell's palsy is a rapid onset of facial weakness with little or no progression beyond 48 to 72 hours. A waxing or waning of symptoms or a prior history of facial weakness raises concern for another cause. The presence of pain, especially in the mastoid process, is not atypical. Lyme disease is suggested by recent outdoor activity in endemic areas. In most cases there will be a spreading rash (erythema migrans) at the site of the tick bite, as well as flulike symptoms such as fever, headache, myalgias, and arthralgias.

On physical examination there should be uniform involvement in all areas of the face. Sparing of the forehead suggests a central lesion because of dual innervation to the frontalis muscle. A weakness localized to one portion of the face suggests a parotid neoplasm involving a segment of the nerve after it has split from the main trunk. The external ear canal, tympanic membrane, and middle ear are examined otoscopically for evidence of infection or middle ear mass. The presence of vesicles in the conchal area is diagnostic for a herpes zoster neuropathy (Ramsey Hunt syndrome). The parotid gland is palpated for any tenderness or mass. A careful neurologic examination is performed looking for evidence of other cranial neuropathies or neurologic deficits. Occasionally, ipsilateral facial hypesthesia is noted in patients with Bell's palsy.

Radiographic and Laboratory Evaluation

In light of the broad differential diagnosis, a plethora of tests could be obtained, including a computed tomography scan or a magnetic resonance image, audiometry, serologies, complete blood cell count and chemistries, and a lumbar puncture. In patients with a classic history for Bell's palsy and an otherwise normal physical examination, the only test I order acutely is an audiogram. This test will help rule out a lesion in the cerebellopontine angle and temporal bone. The acoustic reflex is a routine part of the audiometric evaluation and is helpful in excluding a parotid lesion. The branch to the stapedius muscle exits from the facial nerve in the mastoid process. A viral neuropathy will paralyze this branch because it affects the facial nerve more proximally. A parotid neoplasm, however, affects the facial nerve distal to the stapedial branch and can cause a complete facial paralysis while maintaining an intact stapedial reflex. A radiographic evaluation is not performed acutely, but is ordered if some recovery of facial function is not seen by 3 to 4 months.

TABLE 1. **Causes of Facial Paralysis**

Congenital
Traumatic
  Temporal bone fracture
  Penetrating injury—face, temporal bone
Infectious
  Acute or chronic otitis media
  Malignant otitis externa
  Lyme disease
  Herpes simplex, type 1
  Herpes zoster
  Human immunodeficiency virus
Tumors
  Facial nerve schwannoma
  Facial nerve neurofibroma
  Glomus jugulare
  Cholesteatoma
  Leukemia
  Squamous cell carcinoma—primary or metastatic—temporal bone, parotid
  Parotid tumors—adenoid cystic, mucoepidermoid, etc.
Sarcoidosis
Guillain-Barré syndrome

Electrical Testing

Electrical testing can be used prognostically within the first several weeks of the onset of facial paralysis. The Hilger nerve stimulation test is conducted on the extratemporal portion of the damaged facial nerve. A current up to 10 mA is delivered to the main trunk in an attempt to elicit a motor response. The presence of any facial movement implies that many of the fibers are only in a neuropraxic state (axoplasmic conduction block). The ability to elicit a facial muscle response during the first 2 weeks after onset of Bell's palsy suggests an excellent chance for recovery. Loss of the response within this interval means that most axons have degenerated (axonotmesis) and many may have lost their endoneurial sheath (neurotmesis). Prognosis is more guarded in this group, with only an approximate 50% chance for good return of facial function. Electroneurography (ENOG) is performed in a similar way, but provides quantitative information. A large stimulus is given transcutaneously to the main trunk of the facial nerve near its exit from the temporal bone, and recording electrodes are placed in the nasal labial fold to measure the resulting compound muscle action potation. Each side is tested and a response on the paralyzed side that is less than 10% of the potential on the normal side portends a poor prognosis (chance for recovery approximately 50%). These two prognostic tests have little or no utility beyond the first 2 to 3 weeks after the onset of Bell's palsy. Electrical testing is not necessary in patients with only a paresis because some nerve function is obviously intact and prognosis is excellent. Electromyography testing can be performed many weeks later to provide information on recovery. For example, electromyography can detect reinnervation potentials (polyphasic waves) before visible facial motor function occurs.

FOLLOW-UP VISITS

Patients presenting with weakness or paralysis of their face and suspected Bell's palsy should be observed several times a week for the first 2 to 3 weeks, then every 1 to 2 weeks thereafter until recovery. The more frequent early visits are important to rule out a gradual progression of facial dysfunction in cases presenting with paresis. Such a scenario would be atypical for Bell's palsy. If electrical testing (Hilger or ENOG) is being performed, repeated examinations during the first 2 weeks are important. These data not only provide prognostic information, but are essential in choosing patients who might benefit from surgical intervention (see following section). Close follow-up in the early weeks is also important to confirm that proper eye care is being performed (see following section). Follow-up is continued on a weekly or biweekly basis to make sure that the patient recovers as anticipated. Failure to detect some recovery by 3 months or the development of other symptoms should prompt further diagnostic testing, including radiographic imaging.

TREATMENT

Medical Therapy

Steroids are often used to treat Bell's palsy and the literature is replete with studies arguing for and against such therapy. Recently, a meta-analysis of steroid therapy was published. Three studies (230 total patients) met the following criteria:

1. Prospective with concurrent controls.
2. Treatment within 7 days of paralysis onset using a total dose of prednisone (or equivalent) of at least 400 mg.

The outcome measure was complete recovery of facial function; a good, but incomplete return was considered non-cure. Two of the three studies showed a beneficial affect of approximately 17% (P <0.05). It is possible that this analysis underestimated the beneficial affect of steroids, given the strict outcome measure that was used.

For patients with a complete paralysis (not paresis) seen within 1 week of onset, I prescribe 1.0 mg/kg of prednisone for 3 days, 0.75 mg/kg for 3 days, 0.50 mg/kg for 3 days and then a rapid taper over the next 4 to 6 days.

Given the probable viral cause for Bell's palsy, the use of an antiviral agent seems reasonable. Several studies have suggested improved prognosis for patients given both prednisone and acyclovir versus prednisone alone. Again, early treatment is probably critical. My choice for therapy is either famciclovir or valaciclovir for 1 week.

SURGICAL THERAPY

Surgical decompression of the facial nerve in patients with Bell's palsy has been a subject of controversy for decades. The rationale for surgery is that the inflammatory response within the nerve causes edema, increasing the intraneural pressure. Vascular congestion and insufficiency result from this increased pressure, which in turn causes additional axonal damage. Anatomically, the labyrinthine segment of the facial nerve (especially at the meatal foramen) is particularly vulnerable to vascular compromise and swelling because it represents the most narrow portion of the enclosing bony canal (fallopian canal). Intraoperative observations and electrical studies, as well as histopathologic data, strongly suggest that the labyrinthine segment is the principle site of pathology. Any surgical approach to the facial nerve, therefore, should include this area. Experimental animal studies have shown that to be effective, surgical decompression of the facial nerve should be performed within 2 to 3 weeks of onset of the facial paralysis.

A recent multi-institutional prospective study of surgical decompression of the facial nerve for Bell's palsy has been published. Patients were divided into good and poor prognostic groups based on ENOG data obtained within the first 2 weeks of paralysis. Seventy individuals with less than a 10% response (>90% degeneration) within that time were assigned to either medical treatment (prednisone) or surgery (middle cranial fossa decompression). Surgery was performed within 2 weeks of paralysis onset. Approximately 40% of the patients treated medically had a very good to complete recovery versus 90% who underwent surgery. This was a statistically significant difference. Fifty-four patients who were in the good prognostic group (<90% degeneration on ENOG), given prednisone, and simply observed had the anticipated satisfactory outcome: 90% had very good to complete recovery.

This study confirmed a number of prior observations:

1. ENOG testing within the first 2 weeks of paralysis onset provides important prognostic information.
2. At least half the patients who are in the poor prognostic category based on the ENOG findings will have significant sequelae.
3. Surgical decompression of the facial nerve can be of benefit to patients properly selected. To be effective, this surgery must include a middle cranial fossa approach to the labyrinthine segment of the facial nerve and be performed within 2 weeks of onset of paralysis.

Eye Care

Corneal abrasion or infection is a concern in patients with a facial paralysis. The inability to close the eye completely and to blink is often compounded by decreased tearing and corneal hypesthesia. Frequent use of artificial tears or ophthalmic ointment is recommended. Glasses, particularly when outdoors, diminish air currents around the cornea and help prevent drying. The eye may need to be patched or taped shut, especially at night. If so, care must be exercised that the lid does not open, exposing the cornea to the material covering the eye. Any eye symptoms should be promptly evaluated by an ophthalmologist.

PARKINSONISM

method of
CHRISTOPHER G. GOETZ, M.D., and
STACY HORN, D.O.
Rush-Presbyterian-St. Luke's Medical Center
Chicago, Illinois

Parkinsonism is a term used to describe the clinical constellation of symptoms comprised of bradykinesia, rigidity, tremor, and postural instability. The causes of this constellation of symptoms vary among patients, and parkinsonism may be due to idiopathic Parkinson's disease, other degenerative brain diseases such as multiple system atrophy and progressive supranuclear palsy (collectively called the *Parkinson-plus syndromes*), multiple small-vessel vascular insults, metabolic diseases, and toxin exposure. The diagnosis of Parkinson's disease is made clinically by the confirmation of two of the four major signs either by physical examination or history and a therapeutic response to levodopa/carbidopa therapy. Parkinson's disease and other forms of parkinsonism will be discussed with a focus on accurate diagnosis and contemporary treatment options.

PARKINSON'S DISEASE

James Parkinson first described Parkinson's disease in 1817 in his "Essay on the Shaking Palsy." He detailed the symptoms of six persons, and described cardinal features of the disease, including tremor and postural instability. He did not, however, appreciate the distinction between bradykinesia and rigidity, consolidating these features as weakness (paralysis agitans). The original description impressed Jean Martin Charcot in the late 19th century, and, in his studies, he demonstrated the absence of prominent weakness and separated rigidity from bradykinesia. He called the constellation of symptoms Parkinson's disease.

Idiopathic Parkinson's disease most commonly presents with unilateral symptoms that progress to involve both sides, but some asymmetry persists even in later stages of the disease. Patients often present with a unilateral resting tremor or slowness of an arm or leg. On examination, patients often have masked or expressionless facies with decreased blinking, sialorrhea, cogwheel rigidity, bradykinesia, resting tremor, and postural instability.

Parkinson's disease usually begins in middle-age life and has a peak onset in the sixth decade with a slowly progressive course over about 20 years. Clinicians should not think of Parkinson's disease as a condition that only affects the elderly, and patients with onset in their 40s are common. Parkinson's disease is, by definition, responsive to dopaminergic medications and this helps to confirm the diagnosis.

Patients with mild Parkinson's disease should have some clinical improvement with dopamine agonists such as pergolide (Permax), bromocriptine (Parlodel), pramipexole (Mirapex), and ropinirole (Requip) at therapeutic dosages or levodopa/carbidopa. The typical dosages of the dopamine agonists are listed in Table 1. If patients do not clinically respond with levodopa/carbidopa at dosages greater than 800 mg/d, they most likely do not have idiopathic Parkinson's disease. Parkinson's disease is estimated to affect approximately 1% of the population over the age of 65 years.

The features of Parkinson's disease are due to a loss of neurons in the substantia nigra, specifically the pars compacta of the midbrain. The loss of these neurons causes a deficiency of dopamine in the projection site of these neurons, the putamen and caudate nucleus, collectively known as the *striatum*. Dopamine is essential to the normal nigral-striatal function that assures the production of fluid movement. Dopamine is metabolized by catechol-*O*-methyltransferase (COMT) and monoamine oxidase centrally and dopa decarboxylase and COMT in the periphery.

The cells of the substantia nigra in these patients often contain Lewy bodies, eosinophilic cytoplasmic inclusions with a faint halo. These signs, along with select degeneration of the substantia nigra, are the pathologic hallmarks of the disease. It is important to appreciate that the cells of the substantia nigra normally decline with age, but patients with Parkinson's disease have an accelerated loss for unknown reasons. It is estimated that 70% to 80% of these cells are already lost when patients have symptoms with the first signs of mild Parkinson's disease.

Idiopathic Parkinson's disease is diagnosed based on clinical grounds. There are no confirmatory tests such as laboratory studies or neuroimaging. The final diagnosis is confirmed with pathologic studies, and diagnostic accuracy even with clinical signs and levodopa/carbidopa response is only about 80%. Parkinson's disease has a number of co-morbid factors that may not be present in all patients including sleep disturbances, autonomic dysfunction, constipation, dysphagia, urinary dysfunction, seborrhea, anxiety, dementia, and depression. Table 2 lists some of these problems with their frequency in Parkinson's disease.

TABLE 1. **Dopamine Agonists in the Treatment of Parkinson's Disease**

Dopamine Agonist	Typical Starting Dosage	Typical Therapeutic Dosage
Pergolide (Permax)	0.5 mg/d	0.75–5 mg/d
Bromocriptine (Parlodel)	1.25 mg bid	5–80 mg/d
Pramipexole (Mirapex)	0.125 mg bid or tid	1.5–4.5 mg/d
Ropinirole (Requip)	0.25 mg bid or tid	4–24 mg/d

TABLE 2. **Co-Morbidities of Parkinson's Disease**

Co-Morbid Condition	Incidence (%)
Sleep disturbances	74–98
Constipation	50
Dysphagia	50
Urinary dysfunction	58–71
Depression	40
Anxiety	40
Dementia	7–85 from the literature with a median of 20%

PHARMACOLOGIC TREATMENT OF PARKINSON'S DISEASE

Pharmacologic treatment of Parkinson's disease is approached in two ways: (1) attempt to protect the brain from further nigral cell loss and (2) control the cardinal manifestations, primarily with dopaminergic supplementation.

Attempts to find a neuroprotective agent that slows the degeneration of nigral dopaminergic cells have not yet been definitely successful. A double-blind placebo-controlled trial looking at the possibility of slowing the need for symptomatic treatment through the use of the monoamine oxidase inhibitor (MAOI) selegiline (previously known as deprenyl) (Eldepryl) and vitamin E* was conducted in the 1980s. This study, the DATATOP study, found that the time until treatment with levodopa/carbidopa was required for symptomatic control differed when selegiline was used in the early phase of Parkinson's

*Not FDA approved for this indication.

disease. However, the interpretation of the results was limited due to the fact that selegiline has mild dopaminergic properties and treats some of the early symptoms of Parkinson's disease. Thus, although it certainly delays the clinical need to use levodopa/carbidopa early, selegiline has not been proven to have a neuroprotective effect in people with Parkinson's disease. Further trials with a long washout period would be needed to resolve this issue.

Although the results of this study were inconclusive and no identified neuroprotective agent has yet been established, a number of physicians still initiate selegiline therapy in early Parkinson's disease. The mechanism of selegiline's effect on early Parkinson's disease remains ambiguous, but the drug remains a frequently used monotherapy in the first several months of Parkinson's disease treatment. In this context, it is typically used at dosages of 5 mg in the morning and early afternoon. This medication can be stimulating and cause sleep disturbances if given too late in the evening.

The other agent that may be neuroprotective is coenzyme Q10,* and the efficacy of this medication to slow the progression of early Parkinson's disease is being studied. The usual dosage is 600 mg/d in divided dosages. Other strategies of research interest include use of the MAOI rasagiline,† use of early levodopa at various dosages, and administration of complex molecules collectively called *growth* or *neurotrophic factors.* Access to these protocols requires referral to study centers that are located throughout the United States and Canada. For a listing of these centers, contact the Parkinson's Study Group at www.Parkinson-Study-Group.org.

The second focus of treatment is the control of symptoms of the disease. This strategy is accomplished with a variety of medications that primarily affect the dopaminergic pharmacology with different mechanisms of action. Some increase the amount of dopamine available to the brain, some reduce its breakdown, and others substitute for dopamine. The dopaminergic medications used to treat the symptoms of Parkinson's disease include dopamine agonists, levodopa/carbidopa, and COMT inhibitors. In addition because the neurotransmitter acetylcholine antagonizes dopaminergic activity in the striatum, anticholinergic medications have been used. All of these agents are discussed.

The treatment of Parkinson's disease is complicated because some problems relate directly to the disease and others are effects due to medication treatment and the disease. As previously mentioned, the problems that are part of Parkinson's disease are tremor, rigidity, bradykinesia, and balance difficulty. In addition, as the disease progresses, difficulty with initiating walking and particularly turning or pivoting during walking lead to festination and momentary "freezing" where the feet inexplicably cannot move. If the torso and shoulders move forward or backward at these moments, the patient falls.

Falling is one of the most feared consequences of Parkinson's disease and is associated with increased mortality and disability such as hip fractures. In addition, a progressively shorter therapeutic response to medications characterizes advancing Parkinson's disease with problems of motor fluctuations, most commonly "wearing off" and delayed onset of medication effect. In the most simplistic of terms, medication effects that previously lasted 4 to 8 hours progressively shrink in their duration of effect and leave the patient with a continually shifting clinical state that requires more frequent dosages of medication. Other problems relate to the combination of medications and disease progression. Dyskinesias are hyperkinetic involuntary movements usually seen at the peak medication effect and they are generally considered as overshoot phenomenon from too much dopaminergic stimulation in the context of Parkinson's disease. Hallucinations, psychotic behavior, and delusional thinking can also occur in advancing Parkinson's disease. Although the pharmacology of these behaviors is less clear than that of the dyskinesias, the dopaminergic system is involved because dopaminergic drugs precipitate the behaviors. Drug withdrawal generally improves the behaviors and therapy with dopamine receptor antagonistic drugs reduces these behaviors. In summary, the treatment of moderate and advanced Parkinson's disease involves attention to the cardinal features of the disease, as well as the late-term features of disease progression including motor fluctuations, dyskinesias, and neuropsychiatric symptoms.

Anticholinergic Medications

Anticholinergic medications are the oldest form of therapy for Parkinson's disease and have been used since the 1800s. These medications are typically used to control tremor and are often introduced in early disease when other symptoms of Parkinson's disease are mild and stronger medications may not be needed. The agents are both peripherally and centrally acting medications, so side effects are an important issue. Trihexyphenidyl (Artane) and benztropine (Cogentin) are the most frequently used medications in this class. The typical starting dosage of trihexyphenidyl is 1.0 mg twice daily, which may be optimized to 2 mg thrice daily. The typical starting dosage of benztropine is 0.5 mg twice daily, which may be optimized to a dosage of 2 mg twice daily. The major side effects of these medications include sedation, confusion, hallucinations, dry mouth, blurred vision, constipation, urinary retention, nausea, impaired sweating, and tachycardia. These medications in general are better tolerated by a younger patient population because memory problems can become prominent in older subjects. They are not useful for treating motor fluctuations, dyskinesias, painful dystonic spasms, or hallucinations.

*Not FDA approved for this indication.
†Investigational drug in the United States.

Dopamine Agonists

The dopamine agonists include the ergot agents, pergolide (Permax) and bromocriptine (Parlodel) and the newer non-ergot agents, ropinirole (Requip) and pramipexole (Mirapex). The dopamine agonists are used both in monotherapy and polytherapy with levodopa/carbidopa. They are used as monotherapy in early Parkinson's disease in patients typically younger than 60 to 70 years of age for symptomatic treatment and to help delay the need for levodopa/carbidopa therapy. When used early in the disease process as monotherapy and supplemented with levodopa as symptoms progress over 5 years, agonist therapy is associated with fewer dyskinesias than patients experience when they are treated only with levodopa. In later stages of the disease, these medications may be helpful to control motor fluctuations.

These medications work by directly stimulating the striatal dopamine receptors with a dopamine-like moiety in their chemical structure. The advantages of direct stimulation of the dopamine receptors are multifold and include their independence of action from degenerating dopaminergic neurons, specific targeting of specified classes of dopamine receptors to help limit side effects, and lack of oxidative metabolism that may theoretically induce toxic free radical formation. The typical effective dosages include bromocriptine 5 to 80 mg/d, pergolide 0.75 to 5 mg/d, pramipexole 1.5 to 4.5 mg/d, and ropinirole 4 to 24 mg/d. The side effects of dopamine agonists include nausea, vomiting, orthostatic hypotension, and hallucinations. In addition, the ergot-derived dopamine agonists may rarely cause problems such as retroperitoneal fibrosis, erythromelalgia, pulmonary fibrosis, and Raynaud's-like phenomenon.

These medications need to be started at low dosages and increased until symptom management is attained or limiting side effects occur. Some physicians give the first dose of an agonist in the office and monitor the blood pressure response for 90 minutes to detect orthostatic hypotension that may influence starting dosages. Agonist therapy takes several weeks to reach optimal therapy, so patients and physicians should consider a commitment to agonist therapy for at least 3 months.

Levodopa/Carbidopa

Levodopa/carbidopa is the gold standard of treatment in Parkinson's disease. Levodopa was first administered in the 1960s. It "awakened" parkinsonian patients and allowed previously bedridden individuals to walk. This improvement of motor function was tempered by the high side effect profile including nausea, involuntary movements, orthostatic hypotension, and hallucinations due to the large dosages of oral levodopa that were required.

A major breakthrough in therapy occurred with the addition of peripherally acting inhibitors of dopamine decarboxylase to orally administered levodopa. This inhibitor helped to decrease the amount of dopamine that was converted peripherally and thereby, to increase the central nervous system (CNS) levels of dopamine. This breakthrough lead to greater symptom control and fewer limiting side effects.

In 1975, two dopaminergic medications became commercially available including carbidopa/benserazide (Madopar)* and carbidopa/levodopa. Levodopa/carbidopa is the most effective medication for the symptomatic treatment of Parkinson's disease, but carries long-term risks of motor fluctuations, dyskinesias, and hallucinations. Some symptoms of Parkinson's disease are unresponsive to carbidopa/levodopa therapy: freezing, postural instability, orthostatic hypotension, and dementia. There has been concern that levodopa/carbidopa may be neurotoxic through its oxidative metabolism to a free radical and its generation of hydrogen peroxide. This has been postulated as one of the causes of motor fluctuations and dyskinesias. Another possible cause is that the pulsing dosages of levodopa/carbidopa may be contributing to these problems of long-term treatment.

Concerns about early and high dose levodopa/carbidopa therapy have lead to changes in practice including a usual delay of early treatment with levodopa/carbidopa, the trial of longer acting preparations of levodopa/carbidopa (Sinemet CR), and the use of agonists to permit lower dosages of levodopa/carbidopa without loss of functional motor control. The typical starting dosage and treatment dosages of levodopa/carbidopa vary, but a safe starting dosage is 25/100 mg ½ tablet twice daily, increased as needed for symptomatic control. The side effects of levodopa/carbidopa include nausea, orthostatic hypotension, and hallucinations. The nausea and orthostatic hypotension may be limited by the use of additional carbidopa (Lodosyn) 25 mg given with each dosage of levodopa/carbidopa.

Sustained-release levodopa/carbidopa can be used in both early and late disease. Its main advantage is a less frequent dosing schedule. It has been compared with levodopa/carbidopa to determine the time to onset of motor fluctuations and dyskinesias. Both medications appear to cause motor fluctuations at the same rate. The main disadvantage of sustained-release levodopa/carbidopa is its erratic absorption. The usual starting dosage of sustained-release levodopa/carbidopa 25/100 mg is one tablet twice daily. The tablets can be broken in half, but this physically fractures the pill matrix and destroys some of the formulation's controlled-release effect.

If patients do not show motor improvement to dosages of levodopa/carbidopa greater than 800 mg/d, the diagnosis of idiopathic Parkinson's disease should be reconsidered and the other Parkinson-plus syndromes should be considered.

Enzyme Inhibitors

The addition of COMT inhibitors to the treatment of Parkinson's disease occurred in the 1990s. These

---

*Not available in the United States.

medications are used in conjunction with regular and sustained-release levodopa/carbidopa to increase the amount of levodopa available for transfer into the brain. They are used to enhance levodopa/carbidopa effects and to help control motor fluctuations. These medications work mainly through the peripheral inhibition of the metabolism of levodopa to 3-*O*-methyldopa. As a result of enzyme inhibition, more levodopa remains in the systemic circulation to pass through the blood-brain barrier and become central dopamine. The 3-*O*-methyldopa also competes with levodopa for transport into the circulation. The two COMT inhibitors that are commercially available in the United States include tolcapone (Tasmar) and entacapone (Comtan). Tolcapone is used at dosages of 100 mg to 200 mg thrice daily. This medication has fallen out of favor due to case reports of fatal hepatic toxicity. Patients must sign an informed consent to start this medication and need frequent monitoring of liver enzyme levels. Entacapone is used in dosages of 200 mg with each dosage of levodopa/carbidopa to a maximum dosage of 1600 mg/d. The main side effects of these medications include diarrhea and dyskinesias. The dyskinesias can typically be controlled by a decrease of levodopa/carbidopa dosage by 20% to 30%.

The MAOI selegiline is used in early Parkinson's disease as monotherapy to delay treatment with levodopa/carbidopa and has been proposed but never proven to be a possible neuroprotective agent in early Parkinson's disease. Selegiline works by a variety of possible mechanisms including an increase in striatal dopamine levels through central inhibition of monoamine oxidase-B, a clinically unsuspected antidepressant effect, and an increase in phenylethylamine levels. It has modest effects as monotherapy in improving motor signs of Parkinson's disease. When selegiline is added to levodopa, motor function can be maintained with lower levodopa dosages.

In patients with motor fluctuations, selegiline improves the duration of effectiveness with less end-of-dose wearing off. The symptomatic benefit of selegiline monotherapy may be short-lived and only lasts for months. In contrast, the related selegiline levodopa-sparing effects may be more resistant, and long-term studies looking at patients treated with both selegiline and levodopa/carbidopa showed a diminished dosage of levodopa for symptomatic motor control in the combination group. The combination group also needed a less frequent dosage schedule to control motor symptoms. Use of selegiline in early disease has not been shown to decrease complications of long-term levodopa therapy. The typical dosage of selegiline is 5 mg twice daily. At higher doses, it loses it specificity for the monoamine oxidase-B enzyme system.

Amantadine

The last medication that is helpful in the treatment of Parkinson's disease is the antiviral agent amantadine (Symmetrel). This medication has several mechanisms of action including an increase of dopamine release, the blockade of dopamine reuptake, the stimulation of dopamine receptors, and peripheral anticholinergic properties. Amantadine has been shown to be effective for treating the cardinal features of Parkinson's disease. It is also useful for treating dyskinesias and motor fluctuations later in the disease process possibly due to antiglutamate properties. Amantadine is typically used in divided dosages to a total dosage of 100 to 300 mg/d and is excreted unchanged in the urine. It is important to monitor the renal function of patients on higher dosages of this medication at regular intervals. The main side effects of this medication include confusion, hallucinations, insomnia, nightmares, livedo reticularis, ankle edema, dry mouth, and blurred vision. This medication should be used with care in patients with cognitive dysfunction.

NONPHARMACOLOGIC TREATMENT OF PARKINSON'S DISEASE

The nonpharmacologic treatments for Parkinson's disease are equally important to medical treatment of this disease. These modalities include education, support, exercise, and nutrition.

Education about the disease and its management and progression can provide a sense of control to patients. This information can be gleaned from a variety of sources including national organizations, patient books, and the Internet. Reputable information can be a great source of comfort to patients and their families. On the other hand, information that is delivered out of context can be frightening, so that patients need to review material with their health professional.

Support organizations fulfill a strong role in chronic diseases. These organizations give patients and families the venue to meet with other individuals to discuss similar problems and struggles. Their impact on patients and caregivers can be invaluable but in some instances can be harmful. Patients with early disease may actually be frightened by seeing the effects of late-stage disease, causing more depression and anxiety.

Exercise can be an important factor in the medical and psychological well-being of patients. Exercise increases the patients overall health and functionality. In addition, exercise has a positive impact on mood and energy levels. All of these factors are important aspects of treating chronic disease. It is, however, imperative to help patients find the appropriate type and amount of exercise to decrease mortality due to injuries. Physical therapy can be very helpful for patients in this capacity, both by increasing their overall function and educating patients about availability of exercise programs. Gains from physical therapy only last as long as exercise is maintained, so continuation is essential.

Nutrition is an important part of health education. Patients with Parkinson's disease have decreased muscle mass and more weight loss than healthy control subjects. Patients should be instructed to eat a healthy diet and to take a multiple vitamin with calcium if needed. The calcium is advocated to prevent osteoporosis, which can lead to increased morbidity and mortality especially in patients who are at risk of falling. Patients with Parkinson's disease need to know that if they take their carbidopa/levodopa with a high protein meal, food may interfere with medication absorption and reduce drug efficacy. To maximize levodopa/carbidopa absorption, patients should be advised to take their medications on an empty stomach and avoid eating for 45 minutes. For patients with marked sensitivity to protein, fruits and vegetables should dominate the daytime meals with most protein in the evening. Patients should also be careful about the amount of vitamins and supplements that they consume because hypervitaminosis can be as harmful as deficiencies. Excess vitamin E can cause coagulation problems.

SURGICAL TREATMENT OF PARKINSON'S DISEASE

Surgical treatment of Parkinson's disease can be a useful therapeutic option for patients whose parkinsonism is dominated by motor fluctuations, disabling tremors, or dyskinesias that are unresponsive to medical control. Surgery is reserved for patients without significant co-morbidities. Two types of surgical treatments exist: destructive and constructive. The first can involve ablative procedures or functional inhibition through deep brain stimulation. The second involves transplantation of new cell sources.

In the destructive surgeries, different areas of the brain that are functionally overactive as a result of dopamine loss are targeted to improve specific symptoms. In patients with motor fluctuations and dyskinesias, the globus pallidus interna or the subthalamic nucleus are the preferred sites. In the patient with unilateral tremor predominance, the ventrolateral thalamic nucleus may be the best option. The benefits of an ablative procedure are its reduced need for follow-up, decreased rate of infection, and lower expense. The disadvantages of ablative procedures are the irreversibility of the procedure and inability to perform bilateral procedures due to the high risk of dysarthria and cognitive side effects. The benefits of deep brain stimulation include the ability to control and fine tune the stimulator postoperatively, the ability to perform bilateral procedures, and lack of major destruction to tissue. The disadvantages include expense, need for frequent follow-up and adjustment of the stimulator, hardware failure, and need for battery changes. Both procedures carry a small risk of intracranial hemorrhage. Constructive surgery remains experimental and is confined to specialized research centers. Adrenal medullary cells from the patient's adrenal gland were tested in the 1980s, but current research focuses on human trials of fetal dopamine cells. If successful, these studies will lead to tests of genetically engineered cells and the use of undifferentiated stem cells suitably modified to produce dopamine, levodopa, or neurotrophic factors.

TREATMENT OF THE CO-MORBIDITIES OF PARKINSON'S DISEASE

The major co-morbidities of Parkinson's disease include depression, psychosis, sleep disturbances, and dementia. These may be major factors in disability and should be addressed with patients at each visit.

The depression of patients with Parkinson's disease may range from mild dysthymia to major depression with suicidal ideations. Management strategies range from support and psychotherapy to medical intervention. Treatment of depression with the selective serotonin reuptake inhibitors is often helpful. These medications are typically well tolerated even in elderly patients. Their major side effects include nausea, headache, and loss of libido. Currently available medications and their typical dosages are listed in Table 3.

The psychosis of Parkinson's disease can be frightening to both the patient and the family. The symptoms can include visual, and less commonly, tactile and auditory hallucinations, paranoia, and delusions. The symptoms of psychosis are exacerbated by the dopaminergic medications used to treat the motor symptoms of Parkinson's disease. These neuropsychiatric manifestations may be mild and require no treatment. However, if insight is lost, this can be a significant morbidity that requires treatment. Treatment of neuropsychiatric manifestations is a problem because most of the medications used to treat psychosis work by blocking dopamine. This dopaminergic blockage can cause worsening of patient's motor function. Two strategies can be adopted to help control psychosis. The first is to attempt to decrease the amount of dopaminergic medications without significantly impacting motor function. The second option is to introduce an atypical antipsychotic medication. These medications have the least amount of extrapyramidal side effects and include clozapine (Clozaril), risperidone (Risperdal), and quetiapine (Seroquel). Olanzapine (Zyprexa), although classified as an atypical neuroleptic, has been shown in many reports to aggravate parkinsonism, and hence is not regularly recommended.

The medication that has been most carefully stud-

TABLE 3. **Treatment of Depression in Parkinson's Disease**

Selective Serotonin Reuptake Inhibitors	Typical Starting Dosage	Typical Therapeutic Dosage
Citalopram (Celexa)	20 mg qd	20–60 mg qd
Fluoxetine (Prozac)	20 mg qd	20–80 mg qd
Paroxetine (Paxil)	20 mg qd	20–60 mg qd
Sertraline (Zoloft)	50 mg qd	50–200 mg qd

ied and effectively controls psychosis without exacerbating parkinsonism is clozapine. However, this medication has been associated with bone marrow suppression and requires informed consent for use and weekly complete blood cell counts. Despite these side effects, clozapine remains the our choice for treating psychosis. Olanzapine significantly exacerbates the motor features of Parkinson's disease as compared with clozapine; therefore we do not recommend use of this medication. Besides extrapyramidal side effects, these agents may cause sedation, confusion, and orthostatic hypotension. Lastly, some of these medications are associated with dose-related seizures. These medications should be started at the lowest dosages possible and optimized slowly. Table 4 lists medications with the usual starting dosages and typical therapeutic dosages.

The sleep disturbance associated with Parkinson's disease can include problems with falling and staying asleep. A lack of sleep and chronic fatigue can worsen the motor and psychiatric symptoms of patients and it is important to identify and treat this problem. Attempts to decrease the amount of Parkinson's disease medications taken at nighttime may be extremely useful. Many of these medications disrupt sleep including levodopa/carbidopa, dopamine agonists, amantadine, and selegiline. The first rule of treatment should be to have good sleep hygiene, including having a set time to go to sleep, using the bed only for sleeping, getting up at a designated time each morning, limiting the amount of stimulants such as caffeine taken in the evening, and limiting daytime naps. In patients with sleep disturbances and psychosis, the addition of the antipsychotic medication at bedtime may be helpful to control both problems. In patients who suffer from depression and a sleep disturbance, a medication such as nefazodone (Serzone) or trazodone (Desyrel) at bedtime can be helpful for treating both co-morbidities. The typical starting dosage for nefazodone is 100 mg at bedtime to a maximum dosage of 600 mg/d. The typical starting dosage for trazodone is 50 mg/d to a maximum dosage of 600 mg/d. Other medications that can be used with care to manage sleep problems include benzodiazepines and tricyclic antidepressants.

Dementia of Parkinson's disease is 10 times more frequent than that in age-matched controls. The dementia of Parkinson's disease is marked by dysfunction of the frontostriatal system and is most likely due to cortical involvement with Lewy bodies. Dementia is easily screened for with a Mini-Mental State Examination and abnormalities may be further assessed with formal neuropsychological testing. Dementia of Parkinson's disease typically occurs later in disease duration. Identification of dementia in Parkinson's disease is imperative because these patients may be more sensitive to dopaminergic medications and have neuropsychiatric side effects at lower dosages. Patients with Alzheimer's disease are often treated with centrally acting cholinesterase inhibitors. Studies using these medications in Parkinson's disease to treat dementia are being completed. These studies will need to address the cognitive, as well as the motoric effects of these medications in patients with Parkinson's disease.

TABLE 4. **Medications for the Treatment of Psychosis in Parkinson's Disease**

Medications to Treat Psychosis in Parkinson's Disease	Typical Starting Dosage	Typical Therapeutic Dosage
Clozapine (Clozaril)	12.5 mg qd	12.5–450 mg qd
Quetiapine (Seroquel)	12.5 mg qd	12.5–750 mg qd
Risperidone (Risperdal)	0.5 mg qd	0.5–16 mg qd

INTEGRATION OF PHARMACOLOGIC, NONPHARMACOLOGIC, AND SURGICAL THERAPIES

The physical and emotional priorities of patients with Parkinson's disease are not uniform and the physician and nursing staff will need to understand each patient's primary concerns. In the early phases of the illness, concerns over self-esteem, job security, and sexual dysfunction usually predominate. Psychological counseling, vigilance to diagnosis, treatment of depression, and attention to long-term career planning may be more important than treating mild motor symptoms. In the middle phases of the disease, motor fluctuations and dyskinesias are the major concerns. Lastly, in later stages of the illness, the focus is typically on balance problems, autonomic instability, and cognitive decline. The variability of signs and the interplay between the primary disease and the complications of medication require continual monitoring and neurologic re-evaluation.

OTHER FORMS OF PARKINSONISM

The differential diagnosis of parkinsonism is long and diverse. Because some of these diseases are medically treatable, early identification is essential for good long-term outcomes. The majority of these diseases do not respond well to dopaminergic medications and a trial of levodopa/carbidopa may be helpful in suggesting an alternative diagnosis. The list of problems causing parkinsonism includes medications, toxic substances, postencephalitis, degenerative CNS diseases, hereditary diseases, vascular disease, metabolic diseases, post-traumatic sequelae, and infectious diseases. With the exception of drug-induced parkinsonism, these other conditions have additional neurologic signs that are clearly outside the realm of typical Parkinson's disease. On the other hand in the early phases of these diseases, ancillary signs may not be apparent to the clinician treating the parkinsonism, so vigilance for these diseases is essential.

Medications that block or deplete dopamine can cause a syndrome that is unrecognizable from idiopathic Parkinson's disease. It is important to identify past and present medications in patients who present

TABLE 5. **Medications That Can Induce Parkinsonism**

Antipsychotic medications such as haloperidol (Haldol), trifluoperazine (Stelazine), and fluphenazine (Prolixin)
Gastrointestinal medications that block dopamine include prochlorperazine (Compazine) and metoclopramide (Reglan)
Antihypertensive agents, such as reserpine (Serpasil) and methyldopa (Aldomet)

with classical symptoms of idiopathic Parkinson's disease and to appreciate that neuroleptic medications are excreted very slowly, especially after chronic treatment. These classes of medications and typical examples are listed in Table 5. The parkinsonism is reversible when the offending medication is stopped, although full resolution may be slow. Many elderly patients receive neuroleptics for agitation or insomnia and the widely used gastrointestinal agent metoclopramide (Reglan) can cause parkinsonism.

Toxic substances can also induce a parkinsonian state. The most well-known toxin is methyl-phenyl-tetrahydropyridine. In the 1980s, a group of young patients with parkinsonism were identified and all had self-administered this synthetic analog of meperidine. Methyl-phenyl-tetrahydropyridine is metabolized to 1-methyl-4-phenylpyridium. 1-Methyl-4-phenylpyridum is a highly charged free radical that is taken up into dopamine terminals and blocks the mitochondrial respiratory chain. This blockage causes adenosine triphosphate depletion and eventual nigral cell death. The patients had all of the features of idiopathic Parkinson's disease, although magnified, with typical responses to levodopa/carbidopa, including motor fluctuations and dyskinesias. The only positive aspect of this tragedy was the development of animal models of Parkinson's disease and the resultant advances in research efforts. Several other toxins can cause a parkinsonian syndrome including carbon monoxide, cyanide, and manganese. Carbon monoxide poisoning causes a selective necrosis of the globus pallidus. The patients in whom parkinsonism develops typically have severe carbon monoxide poisoning with coma. Both acute and chronic poisoning with cyanide can induce parkinsonism. The mechanism is unclear, but may be due to selective necrosis of the globus pallidus, putamen, and subthalamic nucleus. Manganese poisoning from inhalation or ingestion can cause bradykinesia, rigidity, and gait disturbance. Dystonia is also a prominent symptom and the tremor that typifies this syndrome is usually of higher amplitude and has more postural enhancement than the typical Parkinson's disease tremor. Manganese intoxication has been described in miners and in patients who require chronic total parenteral nutrition. It is important to recognize this disorder because chelation therapy may be helpful. In the case of patients receiving total parenteral nutrition, an elimination or reduction of manganese from the trace elements of their parenteral solution is important. Lastly, rare chemicals that cause parkinsonism include herbicides such as diquat, carbon disulfide, methanol, n-hexane, and lacquer thinner.

Postencephalic parkinsonism is a disease only rarely seen today. The largest outbreak was of encephalitis lethargica in 1915 to 1928. The parkinsonism was seen in all phases of the disease and following recovery, sometimes many years later. This syndrome was distinguished from idiopathic Parkinson's disease by the presence of oculogyric crisis, marked dystonia, and prominent cognitive features.

Degenerative brain diseases that can mimic Parkinson's disease include progressive supranuclear palsy, multiple system atrophy, diffuse Lewy body disease, and corticobasal degeneration. These are termed the *Parkinson-plus syndromes* and each is identified by the additional clinical signs that accompany parkinsonism. Progressive supranuclear palsy is frequently misdiagnosed as idiopathic Parkinson's disease. It typically presents with rigidity, bradykinesia, and falling. Tremor is rare. Postural instability occurs early in the disease progression. Features that help to distinguish this disease from idiopathic Parkinson's disease include abnormalities of eye movements, pseudobulbar lability, and dystonia. Progressive supranuclear palsy has a more rapid disease progression with an average duration of 5.9 years. Multiple system atrophy includes diseases such as Shy-Drager syndrome, olivopontocerebellar atrophy, and striatonigral degeneration. The clinical features of these diseases include parkinsonism, ataxia, and dysautonomia. The disease duration is 3 to 9 years. Diffuse Lewy body disease typically presents with parkinsonism and cognitive abnormalities. Early agitation, delusions, hallucinations, and cognitive fluctuations are the hallmark of this disease. These patients often respond well to levodopa/carbidopa, but hallucinate on very small dosages. In addition, these patients have an exquisite sensitivity to neuroleptic medications. Corticobasal degeneration has parkinsonian features mixed with cortical sensory loss, dystonia, apraxia, and an alien limb phenomenon. Disease progression is typically 4 to 6 years.

Hereditary diseases that have parkinsonian features include Wilson's disease, the Westphal variant of Huntington's disease, and spinocerebellar ataxia. Wilson's disease is an autosomally recessive inherited disorder that causes an accumulation of copper in the CNS, as well as in the liver. The hallmarks of the disease include tremor, bradykinesia, neuropsychiatric complaints, liver dysfunction, and dystonia. The diagnosis is made most reliably by slit lamp examination for Kayser-Fleischer rings, liver biopsy, serum ceruloplasmin levels, and urinary excretion of copper. This condition is treatable with dietary modifications and copper chelation. Huntington's disease that presents before the age of 20 years often has bradykinesia, rigidity, and parkinsonian features. Huntington's disease is a triplicate repeat disorder located on chromosome 4 and is easily diagnosed with genetic testing. The spinocerebellar ataxias are a group of triplicate repeat disorders that can often have bradykinesia as a central feature of disease. These diseases also have features such as ataxia, dystonia, rigidity, dysarthria, and hyperreflexia.

Vascular disease involving the subcortical white and gray matter due to small vessel occlusion can present with gait disturbances and bradykinesia and is called *lower body parkinsonism.* Progression is typically more rapid with a stepwise progression. The lower extremities are usually more involved than the upper extremities. The coexistence of hypertension and diabetes mellitus are frequent causes of this type of vascular disease. Tremor is typically not a prominent symptom. Neuroimaging of the brain can aid in diagnosis.

The metabolic abnormality most often associated with parkinsonism is hypoparathyroidism. Symptoms occur due to deposition of calcium into the basal ganglia. This syndrome is identifiable by its other features including short stature, obesity, tetany, paresthesias, and short digits. It is easily diagnosed with parathyroid hormone levels. Hypothyroidism and apathetic hyperthyroidism can also mimic parkinsonism with slowness, altered gait, and mental decline. These conditions are easily identified with thyroid stimulating hormone levels, thyroxine levels, triiodothyronine, and levothyroxine levels.

Post-traumatic parkinsonism is seen most often with repeated head injury. This type of abnormality is often seen in boxers and called *dementia pugilistica.* Repeated blows to the head cause nigral degeneration and neurofibrillary tangles. The prominent features of this syndrome include dementia, personality changes, amnesia, ataxia, and tremor. As such, parkinsonian features are one of many other elements of the post-traumatic syndrome. Pure Parkinson's disease caused by head trauma has not been firmly established.

The prion disease Creutzfeldt-Jakob can resemble Parkinson's disease; however, this disease is much more rapidly progressive and may be fatal within months. This disease is marked by rapidly progressive dementia, parkinsonism, and myoclonus. This disorder has a characteristic electroencephalogram with periodic, high-amplitude sharp waves. Brain biopsy specimen shows a spongiform degeneration. No treatment is available. Lastly, infection with HIV can cause symptoms of parkinsonism. This is due to direct viral invasion into the subcortical white matter and basal ganglia. HIV infection can be confirmed with serum testing for the virus in patients with risk factors.

FUTURE PROSPECTIVES

Future advances in the diagnosis and treatment of Parkinson's disease will depend on cooperative efforts between basic science and clinical research teams. Basic scientists are attempting to find the causal agents of Parkinson's disease and test the mechanism of action of toxins on neurons. It is still not entirely clear what factors influence the development of nigral cell loss. An understanding of the basic biochemistry of the steps involved in cell death will greatly aid in developing treatments aimed at disease prevention and symptomatic dopaminergic replacement. In addition, basic and clinical research are attempting to find a definitive test to diagnose Parkinson's disease. Early and accurate diagnosis will be particularly important in targeting future neuroprotective therapies. In clinical research, new drugs to help control the symptoms of Parkinson's disease and the side effects of treatment are being studied. Attempts to understand the possible neurotoxicity and neuroprotection of levodopa/carbidopa at various stages of disease are underway. Surgical procedures to help control the symptoms of Parkinson's disease and the side effects of therapy are being studied in double-blind trials. These studies will help to answer which surgical therapies are best suited to control specific symptoms of the disease and side effects of treatment. Advances are also being made in surgical hardware and techniques. The combination of basic and clinical research has enabled clinicians to offer their patients a wide gamut of therapies. The choice of therapies must be individualized for each patient and guided by an understanding of the scientific role of therapy in the larger context of all possible therapies for Parkinson's disease. Despite remarkable progress, many questions remain unanswered. Government and private funding, the encouragement of young scientists to commit their concerns to the study of Parkinson's disease, and the alliance between clinicians and patients afflicted with Parkinson's disease are pivotal to finding the eventual answers.

PERIPHERAL NEUROPATHY

method of
MATTHEW P. WICKLUND, M.D.
Wilford Hall Medical Center
San Antonio, Texas

and

JERRY R. MENDELL, M.D.
Ohio State University
Columbus, Ohio

Peripheral nervous system disorders may affect motor, sensory, or autonomic neurons to produce weakness, sensory loss, paresthesias, pain, or autonomic dysfunction in varying combinations. Peripheral nerve disorders may be divided into mononeuropathies or polyneuropathies. Mononeuropathies involve damage in the distribution of a single peripheral nerve, often precipitated by compression, entrapment, or trauma. Mononeuropathies will not be addressed in this review; however, multiple mononeuropathies, a pattern often associated with peripheral nerve vasculitis, an important treatable disorder, deserve further discussion. The term *polyneuropathy* describes peripheral nerve disorders eliciting a diffuse, symmetrical, or predominantly symmetrical pattern of involvement. They do not respect the boundaries of individual nerves; the clinical picture simulates a stocking-and-glove distribution.

To properly treat peripheral neuropathies, one must first accurately ascertain the underlying cause, which may pose a challenge because the nerve responds to numerous insults with only a limited repertoire of pathophysiologic responses. Causes of peripheral neuropathy are myriad and include inflammation, vasculitis, dysproteinemia, nutritional deficiencies, endocrine and metabolic disorders, infections, toxins, pharmaceutical agents, and idiopathic conditions. To dissect out the correct cause, one must review the age of onset, course, family history, clinical and anatomic distribution of involvement, spectrum of nerve fibers involved, and concurrent diseases.

Broadly, peripheral neuropathies can be grouped as axonal or demyelinating, and electrophysiologic and pathologic evaluations differentiate these two types. Unfortunately, this distinction often poses difficulties in clinical practice because many chronic neuropathies present the clinician a mixed picture with components of axonal degeneration and demyelination.

The most common form of peripheral nerve disease is *distal axonopathy.* The anatomic uniqueness of the neuron is responsible for this susceptibility. It is the only cell in the entire animal kingdom that sends out a long cytoplasmic process that must be maintained by transport of materials to distal sites. Consider the far-reaching sites of that products synthesized by nuclear DNA must travel. In some species such as the giraffe, elephant, and giant squid, the distance is vast. Even in human beings, the distance from the lumbar spinal cord to the distal end of the lower extremity is significant, especially in view of the dependence of the axon on transported materials to maintain structural integrity (e.g., neurofilaments and neurotubules) and metabolic competence (e.g., mitochondria and enzymes). Well-defined systems are available to shuttle vital constituents to (slow and fast axonal transport) and from (retrograde transport) the periphery. Insult to the cell body can impair transport of many or even selective constituents to the distal axon. On the other hand, the distal axon is also vulnerable to direct insults. For example, certain signals from the nerve terminal must reach the cell body by way of retrograde transport, which can be easily interrupted by physical events and pharmacologic agents. A length-dependent injury is the outcome of this unique anatomic relationship, with clinical manifestations (sensory and motor) affecting the longest axons and leading to initial involvement of the toes and feet with centripetal spread to the more proximal end of the extremity. The term "dying-back neuropathy" was originally applied to this category of neuropathy but has been supplanted by the preferred designation "length-dependent" neuropathy.

The axon also degenerates when the cell body dies (neuronopathy). The process is different, however, and not selective for the distal axon. Instead, the entire axon degenerates within a matter of hours or days. The most common example is the motor neuronopathy designated amyotrophic lateral sclerosis. Sensory neurons are selectively affected in paraneoplastic disease and Sjögren's syndrome, conditions in which cells of the dorsal root ganglion undergo degeneration.

Electrophysiologic studies in axonopathies and neuronopathies show a reduction in the amplitude of motor and sensory action potentials without significant slowing in conduction velocity. These findings stand in contrast to conditions with preferential involvement of the myelin sheaths.

Selective injury to the myelin sheath results in *primary demyelinating neuropathies.* Both inherited processes and acquired injuries, including metabolic or immune attack directed toward the Schwann cell or myelin, promote this injury. Electrodiagnostic studies reveal reduced conduction velocity, prolonged distal latencies and F waves, conduction block, and temporal dispersion, all caused by focal or diffuse loss of myelin-mediated saltatory conduction.

IMMUNE-MEDIATED NEUROPATHIES

Guillain-Barré Syndrome

Guillain-Barré syndrome (GBS) is the eponym applied to a group of immune-mediated peripheral nervous system disorders characterized by a monophasic course, acute onset with progression for less than 4 weeks, areflexia, albuminocytologic dissociation in the spinal fluid, and spontaneous recovery that may take weeks or months, depending on the severity of the disease. Clinical studies over decades have expanded our concept of this entity and thus allow a more complete understanding of the syndrome into several entities, not just one condition (Table 1). The most prevalent subtype, acute inflammatory demyelinating polyradiculoneuropathy (AIDP), involves both motor and sensory findings with prominent demyelination. In the two axonal subtypes, acute motor axonal neuropathy (AMAN) manifests as weakness alone, and acute motor sensory axonal neuropathy (AMSAN) causes weakness with sensory loss. AMSAN is the most devastating form of GBS. The constellation of ophthalmoplegia, ataxia, and areflexia make up the clinical triad of the Fisher syndrome variant. In the Western world, AIDP constitutes over 80% of cases, whereas AMAN, AMSAN, and Fisher syndrome each make up less than 5% of cases. A pure autonomic disorder (acute panautonomic neuropathy) occurs infrequently.

GBS occurs with an incidence of approximately 1 in 100,000 and affects men and women of all ages equally. Two thirds of patients have an antecedent upper respiratory infection (viral, *Mycoplasma pneumoniae, Haemophilus influenzae*, others), diarrheal illness (*Campylobacter jejuni, Escherichia coli*, others), or other provocative event (surgery, pregnancy, immunization, HIV seroconversion). In nearly 90% of cases, evolution of the disease follows a characteristic pattern. Acral paresthesias involving the feet and hands customarily herald the onset of the illness. Over half of all patients complain of pain, which is frequently manifested as a deep aching or throbbing discomfort in the back or as burning, tingling, or shocklike paresthesias. Weakness follows the sensory involvement by a few hours to a few days, classically beginning in the legs and ascending to the arms. Facial muscles are weak in approximately 60% of cases, and eye movement abnormalities are seen in one sixth. Muscle stretch reflexes are absent or reduced in virtually all cases. About one third of patients eventually require mechanical ventilation. In AIDP, most patients reach their nadir within 2 weeks,

TABLE 1. **Variants of Guillain-Barré Syndrome**

Variants with weakness as the predominant manifestation
Acute inflammatory demyelinating polyradiculoneuropathy (AIDP)
Acute motor sensory axonal neuropathy (AMSAN)
Acute motor axonal neuropathy (AMAN)
Variants with other features predominant
Fisher syndrome
Acute panautonomic neuropathy

TABLE 2. **Treatment Options for Guillain-Barré Syndrome (All Variants)**

Therapy	Regimen	Side Effects
Plasma exchange	Remove 200–250 mL/kg	Catheter placement may cause pneumothorax, bleeding, deep vein thrombophlebitis, pulmonary emboli, sepsis Blood removal may cause anemia, low platelet count, coagulation and electrolyte derangements, low calcium and magnesium, hypotension
Intravenous immune globulin	0.4 g/kg/d × 5 d	Fever, chills, myalgias, diaphoresis, fluid overload, hypertension, nausea, vomiting, rash, headaches, aseptic meningitis, neutropenia, acute tubular necrosis, anaphylactic reaction associated with IgA deficiency
Corticosteroids*	No proven benefit	—

*Not FDA approved for this indication.

whereas those with AMAN and AMSAN become maximally weak within 5 to 6 days. The time to maximal functional recovery is 3 months in 70% and 6 months in 82%. Patients with AMSAN frequently experience extended recovery periods (12–18 months) and retain residual severe neurologic deficits.

The diagnosis is made on clinical grounds initially. An elevated cerebrospinal fluid protein (rarely found before the first 7–10 days) with a normal cell count is supportive. A spinal fluid cell count of more than 50 cells/mm^3 suggests infection with HIV. Typical electrophysiologic abnormalities on electromyography and nerve conduction studies may not appear until 2 weeks into the course. In AIDP, nerve conduction studies reveal evidence of demyelination with partial conduction block, prolonged distal and F wave latencies, and subsequently, slow conduction velocities. Reduced compound muscle action potential amplitudes with normal conduction velocity and diffuse denervation by electromyography reflect the changes of AMAN and AMSAN. Increased titers of antibodies to GM_1 or GD_{1a} gangliosides may sometimes be found in the axonal forms, whereas anti-GQ_{1b} antibodies are associated with Fisher syndrome in 95% of cases. These antibodies are postulated to cross-react with the lipopolysaccharides present on infectious organisms and the glycoconjugates present on nerves, a concept called molecular mimicry. Their presence or absence does not influence treatment. Other syndromes that may manifest in a manner similar to GBS and require different treatment include diphtheritic polyneuropathy and acute poliomyelitis (rarely seen in the United States), porphyria, hypophosphatemia, botulism, and tick paralysis.

GBS should be considered a potential medical emergency because respiratory failure may develop quite precipitously. Patients needing assistance ambulating require hospitalization. A mortality rate of 3% to 4% can be expected even with the best medical management. Initial evaluation must include respiratory function with forced vital capacity (FVC) and negative inspiratory force, arterial blood gas determination, an electrocardiogram (ECG), chest radiographs, serum electrolytes, and a complete blood count. Frequent respiratory and continuous ECG monitoring is recommended during the progressive stage. A useful clinical sign of impending respiratory failure is neck flexor weakness less than antigravity (inability to lift the head up from the pillow when supine). Respiratory parameters should be checked every 4 to 6 hours in patients with diminishing strength. Atelectasis and mucous plugging may be minimized with careful pulmonary toilet and incentive spirometry. Transfer to the intensive care unit is mandated if the FVC falls below 20 mL/kg, if the negative inspiratory force is less than 20 cm H_2O, or if oropharyngeal weakness threatens airway control. Intubation should be performed when the FVC falls below 15 mL/kg or the patient can no longer protect the airway. Tracheostomy should be performed to prevent tracheal stenosis if the patient remains ventilator dependent in excess of 14 days.

Autonomic nervous system dysfunction frequently occurs in GBS; manifesting as sinus tachycardia, hypertension (occasionally labile), orthostatic and supine hypotension, vagally mediated bradyarrhythmias, and bladder dysfunction. Continuous ECG and blood pressure monitoring is required for signs of instability. Before ascribing cardiovascular disturbances to dysautonomia, common conditions such as pulmonary embolism, infection, or volume depletion should be excluded. Vasoactive medications with long half-lives should be avoided because impaired blood pressure reflexes may result in exaggerated responses. Occasionally, temporary pacemaker placement is required for atrioventricular block.

Immunomodulatory therapy with two different modalities, plasma exchange and intravenous immune globulin (IGIV), has been documented to be beneficial in treatment of GBS (Table 2). The choice of therapy may be dictated by individual patient considerations. Corticosteroids, as a lone agent, remain contraindicated. A randomized, controlled trial of methylprednisolone* (500 mg/d intravenously for 5 consecutive days) showed no benefit and possibly an increased relapse rate. Six large randomized trials show benefit with plasma exchange in this syndrome. Studies document significantly reduced times to initial improvement and to independent ambulation, as well as fewer days on the ventilator. This benefit extends to patients with mild, moderate, and severe disease. A total of 250 mL/kg cumulative plasma is exchanged, and this exchange should be done within 7 to 14 days of disease onset to achieve maximal benefit. Despite the unequivocal effectiveness of plasma exchange, autonomic instability with labile blood pressure or cardiac dysrhythmias may preclude its use.

IGIV has been shown to have efficacy equal to that of plasma exchange in GBS patients by direct comparison in several controlled trials. The recommended regimen is IGIV* for 5 consecutive days at 0.4 g/kg/d. A common question that arises in clinical practice concerns the potential benefit of tandem therapy, such as plasma exchange followed by IGIV. This combination was addressed in a large trial comparing three modalities of treatment: plasma exchange versus IGIV versus both treatments

*Not FDA approved for this indication.

(plasma exchange followed by IGIV). No significant difference was found between treatment arms. In practice, certain factors may influence the use of IGIV over plasma exchange, including ease of administration, autonomic instability, sepsis, and lack of access to plasma exchange at some sites.

Although generally very well tolerated, IGIV administration may be associated with fever, systemic side effects, hypersensitivity reactions, and aseptic meningitis. Patients with underlying renal compromise, as might be encountered in diabetics with decreased glomerular filtration, are predisposed to acute renal failure with IVIG infusion. This complication can be avoided with a slower rate of infusion. The use of IGIV in patients with IgA deficiency is contraindicated because of the risk of anaphylaxis. The risks for transmission of HIV, hepatitis B, and hepatitis C are not carried in current formulations of IGIV.

A favorable outcome in GBS is ensured by avoiding the complications that accompany the prolonged paralytic phase. Careful surveillance and early treatment of nosocomial respiratory and urinary tract infection remains mandatory. Subcutaneous heparin, 5000 U twice daily and/or pneumatic calf compression devices are standard prophylaxis for deep venous thrombosis and pulmonary emboli. When bulbar dysfunction threatens aspiration, enteric tube feedings should be initiated for airway protection and avoidance of a catabolic state deleterious to muscle strength. Special air-floating beds and frequent position changes help prevent decubitus ulcer formation, whereas twice-daily passive range of motion exercises, in addition to early use of neutral-position hand splints, foot boards, and comfortable ankle-high sneakers, minimize contractures. Attention to limb positioning should help avoid pressure palsies of vulnerable nerves. Pain in GBS may be muscular, skeletal, or neurally mediated and is sometimes responsive to mild analgesics. If severe, tricyclic antidepressants, gabapentin, tramadol, or narcotics may be used. Depression and isolation occur frequently in patients with prolonged paralysis and may be diminished by ensuring adequate time and means for communication, allowing the patient control over some aspects of daily life, arranging visits from recovered GBS patients, and administering judicious pharmacologic treatment in conjunction with counseling.

Overall, complete recovery occurs in over 85% of patients. Permanent disability, usually involving the lower extremities and requiring ankle-foot orthoses, occurs in 10% to 15%. Patients with AMSAN may suffer prolonged ventilator dependence (6 months or longer), profound paraplegia, a recovery phase in excess of 2 years, and greater residual deficit. Poor prognostic factors in GBS include advanced age, rapidly progressive weakness, need for ventilatory support, preceding diarrheal illness, low-amplitude compound motor action potentials, and electrically inexcitable nerves.

Chronic Inflammatory Demyelinating Polyradiculoneuropathy

Chronic inflammatory demyelinating polyradiculoneuropathy (CIDP) is an acquired idiopathic disorder affecting all ages. Proximal as well as distal weakness separates this entity from many chronic distal axonopathies. Patients exhibit generalized hyporeflexia or areflexia and variable sensory deficits. Whereas disease severity reaches its nadir within 4 weeks in GBS, CIDP is differentiated by continued or recurrent progression beyond 8 weeks. In some cases, sensory symptoms may predominate or autonomic manifestations may be prominent. The course of CIDP may be chronic progressive or relapsing and remitting.

Cardinal laboratory features include acellular spinal fluid with elevated protein levels, along with findings of demyelination on electrophysiologic testing. Though not usually required for diagnosis, sural nerve biopsy may reveal combinations of demyelination, remyelination, endoneurial edema, inflammation, and occasionally, axonal degeneration.

Concurrent conditions can complicate diagnosis and treatment. Demyelination of the central nervous system with clinical manifestations similar to those of multiple sclerosis occurs in 5% of patients, and an additional 20% have laboratory features by magnetic resonance imaging or evoked potential testing that demonstrate typical demyelinating central nervous system abnormalities. Approximately 10% of patients carry associated systemic illnesses in addition to CIDP. These conditions include malignancies (Hodgkin's disease, melanoma, and various carcinomas), connective tissue diseases, hepatitis, HIV infection, inflammatory bowel disease, glomerulonephritis, thyrotoxicosis, and diabetes. CIDP may also occur in the setting of a monoclonal gammopathy of undetermined significance (MGUS), with its 25% attendant risk of hematologic malignancy at long-term follow-up. The clinical features of CIDP will sometimes be superimposed on an inherited neuropathy such as Charcot-Marie-Tooth disease (pes cavus, hammer toes). This association reflects a predisposition for an acquired demyelinating disorder to be superimposed on an underlying inherited neuropathy. Recognition of the inflammatory demyelinating component may be difficult, but sudden progression affecting the proximal muscles in the setting of disease previously affecting only the distal muscles is an important clue. Patients improve with immunomodulatory therapy, leaving only the residual distal weakness and sensory loss from the underlying genetic neuropathy.

CIDP responds to treatment with corticosteroids, plasma exchange, and IVIG, all demonstrated by prospective randomized controlled studies (Table 3). Because of its documented effectiveness, ease of administration, and low frequency of side effects, IGIV has emerged as the first therapeutic option for many clinicians in uncomplicated CIDP. A preferred regimen consists of 0.5 g/kg/d for 4 days, with subsequent dosing depending on the clinical response. IGIV seems especially prudent for use as initial treatment in children and in patients with contraindications to corticosteroids (e.g., diabetes, obesity, hypertension, osteoporosis). A clinical response is commonly seen within 1 to 3 weeks from the onset of therapy, and improvement may be maintained with a single dose of 0.4 to 0.5 g/kg every 3 to 4 weeks, the approximate half-life of the immunoglobulin. We will often manage severely affected, nonambulatory patients more aggressively with weekly infusions of 0.2 to 0.25 g/kg after the initial 4-day load. This regimen will continue until significant benefit is achieved, after which it can be tapered to longer intervals.

Prednisone retains an important role in the treatment of CIDP because of its ease of use, lack of expense, prompt onset of action, and physicians' familiarity with the agent. It remains an effective alternative for patients who fail IGIV therapy. In addition, the cost of IGIV can be prohibitory for some patients. We recommend initially administering prednisone at 1.0 to 1.5 mg/kg/d as a single, morning dose and maintaining daily dosing until improvement in strength is documented. Nearly 90% of patients will show improvement within the first 2 months. The intent thereafter is to reduce the dose to an alternate-day regimen if

TABLE 3. **Treatment Options for Chronic Inflammatory Demyelinating Polyradiculoneuropathy**

Therapy	Regimen	Side Effects
Prednisone*	1.0–1.5 mg/kg/d given as a morning dose	Osteoporosis, osteonecrosis of the hip, glucose intolerance, hypertension, cataracts, fluid retention, weight gain, cushingoid appearance, infection
Plasma exchange	Must be individualized to the patient; begin at 2 or 3 exchanges (3 L each) per week for 3 to 6 wk	Catheter placement may cause pneumothorax, bleeding, deep vein thrombophlebitis, pulmonary emboli, sepsis Blood removal may cause anemia, low platelet count, coagulation and electrolyte derangements, low calcium and magnesium, hypotension
Intravenous* immune globulin	Doses individualized to the patient; induction dose, 2 g/kg divided over 2 doses (1 g/kg) or 4 doses (0.5 g/kg); maintenance dose determined by response	Fever, chills, myalgias, diaphoresis, fluid overload, hypertension, nausea, vomiting, rash, headaches, aseptic meningitis, neutropenia, acute tubular necrosis, anaphylactic reaction associated with IgA deficiency

*Not FDA approved for this indication.

possible, followed by a slow taper of 5 mg every 2 weeks, provided that improvement is maintained. Patients with severe disease may benefit when treated with pulse methylprednisolone, 1 g intravenously daily for 5 days, before oral steroids. Long-term corticosteroid therapy carries the risks of weight gain and salt retention, osteoporosis, susceptibility to infection, cataracts and glaucoma, hypertension, glucose intolerance, and aseptic necrosis of joints. Our patients receive dietary counseling in support of a low-sodium, calorie-restricted diet, along with vitamin D supplementation and 1 g of calcium per day. For patients maintained on long-term corticosteroid treatment, we now institute treatment with bisphosphonates (alendronate [Fosamax], 5 mg/d) to minimize bone loss. A tuberculin skin test should be performed before initiation of treatment, and patients must be monitored intermittently thereafter with serum glucose and blood pressure checks along with periodic eye examinations. An exercise regimen tailored to the patient's capabilities is encouraged as a means of retaining strength and offsetting the muscle atrophy caused by the catabolic effects of steroids.

Plasma exchange is also effective in CIDP, but in contrast to GBS, this form of treatment must be used in combination with another immunosuppressive agent (e.g., corticosteroids). We have observed more rapid onset of improvement with plasma exchange than with IGIV in CIDP, and for that reason it is useful in patients with severe weakness or relapsing disease or those refractory to IGIV. The specific regimen of plasma exchange varies, but for severely weak patients, we often recommend an aggressive course of three exchanges weekly for the first 2 weeks, followed by twice-weekly exchanges for the next 3 to 4 weeks. Hypotension, infection secondary to immunosuppression, a transient bleeding diathesis, allergic reactions, and complications related to vascular access are the main contraindications to plasmapheresis.

Other immunosuppressants have been used in this disease as steroid-sparing agents or in refractory cases. Cyclosporine (Sandimmune) and mycophenolate mofetil (CellCept) have been used successfully for immunosuppression after organ transplantation. Their use has been adapted to the refractory CIDP population, along with cyclophosphamide (Cytoxan).

Multifocal Motor Neuropathy

This disorder is characterized by asymmetric weakness, fasciculations, and atrophy affecting the arms more than the legs and is caused by multifocal conduction block of motor axons. Although superficially resembling amyotrophic lateral sclerosis, the lack of upper motor neuron findings on examination and the presence of abnormal nerve conduction studies on electrodiagnostic testing readily distinguish the two conditions. Focal areas of partial conduction block demonstrated by nerve conduction studies are the sine qua non of diagnosis. Increased titers of IgM anti-GM_1 antibodies are usually, but not always detected and do not influence the decision to treat. Patients should be treated with IGIV as described for CIDP (see Table 3). In most patients, the therapeutic response is slow, yet efficacious in this chronic condition requiring prolonged intervention. Unfortunately, the effectiveness of this agent may wane over time in some patients. Corticosteroids and plasma exchange are not effective. Cyclophosphamide may be beneficial, but the use of this agent must be balanced against the severity of the condition in relation to the long-term risks of neoplasia.

Peripheral Nerve Vasculitis

Vasculitic neuropathy may be one of the manifestations of a systemic necrotizing vasculitis accompanying polyarteritis nodosa, microscopic polyangiitis, Wegener's granulomatosis, Churg-Strauss syndrome, collagen vascular disease (lupus erythematosus, rheumatoid arthritis, Sjögren's syndrome), infection (hepatitis B or C, HIV), malignancy, or drug hypersensitivity. A neuropathy in the setting of multiorgan involvement raises a strong suspicion of vasculitis. However, in one third of cases, a vasculitic neuropathy occurs in isolation without accompanying disease and is referred to as isolated peripheral nerve vasculitis or nonsystemic necrotizing vasculitis.

Vasculitic neuropathy has an ischemic pathogenesis evolving from inflammation and necrosis in the vessel walls of the vasa nervorum, with subsequent occlusion of vascular lumina. The features of vasculitic neuropathy may reflect multiple individual nerve involvement (multiple mononeuropathies), overlapping mononeuropathies (which obscure the involvement of single nerves), or a confluent, distal, symmetrical stocking-glove polyneuropathy. Classically associated with burning, dysesthetic, neuropathic pain, peripheral nervous system vasculitis does not cause pain in 20% to 30% of cases. Electrodiagnostic studies may help delineate the pattern of multiple mononeuropathies, and laboratory studies screen for non-neurologic organ involvement and underlying etiologies.

The diagnosis of vasculitis requires biopsy demonstration of transmural inflammatory cell infiltration and fibrinoid necrosis of blood vessels. Biopsy of a cutaneous nerve, such as the sural nerve, with clinical or electrodiagnostic evidence of vasculitic involvement is the procedure of choice. A combined superficial peroneal nerve/peroneus brevis muscle biopsy through a single incision augments the diagnostic yield by allowing evaluation of vessels in both nerve and muscle tissue.

Treatment varies with the cause and centers around several issues: treating the underlying disorder, providing immunosuppressive therapy, minimizing medication side effects, and providing supportive care. Discontinuation of an offending illicit or prescription drug and treatment of an underlying malignancy may stop further vasculitic damage and allow recovery. Patients with hepatitis B– or hepatitis C–associated vasculitis benefit from treatment with interferon alfa, and patients with HIV respond to aggressive multidrug management of the viremia. Most cases of vasculitis will require immunosuppressive therapy. We currently recommend a regimen using prednisone at 1.5 mg/kg/d as a single morning dose, along with cyclophosphamide at 1.5 to 2.5 mg/kg/d orally. In cases with rapid progression or severe disability, the corticosteroid regimen may be initiated with pulse methylprednisolone, 1.0 g intravenously daily or every other day for three to six doses, before switching to oral dosing as described. An alternate-day maintenance dose of prednisone is preferred for long-term administration (1.5 mg/kg/d), but such maintenance is based on individual patient response. When the patient has clearly reached maximal benefit, a slow taper of the prednisone dose by 5 mg every 2 to 4 weeks should be instituted. It has been recommended that cyclophosphamide be continued for 1 year in systemic necrotizing vasculitides, but for patients with isolated peripheral nerve vasculitis, we shorten cyclophosphamide use to 3 months if possible. Alternatives for those intolerant to cyclophosphamide* include cyclosporine,* methotrexate,* chlorambucil,* mycophenolate,* and IGIV.* No regimens have been tested in randomized controlled trials.

Drug toxicities and opportunistic infections complicate the treatment course in nearly 75% of vasculitis patients. Patients are also predisposed to malignancy by long-term cyclophosphamide administration. The litany of complications related to corticosteroid use and appropriate preventive measures have been discussed (see CIDP). Oral hydration and frequent voiding decrease the risk of hemorrhagic cystitis in patients taking cyclophosphamide. Periodic urinalysis to monitor for microscopic hematuria is appropriate. Complete blood counts are obtained monthly and the dosage of cyclophosphamide adjusted to maintain a white blood cell count over 3000/mm^3 and neutrophil count greater than 1000/mm^3. The risk of lymphoma and bladder cancer is increased 10- and 30-fold, respectively, in patients taking cyclophosphamide and generally correlates with the cumulative dose of cyclophosphamide. Recent randomized, controlled studies have used pulsed intravenous cyclophosphamide in doses of 15 mg/kg every 1 to 4 weeks to minimize the risk. Intravenously treated patients had fewer side effects and showed an equivalent response rate, but they relapsed more frequently. Referrals for physical and occupational therapy help maintain range of motion, preserve strength, and increase activities of daily living in patients with substantial neurologic involvement. Orthotic devices along with ambulatory aids such as canes and walkers may improve independence and enhance the quality of life. Appropriate management of neuropathic pain is imperative in these patients (see Painful Sensory Neuropathy later).

*Not FDA approved for this indication.

PARAPROTEINEMIC NEUROPATHIES

Peripheral neuropathies occur in association with monoclonal gammopathies in several disorders, including multiple myeloma, amyloidosis, Waldenstöm's macroglobulinemia, cryoglobulinemia, and MGUS. All adult patients with undiagnosed chronic neuropathy should be screened by serum and urine immunofixation electrophoresis for the presence of an abnormal monoclonal protein (IgG, IgM, or IgA). If a paraprotein exists, further evaluation should include a skeletal survey, bone marrow biopsy with aspiration, and a nerve biopsy where appropriate (see discussion of specific entities in the following sections).

Neuropathy Associated With Myeloma

Neuropathy accompanies multiple myeloma in 5% to 10% of cases and tends to be manifested as a mild distal sensorimotor polyneuropathy. Symptoms of the neuropathy generally do not reverse even with effective treatment of the myeloma. In the less common osteosclerotic variant of myeloma, peripheral neuropathy occurs in 50% to 85% of cases, affects a younger population, and is typically more debilitating. A clue to diagnosis may be some or all of the features of the POEMS syndrome (*p*olyneuropathy, *o*rganomegally, *e*ndocrinopathy, *M* protein, and *s*kin changes) in the setting of a sensorimotor neuropathy. The M protein is typically an IgG or IgA with λ light chains. Nerve conduction studies present a mixed picture of axonal degeneration and demyelination. In two thirds of cases, the skeletal survey demonstrates a solitary myeloma (isolated plasmacytoma) with purely sclerotic radiographic features, whereas in one third, the lesions are mixed sclerotic and lytic. Multiple bone lesions demonstrating varying degrees of sclerosis are seen in 50% of cases. Some patients with isolated plasmacytomas do not have an associated monoclonal gammopathy, thus making diagnosis even more challenging. In these cases, other laboratory features such as an elevated red blood cell count, leukocytosis, or thrombocytosis may lead to the diagnosis.

Solitary myeloma should be treated with local radiation therapy. The neuropathy will usually improve after 3 to 6 months. If no response occurs, other treatment options include prednisone and melphalan in doses appropriate for treating myeloma, as well as surgical excision. For refractory cases, interferon alfa-2b should be considered, as well as chlorambucil.

Primary Amyloid Neuropathy

Acquired amyloid polyneuropathy should be suspected in patients with monoclonal gammopathy and progressive painful peripheral paresthesias, acral loss of pain and temperature sensation, autonomic dysfunction such as orthostatic hypotension or impotence, and carpal tunnel syndrome or other entrapment neuropathies. Approximately 90% of patients with primary systemic amyloidosis have a monoclonal protein detected in serum, urine, or both. It is most often IgG, followed next by IgA; λ light chains are typical. Diagnosis requires tissue demonstration of amyloid filaments by Congo red stain. This stain can be conveniently performed on the bone marrow biopsy, which shows positive staining in nearly 50% of cases. Sural nerve biopsy is positive for amyloid in 80% of patients. Myeloablative chemotherapy with stem cell transplantation has been used successfully in this disease, but with an excessive risk of mortality. The neuropathy remains refractory to the usual chemotherapeutic treatment.

Neuropathy Associated With Monoclonal Gammopathies of Undetermined Significance

Nearly two thirds of patients with neuropathies and monoclonal gammopathies have MGUS. κ Light chains are more common in this group without identifiable plasma cell disorders. In 50% of cases of MGUS neuropathy, the monoclonal protein is an IgM antibody with activity directed against an important myelin constituent, myelin-associated glycoprotein (MAG). The anti-MAG antibodies are thought to play a causative role in development of the neuropathy. Nerve biopsies demonstrate anti-MAG antibody deposited in the uncompacted regions of the myelin sheath along the expected distribution of MAG. In addition, passive transfer experiments in animals leads to a demyelinating neuropathy.

Clinically, the neuropathy associated with anti-MAG antibody is painless and slowly progressive with distal sensory loss and paresthesias, tremor, gait ataxia, distal weakness later in the course, elevated spinal fluid protein, and demyelinating features on electrodiagnostic studies. IgM MGUS neuropathies are usually refractory to treatment, including plasmapheresis and corticosteroids. Pulse cyclophosphamide (1 g/m^2) given monthly may improve function. Newer chemotherapeutic agents such as fludarabine (Fludara)* and rituximab (Rituxan)* hold promise for this recalcitrant neuropathy.

Neuropathies associated with IgG and IgA MGUS but without anti-MAG antibodies have a more heterogeneous clinical profile, yet are more responsive to treatment. In most, a distal, symmetric, sensorimotor polyneuropathy with predominantly sensory symptoms ensues. No clear-cut evidence has emerged that the IgG or IgA is directed against nerve constituents, but the neuropathy is responsive to plasma exchange in many patients. We recommend a therapeutic trial of at least two plasma exchanges per week for 3 to 6 weeks. If an objective benefit can be demonstrated, these patients should continue plasmapheresis. If not, the treatment guidelines for anti-MAG syndrome may be tried. Occasionally, MGUS neuropathies demonstrate findings on examination and electrophysiologic and laboratory studies that are consistent with CIDP or multifocal motor neuropathy and should be treated as discussed in previous sections.

ALCOHOLIC AND NUTRITIONAL NEUROPATHIES

A distal, symmetric polyneuropathy may be associated with alcoholism and nutritional deficiencies. In alcohol abusers, the initial symptoms consist of burning pain in the soles of the feet and aching pains in the calves. Slowly progressive distal weakness and muscle wasting follow. Most experts believe that the neuropathy of alcoholics is due to vitamin deficiencies and not a direct toxic effect of alcohol on nerves. Although a specific vitamin deficiency has not been well demonstrated, a widely held concept is that the neuropathy of alcoholism is related to thiamine (vitamin B_1) deficiency. Treatment of affected patients includes supplementation with B vitamins, including 100 mg thiamine daily. Eating disorders, gastrointestinal bypass procedures, and malabsorption syndromes of various cause also induce nutritional polyneuropathies with deficiencies of vitamin B complex components and are treated with B vitamin supplementation.

Pyridoxine (vitamin B_6) deficiency leads to a peripheral neuropathy, whereas excessive pyridoxine produces a sensory neuronopathy with marked proprioceptive and vibratory sensation loss. The most common cause of pyridoxine deficiency is ingestion of the antituberculous drug isoniazid, which increases the excretion of pyridoxine. A polyneuropathy with sensory greater than motor axonal involvement, occasionally with optic neuritis, can be prevented by the use of 100 mg of daily supplementary pyridoxine. Chronic doses as low as 200 mg/d of pyridoxine or acute ingestion of inordinate amounts (>1 g) may lead to a debilitating syndrome with ataxia and loss of appreciation for where the trunk and limbs are located in space. The neuronopathy associated with chronic doses improves when consumption of pyridoxine ceases.

Vitamin E–deficient neuropathy may occur in patients with autosomal recessive familial isolated vitamin E deficiency or lipid malabsorption (chronic cholestasis, cystic fibrosis, and short-bowel syndrome) and results in a peripheral neuropathy often accompanied by cerebellar ataxia. This condition responds to supplementation tailored to the deficiency, and vitamin E should be monitored to restore normal levels (lower limit, <0.5 mg/dL).

Cobalamin (vitamin B_{12}) deficiency affects the nervous system at all levels and causes peripheral neuropathy, subacute combined degeneration of the spinal cord (dorsal column sensory loss and weakness), and encephalopathy. Common features of this peripheral neuropathy include paresthesias of the hands and feet, lost or diminished ankle muscle stretch reflexes with coexistent hyperreflexia at other joints, and occasionally Babinski signs. Neurologic disease may be seen without macrocytosis and may occur with vitamin B_{12} levels in the low-normal range. Patients with clinical features consistent with cobalamin deficiency and low-normal vitamin B_{12} levels should have their methylmalonic acid levels checked. Elevated levels imply functional cobalamin deficiency because methylmalonic acid is a substrate for an enzymatic reaction catalyzed by vitamin B_{12}. Almost all vitamin B_{12}–deficient patients suffer from an absorptive problem in the gastrointestinal tract, although inadequate dietary intake may be seen in true vegans and in syndromes with hyperemesis. Initial therapy should consist of 1000 μg of cyanocobalamin or hydroxycobalamin administered intramuscularly or subcutaneously for 5 to 7 consecutive days, followed by further injections on a monthly basis or 500 μg of cyanocobalamin delivered intranasally every week. Treatment in cases of decreased absorption must continue for the duration of the patient's life. Because some cases are due to autoantibodies to intrinsic factor or to parietal cells, other autoimmune diseases may be seen in conjunction with cobalamin deficiency.

METABOLIC NEUROPATHIES

Diabetic Neuropathy

Peripheral neuropathies commonly accompany diabetes mellitus and are detectable in 5% to 10% of patients at

*Not FDA approved for this indication.

diagnosis and in over 50% after 25 years of disease. The peripheral neuropathies associated with diabetes are myriad in nature and include cranial neuropathies, limb mononeuropathies, thoracic radiculopathies, diabetic lumbosacral radiculoplexopathy, distal symmetric polyneuropathies, and acute painful sensory neuropathies. Patients often have a mixture of two or more types. Although the cause of neuropathies in diabetes is unknown, a combination of factors involving hyperglycemic hypoxia, dysfunction of ion channel conductance, and vascular injury in nerves may underlie the damage. Multiple mechanisms may be involved, and different mechanisms may lead to the various patterns of involvement.

Cranial neuropathies most often affect the third and sixth cranial nerves and lead to diplopia. The dysfunction generally lasts for 3 to 6 months and resolves spontaneously. Focal compressive neuropathies are generally thought to occur more frequently in diabetic patients. Carpal tunnel syndrome, ulnar nerve entrapment at the elbow, and peroneal nerve palsies at the fibular head also often revert to normal without treatment, but sometimes surgical release is required. Thoracic radiculopathies, though self-limited over months, may subject patients to severe dysesthetic discomfort of the chest wall. Medications for neuropathic pain may help alleviate the pain, but always incompletely. When pain is intractable, we have used hospital-based treatment consisting of intravenous methylprednisolone 1.0 g daily for 5 days, or intravenous immunoglobulin, 0.5 g/kg/d for 4 days.

Patients with diabetic lumbosacral radiculoplexus neuropathy (also called diabetic amyotrophy or Bruns-Garland syndrome) have asymmetric pain in the hip, buttock, or thigh, along with prominent proximal leg weakness of the quadriceps, thigh adductors, and iliopsoas, with little sensory loss. The distal leg muscles are also usually affected, and the other leg is frequently affected after a latency of days to months. This neuropathy affects type 2 diabetics usually after age 50 and is more common in men than woman. No relationship has been noted between the neuropathy and the duration of glucose intolerance. The symptoms progress for weeks or even months after onset. The pain resolves first, with varying degrees of weakness remaining that can be debilitating. At times, the lower extremities can be virtually completely useless. Recovery is slow and depends on nerve regeneration throughout the lower extremities. Complete recovery is possible, but residual weakness is not unusual. The pathogenesis is not known, but some believe that the condition is related to an inflammatory vasculopathy that might be responsive to IGIV. Studies are under way to evaluate this possibility at the present time. The pain should be treated aggressively.

The most common diabetic neuropathy is a diffuse, distal, symmetric, predominantly sensory neuropathy with insidious onset and eventual development of paresthesias and sensory loss in the distal ends of the extremities. Significant weakness rarely occurs until late in the course. Diabetics are more susceptible to CIDP, which should be suspected in patients with symmetrical proximal and distal weakness of the upper and lower limbs. Autonomic dysfunction often coexists as a component of the neuropathy and in some cases may be the predominant symptom. Autonomic neuropathy is manifested as orthostatic hypotension, abnormalities in sweating, diarrhea or constipation, gastroparesis, impotence, or urinary retention. No treatment of diabetic peripheral neuropathy has been shown to reverse the nerve damage, but tight glucose control slows or stalls progression. Symptomatic treatment of the autonomic components can be important in patients with diabetic neuropathy. Orthostatic hypotension is treated initially by teaching patients to change positions slowly, liberalizing fluid and salt intake, using waist-high support stockings, and elevating the head of the bed by 8 to 12 inches. If these conservative measures fail, fludrocortisone (Florinef)* at doses gradually increasing from 0.1 to 0.2 mg once or twice daily is recommended. We also use midodrine (ProAmatine) in doses of 2.5 to 10 mg three to four times daily administered during daytime hours to avoid supine hypertension. Gastroparesis can be treated with 10 mg of metoclopramide before each meal along with restriction of meal size. Cisapride (Propulsid)* was the preferred agent, but it can cause life-threatening cardiac arrhythmias. Newer gastric motility agents are under investigation at the time of this writing and should soon be available. Bladder and erectile dysfunction deserve referral for urologic evaluation. The use of sildenafil citrate (Viagra) is perfectly appropriate.

Hypothyroid Neuropathy

Entrapment neuropathies, particularly carpal tunnel syndrome, are relatively common in patients with hypothyroidism, and a sensory neuropathy with paresthesias and sensory loss in the feet and hands is also common. Although patients may complain of weakness and fatigue, strength generally remains preserved on examination. Muscle stretch reflexes are reduced or absent and may demonstrate the classic "hung-up" response. Cerebrospinal fluid protein may be elevated to over 100 mg/dL, and electrodiagnostic studies show decreased amplitudes of sensory nerve action potentials and mild slowing of both the motor and sensory responses. Once discovered, thyroid replacement reverses the neuropathy, but return to normal may take several months. Hyperthyroidism has not been associated with neuropathy.

Uremic Neuropathy

Seventy percent of patients with renal failure have a peripheral neuropathy; however, it is subclinical in most and noted only on electrophysiologic studies. Weakness is usually the lesser component, with the clinical picture dominated by painful, acral dysesthesias. Electrodiagnostic studies show an axonal sensorimotor polyneuropathy. The cause of uremic neuropathy is not known, but accumulation of a toxic substance is most likely. Although dialysis improves and stabilizes the neuropathy, rarely will the symptoms or electrophysiologic features completely reverse. Successful renal transplantation is an effective treatment that results in progressive improvement and eventual resolution of the neuropathy.

PAINFUL NEUROPATHIES

Painful Sensory Neuropathy

Over the past two decades, neuropathies have been described with normal strength, normal muscle stretch reflexes, and minimal or no abnormalities in large-fiber sensory function (vibration and proprioception). Frequently, clinical findings consist of painful, burning dysesthesias in the distal ends of the extremities and abnormalities only or predominantly in functions mediated by small myelinated or unmyelinated sensory fibers (pain and temperature). Electrodiagnostic studies in these patients are often

---

*Not FDA approved for this indication.

TABLE 4. **Treatment Options for Painful Neuropathies**

Therapy	Regimen	Side Effects
Gabapentin* (Neurontin)	100–1200 mg PO tid	Sedation, dizziness, fatigue
Tramadol* (Ultram)	50–100 mg PO qid	Seizures, dizziness/vertigo, somnolence, pruritis, nausea/vomiting, constipation
Amitriptyline* (Elavil) or nortriptyline* (Aventyl)	10–100 mg PO qhs	Sedation, dry mouth, alopecia, edema, weight gain, constipation, confusion, tremors, seizures, urinary retention, arrythmias
Carbamazepine* (Tegretol)	100–400 mg PO bid–tid	Sedation, disorientation, rash, hepatitis, leukopenia, nausea/vomiting, dizziness, diarrhea, fatigue, diplopia, nystagmus
Topiramate* (Topamax)	50–200 mg PO bid	Dizziness, nervousness, ataxia, weight loss, somnolence, memory problems, psychomotor slowing, paresthesias, language problems
Mexiletine* (Mexitil)	150–300 mg PO bid–tid	Arrhythmias, palpitations, tremor, nausea/vomiting, blurred vision, dizziness, light-headedness

*Not FDA approved for this indication.

normal and thus confuse the picture because of failure to identify objective signs of neuropathy. These patients usually consult with multiple physicians in search for an answer. In many, the symptoms significantly interfere with their quality of life.

Diagnosis in these patients requires acquaintance with the condition, belief in the patient, and confirmation of the diagnosis through specialized testing. We initially evaluate such patients with electromyography and nerve conduction studies, with the realization that even minimal positive findings may be relevant. If these studies fail to detect abnormalities, we assess autonomic function (also mediated by small, unmyelinated nerve fibers). These tests evaluate cutaneous sweating and the response of the heart and blood vessels to changes in posture and deep breathing. In addition, computerized quantitative sensory testing provides objective measures of sensory loss. Algorithms have been established to unequivocally determine sensory loss by applying norms based on age, sex, and site of testing on the extremity. The most sensitive method for establishing the presence of small-fiber neuropathy is skin biopsy with calculation of nerve fiber density in the epidermis. This method can show loss of fibers in the skin, as well as unique pathologic changes affecting these very distal axons. A cause for this small-fiber painful sensory neuropathy is currently discovered in only 10% to 30% of cases. Indicated investigations include evaluation for diabetes, cancer, vasculitis, Sjögren's syndrome, amyloidosis, and monoclonal gammopathies. Recent studies suggest that even mild impairment in the body's utilization of glucose may underlie a large proportion of painful sensory neuropathies. Therefore, these patients should all be evaluated for diabetes with a 3-hour glucose tolerance test. Specialized tests for autoantibodies such as antisulfatide antibodies have not proved beneficial. Recent studies report that painful sensory neuropathy progresses quite slowly and rarely limits ambulation. It is important to reassure patients that this condition will not lead to paralysis because paralysis is a common concern of these patients. The pain needs to be treated aggressively.

Treatment of Painful Neuropathies

Neurogenic pain does not respond well to conventional analgesics, and each individual drug that is effective in neurogenic pain may achieve only a 20% to 30% pain reduction (Table 4). It is important to tell patients of the limited response of any single medication so that expectations are realistic. Thus, if a single agent does not provide enough relief, another drug is added. Multiple medications may be required to adequately subdue the discomfort. We often initiate treatment with gabapentin (Neurontin)* in doses ranging up to 1200 mg three times daily. This medicine has a low side effect profile and does not alter the metabolism or protein binding of other drugs. The biggest problem we encounter in practice is that patients are underdosed with gabapentin. It can be used in doses of up to 3600 mg/d. Tramadol (Ultram),* a mu-opioid receptor agonist, dosed at 50 to 100 mg four times per day, is also very effective. Rare patients experience nausea or sedation, but in general, this agent is well tolerated. Both gabapentin and tramadol have shown efficacy for painful neuropathies in randomized, placebo-controlled trials. The mechanism of action of these drugs is very different, and they are a very good combination in patients with severe pain. Tricyclic antidepressants such as amitriptyline (Elavil)* and nortriptyline (Aventyl)* may be started at low doses of 10 to 25 mg each evening and titrated to effect on a weekly basis up to 50 to 100 mg each evening. Although nortriptyline causes fewer anticholinergic and orthostatic side effects, amitriptyline is helpful for sleep in patients with symptoms at night. Carbamazepine* (Tegretol) and the newer anticonvulsant topiramate (Topamax)* help reduce symptoms, but both require gradual titration over weeks to avoid side effects. Mexiletine (Mexitil),* 300 to 900 mg daily in divided doses, can be surprisingly effective in certain recalcitrant cases. An initial ECG should be obtained to avoid dispensing this agent to patients with cardiac disease or heart block. We have not found topical agents such as capsaicin very helpful. If the pain is very localized, the patient can be taught to apply a 5% lidocaine patch to the affected area. These patches can be changed twice per day and are often effective.

It must be emphasized that most patients require more than one medication to treat painful sensory neuropathy. Each drug should be increased to the maximal tolerated dose before adding another one. If all else fails, narcotic analgesics must be used to treat this condition.

*Not FDA approved for this indication.

ACUTE HEAD INJURIES IN ADULTS

method of
ALEX B. VALADKA, M.D.
Ben Taub General Hospital
Houston, Texas

EPIDEMIOLOGY

Trauma has been described as a silent epidemic. It is the leading cause of loss of years of productive life and the fifth most common cause of death in the United States.

Traumatic brain injury (TBI) is arguably the most important of all types of trauma. Among multiply injured patients, the head is the most frequently injured part of the body, and outcome is determined more by the presence and degree of TBI than by injury to other organ systems. The annual financial impact of TBI in terms of lost economic productivity and lifelong medical care exceeds $25 billion in the United States, fully one third of the total financial impact of all types of trauma.

PATHOLOGY

The most immediate threats to life in patients with TBI are intracranial hematomas and contusions (Figure 1). Patients without such lesions, however, are no less critically ill. In fact, diffuse pathologic processes such as ischemia and diffuse axonal injury probably contribute more to poor outcomes than do mass lesions.

A recently traumatized brain is exquisitely sensitive to deviations from normal homeostasis that would normally be tolerated well. Such secondary insults can have a devastating effect on outcome. Some common secondary insults are listed in Figure 1. Because the primary brain injury caused by the trauma cannot be reversed, the goals of treating TBI are to prevent secondary insults and to correct them as soon as they occur.

EVALUATION

Glasgow Coma Scale

Despite the sophistication of modern imaging techniques, accurate neurologic examination remains the cornerstone of diagnosing TBI. The most widely used evaluation tool is the Glasgow Coma Scale (GCS) (Table 1). This scheme assigns a score to a patient's motor, verbal, and eye-opening responses. The scores in each category are summed to give the overall score. To avoid confusion when components of the GCS cannot be assessed (for example, in patients who are endotracheally intubated), it is best to list the score for each component of the GCS individually, for example, "M 5/E 1/V intubated."

Classification of head injury as mild, moderate, or severe is generally based on a GCS score of 13 to 15, 9 to 12, or 3 to 8, respectively. The percentages of patients who seek medical attention after head injury are 80% with mild, 10% with moderate, and 10% with severe injury. Some recent publications treat patients with a GCS score of 14 or 15 separately from those with a score of 13, which suggests that the definition of moderate TBI may need to be expanded to include those with a GCS of 13.

Pupils

An important part of neurologic assessment besides the GCS is evaluation of pupillary size, symmetry, and reactivity. The parasympathetic fibers that mediate pupillary constriction lie on the surface of the third cranial nerve, so they are susceptible to pressure effects from uncal herniation. Such pressure inactivates these fibers and results in an unopposed dilatory stimulus to the pupil from its sympathetic supply. Ischemia to the midbrain (in which lie the nuclei of the third cranial nerve) may also contribute to pupillary dilation.

Pupils that are fixed (i.e., do not constrict in bright light) and dilated in a patient with TBI indicate the presence of a large intracranial hematoma until proved otherwise. Immediate computed tomography (CT) is mandatory. Even

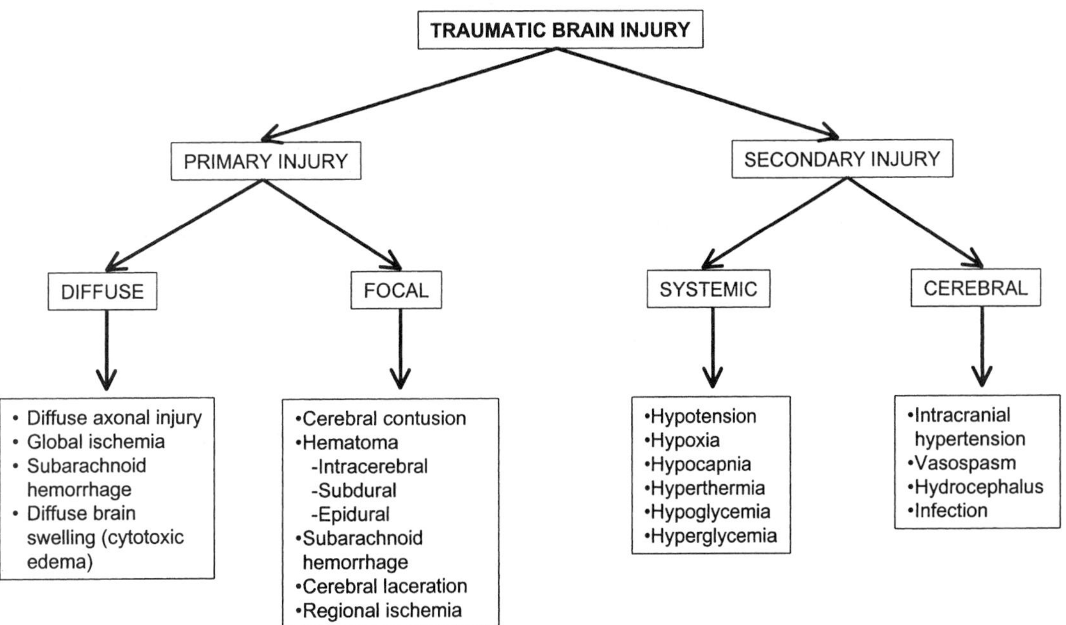

Figure 1. Major pathologic and pathophysiologic entities in traumatic brain injury.

TABLE 1. **Glasgow Coma Scale**

Score	Best Motor Response	Best Verbal Response	Best Eye-Opening Response
6	Obeys commands	—	—
5	Localizes stimulus	Oriented	—
4	Withdraws from stimulus	Conversant but confused	Open spontaneously
3	Flexes arm	States recognizable words or phases	Open to voice
2	Extends arm	Makes unintelligible sounds	Open to painful stimulus
1	No response	No response	Remain closed

if a CT scan demonstrates no mass lesion, prompt treatment of intracranial hypertension and initiation of intracranial pressure (ICP) monitoring must proceed expeditiously.

Radiologic Studies

The gold standard for the radiologic evaluation of TBI is a CT scan of the brain. CT scanning has high sensitivity for revealing fractures and acute intracranial blood. Hospitals that do not have a readily available CT scanner should consider transferring appropriate patients to a center with 24-hour availability of CT scanning, operating rooms, and neurosurgical care.

Skull radiography has little role in evaluating TBI. Some centers have used skull radiography as a screening tool in certain mildly head-injured patients to identify fractures, displacement of the calcified pineal gland, or other abnormalities that can be used to justify ordering a CT scan. However, the recommended low threshold for obtaining a CT scan makes routine skull radiography of little use in most head-injured patients.

Which patients with mild TBI require CT scanning? Certain signs and symptoms, such as those listed in Table 2, indicate a greater likelihood of CT-evident intracranial pathology. In addition to such "laundry lists" of reasons to forego (or obtain) a CT scan, the clinician must also consider such factors as the time since injury, progression of a patient's symptoms, and the reliability and availability of social support structures that will bring the patient back to the hospital if symptoms worsen. In the face of uncertainty about the need for CT scanning, the safest course is to proceed with the study.

It cannot be emphasized too strongly that patients with devastating TBI may have CT scans that demonstrate very little abnormality. Such patients are still extremely vulnerable to secondary insults; thus, they require every bit as much meticulous attention as patients with more dramatic CT results.

Although magnetic resonance imaging has little role in the acute evaluation of TBI, it may be useful later in a patient's course for revealing subtle abnormalities that might not be seen on a CT scan. Such information may uncover an anatomic basis for a patient's unexplained deficits or failure to improve.

TABLE 2. **Common Indications for CT Scanning in Patients With Mild Traumatic Brain Injury**

Headache
Dizziness
Vomiting
Age >60 y
Intoxication with alcohol or other drugs
Seizure
Deficits in short-term memory
Physical evidence of supraclavicular trauma

MANAGEMENT

Mild Traumatic Brain Injury

Patients who demonstrate acute intracranial blood on a CT scan are admitted to the intensive care unit (ICU), even if they have "only" mild TBI. Neurologic deterioration calls for immediate CT scanning to determine whether surgery, placement of an ICP monitor, or other changes in management are required.

At our institution we perform a follow-up CT scan 24 to 48 hours after admission, before transferring patients out of the ICU. Longer ICU stays may be required for progressing intracranial pathology, severe associated injuries, significant underlying medical conditions, or other special circumstances.

Patients with mild TBI often require surgery for systemic injuries. Most may undergo such operations immediately, but if an initial CT scan reveals acute intracranial blood or other worrisome pathology, it may be best to postpone such surgery until the patient has been observed overnight and a CT scan obtained the next day. Before lengthy or complex surgery patients with mild TBI may undergo placement of ICP monitors to detect ICP elevations while they are under general anesthesia.

On discharge from the inpatient unit or emergency center, patients with mild TBI and their familes should be cautioned about the importance of returning to the hospital if worrisome signs or symptoms develop. Such patients should have a responsible adult check on them frequently during the first few days after injury. It is helpful to give these patients and their companions a "head sheet" (Figure 2) that describes warning signs and lists important phone numbers.

Severe and Moderate Traumatic Brain Injury

Initial Assessment and Stabilization

Patients with severe TBI are among the most critically ill of all patients seen in emergency rooms. The highest priority must be given to thorough, yet rapid evaluation and treatment.

Resuscitation and stabilization proceed according to the American College of Surgeons' Advanced Trauma Life Support protocols, which include assess-

DISCHARGE INSTRUCTIONS FOR MILD HEAD INJURY

Our evaluation indicates that your head injury was not serious. However, symptoms can become worse over the next few hours or days. Complications may also develop during this time. A reliable adult companion should remain with you for at least the next 24 hours. This person should call your doctor or bring you back to the emergency room if any of these symptoms develop:

1. Increased sleepiness or difficulty in waking patient up (awaken patient every 2 hours for the first one or two nights).
2. Severe headaches or dizziness.
3. Persistent or severe nausea or vomiting.
4. Seizures.
5. Confusion or abnormal behavior.
6. Bloody or watery drainage from the ear or nose.
7. Weakness or numbness in arms or legs.
8. Problems with vision or the eyes, especially double vision, abnormal eye movements, or the pupil of one eye becoming noticeably larger than the other.
9. Very slow or very rapid pulse.
10. Abnormal breathing, especially very slow or very rapid breathing.

Do not use any pain medicines stronger than acetaminophen (Tylenol) for the next three days. Do not use aspirin or medicines containing aspirin for the next three days. Do not consume alcoholic beverages for at least the next three days.

If you have any questions or if an emergency occurs, our telephone number is ____________________. Your doctor's name is ____________________.

Figure 2. "Head sheet" describing warning signs in patients with mild traumatic brain injury.

ment and stabilization of the ABCs (airway, breathing, and circulation) and a systematic survey to detect other injuries. After basic laboratory and radiographic studies are obtained (Table 3), patients are taken to the CT scanner.

Decisions about performing other emergency radiologic studies, such as an arteriogram or abdominal CT scan, must be individualized. The urgency of such studies must be balanced against the need to avoid exposure to secondary insults by a prolonged stay in the relatively unmonitored environment of a radiology department.

TABLE 3. **Laboratory and Radiologic Studies Obtained in an Emergency Center for Patients With Severe Traumatic Brain Injury**

Laboratory Studies
Complete blood count
Coagulation studies
Electrolytes, blood urea nitrogen, creatinine, glucose
Blood alcohol level
Arterial blood gas
Urinalysis
Toxicology sceen
Pregnancy test in females
Type and crossmatch; notify the blood bank of a possible need for packed red cells, fresh frozen plasma, platelets
Cell counts of diagnostic peritoneal lavage fluid (if performed)
Radiologic Studies
Lateral cervical spine radiograph
Anteroposterior chest radiograph
Anteroposterior pelvic radiograph

Intracranial Pressure

Patients with severe TBI require the same ICU monitoring and support as other critically ill patients. In addition, because the degree and duration of intracranial hypertension have been linked to worse outcome after TBI, these patients require monitoring of ICP and aggressive treatment of its elevations. We insert ICP monitors in all patients who do not obey commands (i.e., Glasgow motor score of 5 or less), as well as in patients with higher GCS scores who may be especially prone to intracranial hypertension. We prefer ventriculostomy catheters over intraparenchymal monitors because the former permit drainage of cerebrospinal fluid (CSF) as a therapeutic intervention.

Figure 3 presents a treatment algorithm for ICP elevations beyond 20 mm Hg. Analgesia reduces pain from associated injuries, whereas pharmacologic paralysis decreases bucking and other movements that can elevate ICP. We use morphine, 2 to 10 mg intravenously every hour as needed, and cisatracurium (Nimbex), up to 10 mg intravenously every hour as needed for these purposes. Others use propofol (Diprivan), but we avoid this agent because of its hypotensive effects and cost. Paralytics should be used only to treat actual ICP elevations; their prophylactic use in all patients (even if ICP is not elevated) may actually cause more problems than it solves.

Persistent intracranial hypertension is treated with CSF drainage if a ventriculostomy catheter is present.

The next step calls for boluses of 20% mannitol.

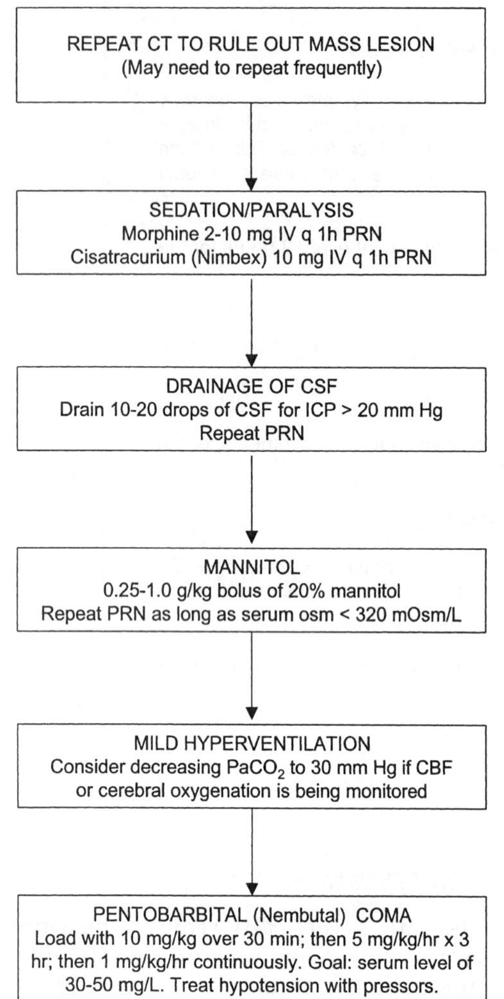

Figure 3. Algorithm for treating elevated intracranial pressure.

This agent has several beneficial effects, including an osmotic effect, which pulls water out of edematous brain tissue, and a rheologic effect, which facilitates vascular constriction (and thus a decrease in cerebral blood volume) by decreasing blood viscosity. Mannitol improves central filling pressures and cerebral blood flow, but subsequent osmotic diuresis may produce systemic hypotension unless volume status is maintained carefully.

ICP elevations refractory to these maneuvers are treated with mild hyperventilation ($Paco_2$ <30 mm Hg) as long as monitors of cerebral blood flow and oxygenation indicate that hyperventilation-induced vasoconstriction is not causing ischemia.

Our final treatment for persistent intracranial hypertension is pentobarbital (Nembutal)-induced coma, which has been shown to lower ICP. Mild hypothermia was not found to be of benefit in a multicenter trial. Currently, renewed interest has been shown in performing decompressive craniectomy, in which a large portion of the skull is removed (to be replaced later) to give the injured brain room to swell. A multicenter trial is being planned to help define the usefulness of this procedure.

Steroids are not recommended in the management of TBI.

Cerebral Perfusion Pressure

Cerebral perfusion pressure (CPP) is defined as mean arterial pressure (MAP) minus ICP. A minumum CPP of 70 mm Hg has been advocated for patients with TBI, but solid data to support this threshold are lacking. More recent investigations suggest the following: the importance of treating ICP elevations above 20 mm Hg should not be overlooked, a CPP of 60 mm Hg may be adequate for most patients, and aggressive use of pressors to maintain a high MAP may increase the incidence of undesirable side effects, especially adult respiratory distress syndrome. The main value of raising MAP may be decreased frequency and severity of arterial hypotension, which is a common and devastating secondary insult.

Systemic Care

Gastric ulceration is prevented by the use of H_2 antagonists. Sequential compression devices prevent lower extremity deep venous thrombosis. Enteral nutrition is initiated within a day or two of admission. We have a low threshold for beginning parenteral nutrition if patients experience persistent problems with enteral feeding. Early physical and occupational therapy help prevent contractures, and skin breakdown is prevented via pneumatic beds and careful positioning.

Cervical Spine Evaluation

Clearance of the cervical spine in patients with TBI is an important but controversial area. We use lateral cervical spine radiography and helical CT scanning with sagittal reconstruction of the entire cervical spine. Others advocate a three-view cervical spine series supplemented by CT scanning through C1–2 and suspicious or nonvisualized areas. Prompt evaluation allows rapid diagnosis and treatment of cervical spine injuries. Early cervical spine clearance expedites mobilization of the patient and avoids complications associated with prolonged use of a rigid cervical collar.

Moderate Traumatic Brain Injury

The management scheme just presented for patients with severe TBI also applies to those with moderate TBI. Although many of the more aggressive steps may not be necessary for moderate TBI, those who deteriorate should be considered to have severe TBI and be treated accordingly.

COMPLICATIONS AND SEQUELAE

Intracranial hematomas may develop or recur during the first few days after injury, as may diffuse brain swelling. Neurologic deterioration or a sustained increase in ICP call for immediate repeat CT scanning.

Infection may have many causes. Penetrating trauma and CSF fistula via skull base fractures may result in meningitis or cerebral abscess. ICP monitors may become infected. Although previous recommendations called for prophylactic replacement of ventriculostomy catheters every few days, recent evidence indicates that such catheters may often be left in place safely for 2 weeks or even longer.

Hydrocephalus may be expected to occur in approximately 5% to 10% of patients with severe TBI. Often, its development is obvious because of persistently high CSF drainage through a ventriculostomy. At other times, its onset may be more insidious. Hydrocephalus is treated by ventriculoperitoneal shunting.

Seizures during the first week after injury can be prevented by prophylactic administration of anticonvulsants. The most frequently used is phenytoin (Dilantin) (18 mg/kg given slowly intravenously; then start with 100 mg intravenously/orally every 8 hours). Beyond the first week, continuation of anticonvulsants seems to have little benefit in patients who did not have a seizure. In those who did have one, the optimal duration of anticonvulsant therapy is not clear. Most authorities recommend treatment for at least several months.

Intellectual and behavioral disturbances are common after TBI. Even mild TBI has been reported to result in postconcussion syndrome in up to 50% of cases. Typical symptoms include headaches, impaired concentration, memory disturbances, impaired abstract reasoning, irritability, dizziness, and blurred vision. Although most cases resolve spontaneously, resolution may require 3 to 6 months or even longer. More severe injuries may produce more serious and prolonged—or even permanent—impairment. Superimposition of new behavioral problems on pre-existing difficulties creates an especially difficult and frustrating problem.

OUTCOME

Outcome after TBI is commonly described via the Glasgow Outcome Scale (Table 4). Patients with severe TBI (i.e., GCS score of 3–8 on admission) can be expected to have a mortality rate of 30% to 36%. A persistent vegetative state occurs in roughly 5%, and severe disability and moderate disability each occur in about 16%. More than 25% of patients, however, eventually have a good recovery.

As one might expect, patients with moderate TBI (initial GCS score of 9 to 12) fare better. Death or a persistent vegetative state occurs in roughly 7%, and another 7% suffer severe disability. Moderate disability is the outcome in approximately 25%. More than 60% of patients with moderate TBI ultimately have a good recovery.

Although scales like the Glascow Outcome Scale are useful for evaluating broad categories of outcome, they lack sensitivity for subtle but important higher level neurologic deficits. Neuropsychological testing may help quantify these problems. Serial neuropsychological testing may be especially important when some sort of "objective" assessment is required for employers, schools, insurance companies, disability applications, and the like.

Rehabilitation aims to maximize a patient's level of functioning in all areas, including physical, psychological, social, and vocational. It remains controversial whether aggressive rehabilitation programs promote more neurologic recovery than would occur otherwise. Nevertheless, these programs are often invaluable for teaching patients how to function maximally within the limits posed by their impairments. Families of patients also receive vital education and training as part of the rehabilitation process.

TABLE 4. **Glasgow Outcome Scale**

Outcome	Score	Description
Good recovery	5	Minor disabilities, but able to resume normal life
Moderate disability	4	More significant disabilities, but can still live independently. Can use public transportation, work in an assisted situation, etc.
Severe disability	3	Conscious but dependent on others for daily care. Often (but not necessarily) institutionalized
Persistent vegetative state	2	Not conscious, but eyes may be open and may "track" movements
Death	1	Self-explanatory

ACUTE HEAD INJURIES IN CHILDREN

method of
ROGER HARTL, M.D.,
BRUCE GREENWALD, M.D., and
JAMSHID GHAJAR, M.D., PH.D.
New York Presbyterian Hospital and Weill Medical College of Cornell University
New York, New York

Head injury and *traumatic brain injury (TBI)* have been used synonymously, with the latter term used commonly as a better descriptor. The general principles of pre-hospital and in-hospital management of TBI in children are similar to those in adults. Maintaining brain perfusion is the guiding principle in treating children with significant TBI. The differences in assessing and treating pediatric patients compared to adults are related to the mode of injury and the subsequent unique pathophysiology. In this article we discuss TBI management in children (<13 years) and emphasize moderate and severe TBI. We point out some of the peculiarities of pediatric trauma that should be recognized by those physicians more familiar with treating adults.

TABLE 1. **Most Important Secondary Insults Causing Poor Outcome**

Secondary Insult	Critical Values in TBI	Main Cause
Arterial hypotension	Systolic blood pressure <65–90 mm Hg, depending on age (see Table 3)	Blood loss, sepsis, cardiac failure, spinal cord injury, brain stem injury
Hypoxemia	Arterial O_2 saturation <90%, PaO_2 <60 mm Hg, apnea, cyanosis	Hypoventilation, thoracic injury, aspiration
Hypocapnia	Sustained $PaCO_2$ <25 mm Hg	Hyperventilation
Intracranial hypertension	ICP >20 mm Hg	Mass lesion, cerebral edema caused by vasodilation and/or increased water content
Cerebral vasospasm	Increased blood flow velocity of intracerebral arteries (transcranial Doppler)	Traumatic subarachnoid hemorrhage

Abbreviations: ICP = intracerebral hemorrhage; TBI = traumatic brain injury.

EPIDEMIOLOGY OF PEDIATRIC HEAD INJURY

TBI or head injury is the most common cause of death and disability in children. Head injury leads to approximately 100,000 pediatric hospitalizations a year, and at least 7000 children die each year from TBI. Mechanisms of trauma frequently differ from those seen in the adult. The mechanism of injury is most likely a pediatric pedestrian struck by a car, unlike adults who are usually car passengers or drivers. Sadly, a common mechanism in the infant population is child abuse. Children often have milder injuries than adults. The frequency of TBI in boys is twice that of girls.

PATHOPHYSIOLOGY

Neurologic injury not only occurs during the impact (*primary injury*) but also evolves over the following hours and days (*secondary brain injury*). Secondary brain damage is the most important cause of in-hospital death. The most important secondary insults contributing to poor outcome in adults and children are listed in Table 1. In a recent study of children with TBI, 13% had a documented hypoxemic episode and 6% were hypercapnic. Patients with early hypotension had a worse neurologic outcome and prolonged hospitalization (Table 2). There are important differences between the adult and the immature brain that affect secondary brain injury in the pediatric age group:

- The infant's skull is soft and thin, allowing it to be easily deformed. Force is easily transferred to the brain. The relatively large size of the head in combination with a less-developed neck musculature renders infants especially vulnerable to acceleration-deceleration trauma, as seen in the shaking impact syndrome.
- The brains of infants and young children have a high water content as compared with adolescents and adults. Experimental studies have shown that the immature blood-brain barrier is much more vulnerable to ischemia. This may facilitate the development of edema following TBI.
- Myelination of the brain continues after birth, and ongoing myelination has been described beyond the first 1 to 2 years of life. Incomplete myelination predisposes babies and toddlers to axonal shear injury.
- Neural plasticity of the young brain accounts for the observation that similar types of injury are better tolerated by the young brain than by the adult brain.
- Increased cerebral blood flow with vascular engorgement has long been believed to be the main reason for cerebral swelling after TBI in children. Based on this concept, hyperventilation and the avoidance of mannitol were recommended for the treatment of malignant brain edema. Recent studies, however, demonstrated that in healthy children between 6 months and 10 years of age, the mean cerebral blood flow is greater than that in adults (Figure 1). Therefore, what was considered hyperemia may in fact have been normal cerebral blood flow for this age group. Therefore, brain swelling may be predominantly due to increased brain water rather than blood volume.

TABLE 2. **Systolic Blood Pressure Associated With a Poor Outcome in Traumatic Brain Injury**

Age (y)	Systolic Blood Pressure (mm Hg)
<1	65
1–5	70–75
5–12	75–80
12–15	80–90

EVALUATION OF CHILDREN WITH HEAD INJURIES

Pre-hospital evaluation and treatment of children with head injury are similar to the protocol in adults. The cornerstones of the resuscitation of severely injured children follow:

- Primary survey with cervical spine control and brief neurologic assessment
- Resuscitation (airway, breathing, circulation)
- Secondary survey with complete neurologic examination and determination of the Glasgow Coma Scale (GCS) score. A modified GCS has been developed to assess children (Table 3)

Be aware that arterial hypotension develops in children after relatively minor blood loss and that their body temperature may drop rapidly after exposure. Scalp wounds should be thoroughly inspected and sutured to prevent blood loss. Intracranial hemorrhage in infants can lead to significant blood loss and hypotension.

The general principles of the TBI workup are similar in children and adults:

- Unless there are signs of cerebral herniation (pupillary asymmetry, dilated/fixed pupils, or extensor posturing or flaccidity to noxious stimuli), patients should not be hyperventilated and the arterial PCO_2 should be maintained at around 35 mm Hg, the lower limit of normocapnia.

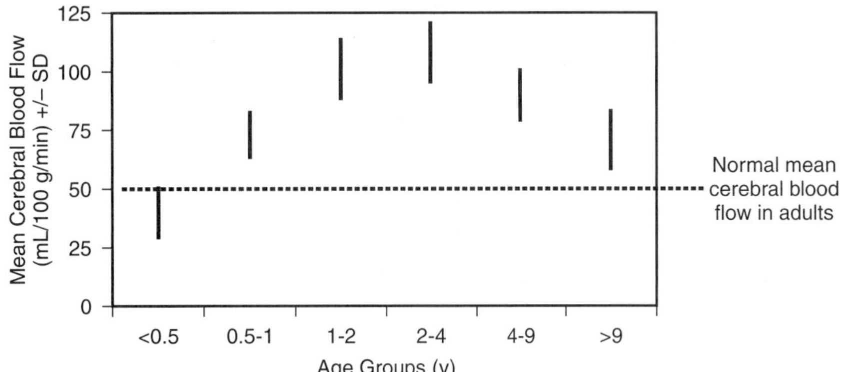

Figure 1. Mean cerebral blood flow in 80 healthy, non-anesthetized children obtained with the xenon 133 method. The normal cerebral blood flow for adults is 50 mL/100 g/min.

- Isotonic fluids should be used for resuscitation to avoid free water overload.
- Computed tomography (CT) is the imaging study of choice to detect skull fractures and intracranial injury with hemorrhage and to assess the necessity of surgical evacuation of a mass lesion. Head CT scan can also demonstrate signs that are closely associated with intracranial hypertension, such as obliterated basal cisterns, compressed cerebral ventricles, and midline shift.
- All comatose patients with abnormal CT scan results and a GCS score of 8 or less should undergo intracranial pressure (ICP) monitoring.
- Plain radiographs of the cervical spine should be obtained as soon as possible along with a CT scan of suspicious areas.
- Once the patient has been stabilized, a careful physical examination should be conducted and child abuse should be ruled out.

TYPICAL FEATURES OF TRAUMATIC BRAIN INJURY IN VARIOUS AGE GROUPS

Children are susceptible to specific types of injuries depending on their age. Overall, mass lesions such as intracerebral hemorrhage, subdural hemorrhage (SDH), epidural hemorrhage, and contusion occur less frequently in children than in adults; however, diffuse axonal injury is seen more commonly in children. Features of diffuse axonal injury on CT scan are petechial hemorrhages at the gray-white matter junction and in the corpus callosum and deep white matter hemorrhage. Shearing injuries include the previous signs and also midbrain lesions. Both shearing injury and diffuse axonal injury are best depicted with magnetic resonance imaging. Diffuse brain swelling occurs approximately twice as frequently in children as adults, and it is associated with a mortality rate as high as 53%.

Newborn

Birth injuries result from trauma during delivery and include cephalohematoma, skull fracture, acute SDH, and contusion. Ping-pong fracture results from an indentation in the cranium and is seen in children younger than 3 years. When seen in the newborn, it is generally attributed to trauma during labor and delivery. This lesion frequently resolves spontaneously. Poor outcome from birth injury is usually related to concomitant hypoxia or ischemia.

Infants

Most injuries are related to falls and child abuse in this group. The so-called growing skull fracture is rare but typically seen during infancy as a late complication after head trauma. In this type of fracture, a depressed skull fracture with injury to the underlying dura leads to herniation of the dura through the defect and slow expansion of the fracture due to cerebrospinal fluid pulsation. Chronic SDH is seen in this age group and frequently remains undetected until patients are evaluated for an enlarging head circumference or for child abuse. This lesion can

TABLE 3. **Glasgow Coma Scale**

Score	Eyes Open	Best Verbal Response in Adults	Best Verbal Response in Children <36 mo	Best Verbal Response in Infants and Preschoolers	Best Motor Response
6	—	—	—	—	Obeys commands
5	—	Oriented and converses	Smiles, interacts	Babbles/gestures	Localizes painful stimuli
4	Spontaneously	Disoriented and converses	Cries, interacts	Cries for needs	Flexion withdrawal
3	To verbal command	Inappropriate words	Consolable, moans	Cries, nonspecific	Flexion-abnormal
2	To painful stimuli	Incomprehensible sounds	Irritable, restless	Sounds	Extension
1	No response	No response	No response	No response	No response

Traumatic brain injury is graded as mild, moderate, or severe on the basis of the Glasgow Coma scale (GCS) after resuscitation. Mild traumatic brain injury (GCS 13–15) in most cases results in concussion and there is full recovery. In moderate head injury the patient is lethargic or stuporous (GCS 9–13), and in severe head injury the patient is comatose and unable to open the eyes (GCS 3–8).

sometimes be treated successfully with percutaneous aspiration by a neurosurgeon. Epidural hematoma is usually related to venous bleeding and can frequently be managed conservatively.

Toddlers and School-Age Children

Falls, bicycle accidents, and pedestrian accidents are the most frequent causes of TBI. Severe trauma results in shearing injury with diffuse axonal injury and SDH. Shearing injury is more commonly seen in children than in adults. Traumatic intracerebral hemorrhage, contusion, epidural hemorrhage, and SDH are seen less frequently in children than adults. Intracranial hemorrhage is sometimes seen in children with hematologic disorders or with excessive drainage of cerebrospinal fluid following ventricular-peritoneal shunt surgery (overshunting).

Adolescents

Adolescents are similar to adults with respect to mechanism and response to TBI.

CHILD ABUSE

Child abuse is the second most frequent cause of death in childhood after motor vehicle accidents; approximately 1500 pediatric deaths are a result of child abuse per year in the United States. The shaking impact syndrome should be suspected in children younger than 3 years of age who present with the following:

- Retinal hemorrhages
- SDH, shearing injury, or localized intracerebral hemorrhage
- Multiple skull fractures, fractures of the ribs and long bones, and bruises in various stages of healing
- History of trauma that does not account for the severity of the actual injury

There does not appear to be a relationship to race, gender, socioeconomic status, or education among victims of shaking impact syndrome. Overall, up to one third of affected children die, one third to one half remain severely disabled, and only one third have a chance of a meaningful recovery.

SEVERE HEAD INJURY IN CHILDREN

After endotracheal intubation, hemodynamic stabilization, and radiographic exclusion of a neurosurgical mass lesion, children with moderate or severe TBI should be admitted to the pediatric intensive care unit. Every child with severe TBI should be evaluated by a neurosurgeon. The recently updated *Guidelines for the Management of Severe Traumatic Brain Injury* provide a helpful reference for physicians treating patients with severe TBI (www.braintrauma.org).

INTRACRANIAL PRESSURE MONITORING AND TREATMENT OF ELEVATED INTRACRANIAL PRESSURE

Elevated ICP is present in the majority of children with severe head injury, and ICP should be monitored in all comatose children with abnormal results on head CT scan. Cerebral perfusion pressure is defined as the mean arterial blood pressure minus ICP. This physiologic variable defines the pressure gradient driving cerebral blood flow and metabolite delivery and is therefore closely related to ischemia. Although no thresholds for cerebral perfusion pressure have been set, an adjustment from the recommended level of 70 mm Hg for adults can be made. Cerebral perfusion pressure should be maintained at a minimum of 50 mm Hg in infants and 60 mm Hg in children. Increased ICP should be treated vigorously.

The treatment of the typical pediatric TBI patient at our institution is outlined in Table 4. Hyperventi-

TABLE 4. **Monitoring Parameters and Management Options in Children With Head Injury**

In All Children With GCS <9 and ICP <15 mm Hg	Add If ICP >15 mm Hg	Add If ICP >25 mm Hg	Add for Persistent ICP >25 mm Hg	Add for Persistent ICP >25 mm Hg or Pupillary Abnormalities
Elevate head of bed 30 degrees	Ventricular CSF drainage	Neuromuscular blockade: vecuronium, atacrurium	Moderate hypothermia, core temperature 34°–36°C	Barbiturates with continuous EEG
Maintain euvolemia and hemodynamic stability, keep CPP 5–10 mm Hg Pa_{O_2} >90 mm Hg Pa_{CO_2} 35–40 mm Hg	Sedation: midazolam or lorazepam Analgesia: fentanyl or morphine	Mannitol 0.25–1 g/kg IV over 5–10 min Q 4–6 h PRN Serum osmolarity 300–320 mOsm/L, serum sodium 150–155 meq/L	Hyperventilation to Pa_{CO_2} 30–35 mm Hg	Hyperventilation to Pa_{CO_2} 25–30 mm Hg Hypertonic saline infusion Decompressive craniectomy
Systolic blood pressure >65 mm Hg in infants, >70 mm Hg in children (see Table 3)	CPP management: Inotropic and pressor support to maintain CPP (dopamine 5–20 μg/kg/min, norepinephrine 0.05–0.5 μg/kg/min)			
CPP >50 mm Hg in infants, >60 mm Hg in children	Repeat head CT to exclude operable mass lesion			

Abbreviations: CPP = cerebral perfusion pressure; CSF = cerebrospinal fluid; CT = computed tomography; EEG = electroencephalography; GCS = Glasgow Coma Scale; ICP = intracranial pressure; IV = intravenous; PRN = as needed.

lation should not be used routinely in these patients because hyperemia is less common than previously thought and a reduction in cerebral blood flow may be harmful for compromised areas of the injured brain. Similarly, there is no reason to avoid mannitol for the treatment of elevated ICP that is unresponsive to cerebrospinal fluid drainage.

Recently, there have been reports of improved ICP control with lumbar drainage in pediatric patients with diffuse brain injuries and ventricular cerebrospinal fluid drainage. More experience is needed before this treatment modality can be recommended. The practice of using propofol instead of barbiturates for the treatment of refractory intracranial hypertension should be viewed with caution because prolonged use of propofol has been associated with adverse reactions in children. Hypertonic saline has been used successfully to control elevated ICP in the pediatric population. Continuous infusion of 3% saline solution to keep serum osmolarity above the normal range was used to treat intracranial hypertension after pediatric TBI. A bolus infusion of 3% to 7.5% hypertonic saline has successfully controlled intracranial hypertension in children and adults. Hyperosmolarity is tolerated as long as euvolemia is maintained. Controlled trials are needed to further evaluate this treatment option before recommending it for routine use. Glucocorticoids are not recommended for the treatment of intracranial hypertension following TBI. Seizures may cause the ICP to increase, and anticonvulsant drugs may be used to prevent early posttraumatic seizures in patients at high risk. Nutritional support should be instituted within a few days following TBI.

OUTCOME FROM HEAD INJURY IN CHILDREN

The overall mortality rate for all pediatric patients with TBI admitted to a hospital is between 10% and 13%. The mortality rate associated with severe TBI in children has recently been reported to be approximately 35% with a good outcome in 31% of patients. Overall, the outcome from severe TBI has been thought to be better for children than for adults. However, very young children do not do as well as school-age children. An admission, postresuscitation GCS score of 3 and 4 has been associated with poor outcome in 75% of patients, whereas children with a GCS score greater than 6 almost always had a good outcome. In contrast to adults, motor and cognitive function in children can significantly improve up to 3 years after trauma. The view that the prognosis after severe TBI is generally better for children has recently been challenged. When comparing patients with the same mechanism of injury (motor vehicle accident), there was no difference in mortality rates between 4041 children and 14,789 adults (33.2% versus 33.5%, respectively). We suggest that previous reports of lower mortality in children may have been due to selection bias in the population.

The general principles of the management of acute TBI in children are similar to those in adults. Differences that exist between age groups relate mainly to the mechanisms and types of injuries that are encountered in the pediatric patient and the response of the immature brain to trauma and blood loss. This article highlights important features of pediatric head injury management and emphasizes that successful treatment is founded upon adherence to the principles of maintaining organ perfusion:

- Oxygenation and hemodynamic resuscitation
- Direct transfer of the patient to a designated trauma center with pediatric intensive care experts
- Head CT scan and cervical spine radiographs
- Neurosurgic evaluation especially for moderate and severe TBI
- Intensive care unit admission for moderate and severe TBI
- ICP and cerebral perfusion pressure monitoring in comatose children with abnormal results on head CT scan and aggressive treatment of intracranial hypertension to maintain cerebral perfusion

BRAIN TUMORS

method of
NINA A. PALEOLOGOS, M.D.
Evanston Northwestern Healthcare
Evanston, Illinois

Roughly 13,000 patients will die each year in the United States of a primary brain tumor. Many more patients with systemic cancer will have brain metastases. In children, primary tumors represent 22% of all childhood neoplasms. In the United States, the incidence of primary brain tumors is approximately 15 per 100,000 and of all intracranial tumors it is approximately 46 per 100,000. Although their frequency may seem small compared with other malignancies, their impact is significant, with most patients dying and many who survive experiencing significant neurologic deficit. The incidence of primary intracranial malignant brain tumors has increased in the past two decades, particularly in the elderly. The incidence of primary central nervous system (CNS) lymphoma has dramatically increased in both the immunocompetent and the immunocompromised populations. Whether these increases are due to improved and more available neuroimaging or reflect a true increase in the incidence is debatable. It appears that the availability of computed tomography (CT) and magnetic resonance imaging (MRI) is partly, but not solely, responsible for the increase in the reported incidence of primary brain tumors. Improvements in the treatment of other illnesses and an increasing survival of the population may also result in emergence of brain tumors that would not have been diagnosed had patients died at earlier ages from other causes.

The histologic classification of most brain tumors is based on its normal cell of origin. The growth rate and the degree of invasiveness vary. Most meningiomas are histologically benign, slowly progressive, and compressive rather than invasive. Glioblastoma multiforme (grade IV astrocytoma) is highly malignant, rapidly progressive, and invasive. Low-grade astrocytomas or oligodendrogliomas are invasive and can be slowly progressive for years but can undergo malignant transformation. These characteristics have clinical implications frequently underlying the presenting symptoms and their evolution and are important in determining prognosis and feasibility of surgical resection. Even a "benign" tumor such as a meningioma may occur in a location that precludes complete surgical resection, and at times these tumors can be very destructive and even fatal.

No proven causal relationship between any environmental factor or behavior and the occurrence of brain tumors has been found. Suggested associations have included certain chemical exposures. Therapeutic ionizing radiation has been shown to cause meningeal and glial neoplasms as a delayed complication. Most patients with brain tumors do not have a known genetic predisposition. Patients with tuberous sclerosis, neurofibromatosis types I and II, von Hippel-Lindau syndrome, and Li-Fraumeni syndrome have an increased incidence of primary brain tumors.

CLINICAL PRESENTATION

A patient with a brain tumor can present with diffuse neurologic impairment or with focal symptoms related to the location of the tumor. Headache occurs in approximately one third of patients. Although most patients with headache alone do not have a brain tumor, any patient presenting with a new persistent or progressive headache should have an MRI of the brain with and without gadolinium enhancement. Headaches that are nocturnal or are present on awakening or after lying supine are particularly worrisome. Headache associated with nausea and vomiting is present in only a small number of patients, particularly those who have large tumors producing raised intracranial pressure, those who have tumors of the posterior fossa, or those who have obstructive hydrocephalus.

Many patients will have no abnormal neurologic signs or symptoms but may present with a seizure. This is particularly true of patients with low-grade gliomas. Seizures may be focal, generalized, or focal with secondary generalization. The occurrence of a seizure for the first time in an adult is suggestive of underlying structural disease and a tumor must be ruled out with gadolinium-enhanced MRI. Focal symptoms and signs such as hemiparesis, aphasia, or a visual field deficit reflect the location of the tumor.

NEUROIMAGING

The neuroimaging method of choice for both diagnosis and follow-up of patients with brain tumors is MRI with and without gadolinium enhancement. CT can miss structural lesions, especially low-grade tumors. FLAIR imaging is particularly useful in diagnosis and follow-up of low-grade gliomas, which do not tend to show enhancement with the administration of gadolinium. Meningiomas are extraparenchymal and usually homogeneously enhancing, glioblastoma multiforme may be ring enhancing, and primary CNS lymphoma may be multifocal and homogenously enhancing. Although these and other neuroimaging characteristics can suggest a particular type of brain tumor, the neuroimaging does not always accurately predict the histology of a tumor. MRI spectroscopy may help differentiate between radiation-induced necrosis and recurrent tumor; however, it is not specific enough or sensitive enough to base treatment decisions on at this point in time.

TREATMENT

Corticosteroids

Dexamethasone (Decadron) is extremely effective in controlling peritumoral edema in patients with primary and secondary brain tumors. It has no oncolytic effect except in primary CNS lymphoma and, perhaps, secondary lymphoma. It has a relatively long half-life, which contributes to its having become the corticosteroid of choice in neuro-oncology. Although there are no prospective trials that have established the best dosage, its usage has become fairly standardized. Large intravenous doses must be given to patients with acute signs and symptoms of raised intracranial pressure. In situations in which the severity of symptoms and their tempo of evolution is less critical, oral dexamethasone at dosages of 4 to 12 mg twice daily is usually adequate. If there is no mass effect or edema, or if a patient has had a complete resection, then dexamethasone may not be necessary.

Surgery

If technically feasible, a complete surgical resection of a brain tumor with maintenance of neurologic function is always the goal. This cannot always be accomplished, but the ability to safely remove tumors from even eloquent areas of brain has improved with the use of stereotactic neurosurgical techniques. Partial tumor "debulking" should be done only if the majority of the tumor can be safely resected or if mass effect requires it. Although it is clear that patients with primary gliomas of the brain do better with gross total resection or large subtotal resections, it is also clear that a small subtotal resection does not add much.

Patients who have tumors that cannot or should not be resected should have stereotactic biopsies for diagnostic purposes. Even if a patient is quite elderly and only palliative radiation is being considered, a stereotactic biopsy should and can almost always be safely done to confirm a neoplastic process and rule out infectious causes, fulminant demyelinating disease, or an inflammatory lesion. Biopsy is not usually necessary (unless abscess or opportunistic infection is being considered) in a patient with known systemic cancer with metastases who presents with multiple enhancing masses in the brain. MRI-guided stereotactic biopsy of tumors in eloquent areas of the brain can usually be done under local anesthesia through a small burr hole. Sampling error can occur because of small sample size and when a biopsy is obtained of an area of the tumor that has less aggressive features than that of another area of the same tumor, which can then lead to undergrading of the neoplasm.

Complete resection alone may be all that is necessary for patients with meningioma, pilocytic astrocytoma, some low-grade gliomas, and some other types of brain tumors. Even those patients with completely resected "benign" or low-grade tumors can have recurrence of tumor and can require adjuvant therapy and they need to be followed closely over time with serial MR images. Complete curative surgical resection is not possible for most high-grade infiltrating gliomas. There is no clear tumor edge, and tumor cells may migrate several centimeters along white matter pathways, where they are unable to be resected and may not be seen on MRI. Even if a gross total resection is accomplished, these patients require adjuvant treatment with radiation, chemotherapy, or both.

Resection of a single metastasis before radiation may maintain or improve neurologic function and may also impact on survival in patients with well-controlled systemic disease.

Most craniotomies are performed under general anesthesia; however, in patients whose tumors are in eloquent areas of the brain, brain mapping of speech and motor areas in patients who are awake during surgery may be performed in an attempt to safely demarcate the tumor from normal brain and preserve neurologic function.

Radiation Therapy

Radiation therapy using external-beam photon irradiation from a linear accelerator is a frequent component of brain tumor therapy. Whether radiation therapy is instituted after surgical resection or biopsy is primarily dependent on the tumor histology. Radiation is used to treat neoplastic cells that remain after the neurosurgical procedure and is therefore usually used for high-grade invasive tumors such as astrocytomas that are impossible to resect completely microscopically. Radiation therapy is the most effective nonsurgical therapy for malignant or high-grade astrocytomas and prolongs survival. Tumors that may have a less aggressive histology but are unresectable owing to location, such as meningiomas of the skull base or low-grade gliomas that are growing, may also at times be treated with radiation.

The primary target of cellular injury is tumor cell nuclear DNA; however, effects on other cellular components may also be important. Radiation has both a direct damaging effect on cellular DNA and an indirect effect on DNA secondary to creation of free radicals. Cells have complex mechanisms for detecting DNA damage caused by radiation and then repairing the injury. Cells that are deficient in these repair mechanisms undergo active DNA destruction and apoptosis. Tumor cell repair mechanisms tend to be more deficient than repair mechanisms of normal cells, and it is this difference that is exploited by using radiation therapy to treat a brain tumor. It cannot be stressed enough, however, that not all normal cells recover, and the effect of radiation therapy on normal cellular elements is what underlies delayed radiation encephalopathy associated with cognitive dysfunction and gait apraxia, radiation necrosis, and radiation-induced vascular injury. These effects can occur months to years after treatment, are usually irreversible, and, at times, are fatal. Careful consideration of these detrimental effects should be made in each case before deciding on radiation therapy as a treatment modality. Although it is clear that radiation therapy is useful in patients with tumors such as anaplastic (grade III) astrocytoma and glioblastoma multiforme (grade IV astrocytoma), it is much less clear whether it is useful in patients with nonprogressing or completely resected low-grade glioma.

The usual dose of focused (to the area of tumor with margins) external-beam radiation therapy for a high-grade glioma is about 60 Gy, with the treatment volume focusing to the tumor location as the dose increases. Treatment is given in divided daily fractions over 5 to 6 weeks. Metastatic tumors are treated with whole-brain radiation therapy to a usual dose of 30 Gy in daily fractions of less than 3 Gy.

Stereotactic radiation using a modified linear accelerator (photon irradiation) or gamma knife (over 200 cobalt sources) is a single-session treatment used to deliver a high dose of ionizing radiation to a precisely defined intracranial target. The target is localized using stereotactic techniques with the goal being to accurately treat the desired target with a minimal amount of radiation delivered to surrounding normal tissue. No prospective studies have shown it to be superior or even equivalent to standard external-beam radiation therapy in the treatment of high-grade gliomas. A major limitation to stereotactic radiation is the volume of tumor that can be treated. If a tumor larger than 3.5 to 4 cm in diameter is treated, there is an increased risk of severe radiation injury. Marked swelling and necrosis may occur. The role of stereotactic radiation is clearer for more benign tumors, such as meningiomas, that are more clearly demarcated from normal tissue than it is for infiltrative, less definable high-grade gliomas.

Chemotherapy

The effectiveness of chemotherapy and immunotherapy in the treatment of brain tumors has been limited by many factors, including difficulty with drug delivery (a function primarily of the blood-brain barrier), tumor cell heterogeneity, and tumor cell drug resistance.

Alkylating agents are the most active agents used for the treatment of malignant astrocytomas, and the addition of these agents to surgery and radiation does increase the likelihood of longer-term survival in patients with grade III and grade IV astrocytomas, with the larger impact probably being in patients with grade III tumors. Carmustine (BCNU) is the agent most studied, with no other agent or agents shown to be superior. A combination of procarbazine (Matulane),* (lomustine (CCNU)), and vincristine (Oncovin) has also been used, especially in grade III astrocytomas, but it is more toxic and probably no better than carmustine alone. More recently, temozo-

*Not FDA approved for this indication.

lamide (Temodar) has shown promise. In a recent study, median progression-free survival in patients with recurrent glioblastoma was 4 weeks longer in patients treated with temozolamide than in similar patients treated with procarbazine. The response rate in patients with recurrent anaplastic astrocytoma was approximately 35%. Overall, survival in patients with recurrent tumor treated with temozolamide was not improved when compared with patients treated with procarbazine*; however, toxicity is usually mild and patients tolerate temozolamide well with maintenance or improvement of quality of life. Chemotherapy-laden biodegradable wafers show modest effect when placed intraoperatively at the time of recurrence and reoperation.

Malignant or aggressive oligodendrogliomas have been shown to be uniquely chemosensitive tumors, with most experience being with the PCV chemotherapeutic regimen. Neoadjuvant (pre-irradiation) chemotherapy is used by many in an effort to differ or delay the cognitive consequences of radiation therapy. Recently, a remarkably strong correlation between the chemosensitivity of these tumors and the loss of heterozygosity at 1p and 19q was found, raising hopes that these cytogenetic losses may be useful in predicting which patients might benefit from chemotherapy. How this chemosensitivity affects survival in this group of patients remains to be seen.

Other regimens that have some activity in malignant gliomas include cisplatin (Platinol)* and etoposide (Toposar),* tamoxifen (Nolvadex),* the topoisomerase inhibitor topotecan (Hycamtin),* paclitaxel (Taxol),* aziridinyl benzoquinone (diaziquone),† carboplatin (Paraplatin),* and methotrexate.* Investigation of angiogenesis inhibitors is ongoing. Chemotherapy has been shown to be of benefit in patients with medulloblastoma (primitive neuroectodermal tumor) using regimens containing cyclophosphamide (Cytoxan)* and vincristine and cisplatin* and etoposide.* Regimens also containing procarbazine and lomustine have been used with some success as well.

Ependymomas may respond to regimens containing vincristine, platinum compounds, and lomustine. Primary CNS lymphoma responds to regimens containing high-dose methotrexate, which penetrates the blood-brain barrier. Primary CNS lymphoma is the only primary tumor of the brain in which corticosteroids produce an oncolytic effect.

Small series have been reported in the literature describing patients with meningioma who have had responses to tamoxifen,* mifepristone (RU-486),* or hydroxyurea (Hydrea).

Unfortunately there has not been much therapeutic advance in the chemotherapeutic treatment of most brain tumors. Novel agents and novel delivery techniques are being studied, including gene therapy, monoclonal antibody–delivered radioisotope, immunomodulators, and differentiation agents. It is hoped that with an increase in our understanding of the molecular biology and mechanisms of tumor resistance there will be improvements in the chemotherapeutic treatment of these diseases.

Symptom Treatment

A number of therapeutic issues are important in the daily management of patients with brain tumors. Seizures may be present in many patients and, if intractable, may be a significant cause of impairment in quality of life. A detailed discussion of the use of various anticonvulsants is beyond the scope of this chapter; however, a few points can be made. Most patients will respond well and tolerate drugs such as phenytoin (Dilantin), carbamazepine (Tegretol), or valproate (Depakote), but drug interactions, liver toxicity, myelosuppression, or allergy can complicate therapy. Phenobarbital, lamotrigine (Lamictal), levetiracetam (Keppra), and other drugs can be used adjuvantly in patients whose seizures are not completely controlled on a single agent or who do not tolerate the usual first-line agents. The prophylactic use of anticonvulsants in patients who have not had seizures is probably unwarranted.

Steroid myopathy is a common side effect of chronic corticosteroid usage and appears to be the most common side effect of corticosteroids in patients with brain tumors. It can be severe, leading to significant morbidity. Using the lowest dose of dexamethasone possible (but as much as needed to control edema) is the goal. Many patients with large or gross total resections or who have lower-grade neoplasms may be able to be tapered off of dexamethasone successfully. Peptic ulcer and gastrointestinal bleeding due to corticosteroid usage is not as significant a problem as is commonly believed. The use of H_2 antagonists usually can be confined to patients who are at particular risk.

Deep vein thrombosis and pulmonary emboli are frequent complications seen in patients with brain tumors, particularly those with significant neurologic disability and immobility. Anticoagulation is probably not as dangerous as once feared, and its judicious use should be considered in appropriate cases.

Attention to the psychosocial needs of brain tumor patients is of utmost importance. The impact of these diseases on the lives of patients and their families cannot be overstated. Social service input and supportive nursing care is vital. Depression and fatigue can be debilitating symptoms in these patients as well, and antidepressants and stimulants may be useful.

Appropriate care of the dying brain tumor patient is equally important to the aggressive treatment at the onset of illness. Hospice groups can be very helpful in managing the final stages and symptoms of these devastating diseases and can provide significant family support. Stopping dexamethasone and other aggressive therapies at the appropriate time and freely treating pain is important in allowing patients and their families to experience death in as peaceful a way as possible.

*Not FDA approved for this indication.
†Not yet approved for use in the United States.

Section 14

The Locomotor System

RHEUMATOID ARTHRITIS

method of
KRISTINE M. LOHR, M.D.
University of Tennessee Health Science Center and VA Medical Center
Memphis, Tennessee

Rheumatoid arthritis (RA) is a chronic, systemic inflammatory disorder mediated primarily by T lymphocytes. The most prominent manifestation is symmetric polyarthritis of diarthrodial joints. The initial stimulus to inflammation remains elusive; however, multiple genetic susceptibility and severity factors and environmental triggers interact to produce a spectrum of clinical features and markers. Viruses implicated include parvovirus B19, human T-lymphotrophic virus type 1, and Epstein-Barr virus. Superantigens from bacteria and viruses and autoantigens (e.g., IgG, epitopes on type II collagen, components of cartilage, products of synoviocytes or chondrocytes, and shared epitopes) are also implicated. The shared epitope, a short sequence of amino acids on DRB1 chains of Class II major histocompatibility complex (MHC) antigens, is associated with genetic susceptibility to and severity of RA. These shared epitopes remain under study and may identify which patients would respond best to a particular combination regimen of drugs.

In the past 2 decades, evidence has accumulated that, once a firm diagnosis is made, early aggressive therapy is indicated. Bony erosions and joint space narrowing occur and progress most rapidly during the first 2 years of disease in most patients. Even if inflammation is controlled early, damaged cartilage may continue to deteriorate. Plain films likely underestimate the damage; magnetic resonance imaging shows focal bone changes in many patients with early RA. In general, the rate of radiographic progression is proportional to the intensity of inflammation and persistence of disease activity. Functional outcome, as measured by health assessment questionnaires, age, and comorbid conditions, best correlates with outcome better than laboratory and radiographic measures. More severe, active disease is associated with increased morbidity and mortality. Thus, a team approach to early, aggressive therapy is best. Close follow-up by a rheumatologist who works with the primary care provider, physical and occupational therapists, and orthopedic surgeon is associated with a better outcome.

GENERAL PROGRAM

The underpinning of the therapeutic regimen should include initial and ongoing education. Educated patients can place their expectations in context and understand the importance of adherence to exercise and pharmacologic regimens and therapeutic monitoring. Many patients search for information on the Internet; thus, the physician should be ready to discuss therapeutic options and, if possible, refer patients to appropriate sites for additional medical information.

Early referral to physical and occupational therapists is crucial. Therapists can do the following:

1. Reinforce the physician's prescription to rest and exercise.
2. Teach optimal joint use to protect the joint.
3. Teach exercise to maintain or increase function and range of motion.
4. Splint inflamed or painful joints to reduce inflammation and trauma.
5. Review, in detail, how patients accomplish activities of daily living, and recommend appropriate assistive devices.
6. Facilitate postoperative recovery after joint surgery.

Furthermore, therapists can devise and recommend an appropriate exercise program tailored to the individual patient.

Regardless of disease activity, most if not all patients require analgesia because pain is what usually initiates their visit to the doctor. Pain limits joint use, interferes with ability to exercise, and contributes to depression and decreased quality of sleep. The mainstay of analgesia in RA is the use of a nonsteroidal anti-inflammatory drug (NSAID) because NSAIDs also suppress symptoms due to inflammation. Choice of NSAID depends on multiple factors. First, determine which over-the-counter and prescription NSAIDs were tried. Second, consider the patient's age and co-morbidities. Prophylactic medications to prevent peptic ulcer and bleeding should be considered when patients are older than 65 years of age, have a history of previous peptic ulcer disease and bleeding, are taking concomitant corticosteroids, or are heavy users of tobacco or alcohol. Misoprostol (Cytotec) may be more cost effective than H_2 blockers and proton pump inhibitors, although perhaps less well tolerated. Alternatively, selective COX-2 inhibitors (e.g., celecoxib [Celebrex], rofecoxib [Vioxx]) or NSAIDs with greater COX-2 than COX-1 inhibition (e.g., etodolac [Lodine], meloxicam [Mobic]) are options in such patients. Third, prescription cost should be balanced with the NSAID requiring the fewest daily doses and the most acceptable toxicity profile.

Addition of medications for chronic pain may be useful adjuncts to improve quality of sleep and treat pain. Tricyclic antidepressant drugs* are usually

*Not FDA approved for this indication.

tried first. However, these may exacerbate symptoms of dry mouth associated with Sjögren syndrome or increased age. Excessive sedation should be avoided, particularly in elderly patients whose risk of falling is increased. In some patients, use of a narcotic analgesic at bedtime avoids unpleasant or unacceptable side effects. In general, judicious use of narcotic analgesics is recommended on weighing the risks and benefits of potential dependence and addiction.

Patients with symptoms of dry eyes can use topical liquid tears daily and lubricant at bedtime. For persistent symptoms, referral to an ophthalmologist is indicated for evaluation and further therapy. Patients with symptoms of dry mouth can try oral lubricants, but these are often unpalatable and inconvenient. Better success may be achieved with anticholinergic drugs, either pilocarpine (Salagen), 5 mg four times daily, or cevimeline (Evoxac), 30 mg three times daily.

PHARMACOLOGIC SUPPRESSION OF INFLAMMATION

From the patient's perspective, control of pain is primary. From the physician's perspective, the goals of therapy are improvement and preservation of functional status, as determined by the health assessment questionnaires, and prevention of cartilage and bone destruction, currently determined by plain radiography. NSAIDs do not alter the natural history of RA, even though they control inflammation and pain through inhibition of proinflammatory prostaglandins. Whether pharmacologic-induced decreases in synovitis and/or bone resorption are responsible for retardation of radiographic progression seen with some drugs remains unknown. Long-term, low-dose corticosteroids (<5 mg/d prednisone) slow the development of new erosions. Unfortunately, some studies demonstrate cumulative toxicity, including osteoporosis, infections, peptic ulcer disease (especially in the presence of NSAIDs), and mortality. Short courses (20 mg/d prednisone with rapid taper over 5 days) are used for RA flares or bridging treatment periods while waiting for a disease-modifying antirheumatic drug (DMARD) to take effect. Intra-articular corticosteroid injection for flares in one or a few joints is effective, provided septic arthritis is ruled out first. Studies are underway to determine cost-effectiveness of newer, expensive drugs associated with retardation of radiographic progression.

Methotrexate

Methotrexate (Rheumatrex) has all but replaced gold salts as the first-line DMARD in moderate or severe RA with poor prognostic features. Its onset of action is rapid, although its disease-modifying ability remains in question. The drug is taken at a dose of 7.5 to 15 mg orally once weekly. A few patients do well on 5 mg, whereas others require as high as 20 to 25 mg weekly. If no response is seen, absorption is questionable, or gastrointestinal side effects limit full dose, then weekly parenteral (intramuscular) therapy is tried. Most patients feel better within 4 to 8 weeks and experience a plateau at 6 months. Approximately 80% respond symptomatically.

Long-term studies demonstrate the effectiveness and safety of methotrexate, especially when combined with folic acid (1–2 mg/d) to reduce the incidence of common side effects. About 10% of patients experience nausea, vomiting, mucositis, and mild alopecia. Elevated serum homocysteine is a risk factor for cardiovascular disease. Folate replacement may decrease this risk by lowering the elevated serum homocysteine levels in methotrexate-treated patients, but it may reduce the drug's efficacy against RA. Patients in Europe appear to do better because the practice of folate supplementation is less common. Macrocytosis can occur with or without folate replacement. Serious hematologic side effects are uncommon and occur more likely in the presence of renal insufficiency, advanced age, or concomitant use of other antifolate medications (e.g., sulfa-containing antibiotics).

Liver biopsies have not validated concerns about long-term use. Alcohol use, obesity, diabetes mellitus, and renal insufficiency are risk factors for hepatic fibrosis and cirrhosis. Pulmonary toxicity, in 3% to 5%, can occur at any time and any dose. Acute cough, fever, and severe dyspnea with bilateral pulmonary infiltrates on chest radiograph can occur. Because of an association between pulmonary toxicity and upper respiratory tract infections, temporary discontinuation of methotrexate may be indicated. Treatment of pulmonary toxicity consists of discontinuation of methotrexate, supportive care, and short-term high-dose corticosteroids. A few patients developed B-cell pseudolymphomas and non-Hodgkin lymphomas that remitted when methotrexate was withdrawn.

Gold Compounds

For decades, parenteral gold salts (gold sodium aurothioglucose [Solganal] and thiomalate [Myochrysine]) were the standard first-line DMARDs. A test dose of 10 mg is given the first week, 25 mg the second week, then 50 mg weekly. When the total dose reaches 1000 mg, the interval can be increased slowly to 50 mg once monthly. Parenteral gold is effective with low toxicity (rash, mucositis, proteinuria, and cytopenia), but erosions still develop. Short-term and intermediate remissions occur. Oral gold (auranofin [Ridaura]) is associated with less severe toxicity but unfortunately less efficacy. Auranofin is taken at 3 to 9 mg/d in a single or divided doses. Gastrointestinal intolerance (i.e., diarrhea) is less if the drug is started at 3 mg/d and the dose increased slowly.

Sulfasalazine

In some studies, the antirheumatic efficacy of sulfasalazine (Azulfidine EN-tabs) is approximate to that of gold and penicillamine; in others, it is comparable to hydroxychloroquine, a less effective drug.

(None of these drugs is as effective as methotrexate.) Some studies showed less radiographic progression with sulfasalazine. Treatment is started at 0.5 to 1.0 g/d with increments to 1.5 to 3 g/d in divided doses. Nausea and upper abdominal discomfort, often associated with headache and dizziness, are common adverse effects usually within the first 2 to 3 months. Use of enteric-coated preparations and starting at a low dose that is gradually increased limits adverse effects. Neutropenia may occur suddenly. Contraindications include sulfa allergy.

D-Penicillamine

D-Penicillamine (Cuprimine, Depen) is used less often in the United States. Its latent onset of 8 to 12 weeks is similar to that of gold, and its profile of adverse effects is similar. It may be useful in patients with extra-articular manifestations. Both subcutaneous nodules and rheumatoid factor titer can decrease, correlating with clinical improvement. Treatment is started at 125 to 250 mg/d for 4 to 8 weeks and raised by similar increments every 1 to 3 months to a maximum of 750 mg/d and occasionally 1000 mg/d.

Hydroxychloroquine

In early, mild RA without poor prognostic features, antimalarial drugs are reasonable additions to NSAID therapy. Hydroxychloroquine (Plaquenil), usually 200 mg twice daily, is well tolerated compared with other agents and is associated with the least incidence of adverse effects. It is often used in combination therapy for moderate to severe RA and may have a beneficial effect on hyperlipidemia associated with corticosteroid use. Chloroquine (Aralen) may be more effective but also more toxic than hydroxychloroquine. Patients should be screened for glucose-6-phosphate dehydrogenase (G6PD) deficiency. The most common side effects are rash, upper abdominal discomfort, nausea and vomiting, headaches, and an uncommon neuromyopathy. Antimalarial retinopathy is less common with hydroxychloroquine; its incidence is increased at higher doses. Routine slit lamp examination at baseline and every 6 to 12 months is required to monitor for this irreversible side effect. Defective accommodation or convergence and corneal deposits, the latter causing halos around lights, are reversible.

Azathioprine

This purine analogue is converted to 6-mercaptopurine in vivo but has a better therapeutic index than 6-mercaptopurine. Azathioprine (Imuran) is initiated at 50 mg/d and increased every 1 to 2 weeks by 50 mg to the maximum of 2 to 2.5 mg/kg. Slower titration using 25 mg and/or an increase every 1 to 2 months is better tolerated. Given current available agents to treat RA, azathioprine is used when other regimens have failed. It is more often used as a corticosteroid-sparing or maintenance agent in other autoimmune diseases. The most important drug interaction is with allopurinol, which inhibits xanthine oxidase-mediated inactivation of 6-mercaptopurine and thus increased cytotoxic effects. Reducing the azathioprine dose by at least two thirds with close monitoring of the complete blood cell count is required. Combination therapy with sulfasalazine and azathioprine may increase the frequency of myelosuppression.

Leflunomide

Leflunomide (Arava) is metabolized to A77 1726, which is responsible for immunomodulation. This compound inhibits dihydroorotate dehydrogenase, an enzyme in the pyrimidine synthesis pathway. B cells appear to be more sensitive than T cells to its effect. A loading dose of 100 mg/d for 3 days is given and then a subsequent dose of 20 mg/d. Some patients may do as well on 10 mg/d. Leflunomide retards radiographic progression and thus is theoretically a logical agent to use in early RA to prevent damage. Adverse effects are mild and include diarrhea, reversible alopecia, hypertension, and elevated liver enzyme levels. Some investigators report clinical improvement when leflunomide is added to methotrexate in patients with incomplete responses, without increased hepatic toxicity. Use it with caution in patients with renal insufficiency. Leflunomide is contraindicated in women who are pregnant or considering pregnancy. Rapid reduction of the active metabolite with cholestyramine in both genders is recommended before planned conception because this may decrease risk to the fetus. There are no human studies to support this approach.

Organ Transplantation Immunosuppressant Drugs

Cyclosporine (Neoral, Sandimmune) is used in organ transplantation and autoimmune diseases, including RA. The newer microemulsion preparation is more bioavailable and associated with less variability in levels. Given its adverse effects with long-term use, cyclosporine is often used only after multiple therapies have failed. Some studies show additional benefit when added to methotrexate.

Gastrointestinal upset is common, as well as hypertrichosis, gingival hyperplasia, tremor, paresthesia, breast tenderness, hyperkalemia, hypomagnesemia, and hyperuricemia. Approximately 20% develop mild hypertension controlled by reduced dosage or antihypertensive medications. Almost all patients develop a small, reversible decrease in renal function. Recent data suggest that, after a year of therapy, serum creatinine rises irreversibly to more than 30% of baseline. To minimize adverse effects, cyclosporine is started at 2.5 mg/kg/d in divided doses, to a maximum of 4 mg/kg/d. Monitoring blood pressure and serum creatinine is required, with reduction of dose if the serum creatinine concentration rises more than 30% above the patient's baseline. Irreversible nephrotoxicity occurs more commonly with higher doses used in transplantation, as does the increased risk of skin cancer and lymphoma. Epstein-Barr virus–induced B-cell lymphoma that reverses with discontinuation of cyclosporine has been reported.

Studies with tacrolimus (FK506; Prograf)* and mycophenolate mofetil (CellCept),* a purine synthesis inhibitor, are underway for use in DMARD-resistant RA. Other immunosuppressants for organ transplantation may be studied in the future. Thalidomide (Thalomid)* is known more for its teratogenic than its immunosuppressive effects. Peripheral neuropathy is a common adverse effect that can develop even after thalidomide is discontinued. Safer, more effective agents for RA are available.

Biologic Agents and Future Therapy

Therapeutic targets for biologic agents in RA are determined by our understanding of the pathogenic process in the synovium. Targets include the following:

1. Upregulation of adhesion molecule, chemokine, and complement expression
2. Expression of T-cell surface activation markers and co-stimulatory molecules
3. MHC Class II/antigen/T-cell receptor complex interactions
4. Secretion and activation of proinflammatory or anti-inflammatory cytokines (interleukins, tumor necrosis factor-α[TNF-α])
5. Synovial cell proliferation and function.

Concerns about long-term use include the potential risk of serious infection and malignancy.

Currently, only TNF-α antagonists are approved by the Food and Drug Administration for therapy for RA. Two preparations are commercially available, with others undergoing human trials and development. The majority of RA patients respond. Although these drugs are effective and well tolerated in early and refractory RA, cost is prohibitive for some patients. These agents retard radiographic progression and thus are theoretically logical agents to use in early RA. However, because of cost, most insurance plans require that patients fail several prior agents before approval for use. Studies of long-term functional joint outcome, safety, and cost-effectiveness are underway to determine the appropriate place of TNF-α antagonists.

Etanercept (Enbrel) is a soluble p75 TNF-α receptor fused to the Fc portion of IgG_1 that neutralizes lymphotoxin-α and TNF-α. Initially recommended to be used in combination with methotrexate, it can be used long term as monotherapy with efficacy and retardation of radiographic progression. The recommended dose is 25 mg subcutaneously twice weekly. Titration or more frequent dosing is not well studied. The most common adverse effect is injection site reaction, followed by upper respiratory tract and other common infections. Autoantibodies and non-neutralizing antibodies occur, but no cases of systemic lupus erythematosus or lymphoproliferative disorders have been reported. Rare cases of central nervous system demyelinating disorders, optic neuritis, and pancytopenia, including aplastic anemia, have been reported.

*Not FDA approved for this indication.

Infliximab (Remicade) is a chimeric IgG1κ monoclonal antibody that specifically neutralizes TNF-α. Current dosage is 3 mg/kg given intravenously at 0, 2, and 6 weeks with subsequent maintenance infusions every 8 weeks, in combination with methotrexate. Its use as a single agent may be approved by the time of publication. This biologic agent at higher, titratable doses has been used for many years to treat refractory Crohn disease. A standard, lower dose is used in RA, but reports of breakthrough symptoms before the 8-week interval suggest that a shorter interval and/or increasing the dosage should be studied. Adverse effects include headache, rash, and upper respiratory and urinary infection. Some infections have been severe. Acute infusion reactions include fever, chills, urticaria, and pruritus. Lupus-like symptoms with anti–double-stranded DNA antibodies have been seen. Hematologic abnormalities are infrequent and transient. Concomitant administration of methotrexate decreases the incidence of human antichimeric antibody responses associated with abrogation of clinical response. At least one patient with Crohn disease developed a lymphoproliferative disorder.

Clinical trials with interleukin-1 (IL-1) receptor antagonist (IL-1Ra)* are ongoing. Preliminary reports suggest IL-1 blockade by IL-1Ra is associated with clinical improvement, reversal of the anemia associated with RA, and retardation of radiographic progression. The drug may be approved for use by the time of publication.

Other Agents

Anecdotal evidence suggested clinical benefit of tetracycline† use in RA. More recent studies using minocycline describe benefit in some patients. It may be useful in early RA or in combination with other drugs. Adverse effects are usually reversible and include gastrointestinal upset, photosensitivity, light-headedness and vertigo, gray-black skin pigmentation, and elevated blood urea nitrogen levels in patients with impaired renal function. Children can develop permanent discoloration of unerupted teeth. Pregnant or nursing women should not take tetracyclines because they retard skeletal development in the fetus and newborn.

Safer, more effective agents have replaced the use of alkylating agents (cyclophosphamide [Cytoxan],† chlorambucil [Leukeran],† and hydroxyurea [Droxia, Hydrea])† in the treatment of RA. Cyclophosphamide in combination with high-dose corticosteroids is used,

*Investigational drug in the United States.
†Not FDA approved for this indication.

however, when RA is complicated by vasculitis. Adverse effects, including malignancy, can be life threatening.

For patients with moderate to severe RA who have failed or are intolerant of DMARDs, use of a protein A immunoadsorption column (Prosorba) entails 12 weekly plasmapheresis treatments. Indications for re-treatment have not been established. Immunosorption removes circulating IgG and IgG-containing immune complexes and releases small but potentially immunomodulatory quantities of staphylococcal protein A into the circulation that may correlate with a clinical response. The most frequent adverse effects include joint pain and swelling, fatigue, paresthesias, headache, hypotension, anemia, nausea, sore throat, edema, abdominal pain, hypertension, rash, dizziness, diarrhea, hematoma, flushing, chills, respiratory difficulties, chest pain, and fever. Sepsis has occurred.

Dapsone,* a sulfone antimicrobial, has been used to treat RA in a few small studies. Initial dosing is 50 mg/d with maintenance at 100 mg/d. Patients should be screened for G6PD deficiency. More standard therapies should be initiated before use of this drug.

Which Disease-Modifying Antirheumatic Drug to Choose First?

In general, starting hydroxychloroquine, oral gold, sulfasalazine, or perhaps minocycline* in patients with mild RA but no poor prognostic features is reasonable. Today most patients with moderately severe or severe RA and poor prognostic features are started on methotrexate. Other choices are parenteral gold, azathioprine, or penicillamine. If cost were irrele-

*Not FDA approved for this indication.

TABLE 1. **Drugs Used in Rheumatoid Arthritis**

Drug	Gastro-intestinal	Mucocu-taneous	Hema-tologic	Liver	Lung	Renal Function	Infection	Terato-genicity	Association With Cancer	Miscellaneous
Azathioprine (Imuran)	+ + +	+	+ +	+ +			+ +	+ +	+ +	Early leukopenia, pancreatitis, interaction with allopurinol
Cyclophosphamide (Cytoxan)*	+ + +	+	+ + +				+ + +	+ + +	+ + +	Hemorrhagic cystitis, bladder cancer, ovarian and testicular failure
Cyclosporine (Sandimmune, Neoral)	+ +	+	+	+		+ + +	+	+	+	Hypertension, neuropathy, lymphoma, ?osteoporosis
Etanercept (Enbrel)			+				+ +	?	?	Rare: multiple sclerosis, optic neuritis, agranulocytosis
Gold, oral (Ridaura)	+ + +	+	+			+		+		Photosensitivity
Gold, parenteral (Solganal)	+	+ + +	+ +	+	+	+ +		+		Photosensitivity
Hydroxychloroquine (Plaquenil)	+ +	+	+					+		Headache; rare retinopathy neuromyopathy
Infliximab (Remicade)	+	+	+				+	?	?	Infusion reaction, headache
Leflunomide (Arava)	+		+	+			+	+ + +	?	
Methotrexate (Rheumatrex)	+ + +	+ + +	+	+ +	+ +		+ +	+ + +	+/+ +	Elevated serum homocysteine, nodulosis, lymphoma, pseudolymphoma, ?osteoporosis
Minocycline (Minocine)*	+	+								Tooth discoloration, skeletal retardation
NSAID	+ + +		+	+				+		Fluid retention and edema, aggravated hypertension
Penicillamine (Cuprimine, Depen)	+ +	+ + +	+ +	+	+ +	+ +		+ +		Rare: myasthenic syndrome, systemic lupus erythematosus, myositis
Sulfasalazine (Azulfidine)	+ + +	+ +	+ +	+	+			+ +		Headache, dizziness, sudden leukopenia

*Not FDA approved for this indication.

TABLE 2. **Recommended Therapeutic Monitoring in Rheumatoid Arthritis**

Drug	Complete Blood Cell Count, Platelets	Aspartate and Alanine Aminotransferases	Albumin	Creatinine	Urine	Other
Azathioprine	Baseline, 1–2 wk with changes in dosage, then every 1–3 mo	Baseline		Baseline		
Cyclophosphamide	Baseline, 1–2 wk with changes in dosage, then every 1–3 mo	Baseline		Baseline	Urinalysis and cytology every 6–12 mo after discontinuation	
Cyclosporine	Baseline, then periodic	Baseline, then periodic		Baseline, every 2 wk until dose stable, then monthly		Baseline potassium, then periodic
Etanercept	Baseline, then periodic					Screen for tuberculosis
Gold, oral	Baseline, then every 4–12 wk			Baseline	Baseline dipstick for protein, then every 4–12 wk	
Gold, parenteral	Baseline, then every 1–2 wk for first 20 wk, then at time of each or every other injection			Baseline	Baseline dipstick for protein, then every 1–2 wk for first 20 wk, then at time of each or every other injection	
Hydroxychloroquine						Screen for G6PD. Funduscopic and visual fields every 6–12 mo (baseline if older than 40 y or previous eye disease)
Infliximab	Baseline, then periodic					Screen for tuberculosis
Leflunomide	Baseline, then every 4–8 wk	Baseline, then every 4–8 wk		Baseline		Screen for hepatitis B and C in patients at risk
Methotrexate	Baseline, then every 4–8 wk	Baseline, then every 4–8 wk	Baseline, then every 4–8 wk	Baseline, then every 4–8 wk		Screen for hepatitis B and C in patients at risk
Minocycline	Baseline, then periodic	Baseline, then periodic		Baseline, then periodic		
NSAID	Baseline, then periodic	Baseline, then periodic		Baseline, then periodic		
Penicillamine	Baseline, then every 2 wk until dose stable, then every 1–3 mo				Dipstick for protein at baseline, then every 2 wk till dose stable, then every 1–3 mo	
Sulfasalazine	Baseline, then every 2–4 wk for first 3 mo, then every 3 mo	Baseline				Screen for G6PD

vant, therapy with leflunomide or a TNF-α antagonist could be first-line.

Failure to respond to multiple DMARDs, often as single agents, is associated with poor prognosis. Combination therapy, akin to that in oncology, has been tried anecdotally and in short-term studies. In general, hydroxychloroquine, oral gold, sulfasalazine, or perhaps minocycline is combined with one or more of those drugs used to treat moderate to severe RA. A common regimen uses methotrexate, hydroxychloroquine, and sulfasalazine. Some argue that combination regimens should be used early and tapered to a single agent when clinical response is noted. More common is the addition of one or more drugs when response to monotherapy (usually hydroxychloroquine, gold, sulfasalazine, or methotrexate) is inadequate.

Therapeutic Monitoring

Patients and physicians should communicate effectively about expectations of clinical response and the importance of monitoring for adverse effects (Tables 1 and 2). The American College of Rheumatology publishes guidelines for frequency of laboratory tests for each drug. In general, periodic complete blood cell count and tests for renal and hepatic function are appropriate for most drugs. Urinalysis is required when using gold. In patients who take daily corticosteroids for prolonged periods, assessment of bone density is necessary, as well as preventive therapy (calcium, vitamin D, estrogen in postmenopausal women and, when indicated, calcitonin or a bisphosphonate). Patients not compliant with monitoring should receive only enough medication until the next monitoring laboratory and/or physician visit. Primary care providers should pay close attention to laboratory results or reliably send results to the consulting/managing rheumatologist.

Complementary Medicine and Diet

Few studies address the use of alternative medicines. Prayer was reported as the most widely used alternative therapy in RA and osteoarthritis. Use of herbs,* supplements,* copper bracelets,* and magnets* occur, but their efficacy remains unknown. The use of omega-3* and omega-6* fatty acids, or fish* rich in these fatty acids, may modulate eicosanoid metabolism to less inflammatory compounds but are not palatable. Many RA patients try glucosamine* and chondroitin,* but use of these supplements has been studied only in the treatment of osteoarthritis.

Surgery

Patients with permanent joint damage and dysfunction benefit from orthopedic surgery. Interventions include carpal tunnel release, tendon rupture repair, total joint replacement, and cervical fusion for myelopathy.

*Not FDA approved for this indication.

JUVENILE RHEUMATOID ARTHRITIS

method of
ILDY M. KATONA, M.D.
Uniformed Services University of the Health Sciences
Bethesda, Maryland

and

LAURA J. MIRKINSON, M.D.
George Washington University School of Medicine
Washington, D.C.

Juvenile rheumatoid arthritis (JRA) encompasses a group of chronic childhood diseases with a common manifestation of inflammatory arthritis that lasts more than 6 weeks with no currently recognizable etiologic factor or factors.

In the European and Canadian literature, these diseases have been referred to as juvenile chronic arthritis, and by a recent nomenclature proposal by the International League Against Rheumatism, they are referred to as juvenile idiopathic arthritis. For the purpose of this article, the term accepted by the American College of Rheumatology, juvenile rheumatoid arthritis, will be used.

JRA is a relatively common chronic disease in childhood with an average incidence of 1 in 100,000 and a prevalence of 1 in 1000. In many patients, the disease exists throughout childhood, and some reports indicate that more than 30% of patients have active disease more than 20 years after onset, well into adulthood. Treatment of chronic arthritis is not only aimed at eliminating symptoms but also seeks to control inflammation, achieve remission, prevent structural damage, and allow normal growth and development of children. Optimal medical care for these children can be provided by a team of health care professionals coordinated by a pediatric primary care provider working with a subspecialist, such as a pediatric rheumatologist with up-to-date knowledge of evidence-based treatment options.

CLASSIFICATION

Classification of JRA is based mainly on the number of joints affected by inflammatory arthritis and on the presence or absence of systemic symptoms. Of note, however, is that patients often do not adhere to the closely defined subtypes. The progression of disease, response to treatment, and overall prognosis of a large number of patients can vary considerably. The American College of Rheumatology continues to define JRA as arthritis occurring at an age of onset of less than 16 years; arthritis in one or more joints; duration of disease of 6 weeks or longer; oligoarticular, polyarticular, or systemic onset; and exclusion of other forms of juvenile arthritis. About 10% to 20% of cases have a systemic onset (prominent systemic symptoms such as fever and rash precede or accompany the arthritis), 40% to 60% are manifested as polyarthritis (five or more joints affected at the time of onset), and 40% to 50% have oligoarticular arthritis (four or fewer joints affected at the time of onset).

Several subtypes of JRA are recognized to have a poorer overall outcome. These subtypes include adolescent girls with erosive, rheumatoid factor–positive polyarticular “adult-like” disease, patients with systemic-onset JRA (SOJRA) with polyarticular disease, and the subgroup of oligoarticular patients in whom involvement of additional joints over time leads to significant polyarticular arthritis. Patients with an oligoarticular onset who are antinuclear antibody (ANA) negative and who do not progress to polyarticular disease seem to have the most favorable outcome. It is important to note that any initial involvement can progress over time to polyarticular disease.

In SOJRA, systemic features predominate in the first phase of the disease. Patients can have a monocyclic, polycyclic, or chronic course. Severe polyarticular involvement eventually develops in many of these patients. They also frequently demonstrate a state of subclinical disseminated intravascular coagulation with increased fibrin split products. These patients are prone to the development of adverse drug reactions and macrophage activation syndrome, which can lead to hepatic failure and central nervous system complications. SOJRA is a diagnosis of exclusion, and patients with persistent febrile illnesses are also evaluated for many possible etiologies, including infectious diseases and malignancy. It is important to recognize that fever, fatigue, weight loss, hepatomegaly, and arthritis are features common to both rheumatic diseases and childhood malignancies. SOJRA can be an extremely aggressive disease, and its significant systemic and articular manifestations can be extraordinarily difficult to control.

Patients with polyarticular JRA (involvement of five or more joints in the first 6 months of their disease) tend to have symmetrical involvement of the large joints, as well as small-joint disease. These patients may manifest systemic symptoms similar to those of SOJRA. They are further subgrouped according to the presence or absence of rheumatoid factor. The rheumatoid factor–positive group has a female preponderance; their arthritis is usually erosive and aggressive, and the prognosis is similar to that of adult-onset rheumatoid arthritis. In the rheumatoid factor–negative group, the disease is generally less symmetrical, affects fewer large joints, and has a less severe course and overall outcome.

In oligoarticular JRA, four or fewer joints are affected in the first 6 months of disease. The large joints are usually involved in an asymmetric distribution, and systemic manifestations (other than uveitis) are rare. This form of JRA is most common in girls younger than 5 years. It is frequently associated with the presence of a positive ANA. Patients with oligoarthritis and positive ANA have the highest risk for development of a chronic anterior uveitis and require very vigorous ophthalmologic surveillance (every 3 months).

Two predominant oligoarticular subgroups are distinguished: girls younger than 5 years with a positive ANA (and a high risk of uveitis) and school-aged and adolescent boys who are often HLA-B27 positive and in whom some form of spondyloarthropathy may later develop. Axial involvement develops in these male patients later in their disease course, but it can initially be extremely difficult to identify them within the overall group of children with oligoarticular JRA.

Pediatric patients with juvenile psoriatic arthritis have articular symptoms similar or identical to those of oligoarticular JRA. Their disease course may closely mimic that of JRA, including pauciarticular or polyarticular arthritis. In these patients, articular symptoms may precede the development of a psoriatic rash by years. Many of them have a positive ANA and are at high risk for the development of chronic anterior uveitis.

Occasionally, patients initially have symptoms of enthesitis, with or without arthritis. In these patients, inflammation, particularly at the site of insertion of tendons and ligaments to bone, produces significant pain that may be difficult to distinguish from the articular pain of patients with JRA. This particular subset of patients is probably part of the larger group of patients in whom recognizable spondyloarthropathies eventually develop.

GENERAL PRINCIPLES OF TREATMENT

The major component of therapy for JRA at the current time is pharmacotherapy. The tremendous advances in basic research, coupled with the rapidity of drug development, have led to a steadily growing number of available drugs. In addition, because of the "Pediatric Rule" of the 1994 Food and Drug Administration (FDA) Modernization Act and the admirable effort of the Pediatric Rheumatology Collaborative Study Group, great interest and effort have been expended in making these drugs available for children. As noted earlier, broad categories of JRA are recognized. Often, a strategy for therapy can be guided by what clinical subgroup best describes a particular patient's features and clinical course. Although a few patients, generally those with mild oligoarticular disease, will respond to first-line therapy of nonsteroidal anti-inflammatory drugs (NSAIDs) alone, most patients with moderate to severe polyarticular JRA require a multidrug regimen. These regimens combine NSAIDs with second-line agents such as methotrexate (MTX), glucocorticoids, immunosuppressants such as cyclosporine* (Sandimmune), and newer biologic drugs such as etanercept (Enbrel). MTX is currently considered the first choice of the second-line agents, and hydroxychloroquine (Plaquenil)* and sulfasalazine (Azulfidine) are often used as a component of a multidrug regimen. In a rare few patients, experimental interventions such as stem cell transplantation are considered. Second-line "disease-modifying" drugs have slower anti-inflammatory action, and their optimal effects may not be seen for several months. Over time, however, they can alter the course of disease and prevent erosive articular changes.

It is the responsibility of health care providers to always be aware that chronic therapy is effective only with good patient and parent compliance. In pediatric patients, optimal dosing at the earliest possible opportunity is an essential component of successful therapy. It is becoming increasingly more difficult to have medications dispensed at schools. Whenever possible, we restrict our dosing regimens to times when our patients are at home. As noted earlier, a combination of drugs is frequently required for the control of moderately severe or severe arthritis. Monitoring for side effects is an intricate part of drug therapy. Even after remission of arthritis is achieved in a given patient, drugs are thought to be necessary for a certain period. A consensus among the physician, patient, and parent determines the exact timing of withdrawal of all medication. Even when the highest caution is exercised, in some patients a flare of disease necessitates re-initiation of therapy.

With more effective medical therapies available, joint function is preserved and the need for additional therapeutic modalities such as physical therapy, occupational therapy, and surgery has decreased notably. In general, the normal lifestyles of children and adolescents with JRA keep them active, and physicians place few, if any restrictions on their activities.

THERAPEUTIC CHOICES

Aspirin, Traditional NSAIDs, and Cyclooxygenase-2 Inhibitors

The use of anti-inflammatory doses of aspirin is negligible and limited to its use in Kawasaki syndrome and rheumatic fever.

*Not FDA approved for this indication.

Increasing numbers of traditional NSAIDs (with inhibitory activity of both isoforms of the cyclooxygenase [COX] enzyme) are being used, such as diclofenac (Voltaren),* ibuprofen (Motrin),* indomethacin (Indocin)*, nabumetone (Relafen), oxaprozin (Daypro),* piroxicam (Feldene),* sulindac (Clinoril),* and tolmentin (Tolectin). Many of these drugs are approved for pediatric use by the FDA, whereas others are sometimes used "off label." In general, the dose of NSAIDs is calculated on a per-kilogram body weight basis for children, and they are started at the low-medium dosage range. The half-life of an NSAID determines its required frequency of administration and indirectly influences patient/parent compliance. Although gastric irritation and the toxic effects of NSAIDs, including gastrointestinal bleeding or perforation, are less frequent in children, they still occur and are likely to increase as children approach adolescence. Patients are advised to take the same precautions as older patients, and we recommend that our patients take these medications with meals. Symptoms of toxicity are treated similarly as in adults, and many patients require concomitant treatment with H_2 blockers and proton pump inhibitors. Of note, NSAIDs (particularly naproxen) have been known to cause an unusual rash seen most prominently on the face. This rash, which was originally described as "pseudoporphyria," starts as small vesicles or blisters and causes small linear scars that may not resolve after use of the medication is discontinued. The use of indomethacin is complicated in some children by its effect on the central nervous system. Among the NSAIDs, only a few choices of liquid preparations (naproxen, ibuprofen, and indomethacin) are used in younger children. Pediatric patients may respond differently to the various NSAIDs; therefore, it is worthwhile changing medications if the response to one is suboptimal after an 8- to 12-week trial in a patient with a mild form of JRA. Laboratory monitoring for children with long-term NSAID use should be performed every 3 to 4 months and should include a complete blood count, urinalysis, and determination of serum creatinine and alanine and aspartate aminotransferase.

Studies involving drugs with selective COX-2–inhibitory properties are currently under way in children. These drugs, such as rofecoxib* (Vioxx) or celecoxib* (Celebrex), have a long half-life that allows daily or twice-daily administration. They may have lower gastrointestinal toxicity than the traditional NSAIDs because of their minimal, if any, effect on the COX-1 enzyme.

Methotrexate

MTX,* an inhibitor of folate metabolism with a potent, multifactorial anti-inflammatory effect, is the most commonly used second-line disease-modifying agent for JRA. Its use in JRA has been shown to lead to an improved clinical and radiologic outcome. MTX is best initiated early in the course of aggressive disease. In addition to its efficacy in treating articular manifestations, it has been demonstrated to be effective in the treatment of uveitis associated with JRA. MTX is available in tablet form (2.5 mg) or in a solution that is ideal for subcutaneous injection or oral administration (25 mg/1.0 mL). MTX is administered once weekly. In our clinic, we advise administering MTX on a day when the patient is at home that is convenient for the family (usually Saturday). Common subjective side effects are gastric upset, nausea, and central nervous system symptoms. These side effects are decreased in some children when folic acid is given either as a single dose (2.5–7.5 mg) 24 hours after MTX or daily in a dose of 1 mg.

The most common organ toxicity of MTX involves the liver and the bone marrow, although most of the side effects seen in adults (among them, hypersensitivity pneumonitis) have been reported in a small number of children. Periodic evaluation (every 4 to 8 weeks), including a complete blood count and assay for serum alanine and aspartate aminotransferase, bilirubin, and albumin, is warranted. Liver fibrosis is extremely rare in children, and routine liver biopsies are not indicated. Given alcohol's hepatic toxicity, we counsel our patients (particularly adolescents) about avoidance of alcohol in general and, specifically, on the day of MTX therapy. Recommendations relating to increased liver enzymes in adults are applicable to pediatric patients as well.

The dose range for MTX is 0.3 to 1 mg/kg/wk. Our most frequent starting dose is 0.5 mg/kg/wk with a maximum dose of 40 mg/wk. The optimal dose of therapy is achieved gradually within a few months. Absorption of orally administered MTX is usually increased linearly up to 0.6 mg/kg/wk. After that, any further increase in absorption of oral MTX is erratic. Therefore, if the clinical response is not maximal once an oral dose of 0.6 mg/kg/wk has been achieved, a trial of subcutaneous MTX may be warranted. The length of therapy with MTX ranges from months to years. Discussion of the overall favorable long-term safety profile of MTX is often reassuring to patients and parents. Once remission has been achieved, discontinuation of MTX therapy can be initiated cautiously. The exact timing and choice of withdrawal (gradual or abrupt) are arbitrary at the current time. Many patients, up to 30% to 50%, relapse after discontinuation of MTX treatment. One group especially vulnerable to relapse consists of children with oligoarticular-onset JRA with a polyarticular course. In teenage patients the teratogenic potential of MTX needs to be discussed repeatedly, and if pregnancy is desired, use of the drug must be stopped several months before impregnation occurs. MTX has been studied and used in combination with sulfasalazine, hydroxychloroquine, and cyclosporine. More recently, tumor necrosis factor-α receptor (TNF-αR) blocking drugs such as etanercept (Enbrel) or infliximab* (Remicade) have been used in combination with MTX.

*Not FDA approved for this indication.

*Not FDA approved for this indication.

Sulfasalazine

Sulfasalazine (Azulfidine) is used frequently in the treatment of spondyloarthropathy. It is also appropriate for treatment of the articular symptoms of JRA. It can be used as a monotherapy or in combination with MTX and/or hydroxychloroquine. The required dosage range is 40 to 60 mg/kg/d (with a maximal dose of 3 g/d), and the drug is administered on a three-times-daily or twice-daily schedule. Administration of sulfasalazine is contraindicated in persons with sulfa allergy or glucose-6-phosphate dehydrogenase deficiency. The ideal dosage should be increased incrementally over a period of 4 to 8 weeks. The most common side effect is gastrointestinal upset, which frequently responds to lowering of the dose and a more gradual series of incremental increases. The use of sulfasalazine in active SOJRA has been reported to be associated with the development of macrophage activation syndrome and should be used only with caution.

Hydroxychloroquine*

The efficacy of hydroxychloroquine (Plaquenil) is limited in children with JRA, but the drug has proved to be useful in certain patients, especially those with mild to moderate arthritis, or as a component of combination therapy. Side effects are very few at the recommended dose of 5 to 7 mg/kg/d, and even its potential retinal toxicity, which warrants regular ophthalmologic examination, is rare.

Cyclosporine*

Cyclosporine (Sandimmune), an inhibitor of T-cell proliferation and cytokine production, has been shown to be beneficial in treating the symptoms and complications of JRA. It is administered orally in a twice-daily regimen in a dose of 3 to 7 mg/kg/d, alone or in combination with weekly doses of MTX. Its potential side effects include hypertrichosis, gingival hyperplasia, and renal toxicity. Frequent measurements of blood pressure and careful monitoring of serum creatinine are recommended.

Biologic Response Modifiers

The standard first- and second-line agents previously described target the inflammatory response at multiple sites. In contrast, the new generation of therapeutic agents, collectively named biologic response modifiers, direct treatment at points thought to be pivotal in the pathogenesis of disease.

TNF is a proinflammatory cytokine that has been shown to play a complex role in the pathogenesis of JRA. Etanercept, an anti-TNF agent, was the first biologic response modifier that received approval from the FDA for the treatment of JRA. It is a dimeric soluble form of the TNF receptor that can bind two TNF molecules and render them biologically ineffective. Etanercept is available in 25-mg single-use vials, and its storage and administration require very specific handling techniques. The effective dosage of etanercept in children is 0.4 mg/kg per dose twice weekly, and it is administered by subcutaneous injection. Parents may administer the drug at home after appropriate training. Except for injection-site reactions, minor side effects of etanercept are rare. Several major side effects have, however, been reported, such as demyelmating neurologic disease, pancytopenia, serious infections, and the development of diabetes mellitus. These side effects should make one cautious with its use, serve as a reminder to balance the benefit–side effect ratio, and advocate its use only in children whose disease cannot be controlled by other, less potentially toxic medications.

Infliximab* is a monoclonal antibody with anti-TNF activity. It is administered in combination with weekly doses of MTX. Infliximab is currently used in the treatment of rheumatoid arthritis in adults, and studies in JRA are under way. Its effectiveness has been shown in Crohn's disease in children. Infliximab is administered as an intravenous infusion in the physician's office at intervals ranging between 2 and 8 weeks.

Cyclophosphamide*

Immunosuppressive drugs such as cyclophosphamide (Cytoxan) are occasionally used in pediatric patients with severe JRA. Monthly pulses of intravenous cyclophosphamide in a dose of 0.5 to 1.0 g/m^2 have been used with success in some patients with systemic-onset, polyarticular JRA whose disease is not controlled with more traditional therapy. The protocol of administration and the precautions recommended are similar to those for other rheumatic diseases, most notably lupus nephritis.

Glucocorticoids

Low-dose (<0.5 mg/kg/d) oral glucocorticoids, given as a single morning dose, have been used as part of the medical management for patients with severe polyarticular arthritis, especially during periods of poor disease control. In young patients, liquid formulations, particularly prednisolone syrup (15 mg/5 mL), are used most frequently.

High-dose (2 mg/kg/d initial dose) oral glucocorticoids, usually given on a split three- or four-times-daily schedule, are used for the initial control of SOJRA. Consolidation to a single daily dose with a subsequent decrease in the total dose is a difficult and challenging task and must be executed with great patience and care.

To completely wean patients with SOJRA from glucocorticoids is a goal that is always difficult to achieve and sometimes unobtainable. During the

*Not FDA approved for this indication.

*Not FDA approved for this indication.

weaning process, the lower dosages are decreased extremely slowly, in the range of 1 mg at a time.

Intravenous pulsed glucocorticoids are used in patients with severe systemic manifestations or life-threatening situations. An intravenous infusion of methylprednisolone at a dose of 30 mg/kg/d can be given. The drug, diluted in 5% dextrose in water is usually given over a period of 1 to 2 hours, and the patient's vital signs are closely monitored during this time. The dose can be repeated for 3 to 5 consecutive days or given once weekly for several weeks.

All patients and their parents need to be counseled about the potential problems of adrenal suppression and the possible need for stress doses of glucocorticoids. We recommend that patients wear a medical alert bracelet as a precaution.

Local delivery of intra-articular glucocorticoids to individual inflamed joints has become a commonly used therapeutic modality. Triamcinolone acetonide (Kenalog) has proved to be a very beneficial preparation in children, probably because of its long half-life. The maximal dose for a peripheral joint (knee) is 40 mg, and for smaller children, 1 mg/kg. For the smaller joints, a half, quarter, or eighth of the total dose (20, 10, or 5 mg) is used. The injection needs to be performed by aseptic technique, and local anesthesia provided by topical and injectable lidocaine makes the procedure considerably more tolerable. Injection of joints in children younger than 7 to 8 years can be a daunting task and is best performed under sedation by a very experienced physician. Restricting physical activity (which requires placement of a walking cast in small children) for 24 to 48 hours after the injection seems to increase the therapeutic benefit. Intra-articular injection leads to only a small amount of transient systemic steroid absorption. The most common side effect of intra-articular glucocorticoid therapy is transient lipolysis in the subcutaneous tissues from leakage of drug into the affected area.

Early Recognition and Treatment of Chronic Anterior Uveitis

Chronic anterior uveitis is a nonarticular complication of JRA, especially of the oligoarticular subtype, and develops most commonly, but not exclusively in the first 5 years of the disease. Routine periodic slit-lamp examination ensures an early diagnosis and most ideal treatment of this potentially blinding disease. Recommendations for the frequency of eye examinations were reviewed and published by the American Academy of Pediatrics in collaboration with the American Academy of Ophthalmology in 1993 and range from every 3 months to once yearly. It is of paramount importance that parents understand the danger of this complication and that they support the health care providers by scheduling the needed periodic slit-lamp examinations.

Treatment of chronic anterior uveitis, including topical glucocorticoids, mydriatics, and systemic anti-inflammatory therapy, depends on the severity of the uveitis. Traditional NSAIDs and MTX* are the most commonly used systemic drugs, but certain patients may also require systemic glucocorticoids. The dosage of MTX used for treatment of uveitis is 1 mg/kg/wk, usually given subcutaneously to prevent potential problems in absorption. Treatment of the uveitis requires a partnership between the ophthalmologist and the rheumatologist. Late complications of uveitis frequently require ophthalmologic surgery.

Other Therapies

Small numbers of selected patients with severe JRA receive treatment with other drugs, including but not limited to intravenous immunoglobulin,* azathiopine* (Imuran), and mycophenolate mofetil* (CellCept). For an occasional patient, injectable gold is still used.

Newer Therapies

Although significant advances have been made in the treatment of JRA, a small group of patients have severe disease that only partially responds or fails to respond to the currently available therapies. One possible hope for these patients is the future availability of new biologic agents, such as new anticytokine or anti–T-cell antibodies or bone marrow ablation with or without stem cell rescue. It is important that patients be carefully selected for these procedures and that the treatment be administered in a randomized fashion to gain insight into its value. In the even more distant future, gene therapy could become available for patients with JRA.

Prevention and Treatment of Macrophage Activation Syndrome

Macrophage activation syndrome, a condition characterized by severe liver involvement, hematologic abnormalities, and a coagulopathy that resembles disseminated intravascular coagulation, is a well-described complication of SOJRA. It commonly occurs during the systemic phase of the disease and is frequently associated with a concurrent viral infection or administration of pharmacotherapeutic agents. Drugs that can be associated with macrophage activation syndrome include, but are not limited to NSAIDs,* sulfasalazine, and MTX.* This syndrome can be successfully treated in most patients by intravenous pulsed methylprednisolone (30 mg/kg/d) alone or in combination with cyclosporine.*

Supportive Therapies

The role of physical therapy, although diminished, is still important to help patients maintain or regain normal joint mobility and normal muscle strength. Physical therapy is especially critical in the very young in whom the disease has interfered with nor-

*Not FDA approved for this indication.

mal motor development. To achieve a normal gait pattern, these children often require an extended length of therapy. Occupational therapy can offer a tremendous contribution to the fine motor development of children with wrist and hand arthritis. Orthotics are needed much less often than a decade or two ago and are intended to preserve range of motion and prevent further deformity.

Leg length discrepancy is a recognized complication of oligoarthritis of the knee. The affected leg has accelerated growth and becomes longer. If the discrepancy is greater than 1 cm, correction is warranted. A shoe lift (internal or external) of 0.5 cm (a 50% correction) is applied to the unaffected shorter leg.

A well-balanced, healthy diet with an adequate caloric count, appropriate vitamins, and 800 to 1200 mg of calcium for children or 1200 to 1500 mg of calcium for adolescents is indicated in patients with JRA. No medical evidence has indicated that any special diet has a positive effect on chronic arthritis, and a restricted diet may well be harmful if it does not provide the nutrients required by the growing and developing child.

Expert general pediatric, dental, orthodontic, and adolescent care are of special importance for children with JRA. Immunizations are optimally given during a period when the disease is well controlled, but they are not withheld except under extreme circumstances. Live-virus vaccines should be avoided in children receiving immunosuppressive therapy.

Exercise, especially weight bearing, is encouraged. It is our general policy to excuse our patients with lower extremity arthritis from vigorous running, but allow them to participate in all other activities as tolerated.

The care of a child with JRA requires an understanding of the many variations of this disease and the unique responses that children with different forms of the disease have to the variety of pharmacologic treatments. JRA is virtually always a nonlethal disease and can be self-limited, but in a large number of cases it can lead to severe eye or joint disability if not appropriately managed. In this group of patients, articular disease is often minimally symptomatic and eye disease is silent. A clinician who does not diligently seek clinical evidence of disease may miss its manifestations. Failure to aggressively treat the articular and extra-articular manifestations of JRA may also fail to prevent its most damaging and late consequences.

ANKYLOSING SPONDYLITIS AND OTHER SPONDYLARTHRITIDES

method of
LARS KOEHLER, M.D., and
HENNING ZEIDLER, M.D.
Hannover Medical School
Hannover, Germany

Ankylosing spondylitis belongs to a group of interrelated diseases termed *spondylarthritides* that are characterized by the lack of rheumatoid factors and rheumatoid nodules and the common features of the sacroiliitis-spondylitis-arthritis syndrome (Table 1). The rationale of grouping these disorders together is based on the sharing of clinical, radiographic, and epidemiologic features as well as the genetic association with the major histocompatibility complex Class I allele HLA-B27. The term *undifferentiated spondylarthritides* was introduced as a nosologic missing link to classify patients failing to meet criteria for definite categories, such as ankylosing spondylitis or psoriatic arthritis.

Histopathologically, two phenomena contribute to the morphologic abnormalities in spondylarthritides. Synovitis and subchondral bone marrow changes result in widespread joint destruction, and an unusual form of chondroid metaplasia progresses to ankylosis. In terms of etiopathophysiology, at least a part of the diseases is related to a persistent bacterial infection that induces and maintains the inflammatory immune response.

CLINICAL FEATURES

Characteristic features of the group of spondylarthritides and the different forms of spondylarthritides are summarized in Tables 2 and 3. The spinal, articular, and extra-articular manifestations can be found in various combinations. For example, a patient with reactive arthritis may present with oligoarthritis of the lower limb or arthritis-conjunctivitis-urethritis syndrome or HLA-B27–positive spondylarthritis with inflammatory back pain.

Axial Involvement

Axial involvement is a common feature of spondylarthritides. Patients usually complain of low back pain of the inflammatory type. The pain begins insidiously, and maximal pain is usually reached in the second half of the night with nocturnal awakening and in the morning. The pain gradually improves with movement, and the patient may be free of pain during the day. The spectrum of disease activity is broad. The spinal involvement can range from recurrent isolated sacroiliitis to progression into the thoracic and cervical regions, leading to complete bony fusion (bamboo spine) and a kyphotic posture.

TABLE 1. **The Spectrum of Spondylarthritides**

Ankylosing spondylitis	Juvenile ankylosing spondylitis
Reactive arthritis	Seronegative enthesopathic arthropathy syndrome
Enteropathic spondylitis (Crohn disease, ulcerative colitis)	Undifferentiated spondylarthritis

TABLE 2. **Common Features of Spondylarthritides**

Absence of

Rheumatoid factors
Subcutaneous ("rheumatoid") nodules

Common Features

Sacroiliitis/spondylitis
Inflammatory peripheral arthritis (often asymmetric)
Enthesopathy
Extra-articular manifestations
- Ocular inflammation (such as conjunctivitis, anterior uveitis)
- Infection of the urogenital or gastrointestinal tract
- Alteration of the skin (psoriasiform skin or nail lesion, erythema nodosum)
- Buccal ulceration of the mouth, small or large intestine, and urogenital tract
- Thrombophlebitis
- Pyoderma gangrenosum

Familial aggregation
Association with HLA-B27

Joints

The most common form of peripheral joint involvement is a nondeforming asymmetric oligoarthritis of the lower limb. The upper limb, especially the wrists, also can be affected.

Enthesitis

Enthesitis is a hallmark of spondylarthritis. The degree of pain can vary from mild to disabling. The plantar or Achilles tendon (heel pain) is frequently involved.

DIAGNOSIS

Diagnosis of each of the spondylarthritides is based primarily on clinical and radiographic findings. The most specific feature is sacroiliitis, detected by imaging techniques. Therefore, in any patient with inflammatory low back pain or suspected spondylarthritis, anteroposterior and lateral radiographs of the lumbar spine that include the sacroiliac joint should be made. The next step depends on the outcome of this radiograph. In the case of grade 2 to 4 sacroiliitis, no further imaging is required. However, plain radiographs may be negative early in disease. Computed tomography, bone scintigraphy, single-photon emission computed tomography, and magnetic resonance imaging are more sensitive in demonstrating inflammatory changes in these joints.

In general, little additional useful information is derived from routinely typing patients with classic ankylosing spondylitis for HLA-B27. However, in monosymptomatic or oligosymptomatic diseases such as peripheral arthritis, enthesitis, dactylitis, acute anterior uveitis, or atrioventricular conduction block, HLA-B27 typing may be useful for early diagnosis of undifferentiated spondylarthritis.

The multiple entry criteria diagnosing spondyloarthropathies (Amor criteria), although developed and evaluated for classification purposes, may also be useful in diagnosis, with the limitation that they do not include the full spectrum of diseases, lack the sensitivity to include patients with milder forms, and show reduced sensitivity in the diagnosis in patients with disease duration of less than 1 year. The Amor criteria are based on a weighted point scale, and a patient is considered as suffering from spondylarthritis if the sum of the 12 criteria values is at least 6 points (Table 4).

TREATMENT

General Principles

The main objectives of therapeutic management of ankylosing spondylitis and the other spondylarthritides are patient education, physical therapy to restore and maintain posture in an upright position and movement, self-management with exercise, and, most importantly, relief of pain and stiffness to facilitate physical therapy.

The association of interrelated diseases to one group, the spondylarthritides, turns out to be extremely useful in terms of therapy because the choice of treatment and combination of therapeutic options, such as physical treatment, drug therapy, and surgical therapy, is determined by the clinical presentation and activity of the disease rather than the precise diagnosis.

The drug therapy should be monitored according to the guidelines of the American College of Rheumatology (http://www.rheumatology.org/research/guidelines/ra-drug/ra-drug.html).

Axial Involvement

The cornerstone of the therapy for axial involvement is physical therapy and nonsteroidal anti-in-

TABLE 3. **Specific Feature of Spondylarthritides**

Feature	Ankylosing Spondylitis	Psoriatic Arthritis	Enteritic Spondylarthritis	Reactive Arthritis
Male:female ratio	3:1	1:1	1:1	1:1
Sacroiliitis/spondylitis	~100%	~20%	<20%	<50%
Symmetry of sacroiliitis	Symmetric	Asymmetric	Symmetric	Asymmetric
Positivity of HLA-B27	95%	50%–70%	—	50%–80%
Peripheral arthritis	~20%	~95%	~15%–20%	~90%
Enthesitis	+ +	+ +	+	+ +
Eye involvement	25%–30%	~20%	<15%	~50%
Cardiac involvement	1%–4%	Rare	Rare	5%–10%
Mucocutaneous lesions	—	~100%	Rare	<40%
Diarrhea	—	—	+ +	+/+ +
Urethritis	(+)	—	—	+ +
Disease triggered by bacteria	(?)	(?)	(+)	+ +

Adapted from Arnett FC Jr, Khan M, Wilkens R: A new look at ankylosing spondylitis. Patient Care, November 30, 1989, (23) 19;82–101 copyright Medical Economics.

TABLE 4. **Amor Criteria for Classification of Spondylarthritides***

	Points
A. Past or current clinical manifestations	
1. Back pain at night and/or back stiffness in the morning	1
2. Asymmetric oligoarthritis	2
3. Gluteal pain without other details	1 or
Alternating gluteal pain	2
4. Sausage-like digit or toe	2
5. Heel pain or other enthesopathy	2
6. Iritis	2
7. Nongonococcal urethritis or cervicitis within 1 month before onset of arthritis	1
8. Diarrhea within 1 month before onset of arthritis	1
9. Past or current psoriasis and/or balanitis and/ or inflammatory bowel disease	2
B. Roentgenographic changes	
10. Sacroiliitis (stage 2 or more if unilateral, stage 3 or more if unilateral)	2
C. Predisposing genetic factors	
11. Presence of the HLA-B27 antigen and/or positive family history for ankylosing spondylitis, Reiter syndrome, psoriasis, uveitis, or chronic bowel disease	2
D. Response to treatment	
12. Improvement within 48 hours after initiation of a nonsteroidal anti-inflammatory drug	2

*Patients with a total score of 6 points or more are classified as having a spondylarthritis.

flammatory drugs (NSAIDs) (Figure 1). Physical therapy modalities are an integral part of management of ankylosing spondylitis. The aims of physiotherapy are to improve mobility and strength and to prevent stiffness and deformities and consists of physical therapy and regular exercise.

NSAIDs are often required for control of inflammation and pain relief to enable physiotherapy. Such medication can be stopped if the patient is free of pain and able to perform physiotherapy on a daily basis. Various NSAIDs have been shown to be effective, including diclofenac, indomethacin, naproxen, piroxicam, and, most recently, meloxicam and celecoxib. NSAIDs improve pain and morning stiffness within 48 hours; discontinuing the drug usually results in a relapse within 48 hours. The time schedule and the dose of the NSAID has to be adapted to the pain profile of the individual patient (Figure 2). The aim of the NSAID therapy is complete suppression of the pain. In case of typical inflammatory back pain with pain in the second half of the night and in the morning, NSAIDs (e.g., diclofenac [Voltaren]) should be administered as a sustained-release preparation at a dose of 100 mg at night. For the morning pain, NSAIDs with a short half-life such as diclofenac (Voltaren), 25 to 50 mg, are required. If the patient complains about a prolonged morning pain, the same NSAID can be given at lunch. An alternative represents the NSAID in a slow-release form (diclofenac SL, 75 mg). If the NSAID used is not sufficient to suppress the symptoms despite adequate administration in relation to the daily pain profile of the patient, the drug has to be changed to another, more potent, NSAID, such as indomethacin. In the case of continuous pain without significant change during daytime, NSAIDs with long half-lives offer the advantage of application only once daily. Meloxicam (Mobic),* 15 mg/d, and piroxicam (Feldene),* 20 mg/d, have shown equivalent efficacy, but patients taking piroxicam had a higher rate of gastrointestinal side effects. In case of treatment failure of the standard NSAIDs, the benefit-risk ratio favors use of phenylbutazone in a daily oral dose of 400 to 600 mg. Close monitoring is required to recognize potentially severe toxicity, such as agranulocytosis.

For patients at risk to develop serious NSAID-induced gastrointestinal side effects such as gastrointestinal bleeding or perforation, cytoprotective strategies are necessary. A proven concept represents the combination of NSAIDs with misoprostol (Cytotec), 200 μg three times a day, or omeprazole (Prilosec), 20 mg/d. Increasing evidence suggests that a new class of NSAIDs, the cyclooxygenase-2 specific inhibitors, have no deleterious effect on the gastrointestinal tract. Initial clinical trials have shown that cyclooxygenase-2 specific inhibitors are as efficacious as conventional NSAIDs.

Refractory spondylarthritis can be defined as the

*Not FDA approved for this indication.

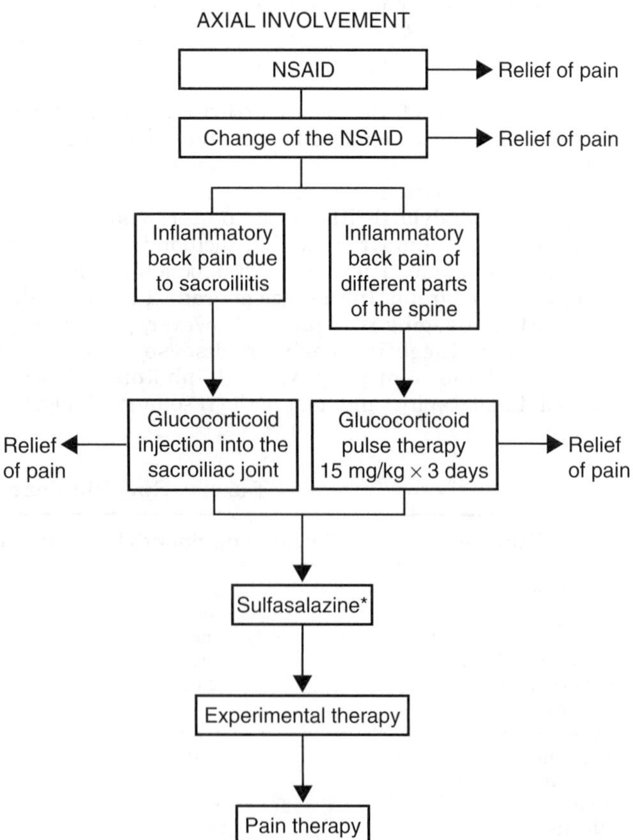

Figure 1. Use of nonsteroidal anti-inflammatory drugs for axial involvement of spondylarthritides. *Not FDA approved for this indication.

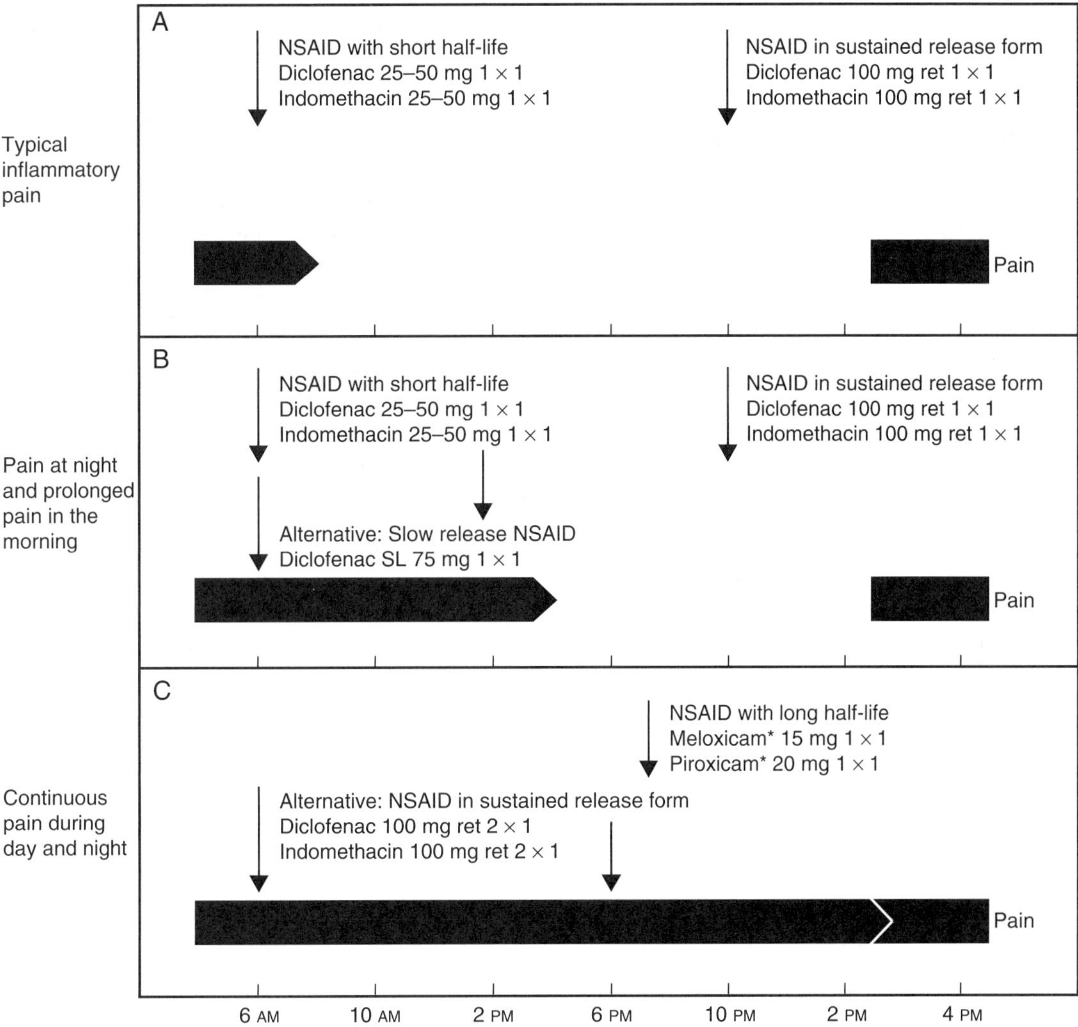

Figure 2. Algorithm for drug therapy for axial involvement of spondylarthritides. *Not FDA approved for this indication.

presence of persistent complaints of rheumatic symptoms despite an optimized NSAID therapy. Before classifying a patient with generalized spondylarthritis refractory to NSAIDs, the dose of the NSAID should be increased to the maximum. Furthermore, a change from one NSAID to another should be considered.

In cases of refractory low back pain due to sacroiliitis, a beneficial effect of intra-articular or periarticular glucocorticoid treatment of the sacroiliac joint has been shown to provide significant improvement. Pulse methylprednisolone therapy may be used in severe NSAID-resistant acute flares involving different parts of the spine. Three pulses of 250 mg prednisolone per day often result in a dramatic improvement in morning stiffness, back pain, and spinal mobility. Improvement is maximal at 1 week and is maintained for 3 to 21 months. Oral glucocorticoid therapy is of little, if any, use in the treatment of spine involvement.

Whether disease-modifying drugs (DMARDs) alter the course of spinal disease has not been clarified unequivocally. Placebo-controlled trials are available only for sulfasalazine but did not show a consistently favorable effect compared with placebo. In clinical practice, sulfasalazine can only be proposed for selected patients with refractory axial involvement, especially in early disease as one treatment option. The efficacy of this therapy should be evaluated after 4 months.

For patients who still complain of spinal pain despite this stepwise approach, experimental therapy modalities with potential benefit are warranted. In pilot studies, infliximab (Remicade),* an antibody directed against tumor necrosis factor-α (TNF-α), as well as etanercept (Enbrel),* a TNF-α receptor antagonist, have provided a profound anti-inflammatory effect with fast relief of back pain in ankylosing spondylitis. With respect to the anti–TNF-α therapy, promising data exist also for undifferentiated spondylarthritis and psoriasis arthritis. Infliximab has to be applied as an intravenous infusion at a dose of 5 mg/kg at day 0, week 2, and week 6, followed by infusions every 6 weeks; and etanercept is given as

*Not FDA approved for this indication.

a subcutaneous injection at a dose of 25 mg twice weekly. Pamidronate (Aredia),* a bisphosphonate given intravenously, also showed beneficial effects in the relief of axial symptoms.

If the anti-inflammatory therapy fails to control spinal pain, the additional use of analgesics (acetaminophen, dextropropoxyphene,† opioids) and/or amitriptyline (Elavil),* 25 mg/d, is indicated to improve pain, sleep, and mobility.

Joints

Indication of the different therapeutic modalities is based on the extent of the articular involvement and the duration of the symptoms. NSAIDs are effective in the therapy for arthritis. Acute flares can be treated with intra-articular or systemic glucocorticoids. DMARDs are indicated for persisting symptoms of at least 3 months, erosive joint disease, or recurrent flares. Sulfasalazine (Azulfidine)* is well tolerated and effective at a dose of 1 g two or three times daily. For other DMARDs hardly any information is available. In clinical practice, methotrexate alone or in combination can be tried in patients refractory to sulfasalazine treatment.

Enthesitis

Therapy for enthesitis consists of NSAIDs, physical therapy, and orthoses. If disease is refractory to this therapy, local corticosteroid injections should be tried. Low dose anti-inflammatory radiotherapy is reserved for those patients with persistent monolocular enthesitis after failure of the therapeutic options mentioned earlier. Because the structures to be treated are usually superficial, orthovoltage irradiation is appropriate. In case of multiple enthesitis in conjunction with elevated acute-phase reactants despite appropriate drug therapy and physiotherapy, treatment with sulfasalazine is recommended. Multiple enthesitis often progresses to a generalized pain syndrome. Therefore, attention to adequate pain therapy is of great importance.

COMPLICATIONS

Iritis

Acute anterior uveitis characterized by unilateral ocular pain, redness, photophobia, or blurred vision should be managed jointly by the rheumatologist and the ophthalmologist. The goal is to resolve the inflammation promptly and to prevent synechiae formation and subsequent glaucoma. Topical corticosteroid drops to suppress inflammation and atropine drops to dilate the pupil are first-line drugs, but occasionally systemic glucocorticoids are needed. For corticosteroid-refractory disease, oral immunosuppressive therapy including methotrexate,* azathioprine (Imuran),* and cyclosporine (Sandimmune)* are used.

*Not FDA approved for this indication.
†Not available in the United States.

Skin/Mucosa

The oral mucosa and genital lesions as well as keratoderma blennorrhagicum are best managed with topical glucocorticoids.

Amyloidosis

Secondary amyloidosis is usually suspected by the finding of proteinuria and should be confirmed by rectal/gastric or renal biopsy. Progression of amyloidosis is prevented by suppression of the inflammation by chlorambucil (Leukeran)* or cyclophosphamide (Cytoxan).* It is the aim of the immunosuppressive therapy to normalize acute phase reactants (erythrocyte sedimentation rate, C-reactive protein).

Spinal Fractures

Spinal fractures can occur in fused segments, even after inadequate trivial trauma. To avoid spinal cord lesions, plain radiographs and (if films are unreliable) computed tomography or magnetic resonance imaging of the suspected area is warranted. A spinal fracture represents an emergency requiring immediate consultation of a trauma surgeon or neurosurgeon.

Cardiac Disease

There is no known medical therapy of aortic valvulitis or heart block. Therefore, the indication for surgical valvular replacement or pacemaker implantation is related to the degree of the respective complication.

*Not FDA approved for this indication.

TEMPOROMANDIBULAR DISORDERS

method of
JEAN-PAUL GOULET, D.D.S., M.S.D.
Université Laval
Québec, Canada

What we thought for many years to be a single disease entity with a diversity of clinical presentations, temporomandibular disorders (TMD) refer nowadays to an array of different biomedical conditions sharing common symptoms and signs involving the musculoskeletal components of the stomatognathic system. More importantly, however, is the heterogeneity of TMD patients from their psychosocial and behavioral features, which may apparently account for different response patterns to treatment. This shift in the appraisal of TMD is the result of a better understanding of pain mechanisms, factors playing a significant role in reports of pain and disability, pain-related behavior, advances in diagnostic imaging techniques, and a more rigorous approach to the diagnosis and management of orofacial pain conditions as a whole.

Jaw and joint pain, alone or combined with temporomandibular joint (TMJ) noises and difficulty in opening, are by far the most frequent reason for the TMD patient to seek care. Other commonly described complaints are joint locking or catching and a variety of nonspecific symptoms, including headaches, earaches, plugged ears, tinnitus, and neckaches. Also reported on rare occasions are bite changes, facial swelling, and transient facial numbness or tingling. As a group, TMD are the first cause of facial pain of nonodontogenic origin and jaw dysfunction. It is important, on the other hand, to realize that not all facial pain of nondental origin is related to masticatory muscles and TMJ problems and that the differential diagnosis goes beyond the scope of TMD. In addition to the teeth, periodontium, major salivary glands, paranasal sinuses, and musculoskeletal structures of the head and neck, orofacial pain may be the result of an intracranial or ear, eye, nose, and throat pathology or may be caused by vascular and neural structures. Finally, besides the psychosocial and behavioral features of patients, no one can neglect the presence of co-morbid conditions such as somatoform, anxiety, and mood disorders, especially depression, as potential contributors to the etiologic construct of chronic facial pain.

TAXONOMY

The whole spectrum of TMD is best captured with the classification adopted by the American Academy of Orofacial Pain (AAOP), which groups conditions specifically involving the masticatory muscles and TMJs (Table 1). However, the diversity of TMD for which patients seek care represents a limited number of conditions. This is why the Research Diagnostic Criteria (RDC) published by Dworkin and LeResche in 1992 are particularly useful. They provide an operational classification using a dual-axis diagnostic system grouping in Axis-I, the most common TMD seen in clinical populations (Table 2). The RDC also integrate in Axis-II the biobehavioral domain that reflects pain intensity and related disability from a psychological and psychosocial perspective that has been shown to be essential to the clinical decision for persistent pain management, independently of the biomedical Axis-I diagnosis. In that regard, the Graded Chronic Pain Scale (GCPS) developed by Von Korff and colleagues is a simple and useful index allowing grading of the current level of psychosocial dysfunction as it relates to the overall severity of chronic face pain and the extent of pain-related interference on the patient's daily life (Table 3). Current evidence indicates that one of five chronic TMD pain patients in tertiary care centers may have grade III or grade IV pain-related disability according to the GCPS and, therefore, a more guarded prognosis. Using the RDC Axis-I biomedical classification requires one to rule out other less common conditions included in the AAOP classification.

TABLE 1. **American Academy of Orofacial Pain Classification of Temporomandibular Disorders**

Masticatory Muscle Disorders

Myofascial pain
Myositis
Myospasm
Local myalgia—unclassified
Myofibrotic contracture
Neoplasia

Temporomandibular Joint Articular Disorders

Congenital or developmental disorders including neoplasia
Disk derangement disorders:
  Disk displacement with reduction
  Disk displacement without reduction
Temporomandibular dislocation
Inflammatory disorders:
  Capsulitis/synovitis
  Polyarthritis
Osteoarthritis (noninflammatory disorders):
  Primary
  Secondary
Infectious arthritis*
Ankylosis
Fracture

*Condition not included in the current classification.
From Okeson JP: Orofacial Pain: Guidelines for Assessment, Diagnosis, and Management. Chicago, Quintessence, 1996.

TABLE 2. **Research Diagnostic Criteria Axis-I Classification of Common Temporomandibular Disorders**

Group I: Muscle Disorders

Myofascial pain
Myofascial pain with limited opening

Group II: Disk Displacement Disorders

Disk displacement with reduction
Disk displacement without reduction, with limited opening
Disk displacement without reduction, without limited opening

Group III: Arthralgia, Arthritis, Arthrosis

Arthralgia (pain in the joint)
Osteoarthritis of the temporomandibular joint
Osteoarthrosis of the temporomandibular joint

From Dworkin SF, LeResche L: Research diagnostic criteria for temporomandibular disorders: Review, criteria, and specifications, critique. J Craniomandib Disord 6:301–334, 1992.

PREVALENCE, DEMOGRAPHIC FEATURES, AND PROGRESSION OF TMD

Available epidemiologic data from population-based studies indicate that as much as 40% of the population would give a positive response if they were asked if they experienced at least one of the three major TMD symptoms in the previous 6 months (i.e., jaw pain, joint clicking, or difficulty in opening). Clearly, the vast majority of people have transient symptoms and do not need any form of treatment. Unfortunately, we do not have any data on the prevalence of specific subsets of TMD. Although people in all age groups from children to the elderly report TMD symptoms, the peak prevalence is among adults between 18 and 45 years old. By age 70, TMD pain will have been experienced at least once by over 80% of the North American population. The proportion of females reporting TMD symptoms generally exceeds that of males by a ratio of 2:1, but females account for at least 80% of the clinical population.

It is estimated that between 5% and 12% of the adult population report TMD pain that is bothersome. Joint clicking is by far the most common TMD symptom, being reported by up to one third of the general population, but its significance in terms of a biopathologic articular condition remains controversial. It is reasonable to say that only a minority of patients with joint clicking will

TABLE 3. **Graded Chronic Pain Scale***

Grade I	Grade III
Characteristic pain intensity <50	Disability points 3 or 4 regardless of characteristic pain intensity
Disability points <3	
Grade II	**Grade IV**
Characteristic pain intensity >50	Disability points 5 or 6 regardless of characteristic pain intensity
Disability points <3	

Characteristic Pain Intensity (CPI) in the Past 6 Months (0–100)

Present, worst, and average pain rated on a 0–10 scale where 0 is "no pain" and 10 is "pain as bad as could be"

CPI = Mean (present pain, worst pain, and average pain) × 10

Disability Points (0–6)

Score for pain interference + score for days lost

Pain Interference Rated on a 0–10 Scale

In the past 6 months, how much has facial pain changed your ability to:

Take part in recreational, social, and family activities where 0 is "no change" and 10 is "extreme change"?

Work (including housework) where 0 is "no change" and 10 is "extreme change"?

In the past 6 months, how much has facial pain interfered with your:

Daily activities where 0 is "no interference" and 10 is "unable to carry on any activities"?

Score for pain interference = Mean (social, work, and daily activities) × 10

0–29 = 0 points
30–49 = 1 point
50–69 = 2 points
70+ = 3 points

Days Lost

How many days in the past 6 months has facial pain kept you from your usual activities?

____(0–180) days

Score for disability days:

0–6 days = 0 points
7–14 days = 1 point
15–30 days = 2 points
31+ days = 3 points

*Included in the Research Diagnostic Criteria Axis-II classification for assessing impact and disability related to TMD pain.

From Dworkin SF, LeResche L: Research diagnostic criteria for temporomandibular disorders: Review, criteria, and specifications, critique. J Craniomandib Disord 6:301–334, 1992.

eventually need some form of treatment because of joint catching, limited jaw function, and joint pain. The prevalence of difficulty in mouth opening is around 5% across population-based studies. It is clear from epidemiologic data that the classic model of TMD progression (i.e., myofascial pain leading to joint clicking, then to joint locking and TMJ degenerative disease) is questionable. The prevalence of TMD pain and related symptoms decreased to dramatically low figures after peaking in middle-aged adults, thus failing to show a build-up of cases in the aging population. This goes against the argument for treating all cases to prevent disease progression because we do not know whose condition is going to deteriorate in terms of physical impairment, disability, and psychosocial dysfunction.

PATIENT ASSESSMENT

The patient assessment process includes a thorough comprehensive history and description of the chief complaint; review of the patient's medical, dental, and personal status; and a comprehensive physical examination. It is important to gather all the relevant information regarding the pain problem, more specifically, about the onset; intensity; character; duration; temporal pattern; location; referral patterns; factors that trigger, aggravate, or alleviate the pain; how the pain has evolved since it started; what are the associated symptoms; and prior treatments. A good review of the general health status and past and current medical treatments allows screening for potential systemic causes or co-morbid conditions. Three important domains need to be covered during the personal history-taking. First is the behaviors that are often indicative of psychological and psychosocial stress or are revealing of difficulty in adapting to home, school, or work-related situations (e.g., oral parafunctional habits such as nocturnal or diurnal tooth clenching and tooth grinding, cheek and nail biting, tics, and mannerisms). The second is the patient's psychological status as it relates to anxiety, depressed moods, and the tendency to somatization, especially when dealing with the chronic TMD-related pain patient. This is best achieved with standardized questionnaires, such as the SLR-90-R Symptom Checklist. Third is interference with psychosocial functioning at the interpersonal and social level. Again, with a chronic pain problem it is important to assess: (1) the impact on the patient's daily activities, behavioral changes, coping capacity, and self-control when the pain is more severe and causes greater dysfunction; (2) the patient's belief model with respect to the weight placed on physical causes; and (3) the reasons for the partial success or failure of prior treatments. In addition to the GCPS the Multidimensional Pain Inventory developed by Kerns and colleagues in 1985 is also a useful standardized tool for such purpose.

To not overlook potential causes of facial pain, the clinical examination should go beyond the sole assessment of musculoskeletal structures. Vital signs should be recorded whenever appropriate. A careful inspection of the head and neck, the eye, ear, nose, and throat structures, and the upper extremities as well as palpation of lymph nodes, major salivary glands, carotid bifurcations, temporal arteries, and neck muscles should be integrated with the RDC examination protocol for the assessment of the masticatory muscles and TMJs (Table 4). The presence of trigger points and radiating pain patterns to the face and jaw should be documented during muscle palpation. A brief intraoral examination must be conducted to rule out tooth pain from a low-grade infection mimicking transient musculoskeletal pain, recent occlusal changes caused by TMJ arthropathy, and excessive tooth wear suggesting past or present nocturnal bruxism. Although occlusal parameters and the relationship between the upper and lower jaw can hardly be overlooked, it is important to remember that no cause-and-effect relationship has been found between any type of malocclusion and subsets of TMD.

Diagnostic imaging of the TMJ and laboratory tests should be used whenever required. Panoramic view radiography and computed tomography (CT) are useful for the detection of bony changes associated with a TMJ arthropathy whereas magnetic resonance imaging (MRI) is best to assess disk derangement disorders. There is no need for using electromyographic recordings of masticatory muscles, ultrasonography and vibratory analysis of TMJ sounds, jaw tracking analysis of mandibular movements, computer-assisted occlusal contact recording, and thermography for diagnostic purposes. These so-called noninvasive instruments and devices have not been rigorously tested in clinical settings where a diversity of facial pain condi-

TABLE 4. **General Guidelines for the Examination of the Masticatory Muscle, Temporomandibular Joint, and Mandibular Motion Based on the Research Diagnostic Criteria for Temporomandibular Disorders**

Muscle and Temporomandibular Joint Palpation

Masticatory muscle and joint palpation are done with the index finger pad using 2 pounds or 1 kg of pressure for extraoral masticatory muscle sites and 1 pound or 0.5 kg for intraoral masticatory muscle sites and the joint. In all instances, palpation is done one side at a time with the examiner asking the patient if the palpation is painful. Palpation includes the following sites:

Extraoral muscle: temporalis; masseter; posterior mandibular region (stylohyoid and posterior digastric); submandibular region (medial pterygoid, suprahyoid, anterior digastric)

Intraoral muscle: lateral pterygoid area; tendon of temporalis

Temporomandibular joint: lateral pole of the condyle; posterior attachment intrameatally

Temporomandibular Joint Sounds

Joint sounds are assessed with the index finger pad during full mouth opening and closing, lateral excursion and protrusion. Sounds that cannot be reproduced two out of three times are called nonreproducible.

Type of sound: clicking, crepitus

Mandibular Range of Motion and Opening Pattern

Mandibular range of motion is measured with a millimeter ruler using the labioincisal edge of the maxillary and opposing mandibular central incisors as reference and includes:

Unassisted opening without pain
Maximum unassisted opening
Maximum assisted opening
Right and left lateral excursion
Protrusion

Opening pattern: straight; lateral deviation without correction; corrected deviation

tions might be confused with TMD. Therefore, they have no proven utility for the diagnosis of TMD subtypes, and, apparently, their use is associated with increased risk of misdiagnosis and overtreatment.

GUIDELINES AND PRINCIPLES FOR TREATMENT DECISION

An accurate biomedical and biobehavioral diagnosis that takes into account the psychological and psychosocial impact of TMD pain is the key to a good treatment selection. This is even more critical given the fact that the vast majority of TMD encounters in clinics are conditions for which the true cause remains unknown. Patients must therefore be made aware that the emphasis is not so much on providing a cure but on finding the proper management strategies through a good understanding of the problem, while taking into account the severity, duration, and impact of the TMD pain and related symptoms on their daily life. The choice is more complicated when patients present with a combination of articular and nonarticular TMD pain problems (myofascial pain and a disk derangement disorder with or without arthralgia) coupled with a co-morbid condition. With complex cases, one must avoid focusing solely on physical parameters, because this may lead to a questionable treatment selection that does not address important biobehavioral issues.

Treatment selection for TMD pain patients must also take into consideration the fact that first it is not unusual for patients to get better with simple reversible treatment after being reassured about the prognosis and self-limiting nature of the problem, being informed about factors that can aggravate the pain, and being provided with means of dealing with flare-ups. Because of the natural history and fluctuating nature of their TMD problem, approximately three of four patients seeking care for the first time are going to get better whatever the type of treatment.

Second, the choice of treatment should be made on a case by case basis because not all patients within a given subset of TMD respond the same way to identical treatments. Each patient is unique in terms of pain severity, temporal patterns (transient pain with frequent rather than infrequent episodes or persistent pain), the extent of the pain (local versus regional), the impact of pain on his or her personal life, co-morbid conditions, and previous experiences with the health care system and treatment failures. No single treatment is appropriate for all, and the patient's preferences should always be taken into account.

Third, no baseline physical signs or symptoms such as the number of masticatory muscle sites tender to palpation, the severity and number of joint sounds, or the magnitude of mandibular movements can predict the course of a TMD and be used to justify preventive treatment or the so-called phase II rehabilitation treatment. Instead, co-morbid conditions such as depression, anxiety, and somatization as well as frequent health care services use have been all associated with persistent TMD pain.

Fourth, a whole spectrum of dental and nondental treatment strategies are offered by a diversity of health care providers and all claim highly successful results. These include occlusal appliances of all sorts, occlusal equilibration, jaw repositioning through occlusal rehabilitation, masticatory muscle spray and stretch techniques, trigger point injections, physical therapy with thermal agents, pharmacotherapy, ultrasound, acupuncture, biofeedback, relaxation, and stress management. Unfortunately, too few well-designed studies have been conducted underscoring a serious lack of available scientific evidence for the effectiveness over the long term of most TMD treatments. Therefore, primary health care providers should always give high priority to safety, cost-effectiveness, and the benefit the patient will get from the treatment selection.

Fifth, the etiology of commonly encountered TMD including intracapsular disk derangement remains obscured, controversial, and, at best, speculative. The structural and functional relationship between the upper and lower teeth, the vertical dimension of occlusions, the position of the condyle in the glenoid fossa as well as jaw and head posture have all been mentioned as potential causes of TMD. So far, no scientific evidence has been published showing a cause-and-effect relationship between any of these factors and subsets of TMD. The fact that TMD symptoms abate after a manipulation of the structural relationship of the jaw or teeth is far from proving that the treatment succeeded by acting on a causal factor. Care providers must avoid the reinforcement of the patient's belief model of a cure through "fixing" physical or structural abnormalities. These patients are at greater risk of having multiple treatment failures and persistent TMD pain.

Sixth, for a subset of TMD patients persistent jaw pain is the predominant focus of the clinical attention, and the resulting impairment and disability are in excess of what would be expected considering the history and clinical findings. When frequent somatic complaints and regional or widespread pain in other parts of the body are also part of the clinical picture, one has to wonder about a "pain disorder" with psychological factors playing an important role in the maintenance and exacerbation of the TMD-related pain.

In summary, a treatment philosophy based on a purely mechanical or anatomical approach or one that addresses only the physical diagnosis is hardly justifiable. Emphasis should be on TMD management rather than on cures using both biomedical and biobehavioral treatment strategies. The general guiding principles for managing a chronic TMD pain patient is not much different from managing other chronic remittent pain conditions. The overall goals are (1) to control or eliminate the TMD pain and learn how to deal and cope with future episodes of similar pain, (2) to improve or restore jaw function, and (3) to improve the quality of life using treatment strategies that are safe, cost-effective, simple, and reversible.

MASTICATORY MUSCLE DISORDERS

Myofascial pain as defined under the RDC classification is by far the most common nonarticular TMD pain condition. It is characterized by a unilateral or bilateral preauricular dull aching pain felt in the jaw muscles. The pain frequently radiates to the temple, ear, and forehead and is exacerbated by jaw function. Besides difficulty experienced when chewing, jaw dysfunction may include limited mandibular opening. Other frequently reported nonspecific symptoms are headaches, plugged ears, tinnitus, and neckaches. Women of child-bearing age represent more than 80% of the clinical population. The typical clinical examination reveals masticatory muscle pain of varying severity on palpation (e.g., temporalis, masseter, lateral pterygoid, posterior digastric, and stylohyoid) with or without limited mandibular opening. Diagnostic criteria include a chief complaint of regional dull aching jaw pain and masticatory muscle pain at three or more muscle sites on the side of the pain complaint. Unless muscle trigger points referring pain and/or provoking autonomic symptoms under sustained pressure are present, the AAOP classification describes this condition under "local myalgia—unclassified." The cause of myofascial pain remains unknown. Malocclusion and related structural abnormalities are frequently mentioned, but no epidemiologic data support such a cause-and-effect relationship. Several studies have reported increased odds of jaw muscle pain among subjects who are aware of their oral parafunctional habits, including bruxism. In addition, there is emerging evidence suggesting that hormonal factors (estrogen) might play a role in the onset of myofascial pain and, therefore, that would explain the gender disparity among the clinical population. This may well go along with the higher proportion of TMD symptoms among patients with fibromyalgia. Because no detectable laboratory abnormalities or biologic markers characterize myofascial pain, the final diagnosis relies on the pain history, examination findings, and the exclusion of other facial pain conditions. As many as 75% of patients improve with reversible conservative treatment, and gradual relief and recovery are usually obtained with simple procedures, including biobehavioral and cognitive therapy. In addition, patients should be made aware that recurring episodes of pain are not uncommon and symptoms may take time to completely abate. Reassurance and explanations about the benign nature of the pain problem are important and management goals should be clearly outlined. Current treatment strategies are summarized in Table 5 and should be used on a case-by-case basis.

LESS COMMON MUSCLE CONDITIONS

Myospasm is an acutely painful muscle condition caused by sudden involuntary prolonged and continuous contraction of a muscle, induced as a protective phenomenon after a sprain, hyperextension, and muscle abuse. Among the etiologic factors are long dental appointments and TMJ dislocation. The main clinical feature is tenderness on palpation of the involved masticatory muscle, which causes severe limitation of jaw movement. Treatment includes avoiding the pain-producing movement, limiting the use of the jaw muscles with a soft nonchewy diet, ice application for 10 minutes repeated several times during the first 24 hours, and, based on the severity, a supportive pharmacologic treatment with a muscle relaxant or nonopioid analgesics.

Myositis as defined by the AAOP refers to a localized acute inflammation involving masticatory muscles after direct trauma or infection. In addition to a sudden onset of unilateral jaw pain that exacerbates during function, patients may also report on and off swelling of the affected muscle. The clinical findings include muscle tenderness on palpation, increased pain during mandibular movements, and a limited range of motion because of pain and edema. Besides ice applications, limiting the use of jaw muscles and the use of nonopioid analgesics such as nonsteroidal anti-inflammatory drugs (NSAIDs) for pain control,

TABLE 5. **Treatment Guidelines for Myofascial Pain of the Masticatory Muscles**

General Guidelines

Reassurance and explanation regarding the pain problem; avoidance of hard and chewy foods for at least 2 weeks and no gum chewing; awareness and self-control of diurnal parafunctional habits.

Physical Therapy to Improve Opening and Masticatory Muscle Function

Home care program with moist heat for 15 minutes over the masseter and temporalis muscles followed by a series of five sustained maximum unforced mandibular openings for 10 seconds before closing (twice a day for 2 weeks and as needed once a day thereafter or more based on improvement of mouth opening). Refer to a physical therapist as needed.

Biobehavioral Treatment

As needed refer to a health psychologist so all psychosocial, behavioral, and psychological contributors are addressed with proper treatment modalities (e.g., biofeedback, stress management techniques, cognitive-behavioral treatment, coping skills).

Pharmacologic Treatment

Short-term use (10–15 days) of either a muscle relaxant (cyclobenzaprine [Flexeril], 10 mg; orphenadrine [Norflex], 100 mg; carisoprodol [Soma], 350 mg) or a benzodiazepine (diazepam [Valium], 5 mg; lorazepam [Ativan], 1 mg) at bedtime to minimize sedation while awake. If longer supportive treatment is needed, tricyclic antidepressants are particularly useful for patients with chronic persistent pain (amitriptyline [Elavil],* or nortriptyline [Pamelor],* 10–25 mg at bedtime).

Nocturnal Parafunction

Interocclusal stabilization splint to wear at night (can also be used for daytime parafunction).

Trigger Points Treatment

Fluori-Methane spray and stretch; injection with 1% lidocaine solution, 1 or 2 mL alone or with 1 mL (40 mg) of hydrocortisone acetate suspension.

*Not FDA approved for this indication.

treatment of the underlying cause should be conducted accordingly.

Myofibrotic contracture is a chronic painless condition characterized by a limited mandibular range of motion due to muscle shortening as a result of fibrosis or scarring of the tendons, ligaments, or muscle fibers. Major causes are prolonged jaw hypomobility after surgery, severe trauma, or neuromuscular disease. Limitation of mandibular opening remains the sole clinical feature with no tenderness during masticatory muscle and joint palpation or intracapsular disk dysfunction accounting for the limited jaw motion. When physical therapy and passive jaw opening exercises aimed at increasing the range of motion have failed, the surgical release of muscle attachment might ultimately be required.

TEMPOROMANDIBULAR JOINT DISORDERS

Disk derangement disorders of the TMJ are essentially a group of intracapsular conditions characterized by abnormal disk position between the condyle and the articular surfaces of the temporal bone. The improper disk position, which is either reducible or nonreducible on full mouth opening, can cause mechanical obstruction and interfere with the normal smooth action of the joint. Disk displacement with reduction (DDwR) is the most common disk derangement disorder. The anteriorly displaced disk moves suddenly into a more normal disk-condyle relationship during opening while a clicking or popping sound occurs, allowing for a full range of jaw motion. The condyle slips off the disk when closing before the teeth move back together. The clinical examination reveals reproducible joint clicking or popping during mandibular movements. Palpation of the TMJ does not elicit any pain unless arthralgia is present. Signs of DDwR are frequent in the general nonpatient population, and the mere identification of clicking or popping does not dictate any treatment because it is sometimes reversible, particularly in teenagers, and most patients with persistent clicking will never experience additional symptoms that will last. Moreover, joint pain when present, is likely related to changes in joint lubrication, an accumulation of inflammatory mediators, and sensitization of the synovial membrane, rather than being caused solely by the displaced disk and impingement of the retrodiskal pad. The use of diagnostic imaging tools such as MRI to confirm a suspected DDwR is only appropriate when there are compelling reasons to believe that the result is going to influence the treatment selection, and invasive irreversible treatment is contemplated on the basis of severe persistent joint dysfunction and pain.

Disk displacement without reduction (DDwoR) or "closed lock" is present when an anteriorly displaced disk stays in front of the condyle during mandibular movements, thus causing a mechanical obstruction and mandibular hypomobility. When present, joint pain is usually exacerbated by joint function. Recent onset of DDwoR is characterized by the sudden disappearance of TMJ clicking coupled with a limited opening. Besides limited maximal unassisted opening, the clinical manifestations include pain during joint palpation, no joint clicking or popping during mandibular motion, uncorrected deviation of the mandible on opening to the affected side, and restriction in the contralateral excursion. On the other hand, a significant number of patients will recover a normal range of mandibular motion and see the pain go away with time, in spite of a nonreducible displaced disk. MRI has become the standard diagnostic imaging technique used to confirm suspected DDwoR. However, it should be used only in selected cases when additional information is needed to confirm the diagnosis and select the proper treatment strategy.

Much has been said about the potential role of malocclusion, occlusal factors, orthodontic treatment, generalized joint laxity, parafunctional habits, and direct trauma to the jaw in the etiology of disk displacement disorders. The literature is replete with anecdotal reports, and although disk displacement disorders can follow direct jaw injury, there is no evidence from well-designed studies showing a cause-and-effect relationship with occlusal factors. In that regard, neither bite adjustment nor more complex dental rehabilitation treatments are justifiable based on the serious lack of evidence showing that disk recapture or a modified jaw position is essential to symptom reduction or to prevent recurrence. Treatment guidelines for disk displacement disorders are outlined in Table 6.

Arthralgia is a clinical diagnosis referring to the presence of localized joint pain that is usually exacerbated by mandibular function. Other terms used to describe this clinical entity are synovitis and capsulitis. The clinical features include pain during function, difficulty in chewing, and limitation of mandibular movements secondary to pain. Occasionally, effusion decreases the ability to close the jaw on the affected side and the patient will complain of an altered bite. The diagnostic criteria for arthralgia are a report of joint pain at rest or during mandibular movements, TMJ pain induced by palpation at rest, and the absence of joint noises and radiographic changes compatible with an arthritic condition (arthritis or osteoarthritis). This condition may be iatrogenic, related to a traumatic event, but frequently no specific cause is uncovered. As for other subtypes of TMD pain, the likelihood of reporting joint pain is greater among subjects aware of parafunctional habits. Symptomatic treatments are summarized in Table 7.

TABLE 6. **Treatment Guidelines for Disk Derangement Disorders of the Temporomandibular Joint**

Disk Derangement With Reduction

General

No specific treatment if no other signs or symptoms of temporomandibular disease. Patient reassurance and explanation regarding joint clicking and popping; awareness and self-control of diurnal parafunctional habits particularly with self-report of joint catching.

TMJ Pain

Avoidance of hard and chewy foods, no gum chewing; short-term pharmacologic treatment with NSAIDs as for arthralgia if not contraindicated.

Disk Derangement Without Reduction

General

Reassurance and explanation regarding the joint problem; awareness and self-control of diurnal parafunctional habits.

Acute Closed-Lock (Days up to Few Weeks)

Mandibular mobilization to force the disk back in place. If not successful, proceed as indicated below.

TMJ Pain

Avoidance of hard and chewy foods as well as wide or forceful opening for at least 2 weeks and no gum chewing; short-term pharmacologic treatment with NSAIDs as for arthralgia if not contraindicated.

Physical Therapy to Improve Joint Translation and Range of Motion

Home care program with jaw mobilization exercises starting with moist heat for 15 minutes over the temporalis and masseter muscles followed by a series of five sustained maximum unforced and painless mandibular openings for 10 seconds before closing (twice a day for 2 weeks and then once a day for 2 additional weeks or more based on improvement of mouth opening). Brief intense icing may be used to reduce postexercise joint pain.

Nocturnal Parafunction and Joint Loading

Interocclusal stabilization splint to wear at night (can also be used for daytime parafunction).

Persistent Joint Hypomobility, Severe Limitation With Pain

In conjunction with biobehavioral treatment (see Table 5) when previous treatment modalities have failed and physical impairment persists, surgical procedures such as arthrocenteses, arthroscopic surgery, or open joint surgery may be contemplated.

Abbreviations: NSAIDs = nonsteroidal anti-inflammatory drugs; TMJ = temporomandibular joint.

TABLE 7. **Treatment Guidelines for Temporomandibular Joint Arthralgia**

General

Reassurance and explanation regarding the joint problem; avoidance of hard and chewy foods and forceful or wide opening for at least 2 weeks and no gum chewing; awareness and self-control of diurnal parafunctional habits

Biobehavioral Treatment

As needed refer to a health psychologist so all psychosocial, behavioral, and psychological factors are addressed with proper treatment modalities (e.g., biofeedback, stress management techniques, cognitive-behavioral treatment, coping skills)

Pharmacologic Treatment

Unless contraindicated, short-term use of nonselective or selective (COX-2 inhibitors) NSAIDs prescribed on a contingency basis for 2 weeks

Nocturnal Parafunction and Joint Loading

Interocclusal stabilization splint to wear at night (can also be used for daytime parafunction)

Abbreviations: COX-2 = cyclooxygenase-2; NSAIDs = nonsteroidal anti-inflammatory drugs.

ARTHRITIC CONDITIONS OF THE TMJ

Osteoarthritis is the most common form of TMJ arthritis. As in the case with other synovial joints, the articular soft tissues break down and remodeling appears to be the result of an imbalance between catabolic and anabolic responses involving biomechanical, biochemical, and enzymatic factors. The main clinical features are preauricular joint pain and joint noise described as grating, grinding, or crunching sounds (e.g., crepitus) occurring during mandibular movements. In addition, patients may also complain of joint stiffness, pain on wide opening, pain on chewing, and limited opening. A diagnosis of TMJ osteoarthritis is made on the basis of radiographic evidence of structural bony changes and joint space narrowing in addition to the main clinical features. However, it may take time before radiographic changes become apparent because in the early stages of TMJ osteoarthritis radiographic evidence typically lags behind articular tissue damage. Diagnostic criteria of TMJ osteoarthritis include self-report of joint pain at rest or during mandibular function, joint pain on palpation, joint crepitus during opening and closing, and radiographic evidence of bony changes of the condylar head or the articular eminence (sclerosis, erosion, flattening, osteophytes, joint space narrowing). It is likely that these patients may also have disk derangement disorders, and the clinical examination may also reveal masticatory muscle tenderness or pain on palpation. Oteoarthritis of the TMJ is secondary when it develops after trauma, intra-articular steroid injections, or disk displacement without reduction. Although strong scientific evidence supporting mechanical loading and microtrauma secondary to partial edentulism and parafunctional habits as playing a major role in osteoarthritis of the TMJ is lacking, these factors need to be addressed when osteoarthritis has indeed developed. Management guidelines of TMJ osteoarthritis summarized in Table 8 include symptomatic treatment of joint pain, control, and reduction of contributory and aggravating factors, and treatment of pathologic sequelae.

Osteoarthrosis of the TMJ is the quiescent form of osteoarthritis. It is characterized by the presence of TMJ crepitus during mandibular movements, radiographic evidence of bony remodeling, and absence of joint pain. Patients will usually seek care because they are concerned by the crunching joint sounds. The clinical examination is negative for pain reported during palpation of the TMJ, and the range of mandibular motion is generally within normal limits. The diagnosis of osteoarthrosis of the TMJ is based on the presence of joint crepitus and imaging information. There is no specific treatment required for osteoarthrosis of the TMJ, and patients need only to be reassured regarding the nature of the joint noises and imaging findings.

TABLE 8. **Treatment Guidelines for Temporomandibular Joint Osteoarthritis**

General

Reassurance and explanation regarding the joint problem; avoidance of hard and chewy foods during the acute phase and no gum chewing; avoidance of excessive mandibular movements; awareness and self-control of diurnal parafunctional habits; brief intense icing may be used to reduce joint pain after eating.

Pharmacologic Treatment

Unless contraindicated, short-term use of nonselective or selective (COX-2 inhibitors) NSAIDs prescribed on a contingency basis for 2 weeks. A short course of oral corticosteroids is reserved for severe joint pain inflammation: methylprednisolone (Depo-Medrol) dose pack for 6 days or 60 mg of prednisolone (Prelone) tapered over 7 to 10 days.

Nocturnal Parafunction and Joint Loading

Intraoral stabilization splint to wear at night and during the day as needed.

Intra-articular Injection

When severe signs of inflammation are nonresponsive to pharmacologic treatment, use methylprednisolone acetate, 1 mL (40 mg), or sodium hyaluronate, 2 mL (16 mg), once a week for 3 consecutive weeks.

Abbreviations: COX-2 = cyclooxygenase-2; NSAIDs = nonsteroidal anti-inflammatory drugs.

Polyarthritis involving the TMJ is not unusual, but it would be extremely rare for the TMJ to be the first joint affected, and most likely when it happens, it is a late manifestation of a generalized systemic polyarthritic condition, such as mixed connective tissue diseases, and autoimmune or metabolic disorders that have already affected other joints in the body. Rheumatoid arthritis is the most common form of polyarthritis involving the TMJ. The main clinical features include joint pain, joint crepitus, difficulty in chewing, pain during mandibular movements, and limited mouth opening. Patients may also report preauricular joint swelling, morning jaw stiffness, masticatory muscle tenderness, and bite changes. Severe cases of TMJ involvement and condylar destruction may lead to anterior open bite. The diagnostic criteria include pain on palpation of the joints, limited range of mandibular movement, joint crepitus, radiographic changes showing bone destruction of the condylar head with alteration of the joint space, other joint involvement, and a positive laboratory serology test for rheumatoid factors. Usually, these patients are already being treated for their systemic condition, but they may be advised of physical therapy and jaw mobilization exercises to maintain the range of motion and informed regarding future need for bite correction. Debilitating sequelae to the TMJ may lead to surgical intervention.

Infectious arthritis of the TMJ is rather uncommon, and usually microbes will reach the joint either through hematogenous spreading or after direct inoculation during TMJ surgery, intracapsular injections, or secondary trauma. Typically, gonococci, staphylococci, streptococci, or pneumococci are most often the etiologic agents of acute bacterial arthritis, but at any age acute arthritis may be associated with infections with viruses (e.g., measles, mumps, parvovirus, HIV, hepatitis B). Patients with polyarthritis chronically affecting the TMJ are more at risk of developing bacterial arthritis. On examination, the patient is likely to complain of joint pain and present with the usual signs of infection (e.g., fever, chills) along with a warm, painful, and swollen joint with evidence of effusion. The diagnosis requires aspiration for synovial fluid examination and cultures for a search of the infecting organism. Successful therapy is achieved with appropriate parenteral antibiotic use, and treatment should be continued for at least 2 weeks after all signs and symptoms have disappeared.

LESS COMMON TEMPOROMANDIBULAR JOINT DISORDERS

Congenital and developmental disorders involving the TMJ include a series of localized conditions (condylar aplasia, hypoplasia, or hyperplasia) that usually cause patients to seek care because of problems with their appearance and/or masticatory dysfunction. Treatment options for debilitating cases may include reconstructive surgery of the joint or orthognathic surgery coupled with orthodontic treatment.

TMJ dislocation occurs when the disk-condyle complex moves in front of the articular eminence and is unable to return to the glenoid fossa. The patient is unable to fully close the mouth and, therefore, the mandible remains in a forward position. Lasting dislocation is accompanied by severe pain, which decreases over time. The mandible is protruded, and the patient will usually need assistance to reduce the dislocation and normalize jaw function. In contrast, TMJ subluxation occurs when on wide opening the disk-condyle complex momentarily passes the articular eminence with a characteristic popping sound and moves back into the glenoid fossae on closing. Clinically, it is manifested by a late joint popping on opening and a very early popping on closing. Patients with joint laxity are more likely to present with TMJ subluxation or dislocation problems. Among the many reported treatment methods advocated for disabling recurrent dislocation (e.g., sclerosing agents, maxillomandibular fixation, capsular plication, botulinum toxin injections into the lateral pterygoid muscle, closed condylotomy, augmentation of the articular eminence, and eminectomy), either augmentation or reduction of the articular eminence seems to have the best long-term success rate.

Ankylosis of the TMJ occurs with soft tissue or bony fusion of the condylar head to the glenoid fossa. It may follow an extended joint immobilization or a traumatic event to the TMJ. The patient will usually complain of a limited opening with a marked deviation to the affected side, a restricted laterotrusion to the contralateral side and, in rare cases, joint pain. Radiographs will show an absence of condylar translation on opening with joint space narrowing and obliteration if it is a bony ankylosis. Appropriate surgical reconstruction of the TMJ is indicated for patients with severe jaw motion disability.

Fractures of the condylar neck or head may result from any significant trauma or blow to the chin. The clinical features are joint swelling, joint pain at rest and during mandibular movement, and restricted opening with deviation toward the affected TMJ. Depending on the type of fracture reduction, surgery may be necessary. Ankylosis, malocclusion, and degenerative joint disease are possible sequelae.

Neoplasia involving the TMJ, either benign or malignant, is rare but has been reported. Synovial chondromatosis, osteoma, osteoblastoma, osteochondroma, osteosarcoma, and chondrosarcoma have been described in the literature as primary neoplasia involving the TMJ. Cases of metastatic disease to the TMJ have also been reported. Clinical findings are variable and may include joint pain, swelling, limited opening, deviation on opening, and bite change. Definitive treatment depends on the type and extent of the neoplastic process.

BURSITIS, TENDINITIS, MYOFASCIAL PAIN, AND FIBROMYALGIA

method of
STEEN E. MORTENSEN, M.D.
Wichita Clinic
Wichita, Kansas

Pain is the body's alert system. A sensation of discomfort generated from tissues in jeopardy of damage is transmitted through the nervous system to nuclei in the central nervous system and finally presented to the cortical centers and our consciousness. Glitches occur in such complex systems, because we often notice when a temporary discomfort or pain catches our attention. These sensations, however, resolve within seconds, occasionally minutes to hours, and, rarely, days.

About one in seven patients or more presenting to the primary care physician's office complains of more chronic pain. Such complaints are commonly related to the musculoskeletal system and may represent a malfunction (as mentioned earlier), actual disease, overuse, trauma, or nerve-signal misinterpretation that may occur in single or multiple sites. Diseases involved include actual arthritis of degenerative or inflammatory type, infection, neoplasia, or other systemic illness. *Bursitis, tendinitis, myofascial* or *regional pain syndromes,* and *fibromyalgia* are terms associated with most of the rest. The human anatomy has over 200 separate bones, over 700 separate muscles, over 150 possible bursae, as well as tendons, ligaments, and fasciae to hold everything together. Any of these may cause symptoms, but certain regions with significant use or application of force are affected more frequently, as outlined later.

BURSITIS AND TENDINITIS

Reducing sheering forces facilitates the body's motions. Synovial membranes located in bursae, tendon sheaths, and joints secrete a lubricating fluid for this purpose. Some bursae are preformed at birth, and some are generated in response to the forces of motion and formed through childhood. The body typically has up to 150 bursae, but only a few are frequently associated with clinical problems such as infections, inflammations, or deposits of material such as calcium, uric acid, hydroxyapatite, calcium pyrophosphate, granuloma, or cholesterol. Tendinitis usually is in the sheaths and other surrounding tissues rather than the tendon itself. Actual trauma with tear or restricted motion does occur in such areas as the rotator cuff, and as stenosing tenosynovitis in the abductor pollicis longus and extensor pollicis brevis (de Quervain disease).

Shoulder

The shoulder function involves three joints, with the glenohumeral joint having the most motion and the least restriction in the body as a whole. Drying after a bath and dressing are actions in which this function is routinely tested, and malfunctions often cause the patient to seek help.

The subdeltoid and subacromial bursae become inflamed through several mechanisms, including overuse, deposits, and spread of inflammation from the adjacent rotator cuff and biceps tendons, which lie in the floor of the structure. The proximal tendon of the biceps muscle's long head traverses the groove between the tubercles on the anterior surface of the humerus in a sheath that may get inflamed. Similarly, the rotator cuff (the confluent tendons of the subscapularis, supraspinatus, infraspinatus, and teres minor muscles), often through use, injury, deposition, or disease, becomes damaged and inflamed. This occurs typically in the superior part made of the supraspinatus and infraspinatus tendons. A tendinitis here may lead to partial or complete rupture of the rotator cuff. Symptoms include pain from impingement on abduction and especially in rotation in the glenohumeral joint. The "drop sign," in which abduction of the arm cannot be maintained against gravity, helps to distinguish between pure bursitis and tendinitis.

Elbow

An infection is not uncommon in the olecranon bursa. It is often caused by *Staphylococcus aureus,* which may enter directly through the skin and often is penicillin resistant. Aggressive treatment with an effective oral, and in immune-compromised hosts intravenous, antibiotic is required. Symptoms include warmth, erythema, swelling, and pain. The skin is often thickened and indurated. Passive and active motion of the elbow is painful. A similar appearance can, however, be caused by crystal-induced inflammation such as gout or pseudogout, and differentiation requires aspiration, microscopy, and culture. Direct trauma through both continued pressure as well as an acute hit on the bursa may cause an effusion with clear, but sometimes bloody, fluid. Symptoms include swelling and discomfort and usually no warmth or erythema. Evaluation of aspirated fluid usually provides the diagnosis.

Hip

Symptoms from bursitis in the pelvis and hip region are often interpreted by the sufferer as relating to the hip joint or sometimes to the spine. Careful examination will usually lead to the correct diagnosis. Plain films may reveal calcium deposits as well as find hidden fractures. Ultrasonography and magnetic resonance imaging can reveal fluid accumulations, such as in the iliopsoas-psoas bursa anterior to the hip joint and sometimes communicating with it. Recently, magnetic resonance imaging has shown tendinitis and even tears in the gluteus medius muscle or tendon, presenting as similar complaints. Trochanteric bursitis, identified by palpation at, behind, and inferior to the trochanter with the hip flexed 90 degrees is a common problem. The ischial bursa is palpated at the same time with the gluteal muscles rolled aside to evaluate for "Weaver's bottom."

Knee

Anserine and prepatellar and infrapatellar bursitis are frequent. A common presentation is that of knee pain initially thought to be secondary to degenerative changes found on plain films. Careful evaluation reveals the pain as coming from a periarticular structure, and appropriate treatment can provide rapid relief. The prepatellar bursa is like the olecranon bursa, being at risk for infection through either penetrating injury or pressure. Early diagnosis and treatment is again important. "Clergyman's knee" or "housemaid's knee," however, is typically due to continued pressure on the tibial tuberosity, the infrapatellar tendon, or the patella itself and can be seen in anyone spending extended time kneeling. Gastrocnemius-semimembranosus bursitis and/or a Baker cyst may cause pressure on the popliteal vein, leading to deep vein thrombosis. Rupture of the cyst can mimic deep venous thrombosis.

Ankle and Foot

The etiology of retrocalcaneal bursitis and Achilles tendinitis includes trauma, overuse, and deposits, and also systemic disease. Exercising without appropriate training or footwear may cause strain and sprain.

Spondyloarthropathies or deposits can cause inflammation of the bursa or tendon. All lead to quite severe pain and often swelling just above the insertion of the tendon on the posterior surface of the calcaneus. It may not be possible clinically to differentiate between the bursitis and tendinitis. Tendinitis of the peroneus longus and brevis tendons is felt behind and below the lateral malleolus. Similarly, pain in the tibialis posterior or flexor hallucis longus behind the medal malleolus can be severe and lead to gait changes, resulting in much more widespread symptoms.

Treatment

Identification and abstinence from triggering activities using rest, splinting, casting, or other supportive means is included in conservative management. Long-term immobilization may cause stiffening or a "frozen shoulder" and should be avoided. Physical therapy with education in biomechanics and exercise is helpful as entry to long-term treatment and prevention. Application of heat or ice, ultrasound, and sometimes iontography with locally applied corticosteroids can provide significant relief.

Anti-inflammatory creams containing salicylic acid are available over the counter and frequently used by patients before visits to health care professionals. Preparations containing ketoprofen (Orudis), naproxen (Naprosyn), or diclofenac (Voltaren) made to order by the pharmacist and applied two to three times daily have been moderately helpful and have little if any systemic effect.

Local injection with a local anesthetic and/or corticosteroid can be necessary in more chronic cases. Repeated use may cause local tissue deterioration. Injection close to major tendons (e.g., the infrapatellar and Achilles) should be avoided, owing to increased risk for rupture.

Nonsteroidal anti-inflammatory drugs (NSAIDs) or, rarely, oral corticosteroids may be necessary in particularly chronic cases. They always carry the risk of significant side effects and should be prescribed in the lowest dose and shortest time span necessary. Three types of NSAIDs are now available:

1. Nonacetylated salicylates with little effect on prostaglandin production and thus fewer side effects, but also less analgesia. These drugs have quite good anti-inflammatory effects in sufficient doses.
2. Aspirin and the long list of compounds more potent and safer than it. All are blocking both cyclooxygenase-1 and -2 and interfere to various degrees in systems dependent on their constitutive expression.
3. Cyclooxygenase-2–specific agents that in phar-

macologic doses block cyclooxygenase-2's constitutive and induced functions.

MYOFASCIAL PAIN

This type of pain is localized in soft tissue and may be caused by repetitive injury. Typical areas involved include the sternomastoid muscles in the neck, causing headaches, face, and neck pains. Suboccipital pains cause the suboccipital neuralgia syndrome. Pains in the trapezius muscle, rhomboids, and levator scapulae generate local, neck, and head pain. Pains in the gluteal muscles and those muscles associated with the trochanter and fascia lata are typically perceived as relating to the hip or low back.

Treatment

A specific diagnosis is important, if possible. Elimination of causing and aggravating factors will improve outcome and hopefully prevent recurrence. Education of the patient with explanation of the nature of the problem is required to avoid recurrence.

Moist heat used over 30 minutes helps to relax the muscle. Muscle relaxants and NSAIDs are often used for pain control. Local injection with local anesthetics is helpful. Passive stretching afterward can release the tension and may be helped by pretreating the skin with a freezing spray such as trichloroethylene. The trigger points may respond favorably to "dry" injections using only the needle. Saline or local anesthetics can be used and give longer benefit. Repeat treatment is often needed every 1 to 2 weeks for a couple of months. Commonly used local anesthetics include lidocaine 0.5% to 1% and bupivacaine 0.25%. The latter may be effective beyond 5 hours. Corticosteroids of various potencies are being used, but they must be carefully managed to avoid local skin atrophy or discoloration, and no studies have demonstrated improvement with their use over that of the anesthetics alone. Triamcinolone hexacetonide (Aristospan) is slow in onset but has a long effect and should be used for deeper or intra-articular injections. Admixing a local anesthetic can effectively block irritation from the microcrystals of the corticosteroid preparation. The use of botulinum toxin has been gaining favor after its successful use in spastic lesions such as blepharospasm and cervical dystonia. Preliminary data suggest that botulinum toxin A is better than botulinum toxin B in myofascial pain syndrome and superior to corticosteroids.

FIBROMYALGIA SYNDROME

The *fibromyalgia syndrome (FMS)* is defined as symmetrical and widespread (above and below diaphragm) pain, involving 11 of 18 possible "tender points," that is chronic (lasting >3 months). In 1992, a group of international researchers published the "Copenhagen declaration," which was adopted by the World Health Organization in 1993. They considered FMS as a component of a much more widespread malfunction.

Tender points are areas of tenderness identified in muscle, muscle-tendon junction, bursa, or fat pad. This is in contrast to *trigger points,* which are areas of muscle painful to palpation, tight areas in the muscle, and a referral pattern of pain. It is now generally accepted that tender points do not represent local pathologic processes as originally suggested in 1904 by Stockman.

Of interest is the fact that the highly reproducible discrete areas we associate with tender points seem to be present in the healthy population as areas of increased sensitivity. In the general population, however, the points are merely uncomfortable when stressed with the standard 4-kg pressure (blanching of the nail of the testing finger) and do not remain painful for hours or even days as do those of the FMS patients.

Known since antiquity, the nonspecific, chronic, and quite severe pains of fibromyalgia affect about 2% of the U.S. population. Some physicians do not presently recognize this syndrome as a legitimate disease, because we still cannot identify any causative pathology. To the sufferers, however, it is a serious reality that interferes with life, performance, and happiness and truly is an illness.

The common complaints include widespread pain, sleep deprivation, central processing problems with memory difficulties and confusion, chronic fatigue, and irritable bowel syndrome. Other complaints include temporomandibular joint pain, sicca syndrome with painful tongue, changed taste and difficulty swallowing, numbness in hands and/or feet, swelling and stiffness, as well as anxiety and depression.

Researchers have attempted to identify the causes for this chronic pain condition throughout the 20th century. In 1904, a report by Ralph Stockman suggested a local inflammatory process and the term *fibrositis* was used. Through the century multiple reports reviewed various aspects of the syndrome, but still without identifying a cause. In 1990, the American College of Rheumatology's revised criteria were published, permitting an organized attempt of gathering the data needed for understanding the pathophysiology and permitting directed therapeutic testing.

Several different theories have been presented and researched as for the cause of the widespread pain:

1. Chronic infection with an unknown agent, because a frequent patient complaint is that of a preceding flulike syndrome continuing into chronicity. No such agent has been identified so far.
2. Sleep disturbance or metabolic anomaly preventing restoration of especially muscle fibers during stage 3 and 4 sleep. Studies by Bennett and coworkers have shown that a subgroup of patients has an apparent decreased presence of growth hormone during sleep. This hormone is thought to be necessary for healing of damaged muscle fibers. In addition, more recent studies have found that at least tempo-

rary improvement can be gained through long-term growth hormone replacement. A number of neurochemical levels or time-release curves are also changed and are being evaluated as to etiologic importance by Russell and others. Excretion of both melatonin and cortisol are changed in female patients. A decreased excretion in the urine of 5-hydroxyindoleacetic acid, seen as a deficiency in levels of serotonin, is associated with FMS but, interestingly, not with the level of pain.

3. Most recent authors seem to agree that the malfunction is in the supraspinal processing of external nerve stimuli. This leads to the patient's so typical complaint of "hurting all over" and the excessive pain perception in tender points and in general.

Treatment

Support, education, and understanding are necessary components in the care of patients with FMS. Patient acceptance and participation in the care is a sine qua non. Education by the physician and other providers is especially needed in this era of information abundance. Providing references to community and Internet resources will enhance the patient's participation in his or her care.

The goals of therapy are reduction of pain and increase in functionality. The two most important treatment issues are improvement of sleep and regulation of daily activities to include aerobic exercise. Walking is accessible and inexpensive, and most patients will accept and follow instructions in a gradually accelerated program. Several studies have evaluated various exercises and found benefits in this approach over the stretching exercises, which do help some.

Pain can be so severe that the patient feels he or she can no longer work. Adjustments in time schedule and environment may permit continuation of gainful employment. Quitting and becoming disabled, often requiring legal action, leads to impaired quality of life and no improvement in symptoms.

Tricyclic antidepressants (TCAs) such as amitriptyline (Elavil)* and nortriptyline (Pamelor)* (dose typically 10–50 mg q hs) as well as the muscle relaxant cyclobenzaprine (Flexeril), 5 to 20 mg 2 hours before bedtime, are the traditional foundation for treatment. They can provide significant pain relief. Improved sleep pattern is gained by giving longer and more coherent sleep periods as well as deeper levels of sleep. Side effects of grogginess and daytime fatigue can be often avoided by giving a daily dose 2 to 4 hours before bedtime and gradually increasing the dose on a weekly basis. Response to these drugs takes 2 to 6 weeks, and perseverance must be encouraged.

Selective serotonin reuptake inhibitors (SSRIs) have been found to be helpful both alone and, in the author's experience, as adjunct therapy to TCAs. They cause less dryness and sleepiness, but occasionally may interfere with sleep; thus they can be more helpful if given in the morning. Again, the dose is increased gradually, and, like the TCAs, the effective dose is usually lower than is needed for treatment of depression.

*Not FDA approved for this indication.

Tramadol (Ultram), with dual affect on both the opiate mu receptor and serotonin receptor systems, has become popular. It works well in some FMS patients and is quite well tolerated. Treatment is begun at 25 mg/d and gradually increased every 3 to 7 days toward a maintenance dose of maximum 300 to 400 mg/d. Side effects include drowsiness and a rare occurrence of seizures. The latter is seemingly more likely if the dose is changed rapidly.

Gabapentin (Neurontin)* is approved for adjunctive therapy of epilepsy and, though similar to γ-aminobutyric acid (GABA), without effect on such receptors. It has been found quite helpful in a number of patients, providing enhanced pain control. It has a very wide therapeutic window and clinically causes few side effects. Here also the dose is gradually increased, beginning with 100 mg/d and then slowly increased to a maintenance level providing satisfactory control. My patients have done very well on 200 to 800 mg/d, but some have only partial pain control on much higher doses.

A newly introduced muscle relaxant, tizanidine (Zanaflex), has been found helpful in reducing pain and providing relaxation. Typical treatment begins with 1 or 2 mg/d about 1 hour before bedtime. The dose is gradually increased 1 to 2 mg every 3 to 7 days. In FMS, a typical maintenance dose is 4 to 12 mg, but for patients with chronic headache several reports have cited effective doses as high as 50 to 60 mg/d (lower doses at mealtime and higher ones 1 hour before bedtime). Side effects include nausea, dizziness, dry mouth, somnolence, constipation, and headaches. The drug is helpful and tolerated in one half to two thirds of patients.

Numerous other compounds and strategies have been tried in this condition, including dextromethorphan. In one study it was added to tramadol and either did not benefit or was not tolerated by the majority of FMS patients studied. However, some 14% of those starting this study experienced an impressive improvement in pain according to the authors and elected to continue to use supplemental dextromethorphan.

CONCLUSION

Patients with chronic pain benefit from the services of an understanding, caring, and knowledgeable physician. Information about pain, its perception and treatment modalities available, is rapidly expanding. Consideration of benefit/risk/cost ratios applied to and personalized for the patient greatly enhances the chance of successful treatment.

*Not FDA approved for this indication.

OSTEOARTHRITIS

method of
GUY TAYLOR, M.B., CH.B.
Wanganui Hospital
Wanganui, New Zealand

and

C. MICHAEL STEIN, M.B., CH.B.
Vanderbilt University School of Medicine
Nashville, Tennessee

Osteoarthritis (OA) results from a complex interaction of cellular, biochemical, and biomechanical factors acting on cartilage, subchondral bone, and the soft tissues of joints, ultimately leading to loss of joint function and symptoms. OA is the most common type of arthritis, and its incidence increases markedly with age. By the age of 65 years more than 80% of the population will have some radiographic evidence of OA and 5% to 10% will be symptomatic. It is one of the most common causes of chronic pain and disability in the elderly and is also of great socioeconomic importance. OA is the most frequent indication for joint replacement surgery, and individuals with OA younger than the age of 65 years incur double the medical costs of non-OA patients. With changing population demographics it is estimated that by the year 2020 the prevalence of OA in the United States will exceed 18%, affecting more than 59 million people.

The most commonly affected joints are the distal (DIP) and proximal (PIP) interphalangeal joints, first carpometacarpal joint, hips, knees, and cervical and lumbar spine. Involvement of wrists, elbows, shoulders or metacarpophalangeal (MCP) joints is unusual and may indicate a predisposing metabolic defect such as hemochromatosis, ochronosis, acromegaly, or calcium pyrophosphate arthropathy. Other well-recognized causes of secondary OA include previous joint infection, inflammation, trauma, surgery (including meniscectomy), and congenital or developmental anatomic abnormality such as hip dysplasia. In primary OA no clear cause can be identified. There are, however, multiple inherited and acquired risk factors. Rare forms of familial premature OA are associated with point mutations in the collagen type II gene (COL2A1) and others with polymorphisms in the gene for aggrecan (cartilage proteoglycan), but the genetics of the more common forms of OA are not known. Generalized nodal OA (multijoint involvement associated with Heberden or Bouchard nodes) appears to be inherited as an autosomal dominant trait in women and an autosomal recessive trait in men. In some studies, genetic factors appear to account for 40% to 65% of the risk for hand and knee OA.

Obesity is an important risk factor for OA in weight-bearing joints. A multivariate analysis showed that obesity contributed 21% to the risk of knee OA, a family history of OA, 9%; previous knee injury, 8%; and meniscectomy, 1%. Obesity is the most common modifiable risk factor for OA with over half of the U.S. population being overweight (body mass index >25). If the heaviest third of the population reduced their weight to that of the middle third, the prevalence of OA would decrease by 20%. Certain occupations or activities may predispose specific joints to OA, for example, fingers in rock climbers, tarsal joints in ballet dancers, knees in builders, and hips in farmers. Recreational exercise in people with normal joints does not appear to be a risk factor for OA, but joint injuries or biomechanical abnormalities do predispose athletes to OA, especially elite athletes.

Cartilage is an avascular, aneural, alymphatic tissue consisting largely of highly hydrated proteoglycans restrained by a fibrillar meshwork of predominantly type II collagen. It was previously thought to be relatively inert. However, embedded in lacunae in this matrix are chondrocytes that respond to both mechanical and chemical stimuli and secrete both matrix macromolecules necessary for regeneration and degradative enzymes such as matrix metalloproteinases, collagenase, stromelysin, and gelatinase. Many enzymes are secreted as inactive precursors, and further regulation occurs in the matrix by, among others, tissue inhibitors of metalloproteinases (TIMPs).

Cartilage is lubricated by synovial fluid. Synovial type B cells produce hyaluronan, which gives synovial fluid its unique viscoelastic properties. This thin layer of fluid is viscous at lower speeds, allowing low-friction sliding during movement such as walking and running, and is elastic at high speed, such as on landing from a jump or suddenly changing direction. OA has traditionally been viewed as a noninflammatory disease, but localized foci of synovitis and the presence of proinflammatory cytokines in OA synovium have been demonstrated. Together, these mechanical, degenerative, and inflammatory processes all contribute to the initial loss of proteoglycans, subsequent loss of collagen integrity, increased matrix hydration, chondrocyte clumping, and, eventually, the fibrillation, erosion, and fissuring of cartilage with subchondral bone remodeling that characterizes OA. Increased understanding of the pathogenesis of OA has stimulated enthusiasm to find chondroprotective or regenerative disease-modifying therapies, in addition to addressing symptoms.

DIAGNOSIS

The diagnosis of OA is clinical, usually supported by appropriate radiology. Radiographic changes of OA are very common in older patients and frequently coexist with other causes of joint pain. Therefore, the radiographic findings of OA are confirmatory rather than diagnostic. Routine laboratory tests will be normal for the patient's age, and significant abnormalities should prompt consideration of an alternative diagnosis or intercurrent illness. Because the presenting symptoms of hemochromatosis are often musculoskeletal, iron saturation or ferritin should be measured in younger patients (<60 years) with OA and those with MCP involvement or chondrocalcinosis. An iron saturation of more than 50% in women or 60% in men should lead to genetic studies for hereditary hemochromatosis. Chondrocalcinosis is more usually a marker of pyrophosphate arthropathy, which in younger patients may be associated with disorders of calcium metabolism. Other flags indicating alternative diagnoses include atypical joint involvement, vasomotor changes (reflex sympathetic dystrophy), acute onset (suggesting injury or crystal-induced arthritis), clinically evident synovitis, systemic symptoms, or a history of significant inflammation (suggesting an inflammatory arthritis such as rheumatoid arthritis), and severe focal rest pain (consider malignancy).

SYMPTOMS

The typical symptoms of OA are pain, crepitus, morning stiffness, gelling (stiffness of a joint after inactivity), instability and loss of function. Pain is usually of gradual onset and described as a mild to moderate ache, intensifying with exercise and relieved by rest. Rest and night pain may occur with advanced disease. Sources of pain in OA include the synovium, joint capsule, periarticular tendons and ligaments, muscle, periosteum, and subchondral bone; and the nature of the pain may therefore vary accordingly. There is a poor relationship between pain and the degree of radiographic change. Partly this may be due to differences in local factors such as proinflammatory cytokine expression or microinfarction in subchondral bone. However, individual variation in peripheral and central pain processing and psychosocially determined response to nociception often plays an important role.

Early morning stiffness and the common gelling that occurs after inactivity in OA usually lasts less than 20 to 30 minutes, unlike the inflammatory arthropathies in which morning stiffness typically lasts several hours. Loss of range of motion results from a combination of loss of cartilage, osteophyte formation, joint capsule fibrosis, and, occasionally, effusion. Typical problems resulting from loss of range of motion and pain include poor grip (interphalangeal joints), difficulty with kneeling or walking down stairs or on rough ground (knees), fastening shoelaces, or getting in and out of cars (hips).

Physical Examination

Examination most often reveals joint line tenderness, bony enlargement, crepitus, pain on movement, reduced range of motion (ROM), instability or malalignment, and, occasionally, effusions, usually with minimal or absent signs of inflammation. In the spine, OA involves predominantly the cervical and lumbar areas. OA of the facet joints and disk degeneration are separate processes but closely linked in that one can cause the other. Bony enlargement of the DIPs are known as Heberden nodes and that of the PIPs as Bouchard nodes. Erosive OA is an uncommon variant that can cause marked deformity at the DIPs and PIPs and occasionally rapid progression at other joints. Occasional patients get intermittent gout that localizes in the joints damaged by OA, causing unusually rapid progression. Deforming OA of the fingers needs to be differentiated from psoriatic arthropathy. The nail changes typical of psoriasis such as onycholysis and pitting may be a clue to that diagnosis.

Pain from hip OA can cause diagnostic difficulty. Typically hip pain is felt in the groin, often in the buttock, sometimes in the anterior thigh and knee, and occasionally just in the knee. Lateral hip pain is usually due to trochanteric bursitis or gluteus medius tendonitis rather than hip OA. With hip arthritis, internal rotation is usually lost first and the patient frequently has a positive Trendelenburg sign. In early disease the patient may only experience pain at the extremes of passive movement. OA of the knee most often affects the medial compartment involvement, either alone or with patellofemoral disease. The natural history of OA is often one of slow progression over many years. However, there may be long periods of stability or even improvement, punctuated by relatively severe exacerbations. Overall, progression is more rapid in the fingers, slower at the knee, and intermediate at the hip.

Imaging

Radiologic investigation should be carried out for a specific purpose. This may be to confirm the clinical findings, to aid decisions about surgical treatment, or to look for complications. The radiographic signs of OA are joint space narrowing (often asymmetric), osteophyte formation, bony sclerosis, cyst formation, and ultimately collapse. Radiographically detectable joint space loss, however, requires loss of 50% or more of the cartilage. Correlation between symptoms and radiographic findings are poor, but some features are more predictive than others. For example, at the hip, loss of joint space correlates better with pain than osteophyte formation.

The correlation between symptoms and radiographic findings is best for hip disease and worst in the hands. Mild to moderate degenerative radiographic changes in the cervical spine are so common after the age of 40 years that they should play little part in deciding if neck pain is due to OA or not. Magnetic resonance imaging is not usually indicated but has the advantage of showing associated soft tissue lesions such as meniscal tears, tendon inflammation or rupture, the extent of bone edema, and stress fractures. Magnetic resonance imaging techniques are available for quantitating cartilage volume but remain a research tool.

MANAGEMENT

Currently, the aims of therapy are to relieve symptoms, maximize function, and retard progression. Disease modification is not yet an attainable goal despite considerable interest and research. Table 1 lists the modalities of therapy in approximate order of sequential use. However, several modalities are typically used concurrently and specific circumstances may dictate a different order.

Nonpharmacologic Therapy

Education of patients and family members is helpful. Patients can be encouraged to contact organizations such as the Arthritis Foundation for written material, self-help groups, exercise classes, and local information about equipment and social support. Support via the telephone by nurses has been shown to improve coping and reduce the frequency of medical consultation. Loss of weight or the use of a walking stick in the contralateral hand reduces the load

TABLE 1. **Management Strategies for Osteoarthritis**

Nonpharmacologic Therapy
Education
Aerobic and joint-specific exercise
Joint protection and unloading
Weight loss
Footwear, orthotics, and appliances
Heat and cold
Self-help groups
Telephone support
Pharmacologic Therapy
Acetaminophen
Topical counterirritants or capsaicin
Nonselective nonsteroidal anti-inflammatory drugs
Misoprostol or proton pump inhibitor if indicated
Cyclooxygenase-2 selective nonsteroidal anti-inflammatory drugs
Weak narcotic analgesics
Intra-articular corticosteroid
Intra-articular hyaluronan
Surgery
Osteotomy
Arthrodesis
Arthroplasty

on weight-bearing joints. Although difficult, weight loss has been shown to both reduce the risk of developing OA and improve pain and function. A simple instruction to lose weight is unlikely to be effective, and patients may require considerable professional counseling, possibly joining a formal weight loss program.

Cushioned insoles soften the impact of walking and orthoses can also be used to correct malalignment or to shift the line of weight bearing (e.g., a lateral heel wedge for knee OA affecting mainly the medial compartment and patellar taping to relieve anterior knee pain). In advanced OA, splints and braces may help control instability and may reduce pain. Assessment by an occupational therapist and supply of appropriate appliances can reduce the patient's disability without impacting on the arthritis itself. Commonly used appliances include jar openers, raised toilet seats, high chairs, rails and "hand extenders" that allow objects to be picked up off the floor without bending. The therapist will also provide individualized joint protection advice. For example, the semi-squat is advised for lifting even moderate weights in patients with low back pain; but if the individual also has knee OA, this position will transmit a force of seven to eight times the body weight through the patellofemoral joint. In this case having a stool at home or work will allow the patient to push the object into a convenient position with his or her feet and sit on the stool in a supported semi-squat to do the lifting. Knowledge of how to use heat, cold, and rest not only provides readily accessible nonpharmacologic pain relief but gives many patients an important sense of control.

Patients should be encouraged to maintain daily activities within the limitations of their pain. All patients with OA, but particularly those with hip and knee involvement, should be prescribed specific exercises. Exercise improves strength and function, reduces pain, and promotes a sense of well being. Stretches help maintain a functional range of movement, prevent contractures, and reduce detrimental compensatory postures. Increased quadriceps strength improves stability of the knee and can be achieved by isometric or resistive exercise. Aerobic exercise such as walking or pool workouts improves function in hip and knee OA without causing flares or increased joint damage. Patients with more than minimal symptoms may benefit from physical therapy.

Pharmacologic Therapy

A large number of products, many controversial, are marketed for and consumed by patients with OA. Drugs are not curative and often only modestly effective in relieving symptoms. Therefore, the risk-benefit ratio of any therapy needs to be considered and patient and physician expectations should be realistic.

Acetaminophen, in conjunction with nonpharmacologic measures, is the drug of first choice. Many patients with mild to moderate pain use an "as required" regimen successfully, but for severe pain regular acetaminophen (e.g., 1 g three to four times a day) is more effective. Nausea is the most common side effect, but the safety profile is excellent and the cost low. In patients with normal hepatic function the risk of hepatic damage with therapeutic doses of acetaminophen is extremely small, but patients should know that over-the-counter and prescription analgesics may also contain acetaminophen and that the total dose should not exceed 4 g/24 h. A number of patients not responding adequately to acetaminophen will benefit from nonsteroidal anti-inflammatory drugs (NSAIDs). These can often be used in low doses on an "as required" basis, but some patients, particularly those with moderate pain or an inflammatory component to their arthritis, benefit from regular, full-dose therapy. Efficacy and toxicity should be assessed after 4 to 6 weeks of therapy and treatment stopped if no additional benefit has been gained. The most serious and frequent adverse effect of NSAIDs is gastrointestinal toxicity. Renal impairment, rashes, antagonism of antihypertensive agents, and liver toxicity occur less often. The strongest risk factors for NSAID-induced upper gastrointestinal bleeding are a previous gastrointestinal hemorrhage and age older than 65 years. The annual rate of hospitalization for peptic ulcer complications in persons 65 years and older taking NSAIDs is 16 per 1000, four times that of non-NSAID users. Other risk factors include concomitant use of corticosteroids or anticoagulants, high doses or combinations of NSAIDs, previous peptic ulcer, and significant co-morbidity.

If patients with one or more of these risk factors require an NSAID, there are two common strategies: (1) treatment with a nonselective NSAID and a gastroprotective drug and (2) treatment with a cyclooxygenase-2 (COX-2) selective NSAID. Such patients receiving a nonselective NSAID should take the lowest effective dose and receive prophylactic gastroprotective therapy. Indomethacin (Indocin) and piroxicam (Feldene) are generally avoided in the elderly because of a greater frequency of side effects. Both misoprostol and the proton pump inhibitors reduce the frequency of serious upper gastrointestinal events in patients taking NSAIDs. Many patients with OA find NSAIDs to be more effective than acetaminophen, but in some studies 60% to 70% of patients receiving NSAIDs chronically could be successfully switched to acetaminophen and appropriate nonpharmacologic interventions. A therapeutic trial of a switch from an NSAID to acetaminophen should be considered in high-risk patients receiving NSAIDs chronically.

The discovery of two forms of cyclooxygenase has led to the emergence of selective COX-2 inhibitors such as celecoxib (Celebrex) 200 mg/d and rofecoxib (Vioxx) 12.5 to 25 mg/d. These drugs have comparable anti-inflammatory and analgesic effects to the nonselective NSAIDs but less upper gastrointestinal toxicity and are therefore useful in elderly patients with OA. As is the case with nonselective NSAIDs, renal toxicity can occur and peripheral edema is relatively common. The COX-2 selective NSAIDs inhibit prostacyclin formation without affecting the constitutive production of proaggregatory thromboxane A_2 by platelets and may theoretically induce a mild proaggregatory state. Patients with known or potential atherosclerotic disease taking low doses of aspirin for cardiovascular prophylaxis should therefore continue to do so. Emerging evidence indicates that combination treatment with low doses of aspirin and a COX-2 selective NSAID may partially abrogate the lower gastrointestinal toxicity seen with COX-2 selective drugs alone. Gastroprotective therapy may be indicated in high-risk patients.

Some patients with pain not controlled by nonpharmacologic measures, simple analgesics, or NSAIDs find occasional use of a weak narcotic analgesic such as tramadol or acetaminophen combined with codeine, hydrocodone, or dextropropoxyphene useful. However, opioid analgesics do not suit all patients, particularly if adverse effects such as dizziness, nausea, and constipation occur without increased analgesia.

Systemic corticosteroids are not recommended in OA, but intra-articular injections (triamcinolone [Kenalog], methylprednisolone [Depo-Medrol]) can be a useful adjunct to treatment, especially in the presence of clinically apparent inflammation or with knee effusions. Because of their potential deleterious effects on connective tissue, corticosteroid injections are best limited to two or three per year in any given joint. Intra-articular injection of hyaluronan provides pain relief comparable to, or greater than, an intra-articular corticosteroid. Two preparations of this glycosaminoglycan, Hyalgan and Synvisc, are approved by the Food and Drug Administration for use in knee OA. These agents, designed to simulate normal synovial fluid but with a poorly understood mode of action, require a course of injections and are expensive but have no systemic reactions and relatively few local reactions. Although the rate of response falls off with increasingly severe OA, some patients with end-stage disease awaiting joint replacement benefit.

Glucosamine* (up to 1.5 g/d) and chondroitin sulfate* (800–1200 mg/d) have achieved much popularity among OA sufferers with relatively little supporting data. Meta-analysis indicates both these agents have modest analgesic effects, and one randomized multicenter trial has suggested that glucosamine may have disease-modifying effects in OA, but the methodology was not optimal and further work is awaited. There is no good evidence to support the use of antioxidants, electromagnetism, vitamin or mineral supplementation, or laser therapy. Research is continuing in several areas, including autologous chondrocyte transplants, gene therapy, and inhibitors of cytokines, TIMPs and other metalloproteinases.

Total joint replacement is an excellent treatment for advanced OA of the hip and knee and for many patients is the intervention that improves function and quality of life most. The surgery is reliable, and, if patients are thoughtfully selected and receive good rehabilitation, the cost-benefit ratio is excellent. Tibial osteotomy can effectively delay joint replacement in younger patients with knee OA that is largely unicompartmental. Arthrodesis, excision of the trapezium, or tendinoplasty all have a role in treating OA at the base of the thumb, which can be very disabling. Arthroscopic débridement and joint lavage are expensive, invasive, and supported by limited uncontrolled data.

*Glucosamine and chondroitin are classified as dietary supplements and have not been evaluated or approved by the FDA for the treatment of osteoarthritis.

POLYMYALGIA RHEUMATICA AND GIANT CELL ARTERITIS

method of
SHAWN L. SLACK, M.D.
The Everett Clinic
Everett, Washington

The term *polymyalgia rheumatica* (PMR) was first used by Barber in 1957 to describe a clinical syndrome of the middle-aged and elderly characterized by pain and stiffness in the shoulder and pelvic girdles and often accompanied by constitutional symptoms. Giant cell arteritis (GCA) is a vasculitis that affects primarily the cranial arteries and occurs most often in the elderly. Approximately 10% of people who present with PMR develop GCA weeks to years later, whereas 50% of people with GCA have coexistent PMR. Both syndromes occur primarily in the sixth to seventh decades of life and are common in people of northern European ancestry.

DIAGNOSIS

PMR is characterized by symmetric proximal muscle pain and stiffness. Stiffness is usually a predominant feature and can be so profound in the morning that patients require help getting out of bed or have to roll themselves out of bed. Polymyalgia is a misnomer; synovial biopsies and magnetic resonance imaging have shown that the symptoms are caused by synovitis and tenosynovitis of the proximal joints and tendons. There is no evidence of myositis. Patients, however, describe pain in the proximal muscles. There is no muscle tenderness or actual muscle weakness, although pain with movement makes strength testing difficult. Systemic features include low-grade fevers, fatigue, and weight loss.

Headache is the most common symptom with GCA. The pain is severe and usually localizes over the temple but can also be occipital or poorly localized. Scalp tenderness is also common and can make it difficult for a patient to lie down or comb his or her hair. Other symptoms may include jaw claudication, dysphagia, fever, and weight loss. Visual disturbances such as blurring, diplopia, and transient visual loss occur in 25% to 50% of patients. Permanent visual loss is the most dreaded complication and occurs in 6% to 10% of patients.

The laboratory hallmark of PMR and GCA is an elevated sedimentation rate. It is usually in excess of 50 mm/h, and may exceed 100 mm/h. Patients may also have a mild anemia. The diagnosis of PMR is primarily clinical, but it is aided by the elevated sedimentation rate and a dramatic response to therapy. The diagnosis of GCA can be confirmed by a temporal artery biopsy. The biopsy specimen must be as long as possible (2–4 cm) and sectioned in multiple areas because the process can be segmental.

TREATMENT

The symptoms of PMR usually respond dramatically to 10 to 20 mg/d of prednisone. The response usually occurs within 24 to 48 hours and always within 1 week. Occasionally, there is only a partial response to a single daily dose, but a complete response can be obtained by splitting the dose, such as 10 mg in the morning followed by 5 mg in the evening. After 1 month at the response dose, a slow taper of no more than 1 mg every 2 weeks should be begun. If symptoms recur, the prednisone dose can be increased by 1 to 2 mg/d. The sedimentation rate should improve with therapy, but symptoms should guide the taper primarily. Once the dose has reached 7 mg/d, the taper should be 1 mg/month. The dose should be reduced to the lowest level required to suppress symptoms. Sixty percent to 70% of patients are able to stop therapy after 2 years. PMR patients should be warned about the symptoms of GCA.

GCA treatment requires 40 to 60 mg/d of prednisone in divided doses. Response is usually rapid; and once corticosteroids are started, blindness is rare. If GCA is suspected, start therapy and arrange for a biopsy within 1 week. Do not withhold therapy if clinical suspicion is strong enough to warrant a biopsy. If visual loss occurs in a patient with GCA, the prognosis for restoring sight is poor. However, in such cases, a course of high-dose corticosteroids should precede prednisone therapy (e.g., 1 g of methylprednisolone [Solumedrol] administered intravenously daily for 3 days). After 1 month of prednisone therapy, the dose should be decreased by 5 mg every week until a dose of 20 mg/d is reached. Thereafter, a conventional PMR taper can be used. Because the sedimentation rate should drop with therapy, a patient's symptoms should guide the taper. Patients should be warned to expect treatment for approximately 2 years.

PMR and GCA patients who are unable to taper their prednisone dosage because of recurring symptoms can be treated with corticosteroid-sparing medications such as hydroxychloroquine (Plaquenil Sulfate),* methotrexate,* or azathioprine (Imuran).* The efficacy of corticosteroid-sparing agents in PMR and GCA is equivocal. Careful monitoring and preventive therapy for corticosteroid-induced osteoporosis is essential for patients on prolonged prednisone therapy.

*Not FDA approved for this indication.

OSTEOMYELITIS

method of
JON T. MADER, M.D.
The University of Texas Medical Branch
Galveston, Texas

and

MARK E. SHIRTLIFF, PH.D.
Montana State University
Bozeman, Montana

Osteomyelitis is characterized by bacterial or fungal infection of the bone, commonly the cortical and/or medullary portions. The terms *osteo* and *myelo* refer to bone and to the marrow cavity, respectively, both of which are involved in the disease. This infectious disease is progressive and results in inflammatory destruction of bone, bone necrosis, and new bone formation.

CONTIGUOUS FOCUS OSTEOMYELITIS WITH *NO* GENERALIZED VASCULAR INSUFFICIENCY

In contiguous focus osteomyelitis, the organism may extend from adjacent soft tissue infections or be directly inoculated into the bone by trauma or pre/intraoperative procedures. Common predisposing conditions include open fractures, surgical reduction and internal fixation of fractures, chronic soft tissue infections, and radiation therapy. In contrast to hematogenous osteomyelitis, multiple bacterial organisms are usually isolated from the infected bone. The bacteriology is diverse, but *Staphylococcus aureus* remains the most commonly isolated pathogen. In addition, aerobic gram-negative bacilli and anaerobic organisms are frequently isolated. Bone necrosis, soft tissue damage, and loss of bone stability occur, often making this form of osteomyelitis difficult to manage. The long bones are most frequently involved.

Therapy

Adequate drainage, thorough débridement, obliteration of dead space, wound protection, and specific antimicrobial coverage are the mainstays of therapy. Loss of bone stability, bone necrosis, and soft tissue damage frequently occur, making this form of osteomyelitis difficult to treat. Surgical débridement of infected bone and soft tissue provides specimens for culture and hastens eradication of the infection. Other steps in the surgical management of contiguous focus osteomyelitis should be tailored to the specific anatomy of the bone infection. Antimicrobial therapy should begin with a broad-spectrum antibiotic regimen. Table 1 outlines initial antibiotic therapy choices. Once the specific organism is identified, the antibacterial activity of different antibiotic classes can be determined by appropriate sensitivity methods. The disk diffusion method is often a sufficient guideline for antibiotic therapy. However, quantitative antibiotic sensitivity testing by the macro-

TABLE 1. **Initial Choice of Antibiotics for Therapy for Infectious Arthritis and Osteomyelitis (Adult Doses)**

Organism	Antibiotics of First Choice	Alternative Antibiotics
Methicillin-sensitive *Staphylococcus aureus*	Nafcillin (Unipen), 2 g q4h, or clindamycin, 900 mg q8h*	Cefazolin (Ancef)
Methicillin-resistant *Staphylococcus aureus*	Vancomycin (Vancocin), 1 g q12h*	Trimethoprim-sulfamethoxazole (Bactrim), or minocycline (Minocin) + rifampin (Rifadin) Quinupristin/dalfopristin (Synercid), linezolid (Zyvox)
S. epidermidis	Vancomycin, 1g q12h,* or nafcillin, 2 g q4h	Cefazolin, clindamycin
Group A *Streptococcus*	Clindamycin (Cleocin), 900 mg q8h	Benzylpenicillin, cefazolin, ampicillin
Group B *Streptococcus*	Clindamycin, 900 mg q8h	Benzylpenicillin, cefazolin, ampicillin
Enterococcus species	Ampicillin, 2 g q6h ± gentamicin, 5 mg/kg/d q8h or qd*	Vancomycin, linezolid (VRE) Quinupristin/dalfopristin (VRE)
Escherichia coli	Cefotaxime (Claforan), 2 g q6h	Cefazolin, levofloxacin (Levaquin), ampicillin
Proteus mirabilis	Ampicillin, 2 g q6h	Cefazolin, levofloxacin, trimethoprim-sulfamethoxazole
P. vulgaris, P. rettgeri, Morganella morganii	Cefotaxime, 2 g q6h, ± gentamicin, 5 mg/kg/d q8h* or qd	Ticarcillin-clavulanic acid (Timentin), levofloxacin
Serratia marcescens	Cefotaxime, 2 g q6h, ± gentamicin, 5 mg/kg/d q8h* or qd	Ticarcillin-clavulanic acid, levofloxacin
Pseudomonas aeruginosa	Ceftazidime (Fortaz), 2 g q8h or cefepime (Maxipime), 2 g q12h	Amikacin (Amikin), ticarcillin-clavulanic acid, ciprofloxacin (Cipro), imipenem (Primaxin)
Bacteroides fragilis group	Clindamycin, 900 mg q8h	Metronidazole (Flagyl), ampicillin-sulbactam (Unasyn)
Peptostreptococcus species	Clindamycin, 900 mg q8h	Metronidazole, ampicillin-sulbactam
Candida species	Amphotericin B (Amphocin, Fungizone), 0.5–0.75 mg/kg/d Fluconazole (Diflucan), 400 mg/d†	
Mycobacterium	Same 12-month antibiotic course as used for pulmonary tuberculosis	
Actinomyces species	Clindamycin, 300 mg qid × 6 months	
Brucella species	Doxycycline + rifampin for 6 to 24 weeks	

*Dose should be individualized with serum level monitoring.
†Increasing reports of fluconazole-resistant *Candida* species, especially *C. krusei* and *C. glabrata.*

dilution or microdilution techniques on all aerobic bone isolates is a prerequisite to determine the minimal concentration of the antibiotic to inhibit (minimal inhibitory concentration [MIC]) and kill (minimal bactericidal concentration [MBC]) the pathogenic organism(s). It is best to choose an antibiotic or antibiotic combination that has a low MIC/MBC relative to its expected serum concentration. The initial antibiotic regimen may be continued or changed on the basis of sensitivity results. The patient is treated for 4 to 6 weeks with appropriate antimicrobial therapy dated from the initiation of therapy or after the last major débridement surgery.

Surgical Management

The principles of treating any infection are equally applicable to the treatment of infection in bone. These include adequate drainage, extensive débridement of all necrotic tissue, obliteration of dead spaces, stabilization, adequate soft tissue coverage, and restoration of an effective blood supply. The number of performed surgical procedures used to achieve these goals increases with the severity of the infection and procedures can be divided into three categories.

Category 1 is removal of necrotic tissue by extensive débridement. Débridement surgery is the foundation of osteomyelitis treatment. It is the most commonly performed procedure, and patients may require multiple débridements. The goal of débridement is to leave healthy, viable tissue. However, even when all necrotic tissue has been adequately débrided, the remaining bed of tissue must be considered contaminated with the responsible organism. Débridement should be direct, atraumatic, and executed with reconstruction in mind. All dead or ischemic hard and soft tissue are excised unless a noncurative procedure has been chosen. Surgical excision of bone must be carried down to uniform haversian or cancellous bleeding termed *the paprika sign* to ensure a positive outcome.

In category 2, there is dead space obliteration with flaps, antibiotic beads, and bone grafts. Adequate débridement may leave a large bony defect termed *dead space*. Appropriate management of dead space created by débridement surgery is mandatory to arrest the disease and to maintain the integrity of the skeletal part. The goal of dead space management is to replace dead bone and scar tissue with durable vascularized tissue. Local tissue flaps or free flaps may be used to fill dead space. An alternative technique is to place cancellous bone grafts beneath local or transferred tissues where structural augmentation is necessary. Careful preoperative planning is critical to conservation of the patient's limited cancellous bone reserves. Open cancellous grafts without soft tissue coverage are useful when a free tissue transfer is not a treatment option and local tissue flaps are inadequate. Complete wound closure should be attained whenever possible. Suction irrigation systems are not recommended because of the high incidence of associated nosocomial infections and the unreliability of these setups. Secondary intention healing is also discouraged because the scar tissue that fills the defect may later become avascular. Antibiotic-impregnated acrylic beads can be used to sterilize and temporarily maintain dead space. The beads are usually removed within 2 to 4 weeks and replaced with a cancellous bone graft. The most commonly used antibiotics in beads are vancomycin (Vancocin), tobramycin (Nebcin), and gentamicin (Septopal). Local delivery of antibiotics (amikacin [Amikin], clindamycin [Cleocin]) into dead space can also be achieved with an implantable pump. Adequate soft tissue coverage of the bone is necessary to arrest osteomyelitis. Most soft tissue defects are closed by primary closure. Small soft tissue defects may be covered with a split-thickness skin graft. In the presence of a large soft tissue defect or an inadequate soft tissue envelope, local muscle flaps and free vascularized muscle flaps may be placed in a one- or two-stage procedure.

Category 3 includes stabilization by external or open reduction and internal fixation. If movement is present at the site of infection, measures must be taken to achieve permanent stability of the skeletal unit. Stability may be achieved with plates, screws, rods, and/or an external fixator. One type of external fixation allows reconstruction of segmental bone defects and difficult infected nonunions. The Ilizarov external fixation method utilizes the theory of distraction histogenesis whereby bone is fractured in the metaphyseal region and slowly lengthened. The growth of new bone in the metaphyseal region pushes a segment of healthy bone into the defect left by surgery. The Ilizarov technique is used for difficult cases of osteomyelitis when stabilization and bone lengthening are necessary. It can also be used to compress nonunions and correct malunions and in a small group of patients for reconstruction of difficult deformities that results from osteomyelitis. However, this technique is labor intensive and requires an extended period of treatment averaging 9 months in the device. The Ilizarov pins usually become infected and the device is painful. Infected pseudarthrosis with segmental osseous defects can be treated by débridement and microvascular bone transfers. Vascularized bone transfer is also useful for the treatment of infected segmental osseous defects of long bones that are more than 3 cm in length. Vascularized bone transfers can be placed after 1 month of inactive sepsis.

Surgical procedures for long bone osteomyelitis can be tailored to the specific anatomy of the bone infection. When the nidus of infection is entirely within the medullary canal of the bone, surgical treatment is usually more straightforward than in other types of bone involvement. Adult patients are surgically treated with a thorough intramedullary reaming, and unroofing is usually performed with or without bone grafting. Soft tissues are reapproximated, and the limb is protected by external means (brace or cast) until the structural integrity of the bone is re-established by normal remodeling. When osteomyelitis is characterized by a full-thickness, cortical sequestration, patients can usually be treated with removal of the dead infected bone (bone saucerization). Bone grafting may be necessary to augment structural support. These patients may require external fixation for structural support while the bone graft incorporates. Complex reconstruction of both bone and soft tissue is frequently necessary. In some cases, osteomyelitis progresses to an infection involving a segmental section of the bone. These patients often require an intercalary resection of the bone to arrest the disease process. Because this advanced stage of osteomyelitis involves an entire through-and-through section of bone, there is a loss of bony stability either before or after débridement surgery. As a result, treatment often must be directed toward establishing structural stability and obliterating débridement gaps by means of cancellous bone grafts or the Ilizarov technique (see earlier). Free flaps and vascularized bone grafts are other possible treatment modalities. All of the modalities previously discussed may have a place in the treatment of this type of osteomyelitis.

After surgery, patients are initially given a broad-spectrum antibiotic that is changed to specific antimicrobial therapy based on meticulous bone cultures taken at débridement surgery or from deep bone biopsy specimens. For a list of antimicrobial regimens for specific pathogens usually associated with osteomyelitis, see Table 1. The authors recommend 2 weeks of intravenous antibiotic therapy followed by 4 weeks of oral therapy except in cases of candidiasis, tuberculosis, actinomycosis, and brucellosis of the bone (also see Table 1 for these antimicrobial regimens).

Host Defect Alteration

If the patient is a compromised host (Table 2), an effort is also made to correct or improve the host defect(s). These include improving the nutritional, medical, and vascular status of the patient and treating any underlying diseases. Host factors are primarily involved with containment of the infection once it is introduced adjacent to or into bone. A systemically and/or locally compromised host does not contain the infection as well as a normal host, and the infection may permeate the bone. Host deficiencies that lead to bacteremia favor the development of hematogenous osteomyelitis.

Exceptions for Obtaining Cultures

Although surgical management is usually initiated before antimicrobial therapy, there are instances when antibiotics are given first. Examples of these situations include delaying surgical treatment when the treatment is worse than the disease or when the patient's condition is serious. Under these conditions,

TABLE 2. **Cierny and Mader Classification System**

Anatomic Type	
Stage 1	Medullary osteomyelitis
Stage 2	Superficial osteomyelitis
Stage 3	Localized osteomyelitis
Stage 4	Diffuse osteomyelitis
Physiologic Class	
A Host	Normal host
B Host	Systemic compromise (Bs) Local compromise (Bl)
C Host	Treatment worse than the disease
Systemic or Local Factors That Affect Immune Surveillance, Metabolism, and Local Vascularity	
Systemic (Bs)	*Local (Bl)*
Malnutrition	Chronic lymphedema
Renal, liver failure	Venous stasis
Diabetes mellitus	Major vessel compromise
Chronic hypoxia	Arteritis
Immune deficiency	Extensive scarring
Malignancy	Radiation fibrosis
Extremes of age	Small vessel disease
Immunosuppression	Complete loss of local sensation
Tobacco abuse	
Intravenous drug use	

patients are treated with antimicrobial therapy until they have stabilized. Antibiotics are then halted for 2 to 3 days, and surgical management is performed.

CONTIGUOUS FOCUS OSTEOMYELITIS WITH GENERALIZED VASCULAR INSUFFICIENCY

The majority of the patients placed into this category of osteomyelitis have diabetes mellitus or peripheral vascular disease from atherosclerosis. The small bones of the feet, talus, calcaneus and distal fibula, and tibia are commonly involved in this category of infection. The infection is usually initiated in soft tissue by minor trauma of the feet, such as infected nail beds, cellulitis, or a trophic skin ulceration. The diminished arterial blood supply has traditionally been considered to be the major predisposing factor. Recent observation suggests that neuropathy is an equally important factor in diabetic patients. Identifiable neuropathy as a complication of diabetes mellitus is present in approximately 80% of patients with foot disease. Multiple organisms are found in patients with osteomyelitis involving the small bones of the feet including *S. aureus*, coagulase-negative *Staphylococcus* species, *Streptococcus* species, *Enterococcus* species, gram-negative bacilli, and anaerobes. Aerobic gram-negative bacilli are usually a part of mixed infection. Cultures obtained by deep bone biopsy or during débridement procedures are indispensable in the diagnosis and choice of directed antimicrobial therapy of contiguous focus osteomyelitis. Culture results not only accurately identify responsible pathogens but also identify those patients with bone lesions that resemble but are not osteomyelitis.

Therapy

Determination of the vascular status of the tissue at the infection site is crucial in the evaluation of these patients. Although several methods can be used to determine the vascular status, measurement of cutaneous oxygen tensions and pulse pressures are the most commonly employed. Cutaneous oxygen tensions are obtained using a modified Clark electrode applied to the skin surface. Cutaneous oxygen tensions provide guidelines for determining the location of adequately perfused tissue. The values are also helpful in predicting the benefit of local débridement surgery and in selecting surgical margins where healing can be expected to occur. Revascularization, if possible, and/or hyperbaric oxygen therapy facilitates healing in areas where borderline oxygen tensions are present.

The patient may be managed with suppressive antibiotic therapy, local débridement surgery, or ablative surgery. The decision regarding treatment options used is based on tissue oxygen perfusion at the infection site, extent of the osteomyelitis and patient preference. The patient can be offered long-term suppressive antibiotic therapy when a definitive surgical procedure would lead to unacceptable patient morbidity or disability, or in cases in which the patient refuses local débridement or ablative surgery. Even with suppressive antibiotic therapy, in time, most of these patients will require an amputation of the involved bone. Local débridement surgery and a 4-week course of antibiotics may be employed in the patient who has osteomyelitis in a bone(s) amenable to débridement. Unless good tissue oxygen tensions are present, the wound will fail to heal and ultimately require an ablative procedure. Digital and ray resections, transmetatarsal amputations, midfoot disarticulations, and Chopart, Lisfranc, and Syme amputations (amputation of the foot with retention of the heel pad) permit the patient to ambulate without a prosthesis. The amputation level is determined by the vascularity and potential viability of the tissues proximal to the site of infection. The patient is given 4 weeks of antibiotics when infected bone is surgically transected. Two weeks of antibiotics are given when the infected bone is completely excised but some residual soft tissue infection remains. When the amputation is performed proximal to the bone and soft tissue infection, the patient is given 1 to 3 days of antibiotic therapy.

HEMATOGENOUS OSTEOMYELITIS

Hematogenous osteomyelitis is caused by microbial seeding of the involved tissue through the host's circulatory system and mainly occurs in infants and children. Because of the abundant vascular supply, the most frequent sites of hematogenous osteomyelitis are the metaphyses of the long bones (tibia, femur). A single pathogenic organism is almost always recovered from the bone in hematogenous osteomyelitis. In the infant, *S. aureus*, group B *Streptococcus*, and *Escherichia coli* are the most frequently recovered bone isolates, whereas in children older than 1 year of age *S. aureus, Streptococcus pyogenes*, and *Haemophilus influenzae* are most commonly isolated. After age 4 the incidence of *H. influenzae* osteomyelitis decreases. However, the overall incidence of *H. influenzae* as a cause of osteomyelitis is decreasing because of the *H. influenzae* vaccine now given to children. In the adult, *S. aureus*, *S. epidermidis,* and aerobic gram-negative organisms account for the majority of the bone or blood isolates.

Therapy

Appropriate therapy for hematogenous osteomyelitis includes correct antimicrobial therapy and, if necessary, adequate drainage, thorough débridement, obliteration of dead space, and wound protection.

Antimicrobial Therapy

Appropriate antimicrobial therapy for osteomyelitis depends on the identification of the causative pathogen and sensitivity results because the infection is usually responsive to specific antimicrobial therapy. Mismanagement with inappropriate antibiotic(s) encourages disease extension, sequestra formation, and the development of a refractory infection. Initially, appropriate culture material must be obtained. A bone biopsy is necessary unless the patient has positive blood cultures along with radiographic or bone scan findings consistent with osteomyelitis. While awaiting sensitivity data, a parenteral antimicrobial regimen is begun presumptuously to cover the clinically suspected pathogens. Table 1 outlines initial antibiotic therapy choices. Once the specific organism is identified, the initial antibiotic regimen may be continued or changed on the basis of sensitivity results. The patient is treated for 4 to 6 weeks with appropriate antimicrobial therapy dated from the initiation of therapy or after the last major débridement surgery. The goal of therapy is to prevent a refractory infection. If the initial medical management fails and the patient is clinically compromised by a recurrent infection, medullary and/or soft tissue débridement will be required in conjunction with another 4 to 6 weeks of antibiotics.

Treatment of Childhood Versus Adult Osteomyelitis

Oral antibiotic therapy can be utilized for treatment of childhood osteomyelitis. However, it is recommended that the patient initially receive 2 weeks of parenteral antibiotic therapy before changing to a 4-week oral regimen. In addition, the patient must be compliant and agree to close outpatient supervision. Absorption and activity of the orally administered antibiotic should be monitored by the measurement of the serum bactericidal activity against the causative pathogen. A peak bactericidal dilution of at least 1:8 or greater should be present and maintained. Oral therapy is possible in pediatric hematogenous osteomyelitis because of an increased bone blood flow and the aggressive mesenchymal and immunologic responses found in this age group. However, patients younger than the age of puberty cannot be given oral antimicrobial therapy with the quinolone class of antibiotics. Although acute hematogenous osteomyelitis in children may primarily be a medical disease, in the adult, débridement surgery, intramedullary reaming, unroofing, and incision and drainage of soft tissue abscesses are often required. Surgical intervention is indicated if the patient has not responded to specific antimicrobial therapy within 48 hours, has evidence of a persistent soft tissue abscess, or is diagnosed or suspected of having joint sepsis.

VERTEBRAL OSTEOMYELITIS

Vertebral osteomyelitis in the adult patient population is usually hematogenous in origin but may occur secondarily to trauma. Clinically, the patient usually presents with vague symptoms and signs consisting of dull constant back pain and spasm of the paravertebral muscles. More specific complaints may localize to a soft tissue abscess. The presence of point tenderness over the involved vertebral body is a characteristic finding. Fever may be low grade or absent.

The lumbar vertebral bodies are most often involved, followed in frequency by the thoracic and cervical vertebrae. The infection is usually monomicrobic when hematogenous in origin. In the normal host, *S. aureus* remains the most commonly isolated organism. However, aerobic gram-negative rods are found in 30% of cases. The primary infection focus of a patient with vertebral osteomyelitis is usually unknown. Intravenous drug abuse shows a high incidence of infection by *Pseudomonas aeruginosa* and *Serratia marcescens*. Unusual pathogens such as fungi may also cause hematogenous osteomyelitis.

Therapy

Antimicrobial Therapy

The therapy for vertebral osteomyelitis requires parenteral antibiotics (see Table 2) and may include early surgery and stabilization. On presentation, the patient should be placed on a broad-spectrum antibiotic regimen for the suspected pathogen. The choice of antibiotic(s) should then be refined based on the biopsy or débridement culture and antibiotic sensitivity results. The antibiotic(s) is given for 4 to 6 weeks and is usually dated from the initiation of therapy or from the last major débridement surgery.

Surgical Intervention and Stabilization

Surgical débridement is usually not necessary when the infection is diagnosed early. The failure rate with bed rest alone is not statistically different from that of patients stabilized with a cast, corset, or brace. Open surgical therapy is usually not necessary, except in cases in which the patient develops an extension of the infection, such as paravertebral or epidural abscesses, when medical management fails, or when instability is pending. The decision to advise an orthosis as opposed to internal fixation or bed rest is best individualized. When epidural and paravertebral abscesses develop, surgical drainage (sometimes emergently) must occur. Fusion of adjacent infected vertebral bodies is a major goal of therapy. Surgical stabilization in the form of vertebrae fusion is not recommended in routine cases because spontaneous bony fusion often occurs after 1 to 2 months with appropriate therapy. Other forms of stabilization, such as plaster body casting, are also usually not necessary because neck or body braces or a molded plastic jacket can usually provide adequate stabilization. In cases in which the infection progresses to the point of neurologic defects, emergent surgical intervention and decompression should be performed. Also, the development or progression of bony destruction or failure of patient improvement with antibiotic treatment often warrants the use of surgical débridement and stabilization.

Monitoring Treatment Success

Erythrocyte sedimentation rates should be monitored to gauge the success of treatment. Using scanning techniques may also provide an indication of patient response to therapy. Although radiographic tests can be useful, favorable therapy response often progresses for a number of weeks before it is detected on plain films. Magnetic resonance imaging is clearly superior in the early detection and evaluation of vertebral osteomyelitis. However, computed tomography is very useful in detecting sequestra and guiding bone biopsy for cultures and histology. Radionuclide scans demonstrate excellent sensitivity usually detecting the infectious process within a few days of infection. However, these scans are not specific and often give false-positive results for noninfectious reactive bone formation such as occurs after trauma or surgery. For patients with vertebral osteomyelitis, magnetic resonance imaging is the most beneficial scan, followed by computed tomography and the gallium-67 citrate scan.

CHRONIC OSTEOMYELITIS

Although both contiguous focus and hematogenous osteomyelitis can progress to a chronic bone infection, no precise criteria distinguish acute from chronic osteomyelitis. Clinically, newly recognized bone infections are considered acute, whereas a relapse of a treated infection represents a chronic process. The hallmark of chronic osteomyelitis is the simultaneous presence of organisms, necrotic bone, and a compromised soft tissue envelope. In addition, the pathologic features of chronic osteomyelitis are the presence of necrotic bone and the exudation of polymorphonuclear leukocytes joined by large numbers of lymphocytes, histiocytes, and occasionally plasma cells. Even after years of apparent eradication of an osteomyelitis infection, success is not ensured. A quiescent focus of bacteria can be reactivated years later and cause a recurrence of infection.

New bone formation is another characteristic of chronic osteomyelitis. New bone forms from the surviving fragments of periosteum, endosteum, and cortex in the region of the infection and is produced by a vascular reaction to the infection. The formation may reach from the periosteum and along the intact periosteal and endosteal surfaces, thereby surrounding the dead bone, forming the involucrum. The involucrum is irregularly shaped and contains openings through which pus may permeate into the surrounding soft tissues. This forms a sinus tract that allows the pus to travel from the involucrum to the skin surfaces. The involucrum may gradually increase in density to form part or all of a new shaft. Depending on the size of the bone and the duration of the infection, the amount and density of the new bone may progressively increase for weeks or months. The formation of new endosteal bone may proliferate and obstruct the medullary canal. Once the sequestrum has been surgically removed, the remaining cavity may be filled with new bone, especially in children. However, in adults the cavity may persist, or the space may be filled with fibrous tissue that connects with the skin surface through a sinus tract.

Multiple species of bacteria are usually isolated from biopsy specimens of infected granulations from deep within the wound. Chronic hematogenous osteomyelitis is the exception to this statement because a single organism is often recovered from these patients even after years of intermittent drainage. The possibility of attenuating the infection is reduced when the integrity of the soft tissue surrounding the infection is poor or the bone itself is unstable secondary to an infected nonunion or a septic joint.

Therapy

The infection will not resolve until the nidus for the persistent contamination is removed. Persistent drainage and/or sinus tract(s) are common, and antibiotic therapy alone is usually unsuccessful in the treatment of chronic osteomyelitis. The components of chronic osteomyelitis treatment include patient evaluation, staging assessment, identification and sensitivity of microorganisms, aggressive débridement surgery, prolonged administration of antibiotics, dead space management, and, if necessary, stabilization (see earlier for descriptions). Reconstruction is considered at the first surgery. In chronic osteomyelitis, there are usually large areas of devitalized cortical and cancellous bone within the wound. The dead areas must be completely débrided, including devitalized scar tissue, marrow, and cortex. The soft tissue covering the area of bone trauma must heal. If healing does not occur, the existing infection will persist or a new infection could form. Compromise of local soft tissue is a major reason for continued drainage.

Hyperbaric oxygen (HBO) therapy should only be

used as an adjunct to standard surgical and antibiotic treatment. Although clinical studies evaluating HBO have been somewhat limited, its use in the treatment of chronic refractory osteomyelitis is generally supported, and it can play an integral role in the effective management of chronic osteomyelitis under the direction of a hyperbaric medical specialist. Historically, treatment pressures of both 2.0 and 2.4 atmospheres absolute (ATA) have been used, with treatment times varying from 2 hours at the lower pressure to 90 minutes at 2.4 ATA. Treatment pressure and duration are the same for monoplace and multiplace chambers. Now the higher pressure of 2.4 ATA is almost universally used. Because experimental evidence suggests that twice-per-day HBO treatment interfere with bone healing, we suggest that HBO treatment be provided on a once-per-day basis for the treatment of osteomyelitis.

PREVENTION

Most cases of long bone osteomyelitis are developed after trauma or pre/intraoperatively. A number of studies have strongly correlated the development of *S. aureus* osteomyelitis with patient nasal carriage. Therefore, patient treatment must also include the elimination of nasal carriage through topical antimicrobial agents. Patients with diabetes mellitus can prevent osteomyelitis by minimizing foot trauma and preventing foot ulcers. This includes education on proper foot care, including daily inspection of the feet. Daily foot washing and the use of moisturizing with creams are necessary to avoid the opening of the skin. Furthermore, patients should avoid activities that might cause unnecessary trauma to avascular, neuropathic feet. This includes walking barefoot or wearing improperly fitted shoes. The only way to reduce the number of contiguous focus osteomyelitis is to prevent the development of diabetic foot ulcers or aggressively prevent diabetic foot ulcers from involving bone by treatment of infection, wound care, and off-loading.

COMMON SPORTS INJURIES

method of
KENNETH B. BATTS, D.O.
Womack Army Medical Center
Fort Bragg, North Carolina

and

FRANCIS G. O'CONNOR, M.D.
Uniformed Services University of the Health Sciences
Bethesda, Maryland

Primary care physicians commonly encounter musculoskeletal injuries. Most of these injuries are due to competitive and/or recreational sports injuries. This article covers the general principles involved in managing common injuries seen among adolescent, younger adult, and adult athletes (Table 1).

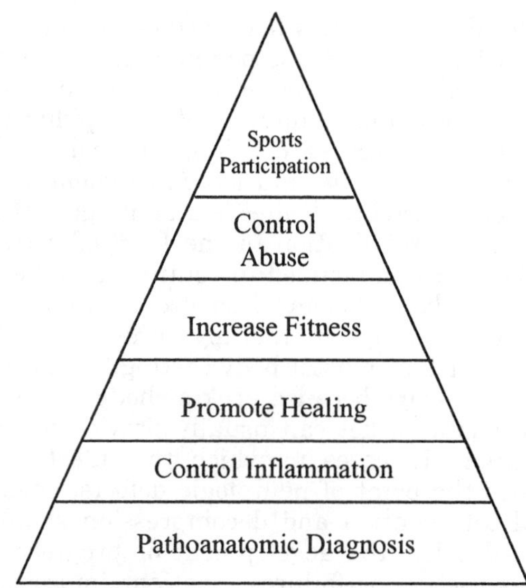

Figure 1. Injury management pyramid.

MANAGEMENT OF ATHLETIC INJURIES

The management of athletic injuries involves a systematic process of diagnosis, rehabilitation, and return to participation. This is accomplished by the application of clinical anatomy with the mechanism of injury. Recognition of all components of an injury allows the clinician to appropriately diagnose and effectively treat an athlete in a stepwise fashion (Figure 1).

The cornerstone of athletic injury management is making an accurate pathoanatomic diagnosis. This requires adept use of a history, physical examination, and selected tests to establish a clear diagnosis. The history attempts to identify the transition that led to the injury. The examination focuses on sorting out victims and culprits. The principle of transition suggests that injury is commonly due to a change in the use of the involved part. The principle of victims and culprits underscores the importance of a biomechanical examination. The presenting injury represents the victim and the subsequent dysfunction represents the culprit (e.g., plantar fasciitis and gastrosoleus inflexibility).

Treatment is initially aimed to control or modify inflammation through protection, rest, ice, compression, elevation, medications, and modalities (PRICEMM). Protection refers to avoiding abusive activity through modifying activity or temporary limb immobilization. Rest alone does not heal, but it allows the body's reparative efforts the opportunity to promote normal healing. Ice is the most effective anti-inflammatory modality used in sports medicine. Ice limits inflammation by causing vasoconstriction and slowing local metabolic activity. An ice cycle, 20

TABLE 1. **Common Athletic Injuries**

Adolescent Athlete	Young Adult Athlete	Adult Athlete
Sever's Disease	Anke sprain	Rotator cuff tendinopathy
Spondylolysis	Patellofemoral pain	Plantar fasciitis
Little league elbow	Medial meniscus tear	Medial gastrocnemius tear
Osgood-Schlatter disease	Anterior cruciate tear	Adhesive capsulitis
Glenohumeral instability		

minutes on and 40 minutes off, can be incorporated into all phases of rehabilitation. Compression limits soft-tissue edema and elevation assists in limiting soft-tissue swelling.

Medications are also used to reduce inflammation and pain. In acute injuries, medications may allow individuals to return to function slightly faster. In chronic, degenerative overuse injuries, the exact role of anti-inflammatory medications in treatment is undefined. Numerous physical modalities are used to treat athletic injury syndromes; however, the role of physical modalities in athletic injury management is undefined.

Healing is promoted through rehabilitative exercise and cardiovascular conditioning. Rehabilitative exercise restores normal strength, endurance, power, flexibility, and function to the area. Exercise enhances tissue oxygenation and nutrition, promotes fibroblast and vascular proliferation, and aligns collagen fibers to meet sports-induced stresses.

When rehabilitative exercise fails to return the athlete to normal function, surgery may be required. Indications for surgery include the failure of a rehabilitative exercise program; an unacceptable quality of life; and persistent pain, weakness, atrophy, or dysfunction.

The next phase of rehabilitation is sport-specific conditioning. This phase of rehabilitation prepares injured tissue to handle increased demands through sport-specific rehabilitative exercise (interval training, plyometrics, interactive eccentric/concentric loading, and anaerobic sprints).

Initial return to play should control force loads on the previously injured tissue by modifying identifiable risk factors. Improving technique, bracing or taping of the injured extremity, controlling the intensity and duration of activity, and appropriately modifying equipment are all effective measures of controlling force loads. Criteria for return to play include the following:

- Full, pain-free range of motion
- Strength equal to 80% to 90% of the uninjured extremity
- Successful demonstration of sport-specific function
- Psychological readiness to return to full participation

COMMON INJURIES OF THE ADOLESCENT ATHLETE

Sever's Disease

Sever's disease is a nonarticular traction apophysitis involving the Achilles tendon and calcaneus. It is most commonly seen in early adolescence, typically presenting as morning heel pain that is aggravated by activity. Heel pain may be unilateral or bilateral and is most commonly identified with sports requiring significant running or jumping (basketball). Physical examination demonstrates tenderness to palpation over the calcaneus as well as tight heel cords. The differential diagnosis includes calcaneal stress fracture, Achilles tendonitis, infection, tumor, and complex regional pain syndromes (reflex sympathetic dystrophy). The diagnosis is clinical. Plain radiographs may demonstrate fragmentation and sclerosis of the secondary ossification center, frequently a normal variant.

Patients should be reassured that this is a growth-related disorder. Most patients can be effectively treated with activity modification, ice after activity, and heel cord flexibility exercises. Some patients may benefit from ¼-inch heel lifts or viscoelastic heel cups. Short-term analgesic therapy, night splints, and/or crutches may be necessary for patients with severe symptoms. In the rare cases that fail to respond to conservative measures, short-term immobilization for 2 to 3 weeks may be beneficial.

Spondylolysis

Back injuries are common in the young athlete, and spondylolysis is frequently diagnosed. Spondylolysis is a mechanical injury that presents commonly as a stress fracture of the pars interarticularis fifth lumbar vertebra. Patients relate an insidious onset of lower back pain exacerbated by activity, especially in sports involving repetitive flexion and extension (e.g., gymnastics). Pain is characteristically worse with rotation and extension and occasionally radiates to the buttocks. Pain can be reproduced on physical examination with the single-leg hyperextension test. Hamstring inflexibility and paraspinous spasm are also seen on examination.

Radiographs are indicated in young athletes with low back pain. Oblique views are unnecessary. Current recommendations are to obtain lumbar anteroposterior and lateral radiographs as well as a single-photon emission computed tomography (SPECT) bone scan in the initial evaluation of the young athlete with back pain exacerbated by lumbar extension. SPECT bone scan imaging may reveal a hot pars interarticularis stress reaction in athletes with unremarkable plain radiographs. The differential diagnosis of spondylolysis includes discogenic disease, spondylolisthesis, atypical Scheuermann's, osteoid osteoma, and infection.

The treatment of spondylolysis is controversial. Orthopedic consultation is recommended. The cornerstone of therapy is activity modification with an aggressive lumbosacral stabilization program avoiding hyperextension. Antilordotic bracing may be required for up to 6 months in patients who fail to respond to initial conservative therapy. In rare, recalcitrant cases, surgical intervention may be warranted for in situ fusion or direct fixation.

Little League Elbow

Little league elbow is the most common injury in young athletes. Throwing creates predictable force loads on the elbow: tension across the medial structures, compression across the lateral structures, and translational forces across the olecranon and humerus. Little league elbow is a combination of various disorders:

1. Medial epicondylar fragmentation and avulsion
2. Delayed or accelerated apophyseal growth of the medial epicondyle
3. Delayed closure of the medial epicondylar growth plate
4. Osteochondritis of the capitellum
5. Deformation and osteochondritis of the radial head
6. Hypertrophy of the ulna
7. Olecranon apophysitis with or without delayed closure of the olecranon apophysis

Pain is the most common complaint. Other symptoms include decreased elbow motion, mild elbow flexion contracture, decreased performance, and localized elbow sensitivity. Physical examination may demonstrate a mild flexion contracture. Tenderness over the medial or lateral epicondyles and the posteromedial and posterolateral aspects of the olecranon fossa is common. Joint stability is assessed at 15 degrees of elbow flexion, and clinical comparison is made with the uninvolved extremity. Plain radiographs, including oblique views, of both the injured and uninjured elbows are needed for comparison. If plain radiographs are inconclusive, a bone scan, computed tomography (CT), or magnetic resonance imaging (MRI) may be useful to determine the extent of the injury. The differential diagnoses include Panner's disease, normal variations, and a possible neoplastic process.

Treatment includes rest and reassurance. Medial stress lesions require 4 to 6 weeks of activity modification, ice, nonsteroidal anti-inflammatory drugs, and a gradual return to activity. In cases in which the medial apophysis is separated by more than 3 mm compared with the unaffected elbow, surgical fixation may be required. Lateral lesions representing osteochondritis dessicans need careful orthopedic follow-up for evidence of radiographic healing. Significant osteochondritic lesions may require surgical intervention for fixation or excision.

Osgood-Schlatter Disease

Osgood-Schlatter disease is the most common lower extremity overuse injury seen in young athletes. This traction apophysitis is a painful enlargement of the anterior tibial tuberosity at the patellar tendon insertion and occurs most commonly during periods of rapid growth. The athlete complains of a painful enlargement of the tibial tuberosity that worsens with running and jumping activities. Physical examination demonstrates a tender tibial tubercle and often a tight extensor mechanism.

The diagnosis is clinical. Radiographs, if obtained, may reveal various stages of fragmentation of the anterior tibial tuberosity. The differential diagnosis includes Sinding-Larsen-Johansson disease, femoral osteochondritis dissecans, osteogenic osteosarcoma, and a bipartite patella. Treatment includes reassurance and activity modification. In some cases, 12 to 24 months may be required for symptom resolution. Ice after activity, an extensor flexibility program, and patellar tendon strapping are useful therapies. For severe cases, short-term immobilization may be required. Surgical ossicle resection can be curative in recalcitrant cases.

Glenohumeral Instability

Instability represents a clinical spectrum from subluxation to frank dislocation. The condition is commonly encountered in athletes involved in repetitive overhead activities producing shoulder microtrauma (e.g., swimming, baseball, tennis). Instability is more common in younger individuals and frequently recurs. Most functional instability is predominately unidirectional.

Physical examination is critical in establishing the diagnosis of glenohumeral instability. Range-of-motion testing may demonstrate increased external rotation, decreased internal rotation, and a tight posterior capsule. Strength testing of the rotator cuff demonstrates weak external rotators and abductors. Special testing should be performed to assess shoulder stability and the integrity of the glenoid labrum. Specifically, the apprehension (fulcrum)/relocation test and the crank test should be performed.

The apprehension/relocation test is performed with the patient supine and the shoulder at 90 degrees of abduction and external rotation. The examiner directs an anterior force across the glenohumeral joint. If the patient complains of pain or apprehension with this maneuver, a posterior directed force should be applied to the proximal humerus to relocate the humeral head into the glenohumeral joint. If pain subsides with this maneuver, and the examiner can continue to externally rotate the shoulder, anterior instability is present.

The crank test is performed with the patient in the seated or supine position. The arm is elevated to 160 degrees in the scapular plane. The examiner then applies a load along the axis of the humerus while maximally circumducting the humerus internally and externally. A positive test result reproducing the patient's symptom of pain or catching suggests labral pathosis.

Diagnostic tests include true anteroposterior and axillary plain radiographs. These views help to identify glenoid and humeral head pathology. MRI with enhancement is the imaging test of choice in cases that fail to improve with conservative therapy, allowing for detection of capsulolabral pathology, as well as concomitant rotator cuff pathology.

Treatment can be guided by clinical subtype (Table 2). Traumatic instability often requires surgical repair. A trial of rehabilitative exercise is appropriate, but individuals who remain symptomatic should be referred for a surgical stabilization procedure. In cases that are caused by overuse or generalized laxity, referral and definitive treatment is required only for those failing a trial of extensive physical therapy. Newer surgical procedures, including capsular thermal shrinkage, offer improved treatment options.

COMMON INJURIES OF THE YOUNG ADULT ATHLETE

Ankle Sprain

Ankle sprain is the most common acute injury involving the lower extremity of athletes who run and jump. During primary weight bearing, the bony structures are the primary stabilizers of the ankle joint. As the ankle dorsiflexes and plantar flexes, the dynamic stabilizers (musculotendinous complex) and the static stabilizers (ligamentous-bony complex) are vulnerable to excessive inversion and eversion motion.

The ankle is at risk for injury in the plantar-flexed, inverted position. Injury commonly occurs when the athlete lands on an opponent's foot, changes direction quickly and decelerates, or steps on an uneven surface. The anterior talofibular ligament is most commonly sprained with inversion. Eversion injuries are less common and involve the medial deltoid ligament as well as the anterior tibiofibular ligament. In these cases, the ankle is dorsiflexed and the talus acts as a wedge between the tibia and fibula. If swelling or ecchymosis occurs above the malleoli, the examiner needs to have a high index of suspicion for a syndesmotic sprain or tear.

In assessing the ability of the athlete to return to competition, key points include the ability to bear weight, the rapid onset of swelling immediately after injury, an audible pop, and a history of chronic ankle sprains. On examination, one must pay attention to pain over bony prominences, indicating a possible fracture/avulsion of the lateral malleolus or the styloid process of the fifth metatarsal. The anterior drawer and the talar tilt (inversion) test the integrity of the anterior talofibular ligament and the calcaneofibular ligament, respectively. The external rotation test is done to assess the anterior and posterior tibiofibular ligaments. The syndesmotic squeeze test assesses the interosseous membrane and the tibiofibular ligaments.

When obtained, anteroposterior, lateral, and mortise radiographs of the ankle and foot may demonstrate avulsion fractures of the medial or lateral malleolus, osteochondral fragments, calcification of ligamentous structures (chronic ankle injuries), or widening of the ankle mortise. Stress radiographs, although sometimes helpful in diagnosing chronic cases, do not offer considerable diagnostic accuracy over the initial physical examination.

Current evidence promotes functional rehabilitation to optimally manage ankle sprains regardless of grade or severity. Initial therapy emphasizes rest, ice, compression, elevation, and nonsteroidal anti-inflammatory drugs to reduce swelling. This is followed by early, protected range of motion; functional bracing; and graduated strength and proprioceptive training. Patients with chronic instability who fail conservative therapy are potential surgical candidates.

Patellofemoral Pain Syndrome

Anatomic and mechanical variations involving the extensor mechanism of the lower extremity have been implicated in producing idiopathic anterior knee pain often referred to as patellofemoral pain syndrome. Malalignment of the patella due to femoral anteversion, genu valgum, tibial torsion, patella alta, tight hamstrings, iliotibial band or rectus femoris, plica, and an insufficient vastus medialis obliquus have all been implicated as causative factors.

The athlete usually complains of multiple symptoms and is nonspecific in distinguishing the location of the pain. Complaints of peripatellar or retropatellar pain after prolonged sitting (theater sign), slipping or subluxation of the patella while descending stairs, or patellofemoral joint pain with increased duration of activity are more common. Physical examination shows a structurally normal knee. Clini-

TABLE 2. **Instability Clinical Presentation Subtypes**

TUBS Mnemonic	AMBRI Mnemonic
Traumatic etiology	***A***traumatic etiology
Unidirectional instability	***M***ultidirectional instability
Bankart ligamentous detachment	***B***ilateral shoulders
Surgical repair	***R***ehabilitation
	Inferior capsular tightening is the surgical procedure for failed conservative therapy

cians should note the position and tracking of the patella, the Q angle, and any muscle imbalance between the quadriceps and hamstrings. The patellar apprehension test, quadriceps inhibition test, and palpation of the patellar facets may reproduce pain around the knee contributing to the diagnosis of patellofemoral pain syndrome.

When obtained, the series of four standard radiographs (anteroposterior, lateral, tunnel, and sunrise) may demonstrate bony abnormalities and an abnormal relation of the patella to the femoral condyles. Treatment is based on patient history and physical assessment. Rehabilitation includes temporary activity modification, ice, nonsteroidal anti-inflammatory drugs, appropriate strengthening and flexibility exercises, and patellar bracing. Reassurance and a modified exercise program are very important in patient outcome. Arthroscopy should be reserved for physical examination abnormalities (recurrent effusion, quadriceps atrophy) or radiographic findings (loose bodies, spurring).

Medial Meniscus Tear

Medial meniscal tears are more common than lateral meniscal tears. Acute valgus stresses during contact sports or sudden cutting and pivoting during noncontact activities are common mechanisms of injury. Acute signs of meniscal injury include pain over the affected joint line, rapid effusion within 24 hours, or the inability to completely extend the knee.

Specific examination focuses on palpation of the joint line, McMurray's test, and Apley's compression test. If the examination is inconclusive, MRI is often helpful in establishing the diagnosis.

Treatment follows the PRICEMM principles. Arthroscopic surgery is indicated for athletes with an acutely locked knee; patients failing to respond to 3 months of conservative therapy; or patients with recurrent effusion, locking, or quadriceps atrophy.

Anterior Cruciate Tear

The majority of anterior cruciate ligament (ACL) tears occur from noncontact sports. Athletes commonly hear a pop, followed by immediate swelling and instability of the knee.

A comparison must be made to the uninjured knee on examination. Lachman's test is more accurate in assessing the integrity of the ACL immediately following the injury. With an intact ACL, the endpoint is solid. In the ACL-deficient knee, translation is increased and the endpoint is soft. The anterior drawer and the pivot shift tests aid in the diagnosis once the patient is relaxed and swelling has diminished. Radiographic indicators of an ACL tear include an avulsion fracture of the lateral tibia, also known as a Segund's fracture. This represents tearing of the lateral capsule and collateral ligament attachments on the proximal tibia. Tibial spine avulsion fractures also occur and may be found on routine radiographs. MRI is useful for identifying complex ligamentous or meniscal injuries where the clinical diagnosis is not conclusive.

Orthopedic consultation for surgical options is critical for active athletes.

Rehabilitation of an ACL tear begins immediately in both nonoperative and operative cases. Regaining full range of motion and strengthening of the quadriceps/hamstring muscle groups with closed-kinetic chain exercises improves the outcome of athletes with reconstructive surgery. Surgical reconstruction of the ACL currently affords the athlete the best opportunity to return to a high level of activity.

COMMON INJURIES OF THE ADULT ATHLETE

Rotator Cuff Tendinopathy

Rotator cuff tendinopathy in adult athletes occurs commonly as a result of overuse degeneration rather than acute trauma. Commonly referred to as subacromial impingement, rotator cuff tendinopathy develops as a progressive pain syndrome involving the supraspinatus tendon impinging beneath the coracoacromial arch. Primary impingement occurs due to acromial variants, spurring, or a tight posterior capsule. In secondary impingement, either glenohumeral instability or degeneration of the rotator cuff compromises the subacromial space. Athletes are unable to actively elevate the arm past 90 degrees without discomfort and commonly complain of night pain or pain when lying on the affected shoulder. The condition is commonly found in sports (baseball, volleyball, swimming, tennis) in which athletes perform repetitive overhead motions.

The primary clinical tests for impingement are the Neer and Hawkin's tests. A diagnostic injection of 5 to 10 mL of 1% lidocaine (Xylocaine) into the subacromial space can help differentiate adhesive capsulitis and rotator cuff tears from impingement syndrome. A positive lidocaine or impingement test relieves approximately 50% of the athlete's pain if there is true impingement. Persistent pain suggests a rotator cuff tear. Radiographs, especially a true lateral scapular view, are important in assessing the subacromial space for morphologic variations of the acromion and subacromial spurring due to osteophyte formation.

Initial therapy focuses on activity modification. Short-term use of nonsteroidal anti-inflammatory drugs or subacromial steroid injections may help athletes with persistent pain. After normal range of motion is restored, the athlete should proceed with progressive rotator cuff strengthening exercises. Patients for whom 3 months of vigorous physical therapy fails to restore normal function are candidates for arthroscopic decompression. MRI can be a useful tool in identifying rotator cuff degeneration as well as assisting in operative planning.

Plantar Fasciitis

Plantar fasciitis is a common overuse injury in runners and jumpers. Abnormalities in foot structure (pes cavus and pes planus) and exertional biomechanical forces (hyperpronation, tight Achilles tendon) increase the risk for this inflammatory condition. The differential diagnosis includes tarsal tunnel syndrome, rheumatoid arthritis, calcaneal stress fracture, and sacral radiculopathy.

The athlete often notices heel pain upon weight bearing early in the morning. The clinical examination may reveal a tight gastrosoleus complex as well as decreased flexibility of the great toe and tautness of the medial arch. The traction spur noticed on 50% of radiographs is not correlated with the clinical course.

Initial inflammation may be relieved by ice massage, nonsteroidal anti-inflammatory drugs, and ultrasound. As inflammation is controlled, the athlete should work on stretching with a heel cord box three to five times per day. Biomechanical support can be obtained with heel pads and cups, low dye taping, orthotics, or tension night splints. Athletes benefiting from low dye taping may also benefit from custom orthotics. Aerobic swimming with flotation devices and bicycling minimizes stress across the plantar fascia. Steroid injections may be used in intractable cases but have been reported to increase the risk for plantar fascial rupture. Recalcitrant cases may require surgical débridement of affected tissue.

Medial Gastrocnemius Tear

A tear or strain of the medial head of the gastrocnemius muscle occurs with the foot plantarflexed and the leg extended in a push-off maneuver. Commonly referred to as tennis leg, the athlete complains of acute pain or soreness after improper warming-up or extreme fatigue. With large tears, the muscle belly will be exquisitely tender and may have a palpable defect. The diagnosis is clinical and treatment is dependent upon the severity of the injury.

Athlete awareness, proper stretching and strengthening are paramount for prevention. Severe tears need to be rested with crutches and may benefit from a short-term lower leg ankle-foot orthosis. Only when the athlete can ambulate without a limp can he or she start active stretching. Minor injuries can be wrapped, actively stretched, and further rehabilitated with heel lifts and calf machine strengthening exercises.

Adhesive Capsulitis

Adhesive capsulitis or frozen shoulder may occur idiopathically or after a sustained period of immobilization due to tendonitis, bursitis, acute injury, or surgery. While the cause of this disorder is unknown, an underlying inflammatory process is suspected. Patients present with progressive pain and loss of motion. Examination reveals initial limited active and passive external rotation, followed by losses in abduction, forward flexion, and internal rotation of the glenohumeral joint. The athlete compensates by increasing the motion of the scapulothoracic joint. Radiographs are indicated to rule out tumor, calcific tendonitis, or degenerative arthritis.

The condition is treated initially with pain control, early passive range of motion (Codman's exercises), and progressive active stretching. Multiple therapeutic modalities to restore shoulder function have been used including nonsteroidal anti-inflammatory drugs, steroid injections, manipulation under anesthesia, ultrasound, and transcutaneous electrical nerve stimulation. In the majority of cases, the condition resolves spontaneously within 6 to 18 months without surgical intervention. Manipulation under anesthesia or arthroscopic surgical release is reserved for patients who fail to show any improvement after 3 to 6 months of conservative therapy.

Section 15

Obstetrics and Gynecology

ANTEPARTUM CARE

method of
KIRK D. RAMIN, M.D., and
GLENN A. GAUNT, M.D.
Mayo Clinic
Rochester, Minnesota

Ideally, antepartum care begins 3 months before actual conception with the recommendation that women who are sexually active and not using contraception should begin daily multivitamin or folic acid supplements. The most convincing trials of this were performed in Europe and China when it was concluded that women of reproductive age should take multivitamin supplements containing 0.4 mg of folate daily. Women with histories of children with neural tube defects or other anomalies should increase this dose to 4 mg of folate in the periconceptional period to reduce risks of recurrence. Preconception counseling should also include an accurate assessment of pre-existing maternal medical conditions. This is the ideal time to stress changes in factors that respond to early intervention: smoking cessation, alcohol or drug abuse, gum disease, and avoidance of teratogens. Alcohol is a known teratogen. Special consideration is given to patients with thyroid disease. Concern focuses on associations with low intelligence quotients in children conceived by hypothyroid mothers.

Consideration for high-risk obstetric referrals may be offered to women with concern for obstetric complications suggested by conditions listed in Table 1. Identification of the high-risk patient is critical to avoiding adverse outcomes.

In most cases, a woman's pregnancy is a normal event that is complicated by potentially dangerous disease in a minority of cases. The physician who manages pregnant patients must follow the normal changes that occur during antepartum care, so that abnormalities can be recognized and treated appropriately. Additionally, routine prenatal care offers multiple opportunities for patient education, primary intervention, and appropriate monitoring of the low-risk pregnancy in the setting of family and/or community. For some women, antepartum care is part of their own continuum in a long-term primary care relationship with caregivers.

TABLE 1. **Potential Indications for High-Risk Referral**

History of preterm delivery
Incompetent cervix
Prior intrauterine fetal demise or stillbirth
Multiple gestation
Third trimester bleeding
Placenta previa after 28 weeks
Current disease involving renal, cardiac, or endocrine systems
Known carrier of genetic disorder
Fetal anomalies
Systemic diseases such as hypertension, diabetes, or asthma
Isoimmunization

TIMELINE OF ROUTINE ANTEPARTUM CARE

First Visit and Early Care

After pregnancy is confirmed, it is extraordinarily important to determine the duration of pregnancy and the estimated date of confinement (EDC). Further care is heavily predicated on this estimate. The history begins with ascertaining the first day of the last menstrual period and calculating the EDC by assuming duration of pregnancy averages 280 days (40 weeks).

The documentation of prior obstetric history includes prior complications, route of delivery, and estimated birth weights. Maternal medical disorders are often exacerbated by pregnancy; cardiovascular, renal, and endocrine disorders require evaluation and counseling concerning possible treatments required. A history of previous gynecologic surgery, including cesarean delivery, is important to consider.

Current medications (prescription and nonprescription) are reviewed. Certain prescription medications are known teratogens and should be discontinued. Examples include isotretinoin (Accutane), tetracycline (Sumycin), quinolone antibiotics (Ciprofloxacin [Cipro] levofloxacin [Levaquin]), and warfarin sodium (Coumadin). Angiotensin-converting enzyme inhibitors should not be used during the third trimester. A family history of twinning, diabetes mellitus, familial disorders, or hereditary disease is relevant.

Honest discussion of substance abuse (alcohol, tobacco, and illicit drugs) is an integral part of the patient interview. Counseling patients about smoking cessation is vital in early pregnancy. Smoking increases the risk of fetal death or damage in utero. It is also associated with increased risk of placental abruption and placenta previa, each of which put both mother and child at risk.

Physical examination begins with a thorough general examination to assess maternal well-being including body mass index (BMI) and blood pressure. The BMI is calculated by dividing weight in kilograms by height in meters squared. The BMI of a patient is categorized as underweight (<19.8), normal weight (19.8–25), overweight (25–30), or obese (>30). A brief fundoscopic examination may reveal signs of hypertension-induced changes. Breast examination may be significant for changes in pregnancy that result from hormonal responses by the mammary ducts. These changes include engorgement and vascular prominence, occasionally resulting in mastodynia. Enlargement of areolar sebaceous glands (Montgomery tubercles) occurs between 6 and 8 weeks' gestation. A pelvic examination is performed with attention to the adequacy of the pelvis and to evaluation for adnexal masses. Numerous changes in the pelvic organs occur in pregnancy. For example, congestion of the pelvic vasculature (Chadwick sign) causes bluish discoloration of the vagina and cervix. Softening of the cervix due to increased vascularity of the cervical tissue (Goodell sign) may occur as early as 4 weeks. The uterus is palpable at the pubic symphysis at 8 weeks. Portable devices using the Doppler effect will reliably detect fetal heart tones at a rate of 120 to 160 beats per minute as early as 8 weeks.

Routine laboratory studies ordered at the first visit include complete blood cell count with differential, ABO and Rh typing, red cell antibody screen, rubella IgG, hepatitis B surface antigen, anti–hepatitis B antibody, syphilis serology, and HIV 1/2 antibody screen. Although some patients may refuse HIV testing, all patients are counseled and offered the option for screening. A midstream urinalysis checks for the presence of protein or glucose. A microscopic examination of the urine is performed to rule out infection or asymptomatic bacteriuria. A Papanicolaou smear is performed in conjunction with cultures for chlamydia and gonorrhea.

Special purpose laboratory studies are also considered in early gestation. Chorionic villus sampling (CVS) may be offered at 9 to 11 weeks for women older than the age of 35 and to those with abnormal pedigrees. From this, placental tissue may be subjected to chromosomal, metabolic, or DNA study. CVS cannot be used for diagnosis of neural tube defects because this requires the measurement of α-fetoprotein levels in maternal serum at a later date. Patients with tuberculosis exposure may be assessed for active tuberculosis with skin testing (if not vaccinated with bacille Calmette-Guérin) and chest radiography. Serologic assessment for toxoplasmosis, cytomegalovirus, and varicella immunity is not routinely indicated. Screening for genetic disorders may be undertaken if concern exists based on racial or ethnic background (hemoglobinopathies, β-thalassemia, α-thalassemia, Tay-Sachs disease) or familial background (cystic fibrosis, fragile X, Duchenne muscular dystrophy).

Follow-up visits are scheduled once monthly until 28 weeks' gestation, and then patients are followed twice monthly until 36 weeks. Care is then scheduled at weekly intervals until delivery. At each visit, weight gain, edema, blood pressure, fundal height, Leopold maneuvers, and fetal heart tones are recorded. Because blood pressure tends to decrease during the second trimester, increases of 30 mm Hg systolic or 15 mm Hg diastolic over first trimester pressures are abnormal. Interval history includes questions about diet, sleeping patterns, and fetal movement. Warning signs such as bleeding, contractions, leaking of fluid, headache, or visual disturbances are reviewed.

15 to 18 Weeks' Gestation

Maternal serum α-fetoprotein (AFP) testing is offered for all pregnancies at 16 to 18 weeks as a means of screening for open neural tube defects or chromosomal trisomy. In pregnancy, AFP is produced in sequence by the fetal yolk sac, the fetal gastrointestinal tract, and, finally, the fetal liver. AFP in the maternal serum occurs through placental exchange and transamniotic diffusion. High levels of AFP are associated with various fetal anomalies, including neural tube defects, multiple gestations, and ventral wall defects. Low levels of AFP are associated with increased risk of Down syndrome. The interpretation of this test is gestational age dependent; even if timed correctly, it is known to have a moderate level of false-positive results. Expanded serum markers of AFP, unconjugated estriol, and beta–human chorionic gonadotropin (β-hCG) are available to more accurately screen for Down syndrome, but detection is only about 60% and false-positive results remain 5%.

A more certain diagnosis is available through ultrasound (US)-guided transabdominal amniocentesis at 16 to 18 weeks. Chromosomes from fetal cells are subjected to fluorescent in-situ hybridization (FISH) analysis, which detects trisomy 13, 18, 21, and abnormal numbers of sex chromosomes.

Interval changes in the physical examination now include the start of colostrum secretion, which may begin as early as 16 weeks' gestation. Chloasma is darkening of the skin over the forehead, bridge of the nose, or cheekbones and is more obvious in those with dark complexions. It can begin to manifest at this time and is intensified by exposure to sunlight. Darkening of the skin in the areola and nipples becomes more accentuated. A darkened line appears in the lower midline of the abdomen from the umbilicus to the pubis (linea nigra). The basis of these changes is stimulation of melanophores by increased melanocyte-stimulating hormone. At 15 to 20 weeks, abdominal enlargement may appear more rapid as the uterus rises out of the pelvis and into the abdomen.

18 to 20 Weeks' Gestation

Increased surveillance for preeclampsia includes testing for urine protein in patients with blood pressure elevations greater than 140/90 mm Hg or in those with weight gains greater than 3 lb per week. Evaluation is also necessary for clinical signs of upper extremity edema, right upper quadrant tenderness, headaches, or vision changes. Proteinuria of more than 300 mg/24 h may indicate renal dysfunction or the onset of preeclampsia.

The mother may detect fetal movements or "quickening" at around 20 weeks. The uterus is palpable at

20 weeks at the umbilicus, and ballottement reveals an occupant floating in amniotic fluid. Measurements that are 2 cm smaller than expected for week of gestation are suggestive of oligohydramnios, intrauterine growth restriction, fetal anomaly, or abnormal fetal lie. Conversely, a measurement 2 cm larger than expected may indicate multiple gestation, polyhydramnios, or fetal macrosomia. These rules apply for the gestational ages of 18 to 32 weeks. Either condition can be fully evaluated with ultrasound (US) examination.

US has long established itself as the single most useful technology in monitoring pregnancy and diagnosing complications. It is for this reason that basic level US is offered at 18 to 20 weeks to evaluate growth, placentation, amniotic fluid volume, and fetal anatomy. If earlier dating of the pregnancy is uncertain, this is an opportunity to confirm or refute prior estimates. If anomalous conditions are discovered, more comprehensive US becomes necessary.

28 Weeks' Gestation

New physical examination findings at this time include the onset of stretch marks, or striae of the breast and abdomen. These are caused by separation of underlying collagen tissue, a response to increased adrenocorticosteroid. The ligamentous structures of the pelvis also undergo slight but definite relaxation of the joints, a progesterone effect. As the uterus enlarges, it often rotates to the right. Fundal size roughly correlates with the estimated gestational age at 26 to 34 weeks. Braxton Hicks contractions, characterized as painless uterine tightening, increase in regularity. The fetal outline can be easily palpated through the maternal abdominal wall.

A complete blood cell count for anemia and a 1-hour glucose tolerance test (after ingestion of 50 g glucose) is scheduled to detect patients at risk of developing gestational diabetes. If the screening test is abnormal, a 3-hour test is performed to confirm the diagnosis. Two or more abnormal values on this test are considered diagnostic of gestational diabetes mellitus. A repeat Rh antibody is checked at this time in Rh-negative mothers. Those who remain unsensitized in the third trimester receive a first dose of RHO immune globulin (RhoGAM) to prevent maternal isoimmunization to fetal red blood cells. A 300-μg dose is sufficient for 15 mL of red cells (equivalent to 30 mL of whole blood).

Return visits at 2-week intervals are now initiated, and the patient is oriented to the labor and delivery ward. Precautions are given regarding the onset of conditions listed in Table 2, any of which should prompt immediate medical attention.

36 Weeks' Gestation

Patients may complain of increased vaginal discharge at this time in their pregnancy, a physiologic consequence of hormone stimulation. The discharge consists mainly of epithelial cells and cervical mucus and is treated with reassurance. Discharge accompanied by itching, burning, or malodor should be evaluated and treated accordingly, however.

TABLE 2. **Warning Signs Prompting Medical Attention**

Vaginal bleeding
Rupture of membranes
Chills or fever
Severe abdominal, pelvic, or back pain
Signs of preeclampsia (headache, edema, upper quadrant pain)
Rhythmic cramping pains (of more than six per hour)
Burning with urination
Prolonged vomiting or inability to keep liquids down
Pronounced decrease in fetal movements

Vaginal and rectal cultures are collected to evaluate for the presence of group B *Streptococcus*. These organisms are implicated in preterm labor, amnionitis, endometritis, and wound infection. If cultures are positive, the patient will be given antibiotic prophylaxis during active labor in efforts to protect the newborn against vertical transmission resulting in newborn sepsis.

Follow-up visits are planned on a weekly basis, with emphasis on weight gain, blood pressure, and signs of preeclampsia. Review of precautions regarding infection, pregnancy loss, and symptoms of preeclampsia completes the visit.

Post-Term Gestation

Three percent to 12% of pregnancies continue beyond 42 weeks of gestation and are considered post term. Although some of these may be due to inaccurate dating, some patients clearly progress to excessively long gestations that are a significant risk to the fetus. Increased antepartum surveillance by cervical examination, fetal heart rate testing (see contraction stress testing), and biophysical profile should be initiated between 41 and 42 weeks. Even if fetal testing is reassuring, patients with reliable dating greater than 41 weeks are candidates for induction of labor.

COMMON CONCERNS OF ANTENATAL PERIOD

Bleeding

About half of pregnant women experience some form of bleeding during their gestation, which often is benign. Patients also have a heightened awareness for symptoms that previously may have gone unnoticed in the nonpregnant state. Efficient and competent evaluation, followed by compassion and reassurance when prudent, will allay many fears and provide clear direction. Spotting due to bleeding at the implantation site may occur from the time of implantation (~6 days after fertilization) until 29 to 35 days after the last menstrual period in many women. Some women have unexplained cyclic bleeding throughout pregnancy. Usually, cardiac activity on ultrasonography in concert with appropriate β-hCG levels confirm a viable early pregnancy. First-trimester bleeding in lieu of these findings may be of concern for spontaneous miscarriage or ectopic pregnancy. Vaginal bleeding in late pregnancy is covered elsewhere.

Nausea

This common symptom occurs in most pregnancies, is heightened before 14 weeks' gestation, and is largely benign. The etiology is not well understood but likely is related to elevating levels of β-hCG. Its moniker "morning sickness" is misleading because nausea of pregnancy may occur at any time during the day. Aggravating factors vary with the individual; success varies with interventions designed to reduce symptoms. Uncomplicated nausea may be responsive to small nonfatty portions at mealtime. Pyridoxine (vitamin B_6) tablets, 12.5 mg orally twice daily, and/or doxylamine (Unisom Nighttime Sleep-Aid), 12.5 mg orally twice daily, are safe in pregnancy and may be helpful. Antiemetic drugs in the outpatient setting are a measure of last resort. Inability to control protracted vomiting in conjunction with clinical dehydration can require hospitalization for intravenous fluids and treatment of hyperemesis gravidarium. Extreme nausea and vomiting or that which persists beyond 18 to 20 weeks' gestation may be a sign of either multiple gestation, thyroid disease, or molar pregnancy.

Nutrition and Weight Gain

The mother's nutrition is a vital factor in the development of the fetus from preconception through the postpartum period. Therefore, the pregnant woman should be advised to eat a balanced diet and informed of the additional 300 kcal/d increase needed during pregnancy. The American College of Obstetricians and Gynecologists (ACOG) recommends a target weight gain of 10 to 12 kg (22–27 lb) during pregnancy. They also advise that underweight women may need to gain more, whereas obese women should gain less. Also, nutritional requirements exist for protein (80 g/d), calcium (1500 mg/d), iron (30 mg/d), and folate (as previously defined). Patients with seizure disorders managed with valproic acid (Depakote) or carbamazepine (Tegretol) are also at risk and may benefit from the higher dose of folate.

Heartburn

Heartburn in the form of reflux esophagitis is caused by the enlarging uterus displacing the stomach and by progesterone's relaxation of the lower esophageal sphincter. Treatment consists of use of antacids, decreasing exacerbating factors such as spicy foods, eating more frequently but in smaller quantity, limiting intake before bedtime, and use of H_2-receptor inhibitors.

Urinary Symptoms

Urinary frequency, nocturia, and bladder irritability are common complaints caused by progesterone-mediated relaxation of smooth muscle and subsequent altered bladder function. Later in pregnancy, urinary frequency becomes even more prominent from pressure on the bladder by the enlarging uterus and the fetal presenting parts, such as when the fetal head descends into the pelvis. Dysuria, however, is often a sign of infection requiring antibiotic treatment. Bacteriuria combined with urinary stasis from altered bladder function predisposes the patient to pyelonephritis. Whereas simple urinary tract infections are treated on an outpatient basis, pyelonephritis remains the most common nonobstetric cause for hospitalization during antenatal care.

Infection

Two infections of special note are HIV infection and bacterial vaginosis. HIV transmission to the newborn can be reduced significantly with appropriate infectious disease and maternal fetal medicine specialty management. Bacterial vaginosis in women at high risk for preterm delivery or recurrent loss, if appropriately treated, can significantly reduce either of these untoward outcomes. Debate exists whether low-risk women should be screened.

Chlamydia trachomatis is an obligate intracellular bacterium and is the most common sexually transmitted bacterial disease in women of reproductive age. It may be associated with urethritis, mucopurulent cervicitis, or acute salpingitis or may be clinically silent. Perinatal transmission is clearly associated with neonatal conjunctivitis (leading to blindness) and pneumonia and likely associated with preterm delivery, premature rupture of membranes, and perinatal mortality. Diagnosis is confirmed by polymerase chain reaction during routine screening. Doxycycline should be avoided in pregnancy and erythromycin is associated with gastrointestinal upset, so treatment with azithromycin (Zithromax) is often appropriate.

Gonococcal infection is associated with concomitant *Chlamydia* infection in about 40% of infected pregnant women. It is usually limited to the lower genital tract, including the cervix, urethra, and periurethral or vestibular glands. Because of an association between gonococcal cervicitis and septic spontaneous abortion, and because preterm delivery, premature rupture of membranes, and postpartum infection are more common with gonococcal infection, routine cultures are appropriate at the first antenatal visit. Because some strains have rendered some β-lactam drugs ineffective for therapy, the recommendation for uncomplicated gonococcal infection is intramuscular ceftriaxone (Rocephin), 125 mg.

Vaginosis due to *Candida albicans* can become symptomatic with caseous white discharge, vaginal itching, or burning and may be associated with red satellite lesions on the vulva. Marked inflammation of the vagina and introitus may be noted. Topical application of over-the-counter antifungal creams such as miconazole nitrate (Monistat-3) or nystatin (Mycostatin) is generally helpful in controlling the imbalance of vaginal flora.

Cytomegalovirus is a ubiquitous DNA herpesvirus that is transmitted horizontally between people by droplet infection. It is transmitted vertically from mother to fetus and is the most common cause of perinatal infection. The virus becomes latent after primary infection with periodic reactivation and viral shedding. Infection is usually clinically silent. Many of the affected infants have died of infection, and most of the survivors have severe handicaps, including mental retardation, blindness, and deafness. Serious sequeale are more common among primary infections. The syndrome of congenital cytomegalovirus infection includes low birth weight, microcephaly, intracranial calcifications, chorioretinitis, mental and motor retardation, sensorineural deficits, hepatosplenomegaly, jaundice, hemolytic anemia, and thrombocytopenic purpura. Confirmation of primary infection is suggested by a fourfold increase of IgG titers in paired acute and convalescent sera or by detecting IgM cytomegalovirus antibodies. There is no effective therapy for maternal infection.

Human parvovirus B19 causes erythema infectiosum, or fifth disease. This is a single-stranded DNA virus that is heralded by the appearance of clinical findings of bright red macular rash and accompanying arthralgias. Acute infection is confirmed by IgM-specific antibody and may prompt adverse pregnancy outcomes, including spontaneous miscarriage and fetal death.

Rubella, also known as *German measles*, is directly responsible for spontaneous miscarriage and severe congenital malformations. Although large epidemics of rubella are nonexistent in the United States because of immunization, the disease can still affect up to 25% of susceptible women. Absence of rubella antibody indicates susceptibility. Vaccination involves an attenuated live virus and therefore is avoided in pregnancy. Vaccination of nonpregnant susceptible women (including those during the postpartum period) and hospital personnel continues to be the mainstay of therapy. Detection by IgM-specific antibody confirms recent infection. Congenital rubella syndrome is a severe example of antenatal infection and includes one or more of the conditions listed in Table 3.

TABLE 3. **Conditions Associated With Congenital Rubella Syndrome**

Eye lesions including cataracts, glaucoma, microphthalmia
Heart disease, including patent ductus arteriosus, septal defects, and pulmonary artery stenosis
Chronic diffuse interstitial pneumonitis
Osseous changes
Sensorineural deafness
Chromosomal abnormalities
Retarded growth
Hepatitis, hepatosplenomegaly, and jaundice
Thrombocytopenia and anemia
Central nervous system defects (meningoencephalitis)

Varicella-zoster virus, the etiologic agent of childhood chickenpox, is a DNA herpesvirus that remains latent in the dorsal root ganglia and may be reactivated years later to cause herpes zoster or shingles. Infection early in pregnancy may lead to severe congenital malformations, including chorioretinitis, cerebral cortical atrophy, hydronephrosis, and cutaneous and bony leg defects. Varicella-zoster immunoglobulin, 125 U/10 kg, can attenuate varicella infection if given within 96 hours.

Genital herpes simplex virus may be confirmed by tissue culture if active lesions are present; in this event cesarean delivery is indicated because the newborn is at risk for acquiring the virus during passage through the birth canal. Oral or topical acyclovir may improve symptoms. If no lesions and no prodromal symptoms are present, then vaginal delivery is recommended.

Trichomonas vaginalis can be found in 20% to 30% of pregnant patients, but only a small number complain of discharge or irritation. This flagellated, oval, motile organism can be seen on normal saline wet prep and is evident clinically by presence of a foamy or greenish discharge accompanied by multiple cervical petechiae. Treatment is with oral metronidazole (Flagyl).

Prenatally acquired infection caused by the protozoan parasite *Toxoplasma gondii* can result in the presence of abnormalities such as microcephalus or hydrocephalus at birth, the development of jaundice with hepatosplenomegaly or meningoencephalitis in early childhood, or the delayed appearance of ocular lesions such as chorioretinitis in later childhood. Cat feces are a common source of this parasite, so expectant mothers should refrain from cleaning the cat's litter box.

Varicose Veins

Pressure by the enlarged uterus on venous return from the legs and progesterone-mediated vasodilatation can lead to prominent varicosities and edema of legs or vulva. Any concern for deep vein thrombosis should be ruled out by examination for erythema, edema, cords, or tenderness. Doppler US may be indicated in equivocal findings of the lower extremity. Benign varicosities almost invariably return to normal post delivery, thus limiting the need for intervention in the anterpartum period. Edema of the lower extremities is common, responds to elevation, and must be differentiated from facial or hand edema accompanying preeclampsia. Hemorrhoids are manifestations of the varicosities of the rectal veins. Treatment focuses on stool softeners, sitz baths, and over-the-counter topical preparations.

Constipation

Bowel transit time and relaxation of intestinal smooth muscle are both increased due to progesterone effects, resulting in overall slowing of bowel function. If pronounced, this can lead to constipation. Dietary management of this condition is centered around recommendations for increased fluids and high-fiber foods. Enemas and laxatives are avoided.

Upper Extremity Discomfort

Periodic numbness and tingling of the fingers is due to exacerbations of carpal tunnel compression exacerbated by tissue edema. Splinting of the affected hand at night is indicated with anticipation of resolution during postpartum diuresis.

Backache and Pelvic Discomfort

Endocrine relaxation of ligamentous structures coupled with an offset center of gravity creates exaggerated spinal curve, joint instability, and compensatory back pain. Most women experience some form of this discomfort as pregnancy progresses. Advice given for improvement in posture, local heat, use of acetaminophen (Tylenol), and massage may be helpful. Minimizing the time spent standing can have a positive effect. Round ligament pain usually occurs during the second trimester and is described as sharp, bilateral, or unilateral groin pain. It may be exacerbated by change in position or rapid movement and may respond to similar measures. These routine aches and pains of pregnancy must be differentiated from rhythmic cramping pains originating in the back. The latter may be a sign of preterm labor requiring appropriate evaluation.

Leg Cramps

Leg cramps in the form of recurrent muscle spasms in pregnancy is thought to be due to lower levels of serum calcium or higher levels of serum phosphorus. The calves are most commonly involved and attacks are more frequent at night and in the third trimester. There are no data from controlled trials to show benefit over placebo for treatment targeted toward reduced phosphate and increased calcium or magnesium intake. Local heat, putting the affected muscle on stretch, acetaminophen, and massage can be helpful in acute events.

Intercourse

In general, intercourse is considered to be safe in pregnancy. The exception to this rule is found in patients who are experiencing uterine bleeding, or postcoital cramps and spotting. It may be wise to avoid intercourse in couples who are at risk for special circumstances. Firmer recommendations can be made in instances of placenta previa or known rupture of membranes; in these instances intercourse should not occur.

Dental Care

Dental procedures under local anesthesia may be carried out at any time during gestation. Use of nitrous oxide inhalants is to be avoided, however. Long procedures should be postponed until the second trimester. Antibiotics are given for dental abscesses and in cases of rheumatic heart disease or mitral valve prolapse.

Radiographs/Ionizing Radiation/Imaging

The adverse effects of ionizing radiation are dose dependent, but there is no single diagnostic procedure that results in a dose of radiation high enough to threaten the fetus or embryo. Diagnostic radiation of less than 5000 mrads is considered by ACOG to have minimal teratogenic risk, and, if medically indicated, radiographic imaging may be performed safely. For example, patients may undergo chest radiographs as indicated; a dose of 0.05 mrad is typical exposure. Radiography in dental procedures requires use of a lead apron as even further protection. Still, the need for radiographs should be evaluated for risks and potential benefits in the individual patient pregnancy to conservatively protect the mother and fetus from theoretical genetic or oncogenic risk. Magnetic resonance imaging is considered safe due to its mechanism of action, which is a nonionizing form of radiation. Use of radioactive iodine is contraindicated in pregnancy.

Immunization

Live virus vaccines must be avoided during pregnancy because of possible effects on the fetus. These include measles, mumps, rubella, and yellow fever. The risks for the fetus from the administration of rabies vaccine are unknown. The varicella vaccine is not recommended in pregnancy.

Diphtheria and tetanus toxoid may be administered in pregnancy if exposure to pathogens is likely. The hepatitis B vaccine series is safe and may be given in pregnancy to women at risk. The influenza vaccine is also recommended in all pregnant women.

TESTS OF FETAL WELL BEING

A primary goal in antepartum care is the competent management of patient care extended to both mother and fetus to (1) reduce risk of fetal demise after 24 weeks, (2) ensure optimal conditions for term delivery after 37 weeks, and (3) intervene for evolving conditions threatening to the well-being of either patient. Any pregnancy that may be at increased risk for antepartum fetal compromise is a candidate for tests of fetal well-being performed weekly beginning at 28 to 32 weeks. Some conditions requiring antepartum testing are listed in Table 4.

Nonstress Test

The nonstress test consists of fetal heart rate monitoring in the absence of uterine contractions. A reactive tracing is one in which heart rate accelerations of 15 beats per minute above the baseline of 120 to

TABLE 4. **Clinical Conditions That Prompt Further Testing**

Post-term pregnancy
Prior loss or stillbirth
Hypertensive disorders
Decreased fetal movements
Oligohydramnios or polyhydramnios
Fetal growth restriction
Insulin-dependent diabetes mellitus
Multiple gestation with discordant fetal growth

160 beats per minute are of at least 15 seconds' duration. Two of these accelerations must be observed in a 20-minute period. False-positive nonreactive tracings are more common before 28 weeks' gestation.

Contraction Stress Test

The just listed requirements for a reactive tracing are combined with tocodynamometer recordings of three contractions of 40 seconds or more duration in a 10-minute period. If no contractions are present, they may be induced via nipple stimulation or intravenously administered oxytocin (Pitocin). Relative contraindications to this test are preterm premature rupture of membranes, classic uterine incision scar, placenta previa, and unexplained vaginal bleeding. The results of the contraction stress test are categorized in Table 5.

Biophysical Profile

The biophysical profile consists of a nonstress test with US observations. A total of 10 points are given for the following elements (2 points each):

1. Reactive nonstress test
2. Presence of fetal breathing movements of 30 seconds or more in 30 minutes
3. Fetal movement defined as three or more discrete body or limb movements within 30 minutes
4. Fetal tone defined as one or more episodes of fetal extremity extension and return to flexion
5. Quantification of amniotic fluid volume, defined as a pocket of fluid that measures at least 2 cm by 2 cm.

ANTEPARTUM HOSPITALIZATION

Pregnant patients with complications requiring hospitalization are admitted to a high-risk antepartum floor in close proximity to the labor and delivery area. Specialists in maternal-fetal medicine are intimately involved in the care plans of these patients.

TABLE 5. **Possible Results of the Contraction Stress Test**

Results	Description
Negative	No late decelerations
Positive	Late decelerations follow 50% of contractions
Equivocal	Intermittent or variable decelerations
Unsatisfactory	Fewer than three contractions in 10 minutes

ECTOPIC PREGNANCY

method of
STEVEN J. ORY, M.D.
University of Miami
Miami, Florida

The incidence of ectopic pregnancy in the United States increased fourfold between 1970 and 1992. In 1992, approximately 108,800 ectopic pregnancies occurred; they accounted for 1.97% of all documented pregnancies. Since 1992, most ectopic pregnancies have been managed on an outpatient basis and are not reported to the Centers for Disease Control and Prevention. Consistent annual increases in the total number of ectopic pregnancies occurred each year before 1992, which has been attributed to earlier and more consistent diagnosis.

There has been a commensurate decline in mortality associated with ectopic pregnancy and a 90% reduction has been documented over the same 22-year interval. Fewer than 50 deaths occur from ectopic pregnancy annually. Major risk factors for ectopic pregnancy include prior tubal pregnancy, history of pelvic infection, and tubal ligation. Tubal pregnancy may occur in up to 50% of patients who conceive following bilateral tubal ligation.

DIAGNOSIS

Traditionally, patients with tubal pregnancy present with pelvic pain and abnormal uterine bleeding; these symptoms occur in over 95% of patients with tubal pregnancy. Often, diagnosis is made after the tube ruptures, when bleeding and pain are most common. Over the past 20 years, the availability of sensitive diagnostic tests and an appreciation of the natural course of ectopic pregnancy have permitted the diagnosis to be made earlier, before tubal rupture.

Human chorionic gonadotropin (hCG) can be detected in more than 99% of ectopic pregnancies. Performing serial hCG assays is the most valuable clinical test in the evaluation of early pregnancy in that it allows confirmation of pregnancy, identification of abnormal pregnancies (failing intrauterine and ectopic pregnancy), and prediction of when an intrauterine gestational sac may be visualized with ultrasonography (US). In a normal viable intrauterine pregnancy, the hCG level doubles every 48 hours through the first 6 to 7 weeks of pregnancy. Approximately 85% of normal intrauterine pregnancies, but only 17% of ectopic pregnancies, have at least a 66% increase in hCG levels. Serial hCG testing is a relatively sensitive test to identify an abnormal pregnancy, but it does not distinguish a failing intrauterine pregnancy from an ectopic pregnancy and has an inherent 48-hour delay. An hCG increase of 50% or less is almost invariably associated with a nonviable pregnancy.

Intrauterine pregnancy can be detected with transvaginal US within 5 weeks of the last menstrual period, but visualization is more closely correlated with hCG levels. The discriminatory hCG zone, which was originally defined with transabdominal US, refers to the range of serum hCG levels above which a normal intrauterine pregnancy can be reliably visualized.

Absence of an intrauterine gestational sac in association with an hCG level exceeding the discriminatory zone is presumptive evidence of ectopic pregnancy. However, this also occurs with failing intrauterine pregnancies and early multiple gestations. The discriminatory zone varies with the specific hCG assay used, the reference standard with which it is calibrated, and the resolution of the available US. Discriminatory zones vary significantly and may be unique for an institution. Currently, almost all hCG assays employ the first or second International Reference Preparation, which generally permits an hCG discriminatory zone between 1000 and 2000 mIU/mL.

The absence of a gestational sac 24 days or more after conception is also presumptive evidence of an abnormal pregnancy when the precise gestational age is known, such as in the case of patients undergoing embryo transfer or receiving hCG for ovulation induction. Identification of an intrauterine gestational sac effectively excludes the diagnosis of ectopic pregnancy. However, *heterotopic pregnancy,* combined intrauterine and ectopic pregnancy, is more common in patients undergoing ovulation induction and in vitro fertilization but does not exceed 1%.

Additional US findings may be useful in establishing the diagnosis, although direct visualization of an ectopic gestation can be accomplished in less than 50% of cases. This finding eliminates the need for additional testing. The presence of an adnexal mass, particularly if it is solid and associated with free fluid in the cul-de-sac, is correlated with ectopic pregnancy in 80% to 90% of cases.

Serum progesterone levels may occasionally be useful in the diagnosis as well. Patients with serum progesterone values less than 5 ng/mL in pregnancy experience spontaneous abortion in 85% of cases, 14% have ectopic pregnancy, and less than 1% have viable intrauterine pregnancies. Serum progesterone levels higher than 20 ng/mL are associated with ectopic pregnancy in 4% of cases, but the risk may be higher when ovulation induction agents are used. Approximately half of tubal pregnancies are associated with serum progesterone levels between 10 and 20 ng/mL, thus limiting the clinical value of this test. Ectopic pregnancy can also be presumptively diagnosed following uterine curettage if products of conception are not recovered and particularly if hCG levels continue to increase.

TREATMENT

Ectopic pregnancy has historically been treated surgically. The surgical treatment of ectopic pregnancy has evolved considerably over the past 30 years. Laparoscopy is favored over laparotomy because it permits outpatient treatment, quicker recovery, reduced needs for analgesia, and comparable safety and efficacy compared with laparotomy. Surgical options include salpingectomy and a variety of conservative procedures in which the tube can be saved. These include *linear salpingostomy,* the removal of the ectopic gestation through a linear incision in the tube; segmental resection with possible later anastomosis; and *fimbrial expression,* the removal of the ectopic pregnancy through the distal end of the fallopian tube. Conservative procedures were previously thought to confer greater future fertility potential, but current evidence suggests that fertility potential is comparable in patients who have undergone conservative surgery and salpingectomy, provided at least one tube remains. A history of infertility before ectopic pregnancy is the strongest predictor of future infertility. Candidates for surgical treatment of ectopic pregnancy include patients in whom laparoscopy is necessary for the diagnosis and those who present with significant pain or hemodynamic instability.

Patients who present earlier with minimal symptoms are candidates for observation or medical therapy. Diagnosis of ectopic pregnancy can be established without laparoscopy by use of serial hCG testing, use of the discriminatory zone, or direct visualization of an ectopic gestation with US.

Spontaneous tubal abortion or resorption is a well-recognized clinical phenomenon. A significant proportion of the increased numbers of ectopic pregnancies has been attributed to improved detection of early tubal pregnancies that previously underwent spontaneous resolution without clinical intervention. Patients with minimal clinical symptoms with early unruptured ectopic pregnancies, usually manifested by hCG levels under 1000 mIU/mL, may be candidates for observation without clinical intervention. They should be observed with measurement of serial hCG levels and should exhibit a consistent decline until levels are undetectable.

Several clinical series have documented the effectiveness of systemic methotrexate* as an alternative treatment for tubal pregnancy. Methotrexate is a folinic acid antagonist that inhibits dihydrofolic acid reductase, blocking DNA synthesis repair and cellular replication. Actively proliferating tissue, such as trophoblast, is particularly susceptible to its effects. Approximately 90% of patients with early ectopic pregnancy can be effectively treated with single-dose methotrexate* therapy without surgical intervention.

A single dose of intramuscular methotrexate,* 50 mg/m^2, is administered. Patients should have a complete blood cell count and a chemistry panel to assess liver function and a quantitative hCG level on the day of treatment. Contraindications to medical therapy include breast-feeding; evidence of immunodeficiency; active liver disease; preexisting blood dyscrasias; active pulmonary disease; peptic ulcer disease; hepatic, renal, or hematologic dysfunction; and sensitivity to methotrexate.* Candidates should be hemodynamically stable without evidence of active intra-abdominal bleeding, desire future fertility, and be available for follow-up care. Ectopic fetal cardiac activity is a relative contraindication to methotrexate therapy. Ideally, the unruptured mass, if visualized by US, should be no greater than 3.5 cm in maximum dimension. Although many investigators have not used a maximum hCG level, results are best if the hCG level is less than 5000 mIU/mL.

After therapy, a follow-up hCG level should be obtained 3 and 6 days later (day 4 and day 7 hCG levels, respectively). Typically, the day 4 hCG level will be greater than the day 1 value, but at least a

*Not FDA approved for this indication.

15% decrease in the level should be noted between the day 4 and day 7 values. Absence of a 15% decline at this point is indicative of lack of response and is an indication for a second dose of methotrexate. Approximately 25% of patients may require a second or third dose. Once a 15% decrease is documented, hCG levels may be measured at weekly intervals until they are no longer detectable. Serial hCG testing is necessary after medical or conservative surgical treatment to identify persistent trophoblastic tissue that has the potential to continue to proliferate and produce tubal rupture and hemorrhage. Treatment for persistent trophoblast is either additional methotrexate or surgery. Adverse effects to methotrexate therapy include nausea, vomiting, stomatitis, diarrhea, gastric distress, and rarely neutropenia, alopecia, and pneumonitis.

Methotrexate* therapy has not been compared in a prospective randomized controlled trial with surgical therapy, but in limited uncontrolled series, the efficacy and patients' future fertility potential appear comparable with both methods.

CONCLUSIONS

Ectopic pregnancy may be diagnosed by monitoring a high-risk group with serial hCG determinations and pelvic US. These patients are candidates for observation and methotrexate therapy if diagnosis can be established early. Many patients still present with pelvic pain and abnormal bleeding and require urgent evaluation and usually require surgery.

*Not FDA approved for this indication.

VAGINAL BLEEDING IN THE THIRD TRIMESTER

method of
RUTH ANNE QUEENAN, M.D.
University of Rochester
Rochester, New York

During pregnancy, the uterus receives 25% of the cardiac output, or approximately 500 mL of blood per minute. Consequently, an obstetric hemorrhage in the third trimester can have disastrous results for the mother and fetus. The physician must be able to implement support for the maternal cardiovascular system quickly, develop a differential diagnosis to ascertain the source of the bleeding, and then provide the best treatment for the mother and fetus.

The first priority is basic life support for the mother: airway, breathing, and circulation. Most patients with third-trimester hemorrhage do not have airway or breathing difficulties. However, administering oxygen (6–8 L by face mask) may forestall the onset of maternal tissue hypoxia and increase oxygen delivery to the fetus. Maintaining adequate intravascular volume is critical in the setting of serious obstetric hemorrhage. Intravenous access should be established immediately with two 18-gauge or larger intravenous catheters to facilitate transfusion of blood products if necessary.

The average pregnant patient can tolerate a 15% volume loss (1000 mL) without any hemodynamic alteration. With a 20% to 25% volume loss (1200–1500 mL), mild tachycardia, a slightly increased respiratory rate, and orthostatic hypotension develop in pregnant patients. The only change in the patient's blood pressure may be a narrow pulse pressure. With 30% to 35% volume loss (about 2 L), the patient will become overtly hypotensive and markedly tachycardic (120–160 beats per minute). When the volume deficit exceeds 40% (2.5 L), the patient may have no discernible blood pressure or pulse in the extremities. Unless volume therapy is quickly initiated, circulatory collapse and cardiac arrest will soon follow. During obstetric hemorrhage, monitoring urine output with a Foley catheter can provide important clinical information. Urine output often decreases as a result of declining renal perfusion before changes in the patient's hemodynamic parameters are noted. In addition, the physician must be mindful of other underlying medical conditions that could alter the response to hemorrhage, such as preeclampsia, anemia, or cardiovascular disease.

To quickly determine whether disseminated intravascular coagulopathy is complicating the clinical picture, blood should be drawn in a red-topped tube. If the blood firmly clots within 7 minutes, the patient is not yet coagulopathic. A type and crossmatch, complete blood count, platelet count, prothrombin time, and partial thromboplastin time should be obtained. In Rh-negative patients, a Kleihauer-Betke test should be ordered and Rh immunoglobin administered accordingly. An arterial blood gas determination can be also useful in managing antepartum hemorrhage. Oxygen tension is usually normal, but the pH and carbon dioxide and bicarbonate levels usually reflect some degree of metabolic acidosis, which may or may not be compensated. A base deficit of −6 to −8 indicates shock and the need for aggressive fluid and blood replacement. Base excesses of greater than −8 usually precede cardiovascular collapse.

The clinician should initially estimate the amount of blood loss that the patient has experienced and develop a plan for volume replacement. Volume replacement can initially be started with crystalloid solutions such as lactated Ringer's or 0.9% normal saline. In general, 3 mL of a crystalloid solution will replace the volume of about 1 mL of whole blood. One milliliter of a colloid solution such as hetastarch or albumin will replace the volume of 1 mL of whole blood. Although both crystalloid and colloids may be used for volume expansion and improved circulation, neither is a substitute for the oxygen-carrying capacity of maternal red blood cells. Consequently, the physician may consider a blood transfusion earlier than in the nonpregnant state to maintain adequate oxygen delivery to the placenta and fetus.

Even though whole blood is the most ideal therapy for antepartum hemorrhage, blood component therapy is almost always more readily available. One unit of packed red blood cells is expected to increase maternal hemoglobin by 1 g/dL. If a transfusion is needed urgently, type-specific blood can be safely administered to a patient with a known negative antibody screen with minimal transfusion risk. Platelets and fresh frozen plasma should be administered for clinical evidence of disseminated intravascular coagulopathy. Automatic prophylactic transfusion with fresh frozen plasma and platelets is no longer recommended.

Only after the mother has been stabilized should the physician focus attention on fetal well-being. All too often a nonreassuring fetal status diagnosed before the mother has been stabilized leads to emergency delivery by cesarean section. Not only is the fetus delivered unnecessarily, but rushing an unstable patient to surgery also further jeopardizes maternal health. Apparent fetal distress often resolves with adequate maternal resuscitation.

The final step in managing third-trimester bleeding is determining the etiology. After the initial assessment of the patient and fetus, an ultrasound (US) should be performed to determine placental location. If the relationship between the placental edge and the internal os is not well visualized, a transvaginal probe may be carefully used. A skilled sonographer can readily detect placenta previa. Visualization of placental abruption is more difficult. A large retroplacental clot must be present before an abruption is detectable by US. Occasionally, a chorionic separation at the edge of the placenta may suggest a retroplacental clot.

Placenta previa is usually associated with painless vaginal bleeding and occurs in 1 in 250 live births. Once the diagnosis of placenta previa is made, management depends on the gestational age, amount of bleeding, fetal condition, and fetal presentation. At term, a major hemorrhage (≥750 mL) or nonreassuring fetal status after adequate maternal volume resuscitation should prompt the physician to consider urgent cesarean delivery. Management decisions are more difficult in a preterm patient. Between 34 and 37 weeks, once the mother and fetus are stabilized, the obstetrician may consider amniocentesis to determine fetal lung maturation before proceeding to delivery. With an immature lung profile or gestational age less than 34 weeks, expectant management is reasonable. In the face of uterine activity and prematurity, tocolysis with either magnesium sulfate or indomethacin may be considered. Although β-mimetics have been used, the associated tachycardia complicates maternal evaluation. Corticosteroid administration to enhance fetal lung development is warranted in patients younger than 34 weeks. Maternal blood transfusion to maintain a hematocrit of greater than 30% provides a margin of safety in expectantly managed patients.

Historically, a double-setup examination has been advocated to determine the possibility of a vaginal delivery. With current high-resolution sonography, we rarely use this approach. A double-setup examination may be useful in patients with marginal previa or a very low-lying placenta. With clear placenta previa, cesarean should be the route of delivery. The type of uterine incision depends on the fetal lie and the position of the previa. For a fetal back-down transverse lie or anterior complete previa, we prefer a low vertical uterine incision. For posterior previa and all other presentations, we prefer a low transverse uterine incision.

The obstetrician should be aware that placenta previa is associated with a higher incidence of placenta accreta, especially if the patient has an anterior previa and one or more previous cesarean sections. Ideally, the patient can be evaluated antenatally by US magnetic resonance imaging to determine whether the placenta is invading the myometrium. If either modality suggests placenta accreta, the positive predictive value is high. However, sensitivity as well as the depth of invasion is underestimated with these radiographic techniques. If placenta accreta is diagnosed before surgery, blood loss can be reduced if the placenta is left in situ while performing either a cesarean hysterectomy or uterine artery embolization in an attempt to preserve the uterus.

Management of placental abruption depends on the degree of placental separation. Grade 1 abruption is associated with minimal uterine bleeding and uterine activity, no signs of hypovolemia, and reassuring fetal status. In a term patient, we would consider oxytocin augmentation because of concern that the abruption may extend. In a preterm patient with uterine activity, tocolysis may be considered. We would follow the same guidelines for tocolysis as discussed in the management of placenta previa. Grade 2 abruption is associated with mild to moderate uterine bleeding, frequent uterine contractions or tetanic uterine contractions, a 20% to 25% volume loss, and evidence of early disseminated intravascular coagulopathy. The fetal heart rate pattern is usually nonreassuring. If vaginal delivery is imminent, it is the preferred mode of delivery. Often, cesarean delivery must be performed because of nonreassuring fetal status remote from delivery. In a patient with early disseminated intravascular coagulopathy, the surgeon should consider a vertical skin incision because such an incision is more hemostatic than a Pfannenstiel incision. Grade 3 abruption is associated with moderate to severe uterine bleeding, maternal hypotension, and fetal death in utero. As with all classifications of abruption, the bleeding may be concealed. The mother must receive vigorous volume replacement with crystalloid, colloids, packed red blood cells, platelets, and fresh frozen plasma after blood for the appropriate laboratory tests has been drawn. Vaginal delivery is the preferred mode of delivery. Cesarean delivery is rarely indicated and should be performed only if the physician cannot maintain adequate maternal blood volume.

A rare cause of vaginal bleeding is vasa previa. This condition occurs when the placenta has a velamentous cord insertion and the vessels, traveling within the membranes, cross the internal cervical os. These fetal vessels can rupture with either spontaneous or artificial rupture of membranes. Because the source of all blood in this case is fetal, abrupt changes in the fetal heart rate tracing occur with hemorrhage from vasa previa. The obstetrician must have a high index of suspicion to diagnose this cause of vaginal bleeding. Immediate delivery by cesarean section is warranted, and the pediatric team must be ready to volume-resuscitate the infant after birth. Fetal blood can be obtained from the placenta under sterile conditions and then filtered and administered to the neonate by the pediatric team. Under the best circumstances, perinatal morbidity and mortality are high.

Although placental abruption and placenta previa account for most significant vaginal bleeding in the third trimester, other causes should be considered. The patient may have lower genital tract trauma, cervical cancer, polyps, or infection. In such cases, the same principles of maternal and fetal evaluation should be applied. Treatment needs to be individualized and based on the source of vaginal bleeding.

HYPERTENSIVE DISORDERS OF PREGNANCY

method of
HELAYNE SILVER, M.D.,
Brown University
Providence, Rhode Island

and

JOHN T. REPKE, M.D.
University of Nebraska
Omaha, Nebraska

Hypertension of one type or another may be expected to complicate up to 10% of human pregnancies. Although pulmonary embolism is the leading cause of maternal mortality in the United States, hypertensive disorders of pregnancy are the leading cause of maternal mortality worldwide and, either directly or indirectly, remain one of the leading causes of perinatal morbidity and mortality. With respect to pregnancy, three generic forms of hypertension are generally described: chronic hypertension, preeclampsia, and gestational hypertension.

Chronic hypertension is hypertension that existed before the pregnancy regardless of whether antihypertensive therapy was initiated. Preeclampsia is a disease characterized by hypertension, proteinuria, and edema that appear in the latter half of pregnancy in an otherwise healthy, nonhypertensive woman. Gestational hypertension is the occurrence of hypertension in the latter half of pregnancy in an otherwise nonhypertensive woman but without the other clinical manifestations associated with preeclampsia. Because of the different roles that each of these diagnoses may play in the clinical management of pregnant women, the conditions are considered as separate entities. Of course, overlap may occur, and these cases present unique challenges to the clinician.

DEFINITIONS AND CLASSIFICATION

Diagnostic criteria for the hypertensive disorders have recently been a subject of great debate, with many committee reports published in the last 5 years outlining varying criteria. Because of this lack of consistency, the National Institutes of Health recently issued a new statement from the National High Blood Pressure Education Program Working Group on High Blood Pressure in Pregnancy to expand and update the recommendations made in the Sixth Report of the Joint National Committee on Prevention, Detection, Evaluation, and Treatment of High Blood Pressure. *Chronic hypertension* is defined as hypertension present before pregnancy or diagnosed before 20 weeks' gestation, with *hypertension* defined as blood pressure equal to or greater than 140 mm Hg systolic or 90 mm Hg diastolic. *Preeclampsia* is defined as onset of hypertension at greater than 20 weeks' gestation, with proteinuria. *Proteinuria* is defined as 300 mg protein or greater per 24-hour specimen. If it is not possible to obtain a 24-hour collection, the group notes that proteinuria usually correlates with 30 mg/dL (1+ dipstick) or greater in a random urine sample without evidence of urinary tract infection. However, random dipsticks of urine for protein are notoriously inaccurate. As many as 66% of patients with negative or trace protein on dipstick will have greater than 300 mg per 24-hour collection, and as many as 12% of patients with 1+ or 2+ protein on dipstick will test negative on a 24-hour collection. Edema is not a good discriminator for preeclampsia because it is very common in normal pregnancy and is therefore no longer part of the diagnostic criteria. *Gestational hypertension* is diagnosed when hypertension is newly diagnosed after 20 weeks and proteinuria does not develop during the course of the pregnancy; therefore, the diagnosis can be finalized only in retrospect. Preeclampsia is superimposed on chronic hypertension with a new onset of proteinuria, sudden increase in pre-existing proteinuria, sudden increase in hypertension, or onset of laboratory abnormalities such as thrombocytopenia (<100,000) or an increase in liver enzymes.

There is some debate about whether systolic blood pressure should be included in the diagnosis of preeclampsia or solely a diastolic blood pressure of greater than 90 mm Hg. The argument for excluding systolic hypertension from the diagnosis of preeclampsia includes the following: it is more variable, and it does not correlate with pregnancy prognosis but diastolic hypertension does. As such, the Australasian Society for the Study of Hypertension in Pregnancy has eliminated systolic hypertension from their recommendations for the diagnosis of preeclampsia.

MEASUREMENT OF BLOOD PRESSURE

Whether the problem is chronic hypertension or preeclampsia, many clinical decisions are based on the absolute measurement of blood pressure. The Joint National Committee on Prevention, Detection, Evaluation, and Treatment of High Blood Pressure concluded that blood pressure measurement should begin after at least 5 minutes of rest. For many years it has been debated whether the fourth or fifth Korotkoff sound should be used in pregnancy in as much as the fifth sound had a very high standard deviation in pregnancy because of the hyperdynamic circulation. More recently, this issue has been resolved, with Korotkoff V being the chosen measurement because it reflects true diastolic pressure more accurately in pregnancy and, importantly, it shows better correlation with outcomes than Korotkoff IV does. An important point must be made, however, with respect to blood pressure measurement during pregnancy. Blood pressure should be measured with patients in the seated position and the sphygmomanometer placed at the level of the heart. Ideally, on a first visit, blood pressure should be measured in both upper extremities. In hospitalized patients, blood pressure may be measured with the patient in the semirecumbent position. Of note, however, is that left-sided blood pressure should not be used to rule in or rule out the diagnosis of a hypertensive disorder regardless of whether the patient is pregnant because raising the cuff above the level of the heart artificially lowers the blood pressure. The many potential causes of artifact in the measurement of blood pressure should be avoided, including the use of an improper cuff size, measurement over clothing, and measurement when the patient is anxious, stressed, or otherwise excited.

CHRONIC HYPERTENSION

Chronic hypertension occurs in 5% to 10% of the adult population. More than 90% of cases will be essential hypertension, with the remaining 10% being secondary hypertension, including but not limited to hypertension from renal disease, endocrine disorders, or collagen vascular diseases. The diagnosis of chronic hypertension is made with the criteria mentioned previously.

Diagnosis

The diagnosis of chronic hypertension is easier to make in the nonpregnant state or in the first trimester. Blood pressure readings in the middle trimester of pregnancy are generally reduced, and thus a blood pressure that is seemingly in the normal range at the middle trimester may in fact be elevated for an individual patient. This variation in blood pressure in pregnancy underlines the importance of preconception and early prenatal care.

The importance of establishing a diagnosis of chronic hypertension is not only to give the patient optimal treatment during pregnancy but also to recognize the potential increased risk of certain medical complications of pregnancy that occur in the setting of underlying chronic hypertension. Such risks include an increased incidence of preeclampsia superimposed on chronic hypertension, as well as an increased risk of abruptio placentae.

Additional high-risk characteristics may be identified during prenatal care. Women older than 40 years, women who have had hypertension for more than 15 years, and women who have uncontrolled hypertension in early pregnancy are at increased risk for an adverse pregnancy outcome. Complicating underlying systemic illnesses such as diabetes, cardiac disease, and collagen vascular diseases also predispose to an adverse pregnancy outcome. In fact, patients who have uncontrolled hypertension in the first trimester have a one in two chance of preeclampsia developing, a perinatal mortality rate approaching 25%, and an incidence of intrauterine growth restriction that approaches 50%. In addition, the risk of premature separation of the placenta, or abruptio placentae, is increased and may occur in up to 10% of pregnancies complicated by chronic hypertension, although it is not clear whether this risk is influenced by the use of antihypertensive medication.

Management

The initial management of a pregnant patient with chronic hypertension includes a thorough evaluation. Ideally, such an evaluation should be done before conception to allow the most flexibility in testing, the most realistic appraisal of baseline blood pressure, and the most comprehensive counseling with respect to the risks of pregnancy. Preconception evaluation also allows the health care provider an opportunity to adjust antihypertensive medications, when indicated, to medications more suited to continuation during pregnancy.

The initial patient evaluation includes a complete history and physical examination and a baseline laboratory evaluation that can be used for comparison as the pregnancy progresses. These baseline studies should include electrolytes, uric acid, liver enzymes, serum creatinine, urinalysis, 24-hour urine collection, and an electrocardiogram. If screening for hyperlipidemia has not previously been done, such screening should also be accomplished at this time. Of course, during this evaluation every attempt should be made to eliminate identifiable causes of hypertension and thus, via exclusion, establish a diagnosis of essential hypertension.

Pharmacotherapy

Once the initial evaluation has been completed, a decision must be made regarding whether pharmacotherapy is indicated. Although the long-term benefits of pharmacotherapy for mild to moderate hypertension have clearly been established, their utility and benefit in pregnancy remains controversial. Blood pressures of up to 150/100 mm Hg may be well tolerated during pregnancy without apparent adverse maternal or fetal effects.

When a decision has been made to proceed with pharmacotherapy, it should be recognized that the primary benefit of pharmacotherapy is to reduce the acute effects of hypertension on the mother. It has not been established that pharmacotherapy for chronic hypertension during pregnancy favorably influences perinatal outcome, the incidence of intrauterine growth restriction, the incidence of superimposed preeclampsia, or the perinatal mortality rate.

When pharmacotherapy is chosen, methyldopa (Aldomet) remains the most widely used medication for the treatment of hypertension during pregnancy because it is the drug that has been most extensively evaluated during pregnancy and has an established safety record for both the mother and fetus. Recommended doses for antihypertensive therapy during pregnancy are given in Table 1. Alternative pharmacotherapy includes β-blockers, specifically, labetalol (Normodyne, Trandate), and in selected cases, calcium channel blockers. β-Blockers compare quite favorably with methyldopa when their use is confined to the latter third of pregnancy. Some suggestion of an association between β-blocker therapy and intrauterine growth restriction has been made specifically, with the β-blocker atenolol (Tenormin), but this potential association should only alert the clinician to the need for close monitoring of fetal growth and not contraindicate the use of these agents in clinically appropriate circumstances. β-Blockers are relatively contraindicated for diabetics or individuals with reactive airway disease.

Calcium channel blockers are effective and probably safe, although they are not generally used as first-line

TABLE 1. **Medical Treatment of a Pregnant Hypertensive Woman**

Drug	Usual Dose	Disadvantages
First-line agents		
Methyldopa (Aldomet)	250 mg bid to 1.5 g bid	Rare: drug-induced hepatitis, positive Coombs' test
β-Blockers: labetalol (Normodyne, Trandate)	100 mg bid to 300 mg qid	Possible: decreased fetal growth, fetal bradycardia
Second-line agents		
Hydralazine (Apresoline)	50 mg qid to 100 mg tid	Postural hypotension, edema, lupus-like syndrome
Calcium channel blockers		Maternal hypotension, uteroplacental insufficiency, IUGR
Nifedipine (Procardia)		
Diuretics: furosemide (Lasix)		Maternal hypovolemia, decreased placental perfusion
ACE inhibitors: enalapril (Vasotec)		Fetal oliguria, renal failure, death

Abbreviations: ACE = angiotensin-converting enzyme; IUGR = intrauterine growth restriction.

therapy in pregnancy. Oral hydralazine (Apresoline) is rarely used for the management of chronic hypertension in pregnancy because more effective choices are available. More controversial is the issue of continued diuretic drugs during pregnancy. In patients who have been maintained on long-standing diuretic therapy, pregnancy does not absolutely contraindicate continuation of diuretic therapy, or at least thiazide diuretic therapy; however, diuretics are associated with subnormal blood volume expansion, so consideration should be made of alternative therapies. Loop diuretics such as furosemide (Lasix) are best discontinued during pregnancy unless absolutely indicated.

Worthy of special mention are the angiotensin-converting enzyme (ACE) inhibitors. Although very effective agents in the management of chronic hypertension, these drugs are contraindicated for use during pregnancy. Fetal renal dysplasia, neonatal renal failure, and decreased fetal calvaria calcification have all been described when these agents have been used during pregnancy. Evidence has also been presented that ACE inhibitors negatively affect uterine blood flow and can increase fetal mortality. The exception for use in pregnancy is patients with severe hypertensive crisis associated with CREST syndrome (calcinosis cutis, Raynaud's phenomenon, esophegeal dysfunction, sclerodactyly, and telangiectasia), where the use of ACE inhibitors may be lifesaving for the mother. Similar precautions apply to use of the newer angiotensin II receptor antagonists, which are Food and Drug Administration category C in the first trimester and category D in the second and third trimesters.

Fetal Surveillance

Although most of the fetal morbidity associated with chronic hypertension in pregnancy is related to superimposed preeclampsia, patients with chronic hypertension during pregnancy have a slightly increased risk of fetal complications, so routine fetal surveillance in the third trimester may be considered. Fetal growth should be monitored closely with ultrasonography, with increased intensity of fetal surveillance indicated if growth restriction is diagnosed. Postpartum, the initial assessment must include a determination of whether continuation of antihypertensive therapy is necessary and then selection of a drug that may be used for long-term hypertension management.

GESTATIONAL HYPERTENSION

Gestational hypertension is worthy of special mention only to reassure clinicians that in and of itself this entity poses no increased risk to the mother or fetus. Preeclampsia will eventually develop in approximately one in five women with gestational hypertension, however, so close surveillance is required. Because of incompletely studied effects of gestational hypertension on fetal-placental function, surveillance of patients with a diagnosis of gestational hypertension is prudent from the time that the diagnosis is made until delivery.

PREECLAMPSIA

Preeclampsia will occur in 4% to 7% of the general obstetric population. It is most common in nulliparous gravidas but can occur in subsequent pregnancies, particularly those complicated by chronic hypertension, renal disease, or diabetes.

TABLE 2. **High-Risk Factors for the Development of Preeclampsia**

Diabetes mellitus
Chronic hypertension
Multiple gestation
Previous preeclampsia
Autoimmune disease (e.g., systemic lupus erythematosus)
Antiphospholipid syndrome
Hyperlipidemia

Pathophysiology

The etiology of preeclampsia remains unknown. Previous hypotheses have included such causes as electrolyte imbalance, maternal malnutrition, and a circulating toxin—hence the name *toxemia of pregnancy.* Although the etiology remains unknown, the pathogenesis of preeclampsia is currently thought to involve a process of uteroplacental ischemia, possibly secondary to disordered trophoblast invasion during implantation, with resultant vascular endothelial cell damage. This endothelial cell damage may account for all the clinical signs and symptoms associated with preeclampsia, including but not limited to intravascular volume constriction, increased vascular tone, edema, capillary leak syndrome, and in severe cases, activation of the coagulation system. An alternative theory relates to long-term increased cardiac output and hyperdynamic circulation leading to vascular endothelial cell damage.

Unlike many diseases, preeclampsia is characterized by having only two categories: mild preeclampsia and severe preeclampsia. Mild preeclampsia was defined earlier. Patients are thought to have severe preeclampsia if they have a blood pressure remaining persistently above 160 mm Hg systolic or 110 mm Hg diastolic, nephrotic proteinuria in excess of 3 g of protein excreted per 24 hours (several sources define ranges from 3 to 5 g of protein excreted per 24 hours in this category; hence, the range is given), persistent oliguria, and a series of clinical signs and symptoms, including but not limited to right upper quadrant or epigastric pain; central nervous system dysfunction, including blurred vision, scotomas, severe headaches, or altered sensorium; the occurrence of pulmonary edema and cyanosis; and eclampsia. *Eclampsia* is defined as the occurrence of a grand mal tonic-clonic seizure in the setting of preeclampsia and in the absence of underlying neurologic disease.

Atypical forms of preeclampsia may also lead to classification of the disease as severe. The most notable of these is the so-called HELLP syndrome, which consists of hemolysis, elevated liver enzymes, and low platelet count.

Prevention

Much work has been devoted to prevention of preeclampsia. These strategies have focused on a variety of therapies, the most popular of which are currently low-dose aspirin* therapy (40–150 mg/d) and calcium supplementation* (2 g elemental calcium per day in four divided doses). Both of these approaches are perhaps best suited for women thought to be at high risk for preeclampsia (Table 2). Recently, however, a completed randomized clinical trial by the National Institute of Child Health and Human Development failed to demonstrate the efficacy of low-dose aspirin in preventing preeclampsia in four specifically identi-

*Not FDA approved for this indication.

fied high-risk groups. These high-risk groups included women with diabetes, women with chronic hypertension, women with a history of preeclampsia, and women with multiple gestations. A subsequent randomized trial of low-risk women similarly showed no benefit to aspirin therapy with respect to the development of preeclampsia.

Another recent trial investigating calcium supplementation for healthy low-risk primigravidas was also disappointing in that it failed to demonstrate a statistically significant reduction in the incidence of preeclampsia in the calcium-supplemented group. Unlike the situation with aspirin, a similar trial of calcium supplementation of equal size has not been performed to date in high-risk women. Other preventive strategies have included zinc supplementation,* magnesium supplementation,* folic acid supplementation* (in an effort to reduce plasma homocysteine levels), and administration of omega-3 fatty acids,* (fish oil) and/or other antioxidants (e.g., ascorbic acid,* α-tocopherol).* At this time, none of these preventive strategies have been conclusively demonstrated to prevent preeclampsia across all populations of pregnant women.

Management

Management of preeclampsia remains a challenge for the clinician. Previous strategies were simple and easy to follow and centered on whether a woman had preeclampsia and whether her disease was mild or severe. In the past, severe preeclampsia was an indication for immediate delivery. More recently, however, studies have demonstrated a potential role for the conservative management of severe preeclampsia when it occurs remote from term. This type of management should occur in a tertiary center under the direct supervision and care of a fetal-maternal medicine specialist. Conservative management is attempted with the goal of maximizing benefit for the fetus by allowing continued gestation and fetal lung maturation with a resultant reduction in neonatal morbidity and mortality. No direct maternal benefits are derived from this approach, but some could be perceived as indirect benefits based on the potential benefits to the woman's unborn child.

MANAGEMENT OF MILD PREECLAMPSIA

Once a diagnosis of mild preeclampsia is made, patients should be hospitalized and evaluated. If the pregnancy is preterm, after a period of initial evaluation, consideration may be given to either close ambulatory monitoring of such patients or continued hospitalization until delivery. After 37 completed weeks of gestation, patients with mild preeclampsia should be considered candidates for delivery, especially if the cervical examination shows a cervix favorable for induction of labor. Patients being expectantly managed with mild preeclampsia should have their platelet count and liver enzymes checked twice weekly and should also have fetal surveillance consisting of at least a nonstress test and determination of the amniotic fluid index two times per week. More complete ultrasound evaluations of the fetus for growth should be performed.

In general, antihypertensive therapy for mild preeclampsia is not indicated. If the blood pressure rises to a level that is dangerous from the perspective of maternal cerebrovascular accident risk, antihypertensive therapy should be initiated, but such therapy should be started in conjunction with a plan for expeditious delivery because this patient would now be categorized as having severe disease.

MANAGEMENT OF SEVERE PREECLAMPSIA

Severe preeclampsia is a potentially life-threatening emergency. All patients with severe preeclampsia should be managed, when feasible, in a tertiary care setting. Severe preeclampsia can be unpredictable in its course and may fulminate quite rapidly. All severe preeclamptic patients beyond 34 weeks of pregnancy should be expeditiously delivered. Between 32 and 34 weeks, the managing perinatologist has room for clinical judgment regarding how expeditiously delivery must be accomplished. Before 32 weeks and certainly before 30 weeks, consideration may be given to expectant management as discussed previously, provided that full informed consent is obtained from the patient and that both the mother and fetus are stable enough to allow for consideration of expectant management (Table 3).

HELLP Syndrome

The HELLP syndrome remains an enigma for practicing obstetricians. Although generally considered to be a variant of preeclampsia, up to one third of patients with signs and symptoms of HELLP syndrome may not, at the time of diagnosis, have evidence of hypertension or proteinuria. Nevertheless, this syndrome is considered part of the spectrum of the disease of preeclampsia and should be managed accordingly.

The occurrence of HELLP syndrome in general necessitates making plans for delivery. An exception may be a patient with minimal elevation of transaminases, thrombocytopenia but with a platelet count of more than 100,000/mm^3, and no clinical symptoms. A diagnosis of HELLP syndrome requires hospitalization of the patient immediately and, when stable, transfer to a tertiary institution. These patients should be given magnesium sulfate, and continuous maternal and fetal surveillance should be initiated. HELLP syndrome is frequently confused with a variety of other illnesses, including but not limited to cholestasis, immune thrombocytopenia, viral illness, acute fatty liver of pregnancy, and autoimmune disease (Table 4). Patients with HELLP syndrome may also be at increased risk for cerebrovascular accidents based on their coagulopathy and on data suggesting that preeclamptic patients may have a disordered capacity for cerebral autoregulation.

It is our practice to aggressively control blood pressure in patients with HELLP syndrome. Administration of intravenous dexamethasone is recommended to stabilize the maternal condition for delivery in antepartum patients and to hasten recovery in postpartum patients. The recommended dosing regimen is 10 mg dexamethasone intravenously every 12 hours antepartum and for two doses postpartum, followed by an additional two doses of 5 mg.

Intrapartum Management

Once a decision for delivery has been made, the mainstay of management in preeclampsia is to control blood pressure and prevent progression of this disease to eclampsia. The latter goal is accomplished by the use of magnesium sulfate. Magnesium sulfate may be administered as a 4- to 6-g bolus over a period of 15 minutes, followed by a continuous infusion at a rate of 2 g/h (Table 5).

Controversy in the past has centered on magnesium sulfate's efficacy as an anticonvulsant. Two large-scale randomized clinical trials have demonstrated magnesium sulfate's superiority in this clinical setting over both phenytoin and diazepam. More recently, there has been

*Not FDA approved for this indication.

TABLE 3. **Guidelines for Expedited Delivery and Conservative Management of Severe Preeclampsia Remote From Term**

Management	Clinical Findings
Maternal guidelines	
Expedited delivery (within 72 h)	One or more of the following Uncontrolled severe hypertension* Eclampsia Platelet count <100,000 with epigastric pain or right upper quadrant tenderness Pulmonary edema Compromised renal function† Persistent severe headache or visual changes
Conservative management	One or more of the following Controlled hypertension Urinary protein >5000 mg/24 h Oliguria (<0.5 mL/kg/h) that resolves with routine fluid or food intake AST or ALT >2 × upper limit of normal without epigastric pain or right upper quadrant tenderness
Fetal guidelines	
Expedited delivery (within 72 h)	One or more of the following Fetal distress as indicated by the fetal heart rate tracing or biophysical profile Amniotic fluid index <5 Ultrasonographically estimated fetal weight ≤5th percentile Reverse umbilical artery diastolic flow
Conservative management	One or more of the following Biophysical profile ≥6 Amniotic fluid index >5 Ultrasonographically estimated fetal weight >5th percentile

*Blood pressure persistently 160 mm Hg systolic or greater or 110 mm Hg diastolic or greater despite maximum recommended doses of two antihypertensive medications.

†Persistent oliguria (<0.5 mL/kg/h) or a rise in serum creatinine of 1 mg/dL over baseline levels.

Abbreviations: ALT = alamine aminotransferase; AST = aspartate aminotransferase.

controversy regarding whether magnesium sulfate prophylaxis should be routinely recommended because the incidence of eclampsia is low and the risk of a witnessed seizure in the hospital is small. This issue is currently the focus of a multicenter randomized trial, so more information should be available in the future. Patients receiving magnesium sulfate must be monitored very closely. Patellar reflexes should be 1+, and the patient should have no evidence of respiratory depression, with a respiratory rate being maintained above 12 per minute. More rarely, arrhythmias may occur with magnesium sulfate therapy. If any evidence of acute magnesium toxicity is present, this toxicity may be treated by administering 1 g of calcium chloride or calcium gluconate intravenously. Because of the statistical probability of seizures in the postpartum period, we recommend continuation of magnesium sulfate therapy for at least 24 hours after delivery. The most common sign of disease reversal is a brisk diuresis. In certain circumstances, continuation of magnesium sulfate therapy for greater than 24 hours may be warranted. It is rare that patients who are otherwise healthy will require invasive hemodynamic monitoring for the management of preeclampsia, but when necessary, it should be performed only by personnel experienced in critical care obstetric medicine.

Eclampsia

Rarely, preeclampsia will progress to eclampsia, which is an obstetric and medical emergency. The hallmarks of management are to protect the patient from injury and protect her airway. Eclampsia has a very predictable course, and in general, aggressive anticonvulsant treatment is not needed. The mainstays of therapy, other than what has been mentioned earlier, include allowing the convulsion to abate and waiting for fetal resuscitation to occur.

TABLE 4. **Clinical Characteristics of HELLP Syndrome, Thrombotic Thrombocytopenic Purpura (TTP), Hemolytic-Uremic Syndrome (HUS), and Acute Fatty Liver of Pregnancy (AFLP)**

Characteristics	HELLP	TTP	HUS	AFLP
Primary organ involved	Liver	Neurologic	Renal	Liver
Gestational age	2nd and 3rd trimester	2nd trimester	Postpartum	3rd trimester
Platelets	↓	↓	↓	N1/↓
PT/PTT	N1	N1	N1	↑
Hemolysis	+	+	+	−/+
Glucose	N1	N1	N1	↓
Fibrinogen	N1	N1	N1	↓↓
Creatinine	N1/↑	↑	↑↑	↑

Abbreviations: ↓ = decreased; ↑ = increased; N1 = normal value; + = present; − = absent; HELLP = hemolysis, elevated liver enzymes, low platelet count; PT = prothrombin time; PTT = partial thromboplastin time.

TABLE 5. **Intravenous Magnesium Sulfate Administration for Seizure Prophylaxis**

6-g bolus over 15-min period
1–3 g/h by continuous infusion pump*
May be mixed in 100 mL crystalloid; if given by IV push, make up as 20% solution; push at maximum rate of 1 g/min (usual rate, 150 mg/min)
40 g $MgSO_4$ in 1000 mL lactated Ringer's solution; run at 25–75 mL/h (1–3 g/h)*

*Made up as a 50% solution.

The course is very predictable, with uterine hypertonus occurring during the convulsion and increased contractility and resting tone lasting from 3 to 15 minutes after cessation of seizure activity. During this time, initial fetal bradycardia is the norm. Gradual recovery should occur as the mother recovers, and in general, many of these patients will be able to undergo vaginal delivery after appropriate stabilization and reassessment of their anticonvulsant medication.

Emergency cesarean section is best avoided because neither the mother nor the fetus may be a suitable candidate for operative delivery during the acute event (Table 6). In cases in which seizures occur despite adequate anticonvulsant therapy, consideration should be given to initiating further neurologic assessment, possibly including imaging studies of the central nervous system to rule out other etiologies for the seizure activity. No consensus has been reached regarding whether magnetic resonance imaging is superior to computed tomography in this setting, and the decision of which method to use may be largely institutional and based on experience, availability, and to a lesser degree, cost.

Postpartum Management

With the current trend toward shorter hospital stays, postpartum management of preeclampsia assumes new importance. A syndrome of late postpartum preeclampsia and eclampsia has been described. Patients with a diagnosis of preeclampsia, when discharged from the hospital, should be carefully educated about the signs and symptoms of preeclampsia and impending eclampsia, such as headache, progressive shortness of breath, visual disturbances, or epigastric pain. These and other signs or symptoms suggestive of preeclampsia should prompt immediate referral to the hospital for evaluation and further management. The long-term prognosis for patients with uncomplicated preeclampsia or eclampsia, even when the disease is severe, is quite good.

TABLE 6. **Management of Eclampsia**

Protect maternal airway; prevent patient injury
Wait for convulsion to abate
Maternal resuscitation
Maximal oxygenation (mask or endotracheal oxygen)
Intravenous access and judicious hydration
Fetal resuscitation
Maternal oxygen, left lateral positioning
Continuous fetal heart rate monitoring
Maternal postictal assessment
Complete blood count, platelets, electrolytes, glucose, calcium, magnesium, toxin screen, blood type, and antibody screen
Careful neurologic examination
Cervical examination
Magnesium sulfate prophylaxis for subsequent seizures
Formulate delivery strategy
Avoid "stat" cesarean section

POSTPARTUM CARE

method of
E. REBECCA PSCHIRRER, M.D.
Eastern Virginia Medical School
Norfolk, Virginia

and

JOAN M. MASTROBATTISTA, M.D.
University of Texas—Houston Medical School
Houston, Texas

NORMAL POSTPARTUM EVENTS

The *postpartum period* is the time from immediately following delivery through the subsequent 6 weeks. The term pregnant uterus weighs approximately 1000 g. Involution begins after placental delivery, and by 6 weeks postpartum, the uterus weighs less than 100 g.

Postpartum vaginal discharge, or *lochia,* is characterized by distinct phases: lochia rubra, serosa, and alba. Lochia consists of red blood cells, decidual tissue, epithelial cells, and bacteria. During the first 3 to 4 days, lochia rubra is predominated by erythrocytes, hence its red color. By postpartum day 4, lochia becomes pale (lochia serosa). A white or yellowish-white color dominates, lochia alba, by day 10, owing to the addition of white blood cells and reduced fluid content. The median duration of lochia serosa is 22 days, although up to 15% of women will still have lochia serosa at their 6-week postpartum examination. Some women experience an increase in bloody discharge 7 to 14 days postpartum, owing to sloughing of the placental site eschar. Regeneration of the endometrium occurs rapidly and is complete by the 16th day postpartum.

Uterine involution in multiparas is often complicated by afterpains: vigorous uterine contractions. Often breastfeeding, owing to oxytocin release, exacerbates these afterpains. If afterpains are of sufficient intensity to require analgesia, nonsteroidal anti-inflammatory agents such as ibuprofen 600 to 800 mg every 4 to 6 hours are helpful. Some women may require narcotic analgesia; alternating narcotic analgesics with nonsteroidal analgesics is often efficacious.

Postpartum weight loss begins immediately with the loss of 10 to 13 pounds from the delivery of the infant, placenta, amniotic fluid, and maternal blood loss. By 6 weeks postpartum, 28% of women achieve their prepregnancy weight. This is often not the case if excessive weight gain (>35 pounds) has occurred during the pregnancy. By 6 months postpartum, the majority of women return to their prepregnancy weight.

Marked hemodynamic changes occur during and after delivery. The average measured blood loss following an uncomplicated spontaneous vaginal delivery is approximately 500 mL and from a cesarean delivery, 1000 mL. Physiologic diuresis occurs in the first week as well as shifting of fluid from the extravascular into the intravascular space. The maternal blood volume returns to its prepregnancy level about 1 week after delivery. The 48 hours following delivery are characterized by continued elevation in cardiac output. By 2 weeks postpartum, the cardiac output returns to nonpregnant levels.

IMMEDIATE POSTPARTUM CARE

Hospital Observation

After a normal vaginal delivery, women are routinely observed for 24 to 48 hours. In the event of a cesarean delivery, the postpartum stay is extended to 72 to 96 hours. Common complications of the immediate postpartum period include hemorrhage and genital tract infection. Vital signs, urine output, and vaginal bleeding should be monitored closely. At our institution, vital signs are obtained every 15 minutes for the first hour, every 30 minutes for 2 hours, and then every 4 hours for 24 hours. Vaginal bleeding is monitored with pad counts; fundal massage of the uterus is performed. Considerable amounts of blood can collect in the uterus without evidence of bleeding. The risk of postpartum hemorrhage (PPH) is greatest in the first hour after delivery; therefore, trained personnel should remain in proximity during this time.

Care of the Perineum

Cleansing of the perineal area after delivery is accomplished with warm water. Application of an ice pack may reduce swelling and discomfort in the hours directly after parturition. In general, pain caused by vaginal laceration or episiotomy repair can be managed with nonsteroidal analgesics such as ibuprofen. These medications are more effective in relieving perineal pain than the alternatives. Additionally, this class of analgesics is safe during lactation. Women with inordinate perineal pain should be examined for evidence of hematoma or infection. Sitz baths are also effective in alleviating tenderness. There is evidence that cool water sitz baths provide greater pain relief than warm water. Topical application of analgesic sprays, emollients, or corticosteroids may also relieve discomfort. Women with third- or fourth-degree episiotomies or lacerations should be given stool softeners, but care should be taken not to induce diarrhea.

Breast Care and Lactation

Breast-feeding should be encouraged in all women, except those who are HIV positive or have active untreated tuberculosis. Endometritis, group B *streptococci* colonization, hepatitis B (after immunoglobulin and vaccine administered to infant), and herpes simplex (excluding active lesions on the breast) are *not* contraindications to breast-feeding. Benefits of breast-feeding include decreased postpartum blood loss, improved mother-infant attachment, optimal infant nutrition, decreased infant infectious morbidity, decreased expense, and convenience. The American Academy of Pediatrics recommends exclusive breast-feeding for the first 6 months of life. Breast-feeding support can be accomplished with the aid of properly trained lactation consultants and successful breast-feeding enhanced through appropriate teaching of mother and infant.

Colostrum production begins immediately after delivery, and milk production begins by day 3 or 4 postpartum. Breast engorgement is common and may be associated with an elevated temperature. In the postpartum woman, any fever should elicit an examination to determine the source. Breast erythema and tenderness, myalgias, and temperature higher than 100.4°F may indicate mastitis. This should be treated without delay but does not necessitate discontinuation of breast-feeding. Dicloxacillin sodium (Dynapen) and clindamycin (Cleocin), if the patient is penicillin allergic, are first-line therapies.

In the rare case when breast-feeding is contraindicated, application of ice packs, wearing a tight-fitting brassiere, and taking nonsteroidal anti-inflammatory drugs may relieve discomfort. Bromocriptine mesylate (Parlodel) therapy is no longer prescribed to suppress lactation because significant maternal morbidity such as symptomatic hypotension, myocardial infarction, and stroke has been reported.

Pain with breast-feeding should be evaluated for inappropriate latch and evidence of infection. Candidiasis, characterized by cherry red nipples and pain that can radiate to the axillary areas, should be treated in both mother and infant. Treatment can be accomplished with application of topical nystatin (Mycostatin), which does not need to be removed before breast-feeding.

Immunizations

Patients who are rubella virus non-immune should be vaccinated before hospital discharge. D-negative women who are non-immune and who delivered an Rh-positive infant should have a Kleihauer-Betke test to determine the proper dose of Rh immune globulin.

Contraception

The immediate postpartum period is an excellent time to address family planning. Combined estrogen and progesterone oral contraceptive pills have been shown to decrease milk production and should therefore not be started until lactation is well established. Progestin-only pills or depot medroxyprogesterone acetate have minimal effects on milk production and may be started before hospital discharge.

POSTPARTUM COMPLICATIONS

Hemorrhage

Early PPH may occur immediately after delivery or within the first 24 hours postpartum. Late PPH occurs after the initial 24 hours but within 6 weeks postpartum. Blood loss of 500 mL or more following the third stage of labor in a vaginal delivery or blood loss greater than 1000 mL during a cesarean delivery constitute a PPH. Health care providers grossly underestimate blood loss. Causes of early PPH include uterine atony, lacerations, retained placenta, uterine rupture or inversion, placenta accreta, and hereditary coagulopathy. Late PPH may be caused by infection, subinvolution of the placental site, retained placental fragments, and coagulopathy. Treatment begins with placement of large bore intravenous lines. Appropriate personnel are summoned, crystalloid infusion begun, and blood products administered as needed.

Uterine atony is initially treated with fundal massage. Bimanual examination and intrauterine exploration may reveal clots in the lower segment, retained placental fragments, or uterine rupture. A Foley catheter monitors urinary output and assists in the contraction of the lower uterine segment. If the uterine fundus is firm and there is no evidence of uterine rupture, examination of the vagina and cervix may reveal lacerations.

Medical management of uterine atony begins with administration of oxytocic agents. Oxytocin (Pitocin),* 20 to 40 U, is added to 1000 mL of crystalloid. A rapid intravascular bolus of oxytocin is contraindicated owing to the risk of circulatory collapse. For women with no intravenous access, 10 U of oxytocin may be given intramuscularly (IM) or intramyometrially (IMM). Methylergonovine maleate (Methergine)* may be administered to women without hypertension in a dose of 200 μg IM or IMM every 2 to 4 hours for six doses. 15-Methylprostaglandin $F_{2\alpha}$ (Hemabate)* may be given IM or IMM in women without asthma; the dose is 250 μg every 15 to 90 minutes, not to exceed eight doses. Dinoprostone (Prostin,* prostaglandin E_2) 20 mg may be administered rectally every 2 hours and should be avoided in the hypotensive patient. Misoprostol (Cytotec),* 400 μg may be given orally or rectally in women without a previous uterine scar.

Infection

Febrile morbidity following delivery is defined as a temperature greater than 100.4°F on two occasions 4 hours apart after the first 24 hours. Endometritis is the most common cause of postpartum fever, complicating 2% of vaginal deliveries and 10% to 15% of cesarean deliveries. Other sources of fever include urinary tract infection, lower genital tract infection, wound infection, pulmonary infection, mastitis, and thrombophlebitis.

Endometritis is a polymicrobial infection that arises from bacterial colonization of the lower genital tract. This infection is associated with prolonged rupture of membranes, prolonged labors, multiple vaginal examinations during labor, cesarean delivery after labor, and anemia. Endometritis is diagnosed by fever, uterine tenderness, and often a foul-smelling discharge. Treatment requires broad-spectrum antibiotics to cover a variety of aerobic and anaerobic organisms. Common pathogens include group A *streptococci* (early, 1–2 days postpartum), *Escherichia coli* or anaerobic organisms (days 3–4 postpartum), and *Chlamydia trachomatis* (late-onset endometritis, days 7–10 postpartum).

Commonly used treatment regimens include an intravenous combination of clindamycin (Cleocin) and gentamicin sulfate (Garamycin), which covers most aerobic and anaerobic organisms. Single-drug therapies include cephalosporins (cefotetan [Cefotan] and cefoxitin sodium [Mefoxin]) and extended-spectrum penicillins (piperacillin sodium [Pipracil] or mezlocillin sodium [Mezlin]) or ampicillin combined with a β-lactamase inhibitor. Triple therapy—ampicillin, gentamicin, and clindamycin—is used if first-line therapy fails. Antibiotics are discontinued when the patient is pain-free and afebrile for 48 hours; subsequent oral therapy is unnecessary. If a woman fails to respond to 3 to 4 days of treatment, other diagnoses should be entertained such as pelvic abscess, wound infection, septic pelvic thrombophlebitis, and pyelonephritis. Pelvic imaging using computed tomography, magnetic resonance imaging, and ultrasound may be useful in evaluation.

Deep Venous Thrombosis

Early ambulation, with assistance, has decreased the occurrence of deep venous thrombosis and pulmonary embolism. These are more common in women who have undergone cesarean delivery or those with inherited thrombophilias. Doppler plethysmography is the initial diagnostic test. If pulmonary embolism is suspected, a ventilation-perfusion scan and spiral computed tomography scan are obtained. If results are inconclusive, pulmonary angiography is the most sensitive test.

Postpartum Blues and Depression

Transient, mild dysphoria is experienced by 50% to 70% of postpartum women. Symptoms include tearfulness, anxiety, irritability, and restlessness. Postpartum blues appear within the first week after delivery and usually resolve by day 10. Because this occurs so frequently, it is likely a normal postpartum event.

True postpartum depression occurs in 8% to 15% of women. This depression continues longer than is usual for postpartum blues and requires appropriate medical and psychiatric intervention. Hypothyroidism may be present with mild dysphoria; therefore, thyroid studies are suggested when evaluating women with postpartum depression. Postpartum psychosis occurs in 0.14% to 0.26% of all women. All women with psychotic symptoms require hospitalization, psychiatric consultation, and initiation of therapy. In subsequent pregnancies, there is a high incidence of recurrent postpartum depression and psychosis.

*Not FDA approved for this indication.

HOSPITAL DISCHARGE

Before hospital discharge, women must tolerate a regular diet and have a return of bladder function, particularly after regional anesthesia. Common discharge medications include prenatal vitamins, iron supplements, and analgesics. Following uncomplicated vaginal deliveries, women usually return for a check-up at 6 weeks postpartum. Commonly, after cesarean delivery, an incisional evaluation is performed 1 to 2 weeks postpartum. Women are encouraged to phone their health care provider if they experience significant vaginal bleeding or pain, temperature higher than 100.4°F, breast erythema or tenderness, serous drainage from a wound, or prolonged crying spells.

RESUSCITATION OF THE NEWBORN

method of
RONALD S. BLOOM, M.D.
University of Utah Health Science Center
Salt Lake City, Utah

The transition from fetus to neonate, involving a series of rapid and dramatic physiologic changes, goes smoothly most of the time. However, in about 10% of births the active intervention of a skilled individual or team is necessary to assist in the transition to prevent, minimize, and/or reverse asphyxia. Because the need for intervention cannot always be predicted, it is a recommendation of the Neonatal Resuscitation Program of the American Academy of Pediatrics and the American Heart Association that "at every delivery there should be at least one person whose primary responsibility is the infant and who is capable of initiating a resuscitation." In addition, "either that person or someone else who is immediately available should have the skills required to perform a complete resuscitation."

PREPARATION

The key elements associated with preparing for a resuscitation are (1) anticipation of the problem, (2) having the appropriate equipment available and in working order, and (3) having trained personnel available.

Anticipations

Not infrequently, problems that put a mother at risk of giving birth to a depressed or asphyxiated infant can be identified by a careful review of the antepartum and intrapartum record (Table 1). Identifying a high-risk situation before delivery provides time for adequate preparation. A cesarean section alone is not a high-risk indication. Only if the cesarean section involves fetal distress or other complications is there any cause for additional concern.

As much as we may desire, it is not possible to anticipate every infant who may need resuscitation. Thus, it is necessary to have the personnel and equipment available at every delivery to initiate a resuscitation along with the capabilities of following through if the initial steps are ineffective.

Equipment

Every delivery room should be fully equipped for a resuscitation in case it is necessary. The equipment must be readily available and in working order. It should not be necessary to have someone leave the delivery area to obtain equipment normally used in a resuscitation.

Personnel

It is essential to have at least one person present who is responsible for the infant and capable of initiating a resuscitation at every delivery. Either that person or others capable of completing a resuscitation should be readily available. Recognize that a full resuscitation requires at least two individuals, if not three. These individuals should be close at hand. Having them on-call at home or at some distance in the hospital is not acceptable. Adequate training involves more than going through a course and receiving a certificate of completion. The Neonatal Resuscitation Program of the American Academy of Pediatrics and the American Heart Association, and similar courses, are excellent starting points. These courses, in and of themselves, do not qualify one to assume independent responsibility. Before being given independent responsibility, an individual must work under the tutelage of experienced personnel in the delivery room.

TABLE 1. **Conditions at High Risk for Resuscitation of the Neonate**

Antepartum Risk Factors	Intrapartum Risk Factors
Previous fetal or neonatal death	Emergency cesarean section
Maternal diabetes	Pre- or post-term gestation
Chronic maternal disease	Abnormal presentation
Hypertension	Forceps- or vacuum-assisted delivery
Anemia or isoimmunization	Rupture of membranes >18 hours before delivery
Thrombocytopenia	Chorioamnionitis
Bleeding—second or third trimester	Prolonged labor >24 hours
Abnormal amniotic fluid volume	Second stage of labor >2 hours
Multiple gestation	Fetal distress
Premature rupture of membranes	Scalp pH <7.2
Size-date discrepancy	Meconium-stained amniotic fluid
Substance abuse	Fetal bradycardia or tachycardia
Fetal malformation	Decreased fetal movement
Decreased fetal activity	Prolapsed cord
No prenatal care	Abruptio placentae
Maternal age <16 or >35	Placenta previa
	Uterine tetany
	Narcotics to mother <4 hours before delivery
	Use of general anesthesia

ROLE OF THE APGAR SCORE

The purpose of the Apgar score is to objectively define the state of the infant at given periods of time after birth, usually 1 and 5 minutes, and every 5 minutes throughout a prolonged resuscitation. It is not used to determine whether or not resuscitation is needed. The initial Apgar score is not assigned until 1 minute of age, yet in many circumstances there is a need for initiating a resuscitation before 1 minute of life. Because an asphyxial episode may begin in utero and extend into the postpartum period, waiting until a 1-minute Apgar score is assigned may delay a resuscitation and increase the chances of damage in the asphyxiated infant. The decision to initiate a resuscitation is based on an ongoing assessment of the infant, not on the Apgar score.

ELEMENTS OF A RESUSCITATION

Rather than a single procedure, a resuscitation can be viewed as a series of individual elements: the initial overview, the initial steps (thermal management, positioning, suctioning, and tactile stimulation), the use of free-flow oxygen, positive-pressure ventilation (PPV), chest compression, and medications. It is not a process that inexorably moves from one element to the next. Rather, it involves an evaluation of the infant, a decision to implement a given element, and a re-evaluation, with the next decision depending on the re-evaluation (Figure 1). For most infants all that is needed is the initial overview and the initial steps. In those who require further resuscitation, PPV is usually all that is necessary. It is the unusual infant who goes on to require chest compression and medications.

Initial Overview

Many parents prefer that the infant be given to the mother immediately after birth and not placed under a radiant warmer unless it is necessary. Because most infants are vigorous, cry at birth, and breathe easily this is usually possible, if desired. It does require an initial overview of the infant to identify potential high-risk situations. If the infant has not passed meconium in utero, is term, is breathing

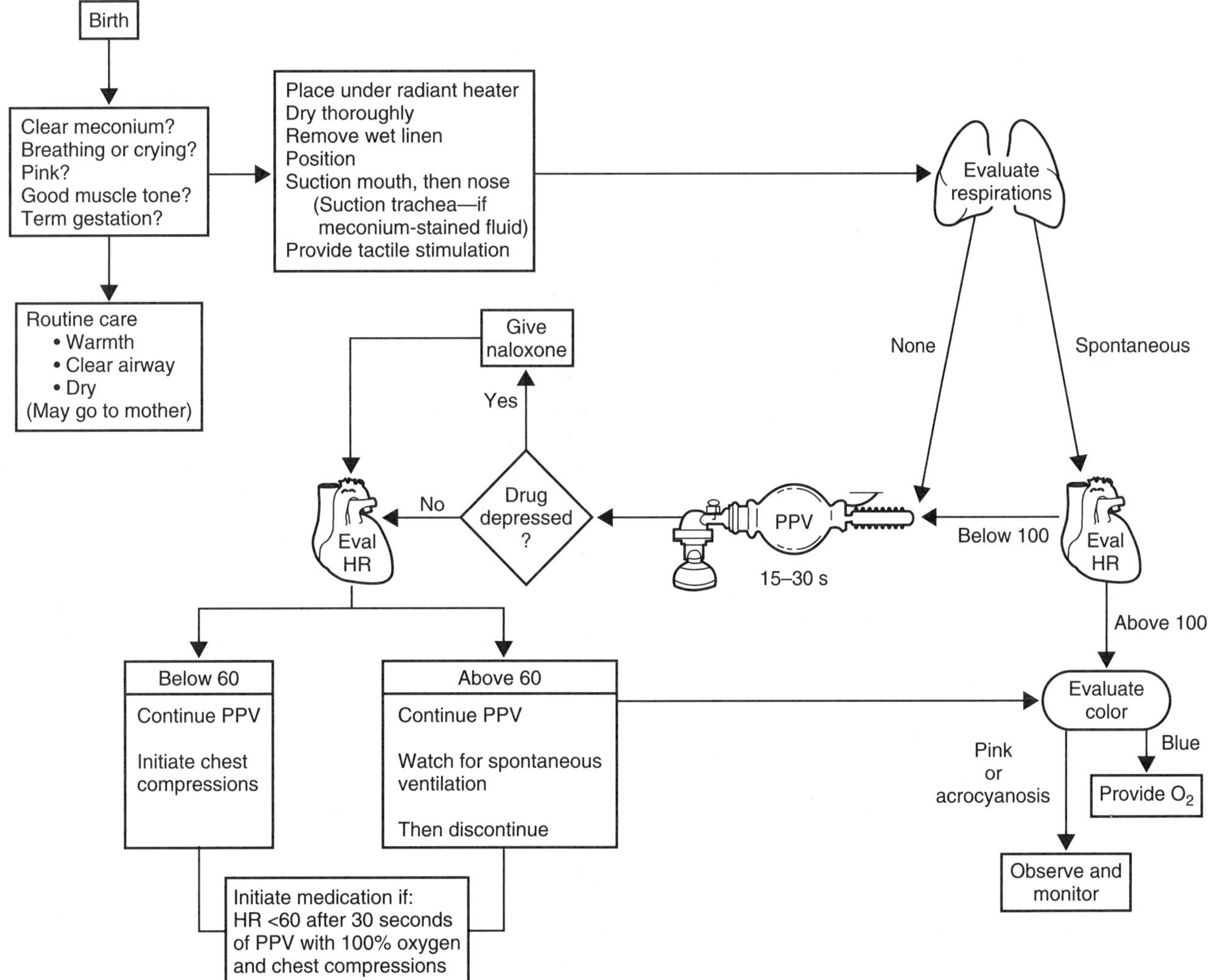

Figure 1. Overview of resuscitation in the delivery room. *Abbreviations:* HR = heart rate; PPV = positive-pressure ventilation. (Adapted from Bloom RS, Cropley C: Textbook of Neonatal Resuscitation. Dallas, American Heart Association, 1996.)

easily, is pink, has good tone, and appears normal and vigorous, it may be appropriate to hand the infant to the mother immediately after birth. A light blanket to prevent evaporative heat loss while the mother holds the infant is useful. However, cover the infant in such a way as to be able to observe for increasing distress. If the infant has passed meconium in utero; is preterm, cyanotic, or pale; has any difficulty breathing or diminished tone; or does not appear normal and vigorous, then the infant should be placed under a radiant warmer and the initial steps of the resuscitative process implemented.

Initial Steps

If not immediately given to the mother, the infant should be placed under a preheated radiant warmer and dried to prevent evaporative heat loss. The airway is cleared using a bulb syringe or suction catheter, suctioning the mouth first and then the nose. Care should be taken not to vigorously suction the infant or stimulate the posterior pharynx because this might induce bradycardia.

Drying and suctioning an infant is usually enough stimulation to initiate breathing. If, after these steps, the infant is not breathing normally, tactile stimulation using a foot slap or flick or a back rub should be done quickly and the infant's respirations and heart rate evaluated. If there is no immediate response to the additional stimulation, and the respirations are not sufficient to sustain the heart rate above 100 beats per minute, PPV should be initiated. Do not continue tactile stimulation in hopes that the infant will breath normally. Prolonged stimulation may simply prolong the time to the use of PPV and prolong the asphyxial episode.

Free-Flow Oxygen

If, after tactile stimulation, the infant is spontaneously breathing, the heart rate is greater than 100 beats per minute, and the infant is cyanotic, free-flow oxygen should be administered. A high concentration of oxygen can be given with an oxygen mask or a flow-inflating bag (anesthesia bag) and mask. When using a bag and mask to deliver free-flow oxygen, caution should be exercised to be sure the mask is not tightly placed over the face to prevent positive pressure to the lungs. Oxygen should be continuously administered until it can be shown that the oxygen concentration can be lowered and the oxygen saturation of the blood remains above 85%, or that lowering the oxygen concentration makes no difference (as with cyanotic congenital heart disease). An oxygen blender and oximeter are useful in determining the amount of oxygen the infant requires.

Positive-Pressure Ventilation

If the infant's respirations are insufficient to sustain the heart rate above 100 beats per minute, PPV with a bag/mask or bag/tube is necessary. A bag and mask, properly used, is capable of ventilating almost all infants and is the most common way to initiate PPV. Both a flow-inflating bag and a self-inflating bag with an attached oxygen reservoir are capable of delivering high concentrations of oxygen and can be used to provide PPV to infants. Regardless of type, the bag should be one designed for neonatal use with a volume of between 200 and 750 mL and generally equal to or less than 500 mL. In general, self-inflating bags are somewhat easier to use and are found in most hospitals. Many, however, prefer the flow-inflating bag because it is believed to be more responsive and permits greater control. However, the flow-inflating bag does require more practice to use than the self-inflating bag. If everyone in the delivery room with responsibilities for resuscitating the infant does not feel comfortable using a flow-inflating bag, then a self-inflating bag should also be available.

The best guide for using PPV is to use enough pressure to cause a gentle rise and fall of the chest. In general, this will require 30 cm H_2O pressure, or higher, for the first breath and pressures of 20 to 40 cm H_2O for subsequent breaths in the immature or diseased lung, with pressures of only 15 to 20 cm H_2O needed in the normal lung. Recognize, however, that the actual pressures may be higher in some infants and lower in others. These pressures are starting points. The rise and fall of the chest is the best guide to adequate pressure. If an adequate rise and fall of the chest is not achieved, the following are the most common causes: inadequate seal, incorrect positioning of the head, blockage of the airway, or insufficient positive pressure. The rate of 40 to 60 breaths per minute is the conventional recommendation when bagging without accompanying chest compression. When prolonged PPV with bag and mask is needed, an orogastric tube should be placed.

Many will feel more comfortable with an endotracheal tube in place of the mask, especially if bag and mask ventilation does not result in a chest rise or there is a prolonged need for PPV or a need for chest compression (Table 2). However, prolonged attempts at placing an endotracheal tube should be avoided. If an endotracheal tube cannot be inserted within a reasonable amount of time (20 seconds, or so) bag and mask ventilation should be used to sustain adequate ventilation between attempts. Multiple unsuccessful attempts should be abandoned unless an endotracheal tube is absolutely necessary.

TABLE 2. **Endotracheal Tube Size and Depth of Insertion**

Birth Weight (approx GA)	Tube Size	Depth of Insertion
<1000 g (<28 wk)	2.5	6.0–7.0
1000–2000 g (28–34 wk)	3.0	7.0–8.0
2000–3000 g (34–38 wk)	3.5	8.0–9.0
>3000 g (38 wk)	3.5–4.0	>9

Abbreviation: GA = gestational age.

Chest Compression

If after 30 seconds of PPV with 100% oxygen and adequate chest rise the heart rate remains low, chest compressions will be needed. The current recommendations are to initiate chest compressions when the heart rate is below 60 beats per minute. Compression of the chest should occur over the lower third of the sternum, just below an imaginary line drawn between the nipples. Each compression should depress the sternum about one third of the anteroposterior diameter of the chest. Compressions should occur 90 times per minute with a ventilation interposed between every third compression. Care should be taken not to ventilate at the same time a chest compression is occurring. If done correctly, the infant will receive 30 ventilations per minute and 90 chest compressions per minute. Within a 2-second period, three compressions and one ventilation would occur.

Once the heart rate has risen to 60 beats per minute, chest compressions can be stopped. If the heart rate remains below 60 beats per minute after 30 seconds of PPV and chest compressions, medications will be required.

Medication

Medication should be used when in spite of PPV and chest compression the heart rate continues to be below 60 beats per minute. Depending on the drug, medications can be administered through an umbilical venous catheter or an endotracheal tube. If an umbilical venous catheter is used, it should be inserted just below the skin. The catheter should be inserted into the umbilical vein until free flow of blood is obtained when the syringe is gently aspirated. This is usually an insertion length of 2 to 4 cm in a cord, which has been cut 1 to 2 cm above the skin. If blood cannot easily be withdrawn from the catheter, it is probably wedged in the liver and should be withdrawn and replaced, preventing direct infusion into the liver. An overview of the medications, including their concentrations, dosages, routes, and precautions, is presented in Table 3.

Epinephrine

Epinephrine is the first drug to be used when chest compressions and PPV do not result in an adequate heart rate. It can be given by means of the umbilical vein catheter or, if venous access has not been established, through the endotracheal tube.

Volume Expanders

Although most asphyxiated infants are not hypovolemic, there are a few circumstances in which volume expanders may be helpful. In the acute circumstance when, after adequate ventilation and oxygenation have been established, poor capillary filling persists, and there is evidence or suspicion of blood loss with signs of hypovolemia, volume expanders should be given. The volume expander of choice is normal saline or lactated Ringer's solution. Previously, 5% albumin was recommended, but increasing data indicate that not only does it not seem to offer an advantage but it may also be associated with some disadvantages. The best volume expander, although rarely available, is whole O-negative blood crossmatched against the mother's blood. With enough notice of an impending problem, this may be attainable.

Sodium Bicarbonate

There may be instances in prolonged resuscitations when a severe metabolic acidosis is suspected or proven when it is reasonable to give sodium bicarbonate. However, this should only be done after establishment of adequate ventilation.

Naloxone (Narcan)

If an infant's respirations are depressed because of a narcotic analgesic within 4 hours of delivery, naloxone may be useful. To ensure a rapid onset of action, it is best administered via an umbilical vein catheter or the endotracheal tube, rather than by intramuscular injection. Recognize, however, that the duration of action of the narcotic may exceed that of naloxone. Thus, the naloxone may wear off before the narcotic, permitting the infant to slip back into respiratory depression. Repeated doses of naloxone may be necessary. The use of naloxone in a mother who is a chronic narcotic user is somewhat dangerous because it may trigger acute withdrawal and seizures in the infant.

MANAGEMENT OF MECONIUM

If there is meconium in the amniotic fluid, the obstetrician should suction the oropharynx and naso-

TABLE 3. **Medications**

Medication	Dose	Delivery	Route
Epinephrine	0.1–0.3 mL/kg (1:10:000 solution)	Rapidly	ET, UV
Volume expanders: normal saline or lactated Ringer's or whole blood	10 mL/kg	Over 5–10 minutes	UV, IV
Sodium bicarbonate	2 mEq/kg	Slowly—1 mEq/kg/min	UV
Naloxone	0.1 mg/kg	Rapidly	ET, UV, IV Can be given IM or SC—onset is delayed

Abbreviations: ET = endotracheal; IM = intramuscular; IV = intravenous; SC = subcutaneous; UV = umbilical vein.

pharynx after the head is delivered and before the shoulders are delivered. The next actions depend on the state of the infant after birth. If the infant is depressed, direct suctioning of the trachea should be done by endotracheal intubation regardless of whether the meconium is thick or thin. If the infant is vigorous (strong respiratory effort, good muscle tone, heart rate of greater than 100 beats per minute), continue with the intital steps. There is no compelling evidence that direct suctioning of the trachea in the vigorous infant provides any advantages.

When a depressed infant who has passed meconium is intubated and direct suctioning is applied, the suction should not be applied for more than 5 seconds. If no meconium is retrieved the first time, do not repeat the process. However, if meconium is retrieved, re-intubate and suction the infant again if there is no bradycardia. If the infant is bradycardic, you may choose to provide PPV without repeat suctioning.

CARE OF THE HIGH-RISK NEWBORN

method of
SUSAN W. AUCOTT, M.D., and
MARILEE C. ALLEN, M.D.
The Johns Hopkins University School of Medicine
Baltimore, Maryland

The neonate, at the time of birth, is undergoing a unique process of transition from the intrauterine environment to extrauterine life. Fluid-filled lungs must rapidly absorb fetal lung fluid and begin providing an appropriate surface for gas exchange. The fetal circulatory pattern must make a rapid transition to extrauterine circulation from directing oxygenated blood from the placenta across the ductus venosus, into the inferior vena cava, and through the foramen ovale and thus into the systemic circulation. This change in pattern requires relaxation of the pulmonary vascular bed to allow adequate blood flow to the lungs and closure of the ductus arteriosus. Additionally, the infant must begin to mobilize its endogenous glucose stores and maintain thermoregulation. Generally, these transitions occur smoothly. In high-risk situations, however, alterations in the normal transition physiology can lead to compromise in the neonate and thus require intervention.

NEWBORN ASSESSMENT

History

Historical data can be essential in the anticipation and evaluation of many conditions in the newborn, and assessment of this begins with the maternal history. Maternal age, parity, past obstetric history, underlying medical problems, and the family history may have direct implications for the current pregnancy. Likewise, the pregnancy history itself yields insight into many issues that directly affect fetal growth and well-being. For example, maternal use of drugs, alcohol, or tobacco can have direct effect on the fetus. Insulin-dependent diabetes mellitus can affect the pregnancy at many stages: increasing the risk of malformations, affecting fetal growth, and increasing the risk in the newborn for multiple complications such as hypoglycemia, polycythemia, hypertrophic cardiomyopathy, and hyperbilirubinemia. The birth history can also provide information regarding risk factors for problems such as sepsis, birth injury, hypoxic-ischemic encephalopathy (HIE), and respiratory distress or apnea secondary to maternal medication.

Apgar Scores

The initial assessment of an infant's transition to extrauterine life is done in the first minutes of life by using the Apgar score. This scoring system, designed by Dr. Virginia Apgar, assesses five components: heart rate, respiratory effort, muscle tone, reflex irritability, and skin color (Table 1). Each component is awarded 0 to 2 points, for a highest possible score of 10. The score is calculated at 1 minute of life and again at 5 minutes. If the score remains 6 or less, additional scores are calculated every 5 minutes until the score reaches 6 or more. The 1-minute score reflects the infant's need for resuscitation, whereas subsequent scores reflect the infant's ongoing transition or response to resuscitation.

Physical Examination

The initial physical examination provides critical information for care of the newborn. Assessing infant size, including birth weight, head circumference, and length, in conjunction with a gestational age assessment such as the revised Ballard examination, gives insight into the infant's condition, allows anticipation of specific complications, and can direct diagnostic evaluation. By comparing the three growth parameters with normative curves for gestational age, one can determine whether the infant's size is appropriate, small (<10th percentile), or large (>90th percentile) for gestational age. Infants small for gestational age are at higher risk for complications such as hypothermia, hypoglycemia, and polycythemia. Likewise, the underlying etiology of their small size may have far-reaching implications. Infants who are symmetrically small have height, weight, and head circumference all less than the 10th percentile, which could be due to a congenital infection or an underlying genetic disorder. Those who are asymmetrically growth restricted have weight most severely affected with more appropriate head growth, which could represent uteroplacental insufficiency resulting from maternal conditions such as hypertension or preeclampsia. Infants large

TABLE 1. **Components of the Apgar Score**

Component	0	1	2
Heart rate	Absent	<100 beats per minute	>100 beats per minute
Respiratory effort	Apneic	Shallow, irregular, gasping	Vigorous cry
Reflex irritability	Absent	Grimace	Active avoidance
Muscle tone	Flaccid	Weak, passive	Active movement
Skin color	Pale, cyanotic	Pale, acrocyanotic	Pink

for gestational age are at increased risk for hypoglycemia and birth injury. Causes of infants being large for gestational age include maternal diabetes, maternal obesity, or familial factors.

Accurate assessment of gestational age is essential for determining whether an infant's growth is appropriate or not. Maternal dates may not be known or may conflict with ultrasound dating. By performing a Ballard examination, which evaluates the maturity of physical as well as neurologic characteristics, an assessment of gestational age can be made (Figure 1). The Ballard examination becomes less accurate in extreme prematurity and in post-term infants.

In addition to assessing growth, the physical examination in a newborn infant should focus on excluding malformations. Recognition of patterns of malformations may allow classification of the infant's condition into a genetic disorder or syndrome, which provides important information regarding prognosis and associated problems not yet appreciated. Early recognition of some conditions may allow for simplification of treatment. For example, congenital hip dislocation, when diagnosed in the newborn period, can be treated by positioning with a harness. If not recognized until later in infancy, surgical correction becomes necessary.

SPECIFIC PROBLEMS OF HIGH-RISK INFANTS

Respiratory

The evaluation of pulmonary processes in the newborn period can be complicated by the normal physiologic transitions that must occur at the time of birth. The infant must expand fluid-filled lungs, subsequently absorb the remaining fluid, and make a transition from the fetal circulatory pattern to a mature circulatory pattern. Signs of respiratory difficulty in newborns include grunting, nasal flaring, intercostal retractions, tachypnea (respiratory rate greater than 60 breaths per minute), cyanosis, and apnea. Mild grunting or flaring may occur in the first hour of life in otherwise healthy infants, but it should not persist or be associated with other signs of distress. When infants have respiratory symptoms, particularly cyanosis or tachypnea, it can be difficult to distinguish pulmonary from cardiac pathology. A chest radiograph may be helpful, with an enlarged or irregular cardiac shadow being consistent with cardiac pathol-

Neuromuscular Maturity

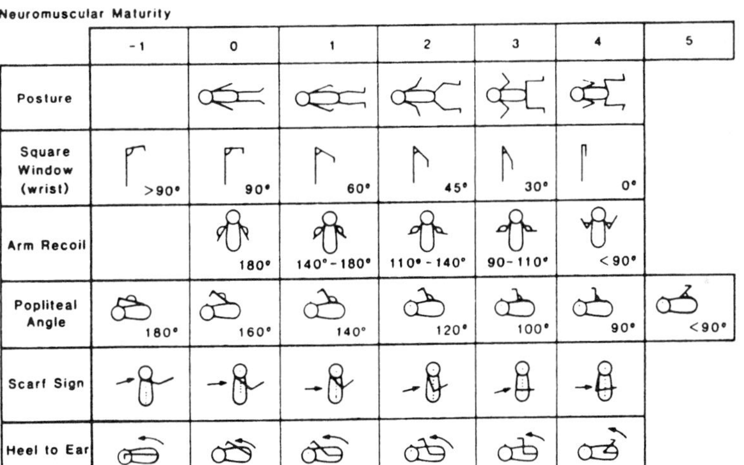

Physical Maturity

	-1	0	1	2	3	4	5
Skin	sticky friable transparent	gelatinous red, translucent	smooth pink, visible veins	superficial peeling &/or rash. few veins	cracking pale areas rare veins	parchment deep cracking no vessels	leathery cracked wrinkled
Lanugo	none	sparse	abundant	thinning	bald areas	mostly bald	
Plantar Surface	heel-toe 40-50 mm: -1 <40 mm: -2	>50mm no crease	faint red marks	anterior transverse crease only	creases ant. 2/3	creases over entire sole	
Breast	imperceptible	barely perceptible	flat areola no bud	stippled areola 1-2mm bud	raised areola 3-4mm bud	full areola 5-10mm bud	
Eye/Ear	lids fused loosely: -1 tightly: -2	lids open pinna flat stays folded	sl. curved pinna; soft; slow recoil	well-curved pinna; soft but ready recoil	formed & firm instant recoil	thick cartilage ear stiff	
Genitals male	scrotum flat, smooth	scrotum empty faint rugae	testes in upper canal rare rugae	testes descending few rugae	testes down good rugae	testes pendulous deep rugae	
Genitals female	clitoris prominent labia flat	prominent clitoris small labia minora	prominent clitoris enlarging minora	majora & minora equally prominent	majora large minora small	majora cover clitoris & minora	

Maturity Rating

score	weeks
-10	20
-5	22
0	24
5	26
10	28
15	30
20	32
25	34
30	36
35	38
40	40
45	42
50	44

Figure 1. Expanded New Ballard Score. (From Ballard JL, Khoury JC, Wedig K, et al: New Ballard Score, expanded to include extremely premature infants. J Pediatr 119:417–423, 1991.)

ogy, or the pulmonary infiltrates of pneumonia, respiratory distress syndrome (RDS), or meconium aspiration can suggest a pulmonic process. When the etiology remains unclear, a hyperoxia test is indicated. The infant is placed in 100% oxygen, and an arterial blood gas determination is obtained. If the oxygen level is less than 100 mm Hg, significant right-to-left shunting is present and suggests cyanotic heart disease or persistent pulmonary hypertension. An oxygen level of greater than 150 mm Hg is consistent with a pulmonary process causing the oxygen requirement. Levels of 100 to 150 mm Hg are equivocal and cannot distinguish between pulmonary and cardiac causes.

A common manifestation of respiratory difficulties is underlying hypoxia. Providing oxygen frequently alleviates the symptoms. Assessment of adequate oxygenation can be accomplished noninvasively by a pulse oximeter, with normal values in the first hour of life in the low 90s, which subsequently rise to the upper 90s. When measured directly, Pa_{O_2} values are 50 to 60 mm Hg at birth and rise to 70 to 90 mm Hg. Repeated sampling of arterial blood can be facilitated by placement of an umbilical arterial catheter. Umbilical arterial catheters can lead to complications, including vasospasm causing loss of perfusion to the lower extremities, clot formation resulting in hypertension, poor renal blood flow or poor blood flow to the lower extremities, and acute blood loss with disconnection or severing of the line. These risks must be weighed against the need for frequent monitoring in an acutely ill infant.

When respiratory distress persists despite provision of oxygen, further support is indicated, particularly in the presence of ongoing hypoxia or hypercarbia. Continuous positive airway pressure can be provided via nasal prongs in conjunction with oxygen. With failure of continuous positive airway pressure to improve ventilation or oxygenation or in the presence of inadequate respiratory effort, assisted ventilation is required. Positive-pressure ventilation is most commonly used in newborns. A disadvantage of assisted ventilation, especially over prolonged periods, is the resultant barotrauma to the lungs. Another form of assisted ventilation is high-frequency ventilation, which allows improved ventilation with lower mean airway pressure and thus less barotrauma.

Transient Tachypnea of the Newborn. A common cause of respiratory symptoms on the first day of life is transient tachypnea of the newborn (TTN). Delayed resorption of amniotic fluid in the lungs impedes adequate gas exchange. The infant has tachypnea, grunting, flaring, retractions, and hypoxia shortly after birth. The history is frequently remarkable for either birth by caesarean section or precipitous vaginal delivery. The infant may have mild symptoms and require only oxygen supplementation, or significant distress may be present and require assisted ventilation. A chest radiograph is not specific, and findings may be indistinguishable from the diffuse infiltrates of pneumonia. Frequently, infants with TTN will have fluid in the right major fissure. The hallmark of TTN is that the symptoms resolve in 24 to 48 hours, and the radiograph returns to normal in the same period. No long-term sequelae are associated with TTN.

Respiratory Distress Syndrome. The most common cause of respiratory problems in preterm infants is RDS which results from pulmonary immaturity and lack of adequate surfactant production. RDS occurs with increasing frequency at decreasing gestational ages. Other risk factors include maternal diabetes and perinatal asphyxia. Infants have respiratory symptoms consisting of tachypnea, grunting, flaring, retracting, and cyanosis either immediately after delivery or within 6 hours of birth. The symptoms can progress and worsen over the first 72 hours of life before improving. Chest radiography can show a hazy, diffuse infiltrate described as a ground-glass appearance, with air bronchograms. Optimally, treatment begins prenatally with administration of glucocorticoids to the mother 24 to 48 hours before delivery. This therapy hastens lung maturity, thus decreasing the incidence of RDS. Postnatally, appropriate support of ventilation and oxygenation must be established. Surfactant administration can decrease the severity of RDS and significantly decreases mortality. It can be given prophylactically in the delivery room, or it can be administered as rescue therapy after documenting the presence of RDS. The disadvantage of surfactant therapy is that it requires placement of an endotracheal tube for administration and can be associated with transient hypoxia or bradycardia during administration. The effect is additive when both antenatal steroids and postnatal surfactant are used. The complications of RDS relate primarily to the need for mechanical ventilation and include pneumothorax, pulmonary interstitial emphysema, and bronchopulmonary dysplasia (BPD).

Bronchopulmonary Dysplasia/Chronic Lung Disease. The combination of oxygen toxicity and barotrauma, particularly when imposed on premature infants, can result in neonatal chronic lung disease or BPD. The original description of BPD occurred after the introduction of mechanical ventilation for the treatment of preterm infants with RDS and applies to all patients who remain oxygen dependent at 28 days of life after mechanical ventilation and have persistent abnormalities on their chest radiograph. With the improved survival of very low birth weight infants, more infants require prolonged mechanical ventilation because of other complications of prematurity such as apnea. This trend has led to a significant increase in a milder form of chronic lung disease despite the use of surfactant. Consequently, a different definition is used in an attempt to describe infants who truly have underlying lung disease, specifically, any infant with a persistent oxygen requirement at 36 weeks' postconceptional age. With either definition, chronic lung disease becomes more prevalent with decreasing birth weight but can occur in any infant who requires mechanical ventilation. The administration of steroids in the presence of

BPD has produced improvement in lung function and facilitates weaning from the ventilator, but it has not enabled a change in the duration of oxygen therapy. The optimal age for starting treatment and the optimal dose schedule and length of treatment are still not clear, with many different protocols being used. The short-term benefits of improved lung function must be weighed against the side effects of the steroids, which include hypertension, hyperglycemia, and poor growth. More recently, concerns of adverse neurologic outcome as a result of poor brain growth have been raised. Mortality in infants with severe BPD is higher than in preterm infants of similar gestational age and can be due to respiratory failure, superimposed infection, or cor pulmonale. Long-term outcomes include an increase in airway hyperreactivity and increased neurodevelopmental impairment.

Pneumothorax. Extrapulmonary extravasation of air occurs more frequently in the neonatal period than at any other time of life. Spontaneous pneumothorax is seen in approximately 1% of all live births. A pneumothorax can be a result of underlying pulmonary pathology, such as pneumonia, meconium aspiration syndrome, or RDS. It can also result from the barotrauma of assisted ventilation on the use of high peak inspiratory pressure during vigorous resuscitation at birth. An infant with a pneumothorax has tachypnea, which may be accompanied by grunting or cyanosis. On physical examination, breath sounds are decreased over the affected side, and the cardiac apex may be shifted. Transillumination can be useful for acutely diagnosing a pneumothorax, with confirmation by chest radiography. Evacuation of a pneumothorax by placement of a chest tube is required if the pneumothorax is under tension or is compromising the infant's ability to ventilate.

Meconium Aspiration Syndrome. Term infants exposed to hypoxic stress in utero may pass meconium before birth and thereby contaminate the amniotic fluid. If hypoxia persists, fetal gasping can occur and draw the meconium-stained fluid into the pharynx and lungs. If further hypoxia has not occurred, the meconium lies predominately in the nose and mouth. When meconium-stained fluid is noted before delivery, the obstetrician suctions the mouth and nose after delivery of the head to prevent the fluid from being drawn into the lungs with the first breaths. Endotracheal suctioning should be done when the infant is depressed and needs resuscitation. Despite these preventive efforts, meconium-stained fluid can enter the lungs, most commonly as a result of in utero fetal gasping. The infant may initially appear well, but symptoms of tachypnea, cyanosis, grunting, and retractions generally develop in the first few hours of life. A chest radiograph may show coarse, patchy infiltrates, frequently with hyperinflation. Treatment consists of respiratory support to maintain adequate oxygenation and ventilation.

Persistent Pulmonary Hypertension of the Newborn. Persistent pulmonary hypertension of the newborn can occur as a primary process or as a complication of other pulmonary processes, such as pneumonia, meconium aspiration syndrome, or congenital diaphragmatic hernia. The normal transition at birth from a fetal circulatory pattern to mature pattern requires a decrease in pulmonary vascular resistance, with subsequent closure of the ductus arteriosus and foramen ovale. This transition is facilitated by air entry into the lungs with a resultant increase in oxygenation, which acts to decrease pulmonary vascular resistance and constrict the ductus. When adequate oxygenation does not occur because of the underlying pulmonary process, pulmonary vascular resistance remains high and a right-to-left shunt occurs across the foramen ovale and through the patent ductus arteriosus. This complication further aggravates the hypoxia, thus resulting in a vicious cycle. Pulmonary vascular pressure remains systemic or suprasystemic. Treatment of persistent pulmonary hypertension includes respiratory support, initially with 100% oxygen to improve oxygenation. Hypotension increases the right-to-left shunt and worsens the hypoxia, so adequate blood pressure must be maintained. Another stimulus for relaxation of the pulmonary vascular bed is alkalosis, which can be accomplished metabolically by giving sodium bicarbonate or with mechanical hyperventilation to drive the $PaCO_2$ down. Hyperventilation with $PaCO_2$ value below 20 mm Hg should be avoided to prevent constriction of cerebral blood flow in an already compromised infant. Additional therapies for persistent pulmonary hypertension in the newborn include nitric oxide, a potent vasodilator, which when inhaled acts selectively on the pulmonary vascular bed. Surfactant has also been used to improve the underlying pulmonary pathology.

Apnea. Apnea is defined as a period during which respiration ceases for at least 10 to 15 seconds and may be associated with cyanosis, pallor, or bradycardia. Apnea must be distinguished from periodic breathing, which occurs in immature infants and consists of pauses in respiration lasting 5 to 10 seconds, followed by 10 to 15 seconds of rapid respiration. Periodic breathing is not a pathologic process and resolves with age. Apnea can be a sign of a systemic process, or it may represent a primary process. Apnea has been described as a symptom in many illnesses, such as sepsis, hypoxia, anemia, seizures, and hypoglycemia, or it may be due to narcotics given to the mother or baby. In a preterm infant in whom these causes of apnea have been excluded, the episodes may be due to apnea of prematurity. Treatment with methylxanthines such as theophylline or caffeine improves apnea by inducing a central stimulatory effect in addition to enhancing diaphragmatic contractility. Apnea of prematurity decreases in frequency with advancing postnatal age.

Cardiology

During the first week of life, the cardiovascular system is undergoing dynamic changes. Pulmonary vascular resistance continues to gradually drop, and the ductus arteriosus constricts and closes, generally on the third day of life. Often, murmurs heard on the first day of life are due to these dynamic processes rather than cardiac pathology. In contrast, significant heart disease may be masked by ductal flow and not become symptomatic until the ductus arteriosus closes. Examples of ductal-dependent lesions are hypoplastic left heart syndrome and critical coarctation of the aorta. Other forms of congenital heart disease that result in excessive left-to-right flow, such as a large ventriculoseptal defect or an endocardial cushion defect, will not produce signs of congestive heart failure until 1 to 2 weeks of age when pulmonary vascular resistance has decreased and allows significantly increased pulmonary flow. Murmurs caused by left-to-right shunting may not be heard on the initial examination and only become apparent after 2 to 3 days of life. Additional features of the cardiac examination, such as a hyperactive precordium or discrepancy of pulses between the upper and lower extremities, are helpful in determining the presence of an underlying cardiac lesion. Cyanotic heart disease is manifested immediately after birth with cyanosis that is unresponsive to the administration of oxygen. Evaluation of possible congenital heart disease should include a hyperoxia test if cyanotic, four extremity blood presence measurements, a chest radiograph to assess cardiac size and the pulmonary vasculature, an electrocardiogram to evaluate the axis, and an echocardiogram.

Patent Ductus Arteriosus. In preterm infants, the ductus arteriosus can reopen, particularly in the presence of fluid overload, hypoxia, or acidosis. Clinically, the infant may have an increasing oxygen requirement, hepatomegaly, tachypnea, and bounding pulses. A wide pulse pressure is noted on blood pressure measurement. A more silent form may occur, with the only manifestation being increased frequency of apneas. The classic machine-like murmur associated with a patent ductus arteriosus in older children is not present. Frequently, a soft systolic murmur is heard along the left sternal border. The murmur may only be heard intermittently. Conservative therapy with fluid restriction may allow some ducts to close, but the closure is often only transient. Indomethacin promotes duct closure and is most effective in the first 2 weeks of life. Indomethacin (Indocin) is contraindicated in acute, severe intraventricular hemorrhage (IVH), in thrombocytopenia, or with evidence of poor renal function. Side effects include decreased urine output and an increased risk of bleeding. In term infants, a patent ductus arteriosus is often asymptomatic and can be monitored for spontaneous closure. When symptoms persist in term or preterm infants despite medical treatment, surgical ligation is required.

Gastroenterology/Nutrition

Fluid and nutrition play an important role in managing an infant. In the first days of life, the focus is on providing appropriate fluid intake with attention to glucose balance. Fluid needs vary depending on the infant's gestational age and day of life. Immature infants have increased insensible losses caused by increased water loss through the immature skin. In contrast, newborns of all gestational ages on the first day of life have a lower glomerular filtration rate, which slowly increases over the first week of life. Weight loss is expected in all infants, for 2 to 3 days in term infants and 5 to 7 days in preterm infants. Weight loss should not exceed 10% of the birth weight. Larger amounts of weight loss are suggestive of inadequate intake and dehydration.

Once the fluid needs have stabilized, attention must shift to providing adequate nutrition to allow growth. Infants will need 100 to 120 kcal/kg/d for growth. Underlying chronic pulmonary or cardiac disease may result in higher caloric demand and could require 120 to 150 kcal/kg/d for growth. If an infant is unable to be fed enterally as a result of either prematurity or an underlying disease process, nutrition should be provided parenterally. Hyperalimentation solutions can provide gradually increasing protein concentrations. Glucose concentrations can also be increased as tolerated. Essential fatty acids must be provided through a lipid emulsion, and fats can also be used to increase caloric intake. Providing parenteral nutrition can lead to complications. Intravenous access with the resultant risk of infection and thrombosis is necessary, and prolonged exposure to hyperalimentation can lead to cholestatic liver disease and possible liver failure.

Optimal nutrition is best provided enterally. It allows higher caloric intake with less risk of fluid overload and avoids the need for intravenous lines. In preterm infants and any term infants who have experienced hypoxia or decreased perfusion, the gastrointestinal tract may not be able to fully digest and absorb the nutrition. When respiratory and cardiac issues have stabilized, enteral feeding is slowly introduced. Many choices are available for providing nutrition. Breast milk provides an excellent source of nutrition along with the addition of maternal antibodies. When breast milk is not available, a variety of commercial formulas can be used and are available as a standard formula or a premature formula. Standard formulas and breast milk provide 20 cal/p 30 mL, whereas preterm formulas have 24 cal/p 30 mL. When using breast milk in preterm infants, fortifiers can be added to increase the caloric density and calcium intake.

Intestinal Obstruction. Infants with intestinal obstruction may have a prenatal history remarkable for polyhydramnios. The fetus normally swallows amniotic fluid, but such swallowing is impaired in an infant with obstruction. Large amounts of oral secretions may be noted in the delivery room. The infant may have emesis and poor feeding shortly after birth. Placement of a nasogastric tube is helpful to decompress the stomach and also assesses the patency of the esophagus. A radiograph showing the tube curled in the upper part of the thorax would suggest esophageal atresia. The classic radiograph of a "double bubble" consisting of a dilated stomach and a dilated proximal duodenum indicates duodenal atresia. Other forms of obstruction include atresia at other sites in the gastrointestinal tract, malrotation with volvulus, meconium ileus, and meconium plug syndrome. Meconium ileus, caused by inspissated meconium, is associated with cystic fibrosis. Meconium plug syndrome, also caused by tenacious plugs of meconium, is diagnosed and treated with a diatrizoate meglumine (Gastrograffin) enema. The hyperosmolar solution allows loosening and passage of the plugs. This syndrome can be associated with cystic fibrosis, but it is more commonly associated with Hirschsprung's disease. All other causes of obstruction require surgical intervention.

Malrotation. When the gastrointestinal tract is formed with inadequate stability of the duodenum, the intestines have increased mobility and can become twisted around the blood supply. This twisting, or volvulus, can lead to ischemia and subsequent necrosis of the bowel if unrecognized. Infants with malrotated intestines can be affected at any time by volvulus. The onset of emesis, particularly when bilious, should alert one to this possibility. Symptoms can appear intermittently or be present shortly after birth. Because of the severity of the outcome, infants with bilious emesis should have an upper gastrointestinal series to assess the position of the duodenum. Malrotation with volvulus requires prompt surgical intervention to minimize the gut ischemia and avoid gut necrosis with a resultant short bowel.

Necrotizing Enterocolitis. Necrotizing enterocolitis (NEC) is a severe bowel disease that can lead to necrosis, perforation, death, or subsequent short-bowel syndrome. NEC is a multifactorial disease that results in bacterial invasion of the intestinal mucosa with gas production. This intramucosal air is called pneumatosis and is the classic diagnostic feature of NEC seen on radiography. More ominous radiographic signs include portal air and pneumoperitoneum, an indication of perforation. Risk factors for NEC include prematurity, previous history of hypoxia or poor gut perfusion, and enteral feeding. Ninety-five percent of all cases of NEC occur in infants who have been fed. The greatest risk is seen in infants who have had their feeding advanced by increments of more than 20 mL/kg/d. The enteral nutrition provides a substrate for bacterial overgrowth.

Clinically, infants may be seen acutely with grossly bloody stools, abdominal distention, and tenderness. More subtle signs and symptoms may include apnea and bradycardia, guaiac-positive stools, and the presence of poor gastric motility manifested by residual gastric contents after feeding. Signs of sepsis such as hypotension, poor perfusion, and lethargy may also occur. Laboratory findings can include neutropenia, thrombocytopenia, anemia, and metabolic acidosis. Treatment of the infant requires stopping all feeding, assessing for sepsis, and treating with antibiotics, with attention to coverage for gastrointestinal flora. Additional supportive care is given as required for stabilization. Frequently, infants require intubation because of hypoventilation resulting from the abdominal distention. Surgery is indicated only when the infant has evidence of perforation or a necrotic bowel. Persistent acidosis and thrombocytopenia despite improving clinical status may be due to a necrotic bowel. Long-term complications include malabsorption, failure to thrive, strictures, and short-bowel syndrome when extensive surgical resections have been required.

Hematology

Anemia. Normal hematocrit values range from 45% to 60% in term infants and from 40% to 50% in preterm infants. Infants born with lower levels are anemic, most commonly because of either acute blood loss or hemolysis. Acute blood loss can result from placenta previa, abruption, cord accidents, or delayed cord damping with the infant elevated from the placenta. Before delivery, the infant can hemorrhage into the placenta and maternal circulation and thereby create a fetal-maternal hemorrhage. This complication should be suspected when the infant has evidence of acute blood loss but no other history of blood loss at delivery. The diagnosis is made by performing a Kleihauer-Betke test on the mother, which quantitates fetal blood on a maternal smear. Hemolytic anemia may be seen at birth, such as with Rh incompatibility, or it may develop in the first 24 to 48 hours of life in other forms of blood group incompatibility. Knowing the maternal blood type and antibody screen results allows one to anticipate significant hemolytic processes. Mothers with the O blood type are at risk for having babies with ABO incompatibility. Additional minor blood group antibodies such as Lewis or Kell antibodies are usually detected on the maternal antibody screen. In all mothers with the O blood type and those with positive antibody screens, cord blood should be sent to determine the infant's blood type in addition to performing a direct Coombs test. A positive direct Coombs test indicates the presence of antibodies in the infant that place the infant at risk for hemolysis. A high reticulocyte count is also suggestive of a hemolytic process. Treatment depends on the severity of the anemia and the associated rise in bilirubin.

Polycythemia. Infants exposed to chronic hypoxia in utero may respond by increasing their hematocrit. This response occurs most commonly in growth-restricted infants and infants of diabetic mothers. A hematocrit greater than 70 in an asymptomatic infant or a hematocrit greater than 65 in a symptomatic infant requires intervention. Symptoms include respiratory distress, cyanosis, hypoglycemia, lethargy, poor feeding, or apnea. The symptoms result from the high viscosity of the blood. The reason for treatment is to avoid the risk of blood vessel occlusion and ischemia. Treatment consists of performing a partial volume, or dilutional, exchange to decrease the hematocrit acutely.

Thrombocytopenia. A platelet count of less than 100,000 denotes thrombocytopenia. The risk of spontaneous hemorrhage becomes a concern when the platelet count is less than 20,000. A theoretical concern of an increased risk of IVH in preterm infants occurs at platelet counts of 20,000 to 50,000. Thrombocytopenia at birth may be caused by a variety of conditions. Infections, particularly bacterial sepsis, can lead to disseminated intravascular coagulation with thrombocytopenia. Autoimmune thrombocytopenia in the mother, such as idiopathic thrombocytopenic purpura, can cause antibody passage across the placenta with resultant thrombocytopenia in the fetus. These infants are at risk of spontaneous IVH in utero. The trauma of the birth process can also place the infant at risk for hemorrhage, particularly intracranial hemorrhage. Maternal treatment with intravenous immune globulin can decrease the antibody load before delivery. Cesarean delivery is frequently recommended to minimize trauma to the infant. Isoimmune thrombocytopenia occurs in mothers who do not express the platelet antigen PLA-1. When the fetus is PLA-1 antigen–positive, the maternal antibodies will cause thrombocytopenia in the fetus, again with the risk of hemorrhage in utero or at delivery. Unlike mothers with idiopathic thrombocytopenic purpura who have a low platelet count, mothers who are PLA-1 antigen–negative are asymptomatic with normal platelet counts and are not aware of their platelet antibody status before birth.

Infants in whom thrombocytopenia is diagnosed should be evaluated for sepsis. Additionally, urine should be sent for cytomegalovirus culture. Maternal platelet counts are reviewed to look for undiagnosed idiopathic thrombocytopenic purpura. If PLA-1 antibodies are suspected, antibody testing on the parents should be performed. Platelet transfusions are initiated for platelet counts of less than 20,000 or for signs of bleeding such as hematuria, guaiac-positive stools, or oozing from puncture sites. In both autoimmune and isoimmune thrombocytopenia, random donor platelets may produce only a small rise in the platelet count, with a subsequent rapid fall. If ongoing platelet transfusion is required, maternal platelets provide sustained platelet levels. In most cases of thrombocytopenia, the platelet count gradually returns to normal.

Hyperbilirubinemia. Hyperbilirubinemia is clinically evident as jaundice. In newborns, jaundice is apparent when the bilirubin level is over 5 mg/dL. A transition in bilirubin metabolism occurs after birth. In utero, bilirubin is eliminated through the placenta. After birth, the onset of hepatic bilirubin metabolism and elimination is delayed. This delay causes a transient, or physiologic, hyperbilirubinemia over the first several days of life. Jaundice appears on the second or third day of life, peaks at 3 to 5 days in term infants and 5 to 7 days in preterm infants, and subsequently resolves. Levels are not generally above 15 mg/dL total and consist of unconjugated, or indirect, bilirubin. Physiologic jaundice must be distinguished from pathologic jaundice. Pathologic jaundice should be suspected when clinical jaundice (a bilirubin level of over 5 mg/dL) occurs in the first 24 hours of life, the rate of rise is greater than 5 mg/dL/d, total bilirubin levels are greater than 15 mg/dL, or the direct bilirubin level is greater than 2 mg/dL. When pathologic jaundice is suspected, total and direct bilirubin levels are measured. The level is elevated if it is greater than 5 mg/dL in the first 24 hours of life, greater than 10 mg/dL at 24 to 48 hours, or greater than 15 mg/dL at over 48 hours.

Etiologies of indirect hyperbilirubinemia can be divided into categories of increased production and decreased elimination. Bilirubin is derived from the breakdown of hemoglobin. Excess destruction of red blood cells leads to increased bilirubin production. One cause of increased red cell breakdown is hemolysis. Reviewing the maternal blood type and antibody screens can determine which infants are at risk for ABO, Rh, or other minor blood group incompatibilities. Further evidence of a hemolytic process includes a low hematocrit, high reticulocyte count, and hemolysis on a blood smear. Performing a blood type and direct Coombs test on the cord or infant blood further determines the presence of incompatibility. When a hemolytic process is suspected but the infant has no predisposing blood group and a negative Coombs test, other causes of hemolysis should be considered, such as red cell membrane and enzyme defects. When the hyperbilirubinemia appears to be nonhemolytic, other sources of excess red cell breakdown are investigated. Polycythemia can cause hyperbilirubinemia as a result of the larger red cell mass. Excessive bruising or large hematomas, particularly large cephalohematomas or IVH, can lead to hyperbilirubinemia. Liver disease that impairs bilirubin uptake or conjugation can increase serum bilirubin levels. Another cause of hyperbilirubinemia occurs in breast-fed infants. Typically, breast milk jaundice develops more gradually, peaks at 10 days, and slowly resolves. Infants are otherwise healthy appearing. Stopping breast milk intake for 24 hours with substitution of formula causes a dramatic decrease in serum bilirubin that does not generally recur after restarting breast milk feeding. Metabolic diseases such as galactosemia or hypothyroidism may be associated with hyperbilirubinemia.

High bilirubin levels can result in bilirubin crossing the blood-brain barrier and causing a form of encephalopathy known as kernicterus. This condition is associated with the later development of choreoathetoid cerebral palsy and hearing impairment. The serum bilirubin level at which kernicterus occurs is unclear. Other factors such as acidosis, hypoxia, hypoalbuminemia, and prematurity can also lead to increased permeability of the blood-brain barrier. Historically, most cases of high bilirubin levels, over 20 mg/dL, with subsequent kernicterus occurred in hemolytic disease, particularly Rh incompatibility. Preterm infants have been found to have kernicterus on autopsy at much lower levels of bilirubin, such as 10 mg/dL in extremely low birth weight infants. With the advent of RhoGAM for prevention of sensitization of Rh-negative women, the incidence of kernicterus has been significantly reduced. This finding has led many to believe that bilirubin levels over 20 mg/dL in nonhemolytic causes of hyperbilirubinemia in term infants are not associated with kernicterus.

Initial treatment for indirect hyperbilirubinemia is phototherapy. Bilirubin absorbs ultraviolet light in the blue-green wavelengths and is converted to a more water-soluble form that is excreted in the urine. Adequate hydration must be maintained because phototherapy increases insensible losses. Phototherapy is indicated for hemolytic hyperbilirubinemia with a rapid rise in bilirubin greater than 5 mg/dL/d or at bilirubin levels of 18 to 20 mg/dL in term infants with nonhemolytic disease. In hemolytic disease with rapidly rising bilirubin levels despite phototherapy, intravenous immune globulin has been shown to lessen the degree of hemolysis. When bilirubin continues to rise despite therapy and bilirubin levels are nearing those associated with kernicterus, an exchange transfusion is performed to remove both bilirubin and the antibodies involved in hemolysis. Exchange transfusions are recommended in term infants at bilirubin levels of over 25 mg/dL in nonhemolytic processes and over 20 mg/dL in hemolytic processes. In preterm infants, exchange transfusion levels are lower because of the increased permeability of the blood-brain barrier, and exchange transfusions should be considered at levels of 12 to 15 mg/dL for 500 to 1000-g infants, at levels of 15 to 18 mg/dL for 1000 to 1500-g infants, and at levels of 18 to 20 mg/dL for 1500 to 2500-g infants. The considerable risk of the procedure must be taken into account when deciding whether to perform the exchange transfusion. An arterial line or umbilical venous line is required to perform the procedure. Complications include hypocalcemia, hypoglycemia, thrombocytopenia, neutropenia, blood pressure instability, and cardiac arrest.

When hyperbilirubinemia is found to have a large direct fraction, with direct bilirubin levels greater than 2 mg/dL, a different course of treatment and evaluation must be undertaken. Direct, or conjugated, bilirubin does not cross the blood-brain barrier and thus does not pose a risk of kernicterus. Likewise, phototherapy is not effective in altering conjugated bilirubin into an excretable form and will not decrease the bilirubin level. Phototherapy causes binding of the direct bilirubin in the skin and results in a bronze color. This cosmetic problem does not harm the baby. Direct hyperbilirubinemia can be associated with urinary tract infections, so a urine culture is recommended as part of the evaluation. Liver disease, such as any viral hepatitis (A, B, C; cytomegalovirus), the presence of α_1-antitrypsin, hepatic injury from hypoxia, or a chemical hepatitis from prolonged hyperalimentation can lead to direct hyperbilirubinemia. Obstruction of the biliary tree such as by gallstones or biliary atresia can lead to direct hyperbilirubinemia.

Renal

Infants have lower glomerular filtration rates at birth that gradually increase over the first week of life. Additionally, preterm infants have immature renal function with a decreased ability to concentrate urine. These factors have direct dosing implications for any renally excreted drug. Doses must be adjusted for the degree of prematurity and age of the infant. Normal urine output for the first 24 hours in an infant can be as low as 1 mL/kg/h. Failure to void in the first 24 hours should prompt an investigation of the urinary tract and renal function.

In utero, poor urine output is manifested as decreased amniotic fluid volume. When prolonged and severe, the fetus is compressed in the uterus, unable to freely move or undergo fetal breathing movements. Contractures develop in the extremities, and lack of fetal breathing leads to pulmonary hypoplasia. The faces of such infants have a characteristic appearance, with a flattened nose and low-set ears. These findings are called Potter syndrome, which is usually lethal because of the pulmonary hypoplasia. Potter syndrome is the end result of any form of renal disease that results in minimal urine output in utero. It can also be seen in prolonged, early, ruptured membranes. Causes of minimal or no urine output in utero include renal agenesis, renal dysplasia, or urinary tract obstruction.

Poor urine output postnatally in the absence of a history of oligohydramnios is most likely due to acute tubular necrosis as a result of hypoxia or hypoperfusion of the kidneys. Clinically, the infant will be oliguric with hematuria or, occasionally, anuric and will have rising urea nitrogen and creatinine levels. Management includes support of oxygenation and perfusion to avoid further injury. Fluid intake must be restricted to compensate for the decreased urinary loss. Close monitoring of electrolytes, particularly potassium, is required. All renally excreted drugs must be monitored by serum level to ensure proper dosing. Commonly, after a period of oliguria, recovery may be preceded by polyuria. Again, fluid and electrolyte balance becomes the focus of management. Most infants have gradual recovery of renal function.

Infectious Disease

Newborn infants are particularly susceptible to a variety of infections as a result of lower levels of activity in their immune system. Additionally, preterm infants have lower levels of antibodies because most maternal antibodies are transferred in the third trimester. Infants can acquire infections prenatally via a hematogenous route through the placenta. Other infections are acquired by ascending through the vaginal canal into the uterine cavity. A maternal history of infections acquired during pregnancy such as herpes or syphilis can alert one to the risk of infection in an infant. Signs of infection in the mother at the time of birth, such as fever, high white blood cell count, or uterine tenderness, place the infant at increased risk of infection. Prolonged rupture of membranes, particularly greater than 24 hours, is associated with increasing risk of infection in the newborn. Additional signs of distress in the fetus, such as fetal tachycardia, meconium-stained fluid, or abnormal fetal heart rate patterns, can be associated with infection. After birth, sepsis can be manifested as fulminant septic shock, or it may have very subtle findings. Infants may have fever, but more commonly they are hypothermic or have temperature instability. Clinical features may include lethargy, poor feeding, irritability, tachypnea, apnea, poor perfusion, and cyanosis. These features are not specific, and infection must frequently be differentiated from a variety of other illnesses. A blood culture is essential for diagnosing bacterial sepsis, but it can be falsely negative in a newborn whose mother was treated with antibiotics more than 4 hours before delivery. A complete blood count can be helpful in distinguishing sepsis from other diseases. Normal white blood cell counts in newborns range from 5000 to 30,000. Both leukocytosis and neutropenia can be seen in sepsis, with neutropenia being a more ominous sign. A differential with a left shift or more immature neutrophil forms is associated with sepsis. Urine cultures are not generally performed in infants younger than 3 days because urinary tract infections are extremely rare in this age group. After 3 days of age, a urine culture is part of the evaluation for sepsis in infants. Chest radiographs are helpful to evaluate for pneumonia, because specific pulmonary findings are often absent on the physical examination. The criteria for performing lumbar puncture remain controversial. Meningitic signs are frequently absent in infants younger than 1 year. Several studies have reviewed historical data and found that spinal fluid cultures were positive in tandem with positive blood cultures. When a reliable blood culture has been performed, many will defer the lumbar puncture. However, in cases of invalid blood culture, such as after maternal antibiotic pretreatment, a spinal tap should be considered.

Bacterial Infection. The most common bacterial pathogens in the newborn period are group B β-hemolytic streptococci, *Escherichia coli*, and *Listeria*. All these pathogens have two clinical manifestations: early-onset sepsis and late-onset sepsis. Early-onset sepsis occurs in the first 3 days of life, the pathogen usually being acquired from the mother perinatally. Infants frequently have respiratory symptoms such as tachypnea, grunting, flaring, and retractions with cyanosis, although most do not have pneumonia as part of the illness. Additional signs of sepsis such as pallor, poor perfusion, and lethargy can develop. Meningitis is uncommon, and early-onset disease is seen more frequently in preterm than term infants. Late-onset disease occurs at 3 to 6 weeks of life. The onset is typically more insidious and characterized by poor feeding and lethargy. Sepsis can be associated with a focus, such as cellulitis, arthritis, osteomyelitis, or meningitis. No predisposition for sepsis is noted in term versus preterm infants. Group B streptococcal disease is by far the most predominant cause of bacterial sepsis, and these organisms can be cultured from 30% of all women.

Attempts to eradicate the organism from the genital tract are frequently unsuccessful because of the reservoir of the organism in the gastrointestinal tract. Identifying women colonized by group B streptococci allows obstetricians to treat these women with penicillin or ampicillin during labor, which has greatly reduced cases of group B streptococcal sepsis. Likewise, aggressive treatment of women in preterm labor with antibiotics has reduced group B streptococcal sepsis. Treatment of suspected sepsis, both early and late onset, must provide excellent coverage for streptococci, *E. coli*, and *Listeria*. When an organism is isolated, therapy can be narrowed on the basis of sensitivity results.

Viral Infection. A number of viral diseases can cause illness in the newborn period. The most severe is due to herpes simplex virus. Herpes is transmitted perinatally and typically occurs at 5 to 10 days of life. In half of all cases of neonatal herpes, the mother has no history of herpes. The highest risk of transmission to the infant occurs with primary herpes infection at the time of delivery, which may be asymptomatic. In women with a known history of genital herpes, transmission rates are very low, most likely because of previous passage of antibodies to the infant and a lower viral load. Herpes infection in infants is divided into three categories: cutaneous, disseminated, and central nervous system (CNS) disease. Infants with cutaneous disease have vesicular lesions. They frequently erupt on the presenting parts or can be at the site of a scalp electrode. The infants will otherwise appear well. Mortality is very low for cutaneous herpes simplex, but when untreated, it can progress to disseminated or CNS disease. Frequent episodes of recurrence without progression of disease are associated with increased morbidity. Disseminated herpes simplex is similar to bacterial sepsis. Only one third of infants have skin lesions at the initial examination, so the clinical picture is often confused with that of bacterial sepsis. Onset of symptoms at 5 to 10 days of life is atypical for both early- and late-onset bacterial sepsis and should thus alert one to the possibility of herpes infection. These infants often have abnormal liver function tests, evidence of disseminated intravascular coagulation, and pneumonia. Associated CNS infection may or may not be seen. Despite supportive care and treatment with acyclovir, mortality remains high at 60%. Herpes can also be manifested as an isolated meningoencephalitis. Infants may have lethargy, poor feeding, or seizures. Mortality is 15%, but significant morbidity is observed, with long-term outcomes including cerebral palsy and mental retardation.

Congenital Infection. Infections occurring in utero can have serious consequences for the developing fetus and frequently result in growth restriction, microcephaly or CNS injury, and other organ system involvement, depending on the infection. Such infections include toxoplasmosis, rubella, cytomegalovirus, herpes, and syphilis.

Neurology

Both preterm and full-term infants are vulnerable to injury to their developing CNS manifested as neurodevelopmental disability. An infant with CNS injury or malformation may have seizures, coma, abnormal muscle tone and reflexes, or various other symptoms that are nonspecific to the CNS (e.g., lethargy, irritability, feeding difficulties, apnea). A fetus with prenatal CNS injury or malformation may have perinatal depression and require resuscitation at birth, possibly leading to a mistaken diagnosis of perinatal asphyxia. On the other hand, a neonate with severe CNS injury or malformation may have few or no neonatal symptoms and not be identified until later in infancy or childhood.

Any infant with perinatal depression and specific or multiple nonspecific neurologic symptoms requires neuroimaging. Preterm infants younger than 32 to 34 weeks' gestation require serial cranial ultrasound because CNS injury may be asymptomatic, even if severe. At least three cranial ultrasounds are recommended for preterm infants: one in the first week to look for IVH, another in the second week to look for ventricular dilation, and one at 3 to 6 weeks to search for evidence of white matter injury. In both preterm and full-term infants, the neonatal neurodevelopmental examination can be used, in addition to neuroimaging, to assess the degree of risk for neurodevelopmental disability. Because many neonates recover function despite CNS injury, disability cannot be diagnosed in the neonatal period. Infants at risk for disability require careful developmental follow-up through infancy and childhood.

Periventricular, Intraventricular, and Intraparenchymal Hemorrhage. The more immature the infant, the greater the risk of CNS injury. A preterm infant's developing cerebral vasculature is more easily disrupted, and especially during labor and delivery, their immature regulatory systems are unable to prevent fluctuations in blood pressure, cerebral blood flow, and tissue oxygenation. The fragile vascular network in combination with inadequate regulatory systems leads to an increased incidence of vascular rupture, infarction, and ischemia. Recent studies have also suggested a role for cytokines released by infection or asphyxia as a cause of CNS injury in both full-term and preterm infants.

Bleeding occurs in the germinal matrix, in the choroid plexus, and into the lateral ventricles in preterm infants. If the hemorrhage is small and self-limited, it is designated a grade 1 hemorrhage. If blood is also found in the ventricles, it becomes a grade 2 IVH. If blood is filling and dilating the ventricles, it is designated a grade 3 IVH. Unilateral or bilateral venous infarction of the brain parenchyma may be associated with IVH and is called an intraparenchymal hemorrhage (IPH) or grade 4 IVH (which is a misnomer). The sickest and most immature preterm infants have a higher incidence of IVH and IPH and greater severity.

The incidence of grade 1 to 4 IVH varies widely from 15% to 45% in preterm infants younger than 32 weeks' gestation. Most (90%) hemorrhages occur in the critical first 3 days after birth. The majority are are silent, but a severe grade 3 to 4 IVH can be catastrophic, with associated pallor, hypotension, metabolic acidosis, anemia, lethargy, apnea, and a full fontanelle. IPH and grade 3 IVH are associated with a high risk of major disability (cerebral palsy and/or mental retardation, 70% to 90% with IPH and 30% to 60% with grade 3 IVH). Posthemorrhagic hydrocephalus (PHH) is a complication of IVH, with progressive ventricular dilation occurring days to weeks after the IVH. Treatment is aimed at reducing the intracranial pressure, with serial lumbar puncture, a trial of medications that decrease cerebrospinal fluid production (i.e., diuretics and acetazolamide [Diamox])* or placement of a reservoir that allows for repeated ventricular taps. The hydrocephalus resolves in as many as 50% of infants with PHH; the rest require a ventriculoperitoneal shunt. Infants recovering from NEC or other conditions that result in scarring of the bowel may require placement of a ventriculoatrial or ventriculopleural shunt. PHH is also associated with a high risk (50% to 70%) of major disability.

Maximal care should be taken with preterm infants to minimize stressors that predispose to IVH, including avoiding hypoxia, fluctuations in blood pressure, decreases in cerebral blood flow (as can occur with hypotension or hypocapnia), and sudden changes in osmolarity (as can occur with rapid infusion with sodium bicarbonate). Many centers treat extremely preterm infants with a high risk of severe IVH and IPH with prophylactic indomethacin for the first 3 days. Indomethacin should not be used in infants with persistent hypotension or unstable blood pressure because it decreases cerebral blood flow. With time, the vascular network and autoregulatory systems mature and the risk of IVH decreases significantly.

White Matter Injury. Injury to the brain's white matter generally results in necrosis, with subsequent absorption of brain parenchyma and the formation of cysts. The classic lesion of white matter injury seen on cranial ultrasound is cyst formation superior and lateral to the ventricles, called periventricular leukomalacia. This lesion may consist of one cyst or multiple cysts or large or small cysts, and it can be unilateral or bilateral. Sometimes the cysts form from injured white matter in the frontal or occipital lobes. When the injured white matter is contiguous with the ventricles, instead of cysts we see enlargement of the lateral ventricles, sometimes with very irregular edges. Ventricular dilation resulting from atrophy of brain tissue is not associated with increased intracranial pressure as is seen with PHH. White matter injury is classically seen in preterm infants 3 to 6 weeks after delivery and has been attributed to CNS ischemia. It may also be seen shortly after delivery in full-term or preterm infants, presumably caused by white matter injury in utero. Recent work suggests that infection (especially chorioamnionitis) and perhaps other insults that result in cytokine release may be an important cause of white matter injury.

*Not FDA approved for this indication.

Other than prompt treatment of hypotension and/or infection, no other method is known for treating or preventing periventricular leukomalacia.

The most common disability associated with white matter injury is spastic diplegia. The incidence of major disability is 10% to 50% if cysts are unilateral, small, and focal. Ventricular dilation, with or without IVH, carries an increased risk of disability. Large bilateral intraparenchymal cysts carry an extremely poor prognosis: as many as 50% to 100% have disability. The type and severity of disability in this group vary, but approximately 50% have severe multiple disability (severe mental retardation, disabling cerebral palsy).

Hypoxic-Ischemic Encephalopathy. HIE is the result of severe and generalized brain injury that occurs around the time of birth (antepartum, intrapartum, or postpartum) in full-term or preterm infants. Acute CNS injury followed by brain edema and swelling and release of cytokines and neurotransmitters leads to secondary CNS injury (which may be even more severe than the acute injury). Infants with HIE have injury to other organ systems as well (see Table 2) and may require life support for survival.

Sarnat and Sarnat (1976) differentiated between mild, moderate, and severe HIE in terms of signs and symptoms. Mild HIE is characterized by a hyperalert state, with jitteriness, overactive and easily elicited reflexes, and increased sympathetic function (e.g., dilated pupils, decreased gastrointestinal motility). Moderate HIE is characterized by lethargy or coma, mild hypotonia, overactive reflexes, seizures, an abnormal electroencephalogram (EEG), and generalized parasympathetic function (e.g., constricted pupils, bradycardia, profuse secretions, diarrhea). Severe HIE is characterized by coma, severe hypotonia or increased extensor tone, intermittent decerebration, decreased or absent reflexes, variable pupil reactivity (often asymmetric pupils), and an abnormal EEG. Mild HIE is generally of short duration (<24 hours), whereas moderate HIE lasts for days and severe HIE can last for weeks.

TABLE 2. **Multisystem Organ Injury With Hypoxic-Ischemic Encephalopathy**

Organ	Signs of Injury
Central nervous system	Seizures, coma, lethargy, abnormal tone, irritability, jitteriness, persistent tremors, feeding problems, apnea, periodic breathing, high-pitched cry, pupillary dilation or constriction
Kidneys	Acute tubular necrosis, oliguria, inappropriate secretion of antidiuretic hormone
Lungs	Pulmonary hemorrhage
Heart	Ventricular dysfunction, tricuspid regurgitation, hypotension, shock
Skin	Dependent pitting edema, sclerema
Gastrointestinal tract	Ileus, necrotizing enterocolitis
Metabolic	Hypoglycemia, hypocalcemia, metabolic acidosis, diabetes insipidus

The prognosis for infants with severe HIE is uniformly poor, with eventual death or major disability. The major disability associated with HIE is generally severe and multiple and includes spastic quadriplegia or mixed cerebral palsy, severe mental retardation, sensory impairment, seizures, and microcephaly. The prognosis for those with mild HIE is generally excellent, although an increase in mild disability may be seen (e.g., language disorders, learning disability). Moderate HIE carries an increased risk of major disability (20%) and mild disability.

For many years, treatment of infants with HIE has been only supportive care: careful monitoring, respiratory support as needed, pressors for hypotension, fluid restriction for oliguria, anticonvulsants for seizure control, and intravenous calcium and glucose for hypocalcemia and hypoglycemia. Some believe that high-dose phenobarbitol, if started immediately regardless of whether seizures are noted, will improve outcome. Several randomized controlled trials of head cooling for infants with severe HIE are under way.

Neonatal Seizures. Although seizures are the most overt sign of CNS symptoms in the neonatal period, very few neonates have the generalized, well-organized, tonic-clonic seizures of older children and adults. Neonatal seizures are classified according to whether they are clonic (e.g., decorticate or decerebrate posturing), tonic (e.g., slow rhythmic jerks), myoclonic (e.g., rapid flexor jerks), or subtle. Subtle seizures are more common in preterm than in full-term infants, and they include eye deviation, chewing movements, lip-smacking, cyclical limb movements, apnea, increase in blood pressure, tachypnea, and bradycardia. Seizures can be distinguished from jitteriness, tremulousness, and clonus in that movements persist despite restraint and cannot be elicited by touch or position change. An EEG is also helpful in making a diagnosis and prognosis.

Because of evidence that seizures per se may cause brain injury, strong efforts should be made to control seizures with anticonvulsants. The recommended first-line anticonvulsant is phenobarbitol, with monitoring of efficacy in seizure control and blood levels (aim for 40 mg/dL). If seizures continue, phenytoin or short-acting benzodiazepines should be added. Seizures that are not accompanied by EEG seizure activity are generally far more difficult to control with anticonvulsants.

Neurodevelopmental outcome is determined by the etiology of the neonatal seizures. HIE, by far the most common cause of seizures in preterm and full-term newborns, generally occurs within 12 to 24 hours and in 60% to 65% of neonates with HIE. Severe HIE, diffuse encephalomalacia on neuroimaging, and a burst suppression pattern on EEG are all associated with an extremely poor prognosis. Neuroimaging can also distinguish between, HIE, intracranial hemorrhage, and CNS malformations. CNS malformations (e.g., holoprosencephaly, lissencephaly, hydranencephaly, schizencephaly), though not very common, indicate severe disability. Seizures can signal meningitis or herpes encephalitis, which must be looked for and treated immediately. Multifocal or focal clonic seizures suggest cerebral infarction or stroke, which lead to long-term focal neurologic deficits. This finding requires diagnostic evaluation to search for causes of the ischemia or a hypercoagulable state (e.g., protein S or C deficiency). Benign causes of neonatal seizures include subarachnoid hemorrhage, hypocalcemia, and hypoglycemia (if treated promptly and not associated with HIE, infection, or inborn errors of metabolism). Narcotic abstinence syndrome can also cause seizures, which generally occur in infants with severe symptoms of withdrawal.

PERINATAL RISK FACTORS

A large number of perinatal risk factors have been identified as being predictive of neurodevelopmental outcome, especially major disabilities (Table 3). The most important risk factors are those associated with CNS abnormalities, including seizures, abnormal neuroimaging, and an abnormal neurodevelopmental examination. When risk factors are multiple, especially when coupled with demographic factors (e.g., low socioeconomic status), the likelihood of disability is even higher. It is important to note that risk factors are not necessarily causative. IVH merely signals CNS injury; blood in the ventricles per se does not damage the brain.

Preterm delivery itself is a risk factor, as is intrauterine growth restriction (IUGR). As many as 5% to 15% of very low birth weight preterm infants with birth weight below 1500 g have cerebral palsy and/or mental retardation. The most common type of cerebral palsy is spastic diplegia, and it tends to be mild. Approximately 50% of infants born at the limit of viability (gestational age, 22 to 25 weeks) have major disability, and severe multiple disabilities are more common in this group. More subtle disorders of CNS function, including language disorders, learning disability, minor neuromotor dysfunction, or attention deficit disorder, occur in as many as 50% of very low birth weight infants and full-term IUGR infants. An infant with both prematurity and IUGR is vulnerable to the complications of both disorders. The risk of major disability in preterm IUGR infants is higher than that of preterm, gestational age–matched, infants with birth weight appropriate for gestational age, and it is more similar to birth weight–matched preterm infants with birth weight appropriate for gestational age. In both cases, it is the etiology of the condition and its complications that cause neurodevelopmental disability, not prematurity or IUGR per se.

TABLE 3. **Perinatal Factors Associated With Significant Risk for Neurodevelopmental Disability**

- Congenital infections
  - Cytomegalovirus
  - Toxoplasmosis
  - Rubella
- Maternal ingestions
  - Alcohol
  - Phenytoin
  - Heroin
  - Cocaine
- Prematurity
- Intrauterine growth restriction
- Poor postnatal growth
- Feeding problems/oromotor dysfunction
- Polycythemia
- Congenital anomalies
- Infection (especially meningitis)
- Chronic lung disease
- Neonatal seizures
- Hypoxic-ischemic encephalopathy
- Cardiopulmonary arrest
- Persistent pulmonary hypertension of the newborn
- Meconium aspiration syndrome
- Cerebral infarction (stroke)
- Intraventricular hemorrhage
- Intraparenchymal hemorrhage
- Ventricular dilation
- Periventricular leukomalacia or intraparenchymal cysts
- Burst suppression pattern on electroencephalography
- Encephalomalacia
- Abnormal neonatal neurodevelopmental examination

NEURODEVELOPMENTAL FOLLOW-UP

All sick neonates need primary care with special attention to growth, health, and development after discharge from the neonatal intensive care unit. Infants with chronic lung disease need careful pulmonary and neurodevelopmental follow-up because of a high risk for rehospitalization, high resource utilization, and neurodevelopmental disability. Infants with a high risk for neurodevelopmental disability (Table 3) need comprehensive developmental follow-up with monitoring and appropriate referral to community early developmental intervention programs. This follow-up should continue through preschool and school age because of the high risk for language disorders, visual perception problems, learning disability, and attention deficit disorder. Careful consideration should be given to a comprehensive multidisciplinary evaluation at school age in all these high-risk infants, and this evaluation is certainly indicated if academic or behavioral problems develop while in school (learning disability and attention deficit disorder are frequently manifested as behavior problems in the classroom).

Development can be monitored during infancy by obtaining a history of language and fine motor and gross motor milestones at each office or clinic visit. Common neuromotor abnormalities on examination include asymmetry of hand or leg use, diffuse hypotonia, extensor hypertonia, marked shoulder retraction, and tight heel cords. If these findings persist or interfere with function (e.g., unable to roll over, difficulty getting into or out of a sitting position), the child should be referred for developmental evaluation. Because CNS injury in infants tends to be diffuse, not focal, delay or abnormality in one stream of development indicates a need for referral for comprehensive multidisciplinary neurodevelopmental evaluation. A child with tight heel cords and persistent toe-walking has mild spastic diplegia. This mild motor impairment often improves with physical therapy and perhaps ankle-foot orthotics. However, associated language or cognitive impairment is frequently present and can be far more handicapping than the initial motor impairment. Each child with any type of developmental delay or persistent neuromotor abnormality should have a comprehensive multidisciplinary evaluation.

NORMAL INFANT FEEDING

method of

KRISTIN E. LAKE, B.S.

Association of Maternal and Child Health Programs
Washington, D.C.

and

ALAN M. LAKE, M.D.

The Johns Hopkins University School of Medicine
Baltimore, Maryland

BREAST-FEEDING

Throughout time, breast milk has been acknowledged as the ideal nutrition for the normal human infant. The introduction of formulas resulted in a significant decline in the number of breast-fed infants, a process reversed in the past decade with more aggressive efforts to educate and support the breast-feeding mother.

Because the majority of first-time mothers were formula fed, the process of education and support must begin in the prenatal period with counseling from the obstetrician, family physician, pediatrician, and lactation consultants. Ideally, one of the prenatal visits is devoted to providing written material emphasizing the advantages of breast-feeding and addressing the common misconceptions of the mother and her family. Procedural instructions for successful breast-feeding can begin at this time and continue through the early postnatal period. A breast examination to identify possible problems with the nipple, areola, or breast itself should be conducted by the obstetrician so that there is ample time to work with the mother to teach helpful techniques to deal with the possible problems early in the breast-feeding experience. Breast care, including the avoidance of strong soaps or ointments in the breast area, should be explained.

Once the baby is born, the mother should be given an opportunity to breast-feed within the first 2 hours after birth. Mothers who have early infant contact tend to breast-feed longer and show more of an attachment to their infant than those who do not have this early contact. The entire health care team must be prepared to address the anticipated early frustrations with nursing; the failure to latch on, the inconsistent interest in proper sucking, and the transient discomfort and engorgement. To achieve the proper grasp and seal, the nipple should be drawn up to the roof of the infant's mouth and the tongue should be stroking under the nipple. The infant's lips should surround the areola and the jaw can then apply pressure, forcing the milk out through the ducts.

To promote successful breast-feeding, mothers benefit from the initiatives of the World Health Organization and its Baby Friendly Hospital Initiative, which encompasses the recommendations noted earlier in addition to an environment of support. This support includes encouraging 24-hour rooming in, avoiding formula supplements and pacifiers, and providing an extended support system after discharge to address the mother's concerns. Mothers of premature infants are encouraged to meet with lactation nurses to develop a program of expressing or pumping milk to be used by the baby until coordinated suck and swallow can be achieved.

In the first 24 to 36 hours, mothers are encouraged to become comfortable with how to initiate the feeding and assist with latching, and they are instructed how to continue long enough to provide the early milk, or *colostrum* and stimulate subsequent milk production. We encourage mothers at home to offer the breast on demand, ideally at 2- to 3 ½-hour intervals.

We encourage the mother to allow the baby 8 to 10 minutes of active sucking on the first breast, stop to burp, and switch to the second breast. Although a small amount of hind milk might remain in the first breast until the next feeding, the baby will usually suck for 10 minutes or longer on the second breast without swallowing as much air or tiring.

All breast-feeding mothers should remain in daily contact with a health care professional until they are comfortable with the act of nursing, the supply of milk, and the number of wet (at least six a day after the third day) and dirty (at least one to three a day after the third day) diapers. All first-time mothers, especially with the short hospital stays, should have a home visit by a health care professional who is trained and comfortable with counseling lactation support. This professional examines the infant and can determine if he or she is not progressing as desired by assessing weight gain and hydration and looking for the presence of jaundice. This professional can also address any concerns the mother has and observe breast-feeding to make sure proper technique for long-term success is being used.

Although we encourage exclusive breast-feeding for the first 6 months and nursing plus formula for the first year, we recognize the many demands on the time and energy of nursing mothers. As a result, we encourage the nursing mother to express the residual milk from the second breast beginning at 3 to 6 weeks to create a "stash" of frozen breast milk that can be offered by another family member once or twice weekly after 6 weeks of age, a process we have determined extends the total duration of the mother's commitment to nursing by freeing her to meet other needs.

The contraindications to breast-feeding are few and listed in Table 1. Prior surgery of the breast may present some special concerns, as do multiple births.

Concerns regarding the transmission of maternal medication through breast milk remains under active investigation but is rarely of concern. For example, concerns in regard to psychotherapeutics such as tricyclics and selective serotonin reuptake inhibitors (SSRIs) appear to be unwarranted.

FORMULA FEEDING

When breast-feeding cannot meet the nutritional needs of the infant, the use of an iron-fortified infant formula can

TABLE 1. **Contraindications to Breast-Feeding**

Maternal HIV/AIDS
Galactosemia
Poorly monitored inborn errors of metabolism
Maternal medications
Antineoplastics: cisplatin (Platinol), cyclophosphamide (Cytoxan)
Street drugs: amphetamines, cocaine, heroin, phencyclidine, methadone, alcohol, marijuana
Ergot alkaloids: ergotamine (Ergomar), ergonovine (Ergotrate)
Benzodiazepines: chronic diazepam (Valium)
Radiopharmaceuticals: pump and discard based on agent used

meet these needs for the first full year of life. The formulas marketed in the United States must meet the strict nutrient requirements of the Food and Drug Administration. For a full review of the nutritional content of formulas, consult the American Academy of Pediatrics *Pediatric Nutrition Handbook,* fourth edition. Parents can be assured of the safety and adequacy of these products, with a special reminder to review the appropriate preparation from powders, concentrates, and water sources.

There are now five categories of infant formulas for infants:

1. Formulas for premature babies
2. Cow milk–based formulas
3. Soy-based formulas
4. Partial protein hydrolysate formulas
5. L-Amino acid based formulas

These are listed and contrasted with regard to nutrient composition in Table 2.

The "preemie" formulas address the needs of the premature infant by increasing the caloric density, using a whey-based protein to enhance gastric emptying, providing a mixture of both lactose and corn syrup starches, and using a mixture of lipids to include both medium chain and long-chain fats. They also contain more calcium. Recent studies suggest that postdischarge weight gain is maximized by extending the use of these formulas past 6 months of age. With a cost that is four times higher than standard formula, families may need assistance in sustaining the use of these products.

The cow milk–based formulas meet the needs of the vast majority of newborns. There is no medical need to use low iron formulas, which are insufficient in iron to meet the needs of the growing infant. The natural sugar in a cow milk formula is lactose, which can be digested by nearly all infants. Nonetheless, a market for lactose-free formulas has been cleverly created to appeal to lactose-intolerant parents to "reduce intestinal gas." Lactose-reduced formulas are appropriate in the early days of acute viral gastroenteritis. Until further information is available, the infant of a parent or first-degree relative with juvenile onset diabetes should avoid cow milk formula in the first 6 months.

The isolated soy protein formulas account for 25% of the market. They are nutritionally complete, are all iron fortified, and have no lactose because the sugars are either sucrose or corn syrup solids. They are appropriate for infants with cow milk allergy, infants with galactosemia, and infants whose parents prefer a vegetarian product.

The hydrolysate formulas are based on enzyme digestion of cow milk proteins. Pregestimil, Nutramigen, and Alimentum are extensively hydrolyzed casein-based and are indicated in infants with cow milk and soy allergy. Carnation Good Start is a partially hydrolyzed whey product that has value in the prevention of cow milk allergy but is not indicated in the infant with established cow milk allergy. Infants with multiple formula intolerance or dietary protein enterocolitis syndromes usually respond to use of the extensively hydrolyzed formulas, often required until 6 to 12 months of age.

Recognizing that some infants with multiple formula protein–intolerance, enterocolitis, and/or severe eczema will not be able to tolerate hydrolyzed protein or breast milk, a category of l-amino acid–based formulas has evolved. At the time this is written, only Neocate is licensed in the first year, although approval of Elecare is anticipated before publication. Both are lactose-free and contain a blend of oils; Elecare also contains medium chain triglycerides. Both formulas are expensive.

Formula-fed babies generally take 30 to 45 mL per feeding in the first 2 days, increasing to 90 to 120 mL every 3 to 4 hours within 10 days. Parents are encouraged to feed on demand but not to wait until the child is crying and upset. Of equal importance is the need to feed the baby when he or she needs to be fed but not to overfeed with every cry. Formulas can be prepared for 24 hours of use, stored in the refrigerator, and warmed as desired in warm water. The use of microwaves is discouraged because uneven heating may lead to high internal temperatures in the bottles. Ready-to-feed formulas contain no flouride. Boiling water from wells may be appropriate in the first few weeks, but there is no need for routine terminal sterilization.

We advise that formula feedings be interrupted routinely to burp the baby. Mild reflux emesis is normal, but the infant who routinely has significant emesis more than 1 hour after a feeding will need evaluation for gastric outlet concerns. Formula intakes by 4 months of age are usually approximately 32 ounces or 1000 mL per day.

SOLID FEEDINGS

After 4 to 5 months of age, thin-textured solids or beikost can be offered. Before this, the extrusion reflex of the tongue prevents the formation of an oral bolus to swallow. Because commercial products no longer contain added sweeteners or salts and have a constant texture that babies prefer with initial feedings, we advise use of commercial cereals, fruits, and yellow vegetables. We begin with 2-ounce (half-jar) servings twice a day, continuing one product for 4 to 6 days to document tolerance.

By 6 months of age, most parents can prepare strained ripe fruits, although commercial vegetables are continued. We prefer use of single ingredient jars to minimize fillers.

We advise against fruit juices because they are of no documented value, contribute to dental decay, and aggravate diarrhea.

VITAMIN AND MINERAL SUPPLEMENTS

Term infants are born with sufficient iron to meet their needs until their birth weight doubles, between 4 and 6 months. Premature infants have lower stores and double their weights faster, meaning that their need for iron occurs younger. We advise iron-fortified cereals be used from 5 months past 1 year of age. Breast-fed infants and infants fed ready-to-feed formula or formula prepared with well water will require fluoride supplementation after 6 months. Vitamin D supplements (400 IU) are advised in breast-fed nonwhite infants, especially those with reduced sun exposure.

Although exclusive breast-feeding past 6 months of age is an admirable goal, the reality is that many nursing

TABLE 2. **Infant Formula Options**

Formula	kcal/mL	Protein	Lipid	Carbohydrate
		Premature Formulas		
Enfamil Enfacare (Mead)	0.75	Nonfat milk	Sunflower, soy	Corn syrup solids
		Whey	Coconut, MCT	Lactose
Similac Neosure (Ross)	0.75	Nonfat milk	Soy, safflower	Corn syrup solids
		Whey	Coconut, MCT	Lactose
		Cow Milk-Based		
Enfamil 20 (Mead)	0.67	Whey	Palm, soy	Lactose
		Casein	Coconut, sunflower	
Enfamil LactoFree (Mead)	0.67	Nonfat milk	Palm, soy, coconut, sunflower	Corn syrup solids
Portagen (Mead)	0.67	Na caseinate	MCT oil (85%)	Corn syrup solids
			Corn oil	Sucrose
Similac (Ross)	0.67	Whey	Safflower, soy	Lactose
		Casein	Coconut	
Similac Lactosefree (Ross)	0.67	Milk protein	Soy, coconut	Corn syrup solids, Sucrose
		Soy-Protein–Based		
Isomil (Ross)	0.67	Soy protein	Soy, coconut	Corn syrup solids
		Methionine	Safflower	Sucrose
ProSobee (Mead)	0.67	Soy protein	Palm olein, soy	Corn syrup solids
		Methionine	Coconut, sunflower	
Carnation Alsoy (Nestle)	0.67	Soy protein	Palm olein, soy	Corn maltodextrin
		Methionine	Coconut, sunflower	Sucrose
		Hydrolyzed Protein		
Carnation Good Start (Nestle)		Partial whey	Palm olein, soy	Lactose
	0.67	Nucleotides	Coconut, safflower	Corn maltodextrin
Pregestimil (Mead)			MCT oil (55%)	Corn syrup, dextrose
	0.67	Casein hydroly safe	Corn oil, soy, safflower	Tapioca starch
Nutramigen (Mead)			Palm olein, soy	Corn syrup solids
	0.67	Casein hydrol safe	Coconut, sunflower	Cornstarch
Alimentum (Ross)			MCT oil (50%)	Sucrose
	0.67	Casein hydrol	Safflower, soy	Tapioca starch
		L-Amino Acid–Based		
Neocate (SHS)			Safflower, soy	Corn syrup solids
	0.67	L-Amino acids	Coconut	
Elecare (Ross)			MCTs, soy, safflower	Corn syrup solids
	1.0	L-Amino acids	Coconut	

Abbreviation: MCT = medium chain triglyceride.

mothers have obligations that preclude expressing milk to meet the child's need. When possible, we encourage mothers away from the home to pump breast milk and store it appropriately for later use. The vast majority can combine breast-feeding with formula supplements. Close follow-up of all infants is mandated during the early months with growth parameters plotted on standard curves to document normal velocities of growth.

BREAST DISORDERS

method of
MARVIN A. DEWAR, M.D.
University of Florida
Gainesville, Florida

Lists of the medical concerns of women rank diseases of the breast at or near the top. Breast complaints are common, and a majority of breast disorders are due to benign processes. Nevertheless, breast cancer must be considered and ruled in or out when evaluating almost all breast complaints. Understanding the evaluation and management of common benign breast disorders and the appropriate workup to diagnose breast cancer is therefore a critical part of the primary care of women.

FIBROCYSTIC DISEASE

Fibrocystic disease of the breast is a term that has been used to characterize a heterogeneous group of disorders that include both pathologic and nonpathologic entities. Probably better referred to as *fibrocystic change,* the clinical syndrome of cyclical tender nodularity is found in up to half of women and histologic findings consistent with fibrocystic change may be found in a majority of women undergoing breast biopsy for benign breast disease. Most of the benign disorders that give rise to this clinical syndrome are probably produced by an imbalance in the developmental and involutional processes that occur in the normal breast.

The relationship between fibrocystic changes and breast cancer has been a source of confusion and concern and depends on the underlying pathologic diagnosis (Table 1). Nonproliferative histologic lesions carry no increased breast cancer risk, whereas proliferative lesions, particularly those with concomi-

TABLE 1. **Benign Breast Disorders: Pathologic Classification**

Nonproliferative Lesions (No Increased Breast Cancer Risk)
Cysts
Mammary duct ectasia
Sclerosing adenosis
Epithelial-related calcifications
Mild hyperplasia
Proliferative Lesions Without Atypia (Slight Increased Breast Cancer Risk)
Moderate or florid hyperplasia
Intraductal papilloma with fibrovascular core
Proliferative Lesions With Atypia (Significant Increased Breast Cancer Risk)
Atypical ductal hyperplasia
Atypical lobular hyperplasia

tant atypia, are associated with increased breast cancer risk. The more common specific breast disorders occurring in fibrocystic disease are dealt with here.

BREAST PAIN

Breast pain is the single most common breast complaint among women. True mastalgia should be distinguished from the physiologic premenstrual breast swelling and tenderness experienced by many women. Premenstrual breast swelling and discomfort are very common and tend to be less severe than mastalgia, occur 3 to 4 days premenstrually, and are associated with a slight increase in the volume of the breasts in the second half of the menstrual cycle. Less commonly, breast discomfort is severe enough to interfere with a woman's daily lifestyle and may require specific therapy. This level of breast pain is referred to as mastalgia.

Mastalgia may be broadly characterized by whether symptoms vary with the menstrual cycle. A daily breast pain calendar that relates breast symptoms to the female reproductive cycle is often helpful in diagnosis and management. Cyclical mastalgia is the most common pattern and is characterized by breast pain most pronounced during the luteal phase and largely relieved with the onset of menses. Cyclical mastalgia usually begins in the third decade and is relatively rare in postmenopausal women who are not on estrogen replacement therapy. The breast pain of cyclical mastalgia is usually poorly localized, often bilateral, and may be described as a tenderness or heaviness most marked in the upper outer quadrant of the breast. Diffuse tender nodularity may be detected on physical examination. Hormonal mechanisms are suspected but have been difficult to elucidate. Currently, the most promising pathophysiologic theories involve alterations in prolactin secretion and/or receptor sensitivity.

Noncyclical mastalgia tends to be more common in women in their 40s or 50s, is often unilateral, and is frequently described as a sharp or burning sensation localized to the subareolar region and inner breast quadrants. No relationship of symptoms to the menstrual cycle is found. Physical examination in noncyclical mastalgia frequently demonstrates "trigger points."

Other causes of breast pain include musculoskeletal discomfort (including costocondritis), C6–C7 cervical radiculopathy, and the late effects of breast trauma or previous surgical scar. Although breast pain is not uncommon in patients with breast cancer, pain is only very rarely the sole presenting symptom of cancer in such women.

Evaluation of women with mastalgia primarily consists of a careful history and physical examination. A breast pain diary (calendar) recorded over two menstrual cycles helps differentiate cyclic from noncyclic mastalgia and provides a baseline for evaluating the effectiveness of subsequent treatment. Mammography is an integral part of the evaluation of mastalgia for women 35 years of age and older but is not necessary for women younger than age 35 who have a negative physical examination of the breasts.

Mild breast pain has a very high spontaneous remission rate and usually does not require specific treatment other than reassurance, over-the-counter as needed analgesics, and advice to wear a well-fitting support bra. Patients with well-localized costocondritis are effectively treated with application of moist heat, nonsteroidal anti-inflammatory agents, and trigger point injection with a lidocaine/corticosteroid mixture. Women with persistent severe mastalgia warrant specific treatment. Evening primrose oil* is a source of highly concentrated polyunsaturated essential fatty acids and has been shown to be an effective treatment in over half of women with cyclical mastalgia and over one third of women with noncyclical mastalgia. Evening primrose oil is given in a dose of 1000 mg three times daily and may take up to 3 months to show effectiveness. Because evening primrose oil has very few side effects it should be considered first-line therapy for women with mastalgia. Bromocriptine mesylate (Parlodel)* in a dose of 1.25 to 5 mg/d is as effective as evening primrose oil but has significant side effects, including nausea, vomiting, headache, dizziness, and fatigue. Danazol (Danocrine) is approved by the Food and Drug Administration (FDA) for the treatment of mastalgia. Dosage ranges from 200 mg/d tapering to 100 mg every other day depending on response. When given for 4 to 6 months, response rates for patients with cyclical mastalgia have been reported to be as high as 80%. Dose-related side effects are significant and include depression, weight gain, irregular menstrual bleeding, hepatic dysfunction, and acne. Danazol is potentially teratogenic, and barrier contraception should be recommended for women with child-bearing potential. Tamoxifen citrate (Nolvadex)* has been shown to be effective in women with severe mastalgia, but its use is limited by safety concerns.

In individual patients, oral contraceptive use may either aggravate or improve cyclical breast pain. Caf-

*Not FDA approved for this indication.

TABLE 2. **Classification of Nipple Discharge**

Milky	Watery
Multicolored	Serous
Purulent	

feine restriction and supplementation of vitamins A, B, and E are of unproven benefit in the treatment of patients with mastalgia. Administration of thyroid hormone,* diuretics,* or progesterone* are of no benefit in the treatment of women with breast pain.

NIPPLE DISCHARGE

Nipple secretion that only occurs with squeezing or milking of the nipple is not usually of clinical significance. Milk discharge related to pregnancy usually resolves within 6 months after the cessation of breast-feeding. Clinically significant nipple discharge is spontaneous, persistent over time, and not lactational. Ten to 15 percent of women with benign breast disease and 2% to 3% of women with breast cancer experience clinically significant nipple discharge. The evaluation and management of nipple discharges depend on specific characteristics shown in Table 2.

Galactorrhea is a milky breast discharge that occurs in the absence of pregnancy or breast-feeding. It tends to be bilateral and can be confirmed as the cause of nipple discharge by staining the milky discharge for fat using Sudan's solution. Some of the underlying pathophysiologic conditions responsible for galactorrhea are shown in Table 3.

Multicolored, thick, and sticky discharges are frequently bilateral, emanate from multiple ducts, and may be red, brown, or green. The underlying cause is usually mammary duct ectasia, a benign process. Infectious diseases of the breasts, usually secondary to gram-positive organisms, cause purulent breast discharges. Watery, serous, serosanguineous, and bloody nipple discharges are seen in a variety of conditions, including mammary duct ectasia, intraductal papilloma, and breast cancer. The risk of an underlying cancer is increased when the discharge is unilateral from a single duct, occurs in perimenopausal or postmenopausal women, and is accompanied by the finding of a breast mass on physical examination. Bloody discharges that occur during pregnancy and lactation are not usually due to cancer and may be followed conservatively with continued breast-feeding if no associated findings suggest breast cancer risk.

Evaluation of women with nipple discharges should focus on characterizing the particular type of discharge present and identifying any underlying breast pathologic process. The presence of blood in the nipple discharge is an important diagnostic finding and can be determined by Hemoccult testing of the discharge material. Red-brown discharges resulting from mammary duct ectasia often appear bloody but produce a brown rather than a red stain on white gauze. Nipple discharges testing positive for the presence of blood should be sent for cytologic examination.

*Not FDA approved for this indication.

TABLE 3. **Galactorrhea: Common Causes**

Anatomic

Chronic nipple stimulation
Chest wall trauma

Endocrine Abnormalities

Hypothyroidism
Anovulatory syndromes

Elevated Prolactin Conditions

Pituitary adenoma
Cushing's disease
Adrenal insufficiency
Cranial pharyngioma
Ectopic prolactin secretion (e.g., lung cancer and hypernephroma)

Medication Related

Psychotropic agents
Oral contraceptives
Metoclopramide
Central α-agonist agents
Tricyclic antidepressants
Chronic opiate use
Amphetamines
Verapamil
Cimetidine

Other Conditions

Renal and liver disease
Chiari-Frommel syndrome (persistent postpregnancy galactorrhea)

In women age 35 and older, mammography should be obtained to look for underlying breast lesions or changes characteristic of duct ectasia. Magnification views of the retroareolar region may be helpful. Galactography (injection of the ductal system) is usually not required and should only be considered after surgical consultation. The workup of abnormal galactorrhea is highlighted in Table 4.

Nonbloody discharges in women with no identifiable underlying breast pathologic process may be managed with reassurance, close clinical follow-up, and regular nipple hygiene using cotton pledgets soaked in hexachlorophene or povidone-iodine. Bloody, serosanguineous, serous, and sticky watery discharges should be referred for surgical evaluation.

TABLE 4. **Evaluation of Abnormal Galactorrhea**

1. Identify causes of local nipple stimulation
2. Careful medication history
3. Pregnancy testing
4. Thyroid-stimulating hormone
5. Liver enzyme testing
6. Renal function tests
7. Serum prolactin levels
8. Magnetic resonance imaging or computed tomography of the pituitary
9. Adrenal testing if indicated

TABLE 5. **Breast Conditions Producing Dominant Masses**

Cysts	Fibrosis
Fibroadenomas	Hamartomas
Cancer	Radial scar
Galactoceles	Intraductal papilloma
Localized sclerosing adenosis	

Associated breast masses are treated as they would be in women without discharge. Women with bloody, serosanguineous, serous, and sticky watery discharges, but without a specifically identifiable underlying lesion may require surgical excision of the involved ductal system. In these cases the most common finding will be an underlying intraductal papilloma. The management of women with abnormal galactorrhea depends on the underlying cause. Bromocriptine* is frequently effective in managing milky discharges in women with galactorrhea and elevated serum prolactin levels.

EVALUATION OF BREAST MASSES

Ruling in or ruling out the presence of breast cancer is a key component of the care of women with all types of breast complaints. This need commonly arises in evaluating women with breast lesions detected either by palpation or imaging studies. Normal glandular breast tissue may reveal cyclical nodularity that tends to be most pronounced in the upper outer quadrant of the breast and does not require specific evaluation. Dominant breast masses persist throughout the menstrual cycle and differ in character from the surrounding breast tissue. Dominant masses require further evaluation and may necessitate tissue diagnosis. Some of the underlying conditions that result in the presence of a breast mass are listed in Table 5.

Fibroadenomas are the most common causes of a dominant breast masses in women younger than age 35. They may be single or multiple and on clinical examination are usually rubbery and very mobile. These masses are hormonally responsive and therefore tend to increase in size during pregnancy and at the end of each menstrual cycle. Fibroadenomas undergo involution at menopause in woman not using estrogen replacement therapy. Usually 1 to 2 cm in diameter, a fibroadenoma that grows to more than 5 cm in diameter is referred to as a "giant fibroadenoma." The presence of fibroadenomas in a patient does not create an increased risk of breast cancer.

Breast cysts are common causes of dominant breast masses in women between the ages of 35 and 50. Clinically, cysts are very firm, mobile, sometimes tender, and difficult to distinguish from solid masses. Breast cysts usually disappear after menopause in the absence of estrogen replacement therapy. Cysts are not a precursor to breast cancer, and their main significance is that they produce a dominant mass that may require evaluation.

Palpable breast cancers are typically firm with indistinct borders and may be affixed to the underlying tissues. A new finding of a nipple retraction, bloody nipple discharge, or skin dimpling due to edema ("peau d'orange") increases the chance that an underlying dominant breast mass is malignant. Even careful physical examination by expert clinicians is frequently unable to differentiate among the many possible causes of dominant breast masses, and further diagnostic workup is frequently warranted.

Office needle aspiration effectively differentiates between cystic and solid breast lesions. Cancer risk is minimal if the cyst aspirant is not bloody and the associated dominant mass lesion completely disappears after aspiration. Nonblood cyst aspiration material can be safely discarded, whereas bloody aspirant should be sent for cytology examination. Clinical re-examination 4 to 6 weeks after cyst aspiration is important to look for recurrence. Surgical referral for biopsy should be obtained if the cyst aspirant is bloody, the underlying mass lesion does not completely resolve with aspiration, or the cyst frequently recurs after repeat aspiration. The interpretation of breast ultrasound or mammography can be confounded by cyst aspiration, and breast imaging should either be obtained before cyst aspiration or be delayed for 2 to 3 weeks after the procedure.

Simple fibroadenomas with classic clinical findings in women younger than age 30 may be safely followed by careful clinical observation. Other noncystic dominant breast masses, however, frequently require a tissue diagnosis to effectively rule out cancer. Mammography or ultrasound imaging correctly identifies a majority of women with malignant breast masses; however, neither is sufficiently sensitive to be solely relied on to rule out breast cancer in many cases.

Open surgical biopsy and/or excision is the traditional gold standard. Because approximately 80% of women undergoing biopsy for breast masses will turn out to have benign disease, there has been considerable interest in identifying safe and effective diagnostic procedures and algorithms that do not always require the expense and morbidity of open surgical biopsy or excision. More recently, fine-needle aspiration (FNA) and fine-needle aspiration biopsy (FNAB) have been used to quickly and accurately diagnose dominant breast masses in the office setting. Although the procedures are simpler, less costly, and associated with less morbidity than open surgical procedures, accuracy and reliability require both an experienced treating physician and a cytopathologist. As with cyst aspiration, breast mammography and ultrasound imaging should be performed before or delayed for several weeks after FNA or FNAB to avoid false-positive images secondary to local hematoma. A number of experts support conservative management and clinical follow-up without requiring open surgical biopsy for patients with dominant breast masses who have a negative "triple test": (1) normal clinical breast examination, (2) breast im-

*Not FDA approved for this indication.

aging study not suggestive of malignancy, and (3) negative FNA or FNAB.

BREAST INFECTIONS

Breast infections can be differentiated by whether they occur in the puerperal/lactational period or whether they occur in the nonpregnant woman. Nonpuerperal breast infections often occur in patients who have underlying mammary duct ectasia, tend to be subareolar, and frequently have a subacute and relapsing course. Patients with nonpuerperal breast infections often do not exhibit systemic toxicity but do experience localized erythema, point tenderness, and induration of the skin surrounding the nipple complex. Oral antibiotics, such as amoxicillin and clavulanate potassium (Augmentin), with coverage for both gram-positive and anaerobic bacteria should be administered. Application of moist heat and careful nipple hygiene with hexachlorophene (pHisoHex) or providone-iodine (Betadine) are also helpful. Breast abscess formation requires drainage using large-bore needle aspiration or open incision. Chronic relapsing nonpuerperal breast infections may require surgical excision of the subareolar duct complex. Breast infections may be difficult to distinguish from inflammatory breast cancer, and biopsy of the involved tissue should be performed in patients who do not respond promptly to antibiotic therapy and local measures.

Lactational breast infections (puerperal mastitis) usually occur in the early weeks of breast-feeding and are manifest by a wedge section of breast tissue that is erythematous, warm, and extremely tender. Fever, chills, and myalgias are common. Moist heat, prevention of breast engorgement, and oral antibiotics such as cephalexin (Keflex) or dicloxacillin sodium (Dynapen) effective against *Staphylococcus aureus* are usually beneficial when begun promptly. Large abscesses may require open surgical drainage and intravenous administration of antibiotics. Weaning the breast-feeding infant is not necessary; and, in fact, continued nursing helps prevent breast engorgement and promotes resolution of the infection. The infant is not adversely affected by nursing from the infected breast.

BREAST IMAGING

Mammography and ultrasonography are the primary imaging studies used to assist in the evaluation of breast disorders. The American Cancer Society recommends annual screening (two-view) mammography and clinical breast examinations for all asymptomatic women older than age 40. Monthly self-breast examination and clinical breast examination every 3 years are also recommended for all women older than age 20. Screening mammography detects 85% to 90% of all breast cancers and is the principal means to detect small preclinical breast cancers that have an excellent prognosis when treated. Twenty to 30 percent of mammographically detected abnormalities referred for biopsy are found to be malignant. Multiple-view diagnostic mammography is used to evaluate women with breast abnormalities and often includes spot compression with magnification views to help elucidate findings.

Mammography reports should be characterized as (1) negative, (2) benign findings, (3) probably benign findings (less than 1%–2% chance of malignancy), (4) suspicious findings (10%–30% chance of malignancy), or (5) findings highly suggestive of malignancy. On mammography, malignant lesions frequently demonstrate spiculated margins, fine irregular microcalcifications, and architectural changes that represent a change from findings on prior mammograms. Benign breast lesions detected by mammography include fat-containing masses, inframammary lymph nodes, and degenerating or calcified fibroadenomas. Probably benign lesions include well-circumscribed masses consistent with fibroadenomas, simple cysts, rounded calcifications, and benign calcifications associated with duct ectasia. Mammographic findings with less clear diagnostic implications can be produced by overlying dense glandular breast tissue, radial scar, underlying postsurgical scar tissue, traumatic fat necrosis, internal breast hematoma, and complex cysts with irregular walls or internal densities.

Probably benign mammographic findings are frequently followed up by careful clinical examination and a repeat mammogram in no more than a 6-month interval. Suspicious and highly suggestive mammography findings should be followed by tissue biopsy. Nonpalpable breast lesions detected by mammography that require tissue diagnosis can be evaluated by mammographically or ultrasound-guided stereotaxic biopsy or open surgical biopsy after needle localization procedures. *Mammography does not detect up to 15% of palpable breast cancers; therefore, a negative imaging study should not dissuade the clinician from pursuing a tissue diagnosis of suspicious lesions.*

Ultrasonography of the breast is primarily useful to distinguish cystic from solid lesions and for directing stereotaxic biopsy efforts of nonpalpable lesions. Because ultrasonography does not detect fine calcifications, it has not proved useful as a screening modality.

BREAST CANCER

Excluding skin cancer, breast cancer is the most common cancer in women and is second only to lung cancer as a cause of cancer-related death in women. In the year 2000, over 180,000 women in the United States were diagnosed with breast cancer and over 40,000 women died of the disease. The lifetime risk of breast cancer among women is 1 in 8, with a risk of 1 in 54 by age 50 and 1 in 23 by age 60. Approximately one half of the cumulative risk of breast cancer occurs in women older than the age of 65, and 75% of breast cancer diagnoses are made in women age 50 or older. Fewer than 5% of breast cancer cases occur in women younger than the age of 40.

Risk Factors

The most important risk factors for the development of breast cancer are female gender and advancing age. Other breast cancer risk factors are listed in Table 6. Breast cancer does occasionally affect men but at a rate of less than 1% of the occurrence in women. The importance of specific genetic markers for the development of breast cancer has been well established. Although women with *BRCA1*, *BRCA2*, and *P53* mutations are at a substantially increased risk of developing breast cancer, they represent cumulatively only 5% to 10% of all breast cancers.

Clinical Presentation and Staging

Early-stage, clinically occult breast cancers (Stage 0) are usually diagnosed based on abnormal findings detected on mammography (particularly suspicious microcalcifications). More advanced breast cancers usually present as specific breast abnormalities such as a palpable mass; change in breast size or shape; new onset of nipple inversion; persistent skin changes such as erythema, edema, or retraction; or nipple discharge, particularly when unilateral, bloody, and spontaneous. Advanced-stage breast cancer may present with evidence of invasion of the skin or chest wall, axillary lymphadenopathy, or distant metastasis to the bone, lung, or liver.

Pathology, Staging, and Prognosis

Breast cancers can be broadly divided into noninvasive and invasive categories. Noninvasive breast cancers include ductal carcinoma in situ (DCIS) and lobular carcinoma in situ (LCIS). DCIS is considered a direct precursor of invasive breast cancer. DCIS frequently produces suspicious microcalcifications detectable by mammography and is responsible for approximately one third of all mammographically detected breast cancers. Women with DCIS have an excellent prognosis when treated, with cure rates of 98% or greater. Lobular carcinoma in situ may be best thought of as a general marker of subsequent breast cancer risk rather than a direct cancer precursor lesion. Women with LCIS have approximately a 1% per year risk of developing subsequent invasive breast cancer, with the risk of breast cancer the same in the biopsied breast and the contralateral breast.

The most common invasive breast cancers are infiltrating ductal carcinoma (75%) and infiltrating lobular carcinoma (10%). Other less common forms of invasive breast cancer include medullary, tubular, and mucinous breast carcinoma. Medullary breast cancer tends to be slow to metastasize and as a result has a better prognosis than other pathologic types.

The classification and clinical staging for breast cancer are shown in Tables 7 and 8. The probability of recurrence and prognosis for patients with breast cancer are most influenced by tumor size and the status of axillary nodes at the time of primary treatment. Overall, patients with negative axillary lymph nodes at the time of diagnosis have lifetime recurrence rates in the range of 25% to 30%. Node-negative patients with small tumors less than 1 cm in

TABLE 6. **Breast Cancer Risk Factors**

Female gender
Advancing age
Family history of breast cancer (particularly when first degree, premenopausal, or bilateral)
Specific genetic mutations
BRCA1
BRCA2
P53
Previous breast cancer
Previous irradiation to the chest
Early age at first menses or late menopause
Never pregnant or first pregnancy after age 30
Obesity
Oral contraceptive use (risk less clear)
Fat intake (risk less clear)
Postmenopausal estrogen replacement (risk less clear)
Alcohol consumption (risk less clear)

TABLE 7. **Breast Cancer TMN Classification**

TX	Primary tumor cannot be assessed
T0	No evidence of primary tumor
Tis	Carcinoma in situ: intraductal carcinoma, lobular carcinoma in situ, or Paget disease of the nipple with no tumor
T1	Tumor ≤2 cm
a	Tumor ≤0.5 cm
b	Tumor >0.5 cm, but not >1 cm
c	Tumor >1 cm, but not >2 cm
T2	Tumor >2 cm, but not >5 cm
T3	Tumor >5 cm
T4	Tumor of any size with direct extension to chest wall or skin
a	Extension to chest wall
b	Edema ulceration of the skin of the breast, or satellite skin nodules confined to the same breast
c	Both of the above
d	Inflammatory carcinoma
NX	Regional lymph nodes cannot be assessed
N0	No regional lymph node metastases
N1	Metastasis to movable ipsilateral axillary nodes
N2	Metastasis to fixed ipsilateral axillary nodes
N3	Metastasis to ipsilateral internal mammary lymph nodes
M0	No evidence of distant metastasis
M1	Distant metastases

TABLE 8. **Breast Cancer Clinical Stage**

Stage	Description
I	T1, N0, M0
IIA	T0, N1, M0
	T1, N1, M0
	T2, N0, M0
IIB	T2, N1, M0
	T3, N0, M0
IIIA	T0 or T1, N2, M0
	T2, N2, M0
	T3, N1 or N2, M0
IIIB	T4, any N, M0
	Any T, N3, M0
IV	Any T, any N, M1

diameter are at even lower risk with long-term recurrence rates of less than 10% after primary treatment.

The prognosis for node-positive breast cancer patients is significantly worse and relates to the number of positive nodes found at the time of primary treatment. Recurrence rates increase as the number of axillary nodes found positive for breast cancer increase. Women who have fewer than four positive axillary nodes have a 5-year recurrence rate of approximately 40%, whereas women with more than four positive axillary nodes have 5-year disease-free rates of less than 25%. Approximately half of the patients with Stage 3 breast cancer will experience recurrence within 2 years after primary treatment. Although 80% of breast cancer recurrences occur during the first 5 years after primary therapy, disease relapse continues to occur for as long as 20 to 30 years after diagnosis. Stage 4 (metastatic) breast cancer has a poor prognosis, with a median survival of approximately 2 years.

Treatment

Noninvasive Breast Cancer

Ductal carcinoma in situ has traditionally been managed with very high cure rates by total mastectomy. Breast-conserving surgery ("lumpectomy") is an appropriate and effective treatment for many women with localized DCIS. Adequate tumor-free surgical margins are important and postexcision mammographic examination of the surgical specimen and postsurgical breast helps ensure complete removal of the lesion. The addition of radiation therapy to lumpectomy reduces the local recurrence rate of DCIS. Because the likelihood of positive axillary nodes is extremely low in DCIS, axillary dissection is usually not performed in these patients.

Lobular carcinoma in situ is treated with local excisional biopsy. Options for addressing the significantly increased risk of subsequent invasive breast cancer in women with LCIS include (1) careful clinical observation with frequent breast physical examination and mammography, (2) chemoprevention with tamoxifen (Nolvadex), and (3) prophylactic bilateral mastectomy.

Invasive Breast Cancer

Surgery and Radiation Therapy. Radical mastectomy (removal of entire breast and immediately adjacent chest wall musculature with axillary dissection) or modified radical mastectomy (removal of entire breast with axillary dissection) has been the traditional surgical approach to Stages 1 and 2 breast cancer. Breast reconstruction after mastectomy can be performed either at the time of primary therapy or delayed until a subsequent procedure. Multiple trials have now convincingly shown that most women with Stages 1 and 2 breast cancer can be safely and effectively surgically treated using breast-conserving therapy (BCS) consisting of primary tumor excision followed by radiation therapy to reduce the chance of local recurrences. BCS may not be appropriate for women with multiple primary tumors, diffuse suspicious microcalcifications, prior breast irradiation, early pregnancy (which would greatly delay radiation therapy), or large tumors in a small breast or for women in whom clear surgical margins cannot be obtained or in whom BCS would produce an unacceptable cosmetic result.

For prognostic reasons, it is important to ascertain the tumor status of the axillary lymph nodes in women undergoing breast-conserving therapy for Stage 1 or 2 breast cancer. Options for accomplishing this include axillary dissection or direct biopsy of the dominant axillary lymph node by an experienced surgeon ("sentinel node biopsy"). In women who undergo sentinel node biopsy, a positive initial biopsy is then followed by complete axillary dissection. Women with Stage 3 breast cancer frequently undergo a course of preoperative chemotherapy or hormone therapy in the hope of gaining sufficient local control of the disease to optimize the subsequent surgical therapy and radiation therapy. The role of surgery in women with metastatic breast cancer is limited, although radiation therapy remains important to treat focal disease sites.

Systemic Therapy. It is widely understood that even women with Stage 1 or 2 breast cancer frequently have clinically nonapparent distant micrometastases at the time of initial diagnosis. As a result, systemic therapy is beneficial both for women with widespread or recurrent breast cancer as well as many women with no apparent metastatic disease at the time of initial diagnosis. Adjuvant hormonal therapy and/or combination chemotherapy should be strongly considered in most women with a diagnosis of invasive breast cancer. Women who are older than the age of 35 and who have a very low risk of recurrence (primary tumor size < 1 cm and positive steroid receptors) may not require adjuvant therapy. Even in this population, the current state of clinical knowledge regarding risks and benefits of adjuvant therapy should be carefully discussed between the physician and patient.

Tamoxifen, a weak estrogen with partial agonist-antagonist properties, improves survival for women with steroid receptor–positive tumors. Tamoxifen produces a survival benefit in both node-negative and node-positive cases and is effective in both premenopausal and postmenopausal women. Tamoxifen is generally given for 5 years, and the survival benefit has been shown to extend beyond the period of drug administration to at least 15 years. Tamoxifen may induce hot flashes in premenopausal women and is associated with an increased risk of endometrial cancer and thromboembolic phenomena.

Combination chemotherapy is used for adjuvant therapy in women with steroid receptor–negative tumors and, in combination with tamoxifen, in women with node-positive, steroid receptor–positive tumors. Node-positive women younger than the age of 50 receive the greatest absolute benefit from combination chemotherapy. Adjuvant chemotherapy is generally administered for a 3- to 6-month course. The classic combination chemotherapy for adjuvant breast cancer treatment has been CMF (cyclophosphamide [Cytoxan], methotrexate [MTX], and fluorouracil [Efudex]). The primary acute adverse effects of CMF protocols include nausea and vomiting, hair loss, bone marrow suppression, induction of menopause, allergic pulmonary infiltrates, and, less commonly, hemorrhagic cystitis and renal failure. Doxorubicin (Adriamycin) is sometimes substituted into the traditional CMF regimen, resulting in slightly greater response rates. This small treatment benefit must be weighed against the increased risk of dose-related cardiac toxicity.

Similarly, a number of clinical trials are evaluating the potential role of paclitaxel (Taxol) and docetaxel (Taxotere) as a part of adjuvant therapy protocols. These agents may produce neurotoxicity in the form of peripheral neuropathy or central nervous system toxicity with seizures.

The treatment of widely metastatic or recurrent breast cancer includes radiation therapy to localized disease sites as well as systemic chemotherapy or hormone therapy. In addition, treatment with the anti-HER-2 monoclonal antibody trastuzumab (Herceptin) is effective in women with HER2-positive metastatic breast cancer. The effectiveness of high-dose chemotherapy combined with autologous bone marrow transplantation in the treatment of women with advanced breast cancer is unclear at this time, and multiple trials are underway to better define the role of this multimodality therapy.

Follow-up After Breast Cancer Treatment

Metastatic breast cancer can occur at almost any body site. Local/regional and skeletal recurrences are most common, followed by lung, liver, and brain metastases. Multiple simultaneous sites of recurrence are frequent. Most cases of recurrent disease occur relatively soon after primary diagnosis and therapy, with 60% to 80% of recurrences occurring within the first 3 years. Although recurrent breast cancer becomes much less likely with increasing time intervals after primary treatment, recurrences can continue to appear for 20 to 30 years after initial diagnosis.

More than three in four patients with recurrent breast cancer are symptomatic at the time of detection. The breast cancer survivor must be followed carefully for signs and symptoms of recurrence such as skin or soft tissue changes around the primary surgical site, abnormalities in the contralateral breast, bone pain, pulmonary symptoms, progressive weight loss, abdominal pain and swelling, jaundice, and focal neurologic symptoms. The physical examination should focus on the primary surgical site, regional lymph nodes, abdomen, and pulmonary areas. Examination of the contralateral breast is crucial.

A history and physical examination should be performed at 3- to 6-month intervals for the first 5 years after primary treatment. Women should be instructed to perform self-breast examinations every month for life. Annual mammography of both breasts in the setting of breast-conserving therapy and the contralateral breast in the setting of mastectomy should be obtained beginning 6 to 9 months after the completion of radiation therapy. Patients with a history of breast cancer have an increased risk for colon, endometrial, and ovarian cancer, and clinicians should be alert to these possibilities.

A number of studies have assessed the potential benefit of more extensive radiologic and laboratory testing in the follow-up of asymptomatic patients after breast cancer treatment. Currently, tests such as routine chest radiographs, bone scans, tumor markers, computed tomography (CT), and magnetic resonance imaging (MRI) are not indicated on a routine basis. Patients with suspected recurrent disease should be evaluated based on specific presenting signs and symptoms. Bone scintigraphy is indicated for patients with bone pain or possible pathologic fractures. Evaluation of potential pulmonary metastasis includes chest radiography, thoracic CT or MRI, and diagnostic thoracentesis for unexplained pleural effusions. CT and MRI are most useful for detecting potential abdominal or central nervous system recurrences. Measurement of specific tumor markers, such as carcinoembryonic antigen and CA 15-3 is sometimes helpful to monitor disease progression and response to therapy.

ENDOMETRIOSIS

method of
ROBERT BARBIERI, M.D.
Harvard Medical School and Brigham and Women's Hospital
Boston, Massachusetts

Endometriosis is the presence of tissue that resembles normal endometrium at sites outside the uterus. The anatomic areas most commonly affected by endometriosis are the ovaries, the pelvic peritoneum, the uterosacral ligaments, the fallopian tubes, the appendix, and the bowel serosa. Endometriomas, or "chocolate cysts," are cysts of endometriosis within the ovary. The gold standard for diagnosing endometriosis is laparoscopy, with visual recognition of endometriosis lesions. The severity of endometriosis is defined by the American Society for Reproductive Medicine using a surgical staging system based on the size and location of endometriosis implants and the severity of pelvic scarring. The stages are stage I—minimal, stage II—mild, stage III—moderate, and stage IV—severe.

The prevalence and incidence of endometriosis have not been well characterized. The prevalence of endometriosis is probably in the range of 5% of women of reproductive age (13–50 years of age). The peak incidence is at 25 to 30 years of age. Hormonal (estrogen), mechanical (retrograde menstruation), and immunologic factors play important roles in the etiology of endometriosis. Endometriosis lesions are absolutely dependent on estrogen for survival and growth. In the absence of estrogen, endometriosis lesions regress. Interventions that reduce estrogen production, such as surgical removal of the ovaries or hormone treatment with a gonadotropin-releasing hormone (GnRH) analogue, are associated with improvement in pelvic pain in most women with endometriosis. Retrograde menstruation of viable endometrial cells from the uterus into the pelvic cavity is believed to be an important "mechanical factor" that is an initiating event in the development of endometriosis. Women with severe stenosis of the cervical os and functioning endometrium menstruate in a retrograde manner back through the fallopian tubes into the pelvic cavity. These women develop endometriosis in almost 100% of cases. In normal women, immunologic mechanisms probably clear the small amount of endometrium that reaches the pelvic cavity from retrograde menstruation. In women with endometriosis there is indirect evidence that abnormalities in the immune system reduce the normal clearance of endometrium that enters the pelvic cavity via retrograde menstruation. A family history of endometriosis is associated with a twofold increased risk, suggesting a genetic predisposition.

Most women with endometriosis present for medical care with a "chief complaint" of *pelvic pain, infertility,* and/or an *adnexal mass* (ovarian endometrioma).

ENDOMETRIOMAS—ENDOMETRIOSIS CYSTS OF THE OVARY

Endometriomas are benign endometriosis cysts of the ovary. The monoclonal nature of endometriomas suggests that they arise from a somatic mutation in a precursor cell. No medical therapy is available. Endometriomas typically present as adnexal masses palpable on physical examination or detected on pelvic ultrasonography. In gynecology, a general rule is that persistent, complex adnexal masses that are larger than 3 cm (as determined by pelvic ultrasonography) should be surgically resected. The basis of this general rule is that surgical removal of all large, persistent, complex, ovarian cysts will increase the detection and effective treatment of ovarian cancer at an early stage. Ovarian cancer, a leading cause of death, can be successfully treated only when it is detected at an early stage. Surgical resection of an endometrioma will treat the tumor and provide definitive pathologic diagnosis (proving that it is not an ovarian cancer). After surgery, about 10% of women develop a second endometrioma. After surgical treatment of an endometrioma, long-term treatment with an estrogen-progestin oral contraceptive reduces the risk of recurrence of endometriosis lesions in the ovary. In women who have not completed their family, prevention of new endometriosis lesions in the ovary protects future fertility by reducing the risk of the need for additional ovarian surgery.

INFERTILITY

Infertility is defined as the inability of a couple to achieve a pregnancy after trying for 12 months. Infertility treatment is complex, and, in most situations, couples with infertility should be referred to infertility specialists for evaluation and treatment. There is evidence that immediate referral of an infertile couple to an infertility specialist results in less resource consumption than a pattern of referral from a primary care physician to a general gynecologist and then finally to an infertility specialist. A standard approach to the initial diagnosis of infertility is to perform a semen analysis, to document ovulation (serum progesterone, basal body temperature chart), and to demonstrate patency of the fallopian tubes (by hysterosalpingography). If the initial workup of the infertile couple demonstrates normal ovulatory function, normal semen analysis, and patent fallopian tubes, there is a 40% chance that the female partner has endometriosis. The sequential treatment of these women often includes one surgical procedure to determine if endometriosis is present. If the laparoscopy demonstrates the presence of endometriosis, then an attempt to resect all the lesions and adhesions can be performed at the same surgery. If surgery is not followed by pregnancy within the next 12 months, then empirical induction of multifollicular ovulation with clomiphene or gonadotropins in combination with intrauterine insemination is commonly recommended. If this approach is not effective, then in vitro fertilization (IVF) is typically recommended (Table 1). This approach to the treatment of infertility associated with endometriosis is described in more detail later.

A large clinical trial demonstrated that surgical treatment (excision or ablation) of endometriosis improves fertility in infertile women with endometriosis. In this study, 341 infertile women with stage I or II endometriosis were randomized to have a diagnostic laparoscopy or a diagnostic laparoscopy combined with surgical resection or ablation of endometriosis lesions. During 36 weeks of postoperative follow-up, 18% of the women in the diagnostic laparoscopy group became pregnant and 31% of the women in the diagnostic laparoscopy plus excision or ablation of endometriosis lesions group became pregnant ($P <$ 0.006). This well-designed clinical trial suggests that surgical resection of endometriosis lesions can improve fertility in infertile women with endometriosis. However, pelvic surgery can cause pelvic adhesions, which can reduce fertility potential. Therefore, I believe that infertile women should not have multiple operations to treat endometriosis lesions that are believed to be causing infertility. If the first adequate and complete operation is not followed by pregnancy during the next 12 months, then empirical induction of multifollicular ovulation with clomiphene (Clomid)

TABLE 1. **Sequential Treatment Approach to the Woman with Infertility and Endometriosis**

Step 1: Surgical diagnosis and treatment. Follow-up for 12 months to see if pregnancy occurs
Step 2: Intrauterine insemination
Step 3: Clomiphene induction of multifollicular ovulation plus intrauterine insemination
Step 4: Follicle-stimulating hormone injections for induction of multifollicular ovulation plus intrauterine insemination
Step 5: In vitro fertilization and embryo transfer

or gonadotropins in combination with intrauterine insemination is commonly recommended.

Clinical trials suggest that treatment of infertility with induction of multifollicular ovulation with clomiphene or gonadotropins in combination with intrauterine insemination is effective in treating infertility associated with endometriosis. Fedele and colleagues randomized 40 women with stage I or stage II endometriosis and infertility to three cycles of human menopausal gonadotropin (luteinizing hormone and follicle-stimulating hormone [LH and FSH]—Pergonal, Repronex) injections plus intrauterine insemination (IUI) or to no treatment. The LH and FSH injections induce multifollicular ovulation. The pregnancy rate per cycle was 4.5% in the no treatment group and 15% in the LH-FSH-IUI group ($P < 0.05$). In a large randomized clinical trial, 932 women with infertility, many of whom had endometriosis, were randomized to receive intracervical sperm insemination (ICI) alone, IUI, FSH (Gonal-F, Follistim) injections plus intracervical sperm insemination, or FSH injections plus IUI. ICI was designed as a "control" that would resemble the effects of natural intercourse. IUI is a commonly used fertility treatment in which an ejaculated semen specimen is treated in the laboratory to concentrate the sperm in a small volume of buffer while removing all the semen. The concentrated sperm pellet is then delivered to the upper portion of the uterine cavity with a small catheter passed through the cervix. ICI and IUI are timed to occur just before ovulation with the use of urine LH detection kits. FSH injections are given to stimulate multifollicular ovulation. After four treatment cycles, the pregnancy rate in each group was FSH plus IUI—33%, FSH plus the control ICI treatment—19%, IUI alone—18%, and the control ICI treatment alone—10% ($P < 0.01$). This study demonstrates that FSH plus IUI, or FSH plus ICI, or IUI alone improves pregnancy rate over an intervention designed to simulate intercourse alone (ICI). A major complication associated with the FSH injections was twin and triplet pregnancy. The maternal and fetal risks associated with triplet pregnancy may diminish the clinical utility of FSH injections in this infertility setting. Compared with FSH, clomiphene (Serophene, Clomid) ovulation induction is associated with fewer twin and triplet pregnancies. Clomiphene plus IUI therapy may result in a better balance of benefits (pregnancy) and risks (triplet pregnancy) than FSH plus IUI therapy.

The infertility treatment that has the greatest efficacy in women with endometriosis is IVF and embryo transfer. IVF and embryo transfer is associated with a 30% per cycle pregnancy rate in the treatment of infertility caused by endometriosis. In many centers, if surgery, followed by IUI alone, followed by multifollicular ovulation induction plus IUI fails to result in a pregnancy, IVF is recommended. In some centers, IVF is offered on a "fast clinical track" as the first intervention in the setting of endometriosis and infertility, especially if the infertile female is older than 37 years of age. In my practice, infertile women younger than 32 years of age have the time to progress in a deliberate manner through all the standard treatment steps: surgery, IUI alone, clomiphene plus IUI, FSH injections plus IUI, and finally IVF. For infertile women older than 37 years of age, rapid progression to IVF is indicated to avoid the possibility that all the "healthy" follicles will be depleted before a pregnancy is achieved.

PELVIC PAIN—THE TRADITIONAL APPROACH

Many women with endometriosis present with pelvic pain, including severe dysmenorrhea, dyspareunia, dyschezia, and lower abdominal pain not related to menses. The standard approach to a woman with severe pelvic pain who has not had significant pain relief when treated with nonsteroidal anti-inflammatory drugs (NSAIDs) and oral contraceptives is to perform laparoscopy to determine the cause of the pain and to see if endometriosis is present. The advantage of placing surgery in a central position in the diagnosis and treatment of women with pelvic pain is that a definitive diagnosis can often be determined; and if endometriosis is demonstrated, surgical resection of lesions can produce significant pain relief for 12 months or more. In one randomized controlled clinical trial, surgical resection of endometriosis lesions was demonstrated to produce pain relief for up to 12 months postoperatively. In this study, the "active" surgical procedure consisted of diagnostic laparoscopy combined with laser ablation of endometriosis lesions plus uterine nerve ablation. The control surgical procedure was a diagnostic laparoscopy plus aspiration of pelvic peritoneal fluid. The physicians who were evaluating the response of the patients and the patients were not informed as to whether the "active" or "control" operation had been performed. In this randomized study, the active surgical procedure resulted in improvement in pain in 63% of women and the control procedure resulted in improvement in pain in 23% of the women at 6 months follow-up ($P < 0.01$). This study suggests that surgical treatment of endometriosis can be effective in the treatment of pain.

Recent clinical trials suggest that after surgical treatment of endometriosis, hormone therapy for 6 months with a GnRH agonist delays the recurrence of pelvic pain by 12 months. In one clinical trial, 109 women with laparoscopically proven endometriosis who had undergone laparoscopic treatment of endometriosis lesions were randomized to receive either a GnRH-agonist analogue, nafarelin (Synarel), 200 μg by nasal insufflation twice daily, or a placebo, by nasal insufflation twice daily for 6 months postoperatively. A major outcome variable was the median time after treatment to initiation of an alternative therapy, which reflects the recurrence of severe pelvic pain. The women who were treated with nafarelin postoperatively had a median time to initiation of an alternative therapy greater than 24 months. In the group treated with placebo the median time to initiation of an alternative therapy was 12 months ($P < 0.001$). This study suggests that the combination of surgery plus postoperative hormone therapy may be helpful in extending the time to recurrence of pelvic pain in women with endometriosis. I offer all women with endometriosis postoperative hormone therapy with either a combination estrogen-progestin oral contraceptive or a GnRH agonist analogue.

PELVIC PAIN—THE USE OF THE "CLINICAL DIAGNOSIS" OF ENDOMETRIOSIS

The current gold standard for the diagnosis of endometriosis is surgical documentation of endometriosis lesions by visual detection. The advantages of this approach are that it is very unlikely that a serious condition, such as ovarian cancer, will be missed or misdiagnosed and that treatment of the endometriosis can take place at the time of surgical visualization. There are a number of clinical disadvantages to using surgical visualization of lesions as the gold standard for the diagnosis of endometriosis. These disadvantages include the requirement for surgery and anesthesia, the possibility that a lesion thought to be endometriosis by visual inspection might not prove to be endometriosis on histologic analysis, and the possibility that some deep endometriosis lesions might be difficult to visualize and consequently not detected. An alternative to surgery is the use of clinical diagnosis, based on history, physical examination, and noninvasive laboratory tests, to make the diagnosis of endometriosis. A recently published study supports the concept of making a clinical diagnosis of endometriosis in certain clinical situations and using empirical hormone treatment for the pelvic pain presumed to be due to endometriosis.

In a recent study, 100 women with chronic pelvic pain met 13 inclusion criteria:

1. Moderate to severe chronic pelvic pain
2. Age 18 to 45 years
3. Regular menstrual cycles
4. No previous diagnosis of endometriosis by a surgical procedure
5. No hormone treatment in past 3 months
6. No evidence for a primary disease of the urinary tract or bowel as the cause of the pain
7. No history of excessive use of alcohol, tranquilizer drugs, or illicit drugs
8. Normal pelvic ultrasound
9. Normal complete blood cell count
10. Normal urinalysis
11. Absence of gonorrhea and chlamydia on tests of an endocervical specimen
12. Negative pregnancy test
13. Failure of NSAIDs and doxycycline treatment to improve the pain symptoms

The women were randomized to receive treatment with depot leuprolide (Lupron Depot), 3.75-mg intramuscular injections every 4 weeks for 12 weeks, or to receive a placebo injection for 12 weeks. Pain was measured with the 4-point Biberoglu and Behrman scale. At the end of 12 weeks of treatment, all of the women underwent laparoscopy to assess the accuracy of the clinical diagnosis of endometriosis. At the end of the study, at laparoscopy, it was determined by surgical visualization of lesions that 87% of the women in the placebo group and 78% of the women in the leuprolide group did have endometriosis. This suggests that the 13-point inclusion criteria listed earlier are relatively effective in identifying women with chronic pelvic pain who have endometriosis as the cause of their pain (at least in this study population). In addition, the study showed that 82% of the women treated with empirical leuprolide had pain relief compared with 39% of the women treated with placebo. This result indicates that in women with a clinical diagnosis of endometriosis, empirical hormone treatment with leuprolide acetate depot, 3.75-mg intramuscular injection every 4 weeks, can be effective in relieving pelvic pain.

This study, and others, support the concept of making the clinical diagnosis of endometriosis based on history, physical findings, and limited laboratory testing. Women clinically diagnosed with endometriosis can then be offered treatment with a GnRH analogue, danazol, or a progestin for their pelvic pain. A recent American College of Obstetricians and Gynecologists technical bulletin, "Medical Management of Endometriosis," discussed this evolving clinical paradigm and concluded that clinical diagnosis of endometriosis and empirical hormone treatment can be efficacious.

HYSTERECTOMY AND BILATERAL OOPHORECTOMY

Hysterectomy and bilateral oophorectomy (TAH-BSO) have been reported to provide long-term pain relief in approximately 85% of women with endometriosis. TAH-BSO treatment is available only to women who have definitely completed their family. After TAH-BSO, hormone replacement therapy with standard regimens can treat vasomotor symptoms without increasing the risk of recurrence of endometriosis and pelvic pain. Large-scale follow-up trials indicate that women with endometriosis and severe pelvic pain who were treated with TAH-BSO have long-term improvement in their pain symptoms and are satisfied with their choice of treatment.

MEDICAL TREATMENT OF PELVIC PAIN CAUSED BY ENDOMETRIOSIS

Women with endometriosis and pelvic pain can be successfully treated with hormone therapy. My practice is to start with hormone treatments with the fewest side effects (NSAIDs used at near maximal doses, oral contraceptives used in a cyclic or continuous manner) and then to progress sequentially to use the more powerful hormone treatments

TABLE 2. **Hormonal Treatments for Pelvic Pain Caused by Endometriosis***

Step 1: Nonsteroidal anti-inflammatory agents at maximal doses
Step 2: Oral contraceptives used in a cyclic manner
Step 3: Oral contraceptives used in "long cycles"
Step 4: GnRH agonist analogue treatment: nafarelin (Synarel, 200 μg by nasal insufflation twice daily) or leuprolide (Lupron Depot, 3.75 mg intramuscularly every 4 weeks)
Step 5: Danazol (Danocrine, 200 mg orally, 2, 3, or 4 times daily)

*Steps 1, 2, and 3 are associated with less severe side effects than steps 4 and 5.

that are associated with significant side effects (GnRH analogues such as nafarelin and leuprolide, danazol). This progression is outlined in Table 2.

The standard combination estrogen-progestin oral contraceptive appears to be effective in the treatment of pelvic pain caused by endometriosis. The standard oral contraceptive pill contains a progestin in every pill. The progestin blocks growth in many endometriosis lesions, in part, by blocking the growth-promoting properties of estrogen. An alternative to the standard schedule (21 hormone pills, followed by 7 days off the pill) for administering combination estrogen-progestin oral contraceptives is to prescribe 63 active hormone pills in a row (3 packs of 21 active pills) followed by 7 days off the pill, followed by 63 active pills in a row. This approach has been described by the author as a "mini-pseudopregnancy" because it often results in menses every 10 weeks rather than every 4 weeks. An even longer cycle can be prescribed by recommending the use of 105 (5 packs of 21 active pills) in a row, followed by 7 days off medication, followed by 105 active pills in a row. In one study, women who were allowed to extend the number of consecutive active pills and avoid the pill-free week reported a high degree of satisfaction with the extended-pill regimen. The major disadvantage to the use of long cycles is that many women develop "breakthrough bleeding" and have a small of amount of uterine bleeding, often reported to be brown in color, many days per week. Breakthrough bleeding is the main reason women using a "mini-pseudopregnancy" discontinue the medication.

If oral contraceptives are not effective, then the patient can be treated with nafarelin, 200 μg twice daily by nasal insufflation, or leuprolide acetate depot, 3.75-mg intramuscular injection every 4 weeks. A standard course of GnRH agonist treatment is 24 weeks, but treatment regimens as short as 12 weeks have been shown to be effective. The GnRH agonist analogues nafarelin and leuprolide initially stimulate pituitary release of LH and FSH, but with chronic use they paradoxically downregulate LH and FSH secretion, resulting in cessation of ovarian follicular growth and suppression of ovarian production of estrogen and progestin. The absence of ovarian production of estrogen and progestin results in amenorrhea and hypoestrogenic side effects such as hot flashes and increased rate of bone resorption. The hypoestrogenism induced by the GnRH agonists is associated with relief of pelvic pain in approximately 85% of women with endometriosis. This strong beneficial effect needs to be balanced against the side effects of hot flashes and bone loss. For some women, the pain relief is so impressive and the side effects are so minimal that they want to stay on the treatment for longer than 6 months. This is safe if the patient is carefully monitored for bone loss. Low-dose steroid "add back" can be added to the GnRH agonist treatment to reduce the rate of bone loss and to treat hot flashes. Add-back regimens that have been demonstrated to be effective are listed in Table 3. After discontinuation of treatment, pelvic pain tends to recur in most women over the next 12 months.

Danazol (Danocrine), an orally active derivative of testosterone, is as effective as nafarelin and leuprolide in the treatment of pelvic pain caused by endometriosis. Danazol is typically prescribed at doses of 200 mg twice daily for up to 6 months. If this dose is not effective in relieving pelvic pain, then the dose can be increased to 200 mg three or four times daily. Danazol is no longer widely used for the treatment of endometriosis because it is associated with significant weight gain (average, 4 kg), deepening of the voice, hirsutism, and musculoskeletal pain. The current use of danazol tends to be as a last resort after NSAIDs, oral contraceptives, and the GnRH agonist analogues have failed to adequately treat pelvic pain caused by endometriosis.

MULTISPECIALTY PAIN PRACTICE

A major challenge in pain treatment is to effectively integrate the psychosocial-mind-brain-body paradigms. The psychosocial paradigm emphasizes the importance of social status and experiences in the family and society on health outcomes. The mind paradigm emphasizes the importance of psychological factors on health. The brain paradigm focuses on neural genes and neurochemistry in the etiology of pain. The body paradigm focuses on the diseased organs that trigger the pain stimulus. There is ample evidence that in women with endometriosis and pelvic pain, factors such as depression, somatization, and past history of sexual or psychological abuse play important roles in modulating the patient's percep-

TABLE 3. **Five Steroidal Add-Back Regimens That Can Reduce the Rate of Bone Loss and Hot Flashes Associated With GnRH Agonist Treatment (Nafarelin or Leuprolide)**

Add-Back Medication	Dose
1. Norethindrone acetate (Aygestin)	5 mg PO daily
2. 17 β-estradiol, transdermal patch plus	25-μg patch
medroxyprogesterone acetate (Provera)	5 mg/d
3. 17 β-estradiol, micronized (Estrace) plus	2 mg PO daily
norethindrone acetate (Aygestin)	1 mg PO daily
4. Conjugated estrogens (Premarin) plus	0.625 mg PO daily
medroxyprogesterone acetate (Provera)	5 mg PO daily
5. Conjugated estrogens (Premarin) plus	0.3 mg PO daily
medroxyprogesterone acetate (Provera)	5 mg PO daily

tion of her pain. For patients with pelvic pain who have not had significant relief from hormonal or surgical treatment, the multispecialty pain practice may prove to be effective.

There are few randomized studies of the efficacy of psychological or psychosocial interventions in the treatment of pelvic pain. In one clinical trial, the effectiveness of a focused organic (surgical) approach to pelvic pain was compared with a multidisciplinary approach to pelvic pain that included surgical, psychological, dietary, and social interventions. The investigators reported that the multidisciplinary approach to pelvic pain resulted in greater long-term improvement in self-reported pain scores than the approach that focused on treating organic disease with surgery. Most large medical centers have an organized pain treatment center that can develop a multidisciplinary treatment plan for the patient with chronic pelvic pain that has failed to respond to surgical intervention and hormone treatment.

Rapid diagnosis is critical to the proper treatment of disease. Two independent studies reported that the average time between onset of the symptoms of endometriosis (pelvic pain) and the definitive diagnosis was over 6 years. The delay between onset of symptoms and definitive diagnosis results in significant frustration for both patients and clinicians. Delay in diagnosis of endometriosis can be reduced if clinicians actively consider the diagnosis in all women with pelvic pain or infertility.

ABNORMAL UTERINE BLEEDING

method of
GREGORY T. FOSSUM, M.D.
Thomas Jefferson University
Philadelphia, Pennsylvania

NORMAL CYCLE

Before you can talk about the etiology of abnormal uterine bleeding, you first have to understand the changes that the endometrium goes through during a normal cycle. The endometrium responds to the serum estradiol and progesterone secreted by the ovary. During the first few days of the cycle, the ovary begins to secrete estradiol. The estradiol stimulates the endometrium to proliferate. An endometrial biopsy done during the proliferative phase will show mitosis in both the stroma and the glandular tissue of the endometrium.

The proliferation continues until ovulation occurs. If ovulation never occurs, the proliferation continues and results in endometrial hyperplasia. At the time of ovulation, the progesterone level starts to rise; this stops all mitotic growth in the endometrium.

The glandular tissue of the endometrium then starts to show secretory changes:

Day 19: The secretion occurs beneath the nuclei.

Day 21: The secretion occurs above the nuclei.

Day 23: The secretion occurs in the lumen. At this time, decidualized changes can be seen in the periarteriolar tissue.

Day 25: As the endometrium progresses, the decidualized changes are seen subcapsular.

Day 27: Finally, decidualized changes are seen throughout the stroma.

The progesterone level by day 27 is already starting to decline. Menstruation then begins. The exact day of the secretory phase from the day of ovulation can be determined when a biopsy is done during different days of the cycle. An endometrial biopsy showing any secretory changes implies that ovulation has occurred.

ABNORMAL UTERINE BLEEDING

The etiology of abnormal uterine bleeding first must be classified as either dysfunctional uterine bleeding or functional uterine bleeding. Dysfunctional uterine bleeding is also known as *anovulation.* Women who ovulate and have abnormal uterine bleeding are known as having *functional uterine bleeding.* Functional uterine bleeding occurs when there is a lesion in the uterus or a blood dyscrasia.

The first task is to determine whether the patient ovulates. Ovulation can be estimated by cycle regularity, but commonly this is not a valid indicator and laboratory determination is necessary.

If an endometrial biopsy is done during the proliferative phase of the menstrual cycle, the pathology report will reveal proliferative endometrium. Similarly, if the patient does not ovulate, the endometrial biopsy will always reveal proliferative endometrium, no matter when the biopsy is done. An endometrial biopsy done during the luteal phase of the menstrual cycle will reveal secretory endometrium. Therefore, the problem is to do the endometrial biopsy at the appropriate time during the cycle, which is not always possible to determine when the bleeding pattern is irregular.

The patient ovulates and has functional uterine bleeding (1) whenever there is abnormal uterine bleeding and a random endometrial biopsy reveals secretory endometrium, and (2) if the serum progesterone level is found to be higher than 2.5 ng/mL.

Anovulation (dysfunctional uterine bleeding) occurs more frequently in younger women (<35 years), and functional uterine bleeding currently occurs more often as the patient ages.

Causes of Functional Uterine Bleeding

The causes of functional uterine bleeding can be further broken down into extrauterine and intrauterine etiologies.

EXTRAUTERINE

Extrauterine causes of abnormal uterine bleeding include chronic medical conditions such as hyperthyroidism, hypothyroidism, diabetes mellitus, dysfunctions of platelets, severe pneumonia, severe liver failure, and congestive heart failure. Coagulation dysfunctions are rare causes of abnormal uterine bleeding.

INTRAUTERINE

Intrauterine causes of abnormal uterine bleeding include pregnancy-related problems, uterine infections, uterine fibroids, endometrial polyps, and genital tract cancers. Estrogen and progesterone supplementation such as hormone replacement therapy (HRT) during menopause or oral contraceptive pills can also result in abnormal uterine bleeding.

History and Physical Examination

The workup of abnormal uterine bleeding should include a thorough history and physical examination. The history should include any possible pattern in the abnormal uterine bleeding, duration of the abnormal uterine bleeding, any changes in the intensity of the bleeding over the past few months, any associated passage of menstrual clots, or associated dysmenorrhea (cramping). The medical history should include any gynecologic surgery and any medications that may include estradiol, progesterone, or testosterone. Any history of blood dyscrasias, epistaxis, or easy bruisability should be obtained. The family medical history also should be explored for blood dyscrasias and gynecologic problems.

The physical examination should include a thorough heart and lung examination. The abdominal examination should look for abdominal masses as well as tenderness. The pelvic examination should include a thorough inspection of the vulva and vagina. Sites of bleeding excoriation or other lesions should be determined. Similarly, the cervix should be examined for possible lesions or bleeding. The uterine size should be determined as well as any irregularities or tenderness of the uterus. Any uterine masses or adnexal masses should be determined.

ENDOMETRIAL BIOPSY

When should the endometrial biopsy be done? Fortunately, endometrial cancer is uncommon. When endometrial biopsies were performed on 111 women who were on tamoxifen (Nolvadex), only 1.4% of the biopsies yielded abnormal results, and only 1 patient was found to have cancer.[1] Endometrial cancer is extremely uncommon for women under age 35. Therefore, endometrial biopsy should be done sparingly in these patients.

After age 35, endometrial biopsy should be routine in the diagnosis of abnormal uterine bleeding. During the Post Menopausal Estrogen/Progesterone Intervention (PEPI) and Health Osteoporosis Progestin Estrogen (HOPE) studies, endometrial biopsy was done before starting HRT and after 6 and 12 months of HRT. Two abnormal biopsies were found. The presence or absence of abnormal bleeding did not increase the risk of finding an abnormality.

ULTRASOUND

Similarly, ultrasound (US) has been used to help diagnose abnormal uterine bleeding. Although 30% of biopsies were found to be abnormal when the endometrial thickness was greater than 8 mm, few of these biopsies showed endometrial cancer.

Two hundred forty-seven women underwent transvaginal US to measure endometrial thickness. This was repeated every 6 months for up to 5 years. Endometrial thickness rose only in the women who were on tamoxifen. One endometrial cancer was found in 1 of 52 asymptomatic women who had abnormal endometrial thickness or morphology by US. Two endometrial cancers were found in asymptomatic women with a normal US measurement. Therefore, Dr. Gerber[2] suggested, "Our results suggest that the transvaginal US is a poor screening tool."

OTHER PROCEDURES

More advanced procedures such as dilation and curettage, hysteroscopy, hysterosalpingogram, and laparoscopy should be reserved for those patients in whom simpler diagnostic procedures are not adequate.

Causes

UTERINE FIBROIDS

Uterine fibroids can cause abnormal uterine bleeding. They are common in women older than 35 years. The physical examination commonly can detect uterine fibroids, but on occasion, US may be necessary to detect a submucous uterine fibroid.

CONTRACEPTIVE PILL

Abnormal uterine bleeding can occur while on the oral contraceptive pill. To have normal uterine bleeding, the three phases of the menstrual cycle must be maintained. The uterus must have a proliferative phase, a secretory phase, and a menstrual phase to have normal uterine bleeding.

The secretory phase occurs while the patient is taking the active pills. The menstrual phase begins when the active pills are stopped. In response to stopping the active pills, the hypothalamus responds by increasing gonadotropin-releasing hormone (GnRH) secretion. This stimulates a rise in follicle-stimulating hormone (FSH) and ultimately a rise in estrogen. The estrogen stimulates proliferation of the endometrium (proliferative phase).

Occasionally, to help control the menstrual cycle for women on the oral contraceptive pill, estrogen needs to be added during the placebo week to stimulate proliferation of the endometrium.

Endometrial Biopsy Results

Proliferative Endometrium

If an endometrial biopsy reveals proliferative endometrium and if it is believed that the patient is anovulatory, the patient should be treated with cyclic progesterone supplementation.

If it is still unknown whether the patient is anovulatory, progesterone serum levels needs to be repeated weekly for 3 weeks. If the progesterone is persistently lower than 2.5 pg/mL, this confirms the diagnosis of anovulation, and the patient needs cyclic progesterone treatment. If the patient is found to be ovulatory, a uterine defect must be investigated such as uterine myomas or polyps.

Occasionally, cyclic therapy with progesterone will decrease menorrhagia but rarely for more than 1 year in women with uterine myomas. A submucous uterine myoma or polyp can be resected with hysteroscopy.

Endometritis

Another cause of abnormal uterine bleeding is endometritis. Broad-spectrum antibiotic therapy should be started for a minimum of 2 weeks. If endometrial cancer or endometrial hyperplasia with atypia is found, hysterectomy is the treatment of choice unless the patient desires future fertility. It is controversial not to perform a hysterectomy in this situation.

Atrophy of the Endometrium

If the biopsy reveals atrophy of the endometrium, estrogen supplementation is necessary. The patient may require 14 to 28 days of unopposed estrogen before starting progesterone. If the endometrial biopsy reveals scant tissue, the biopsy may need to be repeated. If scant tissue is found on the second biopsy, hysteroscopy may be necessary. If in doubt of the diagnosis, hysteroscopy will probably not only give a more accurate diagnosis but also allow potential therapy.

The etiology of abnormal uterine bleeding must be differentiated into functional (ovulatory) or dysfunctional bleeding. If it is dysfunctional uterine bleeding, treat with progesterone. If it is functional uterine bleeding, investigate the etiology.

References

1. Gerber B: J Clin Oncol 18:4359–4363, 2000.
2. Gerber B: J Clin Oncol 18:3464–3470, 2000.

AMENORRHEA

method of
DEBRA A. MINJAREZ, M.D.
Colorado Reproductive Endocrinology
Denver, Colorado

and

BRUCE R. CARR, M.D.
University of Texas Southwestern Medical Center
Dallas, Texas

Amenorrhea is usually defined as the absence or cessation of menstrual flow and is a manifestation of a variety of pathophysiologic disorders. In general, women who fail to menstruate by age 16 in the presence of normal secondary sexual development or by age 14 in the absence of normal secondary sexual development require evaluation. By the age of 16 approximately 98% of all American girls have begun to menstruate, and 2% to 3% of women who previously menstruated become amenorrheic. In a patient who previously menstruated, 3 months of amenorrhea is considered abnormal and warrants further investigation.

Although a number of classifications exist for amenorrhea, one of the more frequently cited categories is primary versus secondary amenorrhea. However, there is considerable overlap in this classification system and it is more useful to differentiate amenorrhea based on the pathophysiologic etiology. Table 1 classifies amenorrhea into three groups: (1) anatomic defects, (2) ovarian failure, and (3) chronic anovulation with or without the presence of estrogen.

EVALUATION OF THE PATIENT
(Figure 1)

In evaluating a patient a thorough history is essential. Information regarding the age at onset of menses, breast and pubic hair development, and growth spurt should be elicited. Other key questions should focus on prior history of uterine surgery, change in weight, psychological stress, medication use, and associated signs such as hirsutism or acne.

The physical examination should target three important areas: (1) the degree of maturation of secondary sex characteristics such as the breasts, the pubic and axillary hair, and the external genitalia; (2) the current estrogen status; and (3) the presence or absence of a uterus. In primary amenorrhea, the presence or absence of secondary sexual development as well as the presence of a normal genital tract will help to differentiate gonadal failure from müllerian anomalies.

Laboratory evaluation should exclude pregnancy, and levels of prolactin, follicle-stimulating hormone (FSH), and thyroid-stimulating hormone (TSH) should be assessed. Estrogen status can be determined by the presence of breast development, and current estrogen secretion is based on the presence of a pink, well-"rugated" moist vagina with clear stretchable cervical mucus. A progestin challenge test can also be used to assess the level of endogenous estrogen. This may consist of orally active medroxyprogesterone acetate (Provera), 10 mg/d for 5 days, micronized progesterone, 300 mg at night, 100 to 200 mg of intramuscular progesterone in oil, or the use of progesterone gel (4% Crinone) intravaginally for 5 days. Within 2 to 7 days after the last dose of the progestational agent, the patient should have the onset of bleeding, establishing the presence of estrogen. If the FSH is low or normal, a progestational challenge will differentiate patients into chronic anovulation with estrogen present (eugonadotropic), chronic anovulation with estrogen deficiency (hypogonadotropic hypogonadism), or anatomic defect. In contrast, patients with normal or low FSH with a disorder of the hypothalamus or pituitary (hypogonadotropic hypogonadism) will not have bleeding. These patients need further evaluation to exclude a central nervous system etiology with magnetic resonance imaging or computed tomography of the head. If the FSH level is elevated, ovar-

TABLE 1. **Classification of Amenorrhea**

I. Anatomic defects
   Labial agglutination/fusion, imperforate hymen, transverse vaginal septum, cervical agenesis, vaginal agenesis, müllerian agenesis, complete androgen insensitivity, Asherman syndrome
II. Ovarian failure (hypergonadotropic hypogonadism)
   A. Gonadal agenesis
   B. Gonadal dysgenesis
      Turner syndrome 45,X, mosaicism
   C. Ovarian enzyme deficiency
      17α-hydroxylase deficiency, 17,20-lyase deficiency
   D. Premature ovarian failure
      Idiopathic, injury (mumps oophoritis, radiation, chemotherapy), resistant ovary, autoimmune, galactosemia
III. Chronic anovulation with estrogen present
   A. Polycystic ovary syndrome
   B. Adrenal disease—Cushing syndrome, late-onset adult adrenal hyperplasia
   C. Ovarian tumors
IV. Chronic anovulation with estrogen absent (hypogonadotropic hypogonadism)
   A. Hypothalamic
      1. Tumors—craniopharyngioma, germinomas, hamartomas, Hand-Schüller-Christian disease, teratomas, endodermal sinus tumors, metastatic carcinoma
      2. Infection and other disorders—tuberculosis, syphilis, encephalitis/meningitis, sarcoidosis
      3. Functional—stress, weight loss/diet, malnutrition, psychological eating disorder, exercise
   B. Pituitary
      1. Tumors—prolactinomas, adrenocorticotropic hormone, thyroid-stimulating hormone, growth hormone, nonfunctional, metastatic carcinoma
      2. Space-occupying lesions—empty sella, arterial aneurysm
      3. Necrosis—Sheehan syndrome, panhypopituitarism
      4. Inflammatory/infiltrative—sarcoidosis, hemochromatosis

From Carr BR: Disorders of the ovary and female reproductive tract. In Wilson JD, Foster DW (eds): Williams Textbook of Endocrinology. Philadelphia, WB Saunders, 1992, pp 733–798.

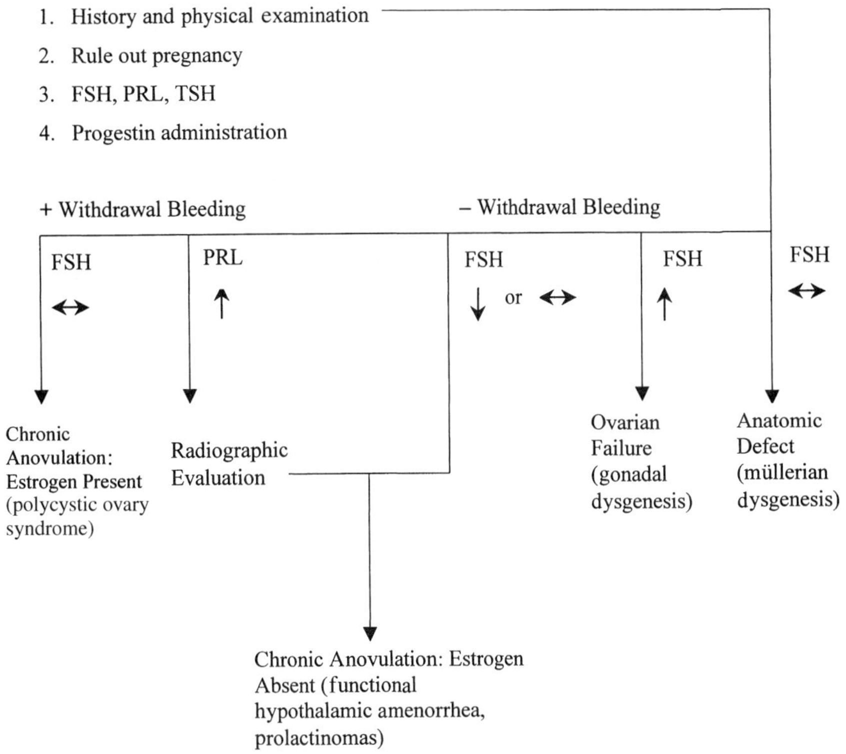

1. History and physical examination
2. Rule out pregnancy
3. FSH, PRL, TSH
4. Progestin administration

+ Withdrawal Bleeding

FSH ↔ → Chronic Anovulation: Estrogen Present (polycystic ovary syndrome)

PRL ↑ → Radiographic Evaluation

– Withdrawal Bleeding

FSH ↓ or ↔

FSH ↑ → Ovarian Failure (gonadal dysgenesis)

FSH ↔ → Anatomic Defect (müllerian dysgenesis)

Chronic Anovulation: Estrogen Absent (functional hypothalamic amenorrhea, prolactinomas)

Figure 1. Suggested flow diagram aiding in the evaluation of women with amenorrhea. *Abbreviations:* FSH = follicle-stimulating hormone; PRL = prolactin; TSH = thyroid-stimulating hormone. (From Carr BR, Wilson JD: Disorders of the ovary and female reproductive tract. In Petersdorf RG, et al [eds]: Harrison's Principles of Internal Medicine, 10th ed. New York, McGraw-Hill, 1983, pp 700–720.)

ian failure (hypergonadotropic hypogonadism) is established.

If the prolactin level is elevated, a detailed history should be elicited for medications that are known to cause hyperprolactinemia. If the TSH is normal, the pituitary should be evaluated further with magnetic resonance imaging or computed tomography to exclude a central nervous system etiology. In patients with an elevated TSH and an elevated prolactin level, the hypothyroid state should be treated first because elevated TSH levels bind to receptors on lactotrophs within the pituitary, stimulating prolactin release.

CAUSES OF AMENORRHEA AND TREATMENT

Anatomic Defects

Anatomic defects of the female genital tract (müllerian anomaly) can prevent the normal egress of menstrual flow. Beginning from the lower genital tract, anatomic defects such as labial agglutination, labial fusion due to sexual ambiguity, imperforate hymen, and congenital defects of the vagina such as transverse septa can result in amenorrhea. These defects will result in accumulation of menstrual blood behind the obstruction, and patients will have cyclic episodes of lower abdominal pain. A müllerian tract anomaly is unlikely in a woman with a vagina and patent cervix determined by uterine sounding and no history of operative procedures on the cervix or uterus.

A more severe anomaly is müllerian agenesis (Mayer-Rokitansky-Hauser syndrome). It is estimated to occur in 1 in 4000 female births and is the second most common cause of primary amenorrhea, the first being gonadal dysgenesis. Women with müllerian agenesis on examination will have an absent or hypoplastic vagina, usually absent uterus and fallopian tubes, functioning ovaries, and normal secondary sex characteristics. If a uterus is present, it may appear as rudimentary bicornuate cords or have functioning endometrium but lack a conduit to the vagina and present with cyclic abdominal pain.

Another similar presentation that should be distinguished from müllerian agenesis is androgen insensitivity (complete testicular feminization). Patients with androgen insensitivity will have normal breast development, a blind-ending vagina, an absent uterus, and a paucity of pubic and axillary hair. These individuals are genetic males, 46XY, with the presence of testes; however, an androgen receptor defect precludes the normal action of testosterone. Karyotyping and measurement of serum testosterone within the male range will confirm the diagnosis. Patients with androgen insensitivity must have their gonads removed after breast development because of the risk of malignant degeneration, which rarely occurs before the age of 20.

Destruction of the endometrium (Asherman syndrome) generally occurs after curettage of the uterine cavity. It is usually associated with postpartum hemorrhage with accompanying curettage, elective abortion with or without infection, or a missed abortion resulting in synechiae. These adhesions can be found in the cervical canal and or the endometrial cavity. Asherman syndrome can also occur after cesarean section, myomectomy, or metroplasty. In a woman with a history of operative procedures and no bleeding or only mild spotting after a progestational test, hysterosalpingography, sonohysterography (fluid contrast ultrasonography), or hysteroscopy is warranted.

Anatomic defects of the outflow tract are successfully treated surgically. Incision or excision of labial fusion, imperforate hymen, or vaginal septum leads to normal menstruation and later fertility. Symptomatic labial adhesions have successfully been treated with estrogen cream. In müllerian agenesis a functional vagina can be created by vaginal dilation of the blind-ending pouch or dimple or by surgical reconstruction using a split-thickness skin graft (McIndoe procedure).

Ovarian Failure

Premature ovarian failure is defined by amenorrhea, hypoestrogenism, and elevated levels of gonadotropins before the age of 40. The most frequent etiology of ovarian failure is gonadal dysgenesis, in which the germ cells undergo accelerated atresia and the ovary is replaced by a fibrous streak. Gonadal dysgenesis can be associated with a variety of abnormal karyotypes but is also found in patients with normal karyotypes. The most common type is due to deletion of genetic material in the X chromosome and accounts for approximately two thirds of gonadal dysgenesis. A 45,X karyotype (Turner syndrome) is found in about half, and most patients will have associated somatic defects such as short stature, webbed neck, shield chest, and cardiovascular defects. The remainder of patients will have chromosomal mosaicism with or without structural abnormalities of the X chromosome. The most common form of mosaicism is 45X,46XX. Presence of a Y chromosome in a cell line requires removal of the gonads because of a 15% to 25% risk of developing a malignant germ cell tumor such as a gonadoblastoma, embryonal cell carcinoma, or seminoma. In patients with gonadal dysgenesis 90% never menstruate and 10% will have sufficient residual follicles to experience menses.

The next largest group of patients with premature ovarian failure have a normal 46,XX or 46,XY karyotype and are characterized as having pure gonadal dysgenesis. These individuals will be of normal or above average stature because of failure of estrogen-mediated epiphyseal closure. Approximately a tenth of patients with a 46,XY karyotype will develop signs of virilization, including clitoromegaly, voice change, and temporal balding.

Other causes of ovarian failure include autoimmune disorders, resistant ovary syndrome, iatrogenic causes (chemotherapy and radiation therapy for malignancy), infection, galactosemia, and 17α-hydroxylase/17,20-hydroxylase deficiency. In autoimmune disorders, premature ovarian failure may be a presenting symptom in polyglandular failure with adrenal insufficiency, hypothyroidism, or other autoimmune disorders. In resistant ovarian syndrome, the ovaries contain many follicles arrested in development before the antral stage, which is thought to be due to resistance of the action of FSH in the ovary. 17α-Hydroxylase deficiency is characterized by primary amenorrhea, sexual infantilism, and hypertension from increased production of deoxycorticosterone, whereas 17,20-lyase deficiency is characterized only by primary amenorrhea and sexual infantilism.

Treatment of ovarian failure is directed at estrogen-progesterone replacement to augment or maintain secondary sexual characteristics and prevent osteoporosis and lower the risk of cardiovascular disease. In women with gonadal dysgenesis (Turner syndrome), an initial regimen of low-dose estrogen should be implemented to provide the necessary estrogen support to initiate breast development without hastening epiphyseal closure. A dose of 0.3 mg of conjugated estrogen (Premarin) daily for 3 to 6 months followed by slow increase to 0.625 mg and finally to 1.25 mg over the same time frame will allow adequate breast development. Progesterone can then be added cyclically to induce final maturation of the breast and withdrawal bleeding. For more convenient dosing regimen, patients can then be switched to an oral contraceptive with the same anti-osteoporotic and cardiovascular benefits.

Chronic Anovulation

The most common causes of amenorrhea are associated with chronic anovulation. The ovaries of women with chronic anovulation do not secrete estrogens in a normal cyclical pattern. It is clinically useful to divide this group into those who produce estrogen in sufficient levels to have withdrawal bleeding after a progestin challenge from those with hypogonadotropic hypogonadism who fail to produce enough estrogen to have withdrawal bleeding.

Chronic Anovulation with Estrogen Present

Women with chronic anovulation and normal or low FSH levels who experience withdrawal bleeding after progestin produce estrogen through extraglandular aromatization of androstenedione. The most common disorder associated with chronic anovulation with estrogen production is polycystic ovarian syndrome (PCOS). PCOS is a complex group of disorders characterized by hirsutism, elevated body mass index, infertility, amenorrhea, oligomenorrhea, or dysfunctional uterine bleeding.

In PCOS menarche occurs at the expected time; however, subsequent uterine bleeding is often unpredictable. When evaluating patients with PCOS, it is important to remember that there is a wide spectrum of clinical features and symptoms. Laboratory evaluation may yield an elevated plasma luteinizing hormone (LH) with normal or low FSH values in a ratio of more than 2:1. The increased LH levels lead to hyperplasia of the ovarian stoma and theca cells and increased androgen production and clinical manifestations, such as hirsutism and acne. However, interpretation of a single LH: FSH ratio can be misleading because only 50% to 60% of patients with PCOS will have an elevated LH level. Alternatively, a normal ratio cannot exclude PCOS.

Ultrasound diagnosis may also be misleading in PCOS. Classically, PCOS ovaries have been described as a "string of pearls" at the periphery of the ovary or the presence of multiple small follicles throughout the ovary. However, it is estimated that 8% to 25% of normal ovulatory women will have polycystic ovaries and only 75% of anovulatory patients will have PCOS. In addition, 14% of patients on oral contraceptives will also have polycystic-appearing ovaries. Thus, the diagnosis of PCOS should not be based on pathologic changes in the ovaries or plasma hormone levels but on the clinical existence of chronic anovulation and varying degrees of androgen excess.

Chronic anovulation with estrogen production may also occur with tumors of the ovary, which can be diagnosed by ultrasonography. Tumors that secrete estrogen or produce androgens, which are then aromatized in extraglandular sites, include granulosa-theca cell tumors, Brenner tumors, cystic teratomas, mucinous cystadenomas, and Krukenberg tumors. Other causes of anovulation with estrogen production include late-onset adrenal hyperplasia, Cushing syndrome, and various thyroid disorders.

Treatment of PCOS depends on the clinical findings and the needs of the individual patient. First-line treatment should be directed toward alleviating predisposing factors such as weight loss to decrease body mass index. If the patient is not hirsute and does not desire pregnancy, monthly withdrawal bleeding should be induced by progestin therapy or oral contraceptive pills to reduce the risk of endometrial hyperplasia. If a patient is hirsute and does not desire pregnancy, excess androgen production can be suppressed with oral contraceptive pills and antiandrogens such as spironolactone (Aldactone).* Once androgen excess is controlled, treatment of previously existing hair growth is accomplished by shaving, depilatories, electrolysis, or laser therapy. If a patient desires pregnancy, ovulation induction with clomiphene citrate (Clomid) will induce ovulation in about 75% of patients. In patients who do not ovulate, treatment with metformin (Glucophage)* has been shown to increase sensitivity to clomiphene citrate. Other alternatives for ovulation induction include treatment with exogenous gonadotropins (Pergonal, Repronex) and laparoscopic ovarian "wedge" by diathermy to reduce the ovarian stroma and thus decrease androgen ovarian production.

Chronic Anovulation Without Estrogen Production

Chronic anovulation without the presence of estrogen is also classified as hypogonadotropic hypogonadism and is characterized by the absence of withdrawal bleeding after progestin treatment. This disorder results from functional or organic disorders that interfere with gonadotropin-releasing hormone (GnRH) or gonadotropin release from the hypothalamic-pituitary axis. Hypothalamic tumors and other destructive or infiltrative hypothalamic disorders are rare, and diagnosis is based on radiographic evaluation such as magnetic resonance imaging of the head.

Another rare cause of hypogonadotropic hypogonadism, which is associated with defects of smell, is Kallmann syndrome. Affected patients are sexually infantile and have a defect in the production of GnRH, are hyposmic or anosmic, may have midline facial defects such as cleft lip, and occasionally have renal agenesis.

More commonly, gonadotropin deficiency leading to chronic anovulation arises from functional disorders such as stress, weight loss from excessive dieting, anorexia or bulimia, or exercise. Women who develop amenorrhea associated with stress, exercise, or dieting exhibit alterations that progress from luteal phase dysfunction and anovulatory cycles to oligomenorrhea and, finally, amenorrhea. In addition, chronic debilitating disease such as end-stage kidney disease, malabsorption syndrome, and acquired immunodeficiency syndrome may lead to hypogonadotropic hypogonadism by means of a central mechanism.

Disorders of the pituitary include tumors, necrosis of the pituitary, empty sella syndrome, and inflammatory or infiltrative disease. The most common cause of amenorrhea associated with pituitary disorders is an increase in the secretion of prolactin. Pituitary tumors comprise approximately 10% of all intracranial tumors and may secrete no hormone, one hormone, or multiple hormones. Prolactin levels are elevated in 50% to 70% of cases as a result of prolactin secretion by prolactinomas or by interference by tumor mass with the normal inhibitory influence of dopamine produced in the hypothalamus on prolactin secretion. The level of plasma prolactin elevation at which radiologic evaluation should be initiated in the absence of amenorrhea is not clear. Some investigators have recommended evaluating all women with elevated levels of prolactin of more than 20 to 30 μg/L, whereas others have recommended evaluating women only when levels exceed 50 to 100 μg/L. Patients with prolactin levels greater than 50 μg/L have a 20% chance of harboring a tumor that can be imaged, patients with levels of 100 μg/L have a 50% chance of having a tumor that can be identified, and patients with levels of 100 to 300 μg/L have a very high frequency of tumor.

Treatment of chronic anovulation due to hypothalamic disorders includes reversal of the underlying cause if possible. Attempts should be made to reverse any stress, to increase weight gain, and to reduce exercise. Estrogen-progestin therapy or an oral contraceptive should be initiated to prevent bone loss and maintain normal secondary sexual characteristics. In patients who do not desire pregnancy, gonadotropin therapy or pulsatile GnRH therapy is successful in inducing ovulation and pregnancy.

*Not FDA approved for this indication.

DYSMENORRHEA

method of
MELISA HOLMES, M.D., and
CHARLES N. LANDEN, Jr., M.D.
Medical University of South Carolina
Charleston, South Carolina

Dysmenorrhea is a common gynecologic disorder characterized by low pelvic pain associated with menses. In addition to pelvic pain, patients may also report low back pain and pain that radiates down the anterior thighs. It may also be accompanied by nausea, vomiting, diarrhea, and rarely syncope. Classically, dysmenorrhea has been subdivided into primary dysmenorrhea, in which there is no underlying pathologic process, and secondary dysmenorrhea, in which a pathologic condition exists that gives discomfort when menses occurs. Each has a prevalence rate of about 75% in menstruating women, although studies of various populations reveal a wide range (12%–95%). Dysmenorrhea is responsible for significant economic costs in lost productivity, physician visits, and medications, and this condition may cause emotional difficulties for women and their families.

PRIMARY DYSMENORRHEA

Primary dysmenorrhea is caused by an increased production of endometrial prostaglandins (primarily $PGF_{2\alpha}$) during the repair process of the late secretory phase. Prostaglandins lead to uterine hypercontractility, local ischemia, increased intrauterine pressure, and sensitization of myometrial nerve endings. Vasopressin levels are also elevated, and the vasospasm induced exacerbates prostaglandin effects.

Primary dysmenorrhea usually affects younger women, presenting within a few years of menarche. This reflects the fact that the first 12 to 24 months of a young woman's menses are usually anovulatory. Symptoms typically begin the day of or before the onset of menses, and last for 3 to 4 days. The physical examination may reveal a mildly tender uterus during menses, but, the examination is otherwise completely normal. The pain may lessen with applied pressure or physical activity.

Treatment of primary dysmenorrhea is directed at the underlying cause, prostaglandin production. Prostaglandin synthetase inhibitors, also called *nonsteroidal anti-inflammatory drugs (NSAIDs),* are effective in up to 80% of patients with primary dysmenorrhea. Ideally, these agents should be initiated before or with the onset of pain and continued for 2 to 4 days at scheduled intervals to prevent re-formation of prostaglandin metabolites and recurrence of pain. Many NSAIDs have been used with success, and the most commonly used are described in Table 1. Mefenamic acid (Ponstel) and naproxen (Naprosyn) have the advantage of a more rapid onset of action in addition to longer duration of activity. A review of randomized trials found that all NSAIDs were more effective than placebo, but ibuprofen gave the most favorable risk-benefit profile. Incomplete pain relief may be improved if NSAIDs are started 1 to 2 days before the expected onset of menses, prophylactically inhibiting prostaglandin production.

Table 1. **Commonly Used Nonsteroidal Anti-Inflammatory Drugs**

Generic Name	Trade Name	Recommended Dose
Ibuprofen	Motrin	400–800 mg q 4–8 h
Naproxen	Naprosyn	250–500 mg q 6–8 h
Naproxen sodium	Anaprox	275–500 mg q 8–12 h
Mefenamic acid	Ponstel	250–500 mg q 6–8 h
Celecoxib*	Celebrex	100 mg q 12 h
Rofecoxib	Vioxx	25–50 mg q 24 h

*Not FDA approved for this indication.

The most recent class of NSAIDs, the cyclooxygenase-2 (COX-2) specific inhibitor, includes two drugs that are approved for treatment of primary dysmenorrhea, celecoxib (Celebrex)* and rofecoxib (Vioxx). Rofecoxib was shown to be as effective as naproxen sodium and superior to a placebo in a double-blind randomized controlled trial. Because these medications do not act on the constitutively produced COX-1 subunit, they have the added benefit of sparing the mucosa of the gastrointestinal (GI) tract. COX-2 inhibitors are therefore recommended for patients with a history of GI bleeding or ulcerations. Given the short course necessary each month to treat primary dysmenorrhea, however, their use in healthy individuals may not be worth the expense, which is higher than traditional NSAIDs.

If NSAIDs prove inadequate or if the patient also has contraceptive needs, combination oral contraceptive pills (OCs) have a 90% success rate in relieving primary dysmenorrhea. Any OC should suffice as long as there are no contraindications, but low dose monophasic OCs with 30 to 35 μg of ethinyl estradiol provide more reliable cycle control and suppression of ovarian cyst formation as well. If OC compliance is an issue, as it often is in young patients, depomedroxyprogesterone acetate (DMPA) (Depo-Provera)* 150 mg intramuscular injection every 3 months may be used. Patient satisfaction with this medication will increase if they are forewarned of the high frequency of irregular bleeding seen with DMPA. Within 9 to 12 months of DMPA therapy, 75% of patients will become amenorrheic or oligomenorrheic. Alternative therapies for primary dysmenorrhea include acupuncture and transcutaneous electrical nerve stimulation, a convenient and noninvasive device that has proven effective but is not widely used.

If neither NSAIDs nor hormonal contraception give adequate relief after 4 to 6 months of therapy, a workup for causes of secondary dysmenorrhea should be undertaken. Referral to a gynecologist is appropriate for consideration of diagnostic laparoscopy or hysteroscopy.

*Not FDA approved for this indication.

SECONDARY DYSMENORRHEA

A variety of conditions may predispose a woman to experiencing discomfort with the onset of menses (Table 2). These problems may begin at any age; therefore, an adolescent should not be assumed to have primary dysmenorrhea. With a thorough history and physical, a specific cause may be suggested. In particular, patients should be asked about other gynecologic complaints because women with *secondary dysmenorrhea* will more often have an abnormal vaginal discharge, irregular bleeding, dyspareunia, GI complaints, and chronic pelvic pain. Women with these problems are also more likely to be survivors of sexual abuse. If pain persists beyond menses, a differential diagnosis for chronic pelvic pain should be explored. If a patient is seen during the first episode of dysmenorrhea, causes of acute pain such as ectopic pregnancy, ovarian torsion, and pelvic inflammatory disease should be ruled out.

The most common cause of secondary dysmenorrhea is endometriosis, which is discussed in more detail elsewhere. Basically, *endometriosis* results from the extrauterine implantation of endometrial tissue that bleeds into the peritoneal cavity and initiates potent peritoneal irritation. The classic triad is dysmenorrhea, dyspareunia, and infertility. Pain often occurs beyond the window of menses; a diagnosis of chronic pelvic pain is made if the pain lasts for 6 months. Dyspareunia characteristically occurs with deep penetration. Dyspareunia and infertility predominantly result from adhesions formed during the frequent glandular implantation and inflammatory response that occur in the pelvis. Pelvic examination may show limited mobility of the uterus, nodularity of the uterosacral ligaments, or adnexal fullness from an endometrioma. Tenderness may be diffuse or focal, but often the uterus is tender with movement due to tension placed on adhesions that then pull on the peritoneal surfaces. Although these characteristics on history and physical are suggestive, the diagnosis of endometriosis can only be made by direct visualization or by presence of implants in a pathologic specimen. If suspected, empiric NSAID and OC therapy may give sufficient relief to patients whose symptoms occur mainly with menses. If relief is incomplete, referral to a gynecologist for laparoscopy or gonadotropin-releasing hormone (GnRH) agonist therapy is appropriate.

TABLE 2. **Causes of Secondary Dysmenorrhea**

Ectopic Foci of Endometrium

Endometriosis
Adenomyosis

Inflammatory

Endometritis/cervicitis
Pelvic adhesive disease
Chronic pelvic inflammatory disease

Structural

Cervical stenosis, transverse vaginal septum, or imperforate hymen
Leiomyomata
Uterine or cervical polyps
Pelvic congestion

Pelvic adhesive disease is suggested when there is a history of abdominal surgery or pelvic infection. Like endometriosis, this diagnosis is frequently one of chronic pelvic pain and is definitively diagnosed by direct visualization. Laparoscopic resection is often performed, but NSAIDs may be adequate. In the setting of chronic NSAID use, COX-2 inhibitors are appropriate to minimize the risk of developing GI ulcerations.

Adenomyosis is another cause of secondary dysmenorrhea. It results from ingrowth of the endometrium into myometrial tissue. The diagnosis can be made with certainty only at the time of pathologic section of the uterus. Most women with adenomyosis remain asymptomatic; however, symptomatic patients typically have pain about 1 week before and throughout menses. Concurrent metrorrhagia, dyschezia, and dyspareunia suggest adenomyosis. It usually occurs in parous women over the age of 40. Pelvic examination may show a diffusely enlarged uterus (up to 14 week size) that is soft and tender to palpation but with normal mobility. Treatment may be conservative in a woman desiring future fertility. Hysterectomy is generally curative but only in about half of cases is the diagnosis confirmed histologically.

Another cause of dysmenorrhea is obstruction of menstrual flow, which leads to uterine or vaginal distention and monthly discomfort. Causes in a patient who has never had menstrual flow include an imperforate hymen and complete transverse vaginal septum, both of which can be diagnosed on physical examination. These require surgical correction. It is important not to attempt aspiration using a needle in potential spaces beyond the obstruction because a serious infection may develop if an open drainage tract is not created. In patients who have established menses, cervical stenosis can occur following cervical procedures such as cryotherapy or cold-knife conization. Dilation with cervical dilators, under ultrasound guidance if necessary, can be both diagnostic and therapeutic. Uterine polyps, if close to the cervical canal, can create a ball-valve effect and intermittently obstruct uterine flow. Fibroids, both submucosal and intramural, can alter the contractile physiology of menstruation and result in painful menses. Saline-instilled sonography is a simple procedure for diagnosing endometrial pathology such as polyps and submucosal fibroids. Treatment varies based on the size and location of myomas but generally is surgical.

Among women with pelvic pain, it is important to assess the timing of the pain with respect to menstruation. A calendar is helpful to prospectively document pain, menses, and other symptoms such as GI disturbances. By definition, dysmenorrhea involves pain that precedes or accompanies the onset of menses but resolves within a few days of menses. Pain outside of that timeframe suggests the need to broaden the differential diagnoses to include other causes of acute and chronic pelvic pain.

PREMENSTRUAL SYMPTOMS AND SIGNS

method of
JERILYNN C. PRIOR, M.D.
University of British Columbia
Vancouver, British Columbia, Canada

Cyclical physical and mood symptoms before flow are often given the name *premenstrual syndrome* (PMS). However, this terminology simplifies what are really several differing, complex hormonal patterns and experiences that have in common only that they all are maximal in the days before menstrual flow. The purpose of this review is to clarify the three very different etiologies of premenstrual symptoms and signs and to indicate approaches to each.

By definition, premenstrual symptoms occur in women who have at least one functioning ovary, regardless of whether they still have a uterus and vaginal bleeding. In addition, although the symptoms and signs may be similar, for clarity, premenstrual symptoms should refer only to experiences in women who have *endogenous* ovarian hormonal patterns. Breast, mood, or bloating experiences in women taking oral contraceptive agents or menopausal ovarian hormone therapy are side effects.

The three different patterns of premenstrual symptoms and signs are shown in Table 1. The first is called *molimina*, or the set of experiences that indicate ovulatory cycles with normal hormonal estrogen and progesterone levels. Typical PMS is characterized by severe mood symptoms, often with breasts that are generally sore, enlarged, and nodular. It may also be associated with bloating and food craving. This type of premenstrual experience occurs in about 1% of the population and is most common in women in their 20s and early 30s. It is now understood to be causally related to higher estrogen levels with or without lower progesterone levels and disturbed ovulation. Increased premenstrual symptoms are characteristic of early perimenopause in women with regular cycles who are in their late 30s or their 40s. These women are experiencing endogenous ovarian hyperstimulation with high ovarian estrogen production and commonly have disturbed ovulation.

HORMONAL AND CLINICAL CHARACTERISTICS OF MOLIMINA

The characteristic and most diagnostic moliminal experience is axillary breast tenderness (without generalized beast soreness). This observation may or may not be associated with mild bloating, sensitivity to emotional stimuli, or increased appetite. The way to assess molimina is by asking an open-ended question called the *molimina question*: "Can you tell, by the way you feel, that your period is coming?" A negative response to the molimina question is related to anovulation as determined by a systematically documented premenstrual progesterone level lower than 18 nmol/L. The lack of molimina predicts anovulation with excellent sensitivity and specificity. A negative response to the molimina question provides a likely diagnosis of anovulation and higher risk for infertility and endometrial and/or breast cancer. The typical hormonal pattern of a cycle with molimina is one with normal ovulatory estradiol and progesterone levels, as shown in Figure 1*A*.

HORMONAL AND CLINICAL CHARACTERISTICS OF *PREMENOPAUSAL* PREMENSTRUAL SYMPTOMS

Typically, in response to the molimina question, a woman with PMS will first describe severe mood symptoms. On further open-ended questioning ("Do you notice anything else?"), they will commonly describe severe breast tenderness. They may also volunteer bloating and craving for chocolate or sweet or salty (high fat) foods.

The hormonal characteristics of cycles that have increased premenstrual symptoms are dominated by higher than usual estradiol levels. As shown in Figure 1*B*, higher estradiol levels begin at the midcycle peak. Ovulation may occur and progesterone levels may be normally high for 10 or more days, or the luteal phase may be short or nonexistent. The key hormonal characteristic is the higher estradiol level, which causes front and generalized breast soreness, amplification of stress responses, and probably fluid retention and increases in appetite.

TABLE 1. **Classification and Descriptive Characteristics of Three Kinds of Premenstrual Symptoms According to the Approach of Jerilynn C. Prior, M.D.**

Characteristic	Molimina	Premenopausal Premenstrual Symptoms	Perimenopausal Premenstrual Symptoms
Age (y)	~22–36	~16 to late 30s	Late 30s to early 50s
Cycle regularity	Usually regular	Usually regular	May be regular or erratic
Cycle type	Ovulatory	Ovulatory or nonovulatory	Ovulatory or nonovulatory
Estradiol levels	Normal	High	Very high
Progesterone levels	Normal	Normal or low	Often low
Flow	Normal Normal, 3–5 d, with 4–8 soaked pads and/or tampons per period	Normal or increased	Often heavy, ≥7 d, with >16 soaked pads and/or tampons per period
Breast symptoms	High lateral mild tenderness	Front and whole-breast tenderness	Persistent, severe breast tenderness
Premenstrual stretchy cervical mucus	Absent	Usually absent	Often present
Migraine headaches	Rare	Sometimes associated	Often present
Sleep disturbance	Usually absent	Sometimes trouble falling asleep	Often early-morning awakening

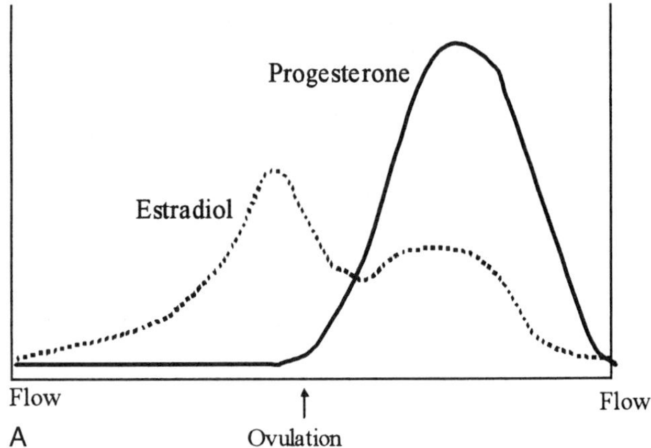

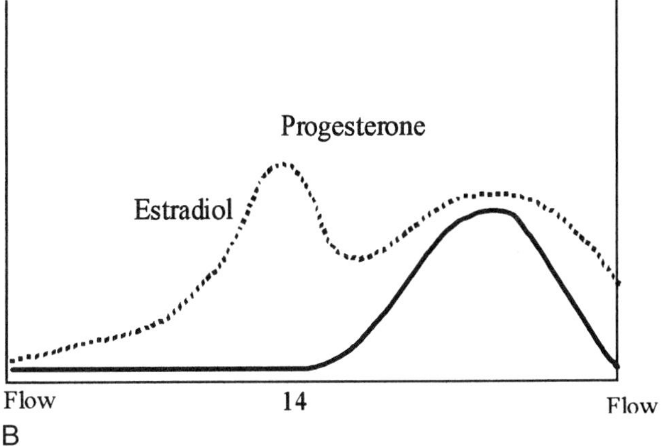

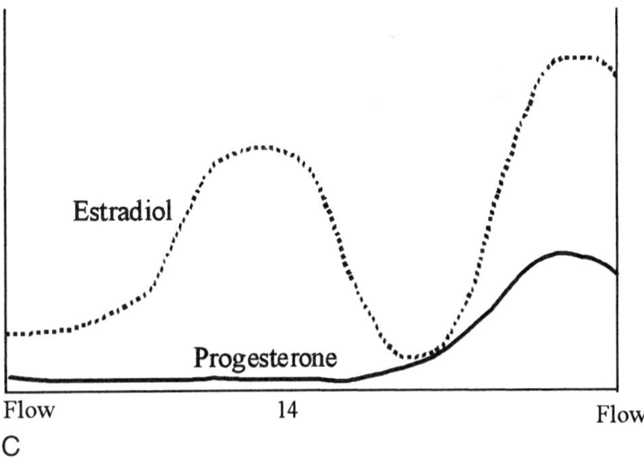

Figure 1. This three-part diagram shows the characteristic hormonal patterns associated with the three types of premenstrual symptoms. *A*, Molimina are associated with normally ovulatory cycles with balanced and cyclical physiologic levels of estradiol and progesterone. *B*, Premenopausal premenstrual symptoms are associated with elevated estradiol levels and normal or decreased progesterone levels in cycles that may be ovulatory or not. *C*, Perimenopausal premenstrual symptoms are associated with high estradiol levels and lack characteristic patterns; cycles are often nonovulatory, with very high hormone levels during prolonged and heavy flow.

HORMONAL AND CLINICAL CHARACTERISTICS OF *PERIMENOPAUSAL* PREMENSTRUAL SYMPTOMS

Perimenopause, the 3 to 10 years of transition before menopause can be defined (i.e., when a year has passed after the last menstrual period) begins gradually in women in their mid 30s to late 40s and often with increased premenstrual symptoms. Increased breast soreness associated with enlargement and nodularity and increased fluid and appetite symptoms with or without changed mood experiences are the first changes that indicate the onset of perimenopause.

Perimenopausal premenstrual symptoms are not initially different from premenopausal ones except that they may be associated with a new onset of heavy flow, sleep disturbances (usually "wee hour" awakening), weight gain, or nighttime hot flashes. The other diagnostic characteristic is that the symptoms do not significantly resolve with increasing exercise and the lifestyle strategies (discussed later) that are so effective for premenopausal women. In addition, the perimenopausal premenstrual symptoms may be much less predictable, and very high estradiol symptoms may last longer, as shown in Figure 1*C*.

Perimenopausal premenstrual symptoms may also be

associated with increased volumes of stretchy cervical mucus (usually clear and like egg white), which is a characteristic and dose-responsive sign of estrogen action at the cervix. Furthermore, as shown in Figure 1*C*, midcycle estradiol peak levels typically occur earlier in the cycle, a situation that is related to higher follicular phase estradiol levels. For women with migraine headaches, rather than being premenstrual, they may move to early in the cycle or follow the midcycle estradiol peak.

THERAPEUTIC APPROACHES TO THE THREE KINDS OF PREMENSTRUAL EXPERIENCE

Molimina

Women with molimina do not need therapy. The symptoms are mild and only reassure a woman and her physician that she is ovulatory. Lack of ovulation even once a year is related to cancellous bone loss in otherwise healthy, physically active, well-nourished women.

Premenopausal Premenstrual Symptoms

A premenopausal woman with severe premenstrual symptoms is often dealing not only with higher estradiol levels but also with increased life stresses and inadequate support. She is also likely to be sedentary, drinking more than three high-caffeine beverages per day (e.g., coffee, colas), eating erratically, and getting less than 8 hours of sleep. Therapy begins with an empathetic ear and the promise that she will improve with changes in her knowledge and improvement in her lifestyle, not with medications.

One key to therapy is a careful, multidimensional record of her hormonal and life experiences across cycles by using a daily Menstrual Cycle Diary. This tool provides assessment of both physiologic and mood experiences and a self-assessment of outside stresses. The second task is to determine whether she is ovulatory. A simple and inexpensive way to determine ovulatory status is to ask her to record her basal temperature at the same time every morning for a few cycles. The daily Menstrual Cycle Diary has a place to record temperature, and the clear instructions describe how to collect the temperature data. When all the temperatures in a given cycle are recorded, it can be determined whether the temperature rises above the average of that cycle's temperatures and consistently stays higher than that average for at least 10 days before flow. If it does, normal ovulation with a normal luteal phase length is confirmed. Temperature elevation lasting less than 10 days indicates ovulation but a short luteal phase cycle.

The only evidence-based maneuvers that relieve premenstrual symptoms are an increase in aerobic exercise and the addition of calcium in a dose of 600 mg twice a day. However, decreasing caffeine intake and committing to healthy well-balanced and regular meals are also important.

Helping patients understand and deal with the stresses in their lives rather than blaming them on PMS is equally important. As shown in Figure 2, women and physicians tend to blame premenstrual emotional symptoms on hormonal changes, but instead, the unresolved day-to-day stresses that become more difficult to ignore or deal with in the days before flow are important. One strategy is for the woman to commit to working on the problem that she feels acutely when she is premenstrual during an easier part of her cycle. Another helpful suggestion is to teach her to say "I feel . . ." rather than the usual accusation. Acknowledging the feeling is the first step toward dealing with it.

For an ovulatory woman with premenstrual symptoms, increasing aerobic exercise is key. This strategy entails starting and gradually increasing an exercise program that raises her heart rate above 130 beats a minute for increasing times per week. The aerobic exercise can be brisk walking for a sedentary woman, jogging for a reasonably fit woman, or running if the woman is already athletic. The key is that it must be training to increasing the aerobic fitness of the woman. This exercise-training strategy seems to work because it decreases hypothalamic ovarian stimuli so that estradiol levels are decreased to normal. Taking 600 mg of elemental calcium twice a day improves premenstrual symptoms, although the mechanism is not clear. Vitamin B_6 (pyridoxine) in doses of 200 to 500 mg/d for the week or two in which most mood and fluid symptoms occur may improve these symptoms through presumed hypothalamic dopamine changes.

A woman who is not consistently ovulating, in addition to the aforementioned strategies, may lessen her symptoms by taking cyclical oral micronized progesterone (Prometrium), 300 mg, at bedtime, or medroxyprogesterone (Provera), 10 mg, on days 14 to 27 of the cycle.

Finally, although some physicians treating pre-

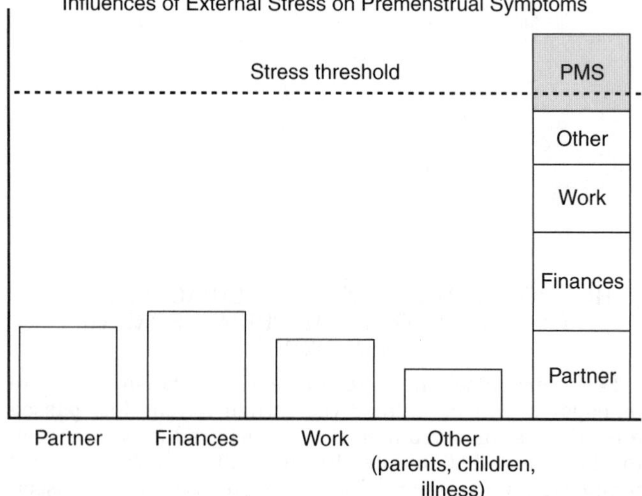

Figure 2. This bar graph shows the separate and usually manageable stressors in a woman's life that all appear to add up during the premenstrual days and are often blamed on premenstrual syndrome.

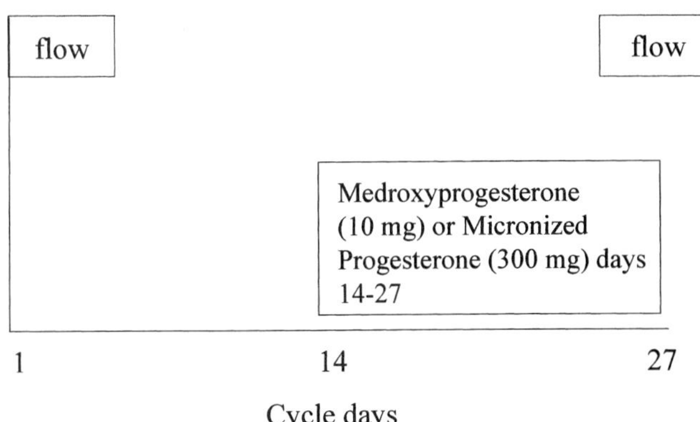

Figure 3. This figure illustrates physiologic "luteal phase replacement" of progesterone or progestin therapy for women with perimenopausal premenstrual symptoms or ovulation disturbances and abnormal flow at any age. Note that the full 14 days of progesterone therapy are continued even though flow may start.

menstrual symptoms rely on fluoxetine (Prozac) or other antidepressants or sedatives, in general, these drugs have more side effects than benefits. The only situations in which I would prescribe them are those in which a woman experiences the mood symptoms more chronically but with premenstrual exacerbation.

Perimenopausal Premenstrual Symptoms

The high estradiol levels in perimenopause occur because the normal ovarian-pituitary feedback loops are disturbed, which makes them not responsive to maneuvers that decrease hypothalamic ovarian stimuli (such as exercise). Typically, low-dose oral contraceptives relieve hot flashes but may make the breast, flow, and mood symptoms worse. The key to dealing with them is to understand that they are normal, to make all the lifestyle changes previously mentioned, and possibly to take cyclical progesterone. The good news is that perimenopausal premenstrual symptoms improve with the onset of oligomenorrhea and disappear with menopause!

It is now understood that premenstrual symptoms, if they are mild (molimina), indicate that the cycle is ovulatory and that the asymptomatic cycle is likely to be anovulatory. Premenopausal premenstrual symptoms are rare and are lessened by increased aerobic exercise and by calcium supplementation, as well as by decreasing caffeine intake, eating healthily, and dealing with life stresses. Perimenopausal premenstrual symptoms, however, are a consequence of the endogenous ovarian hyperstimulation that characterizes the transition to menopause. They are highly resistant to lifestyle therapies but may be managed by understanding and cyclical luteal phase doses of progesterone (Prometrium),* (300 mg at bedtime) or medroxyprogesterone (Provera),* (10 mg) on days 14 to 27 of the cycle (Figure 3).

*Not FDA approved for this indication.

MENOPAUSE

method of
CAROLYN CRANDALL, M.D., and
GAIL A. GREENDALE, M.D.
UCLA National Center of Excellence in Women's Health/Iris Cantor–UCLA Women's Health Center
Los Angeles, California

DEFINITIONS AND PHYSIOLOGY

Menopause is the permanent cessation of menstruation due to loss of ovarian follicular function. Amenorrhea for 12 months in the absence of other causes of secondary amenorrhea defines the diagnosis of menopause. This definition is retrospective, based on the date of final menses. *Perimenopause,* also called the *menopause transition,* is a period of changing ovarian function that precedes menopause. Perimenopause is often, but not always, characterized initially by menstrual cycle irregularity and later by lengthening intermenstrual intervals. The median age at onset of perimenopausal menstrual irregularity is about 47 years. The median age of menopause is 51 years, although current cigarette smokers undergo menopause about 1.5 years earlier than do former or never smokers.

The main estrogen made by the premenopausal ovarian follicle is 17β-estradiol. Inhibin is a sensitive marker of ovarian follicular reserve and exerts negative feedback on pituitary release of follicle-stimulating hormone (FSH). In later reproductive years, the decline in inhibin, reflecting decreased follicular competence, allows an increase in FSH. Decreasing concentrations of estradiol and inhibin contribute to the increase in FSH that accompanies menopause.

DIAGNOSIS

In menstruating women, measurement of FSH is not recommended to confirm perimenopause or to diagnose menopause. During perimenopause, FSH levels fluctuate, reflecting alternating periods of ovarian function and periods of anovulation. Therefore, in the presence of menstrual irregularities or other symptoms consistent with perimenopause, a premenopausal FSH level does not alter the clinical diagnosis of perimenopause. Conversely, FSH may be markedly elevated before the completion of 12 months of amenorrhea, but the diagnosis of menopause should not be made until the menstrual criterion is met.

PERIMENOPAUSAL AND MENOPAUSAL SYMPTOMS AND TREATMENT

Hot Flashes

A *hot flash* is a sensation of increased body heat often followed by a chill. Hot flashes vary in frequency, severity, and duration. About 75% of white women in the United States experience hot flashes during the 2 years before and after the final menses; thus, hot flashes occur commonly in perimenopause

TABLE 1. **Estrogen Alternatives for Hot Flash Suppression***

Medication	Dose	Reduction (%)†
Medroxyprogesterone acetate‡	20 mg/d	74%
Megestrol acetate‡	20 mg bid	85%
Methyldopa‡	375–1125 mg/d	65%
Soy (isolated soy protein or soy extract)	50–75 mg isoflavones/d§	45%
Transdermal clonidine‡	0.1-mg patch	20%

*All listed regimens do not have formal vasomotor indications (off-label use).
†Reduction in hot flashes compared with baseline. On average, placebo produces between 20% and 40% decrease in hot flashes.
‡Not FDA approved for this indication.
§Isoflavones are components of soy that are probably responsible for hot flash suppression.

and early postmenopause. Hot flashes wane in time in most women, although they may persist for many years in some individuals.

Treatment of Hot Flashes

Hot flash frequency is decreased by about 80% after 6 to 8 weeks of treatment with estrogen. However, to achieve satisfactory symptom control, those with severe or frequent flashes may require higher estrogen doses (see Menopause Treatments). The dose of estrogen should be reduced when feasible to minimize potential risks.

Methyldopa (Aldomet),* transdermal clonidine (Catapres),* medroxyprogesterone acetate (Depo-Provera),* megestrol acetate (Megace),* and soy isoflavones* are alternatives to estrogen for hot flash treatment (Table 1). Selective serotonin reuptake inhibitors may be effective, but no placebo-controlled trials are available. Vitamin E,* dong quai,* St. John's Wort,* and ergotamine/phenobarbital preparations* are not effective for this indication. Raloxifene (Evista) may exacerbate or induce hot flashes.

In perimenopausal women with irregular menses, oral contraceptives (OCs) afford quadruple benefits of re-establishment of menstrual regularity, reduction of heavy bleeding, relief from hot flashes, and contraception. The standard contraindications to OCs apply in perimenopausal women, except that OCs especially enhance cardiovascular risk in cigarette smokers over age 35, who should not use OCs.

Vaginal Atrophy

The vaginal epithelium thins after menopause. The epithelial maturation index, which quantifies tissue maturity, is characterized by less mature cell types after menopause; the index, however, does not correlate well with symptoms. Dyspareunia, vaginal dryness, itching, and irritation are considered symptoms of atrophy. Women with these symptoms may have signs of vaginal epithelial pallor, petechiae, friability, and lack of rugae (vaginal tissue folds). However, these signs may be present in the absence of symptoms. Asymptomatic atrophy on physical examination does not mandate treatment. Conversely, women may experience symptoms but have a nonatrophic-appearing examination; a treatment trial is warranted in these women.

*Not FDA approved for this indication.

Treatment of Vaginal Atrophy

Commonly used systemic estrogen doses are generally effective for treatment of vaginal atrophic symptoms, but some women do not have symptom resolution with usual doses. Additional vaginal therapy (hormonal or nonhormonal) may be used in these instances.

Locally administered vaginal estrogens are intended to treat vaginal epithelial tissues without stimulating other estrogen-responsive tissues (e.g., the endometrium or the liver) and without increasing systemic estrogen levels. A low-dose estrogen ring and a low-dose vaginal estrogen tablet are U.S. Food and Drug Administration (FDA)-approved as local treatment. Both appear safe with respect to the endometrium, at most causing weakly proliferative endometrial tissue. However, small but measurable increases in circulating estrogens do occur with estrogen ring use, and effects on estrogen target tissues, such as bone, have not been ruled out. Thus, if *no* systemic exogenous estrogen exposure is desired, vaginal estrogens should be used with caution and vaginal moisturizers should be considered; examples include Astroglide, Moist Again, and Replens.

Urinary Incontinence and Urinary Tract Infection

An association between menopause and urinary tract pathoses is plausible but not definitive. Changes that occur in the genitourinary system that may lead to incontinence or to irritative voiding symptoms (frequency and urgency) include atrophy of the bladder trigone; thinning of the urethral mucosa; diminished sensitivity of the bladder neck and urethral sphincter α-adrenergic receptors; and increasing of the vaginal pH, which promotes vaginal colonization with gram-negative bacteria.

Treatment of Urinary Incontinence and Urinary Tract Infection

Studies using estrogen for urinary incontinence have had mixed results, in part due to methodologic problems. Nonetheless, it is reasonable to offer a trial of estrogen (systemic or topical) for irritative voiding symptoms, stress incontinence, and urge incontinence. The vaginal estrogen produces a 50% reduction in recurrent urinary tract infections.

Sexual Function

Whether sexual function is affected by menopause remains uncertain. Women report diminishing desire and intercourse frequency with increasing age, but the role of menopause per se in the context of other factors such as partner's sexual capability and relationship quality is not known.

Treatment of Sexual Dysfunction

If vaginal atrophy is contributing to poor lubrication or to dyspareunia, estrogen therapy (systemic or vaginal) or nonhormonal vaginal moisturizers will likely produce some benefit. Less certain is whether sexual desire, orgasm, or arousal will similarly improve with estrogen treatment, although an estrogen trial for these conditions is rational. Testosterone treatment to enhance sexual desire, particularly in naturally postmenopausal women, remains debated. After oophorectomy, addition of transdermal testosterone (Androderm; 300 μg) to conjugated equine estrogens (≥0.625 mg/d) treatment may improve sexual function and psychological well-being, but this treatment is not presently FDA approved.

Depression

In the general population, menopause does not cause clinical depression. However, women with a history of depressive illness are at risk for a recurrence during perimenopause. The prevalence of clinical depression in women presenting for medical care of menopause was 45% in one menopause clinic, suggesting that midlife women with depressive symptoms may attribute these to menopause.

Treatment of Depression

Estrogen is inappropriate monotherapy for perimenopausal and postmenopausal women with significant depression; standard therapies for depression should be used. Estrogen may augment responsiveness to fluoxetine and studies attempting to replicate this finding are underway.

MENOPAUSE AND CHRONIC DISEASES

Coronary Heart Disease

Postmenopausal women are at a twofold higher risk for the development of coronary heart disease (CHD) compared to premenopausal women, after accounting for age. Age-adjusted lipid and lipoprotein levels become less favorable in association with menopause; other CHD risk mediators (e.g., insulin resistance and hemodynamic profiles) may also worsen after menopause. Conversely, many intervention studies find salutary effects of various estrogens on lipids and other CHD risk markers.

Prevention of Coronary Heart Disease

Estrogens increase high-density lipoprotein cholesterol and decrease low-density lipoprotein cholesterol; progestins dampen these effects. The effect of exogenous estrogens and estrogens plus progestins on many other proposed mediators of cardiac risk, including insulin resistance, fibrinogen, vascular reactivity, antioxidant function, and blood pressure are generally favorable. Epidemiologic studies attest to about a 50% risk reduction in CHD events and mortality among current users of estrogen. Observational studies similarly find that CHD is decreased by 50% in combination estrogen/progestin users.

The only randomized, controlled trial of combined hormone therapy (0.625 mg of conjugated equine estrogens and 2.5 mg of medroxyprogesterone acetate) and clinical CHD outcomes in women with established CHD had an overall neutral result. However, this study found an increased risk of CHD events and mortality during the first year of treatment and a decreased risk during the third and fourth years of treatment. This temporal pattern makes starting hormone replacement therapy in women with existing CHD inadvisable. However, this study also suggests that risk of CHD may be lowered after several years of hormone use; thus, it is reasonable for women who have CHD and are established postmenopausal hormone users to continue doing so.

Osteoporosis

Osteoporosis as an age-related disorder characterized by low bone mass and loss of microarchitectural stability that makes bone more vulnerable to fracture. Women have about twice as many osteoporotic fractures as do men, owing in large part to lower female peak bone mass, menopause-related bone loss, and less advantageous fall-related risk factor profiles. Whether menopause-related bone loss begins during the perimenopause (before the final menses) remains uncertain.

Prevention of Osteoporosis

Estrogens, alone or in combination with progestins, maintain or modestly increase bone mineral density. Specific doses and formulations of estrogen are U.S. FDA-approved for osteoporosis prevention based on randomized, placebo-controlled clinical trials with bone density outcomes (Table 2). Almost all studies also gave or recommended supplemental calcium. Therefore, women who are taking estrogen for osteoporosis prevention should ensure a total (diet plus supplement) daily intake of 1200 mg of elemental calcium.

In observational studies, postmenopausal estrogen users have about half the risk of all types of osteoporotic fractures compared with women who do not use these hormones. Fracture protection in association with estrogen is largely confined to current or recent users and to those who initiated it within about 5 years of their menopause.

Breast Cancer

Among thinner postmenopausal women, defined as those with a body mass index (BMI) of less than 25, the age-adjusted relative risk of breast cancer declines in relation to menopause. This protective effect of menopause is absent in women with BMI greater than 25.

TABLE 2. **FDA-Approved Estrogen and Estrogen/Progestin Combinations for Treatment of Vasomotor Symptoms and Osteoporosis Prevention**

Route, Formulation, Doses	Trade Name	Minimum Osteoporosis Prevention Dose	Vasomotor Symptom Indication
Oral Route			
CEE (0.3, 0.625, 0.90, 1.25, 2.5 mg)	Premarin	0.625 mg	Yes
0.625 mg CEE/5.0 mg MPA	Premphase	0.625 mg CEE	Yes
0.625 mg CEE/2.5 mg MPA or 0.625 mg CEE/5.0 mg MPA	Prempro	0.625 mg CEE	Yes
EE (0.3, 0.625, 1.25, 2.5 mg)	Estratab, Menest	0.3 mg	Yes
17-β estradiol (E2) with cyclic norgestimate (Nor) (1 mg E_2/0.09 mg Nor)	Ortho-Prefest	1 mg E_2/0.5 mg Nor	Yes
17-β estradiol with NETA (1 mg E_2/0.5 mg NETA)	Activella	1 mg E_2/0.5 NETA	Yes
Estropipate (piperazone estrone sulfate, E_1S)	Ortho-est, Ogen	0.625 mg E_1S	Yes
Ethinyl estradiol (EE)/NETA (5 μg EE/1 mg NETA)	Femhrt	5 μg EE/1 mg NETA	Yes
Micronized estradiol (0.5, 1, 2, mg)	Estrace, Gynodiol	0.5 mg E_2	Yes
Synthetic conjugated equine estrogens (0.625 or 0.9 mg)	Cenestin	NA	Yes*
Esterified estrogens with methyltestosterone (T) (0.625 mg EE/1.25 mg T or 1.25 mg EE/2.5 mg T)	Estratest	NA	Yes*
Ethinyl estradiol (0.02, 0.05, 0.5 mg)	Estinyl	NA	Yes
17-β estradiol reservoir patch (0.05 or 0.1 mg)	Estraderm	0.05 mg E_2	Yes
17-β estradiol patch, others† (0.025, 0.0375, 0.05, 0.075, 0.1 mg)	Alora, Climara, Fempatch, Vivelle, Menorest	0.025 mg	Yes
17-β estradiol and NETA (0.05 mg E2 with either 0.14 mg or 0.25 mg NETA)	Combipatch	NA	Yes

*If vasomotor symptoms are not improved by estrogen alone.

†Of the transdermal estradiol patches listed here, only Climara is specifically approved for osteoporosis prevention at the minimum effective dose of 0.025 mg.

Abbreviations: CEE = conjugated equine estrogens; E_2 = 17β-estradiol; EE = esterified estrogen; MPA = medroxyprogesterone acetate; NA = not specifically approved for osteoporosis prevention; NETA = norethindrone acetate.

Breast Cancer and Postmenopausal Hormone Use

A very large meta-analysis found that thinner postmenopausal women (BMI <~24.5) who were current or recent long-term estrogen users had a 10% increase in breast cancer risk compared with non-users. This increased breast cancer risk associated with current or recent postmenopausal hormone use was absent in women with higher BMI. Another large epidemiologic study found that thin (but not heavier) current or recent estrogen users who had taken estrogen for more than 8 years had a relative risk of breast cancer of 1.5 compared with that in non-users. Combination estrogen and progestin use for 4 or more years was associated with a twofold increase in breast cancer risk, again, only in the thinner women.

TREATMENT

Postmenopausal hormone use can be targeted at symptoms or at prevention of chronic disease. It is important to elicit each patient's goals because therapy directed at some symptoms (e.g., hot flashes) can be short term, whereas treatment for a chronic indication (e.g., osteoporosis prevention) must be long term. Concerns about the potential risks related to prolonged use make this distinction central to the discussion of benefits and risks of treatment.

Some formulations of systemic estrogens or estrogens/progestins are FDA-approved for vasomotor symptoms, whereas others have been tested for their ability to preserve bone mineral density and thus have an osteoporosis indication (see Table 2). Fixed combinations of estrogen/progestin therapy have been evaluated for endometrial safety (i.e., not increasing the incidence of endometrial hyperplasia). Individual progestins are also approved for prevention of endometrial hyperplasia when used in conjunction with estrogen (Table 3).

Estrogen Formulation

Estrogens can be administered by mouth, transdermally, and vaginally. If estrogens (or estrogen/progestin combinations) are being prescribed to prevent osteoporosis, then a dose that has a documented effect on bone density should be used (see Table 2). Lower than bone-protective doses can be tried for hot flash treatment, but as noted, estrogen often must be titrated upward to achieve control of hot flashes. For vaginal and urinary indications, local vaginal administration can minimize systemic exposure to hormones.

Because transdermal estrogen avoids first-pass liver metabolism, it may be particularly useful in women with significant liver function abnormalities or high triglyceride levels. Some 17-β estradiol

TABLE 3. **FDA-Approved Progestogens for Prevention of Estrogen-Related Hyperplasia in Postmenopausal Women**

Schedule	Medication (Trade Names)	Dose	Bleeding Pattern
Cyclical	Medroxyprogesterone acetate (Provera, Amen, Cycrin)	5–10 mg daily for 1st 12–14 days of calendar month	Cyclical bleeding on or after day 9 of progestogen, or no bleeding
	Micronized progesterone (Prometrium)	200 mg daily for 1st 12–14 days of calendar month	
Daily continuous	Medroxyprogesterone acetate Micronized progesterone	2.5 mg daily	Unpredictable light to moderate bleeding for <1 year, or no bleeding

patches use an alcohol-based reservoir system to release estradiol, whereas matrix systems incorporate 17-β estradiol in the patch adhesive, diminishing the occurrence of local rash from 10% (reservoir) to 5% (matrix). Percutaneous estrogen gel or cream preparations are particularly well suited to women who live in a high moisture climate, which increases the rate of skin irritation from patches to about 70%, but there are no U.S. FDA-approved gels currently available.

Side Effects

Although it is widely believed that estrogen causes breast discomfort, the Postmenopausal Estrogen/Progestin Interventions Trial found that this side effect was caused by combination estrogen/progestin therapy and not by estrogen alone; micronized progesterone and medroxyprogesterone acetate (Depo-Provera) produced equivalent reports of pain. The same study also found that women using conjugated equine estrogen alone or in combination with progestin gained less weight over a 3-year period (0.4–0.8 kg) than did placebo-assigned women (1.3 kg).

Unopposed estrogen causes endometrial hyperplasia, but when estrogen is combined with adequate doses of progestin, the rate of hyperplasia is not increased. Importantly, prevention of hyperplasia is well-documented only for the exact doses and durations of the progestins tested in studies; deviation from them is not recommended. There are no long-term tests of daily treatment using low-dose (100 mg) daily micronized progesterone*; this is not an approved or recommended method of hyperplasia prevention. Less-than-monthly progestin dosing is also not approved or recommended; a recent study of quarterly administration of progestin was halted due to unacceptable rates of endometrial cancer development.

Vaginal bleeding is an expected side effect of continuous and cyclical progestin administration. It may take up to 1 year for endometrial atrophy to occur and for bleeding to stop with continuous combined hormone therapy. All cyclical regimens have the same bleeding pattern: if bleeding occurs, it should commence on or after day 9 of the progestin component. Estrogen therapy increases the risk of venous thrombosis and pulmonary embolism; previous deep vein thrombosis or pulmonary embolism is therefore a contraindication to use. In a large randomized trial, clinical gallbladder disease was increased by 40% in women assigned to continuous daily conjugated equine estrogens and medroxyprogesterone acetate.

*Not FDA approved for this indication.

Contraindications

A history of deep venous thrombosis or pulmonary embolism, undiagnosed vaginal bleeding, and undiagnosed breast masses contraindicate estrogen use. Although estrogen administration is not considered appropriate for most patients with breast cancer, the informed breast cancer survivor with debilitating symptoms may elect to use it after detailed discussion with her physician. Hypertension and diabetes mellitus are not contraindications; hormone replacement therapy has a neutral or lowering effect on systolic blood pressure and does not worsen glycemic control.

VULVOVAGINITIS

method of
PAUL NYIRJESY, M.D.
Jefferson Medical College
Philadelphia, Pennsylvania

Vaginitis is one of the most common reasons that women see their physicians. With the advent of over-the-counter antifungal agents, which now account for an estimated $250 million in annual sales, the focus is now on self-treatment instead of accurate diagnosis. However, current data suggest that self-diagnosis and self-treatment are inaccurate and that the best chance at proper diagnosis remains with clinicians.

In the evaluation of a woman with vulvovaginal symptoms, the history should focus not only on vaginal discharge but also on other symptoms such as irritation, itching, burning, and dyspareunia. Both a menstrual and a sexual history may add further insights into the potential etiology. The pelvic examination should include a careful inspection of the vulva, which is often the area with the most notable findings. The laboratory evaluation is often underutilized by clinicians but is essential for proper diagnosis. It should include vaginal pH testing, microscopic examination of saline and 10% potassium hydroxide preparations of vaginal secretions, and sampling of the cervix for chlamydial infection and gonorrhea tests, if appropriate. In cases with a history indicative of vulvovaginal candidiasis (VVC) but negative microscopy, fungal cultures should be considered. The presence of vulvar ulcers should suggest the need for herpes cultures. Other tests, such as vaginal bacterial cultures or *Trichomonas* cultures, are useful only in limited circumstances.

Although the differential diagnosis of vulvovaginal symptoms is broad, most cases of infectious vaginitis will be caused by either bacterial vaginosis (BV), trichomoniasis, or VVC. In those women who fail to meet the criteria for these three conditions, other relatively common causes include irritant dermatitis, atrophic vaginitis, and vulvar non-neoplastic epithelial disorders. Finally, in women whose only complaint is of a vaginal discharge, the possibility that it is physiologic should be entertained.

NORMAL VAGINAL ENVIRONMENT

Essential to an understanding of vaginitis in general is the concept that estrogen plays a crucial role in controlling the normal vaginal environment. In the prepubertal state, the vagina is thinned and hypoestrogenic, with an elevated pH ($\geq$4.7), and culture of the vagina will demonstrate a variety of organisms. With ovarian production of estrogen, growth of lactobacilli is stimulated, and the corresponding production of lactic acid lowers the vaginal pH to less than 4.5. Although lactobacilli are normally the dominant flora of the vagina during the reproductive years, they are part of a heterogeneous microflora. For example, other organisms, such as group B streptococci, the genital mycoplasmas, *Gardnerella vaginalis*, and *Candida albicans* are also commonly found, and their presence on a culture does not necessarily imply the existence of a vaginal infection. In a menopausal woman, the vagina once again becomes thinned, with an elevated pH, and lactobacilli decline in quantity; however, if a woman takes exogenous hormone replacement therapy, the vaginal environment should resemble that of a woman in her reproductive years. Thus, knowing a woman's estrogen status is crucial to understanding findings that may be noted on examination or microscopy.

BACTERIAL VAGINOSIS

BV is believed to be the most prevalent type of vaginitis in women of childbearing age. Reported incident rates for BV have ranged from 5% in the general population to 64% in patients visiting sexually transmitted disease clinics. In the past, many clinicians viewed BV as a nuisance rather than as a serious health problem. Recent research, however, has revealed a link between BV and many other infectious processes of the female genital tract. In pregnant women, BV has been associated with prematurity, preterm premature rupture of membranes, and intra-amniotic fluid infection. In nonpregnant women, it is considered a risk factor for pelvic inflammatory disease, mucopurulent cervicitis, postoperative (hysterectomy, abortion) infections, and urinary tract infections. BV has also been associated in cross-sectional and prospective studies with an increased incidence of HIV seroconversion. Some of these associations may be secondary to the shifts in the vaginal microflora that occur with BV. Women with BV exhibit decreased or absent levels of hydrogen peroxide–producing lactobacilli, which are thought to protect the vagina from infection, and subsequent overgrowth with anaerobic species, *G. vaginalis*, and genital mycoplasmas.

Approximately 50% of women with BV are asymptomatic. When symptomatic, women with BV will generally complain of a fishy odor, an abnormal discharge, or irritation and itching. Examination will reveal a gray, profuse, watery discharge. Other criteria for diagnosis include a vaginal pH of 4.7 or higher, a positive amine or "whiff" test when mixing the secretions with 10% potassium hydroxide, and the presence of clue cells on saline microscopy. If the diagnosis is in doubt, a Gram stain of vaginal secretions may be useful. However, culture for the presence of *G. vaginalis* is not helpful because the mere presence of this organism does not mean that the patient has BV.

Treatment of bacterial vaginosis can be either oral (metronidazole [Flagyl], 500 mg twice daily for 7 days, clindamycin [Cleocin], 300 mg twice daily for 7 days) or topical (metronidazole gel [MetroGel Vaginal], 0.75% at bedtime for 5 days; clindamycin [Cleocin], 2% cream or 100-mg ovules for 3 days). The efficacy of these treatments seems to be similar. In pregnant women with prior preterm deliveries and current BV, treatment with oral metronidazole may decrease the risk of adverse pregnancy outcomes. In a normal pregnancy in which BV is present, treatment does not seem to affect pregnancy outcome.

TRICHOMONIASIS

Vaginal trichomoniasis is a common sexually transmitted disease, with an estimated annual incidence of 3 million in the United States. The prevalence ranges from 5% in family planning clinics to 75% in studies of prostitutes. Female behavioral factors such as number of lifetime and recent sexual partners, history of other sexually transmitted diseases, and nonuse of barrier or oral contraceptives have been associated with infection. Asymptomatic men and women probably represent the primary reservoir for this organism; carriage of the organism may persist for months to years.

In women, trichomoniasis is asymptomatic in 25% to 50% of cases. It may cause an abnormal purulent, frothy, or bloody discharge, often accompanied by malodor, pruritus, and dyspareunia. Other manifestations may include postcoital bleeding, dysuria or urinary frequency, Bartholin gland infection, and pelvic inflammatory disease. Physical findings include varying degrees of vulvar and vaginal inflammation, an abnormal discharge, and punctate hemorrhage of the cervix (strawberry cervix). The classic frothy discharge of *Trichomonas vaginalis* infection is seen in only 12% of cases, and the strawberry cervix occurs in only 2%. Further evaluation of an infected patient may reveal a positive whiff or amine test and an elevated pH. In most cases, the diagnosis rests on the saline smear, in which live motile trichomonads can be identified. However, the wet smear has a sensitivity of 55% to 60%. The Papanicolaou test (Pap smear) has a similar sensitivity but carries with it a false-positive rate of at least 8%. In cases in which the diagnosis remains in question (e.g., suspicious wet smear, abnormal Pap smear but normal evaluation), culture techniques, which can detect as few as 300 trichomonads per milliliter of inoculum, should be considered. The InPouch TV culture system (Biomed Diagnostics, San Jose, CA), a two-chambered bag system, allows wet mount microscopic examination of the culture through the bag and obviates the need for repeat sampling of the culture to detect positive specimens. Polymerase chain reaction tests are presently being used in research settings.

The only approved medication available in the United States for the treatment of trichomoniasis is metronidazole, which can be given as a single 2-g dose or 500 mg twice daily for 7 days. Although case-control studies have failed to reveal an association between birth defects and metronidazole, use of this drug is often avoided in the first trimester because it has mutagenic activity in in vitro assay systems; however, current treatment guidelines for sexually transmitted diseases from the Centers for Disease Control and Prevention do not impose such a restriction on the single 2-g dose. It is important to counsel patients to ensure that their partners receive adequate treatment to avoid reinfection. In cases of metronidazole allergy, desensitization protocols have been shown to permit effective treatment with metronidazole. Resistance to metronidazole is rare but may be increasing. Treatment of patients with metronidazole-resistant trichomoniasis should be done in consultation with an expert; such treatment will often entail courses of higher doses of metronidazole.

VULVOVAGINAL CANDIDIASIS

VVC remains one of the most common infections of the female genital tract. Approximately 20% of reproductive-age women have asymptomatic vaginal colonization with *C. albicans*. By age 25 years, as many as 55% of college women have been diagnosed with symptomatic VVC. Women with uncomplicated VVC have occasional mild to moderate symptomatic episodes with no clear precipitating event. Risk factors for uncomplicated VVC include sexual activity, receptive oral sex, oral contraceptive use, and spermicide use. Although antibiotics have also been implicated as a risk factor, only a few women who take antibiotics will develop VVC, and the mechanism for this association has not been well studied. *C. albicans* is the causative organism in most uncomplicated cases.

An estimated 5% of women suffer complicated VVC. Women who meet this definition have either recurrent (≥4 episodes per year) VVC, severe VVC, or infections caused by species other than *C. albicans*. Women with diabetes or immunosuppression also fall into this category. It is important to differentiate patients with complicated VVC from those with uncomplicated VVC, because women with complicated VVC are more likely to have only transient and incomplete responses to antimycotic therapy and may need more specialized follow-up and attention. The pathogenesis of recurrent VVC remains unclear; current interest has focused on the concept that repeated episodes of VVC are caused by host factors, where normal homeostatic mechanisms are unable to keep *Candida* colonization under control.

Patients with VVC complain primarily of vulvar or vaginal pruritus, irritation, soreness, or burning. Although some patients complain of a thick white discharge, as many as 50% of VVC patients deny a change in their discharge. Examination may reveal varying amounts of vulvar or vaginal erythema or edema, as well as vaginal thrush. In severe cases, fissures may also be noted. The vaginal pH is normal. Diagnosis is made on the basis of hyphae or blastospores on saline or potassium hydroxide microscopy. In patients with a history suggestive of VVC but negative microscopy, or in patients with complicated VVC, fungal cultures will help to clarify the diagnosis and guide therapy.

Clinicians are faced with many choices for antimycotic therapy (Table 1). In general, the mainstay of therapy consists of azole agents, in either topical or oral forms. Topical forms may be taken in a variety of formulations and treatment durations. Overall, no significant differences exist between in vitro and in vivo activity, and the choice of agents with uncomplicated VVC comes down largely to patient preference. Although the trend has been toward shorter courses of therapy, longer follow-up studies have not been performed to look at long-term relapse rates. In general, the main side effect with topical therapy is localized burning in 5% to 10% of patients as an allergic or irritant reaction. Fluconazole (Diflucan), given as a single 150-mg dose, seems to be as effective as a week of topical therapy. Mild side effects, such as headache, nausea, and diarrhea, occur in less than 10% of cases. Insufficient safety data prevent its use in pregnancy. Patients with complicated VVC caused by *C. albicans* may require long-term suppression of their infections to achieve symptomatic relief. Non–*C. albicans* infection may require therapy

TABLE 1. **Choices of Therapy for Vulvovaginal Candidiasis**

Drug (Trade Name)	Formulations	Length of Therapy
Nystatin (Mycostatin)	Vaginal tablet	14 days
Butoconazole (Femstat)	Cream	1–3 days
Clotrimazole (Mycelex)	Cream, suppository, vaginal tablet	1–7 days
Miconazole (Monistat)	Cream, suppository, vaginal tablet	1–7 days
Terconazole (Terazol)	Cream, suppository	3–7 days
Tioconazole (Vagistat)	Cream	1–3 days
Fluconazole (Diflucan)	Oral tablet (150 mg)	1 day

with alternative agents, such as boric acid suppositories (600 mg intravaginally twice daily for 2 weeks, followed by suppressive therapy) or flucytosine cream (Ancobon) (14.5%, 5-g applicator nightly for 2 weeks). Follow-up fungal cultures while the patient is on therapy are quite helpful in this patient population.

CHLAMYDIA TRACHOMATIS

method of
JANET N. ARNO, M.D.
Indiana University School of Medicine
Indianapolis, Indiana

Chlamydia trachomatis remains the most common notifiable disease in the United States, with more than 580,000 cases reported to the Centers for Disease Control and Prevention (CDC) per year in 1998 and 1999. Many cases are asymptomatic and not diagnosed or reported; therefore, its incidence has been estimated to be greater than 4 million cases annually. The most important reasons to treat *C. trachomatis* infection are its relationship to pelvic inflammatory disease (PID), ectopic pregnancy, and enhanced transmission of HIV.

MICROBIOLOGY

C. trachomatis is an obligate intracellular pathogen that can be difficult to isolate in culture, so it is important to obtain optimal specimens. Its unique intracellular dimorphic lifecycle makes it difficult to study. For that reason, antibiotic susceptibility testing requires special laboratories. In contrast to other bacteria, its transformation is elusive, thus slowing identification of virulence factors. Studies have suggested that the tubal scarring that results in obstruction, infertility, and ectopic pregnancy may be due to the immune response to chlamydial heat shock proteins. Sequencing of the chlamydial genome has been done and promises to aid in study.

Strains or serovars of *C. trachomatis*, previously defined serologically, are now identifiable by their major outer membrane protein, a target for vaccine development. Serovars A, B, and C are associated with trachoma, a common cause of blindness in developing countries. Serovars L1, L2, and L3 are associated with lymphogranuloma venereum. Serovars D through K are associated with the common forms of infection, usually confined to the genital tract epithelium. At the present time, identifying the infecting strain of the organism has little day-to-day clinical value, even though certain of the genital serovars have been associated with somewhat more severe symptoms.

CLINICAL MANIFESTATIONS

Approximately 70% of chlamydial endocervical infections are asymptomatic or minimally symptomatic in women. Asymptomatic infections occur in men as well. When symptomatic, patients have cervicitis, urethritis, endometritis, salpingitis, or PID. Cervicitis may be manifested as a vaginal discharge or increased friability, that is, a tendency to bleed from the cervical os when a swab is inserted. Ascending infection occurs commonly and may be asymptomatic. Although acute salpingitis develops in only about 8% of untreated infected women, asymptomatic PID occurs more commonly. Women with chlamydial urethritis may have acute urethral syndrome, defined as the occurrence of dysuria or frequency in the absence of 10^5 organisms/mL of urine. In one study, approximately 25% of individuals with acute urethral syndrome had chlamydial infection as compared with 5% of asymptomatic controls.

Men with urethritis often have a discharge that may vary from scant and watery or mucoid to frankly purulent. Symptoms typically begin 7 to 10 days after a new sexual contact. Nongonococcal urethritis is a syndrome characterized by a mucopurulent or purulent urethral discharge, a Gram stain of the discharge showing more than 5 white blood cells per oil immersion field in the absence of gram-negative diplococci, a positive leukocyte esterase stain, or a microscopic examination of spun urine with 10 or more white blood cells per high-power field. Thirty percent to 50% of cases of symptomatic nongonococcal urethritis are caused by *Chlamydia*. *Ureaplasma histolyticum* (10% to 20%) and *Trichomonas vaginalis* (10%) may also cause the syndrome. Asymptomatic infection occurs in men as well.

For symptomatic patients, empirical treatment is given. Testing is recommended because the sensitivity and specificity of clinical findings are poor. Asymptomatic individuals are detected by screening.

Chlamydia is most common in younger individuals, particularly adolescents, who are single, have multiple partners, use no barrier contraception, and are nonwhite. The CDC currently recommends testing sexually active adolescents for chlamydial infection routinely at the time of their annual examination, even if symptoms are not present. Screening women aged 20 to 24 years is also suggested, particularly for those who have new or multiple sex partners and do not consistently use barrier contraceptives, a recommendation that is not likely to change in the foreseeable future.

DIAGNOSIS

C. trachomatis can be detected by a large variety of diagnostic tests, including culture, enzyme-linked immunoassay, and direct immunofluorescence, or by using amplified DNA technology such as polymerase chain reaction, ligase chain reaction, or an assay based on strand displacement. The sensitivity and specificity of these tests are summarized in Table 1. Amplified DNA tests have often surpassed culture as screening tests of choice in the United

TABLE 1. **Swab Sensitivity and Specificity of Diagnostic Tests for *Chlamydia trachomatis***

	Culture* (%)	EIA (%)	SDA (%)	LCR (%)	DFA (%)	PCR (%)
Chlamydia sensitivity	70–85	70	93–95	85–95	53	90–98
Chlamydia specificity	>99	99	94.8	99.3	99.5	98.3–99.2
Gonorrhea sensitivity	—	No test	96–97	86–96	NA	96–98
Gonorrhea specificity	—	No test	NA	NA	NA	NA

*Sensitivity and specificity are relative to the gold standard of culture or two of three nucleic acid–based tests.

Abbreviations: DFA = direct fluorescent antibody test; EIA = enzyme-linked immunoassay; LCR = ligase chain reaction; NA = not available; PCR = polymerase chain reaction; SDA = strand displacement assay.

Adapted from B van der Pol, Indiana University.

States because of their increased sensitivity. DNA amplification allows urine testing, which greatly simplifies screening, particularly in men. Antigen detection tests such as enzyme-linked immunoassay have the advantage of being inexpensive, and confirmatory tests help make them more specific. Nevertheless, it may be more cost-effective to use the more expensive DNA amplification tests in terms of the number of cases of PID and other complications prevented. To assist in making the decision of whether changing tests makes sense for a given program, the CDC has developed software available through the Internet at the URL *www.cdc.gov/nchstp/dstd/Software/Socrates.htm.*

IMPACT OF SCREENING STRATEGIES

Screening for asymptomatic infection does decrease PID. In a prospective randomized trial published by Scholes in 1996, screening women aged 18 to 34 enrolled in an health maintenance organization resulted in a significant decrease in the development of PID relative to the group that was not screened. Cost analyses have considered different models for screening, including age-based strategies, universal screening, and no screening. Screening by age provided cost savings to the U.S. Army over a 1-year period. Organizations assessing large cohorts of women are likely to benefit from such screening programs, even in the short term.

TREATMENT

Effective treatment regimens for chlamydial genital infection are summarized in Table 2. Two regimens are considered standard for uncomplicated chlamydial cervicitis and urethritis. Azithromycin (Zithromax), 1 g orally,* is often preferred because it is administered as a single dose. Doxycycline (Vibramycin), 100 mg orally twice daily, is equally effective. Tetracycline is effective but less desirable because of its four-times-daily dosing regimen. Ofloxacin (Floxin), 300 mg twice daily for 7 days, is an alternative regimen.

Levofloxacin, the (−)-(S)-entantiomer of ofloxacin that accounts for most of its antibacterial activity, is likely to be at least as effective as ofloxacin but has not been rigorously studied. In one study of Japanese women with cervicitis, levofloxacin (Levaquin)† given at a dose of 500 mg/d resulted in acceptable cure rates when given for 7 days. Shorter regimens were inadequate. Trovafloxacin (Trovan), though effective in women, is not recommended because of potential serious hepatotoxicity.

Treatment in Pregnancy

The treatment of choice for chlamydial genital infection in pregnancy is erythromycin (see Table 2). Because erythromycin is poorly tolerated and doxycycline and quinolones are contraindicated, alternative regimens have been developed. Amoxicillin† appears to be safe and effective as an alternative agent for the treatment of genital chlamydial infections in pregnancy when compared with erythromycin. Azithromycin and clindamycin (Cleocin)* appear to be effective but have not been adequately investigated. A study of 85 evaluable pregnant women found that azithromycin was as effective as erythromycin but had fewer gastrointestinal side effects and was associated with better compliance.

Treatment of chlamydial infection is important because the infection may be transmitted to the infant during delivery and lead to ophthalmia neonatorum or neonatal pneumonia. The degree to which chlamydial infections lead to complications and preterm birth is currently under study.

*Exceeds dosage recommended by the manufacturer.
†Not FDA approved for this indication.

Table 2. **Regimens* for *Chlamydia trachomatis* Genital Infection**

Urethritis or Cervicitis

Recommended:

Azithromycin, 1 g PO in a single dose
or
Doxycycline, 100 mg PO bid for 7 d

Alternative regimens:

Erythromycin base, 500 mg PO qid for 7 d
or
Erythromycin ethylsuccinate, 800 mg PO qd for 7 d
Ofloxacin, 300 mg bid for 7 days (levofloxacin, 500 mg qd for 7 d, is probably effective)

If only erythromycin can be used and a patient cannot tolerate the high-dose regimens, the following can be used:

Erythromycin base, 250 mg PO qid for 14 d, *or* erythromycin ethylsuccinate, 400 mg PO qid for 14 d

Urethritis or Cervicitis During Pregnancy

Recommended:

Erythromycin base, 500 mg PO qid for 7 d
Amoxicillin,† 500 mg PO tid for 7 d

Used by many practitioners:

Azithromycin, 1 g PO in a single dose

Alternative regimens:

Erythromycin ethylsuccinate, 800 mg PO qd for 7 d

If only erythromycin can be used and a patient cannot tolerate the high-dose regimens, the following can be used:

Erythromycin base, 250 mg PO qid for 14 d, *or* erythromycin ethylsuccinate, 400 mg PO qid for 14 d

Pelvic Inflammatory Disease

See article on pelvic inflammatory disease

*Based on 1998 sexually transmitted disease guidelines plus literature from 1998 to 2000.
†Not FDA approved for this indication.

Compliance, Tests of Cure, and Failure Rates

Azithromycin and doxycycline are equally effective at curing infection, with usually greater than a 95% microbiologic cure rate and an 85% to 95% clinical cure rate under study conditions. However, noncompliance with treatment regimens is common, even if

*Not FDA approved for this indication.

full compliance is reported. Luckily, even patients who take less than the prescribed regimen of doxycycline may be cured. In one study of 221 evaluable patients, all 58 patients who took roughly half the medication were cured at 4 weeks.

Currently, tests of cure are not usually recommended. Nevertheless, recurrence of *C. trachomatis* after antibiotic treatment is not infrequent. Because recurrence is common, particularly when partners are not treated, it may be that repeated testing of *Chlamydia*-infected patients is warranted at later time points than the traditional 7 days. A recent study proposed that patients be retested at 12 to 24 weeks. Home sampling may facilitate retesting.

Complications

Although men may occasionally experience pain from ascending infection, most complications of *Chlamydia* infection occur in women. PID will develop in approximately 30% of infected women if untreated, all but 8% asymptomatic. For a discussion of the manifestations of acute PID, including perihepatitis, see the article on PID. Asymptomatic PID results from a chronic inflammatory response and is often detected when tubal factor infertility is diagnosed at laparoscopy. Fallopian tube occlusion is demonstrable. Ectopic pregnancies are also more common in patients with a history of genital infections.

PELVIC INFLAMMATORY DISEASE

method of
KARL E. MILLER, M.D.
University of Tennessee College of Medicine
Chattanooga, Tennessee

Pelvic inflammatory disease (PID) consists of a variety of ascending infections that affect the upper female reproductive tract. This can include any combination of endometritis, salpingitis, oophoritis, tubo-ovarian abscess, and pelvic peritonitis. Sexually transmitted organisms such as *Neisseria gonorrhoeae* and *Chlamydia trachomatis* are the most common causes of this infection; however, multiple other microorganisms have been implicated as well.

Approximately 10% of women will develop PID during their reproductive years. PID is not a reportable disease, but estimates suggest that more than 1 million women receive treatment for this disease in the United States every year. Approximately 25% to 30% of these patients will require hospitalization for treatment. In addition, a significant number of the patients who are hospitalized will undergo a surgical procedure as part of the treatment. Because of these factors, PID has a significant impact on the health and well-being of women during their reproductive years. In addition, this disease adds a considerable cost to the health care system.

PID is almost exclusively a disease of sexually active women. The highest incidence of PID is in the adolescent age group. This age group also has the highest rates of hospitalization and long-term morbidity. Some of the long-term morbidity includes ectopic pregnancy, infertility, dyspareunia, and chronic pelvic pain. One episode of PID can cause these long-term morbidities in approximately 25% of women with PID, and repeated infections increase this percentage dramatically.

ETIOLOGY

The most common causative organisms of PID include *N. gonorrhoeae* and *C. trachomatis*. One of these two organisms can be isolated from the cervix approximately 50% of the time. The other 50% of the time, neither of these organisms is isolated from the cervix or the upper genital tract.

There are other organisms that can cause PID. These include gram-negative and anaerobic organisms such as *Bacteroides* species, *Escherichia coli, Klebsiella* species, *Peptostreptococcus* species, and *Proteus* species. Mycobacteria and the respiratory organisms have been implicated as causative organisms for this infection as well. In addition, organisms that cause bacterial vaginosis have also been suggested as etiologic agents for this ascending infection. This may occur because the breakdown of the cervical mucus barrier secondary to the change in vaginal flora allows these organisms to infect the upper genital tract.

DIAGNOSIS

The difficulty physicians face when diagnosing PID is that it is usually based on clinical impression. Many episodes of PID go undiagnosed because some cases can be asymptomatic and others can have mild or nonspecific signs or symptoms. In order to reduce the potential for missed diagnoses of PID, the Centers for Disease Control and Prevention (CDC) has established minimal, additional, and definitive criteria for when empiric treatment of PID should be initiated (Table 1). In a woman who is sexually active and at risk for PID, empiric treatment should be initiated if all three of the minimum criteria are met. The additional criteria can be used to support the diagnosis of PID. Performing invasive procedures to establish a definitive diagnosis of PID based on the CDC criteria should be used only in select cases in which the diagnosis is in question.

Evaluation for the presence of *N. gonorrhoeae* and *C.*

TABLE 1. **Centers for Disease Control and Prevention Criteria for the Diagnosis of Pelvic Inflammatory Disease**

Minimum Criteria
- Lower abdominal pain
- Adnexal tenderness
- Cervical motion tenderness

Additional Criteria
- Oral temperature >101°F (38.3°C)
- Abnormal cervical or vaginal discharge
- Elevated erythrocyte sedimentation rate
- Elevated C-reactive protein level
- Laboratory documentation of cervical infection with *Neisseria gonorrheae* or *Chlamydia trachomatis*

Definitive Criteria
- Histopathologic evidence of endometritis on endometrial biopsy
- Transvaginal sonography or other imaging abnormalities consistent with PID
- Laparoscopic abnormalities consistent with PID

Abbreviation: PID = pelvic inflammatory disease.

trachomatis cervical infections can be performed using multiple different methods. The easiest is DNA ligase probes. These probes have excellent sensitivities and specificities, and one swab can be used to test for both organisms. Other methods are available but require two separate tests for gonorrhea and chlamydia.

In addition to establishing the diagnosis of PID, patients should be evaluated for other sexually transmitted diseases. This includes offering and counseling about HIV testing. Patients should receive testing for syphilis and hepatitis as well. The patients' partners should also receive testing and treatment based on the results of the tests.

MANAGEMENT

The goal of treatment for PID includes relief of symptoms and reduction of the morbidity that comes from this upper genital tract infection. The treatment should be aimed at all of the potential etiologic organisms. Many regimens have been studied, but the CDC has established antibiotic treatment plans for both outpatient and inpatient management of PID.

Outpatient therapy with oral antibiotics can be used in the majority of PID patients. One important component to outpatient therapy is that follow-up care must be available within 72 hours to evaluate the response to the treatment regimen. In order to provide criteria for determining who can be treated using outpatient therapy, the CDC has established criteria for when it is appropriate to hospitalize patients with PID (Table 2). If patients meet any of these criteria, the appropriate management strategy is hospitalization for parenteral therapy.

The CDC guidelines contain five different parenteral regimens for PID treatment (Table 3). Parenteral infusions of doxycycline can cause discomfort that can be reduced by adding short-acting local anesthesia, heparin, or steroids. Bioavailability of parenteral and oral doxycycline is the same; therefore, oral therapy should be used whenever possible. Parenteral therapy may be changed to oral therapy 24 hours after the patient improves clinically.

There are various outpatient treatment regimens for PID (Table 4). The full course of treatment consists of 14 days. The amoxicillin/clavulanate potassium (Augmentin) plus doxycycline regimen has been shown effective in PID treatment, but the gastrointestinal side effects of this regimen may limit its overall success rate. Azithromycin (Zithromax) has been evaluated in the treatment of PID, but the CDC states that the data are insufficient to recommend this agent in any of the treatment regimens.

TABLE 3. **Parenteral Treatment Regimens for Pelvic Inflammatory Disease**

Regimen A

Cefotetan (Cefotan) 2 g IV every 12 h *or* cefoxitin (Mefoxin) 2 g every 6 h

plus

Doxycycline 100 mg IV or orally every 12 h

Regimen B

Clindamycin (Cleocin) 900 mg every 8 h

plus

Gentamycin loading dose IV or IM (2 mg/kg) followed by maintenance dose (1.5 mg/kg) every 8 h. Single dosing may be substituted.

Alternative Regimens

1. Ofloxacin (Floxin) 400 mg IV every 12 h
   plus
   Metronidazole (Flagyl) 500 mg IV every 8 h
2. Ampicillin/sulbactam (Unasyn) 3 g IV every 6 h
   plus
   Doxycycline 100 mg IV or orally every 12 h
3. Ciprofloxacin (Cipro) 200 mg IV every 12 h
   plus
   Doxycycline 100 mg IV or orally every 12 h
   plus
   Metronidazole 500 mg IV every 8 h

PREVENTION

In order to reduce patients' risks for developing PID, physicians must be able to identify risk factors. The most significant risk factor is multiple sex partners within a short period of time. In addition, the adolescent population is at greater risk for PID than any other age group. Finally, women who have had a prior sexually transmitted disease or prior PID are at increased risk.

Once a risk assessment has been done, a "patient-centered" preventive message should be provided. This includes such issues as appropriate use of barrier methods, the importance of monogamous relationships, and the importance of changing any sexual behaviors that place the patient at risk for PID. In addition, the patient's partner should be evaluated and provided with the same prevention message.

TABLE 2. **Indications for Hospitalization of Patients With Pelvic Inflammatory Disease**

Inability to follow or tolerate an outpatient oral regimen
Severe illness
Nausea and vomiting
High fever
Pregnancy
No response to oral therapy
Immunodeficiency
Tubo-ovarian abscess present
Surgical emergencies that cannot be excluded

TABLE 4. **Outpatient Regimens for Pelvic Inflammatory Disease**

1. Ofloxacin 400 mg orally twice a day
   plus
   Metronidazole 500 mg twice a day
2. Ceftriaxone (Rocephin) 250 mg IM once
   or
   Cefoxitin 2 g IM plus probenecid 1 g orally in a single concurrent dose
   or
   Doxycycline 100 mg orally for 14 days

UTERINE LEIOMYOMA

method of
JOSEPH G. WHELAN III, M.D., and
HOWARD A. ZACUR, M.D., PH.D.
The Johns Hopkins University School of Medicine
Baltimore, Maryland

EPIDEMIOLOGY

Uterine leiomyomas are the most common pelvic tumors in women. Historically they have been described as present in approximately 20% of women older than age 35 years, but their appearance at 50% of postmortem examinations of women suggests a much higher frequency, particularly in African-American women. Because the vast majority of these tumors are benign and usually do not cause significant morbidity, medical or surgical intervention is usually unwarranted. Nevertheless the diagnosis of leiomyoma is given as the most common indication for hysterectomies—the second most frequently performed major surgery for women in the United States. The nomenclature of this common neoplasm is a perpetual problem. The often used term *fibroid* is probably attributed to the tumor's dense fibrous nature, yet this lesion arises not from "fibrous" tissue but from smooth muscle. The term *myoma* is an acceptable substitute for the more histologically correct *leiomyoma* particularly when referring to a pelvic mass of unproven histology.

CLINICAL MANIFESTATIONS

Although most patients with leiomyomas are symptom free, the single most common symptom associated with a leiomyomatous uterus is prolonged or excessive bleeding associated with menstruation. When other symptoms arise they often relate to the location or size of the leiomyoma(s). Interestingly, relatively small tumors are capable of causing significant morbidity (e.g., infarction or infection), whereas very large tumors extending into the abdomen may not cause any noticeable symptoms. Locations for leiomyomas are defined relative to their position in the uterine wall. Leiomyomas may be subserosal (including projections into the broad ligament), intramural, or submucosal. Leiomyomas may be pedunculated on a vascular stalk, arising either from the uterine serosa and located within the abdominal cavity, or from the mucosa lining the uterine cavity. Theoretically, leiomyomas may arise from smooth muscle cells located anywhere in the body, although occurrences outside the müllerian system are rare.

Symptoms of enlarging leiomyomas may be referred to as "pressure" sensations or unexplainable increased abdominal girth. These symptoms develop insidiously and are more commonly encountered than pain. Sharp pain may be experienced as a result of degeneration producing central necrosis of the myoma or by torsion of a myoma attached to a pedicle. Severe menstrual cramps or increased menstrual blood flow may be described by the patient with a submucous myoma as it grows and protrudes into the lower uterine segment. As leiomyomas continue to enlarge, pressure is eventually exerted on adjacent viscera. Pressure on the urinary bladder may provoke urinary frequency whereas external compression of the pelvic ureter may lead to hydroureter and hydronephrosis. Constipation or tenesmus may be associated with a posterior leiomyoma compressing the rectosigmoid.

HISTOPATHOLOGY

Leiomyomas are benign tumors derived from a monoclonal population of smooth muscle cells, usually within uterine myometrium. The histology is characterized microscopically by tightly interlacing bundles of benign smooth muscle cells having uniform-sized rod-shaped nuclei, arranged in a whorl-like pattern and admixed with connective tissue elements. The tumor may contain calcifications as a consequence of tissue necrosis.

Malignant transformation of benign leiomyomas is extremely rare. An often-cited statistic for the incidence of leiomyosarcoma within leiomyomas is 0.5%, although studies have quoted this incidence as low as 0.13%. The microscopic diagnosis of a leiomyosarcoma relies on the number of smooth muscle cell mitotic figures seen per field of high-power magnification. Tumors with 10 or more mitotic figures per 10 high-power fields are considered malignant. Of note is the potential limitation of a "frozen section" histologic evaluation in predicting the presence of a leiomyosarcoma during a surgical resection or biopsy of uterine myomas.

MOLECULAR AND GENETIC ETIOLOGIC FACTORS

Transformation of the smooth muscle cell to a monoclonal neoplasm most likely results from a mutation at the genetic level. Mechanisms involving aberrant expression of bcl 2 (an inhibitor of apoptosis) as well as dysregulation of autocrine growth factors have been studied and have been implicated in the transcription process of proto-oncogenes. Growth factor HMGI-C regulates gene transcription and has been found to be overexpressed in leiomyomas. Mutations causing overexpression of HMGI-C may result in enhanced action of estradiol on myocyte growth. Cytogenetic studies have also identified a significant incidence and variety of chromosomal abnormalities within leiomyomas. It is not believed at this time, however, that these transformation mechanisms constitute a growth continuum between the benign leiomyoma and its malignant counterpart. First-degree female relatives of women with leiomyomas have a higher than background risk of developing leiomyomas, although with such a large incidence of this tumor in the general population it is difficult to prove a clear inheritance pattern. Familial patterns when identified do not follow simple mendelian genetics; therefore, multifactorial issues are implicated.

HORMONAL REGULATION

Significant anecdotal clinical evidence exists supporting gonadal sex steroid stimulation of leiomyoma growth. These tumors become manifest only in the reproductive years when ovaries are functional and are known to regress in menopause when ovarian function has ceased. Leiomyomas may also show marked acute growth during pregnancy when estrogen and progesterone levels are relatively high. Medications that induce hypogonadism are known to reduce leiomyoma volume. Oral contraceptive pills containing significant amounts of estrogen and progestins suppress ovulation, but these agents have not been shown to reliably either shrink or stimulate growth of leiomyomas. Progesterone and synthetic progestogens have been shown to exert an antiestrogen effect on leiomyomas and, in some studies, have been successful in decreasing leiomyoma size. Interestingly, the *anti*progesterone mifepristone (RU486, Mifeprex)* has also been shown to reduce the size of myomas, demonstrating the complexity of gonadal steroid influence on leiomyoma growth patterns. Both estrogen and progesterone receptors have been identified in leiomyomas and have been shown to act in unique ways as compared with actions of those analogous receptors in normal myometrium.

DIAGNOSIS

Usually the myomatous uterus is first detected by pelvic examination, at which time a large or irregularly shaped uterus is appreciated. An intramural or submucosal myoma, however, may cause morbidity without causing a noticeable change in uterine conformation by pelvic examination. When their existence is suspected, uterine imaging by ultrasonography or transvaginal hysterosonography may be performed. These procedures should reveal the number and size of uterine myomas and should also serve to distinguish the ovaries from any irregular masses detected on pelvic examination. If more precise information is needed regarding the size, location, or nature of the myomas, magnetic resonance imaging can provide better image resolution than ultrasonography. Intravenous pyelography is necessary to rule out ureteral compression or obstruction in the case of a myomatous uterus that is tightly compressed against the pelvic walls. A hysterosalpingogram performed under radiologic fluoroscopy can provide information about deformations in the uterine cavity as well as tubal patency. Alternatively, if information is desired regarding only the uterine cavity a saline hysterosonogram can be performed easily in the office. A more definitive description of the myomatous uterus may be afforded by simultaneous laparoscopy and hysteroscopy, although the need for this level of information should warrant the risks of surgery and anesthesia. Ultimately, the definitive diagnosis of a leiomyoma is by histologic identification.

MANAGEMENT

A conservative "observational" approach is the standard management of the asymptomatic myomatous uterus to which no morbidity can be attributed. Physical examination and ultrasound studies performed initially and then again at 3- to 6-month intervals may provide the physician with a reasonable appreciation of whether myomas are enlarging and, if so, at what rate. If the dimensions of the myomas remain unchanged, serial examinations at longer intervals are reasonable. Temporizing is also appropriate if the patient is perimenopausal and not complaining of symptoms.

Uterine myomas that are symptomatic or otherwise causing morbidity require interventional management. The two main approaches to interventional management for uterine myomas are hormonal and surgical. Induction of pseudomenopause with gonadotropin releasing hormone (GnRH) agonists or administration of progestins or estrogen modulating drugs are examples of hormonal treatment. Pseudomenopause may be induced by any of the following GnRH agonist regimens:

*Not FDA approved for this indication.

Leuprolide acetate (Lupron Depot), 3.75 mg every month by intramuscular injection for 2 to 6 months

Goserelin acetate (Zoladex),* 3.6 mg every month by subcutaneous injection for 2 to 6 months

Nafarelin acetate (Synarel),* 200 μg twice daily intranasally for 2 to 6 months

Long-term progestational therapy may be used to suppress myomatous growth by inhibition of ovulation; however, this regimen is not well supported in the current literature as an appropriate treatment for leiomyomas. In fact, basic science studies have shown progesterone to promote activity of some growth factors that are thought to be responsible for leiomyoma growth. In one randomized, double-blind clinical trial medroxyprogesterone acetate was shown to *prevent* shrinkage of uterine myomas when combined with a GnRH agonist as compared with the significant reduction in myoma volume seen with GnRH agonist combined with placebo. GnRH agonist regimens cannot be given indefinitely because long-term hypoestrogenism may irreversibly deplete bone mineralization stores and may cause cardiovascular health risks. In addition, myomas typically regain their previous size within several months after stopping GnRH agonist therapy. GnRH agonist hormonal management may be used as a temporizing measure to shrink leiomyomas in an attempt to convert an abdominal hysterectomy to a vaginal hysterectomy, to ameliorate symptoms in the transition from perimenopause to menopause, or to stop significant menstrual bleeding in the anemic patient in an effort at stabilization before surgery. In the future selective estrogen receptor modulating drugs (e.g., raloxifene [Evista]*) as well as specific growth factor inhibitors (e.g., interferon-alfa [Roferon-A],* pirfenidone†) may find a place in the medical management of leiomyomas.

Surgical therapy for the treatment of the uterine leiomyoma has traditionally involved either myomectomy for those wishing to retain their uterus or hysterectomy as a more permanent treatment. Although submucosal, cervical, or prolapsed lower uterine myomas can be resected from a vaginal or hysteroscopic approach, myomas in the uterine corpus are usually approached by laparotomy. The ideal goal for any myomectomy is complete removal of all palpable uterine myomas through as few uterine incisions as possible. When feasible, uterine incisions should be placed anteriorly and vertically on the uterus to avoid interfering with ovarian-tubal function in the posterior uterine cul-de-sac and to minimize vascular trauma. Deep or extensive incisions in the "contractile" portion of the uterus may necessitate elective cesarean section if childbearing is planned because the scar tissue from the myoma resection may predispose to uterine rupture during labor. Laparoscopic techniques for myomectomy (e.g., electromyolysis, cryomyolysis, laser vaporization) have been de-

*Not FDA approved for this indication.
†Investigational drug in the United States.

scribed; however, the inability to perform meticulous multilayer closure of the uterine wall laparoscopically causes concern for uterine integrity. Patients need to be advised before a myomectomy that there is up to a 30% to 40% recurrence rate of leiomyomas after surgery.

Recently, uterine artery embolization has been studied to treat myomatous uteri by causing transient uterine ischemia. Numerous studies have shown this technique to be successful in reducing myoma volume and improving heavy/irregular bleeding attributed to uterine myomas. These studies, however, have also shown this technique to be complicated by septic shock and/or uterine abscess formation in small but significant percentages. Nontarget ischemia, particularly ovarian ischemia, should be a concern for those patients considering this technique who want to retain ovarian function and fertility potential. The effect of uterine artery embolization on subsequent fertility has not been adequately studied.

One aspect of management of leiomyomas that may cause frustration to the gynecologist is the matter of interventional management for the purpose of optimizing fertility or pregnancy results. In numerous studies uterine leimyomas have been implicated in the following areas of morbidity relating to pregnancy concerns:

- Infertility
- Risk of recurrent pregnancy wastage
- Risk of preterm labor/delivery
- Fetal malpresentation in labor
- Risk for cesarean section
- Risk of hemorrhage during cesarean section
- Risk of emergency hysterectomy during cesarean section

Only if a uterine myoma has caused gynecologic morbidity in the past or is anatomically located in a position that is clearly able to interfere with pregnancy is it reasonable to consider a myomectomy before a patient's plans for attempting pregnancy. The patient in this case should be carefully counseled preoperatively about the possibility of the surgery actually having an untoward effect on uterine or tubal function. A patient with an asymptomatic uterine myoma may express concern about potential complications to her pregnancy. In such cases it is appropriate to reassure the patient that uterine myomas are relatively common and that the vast majority of women with uterine myomas who become pregnant complete their pregnancy without myoma-related complications.

CONCLUSION

Uterine leiomyomas are the most common pelvic tumors in women, although their malignant counterpart, leiomyosarcoma, is extremely rare. These benign tumors may cause gynecologic morbidity that results in the performance of a hysterectomy. However, the majority of myomatous uteri may be managed by conservative clinical surveillance. The two general approaches to this common gynecologic problem, hormonal suppression and surgical resection, will no doubt continue to be used well into the future. Advances will certainly be made in the knowledge of the endocrine function and growth regulation of leiomyomas that will prompt more specific and effective methods of medical treatment. Advances in surgical techniques continue to develop for safer and more efficient removal of myomas from otherwise normal uteri. The recent advent of uterine artery embolization as a definitive therapy for uterine myomas should await further clinical studies before being accepted as a standard option in management.

MANAGEMENT OF ENDOMETRIAL CARCINOMA

method of
HARRISON G. BALL, M.D.
University of Massachusetts Medical School and UMass Memorial Medical Center
Worcester, Massachusetts

EPIDEMIOLOGY

Endometrial cancer is the most common pelvic gynecologic malignancy in the United States. The American Cancer Society estimates that 38,300 new cases will be diagnosed in the United States in 2001 and 6600 women will die of the disease. The lifetime risk for the development of endometrial cancer is 1 in 37 (2.7%). Cancer of the endometrium is uncommon in women younger than 40 years and has an increasing incidence with advancing age.

ETIOLOGY

Women with atypical adenomatous hyperplasia of the endometrium are at greater risk for endometrial cancer. Other risk factors include obesity, unopposed exogenous estrogen therapy, including tamoxifen therapy, late menopause, and nulliparity. Women with hereditary nonpolyposis colorectal cancer have up to a 50% lifetime risk of the development of endometrial cancer. An expert review panel of the American Cancer Society has recommended that women at risk for hereditary nonpolyposis colorectal cancer be offered endometrial biopsy as annual screening for endometrial cancer beginning at age 35.

DIAGNOSIS AND STAGING

Most women with endometrial cancer are perimenopausal or postmenopausal and frequently have intermenstrual bleeding, menorrhagia, or postmenopausal spotting or bleeding. Any amount of bleeding or spotting in a postmenopausal woman requires evaluation of the endometrium. The diagnosis of endometrial cancer is established with an endometrial biopsy or dilation and curettage. Unless the history or physical examination suggests spread of disease beyond the uterus, additional studies are not needed beyond those necessary for evaluation before surgery.

Staging of endometrial cancer is based on findings at the

time of surgery (Table 1). The staging procedure includes peritoneal washings for cytologic examination obtained on entering the peritoneal cavity, evaluation of the uterus for depth of myometrial invasion, determination of histologic grade and involvement of the cervix, and assessment of the fallopian tubes, ovaries, and pelvic and periaortic lymph nodes for metastatic disease. Additionally, careful inspection of the peritoneal cavity should be performed to evaluate the possibility of intraperitoneal dissemination of cancer.

TREATMENT

Most patients with an endometrial cancer have disease confined to the uterus and are candidates for surgery. Surgical options include: total abdominal hysterectomy with bilateral salpingo-oophorectomy and pelvic and periaortic lymph node biopsies; vaginal hysterectomy, preferably with bilateral salpingo-oophorectomy; and more recently, laparoscopic pelvic and periaortic lymph node dissection with bilateral salpingo-oophorectomy and vaginal hysterectomy. Patients who are not candidates for surgery can be treated with either intracavitary radiation therapy or whole-pelvic and intracavitary radiation therapy.

The decision to perform lymph node biopsies in all patients remains controversial. In an effort to minimize lymph node dissection, frozen section of the uterus at the time of hysterectomy can be used to limit more extended surgery to patients who have deep myometrial invasion (>50%), poorly differentiated cancer, and tumor size greater than 2 cm. The accuracy of frozen section evaluation of the uterus varies among institutions. Because the morbidity of pelvic and periaortic lymph node dissection is acceptable in most patients, I favor performing lymph node dissection unless the patient has a relative contraindication to the procedure. The most common reasons that node dissection is not performed include: extreme obesity, advanced age, and coexisting medical problems that would preclude aggressive therapy after surgery if the nodes contain metastatic carcinoma.

After surgery, patients who have adverse prognostic factors are candidates for postoperative radiation therapy. The Gynecologic Oncology Group (GOG) has analyzed prognostic factors in GOG 33 and found histologic grade of the cancer, depth of myometrial invasion, capillary-lymphatic space involvement, gross serosal involvement, positive peritoneal cytology, age older than 50 years, involvement of the fallopian tubes or ovaries, positive peritoneal cytology, and metastatic disease to pelvic or periaortic lymph nodes to be significant factors predictive of recurrence. GOG 99 was a randomized trial of patients with adenocarcinoma of the endometrium and intermediate-risk prognostic factors (stage Ia, Ib, IIa, and IIb occult). Patients with papillary serous and clear cell carcinoma were excluded. Patients were randomized after total abdominal hysterectomy, bilateral salpingo-oophorectomy, and pelvic and periaortic node biopsies to either no further treatment or 5040-cGy whole-pelvic radiation therapy. A statistically significant difference in recurrence-free survival favoring the group that received postoperative radiation therapy was observed. The excess of recurrences in the group that did not receive radiation therapy was at the vaginal apex. What has not been addressed in a prospective study is whether a postoperative vaginal cylinder in patients who have intermediate risk factors for recurrence will result in an equally satisfactory recurrence-free survival as in women who have received whole-pelvic radiation therapy, but with lower morbidity.

The current approach at UMass Memorial Medical Center is for patients to receive postoperative whole-pelvic radiation therapy if they have metastatic disease to pelvic lymph nodes or have not had lymph node biopsies performed and have any of the following: invasion of greater than half of the myometrium, poorly differentiated cancer, involvement of the lower uterine segment or cervix, capillary-lymphatic space involvement, and metastatic disease to the fallopian tubes or ovaries. Patients who have had lymph node biopsies of the pelvic and periaortic nodes and whose biopsies are negative but have greater than 50% myometrial invasion, poorly differentiated cancer, or involvement of the cervical stroma may be considered for either postoperative whole-pelvic radiation therapy or a vaginal cylinder, depending on the risk factors present. Patients with involvement of the serosa of the uterus or with metastatic disease to the fallopian tubes or ovaries receive postoperative whole-pelvic radiation therapy. If positive peritoneal cytology is the only adverse prognostic factor in a patient who has had adequate staging, further therapy is not recommended.

The presence of metastatic disease to periaortic lymph nodes significantly worsens the prognosis, but a subset of these patients can be salvaged with extended-field periaortic radiation therapy in addition to whole-pelvic radiation therapy. The GOG is currently studying women with stage III and IV endometrial cancer with less than 2 cm residual disease confined to the abdomen. GOG 184 randomizes patients to volume-directed radiation therapy, that is,

TABLE 1. **International Federation of Gynecology and Obstetrics Surgical Staging for Carcinoma of the Corpus Uteri**

Stage	Description
Stage Ia	Tumor limited to the endometrium
Stage Ib	Invasion to less than half of the myometrium
Stage Ic	Invasion equal to or more than half of the myometrium
Stage IIa	Endocervical glandular involvement only
Stage IIb	Cervical stromal invasion
Stage IIIa	Tumor invading the serosa of the corpus uteri and/or adnexae and/or positive cytologic findings
Stage IIIb	Vaginal metastases
Stage IIIc	Metastases to pelvic and/or periaortic lymph nodes
Stage IVa	Tumor invasion of bladder and/or bowel mucosa
Stage IVb	Distant metastases, including intra-abdominal metastases and/or inguinal lymph nodes

From Creasman W, Odicino F, Maisonneuve P, et al: Carcinoma of the corpus uteri. J Epidemiol Biostat 3:35–61, 1998.

whole-pelvic radiation therapy with selective use of vaginal brachytherapy for extension to the vagina or involvement of the cervix or lower uterine segment. Radiation therapy to the periaortic lymph nodes is administered if the periaortic nodes are positive. After completion of radiation therapy, patients are randomized to six cycles of either doxorubicin (Adriamycin) plus cisplatin (Platinol) or doxorubicin, cisplatin, and paclitaxel.

RECURRENCE

Local recurrence involving the vaginal apex in patients who have not received previous radiation therapy are usually managed with whole-pelvic radiation therapy, followed by a vaginal cylinder. Patients who have had previous radiation therapy and have an isolated recurrence at the vaginal apex may be candidates for transabdominal resection of the vaginal apex. Patients who are not candidates for radiation therapy or surgery are treated with systemic hormonal therapy or chemotherapy. For patients with well-differentiated cancer with positive progesterone receptors, megestrol acetate (Megace) or tamoxifen (Nolvadex)* alternating with megestrol acetate is used. In other patients or in patients who have failed hormonal therapy, chemotherapy is the treatment of choice. Active chemotherapy agents in the treatment of recurrent endometrial carcinoma include: doxorubicin, cisplatin, carboplatin, and paclitaxel. The GOG has recently completed a trial of cisplatin plus doxorubicin versus cisplatin, doxorubicin, and paclitaxel in patients with advanced or recurrent endometrial adenocarcinoma. The results of this trial have not been published. The GOG has just activated a trial of megestrol acetate alternating with tamoxifen versus doxorubicin, cisplatin, and paclitaxel in patients with advanced or recurrent endometrial adenocarcinoma. With disease progression, patients cross over to the other arm of this study.

POST-THERAPY FOLLOW-UP

After therapy, patients with a low risk for recurrence (stages Ia and Ib, well and moderately differentiated cancer) are seen every 6 months for 3 years and then annually. Patients at higher risk for recurrence are seen every 4 months for 2 years, every 6 months for 3 years, and then annually after 5 years. At each visit, patients should have a physical examination, including pelvic examination and a vaginal Pap smear. Patients who had an elevated serum CA 125 level before therapy may be monitored with serial CA 125 assays. Routine surveillance with computed axial tomography has no role in follow-up.

RESULTS OF THERAPY

Stage I endometrial cancer accounts for more than 70% of cases. The overall 5-year survival rate is 73% and correlates well with surgical stage (Table 2). Patients with recurrence have a poor prognosis, except those with small, isolated recurrence at the vaginal apex who have not previously had radiation therapy. These patients are potentially curable with radiation therapy.

*Not FDA approved for this indication.

TABLE 2. **Five-Year Survival Rate by Surgical Stage**

Stage	Rate
Stage Ia	91%
Stage Ib	88%
Stage Ic	84%
Stage II	72%
Stage III	51%
Stage IV	9%

Adapted from Creasman W, Odicino F, Maisonneuve P, et al: Carcinoma of the corpus uteri. J Epidemiol Biostat 3:35–61, 1998.

CERVICAL CANCER

method of
EILEEN M. SEGRETI, M.D.
Medical College of Virginia Hospitals and Virginia Commonwealth University
Richmond, Virginia

Worldwide, cervical cancer remains a significant problem for women. In developing countries, cervical cancer is one of the most common and deadly malignancies in women. Fortunately, in the United States the incidence and mortality of cervical cancer has fallen from a peak in the 1940s to a current estimated incidence of 12,800 cases in the year 2000. Cervical cancer remains responsible for 4600 deaths a year in the United States. The introduction of the Papanicolaou (Pap) test to examine cervical cytology has been largely responsible for the decline in the incidence of invasive cervical cancer worldwide. Where this test is employed and preinvasive disease treated there has been a significant reduction in cervical cancer mortality.

EPIDEMIOLOGY

Cervical cancer has long been correlated with sexual activity. Women with an early age of first intercourse, multiple sexual partners, a history of sexually transmitted diseases, a history of multiple births, or sexual partners with prior partners with cervical cancer are at an increased risk of developing cervical cancer. Women who abstain from sexual activity are at very low risk of developing cervical cancer. Other factors that are associated with an increased risk of cervical cancer include cigarette smoking, nonuse of barrier contraception, oral contraceptive pills, low socioeconomic status, and, most importantly, infection with the human papillomavirus (HPV). Over 90% of cervical cancers contain HPV DNA.

Cervical dysplasia is a precursor condition of invasive cervical cancer. The classification of cervical dysplasia is based on the thickness of the abnormal cell layers above the basement membrane. Invasive cancer occurs when these abnormal cells escape the confines of the basement membrane and have access to the body of the cervix. Because the cervix is readily visible during pelvic examination, these epithelial cells can be collected and stained to evaluate them for characteristics of dysplasia. Localized and completely visible cervical dysplasia can be treated by surgical excision (scalpel or loop electrosurgical excision procedure), cryotherapy, or laser ablation.

Unfortunately, most women with newly diagnosed cervical cancer in the United States have not had a recent Pap smear, and one half of American women with newly diagnosed cervical cancer have never had a Pap smear. Ten percent of American women with newly diagnosed cervical cancer have not had a Pap smear in the previous 5 years. The American College of Obstetricians and Gynecologists and the American Cancer Society recommend that women have annual Pap smears starting at age 18 or when they become sexually active, whichever comes first. After three consecutive satisfactory annual normal smears in low-risk patients, the interval between screening Pap smears may be increased at the discretion of the physician.

PATHOGENESIS

Most cervical cancers arise from squamous epithelium; however, 15% arise from glandular cells. HPV DNA has been isolated in both squamous and adenocarcinomas. HPV is thought to generate proteins that bind to the cell's natural tumor suppressor genes and inactivate them. This causes uncontrolled cellular growth and division. The "early" proteins E6 and E7 generated by HPV have been found to interact with the tumor suppressor gene products p53 and Rb, respectively, and deactivate them. Investigational therapy to prevent cervical cancer has been directed at interrupting the activity of the oncogenic HPV. It is hoped that development of an effective HPV vaccine will eradicate cervical cancer in the future.

DIAGNOSIS

Cervical cancer may present as a microscopic or a macroscopic lesion. Microscopic lesions are usually detected by a screening Pap smear suggestive of dysplasia. Colposcopically directed cervical biopsies by a skilled clinician are essential in the evaluation of an abnormal Pap test. The cervix is examined after the application of 3% to 5% acetic acid. Dysplasia may appear as acetowhite epithelium, with or without punctation, mosaicism, or abnormal vasculature. A diagram of the colposcopic examination should be drawn. Notes should be made as to whether the lesion and the transformation zone were seen in their entirety. An endocervical curettage should be done to assess the endocervical canal. Directed biopsies should be performed on the worst-looking areas of the ectocervix.

Dysplasia can be removed or ablated if the lesion is seen entirely and the endocervical curettage is negative for dyplasia. Cervical dyplasia in the endocervical scrapings, a lesion not entirely visualized, a transformation zone not entirely visualized, microinvasion on cervical biopsy, marked discrepancy between cytology and histology, or anything suggestive of invasion warrant a cervical conization to exclude more advanced disease.

If a macroscopic lesion is visible on the ectocervix, it is very important to obtain an immediate biopsy, colposcopy being unnecessary. Biopsy is preferable to Pap smear when a visible lesion is present on the cervix. In fact, a Pap smear may show only inflammation and necrotic debris in the presence of an obvious cancer. It is very important not to rely only on a Pap test when there is a visible lesion. The Pap test has a 15% to 20% false-negative rate.

Cervical cancer may be associated with abnormal vaginal bleeding, postcoital bleeding, vaginal discharge, or odor. Advanced disease is often accompanied by back or pelvic pain, but not always. Large endophytic lesions may appear deceptively normal on speculum examination. The mucosa may be intact, but rectovaginal palpation reveals a grossly enlarged and expanded cervix. Rectovaginal examination is mandatory to assess the parametria and posterior pelvis.

STAGING

After the biopsy confirms cancer, further staging evaluation is necessary. Because cervical cancer is so common in underdeveloped countries, only widely available, relatively inexpensive tests are used to assign stage. Cancer of the uterine cervix is staged clinically. These tests include a pelvic examination, a chest radiograph, an intravenous pyelogram, cystoscopy, and proctoscopy. More sophisticated tests (e.g., computed tomography, magnetic resonance imaging, and lymphangiography) are often used, when available, to tailor treatment planning. Findings of distant spread on these studies, however, do not change the stage assignment. The American Joint Committee on Cancer's TNM classification and the Federation Internationale de Gynecologie et d'Obstetrique (FIGO) system are almost identical for cervical cancer. Stage I disease is invasive cancer confined to the uterine cervix. Recently, FIGO has amended the staging system for stage I disease. The definition for microinvasive disease has been altered to more closely align with clinical practice and conservative treatment. Stage IA disease is that diagnosed by microscopy only. If a grossly visible lesion confined to the cervix is present, it is assigned stage IB. Stage IA is divided into stage IA1 and stage IA2. Stage IA1 disease is invasive cancer limited to a depth of invasion 3 mm or less beyond the basement membrane. The lateral spread of the tumor must also be less than or equal to 7 mm. Stage IA2 disease is invasive cancer greater than 3 mm in depth but less than 5 mm in depth as well as less than or equal to 7 mm in lateral spread. Typically, a cervical conization is necessary to assign stage IA disease, because cervical punch biopsies may miss other areas of invasion and mistakenly underestimate the stage. Lymphatic or vascular space invasion does not alter the stage; however, it is a poor prognostic sign. Additionally, the previously large category of stage IB has been subdivided to accommodate cervical volume. Volume of disease has long been known to be an independent risk factor in stage I disease. Additionally, many gynecologic oncologists use tumor size to decide on primary treatment. Hence, stage IB1 disease is 4 cm or less in diameter, whereas stage IB2 disease is greater than 4 cm.

Stage II disease is cancer that has spread locally. When the cancer has spread to the upper two thirds of the vagina, it is classified as stage IIA. When the cancer has spread to the parametria, but not the pelvic sidewall, it is stage IIB. Stage IIIA indicates distal, lower third, vaginal spread. Stage IIIB disease includes pelvic sidewall extension, hydronephrosis, or a nonfunctioning kidney secondary to tumor extension and ureteral obstruction. Stage IVA disease is disease limited to the pelvis; however, the tumor has extended to the bladder or rectal mucosa. Bullous edema of the bladder trigone is not sufficient to be stage IVA. Histologic confirmation by bladder biopsy is necessary to document stage IVA disease. Distant spread, for example, to the lung or pleura, constitutes stage IVB disease.

TREATMENT

Microinvasive squamous cell carcinoma has been successfully treated with cold knife conization in patients desirous of future fertility. If childbearing is completed, however, simple hysterectomy is standard therapy. For stage IB 1 and stage II A disease, radical hysterectomy with complete pelvic lymph node dissection is usually recommended for medically operable patients. Radical hysterectomy and pelvic lymph node dissection is a complex technical procedure that should be attempted only by trained gynecologic oncologists. Radical hysterectomy includes removal of the parametrial tissue, the upper vagina, and a portion of the uterosacral ligaments along with a complete pelvic node dissection. It does not include removal of the ovaries and tubes. In young patients, this allows for a normal duration of endogenous hormones. Larger lesions and those of more advanced stage are often treated with chemoradiation. This therapy will cause premature ovarian failure in premenopausal patients. Radiation therapy consists of 40 to 50 Gy given over 5 to 6 weeks followed by two intracavitary cesium insertions. The brachytherapy has classically been administered by insertion of a uterine tandem and vaginal ovoids under anesthesia. The applicator is carefully packed in the vagina with radiopaque gauze and secured in place. The patient typically then spends 48 hours in the hospital on two separate occasions 1 or 2 weeks apart. Alternatively, high dose rate brachytherapy can be administered to outpatients in the office of the radiation oncologist. This technique delivers a higher dose of radiation in a shorter amount of time but may be associated with a narrowing of the therapeutic window. Recently, randomized clinical trials have shown a better result after the addition of cisplatin (Platinol)* or cisplatin and 5-fluorouracil (Efudex)* to radiation therapy compared with radiation therapy alone.

PROGNOSIS

Prognosis is closely related to stage of disease. Stage IA cervical cancer has a cure rate approaching 100%. Patients with stage IB disease have a 5-year survival of 85% to 90%. Patients with stage IIA disease have a 70% to 80% 5-year survival. Patients with stage IIB disease have a 5-year survival of 60% to 65%. Stage III disease is associated with a 5-year survival of 28% to 60%. The Patterns of Care Outcomes study analysis revealed improved survival in patients treated at radiation oncology centers that treat more than 50 new cervical cancer patients each year. Remarkably, the 5-year survival reported for stage IVA disease is 15% to 30% in expert hands. The treatment of cervical cancer with radiation therapy is best done in radiation oncology centers with a large volume of patients with cervical cancer.

RECURRENCE

Cervical cancer typically recurs in the lung, along the pelvic sidewall, or in the supraclavicular lymph nodes. For patients with distant or unresectable pelvic recurrences, chemotherapy may be offered. Chemotherapy is typically not curative but may provide some prolongation of life. Active agents include cisplatin, paclitaxel, and ifosfamide. Single-agent cisplatin is associated with response rates of 20% to 30%. Combination regimens such as MVAC (methotrexate, vinblastine [Velban],* doxorubicin [Adriamycin],* and cisplatin) are under investigation. MVAC has shown promising results in small single institutional studies. The Gynecologic Oncology Group is currently studying MVAC versus cisplatin versus topotecan (Hycamtin)* and cisplatin in patients with advanced or recurrent cervical cancer.

A pelvic recurrence of cervical cancer is treated with the type of treatment modality not originally used. For example, if a woman underwent a radical hysterectomy, pelvic chemoradiation would be employed. However, if a patient had pelvic chemoradiation initially and cancer recurs in the pelvis, then surgery would be employed to eradicate the recurrence. Typically, surgery would consist of a total pelvic exenteration with urinary conduit formation and creation of a neovagina. Variations on the theme of pelvic exenteration include performing either an anterior exenteration for a small anterior recurrence or a posterior exenteration for a small posterior recurrence. In place of a diverting colostomy, occasionally a very low colorectal anastomosis can be accomplished. Additionally, many gynecologic oncology surgeons are now able to create a continent urinary conduit. The absence of appliances on the abdominal wall surely contributes to an improvement in quality of life. Exenterative surgery is associated with long-term survival in approximately 40% of patients; however, the operation may be associated with significant short- and long-term complications.

*Not FDA approved for this indication.

*Not FDA approved for this indication.

NEOPLASMS OF THE VULVA

method of
GISELLE B. GHURANI, M.D., and
MANUEL A. PENALVER, M.D.
Jackson Memorial Medical Center
Miami, Florida

BENIGN TUMORS OF THE VULVA

Many different nonneoplastic disorders affect the vulva. Most of these are unusual. However, it is important for clinicians to become familiar with these conditions to establish accurate diagnoses and provide adequate treatment. Nonneoplastic tumors can be classified as cystic or solid tumors.

Cystic Vulvar Tumors

Bartholin's duct cyst is the most common large cystic lesion of the vulva, occurring in 2% of women. The etiology is obstruction of the Bartholin's gland duct by nonspecific inflammation, infection, or trauma. Following obstruction, continued glandular secretion of fluid results in cystic dilation of the duct. Treatment is generally not necessary in women younger than 40 years of age unless the cyst becomes infected or symptomatic.

In women over 40 years oif age, enlargement of the gland may rarely be secondary to an adenocarcinoma; therefore, excision of the gland for pathologic evaluation is recommended. For symptomatic women, treatment includes incision and drainage of cyst content with subsequent placement of a Word catheter (a short catheter with an inflatable Foley balloon) left in place for 4 weeks, or marsupialization of the duct, which creates an epithelialized pouch that is sutured open to promote drainage of the gland.

The most common small cysts of the vulva are *epidermal inclusion cysts* that arise from the pilosebaceous apparatus. Typically, multiple nodules appear on the labia majora and are filled with a thick, pale material resulting from desquamation of the cyst lining. These cysts are usually asymptomatic unless they become infected, requiring incision and evacuation.

Mucinous or *ciliated epithelial cysts* occur rarely in the vulva. These cysts usually arise from the urogenital sinus, Gartner's (mesonephric) duct, or müllerian (paramesonephric) embryonic remnants. Usually asymptomatic and located in the vestibule, the cysts require excision only if infected or symptomatic.

Solid Vulvar Tumors

Fibroepithelial polyps (acrochordons, skin tags) are usually small, pedunculated tags of smooth wrinkled skin located on the hair-bearing vulva. They are comprised of fibrovascular stroma lined by keratinizing, stratified squamous epithelium. Treatment by excision is indicated if symptoms develop or if the lesion exceeds 1 to 2 cm in diameter.

Hidradenoma papilliferum is a benign lesion occurring almost exclusively in the genital region. Hidradenomas arise from the apocrine sweat glands of the vulva, representing an intraductal adenoma. Typically, the lesions occur in postpubertal white females. They begin as a single lesion on the labia majus. Most are asymptomatic; however, ulceration and bleeding may occur. Clinically and histologically, these lesions may be mistaken for a malignancy. Excisional biopsy is always required to confirm the diagnosis.

Syringomas are benign tumors of eccrine sweat glands. These lesions occur predominately in adolescent and young adult women. These adenomas of eccrine glands appear as small subcutaneous papules measuring up to 5 mm in diameter. They are symmetrically distributed intradermal lesions occurring predominately in the labia majora. Other common locations include the mons pubis, labia minora, and adjacent thighs. Similar tumors are often found in the eccrine glands of the eyelid. These tumors are usually asymptomatic. Treatment includes excisional biopsy or cryosurgery.

Granular cell myoblastoma is a tumor originating from peripheral nerve sheath cells, the Schwann cells. These tumors, or *schwannomas,* are indolent, solid tumors of the vulva typically located on the labia majora or clitoris. They usually appear as subcutaneous nodules, about 1 to 5 cm in diameter. Furthermore, they can originate in connective tissues throughout the body, most commonly in the skin, tongue, and upper respiratory tract. Although malignant behavior has been described, these tumors are usually benign. Treatment is wide local excision with pathologic evaluation. If resection margins are positive and cells are left behind, these benign tumors tend to recur. Further treatment requires a second operation with wider margins.

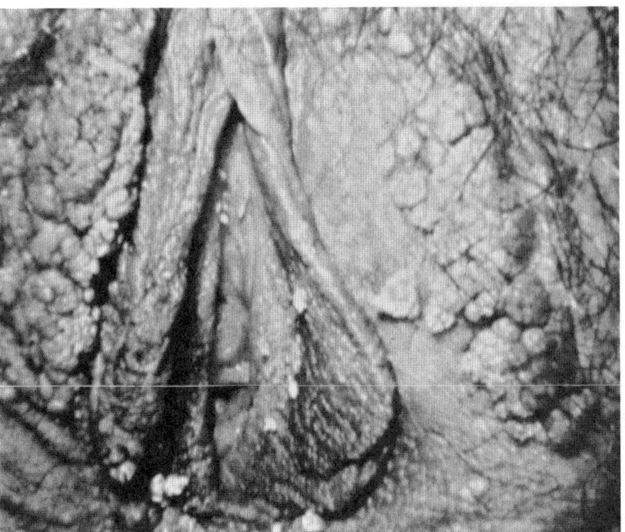

Figure 1. Multiple condylomas of the vulva.

PREMALIGNANT LESIONS AND RELATED DISORDERS OF THE VULVA

Human Papillomavirus

Human papillomavirus (HPV) is a double-stranded DNA virus with many different subtypes of which more than 35 are known to affect the lower genital tract. These highly infectious subtypes of HPV are mucosotropic and cutaneotropic, producing lesions confined to the epithelial layers of the vulva, vagina, cervix, and anal and perianal regions. HPV is the most common viral sexually transmitted disease. Most infections are subclinical, with only about 30% of patients presenting with a clinically apparent, gross lesion. Condyloma acuminata, also known as venereal or anogenital warts, are caused by HPV. Most vulvar condylomata are associated with low oncogenic potential, or low-risk types, HPV types 6 and 11. High oncogenic potential, or high-risk types, HPV 16 and 18, are associated with premalignant changes such as high-grade dysplasias or invasive carcinomas. Predisposition to HPV infection occurs with immunocompromised states such as HIV infection, pregnancy, diabetes, and local trauma.

Vulvar Condyloma

Vulvar condyloma may be single or multiple. The sizes of the warts can vary from tiny papules to large cauliflower-like masses (Figure 1). The diagnosis is usually made by direct inspection of the vulva. Most lesions are asymptomatic, although pruritus may occur. Occasionally, they may become superinfected causing pain, odor, or bleeding. They are highly contagious and spread by skin-to-skin contact. Autoinoculation is also very common.

Treatment includes many different approaches, none of which is completely curative because of the latent virus infection in the surrounding epithelium. Topical chemical treatments include trichloroacetic acid* (TCA) and podophyllin.* TCA, a 50% to 75% solution, is applied directly

*Not FDA approved for this indication.

to the lesions weekly in the office. It coagulates the condylomatous tissue without being absorbed systemically and can therefore be used safely in pregnancy. The physician administers podophyllin as a 10% to 25% solution that is painted weekly on the lesions for 4 to 6 weeks. Podophyllin is absorbed systemically and is associated with neurologic and bone marrow toxicities. Consequently, podophyllin cannot be used during pregnancy or be applied to large surface areas. Podofilox (Condylox),* a 0.5% solution of the active ingredient podophyllotoxin, is now available. Unlike podophyllin, the patient can apply this preparation.

Topical fluorouracil (Efudex),* applied twice daily for 7 days with repetition in 7 to 10 days as needed, has also been used successfully in the treatment of venereal warts. However, systemic absorption is common and ulceration of the vulva can occur. Imiquimod (Aldara 5%)* cream, applied to lesions three times per week for up to 16 weeks, can be used successfully in nonimmunocompromised patients. Imiquimod acts as an immune response modifier that induces cytokine activity, thereby using one's own immune system to battle the infection.

If any form of chemical therapy fails to cause wart regression, biopsy should be performed 1 month after the last treatment to exclude malignancy. Other therapeutic options include laser ablation, electrodesiccation, loop electrosurgical excision procedure (LEEP), or scalpel excision.

Vulvar Intraepithelial Neoplasia

Squamous intraepithelial lesions of the vulva are classified according to the International Society for the Study of Vulvar Diseases (ISSVD). Lesions are categorized as follows:

Vulvar intraepithelial neoplasia I (VIN I) for mild dysplasia, abnormal maturation confined to the lower third of the epithelium

VIN II for moderate dysplasia, abnormal maturation confined to the lower two thirds of the epithelium

VIN III for severe dysplasia or carcinoma in situ; abnormal maturation extends to the upper one third or extends to the entire epithelium

VIN lesions are classically described as occurring in postmenopausal women in their 50s and 60s. However, the frequency of VIN appears to be increasing among younger women. The lesions can be white (Figure 2), red, or pigmented. They can be multifocal or unifocal maculopapular lesions. Most lesions are asymptomatic, although pruritus, dysuria, or bleeding may be a presenting complaint. The labia minora and perineum are the most common locations for VIN. Many of these lesions are associated with HPV, especially types 16 and 18.

The diagnosis is usually made by careful inspection of the vulva at the time of routine gynecologic examinations. The application of 5% acetic acid for at least 5 minutes can aid in identifying subtle lesions. Colposcopy of the entire vulva should be performed once a lesion is identified in order to exclude multifocal disease. Multifocal lesions are more common in premenopausal women and unifocal lesions are usually found in postmenopausal women.

Biopsy of any suspicious areas should be done to confirm the diagnosis. Treatment usually consists of surgical excision with pathologic evaluation. An alternative treatment that is evolving as the modality of choice is laser ablation. Carbon dioxide laser surgery has the advantage of less scarring and less anatomic distortion.

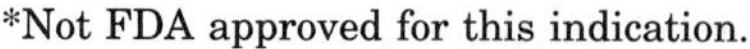

*Not FDA approved for this indication.

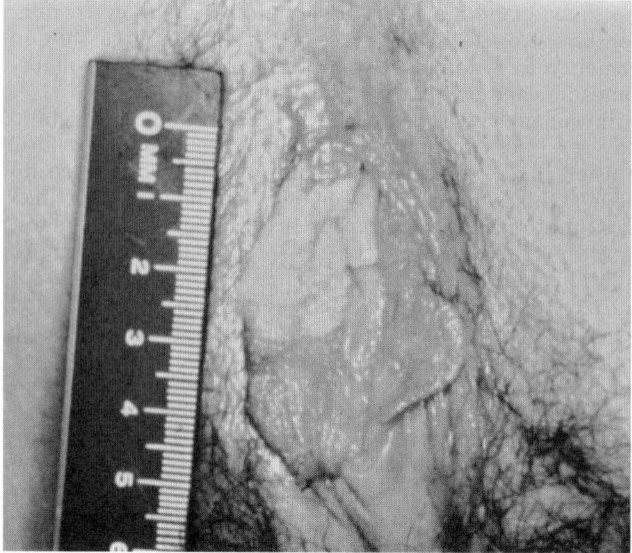

Figure 2. Vulvar intraepithelial neoplasia appears as a white plaque on the labia minus.

Paget's Disease of the Vulva

Paget's disease of the vulva is a rare intraepithelial lesion (adenocarcinoma in situ) that appears grossly as a well demarcated erythematous eczematoid lesion with irregular borders. The finding of hyperemic areas with superficial white coatings has led to the classic description of Paget's disease as "icing on a cake" (Figure 3).

The disease predominantly affects postmenopausal white women. Presenting complaints include pruritus and vulvar soreness. Diagnosis is made by biopsy with the characteristic large eosinophilic Paget cells seen in the

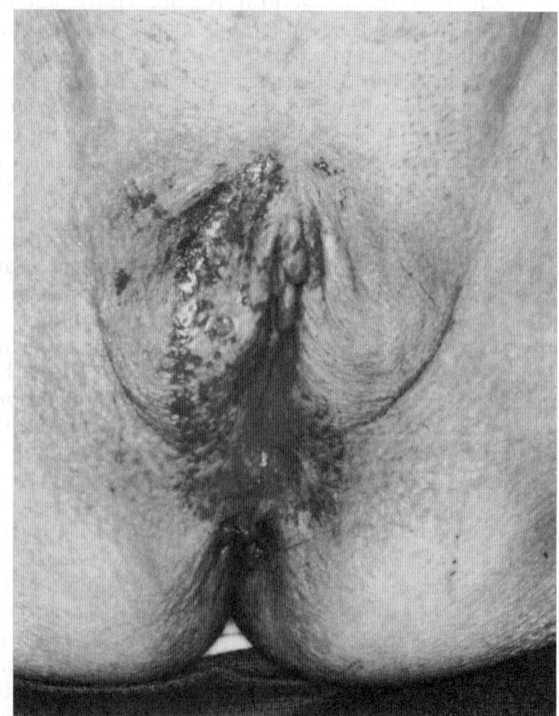

Figure 3. Paget's disease of the vulva with its characteristic red, velvety appearance and overlying white plaques.

basal layer of the epithelium, spread within the epidermis or around dermal appendages. Treatment consists of wide local excision to include the entire lesion. Microscopically, Paget's disease usually extends well beyond the gross lesion, resulting in positive surgical margins and frequent local recurrences. Therefore, some authorities recommend checking the surgical margins with frozen sections to ensure complete excision. Others have abandoned the use of intraoperative frozen section because, unfortunately, recurrences frequently occur even with negative surgical margins.

The importance of Paget's disease of the vulva is the frequent association with invasive carcinomas. An underlying adenocarcinoma of the sweat glands or Bartholin's gland may be present in up to 20% of cases of Paget's disease. Also, a concomitant carcinoma in another site, such as the breast, rectum, colon, or cervix may be present in up to 25% of cases. Therefore, once the diagnosis of Paget's disease of the vulva is made, the clinician should actively exclude the presence of a concomitant invasive carcinoma.

MALIGNANT TUMORS OF THE VULVA

Squamous Cell Carcinoma

Malignant tumors of the vulva account for approximately 4% of all gynecologic cancers. Squamous cell carcinoma is the most common histologic type, accounting for over 90% of vulvar cancer cases (Figure 4). The usual presentation is a postmenopausal woman with a long history of vulvar pruritus who discovers a vulvar mass or lump. It is not uncommon for patients to delay seeking medical attention or for physicians to delay diagnosing the condition.

Predisposing factors include VIN, condyloma acuminata, immunodeficiency, cigarette smoking, and a long history of vulvar dermatoses, especially lichen sclerosus. The majority of squamous carcinomas arise from the labia majora and minora, but they may also appear on the clitoris and perineum. The lymphatic system is the primary route for initial metastasis. The diagnosis is made by biopsy. All suspicious lesions of the vulva, including ulcers, lumps, and pigmented areas, must be biopsied to exclude a carcinoma, even in asymptomatic women.

The International Federation of Gynecology and Obstetrics (FIGO) defines four stages for vulvar cancer, similar to the system used for other gynecologic malignancies. Since 1988, the stages are based on surgical findings, emphasizing the importance of local tumor spread and lymph node metastasis on prognosis. Undoubtedly, the most important prognostic factor for vulvar cancer is lymph node status. The staging system is outlined in Table 1.

Treatment options for vulvar carcinoma have changed dramatically over the past years. Previously, en bloc radical vulvectomy (Figure 5) with bilateral dissection of the groin nodes became the standard treatment for most patients with operable vulvar cancer. Currently, the trend is toward conservation of normal vulva and individualization of treatment depending on the size and location of the primary lesion. For advanced stages of vulvar cancer, treatment usually consists of a combination of surgical excision and radiation therapy.

TABLE 1. **International Federation of Gynecology and Obstetrics Staging of Vulvar Cancer**

Stage I	Tumor ≤2 cm is confined to the vulva and/or perineum, no nodal metastasis
Stage II	Tumor >2 cm confined to the vulva and/or perineum
Stage III	Tumor any size with adjacent spread to the vagina, lower urethra, or anus; and/or unilateral groin node metastasis
Stage IVA	Tumor invades the upper urethra, bladder or rectal mucosa, pelvic bone, and/or bilateral groin node metastasis
Stage IVB	Any distant metastasis, including pelvic lymph nodes

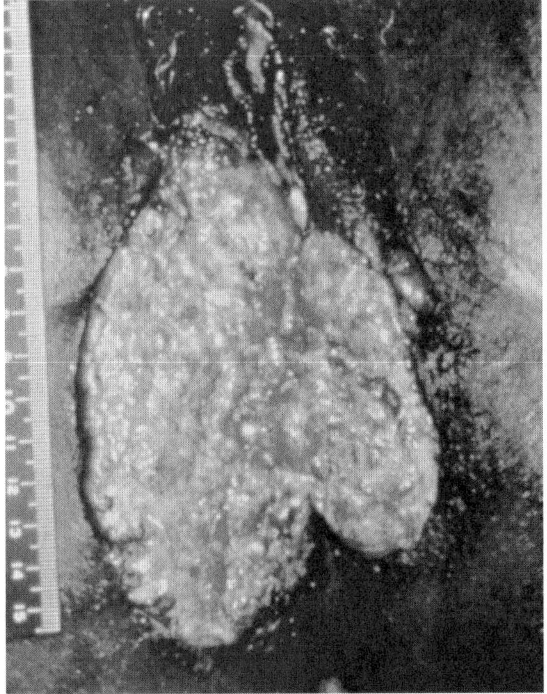

Figure 4. Advanced squamous cell carcinoma of the vulva.

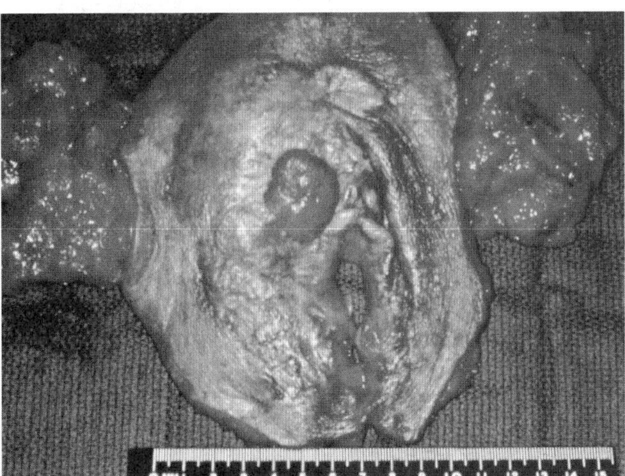

Figure 5. Radical vulvectomy with bilateral groin dissection specimen. The "butterfly" excision is associated with significant postoperative morbidity. Note the carcinoma arising from the right labia majus.

Adenocarcinoma

Adenocarcinoma of the vulva is a rare gynecologic malignancy, accounting for about 1% of all vulvar cancers. Most commonly, adenocarcinomas arise from Bartholin's gland; however, other sites of origin include skin adnexal glands, paraurethral glands, endometriosis, and ectopic breast tissue. Any enlargement of Bartholin's gland in a postmenopausal woman should be considered a malignancy until proven otherwise. Because of the rarity of vulvar adenocarcinoma, an extravulvar primary carcinoma should always be excluded, especially rectal cancer and upper genital tract cancer. Treatment of these tumors is similar to primary squamous cell carcinoma of the vulva and includes radical vulvectomy with bilateral groin lymphadenectomy.

Malignant Melanoma

Although a rare malignancy, vulvar melanoma is the second most common cancer occurring in the vulva. Melanomas arise from junctional or compound nevi. Consequently, some authorities recommend that all pigmented nevi on the vulva should be prophylactically excised. Melanomas usually present as raised, pigmented, or ulcerated lesions, occurring most commonly on the labia minora or clitoris (Figure 6). Prognosis depends on the size of the lesion and the depth of invasion.

The FIGO staging for vulvar carcinoma is not applicable to melanomas. Currently, two classification systems commonly used for melanomas elsewhere on the skin are used to evaluate vulvar melanomas. These include the Clark classification, based on the depth of invasion, and the Breslow classification, based on the thickness of the invasive portion of the lesion. Treatment includes surgical excision, either by wide radical excision or radical vulvectomy, with or without groin dissection depending on the size of the lesion and its depth of invasion.

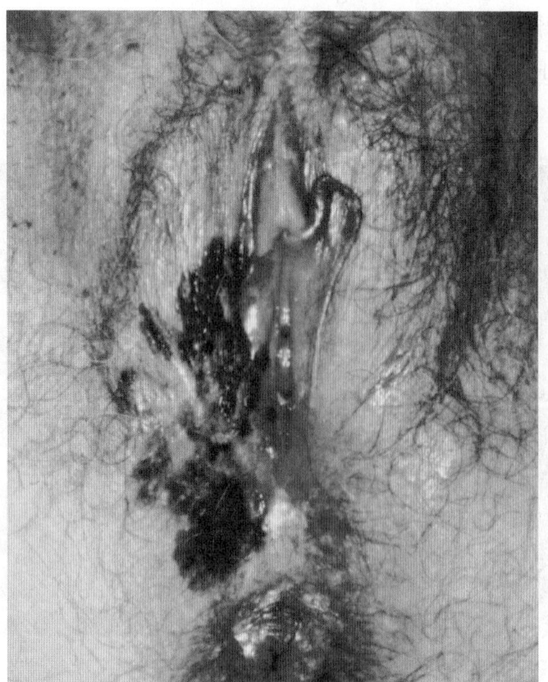

Figure 6. Malignant melanoma of the vulva. The typical pigmented lesion is present.

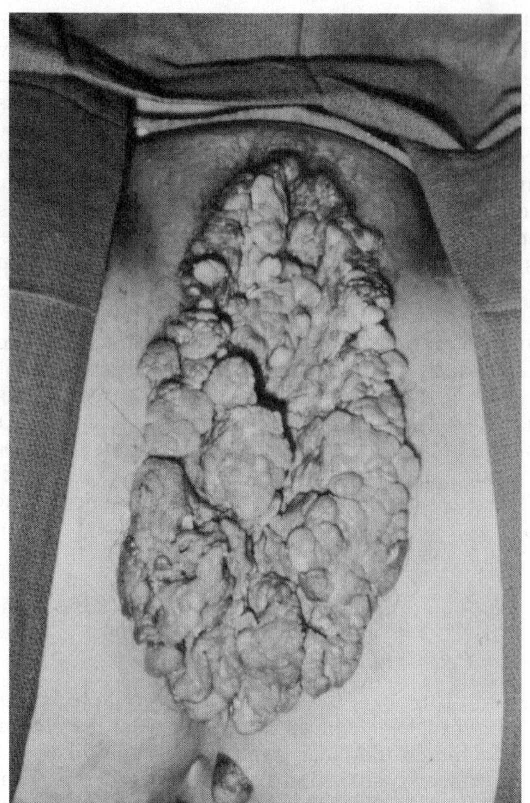

Figure 7. Verrucous carcinoma of the vulva usually grows as exophytic, fungating, condylomatous lesions. These lesions are locally destructive, as illustrated in this advanced case.

Basal Cell Carcinoma

Basal cell carcinomas can arise from the skin or hair follicles of the vulva. They are rare tumors, accounting for 2% of all vulvar cancers. This tumor is an invasive but rarely metastasizing malignancy that usually occurs in white women older than 50 years of age. Typically, the lesions are small with a rolled, pearly border and a central ulceration usually occurring on the labia majora. Treatment is wide local excision. If the surgical margins of resection are negative for tumor, the patient is usually cured.

Verrucous Carcinoma

Verrucous carcinoma, a special variant of squamous cell carcinoma, is also a rare tumor of the vulva. Clinically, patients present with a large cauliflower-like condylomatous mass (Figure 7). It is often necessary to perform multiple biopsies to establish the correct diagnosis. This tumor is invasive but rarely metastasizing, and treatment with wide local excision is recommended. Radiation therapy is ineffective and can actually worsen the patient's prognosis; therefore, it is contraindicated.

Sarcoma

Sarcomas make up only 1% to 2% of all vulvar malignancies. There are more than a dozen histologic types, but the majority are leiomyosarcomas. Patients usually present with a painful mass in the labia majus. The primary treatment is wide surgical excision. Adjuvant radiation therapy may be helpful in decreasing the incidence of local recurrence.

CONTRACEPTION

method of
KURT T. BARNHART, M.D., M.S.C.E., and
MOLINA DAYAL, M.D., M.P.H.
University of Pennsylvania
Philadelphia, Pennsylvania

The need for safe and effective methods of family planning worldwide, and in the United States, is paramount. The world population has surpassed 6 billion—an increase of 1 billion people in just 12 years. It is estimated that another 3 billion people will be added to the global population within the next half century. Globally, millions of women who do not desire pregnancy do not have access to contraception. Moreover, despite widespread access to family planning, more than half of the pregnancies conceived in the United States over the past decade have been unintended. Of these pregnancies, nearly half end in elective abortion. These rates are significantly higher than those reported in other industrialized countries, and many of these unwanted pregnancies are due to contraceptive failures.

A woman's childbearing potential exists for nearly 4 decades. During this time, a woman will pass through numerous life changes with differing health risks and evolving attitudes toward sexual activity and reproduction. No "perfect" family planning method exists for all women at all times in their reproductive life. However, today there are more options available for family planning than ever before. New methods have been developed, and many traditional methods have been improved to enhance safety and effectiveness. This increase in choice will aid the clinician and each couple in choosing among the relative strengths and weaknesses of each method throughout their reproductive years. This article serves as a review of the current family planning methods, with focus on the safety, efficacy, ease of use, side effects, and noncontraceptive benefits of each method.

ASSESSING CONTRACEPTIVE EFFICACY

An objective measure of contraceptive efficacy of each method is necessary to compare methods. Unfortunately, the efficacy of a family planning method is reported in terms of the number of women who become pregnant. Thus, for a given method, the most objective comparison of efficacy is to calculate the number of pregnancies experienced by 100 sexually active fertile women during its first year of use. The number of pregnancies prevented cannot be reported because some women who use no method may not become pregnant. If 100 women use no method of family planning during 1 year, only 85 would become pregnant. It would be incorrect to say that no method has a 15% success rate; instead the numbers are reported to state that the use of no method has an 85% failure rate. Efficacy can be further categorized as theoretical ("perfect use") and actual ("typical use"). Perfect use estimates the effectiveness of the method if it is used correctly and consistently with every act of intercourse. A more realistic measure of efficacy is typical use. This value is derived from studies of actual users, which can be influenced by motivation, frequency of intercourse, and ease of use. Methods that are directly related to coitus are difficult to use and have the largest discrepancy between perfect and typical use.

METHODS

Abstinence

Abstinence is the only 100% effective method of contraception if used 100% of the time. Many couples who abstain choose to avoid intercourse but engage in other forms of sexual intimacy. The health care provider's role is to support the choice of abstinence and teach negotiation skills needed for using abstinence effectively. Because of a high degree of noncompliance, abstinence remains one of the least successful methods overall.

Fertility Awareness

Fertility awareness methods depend on being able to correctly identify fertile days of the menstrual cycle. With proper instruction, couples learn to observe and interpret signs and patterns of fertility that occur during a menstrual cycle, as well as understand how to use this information to avoid (or achieve) a pregnancy. These methods work because of periodic abstinence during the fertile period of a woman's menstrual cycle.

Calendar Calculations. Worldwide, this method is the oldest and most widely practiced method of the fertility awareness methods. Calculation is based on the following assumptions: (1) ovulation occurs on day 14 (± 2 days) before the onset of the next menses, (2) sperm remain viable for about 5 days, and (3) the ovum survives for about 1 day. Past cycle lengths give an estimate of fertile days within a given cycle. Abstaining from intercourse during the fertile time provides contraception.

Basal Body Temperature (BBT). Most ovulatory cycles demonstrate a biphasic BBT pattern: lower in the first half of the cycle, rising to a higher level around the time of ovulation, and remaining at the higher level for the rest of the cycle. It cannot be used to identify the fertile period of a current cycle because ovulation is identified retrospectively. The most effective way of using this method for contraception is to avoid intercourse throughout the first portion of the cycle as well as 2 days after the ovulation-associated temperature rise.

Cervical Secretions. Cervical mucus changes can signal the beginning and end of the fertile period. Secretions during the fertile period are abundant, clear or white, stretchy, and slippery. Ovulation most likely occurs within 1 day before to 1 day after the appearance of the abundant, clear, stretchy, slippery

Text continued on page 1108

TABLE 1. **Methods of Contraception**

Method	Advantages	Disadvantages	Contraindications	Comments	% Women With Unintended Pregnancy Within the First Year		% Women Continuing Use at 1 Year
					Typical Use	*Perfect Use*	
No method					85		
Abstinence	The only 100% effective method No financial cost No risk of STDs	High rate of failure given high degree of noncompliance	None	Clinician must discuss other sexually intimate methods of expression that minimize STD and pregnancy risk	?	0	
Fertility awareness methods	Acceptable to some religions that disapprove other contraceptive methods	Usually requires instruction to use particular method Both partners need to communicate and be committed No protection against STDs			25		63
Calendar method	Involves both partners	No protection against STDs				9	
Ovulation (BBT) method		Cannot be used with irregular menses	Irregular menses	Least reliable of fertility awareness methods		3	
Sympathothermal	No costs beyond that needed for thermometer or LH predictor kits	Women must be able to monitor and interpret temperature and mucus characteristics		Most reliable of fertility awareness methods		3	
Withdrawal/coitus interruptus	Available in any situation No cost No medical side effects	Depends on "control" and trust of partner No protection against STDs		No reinsertion of penis after ejaculation unless washed with soap and water	17	4	
Spermicidal products	Accessible to couples Up to 25% protection against STDs such as gonorrhea and chlamydia (not HIV) Increases efficacy of barrier methods No medical consultation needed	Need to reinsert with each act of intercourse Vary in consistency and percentage of active ingredient Effective for up to 1 hour May increase risk of HIV due to disruption of vaginal epithelium Increased incidence of vaginal candidiasis	Hypersensitivity to spermicidal products	Creams provide better coverage than gels Place 10–60 minutes before intercourse; use additional dose if repeat intercourse or greater than 1 hour Leave in place for >6 hours after intercourse No douching for >6 hours after use Unclear protection from HIV	26	6	40
Sponges	No systemic side effects Continuous protection for 24 hours regardless of number of acts of intercourse Lowers incidence of candidiasis	Increased risk of toxic shock syndrome if in place for >24 hours		Moisten with water before insertion Higher failure rate in parous women	20	9	56
Male condoms	Easily accessible STD protection Allows for male participation Few side effects	Partner dependent Animal-based products do not protect against HIV Condom may break or slip Often not used consistently Coital dependent Oil-based preparations impair condom efficacy and facilitate breakage	Latex allergy Hypersensitivity to spermicidal products	Brands trade off reliability and strength for less thickness to enhance stimulation Lubrication and reservoir tip lower risk of breakage Safe lubricants: egg white, glycerine, nonoxynol 9, saliva, water, aloe-9, K-Y jelly, Astroglide, Gynoll II Prepair, Probe, Ramses Personal Lubricant			

				Less safe lubricants (oil based): conjugated estrogen cream, estradiol cream, baby oil, butter, cocoa butter, cold cream, mineral oil, hand lotion, massage oil, petroleum jelly, vegetable oil, shortening, suntan oil, rubbing alcohol, antifungal medications Should not be used with female condom	14	3	61
Female condom	Not made of latex Three varieties available Can use oil-based products	Does not contain a spermicide Should not be worn with a male condom		Remove immediately after intercourse and before standing Unproven STD benefit	21	5	56
Cervical cap	Spermicide not necessary but improves efficacy Continuous protection for 48 hours (regardless of number acts of intercourse) Additional spermicide not necessary with repeated intercourse	Damaged by oil-based products Abnormal anatomy may preclude use Should not be worn >48 hours Not widely available Few clinicians trained in use	Hypersensitivity to spermicidal products History of toxic shock syndrome	About 6% of women cannot be fitted Failure rate higher in parous women	20	9	56
Diaphragm	Some protection from cervical dysplasia Several varieties available	Must be used with a spermicide Damaged by oil-based products Twice the incidence of urinary tract infection Less efficacy with increased intercourse; repeat dose of spermicide needed	Latex allergy Hypersensitivity to spermicidal products History of toxic shock syndrome	For parous women, diaphragm more effective than sponge or cap May be inserted up to 6 hours before intercourse Should be left in place 6–8 hours after last coitus Should be refit yearly and after pregnancy, miscarriage, abortion, pelvic surgery, or weight change of >10 lb If recurrent UTIs, try smaller diaphragm or different rim or change to a different method	20	6	56
Intrauterine devices	Can be inserted at any time of the menstrual cycle Can prevent and treat Asherman syndrome Does not interfere with lactation Not coital dependent	Uterine perforation possible but very rare	Active pelvic inflammatory disease Pregnancy	Treat vaginal infections before placement Need SBE prophylaxis before insertion if with valvular disease 2%–10% expulsion rate in first year If pregnancy occurs, 5% chance of ectopic pregnancy			

Table continued on following page

TABLE 1. **Methods of Contraception** *Continued*

Method	Advantages	Disadvantages	Contraindications	Comments	% Women With Unintended Pregnancy Within the First Year		% Women Continuing Use at 1 Year
					Typical Use	*Perfect Use*	
Copper T 380A	Effective for 10 years Can be used as emergency contraception Low failure rate (0.6%) Reduces rate of ectopic pregnancy by 90%	Increased bleeding, spotting	Pregnancy Active or history of pelvic inflammatory disease and STD risk Postpartum endometritis or infected AB (within 3 months) Genital actinomycosis Uterine or cervical malignancy Undiagnosed vaginal bleeding Acute vaginitis/cervicitis Wilson disease	Needs easy access to follow-up Need to carefully weigh risks and benefits in immunocompromised women	0.8	0.6	78
Progesterone T	Decreases menstrual flow by 50% Decreases dysmenorrhea	Requires yearly reinsertion Irregular bleeding	Uterine cavity <6 cm, >10 cm *See* Copper T 380A		2	1.5	81
Levonorgestrel IUD	Decreases pelvic inflammatory disease Treats amenorrhea Effective for 5 years	Irregular bleeding	*See* Copper T 380A		0.3	0.3	81
Injectable DMPA	Effective for 12 weeks Useful for effective, temporary contraception Can be used postpartum Can be used with breast-feeding No change in clotting parameters Not coital dependent	Irregular bleeding 50% develop amenorrhea within 1 year of use No STD protection Associated with weight gain (5 lb/y 1; 16 lb/y 2) Contraceptive effects last 4–12 months after discontinuation	Pregnancy Undiagnosed vaginal bleeding Known or suspected breast cancer Acute liver disease or tumors	150 mg IM q12 weeks within 5 d of onset of menses and negative pregnancy test Avoid in women who desire prompt return of fertility	0.3	0.3	70
Norplant (levonorgestrel implants)	Not coital dependent Effective for 5 years No demonstrated increased risk of cervical cancer Lowers risk of endometrial and ovarian cancer, PID, ectopic pregnancy, and anemia No change in cholesterol or coagulation factors	Bloating, mood changes, depression, acne, breast tenderness Weight gain (5 lb) Menstrual irregularity Requires surgical removal and insertion Higher rate of failure with higher weights	Known or suspected breast cancer Undiagnosed vaginal bleeding Acute thrombophlebitis or pulmonary embolism Active liver disease or tumors Pregnancy Use of medications that cause progestins to be metabolized more rapidly (phenytoin, phenobarbital, carbamazepine, rifampin)	Consider addition of conjugated estrogen (1.25 mg) for 1 week for persistent irregular bleeding Each implant contains 36 mg levonorgestrel, released at graduated rates Decreased ovulation in at least half the cycles	0.05	0.05	88

Combined OCPs	Decreases endometrial cancer, ovarian cancer, ovarian cysts, benign breast disease, PMS, dysmenorrhea, hirsutism, acne, pelvic inflammatory disease, uterine fibroid bleeding, endometriosis, menstrual flow Increases bone mass Not coital dependent	Certain medications decrease OCP levels: ampicillin, rifampin, griseofulvin, tetracycline, barbiturates, phenobarbital, phenytoin, primidone May lower anticoagulation effect of warfarin, enhance benzodiazepine effect, reduce prednisolone clearance May increase levels of certain drugs: TCAs, insulin, ibuprofen, oral hypoglycemics, cyclosporine	History of jaundice with pregnancy Undiagnosed vaginal bleeding Known or suspected breast cancer Symptomatic gallbladder disease Thrombophlebitis Cerebrovascular disease Migraine headaches with focal neurologic deficits Personal or family history of thromboembolic disease	Cancer reduction: ovarian cancer reduced by 30% after 4 years, 60% after 5 years, and 80% after 12 years of use; endometrial cancer reduced 40% after 2 years, 60% after 4 years of use No significant risk to fetus if inadvertently taken when pregnant Add condoms for STD protection	5	0.1	71
Progestin only OCP	Compatible with lactation May be tolerated by women who have a contraindication to estrogen Not coital dependent	Irregular bleeding Amenorrhea OCP efficacy lowered with carbamazepine, phenobarbital, phenytoin, primidone, rifampin	Undiagnosed vaginal bleeding Pregnancy Active liver disease or tumors Breast cancer	Increased risk of diabetes if prescribed to patient with gestational diabetes Must be used at the same time each day Consider addition of conjugated estrogen (1.25 mg) for 10–13 days or combined OCPs for breakthrough bleeding	7	0.5	60
Sterilization (female)	No compliance issues Complications <1%	6% regret No STD protection Reversibility difficult		Failure increases with younger women Provide counseling to decrease postprocedure regret If pregnancy occurs, it should be assumed that it is an ectopic until proven otherwise	0.55	0.5–1.9	100
Sterilization (male)	No compliance issues Most cost-effective method <3% complications 0.1%–4% failure rate	Reversibility difficult No STD protection		No impact on prostate cancer Not sterile until >20 ejaculations Success of reversal related to length of time since surgery	0.15	0.1	100
Emergency contraception	Useful backup method No increased risk of congenital abnormalities if pregnancy occurs after treatment	Nausea (30%–50%) and vomiting (15%–25%) common with combined method Ten to 15% will have change in amount, duration, and timing of next menses		More successful the sooner it is initiated Routine antinausea or antiemetic recommended Progestin-only pills associated with less nausea Use pills for less than 72 hours after exposure Insert IUD <5 days after exposure Women with most hormonal contraindications can usually tolerate given short duration Decreases pregnancy rate by 75%	0.25	?	N/A

Abbreviations: AB = abdomen; BBT = basal body temperature; LH = luteinizing hormone; OCP = oral contraceptive pill; SBE = subacute bacterial endocarditis; STD = sexually transmitted disease; TCAs = tricyclic antidepressants; UTIs = urinary tract infections.

discharge. These secretions become thick, cloudy, and sticky after ovulation. It is presumed that the fertile period begins when cervical secretions are first noted until 4 days past the peak day of the clear and slippery discharge.

Symptothermal Method. This approach involves combining both use of cervical secretions and BBT to identify the fertile time. Other indicators of impending ovulation are mittelschmerz (lower abdominal pain or cramping immediately before ovulation) or breast tenderness. Couples using multiple indicators have a better chance of avoiding an undesired pregnancy.

Coitus Interruptus (Withdrawal)

The withdrawal method prevents fertilization by preventing interaction between spermatozoa and ovum. Typically, the couple has vaginal intercourse until ejaculation is impending, at which time the male partner withdraws his penis from the vagina and away from the external genitalia of his female partner. The man relies on his own sensations to determine when ejaculation is imminent. Because sperm is also present in the pre-ejaculate, its deposition can lead to contraceptive failure.

Spermicidal Products

Spermicides consist of two components, namely, their formulation (gel, foam, cream, film, suppository) and their spermicidal chemical. The formulation helps in dispersion of the spermicide and the chemical (nonoxynol 9, octoxynyl 8) destroys the sperm cell membrane. Each formulation delivers a different concentration of spermicide. Spermicides protect against the transmission of chlamydia and gonorrhea. Concern exists regarding the association of existing spermicides and HIV transmission; well-developed studies are needed to answer this important question. More than 30 chemical barrier methods are in various stages of development at the present time. It is anticipated that these formulations can serve to protect a women and her partner from pregnancy and a variety of sexually transmitted infections, including HIV infection.

Vaginal Barriers

Vaginal barriers are easy to use and do not require direct involvement of the male partner for effective use. They can be used intermittently and do not require advance planning.

Male Condom. The male condom remains the most widely available and popular male contraceptive method in the United States. The condom is composed of a thin sheath that is placed over the glans and shaft of the penis. It blocks the passage of semen and is effective only when used from beginning to end of an act of intercourse. Until recently, most condoms were manufactured from latex ("rubber" condoms) whereas a minority were made from the intestinal cecum of lambs ("natural skin" condoms). Natural skin, or nonlatex, condoms, however, contain small pores that permit the passage of viruses such as hepatitis B, herpes simplex, and HIV. Latex condoms can prevent or decrease the transmission of HIV, gonorrhea, chlamydia, human papillomavirus, and herpes simplex virus. Newer condoms manufactured from polyurethane are thinner and stronger than latex condoms; these condoms are more resistant to deterioration, less constricting, and enhance sensitivity. Some condoms contain a spermicide; the dose is much less than that found in separate spermicide preparations. There is no evidence, however, that these condoms are more effective than condoms without spermicide.

Diaphragm. The diaphragm acts as a physical and chemical barrier to sperm. This flexible device is inserted into the vagina so that the dome covers the cervix while the posterior rim sits in the posterior fornix and the anterior rim rests behind the pubic bone. Both latex and nonlatex diaphragms are available. Spermicidal cream/jelly is applied to the inside of its dome before insertion. Additional spermicide is required for repeated acts of intercourse. It provides contraceptive protection for up to 6 hours after placement.

Diaphragms are available in different styles and sizes. The styles differ in the construction of the circular rim. Clinicians can estimate the proper size by measuring the distance between the introitus and the cervix. The diaphragm should be checked for placement after the patient ambulates and performs a Valsalva maneuver. The woman is instructed on insertion and removal and then demonstrates appropriate technique before leaving the office.

Cervical Cap. Like the diaphragm, the cap provides both a physical and chemical barrier to sperm. It is placed in the vagina such that the cap forms a seal between its inner ring and the surface of the cervix. Spermicide is used to fill the dome one third full before insertion. It provides continuous protection for up to 48 hours, regardless of the number of acts of intercourse. Extra spermicide is not needed for repeated acts of intercourse. Use for longer than 48 continuous hours is not recommended to eliminate the increased risk of toxic shock syndrome thereafter.

Female Condom. The female condom provides a physical barrier that lines the entire surface of the vagina and partially shields the perineum. It contains two flexible polyurethane rings, one that serves as an internal anchor while the other ring forms an external, open end that remains outside the vagina. The sheath is coated on the internal and external surfaces by a nonspermicidal lubricant. It can be inserted up to 8 hours in advance. Female and male condoms should not be used together; slippage and displacement of one or both condoms can be caused by adherence. The female condom provides contraceptive protection as well as protection from sexually transmitted diseases.

Intrauterine Device (IUD)

The IUD is one of the most widely used reversible methods of contraception worldwide. Problems in the

1970s led to a negative perception of the IUD; and, according to the 1995 National Survey of Family Growth, less than 1% of women use the IUD in the United States. The IUD works primarily by preventing sperm mobility and oocyte fertilization. Evidence does not support the claim that the IUD is an abortifacient.

Copper (Cu) T 380A (ParaGard). This IUD causes an increase in tubal and uterine fluids containing copper ions, enzymes, macrophages, and prostaglandins that alter and affect sperm and ovum interaction. Changes in the endometrium create a sterile inflammatory response that is spermicidal and prevents viable sperm from reaching the fallopian tubes. The copper IUD is approved for 10 continuous years of use.

Progestin IUD. Two main types include the Progesterone T and the Levonorgestrel Intrauterine System. Both work by a hormonal mechanism of action: cervical mucus is thickened, the endometrium is altered, and both uterine and tubal motility are impaired. Both are thought to interfere with fertilization, although data confirming this are sparse. The Progesterone T is approved for 1 year of contraceptive protection whereas the Levonorgestrel Intrauterine System is effective for up to 5 years. The presence of a progestin in the IUD results in decreased menstrual bleeding and cramps that are associated with the copper IUD.

The IUD is one of the most effective methods of family planning in use today. In some studies it is even more effective than sterilization. The IUD is currently most commonly used in parous women who desire child spacing or a nonpermanent form of family planning. The IUD is safe and is not associated with increased infection outside the first few weeks after insertion. Pelvic inflammatory disease (PID) is not caused by an IUD, but it is caused by the transmission of an infection from an infected partner. An IUD, however, will not lower a woman's risk of PID or other sexually transmitted diseases (STDs), as is the case with some barrier and hormonal methods. Choosing the appropriate candidate for the IUD is critical in reducing the risk of complications. Thus, a woman at risk for an STD (e.g., a woman with multiple sexual partners, a woman whose partner has other sexual partners at risk for an STD, or a woman with a history of endometritis or purulent cervicitis in the past 3 months) should be strongly counseled that the IUD itself will not increase or decrease her risk of future infection. She should be advised that she needs to decrease the risk of infection by also using barrier methods of contraception and by avoiding sexual relations with an infected partner.

Hormonal Methods

Combined Oral Contraceptive Pills

The oral contraceptive pill (OCP) is one of the most extensively studied prescription medications. OCPs effectively prevent pregnancy if used properly. Ideally, fewer than 1 in 100 women would become pregnant in 1 year. With typical use, however, 5 pregnancies per 100 women occur. Failures often occur from missing pills without a backup method of contraception.

Oral contraceptives prevent pregnancy mainly by suppressing ovulation. Ovulation is prohibited by the suppression of follicle-stimulating hormone and luteinizing hormone. The progestational component thickens cervical mucus (preventing transport of sperm), alters tubal motility, and prevents production of a decidualized endometrium, thereby hampering implantation. Estrogen alters the cellular structure of the endometrium such that areas of edema alternate with areas of cellular density; it also causes degeneration of the corpus luteum. Most of the contraceptive efficacy is derived from the progestin effect.

Many varieties of combined OCPs are available. "Monophasic" preparations have a fixed dose of estrogen (usually 20–35 μg of ethinyl estradiol) and a fixed dose of one of several progestins (levonorgestrel [Norplant], norethindrone [Micronor], desogestrel [Desogen], norgestrel [Ovrette], or norgestimate [Ortho-Cyclen]). "Biphasic" OCPs have a constant amount of estrogen with a low dose of progestin during the first half of the cycle and a higher dose of progestin during the second half (mimics a woman's normal progesterone levels). "Triphasic" pills have a constant level of estrogen with a gradually increasing dose of progestin. Both the biphasic and triphasic regimens were developed to decrease the incidence of breakthrough bleeding and progesterone-related side effects but have never been demonstrated to do so.

Both the estrogen and progestin component act on many different organ systems, producing a wide range of contraceptive and other effects. Oral contraceptives have a number of menstrual benefits, including decreased cramping and pain, reduced menstrual flow by at least 60%, and controlled timing of flow. One can avoid menstrual periods on weekends and vacations by skipping the "pill-free" week and continuing active pills; women with dysmenorrhea, severe migraines, or premenstrual syndrome can decrease the frequency of menses in this manner as well. In addition, OCPs can improve acne and hirsutism (by increasing sex hormone binding globulin), prevent functional ovarian cysts, protect against osteoporosis, and treat endometriosis-related pain. The pill has been definitively demonstrated to cut the incidence of ovarian and endometrial cancer in half. Use of OCPs does not confer the same risk of breast cancer as does the use of postmenopausal estrogen replacement therapy. Although there is still a debate regarding the use of the OCP and breast cancer, most new evidence suggests no relationship. Patients with a family history of breast cancer are not at an additional risk and can safely use the OCP. Postmenopausal breast cancer may be reduced in OCP users.

The estrogen component of OCPs can activate blood-clotting mechanisms. Lower-dose pills have fewer cardiovascular effects than did earlier higher-dose pills. In terms of thromboembolic events, it is still overall safer for a woman to use OCPs than to become pregnant. The attributable risk, or the number of venous thromboembolic events (cases) from estrogen in the OCP, is on the order of approximately 6 per 100,000 woman-years. This is in contrast to the estimated 20 cases per 100,000 woman-years if pregnant. In regard to arterial embolic events, there is no evidence to support an increased or decreased risk of myocardial infarction from past or current use of OCPs compared with no use. In addition, the strength of association between OCP use and stroke is weak, with odds ratios ranging from 1.1 to 1.8, most with 95% confidence intervals crossing 1.0. Evidence of a synergistic effect between smoking and OCP use exists for these events. The OCP is contraindicated in women who smoke and are older than 35 years of age or in women with a history of a deep venous blood clot, heart attack, or stroke. The pill should not be used by women with a history of breast cancer, with vaginal bleeding that may suggest the presence of a pregnancy, or who are pregnant. The pill is commonly used in nonsmoking women older than 35 years old and can be used safely until the menopause.

Future trends in OCPs will likely include lower-dose estrogen pills, decreasing the number of placebo pills in each packet of pills, changes in the progestin used in the preparation, and changes in the hormone-free interval, potentially resulting in as few as four menses a year

Other Combination Methods

The Food and Drug Administration (FDA) has approved Lunelle, a monthly contraceptive injection. Lunelle contains a combination of a progestin and estrogen (25 mg medroxyprogesterone acetate and 5 mg estradiol cypionate). The monthly injection improves convenience and contraceptive efficacy. Its phase III trial suggests that the level of contraceptive efficacy is similar to that achieved with surgical sterilization. Its mechanism of action is similar to that of other hormonal methods, is readily reversible (within 3 months), and has fewer side effects.

A combination skin patch is soon to be available as well. The patch releases 20 mg of ethinyl estradiol and 150 mg of 17β-deacetyl norgestimate, providing a week of contraception. This method has a similar profile to combined OCPs but offers the advantage of not requiring a daily dose.

A Silastic vaginal ring that releases 15 μg of ethinyl estradiol and 0.12 mg of 3-keto-desogestrel a day is currently marketed in Europe and may soon be available in the United States. The ring is placed on day 7 of the cycle and removed on day 21. This Silastic ring provides rapid return of fertility after its removal.

Progestin-Only Contraception

These methods offer several effective options to women who cannot use an estrogen-containing contraceptive. These methods, however, do not provide protection against STDs. Progestin-only methods can be administered by mouth, injection, IUDs, implants, or vaginal rings. Their mechanism of action is multifold: (1) inhibition of ovulation, (2) reduction and thickening of cervical mucus (preventing sperm penetration), (3) suppression of the midcycle peaks of luteinizing hormone and follicle-stimulating hormone, and (4) production of a thin and atrophic endometrium. Many of these methods have excellent efficacy rates and can be safely used in women at high risk of estrogen-related side effects. The main disadvantage of these methods is that of poor menstrual cycle control and an increase in irregular vaginal bleeding.

Injectable Progestin (Depo-Provera). This is the most commonly used injectable form of contraception. It is given as an intramuscular injection of 150 mg every 12 weeks. It is expected that less than 1% of women will become pregnant in the first year of use. Menstrual patterns can be irregular, with amenorrhea during the first year of use being very common (50%). The median time to conception from the first omitted dose is 8.5 months. Because this method is so good at suppressing the ovary, concerns have been raised that the use of Depo-Provera may result in a decreased peak bone mass achieved by a women in her early reproductive years. A return to normal bone mineral density is observed after cessation of the medication. Well-developed clinical trials will be published in the near future answering this question.

Implantable Progestin (Norplant). Each of the six implants contains 36 mg of levonorgestrel. The progestin is released at a low, steady rate of 85 μg/d initially, decreasing to 50 μg/d at 9 months, to 35 μg/d at 18 months, and to 30 μg/d thereafter. As with Depo-Provera, irregular menses often occur, as does amenorrhea. An advantage over the injectable progestin is that the median time to conception after removal is approximately 1 month. It is recommended that Norplant be removed after 5 years, given the increase in failure rates thereafter.

Newer implantable methods include Implanon* and Jadelle.* Implanon, a single implantable rod, releases the progesterone keto-desogestrel and is effective for 3 years. Jadelle is composed of two flexible rods (each containing 75 mg levonorgestrel). Both implants have a mechanism of action similar to Norplant. The main advantage of these newer implants over Norplant is less discomfort with insertion and removal. Like Norplant, quick restoration of fertility occurs after their removal.

Minipill. Progestin-only pills need to be taken every day, without a pill-free interval. Because as few as one missed pill can decrease efficacy, they are generally less effective than combined oral contraceptives. The probability of pregnancy in the first year of typical use approximates 5%. In lactating women, the progestin-only pill is nearly 100% effective be-

*Not available in the United States.

cause of the additional effect of breast-feeding. In addition, these pills do not alter the quantity of milk production in lactating women. Menses are often irregular, and the median time to conception after discontinuation is less than 3 months.

Emergency Contraception

Both the IUD and OCPs can be used as emergency contraception. These methods decrease the risk of pregnancy by approximately 75%. There are no medical contraindications to treatment with emergency contraception except pregnancy; a personal or family history of thromboembolism is not a contraindication. These methods prevent pregnancy by causing anovulation or by delaying ovulation; they do not interrupt or disrupt an already established pregnancy.

The most commonly used method is combined estrogen and progestin, which must be taken within 72 hours of unprotected intercourse. After treatment, pregnancy rates are in the range of 0.5% to 2.5%. An antiemetic is often necessary with the use of emergency contraception with the combined estrogen and progestin. With combined therapy, 100 μg of ethinyl estradiol and 1 mg of levonorgestrel in two divided doses 12 hours apart is the standard dose required to reduce the risk of pregnancy by 74% (the "Yupze method"). Progestin-only pills are less likely to have side effects of nausea and vomiting (minimum dose needed is 0.75 mg of levonorgestrel taken 12 hours apart). Taking more pills than specified is not beneficial and may increase the risk of vomiting. "Preven" is a prepackaged kit containing instructions for emergency contraceptive pill use, appropriately dosed pills of estrogen and progestin, a pregnancy test, and product liability insurance. "Plan B" is a prepackaged form of progestin-only pills for emergency contraception use. Recent data suggest that the first dose of medication is the most important one in increasing efficacy with emergency contraception.

Alternatively, a copper IUD can be placed within 5 days of unprotected intercourse. The failure rate is very low, 0.1%. The FDA has approved mifepristone (Mifeprex, RU-486), a progesterone antagonist. In addition to its effect on ovulation, mifepristone also retards endometrial development. A single oral dose (600 mg) is associated with markedly less nausea and an efficacy rate of nearly 100%. A 3-week follow-up should be scheduled to assess the result and to counsel for routine contraception.

Surgical Sterilization

Sterilization has become one of the most widely used methods of family planning worldwide. Both female tubal sterilization and vasectomy are meant to be permanent and are comparable in effectiveness. The failure rates for tubal sterilization range from 0.7% to 5.4% depending on the technique used. Unipolar coagulation and postpartum sterilization result in the lowest cumulative failure rates; unipolar coagulation, however, has been associated with increased morbidity due to bowel injury. Counseling is absolutely essential; approximately 6% of women regret their decision to have permanent sterilization. Regret is more common in women younger than 30 years old and those who have postpartum procedures performed. Vasectomy has a failure rate of 0.1% in the first year.

The high rate of unintended pregnancy in the United States remains a mystery despite widespread availability of highly effective and safe methods of birth control. Although most sexually active couples use a method of contraception, many methods are either ineffective or used incorrectly. Educating couples in regard to consistent and correct contraceptive use while expanding their contraceptive options may significantly decrease unplanned pregnancy rates in the United States.

Section 16

Psychiatric Disorders

ALCOHOLISM

method of
RAY BAKER, M.D.
University of British Columbia
Vancouver, British Columbia, Canada

EPIDEMIOLOGY

The title "Great Impostor," once the nickname for syphilis, is an appropriate moniker for alcohol dependence or alcoholism. Over 20% of hospitalized patients and nearly that proportion of medical office patients are suffering from medical or psychiatric problems caused or exacerbated by excessive alcohol consumption (Table 1). Over 110,000 North Americans die every year as the result of alcohol-related medical conditions, and many more drinkers and their families suffer the medical, psychiatric, and psychosocial toll of problems due to alcohol. Research has repeatedly shown that when primary care physicians screen their patients for heavy drinking and offer brief advice in cutting down or becoming abstinent, there are significant and sustained reductions in alcohol consumption. In spite of this evidence physicians often fail to detect alcohol use disorders in their patients. However, when perceived harm results from illness or injuries due to undiagnosed alcoholism, patients and now their lawyers see detection and management of alcohol use disorders as part of the responsibility of their physicians.

SCREENING

Verbal or pen and paper screening for alcohol problems is more sensitive in detecting alcohol problems than laboratory testing. The AUDIT (Alcohol Use Disorders Identification Test) (Table 2) may be self-administered by patients, and the CAGE questions (Table 3) are easily woven into a diagnostic interview. During very brief patient encounters the following single question is remarkably productive in uncovering alcohol and other substance-related problems, including alcohol-induced family problems: *"Has alcohol or have other drugs ever caused problems in your life?"*

DIAGNOSIS

According to the American Society of Addiction Medicine, alcoholism is "a primary, chronic disease with genetic, psychosocial and environmental factors influencing its development and manifestations. The disease is often progressive and fatal. It is characterized by continuous or periodic impaired control over drinking, preoccupation with the drug alcohol, use of alcohol despite adverse consequences, and distortions in thinking, most notably denial." A useful way to remember the diagnostic criteria of the American Psychiatric Association (Table 4) is with the "3 Cs":

Control: episodic loss of control over ingestion of the drug once ingestion has begun (criteria 3 and 4)

Consequences: continued and recurrent use of the drug despite significant negative consequences (criteria 6 and 7)

Compulsion: an increased preoccupation with, or salience of, the drug use (criteria 4 through 7)

DEFINITION OF ALCOHOL ABUSE

Alcohol abuse simply refers to consumption of ethanol in a potentially hazardous or harmful manner. Unlike the alcohol dependent drinker, the alcohol abuser is able to maintain control and there is not yet a compulsive nature to the drinking.

LABORATORY TESTING

Gamma-Glutamyl Transpeptidase (GGT). During periods of heavy drinking this enzyme is elevated in over 60% of drinkers. It returns to normal within 4 to 6 weeks when excessive drinking stops. This test is less sensitive in adolescents and may be elevated in other conditions (liver disease, biliary tract disease, diabetes, pancreatitis, hyperthyroidism, heart failure, and drug-induced elevation: anticonvulsants, anticoagulants, and protease inhibitors).

TABLE 1. **Conditions Caused by Excessive Alcohol Consumption**

Cardiovascular	**Neurologic**
Hypertension	Wernicke encephalopathy
Cardiomyopathy	Peripheral neuropathy
Arrhythmias	Traumatic injury
Portal hypertension	Seizures
Gastrointestinal	Cerebellar degeneration
Gastritis	Central pontine myelinosis
Reflux esophagitis	Dementia
Peptic ulcer disease	**Immunologic**
Bleeding	Pneumonia
Fatty liver	Sexually transmitted diseases
Alcoholic hepatitis	Infections
Cirrhosis	Gastrointestinal cancers
Pancreatitis	Breast cancer
Metabolic	**Musculoskeletal**
Diabetes	Traumatic injury
Gout	Rhabdomyolysis
Hyperlipidemia	Proximal myopathy
Male feminization	**Sexual/Reproductive**
Psychiatric	Menstrual irregularities
Depression	Impotence
Anxiety	Anovulation
Korsakoff psychosis	Testicular atrophy
Hematologic	Feminization/masculinization
Anemia	Small for dates/prematurity
Thrombocytopenia	Multiple organ system fetal defects
Folate deficiency	
Iron deficiency	

TABLE 2. **Alcohol Use Disorders Identification Test: AUDIT**

1. How often do you have a drink containing alcohol?
- ☐ Never (0)
- ☐ Monthly or less (1)
- ☐ Two to four times a month (2)
- ☐ Two to three times a week (3)
- ☐ Four or more times a week (4)

2. How many drinks containing alcohol do you have on a typical day when you are drinking?
- ☐ 1 (0)
- ☐ 2–3 (1)
- ☐ 4 (2)
- ☐ 5–7 (3)
- ☐ 8 or more (4)

3. How often do you have five or more drinks on one occasion?
- ☐ Never (0)
- ☐ Less than monthly (1)
- ☐ Monthly (2)
- ☐ Weekly (3)
- ☐ Daily or almost daily (4)

4. How often during the last year have you found that you were not able to stop drinking once you had started?
- ☐ Never (0)
- ☐ Less than monthly (1)
- ☐ Monthly (2)
- ☐ Weekly (3)
- ☐ Daily or almost daily (4)

5. How often during the last year have you failed to do what was normally expected of you because of drinking?
- ☐ Never (0)
- ☐ Less than monthly (1)
- ☐ Monthly (2)
- ☐ Weekly (3)
- ☐ Daily or almost daily (4)

6. How often during the last year have you needed a first drink in the morning to get yourself going after a heavy drinking session?
- ☐ Never (0)
- ☐ Less than monthly (1)
- ☐ Monthly (2)
- ☐ Weekly (3)
- ☐ Daily or almost daily (4)

7. How often during the last year have you had a feeling of guilt or remorse after drinking?
- ☐ Never (0)
- ☐ Less than monthly (1)
- ☐ Monthly (2)
- ☐ Weekly (3)
- ☐ Daily or almost daily (4)

8. How often during the last year have you been unable to remember what happened the night before because you had been drinking?
- ☐ Never (0)
- ☐ Less than monthly (1)
- ☐ Monthly (2)
- ☐ Weekly (3)
- ☐ Daily or almost daily (4)

9. Have you or someone else been injured as a result of your drinking?
- ☐ No (0)
- ☐ Yes but not in the past year (2)
- ☐ Yes, during the last year (4)

10. Has a relative or friend, or a doctor or other health worker, been concerned about your drinking or suggested you cut down?
- ☐ No (0)
- ☐ Yes but not in the past year (2)
- ☐ Yes, during the past year (4)

Total Score: ______

A score of 8 or more is considered positive and suggests the need for cutting down and possibly further diagnostic assessment.

From Saunders JB, Aasland OG, Babor TF, et al: Development of the Alcohol Use Disorders Identification Test (AUDIT): WHO Collaborative Project on Early Detection of Persons With Harmful Alcohol Consumption. Addiction 88:791–804, 1993. Taylor & Francis Ltd., http://www.tandf.co.uk/journals.

TABLE 3. **C.A.G.E. Questions**

C: Have you ever felt the need to **C**ut down on your drinking (drug use)?
A: Have people **A**nnoyed you by criticizing your drinking (drug use)?
G: Have you ever felt **G**uilty about your drinking (drug use)?
E: Have you ever needed an **E**ye opener first thing after getting up to steady your nerves or get rid of a hangover?

Positive Screen = 2 positive answers. (Sensitivity: 60%–95%; specificity: 40%–95%)

From Ewing JA: Detecting alcoholism: The CAGE questionnaire. JAMA 252:1905–1907, 1984. Copyright 1984, American Medical Association.

Mean Corpuscular Volume (MCV). Although less sensitive and specific than GGT, the MCV is often elevated because of excessive alcohol consumption. It takes several months to return to normal.

Carbohydrate Deficient Transferring (CDT). Not yet readily available to most clinicians, this test offers both high specificity and sensitivity for excessive alcohol consumption.

NEUROBIOLOGY

Alcohol has been described as a "dirty drug" because it affects many parts of the nervous system and several neuroreceptor systems. In addition to causing nonspecific neuron cell membrane changes, current thinking is that alcohol acts through five separate neuroanatomical-neurochemical systems:

1. *Dopaminergic reward.* Like ingestion of all other addictive drugs, alcohol ingestion results in heightened dopaminergic activity in the mesolimbic reward circuitry in the region of the nucleus accumbens.
2. *Endogenous opioid reward.* The phenomenon of priming (the alcoholic's increase in craving, which triggers loss of control or drinking more than intended) often occurs after one to several alcoholic drinks. Priming is believed to be opiopeptide-mediated, originating in the ventral tegmentum, and can be blocked by opioid antagonists such as naltrexone (ReVia).
3. *Generalized inhibition.* Alcohol activates the gamma-aminobutyric acid (GABA)-ergic system, the most widespread inhibitory neurotransmitter system in the brain, resulting in generalized depression of central nervous system activity. An early effect of relatively low-dose alcohol consumption is to inhibit the cortical areas of the brain responsible for inhibition of behavior and self-consciousness. This results in what appears to be a paradoxical effect—disinhibition of higher risk behaviors, such as unprotected sex, driving while intoxicated, and use of other drugs.
4. *Norepinephrine-induced stimulation.* Acutely, alcohol tends to suppress the effects of the locus ceruleus both on emotions (anxiety, restlessness, irritability, apprehensiveness, and vigilance) and on the parasympathetic nervous system (tachycardia, hypertension, and gastrointestinal hyperactivity).
5. *Glutamate-induced excitation.* Chronic alcohol use and repeated episodes of withdrawal result in heightened sensitivity of NMDA receptors that bind to excitatory amino acids such as glutamate, causing disturbing clinical symptoms such as panic, post-acute withdrawal syndrome, hyperalgesia and "kindling," or heightened susceptibility to seizures.

TABLE 4. **DSM-IV Criteria for Alcohol (Or Other Drug) Dependence**

Definition

A syndrome characterized by a maladaptive pattern of substance use, leading to clinically significant impairment or distress, as manifested by three (or more) of the following, occurring at any time in the same 12-month period:

Diagnostic Criteria

1. Tolerance, as defined by either of the following: a need for markedly increased amounts of the substance to achieve intoxication or desired effect, or, markedly diminished effect with continued use of the same amount of the substance.
2. Withdrawal, as manifested by either of the following: the characteristic withdrawal for the substance or the same (or closely related) substance is taken to relieve or avoid withdrawal symptoms.
3. The substance is often taken in larger amounts or over a longer period than was intended.
4. There is a persistent desire or unsuccessful attempts to cut down or control the substance use.
5. A great deal of time is spent in activities necessary to obtain the substance, use the substance, or recover from its effects.
6. Important social, occupational, or recreational activities are given up or reduced because of substance use.
7. The substance use is continued despite knowledge of having a persistent or recurrent physical or psychological problem that is likely to have been caused or exacerbated by the substance use.

Reprinted with permission from the *Diagnostic and Statistical Manual of Mental Disorders, Fourth Edition, Text Revision.* Copyright 2000 American Psychiatric Association.

Alcohol use creates a trap for alcoholics, who may lack adequate means of comforting themselves during periods of stress. The drug works via the mesolimbic dopamine pathways and the locus ceruleus to provide pleasure (positive reinforcement) while reducing discomfort (negative reinforcement). Yet with continued heavy use the systems responsible for reward, pleasure, or hedonic tone become less effective so that more and more drug is required to achieve the same effect (tolerance). At the same time the excitatory systems become more active in an attempt to reset themselves to pre-drug levels of function, causing agitation and irritability, needing increasing alcohol for suppression. The alcoholic becomes trapped; when alcohol consumption declines, the reward system is almost shut down, resulting in a profound lowering of hedonic tone, whereas the excitatory systems, finally released from inhibition, are free to erupt into unimpeded activity: anxiety, panic, tremulousness, fever, delirium, tachyarrhythmia, hallucination, or even seizures (withdrawal).

MANAGEMENT

Withdrawal

Numerous studies have shown that symptom-driven therapy for alcohol withdrawal, based on the administration of medication when objectively quantified withdrawal signs and symptoms reach a certain level, results in less morbidity and shorter hospital stays, compared with using routine detox standing orders. Anxiety is a large part of the discomfort. Providing comfort in the form of reassurance, social support, and physical measures (warm baths, massage, adequate hydration, and gentle exercise) are highly therapeutic in themselves during the crucial first 96 hours of withdrawal. If symptoms warrant, a sedative-hypnotic drug is needed to provide GABA-ergic inhibition to replace alcohol briefly while neuroadaptation occurs. Effective medication will be cross-tolerant with alcohol, have a long half-life to maintain stable brain levels of the drug, provide seizure prophylaxis, and have an acceptable index of safety. Drugs meeting these criteria include diazepam (Valium, 10–20 mg), phenobarbital, 30 to 60 mg (if given under supervision), chlordiazepoxide (Librium, 50–100 mg), and carbemazepine (Tegretol, 100–200 mg). For elderly patients or those with advanced liver disease, oxazepam (Serax, 30–60 mg) is a preferable drug; although it has a shorter duration of action, because it has a simple metabolic path, it is easier for the liver to metabolize and for the kidneys to excrete. The use of phenytoin in preventing alcohol-withdrawal seizures has been shown to be ineffective. If intravenous fluids with glucose or dextrose are to be administered to the physically dependent alcoholic, thiamine (50–100 mg) must be administered intramuscularly to prevent potentially irreversible Wernicke encephalopathy.

Medications and Alcoholism

Because alcoholism is a complex biopsychosocial disorder, effective treatment must combine psychosocial therapies with whatever adjunctive pharmacotherapy is chosen. Medical detoxification alone, without further psychosocial treatment, will usually be followed by relapse.

Naltrexone (ReVia)

Naltrexone probably blocks opiopeptide-mediated reward mechanisms originating in the ventral tegmental area. Two well-designed randomized controlled studies demonstrated that when a 50-mg tablet of naltrexone daily was combined with psychosocial treatment, alcoholics treated with naltrexone drank significantly less and had fewer relapses than placebo-treated controls receiving psychosocial treatment. Because it is an opioid antagonist, naltrexone is contraindicated in patients requiring opioid medications and can precipitate withdrawal in people using street drugs containing opioids.

Acamprosate

Widely used in Europe but only recently studied in North America, acamprosate (calcium acetyl homotaurinate)* is believed to block the glutamate-NMDA system responsible for much of the prolonged agitation, irritability, and excitability seen in newly abstinent alcohol-dependent patients. It is not associated with significant adverse effects or drug-drug interactions and is not metabolized in the liver, because it is excreted unchanged by the kidney.

*Not available in the United States.

TABLE 5. **Assessment of Alcoholism**

Screening questionnaires: addictions, mental illness
Medical history
Physical examination
Laboratory investigations
Prescription drug review
Structured diagnostic addiction interview
Structured pain evaluation
Comprehensive psychosocial history
Psychiatric history
Mental status examination
Evaluation of current stressors
Collateral interviews

Disulfiram (Antabuse)

Less convincing evidence supports the use of disulfiram, a drug that uncouples the oxidation of ethanol, resulting in temporary accumulation of acetaldehyde, a toxic compound that causes uncomfortable and even dangerous symptoms such as flushing, headache, vomiting, chest pain, dyspnea, and tachycardia. These effects can be life threatening in some patients, especially those with diabetes or serious cardiovascular or hepatic disease.

Importance of Assessment

One size does not fit all. People with alcohol dependence are like jigsaw puzzles with certain missing pieces. The clinician's task is to help these patients discover which pieces are required to reassemble the puzzle. Remember, for much of the patient's drinking career alcohol was not the problem, it was the solution. So, unless the patient is able to develop alternative ways of comforting himself or herself and learn to handle situations in which he or she would usually consume the drug, the alcohol-dependent patient is less likely to remain abstinent. A thorough biopsychosocial assessment will generate a problem list, from which it is straightforward to negotiate a treatment plan to address problem areas identified in the assessment (Tables 5 and 6).

Physician Advice on Abuse Versus Dependence

Management of alcohol abuse, as opposed to dependence, is simply a matter of education and motivation

TABLE 6. **Diagnostic Problem List in Alcoholism**

Addictive or compulsive behaviors: drugs, sex, spending, gambling, eating behaviors, work, exercise
Current level of motivation (stage of change)
Medical co-morbidity
Psychiatric co-morbidity: mood disorders, thought disorders, personality disorders, post-traumatic stress
Absent coping skills: refusal/relapse prevention, identification/management of emotions, handling stress, conflict resolution, boundaries, parenting, money/time management, finding employment
Current stressors/unresolved issues
Global assessment of current function: ability to return to work

so that the alcohol abuser moderates his or her drinking. Although there are documented cases of alcohol-dependent people learning techniques to re-establish control of alcohol consumption, as physicians our recommendations to alcohol-dependent patients should include abstinence, because the risks of drinking far outweigh the potential benefits for the alcoholic. If, however, despite the physician's recommendation for abstinence-based treatment, the alcohol-dependent patient chooses to attempt controlled drinking, there is still a valuable therapeutic opportunity. The doctor may offer to monitor a negotiated behavioral contract; and, whether the patient succeeds or fails in the attempt at regaining control over his or her drinking, he or she is advised and directed to appropriate therapy and support or further treatment.

Alcoholism Counseling

Project MATCH, the largest, most statistically powerful psychotherapy trial ever conducted, resulted in evidence with vital importance to all primary care physicians. The study showed that the actual method of psychosocial treatment for alcohol dependence was not particularly important: all modalities of counseling resulted in dramatic reductions in drinking persisting beyond 15 months. In addition, brief, nonspecialist interventions resulted in results equal to more intensive cognitive-behavioral therapy delivered by highly trained specialist clinicians. The only therapist trait predictive of successful intervention was empathy. Regardless of the counseling method, clinicians demonstrating empathy in their client interactions obtained by far the best outcomes. The essential message for primary care physicians is that empathic, brief, office-based motivational enhancement therapy (moving the patient along the continuum from precontemplative to action) and 12-step facilitation (encouraging them to participate in mutual support group activities such as Alcoholics Anonymous while gently overcoming their resistance to do so) will result in significant rewards for their patients.

When to Refer to Residential Treatment

The American Society of Addiction Medicine patient placement criteria are useful in providing clear clinical criteria to aid in decisions relating to setting and intensity of treatment required for people with substance use disorders. Consider residential treatment for patients who require inpatient supervision for medical or psychiatric safety, lack a home environment conducive to abstinent recovery, work in highly safety-sensitive environments, or have failed at previous outpatient treatment attempts.

Requests for Consultation

Management of the patient with severe or late-stage addiction is complex. Consider getting help from a competent addictionist or (provided he or she has training and experience in addictions) a psychiatrist, psychologist, or pain specialist. Although primary care physicians play a vitally important role in detection, intervention, and supportive follow-up, our addicted patients also require the services of addiction counselors, peer support groups, and, sometimes, mental health professionals.

Relapse Prevention

Physicians have a vital role to play in providing relapse-prevention support, especially during the first 2 years of abstinence. With their permission the physician should provide patients with accountability to help them remain vigilant for the signs and symptoms of impending relapse. Questions for the supportive relapse-prevention visit might include date of last drink, use of other mood-altering activities/drugs ("changing deck chairs on the Titanic"), mutual support group involvement (Alcoholics Anonymous/Narcotics Anonymous meetings, home group, steps, sponsor), nutrition, exercise, sleep, sex, workplace attendance, performance and relationships, spiritual activities, emotional status (look for overconfidence or recurrence of negativity), craving, and, arguably one of the most problematic areas in early recovery, spousal and family relationships.

DRUG ABUSE

method of
NORMAN S. MILLER, M.D.
Michigan State University
East Lansing, Michigan

Drug abuse and dependence continue to be major threats to public health in the United States and throughout the world. The lifetime prevalence of drug abuse and dependence is 7% in the United States, that of alcohol dependence is 15%, and for co-morbid drug and alcohol dependence it is 20%. The concurrent and collaborative use of drugs with alcohol, upwards to 80% in those alcoholics younger than 30, constitutes an epidemic of alarming proportions. For instance, 80% of alcoholics are addicted to nicotine and 80% of cocaine addicts are addicted to alcohol. Each year alcoholism causes 100,000 excess deaths; illicit drug use, 20,000 excess deaths; and nicotine, 400,000 excess deaths. Drug use causes major deleterious psychological and social problems, including family dysfunction, domestic and criminal violence, and child abuse.

Drug and alcohol abuse cost nearly $300 billion annually in the United States or 25% of the national health care budget, and $34 billion is attributed to direct health care costs for hospitals, treatment programs, residential care, and professional services. Drug and alcohol use/addictions are implicated in 25% to 50% of all general hospital admissions and 50% to 75% of psychiatric admissions and contribute substantially to medical complications and costs to those admitted to hospitals for other reasons. According to government surveys, nearly a million individuals are active in specialized treatment for drug and alcohol problems, 29% for drug addiction, 45% for alcoholism, and 26% for both alcoholism and drug addiction.

Physicians are in a unique position to assess and treat individuals who seek evaluation and treatment for medically related health problems associated with drug and alcohol use and addiction. Well-known medical complications from drug disorders are too numerous to cite but prominently include widespread medical and surgical diseases. Physicians can fulfill important roles in the management and treatment of drug disorders in their patients, from identification, diagnosis, treatment, referral, and monitoring. Management of intoxication and withdrawal syndromes is a key service that physicians can provide to reduce morbidity and mortality from drug disorders in their patients. Each drug has a characteristic and predictable intoxication and withdrawal state, based on pharmacokinetic, and pharmacodynamic principles, that require medical evaluation and intervention.

Tolerance is the decreasing effect from, or the need to increase the dose to maintain, an effect. Tolerance develops to most drugs (e.g., 20-fold increase in dose, 2- to 4-fold increase in dose for alcohol) and can be expected as a neuroadaptation to drug and alcohol in repetition and higher doses. Dependence is the stereotypical response to the withdrawal of the drug during elimination after intoxication. Each class of drug possesses its own set of signs and symptoms of withdrawal. Changes in vital signs are not a regular finding in most drug withdrawal except for alcohol. However, behavioral manifestations are usually more informative of drug withdrawal (and intoxication) than physical findings.

Peak periods of duration of withdrawal vary with drug types and half-lives of drugs. In general, the shorter half-life leads to shorter withdrawal and the longer and higher the dose used, the more severe the withdrawal. For instance, opiate and alcohol withdrawal peaks in 3 days, lasts 5 to 7 days, and can be identified by characteristic signs and symptoms. Of importance is that craving or drive to use drugs is prominent in most drug withdrawals, either conscious or unconscious in the individual undergoing withdrawal. Subjective reports of craving are less reliable than objective manifestations such as drug seeking.

Unfortunately, in a study of primary care physicians, 94% of physicians failed to list a drug disorder as one of five possible diagnoses when presented with a case describing a patient with early symptoms of an alcohol disorder. Forty-one percent of pediatricians failed to list drug disorders as one of five possible diagnoses when presented with a case describing classic symptoms of drug disorder in a teenager. Twenty percent of physicians considered themselves "very prepared" to diagnose a substance disorder. This is substantially lower than the 83% who feel "very prepared" to diagnose hypertension, with 82% for diabetes and 44% for depression. Forty-three percent of patients with a drug disorder reported that their physicians never diagnosed the disorder; an additional 10.7% reported their physicians knew about their disorder but did nothing about it. Critically important, almost three fourths of patients reported their primary care physician was not involved in their decision to seek treatment.

Despite these disappointing findings, physicians can use knowledge and develop skills in medical treatment of drug disorders. The physicians can be sanguine about what they can do for their patients if they know that with proper diagnosis, treatment of withdrawal states, and referral for addiction treatment, between 50% and 90% of their patients can achieve abstinence for 1 year or longer.

Management of intoxication and withdrawal by the physician can produce lifesaving measures and compliance with the progression from identification to recovery. The physician can prescribe medications to reduce morbidity and mortality during intoxication and withdrawal and to increase compliance with psychosocial treatments. In addition, the physician can prescribe medications to patients in the subacute and chronic state to reduce relapse to addicting drugs and maintain individuals in the substituted drug or abstinent state.

TREATMENT APPROACHES AND EFFECTIVENESS

The abstinence-based method is commonly used to treat alcohol/drug addiction (95% of programs surveyed). This method utilizes cognitive behavior techniques and referral to 12-step recovery programs, such as Alcoholics Anonymous (AA) and Narcotics Anonymous.

One-year abstinence rates of 80% to 90% were achieved when patients participated in weekly continuing care and/or AA meetings after discharge from the treatment program. Also, 1-year abstinence rates were associated with reduced rates of medical and psychiatric utilization.

According to results of a 1992 survey conducted by AA, the following recovery rates were achieved: (1) of those members sober in AA less than 1 year, 41% will attend AA another year; (2) of those members sober more than 1 year and less than 5 years, 83% will attend AA another year; and (3) of those members sober 5 years or more, 91% will attend AA another year.

Physicians frequently encounter, in addition to alcohol, other drugs such as nicotine, cannabis, cocaine, opiates, sedative-hypnotics and anxiolytics, amphetamines and derivatives, hallucinogens including phencyclidine, inhalants, anticholinergics, and anabolic steroids. Careful assessment, including toxicology and breathalyzer testing and management of intoxication and withdrawal from these classes of drugs can be accomplished according to a rationale based on prescribing pharmacotherapies. Each class of drug has predictable signs and symptoms for intoxication and withdrawal and responds to medications designed to counteract and suppress withdrawal states. The physician can prescribe in a medically safe and effective manner to promote freedom from these adverse drug effects and improvement in overall health. Drug testing for alcohol and drugs should be conducted simultaneously when ordering a chest radiograph or complete blood cell count in diagnosing and treating other medical conditions.

Nicotine

Nicotine is the psychoactive substance and is self-administered in addictive patterns in cigarettes, chewing tobacco, snuff, pipes, and cigars. Individuals self-administer nicotine according to blood levels of nicotine. Nicotine intoxication produces stimulation and depression. Behavioral effects include nausea, euphoria, agitation, and sedation; and physiologic effects include increased heart rate, blood pressure, and motor activity. Significant pharmacologic tolerance and dependence develop to these effects over months and within a given day. Acute withdrawal begins within hours, extends over 3 to 5 days, and can last 1 to 2, or more, weeks. Nicotine withdrawal produces depressed mood, insomnia, irritability, anxiety, difficult concentration, restlessness, decreased heart rate, and increased appetite.

Eighty percent of smokers express a desire to quit, 35% attempt to quit each year, and less than 5% can stop without interventions. Interventions for smoking cessation include pharmacologic and behavioral methods to reduce relapse and promote abstinence from nicotine consumption. Nicotine replacement—nicotine gum, transdermal nicotine, nicotine nasal spray, nicotine inhaler, and antidepressant therapies—are the main pharmacologic therapies. Nicotine polacrilex (Nicorette) gum is nicotine bound to ion-exchange resin. It is available over the counter in 2- and 4-mg doses, several of which are taken per day. The drug is absorbed from buccal mucosa with peak nicotine levels at 30 minutes. Therapy is for 1 to 3 months. Cessation rates of 20% to 40% for 1 year can be achieved if the gum is used in conjunction with behavioral therapies. However, liability for addictive use of nicotine remains a problem in achieving abstinence from cigarettes.

The transdermal patch (Nicoderm) has a lower potential for addictive use because of the controlled sustained release from the skin on the upper body in doses of 7, 14, and 21 mg. The patch is applied each morning and removed in the evening. Peak concentration of nicotine is achieved in 2 to 6 hours, and the steady state is reached in 2 to 3 days after continued patch use. Eight weeks of treatment are suggested, and cessation rates are doubled at 6 months' follow-up.

Nicotine nasal spray delivers nicotine through nasal mucosa, approximating an absorption profile of cigarette smoking. Nicotine reaches peak levels at 5 minutes, and one to two doses are self-administered per hour. Abstinence rates at 1 year from cigarettes were twice those of a placebo. However, the potential for addiction is high because nicotine is delivered at steady and pulsating intervals to the brain.

Nicotine *inhalers* are used similarly to sprays, with peak absorption at 15 minutes from 80 inhalations per 20 minutes, leading to cigarette cessation twice that of placebo at 3 months. However, there is also a high addiction potential.

The antidepressant bupropion (Zyban), in sustained release is given in 150-mg or 300-mg doses over 1 to 2 months. Cigarette smoking ceases at 1 week from starting bupropion, and abstinence rates of twice that of a placebo are achieved at 1 year. The risk for seizure is 1 in 1000 smokers, but the drug is relatively contraindicated in alcohol withdrawal. Bupropion does work by its antidepressant effect because no change in mood was found in studies. Other antidepressants such as nortriptyline (Pamelor)* were found to be efficacious. Antihypertensive clonidine (Catapres)* may be useful in oral or transdermal preparations in 0.1- or 0.2-mg patches or doses every 6 hours for 3 to 5 days. Hypotension and sedation are limiting side effects from clonidine.

*Not FDA approved for this indication.

Sedative Hypnotics and Anxiolytics

Intoxication from this class of drugs (e.g., benzodiazepines, barbiturates, ethchylorvynol [Placidyl], meprobamate) includes slowed mental and physical activities, hypotension, bradycardia, and reduced respiratory rate. Prolonged and severe respiratory depression can lead to acidosis, arrhythmias, arrest, and death. Flumazenil, a benzodiazepine antagonist, can be given intravenously to counter respiratory depression. Withdrawal includes increased psychomotor activity, anxiety, depression, disorientation, agitation, muscular weakness, tremulousness, hyperpyrexia, diaphoresis, seizures, delirium with visual and auditory hallucinations, hypertension, and tachycardia.

Because benzodiazepines have cross-tolerance and dependence with other drugs in this class and a lower potential for respiratory depression, they can be substituted to reduce signs and symptoms of withdrawal. Dose equivalents can be calculated for tapering schedule. A long-acting preparation is generally preferred to produce a smooth suppression of withdrawal, but short-acting preparations should be considered when elimination times are delayed (e.g., significant liver disease). The longer and higher the use, the greater the duration and dose of taper. Generally, 50% of the dose is used to begin the taper over 7 to 10 days for short-acting drugs and 10 to 14 days for long-acting drugs, given three or four times a day. However, for duration of use over a few years, up to 1 to 2 months may be required for the taper. Anticonvulsants such as carbamazepine or valproic acid are effective in conjunction with benzodiazepine taper (conservative approach) or alone in lieu of benzodiazepines. Anticonvulsants are given until therapeutic blood levels are reached, and the dose is maintained for 2 to 4 weeks, followed by a taper.

Opiates

Intoxication from all opiates (heroin, narcotic analgesics, methadone) are similar in producing suppression of the central nervous system. Psychological responses include initial euphoria followed by apathy, dysphoria, depressed mood and affect, psychomotor agitation or retardation, impaired judgment, impaired social or occupational functioning, drowsiness, slurred speech, and impairment in attention and concentration. Physiologic responses include pupillary constriction, hypotension, constipation, respiratory depression, and cardiovascular collapse in large enough doses.

Symptoms of withdrawal from opiates include dysphoria, nausea, vomiting, muscle aches, lacrimination or rhinorrhea, pupillary dilation, sweating, diar-

*Not FDA approved for this indication.

rhea, yawning, fever, insomnia, and an intense drive to use more drugs, particularly opiates. The peak period of withdrawal depends on the half-life of the opiates. For example, for heroin it is 3 days, for opiate analgesics it can vary from 3 to 7 days, and for methadone it is 7 to 14 days. The duration of withdrawal can last up to 7 days for heroin, 7 to 14 days for opiate analgesics, and 14 to 28 days and longer for methadone depending on the duration of use of the opiate and dose; the longer the use and the higher the dose, the more severe and protracted the withdrawal. Withdrawal from opiates is not generally life threatening except when accompanied by co-morbid medical and psychiatric disorders. However, adequate treatment of opiate withdrawal improves compliance with treatments for medical and surgical disorders and for addiction to reduce relapse to opiates.

Pharmacologic therapies for opiate withdrawal are aimed at reducing the drive or "craving" for drugs, high levels of agitation, and somatic and psychological distress accompanying withdrawal. Nonopiate and opiate medications can be used to ameliorate these symptoms, the former more effective in intranasal and lower dosages and the latter more effective in intravenous and higher dosages. However, clonidine can often reduce the symptoms of opiate withdrawal in either instance, particularly when given in an inpatient setting, by 50% to 75%, and more if given in adequate dosages.

Typically, a clonidine* patch (either #1 or #2 patch) is applied on day 1, with 0.1 to 0.2 mg orally four times a day, depending on body weight, for 2 to 3 days, until blood levels from the patch reach equilibrium. In addition, clonidine, 0.1 to 0.2 mg, can be given throughout the withdrawal state up to 1 to 2 weeks, and the clonidine patch may be continued for 2 weeks or longer for protracted withdrawal. Frequent monitoring of blood pressure, pulse, and mental state is indicated because rate-limiting factors include hypotension and sedation from the clonidine. Parameters for withholding clonidine vary with patients, but lower limits are systolic blood pressures of 90 to 100 mm Hg, or pulse of 60 beats per minute. If below these parameters, patch and regular clonidine dosing should be discontinued.

Frequently, because of high levels of agitation and craving for drugs, diazepam (Valium), 5 to 10 mg, orally four times a day is given for 2 to 3 days, and in addition 5 to 10 mg orally four times a day or prn is given to supplement, depending on signs and symptoms. As with clonidine, careful monitoring of vital signs and mental state is indicated to avoid hypotension and oversedation, while balancing against the need to suppress withdrawal to enhance compliance with treatments.

Methadone for short-term detoxification from opiates is initiated with a test dose of 10 mg, and, if tolerated (no excessive sedation or lowering of vital signs), an additional 10 to 20 mg is given for signs and symptoms of withdrawal in a 24-hour period. Typically, 20 to 30 mg/d for 2 to 3 days is sufficient to suppress most withdrawal symptoms from opiates but an additional 5 to 10 mg may be given in unusually severe withdrawal. Because the acute withdrawal period is over in 5 to 7 days, methadone is tapered 5 to 10 mg over 3 to 5 days for approximately 1 week. Clonidine can be initiated during the methadone taper, as outlined earlier in part or wholly to suppress the withdrawal symptoms from methadone during its taper.

Certain patients may be referred to a methadone maintenance program for chronic substitution therapy with methadone or LAAM (*l*-acetyl-α-methadol acetate). Candidates for opiate maintenance therapy should be screened from the population of opiate users. Generally, detoxification and drug-free addiction treatment should be attempted before commitment to long-term opiate substitution therapy. Methadone and LAAM are opiates and addicting themselves, and studies show favorable results shorter term and when combined with psychosocial therapies. Effective doses can range from 20 mg/d to over 100 mg/d, and tolerance develops to methadone, requiring increasing doses and use of other narcotics, including heroin and prescription opiates. A particular limitation of methadone in the longer term is that relapse rates are substantial to heroin and to use of addicting drugs, including benzodiazepines, alcohol, cocaine, and prescription narcotics.

Currently, methadone and LAAM are prescribed in a program setting approved and monitored by the Food and Drug Administration (FDA). However, regulation changes are likely where the Center for Substance Abuse Treatment not only will accredit and monitor methadone and LAAM programs but also allow prescribing in selected office-based physicians. These changes, if they occur, will be implemented over the next few years.

Buprenorphine (Buprenex)* is a newer synthetic agonist/antagonist opiate, which means it has both morphine-like activity (40 times more potent than morphine) and naltrexone-like activity (blocks morphine). Major advantages expected are a ceiling effect on overdose because of antagonist properties but still retaining an agonist effect, which addicts seek in their addictive use of drugs. Buprenorphine is likely to be effective in treatment of opiate withdrawal because of its mixed properties, but its effectiveness in substitution therapies similar to methadone is less clear. Opiate addicts are likely to prefer methadone with its stronger agonist effects than buprenorphine with its antagonist effects. FDA approval is pending.

Pain and Addiction

A substantial movement to increase treatment of acute and chronic pain is underway in the United States. No doubt the concern for unnecessary and debilitating pain is warranted. However, pain is a

*Not FDA approved for this indication.

*Investigational drug in the United States.

normal signal to warn the body, and its protective effects should be considered in treating acute and chronic pain. In addition, those prescribing pain medications should understand not only the benefits but also the untoward effects of prescribing narcotic medications that are addicting.

Addiction to narcotic medications carries with it significant medical morbidity and mortality and is in itself a painful state. Features include depression, decreased mental acuity, decreased energy, preoccupation with acquiring narcotics to exclusion of normal activities, conflict in interpersonal relationships, illicit activities and legal consequences to obtain narcotics, aggravation of underlying sources of pain without guidance from pain, and lethal overdose, either accidental or from suicidal thinking.

Cocaine

Cocaine is a dramatic central nervous system stimulant that produces intense euphoria initially in users, which diminishes with development of tolerance in chronic use, accompanied by increasing levels of anxiety and depression. Common physical effects from cocaine intoxication include elevated blood pressure and pulse, palpitations and cardiac arrhythmias (can be life-threatening), vasoconstriction and ischemia with consequent angina and cerebrovascular stroke, mydriasis, hyperthermia, seizures, tremulousness, hyperactive reflexes, dry mouth, decreased appetite and weight loss, respiratory arrest, and coma. Common psychological effects include euphoria, anxiety, depression, grandiose thinking, delusions, auditory and visual hallucinations, irritability, stereotypical and compulsive behaviors (sometimes self-inflicted or mutilating), and suicidal and homicidal thinking.

Treatment of acute intoxication is aimed at a high level of agitation, hypertension, tachycardia, delusions, and hallucinations: propranolol (Inderal)* in doses to reduce hypertension (20–40 mg orally one to three times daily or as needed and tolerated), haloperidol (Haldol),* 5 to 10 mg orally, as needed, and diazepam, 5 to 10 mg orally. Because cocaine has a short half-life (1–2 hours), treatment of intoxication is brief, except in cases of extreme overdoses. Other supportive measures may be indicated, such as monitoring cardiac and respiratory status.

Cocaine withdrawal characteristically peaks in 2 to 3 days acutely and lasts 5 to 7 days. The major symptoms are anxiety, depression, fatigue and hypersomnia, increased appetite, and generalized malaise. The depth of the depression can be severe, and evaluation for suicidal risk is often necessary, typically lasting only during the acute period of withdrawal. The treatment is supportive, because there is no specific medication that suppresses symptoms of cocaine withdrawal.

Because the hallmark of cocaine withdrawal is irritability, sedatives such as diazepam are effective in reducing discomfort and improving compliance. Diazepam (Valium),* 5 to 10 mg four times a day for 2 to 3 days, will often be sufficient to suppress withdrawal, including craving or a desire to use more cocaine. No particular medication is effective in preventing relapse to cocaine, because studies do not support the use of antidepressants in preventing relapse to cocaine.

*Not FDA approved for this indication.

Amphetamines and Derivatives

Amphetamine and its derivatives share characteristics of intoxication and withdrawal similar to those of other stimulants, particularly cocaine. Their half-lives are short acting, and the course of withdrawal is similar to that of cocaine. Amphetamine drugs include dextroamphetamine, methylphenidate, and other central nervous system stimulants. Amphetamines are highly addicting and produce the greatest propensity for developing addiction when ranked with other addicting drugs. Studies show mortality rates near 90% when animals are allowed to self-administer amphetamines in research paradigms.

Dextroamphetamines and methylphenidate (Ritalin), and similar stimulants, are used to treat attention-deficit disorders and other behavior problems. Careful assessment of pattern of use is indicated to determine if therapeutic effects are still present and to what extent addictive use of these medications has developed. Evaluation of other drug use is indicated as a marker for problematic use of these stimulants. Disturbances of mood, affect, and cognition are common and should be assessed in anyone using these medications chronically.

MDMA (3,4-methylenedioxymethamphetamine), known best as Ecstasy, is a potent amphetamine derivative, highly popular among teenage populations. Ecstasy is used in many settings, but it is particularly prevalent in rave parties, where participants will use Ecstasy and other drugs continuously for 24 hours or more. Significant medical and psychiatric complications ensue, particularly physical and mental exhaustion, disrupted concentration and memory, impaired insight and judgment, depersonalization and derealization, mystical experiences, suspiciousness, and frank paranoid delusions. Perceptual disturbances include loss of boundaries, heightened sensory acuity, overvalued attribution of meaning to ordinary objects, belief that usual thoughts are novel and profound, rage reactions, panic dissociative states, depression, and suicidal thinking and behaviors.

Acute use of MDMA also produces jitteriness, anxiety, depression, jaw clenching, insomnia, sleep disturbances, seizures, hypertension, hyperthermia, dehydration, renal failure, disseminated intravascular coagulation, and rhabdomyolysis. Long-term consequences may include persistent neurotoxicity, at least in animal studies. Careful assessment of people is not yet available.

*Not FDA approved for this indication.

Treatments are directed at the medical and psychiatric complications and can include rehydration, supplementing electrolyte imbalances, sedation with diazepam* and haloperidol,* and a protective and supportive environment during the acute withdrawal period when depression and suicidal thinking may be prominent. Assessment for other drug use, including alcohol, and treatment of withdrawal is mandatory in young populations in whom multiple drug use is the rule.

Cannabis

Cannabis is a poorly understood drug whose pharmacologic properties are generally underestimated and rationalized. Marijuana and hashish are obtained from the plant *Cannabis sativa.* The principal psychoactive constituent is tetrahydrocannabinol (THC), which is a hallucinogenic substance responsible for the psychological and physical effects in humans. In acute doses, cannabis produces a general feeling of well-being; relaxation; emotional disinhibition; drowsiness; distortions of perception of time, body image and distance; increased auditory and visual acuity; and enhanced senses of touch, smell, and taste, as well as body awareness and perceptions. Attention span and ability to process information can be impaired, as well as ability to perform complex motor tasks. Chronic users may display depressed mood and high anxiety levels, including fearfulness and paranoia, misperceptions, and violent and retaliatory behavior. Memory loss and poor judgment frequently accompany regular and chronic cannabis use, and individuals are aware of these deficits at times.

Studies have shown negative effects of cannabis intoxication on driving performance of automobiles, by interfering with motor coordination, tracking, perception, and vigilance, and that actual performance on the road is impaired. The interaction of alcohol and cannabis intensifies the adverse effects on each drug on driving performance.

Studies also confirm personality changes with prolonged use, characterized by diminished drive, lessened ambition, decreased motivation, apathy, shortened attention span, distractibility, poor judgment, impaired communication skills, loss of effectiveness, introversion, magical thinking, derealization and depersonalization, diminished capacity to carry out complex plans or prepare realistically for the future, a peculiar fragmentation in the flow of thought, habit deterioration, and progressive loss of insight.

Physical effects of acute use include increased heart rate, decreased peripheral resistance and increased peripheral blood flow, hypotension, lightheadedness and orthostatic changes, and injected conjunctiva. Other physical effects include increased appetite, dryness of mouth and throat, reduced sex drive, and headaches. Chronic users develop bronchitis, asthma, sore throat and chronic irritation of and damage to sensitive mucous membranes in the respiratory tract, impaired gas exchange, increased signs of airway obstruction, and chronic inflammation changes in the lungs.

Withdrawal from cannabis is subtle and definite and includes malaise, craving for cannabis, mild tachycardia and hypertension, anxiety, and depression. Because cannabis is taken up and stored in muscle and fat, the release can be slow over time and withdrawal symptoms can be protracted over weeks and months. Importantly, patients should be advised that their urine toxicology can be positive in low levels for weeks and months. High levels of THC in the urine are suggestive of recent use; thus, quantification of the amount of THC is important to determine recent use and relapse.

Treatment of cannabis intoxication and withdrawal is supportive and directed at the specific signs and symptoms. Generally, diazepam* in usual doses, 5 to 10 mg orally four times a day and as needed for agitation, over a few days is sufficient, and use of haloperidol,* 5 to 10 mg four times a day and as needed for psychotic and perceptual abnormalities, may be indicated. Often, cannabis users have become addicted to cannabis and other drugs and require evaluation for additional drug use, including alcohol, by clinical interview and urine toxicology. Cannabis addicts often respond to addiction treatment, which is necessary for preventing relapse to cannabis and other drugs.

Hallucinogens and Phencyclidine

The classification *hallucinogens* is a loosely grouped category of drugs related by their ability to produce changes in perceptions, sometimes causing frank hallucinations. The intoxicated state is characterized by alterations in perceptions that affect basically all modalities of sensation, often visual and auditory but less commonly touch and taste. Subtle and marked distortions in time and motion combine to create a sometimes surreal experience for the user, which is an attraction particularly for young users. Clear visual hallucinations of colors and patterns, and even of individuals and objects, accompany intoxication. Also, auditory hallucinations consist of voices and sound clearly audible during drug intoxication.

In sufficient doses, cognitive or memory impairments, disorientation, and confusion often occur. The hallucinogenic experience correlates with changes seen during rapid eye movement sleep and can account for the dreamlike quality of intoxication.

Phencyclidine (PCP) is a prototype drug whose pharmacologic properties are representative of the hallucinogen class of drugs. PCP and the related dissociative anesthetic ketamine are particularly dangerous drugs. Their typical intoxication includes severe impairment in insight and judgment, visual and auditory hallucinations, and paranoid delusions.

*Not FDA approved for this indication.

*Not FDA approved for this indication.

Users appear hyperactive and can be violent as a result of the combined effects of PCP.

Because PCP is an anesthetic, users may be insensitive to pain, which enables them to perform feats of great strength, to break out of restraints, and to overpower others, injuring themselves and making them particularly dangerous. On physical examination, intoxicated individuals show hypertension, tachycardia, eyelid retraction (wide-eyed stare), dry flushed skin, mydriasis, nystagmus, and hyperreflexia.

Many drugs can be classified in this group and include psychedelics, lysergic acid diethylamide (LSD), mescaline, psilocybin, and dimethyltryptamine. Important commonly used hallucinogens include PCP, ketamine, and similar-acting arylcyclohexylamines and anticholinergics, such as scopolamine.

Treatment is directed at the particular constellations of symptoms. Generally, diazepam* is given in usual doses (and higher as needed to sedate agitated users) of between 20 and 60 mg in a 24-hour period either orally or parenterally, depending on the clinical requirements. Haloperidol* may be given for psychotic symptoms in doses ranging from 5 to 20 mg in a 24-hour period, orally or intramuscularly. Addition of an anticholinergic medication to offset extrapyramidal effects such as dystonia, tremors, or rigidity is often indicated. Intoxicated individuals may require physical restraints for their protection, particularly if they are out of control and at risk of harm to themselves or others.

Inhalants

Surveys show that inhalants are the fourth most commonly used drug by adolescents and young adults. Inhalants are commercially available drugs contained in commonly found products, such as gasoline, adhesives, aerosols, cleaning fluids, paint thinners, and lighter fluid. The chemicals are organic hydrocarbon compounds, which are volatile liquids that, when released into air, form gases. Young people are particularly attracted to the exhilarating and hallucinogenic properties that they experience on inhaling the gases. Of critical importance is that these products can be bought over the counter in stores without limitations as glues, butane lighters, gasoline, and food aerosols, for example.

In general, inhalants produce a mixed picture of stimulation and depression and of perceptual and mood distortions. In sufficient doses, respiratory depression, sleep, and anesthesia occurs. Effects are felt rapidly, rendering the individual drowsy and sometimes confused. Memory and cognitive disturbances are common, and at times visual hallucinations and bizarre delusions occur. Long term use is associated with prolonged neurologic impairments, such as cognitive disorders, dysarthria, gait ataxia, nystagmus, loss of hearing and smell, tremors, and cerebral and cerebellar atrophy. Persistent changes occur in personality, such as conduct disorders, antisocial personality, and depressive symptoms.

*Not FDA approved for this indication.

Physical effects, including toxicity, produce increased heart rates, irregular heart beats, fatal arrhythmias, coughing, inflammation of upper respiratory passages, nosebleeds from chronic irritation in sniffing, respiratory depression, nausea, vomiting, diarrhea, liver failure, and renal failure. Organ damage and death occur, and unexplained death in a youth should trigger consideration of inhalant use.

Treatment is directed at identifying the offending organic solvent, conducting a medical and psychiatric assessment, and prescribing medications aimed at symptoms. Diazepam,* haloperidol,* and other selected sedative/hypnotics and antipsychotics can be used according to the clinical indications. Evaluation of other drug use, including alcohol, is essential in populations of young drug users. Referral for acute monitoring of cardiac status and treatment, as well as neurologic and psychiatric evaluations, may be necessary, depending on clinical indications.

Anabolic Steroids

Anabolic steroids are defined as androgenic anabolic steroids, which include testosterone, the male sex hormone, and its derivatives. Body builders and athletes who compete in sports that require strength and power are attracted to the anabolic effects of these steroids. The source of these drugs tend to be from the illicit markets, although physicians remain a source, as they are for other drugs. These compounds can be produced in private and illegally operated laboratories.

The effects of the steroids are to develop male characteristics, such as deepening of male voice, increase in size of penis, body hair, large muscular development, increased vigor, and a feeling of well-being. The psychological effects include euphoria, anxiety, irritability, aggression, reduced or increased fatigue, insomnia, depression and elation, delirium, psychosis, and suicidal or homicidal effects. The physical effects include cardiomegaly, heart failure, myocardial infarction, increased blood pressure, thromboembolic events in extremities, nausea, vomiting, and gastric irritation. Because of suppression of follicle-stimulating hormone and luteinizing hormone, women may have irregular menstrual periods and men may experience decreased sperm production, testicular size, and potency. Women can experience masculinization from testosterone, and men can show feminization from metabolism of testosterone into estrogen. Musculoskeletal problems occur, including tendon rupture and premature closure of long bones, and liver toxicity may include enlargement, hepatitis, and cancer.

Steroids can be used addictively and produce similar psychiatric complications as other drugs. Severe paranoia and suicidality, as well as physical changes, are relatively common in chronic, regular users.

*Not FDA approved for this indication.

Treatment is directed at eliminating its use. Symptomatic treatment includes sedation and, for specific psychosis, medical and psychiatric evaluations and long-term rehabilitation of addiction and psychiatric and medical complications.

Anticholinergics and Antihistamines

These medications are commonly prescribed in many branches of medicine and psychiatry for many indications. What they have in common for abuse and addiction and medical and psychiatric complications are the anticholinergic and antihistaminic effects in a variety of medications. Antidepressants, antipsychotics, antihistamines, and antiextrapyramidal medications contain these properties. These medications can be used addictively and produce significant levels of toxicity, including euphoria, compulsive use, sedation, drowsiness, confusion, paranoia, visual hallucinations, delusions, delirium, coma, tachycardia, arrhythmias, hypotension, constipation, fatigue, mydriasis, blurred vision, dry mouth, and sleep disturbances.

Emergencies that can result from these drugs include life-threatening medical and psychiatric conditions. Rapid diagnosis and treatment, including intensive monitoring, may be required. Pharmacologic treatments are aimed at reducing agitation and psychotic, cardiovascular, gastrointestional, and neurologic complications. Evaluation of other drug use and psychiatric and medical conditions is often indicated.

ANXIETY DISORDERS IN PRIMARY CARE

method of
LAWRENCE R. WU, M.D.
Duke University School of Medicine and Durham Regional Hospital
Durham, North Carolina

Feeling anxious or requests for a "nerve pill" are among the most common chief complaints encountered in a primary care practice. The National Comorbidity Study estimates that 25% of the general population experiences pathologic anxiety at some time during their lifetime. Anxiety disorders are associated with increased medical utilization and expenditures. More often than not patients with anxiety disorders are likely to present with somatic symptoms in the primary care setting. The spectrum of anxiety disorders includes panic disorder and agoraphobia, generalized anxiety disorder (GAD), obsessive-compulsive disorder (OCD), phobic disorder (including social phobia), and post-traumatic stress disorder (PTSD). With the discovery of new psychotropic medications, specific diagnosis within this spectrum is essential because each of these disorders responds to specific pharmacotherapy and psychotherapy.

In many situations anxiety can be adaptive. Some stress is necessary to improve performance in our daily lives, resulting often in personal growth and development. When anxiety interferes with the functions of daily living, causes distress, or is difficult to control, it is pathologic and requires treatment.

The approach to anxiety should recognize that anxiety and depression are often co-morbid conditions. Selective serotonin reuptake inhibitors (SSRIs), which were designed to treat depression, are also effective for many anxiety disorders. In spite of the availability of these medications, psychotherapy is the preferred initial treatment for post-traumatic stress disorder and phobia disorders.

ASSESSMENT AND DIAGNOSIS

Symptoms of anxiety should prompt a mental status examination and brief physical examination to assess for organic causes. Expressing interest and a willingness to listen to the patient are essential for diagnosis and are often therapeutic for the patient. The duration and frequency of symptoms, quality of the distress, precipitating events or cues (if any), associated symptoms, and relieving factors should be elicited from the patient. Associated symptoms can be somatic as well as psychiatric. Asking the patient about any situations that he or she tends to avoid, the effect of the worry on behaviors, and the quality of sleep can clarify the specific type of anxiety present. Intensive feelings of fear or doom suggest a panic disorder, whereas reminders and intrusive thoughts about a terrible event in the past point to PTSD. Avoidance of people or anxiety performing in front of people is the hallmark of social phobia disorder, whereas recurrent thoughts or behaviors that are strange to the patient or others suggest OCD.

As with all psychiatric complaints, patients should be assessed for thoughts of harming self/others and ability to perform the activities of daily living in their current situation. Questioning the patient about signs and symptoms of depression is recommended because depression is often a co-existing or the primary psychiatric disorder.

Assessing for anxiety is also recommended when patients complain of multiple, unexplained somatic symptoms. Concurrent attention to the mental health evaluation is recommended in situations in which the provider is investigating for physical causes of anxiety.

Review of the patient's medicines, use of illicit drugs (and/or alcohol), and past medical history will often reveal physical causes of anxiety. Hyperthyroidism and pulmonary disorders, particularly hypercapnia, can cause symptoms of anxiety. Medications that can cause anxiety include albuterol, theophylline, and sympathetic nervous system agonists. Weight loss, tachycardia, or heat intolerance discovered from the history or physical examination should be a clue to hyperthyroidism.

The diagnoses of specific anxiety disorders are based on clinical criteria adapted from the fourth edition of the American Psychiatric Association's *Diagnostic and Statistical Manual of Mental Disorders* (DSM-IV)—*Primary Care Version* (see Tables 2 through 6). These criteria assume that the provider has made a clinical judgment that the patient's symptoms are not caused by a physical disease and not solely from another mental health disorder. Yet, the patient will often have two or more psychiatric disorders.

APPROACH TO TREATMENT

Successful treatment of anxiety in the primary care setting requires an interested health care provider who is comfortable with the multiple modalities to treat the anxious patient. Reassurance to the patient is necessary. The patient is told that anxiety is common and treatable and is reassured that asking for help is a positive first step. Cognitive restructuring and simple coping techniques can be taught by the interested primary care clinician and are covered in more detail later. Certain aspects of lifestyle have been shown to improve anxiety. Light aerobic exercise improves self-efficacy and can decrease anxiety.

The SSRIs have revolutionized the treatment of anxiety, replacing chronic use of benzodiazepines. SSRIs are effective for OCD, panic disorders, phobias, PTSD, and GAD and are listed in Table 1. Doses of SSRIs for anxiety disorders must be started at lower doses than these used for depression to minimize the short-term agitation sometimes experienced with these medications. The patient should be counseled that side effects often diminish with time and that empirical switching to another SSRI may be necessary. Venlafaxine (Effexor XR), a novel antidepressant, has been approved for the treatment of GAD, and there is now evidence that chronic use of SSRIs is just as effective for GAD as benzodiazepines.

Although tricyclic antidepressants have been used with success in anxiety disorders, drowsiness, anticholinergic side effects, and toxicity have made these medications less popular. Imipramine (Tofranil)* is effective for panic disorder and preferred if a sedating medication is required.

*Not FDA approved for this indication.

Benzodiazepines are the oldest class of medications used to treat anxiety and are listed in Table 1. Although they have the advantage of rapid onset of action, they carry the risk of dependence, sedation, falls in the elderly, and road traffic accidents. Withdrawal syndromes resulting in rebound anxiety, even reactions as severe as delirium tremens, are possible. The prescribing provider must inform the patient and family about these risks. Benzodiazepines should be avoided in patients with a past history of substance abuse, personality disorder, or dosage escalation. These medications are ideal for patients who experience infrequent bouts of anxiety or episodes of anxiety-related insomnia. Shorter-acting benzodiazepines such as lorazepam (Ativan) have been studied for use in specific anxiety disorders, whereas little research has been done using older benzodiazepines (with longer half-lives) in specific anxiety disorders.

Buspirone (Buspar) is a nonbenzodiazepine indicated for generalized anxiety disorder. In head to head trials, it works as well as benzodiazepines for GAD but has a slower onset of action and lacks sedative properties. It is therefore less useful for the anxious patient who needs a sedative. It does not impair alertness and lacks abuse potential.

β-Blockers* are effective and the preferred treat-

*Not FDA approved for this indication.

TABLE 1. **Common Medications Used in the Treatment of Anxiety**

Medication	Starting Dose (mg)	Therapeutic Range (mg/d)	Common Side Effects	Indications*
Selective Serotonin Reuptake Inhibitors				
Citalopram (Celexa)	10	10–60	Nausea, somnolence, dry mouth	PD/AG, OCD, PTSD, SP, GAD
Fluoxetine (Prozac)	5–10	10–80	Nausea, anorexia, insomnia, somnolence	OCD, PD/AG, PTSD, SP, GAD
Fluvoxamine (Luvox)	50	50–300	Nausea, insomnia, somnolence, headache	OCD, PD/AG, PTSD, SP, GAD
Paroxetine (Paxil)	10	10–50	Nausea, somnolence, ejaculation failure	OCD, PD/AG, SP, PTSD, GAD
Sertraline (Zoloft)	25	50–200	Nausea, insomnia, ejaculation failure	OCD, PD/AG, PTSD, SP, GAD
Novel Antidepressants				
Venlafaxine (Effexor XR)	37.5	37.5–225	Nausea, dry mouth, insomnia, dizziness	GAD, PD/AG
Tricyclic Antidepressants				
Clomipramine (Anafranil)	25	25–250	Weight gain, sedation, dry mouth	OCD, PD/AG, PTSD, GAD
Imipramine (Tofranil)	10–25	150–300	Sedation, dry mouth	PD/AG, GAD, PTSD
Other Medications				
Buspirone (Buspar)	5 mg bid	15–60	Dizziness, nausea	GAD
Propranolol (Inderal)	20 mg	20–160	Depression, sedation	Performance anxiety
Benzodiazepines				
Alprazolam (Xanax)	0.25 mg tid	0.25–4	Drowsiness, withdrawal	GAD, PD/AG, PTSD
Clonazepam (Klonopin)	0.25 mg bid	0.25–4	Somnolence, fatigue, depression	PD/AG, GAD, PTSD
Lorazepam (Ativan)	0.5 mg tid	1–6	Sedation, dizziness	GAD, PD/AG, SP

*Underscore indicates FDA approval.

Abbreviations: GAD = generalized anxiety disorder; OCD = obsessive-compulsive disorder; PD/AG = panic disorder/agoraphobia; PTSD = post-traumatic stress disorder; SP = social phobia.

ment for performance anxiety such as fear of public speaking. These medications are taken before the anxiety-provoking event. β-Blockers are rarely effective for other forms of anxiety.

Although monoamine oxidase inhibitors (MAOIs)* have been effective for anxiety, their interaction with common foods (and medicines such as meperidine [Demerol]) may cause malignant hypertension, which has limited their use to psychiatrists familiar with their use and only after other medications have failed.

Other therapies include kava kava (piper methysticum),* an extract of the oceanic kava plant, which is superior to placebo in treating GAD. The most frequent side effects include gastrointestinal complaints and skin reactions.

TREATMENT OF SPECIFIC ANXIETY DISORDERS

The criteria for GAD are listed in Table 2. Although some complain of worry, patients with GAD are most likely to present with somatic symptoms in the primary care setting. Many of these patients will readily admit to worry and stresses, when asked. Most primary care clinicians can provide simple supportive therapy consisting of listening empathetically to the patient's perception of stresses. Disabling episodes of anxiety may require a short course of benzodiazepines for stabilization. Persistent anxiety will require chronic treatment with buspirone (Buspar) or an SSRI, starting at a low dose. Venlafaxine (Effexor XR), a novel antidepressant, is effective and has been FDA approved for GAD. Dosing of venlafaxine starts at 37.5 mg/d and is titrated upward to 225 mg/d. Cognitive behavior therapy (as described later) is helpful and may require referral.

Panic disorder is differentiated from GAD by the panic attack that includes at least four somatic symptoms listed on Table 3. Although these symptoms will often warrant a search for a physical condition, the patient should be concurrently educated about the possibility of panic disorder and its treatment for

*Not FDA approved for this indication.

TABLE 2. **DSM-IV Features of Generalized Anxiety Disorder**

A. Excessive anxiety and worry, occurring >50% days over ≥6 months, causing distress or impairment in social, occupational, or other important areas of functioning
B. Person finds it difficult to control the worry
C. Anxiety and worry are associated with three or more of the following six symptoms:
    1. Restlessness
    2. Fatigue
    3. Difficulty concentrating or mind going blank
    4. Irritability
    5. Muscle tension
    6. Difficulty sleeping or restless unsatisfying sleep

Adapted. Reprinted with permission from the *Diagnostic and Statistical Manual of Mental Disorders, Fourth Edition, Text Revision.* Copyright 2000 American Psychiatric Association.

TABLE 3. **DSM-IV Features of Panic Disorder With Agoraphobia***

A. Recurrent unexpected panic attacks. *Panic attacks* are periods of intense fear or discomfort in which ≥4 of the following symptoms abruptly appear and peak within 10 minutes: palpitations, sweating, trembling, shortness of breath or smothering, feeling of choking, chest pain/discomfort, nausea/abdominal distress, feeling dizzy or faint, feelings of unreality, fear of losing control, fear of dying
B. At least one of the attacks is followed by ≥1 month of ≥1 of the following: worry about having additional attacks, worry about the consequences of the attack, change in behavior related to the attacks
C. *Agoraphobia* is anxiety about being in places or situations from which escape or help may be difficult to obtain, such as being out of the home alone or in crowds.

*Panic disorder without agoraphobia is panic disorder without agoraphobia (C).

Adapted. Reprinted with permission from the *Diagnostic and Statistical Manual of Mental Disorders, Fourth Edition, Text Revision.* Copyright 2000 American Psychiatric Association.

ability. Younger patients with unexplained, recurrent physical symptoms are more likely to have panic. Coexisting depression is common, as is agoraphobia, with panic disorders. Patients with panic disorder benefit from medication with adjunctive psychotherapy. Infrequent panic attacks can be treated with benzodiazepines such as alprazolam (Xanax) or clonazepam (Clonopin). Chronic or frequent attacks can be treated with SSRIs or tricyclic antidepressants. Because side effects of these classes of medications can be particularly troubling to these patients, especially stimulation from SSRIs, initial dosing should begin at significantly lower doses than doses used for depression. Imipramine (Tofranil)* and clomipramine (Anafranil)* are the best studied among tricyclic antidepressants and should be started at 10 mg/d with increases of 10-mg dosing every 3 to 4 days. Among SSRIs, paroxetine (Paxil) should be started at 10 mg/d, fluoxetine (Prozac)* at 10 mg/d, or sertraline (Zoloft) at 25 mg/d. Although MAOIs are effective for panic, severe interactions with foods and other medications limit their use, and they should be used only by psychiatrists. Supportive therapy by the provider can be effective in establishing trust between the provider and the patient. Cognitive behavioral approaches, exposure therapy (if there is a feared stimulus), and relaxation therapy can be helpful in relieving milder panic attacks.

The criteria for a simple phobia are listed in Table 4. An example of a common phobia is anxiety associated with flying. Initial therapy should consist of psychotherapeutic approaches because they provide longer-lasting benefits than medications. Cognitive behavioral therapy consists of reviewing maladaptive automatic thoughts, analyzing assumptions, role playing, and having successful encounters with phobic situations. Social skills training may be required for patients with social phobia. Patients with phobias should be referred for such therapy by experienced providers. SSRIs that have been shown to improve

*Not FDA approved for this indication.

TABLE 4. **DSM-IV Features of Specific Phobia**

A. Marked and persistent fear that is excessive or unreasonable, is recognized as such by the patient, and is cued by a specific precipitant (e.g., flying, heights, enclosed spaces)
B. Exposure to the precipitant invariably provokes an immediate anxiety response, such as a panic attack
C. The phobic situation is avoided and such avoidance interferes significantly with social or occupational or other important areas of functioning
D. Types of phobias may be classified into specific animal type, natural environment type, blood-injection-injury type, situational type, or other type. Social phobia is the fear of one or more social or performance situations in which the person is exposed to unfamiliar people or to scrutiny by others

Adapted. Reprinted with permission from the *Diagnostic and Statistical Manual of Mental Disorders, Fourth Edition, Text Revision.* Copyright 2000 American Psychiatric Association.

social anxiety among patients with social phobia include paroxetine and fluvoxamine (Luvox).*

Lifetime risk of PTSD is estimated to be 1% to 14%. High-risk populations include victims of sexual assault and war veterans. Criteria for PTSD are listed in Table 5. Psychotherapy should be the initial approach to PTSD. Supportive therapy consisting of empathic listening while providing a safe environment can be provided by the primary care physician, even in the context of a short visit. Persistent symptoms require referral to a more experienced therapist. SSRIs have been shown to decrease intrusive recollections and numbing. Medications should also be directed at co-morbid depression, panic, or phobias, if needed.

OCD begins most often in adolescence or early adulthood. The DSM-IV criteria for OCD are listed in Table 6. A combination of behavioral therapy and medication is necessary for this disorder, yielding greater benefit than either modality alone. Behavioral therapy from an experienced therapist is useful for compulsions. Although clomipramine was the first medication useful for OCD, paroxetine, sertraline, and other SSRIs have been shown to be just as useful to decrease compulsions and intrusive obsessions. In OCD, medications may need to be prescribed at higher doses, unlike other forms of anxiety. Often response is not apparent for 3 to 4 months.

Patients should be referred to more experienced mental health providers when the treatment modality exceeds the experience or interest of the primary care provider. Examples of such situations include the need for psychotherapy, a patient threatening harm to self or others, a patient unable to care for self, and failure to respond to pharmacotherapy as expected.

*Not FDA approved for this indication.

TABLE 5. **DSM-IV Features of Post-Traumatic Stress Disorder**

A. Person has experienced a *traumatic event* that involved actual or threatened death/serious injury to self or others with a response of fear, helplessness, or horror.
B. The traumatic event is *persistently re-experienced* in recurrent and intrusive recollections of the event, recurrent distressing dreams, perceptions of reliving such as dissociative flashback episodes, intensive psychological distress, or physiologic reactions when exposed to cues that may represent the event.
C. Persistent *avoidance* of the stimuli associated with the trauma and *numbing* of general responsiveness, as in efforts to avoid thoughts/conversations associated with the trauma, efforts to avoid activities/places/people that arouse recollections, inability to recall an important aspect of the event, markedly diminished interest in significant activities, feeling of detachment or estrangement from others, restricted range of expressed emotions, and/or sense of foreshortened future, such as not expecting to have career
D. Persistent symptoms of increased arousal such as difficulty falling asleep, irritability or outbursts of anger, difficulty concentrating, hypervigilance, exaggerated startle
E. Duration of disturbances in B, C, D is >1 month and interferes with social, occupational, or other important areas of functioning

Adapted. Reprinted with permission from the *Diagnostic and Statistical Manual of Mental Disorders, Fourth Edition, Text Revision.* Copyright 2000 American Psychiatric Association.

TABLE 6. **DSM-IV Features of Obsessive-Compulsive Disorder**

A. Patients may have either obsessions or compulsions. Obsessions are recurrent thoughts, impulses, or images that cause marked anxiety or distress that are experienced as intrusive. Compulsions are ritualistic behaviors or mental acts that are performed in response to an obsession or need to be rigidly carried out.
B. The obsessions or compulsions are excessive, occupy more than 1 h/d, are distressing, and interfere with a person's social, occupational, or other important areas of functioning.

Adapted. Reprinted with permission from the *Diagnostic and Statistical Manual of Mental Disorders, Fourth Edition, Text Revision.* Copyright 2000 American Psychiatric Association.

BULIMIA NERVOSA*

method of
DEAN D. KRAHN, M.D.
William S. Middleton Memorial Veterans Hospital
Madison, Wisconsin

Although bulimia nervosa (BN) and anorexia nervosa (AN) are classified as eating disorders in the fourth edition of the *Diagnostic and Statistical Manual of Mental Disorders* (DSM-IV), the core of these syndromes lies not in aberrant eating but in the pathologic pursuit of thinness. It is in the context of desperate attempts at caloric deprivation and weight loss that seemingly irrational binge-eating and purging behaviors are understandable to the patient, family, and clinician.

Despite the importance of the pursuit of thinness as a basis for understanding BN, the clinical features specific for BN are binge-eating and compensatory behaviors such as vomiting or laxative abuse. The DSM-IV criteria for BN are found in Table 1. Patients diagnosed with BN must binge, on average, twice per week over the last 3 months; use compensatory behaviors at a similar frequency; and have a self-evaluation that is unduly influenced by body shape and weight. Patients with BN might purge by use of self-induced vomiting, laxative use, or diuretic use or

*Supported in part by VA Merit Review Grant.

TABLE 1. **Diagnostic Criteria for Bulimia Nervosa**

A. Recurrent episodes of binge-eating. An episode of binge-eating is characterized by both of the following:
   1. Eating, in a discrete period of time (e.g., within any 2-hour period), an amount of food that is definitely larger than most people would eat during a similar period of time and under similar circumstances.
   2. A sense of lack of control over eating during the episode (e.g., a feeling that one cannot stop eating or control what or how much one is eating).

B. Recurrent inappropriate compensatory behavior in order to prevent weight gain, such as self-induced vomiting; misuse of laxatives, diuretics, enemas, or other medications; fasting; or excessive exercise.

C. The binge-eating and inappropriate compensatory behaviors both occur, on average, at least twice a week for 3 months.

D. Self-evaluation is unduly influenced by body shape and weight.

E. The disturbance does not occur exclusively during episodes of anorexia nervosa.

Specify type:
   1. *Purging type:* During the current episode of bulimia nervosa, the person has regularly engaged in self-induced vomiting or the misuse of laxatives, diuretics, or enemas.
   2. *Nonpurging type:* During the current episode of bulimia nervosa, the person has used other inappropriate compensatory behaviors, such as fasting or excessive exercise, but has not regularly engaged in self-induced vomiting or the misuse of laxatives, diuretics, or enemas.

Reprinted with permission from the *Diagnostic and Statistical Manual of Mental Disorders, Fourth Edition, Text Revision*. Copyright 2000 American Psychiatric Association.

might instead use fasting or excessive exercise to compensate for binges. The purging type has gained far more notoriety and research attention. In general, purging bulimics are more severely ill, have more co-morbid illnesses, and respond less well to treatment than nonpurging bulimics. These criteria state that if AN is present, even if BN criteria are met, then the diagnosis of AN takes precedence. These criteria also exclude from the BN diagnosis subgroups of patients who do not binge-eat but purge frequently. These patients, arguably more ill than the average BN patient, are classified as having an eating disorder, not otherwise specified (EDNOS).

EPIDEMIOLOGY AND CLUES TO ETIOLOGY

Several studies of nonclinical samples of young women in industrialized countries have placed the prevalence of BN at about 2%. The prevalence in women from nonindustrialized countries is clearly much less. The prevalence of BN (and EDNOS) is much higher in societies (or sectors of society) where (1) food is easily obtained by most people; (2) obesity is frequent relative to emaciation due to starvation; and (3) a premium is placed on slimness as a determinant of attractiveness of females. Where these conditions exist there is a high prevalence of dieting (attempted severe caloric restriction). For example, about 90% of college freshman women diet and, whereas only 2% have full-blown BN, nearly 10 times that many are at risk for BN. Interestingly, the more severely a young woman diets, the more likely she is to report symptoms of binge-eating, depressed mood, substance abuse, and multiple gastrointestinal complaints. These symptoms of BN were also reported by a subset of normal male subjects in a study of human semi-starvation done by Keys at the University of Minnesota in 1941. However, these research subjects did not develop a desire to be thin. Thus, caloric restriction is an important proximal cause for most symptoms of BN. However, caloric restriction does not explain why some women develop the drive to pursue thinness to improve their self-evaluation. It also does not explain why caloric restriction ends in anorexic, restrictive, compulsive syndromes in some women and in bulimic, impulsive syndromes in others. Baseline differences in central nervous system serotonergic systems or temperament may be important in determining the symptomatic response to caloric restriction.

PHENOMENOLOGY OF BULIMIA NERVOSA

The first criterion for BN is the presence of recurrent episodes of binge-eating. Although *recurrent* could be defined as more than once, a relatively arbitrary cut-off of "on average, at least twice a week for 3 months" is used. Requiring this level of repetition of both bingeing and compensatory behaviors helps to make the patient group more homogeneous, but the clinician should not assume that a person who binge-eats rarely but purges frequently is less ill. When BN was initially being described in the late 1970s, one frequently heard that bulimics must be exaggerating how much food they had eaten. However, laboratory studies have shown that bulimics who reported binge episodes in the 3000 to 5000 calorie range were, indeed, eating that much. These binges usually contain easily prepared foods that are high in fat and avoided during nonbinge eating. Binges must also be characterized by "loss of control." Most clinicians not specializing in eating disorders take this to mean that food is ingested in a wanton, animal-like manner. But loss of control can also be evidenced by an inability to avoid highly ritualized and predictable binges.

Another important criterion is the performance of purging or other compensatory behaviors, on average, twice per week over the last 3 months. Because people who do not purge find these behaviors repulsive, they often fail to perceive that purging often brings a sense of calm and control as it undoes the panic-inducing consequences of the excessive caloric ingestion. Vomiting or laxative abuse typically follows binges, but sometimes it follows any meal or snack. Because of the loss of large amounts of fluids, these purging mechanisms (as well as the use of diuretics and ipecac) result in large, but short-lived, weight losses. Patients can often understand that diuretics and laxatives create only water loss (not "real" weight loss), but many have a hard time understanding why vomiting is not effective. Vomiting does not work because the average emesis only empties part of the stomach contents. Nonpurging BN patients usually pursue thinness and the avoidance of weight gain due to binges through fasting and excessive exercise. Interestingly, patients are often congratulated for their dedication to exercise and their self-control. However, this is an example where one can have too much of a good thing. These behaviors can result in multiple stress fractures, amenorrhea, decreased bone density, as well as exercising to the point of job loss and relationship breakdown.

Thus, women with BN are often characterized as being trapped in a vicious binge-purge cycle. Their core belief that they can only be acceptable if they achieve a certain degree of thinness leads to severe caloric restriction. However, a certain percentage of all severe dieters will experience (especially during stress or anxiety) a loss of control of food intake, resulting in a binge. A binge episode is sometimes momentarily relieving of the hunger and stress triggering it, but the binge is horrifying to one basing one's self-evaluation on attaining a low weight. This leads to fasting, exercise, or purging. The purging, on one hand, provides a sense of control, relief, and expiation but, on the other hand, leads to a renewed hunger. That hungry, deprived state can lead back to bingeing and an enslaving, vicious cycle of bingeing and purging.

CO-MORBID MENTAL DISORDERS

Patients with BN commonly complain of symptoms of other mental disorders. Most frequent are depressive and anxiety symptoms and syndromes. Complicating the evaluation of these symptoms is that negative moods are increased by starvation and by electrolyte disturbances related to purging. It is important to determine whether these mood and anxiety problems antedated dieting. Patients with BN also have relatively high prevalence of alcohol and other drug abuse (including caffeine and stimulant appetite suppressants), shoplifting and/or kleptomania, and suicide attempts. They suffer from mood instability as well as impulsive behaviors and, therefore, fulfill criteria for borderline personality disorder relatively frequently.

PHYSICAL COMPLICATIONS AND CO-MORBIDITIES

Overweight status is a risk factor for dieting and, thus, for development of BN. However, most physical signs and symptoms in BN patients are direct consequences of dieting, bingeing, or purging. Restriction of food intake results in slowing of multiple physiologic processes, including gastrointestinal transit, thyroid secretion, and cardiac rate. Patients who significantly restrict caloric intake complain of low energy, cold feeling, abdominal pain, and constipation. Excessive dieting in bulimics leads to abnormal luteinizing hormone releasing hormone pulsativity and decreased fertility. Young women presenting for infertility workups or evaluation of irritable bowel syndrome should be questioned closely regarding dieting, bingeing, and purging.

Binge-eating can lead to abdominal pain, diarrhea, and, very rarely, ruptures of the stomach. However, vomiting, laxative abuse, and diuretic abuse are more frequently dangerous. Each of these behaviors leads to fluid and potassium loss. Vomiting causes loss of stomach fluids and potassium, hydrogen, and chloride loss, resulting in hypovolemia and hypokalemic alkalosis. These states, in turn, can cause orthostatic hypotension, syncope, and falls, as well as cardiac arrhythmias, seizures, and either anxiety or mental dulling. Diarrhea induced by laxatives and diuretic abuse also creates hypovolemia and hypokalemia. Chronic hypokalemia can cause kidney failure requiring dialysis or transplant in these patients. Vomiting can also lead to chronic esophagitis and Mallory-Weiss tears with hematemesis. A particularly difficult-to-treat outcome of laxative abuse is the development of a boggy, immobile colon with severe constipation. Repeated use of ipecac for induction of vomiting can lead to cardiomyopathy.

DIAGNOSIS

A high index of suspicion and use of clear, direct questions is the best tool for diagnosis of BN. Young women should be screened for severe dieting and frank BN. Questions should be specific (e.g., What did you have for breakfast yesterday? Lunch yesterday? Dinner yesterday?) as opposed to global (e.g., Are you eating okay?). The general question about "eating okay" will be answered with a "yes" by a dieter satisfied with her food restriction efforts, and the clinician will miss an opportunity for education or intervention.

GOALS AND MOTIVATION

To control BN, the patient must do the following:

1. Stop binges and purges.
2. Eat according to a healthy plan and accept the body that results.
3. Decrease co-morbid symptoms.
4. Decrease the dependence of one's self-esteem on body shape and weight (by presumably finding more meaningful roles/goals).

These goals are often clear to therapists and family. However, prospective patients might be very ambivalent about or frankly opposed to these treatment goals. For example, a patient might believe she is no more worried about weight than her friends. Other than causing others to be concerned, some young women will not have noticed any co-morbid problems. If their weight happens to be going down or is stable, many will believe that purging and dieting is a vital, effective approach to weight management. Thus, BN patients brought to one's clinic because of other problems or family pressure might be unwilling to take action to change their symptoms. In the terms of Prochaska and Di Clemente's Stages of Change Model, these patients are in the precontemplation (unaware of a problem) or contemplation (ambivalent regarding the presence of, significance of, and/or need for action to address a problem) stage. Often, the clinician, family, or friends have the strong desire to plunge ahead with treatment. However, it is problematic to proceed with treatment if the patient has not endorsed treatment goals, even if the person passively attends therapy. Although treatment can begin with such passive or passive-aggressive patients, the initial focus and a recurring theme of treatment must be motivation and commitment to change. Motivational interviewing techniques, originally designed for substance abusers, can be helpful not only in keeping the clinician focused on motivation as a critical goal but also in creating an alliance or contract for future work.

SETTING AND ORDER OF TREATMENT

The majority of BN patients can be treated as outpatients. A small percentage of patients will require episodic hospitalization for suicidal episodes, hypovolemia, and hypokalemia. It is critical that symptoms of eating disorders continue to be addressed during admissions because patients and providers often get deflected onto medical and general psychiatric issues. Although inpatient status is not necessary for most patients, a larger number of patients could benefit from a period of intensive outpatient or partial hospital treatment with specific eating disorder interventions. These settings allow intense psychoeducational and cognitive-behavioral interventions regarding meal planning and eating, mood management, problem-solving, and body image. They also provide for daily exposures to the "real world" so that new skills can be immediately practiced. (See www.psycho.org/clin_res/guide.bk-2.cfm for information on treatment and settings.)

BN patients often have co-morbid states such as alcohol dependence or depression. Clinicians often argue about whether treatment of BN or the co-morbid state should occur first. No definitive studies have clarified these questions, and clinical judgment must be used. However, the decision to treat alcohol dependence, for example, as an initial focus should not distract the providers from the long-term need to address the eating disorder. Cognitive-behavioral, motivational enhancement, and even 12-step approaches often used in substance use or mood and anxiety disorders, can be simultaneously applied to BN symptoms.

SPECIFIC TREATMENT ISSUES

Psychotherapy

When one has determined that the patient is motivated for change, there are clear treatment recommendations to follow. Wilson[1] reviewed the evidence regarding psychotherapy in eating disorders and concluded "Cognitive-behavioral therapy (CBT) for BN stands as one of the most intensively researched and empirically well-established methods in all of CBT for adult clinical disorders (p. 582)." He goes on, "Over 20 randomized controlled trials by different investigators in several countries attest to the efficacy of CBT for BN."

For the clinician, the question is not only "Is CBT efficacious?" but also "How does CBT compare with other treatment?" In general, CBT treatment results in quicker, more complete resolution of symptoms than do other psychotherapies, such as behavioral or interpersonal therapy, or pharmacotherapy. CBT is more likely to result in changes that are maintained after the end of therapy than after cessation of drug treatment. Manualized interpersonal therapy does appear to be as efficacious but slower than CBT. Unfortunately, most therapists do not do CBT for BN. General clinicians can identify appropriate CBT providers by asking about their use of manuals, homework, monitors of behaviors and cognitions, and reconstructions of cognitive distortions. If therapists are not using these techniques, it is fair to assume that they are not doing CBT. Despite the significant findings regarding efficacy of CBT in BN, CBT for BN still fails to fully treat up to half of subjects. Therefore, it is important to note that trials of improved psychotherapies are ongoing.

Pharmacotherapy

A wide variety of antidepressants have been shown to be effective in placebo-controlled, randomized trials. Antidepressant classes efficacious for BN include tricyclic antidepressants, monoamine oxidase inhibitors, and selective serotonin reuptake inhibitors. It is my guess that other types of antidepressants might have efficacy, but these should be saved for patients failing trials on antidepressants proven efficacious. Bupropion is contraindicated in treatment of BN because of the apparent induction of seizures in subjects with BN during a clinical trial.

There are important points that the clinician must understand about use of antidepressants in patients with BN:

1. Antidepressants suppress binge-eating and associated purging even in patients who are not depressed.[2]
2. Antidepressants are not as likely as CBT to induce a complete remission; CBT-treated patients are less likely to relapse than antidepressant-treated patients. Thus, antidepressants are not the treatment of choice nor are antidepressants sufficient treatment for BN by themselves.
3. Fluoxetine (Prozac) is the only antidepressant with FDA approval for treatment of BN. However, in contrast to its use in depression, higher doses of fluoxetine (e.g., 60 mg/d) are more effective than lower doses (e.g., 20 mg/d).
4. Whereas studies of combined antidepressants and CBT have shown few benefits over CBT alone, studies have shown that antidepressants can help patients who have not responded to CBT.
5. Patients who fail to respond to antidepressants should be assessed not only for compliance but also for whether they are vomiting their antidepressants or in such metabolic imbalance that they are unlikely to respond. Relapse clearly occurs even in patients who are compliant with antidepressants.
6. In general, selective serotonin reuptake inhibitors are the favored initial antidepressant choice, owing to safety in overdose and safety in patients at risk for orthostasis or arrhythmia.

In summary, both psychotherapy and antidepressants are effective. Certainly, CBT is the current treatment of choice, but antidepressants can also play an important ancillary role.

NEW DIRECTIONS

Given the paucity of therapists expert in CBT for BN, it is important to achieve the psychoeducational and cognitive restructuring goals by other means (if possible). Self-help manuals and bibliotherapy appear to be effective in at least some BN patients. Especially in areas of "CBT shortage," these interventions might be very valuable. Likewise, many patients unwilling to commit to psychotherapy might be willing to start with this approach. However, it is not yet known how patients likely to benefit from these approaches can be identified. In pharmacotherapy, ondansetron, a medication used for nausea induced by cancer chemotherapy, is reportedly effective in some treatment-resistant BN patients. The place of self-help manuals and ondansetron in the treatment of BN is not yet clear.

REFERENCES

1. Wilson GT: Cognitive behavior therapy for eating disorders: Progress and problems. Behav Res Ther 37:579–595, 1999.
2. Kaye WH, Klump KL, Frank GK, Strober M: Anorexia and bulimia nervosa. Ann Rev Med 31:299–313, 2000.

DELIRIUM

method of
JONATHAN M. FLACKER, M.D.
Emory University School of Medicine
Atlanta, Georgia

Delirium may be the most common complication of illness in older persons, and it is important at the outset to define what is meant by the term delirium. Although *The Diagnostic and Statistical Manual of Mental Disorders*, fourth edition (DSM-IV) includes criteria to define delirium, the Confusion Assessment Method (CAM) (Table 1) is of more use for the average clinician. The diagnosis of delirium by the CAM comprises five features:

1. Acute onset of symptoms
2. Fluctuating course
3. Inattention
4. Altered level of consciousness
5. Disorganized thinking

To diagnose delirium by the CAM the first three symptoms must be present, along with either of the last two. The CAM focuses on the features of the delirium syndrome itself rather than the cause and avoids the diagnostic problems inherent in the assessment of individuals with dementia under DSM-IV criteria.

TABLE 1. **The Confusion Assessment Method**

1. Acute Change in Mental Status

Ask: Is there evidence of an acute change in cognition from the patient's baseline?

In contrast to the insidious deterioration of mental status in progressive dementia, delirium typically occurs over hours to days. Thus, knowledge of the patient's baseline mental status is important.

2. Fluctuating Symptoms

Ask: Does the abnormal behavior fluctuate during the day, that is, does it tend to come and go or increase and decrease in severity?

Delirium may fluctuate over minutes to hours, with waxing and waning symptoms being typical.

3. Inattention

Ask: Does the patient have difficulty focusing attention, for example, being easily distractible or having difficulty keeping track of what was being said?

Attention is usually formally tested by forward digit span (normal is 7 digits forward) or trail-making tests. However, inattention is often obvious after trying to take the history from a delirious patient.

4. Disorganized Thinking

Ask: Was the patient's thinking disorganized or incoherent, such as rambling or irrelevant conversation, unclear or illogical flow of ideas, or unpredictable switching from subject to subject?

5. Altered Level of Consciousness

Ask: Is this patient normally alert?

If mental status is anything besides alert (i.e., vigilant [hyperalert], lethargic [drowsy, easily aroused], stupor [difficult to arouse], or coma [unarousable]), then this feature is present.

The diagnosis of delirium requires the presence of features 1 AND 2 AND 3 AND *either* 4 or 5.

Adapted from Inouye SK, van Dyck CH, Alessi CA, et al: Clarifying confusion: The confusion assessment method: A new method for detection of delirium. Ann Intern Med 113:941–948, 1990.

Delirium is often subtyped by psychomotor features. Delirious patients may be hyperactive, hypoactive, or fluctuate between the two. Normal psychomotor activity is less common.

Some behaviors of those with delirium are commonly observed but not helpful diagnostically. These characteristics include sleep-wake cycle alterations, abnormal psychomotor activity, hallucinations, delusions, abnormal speech patterns, tremor, and emotional lability. The presence of these behaviors should prompt evaluation for the presence of a delirium syndrome.

PREVENTION

The best approach to delirium is to prevent it from occurring in the first place. Initially, one must identify those at greatest risk for delirium. The healthier the patient is, the worse the insult must be to produce delirium. The opposite is also true, however; very frail patients may become delirious with seemingly minor insults.

Infections, fractures, and medications are common contributors to delirium, but a comprehensive list of all possible risk factors and precipitants would be unmanageably long and unusable. More important is the concept that minimizing the physiologic and psychological stresses on patients also minimizes the chances of delirium. As a general rule, anything that can be corrected should be corrected, unless the risks and burdens of such treatments outweigh the potential benefits. Furthermore, medical care should anticipate potential problems before they occur because the prevention of iatrogenic complications will go a long way toward preventing delirium.

Inappropriate medications are an important preventable factor often responsible for delirium. The list of medications associated with delirium is extensive, but common culprits include anticholinergics, neuroleptics, narcotics (especially meperidine [Demerol]), and benzodiazepines (especially long-acting agents). Although interventions such as providing calendars and clocks to all patients for orientation, ensuring that eyeglasses and hearing aids are available, calm reorientation, touch, and reassurance are recommended, their true utility for delirium prevention is not known. However, these measures are low cost, are nontoxic, and seem eminently worthwhile.

RECOGNITION

Delirium may be the first or only sign of acute illness in some patients. Unfortunately, on medical and surgical wards, as well as in the emergency department, in fully two thirds of patients the delirium goes unrecognized. It is important to recognize delirium because unexplained delirium is a medical emergency and requires immediate investigation in search of an explanation.

EVALUATION

The most challenging part of the delirium evaluation is the search for contributing etiologic factors. This search for precipitants should not stop with one identified factor; most hospitalized older persons have many contributors. Management requires attention to each.

A thorough history, physical examination, and medication review is thus the first step in the evaluation of delirium. Medications deserve a careful review, and nutritional supplements and medications taken on an as-needed basis must not be overlooked. A history of alcohol use, and even llicit drug use, should be actively sought. Recent medication withdrawals should be noted. Any medication should be considered as a contributor to delirium if the time course seems right.

The physical examination should pay special attention to any evidence of infection, heart failure, stroke, or fecal impaction. Initial laboratory testing should include a complete blood cell count and determination of electrolytes, blood urea nitrogen, and creatinine. A urinalysis and chest radiograph may be helpful in evaluating for infection, even in the absence of fever. Toxicology screens, oximetry (or blood gas), determination of calcium and thyroid hormone levels, blood cultures, and electrocardiography may be useful to direct the evaluation if clinically indicated or if the etiology of the delirium remains obscure. Asymptomatic strokes are very rarely a cause of delirium. Most such strokes will be nondominant parietal lobe or bilateral occipital lobe infarcts. Computed tomography of the brain is generally not required for the evaluation of delirium in the absence of a history of recent head trauma or abnormal neurologic examination. Similarly electroencephalography and lumbar puncture are usually not necessary unless a cause for delirium cannot be found after initial testing or focal findings such as seizure activity or meningismus are present.

MANAGEMENT

The successful management of delirium as delineated in Table 2 consists of

1. Avoiding complications of hospitalization
2. Treating the primary condition leading to the delirium
3. Removing contributing factors
4. Maintaining behavioral control
5. Supporting the patient and the family during the delirium

A multifaceted approach to delirium is often successful because many factors typically lead to delirium, and thus multiple improvements, even if individually small, may lead to marked clinical improvements.

Review of these recommendations makes it obvious that proper care of the delirious patient is very labor intensive; however, failure to invest the time and effort may result in additional costly and potentially life-threatening complications and long-term loss of function. Physical and pharmacologic restraints are "time savers" that extract a particularly costly toll in accidents, medication side effects, and loss of mobility and should be avoided if possible. When chemical sedation is unavoidable in the elderly delirious patient, low doses of haloperidol (Haldol),* (0.25–0.50 mg), or lorazepam (Ativan),* (0.25–0.50 mg), may be used, with careful reassessment before additional dosing. However, these medications must be used cautiously because they may actually prolong delirium.

The delirious patient is susceptible to a wide range of iatrogenic complications, and careful surveillance is critical. Bowel and bladder function should be watched closely, but urinary catheters, which can lead to urinary tract infection, are to be avoided. Bulk laxatives may help with obstipation, particularly in those who are using narcotic pain medications. Exercise and ambulation avoid the increasing disability and pressure ulcers associated with bed rest. A thick foam mattress overlay can be used as prophylaxis against pressure ulcers when a pressure reduction mattress is not available. Malnutrition can be addressed through nutritional supplements, and careful attention to intake of food and fluids. Some patients may need the staff to assist in feeding.

Treating the primary illness may lead to a resolution of the delirium; however, removing all of the factors that could potentially contribute to the delerium is equally important. Some factors such as age and prior cognitive impairment are not modifiable. Common modifiable contributors are generally either metabolic (e.g., hyponatremia, hypernatremia, and anemia), physiologic (e.g., hypoxemia, dehydration, and uncontrolled pain), or pharmacologic (e.g., anticholinergics, benzodiazepines, narcotics).

Maintaining behavioral control while ensuring both the comfort and safety of the patient can be challenging. Restraints, which can actually increase the risk of falls and injury, should be avoided. The calm reassurance provided by a sitter or family member is usually much more effective than restraints or drugs.

Finally, it is important to stress to family members that delirium is usually not a permanent condition but rather often improves slowly over time. Many cognitive deficits associated with the delirium syndrome can continue to abate even weeks and months after the acute episode.

Older, especially frail patients are at increased risk for delirium with illness. Evaluation and management should focus on the multifactorial nature of delirium. Sedation and restraints should be avoided. In fact, the clinician should begin treating delirium before it begins. Only by understanding delirium, its definition, recognition, predisposing factors, contrib-

TABLE 2. **What to Do About Delirium**

Avoid Iatrogenic Complications
Remove indwelling urinary catheters
Mobilize patient
Use pressure-reducing mattress or overlay
Ensure nutrition and fluids
Treat constipation

Treat the Primary Disease Process

Remove Contributing Factors
Metabolic: anemia, electrolyte abnormalities
Physiologic: hypoxemia, heart failure
Pharmacologic: narcotics, benzodiazepines, neuroleptics

Maintain Behavioral Control
Provide orientation: glasses, hearing aids, clocks, calendars
Social restraint: room near the nursing station, soft light, socialization

Counsel and Support the Patient and Family
Remind everyone that delirium is usually reversible.

*Not FDA approved for this indication.

uting factors, and management, can the clinician hope to prevent it, which may be the best way of avoiding its adverse clinical, functional, and economic sequelae.

MOOD DISORDERS

method of
ROBERT H. HOWLAND, M.D., and
MICHAEL E. THASE, M.D.
University of Pittsburgh School of Medicine
Pittsburgh, Pennsylvania

Major depression is a common clinical condition that is associated with substantial morbidity and mortality around the world. The lifetime prevalence of major depression in the United States is approximately 17%, affecting women twice as often as men. Other depressive disorders, such as dysthymia and minor depression, occur in 4% to 6% of the population. Although dysthymia and minor depression are considered milder forms of depression, a growing body of literature strongly suggests that they also are associated with substantial morbidity and mortality, comparable to major depression and other psychiatric and medical conditions. Hence, the clinical spectrum of depressive disorders represents a significant public health problem.

Clinical, biological, and psychosocial research clearly shows that depression is a heterogeneous syndrome. Despite the heterogeneity, or perhaps because of it, a wide variety of antidepressant therapies have been studied and found effective in the treatment of depression. Although many treatment modalities are available, we will focus on reviewing pharmacotherapy and psychotherapy because these are the most commonly used treatments for depression.

PHARMACOTHERAPY OF DEPRESSION

During the 1950s, the clinical effects of tricyclic antidepressants (TCAs) and monoamine oxidase inhibitors (MAOIs) were first discovered. Since the 1980s, a diverse variety of other medications have been developed and studied for the treatment of depression.

Tricyclic Antidepressants

After their discovery, the TCAs (Table 1) were the cornerstone of pharmacotherapy for depression for nearly three decades. The most commonly used TCAs, so called because of their cyclic chemical structure, include imipramine (Tofranil), desipramine (Norpramin), amitriptyline (Elavil), and nortriptyline (Pamelor). Doxepin (Sinequan), trimipramine (Surmontil), and protriptyline (Vivactil) are less commonly used. Clomipramine (Anafranil) is approved for use in the United States only for the treatment of obsessive-compulsive disorder, but it also is an effective antidepressant. The antidepressant effects of the TCAs are believed to be primarily due to their

TABLE 1. **Tricyclic Antidepressant Drug Dosages**

Drug	Starting Dose (mg)	Dose Range (mg/d)
Amitriptyline (Elavil)	25–50 qhs	150–300
Clomipramine (Anafranil)	25–50 qhs	100–250
Doxepin (Sinequan)	25–50 qhs	150–300
Imipramine (Tofranil)	25–50 qhs	150–300
Trimipramine (Surmontil)	25–50 qhs	150–300
Desipramine (Norpramin)	25–50 qhs	75–300
Nortriptyline (Pamelor)	25 qhs	50–150
Protriptyline (Vivactil)	5 qAM	10–60

inhibition of the reuptake of the neurotransmitters norepinephrine and serotonin. Aside from clomipramine, the TCAs are more active on noradrenergic reuptake inhibition. They also potently block several important postsynaptic neurochemical receptors, which account for most of their typical side effects. Dry mouth, constipation, blurred vision, sinus tachycardia, urinary retention, and memory dysfunction are due to cholinergic receptor blockade. Sedation and weight gain are related to histaminic receptor blockade. Dizziness, hypotension, and reflex tachycardia are caused by their blockade of α_1-adrenergic receptors. The TCAs also have quinidine-like effects on cardiac conduction, which can cause serious cardiotoxic effects, including arrhythmias and conduction abnormalities, that can be fatal with an overdose as small as 7 to 10 times a daily therapeutic dose.

As a group, the TCAs do not differ significantly in their relative antidepressant efficacy. In fact, two TCAs, nortriptyline and desipramine, are secondary amine metabolites of amitriptyline and imipramine, respectively. Nortriptyline and desipramine are often preferred because of less pronounced anticholinergic side effects. Placebo-controlled studies have found them to be effective in adult and geriatric patients. However, antidepressant efficacy has not been established in younger age groups. Higher doses are often associated with greater therapeutic benefit, but this is limited by their greater side effect burden. Measuring plasma levels of imipramine, amitriptyline, desipramine, and nortriptyline is clinically useful for achieving a therapeutic response. Because of their side effects and potential lethality, the use of TCAs has been gradually supplanted by newer-generation antidepressants. The TCAs, however, can be quite effective in treating patients who do not respond to other drugs, and they remain especially effective treatments for more severe melancholic depressions.

Monoamine Oxidase Inhibitors

The pharmacology and presumed mechanism of action of the MAOIs (Table 2) is distinctly different from all other antidepressants. This class includes phenelzine (Nardil), tranylcypromine (Parnate), and isocarboxazid (Marplan). The MAOIs irreversibly inhibit the enzyme monoamine oxidase, which degrades norepinephrine, serotonin, and dopamine,

TABLE 2. **Monoamine Oxidase Inhibitor Drug Dosages**

Drug	Starting Dose (mg)	Dose Range (mg/d)
Phenelzine (Nardil)	15 bid	45–90
Tranylcypromine (Parnate)	10 bid	40–60
Isocarboxazid (Marplan)	10 qAM	30–60

thereby increasing the availability of these neurotransmitters and likely contributing to their antidepressant effects. Typical side effects of the MAOIs include hypotension, dizziness, sedation, weight gain, dry mouth, and sexual dysfunction. Phenelzine is more often associated with these side effects than is tranylcypromine, whereas tranylcypromine may be more likely to cause insomnia. Because the MAOIs inhibit monoamine oxidase in the gut, severe hypertension can occur when foods containing the amino acid tyramine are ingested. (Tyramine stimulates the release of norepinephrine.) As a result, patients treated with MAOIs must follow a tyramine-free diet. In addition, use of the MAOIs is associated with potentially severe and fatal interactions with various other drugs, including antidepressants, narcotics, and sympathomimetics.

Because of their side effect profile and dietary restrictions, the MAOIs have never been commonly used by generalists. However, comparative studies have found the MAOIs to be more effective than the TCAs in the treatment of atypical depression and bipolar depression. In addition, the MAOIs have consistently been found to be effective in 40% to 60% of patients who do not respond to other antidepressants. Like the TCAs, higher doses (within the therapeutic range) also are associated with a greater antidepressant effect if tolerable.

Heterocyclic Antidepressants

Problems with the tolerability and safety of the TCAs and MAOIs led to interest in developing alternative antidepressant drugs. These pharmacologically diverse drugs include amoxapine (Asendin), maprotiline (Ludiomil), and trazodone (Desyrel) (Table 3). Amoxapine is a TCA-like compound that is related to the antipsychotic drug loxapine and can have similar extrapyramidal side effects (e.g., dystonia, akathisia, parkinsonian symptoms, and possibly tardive dyskinesia). As a result, it has not been a commonly used antidepressant, although it is sometimes used as "monotherapy" for the treatment of psychotic depression. Maprotiline is a tetracyclic drug that primarily blocks the reuptake of norepinephrine but is rarely used because of a higher risk of seizures and cardiac toxicity compared with other antidepressants. Trazodone is a phenylpiperazine compound that has weak effects on monoamine reuptake but does block postsynaptic serotonin ($5\text{-}HT_2$) receptors. Trazodone has been used almost exclusively in lower doses as a safe and effective non–habit-forming hypnotic, often in combination with other antidepressants. Higher doses are usually needed to treat severe depression and have been associated with severe hypotension and, rarely, the development of priapism.

TABLE 3. **Heterocyclic Antidepressant Drug Dosages**

Drug	Starting Dose (mg)	Dose Range (mg/d)
Amoxapine (Asendin)	25–50 qhs	200–400
Maprotiline (Ludiomil)	75 qhs	150–250
Trazodone (Desyrel)	50 qhs	300–600

Serotonin Reuptake Inhibitors

The SRIs (Table 4) have become the most commonly used class of antidepressants for the treatment of depression around much of the world. These drugs include fluoxetine (Prozac), paroxetine (Paxil), sertraline (Zoloft), and citalopram (Celexa). A fifth SRI, fluvoxamine (Luvox), is approved in the United States as a treatment for obsessive-compulsive disorder but also is an effective antidepressant. As a class, the SRIs are chemically dissimilar, which accounts for various pharmacologic differences (e.g., different half-lives, active metabolites, and hepatic enzyme inhibitory effects). Despite the pharmacologic differences, these drugs have a similar mechanism of action, which is their potent and specific inhibition of serotonin reuptake. The typical side effects of the SRIs include nausea, diarrhea, insomnia, nervousness, headache, and sexual dysfunction. Additional clinical experience with the SRIs also suggest that some patients may complain of sweating, fatigue, and weight gain. They do not have significant cardiac effects and are much safer than the TCAs in overdose. Several of the SRIs also can inhibit various hepatic enzymes, which are important for drug metabolism and can lead to clinically significant drug interactions, but this limitation has not lessened the utility of the SRIs.

As a group, the SRIs do not differ significantly in their relative efficacy or typical side effect profiles, although there may be subtle differences in the degree of certain side effects. There is some evidence that patients who do not respond to or cannot tolerate one SRI may do better after switching to an

TABLE 4. **Serotonin Reuptake Inhibitor Drug Dosages**

Drug	Starting Dose (mg)	Dose Range (mg/d)
Fluoxetine (Prozac)	20 qAM	10–80
Paroxetine (Paxil)	20 qhs	10–60
Sertraline (Zoloft)	50 qAM	50–200
Fluvoxamine (Luvox)	50 qhs	50–300
Citalopram (Celexa)	20 qAM	20–60

alternative SRI. Comparative studies with the TCAs have generally found similar efficacy rates, although indices of tolerability usually favor the SRIs. There continues to be debate about whether the TCAs are more effective among patients with more severe melancholic depressions. The SRIs have been well studied in other conditions, including several anxiety disorders, eating disorders, and premenstrual dysphoric disorder. Finally, unlike the TCAs, several placebo-controlled studies have found the SRIs to be effective in treating depression in adolescents.

Atypical Antidepressants

The term *atypical antidepressants* (Table 5) is used to group the remaining antidepressant drugs (bupropion, venlafaxine, nefazodone, mirtazapine, and reboxetine), which are chemically unrelated to each other and to the TCAs, MAOIs, and SRIs.

Bupropion

Bupropion (Wellbutrin, Wellbutrin SR, Zyban) is a novel antidepressant that belongs to the aminoketone class of drugs. Its mechanism of action is uncertain, although bupropion appears to facilitate or modulate the effects of norepinephrine and dopamine. Bupropion has virtually no effect on serotonergic, cholinergic, histaminic, or other adrenergic systems. As a result, it lacks the usual side effects seen with the TCAs or SRIs. Typical side effects include restlessness, insomnia, nausea, headache, constipation, and tremors. Bupropion is not associated with sexual dysfunction or weight gain and does not have significant cardiac effects. Bupropion is a modest inhibitor of the hepatic isoenzyme CYP450 2D6 but is not notorious for clinically significant drug interactions. High dosages (>450 mg/d) are associated with an increased risk of seizures, but within the manufacturer's recommended dose range the rate of seizures does not differ from other antidepressant drugs.

Comparative studies of bupropion and other antidepressants in depression have not found any significant differences in efficacy, but bupropion has a different tolerability profile (especially with regard to sexual and weight effects). It is sometimes combined with SRIs to lessen sexual dysfunction or augment antidepressant effects. Bupropion may not be as effective in the treatment of severe anxiety states associated with depression (e.g., obsessive-compulsive or panic anxiety) but might be especially useful in anergic, atypical, seasonal, or bipolar depressions. Bupropion also has a modest, but significant, therapeutic effect for smoking cessation.

TABLE 5. **Atypical Antidepressant Drug Dosages**

Drug	Starting Dose (mg)	Dose Range (mg/d)
Bupropion (Wellbutrin)	100 bid	300–450
Venlafaxine (Effexor)	37.5 qAM	75–375
Nefazodone (Serzone)	100 bid	300–600
Mirtazapine (Remeron)	15 qhs	15–45
Reboxetine (Vestra)	4 bid	8–10

Venlafaxine

Venlafaxine (Effexor, Effexor XR) is a novel antidepressant belonging to the phenylethylamine class of drugs. The primary mechanism of action is the inhibition of serotonin and, at higher doses, norepinephrine reuptake. Typical side effects include nausea, headache, dizziness, dry mouth, constipation, loss of appetite, nervousness, and insomnia. Some patients may complain of fatigue, sweating, and sexual dysfunction. A small proportion of patients may develop increased blood pressure at high doses, but it does not have any other significant cardiac effects. It also does not have any clinically significant effect on hepatic metabolic enzymes and appears to be relatively safe in an overdose.

Some studies directly comparing venlafaxine to the SRI fluoxetine have found it to be more effective and more likely to lead to a full remission, especially at higher doses. In addition, other studies have found it effective in the treatment of refractory depression, including use in patients who had not responded to various antidepressants from different classes. Venlafaxine also has been approved for the treatment of generalized anxiety disorder, but it has not been as well studied as the SRIs in other anxiety disorders.

Nefazodone

Nefazodone (Serzone) is a novel antidepressant that, like trazodone, belongs to the phenylpiperazine class of drugs. Its primary mechanism of action may be blockade of postsynaptic serotonin-2 receptors. It has very weak inhibitory effects on reuptake of norepinephrine or serotonin. Typical side effects include sedation, dry mouth, nausea, headache, constipation, and dizziness. Compared with SRIs and TCAs, it is not associated with sexual dysfunction or weight gain. Although nefazodone is a chemical analogue of the antidepressant trazodone, it is much less sedating initially and has not been found to cause priapism. Hypotension may occur rarely at high doses, but it does not have any other significant cardiac effects and seems to be relatively safe in an overdose. Nefazodone can inhibit the hepatic isoenzyme CYP450 3A4, which has some potential for drug-drug interactions.

Comparative studies have not found any significant difference in efficacy between nefazodone and SRIs or TCAs in the treatment of depression. Across 6 to 8 weeks of treatment, nefazodone appears to have more beneficial effects (than SRIs) on insomnia associated with depression. It is effective in treating anxiety symptoms in depression but has not been as well studied as the SRIs in the treatment of primary anxiety disorders. However, its side effect profile (especially its sexual and weight effects) may be preferable for some patients compared with those of the SRIs.

Mirtazapine

Mirtazapine (Remeron) is a novel, tetracyclic antidepressant belonging to the piperazinoazepine class of drugs. It has a very complicated presumed mechanism of action, involving blockade of several different adrenergic and serotonergic receptors, with the net effect of increasing serotonin and norepinephrine transmission. It also blocks postsynaptic histamine receptors, which causes its most common side effects (i.e., sedation and weight gain). Compared with the SRIs, it is less likely to cause nausea, headache, and sexual dysfunction. In some patients, it can cause dry mouth, constipation, and dizziness. It does not have significant cardiac effects, does not have any clinically significant drug interactions, and appears to be relatively safe in an overdose.

Comparative studies with other antidepressants generally have not found any significant differences in efficacy, although several recent studies found it to be more rapidly effective than SRIs. Its advantage over the SRIs with respect to gastrointestinal and sexual effects must be counterbalanced against its greater degree of sedation and weight gain. However, it may have more rapid and beneficial effects on sleep and anxiety in many patients, compared with the clinical effects of other antidepressants.

Reboxetine

Reboxetine (Vestra)* is a novel antidepressant compound, not yet approved for use in the United States, that is unrelated to the TCAs, MAOIs, SRIs, or other atypical antidepressant drugs. It is a potent and selective norepinephrine reuptake inhibitor and does not bind to serotonin, dopamine, cholinergic, or histamine receptors. As a result, reboxetine is not associated with sedation, weight gain, or sexual dysfunction. Typical side effects include dry mouth, constipation, insomnia, increased heart rate, and urinary hesitancy/retention (in men). It does not have significant cardiac effects, does not have any clinically significant effect on hepatic metabolic enzymes, and appears to be relatively safe in an overdose.

PSYCHOTHERAPY OF DEPRESSION

Historically, before the discovery of effective antidepressant compounds, long-term psychodynamic therapy was considered the treatment of choice for nonpsychotic depressions. This approach, although helpful to patients in many ways, was never studied to determine if it is effective in treating the core symptoms of depression. During the past 30 years, psychological models of depression have been used to develop short-term highly structured forms of psychotherapy specifically for treating depression. Compared with traditional forms of psychotherapy, these depression-focused psychotherapies have been studied in clinical trials and found to be as effective as pharmacotherapy for the treatment of depressed outpatients. Depression-focused psychotherapies should not be considered for treatment of psychotic or bipolar forms of therapy without concomitant pharmacotherapy.

*Not yet approved for use in the United States.

Interpersonal Psychotherapy

Interpersonal psychotherapy (IPT) is a time-limited form of psychotherapy that focuses on difficulties in the patient's intimate and vocational relationships. IPT evolved from the finding that depression is often associated with four types of problems: grief, interpersonal role disputes, role transitions, and interpersonal deficits. IPT has been shown to be an effective and easily used intervention in the treatment of depression. Some studies have found it to be as effective as medication in outpatients with depression.

IPT usually focuses on the "here and now," although past interpersonal problems also are explored to help to understand maladaptive patterns and to identify areas for change. IPT explicitly defines depression as an illness, which allows the patient to assume a "sick" role that requires treatment. Patients are encouraged to examine how their illness has affected their lives and how they can work to become well again.

Techniques that are commonly used in IPT include facilitating affect (e.g., expressing unresolved grief or repressed anger), encouraging activity and socialization, exploring different options for achieving life goals, examining communication problems, clarifying the patient's understanding of his or her interpersonal style, and using the therapy relationship as a model to work through interpersonal problems. The IPT therapist has the flexibility to be directive, offer advice, provide education, and role play appropriate interpersonal behaviors depending on the patient's needs. However, because therapy is time limited, the ultimate goal is to foster more independent and adaptive functioning by the patient so that the therapist can gradually assume a more indirect role as therapy progresses.

Cognitive Therapy

Cognitive therapy (CT) is another time-limited form of psychotherapy that is based on the theory that depression is invariably associated with automatic negative thoughts about oneself, the world, and the future. This therapy employs a number of strategies to help patients recognize the connections between distorted negative thinking and low mood and to challenge the validity of such thoughts. Thus, the goals of CT include both symptomatic improvement of the depression and reduction of cognitive vulnerability.

CT is the best studied form of psychotherapy for depression. Many studies have found it to be as effective a treatment for major depression as TCAs. Several controlled studies have found that the efficacy of CT may be limited in more severe depressions, but this finding has not been observed by a number of other studies.

In CT, therapists often use behavioral techniques to focus on the core features of depression. Therapists define specific problem areas and teach patients to monitor their daily events to identify situations in which they often feel depressed. Graded task assignments and scheduled pleasurable activities help depressed patients to get moving again. Patients also learn to identify the negative and distorted cognitions that automatically arise during such situations and that are linked to the depressed feelings. Then, they examine their beliefs with the help of their therapists, who systematically challenge the beliefs so that patients are able to recognize the distortions and can learn to evaluate thoughts more realistically and accurately. Homework assignments are used to monitor and record the particular problems, situations, automatic thoughts, and feelings that occur outside therapy. As therapy progresses, patients should be better able to use their newly learned cognitive and behavioral strategies to accomplish these tasks and to work through different problem areas more autonomously.

CLINICAL ISSUES IN THE MANAGEMENT OF DEPRESSION

Choice of Antidepressant Therapy

Given the availability of a wide variety of effective antidepressant therapies, how does one choose among these treatments? Because of the delay in onset of action of treatment, adherence to treatment is very important. Hence, patient preference is important to consider. Patients who strongly favor medication or psychotherapy should be offered treatment as such. The choice of psychotherapy will depend, of course, on the availability of a therapist trained in the use of a particular therapy model. The choice of medication also will depend on such factors as patient preference, past treatment history, family treatment history, clinical symptoms, health, and side effect profile.

Response Versus Remission in Depression

The goal of antidepressant treatment should be an optimal outcome, that is, the absence of any depressive symptoms along with a complete recovery of psychosocial function. This type of outcome is referred to as remission. About 50% of patients will have a significant response to the first choice treatment, which is defined as a 50% or greater decrease in their symptoms of depression. Of these responders, however, only about one half to one third attain a full remission. Hence, a significant number of depressed patients are left with residual or persistent symptoms despite adequate antidepressant treatment. For these patients, switching to an alternative antidepressant drug or therapy or combining different antidepressant treatments (e.g., pharmacotherapy and psychotherapy) may lead to a full remission.

Phases of Treatment in Depression

The treatment of depression, whether with pharmacotherapy or psychotherapy, is now provided in three phases, each having different therapeutic goals. The acute phase, which typically lasts 6 to 12 weeks, refers to the initial treatment period, when the treatment is administered with the goal of full-symptom remission. The continuation phase, which typically lasts 4 to 9 months, follows acute phase treatment and is recommended for all patients. The goal of continuation-phase treatment is to prevent early relapse and to allow further symptomatic and psychosocial functional improvement. The goal of maintenance phase treatment is to prevent further recurrences of depression among patients who have a high risk of developing depression again. Such risk factors include three or more previous episodes of major depression, chronic depression, residual or persistent symptoms despite adequate treatment, and severe or disabling episodes of depression. The length of maintenance treatment will depend on the number of risk factors and may range from a year to even life-long treatment.

The Treatment of Nonresponders

For patients who do not have a satisfactory response to their initial antidepressant treatment, various strategies have been advocated. Switching to a different treatment (e.g., an alternative antidepressant drug or psychotherapy) is recommended for patients who have shown no response at all or for those who have intolerable side effects. Augmentation (the strategy of adding a second medication to an antidepressant drug) may be most useful in patients who have shown a partial response to treatment. Although combining pharmacotherapy and psychotherapy is commonly recommended, there is no clear evidence that the combination is more effective than either modality alone in the treatment of uncomplicated depressions. Complicated depressions (e.g., very severe depression, treatment-resistant depression, chronic forms of depression, and partially remitted depression), however, may respond better to the combination of psychotherapy and pharmacotherapy.

BIPOLAR DISORDER

Lithium has been the standard treatment for bipolar disorder for nearly 30 years, but a significant proportion of patients do not respond to or cannot tolerate it. As a result, various anticonvulsant drugs have been actively investigated and are increasingly used in clinical practice in the treatment of bipolar disorder. There is now abundant evidence of the effectiveness of two anticonvulsants, carbamazepine (Tegretol)* and valproate (valproic acid) (Depakene)* and divalproex (Depakote)* is now considered by many physicians to be the most appropriate first-line

*Not FDA approved for this indication.

treatment. For other patients, these anticonvulsants are useful second-line or adjunctive treatments for patients who are intolerant of or do not respond to lithium (e.g., those with rapid-cycling or mixed manic states). More recently, two newer anticonvulsants have become available, gabapentin (Neurontin)* and lamotrigine (Lamictal).* Both were originally approved as adjunctive treatments for patients with poorly controlled partial seizures. During clinical trials of these two drugs in epilepsy, many patients reported positive effects on their mood and emotional well-being. These observations, together with the known effectiveness of valproate and carbamazepine, have led to considerable interest in using them in bipolar disorder.

Carbamazepine* has been the most extensively studied anticonvulsant in bipolar disorder, although it has not been formally approved for this indication. Double-blind placebo-controlled studies have found it to be effective in the acute and prophylactic treatment of mania. Most controlled comparative studies have found that carbamazepine is as effective as lithium, although some have found it slightly less effective. The results from controlled studies also have shown that it is effective in bipolar depression. Similar to lithium, however, it may be relatively more effective in mania than in depression.

Patients with mixed mania, rapid-cycling, or a poor response to lithium often respond well to carbamazepine. Carbamazepine usually is given in divided doses, but many patients can tolerate taking it once a day. The therapeutic range for carbamazepine serum levels is 6 to 12 μg/mL. There is no clinical evidence to support a relationship between serum levels and clinical outcome, however. Thus, in general clinical practice, doses should be increased every 2 to 3 days as tolerated until the patient begins to respond or develops limiting side effects.

Because carbamazepine induces its own metabolism, periodic dose increases may be needed during treatment. Serum levels may therefore be especially useful to assess compliance, distinguish between poor and rapid drug metabolizers, and maintain patients at a steady-state level during long-term treatment. Sedation, dizziness, ataxia, and diplopia are the most common dose-dependent side effects; weight gain frequently occurs during long-term use. Many patients develop benign rashes, mild leukopenia, or transient hepatic enzyme elevations, but the Stevens-Johnson syndrome, agranulocytosis, aplastic anemia, and hepatitis are rare complications. Although monitoring blood cell counts is recommended, this is not needed as frequently as has been suggested in the past. Because carbamazepine induces hepatic enzymes, drug interactions are common. It can significantly decrease levels of other anticonvulsants (including valproate and lamotrigine), neuroleptics, benzodiazepines, tricyclics, and oral contraceptives. Erythromycin, cimetidine, valproate, fluoxetine, fluvoxamine, and calcium channel blockers can increase carbamazepine levels. Therefore, concurrent use of these drugs with carbamazepine may require dose adjustments. Carbamazepine has been found to be relatively safe and often effective when combined with lithium or valproate, although the combinations are more likely to cause side effects than monotherapy with any of these drugs alone.

*Not FDA approved for this indication.

Valproate (divalproex, Depakote) has also been intensively studied in the treatment of bipolar disorder and has an approved indication for the acute treatment of mania. Double-blind placebo-controlled studies have found it to be as effective as lithium in acute mania. Valproate has not been as well studied in the long-term treatment of bipolar disorder, but there is increasing evidence from a number of open studies that it has prophylactic benefits. The results from a recently completed, but unpublished, double-blind placebo-controlled study suggested that it was somewhat more effective than lithium, especially with regard to depressive symptoms. Open-label studies have shown it to be effective in bipolar depression, although it likely has relatively greater antimanic than antidepressant effects. Similar to carbamazepine, mixed mania, rapid cycling, and a poor lithium response tend to predict a positive response to valproate. It is usually given in divided doses, although many patients can tolerate it once a day.

The therapeutic range for valproate serum levels is 50 to 125 μg/mL, although there is no evidence to support a relationship between serum levels and clinical outcome. Doses may therefore be increased every 2 to 3 days as tolerated until a clinical response is seen or limiting side effects develop. Loading doses of 20 to 30 mg/kg/d have been used successfully to treat acute mania and are surprisingly well tolerated. The most common dose-dependent side effects are nausea, sedation, and tremor. Transient hair loss can occur, and weight gain is common with long-term use.

In general, however, valproate appears to be better tolerated than lithium or carbamazepine. Blood dyscrasias, typically thrombocytopenia, are rare. Mild transient hepatic enzyme elevations are somewhat more common with valproate compared with carbamazepine, but hepatotoxicity is rare. Reports of severe hepatitis have been described primarily among young patients with epilepsy taking other anticonvulsants. Drug interactions are less common with valproate compared with carbamazepine, because it is a weak inhibitor of hepatic enzymes, but it can increase serum levels of carbamazepine, lamotrigine, and TCAs. Aspirin and naproxen can increase levels of valproate, whereas carbamazepine can decrease its levels. Therefore, use of these drugs together with valproate may require dose adjustments. Valproate can also be used safely and effectively in combination with lithium or carbamazepine, although side effects will be more common than with monotherapy. The combination of valproate and lithium may be better tolerated than that of carbamazepine and lithium.

Lamotrigine (Lamictal)* has pharmacologic effects that are very different from those of carbamazepine

*Not FDA approved for this indication.

and valproate. The published literature on the use of lamotrigine in bipolar disorder is limited to case reports, uncontrolled open-label studies, and one double-blind trial. The open-label reports found that lamotrigine was effective alone or in combination with other mood stabilizers in the majority of patients, including many who were treatment resistant or had rapid cycling. The antidepressant effects of lamotrigine were demonstrated in one double-blind trial. Antimanic effects have not yet been demonstrated. The most common side effects are nausea, headache, dizziness, ataxia, and diplopia. A benign rash occurs in approximately 10% of patients, and more severe rashes occur in 0.5% to 1.0%; the Stevens-Johnson syndrome has also been reported. Rashes tend to occur more commonly when higher starting doses are used or the dose is rapidly increased, and when it is used together with valproate (which inhibits its metabolism). Lamotrigine does not affect hepatic metabolism. Carbamazepine can increase its metabolism, whereas valproate decreases it. Serum levels are not monitored with lamotrigine, but the usual dose range is 100 to 500 mg/d. Low starting doses of 25 to 50 mg/d, with increases of 50 to 100 mg every 1 to 2 weeks, are recommended to minimize adverse effects, especially when added to valproate.

Gabapentin (Neurontin)* also has pharmacologic effects that differ from all other anticonvulsants. The published literature on the use of gabapentin in bipolar disorder is limited to case reports, uncontrolled open-label studies, and one placebo-controlled trial. The open-label reports found that gabapentin was effective alone or in combination with other mood stabilizers in about 60% to 90% of patients, including those with treatment-resistant or rapid-cycling bipolar disorder. However, the one double-blind study did not find a significant drug-placebo difference. Sedation, dizziness, and ataxia are the most common side effects. Gabapentin is not metabolized, does not affect hepatic metabolism, does not have significant drug interactions, and is not associated with hepatic or hematologic abnormalities. Because it is renally excreted, lower doses may be required in patients with renal disease, but serious toxicity in such patients is unlikely compared with lithium. Serum levels are not monitored with gabapentin. The recommended dose range is 900 to 3600 mg/d, but the effective doses reported in the literature range from 600 to 4800 mg/d. The absorption of gabapentin may be decreased with acute doses greater than 1800 mg, and it may therefore be more effective when given in divided doses rather than once a day. The combination of gabapentin and other mood stabilizers appears to be better tolerated than lamotrigine and other mood stabilizers.

There is now considerable evidence that valproate and carbamazepine are effective alternatives to lithium in the treatment of bipolar disorder. Because valproate is better tolerated and less likely to interact with other drugs, it might be preferred initially to carbamazepine. It is important to realize, however, that carbamazepine and valproate are pharmacologically distinct, and switching or combining them would be a reasonable approach in nonresponders or partial responders. The newer anticonvulsants are a promising addition to the treatment options for bipolar disorder. Gabapentin appears to be better tolerated than lamotrigine, but evidence of efficacy from controlled systematic trials has not been forthcoming.

*Not FDA approved for this indication.

SCHIZOPHRENIA

method of
ROBERT R. CONLEY, M.D.
Maryland Psychiatric Research Center at the University of Maryland
Baltimore, Maryland

The etiology of schizophrenia is an area of active research. The biologic basis for positive symptoms has long been believed to be linked to overactivity of dopamine (DA) neurons, specifically, the DA-producing neurons in the mesolimbic DA pathway. The negative symptoms of schizophrenia may involve regions of the brain other than the DA pathway such as the dorsolateral prefrontal cortex and neurotransmitter systems. The behavioral deficit state suggested by negative symptoms implies an underactivity or even degeneration or developmental arrest of some neuronal systems. Excitotoxic overactivity of the glutamate neurotransmitter system may be involved.

DOPAMINE LINK TO PSYCHOTIC SYMPTOMS AND ADVERSE EFFECTS

It has been known for some time that drugs that increase DA neurotransmission will exacerbate or produce psychotic symptoms whereas drugs that reduce DA neuronal transmission decrease them. All known clinically effective antipsychotic drugs are blockers of DA receptors, particularly the D_2 subtype.

Besides its importance in psychotic symptoms, DA is a critical neurotransmitter in the control of movements. Like the mesolimbic DA pathway, the activity of DA neurons of the nigrostriatal DA pathway is critical to the ability to control movements. When DA receptors are blocked in the postsynaptic projections of the nigrostriatal DA pathway, parkinsonian side effects appear and can be quite severe. These effects include so-called extrapyramidal side effects such as akathisia, dystonia, tremor, rigidity, and akinesia/bradykinesia.

Because D_2-receptor occupancy is believed to be clearly central to both efficacy and tolerability, the association of antipsychotic drugs' D_2-receptor occupancy profile with clinical efficacy, extrapyramidal side effects, and the propensity to produce hyperprolactinemia (another function controlled by blockage of D_2-receptors) has been assessed by positron emission tomography in a study of D_2-receptor occupancy versus clinical response in two cohorts of people in their first episode of schizophrenia. One group in this double-blind study received 1.0 mg/d of haloperidol (Haldol), and the other, 2.5 mg/d of haloperidol for 2 weeks. The study findings confirmed D_2 occupancy to be an important mediator of both clinical response and side effects and, moreover, that the magnitude of receptor occupancy was indeed predictive of clinical improvement, development of hyperprolactinemia, and induction of extrapyramidal side effects. The likelihood of a positive clinical response, development of hyperprolactinemia, and introduction of extrapyramidal side effects increased significantly as D_2 occupancy exceeded 65%, 72%, and 78%, respectively. Although the study was limited to haloperidol, the relationship between D_2 occupancy, efficacy, and side effects in this study helps explain many of the observed clinical differences between conventional (relatively high affinity for D_2 receptors in comparison to other receptor sites) and second-generation antipsychotics (relatively low affinity for D_2 receptors in comparison to other receptor sites).

COMPARATIVE EFFICACY

Each of the second-generation antipsychotics has proved effective for the positive and negative symptoms of schizophrenia in large-scale phase III clinical trials. Although clearly effective for all forms of schizophrenia, clozapine (Clozaril) is approved for use only in patients with treatment-refractory disease because of concern about agranulocytosis and the need for regular blood monitoring. Most early studies comparing clozapine with chlorpromazine (Thorazine) have found clozapine to be as effective or more effective than conventional drugs. This finding was surprising because clozapine has very low affinity for D_2 receptors, a receptor affinity that was thought to be a necessary property for a compound to be an effective antipsychotic. Thus, the clozapine studies were important for two reasons: they demonstrated that antipsychotic drugs could have different efficacy and that direct D_2-receptor blockade was not necessary for a drug to be an effective antipsychotic.

In contrast to clozapine, risperidone (Risperdal), olanzapine (Zyprexa), quetiapine (Seroquel) and ziprasidone (Zeldox) can be used as first-line agents in the treatment of schizophrenia. All of these drugs have fewer parkinsonian side effects associated with their use than seen with the high-potency conventional antipsychotics, such as haloperidol. With regard to efficacy, risperidone has been shown to be more effective than haloperidol for positive and negative symptoms, olanzapine has been shown to be more effective than haloperidol for negative symptoms only, and quetiapine has been shown to have efficacy equivalent to that of haloperidol for positive and negative symptoms. As yet, ziprasidone has few published safety or efficacy data.

The first large clinical trial to demonstrate the efficacy of risperidone was a study that enrolled 523 inpatients with chronic schizophrenia. Each patient was randomly assigned to treatment with 2, 6, 10, or 16 mg/d of risperidone, 20 mg/d of haloperidol, or placebo for 8 weeks. Optimal results were achieved at a dosage of 6 mg/d. Risperidone was found to be significantly more effective than haloperidol for negative symptoms, positive symptoms, disorganized thought, uncontrolled hostility or excitement, and anxiety or depression.

As shown in four double-blind 6-week trials, olanzapine was equally, but not more effective than haloperidol in treating positive symptoms. In the first of these trials, 152 inpatients were randomly assigned to treatment with 1 mg/d of olanzapine, 10 mg/d of olanzapine, or placebo. The second trial compared low-dose, moderate-dose, and high-dose ranges of olanzapine (approximately 5, 10, and 15 mg/d) with haloperidol and placebo in 335 patients. The third trial compared low-dose, moderate-dose, and high-dose ranges of olanzapine with haloperidol and a very low dosage of olanzapine (1 mg/d) in 431 patients. In the last study, 1996 patients were randomly assigned to treatment with haloperidol or 5 to 20 mg/d of olanzapine. Efficacy was assessed by changes in scores on the Brief Psychiatric Rating Scale (BPRS), Positive and Negative Symptom Scale (PANSS), and the Scale for the Assessment of Negative Symptoms (SANS). In both slightly and significantly depressed patients, olanzapine treatment was associated with greater improvement in depressive symptoms than haloperidol was. Olanzapine is also effective for the negative symptoms of schizophrenia. Based on the mean change from baseline in the BPRS negative score, olanzapine was significantly more effective than haloperidol and placebo, but only at the highest dosage range (between 12.5 and 17.5 mg/d).

The efficacy of quetiapine was demonstrated in two double-blind placebo-controlled trials that enrolled a total of 647 patients with chronic or subchronic schizophrenia. One trial was a fixed-dose study comparing multiple dosages of quetiapine (75, 150, 300, 600, and 750 mg/d) with 12 mg/d of haloperidol and placebo. The other trial was a titrated-dose study comparing high doses of quetiapine (maximal daily dose, 750 mg) with low doses of quetiapine (maximal daily dose, 250 mg) and placebo. In each of these trials, quetiapine was significantly more effective than placebo but no more effective than haloperidol for positive and negative symptoms. With regard to positive symptoms, all quetiapine treatment groups in the fixed-dose trial showed improvement in BPRS positive cluster scores, but the difference between quetiapine and placebo was significant only for the groups given 150, 300, and 600 mg/d. Significant improvement in these scores in the titrated-dose trials was seen only in the high-dose group. All treatment groups showed improvement on the SANS. However, only the difference in improvement between the group given 300 mg/d of quetiapine and the placebo group was statistically significant. No statistically significant differences were noted between quetiapine and haloperidol. In the titrated-dose trial, significant improvement was seen only in the high-dose quetiapine group. Quetiapine did not achieve therapeutic superiority on any outcome measure in comparison to haloperidol.

TREATMENT-REFRACTORY SCHIZOPHRENIA

Refractoriness to antipsychotic treatment remains a very significant problem in the clinical management of schizophrenic patients. Unfortunately, as many as one third of patients who are given an adequate trial of a conventional antipsychotic experience a suboptimal response. By definition, treatment refractoriness means that a patient failed to respond to at least two trials in which both the dosage and duration of the trial were considered adequate. Treatment refractoriness implicitly refers to a lack of response in treating positive symptoms; however, having a poor treatment response is not limited to positive symptoms but extends to other symptom domains, including negative symptoms, aggressive behavior, cognitive impairment, and co-morbid mood symptoms.

Clozapine (Clozaril)

Clozapine is the only agent with proven efficacy in the treatment of refractory patients. In the trial by

Kane and colleagues[1] that led to its regulatory approval, 30% of the treatment-refractory patients met the criteria for response by week 6. Since that seminal study, several studies have demonstrated significantly better response rates (approaching 50% to 60%) with longer duration of treatment. Despite its impressive efficacy profile, clozapine remains a treatment of last choice because of an approximate 1% risk of agranulocytosis. Its unfavorable side effect profile, including high anticholinergic activity, sedation, seizures, weight gain, sialorrhea, and orthostasis, further limits its use by adversely affecting patient acceptance and compliance.

The second-generation first-line antipsychotic agents (i.e., risperidone, olanzapine, quetiapine, ziprasidone) share some, but not all of the characteristics that make clozapine so unique. The efficacy of these newer agents in treatment-refractory patients, however, is not as clear. Risperidone and olanzapine have been the most extensively studied, whereas little is known about the efficacy of quetiapine or ziprasidone in treatment-refractory patients.

Risperidone (Risperdal)

Risperidone has demonstrated a response rate in patients refractory to conventional agents. Of note, Bondolfi and colleagues[2] found no difference between the response rates for risperidone and clozapine (approximate response rates of 65%) in an 8-week, randomized, double-blind study of treatment-refractory or treatment-intolerant schizophrenic patients. A 65% response rate is rather high for both drugs and is probably explained by the inclusion in this study of patients who were intolerant of treatment with conventional antipsychotics. Breier and coworkers[3] found a 36% response rate for clozapine and a 20% response rate for risperidone in a prospective 6-week, double-blind trial in patients with refractory schizophrenia. In a recent prospective double-blind study by Wirshing and associates,[4] risperidone was shown to be superior to haloperidol at the end of a 4-week fixed-dose phase (24% response rate for risperidone versus 11% for haloperidol).

Olanzapine (Zyprexa)

Data on the efficacy of olanzapine in treatment-refractory schizophrenia are more mixed. One post hoc analysis of a large outpatient trial reported by Breier and Hamilton[5] found that olanzapine was superior to haloperidol in a subgroup of treatment-refractory patients. Interestingly, in this study, haloperidol significantly attenuated symptoms in about one third of the patients. Such a high rate of response to haloperidol calls into question the degree of treatment refractoriness of the patient cohort and the manner in which refractoriness was defined. In a more scientifically rigorous, 8-week prospective randomized trial in treatment-refractory patients that compared fixed dosages of olanzapine (25 mg/d) and chlorpromazine (1200 mg/d), no advantage was demonstrated for olanzapine over chlorpromazine. In a subsequent trial, patients who had previously failed to respond to olanzapine responded to clozapine at the same rate as had been demonstrated in other trials of clozapine in treatment-refractory patients. As such, failing to respond to olanzapine in no way predicted a subsequent response to clozapine. Sanders and Mossman[6] reported results from 16 treatment-refractory patients whose medication was switched from a conventional antipsychotic to olanzapine. Psychotic symptoms became markedly worse in four patients and improved in two patients. In summary, these studies do not suggest that olanzapine is robustly efficacious in a severely refractory population of patients. The relatively favorable results of the Breier and Hamilton study are probably accounted for by the less stringent definition of treatment refractoriness.

ADVERSE EFFECTS OF ANTIPSYCHOTICS

Second-generation antipsychotics, with their milder side effect profiles, have alleviated the burden of managing many of the adverse side effects associated with the older or conventional antipsychotics. This greater tolerability is a major therapeutic advance. However, the newer drugs are associated with their own side effects, including anticholinergic effects, weight gain, and the more recently identified elevation in plasma glucose and induction of type 2 diabetes mellitus. Because each drug is unique in its risk-benefit profile, antipsychotics must be selected for their efficacy, as well as their side effect profile. Furthermore, when considering the seriousness of a side effect, clinicians should evaluate how commonly it occurs; its impact on morbidity, mortality, and compliance; its reversibility; and the effectiveness of interventions to manage it. This brief review summarizes the literature on the long-term side effects of newer antipsychotics, examines the severity of the problem, and offers recommendations for management.

Short-term side effects such as sedation, extrapyramidal side effects, and orthostatic hypotension can be easily managed by lowering the medication dose or by adding an antiparkinsonian medication. More challenging are the long-term side effects, including hyperprolactinemia, tardive dyskinesia (TD), weight gain, and abnormal glucose metabolism.

Prolactin Elevation

Elevated serum prolactin levels result from blockade of D_2 receptors in the tuberoninfundibular region of the anterior pituitary gland. Many of the conventional antipsychotics and several of the second-generation antipsychotics block this receptor and are associated with elevations in serum prolactin. Transient and modest elevations of prolactin alone are not clinically significant, but high levels—those associated with hyperprolactinemia—may be associated with amenorrhea, galactorrhea, bone loss, or sexual dysfunction. However, assessments to definitively show cause and effect are complicated, particularly with respect to effects on sexuality. Loss of interest in sexual activity is common in patients with psychotic illnesses because of the high association between psychoses and negative and depressive symptoms. Other factors may adversely affect sexuality (e.g., neuroleptic-induced parkinsonism, institutionalization, or the presence of positive symptoms). Psychological causes (e.g., those involving relationship issues) are also factors in sexual dysfunction, as is co-morbid alcohol and substance abuse (i.e., abuses that are highly prevalent in patients with psychotic illnesses). Unfortunately, studies that have shown a link between antipsychotic-induced hyperprolactinemia and sexual dysfunction have not controlled for these or other confounding problems, thus leaving the relationship between cause and effect unclear.

To date, no evidence suggests that antipsychotic-induced hyperprolactinemia is directly linked to efficacy or adverse events. Furthermore, the data appear insufficient to indicate that antipsychotic-induced hyperprolactinemia should be an important consideration in the selection of an antipsychotic.

Tardive Dyskinesia

Second-generation antipsychotics may lower the risk of TD when compared with conventional agents. A significant confounder in any evaluation, however, is that most patients started on the newer drugs have been previously exposed to conventional agents. Therefore, the exact contribution of the newer antipsychotic to TD is often difficult to ascertain. Cases of TD associated with second-generation antipsychotics in patients with no history of exposure to conventional agents are rare but present in the literature.

Numerous studies with clozapine have shown that the incidence of TD actually decreases with clozapine treatment, thus suggesting that it may be an effective treatment of TD. The efficacy of risperidone in treating TD needs further investigation. However, studies have shown that risperidone is associated with a lower incidence of TD than seen with conventional antipsychotics. In a year-long study of risperidone versus haloperidol, the prevalence of TD was 0.6% for risperidone and 2.7% for haloperidol. Olanzapine has also been reported to be associated with a lower rate of TD when compared with conventional antipsychotics. In a large, double-blind, placebo-controlled study, the incidence of new-onset TD was significantly less in patients receiving olanzapine (2.8%) than in haloperidol-treated patients (8.0%). Although no controlled trials have studied olanzapine as therapy for TD, anecdotal reports indicate that olanzapine improves TD. Lower rates of TD with quetiapine than with conventional antipsychotics have also been reported. In a 52-week study involving 85 elderly patients receiving quetiapine, the cumulative incidence of TD was 2.7%, which is much lower than typically reported with conventional antipsychotics.

Weight Gain

The clinical significance of weight gain as a side effect is often underestimated. Excessive weight puts patients at risk for coronary heart disease, hypertension, type 2 diabetes, and dyslipidemia. Most antipsychotic drugs cause some weight gain. Clozapine and olanzapine are associated with the greatest increase in weight. With clozapine, weight gain tends to peak during the first year of treatment. It continues, though at a slower rate, for at least another 3 years. Studies investigating olanzapine also indicate the same magnitude of drug-induced weight gain as with clozapine. The mean weight gain after 1 year was 26 pounds in patients treated with 15 ± 2.5 mg/d of olanzapine. In another double-blind long-term study of olanzapine and haloperidol, the average weight gain with olanzapine was 15 pounds within the first 39 weeks and then appeared to plateau thereafter for the next 2 or more years.

Patients treated with risperidone also gain weight, but not as much as those receiving clozapine or olanzapine. The mean weight gain in one study was 4.6 pounds after 10 weeks of treatment. In the North American trial of risperidone in patients with chronic schizophrenia, treatment resulted in only a 2.2- to 4.4-pound increase in weight. More recently, in a long-term double-blind comparison of risperidone and haloperidol, the average weight gain in risperidone-treated patients after 1 year was in the same range (5.1 pounds), which suggests that weight gain with risperidone plateaus at 10 weeks. Weight gain has also been associated with quetiapine. In a meta-analysis of conventional and novel antipsychotics, quetiapine was associated with a modest mean increase in weight, less than that reported for clozapine and olanzapine and similar to that associated with risperidone. In a large 1-year trial of quetiapine, patients experienced a mean weight gain of 4.9 pounds in the first 5 to 6 weeks of treatment, 4.1 pounds by 6 to 9 months, and 6.1 pounds at 9 to 12 months.

Elevated Glucose and Glucose Deregulation

It is not just weight gain per se that is problematic. Glucose deregulation and diabetes mellitus are increasingly being reported with some antipsychotics. Elevated fasting glucose levels were reported in 7 of 39 patients receiving olanzapine (18%) and 6 of 16 patients (38%) receiving clozapine. Olanzapine also induced new-onset diabetes in seven patients (six patients receiving 10 mg/d, 1 patient receiving 20 mg/d). New cases of diabetes mellitus have been reported in patients receiving olanzapine or clozapine. Interestingly, these patients had little or no weight gain, yet diabetes mellitus developed de novo, thus arguing for a direct effect of olanzapine and clozapine on glucose metabolism and insulin sensitivity. Antipsychotic-induced alterations in glucose regulation might exacerbate the pre-existing glucoregulatory disturbances associated with schizophrenia. The association with antipsychotic-induced diabetes may be a function of drug affinity for serotonin receptors, which are also involved in glucose homeostasis. Recent data confirm that certain antipsychotics can trigger clinically significantly altered glucose metabolism and diabetes and suggest that close monitoring for changes in blood glucose levels is warranted in some cases.

PHARMACOECONOMICS

Psychotic disorders such as schizophrenia are arguably the most serious and disabling psychiatric disorders. They are associated with substantial direct and indirect costs to society, estimated at over $65 billion annually. The annual cost of hospitalizing a single schizophrenic patient is at least $75,000. The government (federal and/or state) pays for 64% of the direct inpatient and outpatient treatment costs of schizophrenia. On any given day, over 100,000 schizophrenic patients are hospitalized, and one third of U.S. hospital beds are devoted to psychiatric illness. There are, of course, additional devastating personal consequences to the afflicted individuals and their families.

The direct costs of managing schizophrenia and related psychoses include primary medical treatments (e.g., inpatient psychiatric hospitalization and outpatient care) and secondary treatments in medical/surgical hospitals or emergency rooms (e.g., for injuries to self or others, concurrent medical problems, or side effects of treatment). Additional costs may also be encountered, such as those related to police, courts, and legal proceedings or imprisonment. The indirect costs, which are considerable, include an inability to work, loss of productivity, suicide, and dependence on others for food, shelter, and subsistence. The family burden of lost wages and caregivers' stress must also be considered. It is interesting to note that despite the availability of first-generation (conventional) antipsychotics since the mid-1950s, the annual cost of schizophrenia has continued to grow. This unexpected increase in cost has been attributed to poor compliance with treatment because of extrapyramidal side effects and other adverse effects associated with these agents. These adverse effects often lead to relapse and rehospitalization (the most expensive item among the direct costs).

The new generation of antipsychotics represents an incremental advance in improving the efficacy and safety of the treatment of psychotic disorders such as schizophrenia. The first-line second-generation antipsychotics risperidone, olanzapine, and quetiapine, as well as clozapine (for refractory patients), have all demonstrated broader efficacy, not only for positive symptoms but also for psychopathology domains such as negative, cognitive, and mood symptoms. Furthermore, newer antipsychotics are associated with fewer extrapyramidal side effects than seen with the older generation of antipsychotics, which has resulted in better compliance, fewer relapses, and improved outcomes (including fewer suicides and increased vocational and social reintegration).

One of the obstacles to the widespread use of antipsychotics, at least initially, has been drug cost, which has been perceived as high. The cost of an annual course of an antipsychotic ranges from $2000 for risperidone to $4000 for olanzapine. This expense stands in contrast to the $50 annual cost for a conventional drug such as haloperidol. However, it soon became apparent that the second-generation antipsychotics, with their broader efficacy and better tolerability, are associated with fewer relapses and dramatically fewer hospital days of care, which more than offset the cost of the medications. In fact, it takes only two or three fewer hospital days to offset the cost of a 1-year supply of a newer antipsychotic, and studies have shown an annual reduction of 10 to 15 hospital days per patient when newer antipsychotics were used instead of the older drugs. Thus, the cost of the second-generation antipsychotics, which represents only 5% of the annual direct cost of managing schizophrenia, has gradually been put in the proper perspective by health care delivery systems. The cost of enforcing compliance (e.g., with injectable depot haloperidol) is in fact equivalent to the cost of oral risperidone, yet without the broader efficacy on negative, cognitive, and other domains and with a 10-fold higher risk of extrapyramidal side effects and TD than with risperidone or other second-generation antipsychotics. As with other branches of medicine, psychiatry is now enjoying an era of safer and more efficacious drugs for severe diseases such as schizophrenia, and these superior drugs are proving to be cost-effective.

Many published studies have documented the cost-effectiveness of antipsychotics by comparing the expenditures per patient before and after conversion from the first-generation to the second-generation antipsychotics. Significant reductions in costs were noted by several studies, primarily as a result of decreased relapse rates and fewer days of hospital care. Studies with clozapine have shown a marked reduction in the care of treatment-refractory patients with chronic schizophrenia who could not even be discharged from the institutional setting before the availability of clozapine. In addition, several studies with risperidone in chronic schizophrenia patients have demonstrated significant reductions in the overall cost of managing psychosis. Similar results from studies with olanzapine and quetiapine are also emerging. However, variations in the per-day cost of medication have been encountered among the newer antipsychotics, with risperidone and quetiapine showing the lowest and olanzapine showing the highest direct medication costs at the mean daily doses used in outpatient or inpatient settings.

REFERENCES

1. Kane J, Honigfeld G, Singer J, Meltzer H: Clozapine for the treatment-resistant schizophrenic: A double-blind comparison with chlorpromazine. Arch Gen Psychiatry 45:789–796, 1988.

2. Bondolfi G, Dufour H, Patris M, et al: Risperidone versus clozapine in treatment-resistant chronic schizophrenia: A randomized double-blind study. The Risperidone Study Group. Am J Psychiatry 155:499–504, 1998.
3. Breier AF, Malhotra AK, Su TP, et al: Clozapine and risperidone in chronic schizophrenia: Effects on symptoms, parkinsonian side effects, and neuroendocrine response. Am J Psychiatry 156:294–298, 1999.
4. Wirshing DA, Marshall BD Jr, Green MF, et al: Risperidone in treatment-refractory schizophrenia. Am J Psychiatry 156:1374–1379, 1999.
5. Breier A, Hamilton SH: Comparative efficacy of olanzapine and haloperidol for patients with treatment-resistant schizophrenia. Biol Psychiatry 45:403–411, 1999.
6. Sanders RD, Mossman D: An open trial of olanzapine in patients with treatment-refractory psychoses. J Clin Psychopharmacol 19:62–66, 1999.

PANIC DISORDER

method of
JACQUES BRADWEJN, M.D., and
DIANA KOSZYCKI, PH.D.
Royal Ottawa Hospital and University of Ottawa
Ottawa, Ontario, Canada

Panic disorder is an anxiety syndrome that is characterized by the presence of recurrent unexpected panic attacks and anticipatory fear of future attacks. Panic attacks, which are the hallmark of panic disorder, are discrete episodes of intense anxiety accompanied by somatic, psychosensorial, and cognitive symptoms. Although panic attacks most often occur unexpectedly, especially in the early stages of the illness, as panic attacks continue to occur, certain situations that have become associated with having a panic attack may also trigger an attack. These types of attacks are called *situational panic attacks*. In some patients, situational panic attacks become the main form of attacks that are experienced. Symptoms frequently experienced during a panic attack are listed in Table 1. By convention, diagnostic criteria for a panic attack are met when symptoms start abruptly, reach a peak very quickly (within 10 minutes), and include at least four symptoms. If fewer than four symptoms occur during an attack, it is called a *limited-symptom attack*. Most patients who experience full-blown panic attacks also suffer from these milder forms of panic. Usually they include only one or two physical symptoms, such as shortness of breath or palpitations, that occur suddenly and for no apparent reason. Panic disorder is often accompanied by agoraphobia, which is characterized by fear and avoidance of situations or places where the dreaded panic may occur. Broadly, these include situations where help may not be readily available in the event of an attack (e.g., being far away from home, being alone), where escape may be difficult in the event of an attack (e.g., elevators, tunnels, public transportation), and where it may be embarrassing to panic (e.g., participating in a meeting). The symptom progression of panic disorder is shown in Table 2.

TABLE 1. **Symptoms Used in the Diagnosis of Panic Attacks**

A panic attack must have an abrupt onset and a rapid crescendo and include at least four of these symptoms:
Palpitations, pounding, or accelerated heart rate
Sweating
Trembling or shaking
Shortness of breath or smothering sensation
Choking sensation
Chest pain or discomfort
Nausea or abdominal distress
Feeling dizzy, unsteady, lightheaded, or faint
Depersonalization (being detached from onself) or derealization (feeling of unreality)
Paresthesia
Chills or hot flushes
Fear of losing control or "going crazy"
Fear of dying

TABLE 2. **Symptom Progression of Panic Disorder**

Recurrent, unexpected panic attacks
↓
Anticipatory fear of future attacks (*anticipatory anxiety* or "fear of fear")
↓
Avoidance of situations in which the feared panic may occur (*agoraphobia*)
↓
Complications: disability, depression, substance abuse

EPIDEMIOLOGY

Panic disorder is common, with a lifetime prevalence of 3.5%. As many as 10% of the population report occasional unexpected panic attacks without meeting full criteria for the disorder. Panic disorder tends to have an early age at onset and a female-to-male ratio of about 2:1. Panic disorder is among the most common presenting problem for people seeking psychiatric treatment and the fifth most common complaint brought to the attention of primary care physicians. Naturalistic follow-up studies indicate that panic disorder is a generally chronic condition with a longitudinal course marked by periods of remission and relapses of varying degrees. Although the number of panic attacks vary from person to person, it is typical to experience one to two attacks a week before seeking treatment. Many patients report that during their worst periods, they can experience panic attacks every day or at least several times a week. Panic disorder, with or without agoraphobia, is associated with high rates of co-morbidity, including depression, alcohol abuse, and another anxiety disorder. Panic disorder has a significant negative impact on social and occupational function and results in high utilization of health care resources and dependence on social welfare. Such data verify that panic disorder is a serious psychiatric illness with tragic costs to the individual, the family, and society.

ETIOLOGY

The cause of panic disorder is still unknown, but most experts agree that multiple factors play a role. Family and twin studies implicate genetic factors, although the mode of inheritance and the specific gene involved remain unknown. Psychological traits with a genetic influence such as anxiety sensitivity, behavioral inhibition, introversion, and neuroticism have also been associated with increased risk for developing panic disorder. Functional and structural brain-imaging studies have found that patients with panic disorder have abnormalities in regions around the hippocampus and other limbic areas. Studies employing pharmacologic probes that provoke or block panic attacks have identified dysregulations in several neurotransmitter-receptor systems, including norepinephrine, serotonin, adenosine, the γ-aminobutyric acid (GABA)-benzodiazepine receptor complex, and several neuropeptide systems. Among the neuropeptides, the involvement of cholecystokinin in the pathophysiology of anxiety and panic has attracted a great deal of interest. Maladaptive cognitions, particularly a tendency to appraise the symptoms of anxiety as being dangerous, have also been implicated in the pathophysiology of panic disorder.

DIAGNOSTIC ASSESSMENT

According to the *Diagnostic and Statistical Manual of Mental Disorders*, fourth edition (DSM-IV), panic disorder is diagnosed if the following three conditions are met:

1. The patient experiences recurrent unexpected panic attacks and either in 1 month worries about subsequent attacks, worries about the implication of the attack, or has a significant change in behavior related to the attacks
2. The attacks are not due to a general medical condition or substance
3. The symptoms are not better accounted for by another mental disorder

Recognition of panic disorder can be difficult. Because of the somatic nature of panic attacks patients will present to hospital emergency departments or to their primary care physician convinced that they are suffering from a serious medical condition. Typically, patients focus on one or two unexplained somatic symptoms that they find alarming and minimize other anxiety symptoms. Failure to recognize that these unexplained somatic symptoms occur with many other symptoms in the context of a panic attack can lead to misdiagnosis and inappropriate intervention. One consequence of an undiagnosed and untreated panic disorder is that patients continue to search for a medical explanation for their unexplained symptoms, with frequent visits to primary care physicians and medical specialists and costly and unnecessary medical tests.

Successful diagnosis of panic disorder depends on the following:

1. Recognition of panic attacks, their recurrence, and complications
2. Familiarity with the diagnostic boundaries of panic disorder and other anxiety syndromes
3. Evaluation of medical conditions that can mimic panic symptoms; this includes hypoglycemia, hyperthyroidism, hyperparathyroidism, pheochromocytoma, seizure disorders, cardiac conditions, and vestibular system dysfunction
4. Evaluation of substances (drugs of abuse or medications) that can mimic panic symptoms; this includes intoxication with central nervous system (CNS) stimulants (cocaine, caffeine, amphetamines) or cannabis, and withdrawal from CNS depressants (alcohol, barbiturates) and benzodiazepines

In short, recognition of panic disorder depends on a good knowledge of the key symptoms of this disorder, a detailed history including determination of the temporal evolution of symptoms, and evaluation of disease or substances in the etiology of panic symptoms. This detailed history should be complemented by a medical examination including laboratory tests aimed at excluding a general medical condition or substance use to illness onset. At a minimum, laboratory tests should include an electrocardiogram and thyroid function test. An electroencephalogram should be performed on patients who experience marked psychosensorial symptoms (i.e., depersonalization or derealization). This complete evaluation will enable the physician to confirm a diagnosis of panic disorder.

TREATMENT

Current approaches for treating the core symptoms of panic disorder include psychotherapy and pharmacotherapy. Among the psychological interventions, cognitive behavior therapy (CBT) is the most effective. A limitation of CBT is a lack of accessibility to trained therapists, especially in rural areas. Pharmacotherapy is universally available through family physicians and for many represents the first choice of treatment. A limitation of medications is that they can produce unpleasant side effects that can affect compliance with treatment. Because patients suffering from panic disorder tend to report more side effects and be more distressed by them than patients with other psychiatric disorders, adherence to treatment recommendations and compliance with medications are significant treatment issues.

Patient Education

Irrespective of choice of treatment, patient education (also known as psychoeducation) is an important component of the therapeutic process. After a review of the symptoms the patient should be informed that he or she suffers from a condition called panic disorder, and that the unexplained physical symptoms being experienced (e.g., increased heart rate, difficulty breathing, sweating, dizziness) are panic attacks and part of the clinical picture of panic disorder. Patients should be told that they do not have a serious medical condition but that some laboratory tests will be carried out to ensure that there is no specific physical cause for their anxiety symptoms. This information not only reassures the patient but also instills a sense of confidence in the physician, which has important implications for treatment compliance. Once the diagnosis of panic disorder is confirmed the patient should be given general information about panic disorder, including its evolution, epidemiology, etiology, and treatment. Patients should be encouraged to educate themselves about their illness. Information about panic disorder can be obtained from a variety of sources, including self-help books, the Internet, or through organizations such as the National Institute of Mental Health or the World Health Organization. Treatment can then be discussed and agreed upon. The goals of treatment should be spelled out. Patients should be informed that panic disorder is a treatable condition but that chronic treatment is often necessary. For many patients, especially those who do not suffer from severe complications of major depression or substance abuse, goals of complete remission (absence of panic attacks, anticipatory anxiety, and agoraphobia) are appropriate and obtainable. This information should

TABLE 3. **Medications for the Treatment of Panic Disorder**

Drug Class	Drug	Dosage Range
Selective serotonin reuptake inhibitor	Fluoxetine (Prozac)*	5–40 mg/d
	Fluvoxamine (Luvox)*	25–150 mg/d
	Paroxetine (Paxil)	10–60 mg/d
	Sertraline (Zoloft)	50–200 mg/d
Tricyclic antidepressant	Clomipramine (Anafranil)*	25–250 mg/d
	Desipramine (Norpramin)*	25–200 mg/d
	Imipramine (Tofranil)*	25–300 mg/d
Benzodiazepine	Alprazolam (Xanax)	1.5–6 mg/d
	Clonazepam (Klonopin)*	1.5–6 mg/d
Monoamine oxidase inhibitor	Phenelzine (Nardil)*	30–90 mg/d

*Not FDA approved for this indication.

be conveyed to patients, and they should be instructed to monitor the frequency and intensity of their symptoms by the use of mental notes or symptom diaries. This helps them understand that a goal of wellness can be aimed for and worked toward.

Pharmacotherapy

Presently, based on efficacy and side effect profiles, the order of use of medication is as follows. Selective serotonin reuptake inhibitors (SSRIs) are used as standard first-line agents followed by tricyclic antidepressants (TCAs)* and benzodiazepines as second- and third-line agents, respectively. In treatment-refractory patients a monoamine oxidase inhibitor may be used. Table 3 describes pharmacotherapeutic agents used in the treatment of panic disorder. Although benzodiazepines have been among the most widely prescribed medicines for panic disorder, problems with sedation, cognitive impairment, and dependence and withdrawal have led to recommendations that their use as a first-line monotherapy be limited. Benzodiazepines may be co-prescribed with an SSRI or a TCA for a time-limited period to decrease symptoms during the treatment period preceding the delayed onset of action of antidepressants. Proper use of first-line medications is often sufficient. SSRIs as well as TCAs should be started at low dosage and increased progressively over a period of 6 to 8 weeks to a therapeutic dosage. Once therapeutic dosage is reached, a trial period of treatment of 4 to 6 weeks is reasonable. Monitoring of symptoms and side effects with the help of the patient's mental or written notes will determine whether the therapeutic goal of remission (zero panic attacks) is achieved. Once this goal is achieved a continuation of treatment for 8 to 12 months is often recommended. However, this is based on clinical consensus rather than hard scientific data. After 8 to 12 months of treatment an attempt can be made to taper medication to determine whether a longer course of treatment is required. Some patients can decrease and even stop medication without experiencing a relapse of symptoms. A majority of patients, however, will require long-term pharmacotherapy to remain symptom free. In short, successful treatment with pharmacotherapy depends on a systematic approach consisting of the following:

1. An order of choice (first-line, second-line, third-line medications)
2. Proper initiation of medication by starting at very low dosages and increasing slowly
3. Optimization of dosage to ensure that a therapeutic dose is achieved

The following sentence can be used to explain the pharmacotherapeutic process to patients: "We start low, go slow, but aim for sufficient."

*Not FDA approved for this indication.

Cognitive Behavior Therapy

CBT can be used alone successfully with many patients suffering from panic disorder, especially if their symptomatology is mild and not complicated. CBT focuses on the role of catastrophic cognitions and fear of anxiety sensations in the psychogenesis and maintenance of panic disorder and associated phobic avoidance. It is a time-limited (i.e., 12 to 16 weekly sessions) manualized treatment that typically includes combinations of strategies such as psychoeducation, symptom monitoring, breathing and relaxation training, cognitive restructuring, and exposure that targets the elimination of fear of anxiety sensations and the associated anticipatory anxiety, vigilance, and avoidance that accompany these fears. Factors associated with good response to CBT include patient perception of therapy as credible, regular attendance of therapy sessions, compliance with homework assignments, and an ability to tolerate some degree of discomfort during exposure exercises. Controlled clinical trials suggest that a high percentage of patients achieve a panic-free state after acute treatment with CBT, with outcome being as good as that obtained with medication. However, follow-up studies have shown that episodic exacerbations of panic symptoms remain after treatment, particularly in patients with a greater severity of illness before treatment onset. Combined CBT and pharmacotherapy may be useful for severely ill patients. A combination of CBT and medications has been found to improve the long-term outcome of panic disorder and reduce relapse after medication discontinuation.

Section 17

Physical and Chemical Injuries

BURN INJURY

method of
JOHN T. SCHULZ III, M.D., PH.D.
Massachusetts General Hospital
Boston, Massachusetts

Despite significant progress in the past 30 years in the care of burned patients, burn injury remains a significant source of morbidity and mortality. Every year 1.5 to 2 million people in the United States are burned. Most can be cared for as outpatients, but up to 100,000 per year require hospitalization. Some are extremely ill and 3000 to 5000 die yearly as a direct consequence of their burn.

Burn care is aimed at saving life, when possible, and at returning burned patients back to their families and to their work. To accomplish this task, the burn center employs surgeons and critical care specialists, dedicated burn nurses, nutritionists, occupational and physical therapists, social workers, psychiatrists, and pastoral care specialists. All of these disciplines are required for the optimal treatment of the broadest range of burned patients.

DEFINITIONS

The terms/acronyms below are widely used and deserve precise definition for the discussion that follows.

- Total body surface area (TBSA): in addition to depth, burn injuries are described in terms of their extent, TBSA, involved in a particular patient. Areas of involvement are approximated in adults by the "rule of 9s" (9% TBSA for each upper extremity, 18% TBSA for each lower extremity, 36% TBSA for the torso, 9% TBSA for the head and neck). For children, the calculation varies with age. A simple rule of thumb is that the surface area of the patient's palm (no fingers) is approximately 1% TBSA.
- *First-degree burn*: a burn that involves the epidermis and does not kill the basal layer of keratinocytes. Dermis is not exposed.
- *Second-degree burn*: a burn that destroys all layers of the epidermis, and from very little to most of the underlying dermis. This classification encompasses a wide range of injury: from a superficial second-degree burn that kills the epidermis and superficially injures the dermis to a deep second-degree burn that kills most of the dermis. The term *partial thickness*, modified as *superficial*, *mid-dermal*, or *deep* is more accurate. A superficial partial-thickness wound heals within days. A deep partial-thickness burn must be excised and grafted like a third-degree burn. All second-degree injuries destroy the epidermis and its barriers to infection, fluid loss, and heat loss. Second-degree burns are usually very painful on exposure to air. They are tender to touch and manipulation. If superficial, they demonstrate blanching with digital or swab pressure.
- *Third-degree burn*: full-thickness skin injury—epidermis and dermis. Burns of this depth do not cause the pain seen in second-degree injuries, because all of the cutaneous sensory nerves in the injured area are destroyed. These areas are insensate to light touch and do not blanch.
- *Fourth-degree burn*: injury extends through the skin into the tissue beneath the dermis (subcutaneous fat, fascia, muscle, bone).
- *Eschar*: dead tissue produced by burn injury.
- *Topical antimicrobial*: substance applied topically to burn eschar to reduce microbial contamination and, consequently, the risk of invasive burn wound infection. Silver sulfadiazene, mafenide acetate, silver nitrate, Acticoat, and collegenase/polysporin are commonly used in the United States. Silver sulfadiazene (Silvadene, Thermazine) is used widely on outpatients and inpatients. It is weaker against *Pseudomonas aeruginosa* than the alternatives. Mafenide acetate (Sulfamylon) is available as a cream or as a solution. It is the only topical agent that penetrates eschar and is consequently used on burned cartilaginous structures (nose, ear). It is weaker against *Staphylococcus* than the alternatives. Silver nitrate (silver ions) kills all bacteria and fungi. Acticoat is a solid-phase fabric that dispenses silver ions.
- *Healing*: denotes epithelialization of the wound with restoration of the epidermal barrier functions. Partial-thickness wounds in which significant dermis remains can heal by expansion of keratinocytes in the epidermal appendages (eccrine and apocrine sweat glands, sebaceous glands, hair follicles). In third-degree burns, the only source of keratinocytes for re-epithelialization is the periphery of the wound. If very small, such wounds can heal by sloughing of the full-thickness eschar, elaboration and contraction of granulation tissue, scar formation, and scar epithelialization. Peripheral keratinocytes can only migrate a few millimeters onto a wound, however, making it unlikely that a full-

thickness wound greater than a few square centimeters in size will heal primarily, even with 90% contraction of the wound bed. For deep partial-thickness wounds, there is insufficient dermis to abrogate granulation (with contraction and scarring) and too few epidermal appendages to promote epithelial regeneration. Consequently, skin grafting is required for deep partial-thickness and third-degree wounds. The standard of care in the United States is to excise and graft any burn wound that is judged unlikely to heal within 3 weeks. For patients with large TBSA burns, the standard of care is operative elimination of burn eschar and coverage with skin grafts or skin substitutes as promptly as possible after acute resuscitation.

- *Escharotomy*: incision through burned skin into subcutaneous tissue. This incision is used to release the tourniquet effect of noncompliant burned skin surrounding an extremity, trunk, or neck in which subcutaneous tissue is filling with edema fluid. It is usually performed with electrocautery.

ACUTE CARE OF THE BURNED PATIENT

Thermal energy denatures protein, causing coagulative necrosis of the skin. Depth of injury is directly related to the temperature and heat index of the agent of injury and to its contact time with the skin and is inversely related to the heat dispersement capability of the skin.

The systemic effect of a patient's burn depends on the TBSA burned (second- plus third-degree burns). In the absence of smoke inhalation injury, otherwise healthy patients with less than 20% TBSA burns are unlikely to become critically ill. Patients with burns between 20% and 40% TBSA are at risk for developing systemic inflammatory response syndrome. Patients with burns of 40% or more TBSA all suffer a profound inflammatory response syndrome accompanied by a diffuse capillary leak in the first 24 hours after injury. These large burns are also accompanied by a persistent hypermetabolic state characterized by increased energy expenditure and muscle wasting despite adequate calorie nutrition.

Transfer Criteria

Guidelines for transfer of a burn patient to a burn center have been developed by the American Burn Association (Table 1).

Patients with burns to the face, hands, feet, perineum, or major joints should be sent to a burn center, whatever the burn size. The reason for triage is that a multidisciplinary approach is necessary to optimize function and cosmesis after burns in these areas (e.g., a patient with partial-thickness burns to the hand and fingers needs to begin occupational therapy immediately under the supervision of a therapist experienced in burn care).

TABLE 1. **American Burn Association Transfer Criteria**

≥10% Total body surface area with second- and third-degree burns in child younger than 10 or adult older than 50
≥20% Total body surface area with second- and third-degree burns in other age groups
Second- and third-degree burns involving face, genitalia, hands, feet, perineum, or major joints
Third-degree burns more than 5% total body surface area in any age group
Electrical burns including lightning injury
Chemical burns
Burns in patients with co-morbidities that could affect management, recovery, or mortality
Patients with concomitant burns and trauma in which the burn is the most significant aspect of injury. Trauma must be evaluated before transfer.
Children should be transferred to a facility with pediatric capabilities
All socially complicated admissions (e.g., when spousal, child, or substance abuse is suspected in the etiology of the burn)

Outpatient Acute Care

Patients with small burns far outnumber those with larger injuries. Many of those with small burns can be cared for as outpatients, and some can be managed in a primary care setting. Wounds in patients that do not meet transfer criteria should be cleansed with sterile saline. Loose epithelium from ruptured blisters should be sharply débrided. If there are intact blisters on a wound that do not appear fragile, they should be left in place as a sterile and painless dressing. Once cleansed and débrided, the wound should be covered with a topical antimicrobial (Acticoat, Silvadene, or Sulfamylon; bacitracin only for very superficial wounds) and dressed with sterile gauze. The dressing should be changed twice daily (less frequently with Acticoat). Most outpatients require a visiting nurse.

Adequate analgesia for dressing changes is essential. Even when there are concerns about abuse potential, opiates are required for adequate analgesia during dressing changes on a partial thickness burn larger than a few square centimeters. Once the burn wound is healed, opiates can be weaned. Newly healed epithelium should be mechanically protected by a dressing for 1 to 2 weeks after full epithelialization, because it is fragile and will blister easily. The patient should be counseled to apply emollients to the healed burn several times per day and to protect any exposed areas with a sunscreen with a high sun protective factor. Itching in the convalescent period can be controlled with antihistamines. Patients who continue to have severe itching or pain in a healed burn long after the wound is epithelialized (chronic pain is fairly common and often neuropathic in origin) should be referred to a burn center.

Wounds are examined periodically until an estimate of depth can be made. Patients with wounds too deep or extensive to heal within 3 or 4 weeks should be seen by a burn surgeon.

Outpatient care may fail due to inadequate analgesia with oral opiates, lack of adequate wound hygiene, failure of family coping mechanisms, and burn wound infection. In such cases the patient should be referred to a burn center for inpatient management.

Large Burn Injuries

The seriously burned patient is approached like other victims of major trauma with special consideration for unique aspects of burn injury.

First, as complete and accurate a history as possible should be obtained and documented, including the circumstances of and mechanism of the burn, the patient's level of consciousness when found, possible associated trauma mechanisms (e.g., a fall, being thrown by an explosion), and the patient's past medical problems, medications, and allergies. Simultaneously, the first caregiver must address the ABCs of **a**irway, **b**reathing, and **c**irculation emphasized in the American College of Surgeons' Trauma Life Support algorithms.

Airway

The patient must have a stable and effective airway. Significant face and neck burns are often accompanied by sufficient hypopharyngeal swelling to occlude the glottis, as are large burn injuries (>35%–40% TBSA), which evoke diffuse capillary leak. Smoke inhalation and carbon monoxide intoxication can depress the level of consciousness and/or elicit airway edema that threatens the airway. Finally, toddlers are at risk of direct scalds to the hypopharynx when they pull hot liquids down onto themselves. Thus, those with burns to the face and neck, as well as those with larger burns of any distribution should be intubated for airway protection unless they are clearly nonstridorous, alert, have no stigmata of smoke inhalation (soot in pharynx, singed facial hair, burned lips and tongue, history of being rescued from a closed, smoke-filled space), and do not have excessive work of breathing. Finally, *any doubt* about the adequacy or future stability of a patient's airway before transport to a burn center should prompt intubation of the patient.

A patient with a large burn, or face and neck burns, who is not intubated should undergo an airway watch in an intensive care unit for at least the first 24 hours after admission. Caregivers must be sure that all tools necessary for intubation and for establishing an emergent surgical airway are at the bedside (including temporizing equipment: appropriate-sized masks for bag ventilation, angiocaths suitable for needle cricothyroidotomy).

Breathing

Once the airway is secure, the patient must have appropriate ventilatory support. In those without premorbid pulmonary problems, smoke inhalation injury, or excessive sedation, pressure support ventilation is usually adequate. Assist-control ventilation (pressure or volume limited) is necessary for the very sedated patient. Those with premorbid or smoke-induced bronchospasm require treatment with bronchodilators. Both pulmonary third spacing of resuscitation fluid and the rigidity of burned truncal skin encircling a subcutaneous space with increasing hydrostatic pressure from edema may significantly decrease pulmonary/chest wall compliance. If the problem is one of restrictive truncal eschar, escharotomy must be performed promptly (minimum acceptable is a bilateral midaxillary incision from axilla to costal margin, connected with two transverse anterior incisions at the costal margin and manubriosternal junction). Finally, chemical paralysis may be necessary to achieve adequate compliance for gas exchange.

Circulation

Adequate circulation must be ensured by fluid resuscitation. Large burns evoke a profound capillary leak syndrome. To support circulation in the face of this sieving effect, *warm* crystalloid is administered in direct proportion to the patient's weight and TBSA burn. The Modified Brook/Parkland Formula (2–4 mL/kg/percent TBSA burn given over 24 hours: one half is given in the first 8 hours, and the remainder is given over the next 16 hours) is used as a starting point for resuscitation with the endpoints being the signs of adequate end organ perfusion listed in Table 2. More than predicted volume may be required in patients with smoke inhalation injury and in those who present with alcohol intoxication.

Peripheral access can be used in a patient with one or more unburned extremities, but central venous access, which provides a route for fluid and medication infusion, blood sampling, and measurement of central venous pressure, is better. Mechanical ventilation is an indication for arterial access, which should be obtained peripherally, if possible (particularly in children, femoral access poses a significant risk of thrombosis and limb loss). All lines should be placed through unburned skin, if possible.

Secondary Survey

Once airway, breathing, and circulation are secured, the secondary survey should be done, including full examination, placement of orogastric/nasogastric (in intubated patients) and urinary catheters. If urine output is sluggish (<0.5 mL/kg/h in adults) and does not respond to increased resuscitation, a pulmonary artery catheter should be considered. Appropriate trauma workup, if indicated, should follow. Any limb that is circumferentially burned should be assessed often for distal perfusion. If there is circulatory compromise, or concern that the limb is becom-

TABLE 2. **Endpoints of Resuscitation**

Urine output 0.5 mL/kg/h in adult; 1–2 mL/kg/h in children
Alert sensorium
Base deficit less than 2
Blood pressure within normal limits for age (systolic blood pressure 90 mm Hg + 2 × age in years for small children)

ing tight as resuscitation continues, escharotomies should be performed with electrocautery (particularly for the hands, feet, forelegs, and forearms as well as sometimes for the neck and the trunk).

In the first 24 hours, fluid resuscitation with crystalloid should be ongoing, urine output should be closely monitored, and the patient should be adequately medicated with amnestics (e.g., benzodiazepines) and opiates (for an intubated adult with a large burn this means the equivalent of 10 to 25 mg of morphine per hour by continuous infusion). Other considerations include prophylaxis for gastric mucosal ulceration with H_2 blockade or equivalent, plans for nutrition through enteral or parenteral routes and deep venous thrombosis prophylaxis with low-molecular-weight heparin.

Finally, patients with large burns lose heat rapidly. Maintenance of normothermia in these patients requires a warm environment (>90°F) and infusion of prewarmed fluids. Before patient transfer, dry gauze dressings are used, because wet dressings increase evaporative heat loss.

Wound Care and Closure

Wounds That Do Not Require Operative Closure. One disadvantage of topical antimicrobial treatment of superficial burn wounds is the pain associated with dressing changes (although for Acticoat the dressing can be at longer intervals, 2 to 4 days for outpatients). A less painful alternative for clean wounds is application of an alloplastic dressing. These dressings share the properties of protecting the wound from contact with air (painful) and from contact with exogenous microbes. Porcine xenograft, nonviable cryopreserved pigskin, provides an effective cover for superficial wounds and vastly reduces the pain of these wounds. A new product, Transcyte, which consists of a bilaminate collagen/nonviable fibroblast/nylon mesh inner layer and a Silastic, selectively permeable, outer layer functions like xenograft and provides a cocktail of fibroblast growth factors that may augment healing. Biobrane, another bilaminate, is sometimes used on superficial partial-thickness wounds.

Alloplastic dressings must be applied to a clean, noninfected wound and examined daily to rule out wound infection. If a patient develops a significant fever after application, the alloplastic material should be removed because these materials effectively trap bacteria onto the wound. Healing beneath the alloplastic dressing occurs by regeneration of the epidermis from epithelial cells in the epidermal appendages of the unburned dermis. Once the epidermis reaches confluence, the alloplastic dressing is easily removed.

Skin Grafting. Patients with burn wounds that will not heal primarily are taken to the operating room, where burn eschar is excised and the resulting wound (which must be well vascularized and free of necrotic material) is closed with autologous split-thickness skin grafts harvested from the patient's unburned skin with dermatomes. Skin grafts can be applied as sheets (typical in patients with small burns and burns to forearm, hand, or face) or meshed and expanded to reduce the necessary donor area. Once the skin grafting procedure is performed, the donor sites are dressed and the newly grafted areas are covered with a dressing that is left in place for 5 to 10 days.

Alternatives to Autologous Skin Grafts. Autologous split-thickness skin grafts are the standard of care, but alternatives are used under specific circumstances. For the patient with large burns and insufficient donor skin to provide coverage, grafting with cadaveric split-thickness skin grafts (allograft, homograft) is often performed. Patients with large burns are somewhat immunosuppressed and accept the allotransplant for 1 or more weeks before rejecting the allokeratinocytes. Allograft provides temporary wound closure while epidermis of donor sites regenerates. Another alternative for patients with limited donor site is Integra, a dermal regeneration matrix (a bilaminate of inner bovine collagen/glycosaminoglycan sponge and outer Silastic sheeting of defined microporosity). Integra is placed on a noncontaminated excised wound bed and left in place for 2 to 3 weeks. During that time, fibroblasts move from the wound bed into the collagen/glycosaminoglycan sponge and replace it with a vascularized "neodermis." Once the neodermis is mature (2 to 3 weeks), the outer layer can be removed and the neodermis covered with ultrathin (1–4/1000 inch) autologous split-thickness skin grafts.

SPECIAL TOPICS

Smoke Inhalation Injury

Smoke inhalation injury contributes substantially to morbidity and mortality in burned patients. Elements of the history consistent with smoke inhalation include flame burns to the face and neck, extensive upper body burns, extensive whole-body flame burns, and being found in a smoke-filled closed space. Physical stigmata of smoke inhalation include singed facial and nasal hair, soot in the oropharynx, and stridor. For the conscious patient who is suspected of having a smoke inhalation injury, endotracheal intubation for airway protection is advisable; if it is not performed, the patient must be watched in an intensive care unit overnight.

Once a patient suspected of inhalation injury is intubated, fiberoptic bronchoscopy should be performed. Carbonaceous material in the airway is diagnostic, but its absence does not exclude inhalation injury because many toxic components of smoke are nonparticulate. No lavage of carbonaceous material should be attempted because this may wash toxins distally. Within 2 to 4 days after smoke inhalation, the carbon, with or without sloughed mucosa, will begin to mobilize in secretions. Corticosteroids have no place in therapy.

Carbon monoxide (carboxyhemoglobin) should be measured in any patient with suspected smoke inhalation. If the value is higher than 20% to 25%, hyperbaric oxygen therapy (i.e., "dive") should be considered, because there are some data that this improves neuropsychiatric outcome. This therapy is usually only safe for the patient who is not otherwise critically ill. Those with carbon monoxide intoxication who are too unstable for a dive should be maintained on 100% inspired oxygen for at least 12 hours.

Manifestation of insult to the lungs is delayed, with peak incidence of onset 5 days after the burn injury. At this time, some patients exhibit a rapid deterioration in gas exchange and lung compliance, with diffuse interstitial infiltrates on chest radiography. Such patients are managed supportively. Extracorporeal membrane oxygenation has not been successful in patients with severe burns because of bleeding complications. Patients with such a dramatic pulmonary decompensation are less frequent than those in whom smoke inhalation promotes ongoing bacterial pneumonitis. Staphylococcal and pseudomonal infections are common in this group of patients. Useful techniques in care are bronchoalveolar lavage to assist with pulmonary toilet and pressure-limited ventilation to control peak airway pressures.

Nutrition

Adequate calorie nutrition is essential. If possible, critically ill patients should be fed enterally to maintain the health of the enteral mucosa with its microbial barrier function. Enterocytes preferentially use glutamine as a nutrient and there is some evidence that glutamine supplementation improves outcome in trauma patients. Hence, it is reasonable to provide enteral glutamine supplements. Care should be exercised in giving enteral feedings to very sick patients with no bowel sounds. Tube-feed bezoars and accompanying peritoneal sepsis have caused the death of several burn and trauma patients in recent years. In patients who do not tolerate gastric feedings, a transpyloric feeding tube can be placed. Prokinetic agents, metoclopramide (Reglan), or erythromycin,* are sometimes useful. Parenteral nutrition should be given to those who do not tolerate tube feedings.

The large burn injury is accompanied by increased basal energy expenditure (1.5–2 times normal) and by muscle wasting despite provision of adequate calories. Patients with large burns should receive 2.5 g of protein/kg/d and sufficient calories to meet their hypermetabolic needs. Patients with smaller burns need adequate nutrition as well and should receive liquid supplements orally or by feeding tube if they are not eating enough.

Infection

The burn wound leaves the patient vulnerable to invasive infection in the burn eschar and surrounding tissue; smoke inhalation creates vulnerability to pulmonary infection by impairing mucosal defense; burns larger than 40% TBSA are invariably accompanied by some element of immunosuppression; and the techniques used to support the critically ill impose risk of iatrogenic infection. Nonetheless, it has been proven that prophylactic antibiotics are of no use (distinct from topical antimicrobials, which are mandatory). Cultures are sent for significant fever or new hemodynamic instability. Antibiotics are administered based on culture results. If a patient's condition is clinically worsening, empirical antibiotics are administered until culture results are back.

Gram-positive infections in newly healed burns can rapidly destroy the new epithelium. Such "infestations" usually respond to antibiotics and topical mupiricin.

Tetanus toxoid boosters should be given on admission. If there is not a clear history of adequate immunization, passive immunization should be performed.

Electrical Burns

Current at less than 1000 volts produces localized skin injuries. More than 1000 volts produces an injury to the skin at entry and exit points and severe injury to deep neuromuscular and skeletal components along the path of the current though the victim. Injury to deep structures probably results from electroporation (laceration of cell membranes) and heat generated by passage of current through bone, which is a powerful resistor. The extremity with clear evidence of severe entry or exit wound should undergo fasciotomy up to the level where the muscle compartments are flaccid to prevent compartment syndrome and limb loss. These wounds must be examined daily or every other day in the operating room and débrided as tissue dies, to prevent progressive microbial myositis and myonecrosis. Serum creatine kinase should be monitored in these patients; and, if elevated, a brisk alkaline diuresis should be maintained to prevent acute renal failure. Radiographic studies sufficient to rule out fractures caused by tetanic contractions should be obtained.

Chemical and Tar Burns

Hot tar sticks to skin. It should be removed with an oil-based emollient, such as petrolatum or bacitracin. Subsequently, the wound should be cared for like any thermal burn.

Acid and alkali burns should be lavaged with lukewarm water for 30 minutes (acid) or 1 hour (alkali). Neutralization should not be attempted because it generates heat, which can further burn the skin. Topical antimicrobial dressings should be applied after adequate lavage.

Hydrofluoric acid is deadly. It is a weak acid and only slowly produces a skin burn, but it is soluble in tissue and the fluoride ion rapidly binds free calcium ion. A few milliliters of concentrated hydrofluoric acid is sufficient to bind all the free calcium in a 70-kg man. The result is refractory arrhythmia, asystole, and death. Victims of hydrofluoric acid contact

*Not FDA approved for this indication.

should be taken to a burn center immediately. Serum ionized calcium should be measured frequently and supplemented as necessary. Cutaneous areas of contact should be infiltrated subcutaneously with 5% to 10% calcium gluconate per square centimeter. Patients should remain monitored in an intensive care unit until their serum calcium level normalizes.

Petroleum distillates (gasoline, jet fuel) cause cutaneous contact burns and have systemic toxicity. Victims of contact must have all clothing removed and affected skin lavaged with water for 30 to 60 minutes. Wounds should then be treated with topical antimicrobial dressings.

Rehabilitation

Attention to rehabilitation needs must start immediately. Critically ill patients should be splinted in safe positions and moved through range of motion daily to prevent contractures. Range of motion exercises should be passive and active as the patient becomes able to participate in therapy. Once ready to leave the intensive care unit, the patient should be mobilized into a chair and rapidly advanced to standing and walking. Those with hand burns require particularly aggressive occupational therapy to maintain function. If necessary, fingers should be pinned with Kirschner wires to prevent extensor tendon contracture. Physical and occupational therapy must be intensive and ongoing until the patient is reintegrated into society.

Scar Management

All significant burn injuries heal with some component of scarring, whether treated with split-thickness skin grafts or not; moreover, scar formation is individual specific, varying from little scarring to keloid-type hypertrophic scars. Understanding of scar physiology is insufficient to allow manipulation of a scar's thickness or compliance as it develops.

Scar and contracture impede optimization of function after a burn injury. One component of scar management is aggressive physical/occupational therapy; often, however, this is insufficient. Although scars do not fully mature for 1 to 2 years after the patient's wounds are closed, if an early scar contracture (in the first 3–12 months post burn) is limiting function of joints or the face, it is addressed surgically. Pressure garments, although unlikely to improve long-term outcome, are worn in the first year after the burn closes to reduce the edema in the scar and thus increase the scar compliance. Hypertrophic scars that remain hyperemic sometimes flatten and soften after injection with corticosteroids (betamethasone [Celestone]). Silicone sheets applied topically sometimes seem to soften scars. Until the human fibroblast is better understood, scar management will remain strictly an art.

Reconstruction

Patients with large burns usually require numerous operative scar releases in the first 2 years after the burn, simply to achieve independence in activities of daily living. Adequate and ongoing scar releases are especially important in growing children, to prevent musculoskeletal deformities. Functional and cosmetic reconstruction of the patient with facial burns is essential if they are to return to society.

Psychiatric Support

Acute care, rehabilitation, scar management techniques, and ongoing assessment of surgical reconstructive needs are essential in empowering the severely burned patient to return to a functional place in his or her family and vocation and in maintaining the function of those with smaller burns in functionally critical locations (e.g., the face and hands). Another component of care not yet discussed that is also critical is psychiatric and social work support. Most burn patients who were conscious at the time of their injury suffer from acute stress disorder in the weeks after their burn. With counseling, psychiatric assessment, and psychotropic medications, many will be able to escape full-blown post-traumatic distress syndrome, which affects 40% of those with significant burn injury. For those who do have some or all of the diagnostic criteria for post-traumatic distress syndrome, psychiatric follow-up is essential. All members of the burn team need to be aware of this. Patients with relatively small burns (<10% TBSA) are also at risk for post-traumatic distress syndrome and need to be screened if they seem to be persistently anxious, depressed, or hypervigilant. With ongoing attention to medical/surgical, emotional, and social needs of burn patients during their acute admission and in the years that follow, many with severe injuries are empowered to return to productive and fulfilling lives.

HIGH-ALTITUDE SICKNESS

method of
JAMES S. MILLEDGE, M.D.
Northwick Park Hospital
Harrow, London, England

High-altitude sickness is caused by hypoxia due to the low barometric pressure of altitude. The same sickness can be induced by lowering the partial pressure in a chamber either by lowering the pressure or the percentage of oxygen in the gas breathed. What is crucial is the partial pressure of oxygen in the inspired air, as was first shown by Paul Bert more than 120 years ago.

Many other clinical conditions may be met with on mountains from cold or infections, for example, and the hypoxia of altitude causes other changes, such as weight loss, psychomotor dysfunction, and reduced physical performance, but these conditions are not considered here. The high-altitude illnesses discussed in this article include the following:

1. Acute mountain sickness (AMS)
   a. Simple or benign
   b. High-altitude cerebral edema (HACE)
   c. High-altitude pulmonary edema (HAPE)
2. Subacute mountain sickness (S-AMS)
   a. Infantile
   b. Adult
3. Chronic mountain sickness (CMS)

ACUTE MOUNTAIN SICKNESS

AMS affects otherwise fit people if they rise to an altitude too fast. If a person goes rapidly to an altitude there is usually a delay of 6 to 24 hours before symptoms are felt. Headache is usually the first symptom, followed by general malaise, loss of appetite, nausea, and vomiting. Sleep is disturbed. The symptoms get worse, typically peaking on the second or third day at altitude and remitting by day 5. Recurrence at that altitude is not seen but may well occur on going to a higher altitude. Treatment is not really necessary, but analgesics can be given for the headache and voluntary hyperventilation helps temporarily.

The incidence of AMS depends on the rate of ascent and the height reached. An incidence of 25% was found in Colorado ski resorts at 1900 to 2940 m where people typically drive in a day from low altitude. In Europe, in climbers walking to mountain huts, an incidence of 9% was found at 2850 m, 13% at 3050 m, and 34% at 3650 m. An incidence of 95% has been reported in tourists flying directly to Shayangboche (3800 m) in the Everest region of Nepal. A history of previous AMS is predictive of likely future trouble and vice versa, but there are many exceptions; and any infection, especially of the respiratory tract, is a risk factor. All ages and races and both sexes can be affected. Older people are possibly at lower risk. Previous altitude experience may be protective to a degree. People born and raised at altitude seem less at risk. Various drugs (Table 1) can mitigate the severity of AMS, of which acetazolamide (Diamox) is the best studied and most used. Acetazolamide probably works by promoting bicarbonate excretion, thus stimulating ventilation and giving a sort of artificial acclimatization. The dose used in trials was 250 mg two or three times a day, but usually a dose of 125 mg twice a day is now recommended so as to lessen side effects. These consist of tingling in the fingers and toes and occasionally around the mouth. Most find this side effect to be unimportant, but a substantial minority find it very unpleasant.

Dexamethasone (Decadron)* (2 to 4 mg orally every 6 hours), which is recommended for cerebral edema, is also protective for simple AMS. Theophylline* has been shown to be beneficial in a dose of 350 mg slow release (250 mg in patients < 70 kg) twice daily. It is best if drugs are started 24 hours before ascent, but some benefit can be gained even if drugs are started after symptoms begin. The best way to prevent AMS is to plan to ascend sufficiently slowly to avoid it. A rule of thumb that has been suggested is when above 3000 m to have each night no higher than 300 m above the last and to have a rest day every 2 to 3 days. However, there is such variability in susceptibility that this rule will be unnecessarily slow for many and too fast for some. An additional rule is needed: do not ascend farther with symptoms of AMS.

*Not FDA approved for this indication.

TABLE 1. **Recommendations for Prevention and Treatment of Acute Mountain Sickness**

Type	Prevention	Treatment
Simple AMS	Gain height slowly.* Go no higher if symptomatic Acetazolamide (Diamox) Dexamethasone (Decadron)†	Self-limiting. If needed, acetaminophen† or acetazolamide or dexamethasone†
High-altitude cerebral edema (HACE)	Same as for simple AMS	DESCENT Dexamethasone,† 4–8 mg q6h Pressure bag
High-altitude pulmonary edema (HAPE)	Same as for simple AMS	DESCENT Nifedipine (Adalat),† 20 mg q6h Pressure bag

*Suggested maximum rate of ascent. Above 3000 m, gain no more than 300 m a day and take a rest day (no height gain) every 2 to 3 days.
†Not FDA approved for this indication.

HIGH-ALTITUDE CEREBRAL EDEMA

A potentially lethal condition, HACE develops from simple or benign AMS. The setting and the initial symptoms are the same, but instead of resolving the symptoms progress, with the addition of more serious neurologic signs. Often the first of these is the development of unsteadiness (ataxia) on walking and later even on sitting. There may be mood changes. In the context of AMS these early signs are all too easily missed because the patient may complain only of a headache and want to be left alone in his or her bedroom or sleeping bag. The patient may then start hallucinating and on examination may be found to have upgoing plantar reflexes and papilledema. Occasionally, ocular palsies occur. In untreated cases coma follows, with death in a few hours or days. The picture is often complicated by HAPE.

Prevention of HACE (see Table 1) is the same as that for AMS: gain altitude slowly, do not go higher with symptoms, and go down if they get worse. As with AMS, all ages and races and both sexes are at risk. The incidence is 1% to 2% of lowlanders going to altitudes above 3000 to 4000 m.

Treatment of HACE is first to get the patient at a

lower altitude as soon as possible. If evacuation is impossible or delayed, dexamethasone* has been shown to be beneficial. The dose suggested is 4 to 8 mg initially, followed by 2 to 4 mg every 6 hours until there is relief of symptoms. Recompression in a portable compression chamber (Gamow or CERTEC bag) for an hour may help and may make it possible for the patient to walk down instead of being carried, a great help in difficult terrain. However, it is stressed that these measures should not take the place of evacuation to lower altitudes.

HIGH-ALTITUDE PULMONARY EDEMA

The other lethal form of AMS is HAPE. It is now thought that some degree of subclinical pulmonary edema may be quite common on arrival at altitude during the period of risk of AMS, but in the majority of people this resolves over the next few days. However, in perhaps 1% to 3% of people the condition becomes progressive. The symptoms of simple AMS usually precede those of HAPE, although these may be quite mild. To these are added increased breathlessness and a cough, which is dry at first and later productive of white frothy sputum that becomes blood tinged as the condition progresses. The patient, if climbing, falls behind his or her companions and is easily exhausted. There may be chest discomfort, a rapid pulse, a fast breathing rate, and a mild pyrexia. The oxygen saturation (on pulse oximetry) is lower than normal for the altitude from an early stage in the condition. On listening at the lung bases, crackles are heard; and as the condition progresses, these are audible without a stethoscope because the patient literally drowns in his or her own secretions. Death can come in a matter of hours from the first symptom.

Patients with HAPE have a very high pulmonary artery pressure, and a loud pulmonary second heart sound may be detected. They have been shown to have a greater than normal pulmonary artery pressor response to hypoxia, and individual susceptibility is marked; that is, once a patient has had one attack, the risk is high for subsequent attacks on going to altitude. All ages, all races, and both sexes are at risk, but possibly youth is a risk factor.

Treatment (see Table 1), as for HACE, is first and foremost to get the patient down. If this is not possible or while awaiting evacuation, nifedipine (Adalat)* 20 mg by mouth, has been shown to be beneficial. This can be repeated every 6 hours if necessary. It is thought to act by reducing the pulmonary artery pressure. Cold, by causing peripheral vasoconstriction and so increasing central blood volume, is a risk factor; thus keeping the patient warm is important. Oxygen, if available, certainly helps, as does treatment in a Gamow or CERTEX recompression bag and, as in HACE, may improve the patient's condition sufficiently to make evacuation easier. Infection may be a factor in causing the condition so that antibiotics are often given but the mechanism is not essentially infective.

Although individual susceptibility is clear and trouble on future altitude trips is likely, it must be said that having had an attack on an expedition and gone down, many climbers have then acclimatized more slowly and succeeded in climbing their peak, such as Denali (Mt. McKinley 6194 m).

*Not FDA approved for this indication.

SUBACUTE MOUNTAIN SICKNESS

Two forms of S-AMS have been reported: adult and infantile. The infantile form was found in Han Chinese babies born in Lhasa (3700 m). They present within the first few months of life with dyspnea, cough, irritability, sleeplessness and signs of cyanosis, edema of the face, oliguria, tachycardia, liver enlargement, crackles in the lungs, and fever. The condition was usually fatal in a few weeks if the infants were kept at altitude. The adult form was reported in Indian soldiers encamped at around 6000 m or higher in Kashmir for more than 6 months. They presented with cough, dyspnea, and effort angina. The signs were of dependent edema. They had cardiomegaly, right ventricular enlargement, and, in most cases, pericardial effusion. The pulmonary artery pressure was elevated. Recovery was rapid on descent to low altitude.

Both forms seem to represent the human form of brisket disease, a condition affecting cattle taken to high altitude. The mechanism seems to be right-sided heart failure from chronic pulmonary hypertension caused by hypoxia.

CHRONIC MOUNTAIN SICKNESS

This is a condition affecting long-term or lifelong residents at high altitude. It was first described in people native to high altitude in the Andes but has since been reported in Tibet and from high-altitude towns in the United States, such as Leadville, Colorado. In Tibet it is much more common in immigrant Han Chinese than Tibetan people.

The symptoms are rather vague and include complaints of headache, dizziness, somnolence, fatigue, and difficulty in concentration and even hallucinations. Poor exercise tolerance is common, but dyspnea is not a prominent complaint. On descending to low altitude the symptoms disappear. The underlying problem is excessive production of red cells with high hemoglobin concentrations. The normal hemoglobin is higher at altitude, but patients with CMS have values much higher than normal for that altitude and this is the cause of their symptoms. Patients are also more hypoxic and so appear markedly cyanotic.

Removal to low altitude is best but often not possible for economic reasons. Repeated venesection of a unit of blood is beneficial and needs to be repeated every 2 to 4 months.

INJURIES DUE TO COLD

method of
MURRAY P. HAMLET, D.V.M.
U.S. Army Research Institute of Environmental Medicine
Natick, Massachusetts

Cold injuries are time and temperature dependent. The longer the tissue is cold, and the colder it gets, the more severe the injury. If cooling does not produce actual freezing of the tissue, then nonfreezing cold injury occurs on rewarming. If ice crystals form in the tissue, then frostbite is the result. The two injuries have different courses but similar sequelae.

The following are injuries caused by cold:

- Nonfreezing Cold Injury
  - Chilblain
  - Pernio
  - Trenchfoot or immersion foot
- Freezing Cold Injury
  - Frostnip
  - Frostbite
- Hypothermia
- Cold Water Near-Drowning (Submersion)

NONFREEZING COLD INJURY

Nonfreezing cold injury has historically been a military problem with little civilian morbidity. Armies have long had significant incidences of nonfreezing cold injury, and many campaigns have been lost because of the loss of manpower associated with cold and wet conditions. However, there are a growing number of cases among three civilian groups: street people, ski slope snowmakers, and rafting crews. These groups put themselves in the threat setting long enough to produce tissue damage.

Chilblain and Pernio

Chilblain, which is mild pain and swelling after cold exposure, and pernio, which is thin, necrotic plaques on the dorsa of the feet, are early, less severe forms of nonfreezing cold injury. The plaques of pernio will slough without scarring, but the area may be extremely painful for years. The time course for these injuries is generally minutes to hours for chilblain and several hours for pernio.

Trenchfoot

Although trenchfoot occurs on the feet, as the name implies, it can also occur on the hands if they are cold and wet for an extended period of time. The combination of cold, wet, tight-fitting footwear with dependent limbs, standing, or walking for long time periods (1–3 days) is the epidemiologic setting. Immersion foot, which results from sitting in a water-logged life boat or from being partially immersed while wearing a life jacket, is the same pathophysiologic injury.

Trenchfoot appears to be a reperfusion injury. It goes through three phases: the prehyperemic phase is typified by being cold and numb; the hyperemic phase is hot and painful; and the post-hyperemic phase is swelling with pain and numbness interspersed, muscle wasting, possible amputation, and very slow healing.

Patients present with swollen, painful extremities and a history of cold and wet exposure for an extended period of time. They have minor discomfort early in the exposure, but as numbness ensues, they typically ignore it and go on. Once in a warm facility, their feet begin to rewarm and become swollen and extremely hot and painful.

Treatment

Treatment is palliative at best. Elevation, nonsteroidal anti-inflammatory drugs, and pain medications give some relief but are not curative. Topical agents have no benefit. If it is a severe injury (true trenchfoot), then liquefaction necrosis will occur distally. Infection, fever, and elevated levels of muscle enzymes call for early surgical débridement. Because the lesion is "wet," rather than the "dry gangrene" of frostbite, infection is a severe and common complication. Closures may not heal, and more proximal closures are often indicated.

Sequelae include cold sensitivity, numbness, paresthesias, and chronic fungal infections from hyperhidrosis. Gait changes occur with a widening stance and a shuffling, shortened stride. Scaling, intermittent nail loss, and recurrent ulcerations of amputation stumps occur. Deep muscle cramps and aching often limit what victims of this injury are able to do for work or recreation. They may never be symptom free. This is a lifelong injury; even relatively minor acute injuries can become long-term disabilities.

FREEZING COLD INJURY

Frostnip is sustained vasoconstriction associated with freezing temperatures. There is no actual freezing of tissue, so there is some pain on rewarming, but little swelling and no bleb formation. Frostnip resolves with no sequelae.

Frostbite, on the other hand, is a significant cellular trauma. There are two types of damage. The first is ice crystal generation, both intercellular and extracellular, which, as ice forms, produces hyperosmolarity and intracellular dehydration. Super-cooled tissue (−13°C) without ice crystal formation shows no histologic damage on rewarming. Tissue cooled to −2°C, tapped to produce crystallization, and then rewarmed shows massive, explosive tissue damage. Endothelial cell damage, destruction of capillary beds, and red cell and platelet sludging compromise the blood flow to the rewarmed extremity. Nerve and transducer damage produces numbness, pain, and paresthesias. Therapy is aimed at dilating constricted vessels, decreasing the sludging of blood, and improving flow distally while tissue survives or demarcates at the freeze front border line.

Frostbite is graded retrospectively as first, second, or third degree. Initially, the tissue is blanched, insensate, and hard. The skin is not mobile over joints. On rewarming, first-degree frostbite results in hyperemia with pain. Rapid rewarming in warm water produces the most pain but the best tissue salvage. Second-degree frostbite shows edema, hyperemia, and blister formation. If the vesicles contain clear fluid and extend to the base of the nails, the injury is second degree. The injury is third degree if the blisters are hemorrhagic and do not extend to the base of the nails and the surrounding tissue is mottled with persistent numbness. The worst injury occurs in a freeze-thaw-refreeze scenario. Much tissue will be lost with this history.

Treatment

All frostbite is best managed with rapid rewarming in warm water (42°–45°C), preferably in a whirlpool. Current practice in Europe is to start at 38°C and warm up to 45°C. It is believed that there is less pain. Failure to rewarm is a bad prognostic sign, signifying potential tissue loss. Full range of motion exercise should be done during thaw and during the twice-daily whirlpool baths (40°C) to prevent flexion contractures. Narcotic pain medication may be necessary during thawing of deep injuries. After thawing, the limbs should be cleaned and exposed to light and air. Then they can be padded dry, and a loose dressing can be applied with pledgets between the digits.

Many compounds have been tried in an attempt to find the "magic treatment" of frostbite; yet none has been found. Compounds that decrease sludging and increase blood flow (Dextran) combined with platelet stabilizers (heparin and aspirin) to prevent clotting have shown some benefit. Nonsteroidal anti-inflammatory agents have some benefit if used early. All medications appear to be more effective if given before thawing. Free radical scavengers allopurinol (Zyloprim)* have been effective in animal models. Frostbite and trenchfoot are generally believed to be reperfusion injuries. New cytokine blocking medications used in pulmonary and cardiac medicine to control reperfusion damage may prove effective in frostbite management. Although chemical sympathectomy (reserpine) was useful, it is no longer available. Surgical sympathectomy should not be done, but sympathetic nerve block may relieve pain if done early in the treatment. Surgical intervention for amputation should be avoided for months. The most common mistake made in frostbite management is early amputation. Surgeons are often surprised at how much tissue actually survives after 3 months of demarcation. Dry mummifying, induration of the digits occurs, and at that point amputation and closures can be done. If the freeze front demarcation line is produced over muscle and the patient develops fever and coagulopathies, then early surgery is indicated. Autoamputation of digits occurs, and granulation closure may suffice. Grafting may be indicated, but graft failures are common if done too early.

Long-term sequelae include cold sensitivity, Raynaud phenomenon, hyperhidrosis, alternating pain and numbness, scaling and cracking of skin, abnormal nail growth, joint pain, and gait modifications. Frostbite victims will be frequent visitors to physicians' offices complaining of these symptoms. They should be encouraged to stop smoking, avoid cold exposure, sleep with socks on, use emollients on their skin, and use nonsteroidal anti-inflammatory drugs. They should be told that complete relief is not possible and that lifestyle modifications may be necessary.

*Not FDA approved for this indication.

HYPOTHERMIA

Hypothermia is a depressed core temperature. If heat production from metabolism, exercise, and shivering is exceeded by heat loss from water immersion, conductive cooling, wet clothing, wind, and cold air, then hypothermia ensues. Assault victims in the cold are not able to protect themselves from cooling because their clothes are often torn or removed and they are unconscious. In an urban setting, hypothermia is often related to drug or alcohol indulgence, accident, or assault. Aged or infirm individuals often become hypothermic. In a wilderness setting, hypothermia results from accidents or being trapped in a storm without sufficient protective gear. Wind, rain, and cold combine to create a high-threat setting, and, therefore, hypothermia occurs as frequently in summer as in winter. Individual body type and clothing will determine the rate of cooling. Physical exertion from heavy exercise that depletes energy stores, for example, hiking and skiing, renders individuals susceptible to hypothermia. They cannot shiver for any period of time and, as a result, their core temperature drops quickly. It is no wonder that lean, dehydrated, exhausted mountaineers with wet clothing routinely succumb to hypothermia. Treatment is determined by one of the three classifications of hypothermia: mild (35°–32°C [95°–89.6°F]), moderate (32° to 28°C [89.6°–82.4°F]), and severe (<28°C [82.4°F]). In mild hypothermia the normal thermoregulatory mechanisms are fully functional. Shivering begins with 0.5°C cooling, followed by ataxia, apathy, and amnesia. In moderate hypothermia, the thermoregulatory system is compromised and will eventually fail. There is a progressive loss of consciousness, and cardiac dysrhythmias occur. In severe hypothermia, victims lose consciousness, shivering ceases, there are significant electrolyte disturbances, and the heart becomes progressively more susceptible to both atrial and ventricular fibrillation. If victims are cooled without rough handling, the heart will eventually stop (asystole).

As core temperature drops, first gross and then fine motor skills are compromised. Muscle strength diminishes, and shivering starts. Peripheral constriction occurs to conserve core heat. As core temperature drops and shivering becomes more intense, victims are unable to do anything constructive to help themselves. They have a stumbling, shuffling gait and slurred speech. They develop a faraway gaze and retreat inward psychologically. If they continue to cool, shivering ceases and they become poikilothermic. Core temperature drops unremittingly.

Although all organ systems slow, the cardiovascular system is the most important system to understand clinically. Initially, heart rate, blood pressure, and respiration rate increase, and as cooling occurs, they diminish. Peripheral resistance increases from vasoconstriction, moving blood to the core, and cold diuresis increases fluid loss. Myocardial contractility decreases, as does cardiac output. Conduction velocities decrease with prolongation of the PR interval and QRS complex and the T waves. P and T waves disappear, and the QRS complex becomes a long sine wave. Progressive bradycardia occurs. If quiet cooling continues, the heart will usually become asystolic. If the individual is bumped or handled roughly during cooling, ventricular fibrillation will occur. If the patient presents asystolic at the hospital, it can generally be assumed that he or she has been slowly cooled for a long time. If the patient is in ventricular fibrillation, he or she may not have been exposed as long and probably did not cool as slowly. These patients are more likely to be successfully resuscitated. Resuscitation has been successful even in victims of complete cardiac arrest with 3 hours of asystole.

As core temperature drops, the tissue demands for oxygen diminish. Although fluid shifts and diuresis increase hematocrit, there is less demand for oxygen at the cellular level. For every 10°C reduction in core temperature, cerebral demand is reduced from 60% to 80% (roughly 7% per degree Celsius). The demand falls much faster than the decrement in cardiac delivery. The end result is that cellular damage to organs and brain does not generally occur in hypothermia. The pancreas is most likely to have lesions, but cardiac lesions and pulmonary hemorrhages have been reported.

A continued drop in core temperature after the victim has been removed from the cold environment is termed *after drop*. It may be due to simple mass action or could occur from countercurrent heat exchange from peripheral cold blood returning to the core as circulation is restored. Peripheral vasoconstriction diminishes. If a 1° or 2° drop in core temperature occurs and the core temperature is 32°C or higher, it is not usually life threatening. However, if this occurs with a core temperature of 28°C or colder, ventricular fibrillation or asystole will ensue. The most critical time for a hypothermic patient is immediately after being removed from the cold. The first 30 minutes are the most unstable and require the most concern for rewarming, fluid replacement, ventilation, and cardiac irritability.

There is a phenomenon termed *paradoxical undressing* that occurs in hypothermia. Victims are often found dead or hypothermic with their clothes in disarray or strewn along their path. The cause of this was initially thought to be assault, but it is now well documented as a result of being hypothermic. The pathophysiology is not completely clear, but it is possible that a paralysis of the peripheral vasoconstriction leading to the warming of the skin and a feeling of being hot could cause such behavior. What little core heat the victim has is shunted to the shell and they cool immediately. Undressing to relieve the feeling of heat is the last thing they do before becoming unconscious.

Clinical Presentation

Mild and moderate hypothermic persons are shivering, dazed, and mildly incoherent. Their fingers and limbs will be stiff and cold to touch. They may have difficulty conversing, and they drift in and out of a sleeplike stupor. If they smell of alcohol, the symptoms of hypothermia may be misread as merely alcohol intoxication. Patients who are shivering and conscious can be assumed to have a core temperature above 30°C (86°F). If unconscious and not shivering, their core temperature is below 30°C. If they are unconscious and above 30°C, then one needs to look for another cause of the lack of consciousness.

Moderate to severe hypothermic individuals appear unconscious and may not be shivering. Their limbs are rigid and snap back when extended. Their skin is pale and mottled blue and rigid. Blood pressure may be unattainable, and the cardiovascular system is highly unstable. If they are handled roughly, then ventricular fibrillation will result. It may be induced during the field rescue of these patients.

Treatment

Field management is best summarized by five steps:

1. Handle patients carefully
2. Ventilate
3. Remove wet clothes and insulate
4. Start intravenous lines
5. Transport

Adding heat by whatever means available, if only to preclude further cooling, adds to potential survival.

The physiologic changes one sees in a patient with a core temperature at 32°, 30°, 28°, or 27°C is normal physiology for that body at that temperature. The physiologic changes, not pathologic changes, are the normal responses to cooling. Only the pancreas shows lesions after hypothermic death. The treatment of the hypothermic patient then is to return the patient's various organ systems to their normal functioning temperature without damaging them. Cardiopulmonary function is most critical. Organ functions return to normal as temperature rises. The basic tenet of treatment is to support the cardiovascular system while core rewarming occurs. Do not rely on medications to manage problems that increased temperature will remedy. Hypothermic patients need few medications, because most drugs have no benefit. While cold, the systems cannot respond to them until the body temperature approaches 37°C (98.6°F).

Patients should be handled carefully to prevent ventricular fibrillation. Bretylium tosylate, 10 mg/kg, has been the drug of choice for hypothermic ventricular arrhythmia, but it is becoming unattainable.

Electrocardiogram, esophageal temperature, blood gases, and potassium and glucose levels are important parameters to measure. Although rectal temperatures are routinely used, there are problems with thermocouple placement. In addition, if peritoneal lavage is used to rewarm, then rectal temperature is no longer valid. Rectal temperature is warmer than esophageal temperature while cooling occurs, and it warms slower than the heart with external rewarming.

Ventilation in the field, during transport, and in the emergency department raises the fibrillatory threshold. This changes the cardiac sensitivity and is perhaps the most valuable piece of the management strategy.

Intravenous fluids (crystalloid and two large-bore lines) decrease viscosity and increase cardiac output. These fluids should be warmed to 42°C to enhance endothelial cell function. Endothelial cells below 30°C in an acid medium lose their cell contact integrity. Fluids allow extravasation into the third space. It is essential to maintain a central venous pressure early in resuscitation to preclude this extravasation. As temperature rises, so also can the central venous pressure.

Coagulation factor activity is independently depressed by cold temperature. Below 31°C (87.8°F) most are not active, which explains why hypothermic trauma victims bleed profusely. Hypothermics are routinely thrombocytopenic from sequestration of platelets in the liver, spleen, and lungs. The hypoglycemia that is present may be treated cautiously with bicarbonate, calcium, and insulin. Insulin is nonfunctional below 30°C. Therefore, give insulin very cautiously to hypothermic diabetics. As the patient warms, the insulin becomes active.

Rewarming Temperatures

Treatment and various rewarming methods revolve around the initial temperature of the patient. If the patient is above 32°C and semiconscious, external methods can be used, including heated air, warm blankets, and water immersion. If the patient is unconscious with a temperature above 32°C, which may be due to drug overdose or stroke, then heated air, water immersion, and more aggressive core rewarming methods may be indicated. If the patient's temperature is below 32°C and the person is unconscious, then core rewarming with peritoneal dialysis or arteriovenous shunt is indicated. If the temperature is below 27°C and the patient is asystolic, then cardiopulmonary bypass is the method of choice. The colder the patient and the less responsive, the more aggressive and invasive the warming methods needed. Although various lavage methods have been used (including gastric, colonic, or bladder), they have too small a surface area for effective heat exchange. Pericardial lavage is much too invasive, and pleural lavage, although effective, is quite invasive. If one has good reason to put in one chest tube, then a second lower chest tube might be indicated to use as a rewarming avenue. Peritoneal lavage, however, has been used effectively for 35 years and has many advantages for rewarming. It is easy, the equipment is readily available, it produces high heat transfer to the core, it does not compromise cardiac manipulation, and it gives the widest potential range of core temperature for resuscitation. Initially, 2 L of 45°C saline is instilled rapidly into the abdomen. This is followed by the placement of one 14 French catheter in each of the abdominal gutters. Saline or other dialysis fluid at 42° to 45°C is instilled in one side and gravity-drained from the other. A short dwell time is indicated early in resuscitation, but as patients rewarm a longer dwell time is necessary for heat exchange. The added benefits of peritoneal lavage include selective removal of some potassium and drugs, heating the pancreas for increased production of insulin, and warming the liver for increased clotting factor production.

Patients may be acidotic or alkalotic, but most commonly they are metabolically acidotic. Shivering induces lactic acidosis, and hypoperfusion leading to cellular hypoxia also contributes to the acidosis. Decreased ventilation also decreases oxygen saturation throughout the body. Blood gases should not be corrected for temperature. Adding carbogen, 1% to 2% carbon dioxide, to the ventilation gases will help maintain a relatively mild alkalosis, which appears to be protective during rewarming.

For severe, 27°C or colder, asystolic patients, there is growing support for cardiopulmonary bypass. Oxygenation, warming, and perfusion rates can be tightly controlled. Dramatic successes have been claimed after 3 hours of asystole. Standard femorofemoral bypass with 5° to 10°C gradient temperatures is sufficient to produce rapid core rewarming without large transmural temperature gradients. Hospitals with cardiac bypass capability need to include the emergency department staff in the bypass team in a protocol to handle patients with severe hypothermia.

COLD WATER NEAR-DROWNING (SUBMERSION)

Cold water near-drowning produces rapid core cooling combined with hypoxemia. Cold protects the brain from the hypoxemia of submersion. This is most commonly beneficial in small children in whom body mass is small, there is a high surface area, and cooling can occur rapidly. Although successful neurologic survival has occurred in young adults, most have been in small children.

Much controversy exists as to why cold water submersion is survivable. Control studies are not ethically possible, and animals may not drown the way humans do. One theory holds that the mammalian dive reflex from facial cooling causes bradycardia and a shunting of blood from the skin and organs to the brain-heart-lung loop. The laryngeal spasm caused by aspirating water traps air in the lungs and is available to oxygenate the brain. The second theory is that the rapid cooling of the head and torso decreases the metabolic demands of the brain and allows for neurologic survival. A third theory suggests that repeated aspiration of cold water with the dive reflex in place causes rapid internal cooling of the brain. In fact, all may play a role in survival. The wide range of response to resuscitation indicates that many variables must come together to allow for a successful outcome.

Clinical Presentation

Patients may present cold, either in complete cardiac arrest or with some cardiac function. Warm water submersions of more than 5 minutes are almost universally untreatable. Successful outcomes have been accomplished after ice water submersions of 60 minutes. A hypothermic, submersed child, with a functional heart has a fair chance of success when presented at the emergency department. A similar child, asystolic on presentation, has little or no chance of being completely neurologically intact after resuscitation.

Intubation, cardiopulmonary resuscitation, and mild rewarming are indicated. Warming should only be to the point of cardioversion. Slow rewarming should follow as perfusion of the brain occurs. Recovery from drowning is also a reperfusion injury of the brain. Once on a ventilator and with increased cardiac output, medications to move fluid out of the brain (mannitol, 7.5% saline) and diuretics (Furosemide [Lasix] or dexamethasone [Decadron]) are indicated. The goal of treatment is to raise the oxygen saturation of the brain, maintain circulation and perfusion at a low pressure to minimize extravasation, pull fluids from the tissues, and produce diuresis to remove the fluid. Treatment is time compressed. Every decision has to be the right one.

Controversy exists about the use of extracorporeal perfusion (ECP) in the submersion victim. One school holds that ECP has everything the patient needs (e.g., oxygen, perfusion, pressure control, volume management). The other believes that there will be many more bad outcomes if cold, asystolic children are put on ECP. There have been some dramatic successes with ECP, but there may also be many more neurologically damaged survivors. This conundrum of withholding a potentially lifesaving treatment modality to avoid a bad outcome will not be solved easily. A rational, thought-out algorithm for placing submersion victims on ECP must be established in each treatment facility. More importantly, a set of criteria for cessation of ECP in potentially bad outcomes needs to be in place. This medical, ethical, legal, and moral dilemma needs to be addressed by hospital staff before the admission of a nearly drowned child.

DISTURBANCES DUE TO HEAT

method of
WILLIAM O. ROBERTS, M.D., M.S.
MinnHealth Family Physicians
White Bear Lake, Minnesota

DEFINITION

Hyperthermia and heat stroke are the major disturbances of body homeostasis associated with hot environments and can affect all body systems. *Hyperthermia* is defined as a rectal temperature greater than 104°F (40°C). Heat stroke is a potentially fatal disorder and is classified as either exertional or nonexertional (classic) heat stroke when hyperthermia is associated with organ system dysfunction. *Exertional hyperthermia* implies that a rapid core temperature elevation is due to muscle work with failure to remove heat from the body, whereas the hyperthermia of *classic heat stroke* is generally due to slow accumulation of environmental heat with restricted heat dissipation. Untreated or unrecognized exertional heat stroke can progress to hypothalamic failure and present as the "classic" clinical picture.

RISK FACTORS

Classic heat stroke usually occurs during heat waves with prolonged day and night exposure to high ambient temperature and relative humidity. Classic heat stroke victims are often elderly with multifactorial risks of chronic disease, malnutrition, and poor socioeconomic status. Chronic cardiovascular or neurologic diseases, and diabetes mellitus with impaired autonomic control, impede the ability of the body to remove excess heat. Infants and children with an increased surface area to mass ratio; the elderly with decreased maximum heart rate; and obese people with lower physical fitness, decreased cardiovascular capacity, greater energy expenditure for given task, and a thicker insulation layer are prone to classic heat stroke. Drugs and medications that affect fluid and electrolyte balance, vascular tone, sweating mechanism, cardiac output, and central nervous system (CNS) function increase the risk of exertional and classic heat stroke.

COMPLICATIONS

Heat stroke can lead to complications of death, seizure, rhabdomyolysis, renal failure, lactic acidosis, disseminated intravascular coagulation, adult respiratory distress syndrome, cerebellar syndrome, cardiac damage, and immune system suppression leading to increased post–heat stroke pulmonary bacterial and systemic fungal infections. Exertional heat stroke that is promptly recognized and rapidly treated on site rarely leads to these complications. However, complications do occur in high school football players, who probably go unrecognized and untreated beyond the "golden hour"

INCIDENCE

Both exertional and classic heat stroke are true emergencies with potential for multisystem failure, as demonstrated by the list of potential complications. The incidence in athletics is variable with less than 0.5% of entrants in "hot humid" short (5–20 km) road races and less than 0.005% of entrants in "cool" long (42 km) road races. There were deaths during high school football practices in both the 1995 and 1998 heat waves. The incidence in the general population is difficult to assess, but heat stroke usually occurs in clusters after 2 to 4 days of continuous exposure to hot, humid conditions.

PATHOPHYSIOLOGY

The basic pathophysiology of heat illness reflects the rise in core body temperature as the summation of body heat gained from muscle activity and/or passively accumulated from the environment. Environmental heat is added to the body when the ambient temperature is greater than skin temperature and is stored in the body when high humidity limits evaporation or the temperature gradient to the environment limits conduction, convection, and radiation losses.

Dehydration limits the cardiovascular heat transport to the skin and limits sweat production, increasing the risk of heat stroke. As cells store heat and cellular mechanisms fail, each organ system begins to lose normal function. Cell membranes leak and toxic intracellular contents enter the intracellular and intravascular spaces, causing damage to other organs. The brain is particularly heat sensitive and begins to malfunction early in the cascade of organ system failures.

DIAGNOSIS

Recognition of exertional hyperthermia, exertional heat stroke, and classic heat stroke is simple with a core temperature measurement in hot conditions or when the clinical picture is consistent with the condition. Beyond temperature measurement, assessing CNS status is the most telling of the clinical parameters. Exertional hyperthermia will present as an elevated core temperature but no CNS symptoms. Heat stroke has several nonspecific symptoms, including confusion, fatigue, impaired judgment, weakness, flushing, chills, hyperventilation, and dizziness. Vital signs include an elevated body temperature greater than 104°F, pulse rate in the 100 to 120 beats per minute range, and a decreased blood pressure. The core temperature may be less than 104°F if spontaneous cooling has occurred since the initial collapse. Temperature measurement must give an accurate core estimate. The preferred measurement site in athletic settings is the rectum. Oral, aural canal (tympanic membrane), and axillary temperatures are inadequate for diagnosis of hyperthermia in athletes, because these temperatures are heavily influenced by the skin temperature and will be cooler than core if the skin is wet with sweat. If the shell temperature is elevated, then all temperature measurement techniques can be accurate and lead to the diagnosis of classic heat stroke.

CNS depression is the hallmark of heat stroke, demonstrated by bizarre behavior, loss of hind limb function, memory loss, collapse, delirium, and, in very severe cases, stupor and coma. The skin is ashen, sweaty, and cool to touch in early exertional heat stroke and progresses to dry, pink, and hot in classic heat stroke. Seizure can occur and should be controlled because the muscle work can increase the core temperature. Both seizure and muscle cramping can be controlled with diazepam (Valium) 1 to 5 mg intravenous (IV) push or magnesium sulfate, 1 to 5 g IV push (off label use). In the athletic setting, hyponatremia should be considered as the reason for seizure if the rectal temperature is not elevated.

TREATMENT

The treatment of hyperthermia is immediate body cooling and should begin in the field. Suspected victims should discontinue activity to stop intrinsic heat production and be moved to a cooler environment. First aid cooling consists of applying ice packs to the high heat loss areas of the body—the neck, axilla, and groin. The fastest and most effective means of body cooling is immersion of the trunk, or trunk and limbs, in 32° to 65°F water, producing an average cooling rate of 17°F/h. The advantages of fluid immersion are the rapid conduction of heat from the body and the blood pressure augmentation from the hydrostatic pressure. Cool towels or ice packs to neck, axilla, and groin cool the body at a slower rate of 6° to 8°F/h and can be used when a shallow tub is not available or the patient requires more intensive monitoring than can be accomplished while immersed in water. The rectal temperature (intermittent or continuous), CNS status, and vital signs should be monitored every 5 to 10 minutes, and cooling measures should be discontinued when the core temperature is lowered to 102°F. There is a golden hour in the management of heat stroke. In athletic settings, with medical teams skilled in the recognition and treatment of exertional heat stroke, athletes are often released from the medical area without hospitalization, unless complicating factors such as medication use, dysrhythmia, rhabdomyolysis, or hyponatremia are suspected. All victims of classic heat stroke should be admitted to a hospital for observation and treatment of associated disorders.

Hospital care of classic and severe exertional heat stroke may require intensive management of the organ systems damaged by prolonged hyperthermia. Careful fluid replacement is required because fluid is returned to intravascular space during cooling. Intravenous fluids should be limited to 1 liter in the first hour unless severe dehydration is suspected or central venous pressure is monitored. Repeated laboratory assessment should include glucose, aspartate aminotransferase, sodium, potassium, blood urea nitrogen, creatinine, blood cell counts, coagulation studies, lactic acid, blood gas analysis and creatine kinase screens for organ damage and system dysfunction. The prognosis is poor if there is renal failure before 48 hours, persistent coma after cooling, or an aspartate aminotransferase elevation of more than 1000 IU/L after 72 hours.

PREVENTION

Prevention of hyperthermia is possible with activity modifications, hydration, and acclimatization in athletic settings. As little as 30 minutes in air conditioning per day made a difference between life and death in elderly shut-ins during the 1995 heat wave in Chicago. A little time away from heat stress for the elderly, and even athletes, may be worth the extra effort. One should be leery of the second and third day in the heat for both forms of heat stroke.

The morbidity and mortality of heat stroke is probably related to the area under the core temperature versus the time curve above some critical level beginning in the 104°F to 106°F range. Immediate recognition and rapid cooling by immersion of increased core temperature minimizes the risk of organ damage and death. Exertional heat stroke casualties treated immediately with full return of mental status and stable vital signs may be discharged from the medical area without hospitalization, in contrast to classic heat stroke victims. The ill and elderly should be moved to air-conditioned environments for at least a part of each day during a heat wave as a public health intervention to decrease the risk of heat stroke.

SPIDER BITES AND SCORPION STINGS

method of
JEFFREY R. SUCHARD, M.D.
University of California Irvine Medical Center
Orange, California

SPIDER BITES

For reasons that remain obscure to me, patients will ascribe a wide variety of lesions to spider bites. From both the medical and legal perspectives, clinicians should approach any complaint of a spider bite with caution. The evidence is circumstantial, at best, unless the patient does at least one of the following:

1. Gives a reliable eye-witness history
2. Produces the offending animal for identification (not just any spider found around the house)
3. Exhibits systemic manifestations that clearly demonstrate a spider bite

Most complaints of "spider bites" have, on further investigation, been attributed to other arthropods (e.g., fleas, ticks, bedbugs, and so on) or to various dermatologic or systemic conditions (e.g., erythema chronicum migrans, toxic epidermal necrolysis, diabetic ulcers, herpes simplex, or purpura fulminans). I have seen a classic case of angiotensin-converting enzyme (ACE) inhibitor–induced angioedema presenting as a spider bite; of course, no spider was ever seen, and no bite was ever felt.

Nevertheless, real spider bites do occur infrequently. Many species are capable of biting and envenomating human beings. What typically results, however, is simply local pain and inflammation, sometimes with an allergic component. Treatment of these bites consists of reassurance, symptomatic therapy, attention to tetanus immunization status, and occasional antibiotics for cellulitis. Systemic effects from envenomation are unusual if the offending spider is not a black widow or one of the brown spiders.

Tarantulas may be kept as pets, and because of their size can inflict a painful, yet nonvenomous, bite. Tarantulas also bear highly urticarious hairs that they can flick at predators, which have caused cases of ophthalmia nodosa among people who handle these spiders or clean their cages. The spiders most commonly implicated in serious envenomations in the United States are discussed in more detail next.

Latrodectus *Species (Black Widow Spiders)*

Latrodectus species are found worldwide. The chief black widow spider (BWS) species in the United States are *Latrodectus mactans* in the East and *Latrodectus hesperus* in the West. The adult female BWS has a shiny, black, globular abdomen with an orange or red marking shaped like an hourglass on the ventral surface. In captivity, the female spider will eat the male after mating, although this is rare in the wild. The BWS often builds its chaotic web in dark places, including manufactured structures such as garages, wood piles, outdoor toilets, and patio furniture.

Latrodectus venom induces release of neurotransmitters at noradrenergic and cholinergic synapses. A bite is usually felt as a brief, sharp pain. Over the next several minutes to hours, a deep, severe pain may develop and radiate to contiguous areas: a bite on the arm may produce chest pain, whereas a bite on the thigh or buttock can produce abdominal pain.

The bitten area may show tiny puncture wounds without necrosis or swelling. A dime-sized halo lesion of pallor surrounded by erythema may be seen due to local vasoactive effects. With severe envenomations, the symptoms may not peak for 12 to 18 hours and can last for several days; milder symptoms may persist for 2 to 3 weeks. Cholinergic venom effects cause muscle cramping and pain in major muscle groups. Noradrenergic venom effects include localized or generalized diaphoresis and hypertension. The pain from BWS envenomation may mimic renal colic, an acute abdomen, or myocardial ischemia.

The primary goal in treating BWS bites is pain control. Mild pain may be treated with oral analgesics. More severe envenomations warrant parenteral analgesics, such as morphine or fentanyl (Sublimaze), and possibly benzodiazepine sedation as well. The pain may wax and wane for some time; discharged patients should be prescribed adequate analgesics lest they return or seek help elsewhere.

An effective horse serum–derived antivenom is available. Antivenom is indicated for complications due to hypertension, due to severe pain resistant to parenteral analgesics, or in symptomatic pregnant women because the venom may induce abortion. Antivenom should only be given in controlled and monitored clinical settings after screening the patient for contraindications. Deaths from BWS bites are exceedingly rare, and the last reported fatality in the United States was actually from antivenom-induced anaphylaxis. Intravenous calcium and centrally acting muscle relaxants (e.g., methocarbamol [Robaxin]) are no longer recommended.

Loxosceles *Species (Brown Spiders)*

People commonly know that brown recluse spider (*Loxosceles reclusa*) bites can produce chronic, slow-healing ulcers. Some patients, therefore, ascribe their skin lesions to brown recluse spider bites, even if this is geographically impossible or an obvious alternative diagnosis is evident (e.g., venous stasis ulcers, active parenteral drug abuse). Several spiders, including non-*Loxosceles* species, may produce such lesions of "necrotizing arachnidism," but the brown recluse gets the bum rap.

Loxosceles spiders have a violin-shaped dark marking on the dorsum of the cephalothorax, so they are sometimes called *fiddleback* spiders. At least 10 species have been found in the United States. *L. reclusa* is found mostly in the South and Midwest, where real brown recluse bites are an endemic problem. In the Southwest, *Loxosceles arizonica*, *Loxosceles deserta*, and a few other species predominate.

The actual bite often remains unnoticed. Within a few hours, localized burning, stinging pain ensues with erythema and a surrounding pale halo from vasospasm. The lesion soon develops into a dark vesicle or bulla that ruptures, leaving an ulcerated lesion that may take up to 6 to 8 weeks to heal. Systemic effects (malaise, myalgias, diffuse rash, intravascular hemolysis, risk for renal failure) are relatively rare but are more common in children. These effects are evident within 72 hours if they occur at all; patients who exhibit these systemic effects should be admitted. *Loxosceles* venom contains sphingomyelinase, an enzyme responsible for dermal necrosis-inducing and hemolytic effects.

The great majority of brown spider bites will respond well to local wound care. Surgical referral is rarely indicated and only for lesions that fail to heal as expected. Antibiotics should be used if there is concern about wound infection. Several treatment regimens of unclear efficacy have been proposed for *Loxosceles* bites, including dapsone, hyperbaric oxygen, immediate lesion excision, and experimental antivenom.

SCORPION STINGS

Several hundred species of scorpions are found worldwide, the vast majority of which are not especially dangerous to human beings. Stings from most scorpion species result only in local pain and inflammation that respond well to minimal supportive measures. However, a few dozen species, almost all from the Buthidae family, cause significant morbidity and mortality. Scorpion envenomation is a serious endemic problem in many parts of the world: *Buthus* and *Leiurus* species in North Africa and the Middle East, *Mesobuthus* in India, *Parabuthus* in Southern Africa, *Tityus* in South America and around the Caribbean, and *Centruroides* species in Mexico. Death in up to one third of patients has been reported in the past, although this was mostly due to lack of adequate supportive care and monitoring capabilities. Fatality rates still amount to 1% to 3% for some foreign scorpion stings, even in places where intensive care unit care is available.

Envenomation by the most dangerous scorpion species produces a characteristic clinical picture with autonomic instability and neuromuscular hyperactivity. The venom opens sodium channels on nerve cell membranes, resulting in repetitive firing and excessive release of endogenous neurotransmitters. Cholinergic effects (hypersalivation, diaphoresis, bronchorrhea) may briefly be seen, followed by a prolonged state of sympathomimetic excess, often characterized by hypertensive crises with encephalopathy, pulmonary edema, and/or cardiac injury. The most severely affected victims are usually children, not only owing to a higher venom dose per kilogram but also because children are more likely to encounter scorpions while roaming outdoors barefooted.

Only one scorpion species in the United States is considered truly dangerous, the bark scorpion *Centruroides exilicauda* (sometimes called *C. sculpturatus*), which is found in Arizona and neighboring areas of adjacent states. The bark scorpion is relatively small (<10 cm) and sleek with thin pincers and tail segments, colored uniformly yellow to tan. Larger, uglier, bristled, or dark scorpions found in the United States may appear more fearsome, but their stings do not produce significant systemic effects.

The most common clinical effects from bark scorpion stings are local pain and paresthesias. A local inflammatory response, mark, or lesion is almost never seen. Nonetheless, tapping the sting area exacerbates pain and paresthesias and may be diagnostic in questionable cases. Sometimes the paresthesias generalize and can be accompanied by neuromuscular hyperactivity and cholinergic/parasympathetic effects such as excessive oral and airway secretions. Serious signs of sympathetic excess are rarely if ever seen from *C. exilicauda* stings.

Neuromuscular hyperactivity may manifest as unusual writhing or jerking that can be mistaken for seizures. Muscles controlled by the bulbar nerves may also be affected, resulting in roving, random eye movements and poor airway control. Small children are generally the most seriously affected and they may present with writhing, drooling, and inconsolable crying, sometimes without any clear precipitating event if the scorpion is not seen: a dramatic and challenging clinical picture. Larger children and adults may be discomforted by neuromuscular effects but are rarely in any life-threatening danger.

With proper attention to airway control and supportive care measures, bark scorpion sting victims should recover completely. Serious effects last only a few hours to a day, although complaints of residual paresthesias may last days to weeks. Patients with only local effects need no specific treatment, only reassurance, pain control, and attention to tetanus immunization status.

Debate remains regarding the optimal treatment of advanced-grade envenomations, most often seen in small children. Some advocate admitting to an intensive care unit, administering sedatives to control agitation, and monitoring for respiratory distress. This approach is certainly safe but may increase the risk of airway compromise, need for intubation, hospitalization time, and cost. In Arizona, a goat-derived *Centruroides* antivenom is available that is remarkably efficacious in reversing serious neurologic effects.

Nearly all patients receiving antivenom can be discharged home with minimal residual symptoms within a few hours. Antivenom carries risk for allergic reactions, both immediate and delayed. Before dosing, patients should be screened for goat allergies and other relative contraindications. Up to 60% of patients receiving antivenom develop serum sickness within a few weeks, which responds well to oral antihistamines and corticosteroids. Consultation with toxicologists familiar with *Centruroides* antivenom can be obtained by calling the Samaritan Regional Poison Center in Phoenix, Arizona at 602-253-3334.

SNAKEBITE

method of
MIGUEL C. FERNÁNDEZ, M.D.
University of Texas Health Sciences Center
San Antonio, Texas

Crotalidae and Elapidae are the two groups of snakes native to the United States that cause significant human envenomation. The (sub)family Crotalinae, formerly Crotalidae, includes three genera of native snakes: *Crotalus* (rattlesnakes), *Sistrurus* (massasaugas and pygmy rattlesnakes), and *Agkistrodon* (copperheads and cottonmouths/water moccasins). Crotalines are known as pit vipers because of a thermosensory organ located in a pit between each eye and naris that aids in detecting warm-blooded prey and predators. The only native elapids north of the U.S.-Mexican border are *Micrurus fulvius fulvius* (eastern coral), the closely related *Micrurus fulvius tenere* (Texas coral), and the rarely encountered *Micruroides euryxanthus* (Sonoran or Arizona coral).

Current and reliable statistics about the incidence of snakebite in the United States are nonexistent. An estimated tens of thousands of bites occur each year, with about one fifth of these bites by venomous snakes. It is presumed that only a fraction of them are reported to U.S. poison control centers. Only 3984 bites were reported in 1999, including two deaths. Just seven fatalities associated with snakebite were reported from 1993 to 1999, although up to a dozen fatalities may actually occur per year. Roughly half of venomous bites occur because of a careless or inadvertent encounter with a snake and are thus termed "innocent bites." The other half result from direct provocation or handling. Killing a snake does not prevent the potential for envenomation because postmortem venom can remain active and capable of causing harmful effects for an undetermined time. At a "rattlesnake roundup" cook-off one might witness the eerie sight of dozens of rattlesnake jaws reflexively opening and closing after decapitation. Likewise, one may encounter fresh rattlesnake roadkill with a partially intact nervous system still possessing the capability to strike on stimulation. Although usually quite docile, coral snakes are capable of striking quickly when provoked. It is thus unwise to try to capture or handle any potentially venomous snake in an attempt to identify it unless one is a well-equipped expert. Snakebites are most likely to occur in warm weather during the warmer time of the day and most often in the warmer southwest, south central, and southeastern states. Snakebites occur most often in young males, with over 95% of bites to an extremity. Roughly 70 to 100 exotic venomous snakebites are reported each year, usually in those who own or handle snakes intentionally.

DIAGNOSIS

The diagnosis of snakebite envenomation is clinical and based on the history, signs, and symptoms. The diagnosis may be difficult initially because some bites may show little to no apparent effects in the early stages. The history may not be clear, especially in the case of young children, impaired individuals, or others who may not be able to effectively communicate an unusual occurrence because of intoxication, some other cause of altered mental status, or language barrier.

Although most crotaline envenomations result in the early development of symptoms, the onset or recognition of significant venom effects may be delayed in both crotaline and elapid bites for up to 12 to 24 hours, respectively. Patients bitten by venomous snakes that do not exhibit significant venom effects are said to have experienced a "dry bite." The incidence of dry bites reported by various authors ranges from 1% to 27% of all bites. The 1999 report of the American Association of Poison Control Centers showed that no effect occurred in 3.3% of those bitten by known native venomous species and 27% experienced only minor symptoms.

The venom of pit vipers is delivered directly through hinged, hollow upper fangs when provoked or when attacking prey. Elapid venom is delivered via short, rigid, longitudinally grooved fangs and dental abrasion of the skin. Coral snake envenomation probably requires chewing for several seconds to be effective. Elapid envenomation leads to relatively few local tissue effects other than pain, but it may cause life-threatening neurologic toxicity, including prolonged respiratory paralysis.

Unlike the neurotoxic elapids, most crotalines primarily depend on their venom to immobilize their prey by causing hypovolemic shock. Crotaline venom is chiefly composed of water and numerous polypeptides that damage endothelial cells, thereby allowing extravasation and sometimes massive third-spacing of blood and plasma into adjacent tissue, alter coagulation, and digest tissue. The exception to this generalization is the Mohave rattlesnake (*Crotalus scutulatus scutulatus*) with type A venom, which contains relatively large proportions of the potent Mohave toxin that immobilizes prey through neuromuscular blockade. Venom composition may show not only interspecies but also intraspecies variation, even in a single snake throughout its life, and thus its effects on human tissue may vary correspondingly.

Significant coagulopathy may be produced by crotaline envenomation, occasionally including marked platelet aggregation and consumption. However, true disseminated intravascular coagulation (DIC) does *not* occur. A DIC-like syndrome may occur but differs from DIC in several important ways. Enzymatic thrombin-like venom glycoproteins produce non–cross-linked fibrin monomers that are rapidly degraded into fibrin split products. Because the victim's endogenous thrombin is not consumed and pathologic activation of factor XIII does not occur, cross-linked fibrin is not formed and D dimer is not commonly formed. In contradistinction, true DIC involves pathologic thrombin production and activation of factor XIII, which produces cross-linked fibrin. Antithrombin III is depleted, and on fibrinolysis, D dimer is formed. DIC causes intravascular thrombosis, microangiopathic hemolysis, and platelet consumption.

Therapeutically, the difference between DIC and DIC-like syndrome is huge and poorly recognized. In crotaline envenomation, circulating venom destroys transfused blood product coagulation factors and platelets. Therefore, unless a patient is actively exsanguinating, blood product transfusions are not helpful and may unnecessarily expose the patient to associated risks. Likewise, heparin therapy has no place in the treatment of crotaline venom–induced coagulopathy because heparin's efficacy is dependent on that of antithrombin III, which has no effect on crotaline thrombin-like enzymatic glycoproteins. Crotaline antivenom is effective in treating venom-induced coagulopathy by binding to and disabling coagulopathy-causing venom components.

Although crotaline venom may also possess significant neurotoxins and other components that produce systemic toxicities, it is more likely to cause local tissue effects. Crotaline fang marks may be present with sometimes just one puncture or abrasion wound apparent, often oozing blood. Other bites exhibit multiple wounds from repeated strikes or more indistinct abrasions or toothmarks from smaller rear teeth. Ecchymosis and sometimes hemorrhagic blebs may form at or adjacent to the bite site. Besides pain, local swelling, and oozing, the patient may exhibit or complain of anxiety and fear, perioral and peripheral paresthesias, weakness, lightheadedness, nausea, vomiting, gustatory alteration, diaphoresis, and chills. Envenomation effects are often progressive, and the clinician must remain vigilant in monitoring the patient's condition so that significant changes are not missed. Changes may occur over minutes to hours. Because venom primarily spreads lymphatically, induration and elicited tenderness progress along lymphatic lines. Lymphatic channels and regional lymph nodes may be tender in advance of induration. The leading edge of induration may also progress on one aspect of an affected limb related to lymphatic drainage from the bite site and is a better indicator of the progression of envenomation than is serial measurement of limb diameter. Local wound erythema or other discoloration often does not progress to the leading edge of induration and is therefore not considered to be a good indicator of the severity of envenomation.

In severe envenomation, respiratory distress leading to arrest may occur, as well as an altered level of consciousness, lethargy, ptosis, muscle fasciculations, myokymia, and anaphylactoid or anaphylactic shock secondary to venom exposure. Hypovolemic shock from massive third-spacing of fluid and blood may lead to renal failure from decreased glomerular filtration. Renal failure may also result from hemoconcentration, hemolysis, coagulopathic by-product deposition, or venom nephrotoxins. Rhabdomyolysis resulting from the development of compartment syndrome has not been reported as a cause of renal failure in American snakebite. In general, systemic extravasation may lead to end-organ failure. Envenomation by the coral snake may lead to many neurologic findings and complaints, including minor to no local pain or tissue injury and cranial nerve abnormalities. By far the most important effects are related to paralysis of the oropharyngeal and hypopharyngeal muscles and hypersalivation, which may compromise the airway, and respiratory paralysis leading to aspiration and respiratory arrest.

Although greatly feared because of the potentially devastating sequelae of systemic toxicity, including renal failure, the development of a compartment syndrome does not commonly occur. When compartment syndrome is diagnosed, it is often without objective measurements of compartment pressure. Most snakebites are subcutaneous and do not involve the muscle compartment directly. Crotaline snakebite envenomation can be a confusing mimic of compartment syndrome in that both exhibit the clinical findings of pain, pain on passive extension, hypoesthesia, edema, and tenseness of the tissue. Distinguishing between the two must be accomplished through objective measurements of serial compartment pressure to avoid the deforming and potentially disabling sequelae of fasciotomy.

PREHOSPITAL TREATMENT

Rapid delivery of a snakebitten patient to a health care facility and supportive care are the safest and most efficacious forms of prehospital care. The patient should be reassured and kept calm. The extremity should be kept at rest and level with the heart. In anticipation of the development of edema, all jewelry and constrictive clothing should be removed. If available, surface wound cleansing may remove venom that could otherwise continue to be absorbed through wound openings. It is inadvisable to add additional insult to injury in the form of unproven and potentially deleterious methods of field therapy such as cryotherapy, incisions, mouth suction, tourniquet, or electric shock. No studies have proved the efficacy of any of these therapies in humans. These interventions may lead to disastrous consequences and to additional structural damage, infection, and gangrene by increasing tissue ischemia, further compromising the wound and increasing the likelihood of surgical intervention. Immediate application of a wound extractor device that produces strong local suction may be considered, but the efficacy of this method is controversial. In coral snakebite, an exception is made for the application of a constrictive band, not a tourniquet, to be applied to the proximal portion of the extremity. Coral bites do not carry the risk of local tissue destruction, so inhibiting proximal lymphatic flow may aid in preventing the central spread of neurotoxins before antivenom administration. At least one large-bore peripheral intravenous line should be placed in an unaffected extremity and intravenous fluids administered. Prehospital administration of antivenom therapy is not currently advised because of concern over the possible development of allergic reactions and the length of time necessary to reconstitute antivenom.

HOSPITAL TREATMENT

It is a generally accepted view of medical toxicologists that the mainstays of treatment of snakebite envenomation are proper evaluation, stabilization, and administration of antivenom. Although this sequence may seem straightforward, few practitioners have adequate experience in the treatment of snakebite envenomation to help them avoid medical and legal complications. It is strongly advised that one contact a local expert through a regional poison control center for assistance in case management (800–222–1222).

Patient evaluation and management should begin with a thorough history of symptoms and the circumstances and time interval since the bite. A description of the snake and all field interventions should be obtained, as well as a history of any allergy to medications, sheep, horses, or animal products. The physical examination should focus on both local and systemic signs of toxicity, with attention paid first to protection and maintenance of the airway, breathing, and circulation. Two large-bore intravenous lines should be established in nonaffected extremities and a copious colloid infusion initiated to compensate for extravasation and renal protein load. Tetanus immunization should be given if not current.

Laboratory examination should include a complete blood count, platelet count, prothrombin time, partial thromboplastin time, international normalized ratio, fibrinogen, fibrin degradation products, D dimer, creatinine phosphokinase, electrolytes, renal functions, and urinalysis. Serial examinations of the hematocrit and coagulation profiles are recommended at frequent intervals initially (2–4 hours) and decreased in frequency after stabilization. It is newly recognized that late coagulopathy, as remote as 1 week, may occur in crotaline envenomation. The clinical significance of late coagulopathy is dependent on its degree of severity and patient activity and co-morbidities.

It is recommended that the wounded extremity not be circumferentially wrapped or bound in any manner, although a lightly applied sterile dressing may be used after wound cleansing with a mild soap and rinse. Prophylactic antibiotics are unnecessary and should be reserved for wounds that have had mouth contact or are otherwise severely contaminated. Unless signs of infection develop, prophylactic use of antibiotics may complicate therapy if an adverse drug reaction should occur and an antibiotic-related allergic response is mistakenly attributed to antivenom. Fasciotomy should be considered only after compartment pressures are consistently elevated above 30 mm Hg for several hours, during which time the extremity has been elevated and copious intravenous fluid and adequate doses of antivenom administered.

The severity of envenomation should be graded according to a uniform scoring system to help guide therapy. One example of such a system is shown in Table 1. Progression of signs and symptoms is to be expected, and thus grading the envenomation is a continuous process. No scoring system is adequate to describe the variable and temporally related constellation of effects that may develop in a particular patient.

Antivenom therapy is indicated in patients with at least mild envenomation and a history of progressive signs and symptoms or the presence of moderate to severe envenomation with or without systemic manifestations. Antivenom cannot reverse tissue damage, but rather binds to venom components to prevent further damage. It may also act to disaggregate sequestered platelets and thereby lead to a relatively rapid rebound in the platelet count. Antivenom shows a temporally related ability to reverse both the anticoagulant and procoagulant effects of venom. Pain should be managed with judicious use of opioids rather than nonsteroidal anti-inflammatory drugs to avoid interference with platelet function.

Two Food and Drug Administration–approved polyvalent antivenoms are currently available for crotaline envenomation in the United States. Wyeth-Ayerst has produced an equine-derived antivenom that has been used for decades. Savage Laboratories recently released CroFab, an ovine-derived antivenom consisting of purified fragmented antibodies (Fabs) that has been approved for use in mild to moderate Crotalidae (Crotalinae) envenomation. The availability of each of these products is currently in flux. The two antivenoms are distinct and not interchangeable in terms of reconstitution, number of vials recommended, and administration interval. Small preliminary studies support the theoretical presumption that Fab antivenom is less antigenic. The reluctance to administer antivenom is often based on fear of the risk of producing anaphylactoid, anaphylactic, or delayed (serum sickness) reactions. Although serum sickness commonly occurs after use of the Wyeth product, the true incidence of adverse reactions to the Fab product will not be known for some time. No head-to-head studies published to date have compared the two antivenoms with regard to relative safety, efficacy, and adverse reactions. Table 2 summarizes the limited comparisons that may be made currently. In January 2001, Wyeth Laboratories released its plan to halt production of its antivenoms for both crotaline and coral snakes. It is unknown for how long current supplies will remain available.

If antivenom is indicated and available, either product is recommended over no treatment at all. In the case of the Wyeth product, the skin test that is recommended by the package insert does not reliably predict development of an allergic response. Therefore, a positive skin test does not preclude treatment with their antivenom. Administration of CroFab is not preceded by a skin test, and the Wyeth skin test bears no relevance to this product. To avoid anaphylactic/anaphylactoid reactions in those with a history of an allergic response to antivenom or its particular animal derivation, one may pretreat the patient with standard doses of intravenous H_1 and H_2 blocking agents. CroFab is produced with papain and could theoretically produce an allergic response in those allergic to papaya. Severe anaphylactic/anaphylactoid reactions should be treated with standard interventions, including airway, breathing, and circulatory support, epinephrine, and corticosteroids.

TABLE 1. **Crotalid Envenomation: Determining the Degree of Envenomation**

Degree of Envenomation	Contiguous Manifestations	Systemic Manifestations	Laboratory Abnormalities
None or trivial ("dry bite")	Punctures or abrasions; pain and tenderness at the bite	None	None
Mild or minimal	Punctures or abrasions; pain, tenderness, edema, and erythema at and adjacent to the bite	Perioral paresthesias	None
Moderate	Punctures or abrasions; pain, tenderness, edema, and erythema beyond the area adjacent to the bite	Perioral paresthesias, peripheral paresthesias, gustatory changes, nausea, emesis, diarrhea, weakness, lightheadedness, diaphoresis, chills	↑ PT, ↑ PTT, ↓ platelets, ↓ fibrinogen, ↑ hemoglobin
Severe	Punctures or abrasions; pain, tenderness, edema, and erythema of an entire extremity	Ventilatory insufficiency, hypotension, shock, bleeding, altered mental status, fasciculations, seizures	↑ ↑ PT, ↑ ↑ PTT, ↓ ↓ platelets, ↓ ↓ fibrinogen, ↑ ↑ hemoglobin

Abbreviations: PT = prothrombin time; PTT = partial thromboplastin time.

From Walter FG, Fernández MC, Haddad LM: North American venomous snakebite. In Haddad LM, Shannon MW, Winchester JF (eds): Clinical Management of Poisoning and Drug Overdose, 3rd ed. Philadelphia, WB Saunders, 1998, p 339.

TABLE 2. **Comparison of Polyvalent Crotaline Antivenoms**

Comparative Concept	Wyeth Antivenin (Crotalidae) Polyvalent (Wyeth-Ayerst)	CroFab (Crotalidae Polyvalent Immune Fab [Ovine]) (Savage)
Animal origin	Horse	Sheep
Snake venoms used to inoculate animals to obtain antibodies	*Crotalus adamanteus* *Crotalus atrox* *Crotalus durissus terrificus* *Bothrops atrox (fer-de-lance)*	*C. adamanteus* *C. atrox* *Crotalus scutulatus* *Agkistrodon piscivorus*
Initial dose (vials) in mild to moderate envenomation	5–10	4–6
Initial dose (vials) in severe envenomation	10–20	Not FDA approved
Potential allergenicity	Yes	Yes
Product availability	Uncertain, production discontinuance is planned	In production, limited distribution

Likewise, these interventions may be used to treat newly developing or delayed reactions, including serum sickness, depending on the severity of the reaction. Because of the potential for severe reactions to antivenom and the need for continuous monitoring, snakebite is best treated in the intensive care unit.

Dosing for either antivenom depends on the degree of envenomation and is not adjusted to the weight or age of the patient. A starting dose of 5 to 10 vials of Wyeth polyvalent antivenom is commonly recommended for mild to moderate envenomation and 20 vials for severe cases. Mixing of this antivenom can take 30 to 60 minutes. Each vial of the lyophilized protein is mixed with 10 mL of sterile water and rocked until solubilized. Rapid agitation of the mixture causes denaturation and compromises the efficacy of the antivenom while preserving the risk of an adverse reaction. The solution is then diluted into 1 L of normal saline, or 20 mL/kg in children, with the goal of infusion over a 1-hour period at a gradually increasing rate. Additional doses are given to treat continued progression of venom effects. CroFab is also reconstituted with 10 mL of sterile water, mixed by gentle swirling, and then further diluted in 250 mL of normal saline. Initial gradual infusion of four to six vials over a 1-hour period is performed, as with the Wyeth product, and may be repeated as needed. Optimal dosing of CroFab is still evolving. The package insert instructions should be followed unless new data support a change in these recommendations. Delayed coagulopathy may indicate a need for retreatment after the use of either antivenom.

The indication for antivenom treatment in coral snake envenomation is a history of a bite by a coral snake. Unlike the case of pit viper envenomation, treatment is ideally begun before the onset of symptoms. Initial dosing with five vials (Wyeth) should be followed by additional doses if neurotoxicity develops. A confirmed case of Sonoran coral snakebite has not been reported in many years, and no treatment is available for it other than supportive care. Exotic snakebite treatment also begins with good supportive care and a call to the local zoo, which may have access to exotic antivenom. In all cases, the regional poison control center will be most helpful in providing current information and guidance in the treatment of envenomation.

MARINE STINGS, BITES, AND POISONING

method of
PETER J. FENNER, M.D.
James Cook University
Townsville, Queensland, Australia

Medical problems and injuries resulting from envenomation by marine animals are common and occur worldwide, although more commonly in tropical and subtropical waters. *Envenomation* is the introduction of venom from an animal to a human or another animal, primarily by biting or stinging. Research into the large variety of marine toxins is becoming more common, but overall knowledge remains sparse. Much of the current research occurs in Australia because most of these marine hazards are common to its waters, especially the Australian tropics.

Morbidity and even mortality is frequently underestimated in some cases and overestimated in others. Knowledge of first aid and medical treatment for marine stings is lacking, with only one international postgraduate course and no undergraduate medical instruction worldwide. Physicians unfamiliar with these cases, particularly those involving immediate, life-threatening incidents, may misdiagnose, reducing the chance of successful intervention. For less severe cases, tourists returning home from the tropics may find their doctors mystified by the malady and therefore uncertain of the treatment.

ASSESSMENT AND TREATMENT OF MARINE ENVENOMATION

Treatment of marine envenomation is the most common first aid procedure provided by lifesaving and first aid organizations caring for those injured in the beach environment. First aid treatments for marine envenomation are somewhat standard, but most are largely unproven and recommended from experience of other, similar envenomations. Because marine envenomation usually occurs in areas remote from immediate medical care, and because their systemic effects occur so rapidly, critical assessment of efficacy of the recommended first aid treatments is typically based on case reports and not scientific research. Treatment is usually effective but may be improved. Much work remains to be done in this area.

First aid treatment effectively divides marine animal envenomation into three groups:

1. For stings from marine animals with venomous spines, for which local heat treatment is effective, the envenomated area can be placed in hot water. This includes injuries from stingrays and stonefish, as well as spiny fish (aquarium specimens) and even spiky echinoderms. The water temperature should be as hot as can be tolerated, usually about 43°C, but it should first be tested by the first aider or by a trial on a nonenvenomated limb of the victim. This treatment may be used, and remains effective, for many hours if medical aid is not close at hand; however, the water has to be continually "topped up" to maintain the required temperature to prevent local pain. It is often mistakenly suggested that the heat denatures the venom protein because research has demonstrated that these marine venoms are usually only denatured by much higher temperatures than those used in first aid treatment.
2. Jellyfish envenomation, where almost every sting causes a degree of localized skin pain, responds to localized cold treatment. The simplest methods of providing this treatment involves the use of ice, wrapped in a polyethylene bag, or special cold packs, kept in the freezer (which must be covered with a cloth before application to prevent skin damage). Either will stop or greatly reduce skin pain in almost 90% of the cases without other analgesia being necessary. They are first applied for 5 to 15 minutes and then reapplied, if necessary. When reapplication is required, pain relief occurs in an additional 6% of cases. Thus, cold treatment is effective in some 96% of cases.
3. Some marine animals deposit a large amount of venom into one area. In these cases, compression/immobilization bandaging should be effective in local retention of venom, delaying absorption and the systemic effects of the poison and allowing safer transport to medical aid. Examples of marine mammals that envenomate in this manner include the blue-ringed octopus, sea snakes, and cone shells. While recommended treatment is presumed to be efficacious, it is based on work by Sutherland in land snakes and is, as yet, unproven for these other envenomations.

Prevention of further envenomation from marine stings and bites is also essential and is usually achieved by (1) removal of any remaining venom apparatus (e.g., the use of vinegar to remove remaining adherent tentacles by the potentially lethal box jellyfish—see later) and (2) compression bandaging and limb immobilization. Further medical treatment in the emergency department and after admission, if necessary, is more standard, based on accepted treatment protocols.

CNIDARIAN (JELLYFISH) STINGS

Cnidarian Venoms

Cnidarian venoms are complex groups of proteins, polypeptides, and enzymes, with dermatonecrotic, hemolytic, pruritic, cardiopathic, and neurotoxic properties. Because of their thermolability they are difficult to study and isolate. Consequently, laboratory and animal research has provided both confusing and contradictory pharmacologic results. Recent work has been more predictable, and ion channel pharmacokinetic study is a current research direction. In October 2000 two carybdeid jellyfish (*Carybdea alata* and *C. rastoni*) had their DNA sequenced.

Clinical Effects

Clinical effects can be roughly divided into several main categories, which can also be treated by the suggested guidelines. Some syndromes contain more than one of the following subgroups of signs, symptoms, and treatments.

Life-threatening Effects

Effects that may be life-threatening result from the following:

- Cardiotoxins causing cardiovascular collapse or decompensation (e.g., massive chirodropid [multitentacled box jellyfish] and other massive jellyfish stings [including *Physalia* and *Stomolophus* stings])
- Neurotoxins affecting neurotransmission and causing hypoxia and other serious systemic effects
- Secondary infection with pathogenic marine bacteria
- Renal failure from myotoxicity (one report after a *Physalia* jellyfish sting)
- Anaphylaxis (one report—*Pelagia* species in the Mediterranean)

Death may occur rapidly, but these cases have often been exaggerated and exact figures are difficult to obtain, as are facts to confirm the accuracy of such reports. Morbidity data, both acute and chronic, are even more difficult to obtain and are thus greatly underestimated.

Other Effects

Pain occurs with many forms of marine envenomation. It may be localized, regionalized, or systemic, with effective first aid sometimes inadequate. Most jellyfish and marine animal envenomations cause obvious, and often painful, skin markings. Occasionally, delayed allergic rashes appear 10 to 16 days after original envenomation (especially in chirodropid stings). Rarely, bizarre and varied lesions may appear at distal skin sites (often with *Physalia* species stings) and include a distal granuloma. Gastrointestinal effects may occur. These include nausea, vomiting, diarrhea, and abdominal pain. Peripheral vascular compromise is rare, but acute blockage or compromise to limb or finger circulation has occurred after some jellyfish stings (notably *Physalia* species in the Indian Ocean). Neurotoxic effects include peripheral neuritis, mononeuritis multiplex, autonomic neurotoxicity, and central neurotoxic effects; rarely, reactive arthralgia and hallucinatory fits may occur.

Scyphozoan Jellyfish

Severe and Fatal Envenomations

There have been at least eight documented deaths from *Stomolophus nomurai* (sand jellyfish) in the Yellow Sea near Qingdao, southeast of Beijing (from acute pulmonary edema) and three deaths documented in the southeastern United States from *Physalia physalis* (Portuguese man-o'-war) from circulatory collapse. No antivenin is available. Other severe envenomations, including unconsciousness and delirium, occurred in the west Atlantic Ocean; and bilateral upper limb gangrene has occurred in the Indian Ocean, with *Physalia* strongly implicated in both areas after serologic studies, although it was not confirmed histologically or morphologically.

Pelagia noctiluca (the mauve stinger) in the Mediterranean, on one occasion only, has produced life-threatening anaphylaxis from its sting, with the victim only saved by prompt medical intervention. Other scyphozoan stings with severe morbidity have occurred around the world. The reader is referred to more specialized sources.

Cubozoan (Box) Jellyfish

Box jellyfish species, which are mainly present in tropical oceans in summer (particularly the Indo-west-Pacific including Australia and the Philippines), cause more human death and serious morbidity than any other marine species. Their bell diameter size ranges from 300 mm to a few millimeters. Unlike scyphozoan jellyfish, tentacles arise in four corners, and they can be divided into two groups: multitentacled chirodropids (including the *Chironex* box-jellyfish—*Chironex fleckeri*) in Australia and four-tentacled carybdeids (e.g., the "Irukandji" jellyfish group). All known box jellyfish have nematocysts that are totally inactivated by household vinegar (4%–6% acetic acid in water). Vinegar does not stop the pain.

Severe and Fatal Envenomations

The Australian *Chironex* box jellyfish has caused at least 63 documented human deaths since 1884. Similar box jellyfish (*Chiropsalmus quadrigatus*) have caused thousands of deaths over the years throughout the tropical and subtropical Indo-Pacific Ocean, including some 20 to 50 deaths per year in the Philippines. There has been one box jellyfish death in Texas on the Gulf of Mexico (*Chiropsalmus quadrumanus*).

Chirodropid venom is a complex mixture containing powerful dermatonecrotic, pain-producing, neurotoxic, and cardiotoxic effects in humans. Fortunately, most chirodropid stings, although causing severe skin pain, are small and not life threatening. Massive stings cause immediate and severe skin pain, with respiratory or cardiac arrest occurring within minutes, while still by the water's edge.

First Aid and Medical Treatment of Major Jellyfish Stings

Major jellyfish stings often require resuscitation (expired air or cardiopulmonary resuscitation). Further measures include supplemental oxygen IV access, and plasma expanders, preferably before moving the victim off the beach. *Chironex* box jellyfish stings need immediate vinegar dousing for 30 seconds to prevent further envenomation from remaining adherent tentacles, and larger stings may need specific box jellyfish Commonwealth Serum Laboratories (CSL) antivenin, which can be given intramuscularly by ambulance officers or IV by paramedics in some areas of tropical Australia. Minor stings can be treated with vinegar to inactivate stinging cells in remaining tentacular material, followed by ice or cold packs applied to the sting area.

Hospital treatment includes cardiographic monitoring, continued resuscitation with an endotracheal tube, if necessary, and inotropes, if needed. Pulmonary edema is treated conventionally with oxygen, diuretics, opiates, and sublingual or intravenous nitrates. Continuous positive airway pressure (CPAP) by mask with up to 14 L of oxygen may be required or even intermittent positive-pressure ventilation (IPPV) and positive end-expiration pressure (PEEP) for continuing, or developing, arterial hypoxia. Further medical care follows the usual protocols of investigation and treatment.

Carybdeids—Four-Tentacled Box-Jellyfish

These include both large (*Tamoya* and *Carybdea* species) and small (*Carukia barnesi*—the "Irukandji") jellyfish. Most occur widely in many oceans of the world and cause nuisance stings, which may be more serious on occasions. *Carukia*, the "Irukandji," warrants special mention because although it is small (12-mm bell diameter), it causes severe systemic symptoms that may be life threatening.

The Irukandji Syndrome

The classic Irukandji syndrome is well documented. After an initial mild skin sting, a bizarre set of delayed symptoms presents 20 to 40 minutes later. These include severe back and limb pains, severe headache, nausea, vomiting, sweating, restlessness, and an anxiety with a sense of "impending doom." Severe systemic hypertension may occur (up to 250/

150 mm Hg in previously fit young adults). Occasionally, some 10 to 12 hours later, these individuals may become severely dyspneic from acute toxic myocardial dilation and pulmonary edema. Ventilation may be necessary.

Treatment includes IV narcotic pain relief, oxygen, and antiemetics. Phentolamine (Regitine) 5 to 10 mg, is given intravenously, is repeated when necessary, and will usually reduce the catecholamine-like symptoms. Pulmonary edema is treated as described earlier with medication, CPAP, or IPPV, and with PEEP for continuing, or developing, arterial hypoxia. Further medical care follows the usual protocols of investigation and treatment. Antivenin is not available at present, but current research is underway.

Other jellyfish causing a similar "Irukandji-like" syndrome include some stings from *Physalia physalis* (Portuguese-man-o'-war), *Stomolophus nomurai* (sand jellyfish) in China, large carybdeids (e.g., *Tamoya*) in tropical world oceans, and *Gonionemus*, a small hydroid in the north of Japan and around Vladivostock.

Miscellaneous Jellyfish Reactions

Sea Bathers' Eruption

Sea bathers' eruption, also known as "swimmers' itch," "sea lice," and a number of "local" names, is an itchy skin irritation having many causes. These include small jellyfish medusae, sea anemone larvae, marine algae, crab larvae, small crustaceans, and "fluke" (schistosome) dermatitis. The main offender is the larval phase of *Linuche unguiculata* (thimble jellyfish), which is especially common in the Caribbean at certain times of the year, where it is often known as "el Caribe." A swimsuit or other clothing offers little or no protection because the tiny organisms are sucked in under clothing when entering the water and then are compressed against the skin by the clothing as it drains when the swimmer exits the water. Treatment is largely ineffective, but ultrapotent corticosteroid creams and antihistamines are used to give some relief. The condition may last up to 3 weeks. Unrelieved scratching can lead to secondary infection.

Jellyfish Ophthalmologic Stings

Jellyfish stings of the cornea or around the eye require ophthalmologic referral and assessment. They may produce eye pain, photophobia, and decreased visual acuity. Topical anesthesia will ease corneal pain, but specialist slit lamp examination with removal of impacted nematocysts may be necessary, possibly with drops to control intraocular pressure, inflammation, or secondary infection.

PENETRATING MARINE INJURIES

Spiny Fish

Envenomations and Injuries

Many marine and some freshwater fish are equipped with defensive spines with a venom apparatus. The most common of these are the stingray and stonefish, but this group includes many varieties worldwide, including weeverfish and catfish. The initial local pain varies in intensity among species, but general systemic effects, first aid, and medical treatments are similar for most spiny fish injuries.

Appearance

Stingrays are large flat fish with "wings" and a long whiplike tail that is equipped with one to six sharp barbs. Distribution is worldwide in tropical and subtropical waters. Contact with humans is usually in shallow water, where stingrays burrow under the sand and are stepped on by the unwary wader. The stingray stings defensively by a reflex forward whip of the tail, causing cuts, grazes, or embedding of one or more of the barbs that are situated on its tail.

Stonefish are usually 20 to 30 cm long and found on rocks and reefs in the tropical and subtropical Indo-Pacific waters. They have tough, warty skin, which may be covered with slime and is usually the color of the surrounds (frequently dark brown). On the back there are 13 sharp spines that penetrate the skin of the victim and inject venom. They will pierce thin soles of shoes.

First Aid and Medical Treatment

The puncture wound area is immersed in hot water—about 43°C (remember to first test the water). The glancing blow from a stingray barb occasionally causes open wounds, which may bleed profusely: a compression dressing and bandage or, rarely, a tourniquet may be necessary to control hemorrhage.

In stingrays, during penetration of the integument of the victim, the barb sheath ruptures, leaving tissue and venom in the wound, which will cause necrosis and infection. The whole tract should be carefully explored and even excised if possible, to remove remaining foreign material. The crater can then be packed with an alginate-based wick. This is then ejected around the tenth day after envenomation, allowing healing by secondary intention.

With all penetrating injuries, tetanus immunization is advised and treatment of secondary infection may be necessary. A skilled medical team must evaluate wounds to the chest or abdomen as soon as possible, using advanced imaging.

In stonefish envenomation, the victims suffer immediate, severe pain, which may cause them to become frantic or delirious. A bluish discoloration occurs around the puncture site, and the area often becomes edematous. Local limb paralysis, nausea and vomiting, as well as faintness may occur. Stonefish antivenin may be necessary to control severe pain.

Fatalities

At least 17 fatalities from stingrays have occurred worldwide. Trunk wounds cause most of the fatalities, but acute exsanguination has caused at least two; and one death occurred from tetanus complicating a lower leg wound.

Worldwide, deaths from stonefish envenomation are rare and difficult to actually confirm scientifically. Just five deaths have been reported, and those were described in very poor detail.

Sea Snakes

Sea snakes are similar in appearance to land snakes except they have a flattened tail to assist swimming. They have no gills because they are air breathers. Sea snakes are common in all oceans except for the Atlantic. They are inquisitive but not usually aggressive unless trapped in fishing nets.

Envenomation

Most bites are "dry": less than 10% of sea snakes actually inject any venom. The bite is relatively painless; and if venom is injected, it may be followed by symptoms including drowsiness, nausea and vomiting, weakness, visual disturbances, breathing problems, and muscle pains or stiffness. Myolysis may cause renal impairment.

Fatalities

Thousands of fatalities from sea snake envenomation have occurred in the Indo-West Pacific. Current estimates of the fatality rates worldwide are becoming less common.

First Aid and Medical Treatment

Compression/immobilization bandaging and cardiopulmonary resuscitation are applied, if necessary. This may be followed by intravenous antivenin (Australian or Japanese). The role of antivenin in reducing developing myolysis is uncertain. Good hydration and the maintenance of a good urinary output will help reduce myolysis. Renal failure and/or respiratory failure should be treated along standard lines. Primary coagulopathy does not occur in sea snake envenomation. Tetanus immunization should be considered, and follow-up to exclude secondary infection may be necessary.

The Venoms

The toxic effects are postsynaptic neurotoxic paralysis and myolysis. Either can predominate clinically, but the latter effect does so more commonly. Sea snake venoms, in contrast to many terrestrial venomous snake venoms, exhibit no clinical coagulopathic properties. The myotoxins act similarly to the phospholipase A_2 myotoxins seen in elapid and viper venoms. Secondary renal damage (distal tubular necrosis) is a danger in severe myolysis and has proved fatal. Muscle regeneration can occur slowly and will commence 1 to 2 weeks after envenomation. The postsynaptic protein neurotoxins bind to acetylcholine receptors at the neuromuscular junction, particularly of skeletal muscle. Binding is slow, but release is far slower.

Clinical Picture of Envenomation

Onset is from 30 minutes to about 4 hours after the bite. Anxiety symptoms may be early and can confuse the clinical picture. Muscle aches and pains usually occur early (myolysis). Headache, sweating, nausea, and vomiting usually follow, along with signs of true paresis, including blurred vision, ptosis, drooling, dysphagia, and dysarthria, and signs of respiratory insufficiency and airway compromise. Urine should be checked for myoglobinuria, plasma/serum creatine kinase, and aspartate aminotransferase. Hyperkalemia should be assessed for and corrected if necessary.

First Aid and Medical Management

The patient is immobilized completely with a compression/immobilization bandage and transported to a hospital. Intravenous access is needed for rehydration (adequate urine output monitoring), as may be analgesia for myalgia and early antivenin administration in diagnosed cases. Intubation with respiratory support may be necessary. Tetanus immunization should be ensured if appropriate.

Cone Shells

Envenomation and Conotoxins

The envenomation occurs by the forcible ejection of a venom-armed radula "tooth" and fired from a proboscis rather like a poisonous dart. The envenomation is usually immediately painful, with the injection of a potent peptide toxin mix, whose most important action is postsynaptic neuromuscular blockade of skeletal muscle contraction. Other conotoxin components have ion channel blocking and other disruptive ion channel effects. Death occurs in seriously envenomated patients from the hypoxia of respiratory failure but is completely preventable by respiratory resuscitation. The clinical situation is similar to a blue-ringed octopus envenomation, although their toxins differ considerably.

First Aid and Medical Treatment

The following steps should be taken:

1. Immediately apply a compression/immobilization bandage.
2. Keep the patient strictly immobilized before medical handover.
3. Establish intravenous cannulation, with monitoring of the central venous pressure if necessary.
4. Provide respiratory assistance: expired air resuscitation and subsequent IPPV as indicated. Respiratory support may be required for several hours in severe cases.
5. Provide analgesia if necessary.
6. Know that symptomatic treatment is all that is available but is effective.
7. Ensure tetanus prophylaxis.

Despite the antigenic nature of the toxin and some previous attempts at antivenin production, studies have never proceeded beyond the animal experimental stage. No antivenin is presently available, although research is continuing in Queensland, Australia.

SECONDARY INFECTION OF MARINE WOUNDS

Unlike usual skin infections, marine stings may become infected with unusual organisms, including *Vibrio, Aeromonas*, and *Pseudomonas*, among others. Swabs for culture and sensitivity need a saline-based culture medium, which the person ordering the test should specify. First-line therapy for marine organisms includes co-trimoxazole, ciprofloxacin, or doxycycline. Diabetic and immunosuppressed patients are particularly vulnerable to marine wound infections.

Almost all penetrating wounds (e.g., spiny fish) will become infected unless thorough cleansing of the wound is achieved (see earlier). Even cuts and scratches from oyster rocks and coral grazes frequently become infected. Thorough wound cleansing and early antibiotics, when antibiotics appear necessary, can avoid significant morbidity.

MARINE POISONING

Marine poisoning includes poisoning, which is sometimes fatal, from many sources. The most common of these are paralytic shellfish poisoning, putrefied fish flesh poisoning (scombroid), tropical fish poisoning (ciguatera), and tetrodotoxin poisoning ("fugu"). Others include various poisoning effects caused from ingestion of toxic marine animal flesh. Further information can be gained from specialized texts on such poisonings as clupeotoxism, ichthyotoxism, gempylotoxism, and Arctic animal flesh poisoning (hypervitaminosis A).

Toxic Shellfish Poisoning

Toxic shellfish poisoning is a large and important cause of morbidity and mortality, particularly in children. Classification is based on clinical effects:

- Paralytic shellfish toxins (saxitoxin group)
- Neurotoxic shellfish toxins (brevetoxin group)
- Diarrhetic shellfish toxins (okadaic acid group)
- Amnesic shellfish toxin (domoic acid)

These toxin groups appear to block nerve/muscle sodium channels, with brevetoxins stimulating sodium channels in autonomic nerves and domoic acid being a potent depolarizer of spinal ventral root neurons.

Clinical Features

Paralytic shellfish poisoning causes, within hours, paresthesia of lips, mouth, and throat; disequilibrium; limb weakness; and nausea and vomiting. This may last 2 to 5 days. Respiratory failure may occur, and mortality has reached 44%.

Neurotoxic shellfish poisoning causes gastrointestinal effects, paresthesia, ataxia, bradycardia, bronchospasm, and convulsions. It lasts 2 to 3 days.

Diarrhetic shellfish poisoning causes severe gastrointestinal illness for about 3 days, which may cause hypovolemic shock.

Amnesic, or "encephalopathic," shellfish poisoning causes gastrointestinal tract symptoms, ophthalmoplegia, cognitive impairment, pareses, coma, and memory loss.

Treatment

Management includes respiratory and circulatory support, rehydration, gastric emptying with airway protection, activated charcoal, and anticonvulsants. Hemodialysis has been used with some success. No specific antidotes or antivenins are available.

Scombroid Fish Poisoning

Scombrotoxism results from the ingestion of improperly preserved fish (putrefaction), in which the enzymatic production by contaminating bacteria of histamine from histidine has occurred. *Proteus, E. coli, Salmonella*, and *Klebsiella* species all possess histidine decarboxylase and convert histidine to histamine under warm conditions. Popular fish such as mackerel, tuna, bonito, sardines, and anchovies may be involved. Australian salmon have been implicated. The taste is unaffected or may be "peppery."

Clinical Features

Onset is usually within 1 hour with gastrointestinal symptoms, hot flushing and sweating, bright red rash, burning in mouth, respiratory symptoms, chest tightness, dizziness, and, in serious cases, swelling of tongue, mouth blistering, and dyspnea. The duration may be from hours to several days. This is not an allergic reaction but is intoxication by exogenous histamine.

Treatment

The victim is observed for about 2 hours. If there is no improvement or the patient's condition worsens, parenteral antihistamines and H_2 receptor antagonists may help. In severe cases, orogastric lavage and activated charcoal with respiratory and circulatory support and epinephrine may be necessary.

Ciguatera—Tropical Fish Poisoning

Occurrence and Distribution

Ciguatera is common in the Indo-West Pacific, southwest coast of north America, Indian Ocean, and Caribbean regions. Fatalities have occurred in the Indian and Pacific Oceans and the Caribbean, but inaccurate reporting and false diagnoses make statistics difficult to validate. Fatalities seem to be much less common than once thought, although morbidity is severe in some areas where total reliance on seafood in endemic areas causes great problems (e.g., Marshall Islands).

Toxins

Ciguatoxins (CTX) include P-CTX-1, a potent sodium channel toxin. All CTX seem to arise from strains of the benthic (bottom-dwelling) dinoflagellate *Gambierdiscus toxicus*. Blooms of *G. toxicus* cause CTX to accumulate in small fish, which are prey to larger fish consumed by humans. This human consumption can cause ciguatera. Cooking, boiling, marination, freezing, desiccation, or storage does not affect CTX in fish.

Tests have now been developed for CTX in freshly caught fish flesh but are not yet in common use. Do not feed suspect fish to pets because it may cause hind leg paralysis, seizures, and death.

Clinical Features

Clinical signs and symptoms of CTX are dose dependent. Two main clinical patterns of ciguatera are gastrointestinal and neurologic, with some cases showing some of both patterns and gastrointestinal patterns dominant, including diarrhea (approximately 60% cases), nausea (50%), vomiting (30%), and abdominal pain. Other symptoms include profound lassitude (90%); myalgia (80%); burning/pruritus sensation with difficulty in an apparent "temperature sense" reversal (70%); arthralgia (70%); paresthesia—hands, feet, mouth, and lips (60%); mood changes—depression, irritability, anxiety (50%); ataxia and vertigo (40%); systemic "chills" (40%); tooth pain (30%); rashes and dysuria (20%); weakness in specific muscle groups (20%); and, less commonly, bradycardia and hypotension. Gastrointestinal problems usually last a few days, but neurologic signs and symptoms may persist for months, causing severe disruption of daily life. Ciguatera has also been passed sexually and from breast milk.

Differential Diagnosis

There are no specific investigations and diagnosis is clinical. With a plethora of symptoms, misdiagnosis is common and physicians need a heightened awareness of this poisoning.

Treatment

IV fluids to correct fluid imbalance may be necessary, as well as the usual treatments for diarrhea and vomiting. Intravenous mannitol (Osmitrol)* has often been used successfully. The mechanisms of action are unclear. Chronic symptoms may need treatment with antiemetics, antidiarrheals, antipruritics, tranquilizers, and antidepressants. Counseling may be of benefit.

Tetrodotoxication Poisoning

Tetrodotoxin (TTX) is the same in pufferfish poisoning, where it is ingested, and the blue-ringed octopus, where it is injected by a bite. TTX poisoning from pufferfish ingestion has caused many human fatalities worldwide, especially in Japan where pufferfish flesh ("fugu") is a delicacy.

Three Australian deaths and at least two "near misses" are documented from the bite of the blue-ringed octopus (*Hapalochlaena* species), and one death has occurred in Singapore. Serious envenomation from this commonly occurring octopus is rare.

Distribution of Animals

Pufferfish are present in marine environments worldwide with a predominance in tropical waters. They average 20 to 50 cm in length. They have a water-inflating mechanism that is used for defensive purposes. The blue-ringed octopus is small (few centimeters) with dark brown markings and blue "rings" that become iridescent when the animal is irritated. A bite from its beak underneath the body injects venom (TTX) and is relatively painless.

Clinical Features of Tetrodotoxication

Circumoral paresthesia is followed in severe cases by dysphagia, dysarthria, visual disturbance, general weakness, respiratory difficulty, and hypoxia with hypotension and fixed and dilated pupils and possibly fatal respiratory depression.

First Aid and Medical Management

A compression/immobilization bandage is applied. Airway protection should be ensured and expired air resuscitation provided with oxygen, if available. Intravenous access and IPPV will be necessary until spontaneous breathing commences (up to 12 to 24 hours). Anticholinesterase therapy has been effective for some TTX poisoning.

Marine Bites

Marine bites include massive tissue trauma caused by saltwater crocodiles (*Crocodylus porosus*) in the Indo-Pacific area and shark attacks, which occur worldwide. There were fewer than 75 shark attacks per year worldwide during the 1990s, with 10 or fewer deaths each year. There have been 27 fatal and 31 nonfatal crocodile attacks in Australia in the past 100 years. Accurate figures are not available from other sources.

The most common shark causing injury and death is the great white shark (*Carcharodon carcharias*), although others have been implicated, including the mako shark and the tiger shark. Shark injuries often occur when the shark mistakes a swimmer for a seal and inflicts an initial bite designed to be debilitating; this frequently involves traumatic amputation of a limb. When the potential meal (the human victim in these cases) becomes exsanguinated, then the shark may return more leisurely. Surviving victims suffer major tissue loss and frequently severe infection (see earlier discussion on marine bacteria). First aid includes the use of tourniquets, supplemental oxygen, and intravenous access with large volumes of colloid, often before the victim is moved from the scene. Further treatment consists of correction of blood loss,

*Not FDA approved for this indication.

massive doses of appropriate antibiotics (see earlier), tetanus injections, and hyperbaric treatment, if available.

ACUTE POISONINGS

method of
HOWARD C. MOFENSON, M.D.,
THOMAS CARACCIO, PHARM.D.,
MICHAEL A. MCGUIGAN, M.D., and
JOSEPH GREENSHER, M.D.
Long Island Regional Poison and Drug Information Center
Mineola, New York

COMMON ABBREVIATIONS

ABG = arterial blood gas
AC = activated charcoal
AG = anion gap
ALT = alanine aminotransferase
AST = aspartate aminotransferase
AV = atrioventricular
BUN = blood urea nitrogen
BZP = benzodiazepine
CDC = Centers for Disease Control and Prevention
CNS = central nervous system
ECG = electrocardiogram
EEG = electroencephalogram
FDA = Food and Drug Administration
GABA = γ-aminobutyric acid
GI = gastrointestinal
HIV = human immunodeficiency virus
ICU = intensive care unit
MAOI = monoamine oxidase inhibitor
MDAC = multiple-dose activated charcoal
NAC = *N*-acetylcysteine
OSHA = Occupational Safety and Health Administration
$Paco_2$ = arterial carbon dioxide tension
Pao_2 = arterial oxygen tension
PEEP = positive end-expiratory pressure
PEG = polyethylene glycol
pK_a = negative logarithm of dissociation constant
PTZ = phenothiazine
SG = specific gravity
$t_{1/2}$ = half-life
Vd = volume of distribution

MEDICAL TOXICOLOGY (INGESTIONS, INHALATIONS, DERMAL AND OCULAR ABSORPTIONS)

Epidemiology

An estimated 5 million potentially toxic exposures occur each year in the United States. Poisoning is responsible for almost 12,000 deaths (including those caused by carbon monoxide) and more than 200,000 hospitalizations.

Poisoning accounts for 2% to 5% of pediatric hospital admissions, 10% of adult admissions, 5% of hospital admissions in the elderly population (older than 65 years), and 5% of ambulance calls. The largest number of fatalities resulting from poisoning are caused by carbon monoxide (CO).

Pharmaceutical preparations are involved in 40% of poisonings. The most frequent pharmaceutical toxic exposure is to acetaminophen. The leading pharmaceuticals causing fatalities were: analgesics, antidepressants, sedative hypnotics or antipsychotic drugs, stimulants and street drugs, cardiovascular agents, and alcohols.

The severity of the manifestations of acute poisoning varies greatly, depending on whether the poisoning was accidental or intentional.

Unintentional (accidental) exposure makes up 87% of all cases of poisoning. Most are acute, involve children younger than 5 years, occur in the home, and result in no or minor toxicity. Many ingestions consist of relatively nontoxic substances that necessitate minimal medical care.

Intentional (suicidal) ingestions constitute 10% to 15% of poisonings, often involve multiple substances, and frequently include ethanol, acetaminophen, and aspirin. Suicides make up 60% to 90% of reported poisoning fatalities. About 25% of suicides are attempted with drugs.

ASSESSMENT AND MAINTENANCE OF VITAL FUNCTIONS

Initial assessment of all medical emergencies follows the principles of basic and advanced cardiac life support. The adequacy of the patient's airway, degree of ventilation, and circulatory status should be determined. Vital functions should be established and maintained. Vital signs, as well as core body temperature, should be measured frequently. Evaluation of vital functions should include not only rates but also effective function (e.g., respiratory rate and depth and air exchange). See Table 1 for important measurements and vital signs.

The level of consciousness should be assessed by noting immediate AVPU signs (*a*lert, responds to *v*erbal stimuli, reacts to *p*ainful stimuli, or *u*nconscious). If the patient is unconscious, the severity is assessed by the Reed classification (Table 2) or the Glasgow Coma Scale (Table 3).

If the patient is comatose, management requires administering 100% oxygen, establishing vascular access, obtaining blood for pertinent laboratory studies, and administering glucose, thiamine, and naloxone (Narcan); intubation to protect the airway should also be considered. Pertinent laboratory studies include ABGs, electrocardiography, determination of glucose and electrolyte concentrations, renal and liver tests, and for all intentional ingestions, determination of the acetaminophen plasma concentration

TABLE 1. **Important Measurements and Vital Signs**

Age	BSA (m²)	Weight (kg)	Height (cm)	Pulse (bpm), Resting	Blood Pressure (mm Hg)			RR (rpm)
						Hypertension		
					Hypotension	SIGNIFICANT	SEVERE	
NB	0.19	3.5	50	70–190	<40/60	>96	>106	30–60
1–6 mo	0.30	4–7	50–65	80–160	<45/70	>104	>110	30–50
6 mo–1 y	0.38	7–10	65–75	80–160	<45/70	>104	>110	20–40
1–2 y	0.50–0.55	10–12	75–85	80–140	<47/74	>74/112	>82/118	20–40
3–5 y	0.54–0.68	15–20	90–108	80–120	<52/80	>76/116	>84/124	20–40
6–9 y	0.68–0.85	20–28	122–133	75–115	<60/90	>82/122	>86/130	16–25
10–12 y	1.00–1.07	30–40	138–147	70–110	<60/90	>82/126	>90/134	16–25
13–15 y	1.07–1.22	42–50	152–160	60–100	<60/90	>86/136	>92/144	16–20
16–18 y	1.30–1.60	53–60	160–170	60–100	<60/90	>92/142	>98/150	12–16
Adult	1.40–1.70	60–70	160–170	60–100	<60/90	>90/140	>120/210	10–16

Abbreviations: bpm = beats per minute; BSA = body surface area; NB = newborn; rpm = respirations per minute; RR = respiratory rate.
Data from Nadas A: Pediatric Cardiology, 3rd ed. Philadelphia, WB Saunders, 1976; Blumer JL (ed): A Practice Guide to Pediatric Intensive Care. St Louis, CV Mosby, 1990; AAP and ACEP Respiratory Distress in APLS Pediatric Emergency Medicine Course, 1993, p 5; Second Task Force on blood pressure control in children—1987. Pediatrics *79:*1, 1987; Linakis JG: Hypertension. In Fleisher GR, Ludwig S (eds): Textbook of Pediatric Emergency Medicine, 3rd ed. Baltimore, Williams & Wilkins, 1993, p 249.

(APC). Radiography of the chest and abdomen may be useful.

The severity of a stimulant's effects can also be assessed (Table 4). The assessment should be recorded to monitor the trend.

Exposure: Completely expose the patient by removing clothes and other items that interfere with a thorough evaluation. Look for clues to etiology in the clothes, including the hat and shoes.

Prevention of Toxin Absorption and Reduction of Local Damage

Routes

Poisoning exposure routes include: ingestion (80%), dermal contact (7%), ophthalmic exposure (5%), inhalation (5%), insect bites and stings (2.7%), and parenteral injections (0.3%). The effect of the toxin may be local, systemic, or both.

Local effects (skin, eyes, mucosa of the respiratory or GI tract) occur in areas of contact with the poisonous substance. Local effects are nonspecific chemical reactions that depend on the chemical properties (e.g., pH), concentration, contact time, and type of exposed surface.

Systemic effects occur when the poison is absorbed into the body and depend on the dose and distribution of the toxin and the functional reserve of the organ systems. Complications resulting from shock, hypoxia, chronic exposure, and existing illness may also influence systemic toxicity.

Delayed Toxic Action

Most pharmaceuticals are absorbed within 90 minutes. However, patients exposed to a potential toxin may be asymptomatic at the time of examination for several reasons: the substance may be nontoxic, an insufficient amount of the toxin may have been involved, or a sufficient amount may not yet have been absorbed or metabolized to produce toxicity.

Absorption may be significantly delayed for several reasons:

- A drug with anticholinergic properties is involved (e.g., antihistamines, belladonna alkaloids, diphenoxylate with atropine [Lomotil], PTZs, cyclic antidepressants).

TABLE 2. **Classification of the Level of Consciousness**

Stage	Status	Level of Consciousness	Pain Response	Reflexes	Respiration	Circulation
0	Lethargic, able to answer questions and follow commands	Asleep	Arousable	Intact	Normal	Normal
I	Responsive to pain, brainstem and deep tendon reflexes intact	Comatose	Withdraws	Intact	Normal	Normal
II	Unresponsive to pain	Comatose	None	Intact	Normal	Normal
III	Unresponsive to pain, most reflexes absent, respiratory depression	Comatose	None	Absent	Depressed	Normal
IV	Unresponsive to pain, all reflexes absent, cardiovascular and respiratory depression	Comatose	None	Absent	Cyanosis	Shock

Modified from Reed CE, Driggs MF, Foote CC: Acute barbiturate intoxication: A study of 300 cases based on a physiologic system of classification of the severity of the intoxication. Ann Intern Med *37:*290, 1952.

TABLE 3. **Glasgow Coma Scale**

Scale	Adult Response	Score	Pediatric Response (0–1 y)*
Eye opening	Spontaneous	4	Spontaneous
	To verbal command	3	To shout
	To pain	2	To pain
	None	1	No response
Motor response			
To verbal command	Obeys	6	
To painful stimuli	Localized pain	5	Localized pain
	Flexion withdrawal	4	Flexion withdrawal
	Decorticate flexion	3	Decorticate flexion
	Decerebrate extension	2	Decerebrate extension
	None	1	None
Verbal response, adult	Oriented and converses	5	Cries, smiles, coos
	Disoriented but converses	4	Cries or screams
	Inappropriate words	3	Inappropriate sounds
	Incomprehensible sounds	2	Grunts
	None	1	Gives no response
Verbal response, child	Oriented	5	
	Words or babbles	4	
	Vocal sounds	3	
	Cries or moans to stimuli	2	
	None	1	

*From Seidel J: Preparing for pediatric emergencies. Pediatr Rev *16*:466–472, 1995.
Modified from Teasdale G, Jennett B: Assessment of coma and impaired consciousness. Lancet *2*:81–84, 1974; Simpson D, Reilly P: Pediatric coma scale. Lancet *2*:450, 1982.

- Sustained-release and enteric-coated preparations, which have delayed and prolonged absorption, are involved.
- Concretions may form (e.g., with the ingestion of salicylates, iron, glutethimide, or meprobamate [Equanil]) and can delay absorption and prolong the action.
- Substances must be metabolized to a toxic metabolite or time is required to produce a toxic effect on the organ system (e.g., acetaminophen [Tylenol], *Amanita phalloides* mushrooms, acetonitrile, carbon tetrachloride, colchicine, digoxin [Lanoxin], ethylene glycol, heavy metals, methanol, methylene chloride, MAOIs, oral hypoglycemic agents, parathion, paraquat).

Decontamination

Decontamination procedures should be considered for an asymptomatic patient if the exposure involves potentially toxic substances in toxic amounts.

TABLE 4. **Classification of Severity of Effects of Stimulants**

Severity	Manifestations
Grade 1	Diaphoresis, hyperreflexia, irritability, mydriasis, tremors
Grade 2	Confusion, fever, hyperactivity, hypertension, tachycardia, tachypnea
Grade 3	Delirium, mania, hyperpyrexia, tachydysrhythmia
Grade 4	Coma, convulsions, cardiovascular collapse

Adapted with permission from Espelin DE, Done AK: Amphetamine poisoning. Effectiveness of chlorpromazine. N Engl J Med *278*:1361–1365, 1968.

Ocular exposure should be treated immediately with water or saline irrigation for 15 to 20 minutes with the eyelids fully retracted. The use of neutralizing chemicals is contraindicated. All caustic and corrosive injuries should be examined by an ophthalmologist after the instillation of fluorescein dye.

Dermal exposure is treated immediately with copious irrigation for 30 minutes. Shampooing the hair, cleansing the fingernails, navel, and perineum, and irrigating the eyes are necessary with extensive exposure. The clothes should be specially bagged and may have to be discarded. Leather goods can be irreversibly contaminated and must be abandoned. Caustic (alkali) exposure can require hours of irrigation. Dermal absorption can occur with such substances as pesticides, hydrocarbons, and cyanide.

Injection of drugs and toxins can involve envenomation. Cold packs and tourniquets should not be used, and incision is not generally recommended. Venom extractors may be used within minutes of envenomation, and proximal lymphatic constricting bands or elastic wraps may be used to delay lymphatic flow and immobilize the extremity.

Inhalation of toxic substances is managed by immediately removing the victim from the contaminated environment, if necessary, by protected rescuers.

GI exposure is the most common route of poisoning. GI decontamination may be performed by gastric emptying (induction of emesis, gastric lavage), adsorption by administering single or multiple doses of AC, or whole-bowel irrigation. No procedure is routine; the procedure should be individualized on the basis of the patient's age, properties of the substance ingested, and time since ingestion. If no attempt is made to decontaminate the patient, the reason should be clearly documented in the medical record (e.g., time elapsed, past peak of action, ineffectiveness, or risk of procedure).

Gastric-Emptying Procedures. The technique used is influenced by the patient's age and the procedure's effectiveness (the size of the orogastric tube used in a small child may not be large enough for adequate lavage, e.g., with iron tablets), time of ingestion (gastric emptying is usually ineffective more than 1 hour after ingestion), clinical status (asymptomatic and the time to peak effect has elapsed or the patient's condition is too unstable), formulation of the substance ingested (regular release, sustained release, enteric coated), amount ingested, caustic action, and rapidity of onset of CNS depression or stimulation (convulsions). Most studies show that gastric emptying removes only about 30% (19%–62%) of the ingested toxin under optimal conditions, and it has not been demonstrated that the procedure improved the outcome.

The clinician should attempt to obtain ample information about the patient, including the patient's intent.

The regional poison control center should be consulted for the exact ingredients and the latest management. The first-aid information on product labels is notoriously inaccurate, and product ingredients change.

Syrup of Ipecac–Induced Emesis. Syrup of ipecac–induced emesis is most useful in young children within 1 hour of a witnessed ingestion of a toxic amount of a known agent. The poison control center should be called before inducing emesis. It is not considered useful in the emergency department setting.

Contraindications or situations in which induction of emesis is inappropriate include the following:

- Ingestion of caustic substances
- Loss of airway protective reflexes, for example, with substances that can produce rapid onset of CNS depression or convulsions
- Ingestion of low-viscosity petroleum distillates
- Significant vomiting before examination or hematemesis
- Age younger than 6 months
- Foreign bodies (emesis is ineffective and may lead to aspiration)
- Clinical conditions: pregnancy, neurologic impairment, hemodynamic instability, increased intracranial pressure, and hypertension
- Delay in evaluation (more than 1 hour after ingestion)

The patient cannot tolerate oral intake for a mean of 2 to 3 hours after ipecac-induced emesis.

The dose of syrup of ipecac for a 6- to 9-month-old infant is 5 mL; for a 9- to 12-month-old, 10 mL; and for a 1- to 12-year-old, 15 mL. For children older than 12 years and for adults, the dose is 30 mL. The dose may be repeated once if the child does not vomit in 15 to 20 minutes. The vomitus should be inspected for remnants of pills or toxic substances, and the appearance and odor should be documented.

Gastric Aspiration and Lavage. This procedure is recommended only if life-threatening amounts of substances are involved, if the benefits outweigh the risks, if performed within 1 hour after ingestion, and if no known contraindications exist. Contraindications are similar to those for ipecac-induced emesis. The procedure can be accomplished after the insertion of an endotracheal tube in patients with CNS depression or controlled convulsions. The patient should be placed with the head lower than the hips in a left lateral decubitus position. The location of the tube should be confirmed by radiography, if necessary, and suctioning equipment should be available.

Contraindications to gastric aspiration and lavage include the following:

- Caustic ingestions because of the risk of esophageal perforation
- Uncontrolled convulsions because of the danger of aspiration and injury during the procedure
- High-viscosity petroleum distillate products
- CNS depression or absence of protective airway reflexes without endotracheal tube protection
- Significant cardiac dysrhythmias, which should be controlled
- Either significant emesis before examination or hematemesis
- Delay in evaluation (more than 1 hour after ingestion)

For adults, a large-bore orogastric Lavacuator hose or a No. 42 French Ewald tube is used. For children, a No. 22 to No. 28 French orogastric-type tube is used, but this technique is usually ineffective in solid ingestions (e.g., iron tablets).

The amount of fluid used for lavage varies with the patient's age and size. In general, aliquots of 50 to 100 mL per lavage are used for adults and 5 mL/kg up to 50 to 100 mL per lavage for children. Lavage fluid is 0.89% saline.

Activated Charcoal. Recent guidelines indicate that there is insufficient evidence to recommend the routine use of AC. AC is indicated only if it can be administered within 1 hour of ingestion of a toxic amount of substance. Oral AC adsorbs the toxin onto its surface before GI absorption and interrupts enterogastric and enterohepatic circulation of toxic metabolites. AC is a stool marker indicating that the toxin has passed through the GI tract.

AC does not effectively adsorb small molecules or molecules lacking carbon, as listed in Table 5. AC adsorption may be diminished by the concurrent presence in the stomach of milk, cocoa powder, or ice cream.

Relative contraindications to the use of AC include the following:

- It does not interfere with the effectiveness of NAC in acetaminophen overdose.
- It does not effectively adsorb caustics and corro-

TABLE 5. **Substances Poorly Adsorbed by Activated Charcoal**

C—Caustics and corrosives
H—Heavy metals (arsenic, iron, lead, lithium, mercury)
A—Alcohols (ethanol, methanol, isopropyl) and glycols (ethylene glycol)
R—Rapid onset or absorption of cyanide and strychnine
C—Chlorine and iodine
O—Others insoluble in water (substances in tablet form)
A—Aliphatic and poorly absorbed hydrocarbons (petroleum distillates)
L—Laxatives, sodium, magnesium, potassium

sives, may produce vomiting or cling to the mucosa, and may falsely appear as a burn at endoscopy.

- It should not be given to a comatose patient without securing the airway.
- It should not be given in the absence of bowel sounds.

The usual initial adult dose is 60 to 100 g, and the dose for children is 15 to 30 g. It is administered orally as a slurry mixed with water or by nasogastric or orogastric tube. *Caution*: The clinician must be sure that the tube is in the stomach. Cathartics are not necessary.

MULTIPLE-DOSE ACTIVATED CHARCOAL. Repeated dosing with AC decreases the half-life and increases the clearance of phenobarbital, dapsone, quinidine, theophylline, and carbamazepine. Recent guidelines indicate there is insufficient evidence to support the use of MDAC unless a life-threatening amount of one of the substances mentioned previously is involved. Cathartics are no longer recommended. At present, no controlled studies have demonstrated that MDAC or cathartics alter the clinical course of an intoxication. The MDAC dosage varies from 0.25 to 0.50 g/kg every 1 to 4 hours, and continuous nasogastric tube infusion of 0.25 to 0.5 g/kg/h has been used to decrease vomiting.

GI dialysis involves diffusion of the toxin from the higher concentration in the serum of the mesenteric vessels to the lower levels in the GI tract mucosal cells and subsequently into the GI lumen, where the concentration has been lowered by intraluminal AC adsorption.

Complications of AC use have been reported in at least a dozen cases, but many cases of pulmonary aspiration and "charcoal" lung go unreported.

Catharsis. Cathartics were used in the past to hasten the elimination of any remaining toxin in the GI tract. However, no studies have demonstrated the effectiveness of cathartics, and they are no longer recommended as a form of GI decontamination.

Whole-Bowel Irrigation. In whole-bowel irrigation, solutions of PEG with balanced electrolytes are used to cleanse the bowel without causing shifts in fluids or electrolytes.

Indications (not approved by the FDA): The procedure has been studied and used successfully in iron overdose when abdominal radiographs reveal incomplete emptying of excess iron. Additional indications include ingestions such as body packing of illicit drugs (e.g., cocaine, heroin). The procedure is to administer, orally or by nasogastric tube, the solution (GoLYTELY or Colyte) at 0.5 L/h in children younger than 5 years, 1 L/h in children aged 6 to 12 years, or 1.5 to 2 L/h in adolescents and adults for 5 hours. The endpoint is reached when the rectal effluent is clear or radiopaque material can no longer be seen in the GI tract on abdominal radiographs.

Contraindcations: These measures should not be used if extensive hematemesis, ileus, or signs of bowel obstruction, perforation, or peritonitis are present.

Dilution. Dilutional treatment is indicated for the immediate management of caustic and corrosive poisonings but is otherwise not useful. Administration of diluting fluid—more than 30 mL in children and 250 mL in adults—may produce vomiting and reexpose the vital tissues to the effects of local damage and possible aspiration.

Neutralization. Neutralization has not been proved to be safe or effective.

Endoscopy and Surgery. Surgery has been required in the management of body packer's obstruction, intestinal ischemia produced by cocaine ingestion, and the local caustic action of iron.

Differential Diagnosis Based on Central Nervous System Manifestations of Poisoning

Neurologic parameters help in classifying and assessing the need for supportive treatment and may provide diagnostic clues to the etiology. See Tables 6 through 9.

Use of Antidotes

Antidotes are available for only a relatively small number of poisons and should be administered only after the integrity of vital functions has been established. Table 10 summarizes the commonly used antidotes, their indications, and methods of administration. The regional poison control center should be consulted for further information on these antidotes.

Enhancement of Elimination

Medical methods for elimination of absorbed toxic substances are diuresis, dialysis, hemoperfusion, exchange transfusion, plasmapheresis, enzyme induction, and inhibition. Methods of increasing urinary excretion of toxic chemicals and drugs have been studied extensively, but the other modalities have not been well evaluated.

In general, these methods are needed in only a minority of instances and should be reserved for life-threatening circumstances or when a definite benefit is anticipated.

Diuresis

Diuresis increases the renal clearance of compounds that are eliminated primarily by the renal

Text continued on page 1185

TABLE 6. **Toxic Effects of Central Nervous System Depressants***

General Manifestations	CNS Depressants
Bradycardia	Alcohols and glycols (S-H)
Bradypnea†	Anticonvulsants (S-H)
Shallow respirations	Antidysrhythmics (S-H)
Hypotension	Antihypertensives (S-H)
Hypothermia	Barbiturates (S-H)
Flaccid coma	Benzodiazepines (S-H)§
Miosis	Butyrophenones (Syly)
Hypoactive bowel sounds	β-Adrenergic blockers (Syly)
Frozen addict syndrome‡	Calcium channel blockers (Syly)
	Digitalis (Syly)
	Opioids (O)‖¶
	Lithium (mixed)
	Muscle relaxants
	Phenothiazines (Syly)
	Nonbarbiturate, benzodiazepine sedative hypnotics (S-H)‖ (chloral hydrate, glutethimide, methaqualone, methyprylon, ethchlorvynol, bromide)
	Tricyclic antidepressants (late) (Syly)

*CNS depressants are cholinergics (C), opioids (O) and sedative hypnotics (S-H), and sympatholytic agents (Syly). The hallmarks of CNS depressant activity are lethargy, sedation, stupor, and coma.

†Barbiturates may produce an initial tachycardia.

‡The "frozen addict" syndrome is due to a neurotoxin resulting from improper synthesis of an analogue of meperidine. Its manifestations are similar to those of the permanent type of parkinsonism.

§Benzodiazepines rarely produce coma that interferes with cardiorespiratory function.

‖Convulsions are produced by codeine, propoxyphene (Darvon), meperidine (Demerol), glutethimide, phenothiazines, methaqualone, and tricyclic or other cyclic antidepressants.

¶Pulmonary edema is common with opioids and sedative hypnotics.

TABLE 8. **Toxic Effects of Hallucinogens***

General Manifestations	Hallucinogens
Tachycardia and dysrhythmias	Amphetamines
	Anticholinergics
Tachypnea	Carbon monoxide
Hypertension	Cardiac glycosides
Hallucinations, usually visual	Cocaine
	Ethanol
Disorientation	Hydrocarbon inhalation: abuse or occupational
Panic reaction	
Toxic psychosis	Lysergic acid diethylamide (LSD)
Moist skin	Marijuana
Mydriasis (reactive)	Mescaline (peyote)
Hyperthermia	Mescaline-amphetamine hybrids†
Flashbacks	Metals (chronic mercury, arsenic)
	Mushrooms (psilocybin)
	Phencyclidine
	Plants (morning glory seeds, nutmeg)

*Considerable overlap occurs in this category; however, the major hallmark is hallucinations.

†The mescaline-amphetamine hybrids are methylene dioxymethamphetamine (MDMA, Ecstasy, Adam) and methylene dioxyamphetamine (MDA, Eve), which have been associated with deaths.

TABLE 7. **Toxic Effects of Central Nervous System Stimulants***

General Manifestations	CNS Stimulants
Tachycardia	Amphetamines (Sy)
Tachypnea and dysrhythmias	Anticholinergics (Ach)‡
	Cocaine (Sy)
Hypertension	Camphor (mixed)
Convulsions	Ergot alkaloids (Sy)
Spastic coma†	Isoniazid (mixed)
Toxic psychosis	Lithium (mixed)
Mydriasis (reactive)	Lysergic acid diethylamide (LSD) (H)
Agitation and restlessness	
Moist skin	Hallucinogens (H)
Tremors	Mescaline and synthetic analogues
	Metals (arsenic, lead, mercury)
	Methylphenidate (Ritalin) (Sy)
	MAOIs (Sy)
	Pemoline (Cylert) (Sy)
	Phencyclidine (H)§
	Salicylates (mixed)
	Strychnine (mixed)
	Sympathomimetics (Sy) (phenylpropanolamine, theophylline, caffeine, thyroid)
	Withdrawal from ethanol, β-adrenergic blockers, clonidine, opioids, sedative hypnotics (W)

*CNS stimulants are anticholinergics (Ach), hallucinogens (H), sympathomimetics (Sy), and withdrawal (W). The hallmarks of CNS stimulant activity are convulsions and hyperactivity.

†Flaccid coma eventually develops after seizures.

‡Anticholinergics produce dry skin and mucosa and decreased bowel sounds.

§Phencyclidine may produce miosis.

TABLE 9. **Effects of Toxins on the Autonomic Nervous System**

General Manifestations	Agents
Anticholinergic	
Tachycardia, dysrhythmias (rare)	Antihistamines
	Antispasmodic GI preparations
Tachypnea	Antiparkinsonian preparations
Hypertension (mild)	Atropine
Hyperthermia	Cyclobenzaprine (Flexeril)
Hallucinations	Mydriatic ophthalmologic agents
Mydriasis (unreactive)	Over-the-counter sleep agents
Flushed skin	Plants (*Datura* species), mushrooms
Dry skin and mouth	
Hypoactive bowel sounds	Phenothiazines (early)
Urinary retention	Scopolamine
Lilliputian hallucinations	Tricyclic or other cyclic antidepressants (early)
Cholinergic	
Bradycardia (muscarinic)	Bethanechol
Tachycardia (nicotinic)	Carbamate insecticides (carbaryl)
Miosis (muscarinic)	
Diarrhea (muscarinic)	Edrophonium
Hypertension (variable)	Organophosphate insecticides (malathion, parathion)
Hyperactive bowel sounds	
Excess urination (muscarinic)	Parasympathetic agents (physostigmine, pyridostigmine)
Excess salivation (muscarinic)	
Lacrimation (muscarinic)	
Bronchospasm (muscarinic)	Toxic mushrooms (*Amanita muscaria, Clitocybe* species)
Muscle fasciculations (nicotinic)	
Paralysis (nicotinic)	

Table 10. **Initial Doses of Antidotes for Common Poisonings, Alphabetically Arranged**

Antidote	Use	Dose	Route	Adverse Reactions (AR) and Comments
***N*-Acetylcysteine** (NAC, Mucomyst) Stock level to treat 70-kg adult for 24 h: 7 vials, 20%, 30 mL	Acetaminophen, carbon tetrachloride (experimental)	140 mg/kg loading, followed by 70 mg/kg q4h for 17 doses	PO	Nausea, vomiting Dilute to 5% with sweet juice or flat cola
Atropine. Stock level to treat 70-kg adult for 24 h; 1 g (1 mg/mL in 1 or 10 mL)	Organophosphate and carbamate pesticides	*Child:* 0.02–0.05 mg/kg repeated q5–10min to maximum of 2 mg as necessary until cessation of secretions. *Adult:* 1–2 mg q5–10min as necessary. Dilute in 1–2 mL of 0.89% saline for endotracheal instillation *IV infusion dose:* Place 8 mg of atropine in 100 mL of D5W or saline. Concentration = 0.08 mg/mL. Dose range = 0.02–0.08 mg/kg/h or 0.25–1 mL/kg/h. Severe poisoning may require supplemental IV atropine intermittently in doses of 1–5 mg until drying of secretions occurs	IV or ET	Tachycardia, dry mouth, blurred vision, and urinary retention Ensure adequate ventilation before administration
Calcium chloride (10%). Stock level to treat 70-kg adult for 24 h: 5–10 vials, 1 g (1.35 mEq/mL)	Hypocalcemia, fluoride, calcium channel blockers	0.1–0.2 mL/kg (10–20 mg/kg) slow push q 10 min up to maximum of 10 mL (1 g). Because calcium response lasts 15 min, some patients may require continuous infusion of 0.2 mL/kg/h up to maximum of 10 mL/h during monitoring for dysrhythmias and hypotension	IV	Administer slowly with BP and ECG monitoring and have magnesium available to reverse calcium effects **AR:** Tissue irritation, hypotension, dysrhythmias resulting from rapid injection Contraindication: Digitalis glycoside intoxication
Calcium gluconate (10%). Stock level to treat 70-kg adult for 24 h: 5–10 vials, 1 g (0.45 mEq/mL)	Hypocalcemia, fluoride, calcium channel blockers, hydrofluoric acid, black widow envenomation	0.3–0.4 mL/kg (30–40 mg/kg) slow push; repeat as needed up to maximum dose of 10–20 mL (1–2 g)	IV	Same as for calcium chloride
Calcium gluconate gel. Stock level: 3.5 g	Hydrofluoric acid	2.5 g of USP powder added to 100 mL of water-soluble lubricating jelly (e.g., K-Y Jelly, Lubafax) (or 3.5 g into 150 mL). Some use 6 g of calcium carbonate in 100 g of lubricant. Place injured hand in surgical glove filled with gel, or apply q4h. If pain persists, calcium gluconate injection may be needed (after)	Dermal	Powder is available from Spectrum Pharmaceutical Company in California: 1-800-772-8786. Commercial preparation of calcium gluconate gel is available from Pharmascience in Montreal, Quebec: 514-340-1114
Infiltration of calcium gluconate	Hydrofluoric acid	Dose: Infiltrate each square cm of affected dermis or subcutaneous tissue with about 0.5 mL of 10% calcium gluconate with a 30-gauge needle. Repeat as needed to control pain	Infiltrate	

Table continued on following page

TABLE 10. **Initial Doses of Antidotes for Common Poisonings, Alphabetically Arranged** *Continued*

Antidote	Use	Dose	Route	Adverse Reactions (AR) and Comments
Cyanide antidote kit. Stock level to treat 70-kg adult for 24 h: 2 Lilly Cyanide Antidote kits	Cyanide; hydrogen sulfide (nitrites only are given; do not use sodium thiosulfate for hydrogen sulfide) Individual portions of the kit can be used in certain circumstances (consult PCC)	Amyl nitrite: 1 crushable ampule for 30 s of every minute. Use new ampule q3min. May omit step if venous access is established	Inhalation	If methemoglobinemia occurs, do not use methylene blue to correct this condition because it releases cyanide
		Sodium nitrite: *Child:* 0.33 mL/kg of 3% solution if hemoglobin level is not known, otherwise follow tables with product. *Adult:* up to 300 mg (10 mL). Dilute nitrite in 100 mL of 0.9% saline, administer slowly at 5 mL/min. Slow infusion if fall in BP	IV	
		Sodium thiosulfate: *Child:* 1.6 mL/kg of 25% solution; may be repeated q 30–60 min to a maximum of 12.5 gm or 50 mL in *adult.*	IV	**AR:** Nausea, dizziness, headache; tachycardia, muscle rigidity, and bronchospasm (rapid administration)
Dantrolene sodium (Dantrium). Stock level to treat 70-kg adult for 24 h: 700 mg in 35 vials (20 mg per vial)	Malignant hyperthermia	Administer over 20-min period 2–3 mg/kg IV rapidly Repeat loading dose q 10 min, if necessary up to a maximum total dose of 10 mg/kg. When temperature and heart rate decrease, slow the infusion to 1–2 mg/kg q6h for 24–48 h until all evidence of malignant hyperthermia syndrome has subsided. Follow with oral doses of 1–2 mg/kg qid for 24 h as necessary	IV or PO	Available as 20-mg lyophilized dantrolene powder for reconstitution; the powder contains 3 g of mannitol and sodium hydroxide in 70-mL vials. Mix with 60 mL of sterile distilled water without a bacteriostatic agent and protect from light. Use within 6 h after being reconstituted **AR:** Hepatotoxicity occurs with cumulative dose of 10 mg/kg; thrombophlebitis (best given in central line)
Deferoxamine (DFO, Desferal). Stock level to treat 70-kg adult for 24 h: 12 vials (50 mg per ampule)	Iron (100 mg of DFO binds 8.5–9.3 mg of iron)	IV infusion of 15 mg/kg/h (3 mL/kg/h: 500 mg in 100 mL D5W), maximum of 6 g/d. Rates of >45 mg/kg/h if conc. >1000 μg/dL.	IV preferred; avoid therapy >24 h	Hypotension (minimized by avoiding rapid infusion) DFO challenge test (50 mg/kg) is unreliable if negative
Diazepam (Valium). Stock level to treat 70-kg adult for 24 h: 200 mg	Any intoxication that provokes seizures when specific therapy is not available, e.g., amphetamines, PCP, barbiturate and alcohol withdrawal, chloroquine poisoning	*Adult:* 5–10 mg (maximum of 20 mg) at a rate of 5 mg/min until seizure is controlled. May be repeated 2 or 3 times *Child:* 0.1–0.3 mg/kg up to 10 mg slowly over 2-min period	IV	**AR:** Confusion, somnolence, coma, hypotension Intramuscular absorption is erratic. Establish airway and administer 100% oxygen and glucose

Digoxin-specific Fab antibodies (Digibind). Stock level to treat 70-kg adult for 24 h: 20 vials	Digoxin, digitoxin, oleander tea with any of the following: (1) imminent cardiac arrest or shock, (2) hyperkalemia of >5.0 mEq/L, (3) serum digoxin of >10 ng/mL (adult) or >5 ng/mL (child) at 8–12 h after ingestion in adults, (4) digitalis delirium, (5) ingestion of more than 10 mg in adult or 4 mg in child, (6) bradycardia or second- or third-degree heart block unresponsive to atropine, (7) life-threatening digitoxin or oleander poisoning	1. *Amount (total mg) ingested known* multiplied by bioavailability (0.8) = body burden. The body burden divided by 0.6 (0.6 mg of digoxin is bound by 1 vial of 40 mg of Fab) = number of vials needed 2. *If amount is unknown but the steady-state serum concentration is known in ng/mL:* *Digoxin:* ng/mL × (Vd = 5.6 L/kg) × wt (kg) = μg body burden. Body burden divided by 1000 = mg body burden/0.6 = number of vials needed 3. *If the amount is not known,* agent is administered in life-threatening situations as 10 vials (400 mg) IV in saline over 30-min period in adults. If cardiac arrest is imminent, administer 20 vials (adult) as a bolus	IV	Administer by infusion over 30-min period through a 0.22-μm filter. If cardiac arrest is imminent, may administer by bolus injection. Consult PCC for more details **AR:** Allergic reactions (rare), return of condition being treated with digitalis glycoside
Dimercaprol (BAL in Oil). Stock level to treat 70-kg adult for 24 h: 1200 mg (4 ampules, 100 mg/mL of 10% solution in oil in 3-mL ampule)	Chelating agent for arsenic, mercury, lead, antimony, bismuth, chromium, copper, gold, nickel, tungsten, and zinc	3–5 mg/kg q4h, usually for 5–10 d	Deep IM	**AR:** Local injection site pain and sterile abscess, nausea, vomiting, fever, salivation, hypertension, and nephrotoxicity (alkalize urine)
Diphenhydramine (Benadryl). Antiparkinsonian action. Stock level to treat 70-kg adult for 24 h: 5 vials (10 mg/mL, 10 mL each)	Used to treat extrapyramidal symptoms and dystonia induced by phenothiazines, PCP, and related drugs	*Child:* 1–2 mg/kg IV slowly over 5-min period up to maximum of 50 mg, followed by 5 mg/kg per 24 h PO divided q6h, up to 300 mg/ 24 h *Adult:* 50 mg IV followed by 50 mg PO qid for 5–7 d. Note: Symptoms abate within 2–5 min after IV administration	IV and PO	Fatal dose, 20–40 mg/kg **AR:** Dry mouth, drowsiness
Ethanol (ethyl alcohol). Stock level to treat 70-kg adult for 24 h: 3 bottles, 10% (1 L each)	Methanol, ethylene glycol	10 mL/kg loading dose concurrently with 1.4 mL/kg (average) infusion of 10% ethanol. (Consult PCC for more details.)	IV	**AR:** Nausea, vomiting, sedation. Use 0.22-μm filter if preparing from bulk 100% ethanol
Flumazenil (Romazicon). Stock level to treat 70-kg adult for 24 h: 10 vials (0.1 mg/mL, 10 mL)	Benzodiazepines	Administer 0.2 mg (2 mL) over 30-s period. (Pediatric dose not established, 0.01 mg/kg.) Wait 3 min for a response. If desired consciousness is not achieved, administer 0.3 mg (3 mL) over 30-s period Wait 3 min for response. If desired consciousness is not achieved, administer 0.5 mg (5 mL) over 30-s period at 60-s intervals up to a maximal cumulative dose of 3 mg (30 mL) (1 mg in children) Because effects last only 1–5 h, if there is a response, monitor carefully over next 6 h for resedation. If multiple repeated doses, consider a continuous infusion of 0.2–1 mg/h	IV	It is not recommended to improve ventilation. Its role in CNS depression needs to be clarified. It should not be used routinely in comatose patients. It is *contraindicated* in cyclic antidepressant intoxications, stimulant overdose, in long-term benzodiazepine use (may precipitate life-threatening withdrawal), if benzodiazepines are used to control seizures, in head trauma **AR:** Nausea, vomiting, facial flushing, agitation, headache, dizziness, seizures, death

Table continued on following page

TABLE 10. **Initial Doses of Antidotes for Common Poisonings, Alphabetically Arranged** *Continued*

Antidote	Use	Dose	Route	Adverse Reactions (AR) and Comments
Folic acid (Folvite). Stock level to treat 70-kg adult for 24 h: two 100-mg vials	Methanol or ethylene glycol (investigational)	1 mg/kg up to 50 mg q4h for 6 doses	IV	Uncommon
Fomepizole (4-MP, Antizole) Stock level to treat 70 kg adult: four–1.5 mL vials (1 g/mL)	Ethylene glycol (Methanol)	Loading dose: 15 mg/kg (0.015 mL/kg) IV followed by maintanence dose of 10 mg/kg (0.010 mL/kg every 12 h for 4 doses, then 15 mg/kg every 12 h until ethylene glycol levels are <20 mg/dL Fomepizole can be given to patients undergoing hemodialysis; see text Antizol should be diluted in 100 mL 0.9% saline or D5W and mixed well	IV	Suggested: co-administer folate, 50 mg IV (*child:* 1 mg/kg), thiamine, 100 mg/day (*child:* 50 mg), and pyridoxine, 50 mg IV or q6h, until intoxication is resolved Monitor for urinary oxalate crystals **AR:** headache, nausea, dizziness
Glucagon. Stock level to treat 70-kg adult for 24 h: 100 mg (10 vials, 10 U)	β-blockers, calcium channel blockers, hypoglycemic agents	*Adult:* 5–10 mg, then infuse 1–5 mg/h *Child:* 0.05–0.1 mg/kg, then infuse 0.07 mg/kg/h. Large doses up to 100 mg/24 h have been used	IV	**AR:** Hyperglycemia, nausea, vomiting Dissolve in D5W, not in 0.9% saline. Do not use diluent in package because of possible phenol toxicity
Magnesium sulfate. Stock level to treat 70-kg adult for 24 h: approximately 25 g (50 mL of 50% or 200 mL of 12.5%)	Torsades de pointes	*Adult:* 2 g (20 mL of 20% solution) over 20-min period. If no response in 10 min, repeat and follow by continuous infusion at 1 g/h *Child:* 25–50 mg/kg initially, maintenance with 30–60 mg/kg per 24 h (0.25–0.50 mEq/kg per 24 h) up to 1000 mg per 24 h. (Dose not studied in controlled fashion.)	IV	Use with caution if there is renal impairment
Methylene blue. Stock level to treat 70-kg adult for 24 h: five ampules (10 mg per 10 mL)	Methemoglobinemia	0.1–0.2 mL/kg of 1% solution, slow infusion, may be repeated q 30–60 min	IV	**AR:** Nausea, vomiting, headache, dizziness
Nalmefene (Revex). Stock level: not established	Narcotic antagonist	The dose for opioid overdose as bolus in adults is 0.5–1 mg q2min up to a total of 2 mg IV. May also be given IM or SC. In patients with renal failure, administer over a 1-min period. In postoperative opioid depression reversal, 0.1–0.5 μg/kg IV q2min as needed and may be repeated up to total dose of 1 μg/kg	IV, IM, SC	Role in comatose patients and opioid overdose is not clear. It is 16 times more potent than naloxone; duration of action is up to 8 h (half-life, 10.8 h; versus naloxone, 1 h). Clinical trials in more than 1750 patients have not shown significant adverse reactions

Naloxone (Narcan). Stock level to treat 70-kg adult for 24 h: 3 vials (1 mg/mL, 10 mL)	Comatose patient; ineffective ventilation or adult respiratory rate <12 rpm; opioids	In suspected overdose, administer 0.1 mg/kg IV in child younger than 5 y, up to 2 mg. In older children and adults, administer 2 mg q2min up to a total of 10–20 mg. Can also be administered into the ET tube. If no response by 10 mg, pure opioid intoxication is unlikely If opioid abuse is suspected, restraints should be in place before administration; initial dose, 0.1 mg to avoid withdrawal and violent behavior. The initial dose is then doubled every minute progressively to a total of 10 mg Continuous infusion has been advocated because many opioids outlast the short half-life	IV, ET	Larger doses of naloxone may be required for more poorly antagonized synthetic opioid drugs: buprenorphine, codeine, dextromethorphan, fentanyl, pentazocine, propoxyphene, diphenoxylate, nalbuphine, new and potent designer drugs, or long-acting opioids such as methadone **Complications:** Although naloxone is safe and effective, there are rare reports of complications (in <1% of cases) of pulmonary edema, seizures, hypertension, cardiac arrest, and sudden death The infusions are titrated to avoid respiratory depression and opioid withdrawal manifestations Tapering of infusions can be attempted after 12 h and when the patient's condition has been stabilized
Physostigmine (Antilirium). Stock level to treat 70-kg adult for 24 h: 10 ampules (2 mL each)	Anticholinergic agents (not routinely used, indicated only with life-threatening complications)	*Child:* 0.02 mg/kg slow push to maximum of 2 mg q30–60min *Adult:* 1–2 mg q5min to maximum of 6 mg	IV	**AR:** Bradycardia, asystole, seizures, bronchospasm, vomiting, headaches. Do not use for cyclic antidepressants
Pralidoxime (2-PAM, Protopam). Stock level to treat 70-kg adult for 24 h: 12 vials (1 g/20 mL)	Organophosphates	*Child ≤12 y:* 25–50 mg/kg maximum (4 mg/kg/min); *older than 12 y:* 1–2 g per dose in 250 mL of 0.89% saline over period of 5–10 min. Maximal dose 200 mg/min. Repeat q6–12h for 24–48 h. Maximal adult dose, 6 g/d Alternative: Main infusion of 1 g in 100 mL of 0.9% saline at 5–20 mg/kg/h (0.5–12 mL/kg/h) up to maximum of 500 mg/h or 50 mL/h. Titrate to desired response. Endpoint is absence of fasciculations and return of muscle strength	IV	**AR:** Nausea, dizziness, headache; tachycardia, muscle rigidity, bronchospasm (rapid administration)
Pyridoxine (vitamin B_6). Stock level to treat 70-kg adult for 24 h: 100 mg/mL of 10% solution 20 vials	Seizures caused by isoniazid or *Gyromitra* mushrooms; ethylene glycol (investigational)	Isoniazid (INH): *Unknown amount ingested:* 5 g (70 mg/kg) in 50 mL of D5W over 5-min period with diazepam, 0.3 mg/kg IV, at rate of 1 mg/min in child or 10 mg per dose at rate up to 5 mg/min in adults. Use different site (synergism). May repeat q5–20min until seizure controlled. Up to 375 mg/kg has been given (52 g). *Known amount ingested:* 1 g for each gram of INH ingested over 5-min period with diazepam (dose above) *Gyromitra* mushrooms: 25 mg/kg for child or 2–5 g for adult over period of 15–30 min to maximum of 20 gm Ethylene glycol: 100 mg/d	IV	After seizure is controlled, administer remainder of pyridoxine at 1 g per 1 g of INH or total of 5 g as infusion over 60-min period **AR:** Uncommon; do not administer in same bottle as sodium bicarbonate For *Gyromitra* mushrooms, some use 25 mg/kg PO early when mushroom is suspected

Table continued on following page

TABLE 10. **Initial Doses of Antidotes for Common Poisonings, Alphabetically Arranged** *Continued*

Antidote	Use	Dose	Route	Adverse Reactions (AR) and Comments
Sodium bicarbonate ($NaHCO_3$). Stock level to treat 70-kg adult for 24 h: 10 ampules or syringes (500 mEq)	Tricyclic antidepressant (TCA) cardiotoxicity (wide QRS >0.10 s, ventricular tachycardia, severe conduction disturbances), metabolic acidosis, phenothiazine cardiotoxicity	1–2 mEq/kg undiluted as a bolus. If no effect on cardiotoxicity, repeat twice a few minutes apart	IV	Monitor serum sodium and potassium and blood pH because fatal alkalemia and hypernatremia have been reported. Continuous infusion of bicarbonate by itself is of limited usefulness in setting of TCA intoxication because of delayed onset. Prophylactic $NaHCO_3$ has not been encouraged
	Salicylate: To keep blood pH at 7.5–7.55 (not >7.55) and urine pH at 7.5–8.0. Alkalization is recommended if salicylate concentration >40 mg/dL in acute poisoning and at lower levels if symptomatic in chronic intoxication. 2 mEq/kg raises blood pH 0.2 U	*Adult* with clear physical signs and laboratory findings of acute moderate or severe salicylism: bolus of 1–2 mEq/kg followed by infusion of 100–150 mEq $NaHCO_3$ added to 1 L of 5% dextrose at rate of 200–300 mL/h *Child:* Bolus same as for adult, followed by 1–2 mEq/kg in infusion of 20 mL/kg/h 5% dextrose in 0.45% saline. Add potassium when patient voids Rate and amount of the initial infusion if patient is volume depleted: 1 h to achieve urine output of 2 mL/kg/h and urine pH of 7–8 In mild cases without acidosis and with urine pH >6, administer 5% dextrose in 0.9% saline with 50 mEq/L or 1 mEq/kg $NaHCO_3$ as maintenance to replace ongoing renal losses. If acidemia is present and pH <7.2, add 2 mEq/kg as loading dose followed by 2 mEq/kg q 3–4 h to keep pH at 7.5–7.55. If acidemia is present, recommend isotonic $NaHCO_3$, 3 ampules to 1 L of D5W at 10–15 mL/kg/h or sufficient to produce normal urine flow and urine pH of 7.5 or higher	IV	Monitor both urine pH and blood pH. Do not use urine pH alone to assess the need for alkalization because of the paradoxical aciduria that may occur Adjust the urine pH to 7.5–8 by $NaHCO_3$ infusion After urine output established, add potassium, 40 mEq/L
	Long-acting barbiturates: phenobarbital, mephobarbital (Mebaral), metharbital (Gemonil), primidone (Mysoline) *Note:* Alkalization is not effective for the short- and intermediate-acting barbiturates	2 mEq/kg during the first hour or 100 mEq in 1 L of D5W with 40 mEq/L potassium at rate of 100 mL/h in adults Adequate potassium is necessary to accomplish alkalization	IV	Additional $NaHCO_3$ and potassium chloride may be needed Adjust the urine pH to 7.5–8 by $NaHCO_3$ infusion

Abbreviations: BP = blood pressure; D5W = 5% dextrose in water; ET = by endotracheal route; PCC = poison control center; PCP = phencyclidine; rpm = respirations per minute; USP = U.S. Pharmacopeia.

route, are significantly reabsorbed in the renal tubules, and have a small Vd and low protein binding (PB). Acid diuresis is not recommended and may precipitate myoglobin in the renal tubules. Alkalization without diuresis with sodium bicarbonate ($NaHCO_3$) at 1 to 2 mEq/kg in 15 mL of 5% dextrose in water (D5W) per kilogram may be used in the treatment of weak acid intoxications, such as with salicylates (severe salicylate poisoning can necessitate hemodialysis) and long-acting barbiturates (LABs) (e.g., phenobarbital). Additional boluses of 0.5 mEq/kg can be administered to maintain alkalization, but blood pH values higher than 7.55 should be avoided. Many clinicians use alkalization without diuresis because of the danger of fluid overload.

Dialysis

Dialysis is an extrarenal means of removing certain substances from the body and can substitute for the kidneys when renal failure occurs. Dialysis is not the first measure instituted; however, it may be lifesaving later in the course of severe intoxication. It is needed in only a minority of intoxicated patients.

Peritoneal dialysis uses the peritoneum as the membrane for dialysis. Although only one twentieth as effective as hemodialysis, it is easier to use and less hazardous to the patient, but also less effective in removing the toxin; thus, it is seldom used except in small infants.

Hemodialysis is the most effective means of dialysis but requires experience with sophisticated equipment. Blood is circulated past a semipermeable membrane by an extracorporeal method. Substances are removed by diffusion down a concentration gradient. Anticoagulation with heparin is necessary.

Hemodialysis is contraindicated when (1) the substance is not dialyzable, (2) hemodynamic instability (e.g., shock) is present, and (3) coagulopathy is present.

Patient-related criteria for dialysis include the following: (1) anticipated prolonged coma and the likelihood of complications, (2) renal compromise (toxin excreted or metabolized by the kidneys and the presence of dialyzable chelating agents in heavy metal poisoning), (3) laboratory confirmation of a lethal blood concentration, (4) lethal dose poisoning with an agent that has delayed toxicity or is known to be metabolized into a more toxic metabolite (e.g., ethylene glycol, methanol), and (5) hepatic impairment when the agent is metabolized by the liver and clinical deterioration occurs despite optimal supportive medical management.

Dialyzable substances diffuse easily across the dialysis membrane and have the following characteristics: (1) a low molecular weight (less than 500 and preferably less than 350), (2) a Vd of less than 1 L/kg, (3) low PB (less than 50%), (4) high water solubility (low lipid solubility), and (5) high plasma concentration and a toxicity that reasonably correlates with the plasma concentration (Tables 11 and 12).

Hemodialysis also has a role in correcting disturbances that are not amenable to appropriate medical

TABLE 11. **Considerations for Hemodialysis or Hemoperfusion**

Serious Ingestions

Immediately notify the nephrologist. Compounds that are ingested in potentially lethal doses in which rapid removal may improve the prognosis include:
- Amatoxins from *Amanita phalloides* mushroom: any amount with symptoms
- Arsenic trioxide: 120 mg in adults
- Ethylene glycol: 1.4 mL/kg of a 100% solution or equivalent
- Methanol: 6 mL/kg of a 100% solution or equivalent
- Paraquat: 1.5 g in adults
- Diquat: 1.5 g in adults
- Mercuric chloride: 1.0 g in adults

Dialyzable Substances

Alcohol*	Isoniazid
Ammonia	Lithium*
Amphetamines	Meprobamate
Anilines	Paraldehyde
Antibiotics	Potassium*
Barbiturates (long-acting)*	Procainamide
Boric acid	Quinidine
Bromides*	Quinine*
Calcium	Salicylates*
Chloral hydrate*	Strychnine
Fluorides	Thiocyanates
Iodides	

Nondialyzable Substances

Anticholinergics	Glutethimide
Antidepressants (cyclic and MAOIs)	Hallucinogens
	Methaqualone†
Barbiturates (short-acting)	Opioids including heroin
Benzodiazepines	Phenothiazines
Digitalis and related drugs	Phenytoin
Ethchlorvynol	

*Most useful.
†Controversial.

management. These roles are easily remembered by the "vowel" mnemonic:

A = refractory *a*cid-base disturbances
E = refractory *e*lectrolyte disturbances
I = *i*ntoxication with dialyzable substances (see Tables 11 and 12)
O = *o*verhydration
U = *u*remia (renal failure)

Complications of dialysis include hemorrhage, thrombosis, air embolism, hypotension, infections, electrolyte imbalance, thrombocytopenia, and removal of therapeutic medications.

Hemoperfusion

Hemoperfusion is the parenteral form of oral AC therapy. Heparinization is necessary. The patient's blood is routed extracorporeally through an outflow arterial catheter and then through a filter-adsorbing cartridge (charcoal or resin) and returned through a venous catheter. High flow rates (e.g., 300 mL/min) through the filter are used to maximize efficient use of the filter. Cartridges must be changed every 4 hours. Blood glucose, electrolytes, calcium, albumin, complete blood cell count (CBC), platelets, and serum and urine osmolarity must be carefully monitored.

TABLE 12. **Plasma Drug Concentrations Above Which Removal by Extracorporeal Measures May Be Indicated***

Drug	Plasma Concentration	Protein Binding (%)	Vd (L/kg)	Method of Choice
Amanitine	Not available	25	1.0	HP
Ethanol	500–700 mg/dL	0	0.3	HD
Ethchlorvynol	150 μg/mL	35–50	3–4	HP
Ethylene glycol	25–50 μg/mL	0	0.6	HD
Glutethimide	100 μg/mL	50	2.7	HP
Isopropyl alcohol	400 mg/dL	0	0.7	HD
Lithium	4 mEq/L	0	0.7	HD
Meprobamate	100 μg/mL	0	NA	HP
Methanol	50 mg/dL	0	0.7	HD
Methaqualone	40 μg/dL	20–60	6.0	HP
Other barbiturates	50 μg/dL	50	0–1	HP
Paraquat	0.1 mg/dL	Poor	2.8	HP > HD
Phenobarbital	100 μg/dL	50	0.9	HP > HD
Salicylates	80–100 mg/dL	90	0.2	HD > HP
Theophylline		0	0.5	
Chronic	40–60 μg/mL			HP
Acute	80–100 μg/mL			HP
Trichloroethanol	250 μg/mL	70	0.6	HP

*In mixed or chronic drug overdoses, extracorporeal measures may be considered at lower drug concentrations.

Abbreviations: HD = hemodialysis; HD < HP = hemodialysis preferred over hemoperfusion; HP = hemoperfusion; HP > HD = hemoperfusion preferred over hemodialysis.

Modified from Winchester JF: Active methods for detoxification. In Haddad LM, Winchester JF (eds): Clinical Management of Poisoning and Drug Overdose, 2nd ed. Philadelphia, WB Saunders, 1990, pp 148–167; Balsam L, Cortitsidis GN, Fienfeld DA: Role of hemodialysis and hemoperfusion in the treatment of intoxications. Contemp Manage Crit Care 61–71, 1990.

This procedure has extended extracorporeal removal to a large range of substances that were formerly either poorly dialyzable or nondialyzable. It is not limited by molecular weight, water solubility, or PB. However, hemoperfusion is limited by a Vd greater than 400 L, by plasma concentration, and by rate of flow through the filter. AC cartridges are used primarily for hemoperfusion in the United States. Analysis of studies using hemodialysis and hemoperfusion indicates that the use of these techniques does not substantially reduce morbidity or mortality except in certain cases (e.g., with theophylline). Hemoperfusion may be recommended in combination with hemodialysis (e.g., for paraquat, electrolyte disturbances). Contraindications are similar to those for hemodialysis.

Patient-related criteria for the use of hemoperfusion include the following: (1) anticipated prolonged coma and the likelihood of complications, (2) laboratory confirmation of lethal blood concentrations, (3) lethal dose poisoning with an agent that has delayed toxicity or is known to be metabolized into a more toxic metabolite, and (4) hepatic impairment when an agent is metabolized by the liver and clinical deterioration is evident despite optimal supportive medical management.

Limited data are available to determine which toxicities are best treated with hemoperfusion. However, hemoperfusion has proved useful in glutethimide intoxication, barbiturate overdose, even with short-acting barbiturates (SABs), carbamazepine, phenytoin, theophylline, and chlorophenothane (DDT). See Tables 11 and 12.

Complications include hemorrhage, thrombocytopenia, hypotension, infection, leukopenia, depressed phagocytic activity of granulocytes, decreased immunoglobulin levels, hypoglycemia, hypothermia, hypocalcemia, pulmonary edema, and air and charcoal embolism.

Plasmapheresis

Plasmapheresis consists of removal of a volume of blood. All the extracted components are returned to the blood except the plasma, which is replaced with a colloidal protein solution. Clinical data related to guidelines and efficacy in toxicology are limited.

Supportive Care, Observation, and Therapy for Complications

Comatose Patients or Patients With Altered Mental Status

If airway protective reflexes are absent, endotracheal intubation is indicated. If respirations are ineffective, ventilation with 100% oxygen is instituted. If a cyanotic patient fails to respond to oxygen, the presence of methemoglobinemia should be suspected. A reagent strip test for blood glucose should be performed to detect hypoglycemia and the specimen sent to the laboratory for confirmation.

Glucose. Glucose is administered if the glucose reagent strip visually reads less than 150 mg/dL. Venous rather than capillary blood should be used for the reagent strip if the patient is in shock or is hypotensive.

Hypoglycemia accompanies many poisonings, including those with ethanol (especially in children), clonidine (Catapres), insulin, organophosphates, salicylates, sulfonylureas, and the unripened fruit or seed of a Jamaican plant called ackee. If hypoglycemia is present or suspected, glucose is administered immediately as an intravenous (IV) bolus in the following doses: for a neonate, 10% glucose (5 mL/kg); for a child, 25% glucose at 0.25 g/kg (2 mL/kg); and for an adult, 50% glucose at 0.5 g/kg (1 mL/kg).

Thiamine. This agent is administered to avoid precipitating thiamine deficiency encephalopathy (Wernicke-Korsakoff syndrome) in alcohol abusers and malnourished patients. The overall incidence of thiamine deficiency in ethanol abusers is 12%. Thiamine at 100 mg IV should be administered around the time of glucose administration but not necessarily before the glucose because it is more important to correct the hypoglycemia. The clinician should be prepared to manage anaphylaxis associated with thiamine allergy, but this complication is extremely rare.

Naloxone. This agent reverses CNS and respiratory depression, miosis, bradycardia, and decreased GI peristalsis caused by opioids acting through mu, kappa, and delta receptors.

In suspected overdose in a child younger than 5 years, naloxone is administered IV in a dose of 0.1 mg/kg up to 2 mg; in older children and adults, 2 mg should be administered every 2 minutes for 5 doses up to a total of 10 mg. Naloxone can also be administered into an endotracheal tube. If no response is seen after 10 mg has been given, pure opioid intoxication is unlikely. If opioid abuse is suspected, restraints should be in place before the administration of naloxone, and it is recommended that the initial dose be 0.1 to 0.2 mg to avoid withdrawal and violent behavior. The initial dose is then doubled every minute progressively to a total of 10 mg. Naloxone may unmask concomitant sympathomimetic intoxication, as well as withdrawal.

Larger doses of naloxone may be required for more poorly antagonized synthetic opioid drugs: buprenorphine (Buprenex), codeine, dextromethorphan, fentanyl, pentazocine (Talwin), propoxyphene (Darvon), diphenoxylate, nalbuphine (Nubain), new potent "designer" drugs, or long-acting opioids such as methadone.

Indications for continuous infusion include a second dose for recurrent respiratory depression, exposure to poorly antagonized opioids, a large overdose, and decreased opioid metabolism (e.g., in impaired liver function). Continuous infusion has been advocated because many opioids outlast the short $t_{1/2}$ of naloxone (30 to 60 minutes). The naloxone infusion hourly rate is equal to the effective dose required to produce a response (improvement in ventilation and arousal). An additional dose may be needed in 15 to 30 minutes as a bolus. The infusions are titrated to avoid respiratory depression and manifestations of opioid withdrawal. Tapering of infusions can be attempted after 12 hours and when the patient's condition has stabilized.

Complications: Although naloxone is safe and effective, pulmonary edema, seizures, hypertension, cardiac arrest, and sudden death have been reported rarely (in less than 1% of cases).

Agents Whose Role Is Not Clarified

Nalmefene. (Revex.) This long-acting parenteral opioid antagonist, approved by the FDA, is undergoing investigation, but its role in comatose patients and opioid overdose is not clear. It is 16 times more potent than naloxone, and its duration of action is up to 8 hours ($t_{1/2}$ of 10.8 hours, in comparison to 1 hour for naloxone).

Flumazenil. (Romazicon.) This agent is a pure competitive BZP antagonist. It has been demonstrated to be safe and effective for BZP-induced sedation, but it is not recommended for improving ventilation. Its role in CNS depression needs to be clarified. It should not be used routinely for comatose patients and is not an essential ingredient of the coma therapeutic regimen. Flumazenil is contraindicated in cyclic antidepressant intoxications, in stimulant overdose, in long-term BZP use (may precipitate life-threatening withdrawal), in cases in which BZPs are used to control seizures, and in head trauma. Seizures, dysrhythmias, and death have been reported in the contraindicated scenarios.

Laboratory and Radiographic Studies

Initial studies should include an ECG to assess for dysrhythmias or conduction delays (resulting from cardiotoxic medications), a chest radiograph for aspiration pneumonia (if the patient has loss of consciousness, is unarousable, or has vomited) or noncardiac pulmonary edema, and measurement of electrolyte and glucose concentrations in the blood. The AG should be calculated, and acid-base and ABG profiles (if the patient has respiratory distress or altered mental status) and a serum osmolality assay should be obtained. See Table 13 for appropriate testing on the basis of clinical toxicologic findings. All laboratory specimens should be carefully labeled, timed, and dated. For potential legal cases, a "chain of custody" must be established. Assessment of the laboratory studies may give a clue to the etiologic agent.

Electrolyte, Acid-Base, and Osmolality Disturbances

Electrolyte and acid-base disturbances are evaluated and corrected. Metabolic acidosis (low Pa_{CO_2} and low HCO_3^-) with an increased AG is seen with many agents in overdose.

Metabolic Acidosis and the Anion Gap. The AG is an estimate of the anions other than chloride and HCO_3^- that are necessary to counterbalance the positive charge of sodium. The AG gives a clue to the underlying disorder, compensation, and complications.

The AG is calculated from the standard serum electrolytes by subtracting total carbon dioxide (which reflects the actual measured HCO_3^-) and chloride from sodium: $Na^+ - (Cl^- + HCO_3^-) = AG$.

TABLE 13. **Patient Condition/Systemic Toxin and Appropriate Tests**

Condition/Toxin	Tests
Comatose	Toxicologic tests (acetaminophen, sedative hypnotics, ethanol, opioids, benzodiazepines) Glucose, ammonia, CT, CSF analysis
Respiratory toxin	Spirometry, ABGs, chest radiography, monitoring O_2 saturation
Cardiac toxin	ECG 12-lead and monitoring, echocardiogram, serial cardiac enzymes, hemodynamic monitoring
Hepatic toxin	Enzymes (AST, ALT, GGT), ammonia, albumin, bilirubin, glucose, PT, APTT, amylase
Nephrotoxin	BUN, creatinine, electrolytes (Na^+, K^+, Mg^{2+}, Ca^{2+}, PO_4^{3-}), serum and urine osmolarity, 24-h urine for heavy metals, CK, serum and urine myoglobin, urinalysis, and urinary sodium
Bleeding	Platelets, PT, APTT, bleeding time, fibrin split products, fibrinogen type and match blood

Abbreviations: APTT = activated partial thromboplastin time; CK = creatine kinase; CSF = cerebrospinal fluid; CT = computed tomography; GGT = γ-glutamyltransferase; PT = prothrombin time.

TABLE 15. **Blood Chemistry Derangements in Toxicology**

Derangement	Toxin or Disease
Acetonemia without acidosis	Acetone or isopropyl alcohol
Hypomagnesemia	Ethanol, digitalis
Hypocalcemia	Ethylene glycol, oxalate, fluoride
Hyperkalemia	β-Blockers, acute digitalis, renal failure
Hypokalemia	Diuretics, salicylism, sympathomimetics, theophylline, corticosteroids, chronic digitalis
Hyperglycemia	Diazoxide, glucagon, iron, isoniazid, organophosphate insecticides, phenylurea insecticides, phenytoin, salicylates, sympathomimetic agents, thyroid vasopressors
Hypoglycemia	β-Blockers, ethanol, insulin, isoniazid, oral hypoglycemic agents, salicylates
Elevated creatine kinase	Amphetamines, ethanol, cocaine, phencyclidine
Elevated creatinine and normal BUN	Isopropyl alcohol, diabetic ketoacidosis

Potassium is not generally used in the calculation because it may be hemolyzed and is an intracellular cation. The lack of an AG disturbance does not exclude a toxic basis for the disorder.

The normal gap was found to be 8 to 12 mEq/L by flame photometry. However, a lower normal AG of 7 ± 4 mEq/L has been determined by newer techniques (e.g., use of ion-selective electrodes or colorimetric titration). Some studies have found the AG to be relatively insensitive for determining the presence of toxins.

It is important to recognize the AG toxins salicylates, methanol, and ethylene glycol because they have specific antidotes and hemodialysis is effective in management.

A list of the potential causes of increased AG, decreased AG, or no change in AG is presented in Table 14. The most common cause of a decreased AG is laboratory error. Lactic acidosis produces the largest AG and can result from any poisoning that causes hypoxia, hypoglycemia, or convulsions.

Other blood chemistry derangements that suggest certain intoxications are shown in Table 15.

Serum Osmolal Gaps. The serum *osmolality* is a measure of the number of molecules of solute per kilogram of solvent, or mOsm/kg of water. The *osmolarity* is solute per liter of solution, or mOsm/L of water at a specified temperature. Osmolarity is usually a calculated value, and osmolality is generally a measured value. They are considered interchangeable when 1 L equals 1 kg. Normal serum osmolality is 280 to 290 mOsm/kg. Serum for the freezing point osmolarity measurement and serum for electrolyte calculation should be drawn simultaneously.

The serum osmolal gap is defined as the difference between the measured osmolality determined by the

TABLE 14. **Potential Causes of Metabolic Acidosis**

No Gap, Hyperchloremic	Increased Gap, Normochloremic	Decreased Gap
Acidifying agents	Methanol	Laboratory error†
Adrenal insufficiency	Uremia*	Intoxication (bromine, lithium)
Anhydrase inhibitors	Diabetic ketoacidosis*	Protein abnormal
Fistula	Paraldehyde,* phenformin	Mafenide (sodium low)
Osteotomies	Isoniazid	
Obstructive uropathies	Iron	
Renal tubular acidosis	Lactic acidosis†	
Diarrhea, uncomplicated*	Ethanol,* ethylene glycol*	
Dilutional hyperchloremia	Salicylates, starvation, solvents	
Mafenide Sulfamylon		

*Indicates a hyperosmolar situation. Studies have found that the anion gap may be relatively insensitive for determining the presence of toxins.
†Lactic acidosis caused by carbon monoxide, cyanide, hydrogen sulfide, hypoxia, ibuprofen, iron, isoniazid, ischemia, phenformin, salicylates, seizures, or theophylline.

freezing point method and the calculated osmolarity determined as follows: the serum sodium value multiplied by 2 plus the BUN divided by 3 plus the blood glucose value divided by 20. This gap estimate is usually within 10 mOsm of the simultaneously measured serum osmolality. Ethanol, if present, may be included in the equation to eliminate its influence on osmolality; the ethanol concentration divided by 4.6 is added to the equation. See Table 16.

Calculated mOsm =

$$2Na^+ + \frac{\text{BUN (mg/dL)}}{3} + \frac{\text{Blood Glucose (mg/dL)}}{20} + \frac{\text{Ethanol (mg/dL)}}{4.6}$$

The osmolal gap is valid for a hemodynamically intact individual; it is not valid in shock and the postmortem state. Metabolic disorders such as hyperglycemia, uremia, and dehydration increase the osmolarity but do not usually cause gaps greater than 10 mOsm/kg.

A gap greater than 10 mOsm/kg suggests that unidentified osmolal-acting substances are present: acetone, ethanol, ethylene glycol, ethchlorvynol, glycerin, isopropyl alcohol, isoniazid, ethanol, mannitol, methanol, $NaHCO_3$ (1 mEq/kg raises osmolality by 2 mOsm/L), and trichloroethane. Assessment for alcohol and glycol ingestion should be made when the degree of obtundation exceeds that expected from the blood ethanol concentration (BEC) or when other clinical conditions exist, such as visual loss (methanol), metabolic acidosis (methanol and ethylene glycol), and renal failure (ethylene glycol).

A falsely elevated osmolal gap may be produced by other low-molecular-weight un-ionized substances (acetone, dextran, dimethyl sulfoxide, diuretics, ethyl ether, mannitol, sorbitol, trichloroethane) or in conditions such as diabetic ketoacidosis, hyperlipidemia, and an excess of unmeasured electrolytes (e.g., magnesium).

False-negative results can occur when a normal osmolal gap is reported in the presence of alcohol or glycol poisoning if the parent compound is already metabolized—as, for example, when the osmolal gap is measured after a significant time has elapsed since ingestion. In alcohol and glycol intoxications, an early osmolar gap is due to the relatively nontoxic parent drug, and delayed metabolic acidosis and an increased AG are due to the more toxic metabolites.

Serum Concentration (mg/dL) =

$$\frac{\text{mOsm Gap} \times \text{Molecular Weight of Substance.}}{10}$$

See Table 16.

Radiographic Studies

Chest and neck radiographs are obtained to detect pathologic conditions such as aspiration pneumonia and pulmonary edema, for localization of foreign bodies, and to determine the location of the endotracheal tube.

Abdominal radiographs are obtained to detect radiopaque substances. A mnemonic for radiopaque substances seen on abdominal radiographs is CHIPES: *c*hlorides and *c*hloral hydrate; *h*eavy metals (arsenic, barium, iron, lead, mercury, zinc); *i*odide; *P*lay Doh, *P*epto-Bismol, or *p*henothiazine (which does not always show up on an abdominal radiograph if already dissolved); *e*nteric-coated tablets; and *s*odium, potassium, and other elements in tablet form (bismuth, calcium, potassium) and *s*olvents containing chlorides (e.g., carbon tetrachloride).

Toxicologic Studies

In the average toxicology laboratory, false-negative results occur at a rate of 10% to 30% and false-positive results at a rate of 0% to 10%.

The predictive value of a positive result is about 90%. A negative result of a toxicology screen does not exclude poisoning. The negative predictive value of toxicologic screening is about 70%. For example, the following BZPs may not be detected by routine screening tests for BZP: alprazolam (Xanax), clonazepam (Klonopin), temazepam (Restoril), and triazolam (Halcion).

The "toxic" urine screen is a qualitative urine test for several common drugs, usually substances of abuse (cocaine and metabolites, opioids, amphetamines, BZPs, barbiturates, phencyclidine [PCP]). Results are usually available within 2 to 6 hours. Because these tests may vary in different hospitals and communities, the physician should determine exactly which substances are included in the toxic urine screen of the laboratory used.

TABLE 16. **Alcohols and Glycols**

Alcohol or Glycol	**1 mg/dL in Blood Raises Osmolality (mOsm/L) by**	**Molecular Weight**	**Conversion Factor***
Ethanol	0.228	40	4.6
Methanol	0.327	32	3.2
Ethylene glycol	0.190	62	6.2
Isopropanol	0.176	60	6.0
Acetone	0.182	58	5.8
Propylene glycol	Not available	72	7.2

*Example: Methanol osmolality: Subtract the calculated osmolarity from the measured serum osmolality (freezing point method) = osmolar gap × 3.2 (0.1 molecular weight) = estimated serum methanol concentration.

The detection time is the number of days after intake of a substance during which a person would be expected to excrete detectable levels of the substance or metabolite in urine. In general, urine detection is possible for 1 to 3 days after cocaine exposure, 2 to 4 days after heroin (the presence of monoacetylmorphine is diagnostic of heroin use but is detectable for only 12 hours after use), and 2 to 4 days after PCP; if use is chronic, the time is doubled.

COMMON POISONS

Acetaminophen. (*N*-acetyl-*p*-aminophenol [APAP], Tylenol, called paracetamol in the United Kingdom.) *Toxic mechanism.* Of therapeutic doses of APAP, less than 5% is metabolized by cytochrome P-450IIE1 to a toxic reactive oxidizing metabolite, *N*-acetyl-*p*-benzoquinonimine (NAPQI). In overdose, sufficient glutathione is not available to reduce the excess NAPQI into a nontoxic conjugate, and it forms covalent bonds with hepatic intracellular proteins to produce centrilobular necrosis and, by a similar mechanism, renal damage. *Toxic dose*: The therapeutic dosage is 10 to 15 mg/kg per dose, with a maximum of five doses per 24 hours and a maximal total daily dose of 2.5 g. An acute single toxic dose is greater than 140 mg/kg, possibly greater than 200 mg/kg in children. Factors affecting the cytochrome P-450 enzymes (enzyme inducers such as anticonvulsants [barbiturates, phenytoin], isoniazid, alcoholism) and factors that decrease glutathione stores (e.g., alcoholism, malnutrition, HIV infection) contribute to the toxicity of APAP. Patients with chronic alcoholism who ingest APAP at 3 to 4 g/d for a few days can have depleted glutathione stores and require NAC therapy at blood APAP levels 50% below hepatotoxic levels on the nomogram (Figure 1). *Kinetics*: Onset of action occurs in 0.5 to 1 hour, the peak plasma concentration occurs in 20 to 90 minutes, but usually 2 to 4 hours after an overdose, and the duration is 4 to 6 hours. The Vd is 0.9 L/kg. PB is low, less than 50% (albumin); the $t_{1/2}$ is 1 to 3 hours. The route of elimination is hepatic metabolism to an inactive nontoxic glucuronide conjugate and an inactive nontoxic sulfate metabolite by two saturable pathways, and less than 5% is metabolized to the reactive metabolite NAPQI. In children younger than 6 years, metabolic elimination occurs to a greater degree by conjugation with the sulfate pathway, which may be hepatoprotective. *Manifestations*: The four phases of the intoxication's clinical course may overlap, and the absence of a phase does not exclude toxicity. Phase I occurs within 0.5 to 24 hours after ingestion and may consist of a few hours of malaise, diaphoresis, nausea, and vomiting, or symptoms may be absent. CNS depression or coma is not a feature. Phase II occurs 24 to 48 hours after ingestion and is a period of diminished symptoms. The liver enzymes AST (earliest) and ALT may increase as early as 4 hours or as late as 36 hours after ingestion. Phase III occurs in 48 to 96 hours, with peak liver function abnormalities at 72 to 96 hours. The degree of elevation of hepatic enzyme values does not correlate with outcome. Recovery starts in about 4 days unless hepatic failure develops. Fulminant hepatotoxicity develops in less than 1% of patients. Phase IV occurs in 4 to 14 days, with hepatic enzyme abnormalities reaching resolution. If extensive liver damage has occurred, sepsis and disseminated intravascular coagulation may ensue. Death can occur at 7 to 14 days. Transient renal failure may develop at 5 to 7 days with or without evidence of hepatic damage. Rare cases of myocarditis and pancreatitis have been reported.

Management: (1) For GI decontamination, emesis may be useful within 30 minutes. However, it may interfere with the retention of AC and NAC. Gastric lavage is not necessary if AC is administered early. Studies have indicated that AC is useful within 4 hours after ingestion. MDAC has not been well studied. AC does adsorb NAC if they are given together, but such adsorption is not clinically important. However, if AC must be given along with NAC, the administration of AC must be separated from that of NAC by 1 to 2 hours to avoid vomiting. Use of a saline sulfate cathartic in adults is recommended because it can enhance the activity of the sulfate metabolic pathway, which may be hepatoprotective. (2) NAC (Table 17; also see Table 10), a derivative of the amino acid cysteine, acts as a sulfhydryl donor for glutathione synthesis and may enhance the nontoxic sulfation pathway and result in conjugation of NAPQI. Oral NAC should be administered within the first 8 hours after a toxic amount of APAP has been ingested. NAC may be started while the results of blood tests for the APC are awaited, but there is no advantage to giving it before 8 hours. If the APC at more than 4 hours after ingestion is above the

TABLE 17. **Protocol for *N*-Acetylcysteine Administration**

Route	Loading Dose	Maintenance Dose	Course Duration (h)	FDA Approval
Oral	140 mg/kg	70 mg/kg q4h	72	Yes
Intravenous—England, Canada	150 mg/kg over 15-min period	50 mg/kg over 4-h period, followed by 100 mg/kg over 16-h period	20	No
Intravenous—investigational in United States	140 mg/kg	70 mg/kg q4h	48	No

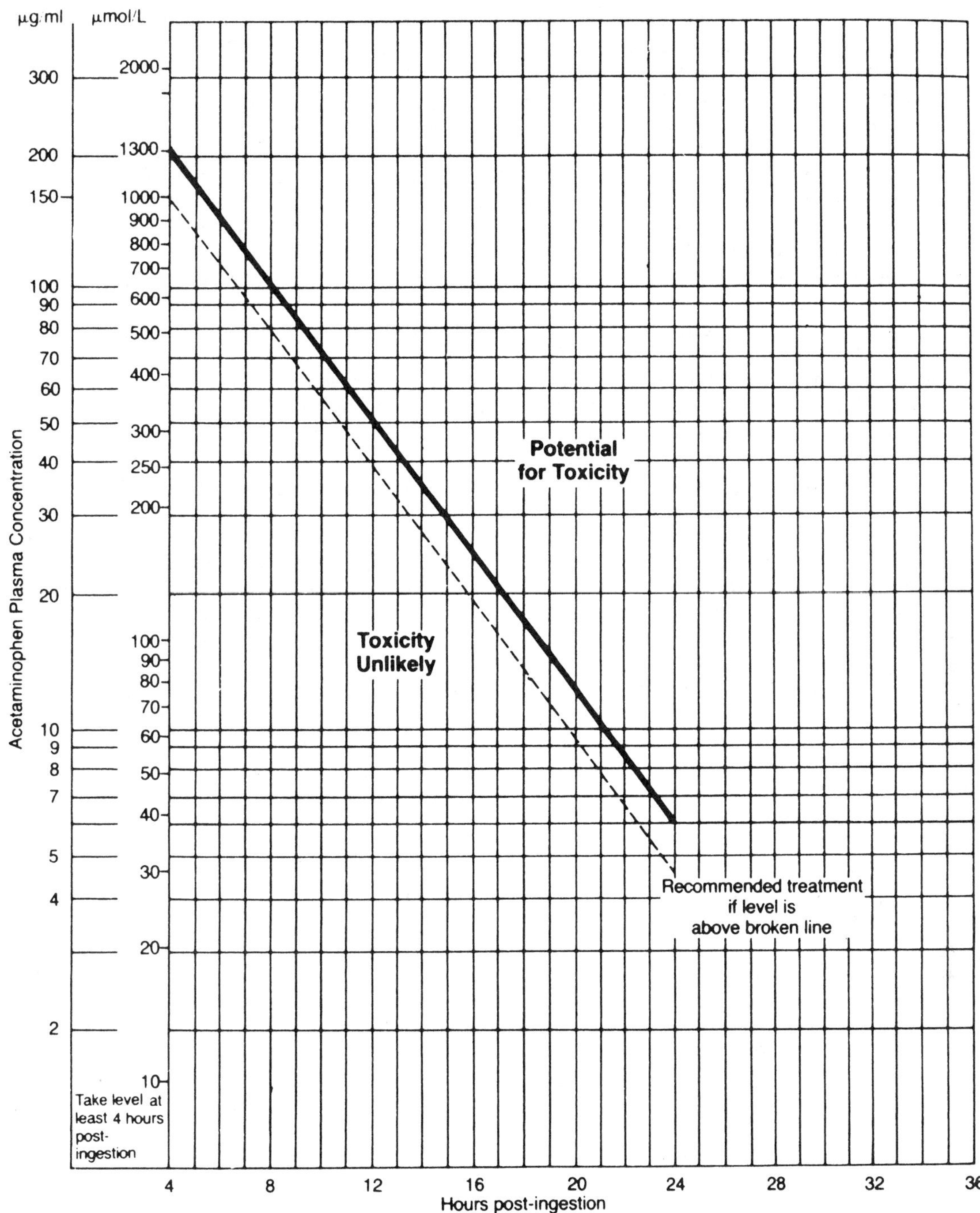

Figure 1. Nomogram for acetaminophen intoxication. Start *N*-acetylcysteine therapy if levels and time coordinates are above the lower line on the nomogram. Continue and complete therapy even if subsequent values fall below the toxic zone. The nomogram is useful only in acute single ingestions. Levels in serum drawn before 4 hours may not represent peak levels. (From Rumack BH, Matthew H: Acetaminophen poisoning and toxicity. Reproduced with permission from *Pediatrics*, Vol 55, Page 871, Figure 2, Copyright 1975.)

lower line on the modified Rumack-Matthew nomogram (see Fig. 1), the full 17-dose maintenance course should be continued. Repeated blood specimens should be obtained 4 hours after determination of the initial level if it is greater than 20 µg/mL because of unexpected delays in the peak caused by food and co-ingestants. An IV preparation (see Table 17) has been used in Europe and Canada since the late 1970s but is not approved in the United States (studies are in progress). A few anaphylactoid reactions and deaths have occurred with the IV route. *Variations in NAC therapy*: (a) In patients with chronic alcoholism, it is recommended that NAC be administered at 50% below the lower toxic line on the nomogram. (b) If emesis occurs within 1 hour after NAC administration, the dose should be repeated. To help prevent emesis, the proper dilution from 20% to 5% NAC should be served in a palatable vehicle in a covered container with a straw. If this technique is unsuccessful, NAC should be administered through a nasogastric tube or a fluoroscopically placed nasoduodenal tube by a slow drip over a period of 30 to 60 minutes. Antiemetics may be used if necessary: metoclopramide (Reglan) at 10 mg per dose IV a half-hour before NAC (in children, 0.1 mg/kg with a maximum of 0.5 mg/kg/d) or, as a last resort, ondansetron (Zofran) at 32 mg (0.15 mg/kg) by infusion over a 15-minute period, repeated for three doses if necessary. The potential side effects of ondansetron are anaphylaxis and increases in liver enzyme values. (c) Some investigators recommend variable durations of NAC therapy and stop treatment if the APC becomes nondetectable in serial determinations and the liver enzymes (ALT and AST) remain normal after 36 hours. (d) Time of administration: A loss of efficacy occurs if NAC is initiated more than 8 to 10 hours after ingestion, but the loss is not complete, and NAC may be initiated 36 or more hours after ingestion. Late treatment (after 24 hours) has been shown to decrease the rates of morbidity and mortality in fulminant liver failure caused by acetaminophen and other etiologic agents. (e) An extended-release caplet ("ER" is embossed on the caplet) contains 325 mg of immediate-release and 325 mg of delayed-release formulations. A single serum APAP determination 4 hours after ingestion can underestimate the dose because the extended-release formulation can yield secondary delayed peaks. In overdoses of an extended-release formulation, it is recommended that additional APAP levels be obtained at 4-hour intervals after the initial level. If any peak is in the toxic zone, therapy should be initiated. (3) Pregnancy: It is recommended that pregnant patients with toxic plasma concentrations of APAP receive NAC therapy to prevent hepatotoxicity in both the fetus and mother. The available data suggest no teratogenicity caused by NAC or APAP. (4) Chronic intoxication: Indications for NAC therapy are a history of ingestion of 3 to 4 g for several days, elevated liver enzyme (AST and ALT) values, and chronic alcoholism or use of chronic enzyme inducers. (5) Specific supportive care may be needed to treat liver failure, pancreatitis, transient renal failure, and myocarditis. (6) Liver transplantation has a definite but limited role in acute APAP overdose. According to a retrospective analysis, a continuing rise in the prothrombin time (4-day peak, 180 seconds), pH less than 7.3 (2 days after overdose), a serum creatinine level greater than 3.3 mg/dL, severe hepatic encephalopathy, and a disturbed coagulation factor VII/V ratio of more than 30% suggest a poor prognosis and may be indicators for hepatology consultation for consideration of orthotopic liver transplantation. (7) Extracorporeal measures are not expected to be of benefit.

Laboratory investigations: The therapeutic reference range is 10 to 20 μg/mL. For toxic levels, see the nomogram in Figure 1. Appropriate, reliable methods for analysis are radioimmunoassay, high-performance liquid chromatography (HPLC), and gas chromatography. Spectroscopic assays often give falsely elevated values. *Cross-reactions*: Bilirubin, salicylate, salicylamide, diflunisal, phenols, and methyldopa increase the APAP level. Each 1 mg/dL increase in creatinine increases the APAP plasma level 30 μg/mL. *Monitoring*: If a toxic APAP level is present, monitor the liver profile (including AST, ALT, bilirubin, prothrombin time), serum amylase, blood glucose, CBC, platelet count, phosphate, electrolytes, bicarbonate, ECG, and urinalysis. *Disposition*: All cases of intentional ingestion require determination of a serum APAP level 4 hours or more after ingestion. Patients who ingest more than 140 mg/kg should receive therapy within 8 hours after ingestion or until the results of the APC determination 4 hours after ingestion are known.

Amphetamines. (Illicit methamphetamine ["ice"], diet pills, various trade names.) *Analogues*: 3,4-Methylenedioxymethamphetamine (MDMA; known as Ecstasy, XTC, Adam), and 3,4-methylenedioxyamphetamine (MDEA; known as Eve). MDMA is a common hallucinogenic and euphoriant "club drug" used at "raves," which are dances initially popularized in Europe and now commonplace in the United States where adolescents dance in overcrowded, hot, noisy locations, usually all night long. Use of methamphetamine and designer analogues of "meth" is on the rise, especially in young people between the ages of 12 and 25. Other similar stimulants are phenylpropanolamine and cocaine. *Toxic mechanism*: Amphetamines have a direct CNS stimulant effect and a sympathetic nervous system effect by releasing catecholamines from α- and β-adrenergic nerve terminals but inhibiting their reuptake. MDMA has the additional hazard of a serotonin effect (refer to the serotonin syndrome in the selective serotonin reuptake inhibitor [SSRI] section). MDMA also affects the dopamine system in the brain. Because of its effects on serotonin, dopamine, and norepinephrine, MDMA can lead to serotonin syndrome (associated with malignant hyperthermia and rhabdomyolysis), which has contributed to the potentially life-threatening hyperthermia observed in several patients who used MDMA. Phenylpropanolamine stimulates only the β-adrenergic receptors. *Toxic dose*: In children, 1 mg/kg dextroamphetamine; in adults, 5 mg/kg. A dose of 12 mg/kg has been reported to be lethal. *Kinetics*: Amphetamine is a weak base with a pK_a of 8 to 10. Onset of action is in 30 to 60 minutes. Peak effects occur at 2 to 4 hours. The $t_{1/2}$ is pH dependent; it is 8 to 10 hours with acidic urine (pH <6.0) and 16 to 31 hours with alkaline urine (pH >7.5). The Vd is 2 to 3 L/kg. Elimination is 60% hepatic to a hydroxylated metabolite that may be responsible for the psychotic effects of amphetamines. Excretion by the kidney is 30% to 40% at an alkaline urine pH and 50% to 70% of an acidic urine pH. *Manifestations*: Effects are seen within 30 to 60 minutes after ingestion. Restlessness, irritation and agitation, tremors and hyperreflexia, and auditory and visual hallucinations occur. Dilated but reactive pupils, cardiac dysrhythmias (supraventricular and ventricular), tachycardia, and hyperpyrexia may precede seizures, convulsions, hypertension, paranoia, violence, intracranial hemorrhage, rhabdomyolysis, myoglobinuria, psychosis, and self-destructive behavior. Paranoid psychosis and cerebral vasculitis occur with chronic abuse. MDMA is often adulterated with cocaine, heroin, and/or ketamine to create a variety of mood alterations. Such adulterations must be taken into consideration when managing these patients because the symptom complex may reflect both CNS stimulation and depression.

Management (similar to that for cocaine): (1) Provide supportive care: blood pressure and cardiac thermal monitoring and seizure precautions. Diazepam is also administered (see Table 10). (2) GI decontamination: Administer AC. (3) Treat anxiety, agitation, and convulsions with diazepam. If diazepam fails to control seizures, use neuromuscular blockers and monitor the EEG for nonmotor seizures. Avoid neuroleptics (PTZs and butyrophenones), which can lower the seizure threshold. (4) Cardiovascular disturbances: Hypertension and tachycardia are usually transient and can be managed by titration of diazepam. Nitroprusside may be used for hypertensive crisis; use a maximal infusion rate of 10 μg/kg/min for 10 minutes, followed by 0.3 to 2 μg/kg/min. Myocardial ischemia is managed by oxygen, vascular access, BZPs, and nitroglycerin. Aspirin and thrombolysis are not routinely recommended because of the danger of intracranial hemorrhage. Delayed hypotension can be treated with fluids and vasopressors if needed. Life-threatening tachydysrhythmias may respond to an α-blocker (e.g., phentolamine at 5 mg IV for adults and 0.1 mg/kg IV for children) and a short-acting β-blocker (esmolol at 500 μg/kg IV over a 1-minute period for adults and 300 to 500 μg/kg IV over a 1-minute period for children). Ventricular dysrhythmias may respond to lidocaine or, in a severely hemodynamically compromised patient, immediate synchronized electrical cardioversion. (5) Treat rhabdomyolysis and myoglobinuria with fluids, alkaline diuresis, and diuretics. (6) Treat hyperthermia with external cooling and cool 100% humidified oxygen. (7) If focal neurologic symptoms are present, consider a diagnosis of cerebrovascular accident and perform computed tomography (CT) of the head. (8) Treat paranoid ideation and threatening behavior with rapid tranquilization. (9) Observe the patient for suicidal depression, which may follow intoxication and may require suicide precautions. (10) Extracorporeal measures are of no benefit.

Laboratory investigations: ECG and cardiac monitoring is instituted, and monitoring is also indicated for ABGs and oxygen saturation, electrolytes, blood glucose, BUN, creatinine, creatine kinase and cardiac fraction (if chest pain is present), and liver profile; evaluate for rhabdomyolysis, and check the urine for myoglobin, cocaine and metabolites, and other substances of abuse. The peak plasma concentration is 10 to 50 ng/mL 1 to 2 hours after the ingestion of 10 to 25 mg. The toxic plasma concentration is 200 ng/mL. Cross-reactions occur with amphetamine derivatives (e.g., MDMA, also known as Ecstasy), brompheniramine, chlorpromazine, ephedrine, phenylpropanolamine, phentermine, phenmetrazine, ranitidine, and Vicks Inhaler (L-desoxyephedrine) and may give false-positive results. *Disposition*: Symptomatic patients should be observed in a monitored unit until the symptoms resolve and then observed for a short time after resolution for relapse.

Anticholinergic Agents. Drugs with anticholinergic properties include antihistamines (H_1 blockers); neuroleptics (PTZs); tricyclic antidepressants; antiparkinsonism drugs (trihexyphenidyl [Artane], benztropine [Cogentin]); over-the-counter sleep, cold, and hay fever medicines (methapyrilene); ophthalmic products (atropine); products of common plants, including jimsonweed *(Datura stramonium)*, deadly nightshade *(Atropa belladonna)*, and henbane *(Hyoscyamus niger)*; and antispasmodic agents for the bowel (atropine derivatives). *Toxic mechanism*: By competitive inhibition, anticholinergic agents block the action of acetylcholine on postsynaptic cholinergic receptor sites. The mechanism involves primarily peripheral and CNS muscarinic receptors. *Toxic dose*: Toxic amounts of atropine are 0.05 mg/kg in children and greater than 2 mg in adults. The minimal estimated lethal dose of atropine is greater than 10 mg in adults and greater than 2 mg in 2-year-old children. Other synthetic anticholinergic agents are less toxic, the fatal dose varying from 10 to 100 mg. *Kinetics*: The onset of action with IV administration occurs in 2 to 4 minutes; peak effects on salivation after an IV or intramuscular (IM) dose occur in 30 to 60 minutes. Onset after ingestion is in 30 to 60 minutes, peak action occurs in 1 to 3 hours, and the duration is 4 to 6 hours, but symptoms are prolonged with overdose or sustained-release preparations. *Manifestations*: Anticholinergic signs: hyperpyrexia ("hot as a hare"), mydriasis ("blind as a bat"), flushing of skin ("red as a beet"), dry mucosa and skin ("dry as a bone"), "Lilliputian-type" hallucinations and delirium ("mad as a hatter"), coma, dysphagia, tachycardia, moderate hypertension, and, in rare instances, convulsions and urine retention.

Management: (1) If respiratory failure occurs, use intubation and assisted ventilation. (2) For GI decontamination, emesis should be avoided in a patient with diphenhydramine overdose because of rapid onset of action and the possibility of seizures. Use AC if bowel sounds are present; MDAC is not recommended. (3) Control seizures with BZPs (diazepam or lorazepam). (4) Use of physostigmine (see Table 10) is not routine and is reserved for reversal of life-threatening anticholinergic effects refractory to conventional treatments. This drug should be administered with adequate monitoring and resuscitative equipment available; it should be avoided if a tricyclic antidepressant is present in the patient's system. (5) Relieve urine retention by catheterization to avoid reabsorption. (6) If cardiac dysrhythmias are present, treat supraventricular tachycardia only if the patient is unstable. Control ventricular dysrhythmias with lidocaine or cardioversion. (7) Control hyperpyrexia by external cooling. (8) Hemodialysis and hemoperfusion are not effective.

Laboratory investigations: Monitor ABGs (in respiratory depression), electrolytes, glucose, and the ECG. Anticholinergic drugs and plants having anticholinergic effects are not routinely included in screens for substances of abuse. *Disposition*: Symptomatic patients should be observed in a monitored unit until the symptoms resolve and then observed for a short time after resolution for relapse.

Antihistamines. (H_1-receptor antagonists.) Antihistamines include the H_1-blocker "sedating anticholinergic" type. A single adult dose includes the following:

1. Ethanolamines: diphenhydramine (Benadryl), 25 to 50 mg (1 mg/kg in a child); dimenhydrinate (Dramamine), 50 mg; and clemastine (Tavist), 1.34 to 2.68 mg.
2. Ethylenediamines: tripelennamine (pyribenzamine), 25 to 50 mg (1 mg/kg in a child).
3. Alkylamines: chlorpheniramine (Chlor-Trimeton), 4 to 8 mg (0.9 mg/kg in a child), and brompheniramine (Dimetane), 4 to 8 mg (0.125 mg/kg in a child).
4. Piperazines: cyclizine (Marezine), 50 mg; hydroxyzine (Atarax), 50 to 100 mg (0.6 mg/kg in a child); and meclizine (Antivert), 50 to 100 mg.
5. Promethazine (Phenergan), 12.5 to 25 mg (0.1 mg/kg in a child).

THE H_1-BLOCKER SEDATING ANTIHISTAMINES. Many of these agents are used in combination with other medications such as acetaminophen, aspirin, codeine, dextromethorphan, ephedrine, phenylephrine, phenylpropanolamine, and pseudoephedrine. *Toxic mechanism*: H_1-sedating–type antihistamines produce blockade of cholinergic muscarinic receptors (anticholinergic action) and depress or stimulate the CNS; in large overdoses, some have a cardiac membrane–depressant effect (e.g., diphenhydramine) and cause α-adrenergic receptor blockade (e.g., promethazine). *Toxic dose*: For diphenhydramine, the estimated toxic oral amount in a child is 15 mg/kg, and the potential lethal amount is 25 mg/kg. In an adult, the potential lethal amount is 2.8 g. Ingestion of five times the single dose of an antihistamine is toxic. *Kinetics*: Onset is in 15 to 30 minutes to 1 hour, and peak effects occur in 1 to 4 hours; PB is 75% to 80%; Vd is 3.3 to 6.8 L/kg and $t_{1/2}$ is 3 to 10 hours. Elimination is 98% hepatic by *N*-demethylation. Interactions with erythromycin, ketoconazole (Nizoral), and derivatives produce excessive blood levels and ventricular dysrhythmias. *Manifestations*: Exaggerated anticholinergic effects, jaundice (cyproheptadine), coma, seizures, dystonia (diphenhydramine), rhabdomyolysis (doxylamine), and, with large doses, cardiotoxic effects (diphenhydramine) may be seen. *Management and disposition* (see "Anticholinergic Agents"): $NaHCO_3$ at 1 to 2 mEq/kg IV may be useful for myocardial depression and QRS prolongation.

THE NONSEDATING SINGLE-DAILY-DOSE ANTIHISTAMINES. Single adult doses include loratadine (Claritin), 10 mg; fexofenadine (Allegra), 60 mg; and cetirizine (Zyrtec), 5 and 10 mg. *Toxic mechanism*: These agents produce peripheral H_1 blockade and do not possess anticholinergic and sedating actions. The original agents terfenadine (Seldane) and astemizole (Hismanal) were recently removed from the market because of the severe cardiac dysrhythmias associated with their use, especially in combination with macrolide antibiotics and certain antifungal agents that inhibit hepatic metabolism or excretion, such as ketoconazole. The newer, nonsedating single-daily-dose antihistamines (NSDDs), including loratadine, fexofenadine, and cetirizine, have not been reported to cause the severe drug interactions associated with terfenadine and astemizole. *Toxic dose*: In an adult with an overdose of 3360 mg of terfenadine, ventricular tachycardia and fibrillation developed but responded to lidocaine and defibrillation; a 1500-mg overdose produced hypotension. Cases of delayed, serious dysrhythmias (torsades de pointes) have been reported with more than 200 mg of astemizole. *Kinetics*: Onset occurs in 1 hour, peak effects occur in 4 to 6 hours, and duration is greater than 24 hours. These drugs are more than 90% protein bound. Plasma $t_{1/2}$ is 3.5 hours. Metabolism is in the GI tract and liver. Only 1% is excreted unchanged, 60% in feces and 40% in urine. The chemical structure of these medications prevents entry into the CNS. *Manifestations*: Overdose produces headache, nausea, confusion, and serious dysrhythmias (e.g., torsades de pointes). *Management*: (1) Obtain an ECG and establish cardiac monitoring. Treat dysrhythmias with standard agents. Torsades de pointes is best treated with magnesium sulfate at 4 g or 40 mL of a 10% solution given IV over a period of 10 to 20 minutes (see Table 10) and countershock if the patient fails to respond. (2) GI decontamination with AC is advised. *Disposition*: All asymptomatic children who acutely ingest more than the maximal adult dose and all symptomatic children should be referred to a health care facility for a minimum of 6 hours' observation, as well as cardiac monitoring. Asymptomatic adults who acutely ingest more than the maximal adult daily dose (twice the maximal daily dose of the new NSDDs) should be monitored for a minimum of 6 hours. All symptomatic patients should be monitored for as long as symptoms are present.

Barbiturates. Barbiturates are used as sedatives, anesthetic agents, and anticonvulsants. *Toxic mechanism*: Barbiturates are GABA agonists (they increase chloride flow and inhibit depolarization). They enhance the CNS depressant effect and depress the cardiovascular system. *Toxic dose*: (1) The SABs (including the intermediate-acting agents) and their hypnotic doses are amobarbital (Amytal), 100 to 200 mg; aprobarbital (Alurate), 50 to 100 mg; butabarbital (Butisol), 50 to 100 mg; butalbital (Sandoptal), 100 to 200 mg; pentobarbital (Nembutal), 100 to 200 mg; and secobarbital (Seconal), 100 to 200 mg. They cause toxicity at lower doses than LABs do, and the minimal toxic dose is 6 mg/kg, the fatal adult dose is 3 to 6 g. (2) The LABs include mephobarbital (Mebaral), 50 to 100 mg, and phenobarbital (Luminal), 100 to 200 mg. The minimal toxic dose of these agents is greater than 10 mg/kg; the fatal adult dose is 6 to 10 g. A general rule is that an amount 5 times the hypnotic dose is toxic and 10 times the hypnotic dose is potentially fatal. Methohexital and thiopental are ultra–short-acting parenteral preparations and are not discussed in detail here. *Kinetics*: Barbiturates are enzyme inducers. (1) SABs are highly lipid soluble, penetrate the brain readily, and have shorter elimination times. Onset is in 10 to 30 minutes, with the peak effect occurring in 1 to 2 hours, and the duration is 3 to 8 hours. The Vd is 0.8 to 1.5 L/kg. The pK_a is about 8, and the mean $t_{1/2}$ varies from 8 to 48 hours. (2) LABs have longer elimination times and may be used as anticonvulsants. Onset is in 20 to 60 minutes, the peak occurs in 1 to 6 hours or, in an overdose, 10 hours, and the duration is greater than 8 to 12 hours. The Vd is 0.8 L/kg. The pK_a of phenobarbital is 7.2, and alkalization of urine promotes its excretion. The $t_{1/2}$ is 11 to 120 hours. *Manifestations*: In mild intoxication, the initial symptoms resemble those of alcohol intoxication and include ataxia, slurred speech, and depressed cognition. Severe intoxication causes slow respirations, coma, and loss of reflexes (except pupillary light reflex). Hypotension (venodilation), hypothermia, and hypoglycemia occur, and death is by respiratory arrest. Bullous skin lesions ("barb burns") over pressure points may be present. Barbiturates can precipitate an attack of acute intermittent porphyria. *Management*: (1) Establish and maintain vital functions. Intense supportive care, including intubation and assisted ventilation, should dominate the management. All stuporous and comatose patients should have glucose, thiamine, and naloxone given IV and be admitted to the ICU. (2) GI decontamination: Avoid emesis, especially in SAB ingestions. AC followed by MDAC (0.5 g/kg) every 2 to 4 hours has been shown to reduce the serum $t_{1/2}$ of phenobarbital by 50%, but its effect on the clinical course is undetermined. (3) Fluid management: Administer fluids to correct dehydration and hypotension. Vasopressors may be necessary to correct severe hypotension, and hemodynamic monitoring may be needed. Observe carefully for signs of fluid overload. (4) Alkalization (ion trapping) is used for phenobarbital (pK_a of 7.2) but not for SABs. $NaHCO_3$, 1 to 2 mEq/kg IV in 500 mL of 5% dextrose for adults or 10 to 15 mL/kg for children during the first hour, followed by sufficient bicarbonate to keep the urine pH at 7.5 to 8.0, enhances the excretion of phenobarbital and shortens the $t_{1/2}$ by 50% (see Table 10). Diuresis is not advocated because of the danger of cerebral or pulmonary edema. (5) Hemodialysis shortens the $t_{1/2}$ to 8 to 14 hours, and charcoal hemoperfusion shortens the $t_{1/2}$ to 6 to 8 hours. Both may be effective for LABs and SABs. If the patient does not respond to supportive measures or if the phenobarbital plasma concentration is greater than 150 μg/mL, both procedures may be used in an attempt to shorten the $t_{1/2}$. (6) Treat any bullae as local second-degree skin burns. (7) Treat hypothermia. *Laboratory investigations*: Most barbiturates are detected by routine drug screens and can be measured in most hospital laboratories. Monitor barbiturate levels, ABGs, a toxicology screen including acetaminophen and ethanol, glucose, electrolytes, BUN, creatinine, creatine kinase, and urine pH. Minimal toxic plasma levels are greater than 10 μg/mL for SABs and greater than 40 μg/mL for LABs. Fatal levels are 30 μg/mL for SABs and greater than 80 to 150 μg/mL for LABs. SABs and LABs can be detected in urine 24 to 72 hours after ingestion and LABs up to 7 days. *Disposition*: All comatose patients should be admitted to the ICU. Awake and oriented patients with a SAB overdose should be observed for at least 6 asymptomatic hours, and those with an LAB overdose for at least 12 asymptomatic hours. In an intentional overdose, psychiatric clearance is needed before discharge. Chronic use can lead to tolerance, physical dependence, and withdrawal and necessitates follow-up.

Benzodiazepines. BZPs are used as anxiolytics, sedatives, and relaxants. *Toxic mechanism*: GABA agonists produce CNS depression and increase chloride flow, thereby inhibiting depolarization. Flunitrazepam (Rohypnol), street name "roofies," is a long-acting benzodiazepine agonist sold by prescription in more than 60 countries worldwide but not legally available in the United States. *Toxic dose*: In the elderly, the therapeutic dose should be reduced by 50%. BZPs have an additive effect with other CNS depressants. (1) For long-acting BZPs ($t_{1/2}$ greater than 24 hours), the maximal therapeutic doses are chlordiazepoxide (Librium), 50 mg; clorazepate (Tranxene), 30 mg; clonazepam, 20 mg; diazepam (Valium), 10 mg (0.2 mg/kg for children); and flurazepam (Dalmane), 30 mg. (2) Short-acting BZPs ($t_{1/2}$ of 10 to 24 hours) include alprazolam, 0.5 mg, and lorazepam, 4 mg or 0.05 mg/kg for children, which act similar to the long-acting BZPs. (3) The BZPs that are ultra short acting ($t_{1/2}$ less than 10 hours) are more toxic and include temazepam, 30 mg; triazolam, 0.5 mg; midazolam, 0.2 mg/kg; and oxazepam (Serax), 30 mg. (4) In overdoses: Ingestion of 10 to 20 times the therapeutic dose (greater than 1500 mg of diazepam or 2000 mg of chlordiazepoxide) of long-acting BZPs has resulted in mild coma without respiratory depression. Fatalities are rare, and most patients recover within 24 to 36 hours after overdose with long- and short-acting BZPs. Asymptomatic patients who have taken nonintentional overdoses of less than five times the therapeutic dose may be observed. The ultra–short-acting BZP triazolam has produced respiratory arrest and coma within 1 hour after the ingestion of 5 mg and death with the ingestion of as little as 10 mg. Midazolam and diazepam administered by rapid IV injection have produced respiratory arrest. *Kinetics*: The onset of CNS depression is usually in 30 to 120 minutes, and the peak generally occurs within 1 to 3 hours with the oral route. The Vd is 0.26 to 6 L/kg (for long-acting BZPs, 1.1 L/kg). PB is 70% to 99%. Flunitrazepam has an onset of 1/2 to 2 hours, oral peak at 2 hours, a duration of 8 hours or more, and a $t_{1/2}$ of 20 to 30 hours. The Vd is 3.3 to 5.5 L/kg; it is 80% protein bound. Flunitrazepam can be identified in urine for 4 to 30 days after ingestion. *Manifestations*: Ataxia, slurred speech, and CNS depression may be seen. Deep coma leading to respiratory depression suggests the presence of short-acting BZPs or should prompt a search for other causes. *Management*: (1) GI decontamination: Emesis should be avoided. Gastric lavage (within 1 hour) and AC are advised if the ingestion was recent. (2) Supportive treatment should be provided, but intubation and assisted ventilation are rarely required. (3) Flumazenil (see Table 10) is a specific BZP receptor antagonist that blocks chloride flow and is an inhibitor of neurotransmitters. It reverses the sedative effects of BZPs, zolpidem (Ambien), and endogenous BZPs associated with hepatic encephalopathy. It is not recommended for reversing BZP-induced hypoventilation. It should be used with caution in overdoses if BZP dependence is a possibility (because it can precipitate life-threatening withdrawal), if a cyclic antidepressant is suspected, or if the patient has a known seizure disorder. *Laboratory investigations*: Most BZPs can be detected in urinary drug screens. Quantitative blood levels are not useful. BZPs not usually detected in urinary screens include alprazolam, clonazepam, flunitrazepam,* lorazepam, lormetazepam,* midazolam, oxazepam, temazepam, and triazolam. BZPs may not be detected if the dose is less than 10 mg, elimination is rapid, or different or no metabolites are present. Cross-reactions occur with nonsteroidal anti-inflammatory drugs (NSAIDs) (tolmetin, naproxen, etodolac, and fenoprofen). In cases in which "date rape" drugs such as flunitrazepam are suspected, contact a police crime or reference laboratory for testing. *Disposition*: Comatose patients should be admitted to the ICU. If the overdose was intentional, psychiatric clearance is needed before discharge. Chronic use can lead to tolerance, physical dependence, and withdrawal.

β-Adrenergic Blockers. (β-Blockers.) β-Blockers are used in the treatment of hypertension and a number of systemic and ophthalmic disorders. Lipid-soluble drugs have CNS effects, active metabolites, a longer duration of action, and interactions with other drugs (e.g., propranolol). Cardioselectivity is lost in overdoses. Intrinsic partial agonist agents (e.g., pindolol) may initially produce tachycardia and hypertension. A cardiac membrane–depressive effect (quinidine-like) occurs with overdose but not therapeutic doses (e.g., metoprolol, sotalol). The α-blocking effect is weak (e.g., labetalol). Properties of β-blockers include the factors listed in Table 18. *Toxic mechanism*: β-Blockers compete with the catecholamines for receptor sites and block receptor action in the bronchi and the vascular smooth muscle and myocardium. *Toxic dose*: Ingestion of more than twice the maximal recommended daily therapeutic dose is considered toxic (see Table 18). Ingestion of propranolol at 1 mg/kg by a child may produce hypoglycemia. Fatalities have been reported in adults who ingested 7.5 g of metoprolol. The most toxic agent is sotalol, and the least toxic, atenolol. *Kinetics*: Regular release usually causes symptoms within 2 hours. Propranolol's onset of action occurs in 20 to 30 minutes; the peak is at 1 to 4 hours but may be delayed with co-ingestants and sustained-release preparations. The duration of effect is 4 to 6 hours but may be 24 to 48 hours in overdoses and longer with the sustained-release type. With sustained-release preparations, the onset may be delayed 6 hours and the peak 12 to 16 hours; the duration of effect may be 24 to 48 hours. The regular preparation with the longest $t_{1/2}$ is nadolol (12 to 24 hours), and that with the shortest is esmolol (5 to 10 minutes). PB is variable and ranges from 5% to 93%. The Vd is 1 to 5.6 L/kg. Atenolol, nadolol, and sotalol have enterohepatic recirculation. *Manifestations*: See toxic properties and Table 18. Lipid-soluble agents produce coma and seizures. Bradycardia and hypotension are the major clinical signs and may lead to cardiogenic shock. Intrinsic partial agonists may initially cause tachycardia and hypertension. Bronchospasm may occur in patients with reactive airway disease with any β-blocker because the selectivity is lost in overdoses. ECG changes include AV conduction delay and frank asystole. Membrane-depressant effects produce prolonged QRS and QT intervals, which may result in torsades de pointes. Sotalol produces a prolonged QT. Hypoglycemia (blocking of catecholamine counterregulatory mechanisms) and hyperkalemia may occur, especially in children.

Management: (1) Establish and maintain vital functions. Establish vascular access, obtain a baseline ECG, and institute continuous cardiac and blood pressure monitoring. Have a pacemaker available. Hypotension is treated with fluids initially, although it does not usually respond. Frequently, glucagon and cardiac pacing are needed. Cardiology consultation should be sought. (2) GI decontamination is performed initially with AC. MDAC is not recommended for symptomatic patients. Gastric lavage is done at less than 1 hour after ingestion. If gastric lavage is performed, use of prelavage atropine (0.02 mg/kg for a child and 0.5 mg for an adult) and cardiac monitoring is recommended. Whole-bowel irrigation should be considered in large overdoses with sustained-release preparations (although no studies have been conducted). (3) Cardiovascular disturbances: A cardiology consultation should be obtained. Class IA (procainamide, quinidine) and class III (bretylium) antidysrhythmic agents are not recommended. Bradycardia in asymptomatic, hemodynamically stable patients necessitates no therapy. It is not predictive of the future course. If the patient is unstable (has hypotension or high-degree AV block), use atropine (0.02 mg/kg up to 2 mg in adults), glucagon, and a pacemaker. In ventricular tachycardia, use overdrive pacing. A wide QRS interval may respond to $NaHCO_3$ (see Table 10). Torsades de pointes (associated with sotalol) may respond to magnesium sulfate (see Table 10) and overdrive pacing. Prophylactic

*Not available in the United States.

TABLE 18. **Pharmacologic and Toxic Properties of β-Blockers***

Name	Dose	Lipid Solubility	Intrinsic Sympathomimetic Activity (Partial Agonist)	Membrane-Stabilizing Effect	Cardiac Selectivity (Beta-Selective)	Alpha Blocker
Acebutolol (Sectral)	Maximum daily dose, 800 mg; therapeutic plasma level, 200–2000 ng/mL	Moderate	+	+	+	+
Alprenolol†	Maximum daily dose, 800 mg; therapeutic plasma level, 50–200 ng/mL	Moderate	2+	+	–	–
Atenolol (Tenormin)	Maximum daily dose, 100 mg; therapeutic plasma level, 200–500 ng/mL	Low	–	–	2+	–
Betaxolol (Kerlone)	Maximum daily dose, 20 mg; therapeutic plasma level, NA	Low	+	–	+	–
Carteolol (Cartrol)	Maximum daily dose, 10 mg; therapeutic plasma level, NA	No	+	–	–	–
Esmolol (Brevibloc) (class II antidysrhythmic, by intravenous route only)		Low	–		+	–
Labetalol (Trandate)	Maximum daily dose, 800 mg; therapeutic plasma level, 50–500 ng/mL	Low	+	±	–	+
Levobunolol (eye drops 0.25% and 0.5%)	Maximum daily dose, 20 mg; therapeutic plasma level, NA	No	–	–	–	–
Metoprolol (Lopressor)	Maximum daily dose, 450 mg; therapeutic plasma level, 50–100 ng/mL	Moderate	–	–	2+	–
Nadolol (Corgard)	Maximum daily dose, 320 mg; therapeutic plasma level, 20–400 ng/mL	Low	–	–	–	–
Oxprenolol†	Maximum daily dose, 480 mg; therapeutic plasma level, 80–100 ng/mL	Moderate	2+	+	–	–
Pindolol (Visken)	Maximum daily dose, 60 mg; therapeutic plasma level, 50–150 ng/mL	Moderate	3+	±	–	–
Propranolol (Inderal) (class II antidysrhythmic)	Maximum daily dose, 360 mg; therapeutic plasma level, 50–100 ng/mL	High	–	2+	–	–
Sotalol (Betapace) (class III antidysrhythmic)	Maximum daily dose, 480 mg; therapeutic plasma level, 500–4000 ng/mL	Low	–	–	–	–
Timolol (Blocadren)	Maximum daily dose, 60 mg; therapeutic plasma level, 5–10 ng/mL	Low	–	±	–	–

*– indicates no effect; + indicates mild effect; 2+ indicates moderate effect; 3+ indicates severe effect; ± indicates no effect or mild effect; NA indicates not available.

†Not available in the United States.

magnesium for a prolonged QT interval has been suggested, but supporting data are lacking. Do not use epinephrine because an unopposed α-adrenergic effect may occur. Hypotension and myocardial depression are managed by correction of dysrhythmias, use of the Trendelenburg position, and administration of fluids, glucagon, and/or amrinone (Inocor). Hemodynamic monitoring may be needed to manage fluid therapy. Glucagon (see Table 10) is the initial drug of choice. It works through adenylate cyclase and bypasses catecholamine receptors, so it is not affected by β-blockers. It increases cardiac contractility and the heart rate. Glucagon is given as an IV bolus of 5 to 10 mg* over a 1-minute period, followed by a continuous infusion at 1 to 5 mg/hour (in children, 0.15 mg/kg followed by 0.05 to 0.1 mg/kg/h). In large doses and in infusion therapy, use D5W, sterile water, or saline as the diluent to reconstitute glucagon in place of the 0.2% phenol diluent provided with some drugs. Effects are seen within minutes. Glucagon can be used with other agents such as amrinone. Amrinone inhibits the enzyme phosphodiesterase, which metabolizes cyclic adenosine monophosphate. A bolus of 0.15 to 2 mg/kg (0.15 to 0.4 mL/kg) is administered IV, followed by infusion of 5 to 10 μg/kg/min. (4) Treat hypoglycemia with IV glucose and emergency hyperkalemia with calcium (avoid if digoxin is present), bicarbonate, and glucose. (5) Control convulsions with diazepam or phenobarbital. (6) If bronchospasm is present, give β_2 nebulized bronchodilators and aminophylline. (7) Extraordinary measures include intra-aortic balloon pump support. (8) Extracorporeal measures: Hemodialysis for poisonings with atenolol, acebutolol, nadolol, and sotalol (low Vd, low PB) may be helpful, particularly with evidence of renal failure. It is not effective for intoxication with propranolol, metoprolol, or timolol. (9) Investigational: Prenalterol† has successfully reversed both bradycardia and hypotension.

Laboratory investigations: Measurement of blood levels is not readily available or useful. (For propranolol the toxic level is greater than 2 ng/mL.) *Monitoring*: ECG and cardiac monitoring is recommended, as well as monitoring of blood glucose and electrolytes, BUN and serum creatinine, and ABGs if respiratory symptoms are present. *Disposition*: Asymptomatic patients with a history of overdose require a baseline ECG and continuous cardiac monitoring for at least 6 hours with regular-release preparations and for 24 hours with sustained-release preparations. Symptomatic patients should be observed with cardiac monitoring for 24 hours. If seizures, abnormal rhythm, or vital signs indicate, the patient should be admitted to the ICU.

Calcium Channel Blockers. These agents are used in the treatment of effort angina, supraventricular tachycardia, and hypertension. *Toxic mechanism*: Calcium channel blockers reduce the influx of calcium through the slow channels in membranes of the myocardium, the AV nodes, and vascular smooth muscles, thereby resulting in peripheral, systemic, and coronary vasodilation, impaired cardiac conduction, and depression of cardiac contractility. All calcium channel blockers have vasodilatory action, but only bepridil, diltiazem, and verapamil depress myocardial contractility and cause AV block. *Toxic dose*: Any ingested amount greater than the maximal daily dose has the potential of being severely toxic. Maximal oral daily doses are as follows: for amlodipine (Norvasc), 10 mg (children <0.25 mg/kg); for bepridil (Vascor), 400 mg (children <5.7 mg/kg); for diltiazem (Cardizem), 360 mg (toxic dose <2 g) (children <6 mg/kg); for felodipine (Plendil), 10 mg (children <0.56 mg/kg); for isradipine (DynaCirc), 40 mg (children <0.4 mg/kg); for nicardipine (Cardene), 120 mg (children <0.85 mg/kg); for nifedipine (Procardia), 120 mg (children <2 mg/kg); for nimodipine (Nimotop), 360 mg (children <0.85 mg/kg); for nitrendipine (Baypress*), 80 mg (children <1.14 mg/kg); and for verapamil (Calan), 480 mg (children <15 mg/kg). *Kinetics*: The onset of action of regular-release preparations varies: for verapamil, 60 to 120 minutes; for nifedipine, 20 minutes; and for diltiazem, 15 minutes after ingestion. The peak effect is at 2 to 4 hours for verapamil, 60 to 90 minutes for nifedipine, and 30 to 60 minutes for diltiazem; however, the peak action may be delayed for 6 to 8 hours. The duration is up to 36 hours. With sustained-release preparations, the onset is usually at 4 hours but may be delayed; the peak effect is at 12 to 24 hours, and concretions and prolonged toxicity can develop. The $t_{1/2}$ for hepatic elimination varies from 3 to 7 hours. The Vd varies from 3 to 7 L/kg. *Manifestations*: Hypotension, bradycardia, and conduction disturbances occur 30 minutes to 5 hours after ingestion. A prolonged PR interval is an early and constant finding and may occur at therapeutic doses. Torsades de pointes has been reported. All degrees of blocks may occur and may be delayed 12 to 16 hours. Lactic acidosis may be present. Calcium channel blockers do not affect intraventricular conduction, so the QRS interval is not usually affected. Hypocalcemia is rarely present. Hyperglycemia may be present because of calcium-dependent insulin release. Mental status changes, headaches, seizures, hemiparesis, and CNS depression may occur. Calcium channel blockers may precipitate respiratory failure in patients with Duchenne's muscular dystrophy.

Management: (1) Establish and maintain vital functions. Obtain a baseline ECG, and institute continuous cardiac and blood pressure monitoring. A pacemaker should be available. Cardiology consultation should be sought. (2) GI decontamination: AC is recommended. MDAC is not advised (no data are available). If a large sustained-release preparation is involved, whole-bowel irrigation may be useful, but its effectiveness has not been investigated. (3) If the patient is symptomatic, immediate cardiology consultation should be obtained because a pacemaker and

*Exceeds dosage recommended by the manufacturer.
†Not available in the United States.

*Not available in the United States.

hemodynamic monitoring may be needed. (4) In the presence of heart block, atropine is rarely effective and isoproterenol may produce vasodilation. Consider the use of a pacemaker early. (5) Treat hypotension and bradycardia with positioning, fluids, calcium gluconate or calcium chloride, glucagon, amrinone, and ventricular pacing. Calcium gluconate or calcium chloride (see Table 10): Avoid calcium salts if digoxin is present. Calcium usually reverses depressed myocardial contractility but may not reverse nodal depression or peripheral vasodilation. Calcium chloride is used as a 10% solution at 0.1 to 0.2 mL/kg up to 10 mL in an adult or calcium gluconate as a 10% solution at 0.3 to 0.4 mL/kg up to 20 mL in an adult, administered IV over a period of 5 to 10 minutes. Monitor for dysrhythmias, hypotension, and serum calcium. The aim is to increase the calcium value 4 mg/dL to a maximum of 13 mg/dL. The calcium response lasts 15 minutes, and repeated doses or a continuous calcium gluconate infusion (0.2 mL/kg/h, up to a maximum of 10 mL/h) may be necessary. If calcium fails, try glucagon (see Table 10) for its positive inotropic or chronotropic effect or both. Amrinone, an inotropic agent, may reverse calcium channel blockers. The effective dose is 0.15 to 2 mg/kg (0.15 to 0.4 mL/kg) by IV bolus, followed by infusion at 5 to 10 μg/kg/min. (6) Hypotension: Fluids, norepinephrine, and epinephrine may be required for hypotension. Amrinone and glucagon have been tried alone and in combination. Dobutamine and dopamine are often ineffective. (7) Extracorporeal measures (e.g., hemodialysis and charcoal hemoperfusion) are not considered useful. (8) Patients receiving digitalis and calcium channel blockers run the risk of digitalis toxicity because calcium channel blockers increase digitalis levels. (9) Extraordinary measures such as intra-aortic balloon pump and cardiopulmonary bypass have been used successfully. (10) For patients with calcium channel blocker toxicity that fails to respond to aggressive symptomatic and supportive management, including calcium gluconate or chloride, recent studies demonstrate that insulin and glucose have therapeutic value in the treatment of these patients. The suggested dose range for insulin is an infusion of insulin at greater than 0.5 IU/kg/h with a simultaneous glucose infusion at 1 g/kg/h, with glucose monitoring every 30 minutes for at least the first 4 hours of administration and subsequent glucose adjustment to maintain euglycemia. Potassium should be monitored regularly because levels may shift in response to the insulin.

Laboratory investigations: Specific drug levels are not easily available and are not useful. Monitor blood glucose, electrolytes, calcium, ABGs, pulse oximetry, creatinine, BUN, hemodynamics, ECG, and cardiac function. *Disposition*: With intoxications involving regular-release preparations, monitoring is indicated for at least 6 hours, and with those involving sustained-release preparations, for 24 hours after the alleged ingestion. For patients with intentional overdose, psychiatric clearance is needed. Symptomatic patients should be admitted to the ICU.

Carbon Monoxide. CO is an odorless, colorless gas produced by incomplete combustion; it is an in vivo metabolic breakdown product of the methylene chloride used in paint removers. *Toxic mechanism*: The affinity of CO for hemoglobin is 240 times greater than that of oxygen; it shifts the oxygen dissociation curve to the left, which impairs hemoglobin release of oxygen to tissues and inhibits the cytochrome oxidase system. *Toxic dose and manifestations*: See Table 19. CO exposure and manifestations: Exposure to 0.5% for a few minutes is lethal. Contrary to popular belief, the skin rarely turns cherry-red in a living patient. Sequelae correlate with the level of consciousness at initial evaluation. ECG abnormalities may be noted. The creatine kinase level is often elevated;

TABLE 19. **Carbon Monoxide Exposure and Possible Manifestations**

CO in Atmosphere (%)	Duration of Exposure (h)	COHb Saturation (%)	Manifestations
<0.0035 (35 ppm)	Indefinite	3.5	None
0.005–0.01 (50–100 ppm)	Indefinite	5	Slight headache, decreased exercise tolerance
Up to 0.01 (100 ppm)	Indefinite	10	Slight headache, dyspnea on vigorous exertion; driving skills may be impaired
0.01–0.02 (100–200 ppm)	Indefinite	10–20	Dyspnea on moderate exertion; throbbing, temporal headache
0.02–0.03 (200–300 ppm)	5–6	20–30	Severe headache, syncope, dizziness, visual changes, weakness, nausea, vomiting, altered judgment
0.04–0.06 (400–600 ppm)	4–5	30–40	Vertigo, ataxia, blurred vision, confusion, loss of consciousness
0.07–0.10 (700–1000 ppm)	3–4	40–50	Confusion, tachycardia, tachypnea, coma, convulsions
0.11–0.15 (1100–1500 ppm)	1.5–3	50–60	Cheyne-Stokes respirations, coma, convulsions, shock, apnea
0.16–0.30 (1600–3000 ppm)	1.0–1.5	60–70	Coma, convulsions, respiratory and heart failure, death
> 0.40 (> 4000 ppm)	Few minutes		Death

Abbreviation: COHb = carboxyhemoglobin.

rhabdomyolysis and myoglobinuria may occur. The carboxyhemoglobin (COHb) level expresses as a percentage the extent to which CO has bound with the total hemoglobin. This value may be misleading in an anemic patient. The patient's initial symptoms are more reliable than the COHb level. In Table 19, the manifestations listed for each level are in addition to those already listed at the preceding level. Note that 0.01% = 100 parts per million (ppm). A level greater than 40% is usually associated with obvious intoxication. The COHb may not reliably correlate with the severity of the intoxication, and attempts to link symptoms to specific levels of COHb are frequently inaccurate. *Kinetics*: The natural metabolism of the body produces small amounts of COHb: less than 2% for nonsmokers and 5% to 9% for smokers. CO is rapidly absorbed through the lungs, the rate of absorption being directly related to alveolar ventilation. Elimination occurs through the lungs. The $t_{1/2}$ of COHb in room air (21% oxygen) is 5 to 6 hours; in 100% oxygen, 90 minutes; and in hyperbaric oxygen (HBO) at 3 atm of oxygen, 20 to 30 minutes.

Management: (1) Adequately protect the rescuer. Remove the patient from the contaminated area, and establish vital functions. (2) The mainstay of treatment is administration of 100% oxygen via a nonrebreathing mask with an oxygen reservoir or endotracheal tube. Give 100% oxygen to the patient until the COHb level is 2% or less. Assisted ventilation may be necessary. (3) Monitor ABGs and COHb. Determine the current COHb level and extrapolate to the COHb level at the time of exposure by using the $t_{1/2}$ of COHb in different percentages of ambient oxygen (see *Kinetics* just discussed). *Note*: A near-normal COHb level does not exclude significant CO poisoning, especially if measured several hours after the termination of exposure or if oxygen has been administered before the sample is obtained. (4) An exposed pregnant woman should be kept in 100% oxygen for several hours after the COHb level is almost zero because COHb concentrates in the fetus and oxygen is needed longer to ensure elimination of CO from the fetal circulation. Monitor the fetus. CO and hypoxia are teratogenic. (5) Metabolic acidosis should be treated with sodium bicarbonate only if the pH is below 7.2 after correction of the hypoxia and adequate ventilation. Acidosis shifts the oxygen dissociation curve to the right and facilitates oxygen delivery to the tissues. (6) Use of the HBO chamber: The decision must be made on the basis of the availability of a hyperbaric chamber, the ability to handle other acute emergencies that may coexist, the extrapolated COHb level, and the severity of the poisoning. The standard of care for persons exposed to CO has yet to be determined, but most authorities recommend HBO therapy with any of the following guidelines: (a) if HBO therapy is not readily available, a COHb greater than 40%, or if HBO therapy is readily available, a COHb greater than 25%; (b) if the patient is unconscious or has a history of loss of consciousness or seizures; (c) if cardiovascular dysfunction (clinical ischemic chest pain or ECG evidence of ischemia) is present; (d) the patient has metabolic acidosis; (e) if symptoms persist despite 100% oxygen therapy; (f) if the initial COHb level is greater than 15% in a child, in a patient with cardiovascular disease, or in a pregnant woman; or (g) if signs of maternal or fetal distress are noted, regardless of the COHb level. Management of CO toxicity in infants and fetuses is a special problem because fetal hemoglobin has greater affinity for CO than adult hemoglobin does. A neurologic-cognitive examination has been used to help determine which patients with low CO levels should receive more aggressive therapy. Testing should include the following: general orientation memory testing (address, phone number, date of birth, present date) and cognitive testing (serial 7s, digit span, forward and backward spelling of three- and four-letter words). Patients with delayed neurologic sequelae or recurrent symptoms for up to 3 weeks may benefit from HBO treatment. (7) Treat seizures and cerebral edema.

Laboratory investigations: ABGs may show metabolic acidosis and normal oxygen tension. If the patient has significant poisoning, monitor the ABGs, electrolytes, blood glucose, serum creatine kinase and cardiac enzymes, renal function, and liver function. Obtain a urinalysis and test for myoglobinuria. Obtain a chest radiograph if smoke has been inhaled or if use of an HBO chamber is being considered. ECG monitoring is needed especially if the patient is older than 40 years, has a history of cardiac disease, or has moderate to severe symptoms. Determine the blood ethanol level, and conduct toxicology studies on the basis of symptoms and circumstances. Monitor COHb during and at the end of therapy. The pulse oximeter has two wavelengths and overestimates oxyhemoglobin saturation in CO poisoning. The true oxygen saturation is determined by blood gas analysis and measuring the oxygen bound to hemoglobin. The co-oximeter measures four wavelengths and separates out COHb and the other hemoglobin-binding agents from oxyhemoglobin. Fetal hemoglobin has a greater affinity for CO than adult hemoglobin does, and the COHb may be falsely elevated as much as 4% in young infants. *Disposition*: Patients with no or mild symptoms (after exposure of less than 5 minutes) who become asymptomatic after a few hours of oxygen therapy and have a CO level below 10%, normal findings on physical examination and on neurologic-cognitive examination, and normal ABG parameters, may be discharged but instructed to return if any signs of neurologic dysfunction arise. Patients with CO poisoning necessitating treatment need follow-up neuropsychiatric examination.

Caustics and Corrosives. The U.S. Consumer Products Safety Commission labeling recommendations on containers for acids and alkalis indicate the potential for producing serious damage: caution (weak irritant), warning (strong irritant), danger (corrosive). Some common acids with corrosive potential are acetic acid (>50%), calcium oxide, formic acid, glycolic acid (>10%), hydrochloric acid (>10%), mercuric chloride, nitric acid (>5%), oxalic acid (>10%), phosphoric acid (>60%), sulfuric acid (battery acid) (>10%), zinc chloride (>10%), and zinc sulfate (>50%). Some common alkalis with corrosive potential include ammonia (>5%), calcium carbide, calcium hydroxide (dry), potassium hydroxide (lye) (>1%), and sodium hydroxide (lye) (>1%). *Toxic mechanism*: Acids produce mucosal coagulation necrosis and an eschar and may be systemically absorbed, but with the exception of hydrofluoric acid, they do not penetrate deeply. Injury to the gastric mucosa is more likely, although specific sites of injury for acids and alkalis are not clearly defined. Alkalis produce liquefaction necrosis and saponification and penetrate deeply. The esophageal mucosa is more likely to be damaged. Oropharyngeal and esophageal damage is more frequently caused by solids than by liquids. Liquids produce superficial, circumferential burns and gastric damage. *Toxic dose*: The toxicity is determined by concentration, contact time, and pH. Significant injury is more likely at pH values less than 2 or greater than 12 and stricture at pH 14, prolonged contact time, and large volumes. *Manifestations*: The absence of oral burns does not exclude the possibility of esophageal or gastric damage. General clinical findings include stridor; dysphagia; drooling; oropharyngeal, retrosternal, and epigastric pain; and ocular and oral burns. Alkali burns are yellow, soapy, frothy lesions. Acid burns are gray-white and later form an eschar. Abdominal tenderness and guarding may be present if the abdomen is perforated.

Management: Bring the container; the substance must be identified and the pH of the substance, vomitus, tears, and saliva tested. *Ingestion, ocular, and dermal management*: (1) Prehospital and initial hospital management: If ingestion occurs, all GI decontamination procedures are contraindicated except for immediate rinsing, removal of the substance from the mouth, and then dilution with small amounts (sips) of milk or water. Check for ocular and dermal involvement. Contraindications to oral dilution are dysphagia, respiratory distress, obtundation, and shock. If ocular involvement occurs, immediately irrigate with tepid water for at least 30 minutes, perform fluorescein staining of the eye, and consult with an ophthalmologist. If dermal involvement occurs, immediately remove contaminated clothes and irrigate the skin with tepid water for at least 15 minutes. Consult with a burn specialist. (2) For acid ingestion, some authorities advocate placement of a small, flexible nasogastric tube and aspiration within 30 minutes after ingestion. (3) The patient should receive only IV fluids after dilution until endoscopic consultation is obtained. (4) Endoscopy is valuable for predicting damage and the risk of stricture. The indications are controversial: some authorities recommend its use in all caustic ingestions regardless of symptoms, whereas others are selective and use clinical features such as vomiting, stridor, drooling, and oral or facial lesions as criteria. Endoscopy is indicated for all symptomatic patients or those with intentional ingestion. Endoscopy may be performed immediately if the patient is symptomatic but is usually done 12 to 48 hours after ingestion. After 72 hours the risk of perforation is increased. (5) Corticosteroids may be ineffective and are considered mainly for second-degree circumferential burns. If a corticosteroid is used, start hydrocortisone sodium succinate IV at 10 to 20 mg/kg/d within 48 hours and change to oral prednisolone at 2 mg/kg/d. Continue prednisolone for 3 weeks and then taper the dose. (6) Provide tetanus prophylaxis. Antibiotics are not useful prophylactically. (7) An esophagogram is not useful in the first few days and may interfere with endoscopic evaluation; later, it may be used to assess the severity of damage. (8) Investigative therapy includes agents to inhibit collagen formation and the use of intraluminal stents. (9) Esophageal and gastric outlet dilation may be needed if evidence of stricture is noted. Bougienage of the esophagus has, however, been associated with brain abscess. Interposition of a colon segment may be necessary if dilation fails to provide a passage of adequate size. *Inhalation management* requires immediate removal of the patient from the environment, administration of humid supplemental oxygen, and observation for airway obstruction and noncardiac pulmonary edema. Obtain radiographic and ABG evaluation when appropriate. Intubation and respiratory support may be required. Certain caustics produce systemic disturbances: formaldehyde, metabolic acidosis; hydrofluoric acid, hypocalcemia and renal damage; oxalic acid, hypocalcemia; phenol, hepatic and renal damage; and pitric acid, renal injury.

Laboratory investigations: If acid has been ingested, determine the acid-base balance and electrolytes. If pulmonary symptoms are present, use chest radiography, ABGs, and pulse oximetry. *Disposition*: Infants and small children should be medically evaluated and observed. Admit all symptomatic patients to the hospital. Admit to the ICU if the patient has severe symptoms or danger of airway compromise. After endoscopy, if no damage is seen, the patient may be discharged when oral feedings are tolerated. Intentional exposure necessitates psychiatric evaluation before discharge.

Cocaine. (Benzoylmethylecgonine.) Cocaine is derived from the leaves of *Erythroxylon coca.* A body packer is a person who conceals many small packages of cocaine contraband in the GI tract or other areas for illicit transport. A body stuffer spontaneously ingests substances for the purpose of hiding evidence. *Toxic mechanism*: Cocaine directly stimulates CNS presynaptic sympathetic neurons to release catecholamines and acetylcholine, blocks presynaptic reuptake of the catecholamines, blocks the sodium channels along neuronal membranes, and increases platelet aggregation. Long-term use depletes the CNS of dopamine. *Toxic dose*: The maximal mucosal local anesthetic therapeutic dose is 200 mg, or 2 mL of a 10% solution. Psychoactive effects occur at 50 to 95 mg; cardiac and CNS effects occur at 1 mg/kg. The potential fatal dose is 1200 mg intranasally, but death has occurred with 20 mg parenterally. *Kinetics*: See Table 20. Cocaine is well absorbed by all routes, including nasal insufflation and oral, dermal, and inhalation routes. It is metabolized by plasma and liver cholinesterase to the inactive metabolites ecgonine methyl ester and benzoylecgonine. Plasma pseudocholinesterase is congenitally deficient in 3% of the population and decreased in fetuses, young infants, elderly persons, pregnant women, and patients with liver disease. Persons with this enzyme deficit are at increased risk for life-threatening cocaine toxicity. PB is 8.7%, the Vd is 1.2 to 1.9 L/kg, and 10% of cocaine is excreted unchanged. Cocaine and ethanol undergo liver synthesis to form cocaethylene, a metabolite with a $t_{1/2}$ three times longer than that of cocaine. This metabolite may account for some of cocaine's cardiotoxicity and appears to be more lethal than cocaine or ethanol alone. *Manifestations*: (1) CNS: euphoria, hyperactivity, agitation, convulsions, intracranial hemorrhage; (2) eye-ear-nose-throat: mydriasis, septal perforation; (3) cardiovascular: cardiac dysrhythmias, hypertension and hypotension (in severe overdose), chest pain (occurs frequently, but only 5.8% of affected patients have true myocardial ischemia and infarction); (4) hyperthermia (vasoconstriction, increased metabolism); (5) GI: ischemic bowel perforation if the drug was ingested; (6) rhabdomyolysis, myoglobinuria, and renal failure; (7) premature labor and abruptio placentae; (8) in prolonged toxicity, suspect body cavity packing; and (9) mortality resulting from cerebrovascular accidents, coronary artery spasm and myocardial injury, and lethal dysrhythmias.

Management: (1) Supportive care: Blood pressure, cardiac, and thermal monitoring and seizure precautions are instituted. Diazepam is the agent of choice for treatment of cocaine toxicity with agitation, seizures, and dysrhythmias; the dose is 10 to 30 mg IV at 2.5 mg/min for an adult and 0.2 to 0.5 mg/kg at 1 mg/min up to 10 mg for a child. (2) GI decontamination: If cocaine is ingested, administer AC. MDAC may absorb cocaine leakage in body stuffers or body packers. Whole-bowel irrigation with PEG solution has been used in body packers and stuffers if the contraband is in a firm container. If packages are not visible on an abdominal radiograph, a contrast study and/or ultrasonography can help confirm successful passage. PEG may desorb the cocaine from AC. Cocaine in the nasal passage can be removed with an applicator dipped in a non–water-soluble product (lubricating jelly). (3) In body packers and stuffers, secure venous access and have drugs readily available to treat life-threatening manifestations until the contraband is passed in the stool. Surgical removal may be indicated if a packet does not pass the pylorus, in a symptomatic body packer, or for intestinal obstruction. (4) Cardiovascular disturbances: Hypertension and tachycardia are usually transient and can be managed by careful titration of diazepam. Nitroprusside may be used for the treatment of hypertensive crisis. Myocardial ischemia is managed by oxygen, vascular access to administer IV medications, BZPs, and nitroglycerin. Use of aspirin and thrombolytic agents is not routinely recommended because of the danger of intracranial hemorrhage. Dysrhythmias are usually supraventricular tachycardias and do not mandate specific management. Adenosine is ineffective. Life-threatening tachydysrhythmias may respond to phentolamine in a dose of 5 mg given as an IV bolus in adults or 0.1 mg/kg in children at 5- to 10-minute intervals. Phentolamine also relieves coronary artery spasm and myocardial ischemia. Electrical synchronized cardioversion should be considered for hemodynamically unstable dysrhythmias. Lidocaine is not recommended initially but may be used after 3 hours for ventricular tachycardia. Wide-complex QRS ventricular tachycardia may be treated with $NaHCO_3$ at 2 mEq/kg as a bolus. β-Adrenergic blockers are not recommended. (5) Treat anxiety, agitation, and convulsions with diazepam. If diazepam fails to control seizures, use neuromuscular blockers and monitor the EEG for nonmotor seizures. (6) Hyperthermia: Administer external cooling and cool humidified 100% oxygen. Neuromuscular paralysis to control seizures reduces body temperature. Dantrolene and antipyretics are not recommended. (7) Treat rhabdomyolysis and myoglobinuria with fluids, alkaline diuresis, and diuretics. (8) If the patient is pregnant, monitor the fetus and observe for threatened spontaneous abortion. (9) Treat paranoid ideation and threatening behavior with rapid tranquilization. Observe the patient for suicidal depression, which may follow intoxication and necessitate suicide precautions. (10) If focal neurologic manifestations are present, consider a diagnosis of cerebrovascular accident and perform CT. (11) Extracorporeal measures are of no benefit.

Laboratory investigations: Monitoring: ECG and cardiac monitoring is instituted, as is monitoring of ABGs and oxygen saturation, electrolytes, blood glu-

TABLE 20. **Different Routes and Kinetics of Cocaine**

Type	Route	$t_{1/2}$ (min)	Onset	Peak (min)	Duration (min)
Cocaine leaf	Oral, chew	NA	20–30 min	45–90	240–360
Hydrochloride	Insufflation	78	1–3 min	5–10	60–90
	Ingested	54	20–30 min	50–90	Sustained
	Intravenous	36	30–120 s	5–11	60–90
Freebase, crack	Smoked	—	5–10 s	5–11	Up to 20
Coca paste	Smoked	—	Unknown		

cose, BUN, creatinine, creatine kinase and cardiac function if chest pain is present, liver profile, rhabdomyolysis and urine for myoglobin, and urine for cocaine and metabolites and other substances of abuse. Abdominal radiography or ultrasonography is performed for assessment in body packers. A urine sample collected more than 12 hours after cocaine intake contains little or no cocaine. If cocaine is present, it has been used within the past 12 hours. Cocaine's metabolite benzoylecgonine may be detected within 4 hours after a single nasal insufflation and as long as 48 to 114 hours after use. IV drug users should have HIV and hepatitis virus testing. Cross-reactions with herbal teas, lidocaine, and droperidol may give false-positive results with some laboratory methods. *Disposition*: Patients with mild intoxication or a brief seizure that does not necessitate treatment who become asymptomatic may be discharged after 6 hours with appropriate psychosocial follow-up. If cardiac or cerebral ischemia manifestations are noted, monitor in the ICU. Body packers and stuffers require ICU care until passage of the contraband.

Cyanide. Some sources of cyanide: (1) Hydrogen cyanide (HCN) is a byproduct of burning plastic and wool and is produced in residential fires and salts in ore extraction. (2) Nitriles, such as acetonitrile (present in artificial nail removers), are metabolized in the body to produce cyanide. (3) Cyanogenic glycosides in the seeds of fruit stones (as amygdalin in apricots, peaches, and apples) in the presence of intestinal β-glucosidase form cyanide (the seeds are harmful only if the capsule is broken). (4) Sodium nitroprusside, the antihypertensive vasodilator, contains five cyanide groups. *Toxic mechanism*: Cyanide blocks the cellular electron transport mechanism and cellular respiration by inhibiting the mitochondrial ferricytochrome oxidase system and other enzymes. This action results in cellular hypoxia and lactic acidosis. *Toxic dose*: The ingestion of 1 mg/kg or 50 mg of HCN can produce death within 15 minutes. The lethal dose of potassium cyanide is 200 mg. Five to 10 mL of 84% acetonitrile is lethal. The permissible exposure limit for volatile HCN is 10 ppm, and 300 ppm is fatal in minutes. *Kinetics*: Cyanide is rapidly absorbed by all routes. In the stomach it forms hydrocyanic acid. PB is 60%; the Vd, 1.5 L/kg. Cyanide is detoxified by metabolism in the liver via the mitochondrial endogenous thiosulfate-rhodanese pathway; this pathway catalyzes the transfer of sulfur to cyanide to irreversibly form the less toxic thiocyanate, which is excreted in the urine. The $t_{1/2}$ for cyanide elimination from the blood is 1.2 hours. Cyanide is also detoxified by reacting with hydroxocobalamin (vitamin B_{12a}) to form cyanocobalamin (vitamin B_{12}). Elimination is through the lungs. *Manifestations*: HCN has the distinctive odor of bitter almonds (odor of silver polish). The clinical findings are flushing, hypertension, headache, hyperpnea, seizures, stupor, cardiac dysrhythmias, and pulmonary edema. Cyanosis is absent or appears late. Various ECG abnormalities may be present.

Management: (1) Protect rescuers and attendants. Immediately administer 100% oxygen and continue during and after the administration of the antidote. If cyanide is inhaled, remove the patient from the contaminated atmosphere. Attendants should not administer mouth-to-mouth resuscitation. (2) Cyanide antidote kit (see Table 10): The clinician must decide whether to use any or all components of the kit. The mechanism of action of the antidote kit is to form methemoglobin (MetHb), which has a greater affinity for cyanide than does the cytochrome oxidase system and forms cyanomethemoglobin. The cyanide is transferred from MetHb by sodium thiosulfate, which provides a sulfur atom that is converted by the rhodanese-catalyzed enzyme reaction (thiosulfate sulfurtransferase) to convert cyanide into the relatively nontoxic sodium thiocyanate, a form excreted by the kidney. Procedure for using the antidote kit: Step 1, use of amyl nitrite inhalant Perles, is only a temporizing measure (forms only 2% to 5% MetHb) and can be omitted if venous access is established. Administer 100% oxygen and the inhalant for 30 seconds of every minute. Use a new Perles every 3 minutes. Step 2, administration of a sodium nitrite ampule, is not necessary in poisonings associated with residential fires, smoke inhalation, nitroprusside, or acetonitrile. Sodium nitrite is administered IV to produce a MetHb concentration of 20% to 30% at 35 to 70 minutes after administration. For adults, 10 mL of a 3% solution of sodium nitrite (0.33 mL/kg of a 3% solution for children) is diluted to 100 mL with 0.9% saline and administered slowly IV at 5 mL/min. If hypotension develops, slow the infusion. Step 3, administration of sodium thiosulfate, is useful alone in smoke inhalation, nitroprusside toxicity, and acetonitrile toxicity and should not be used at all in hydrogen sulfide poisoning. For adults, administer 12.5 g of sodium thiosulfate or 50 mL of a 25% solution (for children, 1.65 mL/kg of a 25% solution) IV over a period of 10 to 20 minutes. If cyanide-related symptoms recur, repeat the antidotes in 30 minutes as half of the initial dose. The dosage regimen for children on the package insert must be carefully followed. One hour after the antidotes are administered, the MetHb level should be obtained and should not exceed 20%. Methylene blue should not be used to reverse excessive MetHb. (3) GI decontamination after oral ingestion by gastric lavage and AC is recommended but not very effective (1 g of AC binds only 35 mg of cyanide). (4) Treat seizures with IV diazepam. Correct acidosis with $NaHCO_3$ if it does not resolve rapidly with therapy. (5) Treat metabolic acidosis with $NaHCO_3$. (6) The HBO chamber, hemodialysis, or hemoperfusion has no role in treatment. (7) Other antidotes: In France, hydroxocobalamin (vitamin B_{12a}) is used (it exchanges its hydroxyl with free cyanide to form cyanocobalamin). It has proved effective when given immediately after exposure in large doses of 4 g (50 mg/kg) or 50 times the amount of cyanide in the exposure with 8 g of sodium thiosulfate (it has FDA orphan drug approval).

Laboratory investigations: Obtain and monitor ABGs, oxygen saturation, blood lactate (which takes

0.5 hour), blood cyanide (which takes hours), hemoglobin, blood glucose, and electrolytes. Lactic acidemia, a decrease in the arterial-venous oxygen difference, and bright red color of the venous blood are manifestations of toxicity. If smoke inhalation is the possible source of exposure, obtain COHb and MetHb concentrations. The cyanide level in whole blood for a smoker is less than 0.5 μg/mL; with exposure plus flushing and tachycardia, 0.5 to 1.0 μg/mL; with obtundation, 1.0 to 2.5 μg/mL; and with coma and death, greater than 2.5 μg/mL. *Disposition*: Asymptomatic patients should be observed for a minimum of 6 hours. Patients who ingest nitrile compounds must be observed for 24 hours. Patients requiring antidote administration should be admitted to the ICU.

Digitalis. Cardiac glycosides are found in cardiac medications, common plants, and the skin of *Bufo* species of toad. More than 1 to 3 mg may be found in a few leaves of oleander or foxglove. *Toxic mechanism*: Cardiac glycosides inhibit the enzyme Na^+, K^+-ATPase, which leads to intracellular potassium loss, increased intracellular sodium-producing phase 4 depolarization, increased automaticity, and ectopy. Increased intracellular calcium and potentiation of contractility occur. Pacemaker cells are inhibited and the refractory period is prolonged, effects leading to AV block. Vagal tone is increased. *Toxic dose*: The digoxin total digitalizing dose is 0.75 to 1.25 mg, or 10 to 15 μg/kg in patients older than 10 years and 40 to 50 μg/kg in those younger than 2 years; 30 to 40 μg/kg at 2 to 10 years of age produces a therapeutic serum concentration of 0.6 to 2.0 ng/mL. The acute single toxic dose is more than 0.07 mg/kg, or more than 2 to 3 mg in adults; however, 2 mg in a child or 4 mg in an adult usually produces mild toxicity. Serious and potentially fatal overdoses are produced by the ingestion of greater than 4 mg in a child and greater than 10 mg in an adult. Digoxin clinical toxicity is usually associated with serum digoxin levels of 3.5 mg/mL or more in adults. Patients at greatest risk of overdose include those with cardiac disease, electrolyte abnormalities (low potassium, low magnesium, low thyroxine, high calcium), or renal impairment and those receiving amiodarone, quinidine, erythromycin, tetracycline, calcium channel blockers, and β-blockers. *Kinetics*: Digoxin is a metabolite of digitoxin. With oral ingestion, onset occurs within 1 to 2 hours, peak levels occur at 2 to 3 hours, and peak effects are seen at 3 to 4 hours; the duration is 3 to 4 days. In overdose, the typical onset is at 30 minutes, with peak effects in 3 to 12 hours. With intoxication from IV use, onset is in 5 to 30 minutes, the peak level occurs immediately, and the peak effect occurs at 1.5 to 3 hours. Elimination is 60% to 80% renal. The Vd is 5 to 6 L/kg. The cardiac-to-plasma ratio is 30:1. The elimination $t_{1/2}$ is 30 to 50 hours. After an acute ingestion overdose, the serum concentration does not reflect the tissue concentration for at least 6 hours or more, and steady state is reached 12 to 16 hours after the last dose. *Manifestations*: Effects may be delayed 9 to 18 hours. (1) GI effects: Nausea and vomiting are always present in acute ingestion and may occur in chronic ingestion. (2) Cardiovascular effects: The "digitalis effect" on the ECG consists of scooped ST segments and PR prolongation. In overdose, any dysrhythmia or block is possible, but none is characteristic. Bradycardia occurs in acute overdose in patients with healthy hearts or tachycardia with existing heart disease or in chronic overdose. Ventricular tachycardia is seen only in severe poisoning. (3) CNS effects are headaches, visual disturbances, and colored-halo vision. (4) Potassium disturbances: Hyperkalemia is a predictor of serum digoxin concentrations greater than 10 ng/mL and is associated with a 50% mortality rate without treatment. In one review, if serum potassium was less than 5.0 mEq/L, the survival rate was 100%; if 5 to 5.5 mEq/L, 50% of the patients survived; and if greater than 5.5 mEq/L, all died. Hypokalemia is commonly seen with chronic intoxication. Patients with normal digitalis levels may have toxicity in the presence of hypokalemia. (5) Chronic intoxications are more likely to produce scotoma, color perception disturbances, yellow vision, halos, delirium, hallucinations or psychosis, tachycardia, and hypokalemia.

Management: Obtain a cardiology consultation and have a pacemaker readily available. (1) GI decontamination: Use caution with vagal stimulation, and avoid emesis and gastric lavage. Administer AC; if a nasogastric tube is required for AC therapy, consider pretreatment with atropine (0.02 mg/kg for a child and 0.5 mg for an adult). MDAC may interrupt the enterohepatic recirculation of digitoxin and adsorb active metabolites but is not routinely recommended. (2) Digoxin-specific antibody fragment (Fab, Digibind), 38 mg, binds with 0.5 mg of digoxin and is then excreted through the kidneys. It decreases digoxin levels 50-fold (see Table 10). Indications include life-threatening, hemodynamically unstable dysrhythmias (ventricular dysrhythmias or rapid deterioration of clinical findings); ingestion greater than 4 mg in a child and 10 mg in an adult; serum potassium greater than 5.0 mEq/L produced by cardiac glycoside toxicity; serum digoxin toxicity (more than 10 ng/mL in adults or more than 5 ng/mL in children) 6 to 8 hours after acute ingestion; and unstable, severe bradycardia or second- or third-degree block unresponsive to atropine. This agent is also useful in digitalis delirium with thrombocytopenia and in the treatment of life-threatening digitoxin and oleander poisoning. Empirical digoxin-specific Fab fragment therapy may be administered as a bolus through a 22-μm filter in a critical emergency. If the clinical situation is less urgent, administer over a period of 30 minutes. The empirical dose is 10 vials for adults and 5 vials for children. *Calculation of dose*: The amount (total milligrams) of digoxin known to have been ingested multiplied by 80% bioavailability (0.8) = body burden. If the agent was given as liquid capsules or IV, do not multiply by 0.8. The body burden divided by 0.5 (0.5 mg of digoxin is bound by 1 vial of 38 mg of Fab) = number of vials needed. If the amount is unknown but the steady-state serum concentration is known, for digoxin:

$$\text{Digoxin (ng/mL)} \times \text{Vd (5.6 L/kg)} \times \text{Weight (kg)} = \text{Body Burden } (\mu g)$$

$$\text{Body Burden/1000} = \text{Body Burden (mg)}$$

$$\text{Body Burden/0.5} = \text{Number of Vials Needed}$$

For Digitoxin:

$$\text{Digitoxin (ng/mL)} \times \text{Vd (0.56 L/kg)} \times \text{Weight (kg)} = \text{Body Burden } (\mu g)$$

$$\text{Body Burden/1000} = \text{Body Burden (mg)}$$

$$\text{Body Burden/0.5} = \text{Number of Vials Needed}$$

(3) Antidysrhythmic agents and a pacemaker should be used only if Fab therapy fails. The onset of action is within 30 minutes. Complications of Fab therapy are related mainly to withdrawal of digoxin and worsening heart failure and include hypokalemia, decreased glucose levels (if glycogen stores are low), and allergic reactions (rare). Digitalis administered after Fab therapy is bound and may be inactivated for 5 to 7 days. (4) For ventricular tachydysrhythmias, correct electrolyte disturbances and administer lidocaine or phenytoin. For torsades de pointes, administer 20 mL of 20% magnesium sulfate, given IV slowly over a period of 20 minutes, to an adult or 25 to 50 mg/kg to a child, and titrate to control the dysrhythmia. Discontinue magnesium if hypotension, heart block, or a decrease in deep tendon reflexes occurs. Magnesium should be used with caution if renal impairment is present. Ventricular pacing should be reserved for patients who fail to respond to Fab. (5) Do not use antidysrhythmics of classes IA, IC, II, and IV or agents that increase conduction time (e.g., procainamide, bretylium, diltiazem, β-blockers). Class IB drugs can be used. (6) Cardioversion should be used with caution; start at a setting of 5 to 10 J and pretreat with lidocaine, if possible, because cardioversion may precipitate ventricular fibrillation or asystole. (7) Treat unstable bradycardia and second- and third-degree AV block with atropine. If the patient is unresponsive, use Fab. A pacemaker should be available if the patient fails to respond. Avoid isoproterenol, which causes dysrhythmias. (8) Electrolyte disturbances: Potassium disturbances are due to a shift, not a change in total body potassium. Treat hyperkalemia (potassium level greater than 5.0 mEq/L) with Fab only. Never use calcium, insulin, or glucose. Do not use $NaHCO_3$ concomitantly with Fab because it may produce severe, life-threatening hypokalemia. Sodium polystyrene sulfonate (Kayexalate) should not be used. Treat hypokalemia with caution because this condition may be cardioprotective. (9) Extracorporeal procedures are ineffective. Hemodialysis is used for severe or refractory hyperkalemia.

Laboratory investigations: Monitor baseline ECG and continuous cardiac function and blood glucose, electrolyte, calcium, magnesium, BUN, and creatinine levels. Measure initial digoxin levels more than 6 hours after ingestion because earlier values do not reflect the tissue distribution. Obtain free (unbound) serum digoxin concentrations after Fab therapy because the free (unbound) digoxin decreases and reflects the true level. *Cross-reactions*: An endogenous digoxin-like substance cross-reacts in most common immunoassays (not with HPLC), and values as high as 4.1 ng/mL have been reported in newborns, in patients with chronic renal failure or abnormal immunoglobulins, and in women in the third trimester of pregnancy. *Disposition*: Consult with a poison control center and cardiologist experienced with the use of digoxin-specific Fab fragments. All patients with significant dysrhythmias, symptoms, an elevated serum digoxin concentration, or elevated serum potassium level should be admitted to the ICU. Fab and pacemaker therapy should be readily available. Asymptomatic patients with nontoxic levels should have studies repeated in 12 hours.

Ethanol. (Grain alcohol.) See Table 21. *Toxic mechanism*: Ethanol has CNS hypnotic and anesthetic effects produced by a variety of mechanisms, including membrane fluidity and effect on the GABA system. It promotes cutaneous vasodilation (contributing to hypothermia), stimulates secretion of gastric juice (potentially causing gastritis), inhibits secretion of antidiuretic hormone, inhibits gluconeogenesis (potentially causing hypoglycemia), and influences fat metabolism (potentially causing lipidemia). *Toxic dose*: 1 mL/kg of absolute or 100% ethanol or 200-proof ethanol (proof defines alcohol concentration in beverages) results in a BEC of 100 mg/dL. The potentially fatal dose is 3 g/kg for children or 6 g/kg for adults. Children frequently have hypoglycemia at a BEC greater than 50 mg/dL. *Kinetics*: Onset of action occurs 30 to 60 minutes after ingestion, peak action is at 90 minutes on an empty stomach, and the Vd is 0.6 L/kg. The major route of elimination (more than 90%) is by hepatic oxidative metabolism. The first step involves the enzyme alcohol dehydrogenase (ADH), which converts ethanol to acetaldehyde. The kinetics in this step are zero order at a constant rate (regardless of the level) of 12 to 20 mg/dL/h (12 to 15 mg/dL/h in nonalcoholic drinkers, 15 mg/dL/h in social drinkers, 30 to 50 mg/dL/h in alcoholics, and 28 mg/dL/h in children). At a low BEC (less than 30 mg/dL), the metabolism is by first-order kinetics. In the second step of metabolism, the acetaldehyde is metabolized by acetaldehyde dehydrogenase to acetic acid. In subsequent steps, acetic acid is metabolized via the Krebs citric acid cycle to carbon dioxide and water. The enzyme steps are dependent on nicotinamide adenine dinucleotide, which interferes with gluconeogenesis. Only 2% to 10% of ethanol is excreted unchanged by the kidneys. BEC and the

TABLE 21. **Summary of Alcohol and Glycol Features***

Feature	Alcohol			Ethylene Glycol
	Methanol	*Isopropanol*	*Ethanol*	
Principal uses	Gas line Antifreeze Sterno Windshield wiper de-icer	Solvent Jewelry cleaner Rubbing alcohol	Beverage Solvent	Antifreeze De-icer
Odor	None	None	Yes	None
Specific gravity	0.719	0.785	0.789	1.12
Fatal dose	1 mL/kg	3 mL/kg	5 mL/kg	1.4 mL/kg
Hepatic enzyme	Alcohol dehydrogenase	Alcohol dehydrogenase	Alcohol and acetaldehyde dehydrogenases	Alcohol dehydrogenase
Toxic metabolite(s)	Formate, formaldehyde	Acetone	Acetaldehyde	Glyoxylic acid, oxalate
Drunkenness	±	2+	2+	1+
Metabolic change		Hyperglycemia	Hypoglycemia	Hypocalcemia
Metabolic acidosis	4+	0	1+	2+
Anion gap	4+	±	2+	4+
Ketosis	Ketobutyric acid	Acetone	Hydroxybutyric acid	None
GI tract	Pancreatitis	Hemorrhagic gastritis	Gastritis	
Visual	Blindness, pink optic disk			
Crystalluria	0	0	0	+
Pulmonary edema				+
Renal failure				+
Molecular weight	32	60	46	62
Osmolality†	0.337	0.176	0.228	0.190

*0 indicates no effect; + indicates mild effect; ± indicates no effect or mild effect; 2+ indicates moderate effect; 4+ indicates severe effect.
†A concentration of 1 mL/dL of substances raises the freezing point osmolarity of serum. The validity of the correlation of osmolality with blood concentrations has been questioned. Inebriation index: methanol < ethanol < ethylene glycol < isopropanol.

amount ingested can be estimated by the following equations:

$$\text{BEC (mg/dL)} = \frac{\text{Amount Ingested (mL)} \times \text{\% Ethanol in Product} \times \text{SG (0.79)}}{\text{Vd (0.6 L/kg)} \times \text{Body Weight (kg)}}$$

$$\text{Dose (amount ingested)} = \frac{\text{BEC (mg/dL)} \times \text{Vd (0.6 L/kg)} \times \text{Body Weight (kg)}}{\text{\% Ethanol} \times \text{SG (0.79)}}$$

Manifestations: See Table 22. (1) Acute: BECs over 30 mg/dL produce euphoria; over 50 mg/dL, incoordination and intoxication; over 100 mg/dL, ataxia; over 300 mg/dL, stupor; and over 500 mg/dL, coma. Levels of 500 to 700 mg/dL may be fatal. Children frequently have hypoglycemia at a BEC above 50 mg/dL. (2) Patients with chronic alcoholism tolerate a higher BEC, and correlation with manifestations is not valid. A rapid interview for alcoholism uses the CAGE questions: C, Have you felt the need to *c*ut down? A, Have others *a*nnoyed you by criticizing your drinking? G, Have you felt *g*uilty about your drinking? E, Have you ever had a morning *e*ye-opening drink to steady your nerves or get rid of a hangover? Two affirmative answers indicate probable alcoholism.

Management: Inquire about trauma and disulfiram (Antabuse) use. (1) Protect from aspiration and hypoxia. Establish and maintain vital functions. The patient may require intubation and assisted ventila-

TABLE 22. **Clinical Signs in an Intolerant Ethanol Drinker**

Ethanol (mg/dL)	Blood (μg/mL)	Concentration* (mmol/L)	Manifestations† in Nonalcoholics
>25	>250	>5.4	Euphoria
>47	>470	>10.2	Mild incoordination, sensory and motor impairment
>50	>500	>10.8	Increased risk of motor vehicle accidents
>100	>1000	>21.7	Ataxia (legal toxic level in many localities)
>150	>1500	>32.5	Moderate incoordination, slow reaction time
>200	>2000	>43.4	Drowsiness and confusion
>300	>3000	>65.1	Severe incoordination, stupor, blurred vision
>500	>5000	>108.5	Flaccid coma, respiratory failure, hypotension; may be fatal

*Ethanol concentrations are sometimes reported as percentages. Note that mg% is not equivalent to mg/dL because ethanol weighs less than water (SG, 0.79). A 1% ethanol concentration is 790 mg/dL and 0.1% is 79 mg/dL.
†Great variation is seen in individual behavior at particular blood ethanol levels. Behavior is dependent on tolerance and other factors.

tion. (2) GI decontamination plays no role. (3) If the patient is comatose, administer 50% glucose IV at 1 mL/kg in adults and 25% glucose at 2 mL/kg in children. Thiamine, 100 mg IV, is administered if the patient has a history of chronic alcoholism, malnutrition, or suspected eating disorders and to prevent Wernicke-Korsakoff syndrome. Naloxone has produced a partially inconsistent response and is not recommended for known alcoholics taking CNS depressants. (4) General supportive care: Administer fluids to correct hydration and hypotension; correct electrolyte abnormalities and acid-base imbalance. Vasopressors and plasma expanders may be necessary to correct severe hypotension. Hypomagnesemia is frequently present in chronic alcoholics. For hypomagnesemia, administer a loading dose of 2 g of a 10% magnesium sulfate solution given IV over a 5-minute period in the ICU with blood pressure and cardiac monitoring and have 10% calcium chloride on hand in case of overdose. Follow with a constant infusion of 6 g of 10% magnesium sulfate over a period of 3 to 4 hours. Be cautious with magnesium administration if renal failure is present. (5) Hypothermic patients should be warmed. See general treatment of poisoning. (6) Hemodialysis may be used in severe cases when conventional therapy is ineffective (rarely needed). (7) Treat repeated or prolonged seizures with diazepam. Brief "rum fits" do not necessitate long-term anticonvulsant therapy. Repeated seizures or focal neurologic findings may warrant skull radiography, lumbar puncture, and CT of the head, depending on the clinical findings. (8) Treat withdrawal with hydration and large doses of chlordiazepoxide (50 to 100 mg) or diazepam (2 to 10 mg) IV; these medications may be repeated in 2 to 4 hours. Large doses of BZPs may be required for delirium tremens. Withdrawal can occur in the presence of an elevated BEC and can be fatal if untreated.

Laboratory investigations: The BEC should be specifically requested and monitored. (Gas chromatography or a breathalyzer test gives rapid, reliable results in the absence of belching or vomiting; enzymatic methods do not differentiate between the alcohols.) Monitor ABGs, electrolytes, and glucose; determine the anion and osmolar gap (measure by freezing point depression, not vapor pressure); and check for ketosis. See discussion of general management. The AG increases 1 mg/kg for each 4.5-mg/dL increase in BEC. Obtain a chest radiograph to determine whether aspiration pneumonia is present. Perform renal and liver function tests and obtain bilirubin levels. *Disposition*: Clinical severity (e.g., whether intubation or assisted ventilation is needed or aspiration pneumonia is present) should determine the level of hospital care needed. Young children with significant accidental exposure to alcohol (calculated to reach a BEC of 50 mg/dL) should have their BEC measured and blood glucose levels monitored for hypoglycemia frequently for 4 hours after ingestion. Patients with acute ethanol intoxication seldom require admission unless a complication is present. However, intoxicated patients should not be discharged until they are fully functional (can walk independently, talk and think coherently), have had their suicide potential evaluated, have a proper environment to which they can be discharged, and have a sober escort. Extended liability means that a physician can be held liable for subsequent injuries or death of an intoxicated patient who has been allowed to sign out against medical advice. No patient with an altered mental status can sign out.

Ethylene Glycol. Ethylene glycol is found in solvents, windshield de-icer, antifreeze (95%), and air-conditioning units and has contaminated imported wines. Ethylene glycol is a sweet-tasting, colorless, water-soluble liquid with a sweet aromatic aroma. *Toxic mechanism*: Ethylene glycol is oxidized by ADH to glycolaldehyde and then metabolized to glycolic acid and glyoxylic acid. Glyoxylic acid is metabolized to oxalic acid. Ethylene glycol metabolites are metabolized via pyridoxine-dependent pathways to glycine, benzoic acid, and hippuric acid and by thiamine- and magnesium-dependent pathways to α-hydroxyketoadipic acid. The metabolites of ethylene glycol produce a profound metabolic acidosis, increased AG, hypocalcemia, deposition of oxalate crystals in tissues, and renal damage. *Toxic dose*: The ingestion of 0.1 mL of 100% ethylene glycol per kilogram can result in a toxic serum ethylene glycol concentration (SEGC) of 20 mg/dL, a level that necessitates ethanol therapy, the antidote. Ingestion of 3.0 mL of a 100% solution by a 10-kg child or 30 mL of 100% ethylene glycol by an adult produces an SEGC of 50 mg/dL (8.1 mmol/L), a concentration that requires hemodialysis. The fatal amount is 1.4 mL of a 100% solution per kilogram. *Kinetics*: Absorption is by dermal, inhalation, and ingestion routes. Ethylene glycol is rapidly absorbed from the GI tract. Onset is in 30 minutes to 12 hours, and the peak level usually occurs at 2 hours. Without ethanol, the $t_{1/2}$ is 3 to 8 hours; with ethanol, 17 hours; and with hemodialysis, 2.5 hours. The Vd is 0.65 to 0.8 L/kg. For metabolism, see the toxic mechanism discussion. Renal clearance is 3.2 mL/kg/min. About 20% to 50% is excreted unchanged in the urine. The following equations can be used for calculating SEGC and the amount ingested (EG is ethylene glycol):

Calculation of SEGC:

$$0.12 \text{ mL/kg of 100\% EG} = \text{SEGC of 10 mg/dL}$$

$$\text{SEGC (mg/dL)} = \frac{\text{Amount Ingested (mL)} \times \text{\% EG} \times \text{SG (1.12)}}{\text{Vd (0.65 L/kg)} \times \text{Weight (kg)}}$$

$$\text{Amount Ingested (mL)} = \frac{\text{SEGC (mg/dL)} \times \text{0.65 L/kg} \times \text{Weight (kg)}}{\text{\% EG} \times \text{SG (1.12)}}$$

Manifestations: Phase I: The onset is 30 minutes to 12 hours after ingestion or longer with concomitant ethanol ingestion. The patient acts inebriated at an SEGC of 50 to 100 mg/dL. Hypocalcemia, tetany, and calcium oxalate and hippuric acid crystals in the urine may be observed within 4 to 8 hours but are not always present. Early, before metabolism of ethylene glycol, an osmolal gap may be present. Later, the metabolites of ethylene glycol produce changes starting 4 to 12 hours after ingestion, including an AG, metabolic acidosis, coma, convulsions, cardiac disturbances, and pulmonary and cerebral edema. Fluorescent urine is not an indicator of ethylene glycol ingestion and should not be used as a screen. Phase II: After 12 to 36 hours, cardiopulmonary deterioration occurs with pulmonary edema and congestive heart failure. Phase III: In 36 to 72 hours, oliguric renal failure resulting from oxalate crystal deposition and from tubular necrosis predominates, and pulmonary edema occurs. Phase IV: Neurologic sequelae occur 6 to 10 days after ingestion and include facial diplegia, hearing loss, bilateral visual disturbances, elevated cerebrospinal fluid pressure with or without elevated protein and pleocytosis, vomiting, hyperreflexia, dysphagia, and ataxia.

Management: (1) Establish and maintain vital functions. Protect the airway and use assisted ventilation, if necessary. (2) GI decontamination has a limited role, with only gastric lavage within 30 to 60 minutes after ingestion. AC is not effective. (3) Obtain baseline serum electrolyte, calcium, and glucose levels, ABGs, ethanol concentration, SEGC (difficult to obtain and often takes more than 48 hours), and methanol concentration. In the first few hours, determine the measured serum osmolality and compare it with the calculated osmolarity (see "Serum Osmolal Gaps"). (4) If seizures occur, exclude hypocalcemia and treat with IV diazepam. If hypocalcemic seizures occur, treat with 10 to 20 mL of 10% calcium gluconate (0.2 to 0.3 mL/kg for children) slowly IV and repeat as needed. (See Table 10.) (5) Correct metabolic acidosis with $NaHCO_3$ given IV. (6) Fomepizole (Antizol) inhibits the enzyme ADH. Unlike ethanol, it does not require constant monitoring of ethanol levels or attendant titration to achieve a concentration greater than 100 mg/dL; additionally, it does not cause CNS depression. It is available in 1.5-mL vials (1 g/mL). The loading dose is 15 mg/kg (0.015 mL/kg) given IV. The maintenance dose is 10 mg/kg (0.010 mL/kg) IV every 12 hours for 4 doses, then 15 mg/kg every 12 hours until ethylene glycol levels are less than 20 mg/dL. The solution is prepared by injecting 100 mL of 0.9% saline or D5W and mixing well. Fomepizole can be given to patients undergoing hemodialysis but should be dosed as follows:

- Fomepizole (Antizol) dosing in patients requiring hemodialysis
  - Dose at the beginning of hemodialysis
    - If less than 6 hours since the last Antizol dose—do not administer a dose
    - If more than 6 hours since the last dose—administer the next scheduled dose
  - Dosing during hemodialysis
    - Dose every 4 hours
  - Dosing at the time that hemodialysis is completed
    - Time between the last dose and the end of dialysis less than 1 hour—do not administer a dose at the end of dialysis
    - 1 to 3 hours—administer half of the next scheduled dose
    - More than 3 hours—administer the next scheduled dose
  - Maintenance dosing while not undergoing hemodialysis
    - Give the next scheduled dose 12 hours from the last dose administered

(7) Ethanol therapy should be initiated immediately if 4-methylpyrazole is not readily available or if a delay is anticipated in obtaining fomepizole. The enzyme ADH has 100 times greater affinity for ethanol than for ethylene glycol. Therefore, ethanol blocks the metabolism of ethylene glycol at BECs of 100 to 150 mg/dL. Initiate therapy if the patient has ingested 100% ethylene glycol at 0.1 mL/kg, if the SEGC is more than 20 mg/dL, if an osmolar gap is present that is not accounted for by other alcohols or factors (e.g., hyperlipidemia) (see "Serum Osmolal Gaps"), if the patient has metabolic acidosis with an increased AG, or if oxalate crystals are present in the urine while awaiting hemodialysis. Ethanol should be administered IV (the oral route is less reliable) to produce a BEC of 100 to 150 mg/dL. The loading dose is derived from the formula: 1 mL of 100% ethanol per kilogram = a BEC of 100 mg/dL (which protects against metabolism of ethylene glycol). Therefore, 10 mL of 10% ethanol is administered IV concomitantly with a maintenance dose of 10% ethanol of 2.0 mL/kg/h (alcoholic), 0.83 mL/kg/h (nondrinker), or 1.4 mL/kg/h (social drinker). Increase the infusion rate of 10% ethanol to 2 to 3.5 mL/kg/h when the patient is receiving hemodialysis. (8) Hemodialysis: Obtain a nephrology consultation. Early hemodialysis is indicated if the ingestion is potentially fatal, if the SEGC is more than 50 mg/dL (some authorities recommend hemodialysis at levels of more than 25 mg/dL), if severe acidosis or electrolyte abnormalities occur despite conventional therapy, or if congestive heart failure or renal failure is present. Hemodialysis reduces the ethylene glycol $t_{1/2}$ from 17 hours with ethanol therapy to 3 hours. Continue therapy (ethanol and hemodialysis) until the SEGC is less than 10 mg/dL or undetectable, the glycolate level is undetectable, the acidosis has cleared, no mental disturbances are present, the creatinine level is normal, and urine output is adequate. This process may require 2 to 5 days. (9) Adjunctive therapy: Thiamine (100 mg/day [children, 50 mg] slowly over a 5-minute period IV or IM and repeated every 6 hours) and pyridoxine (50 mg IV or IM every 6 hours) have been recommended until the intoxication is resolved but have not been extensively studied. Folate may be given at 50 mg IV (in children, 1 mg/kg)* every 4 hours for six doses. (10) Therapy with 4-methylpyrazole given orally at 15 mg/kg, followed by 5 mg/kg in 12 hours and then 10 mg/kg

*Exceeds dosage recommended by the manufacturer.

every 12 hours until levels of the toxin are not detectable, blocks ADH without causing inebriation.

Laboratory investigations: Monitor blood glucose, electrolytes, urinalysis (look for oxalate ["envelope"] and monohydrate ["hemp seed"] crystals; urine fluorescence should not be used as a screen), and ABGs. Obtain ethylene glycol and ethanol levels and determine plasma osmolarity (use the freezing point depression method) and calcium, BUN, and creatinine levels. An SEGC of 20 mg/dL is toxic (ethylene glycol levels are difficult to obtain). If possible, obtain a glycolate level. *Cross-reactions*: Propylene glycol, a vehicle in many liquids and IV medications (phenytoin, diazepam), other glycols, and triglycerides, may produce spurious ethylene glycol levels. *Disposition*: All patients who ingest significant amounts of ethylene glycol should be referred to the emergency department. If the SEGC cannot be obtained, follow-up for 12 hours with monitoring of the osmolal gap, acid-base parameters, and electrolytes is recommended to rule out the development of metabolic acidosis with an AG.

Hydrocarbons. The lower the viscosity and surface tension or the greater the volatility, the greater the risk of aspiration. Volatile substance abuse has resulted in the "sudden sniffing death syndrome," most likely caused by dysrhythmias. *Toxicologic classification and toxic mechanism*: All systemically absorbed hydrocarbons can lower the myocardial threshold for the development of dysrhythmias produced by endogenous and exogenous catecholamines. (1) Petroleum distillates are aliphatic hydrocarbons. *Toxic dose*: Aspiration of a few drops produces chemical pneumonitis, but these substances are poorly absorbed from the GI tract and produce no systemic toxicity by this route. Examples are gasoline, kerosene, charcoal lighter fluid, mineral spirits (Stoddard's solvent), and petroleum naphtha. (2) Aromatic hydrocarbons are six-carbon ringed structures that produce CNS depression and, in chronic abuse, may have multiple organ effects. Examples are benzene (which in chronic intoxication produces leukemia), toluene, styrene, and xylene. The ingested, seriously toxic dose is 20 to 50 mL in an adult. (3) Halogenated hydrocarbons are aliphatic hydrocarbons with one or more halogen substitutions (Cl, Br, Fl, or I). They are highly volatile and abused as inhalants. They are well absorbed from the GI tract, produce CNS depression, and have metabolites that can damage the liver and kidneys. Examples are methylene chloride (which may be converted to CO in the body), dichloroethylene (which also causes a disulfiram-like reaction ["degreaser's flush"] when associated with consumption of ethanol), and 1,1,1-trichloroethane (Glamorene Spot Remover, Scotchgard, typewriter correction fluid) (the acute lethal oral dose is 0.5 to 5 mL/kg). (4) Dangerous additives to the hydrocarbons include those in the mnemonic CHAMP: *c*amphor (demothing agent), *h*alogenated hydrocarbons, *a*romatic hydrocarbons, *m*etals (heavy), and *p*esticides. Exposure to these agents may warrant gastric emptying with a small-bore nasogastric lavage tube. (5) Heavy hydrocarbons have high viscosity, low volatility, and minimal GI absorption, so gastric decontamination is not necessary. Examples are asphalt (tar), machine oil, motor oil (lubricating oil, engine oil), home heating oil, and petroleum jelly and mineral oil. (6) Mineral seal oil (e.g., signal oil), found in furniture polishes, is a low-viscosity, low-volatility oil with minimal absorption that never warrants gastric decontamination. It can produce severe pneumonia if aspirated.

Management: (1) Asymptomatic patients who have ingested small amounts of petroleum distillates may be observed at home by reliable caretakers for the development of signs of aspiration (cough, wheezing, tachypnea, and dyspnea), with periodic telephone contact for 4 to 6 hours. (2) Inhalation of any hydrocarbon vapors in a closed space can produce intoxication. Remove the victim from the environment and administer oxygen and respiratory support. (3) GI decontamination is not advised for the ingestion of hydrocarbons that do not usually cause systemic toxicity (petroleum distillates, heavy hydrocarbons, mineral seal oil). For hydrocarbons that cause systemic toxicity in small amounts (aromatic hydrocarbons, halogenated hydrocarbons), pass a small-bore nasogastric tube (these substances are liquids) and aspirate if appropriate time has not elapsed (absorption with aromatic and halogenated hydrocarbons is complete in 1 to 2 hours) and spontaneous vomiting has not occurred. Patients with altered mental status should have their airway protected because of concern over uncontrolled vomiting. Although some toxicologists advocate ipecac-induced emesis under medical supervision instead of small-bore nasogastric gastric lavage, we do not. AC is suggested, but no reliable data concerning its effectiveness have been presented and it may produce vomiting. AC may, however, be useful for adsorbing toxic additives or co-ingestants. (4) A symptomatic patient who is coughing, gagging, choking, or wheezing on arrival has probably already aspirated. Offer supportive respiratory care: maintain the airway, provide assisted ventilation, and offer supplemental oxygen with monitoring of pulse oximetry; also measure ABGs, obtain a chest radiograph and ECG, and admit the patient to the ICU. A chest radiograph for aspiration may be positive as early as 30 minutes, and almost all are positive within 6 hours. If bronchospasm occurs, administer a nebulized β-adrenergic agonist and IV aminophylline if necessary. Avoid epinephrine because of the susceptibility to dysrhythmias. If cyanosis is present that does not respond to oxygen and the PaO_2 is normal, suspect methemoglobinemia, which may necessitate therapy with methylene blue (see Table 10). Corticosteroids and prophylactic antimicrobial agents have not been shown to be beneficial. (Fever or leukocytosis may be produced by the chemical pneumonitis itself.) It is not necessary to surgically treat pneumatoceles that develop because they usually resolve. Most infiltrations resolve spontaneously in 1 week, except for lipoid pneumonia, which may last up to 6 weeks. Dysrhythmias may necessitate α- and β-adrenergic antagonists or cardioversion. (5) Enhanced elimination procedures have no role in hydrocarbon toxicity. (6) Methylene chloride is metabolized in several hours to CO. See the section on treatment of CO poisoning. Give 100% oxygen, and monitor serial COHb levels, ECG, and pulse oximetry. (7) Halogenated hydrocarbons are hepatorenal toxins; therefore, monitor liver and kidney function. NAC therapy may be useful if the patient has evidence of hepatic damage. (8) Investigational: Surfactant was used for hydrocarbon aspiration in an animal study of aspirated hydrocarbons and found to be detrimental. Extracorporeal membrane oxygenation has been used successfully in a few patients with life-threatening respiratory failure.

Laboratory investigations: Monitor ECG continuously; ABGs; liver, pulmonary, and renal function; serum electrolytes; and serial chest radiographs. *Disposition*: Asymptomatic patients who have ingested small amounts of petroleum distillates can be managed at home. Symptomatic patients with abnormal chest radiography, oxygen saturation, or ABG results should be admitted to the hospital. If the patient becomes asymptomatic, oxygenation is normal, and repeated radiographs are normal, the patient can be discharged.

Iron. More than 100 over-the-counter iron preparations are available for supplementation and treatment of iron deficiency anemia. *Toxic mechanism*: Toxicity depends on the amount of elemental (free) iron available in various salts (gluconate, 12%; sulfate, 20%; fumarate, 33%; lactate, 19%; and chloride, 21% of elemental iron), not on the amount of the preparation. Locally, iron is corrosive and may cause fluid loss, hypovolemic shock, and perforation. Excessive free iron in the blood is directly toxic to the vasculature and leads to the release of vasoactive substances that produce vasodilation. In overdose, iron deposits injure mitochondria in the liver, the kidneys, and the myocardium. The exact mechanism of cellular damage is not clear. *Toxic dose*: The therapeutic dose of elemental iron is 6 mg/kg/d. Elemental iron at 20 to 40 mg/kg per dose may produce mild self-limited GI symptoms, a dose of 40 to 60 mg/kg produces moderate toxicity, more than 60 mg/kg produces severe toxicity and is potentially lethal, and more than 180 mg/kg is usually fatal without treatment. Children's chewable vitamins with iron have 12 to 18 mg of elemental iron per tablet or per 0.6 mL of liquid drops. These preparations rarely produce toxicity unless extremely large quantities are ingested. The following equation can be used to calculate the amount of elemental iron ingested:

$$\text{Elemental Iron (mg/kg)} = \frac{\text{Number of Tablets Ingested} \times \text{\% Elemental Iron}}{\text{Body Weight (kg)}}$$

Kinetics: Absorption occurs chiefly in the upper part of the small intestine, usually with iron in the ferrous (2+) state absorbed into the mucosal cells, where it is oxidized to the ferric (3+) state and bound to ferritin. Iron is slowly released from ferritin into plasma to become bound to transferrin and then transported to specific tissues for production of hemoglobin (70%), myoglobin (5%), and cytochrome. About 25% of iron is stored in the liver and spleen. In overdoses, larger amounts of iron are absorbed because of direct mucosal corrosion. No mechanism is available for additional elimination of iron (normal elimination is 1 to 2 mg/d), except through bile, sweat, and blood loss. *Manifestations*: Serious toxicity is unlikely if the patient remains asymptomatic for 6 hours, has a normal white blood cell count and glucose level, and has a negative abdominal radiograph. Iron intoxication usually follows a multiphasic course. A phase may be omitted entirely. Phase I: GI mucosal injury occurs 30 minutes to 12 hours after ingestion. Vomiting starts 30 minutes to 1 hour after ingestion and is persistent. Hematemesis and bloody diarrhea, abdominal cramps, fever, hyperglycemia, and leukocytosis occur. Enteric-coated tablets may pass through the stomach without causing symptoms. Acidosis and shock can occur within 6 to 12 hours. Phase II is a latent period of apparent improvement spanning the 8 to 12 hours after ingestion. Phase III is the systemic toxicity phase (12 to 48 hours after ingestion), with cardiovascular collapse and severe metabolic acidosis. Phase IV (2 to 4 days after ingestion) is characterized by hepatic injury associated with jaundice, elevated liver enzymes, prolonged prothrombin time, and kidney injury with proteinuria and hematuria. Pulmonary edema, disseminated intravascular coagulation, and *Yersinia enterocolitica* sepsis can occur. In phase V (4 to 8 weeks after ingestion), sequelae affecting the pyloric outlet or intestinal stricture may cause obstruction or anemia secondary to blood loss.

Management: (1) GI decontamination: Induce emesis immediately with ingestion of elemental iron greater than 40 mg/kg if the patient has not already vomited. Gastric lavage with 0.9% saline is less effective than emesis because of the large size of the tablets, but it may be useful if chewed tablets and liquid preparations are involved. AC is ineffective. Obtain an abdominal radiograph after emesis or lavage to determine the success of gastric-emptying procedures. Children's chewable vitamins and liquid iron are not radiopaque. If radiopaque iron is still present, consider whole-bowel irrigation with a PEG solution (see the section on evaluation and general management). (2) In extreme cases, removal by endoscopy or surgery may be necessary because coalesced iron tablets can produce hemorrhagic infarction in the bowel and perforation peritonitis. (3) Deferoxamine (DFO) (see Table 10): About 100 mg of DFO binds only 8.5 to 9.35 mg of free iron in the serum in transit. The DFO infusion rate (the IV route is preferred) should not exceed 15 mg/kg/h or 6 g daily, but higher rates (up to 45 mg/kg/h) and larger daily amounts have been administered and tolerated in extreme cases of iron poisoning (greater than 1000 μg/dL). The DFO-iron complex is hemodialyzable if renal failure develops. Indications for chelation therapy are any of the following: serious clinical intoxication (severe vomiting and diarrhea [often bloody], severe abdominal pain, metabolic acidosis, hypotension, or shock), symptoms that persist or become worse, an estimate of elemental iron ingestion that is quite high and the presence of symptoms, and serum iron (SI) levels greater than 500 μg/dL. Chelation should be performed as early as possible, within 12 to 18 hours, to be effective. Start the infusion slowly and gradually increase to avoid hypotension. Successful chelation results in a urine color change from a positive vin rosé color to a normal color. Adult respiratory distress syndrome has developed in patients receiving high doses of DFO for several days; therefore, avoid prolonged infusions over 24 hours. Endpoints of treatment are absence of symptoms and clearing of urine that was originally a positive vin rosé color. In a diagnostic chelation test, DFO, 50 mg/kg in children or 1 g in adults IM, produces a vin rosé color (ferroxime-iron complex) of the urine within 3 hours. This test is not reliable for elevated SI levels; however, obtain a baseline urine sample for comparison with subsequent specimens. (4) Supportive therapy: IV bicarbonate may be needed to correct the metabolic acidosis. Hypotension and shock treatment may necessitate fluid volume expansion, vasopressors, and blood transfusions. Attempt to keep the urine output at more than 2 mL/kg/h. Coagulation abnormalities and overt bleeding necessitate infusion of blood products and vitamin K. (5) Treatment in pregnant patients is similar to that in any others with iron poisoning. (6) Extracorporeal measures: Hemodialysis and hemoperfusion are not effective. Exchange transfusion has been used in single cases of massive poisoning in children.

Laboratory investigations: Iron poisoning produces AG metabolic acidosis. Monitor the CBC, blood glucose, SI, stools and vomitus (for occult blood), electrolytes, acid-base balance, urinalysis results and urine output, liver function tests, BUN, and creatinine. If GI bleeding occurs, obtain and match the blood type. SI measured at the proper time correlates with the clinical findings. The lavender-topped Vacutainer tube contains ethylenediaminetetraacetic acid (EDTA), which falsely lowers the SI. Obtain the SI before administering DFO. SI levels at 2 to 6 hours of less than 350 μg/dL predict an asymptomatic course, levels of 350 to 500 μg/dL are usually associated with mild GI symptoms, and levels above 500 μg/dL predict a 20% risk of shock and serious iron intoxication with phase III manifestations. A follow-up SI level after 6 hours may not be elevated, even in severe poisoning; however, an SI level at 8 to 12 hours is useful for excluding delayed absorption from a bezoar or sustained-release preparation. Determination of the total iron-binding capacity is not necessary. Abdominal radiographs can visualize adult iron tablet preparations before they dissolve. A negative radiograph does not exclude iron poisoning. Iron sepsis: Patients in whom high fever and signs of sepsis develop after iron overdose should have blood and stool cultures checked for *Y. enterocolitica*. *Disposition*: Observe patients who are asymptomatic or have minimal symptoms for persistence and progression of symptoms or the development of signs of toxicity (GI bleeding, acidosis, shock, altered mental state). A patient with mild self-limited GI symptoms who becomes asymptomatic or has no signs of toxicity for 6 hours is unlikely to have serious intoxication and can be discharged after psychiatric clearance, if needed. Patients with moderate or severe toxicity should be in the ICU.

Isoniazid. (Isonicotinic acid hydrazide [INH], Nydrazid.) INH is a hydrazide derivative of vitamin B_3 (nicotinamide) used as an antituberculosis drug. *Toxic mechanism*: INH produces pyridoxine deficiency by doubling the excretion of pyridoxine (vitamin B_6) and by inhibiting the interaction of pyridoxal 5-phosphate (the active form of pyridoxine) with L-glutamic acid decarboxylase to form GABA, the major CNS neurotransmitter inhibitor, and it may result in seizures and coma. INH blocks the conversion of lactate to pyruvate and thereby causes profound lactic acidosis. *Toxic dose*: The therapeutic dose is 5 to 10 mg/kg (maximum of 300 mg) daily. A single acute dose of 15 mg/kg lowers the seizure threshold, 35 to 40 mg/kg produces spontaneous convulsions, more than 80 mg/kg produces severe toxicity, and 200 mg/kg is an obligatory convulsant. Malnourished persons, those with a previous seizure disorder or alcoholism, and slow acetylators are more susceptible to INH toxicity. In chronic intoxication, 10 mg/kg/d produces hepatitis in 10% to 20% of patients, but doses of 3 to 5 mg/kg/d affect less than 2%. *Kinetics*: Rapid absorption from the intestine occurs in 30 to 60 minutes, onset is in 30 to 120 minutes, and the peak level of 5 to 8 μg/mL is reached within 1 to 2 hours. The Vd is 0.6 L/kg; PB is minimal. Elimination is by liver acetylation to a hepatotoxic metabolite, acetylisoniazid, which is then hydrolyzed to isonicotinic acid. Slow acetylators show a $t_{1/2}$ of 140 to 300 minutes (mean of 5 hours) and eliminate 10% to 15% of the drug unchanged in the urine. Forty-five percent to 75% of whites and 50% of African blacks are slow acetylators, and with chronic use (without pyridoxine supplements), peripheral neuropathy may develop. Fast acetylators show a $t_{1/2}$ of 35 to 110 minutes (mean of 80 minutes) and excrete 25% to 30% of the drug unchanged in the urine. About 90% of Asians and patients with diabetes mellitus are fast acetylators, and hepatitis may develop with chronic use. In overdose and hepatic disease, the serum $t_{1/2}$ may increase. INH inhibits the metabolism of phenytoin, diazepam, phenobarbital, carbamazepine, and prednisone. These drugs also interfere with the metabolism of INH. Ethanol may decrease the INH $t_{1/2}$ but may also increase its toxicity. *Manifestations*: Within 30 to 60 minutes, nausea, vomiting, slurred speech, dizziness, visual disturbances, and ataxia are present. Within 30 to 120 minutes, the major clinical triad of severe overdose develops: (1) refractory convulsions (90% of overdose patients have one or more seizures), (2) coma, and (3) resistant, severe AG lactic acidosis (secondary to convulsions), often with pH of 6.8.

Management: (1) Control seizures by administering pyridoxine, 1 g for each gram of isoniazid ingested (see Table 10). If the dose ingested is unknown, give at least 5 g of pyridoxine IV. Pyridoxine is administered in 50 mL of D5W or 0.9% saline over a period of 5 minutes IV. Do not administer in the same bottle as for $NaHCO_3$. Repeat IV pyridoxine every 5 to 20 minutes until seizures are controlled. Total doses of pyridoxine up to 52 g have been safely administered. However, a persistent crippling sensory neuropathy has developed in patients given 132 and 183 g of pyridoxine. Some authorities recommend prophylactic pyridoxine if the patient has ingested 80 mg of INH per kilogram. Administer diazepam concomitantly with pyridoxine, but at a different site. They work synergistically. Administer diazepam IV at 0.3 mg/kg slowly at a rate of 1 mg/min in children or 10 mg per dose slowly at a rate of 5 mg/min in adults. After the seizures are controlled, administer the remainder of the pyridoxine (1 g per gram of INH), or a total dose of 5 g, as an infusion drip over a 60 minute period. Do not use phenobarbital or phenytoin because they are ineffective. (2) In asymptomatic patients or patients without seizures, pyridoxine should be considered prophylactically in gram-for-gram doses with large overdoses (80 mg/kg per dose or more) of INH (there are no supporting studies, however). (3) In comatose patients, pyridoxine administration may result in rapid regaining of consciousness. (4) Correction of the acidosis and control of the seizures may occur spontaneously with pyridoxine administration. Administer $NaHCO_3$ if acidosis persists. (5) GI decontamination: After the patient is stabilized or if the patient is asymptomatic, gastric lavage may be performed after recent (less than 1 hour) ingestion, with protection of the airway if necessary. AC may be administered. (6) Hemodialysis is rarely needed because of antidotal therapy and the short $t_{1/2}$, but it may be used as adjunctive therapy for uncontrollable acidosis and seizures. Hemoperfusion has not been adequately evaluated. Diuresis is ineffective.

Laboratory investigations: INH produces AG metabolic acidosis. Therapeutic levels are 5 to 8 μg/mL, and acute, toxic levels are more than 20 μg/mL. Monitor blood glucose (hyperglycemia is common), electrolytes (hyperkalemia is frequent), bicarbonate, ABGs, liver function tests (elevations occur with chronic exposure), BUN, and creatinine. *Disposition*: Asymptomatic or mildly symptomatic patients who become asymptomatic may be observed in the emergency department for 4 to 6 hours. Larger amounts of INH may warrant pyridoxine and longer periods of observation. Patients with intentional ingestion require psychiatric evaluation before discharge. Patients with convulsions or coma should be admitted to the ICU.

Isopropanol. (Rubbing alcohol, solvents, lacquer thinner.) Coma has occurred in children sponged for fever with isopropanol. See Table 21. *Toxic mechanism*: Isopropanol is a gastric irritant. It is metabolized to acetone, a CNS and myocardial depressant. It inhibits gluconeogenesis. Normal propyl alcohol is related to isopropanol but is more toxic. *Toxic dose*: The toxic dose is 0.5 to 1 mg of 70% isopropanol per kilogram (1 mL of 70% isopropanol per kilogram produces a blood isopropanol concentration [BIPC] of 70 mg/dL). The CNS depressant effect is twice that of ethanol. *Kinetics*: Onset is within 30 to 60 minutes, and the peak effect occurs 1 hour after ingestion. Elimination is renal. Isopropanol is metabolized to acetone. The Vd is 0.6 L/kg. The BIPC and amount ingested can be estimated by using equations in ethanol kinetics and an SG of 0.785 for isopropanol:

$$\text{BIPC (mg/dL)} = \frac{\text{Amount Ingested (mL)} \times \text{\% Isopropanol in Product} \times \text{SG (0.79)}}{\text{Vd (0.6 L/kg)} \times \text{Body Weight (kg)}}$$

$$\text{Dose (Amount ingested)} = \frac{\text{BIPC (mg/dL)} \times \text{Vd (0.6 L/kg)} \times \text{Body Weight (kg)}}{\text{\% Ethanol} \times \text{SG (0.79)}}$$

Manifestations: Ethanol-like inebriation with an acetone odor of the breath, gastritis occasionally with hematemesis, acetonuria, and acetonemia without systemic acidosis are seen. CNS depressant effects include lethargy at 50 to 100 mg/dL and coma at 150 to 200 mg/dL; ingestion of more than 240 mg/dL is potentially fatal in adults. Hypoglycemia and seizures may occur. *Management*: (1) Protect the airway with intubation and administer assisted ventilation if necessary. If the patient is hypoglycemic, administer glucose. Supportive treatment is similar to that for ethanol. (2) GI decontamination has no role in treatment. (3) Hemodialysis in cases of life-threatening overdose is rarely needed. Consult a nephrologist if the BIPC is greater than 250 mg/dL. *Laboratory investigation*: Monitor isopropanol levels, acetone, glucose, and ABGs. The osmolal gap increases 1 mOsm per 5.9 mg/dL of isopropanol and 1 mOsm per 5.5 mg/dL of acetone. Absence of excess acetone in the blood (normal, 0.3 to 2 mg/dL) within 30 to 60 minutes or excess acetone in the urine within 3 hours excludes the possibility of significant isopropanol exposure. *Disposition*: Symptomatic patients with concentrations greater than 100 mg/dL require at least 24 hours of close observation for resolution and should be admitted to the hospital. If the patient is hypoglycemic, hypotensive, or comatose, admit to the ICU.

Lead. Lead is an environmental toxin. Acute lead intoxication is rare and usually caused by inhalation of lead, which results in severe intoxication and often death. It may be produced by burning lead batteries or using a heat gun to remove lead paint. It also results from exposure to high concentrations of organic lead (e.g., tetraethyl lead). Chronic lead poisoning occurs most often in children 6 months to 6 years of age who are exposed in their environment and in adults in certain occupations. See Table 23. In the United States, the percentage of children 1 to 5 years of age with a venous blood lead level (VBPb) greater than 10 μg/dL decreased from 88.2% in a survey from 1976 to 1980 to 8.9% in a survey from 1988 to 1991 as a result of measures to reduce lead in the environment, particularly by reducing leaded gasoline. However, an estimated 1.7 million children between 1 and 5 years old have blood lead levels greater than 10 μg/dL, and more than 1 million workers in over 100 different occupations are exposed to lead. *Toxic dose in chronic lead poisoning*: An intake of more than 5 μg/kg/d in children or more than 150 μg/d in adults can give toxic levels of lead on screening. In 1991, the CDC recommended routine screening consisting of a VBPb or a capillary blood lead determination for all children. In children a VBPb greater than 10 μg/dL was determined by the CDC to be a threshold of concern (it was 25 μg/dL in 1985). The average VBPb in the United States is 4 μg/dL. In occupational exposure (see Table 23), a VBPb greater than 40 μg/dL is indicative of increased lead absorption in adults. *Toxic mechanism*: Lead affects the sulfhydryl enzyme systems of proteins, the immature CNS, the enzymes of heme synthesis, vitamin D conversion, the kidneys, the bones, and growth. Lead alters the tertiary structure of cell proteins by denaturing them and causes death. Risk factors are mouthing behavior of infants and children and excessive oral behavior (pica), living in a run-down neighborhood, a poorly maintained home, and poor nutrition (e.g., low calcium and iron). Use of the CDC questionnaire is recommended at every pediatric visit. See Table 24. If any answers to the CDC questionnaire are positive, obtain a blood screening test for lead. However, studies have suggested that to be more accurate in identifying lead exposure, the questionnaire would have to be modified for each community because it has had poor sensitivity (40%) and specificity (60%). *Sources of lead* (Table 25): (1) The primary source of lead is deteriorating lead-based paint, which forms leaded dust. Lead concentrations in indoor paint were not reduced to safer levels (0.06%) until 1978. Lead can also be produced by improper interior or exterior home renovation (scraping or demolition). (2) The use of leaded gasoline (limited in 1973) resulted in residues from leaded motor vehicle emissions. Lead persists in the soil near major highways and deteriorating homes and buildings. Vegetables grown in contaminated soil may contain lead. (3) Oil refineries and lead-processing smelters are other sources. (4) Food cans produced in Mexico contain lead solder (95% of those produced in the United States do not). (5) Lead pipes (manufactured until 1950) and pipes with lead solder (manufactured until 1986) deliver lead-containing drinking water (calcium deposits, however, may offer some protection). Water at the consumer's tap should have a lead level less than 15 ppb (parts per billion). See Table 26. (6) Occupational exposure (see Table 23): OSHA standards require employers to provide showering and clothes-changing facilities for persons working with lead; however, businesses with fewer than 25 employees are exempt from this regulation. The OSHA lead standard of 1978 set a limit of 60 μg/dL for occupational exposure to lead. At a blood lead level of 60 μg/dL, a worker should be removed from lead exposure and not allowed back until the level is below 40 μg/dL. Many authorities think that this level should be lower. The lead residue on workers' clothes may represent a hazard to their families. Others occupationally exposed to lead include plumbers, pipefitters, lead miners, auto repairers, shipbuilders, printers, steel welders and cutters, construction workers, and those in rubber product manufacturing. (7) Other sources are leaded pots to make molds and "kusmusha" tea. (8) Hobbies (see Table 27) associated with lead exposure include mak-

TABLE 23. **Occupations Associated With Lead Exposure**

Lead production or smelting	Instructor or janitor at firing range
Production of illicit whiskey	Demolition of ships and bridges
Brass, copper, and lead foundries	Battery manufacturing
Radiator repair	Machining or grinding lead alloys
Scrap handling	Welding of old painted metals
Sanding of old paint	Thermal paint stripping of old buildings
Lead soldering	Ceramic glaze and pottery mixing
Cable stripping	

Modified from Rempel D: The lead-exposed worker. JAMA *262*:532–534, 1989. Copyright 1989, American Medical Association.

TABLE 24. **CDC Questionnaire: Priority Groups for Lead Screening**

1. Children 6–72 mo old (was 12–36 mo) who live in or are frequent visitors to older deteriorated housing built before 1960
2. Children 6–72 mo old who live in housing built before 1960 with recent, ongoing, or planned renovation or remodeling
3. Children 6–72 mo old who are siblings, housemates, or playmates of children with known lead poisoning
4. Children 6–72 mo old whose parents or other household members participate in a lead-related industry or hobby
5. Children 6–72 mo old who live near active lead smelters, battery recycling plants, or other industries likely to result in atmospheric lead release

TABLE 25. **Product Lead Content by Dry Weight**

Product	Lead (%)	Product	Lead (%)
Plastic additives	2.0	Construction material	0.1
Priming inks	2.0	Fertilizers	0.1
Plumbing fixtures	2.0	Toys and recreational games	0.1
Solder	0.6	Curtain weights	0.1
Pesticides	0.1	Fishing weights	0.1
Stained glass came	0.1	Glazes, enamels, frits	0.06
Wine bottle foil	0.1	Paint	0.06

TABLE 26. **Agency Regulations and Recommendations for Lead Content**

Agency	Specimen	Acceptable Level	Comments
CDC	Blood, child	10 μg/dL	Investigate community
OSHA	Blood, adult	60 μg/dL	Medical removal from work
OSHA	Air	50 μg/m^3	PEL
	Air	0.75 mg/m^3	Tetraethyl or tetramethyl
ACGIH	Air	150 μg/m^3	TWA
EPA	Air	1.5 μg/m^3	3-mo average
EPA	Water	15 μg/L (ppb)	5 ppb circulating
EPA	Food	100 μg/d	Advisory
FDA	Wine	300 ppm	Plan to reduce to 200 ppm
EPA	Soil and dust	50 ppm	
CPSC	Paint	600 ppm (0.06%)	By dry weight

Abbreviations: ACGIH = American Conference of Governmental Industrial Hygienists; CDC = Centers for Disease Control and Prevention; CPSC = Consumer Products Safety Commission; EPA = Environmental Protection Agency; FDA = Food and Drug Administration; OSHA = Occupational Safety and Health Administration; PEL = permissible exposure limit (highest level over 8-hour workday); ppb = parts per billion; ppm = parts per million; TWA = time-weighted average (air concentration for 8-h workday and 40-h workweek).

ing stained glass windows, lead fish sinkers, and curtain weights, which may pose additional hazard if ingested and retained by children; imported pottery with ceramic glaze can leach large amounts of lead into acids (e.g., citrus fruit juices). (9) Some "traditional" folk remedies or cosmetics contain lead: "Azarcon por empacho" ("Maria Louisa," 90% to 95% lead trioxide), a bright orange powder (used in Hispanic culture, especially Mexican, for digestive problems and diarrhea); "Greta" (4% to 90% lead), a yellow powder for "empacho" ("empacho" refers to a variety of GI symptoms; used in Hispanic cultures, especially Mexican); "Payloo-ah," an orange-red powder for rash and fever (used in Southeast Asian cultures, especially northern Laotian Hmong immigrants); "Alkohl" (kohl, suma, 5% to 92% lead), a black powder (used in Middle Eastern, African, and Asian cultures as a cosmetic and umbilical stump astringent); "Farouk," an orange granular powder with lead (Saudi Arabian); "Bint Al Zahab," used to treat colic (Saudi Arabian); "Surma" (23% to 26% lead), a black powder used in India as a cosmetic and to improve eyesight; and "Bali goli," a round black bean that is dissolved in "grippe water" (used by Asian and Indian cultures to aid digestion). (10) Substance abuse: The synthesis of amphetamines includes lead acetate, which may not be removed before use. Lead poisoning as a result of sniffing organic leaded gasoline has been reported. *Kinetics*: Absorption of lead is 10% to 15% of the ingested dose in adults; in children, up to 40% is absorbed, especially when iron deficiency anemia is present. Inhalation absorption is rapid and complete. The Vd in blood (0.9% of the total body burden) is 95% in red blood cells. The $t_{1/2}$ of lead in blood is 35 to 40 days; in soft tissue, 45 days; and in bone (99% of the lead), 28 years. Lead is eliminated via the stool (80% to 90%), kidneys (10%; 80 μg/day), and hair, nails, sweat, and saliva. Organic lead is metabolized in the liver to inorganic lead; 9% is excreted in the urine per day. Lead passes through the placenta to the fetus and is present in breast milk. *Manifestations*: See Table 28. Adverse health effects include the following: (1) Hematologic: Lead inhibits δ-aminolevulinic acid dehydratase early in the synthesis of heme (which has been associated with CNS symptoms) and ferrochelatase (which transfers iron to ferritin for iron incorporation into protoporphyrin to produce heme); anemia is a late finding. Decreased heme synthesis starts at a VBPb of more than 40 μg/dL. Basophilic stippling occurs in 20% of persons with severe lead poisoning. (2) Neurologic: Segmental demyelination and peripheral neuropathy, usually of the motor type (wrist and ankle drop), occur in workers. A VBPb greater than 70 μg/dL (usually greater than 100 μg/dL) produces encephalopathy in children (a symptom mnemonic is PAINT: *p*ersistent forceful vomiting and papilledema, *a*taxia, *i*ntermittent stupor and lucidity, *n*eurologic coma and refractory convulsions, *t*ired and lethargic). Decreased cognitive abilities have been associated with a VBPb higher than 10 μg/dL; behavior problems and decreased attention span and learning abilities have been reported. IQ scores may begin to decrease at 15 μg/dL. In adults, peripheral neuropathies and "lead gum lines" at the dental border of the gingiva occur. Encephalopathy is rare in adults. (3) Renal nephropathy with damaged capillaries and glomeruli is seen at a VBPb greater than 80 μg/dL, but renal damage and hypertension have also been observed with low VBPb values. Lead reduces the excretion of uric acid, and high-level exposure is associated with hyperuricemia and "saturnine gout," Fanconi's syndrome (aminoaciduria and renal tubular acidosis), and tubular fibrosis. A linear association between hypertension and a VBPb of 30 μg/dL has been reported. (4) Reproductive system effects include spontaneous abortion, transient delay in devel-

TABLE 27. **Hobbies Associated With Lead Exposure**

Casting of ammunition
Collecting antique pewter
Collecting or painting lead toys (e.g., soldiers and figures)
Ceramics or glazed pottery
Refinishing furniture
Making fishing weights
Home renovation
Jewelry making (lead solder)
Glass blowing (lead glass)
Bronze casting
Printmaking and other fine arts (when lead white, flake white, chrome yellow pigments are involved)
Liquor distillation
Hunting and target shooting
Painting
Car and boat repair
Restoring old houses or furniture
Making stained lead glass
Copper enameling

TABLE 28. **Summary of Lead-Induced Health Effects in Adults and Children**

Blood Lead Level (μg/dL)	Age Group	Health Effect
>100	Adult	Encephalopathic signs and symptoms
>80	Adult	Anemia
	Child	Encephalopathy
		Chronic nephropathy (e.g., aminoaciduria)
>70	Adult	Clinically evident peripheral neuropathy
	Child	Colic and other GI symptoms
>60	Adult	Female reproductive effects
		CNS disturbances and symptoms (i.e., sleep disturbances, mood changes, memory and concentration problems, headaches)
>50	Adult	Decreased hemoglobin production
		Decreased performance on neurobehavioral tests
		Altered testicular function
		GI symptoms (i.e., abdominal pain, constipation, diarrhea, nausea, anorexia)
	Child	Peripheral neuropathy
>40	Adult	Decreased peripheral nerve conduction
		Hypertension, age 40–59 y
		Chronic neuropathy
>25	Adult	Elevated erythrocyte protoporphyrin in males
15–25	Adult	Elevated erythrocyte protoporphyrin in females
	Child	Decreased intelligence and growth
>10	Fetus/child	Preterm delivery
		Impaired learning
		Reduced birth weight
		Impaired mental ability

From Implementation of the Lead Contamination Control Act of 1988. MMWR Morb Mortal Wkly Rep 41:288–290, 1992.

opment (catch-up age, 5 to 6 years), decreased sperm count, and abnormal sperm morphology. Lead is transmitted across the placenta in 75% to 100% of cases and is teratogenic. (5) Metabolic: Decreased cytochrome P-450 (which alters the metabolism of drugs and endogenously produced substances), decreased activation of cortisol, and decreased growth caused by interference with vitamin conversion (25-hydroxyvitamin D to 1,25-dihydroxyvitamin D) have been seen at a VBPb of 20 to 30 μg/dL. (6) Other abnormalities in thyroid, cardiac, and hepatic function occur in adults. Abdominal colic is seen in children with a VBPb greater than 50 μg/dL.

Management: The basis of treatment is removal of the source. Cases of poisoning in children should be reported to the local health department and cases of occupational poisoning to OSHA. Control the exposure by identifying and abating the source, improving housekeeping by wet mopping and using a high-phosphate detergent solution, allowing cold water to run for 2 minutes before using it for drinking, and planting shrubbery in contaminated soil to keep children away. (1) GI decontamination: Lead does not bind to AC. Do not delay chelation therapy for complete GI decontamination in severe cases. Whole-bowel irrigation has been used before treatment. Some authorities recommend abdominal radiography followed by GI decontamination, if necessary, before switching to oral therapy. (2) Supportive care includes measures to deal with refractory seizures (continue antidotal therapy, diazepam, and possibly neuromuscular blockers), hepatic and renal failure, and intravascular hemolysis. Treat seizures with diazepam, followed by neuromuscular blockers if needed. (3) Chelation therapy is used for children with levels above 45 μg/dL and adults with levels above 80 μg/dL or at lower levels with a positive lead mobilization test. See Table 29. Dimercaprol (BAL, British antilewisite) is a peanut oil–based dithiol (two sulfhydryl molecules) that combines with one atom of lead to form a heterocyclic stable ring complex. It is usually reserved for cases in which VBPb is above 70 μg/dL. It chelates red blood cell–bound lead and enhances its elimination through the urine and bile. It also crosses the blood-brain barrier. About 50% of patients have adverse reactions, including an unpleasant metallic taste in the mouth, pain at the injection site, sterile abscesses, and fever. Edetate calcium disodium (EDTA, $CaNa_2EDTA$, Calcium Disodium Versenate) is a water-soluble chelator given IM (with 0.5% procaine) or IV. The calcium in the compound is displaced by divalent and trivalent heavy metals, which form a soluble complex that is stable at physiologic pH (but not at acid pH) and enhances clearance in the urine. It is usually administered IV, especially in severe cases. It must not be administered until adequate urine flow is established. It may redistribute lead to the brain; therefore, BAL is started at a VBPb exceeding 55 μg/dL in children and 100 μg/dL in adults. Phlebitis occurs at concentrations above 0.5 mg/mL. Alkalization of the urine may be helpful (see Table 10). $CaNa_2EDTA$ should not be confused with sodium EDTA (disodium edetate), which is used to treat hypercalcemia; inadvertent use may produce severe hypocalcemia. Succimer (dimercaptosuccinic acid [DMSA], Chemet), a derivative of BAL, is an oral agent approved by the FDA in 1991 for chelation in children with a VBPb above 45 μg/dL. The recom-

TABLE 29. **Pharmacologic Chelation Therapy for Lead Poisoning**

Drug	Route	Dose	Duration	Precautions	Monitor
Dimercaprol (BAL in Oil)	IM	3–5 mg/kg q 4–6 h	3–5 d	G6PD deficiency Concurrent iron therapy	AST and ALT
$CaNa_2EDTA$ (Calcium Disodium Versenate)	IM or IV	50 mg/kg/d	5 d	Inadequate fluid intake Renal impairment	Urinalysis BUN Creatinine
D-Penicillamine (Cuprimine)	PO	10 mg/kg/d; increase to 30 mg/kg over 2-wk period	6–20 wk	Penicillin allergy Concurrent iron therapy Lead exposure Renal impairment	Urinalysis BUN Creatinine CBC
2,3-Dimercaptosuccinic acid (DMSA; succimer)	PO	10 mg/kg per dose tid for 5 d 10 mg/kg per dose bid for 14 d	19 d	AST and ALT elevations Concurrent iron therapy G6PD deficiency Lead exposure	AST and ALT

Abbreviations: BAL = British antilewisite; CBC = complete blood count; EDTA = ethylenediaminetetraacetic acid; G6PD = glucose-6-phosphate dehydrogenase.

mended dose is 10 mg/kg given every 8 hours for 5 days and then every 12 hours for 14 days (see Table 10). DMSA is under investigation to determine its role in children with a VBPb less than 45 μg/dL. Although not approved for adults, it has been used in adults at the same dosage. Monitor the CBC, liver transaminases, and urinalysis for toxicity. D-Penicillamine is given at 20 to 40 mg/kg/d, not to exceed 1 g/d. It is an oral chelator used to enhance the urinary elimination of lead; it is not FDA approved and has a 10% adverse reaction rate. Succimer is preferred. D-Penicillamine is used in adults with minimal symptoms but high VBPbs. A VBPb above 70 μg/dL or clinical symptoms suggesting encephalopathy in children indicate a potentially life-threatening emergency. Management should be accomplished in a medical center with a pediatric ICU by a multidisciplinary team that includes a critical care specialist, toxicologist, neurologist, and neurosurgeon, with careful monitoring of neurologic parameters, fluid status, and intracranial pressure if necessary. These patients need close monitoring for hemodynamic instability. Adequate hydration should be maintained to ensure renal excretion of lead. Monitor fluids, renal and hepatic function, and electrolytes. While measures to ensure adequate urine flow are implemented, therapy should be initiated with IM dimercaprol (BAL) only (25 mg/kg/d divided into six doses). Four hours later, a combination of a second dose of BAL given IM with $CaNa_2EDTA$ (50 mg/kg/d) given IV as a single dose infused over a period of several hours or as a continuous infusion is administered. The double therapy is continued until VBPb is less than 40 μg/dL. Therapy is continued for 72 hours and followed by one of two alternatives: either parenteral therapy with the two drugs ($CaNa_2EDTA$ and BAL) for 5 days or continued therapy with $CaNa_2EDTA$ alone if the patient has a good response and VBPb is below 40 μg/dL. If a report on VBPb has not been obtained, continue therapy with both BAL and EDTA for 5 days. In cases of lead encephalopathy, parenteral chelation should be continued with both drugs until the patient is clinically stable before therapy is changed. Mannitol and dexamethasone can reduce the cerebral edema, but removal of the lead is essential, and the role of these agents in lead encephalopathy is not clear. Avoid surgical decompression to reduce cerebral edema. If BAL and $CaNa_2EDTA$ are used together, a minimum of 2 days with no treatment should elapse before another 5-day course of therapy is considered. Repeat the 5-day course with $CaNa_2EDTA$ alone if the blood lead level remains above 40 μg/dL or in combination with BAL if it is above 70 μg/dL. If a third course is required, unless there are compelling reasons, wait at least 5 to 7 days before administration. Continue chelation therapy at all costs. After chelation therapy, a period of equilibration of 10 to 14 days should be allowed and repeated determinations of VBPb concentrations obtained. If the patient is stable enough for oral intake, oral succimer at 30 mg/kg/d in three divided doses for 5 days, followed by 20 mg/kg/d in two divided doses for 14 days, has been suggested, but data are limited. Continue therapy until VBPb is less than 20 μg/dL in children or 40 μg/dL in adults. Chelators combined with lead are hemodialyzable in the event of renal failure.

Laboratory investigations: (1) A classification of blood lead concentrations in children is given in Table 30. (2) The lead mobilization test is used to determine the chelatable pool of lead. It consists of the administration of 25 mg of $CaNa_2EDTA$ per kilogram in children or 1 g in adults as a single dose deeply IM, with 0.5% procaine diluted 1:1, or as an infusion. Empty the bladder and collect the urine for 24 hours (3 days with renal impairment). A modified 8-hour collection may be obtained. If the ratio of micrograms of lead excreted in the urine to milligrams of $CaNa_2EDTA$ administered is greater than 0.6, it represents an increased lead body burden, and therapeutic chelation is indicated. However, many authorities consider this test of little importance in making

TABLE 30. **Classification of Blood Lead Concentrations in Children**

Blood Lead Level (μg/dL)	Classification	Recommended Interventions
<9	I	None
10–14	IIa	Community intervention Repeat blood lead determination in 3 mo
15–19	IIb	Individual case management Environmental counseling Nutritional counseling Repeat blood lead determination in 3 mo
20–44	III	Medical referral Environmental inspection and/or abatement Nutritional counseling Repeat blood lead determination in 3 mo
45–69	IV	Environmental inspection and/or abatement Nutritional counseling Pharmacologic therapy: oral succimer or parenteral $CaNa_2EDTA$ Repeat q2wk for 6–8 wk, monthly for 4–6 mo
>70	V	Hospitalization in ICU Environmental inspection and/or abatement Pharmacologic therapy: dimercaprol given IM alone initially, then dimercaprol given IM and $CaNa_2EDTA$ together; repeat every wk

Abbreviation: EDTA = ethylenediaminetetraacetic acid.

the decision about chelation. The use of x-ray fluorescence of bone as an alternative to determine the lead burden is being tested. (3) Evaluate the CBC, serum ferritin, VBPb, erythrocyte protoporphyrin (greater than 35 μg/dL indicates lead poisoning, as well as iron deficiency and other causes), electrolytes, serum calcium and phosphorus, urine, BUN, and creatinine. Abdominal and long-bone radiographs are not routine but may be useful in certain circumstances for identifying radiopaque material in the bowel and lead lines in proximal end of the tibia (these effects occur after prolonged exposure in association with VBPb above 50 μg/dL). Serial VBPb measurements are obtained on days 3 and 5 during treatment, 7 days after chelation therapy, then every 1 to 2 weeks for 8 weeks, and then every month for 6 months. Stop the IV infusion at least 1 hour before obtaining blood for lead determination. (4) Neuropsychological tests are difficult to conduct in young children but should be considered at the end of treatment, especially to determine auditory dysfunction. *Disposition*: All patients with VBPb above 70 μg/dL or who are symptomatic should be admitted to the hospital. If a child is hospitalized, all lead hazards must be removed from the home before the child is allowed to return. The source must be eliminated by conducting environmental and occupational investigations. The local health department should be involved in the management of children with lead poisoning; OSHA should be involved in occupational lead poisoning. Consultation with the poison control center and/or an experienced toxicologist is necessary when chelation therapy is used. Follow-up VBPb concentrations should be obtained within 1 to 2 weeks, then every 2 weeks for 8 weeks, and then monthly for 6 months if the patient requires chelation therapy. All patients with VBPb values above 10 μg/dL should undergo follow-up evaluation at least every 3 months until two serial measurements are 10 μg/dL or three serial measurements are less than 15 μg/dL.

Lithium. (Li, Eskalith, Lithane.) Lithium is an A-1 alkali metal whose primary use is in the treatment of bipolar psychiatric disorders. Most intoxications are chronic overdoses. One gram of lithium carbonate contains 189 mg of lithium; a regular tablet, 300 mg or 8.12 mEq; and a sustained-release preparation, 450 mg or 12.18 mEq. *Toxic mechanism*: The brain is the primary target organ of toxicity, but the mechanism is unclear. Lithium may interfere with physiologic functions by acting as a substitute for cellular cations (sodium and potassium) and in this manner depresses neural excitation and synaptic transmission. *Toxic dose*: A lithium dose of 1 mEq/kg (40 mg/kg) results in a serum lithium concentration of about 1.2 mEq/L. The therapeutic serum lithium concentration in acute mania is 0.6 to 1.2 mEq/L; for maintenance, it is 0.5 to 0.8 mEq/L. Serum lithium levels are usually obtained 12 hours after the last dose. The toxic dose is determined by clinical manifestations and serum levels after the distribution phase. Acute ingestion of twenty 300-mg tablets (300 mg increases the serum lithium concentration by 0.2 to 0.4 mEq/L) in adults may produce serious intoxication. Chronic intoxication is produced by any state that increases lithium reabsorption. Risk factors that predispose to chronic lithium toxicity are febrile illness, impaired renal function, hyponatremia, advanced age, lithium-induced diabetes insipidus, dehydration, vomiting and diarrheal illness, concomitant drugs (thiazide and spironolactone diuretics, NSAIDs, salicylates, angiotensin-converting enzyme inhibitors [captopril], and SSRIs [e.g., fluoxetine and antipsychotic drugs]). *Kinetics*: GI absorption is rapid and peaks in 2 to 4 hours after the ingestion of regular-release preparations, and complete absorption occurs by 6 to 8 hours. Absorption may be delayed 6 to 12 hours after the ingestion of sustained-release preparations. The onset of toxicity may occur 1 to 4 hours after an acute overdose but is usually delayed because lithium enters the brain slowly. The Vd is 0.5 to 0.9 L/kg. Lithium is not protein bound. The $t_{1/2}$ after a single dose is 9 to 13 hours; at steady state it may be 30 to 58 hours. Renal handling of lithium is similar to that of sodium: by glomerular filtration and reabsorption (80%) in the proximal renal tubules. Adequate sodium must be present to prevent lithium reabsorption. More than 90% of lithium is excreted by the kidney unchanged, 30% to 60% within 6 to 12 hours. Alkalization of the urine increases clearance. *Manifestations*: It is important to distinguish among side effects, acute toxicity in a patient receiving chronic therapy, and chronic intoxication. Chronic is the most common and dangerous type of intoxication. (1) Side effects of lithium include fine tremor, GI upset, hypothyroidism, polyuria and frank diabetes insipidus, dermatologic manifestations, and cardiac conduction deficits. Lithium is also teratogenic. (2) Toxic effects: Patients with acute poisoning may be asymptomatic, with an early high serum lithium concentration of 9 mEq/L, and deteriorate as the serum level falls 50% and lithium is distributed to the brain and other tissues. Nausea and vomiting may begin within 1 to 4 hours, but systemic manifestations are usually delayed several more hours. It may take as long as 3 to 5 days for serious symptoms to develop. Acute toxicity is manifested by neurologic findings, including weakness, fasciculations, altered mental state, myoclonus, hyperreflexia, rigidity, coma, and convulsions with limbs in hyperextension. Its cardiovascular effects are nonspecific and occur at therapeutic doses: flat T or inverted T waves, AV block, and a prolonged QT interval. Lithium is not a primary cardiotoxin. Cardiogenic shock is secondary to CNS toxicity. (3) Chronic intoxication is associated with manifestations at lower serum lithium concentrations. Some correlation with manifestations is seen, especially at higher serum lithium concentrations. See Table 31. Permanent neurologic sequelae can result from lithium intoxication.

TABLE 31. **Classification of Severity of Chronic Lithium Intoxication**

Classification	Manifestations	Blood Concentration (mEq/L)*
Subacute or pretoxic	Apathy, fine tremor, vomiting and diarrhea, weakness	<1.2
Mild intoxication	Lethargy, drowsiness; hypertonia, hyperreflexia; muscle rigidity, dysarthria; ataxia, apathy, nystagmus	1.2–2.5
Moderate intoxication	Impaired consciousness; severe fasciculations; coarse tremor, severe ataxia; myoclonus, paresthesias; diabetes insipidus; electrocardiographic changes; renal tubular acidosis; paralysis, blurred vision	2.5–3.5
Severe intoxication	Muscle twitching, coma; severe myoclonic jerking; cardiac dysrhythmias; seizures, spasticity, shock	>3.5

*Plasma lithium concentrations (not an absolute correlation).
Modified from El-Mallakh RS: Treatment of acute lithium toxicity. Vet Hum Toxicol *26*:31–35, 1984.

Management: (1) Establish and maintain vital functions. Institute seizure precautions and treat seizures, hypotension, and dysrhythmias. Restore normothermia. (2) Evaluation: Examine for rigidity and signs of hyperreflexia, and monitor hydration status, renal function (BUN, creatinine), and electrolytes, especially sodium. Inquire about the use of diuretics and other drugs that increase serum lithium concentrations, and have the patient discontinue their use. If the patient has been receiving chronic therapy, discontinue such treatment. Obtain serial serum lithium concentrations every 4 hours until the concentration peaks and there is a downward trend toward an almost therapeutic range, especially with sustained-release preparations. Monitor vital signs, including temperature and ECG; conduct serial neurologic examinations, including mental status testing; and measure urine lithium output. Obtain a nephrology consultation if the serum lithium level is chronic and elevated (above 2.5 mEq/L), if a large amount of lithium has been ingested, or if the patient has an altered mental state. (3) Fluid and electrolyte therapy: An IV line should be established and hydration and electrolyte balance restored. Determine the serum sodium level before administration of 0.89% saline fluid in chronic overdoses because hypernatremia may be present as a result of diabetes insipidus. Although current evidence indicates that an initial 0.89% saline infusion (at 200 mL/hr) enhances the excretion of lithium, once hydration, output, and normonatremia are established, administer 0.45% saline and slow the infusion (to 100 mL/h). (4) GI decontamination: Gastric lavage is questionable because of the size of these tablets. AC is ineffective. With slow-release preparations, whole-bowel irrigation may be useful, but the efficacy of such decontamination has not been proved. Sodium polystyrene sulfonate, an ion exchange resin, is difficult to administer and has been used only in a few uncontrolled studies. We do not recommend it. (5) Hemodialysis is the most efficient method of removing lithium from the vascular compartment. It is the treatment of choice for severe intoxication with an altered mental state and seizures and in anuric patients. Long "runs" are used until the serum lithium level is below 1 mEq/L because of extensive re-equilibration. Monitor the serum lithium level every 4 hours after dialysis for rebound. Repeated and prolonged hemodialysis may be necessary. Expect a lag in neurologic recovery.

Laboratory investigations: Monitor the CBC (lithium causes significant leukocytosis), renal dysfunction, thyroid dysfunction (chronic intoxication), ECG, and electrolytes. Determine the serum lithium concentrations every 4 hours until a downward trend to near the therapeutic range is observed. The levels do not always correlate with the manifestations but are more predictive in severe intoxication. A value above 3.0 mEq/L with chronic intoxication and an altered mental state indicates severe toxicity. Patients with a value above 9 mEq/L after an acute overdose may be asymptomatic. *Cross-reactions*: The green-topped

Vacutainer specimen tube containing heparin spuriously elevates the serum lithium value by 6 to 8 mEq/L. *Disposition*: An acute, asymptomatic lithium overdose cannot be medically cleared on the basis of a single lithium level. Patients should be admitted to the hospital if they have any neurologic manifestations (altered mental status, hyperreflexia, stiffness, or tremor). Patients should be admitted to the ICU if they are dehydrated, have renal impairment, or have a high or rising lithium level.

Methanol. (Wood Alcohol.) The concentration of methanol in Sterno fuel is 4% (it also contains ethanol); in windshield washer fluid, 30% to 60%; and in gas line antifreeze, 100%. *Toxic mechanism*: Methanol is metabolized by hepatic ADH to formaldehyde and formate. Formate produces tissue hypoxia, metabolic lactic acidosis, and retinal damage. Formate is converted by folate-dependent enzymes to carbon dioxide. *Toxic dose*: The minimum toxic amount is approximately 100 mg/kg. One tablespoonful (15 mL) of 40% methanol was lethal for a 2-year-old child and can cause blindness in an adult. The lethal oral dose is 30 to 240 mL of 100% methanol (20 to 150 g). The toxic blood methanol concentration (BMC) is above 20 mg/dL; the very serious toxic and potentially fatal level is greater than 50 mg/dL. The BMC and amount ingested can be estimated from the following equations and an SG for methanol of 0.719:

$$\text{BMC (mg/dL)} = \frac{\text{Amount Ingested (mL)} \times \text{\% Methanol in Product} \times \text{SG (0.719)}}{\text{Vd (0.6 L/kg)} \times \text{Body Weight (kg)}}$$

$$\text{Dose (amount ingested)} = \frac{\text{BMC (mg/dL)} \times \text{Vd (0.6 L/kg)} \times \text{Body Weight (kg)}}{\text{\% Ethanol} \times \text{SG (0.719)}}$$

Kinetics: The onset of effect can be within 1 hour but is typically delayed 12 to 18 hours by metabolism to toxic metabolites. It may be delayed longer if ethanol is ingested concomitantly. Onset may be up to 72 hours in infants. The peak BMC occurs at 1 hour. The Vd is 0.6 L/kg (total body water); $t_{1/2}$ is 8 hours (with ethanol blocking it is 30 to 35 hours, and with hemodialysis, 2.5 hours). For metabolism, see the section on toxic mechanism. Elimination is renal. *Manifestations*: Slow metabolism may delay the onset for 12 to 18 hours or longer if ethanol is ingested concomitantly. Methanol may produce inebriation, a formaldehyde odor on the breath, hyperemia of the optic disk, violent abdominal colic, "snow" vision, blindness, and shock. Later, worsening acidosis, hypoglycemia, and multiple organ failure develop; death results from the complications of intractable acidosis and cerebral edema. Methanol produces an osmolal gap (early), and its metabolite formate produces AG metabolic acidosis (later). Absence of an osmolar gap or AG disturbance does not always rule out methanol intoxication.

Management: (1) Protect the airway by intubation to prevent aspiration, and administer assisted ventilation as needed. Administer 100% oxygen if needed. Consult with a nephrologist early regarding the need for hemodialysis. (2) GI decontamination procedures have no role in management. (3) Treat metabolic acidosis vigorously with $NaHCO_3$ at 2 to 3 mEq/kg IV. Large amounts may be needed. (4) Ethanol or fomepizole therapy and hemodialysis (see Table 10): Classically, ethanol therapy was started if the BMC was above 20 mg/dL, and hemodialysis was added if the concentration was above 50 mg/dL, but values less than 25 mg/dL are currently used as an indication for hemodialysis. Ethanol therapy: ADH has 100 times greater affinity for ethanol than methanol. Therefore, ethanol blocks the metabolism of methanol at a BMC of 100 to 150 mg/dL. Initiate therapy to block metabolism if the patient has ingested 0.4 mL of 100% methanol per kilogram, if the blood methanol level is above 20 mg/dL or the patient has an osmolar gap that is not accounted for, or if the patient is symptomatic or acidotic with an increased AG and/or hyperemia of the optic disk. (See Table 10.) *Hemodialysis*: Hemodialysis increases the clearance of both methanol and formate 10-fold over renal clearance. Continue to monitor methanol levels and/or formate levels for rebound every 4 hours after the procedure. Toxicologists and nephrologists have recommended early hemodialysis at blood methanol levels greater than 25 mg/dL because it significantly shortens the course of the intoxication and provides better outcomes. Other indications for early hemodialysis are significant metabolic acidosis, electrolyte abnormalities despite conventional therapy, and the presence of visual or mental symptoms. A serum formate level greater than 20 mg/dL has also been used as a criterion for hemodialysis. If hemodialysis is performed, increase the infusion rate of 10% ethanol to 2.0 to 3.5 mL/kg/h. Obtain the BEC and glucose concentration every 2 hours. Continue therapy with both ethanol and hemodialysis until a blood methanol level is undetectable, no acidosis is present, and the patient has no mental or visual disturbances. This process may require 2 to 5 days. (5) Treat hypoglycemia with IV glucose. (6) A bolus of folinic acid and folic acid has been used successfully in animal investigations to enhance formate metabolism to carbon dioxide and water. Administer leucovorin (Wellcovorin) at 1 mg/kg up to 50 mg IV every 4 hours for several days. (7) Obtain ophthalmologic consultation initially and at follow-up.

Laboratory investigations: Methanol is detected on drug screens if specified. Monitor methanol and ethanol levels every 4 hours, electrolytes, glucose, BUN, creatinine, amylase, and ABGs. Formate levels correlate more closely than do blood methanol levels with the severity of intoxication and should be obtained if possible. If methanol levels are not available, the osmolal gap × 3.2 can be used to estimate the blood methanol levels in milligrams per deciliter. *Disposition*: All patients who ingest significant amounts of methanol should be referred to the emergency department for evaluation and BMC determination. Ophthalmologic follow-up of all intoxications should be arranged.

Monoamine Oxidase Inhibitors. MAOIs include MAO-A inhibitors, the hydrazine phenelzine sulfate (Nardil; dose, 60 to 90 mg/d), isocarboxazid (Marplan; 10 to 30 mg/d), and the nonhydrazine tranylcypromine (Parnate; 20 to 40 mg/d). The MAO-B inhibitor selegiline (deprenyl, Eldepryl; 10 mg/d), an antiparkinsonism agent, does not have toxicity similar to that of MAO-A and is not discussed. MAOIs are used to treat severe depression. *Toxic mechanism*: MAO enzymes are responsible for the oxidative deamination of both endogenous and exogenous catecholamines. MAO-A in the intestinal wall also metabolizes tyramine in food. MAOIs permanently inhibit MAO enzymes until a new enzyme is synthesized at 14 days or later. The toxicity results from accumulation, potentiation, and prolongation of catecholamine action, followed by profound hypotension and cardiovascular collapse. *Toxic dose*: Toxicity begins at 2 to 3 mg/kg, and fatalities occur at 4 to 6 mg/kg. Death has occurred after a single 170-mg dose of tranylcypromine in an adult. *Kinetics*: Structurally, MAOIs are related to amphetamines and catecholamines. The hydrazine peak level occurs at 1 to 2 hours; elimination is by hepatic acetylation metabolism and excretion of inactive metabolites in the urine. The nonhydrazine peak level occurs at 1 to 4 hours, and elimination is by hepatic metabolism to active amphetamine-like metabolites. The onset of symptoms in overdoses is delayed 6 to 24 hours after ingestion, peak activity occurs at 8 to 12 hours, and the duration is 72 hours or longer. Peak MAOI effect occurs in 5 to 10 days, and effects last as long as 5 weeks. *Manifestations* (for MAO-A inhibitors, not MAO-B inhibitors): (1) Acute ingestion overdose: Phase I consists of an adrenergic crisis in which the onset of effects is delayed for 6 to 24 hours and the peak may not be reached until 24 hours. Initial manifestations are hyperthermia, tachycardia, tachypnea, dysarthria, transient hypertension, hyperreflexia, and CNS stimulation. Phase II consists of neuromuscular excitation and sympathetic hyperactivity with an increased temperature (above 104°F [40°C]), agitation, hyperactivity, confusion, fasciculations, twitching, tremor, masseter spasm, muscle rigidity, acidosis, and electrolyte abnormalities. Seizures and dystonic reactions may occur. The pupils are mydriatic and sometimes nonreactive, with a "Ping-Pong gaze." Phase III, CNS depression and cardiovascular collapse, occurs in severe overdose as the catecholamines are depleted. Symptoms usually resolve within 5 days but may last 2 weeks. Phase IV consists of secondary complications: rhabdomyolysis, cardiac dysrhythmias, multiple organ failure, and coagulopathies. (2) Biogenic interactions usually occur while therapeutic doses of MAOIs are given or shortly after they are discontinued, before the new MAO enzyme is synthesized. Onset occurs within 30 to 60 minutes after exposure. The following substances have been implicated: indirect-acting sympathomimetics (e.g., amphetamines); serotonergic drugs, opioids (e.g., meperidine, dextromethorphan), tricyclic antidepressants, and SSRIs; tyramine-containing foods (wine, beer, avocado, cheese, caviar, chocolate, chicken liver); and L-tryptophan. SSRIs should not be started for at least 5 weeks after MAOI use has been discontinued. In mild cases, usually caused by foods, headache and hypertension develop and last for several hours. In severe cases, malignant hypertension and malignant hyperthermia syndromes consisting of hypertension or hyperthermia, altered mental state, skeletal muscle rigidity, shivering (often beginning in the masseter muscle), and seizures may occur. The serotonin syndrome, which may be due to inhibition of serotonin metabolism, has clinical manifestations similar to those of malignant hyperthermia and may occur with or without hyperthermia or hypertension. (3) Clinical findings in chronic toxicity include tremors, hyperhidrosis, agitation, hallucinations, confusion, and seizures and can be confused with withdrawal syndromes.

Management: (1) MAOI overdose: GI decontamination with ipecac-induced emesis should not be used because it may aggravate the food-MAOI interaction and cause hypertension. Use gastric lavage and AC or AC alone. If the patient is admitted to the hospital and is well enough to eat, order a nontyramine diet. Extreme agitation and seizures can be controlled with BZPs and barbiturates. Phenytoin is ineffective. Nondepolarizing neuromuscular blockers (nondepolarizing succinylcholine) may be needed in severe cases of hyperthermia and rigidity. If severe hypertension (catecholamine-mediated) is present, use phentolamine, a parenteral α-blocking agent, at 3 to 5 mg IV, or labetalol, a combination of an α-blocking agent and β-blocker, as a 20-mg IV bolus. If malignant hypertension with rigidity occurs, use short-acting nitroprusside and BZP. Hypertension is often followed by severe hypotension, which should be managed with fluid and vasopressors. *Caution*: Vasopressor therapy should be administered at lower doses than usual because of an exaggerated pharmacologic response. Norepinephrine is preferred over dopamine, which requires release of intracellular amines. Cardiac dysrhythmias are treated with standard therapy but are often refractory, and cardioversion and pacemakers may be needed. For malignant hyperthermia, administer dantrolene (see Table 10), a nonspecific peripheral skeletal relaxing agent that inhibits the release of calcium from the sarcoplasm. Dantrolene is reconstituted with 60 mL of sterile water without bacteriostatic agents; do not use glass equipment, protect from light, and use within 6 hours. The loading dose of dantrolene is 2 to 3 mg/kg given IV as a bolus, which is repeated until the signs of malignant hyperthermia (tachycardia, rigidity, increased end-tidal carbon dioxide, and increased temperature) are controlled. The maximal total dose is 10 mg/kg to avoid hepatotoxicity. When malignant hyperthermia subsides, give 1 mg dantrolene per kilogram IV every 6 hours for 24 to 48 hours; then give 1 mg/kg orally every 6 hours for 24 hours to prevent recurrence. Because of the danger of thrombophlebitis after peripheral dantrolene administration, it should be given through a central line if possible. In addition, provide external cooling and correct metabolic acidosis and electrolyte disturbances. BZP can be used for sedation. Dantrolene does not reverse central dopamine blockade; therefore, give bromocriptine mesylate at 2.5 to 10 mg orally or through a nasogastric tube three times a day. Treat rhabdomyolysis and myoglobinuria with fluid diuresis, furosemide, and alkalization. Hemodialysis and hemoperfusion are of no proven value. (2) Biogenic amine interactions are managed symptomatically as for overdose. For the serotonin syndrome, cyproheptadine, a serotonin blocker, may be given orally at 4 mg/h for three doses, or methysergide (Sansert) at 2 mg orally every 6 hours for three doses may be used, but their efficacy is not proven.

Laboratory investigations: Monitor the ECG, cardiac parameters, creatine kinase, ABGs, pulse oximetry, electrolytes, blood glucose, and acid-base balance. *Disposition*: All patients who ingest more than 2 mg/kg should be admitted to the hospital for 24 hours of observation and monitoring in the ICU because the life-threatening manifestations may be delayed. Patients with drug or dietary interactions that are mild may not require admission if symptoms subside within 4 to 6 hours and they remain asymptomatic. Patients with symptoms that persist or require active intervention should be admitted to the ICU.

Opioids. (Narcotic Opiates.) Opioids are used for analgesia, as antitussives, and as antidiarrheal agents, and illicit forms (heroin, opium) are used in substance abuse. Tolerance, physical dependence, and withdrawal may develop. *Toxic mechanism*: At least four main opioid receptors have been identified. Mu is considered the most important for central analgesia and depression, kappa and delta are predominant in spinal analgesia, and sigma receptors may mediate dysphoria. Death is due to dose-dependent CNS respiratory depression or is secondary to apnea, pulmonary aspiration, or noncardiac pulmonary edema. The mechanism of noncardiac pulmonary edema is unknown. *Toxic dose*: The toxic dose depends on the specific drug, route of administration, and degree of tolerance. For therapeutic and toxic doses, see Table 32. In children, respiratory depression has been produced by 10 mg of morphine or methadone, 75 mg of meperidine, and 12.5 mg of diphenoxylate. Because infants younger than 3 months are more susceptible to respiratory depression, the dose should be reduced by 50%. *Kinetics*: Onset of the analgesic effect of morphine after oral ingestion is at 10 to 15 minutes; the effect peaks in 1 hour, and the duration is 4 to 6 hours, but with sustained-release preparations (e.g., MS Contin), the duration is 8 to 12 hours. Opioids are 90% metabolized in the liver by hepatic conjugation and 90% excreted in the urine as inactive compounds. The Vd is 1 to 4 L/kg; PB is 35% to 75%. The typical plasma $t_{1/2}$ of opiates is 2 to 5 hours, but that of methadone is 24 to 36 hours. Morphine metabolites include morphine-3-glucuronide (M3G) (inactive), morphine-6-glucuronide (M6G) (active), and normorphine (active). Meperidine is rapidly hydrolyzed by tissue esterases into the active metabolite normeperidine, which has twice the convulsant activity of meperidine. Heroin (diacetylmorphine) is deacetylated within minutes to the metabolite 6-monacetylmorphine (6MAM), the presence of which is diagnostic of heroin use, and morphine. Propoxyphene (Darvon) has a rapid onset, and death has occurred within 15 to 30 minutes after a massive overdose. Propoxyphene is metabolized to norpropoxyphene, an active metabolite with convulsive, cardiac dysrhythmic, and heart block effects. Symptoms of diphenoxylate (Lomotil) intoxication appear within 1 to 4 hours. It is metabolized into the active metabolite difenoxin, which is five times more active as a recurrent respiratory depressant. Death has been reported in children after a single tablet. *Manifestations*: (1) Initial or mild intoxication produces miosis, a dull facial expression, drowsiness, partial ptosis, and "nodding" (head drops to the chest and then bobs up). Larger amounts produce the classic triad of miotic pupils (exceptions follow), respiratory depression, and depressed level of consciousness (flaccid coma). The blood pressure, pulse, and bowel sounds are decreased. (2) The presence of dilated pupils does not exclude opioid intoxication. Some exceptions to miosis include dextromethorphan (which paralyzes the iris), fentanyl, meperidine, and diphenoxylate (rarely). Physiologic disturbances, including acidosis, hypoglycemia, hypoxia, and a postictal state or those caused by a co-ingestant, may also produce mydriasis. (3) Usually, the muscles are flaccid, but increased muscle tone may be produced by meperidine and fentanyl (chest rigidity). (4) Seizures are rare but can occur with codeine, meperidine, propoxyphene, and dextromethorphan. Hallucinations and agitation have been reported. (5) Pruritus and urticaria caused by histamine release after the use of some opioids or by sulfites may be present. (6) Noncardiac pulmonary edema often occurs after resuscitation and naloxone administration, especially with IV abuse. (7) Cardiac effects include vasodilation and hypotension. A heart murmur in a person who is addicted to an IV drug suggests endocarditis. Propoxyphene can produce delayed cardiac dysrhythmias. (8) Fentanyl is 100 times more potent than morphine and can cause chest wall muscle rigidity. Some of its derivatives are 2000 times more potent than morphine.

Management: (1) Provide supportive care, particularly an endotracheal tube and assisted ventilation. Temporary ventilation may be provided by a bag-valve mask with 100% oxygen. Begin cardiac monitoring, establish IV access, and obtain specimens for ABGs, glucose, electrolytes, BUN, creatinine, CBC, a coagulation profile, liver function determination, a toxicology screen, and urinalysis. (2) GI decontamination: Do not induce emesis. Administer AC if bowel sounds are present. Cathartics may be needed because of opioid-induced decreased GI mobility and

TABLE 32. **Doses, Onset, and Duration of Action of Common Opioids**

Drug	Oral Dose		Onset of Action (min)	Duration of Action (h)	Adult Fatal Dose
	Adult	*Child*			
Camphored tincture of opium (0.4 mg/mL), paregoric	25 mL	0.25–0.50 mL/kg	15–30	4–5	NA
Codeine	30–180 mg (>1 mg/kg is toxic in a child, above 200 mg in an adult; >5 mg/kg is fatal in a child)	0.5–1 mg/kg	15–30	4–6	800 mg
Dextromethorphan	15 mg 10 mg/kg is toxic	0.25 mg/kg	15–30	3–6	NA
Diacetylmorphine (heroin)	60 mg Street heroin is less than 10% pure	NA	15–30	3–4	100 mg
Diphenoxylate (Lomotil)	5–10 mg 7.5 mg is toxic in a child, 300 mg in an adult	NA	120–240	14	300 mg
Fentanyl (Sublimaze, Duragesic transdermal)	0.1–0.2 mg	0.001–0.002 mg/kg	7–8	0.5–2	1.0 mg
Hydrocodone (Hycodan, Vicodin)	5–30 mg	0.15 mg/kg	30	3–4	100 mg
Hydromorphone (Dilaudid)	4 mg	0.1 mg/kg	15–30	3–4	100 mg
Meperidine (Demerol)	100 mg	1–1.5 mg/kg	10–45	3–4	350 mg
Methadone (Dolophine)	10 mg	0.1 mg/kg	30–60	4–12	120 mg
Morphine	10–60 mg Oral dose is 6 times the parenteral dose; MS Contin (sustained release)	0.1–0.2 mg/kg	< 20	4–6	200 mg
Oxycodone (Percodan)	5 mg	NA	15–30	4–5	NA
Pentazocine (Talwin)	50–100 mg	NA	15–30	3–4	NA
Propoxyphene (Darvon)	65–100 mg 100 mg hydrochloride = 65 mg of napsylate, toxic at 10 mg/kg	NA	30–60	2–4	700 mg

Abbreviation: NA = not available.

constipation. (3) Naloxone (Narcan) (see Table 10): If addiction is suspected, restrain the patient first; then administer 0.1 mg of naloxone and double the dose every 2 minutes until the patient responds or 10 to 20 mg has been given. If addiction is not suspected, give 2 mg every 2 to 3 minutes to a total of 10 to 20 mg. It is essential to determine whether the patient has a complete response to naloxone (mydriasis, improvement in ventilation) because administration of this drug is a diagnostic therapeutic test. A continuous naloxone infusion may be appropriate, with administration of the "response dose" every hour. Repeated doses of naloxone may be necessary because the effects of many opioids can last much longer than that of naloxone (30 to 60 minutes). Methadone intoxication may necessitate naloxone infusion for 24 to 48 hours. Half of the response dose may have to be repeated in 15 to 20 minutes after the infusion is started. Acute iatrogenic withdrawal on administration of naloxone to a dependent patient should not be treated with morphine or other opioids. Naloxone's effects are limited to 30 to 60 minutes (shorter than those of most opioids), and withdrawal effects subside in a short time. (4) Nalmefene (Revex), an FDA-approved long-acting (4 to 8 hours) pure opioid antagonist, is being investigated, but its role in acute intoxication is unclear. It may have a role in place of naloxone infusion but could produce prolonged withdrawal. (5) Noncardiac pulmonary edema does not respond to naloxone, and the patient requires intubation, assisted ventilation, PEEP, and hemodynamic monitoring. Fluids should be given cautiously in opioid overdose because they stimulate antidiuretic hormone. (6) If the patient is comatose, give 50% glucose (3% to 4% of comatose opioid overdose patients have hypoglycemia) and thiamine before naloxone. If the patient has seizures unresponsive to naloxone, administer diazepam and examine for other metabolic (hypoglycemia, electrolyte disturbances) and structural disorders. (7) Hypotension is rare and should prompt a search for another cause. (8) If the patient is agitated, exclude hypoxia and hypoglycemia before considering opioid withdrawal. (9) Complications to consider include urine retention, constipation, rhabdomyolysis, myoglobinuria, hypoglycemia, and withdrawal. Dextromethorphan can interact with MAOIs and cause severe hyperthermia and, possibly, the serotonin syndrome (refer to the SSRI section). Dextromethorphan inhibits the metabolism of norepinephrine and serotonin and blocks the reuptake of serotonin. It is found as a component in a large number of nonprescription cough and cold remedies.

Laboratory investigations: For overdoses, monitor ABGs, blood glucose, and electrolytes; obtain chest radiographs and an ECG. For drug abusers, consider testing for hepatitis B, syphilis, and HIV antibody (HIV testing usually requires consent). Blood opioid concentrations are not useful. They confirm the diagnosis (morphine therapeutic levels are 65 to 80 ng/mL; toxic levels are greater than 200 ng/mL) but are not useful for making a therapeutic decision. Cross-reactions can occur with Vicks Formula 44, poppy seeds on baked goods, and other opioids (codeine and heroin are metabolized to morphine). Naloxone in a dose of 4 mg IV was not associated with a positive enzyme multiple immunoassay technique (EMIT) urine screen at 60 minutes, 6 hours, or 48 hours. *Disposition*: If a patient responds to IV naloxone, careful observation for relapse and the development of pulmonary edema is required, with cardiac and respiratory monitoring for 6 to 12 hours. Patients who need repeated doses of naloxone or an infusion or in whom pulmonary edema develops require ICU admission and cannot be discharged from the ICU until they are symptom-free for 12 hours. With IV administration, complications are expected to be present within 20 minutes after injection, and discharge after 4 symptom-free hours has been recommended. Adults with an oral overdose have a delayed onset of toxicity and require observation for 6 hours. Children with an oral opioid overdose should be admitted to the hospital for 24 hours of observation because of delayed toxicity. Restrain any patient who attempts to sign out against medical advice after treatment with naloxone, at least until psychiatric evaluation.

Organophosphates and Carbamates. Sources of cholinergic intoxication are insecticides, medicinals (carbamates), and some mushrooms. Examples of organophosphate (OP) insecticides are malathion (Cythion; low toxicity, median lethal dose [LD_{50}] is 2800 mg/kg), chlorpyrifos (Dursban [removed from the market]; moderate toxicity, LD_{50} is 250 mg/kg), and parathion (high toxicity, LD_{50} is 2 mg/kg); carbamate insecticides are carbaril (Sevin; low toxicity, LD_{50} is 500 mg/kg), propoxui (Baygon; moderate toxicity, LD_{50} is 95 mg/kg), and aldicarb (Temik; high toxicity, LD_{50} is 0.9 mg/kg). Carbamate medicinals include neostigmine and physostigmine (Antilirium). Cholinergic compounds also include the dreaded "G" nerve war weapons Tabun (GA), sarin (GB), soman (GB), and VX. *Toxic mechanism*: (1) OPs phosphorylate the active site on red blood cell acetylcholinesterase and pseudocholinesterase in the serum (3% of the general population have a deficiency) and other organs and cause irreversible inhibition. The two types of OP action are direct action by the parent compound (e.g., tetraethyl pyrophosphate) and indirect action by the toxic metabolite (e.g., paraoxon or malaoxon). (2) Carbamates (esters of carbonic acid) cause reversible carbamylation of the active site of the enzymes. When a critical amount of cholinesterase is inhibited (more than 50% from baseline), acetylcholine accumulates and causes transient stimulation of conduction and, soon after, paralysis of conduction through cholinergic synapses and sympathetic terminals (muscarinic effect), the somatic nerves, the autonomic ganglia (nicotinic effect), and CNS synapses. (3) Major differences of the carbamates from OPs: Carbamate toxicity is less severe and the duration is shorter. Carbamates rarely produce overt CNS effects (poor CNS penetration); with carbamates, the acetylcholinesterase returns to normal rapidly, so blood values are not useful even in confirming the diagnosis. With carbamates, pralidoxime, the enzyme regenerator, may not be necessary in the management of mild intoxication (e.g., carbaril), but atropine is required. *Toxic dose*: Parathion's minimum lethal dose is 2 mg in children and 10 to 20 mg in adults. The lethal dose of malathion is greater than 1375 mg/kg (it is 1000 times less toxic than parathion) and that of chlorpyrifos is 25 g, but such high amounts are rarely ingested. *Kinetics*: Absorption is by all routes. The onset of acute toxicity after ingestion occurs as early as 3 hours, usually before 12 hours, and always before 24 hours. The onset with lipid-soluble agents absorbed by the dermal route (e.g., fenthion) may be delayed more than 24 hours after exposure. Inhalation toxicity occurs immediately after exposure. Massive ingestion can produce intoxication within minutes. The effects of the thions (e.g., parathion, malathion) are delayed because they undergo hepatic microsomal oxidative metabolism to their toxic metabolites, the oxons (e.g., paraoxon, malaoxon). The $t_{1/2}$ of malathion is 2.89 hours; that of parathion is 2.1 days. The metabolites are eliminated in the urine, and the presence of *p*-nitrophenol in the urine is a clue up to 48 hours after exposure. *Manifestations*: Many OPs produce a garlic odor on the breath or in the gastric contents or the container. Diaphoresis, excessive salivation, miosis, and muscle twitching are helpful clues. (1) Early, a cholinergic (muscarinic) crisis develops and consists of parasympathetic nervous system activity. DUMBELS is a mnemonic for the manifestations of *d*efecation, cramps, and increased bowel mobility; *u*rinary incontinence; *m*iosis (mydriasis may occur in 20%); *b*ronchospasm and bronchorrhea; *e*xcess secretion; *l*acrimation; and *s*eizures. Bradycardia, pulmonary edema, and hypotension may be present. (2) Later, sympathetic and nicotinic effects occur and consist of *m*uscle weakness and fasciculations (eyelid twitching is often present), *a*drenal stimulation and hyperglycemia, *t*achycardia, *c*ramps in muscles, and *h*ypertension (mnemonic, MATCH). Finally, paralysis of the skeletal muscles ensues. (3) CNS effects are headache, blurred vision, anxiety, ataxia, delirium and toxic psychosis, convulsions, coma, and respiratory depression. Cranial nerve palsies have been noted. Delayed hallucinations may occur. (4) Delayed respiratory paralysis and neurologic and neurobehavioral disorders have been described after exposure to certain OPs or with dermal exposure. The "intermediate" syndrome consists of paralysis of the proximal and respiratory muscles developing 24 to 96 hours after the successful treatment of OP poisoning. A delayed distal polyneuropathy has been described with certain OPs (e.g., tri-*o*-cresyl phosphate [TOCP], bromoleptophos, methomidophos). (5) Complications include aspiration, pulmonary edema, and adult respiratory distress syndrome.

Management: (1) Safeguard health care personnel with protective clothing (masks, gloves, gowns, goggles, and respiratory equipment or hazardous material suits, as necessary). General decontamination consists of isolation, bagging, and disposal of contaminated clothing and other articles. Establish and maintain vital functions. Institute cardiac and oxygen saturation monitoring. Intubation and assisted ventilation may be needed. Suction secretions until atropinization drying is achieved. (2) Specific decontamination: Dermal: Prompt removal of clothing and cleansing of all affected areas of skin, hair, and eyes are indicated. Ocular: Irrigation with copious amounts of tepid water or 0.9% saline is performed for at least 15 minutes. GI: If ingestion is recent, use gastric lavage with airway protection, if necessary, and administer AC. (3) Antidotes: Atropine sulfate (see Table 10) is both a diagnostic and a therapeutic agent. Atropine counteracts the muscarinic effects but is only partially effective for the CNS effects (seizures and coma). Use preservative-free atropine (no benzyl alcohol). If the patient is symptomatic (bradycardia or bronchorrhea may be present), administer a test dose of 0.02 mg/kg for a child or 1 mg for an adult IV. If no signs of atropinization (tachycardia, drying of secretions, and mydriasis) are seen, immediately administer atropine at 0.05 mg/kg for a child or 2 mg for an adult every 5 to 10 minutes as needed to dry the secretions and clear the lungs. Beneficial effects are seen within 1 to 4 minutes, and the maximal effect occurs in 8 minutes. The average dose in the first 24 hours is 40 mg, but 1000 mg or more has been required in severe cases. Glycopyrrolate (Robinul) may be used if atropine is not available. Maintain the maximal dose for 12 to 24 hours; then taper it and observe for relapse. Poisoning, especially with lipophilic agents (e.g., fenthion, chlorfenthion), may necessitate weeks of atropine therapy. The alternative is a continuous infusion of 8 mg of atropine in 100 mL of 0.9% saline at a rate of 0.02 to 0.08 mg/kg/h (0.25 to 1.0 mL/kg/h), with additional 1- to 5-mg boluses as needed to dry the secretions. Pralidoxime chloride (2-PAM) has antinicotinic, antimuscarinic, and possibly CNS effects. Concomitant use of this agent may require a reduction in the dose of atropine (see Table 10). It acts to reactivate the phosphorylated cholinesterases by binding the phosphate moiety on the esteric site and displacing it. It should be given early before "aging" of the phosphate bond produces tighter binding. However, reports indicate that 2-PAM is beneficial even several days after the poisoning. Improvement is seen within 10 to 40 minutes. The initial dose of 2-PAM is 1 to 2 g in 250 mL of 0.89% saline over a period of 5 to 10 minutes, for a maximum of 200 mg/min (in adults), or 25 to 50 mg/kg (in children younger than 12 years), for a maximum of 4 mg/kg/min. Repeat every 6 to 12 hours for several days. An alternative is a continuous infusion of 1 g in 100 mL of 0.89% saline at 5 to 20 mg/kg/h (0.5 to 12 mL/kg/h) up to 500 mg/h, with titration to the desired response. The maximal adult daily dose is 12 g. Cardiac and blood pressure monitoring is advised during and for several hours after the infusion. The endpoint is absence of fasciculations and return of muscle strength. (4) Contraindicated drugs: Do not use morphine, aminophylline, barbiturates, opioids, phenothiazine, reserpine-like drugs, parasympathomimetics, or succinylcholine. (5) Noncardiac pulmonary edema may necessitate respiratory support. (6) Seizures may respond to atropine and 2-PAM, but the effect is not consistent and anticonvulsants may be required. (7) Cardiac dysrhythmias may necessitate electrical cardioversion or antidysrhythmic therapy if the patient is hemodynamically unstable. (8) Extracorporeal procedures are of no proven value.

Laboratory investigations: Monitor the chest radiograph, blood glucose (nonketotic hyperglycemia occurs frequently), ABGs, pulse oximetry, ECG, blood coagulation status, liver function, hyperamylasemia (pancreatitis has been reported), and the urine for the metabolite alkyl phosphate *p*-nitrophenol. Draw blood for red blood cell cholinesterase determination before giving pralidoxime. In mild poisoning, this value is 20% to 50% of normal; in moderate poisoning, 10% to 20% of normal; and in severe poisoning, 10% of normal (more than 90% depressed). A postexposure rise of 10% to 15% in the cholinesterase level determined at least 10 to 14 days after exposure confirms the diagnosis. *Disposition*: Asymptomatic patients with normal examination findings after 6 to 8 hours of observation may be discharged. If intentional poisoning occurs, psychiatric clearance is required for discharge. Symptomatic patients should be admitted to the ICU. Observation of patients with milder carbamate poisoning, even those requiring atropine, for 6 to 8 hours without symptoms may be sufficient to rule out significant toxicity. If workplace exposure occurs, notify OSHA.

Phencyclidine. (PCP, "angel dust," "peace pill," "hog.") PCP is an arylcyclohexylamine related to ketamine and is chemically related to the PTZs. It is a "dissociative" anesthetic that has been banned in the United States since 1979 and is now an illicit substance; at least 38 analogues exist. It is inexpensively manufactured by "kitchen" chemists and is mislabeled with the names of other hallucinogens. Improperly synthesized PCP may release cyanide when heated or smoked and can cause explosions. *Toxic mechanism*: PCP action is complex and not completely understood. It inhibits neurotransmitters and causes loss of pain sensation without depressing the CNS respiratory status. It stimulates α-adrenergic receptors and may act as a "false" neurotransmitter. The effects are sympathomimetic, cholinergic, and cerebellar stimulation. *Toxic dose*: The usual dose in "joints" is 100 to 400 mg; weight; joints or leaf mixture, 0.24% to 7.9%, 1 mg per 150 leaves; tablets, 5 mg (usual street dose). CNS effects at 1 to 6 mg are hallucinations and euphoria; 6 to 10 mg produces toxic psychosis and sympathetic stimulation, 10 to 25 mg produces severe toxicity, and more than 100 mg has resulted in fatality. *Kinetics*: PCP is a lipophilic weak base with a pK_a of 8.5 to 9.5. It is rapidly absorbed when smoked and snorted, poorly absorbed from the acid stomach, and rapidly absorbed from the alkaline medium of the small intestine. It is secreted enterogastrically and is reabsorbed in the small intestine. The onset of action when smoked is at 2 to 5 minutes, with a peak in 15 to 30 minutes. The onset is at 30 to 60 minutes when taken orally and immediate when taken IV. Most adverse reactions in overdose begin within 1 to 2 hours. Its duration of action at low doses is 4 to 6 hours, and normality returns in 24 hours; in large overdoses, fluctuating coma may last 6 to 10 days. The $t_{1/2}$ is 1 hour (in overdose, 11 to 89 hours). The Vd is 6.2 L/kg, and PB is 70%. It is eliminated by gastric secretion, liver metabolism, and 10% urinary excretion of conjugates and free PCP. Renal excretion may be increased 50% with urinary acidification. PCP concentrates in brain and adipose tissue. *Manifestations*: The classic picture is one of bursts of horizontal, vertical, and rotary nystagmus, which is a clue (occurs in 50% of cases); miosis; hypertension; and fluctuating, altered mental state. A wide spectrum of clinical manifestations are observed: (1) Mild intoxication: A dose of 1 to 6 mg produces drunken and bizarre behavior, agitation, rotary nystagmus, and a blank stare. Violent behavior and sensory anesthesia make these patients insensitive to pain, self-destructive, and dangerous. Most are communicative within 1 to 2 hours, are alert and oriented in 6 to 8 hours, and recover completely in 24 to 48 hours. (2) Moderate intoxication: A dose of 6 to 10 mg produces excess salivation, hypertension, hyperthermia, muscle rigidity, myoclonus, and catatonia. Recovery of consciousness occurs in 24 to 48 hours and complete recovery in 1 week. (3) Severe intoxication: A dose of 10 to 25 mg results in opisthotonos, decerebrate rigidity, convulsions, prolonged fluctuating coma, and respiratory failure. This category involves a high rate of medical complications. Recovery of consciousness occurs in 24 to 48 hours, with complete normality in 1 month. (4) Medical complications include apnea, aspiration pneumonia, cardiac arrest, hypertensive encephalopathy, hyperthermia, intracerebral hemorrhage, psychosis, rhabdomyolysis and myoglobinuria, and seizures. Flashbacks and loss of memory last for months. PCP-induced depression and suicide have been reported. (5) Fatalities occur with ingestions greater than 100 mg and with serum levels higher than 100 to 250 ng/mL.

Management: Observe the patient for violent, self-destructive, bizarre behavior and paranoid schizophrenia. Patients should be placed in a low-sensory environment and dangerous objects removed from the area. (1) GI decontamination is not effective because PCP is rapidly absorbed from the intestines. Avoid overtreating mild intoxication. Initially, administration of AC should be considered. Insufficient evidence is available to support the use of MDAC. Continuous gastric suction is not routine but may be useful (with protection of the airway) in severe toxicity (stupor or coma) because the drug is secreted into the gastric juice. (2) Protect patients from harming themselves or others. Physical restraints may be necessary, but use them sparingly and for the shortest time possible because they increase the risk of rhabdomyolysis. Avoid metal restraints such as handcuffs. For behavioral disorders and toxic psychosis, diazepam is the agent of choice. Pharmacologic intervention includes diazepam in a dose of 10 to 30 mg orally or 2 to 5 mg IV initially; titrate upward to 10 mg, but up to 30 mg may be required. The "talk-down" technique is usually ineffective and dangerous. Avoid PTZs and butyrophenones in the acute phase because they lower the convulsive threshold; however, they may be needed later for psychosis. Haloperidol (Haldol) administration has been reported to produce catatonia. (3) Seizures and muscle spasms are controlled with diazepam in a dose of 2.5 mg, up to 10 mg. (4) Hyperthermia (temperature above 38.5°C [101.3°F]) is treated with external cooling measures. (5) Hypertension is usually transient and does not mandate treatment. In an emergency hypertensive crisis (blood pressure above 200/115 mm Hg), use nitroprusside, 0.3 to 2 μg/kg/min. The maximal infusion rate is 10 μg/kg/min for only 10 minutes. (6) Acid ion–trapping diuresis is not recommended because of the danger of myoglobin precipitation in the renal tubules. (7) Rhabdomyolysis and myoglobinuria are treated by correcting volume depletion and ensuring a urine output of at least 2 mL/kg/h. Alkalization is controversial because of PCP reabsorption. (8) Hemodialysis is beneficial if renal failure occurs; otherwise, the extracorporeal procedures are not beneficial.

Laboratory investigations: Marked elevation of the creatine kinase level may be a clue to PCP intoxication. Values greater than 20,000 U have been reported. Monitor results of urinalysis and test urine for myoglobin with *o*-toluidine blood reagent strip. A 3+ or 4+ test result and less than 10 red blood cells per high-power field on microscopic examination suggest myoglobinuria. Measure for PCP in the gastric juice, where it is concentrated 10 to 50 times higher than in blood or urine. Monitor blood for creatine kinase, uric acid (an early clue to rhabdomyolysis), BUN, creatinine, electrolytes (hyperkalemia), and glucose (20% of intoxications involve hypoglycemia); also monitor urine output, liver function, ECG, and ABGs if any respiratory manifestations are noted. PCP blood concentrations are not helpful. A level of 10 ng/mL produces excitation, 30 to 100 ng/mL produces coma, and more than 100 ng/mL produces seizures and fatalities. PCP may be detected in the urine of the average user for 10 to 14 days or up to 3 weeks after the last dose. With chronic use it can be detected for more than 1 month. The analogue of PCP may not test positive for PCP in the urine.

Cross-reactions: Bleach and dextromethorphan may cause false-positive urine test results on immunoassay, and doxylamine, a false-positive result on gas chromatography. *Disposition*: All patients with coma, delirium, catatonia, violent behavior, aspiration pneumonia, sustained hypertension (blood pressure above 200/115 mm Hg), or significant rhabdomyolysis should be admitted to the ICU until they are asymptomatic for at least 24 hours. If patients with mild intoxication are mentally and neurologically stable and become asymptomatic (except for nystagmus) for 4 hours, they may be discharged in the company of a responsible adult. All patients must be assessed for the risk of suicide before discharge. Drug counseling and psychiatric follow-up should be arranged. Patients should be warned that episodes of disorientation and depression may continue intermittently for 4 weeks or more.

Phenothiazines and Nonphenothiazines: Neuroleptics. *Toxic mechanism*: Neuroleptics have complex mechanisms of toxicity, including (1) block of postsynaptic dopamine receptors, (2) block of peripheral and central α-adrenergic receptors, (3) block of cholinergic muscarinic receptors, (4) a quinidine-like antidysrhythmic and myocardial depressant effect in large overdose, (5) a lowered convulsive threshold, and (6) an effect on hypothalamic temperature regulation. See Table 33. *Toxic dose*: Extrapyramidal reactions, anticholinergic effects, and orthostatic hypotension may occur at therapeutic doses (see Table 33). The toxic amount is not established, but the maximal daily therapeutic dose may result in significant side effects, and twice this amount is potentially fatal. Chlorpromazine (Thorazine), the prototype, may produce serious hypotension and CNS depression at doses above 200 mg (17 mg/kg) in children and 3 to 5 g in adults. Fatalities have been reported after the ingestion of 2.5 g of loxapine and mesoridazine and 1.5 g of thioridazine. *Kinetics*: These agents are lipophilic and have unpredictable GI absorption. Peak levels occur 2 to 6 hours after ingestion, and the drugs undergo enterohepatic recirculation. The mean serum $t_{1/2}$ in phase I is 1 to 2 hours, and the biphasic $t_{1/2}$ is 20 to 40 hours. PB is 92% to 98%. Oral chlorpromazine has an onset at 30 to 60 minutes, peak effect at 2 to 4 hours, and a duration of 4 to 6 hours. With sustained-release preparations, the onset is at 30 to 60 minutes and the duration is 6 to 12 hours. PB is 95%; Vd, 10 to 40 L/kg. Elimination is by hepatic metabolism, which results in multiple metabolites (some are active). Metabolites may be detected in urine months after chronic therapy. Only 1% to 3% is excreted unchanged in the urine. *Manifestations*: (1) PTZ overdose effects: Anticholinergic symptoms may be present early but are not life-threatening. Miosis is usually present (80%) if the PTZ has a strong α-adrenergic blocking effect (e.g., chlorpromazine), but if it has strong anticholinergic activity, mydriasis may occur. Agitation and delirium rapidly progress to coma. Major problems are cardiac toxicity and hypotension. The cardiotoxic effects are seen more commonly with thioridazine and its metabolite mesoridazine. These agents have produced the largest number of fatalities in PTZ overdoses. Cardiac conduction disturbances include prolonged PR, QRS, and QT_c intervals; U and T wave abnormalities; and ventricular dysrhythmias, including torsades de pointes. Seizures occur mainly in patients with convulsive disorders or loxapine overdose. Sudden death in children and adults has been reported. (2) Idiosyncratic dystonic reactions are most common with the piperidine group. The reaction is not dose dependent and consists of opisthotonos, torticollis, orolingual dyskinesia, and oculogyric crisis (painful upward gaze). It occurs more frequently in children and women. (3) Neuroleptic malignant syndrome occurs in patients receiving chronic therapy and is characterized by hyperthermia, muscle rigidity, autonomic dysfunction, and altered mental state. One case of this syndrome has been reported with acute overdose. (4) The loxapine syndrome consists of seizures, rhabdomyolysis, and renal failure.

Management: (1) Establish and maintain vital functions. All patients with overdose require venous access, 12-lead ECG (to measure intervals), cardiac and respiratory monitoring, and seizure precautions. Monitor core temperature to detect a poikilothermic effect. A comatose patient may require intubation and assisted ventilation, 100% oxygen, IV glucose, naloxone, and 100 mg of thiamine. (2) GI decontamination: Emesis is not recommended. Gastric lavage may be useful but is not necessary if AC or a cathartic is administered promptly. MDAC has not proved beneficial. A radiograph of the abdomen may be useful if the PTZ is radiopaque. Haloperidol and trifluoperazine are most likely to be radiopaque. Whole-bowel irrigation may be useful when a large number of pills are visualized on a radiograph or sustained-release preparations are involved, but this modality has not been investigated for management of PTZ toxicity. (3) Treat convulsions with diazepam or lorazepam. A loxapine overdose may result in status epilepticus. If nondepolarizing neuromuscular blockade is required, use pancuronium (Pavulon) or vecuronium (Norcuron) (not succinylcholine [Anectine], which may cause malignant hyperthermia), and monitor the EEG during paralysis. (4) Dysrhythmias: Monitor with serial ECG. Treat unstable rhythms with electrical cardioversion. Avoid class IA antidysrhythmic drugs (procainamide, quinidine, and disopyramide). Hypokalemia predisposes to dysrhythmias and should be corrected aggressively. Supraventricular tachycardia with hemodynamic instability is treated with electrical cardioversion. The role of adenosine has not been defined. Avoid calcium channel blockers and β-blockers. QRS interval prolongation is treated with $NaHCO_3$ at 1 to 2 mEq/kg by IV bolus given over a period of a few minutes. Torsades de pointes is treated with 2 g of a 20% magnesium sulfate solution given IV over a 2- to 3-minute period; if no response is seen in 10 minutes, the treatment is repeated and followed by a continuous infusion of 5 to 10 mg/min, or an infusion of 50 mg/min is given for 2 hours, followed by an infusion

TABLE 33. **Neuroleptic Daily Doses and Properties: Comparison of Effects***

Compound/Dose	Effects: Antipsychotic	Anticholinergic	Extrapyramidal	Hypotensive and Cardiotoxic	Sedative
PHENOTHIAZINE					
Aliphatic†	1+	3+	2+	2+	3+
Chlorpromazine (Thorazine), 20–50 mg adult dose; range, 20–2000 mg/24 h					
Promethazine (Phenergan), 25–50 mg adult dose; range, 25–200 mg/24 h					
Piperazine‡	3+	1+	3+	1+	1+
Fluphenazine (Prolixin), 2.5–10 mg adult dose; range, 2.5–20 mg/24 h					
Perphenazine (Trilafon), 4–16 mg adult dose; range, 10–30 mg/24 h					
Prochlorperazine (Compazine), 5–10 mg adult dose; range, 15–40 mg/24 h					
Trifluoperazine (Stelazine), 2–5 mg adult dose; range, 15–40 mg/24 h					
Piperidine†	1+	2+	1+	3+	3+
Mesoridazine (Serentil), 25–100 mg adult dose; range, 150–400 mg/24 h					
Thioridazine (Mellaril), 25–100 mg adult dose; range, 150–300 mg/24 h					
NONPHENOTHIAZINE					
Butyrophenone‡	3+	1+	3+	1+	1+
Haloperidol (Haldol), 0.5–5.0 mg adult dose; range, 1–100 mg/24 h					
Dibenzoxazepine‡	3+	1+	3+	1+	2+
Loxapine (Loxitane), 10–50 mg adult dose; range, 60–100 mg/24 h					
Dihydroindolone‡	3+	1+	3+	1+	1+
Molindone (Moban), 5–25 mg adult dose; range, 50–225 mg/24 h					
Thioxanthenes‡	3+	1+	3+	3+	1+
Thiothixene (Navane), 2–15 mg adult dose; range, 5–80 mg/24 h					
Chlorprothixene (Taractan), 5–60 mg adult dose; range, 75–200 mg/24 h					

*1+ indicates very low activity; 2+, moderate activity; 3+, very high activity. Equivalent doses: 100 mg of chlorpromazine or thioridazine = 50 mg of mesoridazine = 15 mg of loxapine or prochlorperazine = 10 mg of molindone or perphenazine = 5 mg of thiothixene = 2 mg of fluphenazine or haloperidol.
†Low antipsychotic potency.
‡High antipsychotic potency.

of 30 mg/min given over a period of 90 minutes twice a day for several days, as needed. The dose in children is 25 to 50 mg/kg initially with a maintenance dose of 30 to 60 mg/kg per 24 hours (0.25 to 0.50 mEq/kg per 24 hours), up to 1000 mg per 24 hours. Monitor serum magnesium. Ventricular tachydysrhythmias: If the patient is stable, lidocaine is the agent of choice. If the patient is unstable, electrical cardioversion is performed. Heart blocks with hemodynamic instability should be managed with temporary cardiac pacing. (5) Hypotension is treated with the Trendelenburg position, 0.89% saline, and in refractory cases or if fluid overload is a possibility, administration of vasopressors. The vasopressor of choice is the α-adrenergic agonist norepinephrine, 0.1 to 0.2 μg/g/min and titrated to response. Epinephrine and dopamine should not be used because β-receptor stimulation in the presence of α-receptor blockade may provoke dysrhythmias and PTZs are antidopaminergic. (6) Treat hypothermia or hyperthermia with external warming or cooling measures. Do not use antipyretic drugs. (7) Management consists of the following: (a) Immediately discontinue use of the offending agent. (b) Hyperventilate the patient with 100% humidified, cooled oxygen at high gas flow (at least 10 L/min). (c) Administer a benzodiazepine to control convulsions, and facilitate cooling measures. (d) Initiate appropriate mechanical cooling measures, which may include IV cold saline (*not* Ringer's lactate); ice baths, cold lavage of the stomach, bladder, and rectum; and a hypothermic blanket. (e) Correct acid-base and electrolyte disturbances. Treat significant hyperkalemia with hyperventilation, calcium, sodium bicarbonate, IV glucose, and insulin. Hemodialysis may be necessary. (f) Dysrhythmias usually respond to correcting the underlying acid-base disturbances and hyperkalemia. If antidysthymic agents are required, *avoid* calcium channel blockers, which may precipitate hyperkalemia and cardiovascular collapse. (g) Dantrolene sodium (Dantrium), which is a phenytoin derivative, inhibits calcium release from the sarcoplasmic reticulum and results in decreased muscle contraction. Dantrolene acts peripherally and does not reverse the rigidity or psychomotor disturbances resulting from the central dopamine blockade; therefore, it is often used in combination with bromocriptine (Parlodel). Bromocriptine mesylate acts centrally as a dopamine agonist, as does amantadine hydrochloride (Symmetrel). Bromocriptine and dantrolene have been reported to be successful in combination with cooling and good supportive measures in malignant hyperthermia. *Dosing: Dantrolene sodium*, 2 to 3 mg/kg IV, should be given as a bolus, followed by 1 mg/kg per dose. To prevent symptom recurrence, administer 1 mg/kg every 6 hours for 24 to 48 hours after the episode. After that time, oral dantrolene can be used at a dose of 1 mg/kg every 6 hours for 24 hours as necessary. Observe for thrombophlebitis after IV dantrolene. It is best administered via a central line. *Bromocriptine mesylate*, 2.5 to 10 mg orally or via a nasogastric tube three times a day, should be used in combination with dantrolene. (8) Idiosyncratic dystonic reaction can be treated with diphenhydramine at 1 to 2 mg/kg per dose given IV over a 5-minute period up to a maximum of 50 mg; a response is noted within 2 to 5 minutes. Follow with oral doses for 5 to 7 days to prevent recurrence. (9) Extracorporeal measures (hemodialysis, hemoperfusion) are not effective in enhancing removal of these agents.

Laboratory investigations: Monitor ABGs, renal and hepatic function, electrolytes, blood glucose, and creatine kinase and assess for myoglobinemia in neuroleptic malignant syndrome. Most of these agents are detected by routine screens. A positive ferric chloride test of the urine occurs with a sufficient blood level; however, it is not specific (salicylates and phenolic compounds also produce a positive result). Quantitative serum levels are not useful in management. Cross-reactions with EMIT tests occur with cyclic antidepressants. PTZs produce false-negative results of pregnancy urine tests in which human chorionic gonadotropin is used as the indicator and false-positive results of tests for urinary porphyrins, the indirect Coombs test, and urobilinogen and amylase tests. *Disposition*: Asymptomatic patients should be observed for at least 6 hours after gastric decontamination. Symptomatic patients with cardiotoxicity, hypotension, or convulsions should be admitted to the ICU and monitored for 48 hours.

Salicylates. (Acetylsalicylic acid, aspirin, salicylic acid.) *Toxic mechanism*: The primary toxic mechanisms include (1) direct stimulation of the medullary chemoreceptor trigger zone and respiratory center, (2) uncoupling of oxidative phosphorylation, (3) inhibition of the Krebs cycle enzymes, (4) inhibition of vitamin K–dependent and –independent clotting factors, (5) alteration of platelet function, and (6) inhibition of prostaglandin synthesis. *Toxic dose*: Acute mild intoxication occurs at a dose of 150 to 200 mg/kg (tinnitus, dizziness), moderate intoxication at 200 to 300 mg/kg, and severe intoxication at 300 to 500 mg/kg (CNS manifestations). An acute salicylate plasma concentration (SPC) higher than 30 mg/dL (usually over 40 mg/dL) may be associated with clinical toxicity. Chronic intoxication occurs at ingestions of more than 100 mg/kg/d for more than 2 days because of cumulative kinetics. Methyl salicylate (oil of wintergreen) is the most toxic form of salicylate; 1 mL of 98% methyl salicylate contains 1.4 g of salicylate. Fatalities have occurred with the ingestion of 1 teaspoonful in a child and 1 ounce in adults. It is found in topical ointments and liniments (18% to 30%). *Kinetics*: Acetylsalicylic acid is a weak acid with a pK_a of 3.0. Salicylic acid is absorbed from the stomach and small bowel and dermally. Onset of action is within 30 minutes. Methyl salicylate and effervescent tablets are absorbed more rapidly. An SPC is detectable within 15 minutes after ingestion, and the peak occurs in 30 to 120 minutes but may be delayed 6 to 12 hours in large overdoses, in overdoses with enteric-coated and sustained-release preparations, and if concretions develop. The therapeutic duration of action is 3 to 4 hours but is markedly prolonged in an overdose. The $t_{1/2}$ of salicylic acid is 3 hours after a 300-mg dose, 6 hours after a 1-g overdose, and over 10 hours after a 10-g overdose. The Vd is 0.13 L/kg for salicylic acid but increases as the SPC increases. PB is up to 90% for salicylic acid at pH 7.4 at a therapeutic SPC, 75% at an SPC above 40 mg/dL, 50% at an SPC of 70 mg/dL, and 30% at an SPC of 120 mg/dL. Elimination includes Michaelis-Menten hepatic metabolism by three saturable pathways: (1) glycine conjugation to salicyluric acid (75%), (2) saturable glucuronyl transferase to salicyl phenol glucuronide (10%), and (3) salicyl aryl glucuronide (4%). Nonsaturable pathways involve hydrolysis to gentisic acid (<1%), and 10% is excreted unchanged. Acidosis increases the severity by increasing the nonionized salicylate that can move into the brain cells. In the kidneys, the un-ionized salicylic acid undergoes glomerular filtration, and the ionized portion undergoes secretion in the proximal tubules and passive reabsorption in the distal tubules. Renal excretion of salicylate is enhanced by alkaline urine. *Manifestations*: Ingestion of concentrated topical salicylic acid preparations (e.g., Compound W) can cause caustic mucosal injury to the GI tract. The possibility of an occult salicylate overdose should be considered in any patient with an unexplained acid-base disturbance. Acute overdose: (1) Minimal symptoms—tinnitus, dizziness, and difficulty hearing—may occur at a high therapeutic SPC of 20 to 30 mg/dL. Nausea and vomiting may occur immediately as a result of local gastric irritation. (2) Phase I consists of mild manifestations (1 to 12 hours after ingestion at a 6-hour SPC of 45 to 70 mg/dL). Nausea and vomiting followed by hyperventilation are usually present within 3 to 8 hours after an acute overdose. Hyperventilation with an increase in both rate (tachypnea) and depth (hyperpnea) is present but may be subtle. It results in mild respiratory alkalosis (serum pH greater than 7.4 and urine pH greater than 6.0). Some patients may have lethargy, vertigo, headache, and confusion. Diaphoresis is prominent. (3) Phase II involves moderate manifestations (12 to 24 hours after ingestion at a 6-hour SPC of 70 to 100 mg/dL). Serious metabolic disturbances, including marked respiratory alkalosis followed by AG metabolic acidosis, and dehydration occur. The pH may be normal, elevated, or depressed, with a urine pH less than 6.0. Other metabolic disturbances may include hypoglycemia or hyperglycemia, hypokalemia, decreased ionized calcium, and increased BUN, creatinine, and lactate. Mental disturbances (confusion, disorientation, hallucinations) may occur. Hypotension and convulsions have been reported. (4) Phase III involves severe intoxication (more than 24 hours at a 6-hour SPC of 100 to 130 mg/dL). In addition to the preceding clinical findings, coma and seizures develop and indicate severe intoxication. Pulmonary edema may occur. Metabolic disturbances include metabolic acidemia (pH less than 7.4) and aciduria (pH less than 6.0). In adults, alkalosis may persist until terminal respiratory failure occurs. (5) In children younger than 4 years, a metabolic or mixed metabolic acidosis and respiratory alkalosis develop within 4 to 6 hours because these children have less respiratory reserve and accumulate lactate and other organic acids. Hypoglycemia is more common in children. (6) Fatalities occur at a 6-hour SPC greater than 130 to 150 mg/dL and result from CNS depression, cardiovascular collapse, electrolyte imbalance, and cerebral edema. Chronic salicylism is more serious than acute intoxication, and the 6-hour SPC does not correlate with the manifestations. It usually occurs with therapeutic errors in young children or the elderly with underlying illness, and the diagnosis is delayed because it is not recognized. Noncardiac pulmonary edema is a frequent complication in the elderly. The mortality rate is about 25%. Chronic salicylate poisoning in children may mimic Reye's syndrome. It is associated with exaggerated CNS findings (hallucinations, delirium, dementia, memory loss, papilledema, bizarre behavior, agitation, encephalopathy, seizures, and coma). Hemorrhagic manifestations, renal failure, and pulmonary and cerebral edema may occur. The metabolic picture is that of hypoglycemia and mixed acid-base derangements. A chronic SPC higher than 60 mg/dL with metabolic acidosis and an altered mental state is extremely serious.

Management: Treatment is started on the basis of clinical and metabolic findings, not on the basis of salicylate levels. Continuous monitoring of urine pH is essential for successful alkalization treatment. Always obtain an acetaminophen plasma level. (1) Establish and maintain vital functions. If the mental state is altered, administer glucose, naloxone, and thiamine in standard doses. Depending on the severity, the initial studies include an immediate and a 6-hour postingestion SPC, ECG and cardiac monitoring, pulse oximetry, urine assays (analysis, pH, SG, and ferric chloride test), chest radiography, ABGs, blood glucose, electrolytes and AG calculation, calcium (ionized), magnesium, renal and liver profiles, and prothrombin time. Test gastric contents and stool for occult blood. Bismuth and magnesium salicylate preparations may be radiopaque on radiographs. A nephrologist should be consulted for moderate, severe, or chronic intoxication. (2) GI decontamination: Gastric lavage and AC are useful up to 1 hour after ingestion if a toxic dose was ingested (each gram of AC binds 550 mg of salicylic acid). MDAC is not recommended for routine use. Concretions may occur with massive (usually 300 mg/kg) ingestions, and if blood levels fail to decline, prompt contrast radiography of the stomach may reveal concretions that must be removed by repeated lavage, whole-bowel irrigation, endoscopy, or gastrostomy. (3) Fluids and electrolytes (Table 34): Shock: Establish perfusion and vascular volume with 5% dextrose in 0.89% saline; then proceed with correction of dehydration and alkalization. Fluids and bicarbonate: In acute moderate or severe salicylism (see Table 34), adults should receive a bolus of 1 to 2 mEq of $NaHCO_3$ per kilogram, followed by an infusion of 100 to 150 mEq of $NaHCO_3$ added to 500 to 1000 mL of 5% dextrose and administered over a 60-minute period. Children should receive a bolus of 1 to 2 mEq of $NaHCO_3$ per kilogram, followed by an infusion of 1 to 2 mEq/kg added to 20 mL/kg of 5% dextrose administered over

TABLE 34. **Fluid and Electrolyte Treatment of Salicylate Poisoning**

Type of Salicylism	Metabolic Disturbance	Blood pH	Urine pH	Hydrating Solution	Amount of $NaHCO_3$ (mEq/L)	Amount of Potassium (mEq/L)
Mild	Respiratory alkalosis	>7.4	>6.0	5% dextrose 0.45% saline	50 (adult) 1 mEq/kg (child)	20
Moderate						
Chronic	Respiratory alkalosis	>7.4	<6.0	D5W	100 (adult)	40
Child younger than 4 y	Metabolic acidosis	<7.4			1–2 mEq/kg (child)	
Severe						
Chronic	Metabolic acidosis	<7.4	<6.0	D5W	150 (adult)	60
Child younger than 4 y	Respiratory alkalosis				2 mEq/kg (child)	
CNS depressant co-ingestant	Respiratory acidosis	<7.4	<6.0	D5W	100–150*	60

*Hypoventilation must be corrected.

Abbreviation: D5W = 5% dextrose in water.

Modified from Linden CH, Rumack BH: The legitimate analgesics, aspirin and acetaminophen. *In* Hansen W Jr (ed): Toxic Emergencies. New York, Churchill Livingstone, 1984, p 118.

a 60-minute period. Add potassium to the IV infusion after the patient voids. Attempt to achieve a target urine output of more than 2 mL/kg/h and a target urine pH of more than 7. The initial infusion is followed by subsequent infusions (two to three times normal maintenance) of 200 to 300 mL/h in adults or 10 mL/kg/h in children. If the patient is acidotic and the serum pH is less than 7.15, an additional 1 to 2 mEq $NaHCO_3$ per kilogram is given over a period of 1 to 2 hours, and persistent acidosis may necessitate $NaHCO_3$ at 1 to 2 mEq/kg every 2 hours. Adjust the infusion rate, the amount of bicarbonate, and the electrolytes to correct serum abnormalities and maintain the targeted urine output and urinary pH. Most authorities believe that the diuresis is not as important as the alkalization or MDAC. Carefully monitor for fluid overload in those at risk of pulmonary and cerebral edema (e.g., the elderly) and because of inappropriate secretion of antidiuretic hormone. In patients with mild intoxication who are not acidotic and whose urine pH is greater than 6, administer 5% dextrose in 0.45% saline, with $NaHCO_3$ at 50 mEq/L or 1 mEq/kg as maintenance to replace ongoing renal losses. (4) Alkalization: $NaHCO_3$ is administered to produce a serum pH of 7.4 to 7.5 and urine pH above 7. Carbonic anhydrase inhibitors (e.g., acetazolamide [Diamox]) should not be used. If the patient is acidotic, additional bicarbonate may be required. About 2 mEq/kg raises the blood pH by 0.1. In children, alkalization may be a difficult problem because of the organic acid production and hypokalemia. Hypokalemic and fluid-depleted patients cannot undergo adequate alkalization. Alkalization is usually discontinued in asymptomatic patients with an SPC below 30 to 40 mg/dL but is continued in symptomatic patients regardless of the SPC. A decreased serum bicarbonate level with a normal or high blood pH indicates respiratory alkalosis predominating over metabolic acidosis, and bicarbonate should be administered cautiously. Alkalemia (pH of 7.40 to 7.50) is not a contraindication to bicarbonate therapy because these patients have a significant base deficit in spite of the elevated blood pH. (5) Potassium is added (20 to 40 mEq/L) to the infusion after the patient voids. In severe, late, and chronic salicylism, potassium at 60 mEq/L may be needed. When the serum potassium level is below 4.0 mEq/L, add 10 mEq/L during the first hour. If the patient has hypokalemia (less than 3 mEq/L), flat T waves, and U waves, administer 0.25 to 0.5 mEq/kg up to 10 mEq/h. Administer potassium with ECG monitoring. Recheck the serum potassium value after each rapidly administered dose. A paradoxical urine acidosis (alkaline serum pH and acidic urine pH) indicates that potassium is probably needed. (6) Convulsions are treated with diazepam or lorazepam, but rule out hypoglycemia, a low ionized calcium concentration, cerebral edema, or hemorrhage with CT. If tetany develops, discontinue the $NaHCO_3$ therapy and administer 10% calcium gluconate at 0.1 to 0.2 mL/kg. (7) Pulmonary edema management consists of fluid restriction, high forced inspiratory oxygen (FIO_2), mechanical ventilation, and PEEP. (8) Cerebral edema management consists of fluid restriction, elevation of the head, hyperventilation, osmotic diuresis, and dexamethasone. (9) Administer vitamin K_1 parenterally to correct an increased prothrombin time of more than 20 seconds and coagulation abnormalities. If active bleeding is noted, administer fresh plasma and platelets as needed. (10) Hyperpyrexia is managed by external cooling measures, not antipyretics. (11) Hemodialysis is the method of choice for removing salicylates because it corrects the acid-base, electrolyte, and fluid disturbances as well. Indications for hemodialysis include acute poisoning with an SPC greater than 100 to 130 mg/dL without improvement after 6 hours of appropriate therapy; chronic poisoning with cardiopulmonary disease and an SPC as low as 40 mg/dL with refractory acidosis, severe CNS manifestations (coma and seizures), and progressive deterioration, especially in the elderly; impairment of vital organs of elimination; clinical deterioration in spite of good supportive care, repeated doses of AC, and alkalization; and severe refractory acid-base or electrolyte disturbances despite appropriate corrective measures.

Laboratory investigations: In all intentional salicylate overdoses, the acetaminophen plasma level should be determined after 4 hours. (1) Continuously monitor ECG, urine output, urine pH, and SG. Every 2 to 4 hours in severe intoxication, monitor SPC; glucose (in salicylism, CNS hypoglycemia may be present despite a normal serum glucose level); electrolytes; ionized calcium, magnesium, and phosphorus; AG; ABGs; and pulse oximetry. Daily, monitor BUN, creatinine, liver function tests, and the prothrombin time. (2) In the *ferric chloride test*, 1 mL of boiled urine containing 2 or 3 drops of 10% ferric chloride turns purple if salicylates are present. This test is nonspecific and is positive for ketones (if the sample is not boiled), PTZs, and phenolic compounds in urine. (3) SPC: The therapeutic value is less than 10 mg/dL for analgesia and 15 to 30 mg/dL for an anti-inflammatory effect. Mild toxicity occurs at values above 30 mg/dL (tinnitus, dizziness) and severe toxicity at concentrations above 80 mg/dL (CNS changes). *Cross-reaction*: Diflunisal (Dolobid) results in a falsely high SPC. The Done nomogram (Figure 2) was used as a predictor of expected severity after an acute single ingestion. It is not considered accurate in evaluating acute or chronic salicylate intoxication. *Disposition*: Because of the limitations of SPCs, patients are managed on the basis of clinical and laboratory findings. Patients who are asymptomatic should be monitored for a minimum of 6 hours and longer if ingestion of enteric-coated tablets, a massive overdose, or suspicion of concretions is involved. Those who remain asymptomatic with an SPC below 35 mg/dL may be discharged after psychiatric evaluation, if indicated. Patients with chronic salicylate intoxication, acidosis, and an altered mental state should be admitted to the ICU. Patients with acute ingestion, an SPC below 60 mg/dL, and

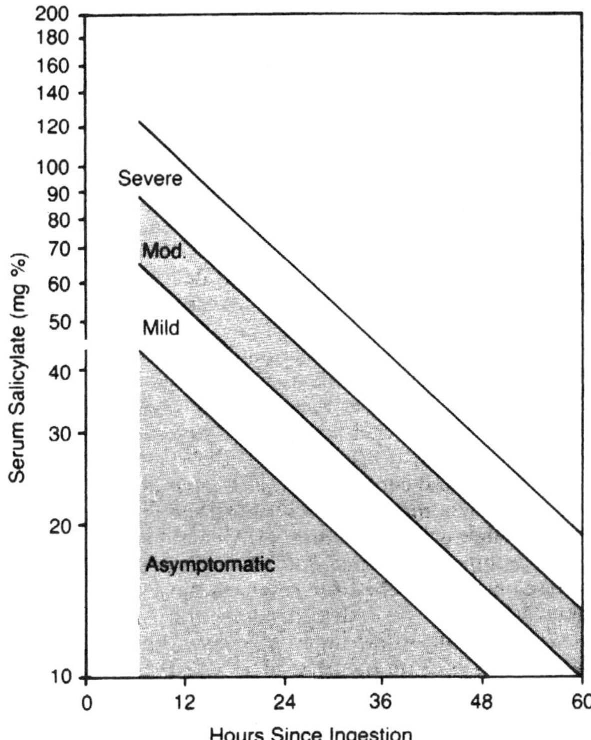

Figure 2. The Done nomogram for salicylate intoxication. (Redrawn from Done A: Salicylate intoxication: Significance of measurements of salicylate in blood in cases of acute ingestion. Reproduced with permission from *Pediatrics*, Vol 26, Page 800, Figure 3, Copyright 1960.)

mild symptoms may be able to receive adequate treatment in the emergency department. Patients with moderate or severe intoxications should be admitted to the ICU.

Selective Serotonin Reuptake Inhibitors. (SSRIs; antidepressants.) SSRIs are primarily prescribed as antidepressants. SSRIs include the prototype fluxetine (Prozac, 10-, 20-mg tablets), paroxetine (Paxil, 20-, 30-, 40-mg tablets), and sertraline (Zoloft, 25-, 50-, 100-mg tablets). *Toxic mechanism*: SSRIs interfere with neuron reuptake of serotonin (5-hydroxytryptamine, or 5-HT) at presynaptic ganglia sites in the brain and thereby increase the activity of serotonin. SSRIs should not be used until 5 weeks after an MAOI is given, nor should MAOI therapy be initiated or discontinued within 5 weeks of administration of an SSRI. *Toxic dose*: The therapeutic oral dose for fluoxetine is 20 to 80 mg/d. No toxicity in children has occurred with an oral dose of 3.5 mg/kg. A fatal dose for adults is 6 g. The therapeutic dose of paroxetine is 20 to 50 mg/d. In 35 adult patients, serious side effects did not develop in any after the ingestion of 10 to 1000 mg, and a study involving 35 children failed to demonstrate serious adverse effects at doses less than 180 mg. *Kinetics*: Fluoxetine is well absorbed from the GI tract and has a peak plasma concentration lasting 6 to 8 hours. The 95% protein-bound $t_{1/2}$ is 4 days (for the demethylated active metabolite norfluoxetine, $t_{1/2}$ is 7 to 15 days). Elimination is 80% renal, and Vd is 20 to 42 L/kg. Fluoxetine and other serotonin inhibitors arrest the action of cytochrome P-450IID6. Therefore, interactions may occur with many other medications, such as antidysrhythmic class IC drugs (quinidine), phenytoin (Dilantin), haloperidol, lithium, tricyclic antidepressants, β-blockers, codeine, and carbamazepine (Tegretol). Paroxetine is almost completely absorbed from the GI tract; it undergoes extensive first-pass liver metabolism by oxidation and methylation to inactive metabolites. The peak is from 2 to 8 hours. Paroxetine inhibits the P-450 system; it may increase the incidence of bleeding with warfarin (Coumadin) and decrease the availability of phenytoin, phenobarbital, and digoxin. PB is greater than 90%, and Vd = 13 L/kg. The average $t_{1/2}$ is 21 hours. Sertraline levels peak between 8 and 12 hours, and the Vd is 20 L/kg. The average $t_{1/2}$ is 26 hours, and PB is 98%. Sertraline is metabolized to form the less active metabolite *N*-desmethylsertraline ($t_{1/2}$ of 62 to 104 hours.) *Manifestations*: All SSRIs may cause *serotonin syndrome, a potentially life-threatening reaction*, if they are administered concurrently with an MAOI. Serotonin syndrome is a result of cerebral serotonergic stimulation and can cause severe hyperthermia, myoclonus, rhabdomyolysis, confusion, tremors, and a variety of psychological disturbances, in addition to cardiovascular complications and extrapyramidal side effects, which include akathisia, dyskinesia, and parkinsonian-like syndromes. Additional side effects are increased suicidal ideation, seizures, sexual disorders, and hematologic disorders (platelet serotonin activity blockade leading to prolonged bleeding times). Inappropriate secretion of antidiuretic hormone resulting in hyponatremia may occur if SSRIs are administered to elderly patients. This effect is usually seen within the first week of therapy. Overdose effects are similar to those seen in serotonin syndrome. *Management*: No specific antidote is available. Initial management consists of stabilizing vital functions, including thermoregulation. Therapy is supportive, and it is essential to anticipate potential life-threatening manifestations, including hypotension, hyperthermia, seizures, coma, disseminated intravascular coagulation, ventricular tachycardia, and metabolic acidosis. Vital signs should be monitored, and EEG, creatine kinase, and blood chemistry studies should be obtained. BZPs should be given to prevent/control muscle hyperactivity (diazepam [Valium] for seizures and clonazepam [Klonopin] for myoclonus). If BZP therapy fails to control muscle activity or seizures, anesthesia or nondepolarizing neuromuscular blockade may be necessary. Electrolyte abnormalities should be corrected and acid-base balance restored. Fluids should be given to maintain urine output greater than 2 mL/kg/h in patients with a risk of myoglobinuria. No data support the use of GI decontamination, although AC may be used if ingestion has occurred within 1 hour, with attention to airway protection. Hemodialysis and charcoal hemoperfusion are unlikely to be beneficial. Haloperidol, phenothiazines, and other highly protein-bound drugs should be avoided. BZP and cooling therapy should be used for patients with hyperthermia. Serotonin antagonists such as cyproheptadine (Periactin) may be useful in patients with serotonin syndrome, although no controlled data are available. Dantrolene and bromocriptine are not recommended and may actually precipitate serotonin syndrome. *Laboratory investigations*: Blood serum CBC, electrolytes (acidosis, hyponatremia), glucose, coagulation profile (disseminated intravascular coagulation may occur), liver function tests, and creatine kinase should be obtained. SSRIs may increase cholesterol and triglycerides and decrease uric acid. An ECG should be obtained. *Disposition*: Children 5 years old or younger who ingest less than 180 mg of paroxetine, 3.5 mg/kg of fluoxetine, or 100 mg of sertraline may be observed at home. Symptomatic patients should be admitted to the ICU until they are asymptomatic for 24 hours. Asymptomatic patients should be observed for 6 hours. All patients should be assessed for the risk of suicide before discharge.

Sildenafil. (Viagra, 25-, 50-, and 100-mg tablets.) *Toxic mechanism*: Normal penile erection depends on relaxation of smooth muscle in the corpus cavernosum. Sildenafil is a selective inhibitor of cyclic guanosine monophosphate type 5 catabolism in the corpus, which causes erections to subside and enhances the vasodilating effect of nitric oxide (NO) produced during sexual stimulation. The source of NO is the vascular endothelium. Normal circulating levels of NO are low, except when patients are receiving nitrate therapy. *Toxic dose*: The therapeutic dose is 25 to 50 mg in tablet form taken 1 hour before sexual activity. Men with renal dysfunction or severe hepatic impairment who are taking cytochrome P-450 inhibitors (erythromycin, ketoconazole, itraconazole) or older than 65 years should take lower doses. *Interactions*: Any individual who takes nitrate donors, such as nitroglycerin, faces the risk of hypotension, syncope, and exacerbation of underlying coronary disease. Nitroprusside use is a contraindication. *Kinetics*: Sildenafil is rapidly absorbed after oral administration. The peak concentration occurs within 1 hour, with a $t_{1/2}$ of 3 to 5 hours. The duration of action is 15 to 25 hours. *Manifestations*: Chest pains, dizziness, lightheadedness, or myocardial ischemia can occur, especially if sildenafil is taken concomitantly with nitrates. Patients report mild to moderate headache, indigestion, and facial flushing. A small percentage have a bluish tinge to their vision that makes it difficult to distinguish blue from green.

Management: Before administering an organic nitrate, emergency room physicians and health care providers should ask male patients who have chest pain if they have been taking sildenafil. If the answer is affirmative, symptomatic and supportive care should be initiated. ECG monitoring, as well as vital signs, should be obtained. Treatment with nitrates should be avoided. Because of the rapidity of onset, GI decontamination procedures are not helpful.

Laboratory investigations: In addition to ECG and monitoring vital signs, a complete cardiac workup should be performed, including the MB isoenzyme of creatine kinase, troponin levels, and cardiology consultation. *Disposition*: Patients who manifest cardiac symptoms should be observed in the cardiac care unit for 24 hours. If they remain clinically stable and are asymptomatic for 24 hours, and if myocardial infarction has been excluded, these patients can be sent home with responsible adult caregivers and scheduled for appropriate follow-up.

Tricyclic and Other Cyclic Antidepressants. Traditionally, tricyclic antidepressants have been an important cause of pharmaceutical overdose fatalities (more than 100 in 1992). The mortality has been reduced from 15% in the 1970s to less than 1% in the 1990s through a better understanding of their pathophysiology and improvements in management. See Table 35. *Toxic mechanism*: The major mechanisms of toxicity of the tricyclic antidepressants are central and peripheral anticholinergic effects, peripheral α-adrenergic blockade, quinidine-like cardiac membrane–stabilizing action blocking the fast inward sodium channels, and inhibition of synaptic neurotransmitter reuptake in the CNS presynaptic neurons. The tetracyclic, monocyclic aminoketone dibenzoxazepine possesses convulsive activity and less cardiac toxicity in overdoses. Triazolopyridine has less serious cardiac and CNS toxicity. *Toxic dose*: The therapeutic dose of imipramine (Tofranil) is 1.5 to 5 mg/kg; a dose greater than 5 mg/kg may be mildly toxic; 10 to 20 mg/kg may be life-threatening, although doses of less than 20 mg/kg have produced a few fatalities; more than 30 mg/kg is associated with 30% mortality; and at doses higher than 70 mg/kg, survival is rare. Doses of 375 mg in a child and as little as 500 to 750 mg in an adult have been fatal. In adults, 5 times the maximal daily dose is toxic, and 10 times the maximal daily dose is potentially fatal. Although major overdose symptoms are associated with plasma concentrations above 1 μg/mL (1000 ng/mL), plasma tricyclic levels do not necessarily correlate with toxicity; therefore, clinical signs and symptoms should guide therapy. Relative dosage equivalents are as follows: 100 mg of amitriptyline = 125 mg of amoxapine = 75 mg of desipramine = 100 mg of doxepin = 75 mg of imipramine = 75 mg of maprotiline = 50 mg of nortriptyline = 200 mg of trazodone. See Table 35. *Kinetics*: Cyclic antidepressants are lipophilic. They are rapidly absorbed from the alkaline small intestine, but absorption may be prolonged and delayed in massive overdose because of anticholinergic action. Onset varies from less than 1 hour (30 to 40 minutes) and rarely to 12 hours. Peak serum levels are reached in 2 to 8 hours, and the peak effect occurs in 6 hours but may be delayed 12 hours as a result of erratic absorption. The clinical effects correlate poorly with plasma levels. Cyclic antidepressants are highly protein bound to plasma glycoproteins (98% at pH 7.5 and 90% at pH 7.0); the Vd is 10 to 50 L/kg. The $t_{1/2}$ varies from 10 hours for imipramine to 81 hours for amitriptyline and 100 hours for nortriptyline. The active metabolites have considerable $t_{1/2}$ values. Elimination is by hepatic

TABLE 35. **Cyclic Antidepressants: Daily Doses and Major Properties***

Generic Name	Adult Daily Dose (mg)	Therapeutic Range (ng/mL)	Half-Life (h)	Toxicity		
				Antichol	*CNS*	*Cardiac*
TRICYCLIC ANTIDEPRESSANTS						
Major toxicity is cardiac						
Tertiary amines demethylated into secondary active amine metabolites						
Amitriptyline (Elavil)	75–300	120–250	31–46	3+	3+	3+
Imipramine (Tofranil)	75–300	125–250	9–24	3+	3+	2+
Doxepin (Sinequan)	75–300	30–150	8–24	3+	3+	2+
Trimipramine (Surmontil)	75–200	10–240	16–18	3+	3+	2+
Secondary amines metabolized into inactive metabolites						
Nortriptyline (Pamelor)†	75–150	50–150	18–93	2+	3+	3+
Desipramine (Norpramin)	75–200	75–160	14–62	1+	3+	3+
Protriptyline (Vivactil)	20–60	70–250	54–198	2+	3+	3+
NEWER CYCLIC ANTIDEPRESSANTS						
Tetracyclic agent produces a high incidence of cardiovascular disturbances and seizures						
Maprotiline (Ludiomil)	75–300	—	30–60	1+	2+	3+
Triazolopyridine, a noncyclic agent, produces less serious cardiac and CNS toxicity						
Trazodone (Desyrel)	50–600	700	4–7	1+	1+	1+
Monocyclic aminoketone produces seizures in doses > 600 mg						
Bupropion (Wellbutrin)	200–400	—	8–24	1+	3+	1+
Dibenzazepine						
Clomipramine (Anafranil)	100–250	200–500	21–32	2+	2+	2+
Dibenzoxazepine produces syndrome of convulsions, rhabdomyolysis, and renal failure						
Amoxapine (Asendin)	150–300	200–500	6–10	1+	3+	2+

*Other drugs with similar structures are cyclobenzaprine (Flexeril), a muscle relaxant (similar to amitriptyline), and carbamazepine (Tegretol), an anticonvulsant (similar to imipramine); however, they cause less cardiac toxicity. 1+ indicates mild effect, 2+ indicates moderate effect, and 3+ indicates severe effect.

†Not available in the United States.

Abbreviations: Antichol = anticholinergic effect; Cardiac = cardiac effect; CNS = central nervous system effect (primarily seizures).

metabolism. The tertiary amines are metabolized to active demethylated secondary amine metabolites. The active secondary amine metabolites undergo 15% enterohepatic recirculation and are metabolized over a period of days to nonactive metabolites. The intestinal bacterial flora may reconstitute the active metabolites. Only 3% of an ingested dose is excreted in the urine unchanged. *Manifestations*: On arrival at the hospital, previously alert, oriented patients may suddenly become comatose, have a seizure, suffer hemodynamically unstable dysrhythmias within minutes, and die. In most patients with severe toxicity, symptoms develop within 1 to 2 hours, but onset may be delayed 6 hours after an overdose. (1) Small overdoses produce early anticholinergic effects, agitation, and transient hypertension, which are not life-threatening. (2) Large overdoses produce depression of the CNS and myocardium, convulsions, and hypotension. Death usually occurs within the first 2 to 6 hours after ingestion. (3) ECG screening tools for use in tricyclic antidepressant toxicity include a QRS greater than 0.10 second (seizures are likely) and a QRS greater than 0.16 second (50% of patients had ventricular dysrhythmias—life-threatening in 20% of cases—and seizures), a terminal 40 ms of the QRS axis greater than 120 degrees in the right frontal plane, and an R wave greater than 3 mm as measured by the right arm lead. The quinidine cardiac membrane–stabilizing effect produces depression of myocardium, conduction disturbances, and ECG changes. The peripheral α-adrenergic blockade produces hypotension.

Management: (1) Establish and maintain vital functions. Even if the patient is asymptomatic, establish IV access, monitor vital signs and neurologic status, obtain a baseline 12-lead ECG, and continue cardiac monitoring for at least 6 hours from admission or 8 to 12 hours after ingestion. Measure the

QRS interval every 15 minutes. (2) GI decontamination: Do not induce emesis, and omit gastric lavage if AC is available. If the mental state is altered, protect the airway. AC at 1 g/kg is recommended up to 1 hour. Clinical benefit of MDAC has not been demonstrated. (3) Control seizures. Alkalization does not control seizures; use diazepam or lorazepam. Status epilepticus (as may occur with amoxapine) may necessitate high-dose barbiturates or neuromuscular blockers with IV diazepam. If this treatment is not successful, paralysis is induced by short-acting, nondepolarizing neuromuscular blockers such as vecuronium, along with intubation and assisted ventilation. A bolus of $NaHCO_3$ is recommended as an adjunct to correct the acidosis produced by the seizures. (4) Cardiovascular management consists of administration of $NaHCO_3$ (see Table 10). A dose of 1 to 2 mEq/kg is given undiluted as a bolus and repeated twice a few minutes apart, if needed, for sodium loading and alkalization, which increases PB. The sodium loading overcomes the sodium channel blockage and is more important than the alkalization, which increases PB from 90% to 98%. Indications include a QRS complex greater than 0.12 second, ventricular tachycardia, severe conduction disturbances, metabolic acidosis, coma, and seizures. An infusion of $NaHCO_3$ by itself is of limited use in controlling dysrhythmias because of its delayed onset of action. Bolus therapy is given as needed. Hyperventilation alone has been advocated, but the pH elevation is not so instantaneous and compensatory renal excretion of bicarbonate occurs; therefore, it is not recommended. The combination of hyperventilation and $NaHCO_3$ has produced fatal alkalemia and is not recommended. Monitor serum potassium (the sudden increase in blood pH can aggravate or precipitate hypokalemia), serum sodium, ionized calcium (hypocalcemia may occur with alkalization), and blood pH. (5) Specific cardiovascular complications should be treated as follows: For management of hypotension, norepinephrine, a predominantly α-adrenergic drug, is preferred over dopamine. Hypertension that occurs early rarely necessitates treatment. Sinus tachycardia does not usually necessitate treatment. Supraventricular tachycardia with hemodynamic instability necessitates synchronized electrical cardioversion, starting at 0.25 to 1.0 watt-second/kg, after sedation. Ventricular tachycardia that persists after alkalization mandates IV lidocaine or countershock if the patient is hemodynamically unstable. Ventricular fibrillation should be treated with defibrillation. Torsades de pointes is treated with a 20% magnesium sulfate solution given IV, 2 g over a period of 2 to 3 minutes, followed by a continuous infusion of 1.5 mL of a 10% solution or 5 to 10 mg/min (see Table 10). For bradydysrhythmias, atropine is contraindicated because of the anticholinergic activity. Isoproterenol at 0.1 μg/kg/min with caution may produce hypotension. If the patient is hemodynamically unstable, use a pacemaker. (6) Extraordinary measures such as intra-aortic balloon pumping and cardiopulmonary bypass have been successful. (7) Investigational: Use of Fab specific for tricyclic antidepressants has been successful in animals. Prophylactic $NaHCO_3$ to prevent dysrhythmias is being investigated. (8) Contraindicated: Physostigmine has produced asystole. Flumazenil has produced seizures.

Laboratory investigations: Monitoring: If altered mental status or ECG abnormalities are present, obtain ABGs, institute ECG monitoring, perform chest radiography, and determine blood glucose, serum electrolytes, calcium, magnesium, BUN and creatinine, liver profile, creatine kinase, and urine output; in severe cases, hemodynamic monitoring is indicated. Levels of tricyclic and other cyclic antidepressants below 300 ng/mL are therapeutic, levels above 500 ng/mL indicate toxicity, and levels above 1000 ng/mL indicate serious poisoning and are associated with QRS widening. *Disposition*: Admission to the ICU for 12 to 24 hours is essential for any patient with an antidepressant overdose who meets any of the following criteria: ECG abnormalities (except sinus tachycardia), altered mental state, seizures, respiratory depression, or hypotension. Low-risk patients are those who do not have the preceding symptoms 6 hours after ingestion, those with minor transient manifestations such as sinus tachycardia who subsequently become and remain asymptomatic for a 6-hour period, and asymptomatic patients who remain asymptomatic for 6 hours. These patients may be discharged if the ECG remains normal and they have normal bowel sounds, have AC therapy repeated once, and undergo psychiatric counseling. Even if the patient is asymptomatic on arrival at the health care facility, IV access should be established, vital signs and neurologic status should be monitored, a baseline 12-lead ECG should be obtained, and cardiac monitoring should be continued for at least 6 hours. *Caution*: In 25% of fatal cases, the patients were initially alert and awake during evaluation. However, on re-examination, most patients with fatalities that were initially deemed sudden cardiac death actually had symptoms that were missed. Children younger than 6 years with nonintentional (accidental) exposure to amitriptyline (Elavil), desipramine (Norpramin), doxepin (Sinequan), imipramine, or nortriptyline (Aventyl) in a dose less than 5 mg/kg who are asymptomatic and have caregivers considered to be reliable can be observed at home with close poison control follow-up for 6 hours. Parents or caregivers should be given instructions regarding signs and symptoms to watch for. Children who are symptomatic or who ingest more than 5 mg/kg should be referred to the emergency department for monitoring, observation, and treatment with AC.

Section 18

Appendices and Index

REFERENCE INTERVALS FOR THE INTERPRETATION OF LABORATORY TESTS

method of
WILLIAM Z. BORER, M.D.
Thomas Jefferson University Hospital
Philadelphia, Pennsylvania

Most of the tests performed in a clinical laboratory are quantitative in nature. That is, the amount of a substance present in blood or serum is measured and reported in terms of concentration, activity (e.g., enzyme activity), or counts (e.g., blood cell counts). The laboratory must provide reference intervals to assist the clinician in the interpretation of laboratory results. These reference intervals comprise the physiologic quantities of a substance (concentrations, activities, or counts) to be expected in healthy persons. Deviation above or below the reference range may be associated with a disease process, and the severity of the disease process may be associated with the magnitude of the deviation. Unfortunately, a sharp demarcation rarely exists to distinguish between physiologic and pathologic values, and the time of transition between the two is often gradual as the disease process progresses.

The terms *normal* and *abnormal* have been used to describe the laboratory values that fall inside and outside the reference range, respectively. Use of these terms is inappropriate, because no good definition of normality exists in the clinical sense and because the term *normal* may be confused with the statistical term *gaussian*. Reference ranges are established from statistical studies in groups of healthy volunteers. These study subjects must be free of disease, but they may have lifestyles or habits that result in variations in certain laboratory values. Examples of these variables include diet, body mass, exercise, and geographic location. Age and gender may also affect reference values.

When the data from a large cohort of healthy subjects fit a gaussian distribution, the usual statistical approach is to define the reference limits as two standard deviations above and below the mean. By definition, the reference range excludes the 2.5% of the population with the lowest values and the 2.5% with the highest values. Nongaussian distributions are handled by different statistical methods, but the result is similar in that the reference range is defined by the central 95% of the population. In other words, the probability that a healthy person will have a laboratory result that falls outside the reference

TABLE 1. **Base SI Units**

Property	Base Unit	Symbol
Length	meter	m
Mass	kilogram	kg
Amount of substance	mole	mol
Time	second	s
Thermodynamic temperature	kelvin	K
Electrical current	ampere	A
Luminous intensity	candela	cd
Catalytic amount	katal	kat

TABLE 2. **Derived SI Units and Non-SI Units Retained for Use With SI Units**

Property	Unit	Symbol
Area	square meter	m^2
Volume	cubic meter liter	m^3 L
Mass concentration	kilogram/cubic meter gram/liter	kg/m^3 g/L
Substance concentration	mole/cubic meter mole/liter	mol/m^3 mol/L
Temperature	degree Celsius	$C = K - 273.15$

TABLE 3. **Standard Prefixes**

Prefix	Multiplication Factor	Symbol
yocto	10^{-24}	y
zepto	10^{-21}	z
atto	10^{-18}	a
femto	10^{-15}	f
pico	10^{-12}	p
nano	10^{-9}	n
micro	10^{-6}	μ
milli	10^{-3}	m
centi	10^{-2}	c
deci	10^{-1}	d
deca	10^{1}	da
hecto	10^{2}	h
kilo	10^{3}	k
mega	10^{6}	M
giga	10^{9}	G
tera	10^{12}	T

range is 1 in 20. If 12 laboratory tests are performed, the probability that at least one of the results will be outside the reference range increases to about 50%. This means that all healthy persons are likely to have a few laboratory results that are unexpected. The clinician must then integrate these data with other clinical information, such as the history and physical examination, to arrive at an appropriate clinical decision.

The reference intervals for many tests (especially enzyme and immunochemical measurements) vary with the method used. Accordingly, each laboratory must establish reference intervals that are appropriate for the methods used.

SI UNITS

During the 1980s a concerted effort was made to introduce SI units (le Système International d'Unités). The rationale for conversion to SI units is sound. Laboratory data are scientifically more informative when the units are based on molar concentration rather than on mass concentration. For example, the conversion of glucose to lactate and pyruvate or the binding of a drug to albumin is more easily understood in units of molar concentration. Another example is illustrated as follows:

Conventional Units

1.0 g of hemoglobin:

- Combines with 1.37 mL of oxygen
- Contains 3.4 mg of iron
- Forms 34.9 mg of bilirubin

SI Units

4.0 mmol of hemoglobin:

- Combines with 4.0 mmol of oxygen
- Contains 4.0 mmol of iron
- Forms 4.0 mmol of bilirubin

The use of SI units would also enhance the standardization of nomenclature to facilitate global communication of medical and scientific information. The units, symbols, and prefixes employed in the international system are shown in Tables 1, 2, and 3.

Unfortunately, problems have arisen with the implementation of SI units in the United States. Their introduction in 1987 prompted many medical journals to report laboratory values in both SI and conventional units in anticipation of complete conversion to SI units in the early 1990s. The lack of a coordinated effort toward this goal has forced a retrenchment on the issue. Physicians continue to think and practice with laboratory results expressed in conventional units, and few, if any, American hospitals or clinical laboratories use SI units exclusively. Complete conversion to SI units is not likely to occur in the foreseeable future, but most medical journals will probably continue to publish both sets of units. For this reason, the values in the tables of reference ranges in this appendix are given in both conventional units and SI units.

TABLES OF REFERENCE INTERVALS

Some of the values included in the tables that follow have been established by the Clinical Laboratories at Thomas Jefferson University Hospital, Philadelphia, Pennsylvania, and have not been published elsewhere. Other values have been compiled from the sources cited in the references. These tables are provided for information and educational purposes only. Laboratory values must always be interpreted in the context of clinical data derived from other sources, including the medical history and physical examination. Users must exercise individual judgment when employing the information provided in this appendix.

Reference Intervals for Hematology

Test	Conventional Units	SI Units
Acid hemolysis (Ham test)	No hemolysis	No hemolysis
Alkaline phosphatase, leukocyte	Total score 14–100	Total score 14–100
Cell counts		
Erythrocytes		
Males	4.6–6.2 million/mm^3	4.6–6.2 × 10^{12}/L
Females	4.2–5.4 million/mm^3	4.2–5.4 × 10^{12}/L
Children (varies with age)	4.5–5.1 million/mm^3	4.5–5.1 × 10^{12}/L
Leukocytes, total	4500–11,000/mm^3	4.5–11.0 × 10^9/L
Leukocytes, differential counts*		
Myelocytes	0%	0/L
Band neutrophils	3%–5%	150–400 × 10^6/L
Segmented neutrophils	54%–62%	3000–5800 × 10^6/L
Lymphocytes	25%–33%	1500–3000 × 10^6/L
Monocytes	3%–7%	300–500 × 10^6/L
Eosinophils	1%–3%	50–250 × 10^6/L
Basophils	0%–1%	15–50 × 10^6/L
Platelets	150,000–400,000/mm^3	150–400 × 10^9/L
Reticulocytes	25,000–75,000/mm^3 (0.5%–1.5% of erythrocytes)	25–75 × 10^9/L

Reference Intervals for Hematology *Continued*

Test	Conventional Units	SI Units
Coagulation tests		
Bleeding time (template)	2.75–8.0 min	2.75–8.0 min
Coagulation time (glass tube)	5–15 min	5–15 min
D Dimer	<0.5 μg/mL	<0.5 mg/L
Factor VIII and other coagulation factors	50%–150% of normal	0.5–1.5 of normal
Fibrin split products (Thrombo-Welco test)	<10 μg/mL	<10 mg/L
Fibrinogen	200–400 mg/dL	2.0–4.0 g/L
Partial thromboplastin time, activated (aPTT)	20–35 s	20–35 s
Prothrombin time (PT)	12.0–14.0 s	12.0–14.0 s
Coombs' test		
Direct	Negative	Negative
Indirect	Negative	Negative
Corpuscular values of erythrocytes		
Mean corpuscular hemoglobin (MCH)	26–34 pg/cell	26–34 pg/cell
Mean corpuscular volume (MCV)	80–96 μm^3	80–96 fL
Mean corpuscular hemoglobin concentration (MCHC)	32–36 g/dL	320–360 g/L
Haptoglobin	20–165 mg/dL	0.20–1.65 g/L
Hematocrit		
Males	40–54 mL/dL	0.40–0.54
Females	37–47 mL/dL	0.37–0.47
Newborns	49–54 mL/dL	0.49–0.54
Children (varies with age)	35–49 mL/dL	0.35–0.49
Hemoglobin		
Males	13.0–18.0 g/dL	8.1–11.2 mmol/L
Females	12.0–16.0 g/dL	7.4–9.9 mmol/L
Newborns	16.5–19.5 g/dL	10.2–12.1 mmol/L
Children (varies with age)	11.2–16.5 g/dL	7.0–10.2 mmol/L
Hemoglobin, fetal	<1.0% of total	<0.01 of total
Hemoglobin A_{1C}	3%–5% of total	0.03–0.05 of total
Hemoglobin A_2	1.5%–3.0% of total	0.015–0.03 of total
Hemoglobin, plasma	0.0–5.0 mg/dL	0.0–3.2 μmol/L
Methemoglobin	30–130 mg/dL	19–80 μmol/L
Sedimentation rate (ESR)		
Wintrobe: Males	0–5 mm/h	0–5 mm/h
Females	0–15 mm/h	0–15 mm/h
Westergren: Males	0–15 mm/h	0–15 mm/h
Females	0–20 mm/h	0–20 mm/h

*Conventional units are percentages; SI units are absolute cell counts.

Reference Intervals* for Clinical Chemistry (Blood, Serum, and Plasma)

Analyte	Conventional Units	SI Units
Acetoacetate plus acetone		
Qualitative	Negative	Negative
Quantitative	0.3–2.0 mg/dL	30–200 μmol/L
Acid phosphatase, serum (thymolphthalein monophosphate substrate)	0.1–0.6 U/L	0.1–0.6 U/L
ACTH (see Corticotropin)		
Alanine aminotransferase (ALT) serum (SGPT)	1–45 U/L	1–45 U/L
Albumin, serum	3.3–5.2 g/dL	33–52 g/L
Aldolase, serum	0.0–7.0 U/L	0.0–7.0 U/L
Aldosterone, plasma		
Standing	5–30 ng/dL	140–830 pmol/L
Recumbent	3–10 ng/dL	80–275 pmol/L
Alkaline, phosphatase (ALP), serum		
Adult	35–150 U/L	35–150 U/L
Adolescent	100–500 U/L	100–500 U/L
Child	100–350 U/L	100–350 U/L
Ammonia nitrogen, plasma	10–50 μmol/L	10–50 μmol/L
Amylase, serum	25–125 U/L	25–125 U/L
Anion gap, serum, calculated	8–16 mEq/L	8–16 mmol/L
Ascorbic acid, blood	0.4–1.5 mg/dL	23–85 μmol/L
Aspartate aminotransferase (AST) serum (SGOT)	1–36 U/L	1–36 U/L
Base excess, arterial blood, calculated	0 ± 2 mEq/L	0 ± 2 mmol/L

Table continued on following page

Reference Intervals* for Clinical Chemistry (Blood, Serum, and Plasma) *Continued*

Analyte	Conventional Units	SI Units
Bicarbonate		
Venous plasma	23–29 mEq/L	23–29 mmol/L
Arterial blood	21–27 mEq/L	21–27 mmol/L
Bile acids, serum	0.3–3.0 mg/dL	0.8–7.6 μmol/L
Bilirubin, serum		
Conjugated	0.1–0.4 mg/dL	1.7–6.8 μmol/L
Total	0.3–1.1 mg/dL	5.1–19.0 μmol/L
Calcium, serum	8.4–10.6 mg/dL	2.10–2.65 mmol/L
Calcium, ionized, serum	4.25–5.25 mg/dL	1.05–1.30 mmol/L
Carbon dioxide, total, serum or plasma	24–31 mEq/L	24–31 mmol/L
Carbon dioxide tension (P_{CO_2}), blood	35–45 mm Hg	35–45 mm Hg
β-Carotene, serum	60–260 μg/dL	1.1–8.6 μmol/L
Ceruloplasmin, serum	23–44 mg/dL	230–440 mg/L
Chloride, serum or plasma	96–106 mEq/L	96–106 mmol/L
Cholesterol, serum or EDTA plasma		
Desirable range	<200 mg/dL	<5.20 mmol/L
LDL cholesterol	60–180 mg/dL	1.55–4.65 mmol/L
HDL cholesterol	30–80 mg/dL	0.80–2.05 mmol/L
Copper	70–140 μg/dL	11–22 μmol/L
Corticotropin (ACTH), plasma, 8 AM	10–80 pg/mL	2–18 pmol/L
Cortisol, plasma		
8:00 AM	6–23 μg/dL	170–630 nmol/L
4:00 PM	3–15 μg/dL	80–410 nmol/L
10:00 PM	<50% of 8:00 AM value	<50% of 8:00 AM value
Creatine, serum		
Males	0.2–0.5 mg/dL	15–40 μmol/L
Females	0.3–0.9 mg/dL	25–70 μmol/L
Creatine kinase (CK), serum		
Males	55–170 U/L	55–170 U/L
Females	30–135 U/L	30–135 U/L
Creatine kinase MB isoenzyme, serum	<5% of total CK activity <5% ng/mL by immunoassay	<5% of total CK activity <5% ng/mL by immunoassay
Creatinine, serum	0.6–1.2 mg/dL	50–110 μmol/L
Estradiol-17β, adult		
Males	10–65 pg/mL	35–240 pmol/L
Females		
Follicular	30–100 pg/mL	110–370 pmol/L
Ovulatory	200–400 pg/mL	730–1470 pmol/L
Luteal	50–140 pg/mL	180–510 pmol/L
Ferritin, serum	20–200 ng/mL	20–200 μg/L
Fibrinogen, plasma	200–400 mg/dL	2.0–4.0 g/L
Folate, serum	3–18 ng/mL	6.8–41 nmol/L
Erythrocytes	145–540 ng/mL	330–1220 nmol/L
Follicle-stimulating hormone (FSH), plasma		
Males	4–25 mU/mL	4–25 U/L
Females, premenopausal	4–30 mU/mL	4–30 U/L
Females, postmenopausal	40–250 mU/mL	40–250 U/L
Gamma-glutamyltransferase (GGT), serum	5–40 U/L	5–40 U/L
Gastrin, fasting, serum	0–100 pg/mL	0–100 mg/L
Glucose, fasting, plasma or serum	70–115 mg/dL	3.9–6.4 nmol/L
Growth hormone (hGH), plasma, adult, fasting	0–6 ng/mL	0–6 μg/L
Haptoglobin, serum	20–165 mg/dL	0.20–1.65 g/L
Immunoglobulins, serum (see table of Reference Intervals for Tests of Immunologic Function)		
Iron, serum	75–175 μg/dL	13–31 μmol/L
Iron binding capacity, serum		
Total	250–410 μg/dL	45–73 μmol/L
Saturation	20%–55%	0.20–0.55
Lactate		
Venous whole blood	5.0–20.0 mg/dL	0.6–2.2 mmol/L
Arterial whole blood	5.0–15.0 mg/dL	0.6–1.7 mmol/L
Lactate dehydrogenase (LD), serum	110–220 U/L	110–220 U/L
Lipase, serum	10–140 U/L	10–140 U/L

Reference Intervals* for Clinical Chemistry (Blood, Serum, and Plasma) *Continued*

Analyte	Conventional Units	SI Units
Lutropin (LH), serum		
Males	1–9 U/L	1–9 U/L
Females		
Follicular phase	2–10 U/L	2–10 U/L
Midcycle peak	15–65 U/L	15–65 U/L
Luteal phase	1–12 U/L	1–12 U/L
Postmenopausal	12–65 U/L	12–65 U/L
Magnesium, serum	1.3–2.1 mg/dL	0.65–1.05 mmol/L
Osmolality	275–295 mOsm/kg water	275–295 mOsm/kg water
Oxygen, blood, arterial, room air		
Partial pressure (PaO_2)	80–100 mm Hg	80–100 mm Hg
Saturation (SaO_2)	95%–98%	95%–98%
pH, arterial blood	7.35–7.45	7.35–7.45
Phosphate, inorganic, serum		
Adult	3.0–4.5 mg/dL	1.0–1.5 mmol/L
Child	4.0–7.0 mg/dL	1.3–2.3 mmol/L
Potassium		
Serum	3.5–5.0 mEq/L	3.5–5.0 mmol/L
Plasma	3.5–4.5 mEq/L	3.5–4.5 mmol/L
Progesterone, serum, adult		
Males	0.0–0.4 ng/mL	0.0–1.3 mmol/L
Females		
Follicular phase	0.1–1.5 ng/mL	0.3–4.8 mmol/L
Luteal phase	2.5–28.0 ng/mL	8.0–89.0 mmol/L
Prolactin, serum		
Males	1.0–15.0 ng/mL	1.0–15.0 μg/L
Females	1.0–20.0 ng/mL	1.0–20.0 μg/L
Protein, serum, electrophoresis		
Total	6.0–8.0 g/dL	60–80 g/L
Albumin	3.5–5.5 g/dL	35–55 g/L
Globulins		
$Alpha_1$	0.2–0.4 g/dL	2.0–4.0 g/L
$Alpha_2$	0.5–0.9 g/dL	5.0–9.0 g/L
Beta	0.6–1.1 g/dL	6.0–11.0 g/L
Gamma	0.7–1.7 g/dL	7.0–17.0 g/L
Pyruvate, blood	0.3–0.9 mg/dL	0.03–0.10 mmol/L
Rheumatoid factor	0.0–30.0 IU/mL	0.0–30.0 kIU/L
Sodium, serum or plasma	135–145 mEq/L	135–145 mmol/L
Testosterone, plasma		
Males, adult	300–1200 ng/dL	10.4–41.6 nmol/L
Females, adult	20–75 ng/dL	0.7–2.6 nmol/L
Pregnant females	40–200 ng/dL	1.4–6.9 nmol/L
Thyroglobulin	3–42 ng/mL	3–42 μg/L
Thyrotropin (hTSH), serum	0.4–4.8 μIU/mL	0.4–4.8 mIU/L
Thyrotropin-releasing hormone (TRH)	5–60 pg/mL	5–60 ng/L
Thyroxine (FT_4), free, serum	0.9–2.1 ng/dL	12–27 pmol/L
Thyroxine (T_4), serum	4.5–12.0 μg/dL	58–154 nmol/L
Thyroxine-binding globulin (TBG)	15.0–34.0 μg/mL	15.0–34.0 mg/L
Transferrin	250–430 mg/dL	2.5–4.3 g/L
Triglycerides, serum, after 12-hour fast	40–150 mg/dL	0.4–1.5 g/L
Triiodothyronine (T_3), serum	70–190 ng/dL	1.1–2.9 nmol/L
Triiodothyronine uptake, resin (T_3RU)	25%–38%	0.25–0.38
Urate		
Males	2.5–8.0 mg/dL	150–480 μmol/L
Females	2.2–7.0 mg/dL	130–420 μmol/L
Urea, serum or plasma	24–49 mg/dL	4.0–8.2 nmol/L
Urea nitrogen, serum or plasma	11–23 mg/dL	8.0–16.4 nmol/L
Viscosity, serum	1.4–1.8 × water	1.4–1.8 × water
Vitamin A, serum	20–80 μg/dL	0.70–2.80 μmol/L
Vitamin B_{12}, serum	180–900 pg/mL	133–664 pmol/L

*Reference values may vary depending upon the method and sample source used.

Reference Intervals for Therapeutic Drug Monitoring (Serum)

Analyte	Therapeutic Range	Toxic Concentrations	Proprietary Name(s)
Analgesics			
Acetaminophen	10–20 μg/mL	>250 μg/mL	Tylenol Datril
Salicylate	100–250 μg/mL	>300 μg/mL	Aspirin Bufferin
Antibiotics			
Amikacin	25–30 μg/mL	Peak >35 μg/mL Trough >10 μg/mL	Amikin
Gentamicin	5–10 μg/mL	Peak >10 μg/mL Trough >2 μg/mL	Garamycin
Tobramycin	5–10 μg/mL	Peak >10 μg/mL Trough >2 μg/mL	Nebcin
Vancomycin	5–35 μg/mL	Peak >40 μg/mL Trough >10 μg/mL	Vancocin
Anticonvulsants			
Carbamazepine	5–12 μg/mL	>15 μg/mL	Tegretol
Ethosuximide	40–100 μg/mL	>150 μg/mL	Zarontin
Phenobarbital	15–40 μg/mL	40–100 ng/mL (varies widely)	Luminal
Phenytoin	10–20 μg/mL	>20 μg/mL	Dilantin
Primidone	5–12 μg/mL	>15 μg/mL	Mysoline
Valproic acid	50–100 μg/mL	>100 μg/mL	Depakene
Antineoplastics and Immunosuppressives			
Cyclosporine	50–400 ng/mL	>400 ng/mL	Sandimmune
Methotrexate, high-dose, 48-hour	Variable	>1 μmol/L, 48 h after dose	
Tacrolimus (FK-506), whole blood	3–10 μg/L	>15 μg/L	Prograf
Bronchodilators and Respiratory Stimulants			
Caffeine	3–15 ng/mL	>30 ng/mL	
Theophylline (aminophylline)	10–20 μg/mL	>20 μg/mL	Elixophyllin Quibron
Cardiovascular Drugs			
Amiodarone (obtain specimen more than 8 hours after last dose)	1.0–2.0 μg/mL	>2.0 μg/mL	Cordarone
Digitoxin (obtain specimen 12–24 hours after last dose)	15–25 ng/mL	>35 ng/mL	Crystodigin
Digoxin (obtain specimen more than 6 hours after last dose)	0.8–2.0 ng/mL	>2.4 ng/mL	Lanoxin
Disopyramide	2–5 μg/mL	>7 μg/mL	Norpace
Flecainide	0.2–1.0 ng/mL	>1 ng/mL	Tambocor
Lidocaine	1.5–5.0 μg/mL	>6 μg/mL	Xylocaine
Mexiletine	0.7–2.0 ng/mL	>2 ng/mL	Mexitil
Procainamide	4–10 μg/mL	>12 μg/mL	Pronestyl
Procainamide plus NAPA	8–30 μg/mL	>30 μg/mL	
Propranolol	50–100 ng/mL	Variable	Inderal
Quinidine	2–5 μg/mL	>6 μg/mL	Cardioquin Quinaglute
Tocainide	4–10 ng/mL	>10 ng/mL	Tonocard
Psychopharmacologic Drugs			
Amitriptyline	120–150 ng/mL	>500 ng/mL	Elavil Triavil
Bupropion	25–100 ng/mL	Not applicable	Wellbutrin
Desipramine	150–300 ng/mL	>500 ng/mL	Norpramin
Imipramine	125–250 ng/mL	>400 ng/mL	Tofranil
Lithium (obtain specimen 12 hours after last dose)	0.6–1.5 mEq/L	>1.5 mEq/L	Lithobid
Nortriptyline	50–150 ng/mL	>500 ng/mL	Aventyl Pamelor

Reference Intervals* for Clinical Chemistry (Urine)

Analyte	Conventional Units	SI Units
Acetone and acetoacetate, qualitative	Negative	Negative
Albumin		
Qualitative	Negative	Negative
Quantitative	10–100 mg/24 h	0.15–1.5 μmol/d
Aldosterone	3–20 μg/24 h	8.3–55 nmol/d
δ-Aminolevulinic acid (δ-ALA)	1.3–7.0 mg/24 h	10–53 μmol/d
Amylase	<17 U/h	<17 U/h
Amylase/creatinine clearance ratio	0.01–0.04	0.01–0.04
Bilirubin, qualitative	Negative	Negative
Calcium (regular diet)	<250 mg/24 h	<6.3 nmol/d
Catecholamines		
Epinephine	<10 μg/24 h	<55 nmol/d
Norepinephine	<100 μg/24 h	<590 nmol/d
Total free catecholamines	4–126 μg/24 h	24–745 nmol/d
Total metanephines	0.1–1.6 mg/24 h	0.5–8.1 μmol/d
Chloride (varies with intake)	110–250 mEq/24 h	110–250 mmol/d
Copper	0–50 μg/24 h	0.0–0.80 μmol/d
Cortisol, free	10–100 μg/24 h	27.6–276 nmol/d
Creatine		
Males	0–40 mg/24 h	0.0–0.30 mmol/d
Females	0–80 mg/24 h	0.0–0.60 mmol/d
Creatinine	15–25 mg/kg/24 h	0.13–0.22 mmol/kg/d
Creatinine clearance (endogenous)		
Males	110–150 mL/min/1.73 m^2	110–150 mL/min/1.73 m^2
Females	105–132 mL/min/1.73 m^2	105–132 mL/min/1.73 m^2
Cystine or cysteine	Negative	Negative
Dehydroepiandrosterone		
Males	0.2–2.0 mg/24 h	0.7–6.9 μmol/d
Females	0.2–1.8 mg/24 h	0.7–6.2 μmol/d
Estrogens, total		
Males	4–25 μg/24 h	14–90 nmol/d
Females	5–100 μg/24 h	18–360 nmol/d
Glucose (as reducing substance)	<250 mg/24 h	<250 mg/d
Hemoglobin and myoglobin, qualitative	Negative	Negative
Homogentisic acid, qualitative	Negative	Negative
17-Ketogenic steroids		
Males	5–23 mg/24 h	17–80 μmol/d
Females	3–15 mg/24 h	10–52 μmol/d
17-Hydroxycorticosteroids		
Males	3–9 mg/24 h	8.3–25 μmol/d
Females	2–8 mg/24 h	5.5–22 μmol/d
5-Hydroxyindoleacetic acid		
Qualitative	Negative	Negative
Quantitative	2–6 mg/24 h	10–31 μmol/d
17-Ketosteroids		
Males	8–22 mg/24 h	28–76 μmol/d
Females	6–15 mg/24 h	21–52 μmol/d
Magnesium	6–10 mEq/24 h	3–5 mmol/d
Metanephines	0.05–1.2 ng/mg creatinine	0.03–0.70 mmol/mmol creatinine
Osmolality	38–1400 mOsm/kg water	38–1400 mOsm/kg water
pH	4.6–8.0	4.6–8.0
Phenylpyruvic acid, qualitative	Negative	Negative
Phosphate	0.4–1.3 g/24 h	13–42 mmol/d
Porphobilinogen		
Qualitative	Negative	Negative
Quantitative	<2 mg/24 h	<9 μmol/d
Porphyrins		
Coproporphyrin	50–250 μg/24 h	77–380 nmol/d
Uroporphyrin	10–30 μg/24 h	12–36 nmol/d
Potassium	25–125 mEq/24 h	25–125 mmol/d
Pregnanediol		
Males	0.0–1.9 mg/24 h	0.0–6.0 μmol/d
Females		
Proliferative phase	0.0–2.6 mg/24 h	0.0–8.0 μmol/d
Luteal phase	2.6–10.6 mg/24 h	8–33 μmol/d
Postmenopausal	0.2–1.0 mg/24 h	0.6–3.1 μmol/d
Pregnanetriol	0.0–2.5 mg/24 h	0.0–7.4 μmol/d

Table continued on following page

Reference Intervals* for Clinical Chemistry (Urine) *Continued*

Analyte	Conventional Units	SI Units
Protein, total		
Qualitative	Negative	Negative
Quantitative	10–150 mg/24 h	10–150 mg/d
Protein/creatinine ratio	<0.2	<0.2
Sodium (regular diet)	60–260 mEq/24 h	60–260 mmol/d
Specific gravity		
Random specimen	1.003–1.030	1.003–1.030
24-h collection	1.015–1.025	1.015–1.025
Urate (regular diet)	250–750 mg/24 h	1.5–4.4 mmol/d
Urobilinogen	0.5–4.0 mg/24 h	0.6–6.8 μmol/d
Vanillylmandelic acid (VMA)	1.0–8.0 mg/24 h	5–40 μmol/d

*Values may vary depending on the method used.

Reference Intervals for Toxic Substances

Analyte	Conventional Units	SI Units
Arsenic, urine	<130 μg/24 h	<1.7 μmol/d
Bromides, serum, inorganic	<100 mg/dL	<10 mmol/L
Toxic symptoms	140–1000 mg/dL	14–100 mmol/L
Carboxyhemoglobin, blood:	saturation	
Urban environment	<5%	<0.05
Smokers	<12%	<0.12
Symptoms		
Headache	>15%	>0.15
Nausea and vomiting	>25%	>0.25
Potentially lethal	>50%	>0.50
Ethanol, blood	<0.05 mg/dL <0.005%	<1.0 mmol/L
Intoxication	>100 mg/dL >0.1%	>22 mmol/L
Marked intoxication	300–400 mg/dL 0.3%–0.4%	65–87 mmol/L
Alcoholic stupor	400–500 mg/dL 0.4%–0.5%	87–109 mmol/L
Coma	>500 mg/dL >0.5%	>109 mmol/L
Lead, blood		
Adults	<25 μg/dL	<1.2 μmol/L
Children	<15 μg/dL	<0.7 μmol/L
Lead, urine	<80 μg/24 h	<0.4 μmol/d
Mercury, urine	<30 μg/24 h	<150 nmol/d

Reference Intervals for Tests Performed on Cerebrospinal Fluid

Test	Conventional Units	SI Units
Cells	<5/mm³; all mononuclear	$<5 \times 10^6$/L, all mononuclear
Protein electrophoresis	Albumin predominant	Albumin predominant
Glucose	50–75 mg/dL (20 mg/dL less than in serum)	2.8–4.2 mmol/L (1.1 mmol less than in serum)
IgG		
Children under 14	<8% of total protein	<0.08 of total protein
Adults	<14% of total protein	<0.14 of total protein
IgG index		
$\left(\frac{\text{CSF/serum IgG ratio}}{\text{CSF/serum albumin ratio}}\right)$	0.3–0.6	0.3–0.6
Oligoclonal banding on electrophoresis	Absent	Absent
Pressure, opening	70–180 mm H_2O	70–180 mm H_2O
Protein, total	15–45 mg/dL	150–450 mg/L

Abbreviation: CSF = cerebrospinal fluid.

Reference Intervals for Tests of Gastrointestinal Function

Test	Conventional Units
Bentiromide	6-h urinary arylamine excretion greater than 57% excludes pancreatic insufficiency
β-Carotene, serum	60–250 ng/dL
Fecal fat estimation	
Qualitative	No fat globules seen by high-power microscope
Quantitative	<6 g/24 h (>95% coefficient of fat absorption)
Gastric acid output	
Basal	
Males	0.0–10.5 mmol/h
Females	0.0–5.6 mmol/h
Maximum (after histamine or pentagastrin)	
Males	9.0–48.0 mmol/h
Females	6.0–31.0 mmol/h
Ratio: basal/maximum	
Males	0.0–0.31
Females	0.0–0.29
Secretin test, pancreatic fluid	
Volume	>1.8 mL/kg/h
Bicarbonate	>80 mEq/L
D-Xylose absorption test, urine	>20% of ingested dose excreted in 5 h

Reference Intervals for Tests of Immunologic Function

Test	Conventional Units	SI Units
Complement, serum		
C3	85–175 mg/dL	0.85–1.75 g/L
C4	15–45 mg/dL	150–450 mg/L
Total hemolytic (CH_{50})	150–250 U/mL	150–250 U/mL
Immunoglobulins, serum, adult		
IgG	640–1350 mg/dL	6.4–13.5 g/L
IgA	70–310 mg/dL	0.70–3.1 g/L
IgM	90–350 mg/dL	0.90–3.5 g/L
IgD	0.0–6.0 mg/dL	0.0–60 mg/L
IgE	0.0–430 ng/dL	0.0–430 μg/L

Lymphocyte Subsets, Whole Blood, Heparinized

Antigen(s) Expressed	Cell Type	Percentage	Absolute Cell Count
CD3	Total T cells	56%–77%	860–1880
CD19	Total B cells	7%–17%	140–370
CD3 and CD4	Helper-inducer cells	32%–54%	550–1190
CD3 and CD8	Suppressor-cytotoxic cells	24%–37%	430–1060
CD3 and DR	Activated T cells	5%–14%	70–310
CD2	E rosette T cells	73%–87%	1040–2160
CD16 and CD56	Natural killer (NK) cells	8%–22%	130–500

Helper/suppressor ratio: 0.8–1.8

Reference Values for Semen Analysis

Test	Conventional Units	SI Units
Volume	2–5 mL	2–5 mL
Liquefaction	Complete in 15 min	Complete in 15 min
pH	7.2–8.0	7.2–8.0
Leukocytes	Occasional or absent	Occasional or absent
Spermatozoa		
Count	60–150 × 10^6 mL	60–150 × 10^6 mL
Motility	>80% motile	>0.80 motile
Morphology	80%–90% normal forms	>0.80–0.90 normal forms
Fructose	>150 mg/dL	>8.33 mmol/L

SELECTED REFERENCES

Bick RL (ed): Hematology—Clinical and Laboratory Practice. St Louis, Mosby–Year Book, 1993.
Borer WZ: Selection and use of laboratory tests. In Tietz NW, Conn RB, Pruden EL (eds): Applied Laboratory Medicine. Philadelphia, WB Saunders, 1992, pp 1–5.
Campion EW: A retreat from SI units. N Engl J Med 327:49, 1992.
Drug Evaluations Annual. Chicago, American Medical Association, 1994.
Friedman RB, Young DS: Effects of Disease on Clinical Laboratory Tests, 3rd ed. Washington, DC, AACC Press, 1997.
Henry JB: Clinical Diagnosis and Management by Laboratory Methods, 19th ed. Philadelphia, WB Saunders, 1996.
Hicks JM, Young DS: DORA 97–99: Directory of Rare Analyses. Washington, DC, AACC Press, 1997.
Jacob DS, Demott WR, Grady HJ, et al (eds): Laboratory Test Handbook, 4th ed. Baltimore, Williams & Wilkins, 1996.
Kaplan LA, Pesce AJ: Clinical Chemistry—Theory, Analysis, and Correlation, 3rd ed. St Louis, Mosby–Year Book, 1996.
Kjeldsberg CR, Knight JA: Body Fluids: Laboratory Examination of Amniotic, Cerebrospinal, Seminal, Serous and Synovial Fluids, 3rd ed. Chicago, ASCP Press, 1993.
Laposata M: SI Unit Conversion Guide. Boston, NEJM Books, 1992.
Scully RE, McNeely WF, Mark EJ, McNeely BU: Normal reference laboratory values. N Engl J Med 327:718–724, 1992.
Speicher CE: The Right Test: A Physician's Guide to Laboratory Medicine, 3rd ed. Philadelphia, WB Saunders, 1998.
Tietz NW (ed): Clinical Guide to Laboratory Tests, 3rd ed. Philadelphia, WB Saunders, 1995.
Wallach J: Interpretation of Diagnostic Tests: A Synopsis of Laboratory Medicine, 6th ed. Boston, Little, Brown, 1996.
Young DS: Implementation of SI units for clinical laboratory data. Ann Intern Med 106:114–129, 1987.
Young DS: Determination and validation of reference intervals. Arch Pathol Lab Med 116:704–709, 1992.
Young DS: Effects of Drugs on Clinical Laboratory Tests, 4th ed. Washington, DC, AACC Press, 1995.
Young DS: Effects of Preanalytical Variables on Clinical Laboratory Tests, 2nd ed. Washington, DC, AACC Press, 1997.

SOME POPULAR HERBAL PRODUCTS

method of

MIRIAM M. CHAN, R.PH., PHARM.D.
Riverside Family Practice Residency Program
Columbus, Ohio

Herb	Common Uses	Precautions and Drug Interactions
Black cohosh	Commonly used to relieve menopausal symptoms, such as hot flashes Also used to treat premenstrual discomfort and dysmenorrhea	Black cohosh has estrogen-like action and has been shown to decrease luteinizing hormone. Large doses of the plant may induce miscarriage, and it is contraindicated during pregnancy. It may cause gastrointestinal disturbances, headache, and hypotension. Long-term studies have not been conducted on the herb; therefore, its use should be limited to 6 months.
Chamomile	Used orally to calm nerves and treat gastrointestinal spasms and inflammatory disease of the gastrointestinal tract Used topically to treat wounds, skin infections, and skin/mucous membrane inflammations	Chamomile may cause an allergic reaction, especially in people with severe allergies to ragweed or other members of the daisy family (e.g., echinacea, feverfew, and milk thistle). It should not be taken concurrently with other sedatives, such as alcohol, or benzodiazepines.
Echinacea	As an immune stimulant, particularly for the prevention and treatment of cold and influenza Supportive therapy for lower urinary tract infections Used topically to treat skin disorders and promote wound healing	Echinacea should not be used in patients with autoimmune disease. Long-term use (>8 weeks) may suppress immunity and therefore is not recommended. Allergic reaction to echinacea has been reported. Adverse events are rare and may include mild gastrointestinal effects.
Ephedra (Ma Huang)	For diseases of the respiratory tract with mild bronchospasms Commonly found in weight-loss products Also marketed as a stimulant for performance enhancement	Ephedra contains ephedrine, which has sympathomimetic activities. Consequently, it should not be used in patients who have cardiovascular disease, diabetes, glaucoma, hypertension, hyperthyroidism, prostate enlargement, psychiatric disorders, or seizure. Serious adverse effects including seizures, arrhythmias, heart attack, stroke, and death have been associated with the use of ephedra. Concurrent use of ephedra and digitalis, guanethidine, MAOIs, or other stimulants, including caffeine, is not recommended.
Feverfew	For migraine headache prophylaxis For treatment of fever, menstrual problems, and arthritis	Feverfew may induce menstrual bleeding and is contraindicated in pregnancy. Fresh leaves may cause oral ulcers and gastrointestinal irritation. Sudden discontinuation of feverfew can precipitate rebound headache. Feverfew may interact with anticoagulants and potentiate the antiplatelet effect of aspirin.

Herb	Common Uses	Precautions and Drug Interactions
Garlic	To lower blood pressure and serum cholesterol To prevent artherosclerosis	The intake of large quantities can lead to stomach complaints. Garlic has antiplatelet effects and may interact with anticoagulants.
Ginger	As an antiemetic For prevention of motion sickness	Ginger should not be used in patients with gallstones because of its cholagogic effect. It may inhibit platelet aggregation. Cases of postoperative bleeding have been reported. Large doses of ginger may increase bleeding time in patients taking antiplatelet agents.
Ginkgo biloba	For dementia to slow cognitive deterioration For claudication to increase peripheral blood flow	Adverse effects are rare and may include mild stomach or intestinal upsets, headache, or allergic skin reaction. Ginkgo can inhibit platelet aggregation. Reports of spontaneous bleeding have been published. Concurrent use of ginkgo and anticoagulants, antiplatelet agents, vitamin E, or garlic may increase risk of bleeding.
Ginseng	As a tonic in time of stress, fatigue, and debility, and during convalescence To improve physical performance and stamina	Ginseng has a mild stimulant effect and should be avoided in patients with cardiovascular disease. Tachycardia and hypertension can occur. Overdosages can lead to "ginseng abuse syndrome," which is characterized by insomnia, hypotonia, and edema. Ginseng has estrogenic effects and may cause vaginal bleeding and breast tenderness. Ginseng should not be used with other stimulants. Patients taking antidiabetic agents and ginseng should be monitored to avoid hypoglycemic effects of ginseng. Ginseng may interact with warfarin, causing decreased INR. Siberian ginseng may increase digoxin levels. There have been reports of drug interaction between ginseng and phenelzine (an MAOI) resulting in insomnia, headache, tremulousness, and manic-like symptoms.
Kava-kava	Anxiolytic for nervous anxiety, stress, and restlessness Sedative to induce sleep	Contraindications include patients with depression, pregnancy, and nursing mothers. Kava may affect motor reflexes and judgment for driving and/or operating heavy machinery. Accommodative disturbances have been reported. Kava may cause exacerbation of Parkinson's disease. Extended use can cause a temporary yellow discoloration of skin, hair, and nails. Kava has been shown to have additive CNS effects with other CNS depressants (e.g., benzodiazepines, alcohol) or herbal tranquilizers.
Milk thistle	As a hepatoprotectant and antioxidant, particularly for the treatment of hepatitis, cirrhosis, and toxic liver damage Used in Europe for the treatment of hepatotoxic mushroom poisoning from *Amanita phalloides*	Adverse effects are rare but may include diarrhea and allergic reactions. Patients taking antidiabetic agents and milk thistle should be monitored to avoid hypoglycemia.
Saw palmetto	To treat urination problem in benign prostatic hyperplasia For irritable bladder	Adverse effects are rare but may include headache, nausea, and upset stomach. High doses can cause diarrhea.
St. John's wort	Effective for mild to moderate depression May have anti-inflammatory and anti-infective activities	St. John's wort should not be used in pregnancy. Side effects include dry mouth, gastrointestinal upset, dizziness, fatigue, and constipation. St. John's wort may induce photosensitivity, especially in fair-skinned individuals. Caution advised if used with other antidepressants, including SSRIs or serotonergic drugs because it may cause serotonin syndrome. St. John's wort has been shown to induce the P450 isoenzymes and decrease the blood levels of many drugs such as indinavir, cyclosporine, digoxin, theophylline, oral contraceptive pills, and warfarin.
Valerian	Mild sedative for insomnia Minor tranquilizer for nervousness	Valerian can cause morning drowsiness. Long-term administration may lead to paradoxic stimulation, including restlessness and palpitations. It may potentiate the sedative effect of CNS depressants (e.g., benzodiazepines, alcohol) and other herbal tranquilizers.

Abbreviations: CNS = central nervous system; MAOI = monoamine oxidase inhibitor; SSRIs = selective serotonin reuptake inhibitors.

NEW DRUGS FOR 2000

method of
GRACE M. KUO, PHARM.D.
Baylor College of Medicine
Houston, Texas

Generic Name/ Active Ingredient(s)	Trade Name (Manufacturer)	Strength	Dosage Form	Dosage Range	FDA Rating	Pregnancy Rating	Cytochrome	FDA Approval Date	Indication	Classification
Alosetron HCl	Lotronex (Glaxo Wellcome)	1 mg	Tablet	1 mg PO bid	1-P	B	(−) 1A2 (−) 2E1	02-09-00 (withdrew from market on 11-29-00)	Treatment of irritable bowel syndrome in women whose predominant bowel symptom is diarrhea	Gastrointestinal
Arsenic trioxide	Trixenox (Cell Therapeutics, Inc.)	10 mg/mL × 10 mL vial	Injectable	Diluted with 100–250 mL D5W or NS IV over 1–2 h	1-P	D	None	09-25-00	Induction of remission and consolidation in patients with acute promyelocytic leukemia	Antineoplastic
Bivalirudin	Angiomax (The Medicines Co.)	250 mg per vial	Injectable	1.0 mg/kg IV bolus, then IV infusion of 2.5 mg/kg/h × 4 h. See package insert for dosing guidelines.	1-S	B	None	12–15-00	In conjunction with aspirin in patients with unstable angina undergoing percutaneous transluminal coronary angioplasty	Anticoagulant
Cetrorelix	Cetrotide (Asta Medica)	0.25, 3 mg	Injectable	Dose adjusted according to individual response	1-S	X	None	08-11-00	Prevention of premature luteinizing hormone surges in women undergoing controlled ovarian stimulation	Hormone
Cevimeline HCl	Evoxac (SnowBrand)	30 mg	Capsule	30 mg PO bid	1-S	C	(−) by 2D6 (−) by 3A3/4	01-11-00	Treatment of symptoms of dry mouth in patients with Sjögren's syndrome	Mouth product
Insulin glargine	Lantus (Aventis)	100 U 5, 10 mL 3 mL cartridge	Injectable vials Package of 5	Individualized dosing	1-S	C	None	04-20-00	Once-daily SC administration in the treatment of adult and pediatric patients with type 1 diabetes mellitus, and of adult patients with type 2 diabetes mellitus who require basal (long-acting) insulin for the control of hyperglycemia	Antidiabetic
Mifepristone (RU-486)	Mifeprex (Danco Laboratories)	200 mg	Tablet	600 mg PO × 1 on day 1 followed by misoprostol 400 μg on day 3	1-P	X	3A4	09-28-00	Medical termination of intrauterine pregnancy through 49th d of pregnancy, followed by misoprostol after 2 d	Abortifacient
Oxcarbazepine	Trileptal (Novartis)	150, 300, 600 mg	Film-coated tablet	300 mg PO bid (recommended dose = 1200 mg/d)	1-S	C	(−) 2C19 (+) 3A4/5	01-14-00	Treatment of partial seizures in children ages 4–16 y with epilepsy	Anticonvulsant

Pantoprazole sodium	Protonix (Wyeth Ayerst)	40 mg	Tablet	40 mg PO q d up to 8 wk	1-S	B	By 2C19, and 3A4, 2D6, 2C9	02-02-00	Short-term treatment (up to 8 wk) in the healing and symptomatic relief of erosive esophagitis	Gastrointestinal
Rivastigmine tartrate	Exelon (Novartis)	1.5, 3, 4.5, 6 mg 2 mg/mL	Capsule Solution	Start with 1.5 mg PO bid, then titrate to 3–6 mg PO bid	1-S	B	None	04-21-00	Treatment of mild to moderate dementia of the Alzheimer type	CNS Agent
Tinzaparin sodium	Innohep (Dupont)	2 mL 20,000 anti-Xa IU/mL	Injectable	175 anti-Xa IU/kg SC q d × at least 6 d until patient is adequately anticoagulated with warfarin	1-S	B	07-14-00	Treatment of acute symptomatic deep vein thrombosis with or without pulmonary embolism when administered in conjunction with warfarin sodium	Thrombin inhibitor	
Triptorelin pamoate	Trelstar Depot (Debio/Pharmacia & Upjohn)	3.75 mg	Injectable	3.75 mg IM monthly	1-S	X	None	06-15-00	Palliative treatment of advanced prostate cancer	Antineoplastic
Isopropyl unoprostone	Rescula (Ciba Vision Corp Div Novartis Co.)	0.15%	Ophthalmic solution eye drops	1 drop in affected eye(s) twice daily	1-P	C	None	08-03-00	Lowering of intraocular pressure in patients with open-angle glaucoma or ocular hypertension	Glaucoma
Verteporfin	Visudyne (QLT Photo Therapeutics, Inc.)	15 mg	Injectable	2-step process with both drug (6 mg/m² in D5W, 30 mL total) and light	1-P	C	None	04-12-00	Treatment of age-related macular degeneration in patients with predominantly classic subfoveal choroidal neovascularization	Ophthalmic phototherapy
Zonisamide	Zonegran (Elan)	100 mg	Capsule	100—600 mg/d (titration)	1-S	C	3A4	03-27-00	Adjunctive therapy in the treatment of partial seizures in adults with epilepsy	Anticonvulsant

FDA rating refers to the chemical type (1 = new molecular entity) and therapeutic potential (P = priority drug review; S = standard drug review).
FDA Pregnancy Categories:
A = Adequate studies in pregnant women have not demonstrated a risk to the fetus in the first trimester of pregnancy, and there is no evidence of risk in later trimesters.
B = Animal studies have not demonstrated a risk to the fetus, but there are no adequate studies in pregnant women . . . *or* . . . Animal studies have shown an adverse effect, but adequate studies in pregnant women have not demonstrated a risk to the fetus during the first trimester of pregnancy and there is no evidence of risk in later trimesters.
C = Animal studies have shown an adverse effect on the fetus but there are no adequate studies in human beings; the benefits from the use of the drug in pregnant women may be acceptable despite its potential risk . . . *or* . . . There are no animal reproduction studies and no adequate studies in human beings.
D = There is evidence of human fetal risk, but the potential benefits from the use of the drug in pregnant women may be acceptable despite its potential risks.
X = Studies in animals or human beings demonstrate fetal abnormalities or adverse reaction reports indicate evidence of fetal risk. The risk of use in a pregnant woman clearly outweighs any possible benefit.
Regardless of the designated Pregnancy Category or presumed safety, no drug should be administered during pregnancy unless it is clearly needed and potential benefits outweigh potential hazards to the fetus.

NOMOGRAM FOR THE DETERMINATION OF BODY SURFACE AREA OF CHILDREN AND ADULTS

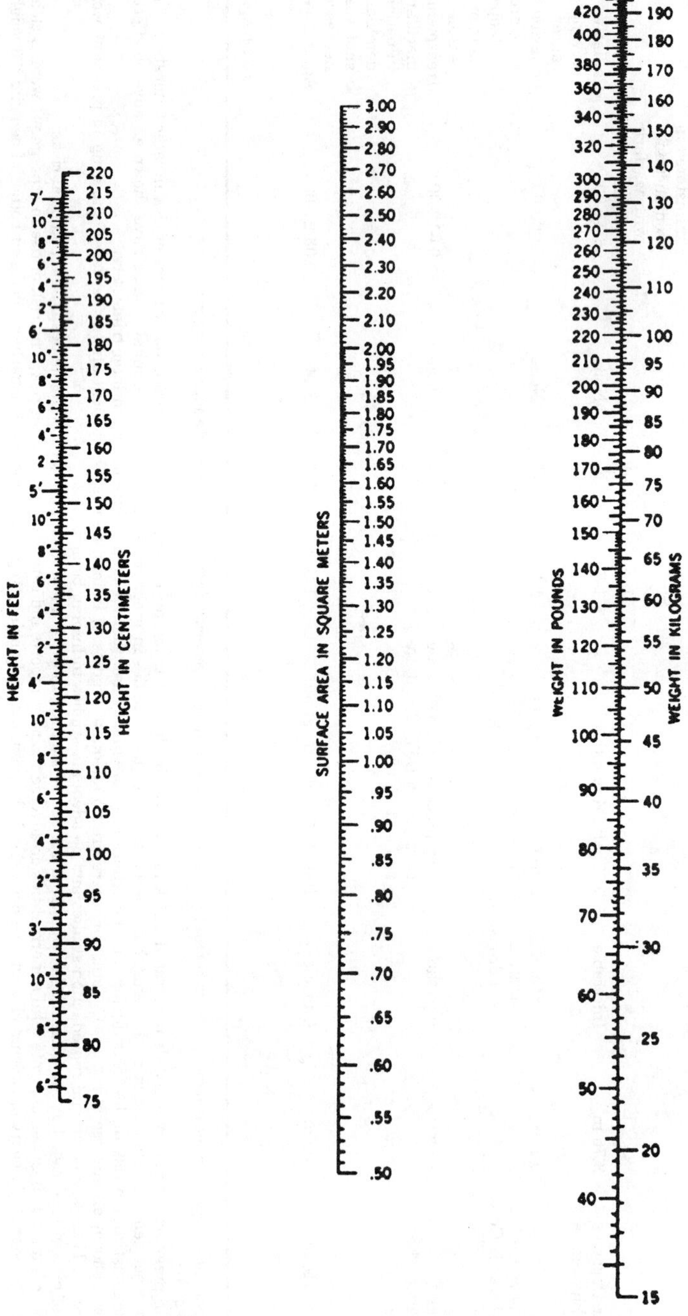

From Boothby WM, Sandiford RB: Boston Med Surg J 185:337, 1921.

Index

Note: Page numbers followed by f indicate figures; those followed by t indicate tables. Drugs are listed under the generic name.